AF664376

Glasscock-Shambaugh
SURGERY of the EAR

6 EDITION

EDITORS

AINA JULIANNA GULYA, MD, FACS (Editor-in-Chief)
Clinical Professor of Otolaryngology—Head and Neck Surgery
The George Washington University
Washington, D.C.
Former Chief of Clinical Trials Branch
National Institute on Deafness and Other Communication Disorders
Bethesda, Maryland

LLOYD B. MINOR, MD, FACS
Provost and Senior Vice President for Academic Affairs
The Johns Hopkins University
University Distinguished Service Professor of Otolaryngology—Head & Neck Surgery
The Johns Hopkins University School of Medicine
Baltimore, Maryland

DENNIS S. POE, MD, FACS
Associate Professor, Department of Otology and Laryngology
Harvard Medical School
Department of Otolaryngology at Children's Hospital
Boston, Massachusetts
Visiting Professor, Department of Otolaryngology
Tampere University Medical School, Tampere, Finland

2010
PEOPLE'S MEDICAL PUBLISHING HOUSE-USA
SHELTON,CONNECTICUT

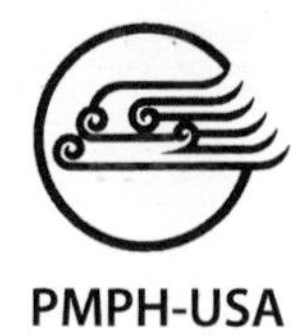

This edition has been published by special arrangement with People's Medical Publishing House, USA

CBS ISBN: 9788123920481

Reprint: 2012

Published by:
Satish K. Jain for CBS Publishers & Distributors Pvt. Ltd.,
4819/XI Prahlad Street, 24 Ansari Road, Daryaganj, New Delhi - 110002, India.
e-mail: cbspubs@vsnl.com, delhi@cbspd.com • www.cbspd.com

Branches:
- ***Bengaluru:*** Seema House, 2975, 17th Cross, K.R. Road, Bansankari 2nd Stage, Bengaluru - 560070 Ph.: +91-80-26771678/79 Fax: +91-80-26771680 • E-mail: cbsbng@gmail.com, bangalore@cbspd.com
- ***Pune:*** Bhuruk Prestige, Sr. No. 52/12/2+1+3/2, Narhe, Haveli (Near Katraj-Dehu Road By-pass), Pune - 411051 Ph.: +91-20-64704058/59, 32342277 • E-mail: pune@cbspd.com
- ***Kochi:*** 36/14, Kalluvilakam, Lissie Hospital Road, Kochi - 682018, Kerala • Ph.: +91-484-4059061-65 Fax: +91-484-4059065 • E-mail: cochin@cbspd.com
- ***Chennai:*** 20, West Park Road, Shenoy Nagar, Chennai - 600030 Ph.: +91-44-26260666, 26208620 • Fax: +91-44-42032115 E-mail: chennai@cbspd.com

Printed at : Goyal Offset Works Pvt. Ltd. Haryana (INDIA)

Dedications

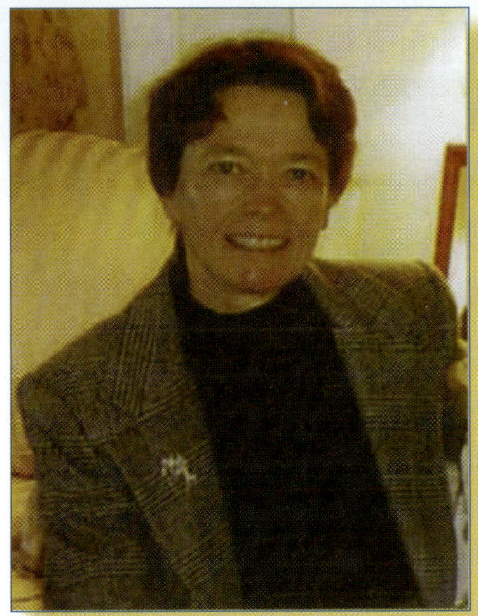

With many thanks to my ever-supportive husband, William R. Wilson, MD, FACS.

A. JULIANNA GULYA, MD, FACS

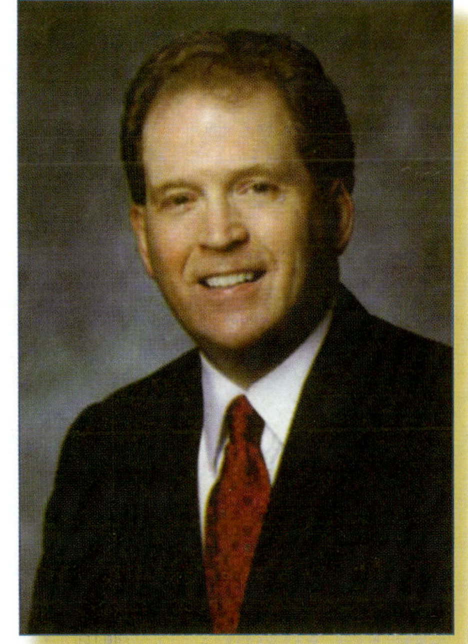

With love and appreciation to my constantly supportive wife, Lisa, and our children, Emily and Sam. I also thank my mentors for their wisdom and skill; my patients for their insights and partnerships with us in our collective quest to improve their lives; and my colleagues and students for their keen insights and dedication as we pursue together the goal of increasing scientific knowledge and advancing clinical care.

LLOYD B. MINOR, MD, FACS

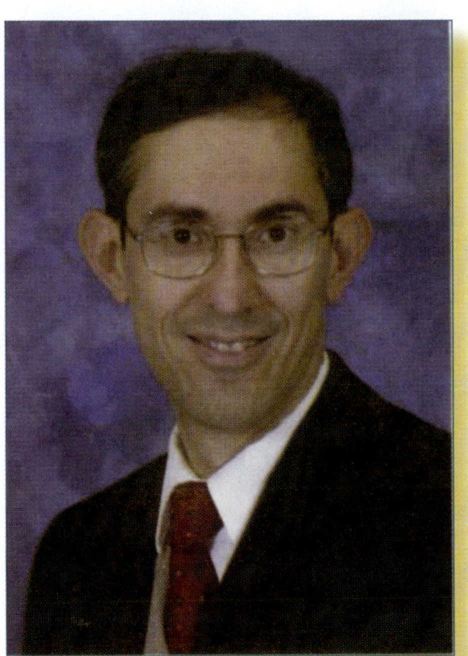

To my loving and wonderfully supportive wife, Milja-Riitta and children Lara, Daniel, and Sonja. Also to our teachers, who gave us the foundations to serve our patients and to our patients, who have been our ultimate educators.

DENNIS S. POE MD, FACS

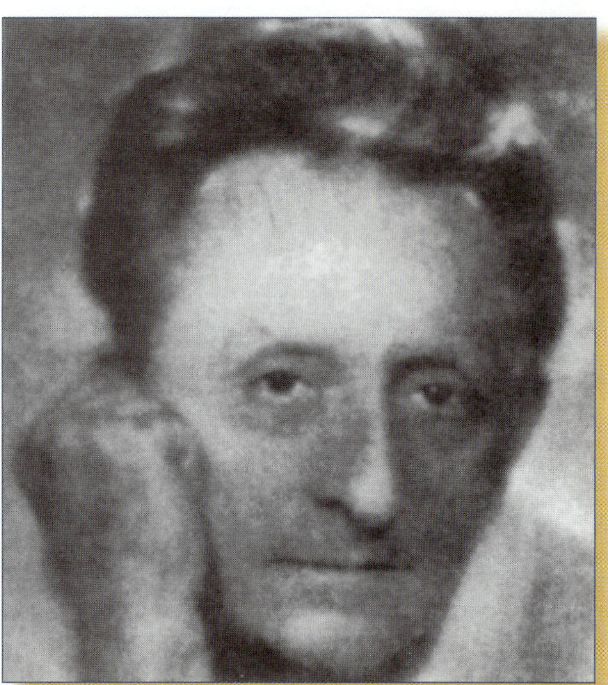

JULIUS LEMPERT (1890-1968) • Foremost advocate of the endaural approach to the temporal bone. His one-stage fenestration operation led to the renaissance of reconstructive surgery for conductive hearing loss.

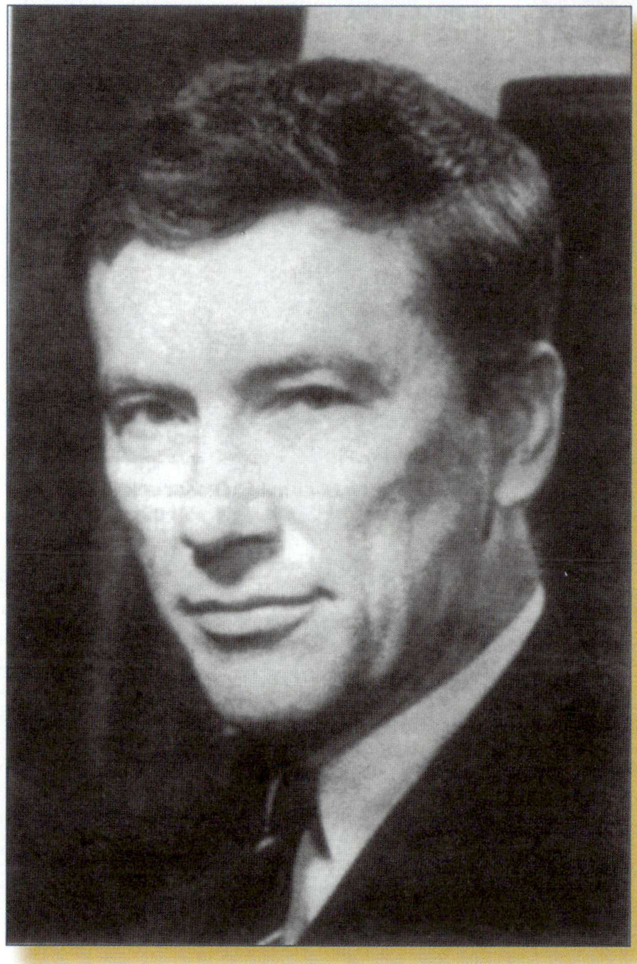

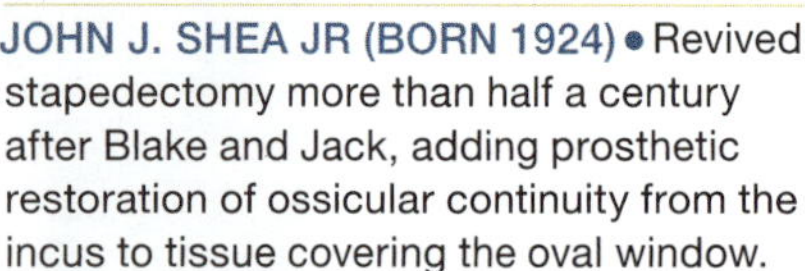

JOHN J. SHEA JR (BORN 1924) • Revived stapedectomy more than half a century after Blake and Jack, adding prosthetic restoration of ossicular continuity from the incus to tissue covering the oval window.

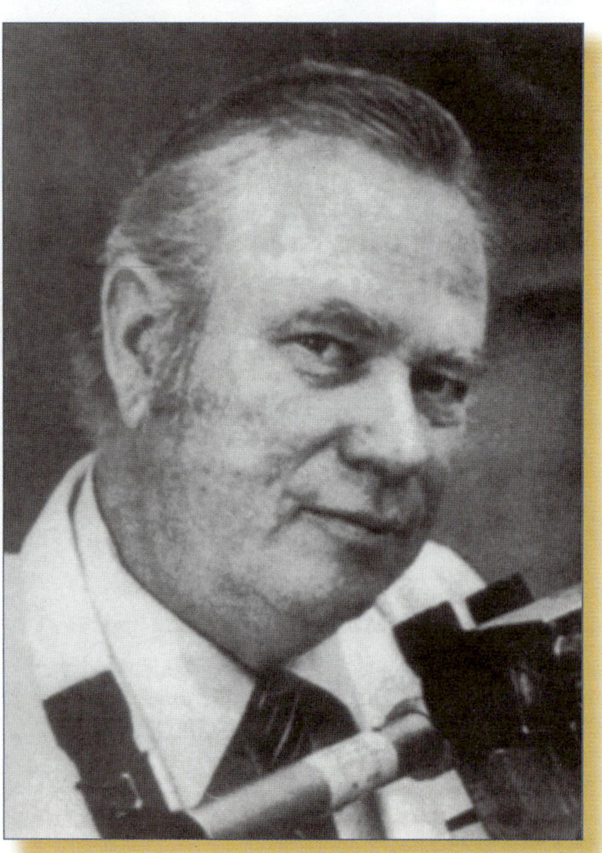

WILLIAM F. HOUSE, MD (BORN 1923) • The "father of neurotology." He pioneered the early diagnosis and translabyrinthine removal of vestibular schwannomas and the development of the cochlear implant.

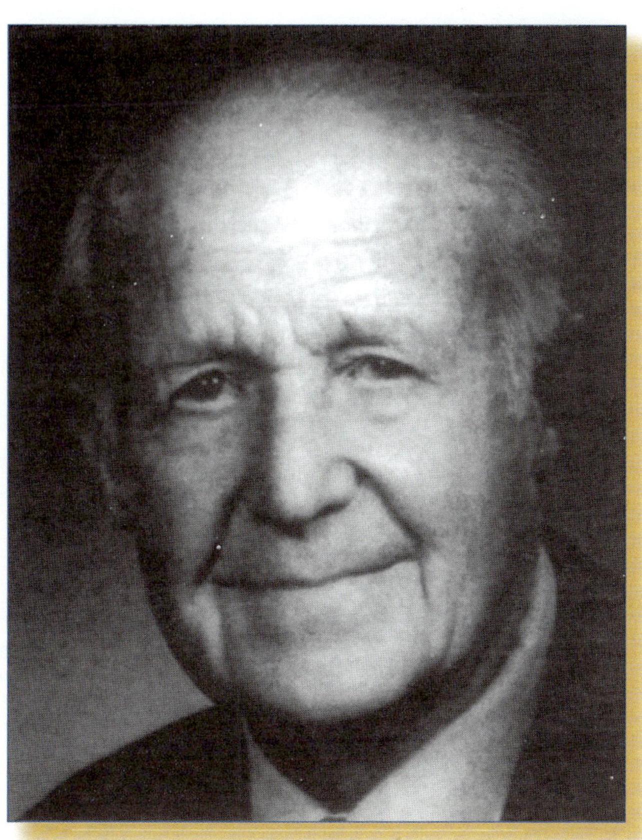

GEORGE E. SHAMBAUGH JR, MD (1903-1999) • Author of the first and second editions of Surgery of the Ear and senior coauthor of the third edition.

MICHAEL E. CLASSCOCK III. MD, FACS • Editor of the fourth edition of *Surgery of the Ear* and co-editor of the fifth.

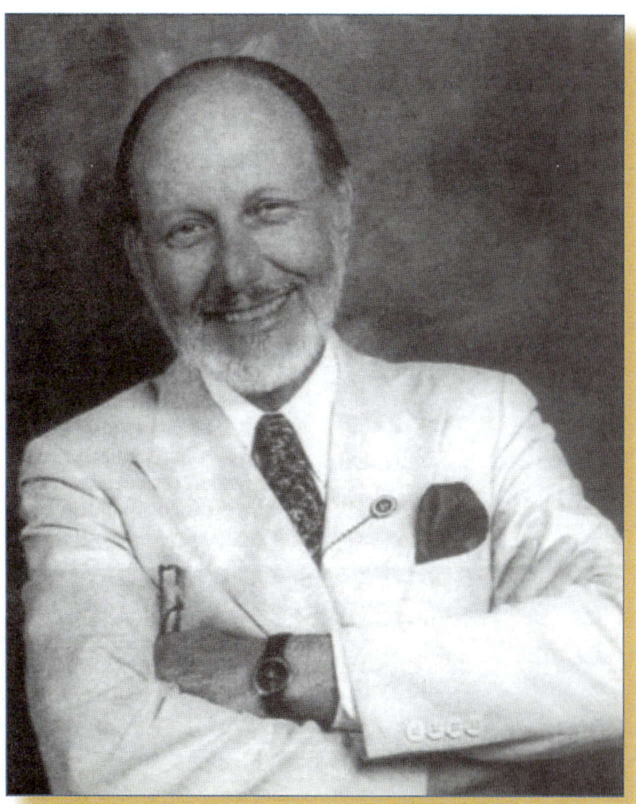

Contents

SECTION III. FUNDAMENTALS OF OTOLOGIC AND NEUROTOLOGIC SURGERY

SECTION IV. SURGERY OF THE EXTERNAL EAR

SECTION V. SURGERY OF THE TYMPANOMASTOID COMPARTMENT

SECTION VI. SURGERY OF THE INNER EAR

SECTION VII. SURGERY OF THE INTERNAL AUDITORY CANAL/ CEREBELLOPONTINE ANGLE/ PETROUS APEX

SECTION VIII. SURGERY OF THE SKULL BASE

Foreword

When George Shambaugh Jr. took 6 months off from his busy private practice of otology in the late 1950s to write the first edition of *Surgery of the Ear*, I doubt he had any idea that the book would become a classic text studied by generations of young surgeons.

A span of 50 years sees a multitude of advances in any medical specialty, and otology is no exception. That first edition was published in 1959 at the beginning of a new era in otology ushered in by the likes of Samuel Rosen, John J. Shea Jr., and William F. House. Rosen's stapes mobilization led to Shea's stapedectomy, which galvanized the imagination of every otolaryngologist in the world. Then in 1960, William F. House began his monumental work on acoustic neuromas (vestibular schwannomas), establishing neurotology as a subspecialty now recognized by the American Board of Otolaryngology—Head and Neck Surgery.

House's contributions dominated the literature in the following decades. He developed the intact canal wall mastoidectomy, introduced the use of canal skin for tympanoplasty, established the endolymphatic shunt procedure for the control of the symptoms of Ménière's disease, and finally crowned his accomplishments with his pioneering work on the first cochlear and brainstem implants.

In 1959 children born with profound hearing loss were destined to spend their life in the deaf culture. They had to rely on American Sign Language to communicate with each other and essentially never integrated into the hearing world. Now these children are provided with a cochlear implant at an early age, learn to speak, and do remarkably well in a normal hearing environment.

Technology was vastly different back then. The Zeiss operating microscope of 1959 had no viewing tube, TV, or 16-mm movie camera. These all came later through the efforts of Jack Urban, an engineer who worked directly with House in Los Angeles. There were no CT, MRI, or PET scans and no surgical lasers. Audiology was limited to air and bone conduction, speech discrimination, and the tone decay test. The ABR and acoustic emissions had yet to be discovered. The internet was decades away, as were personal computers, laptops, cell phones, fax machines, and the multitude of other high-tech devices we take for granted today. So in reviewing that first edition, I am struck by how simple it was at the time. We couldn't imagine what was to come. And as a resident and later in my fellowship, it all appeared a little daunting.

It is important to update any medical text on a regular basis because science is not a static field. This current edition is far different from the 1959 one that I cut my teeth on. It has been edited by three fine otologists, Julianna Gulya, Dennis Poe, and Lloyd Minor. I'm grateful to have had the opportunity to work with each one of them as part of my fellowship program in Nashville. This sixth edition reflects the current state of the art in our specialty and includes a DVD with 30 video clips of current diagnostic procedures and surgical techniques. W. B. Saunders published the first few editions, B. C. Decker transitioned it into the 21st century and now a new publisher, PMPH-USA, Ltd, is taking it forward. This is a classic that should continue on a regular basis.

I am grateful for the many contributors who have made this edition so outstanding. At this point in time, I simply sit back and marvel at the intelligence and commitment of my younger colleagues. So, I dedicate this text to them. As Howard House was fond of saying, "our specialty is in the good hands of modern day Otonauts."

Michael E. Glasscock III, MD, FACS
Austin, TX
May 2009

Preface

In his Preface to the Fifth Edition of *Surgery of the Ear*, Michael E. Glasscock III was indeed prescient in his prediction that updating would be needed within 6 to 8 years. Much has changed in otology/neurotology since the last edition, and to remain relevant, this text required change as well.

One major change, apparent on even the most casual inspection, is the addition of color illustrations. Also updated and enhanced is the video DVD that accompanies the book—including 30 videos of important diagnostic and surgical procedures. The "Temporal Bone Dissection Guide Appendix" is updated with several new illustrations.

Several new chapters have been added, for example, "Hearing Aids," "Vestibular Rehabilitation," and "Tinnitus Rehabilitation," reflecting the importance of these management options in the armamentarium of the neurotologist. Two other new chapters, "Tumor Biology" and "The Prevention and Management of Cerebrospinal Fluid Leaks," now consolidate information that was previously scattered across several chapters, enabling more efficient, targeted use of that information. Acknowledging the explosion of options available to the surgeon, "Ossicular Reconstruction" and "Tympanoplasty" are now addressed in two distinct chapters. Many other chapters have been extensively updated, incorporating the advances of the past 6 years.

We aspired to maintain the historic heritage of this classic text and continue the tradition established by Drs. Glasscock and Shambaugh while updating chapters. This sixth edition remains a practical and comprehensive, yet manageable, reference in otology/neurotology that promises to be of great value to both experienced surgeons and trainees preparing for board exams.

A. Julianna Gulya, MD, FACS
Lloyd B. Minor, MD, FACS
Dennis S. Poe, MD, FACS

Contributors

Stephanie Moody Antonio, MD
Assistant Professor, Department of Otolaryngology—Head & Neck Surgery
Eastern Virginia Medical School
Norfolk, VA
* *Diseases of the Auricle, External Auditory Canal, and Tympanic Membrane*

Ben J. Balough, MD
Captain, Medical Core, United States Navy
Sherman Department of Otolaryngology
Naval Medical Center
San Diego, CA
* *Surgical Anatomy of the Temporal Bone and Dissection Guide*

Sanjay A. Bhansali, MD, FACS
Ear Consultants of Georgia
Atlanta, GA
* *Vestibular Testing*

Dennis I. Bojrab, MD
Michigan Ear Institute, Farmington Hills, MI
Chairman, Department of Otolaryngology, Beaumont Hospital, Royal Oak, MI
Oakland University School of Medicine
Rochester, MI
Director, Neuroscience Center, Providence Park Hospital, Novi, MI
Clinical Professor, Department of Otolaryngology and Neurosurgery, Wayne State University
Farmington Hills, MI
* *Vestibular Testing*
* *Surgical Anatomy of the Temporal Bone and Dissection Guide*

Derald E. Brackmann, MD
Clinical Professor of Otolaryngology—Head and Neck Surgery/Neurological Surgery
University of Southern California School of Medicine
President and Board of Directors
House Ear Institute
Los Angeles, CA
* *Auditory Brainstem Implant*

John P. Carey. MD
Associate Professor, Department of Otolaryngology—Head & Neck Surgery
Johns Hopkins Medical Center
Baltimore, MD
* *Surgical Treatment of Peripheral Vestibular Disorders*

Keith A. Casper, MD
Assistant Professor, Department of Otolaryngology—Head & Neck Surgery
University of Cincinnati Academic Health Center
Cincinnati, OH
* *Surgery for Cancer of the External Ear*
* *Surgery for Malignant Lesions*

Martin J. Citardi, MD
Professor and Chair, Department of Otorhinolaryngology—Head & Neck Surgery
University of Texas Medical School
Houston, TX
* *Surgery for Cystic Lesions of the Petrous Apex*

Benjamin T. Crane, MD, PhD
Assistant Professor, Department of Otolaryngology
University of Rochester Medical Center
Rochester, NY
* *Surgical Treatment of Peripheral Vestibular Disorders*
* *Surgical Anatomy of the Temporal Bone and Dissection Guide*

Boberto A. Cueva, MD, FACS
Regional Neurotologist/Skull Base Surgeon, Southern California Permanente Medical Group
Associate Clinical Professor/Voluntary and Co-Director of Neurotology Fellowship
University of California
San Diego, CA
* *Principles of Temporal Bone and Skull Base Surgery*
* *Neurophysiologic Monitoring in Otologic/Neurotologic Surgery*
* *Prevention and Management of Cerebrospinal Fluid Leaks*

Christopher J. Danner, MD
Director of Clinical Research, Tampa Bay Hearing & Balance Disorder Center
Associate Clinical Professor
Department of Communicative Disorders
University of South Florida, Tampa, FL
Associate Director of Prosper Ménière Society
Little Rock, AR
* *Prevention and Management of Cerebrospinal Fluid Leaks*

Charles C. Della Santina, MD, PhD
Associate Professor of Otolaryngology—Head & Neck Surgery and Biomedical Engineering
Director, Johns Hopkins Vestibular Neuroengineering Lab
Johns Hopkins School of Medicine
Baltimore, MD
* *Implantable Middle Ear and Bone Conduction Hearing Devices*

Chris De Souza, MD, FACS
Visiting Assistant Professor of Otolaryngology, State University of New York—Downstate Medical Center
Brooklyn, NY
Consultant Otology Surgeon, Tata Memorial Hospital
Mumbai, India
* *Intracranial Complications of Otitis Media*

David R. Friedland, MD, PhD
Associate Professor and Chief, Division of Otology and Neuro-otologic Skull Base Surgery
Department of Otolaryngology and Communication Sciences
Medical College of Wisconsin
Milwaukee, WI
* *Stereotactic Radiosurgery and Radiotherapy for Temporal Bone Tumors*

Lendra M. Friesen, MS
Director of Cochlear Implant Research, Department of Otolaryngology, Sunnybrook Health Sciences Centre
Associate Scientist, Sunnybrook Research Institute
Associate Professor, Department of Otolaryngology
University of Toronto
Toronto, ON, Canada
* *Auditory Brainstem Implant*

Bruce J. Gantz, MD
Professor and Chair, Department of Otolaryngology—Head & Neck Surgery
University of Iowa Hospitals and Clinics
Iowa City, IA
* *Surgery of the Facial Nerve*

M. Miles Goldsmith, MD, FACS
Georgia Ear Institute
Savannah, GA
* *Image-Guided Systems in Neurotology/Skull Base Surgery*

Quinton Gopen, MD
Instructor, Department of Otology and Laryngology
Harvard Medical School
Department of Otolaryngology, Children's Hospital
Boston, MA
* *Endoscopic Diagnosis and Surgery of Eustachian Tube Dysfunction*
* *Pathology and Clinical Course Inflammatory Diseases of the Middle Ear*

Samuel P. Gubbels, MD
Assistant Professor, Department of Surgery, Division of Otolaryngology
University of Wisconsin
Madison, WI
* *Surgery of the Facial Nerve*

Aina Julianna Gulya, MD, FACS
Clinical Professor of Otolaryngology—Head & Neck Surgery
The George Washington University
Washington, DC
Former Chief of Clinical Trials Branch, National Institute on Deafness and Other Communication Disorders
Bethesda, MD
* *Developmental Anatomy of the Temporal Bone and Skull Base*
* *Anatomy of the Temporal Bone and Skull Base*

Ophir Handzel, MD, LLB
Department of Otolaryngology—Head & Neck Surgery
Tel-Aviv Sourasky Medical Center
Tel-Aviv, Israel
Surgery for Otosclerosis

David S. Haynes, MD
Director, Division of Otology and Neurotology
The Otology Group of Vanderbilt
Neurotology Fellowship Program Director, Associate Professor, Department of Otolaryngology
Associate Professor, Department Hearing and Speech Sciences
Vanderbilt University Medical Center
Nashville, TN
* *Clinical Diagnosis*
* *Canal-Wall-Up Mastoidectomy*

Stefan Heller, PhD
Associate Professor, Department of Otolaryngology—Head & Neck Surgery
Stanford University School of Medicine
Stanford, CA
* *Auditory Physiology: Inner Ear*

Masoud Hemmati, MD
Professor and Chairman, Department of Radiology
University of Illinois
Chicago, IL
* *Imaging of the Temporal Bone*

Gayle E. Hicks, PhD, DABNM
Diplomat of the American Board of Neurophysiologic Monitoring, American Board of Audiology, Board Certification
Neurodynamics, Inc.
San Diego, CA
* *Neurophysiologic Monitoring in Otologic/ Neurotologic Surgery*

William E. Hitselberger, MD
Neurosurgeon
Los Angeles, CA
* *Auditory Brainstem Implant*

Gordon B. Hughes, MD
Program Director—Clinical Trials, Division of Scientific Programs
National Institute on Deafness & Other Communication Disorders
National Institutes of Health
Bethesda, MD
* *Surgery for Cystic Lesions of the Petrous Apex*

Timothy E. Huller, MD, FACS
Assistant Professor, Department Otolaryngology—Head & Neck Surgery
Department of Anatomy and Neurobiology, Program in Audiology & Communication Sciences
Washington University School of Medicine
St. Louis, MO
* *Vestibular Physiology and Disorders of the Labyrinth*

C. Gary Jackson, MD, FACS
Nashville, TN
* *Principles of Temporal Bone and Skull Base Surgery*
* *Surgery for Benign Tumors of the Temporal Bone*

Robert A. Jahrsdoerfer, MD
Professor, Department of Otolaryngology—Head & Neck Surgery
University of Virginia School of Medicine
Charlottesville, VA
* *Surgery for Congenital Aural Atresia*

Pawal J. Jastreboff, PhD, ScD, MBA
Professor, Department of Otolaryngology—Head & Neck Surgery
Emory University School of Medicine
Atlanta, GA
* *Tinnitus*

Elina Kari, MD
Department of Otolaryngology—Head & Neck Surgery
Emory University School of Medicine
Atlanta, GA
* *Tinnitis*

B. Maya Kato, MD
Michael R. Gatto & Associates
Palm Springs, CA
* *Vestibular Testing*

Bradley W. Kesser, MD
Associate Professor, Department of Otolaryngology—Head & Neck Surgery
University of Virginia Health System
Charlottesville, VA
* *Surgery for Congenital Aural Atresia*

Arvind Kumar, MD, FRCS
Emeritus Professor, Department of Otolaryngology
University of Illinois
Adjunct Professor, Department of Otolaryngology
Northwestern University
Chicago, IL
Ear Institute of Chicago
Hinsdale, IL
* *Aural Complications of Otitis Media*

John F. Kveton, MD, FACS
Clinical Professor of Surgery (Otolaryngology) & Neurosurgery
Yale University School of Medicine
New Haven, CT
* *Open Cavity Mastoid Operations*

Anil K. Lalwani, MD
Professor, Department of Otolaryngology, Pediatrics, Physiology & Neuroscience
New York University School of Medicine
New York, NY
* *Genetics in Otology and Neurotology*

Joung Lee, MD
Professor of Surgery, Department of Neurosurgery
The Cleveland Clinic—Lerner College of Medicine
Cleveland, OH
* *Surgery for Cystic Lesions of the Petrous Apex*

John P. Leonetti, MD
Professor and Vice-Chairman, Department of Otolaryngology, Neurotology, Otology, and Skull Base Surgery
Co-director of the Loyola Center for Cranial Base Surgery
Loyola University Medical Center
Maywood, IL
* *Surgery for Benign Tumors of the Temporal Bone*

S. George Lesinski, MD
Otologist, Queen City Ear/Nose/Throat Association
Director, Midwest Ear Foundation
Cincinnati, OH
* *Lasers in Otology*

Samuel C. Levine, MD, FACS
Professor, Otolaryngology and Neurosurgery
University of Minnesota
Minneapolis, MN
* *Intracranial Complications of Otitis Media*

Charles Limb, MD
Associate Professor, Department of Otolaryngology—Head and Neck Surgery
Johns Hopkins University School of Medicine
Baltimore, MD
* *Neurophysiology: The Central Auditory System*

Lawrence R. Lustig, MD
Francis A. Sooy Professor, Department of Otolaryngology—Head & Neck Surgery
University of California—San Francisco
San Francisco, CA
* *Implantable Middle Ear and Bone Conduction Hearing Devices*

Sam J. Marz, MD
Professor, Department of Otolaryngology, Otology, Neurotology, and Skull Base Surgery
Residency Program Director
Director of the Loyola Hearing Center
Loyola University Medical Center
Maywood, IL
* *Surgery for Benign Tumors of the Temporal Bone*

Kinuko Masaki, PhD
Department of Otolaryngology—Head & Neck Surgery
Stanford University School of Medicine
Stanford, CA
* *Auditory Physiology: Inner Ear*

Douglas E. Mattox, MD
Professor and William Chester Warren, Jr, MD Chairman, Department of Otolaryngology—Head & Neck Surgery
Emory University School of Medicine
Atlanta, GA
* *Tinnitis*

Bradford J. May, PhD
Professor, Department of Otolaryngology—Head & Neck Surgery
Johns Hopkins University School of Medicine
Baltimore, MD
* *Neurophysiology: The Central Auditory System*

Michael J. Mckenna, MD
Professor, Department of Otology & Laryngology
Massachusetts Eye & Ear Infirmary
Boston, MA
* *Surgery for Otosclerosis*

Saumil N. Merchant, MD
Eliasen Professor of Otology and Laryngology
Harvard Medical School
Director, Otopathology Laboratory and Co-director Wallace Middle Ear Research Unit
Massachusetts Eye and Ear Infirmary
Boston, MA
* *Acoustics and Mechanics of the Middle Ear*

Anand N. Mhatre, PhD
Assistant Professor, Department of Otolaryngology, and Physiology & Neuroscience
New York University School of Medicine
New York, NY
* *Genetics in Otology and Neurotology*

Lloyd B. Minor, MD, FACS
Provost and Senior Vice President for Academic Affairs
The Johns Hopkins University
University Distinguished Service Professor of Otolaryngology—Head & Neck Surgery
The Johns Hopkins University School of Medicine
Baltimore, MD
* *Vestibular Physiology and Disorders of the Labyrinth*
* *Surgical Treatment of Peripheral Vestibular Disorders*

Matthew R. O'Malley, MD
Midwest Ear Institute
Indianapolis, Indiana
* *Clinical Diagnosis*

Steven R. Otto, MA
Senior Research Associate, Department of Communication and Auditory Neuroscience
House Ear Institute
Los Angeles, CA
* *Auditory Brainstem Implant*

Mark D. Packer, MD
Assistant Clinical Professor, Otolaryngology
University of Texas Medical School at San Antonio
Director of Otology and Neurotology, Wilford Hall Medical Center, Lackland Air Force Base
San Antonio, TX
* *Tumor Biology, Vestibular Schwannoma*

Nathan C. Page, MD
Department of Otolaryngology
Rady Children's Hospital
San Diego, CA
* *Vestibular Physiology and Disorders of the Labyrinth*

Myles Pensak, MD, FACS
H.B. Broidy Professor and Chairman, Department of Otolaryngology—Head & Neck Surgery
University of Cincinnati Academic Health Center
Cincinnati, OH
* *Surgery for Cancer of the External Ear*
* *Surgery for Malignant Lesions*

Travis J. Pfannenstiel, MD
Major, United States Army
Otology, Neurotology and Skull Base Surgery
Naval Medical Center
San Diego, CA
* *Vestibular Testing*

Dennis S. Poe, MD, FACS
Associate Professor, Department of Otolaryngology and Laryngology, Harvard Medical School
Department of Otolaryngology at Children's Hospital
Boston, MA
Visiting Professor, Department of Otolaryngology
Tampere University Medical School
Tampere, Finland
* *Endoscopic Diagnosis and Surgery of Eustachian Tube Dysfunction*
* *Endoscope-Assisted Ear Surgery*
* *Ossicular Chain Reconstruction*

Virginia Ramachandran, AuD
Senior Staff Audiologist, Division of Audiology
Department of Otolaryngology—Head and Neck Surgery
Henry Ford Hospital
Detroit, MI
* *Hearing Aids*

Peter S. Roland, MD
Professor and Chairman, Otolaryngology—Head & Neck Surgery
Professor, Neurological Surgery
Chief, Pediatric Otology
University of Texas Southwestern Medical Center
Dallas, TX
* *Cochlear Implants in Adults and Children*

John J. Rosowski, PhD
Professor of Otology & Laryngology and Health Sciences & Technology
Harvard Medical School
Principal Investigator, Eaton Peabody Laboratory of Auditory Physiology, Massachusetts Eye & Ear Infirmary
Boston, MA
Affiliate Faculty Member, Division of Health Sciences & Technology
Harvard University—Massachusetts Institute of Technology
Cambridge, MA
* *Acoustics and Mechanics of the Middle Ear*

Paul M. Ruggieri, MD
Head, Sections of Neuroradiology and MRI
Imaging Institute
The Cleveland Clinic, Cleveland, OH
* *Surgery for Cystic Lesions of the Petrous Apex*

Christina L. Runge- Samuelson, MD, PhD
Associate Professor, Department of Otolaryngology and Communication Sciences
Medical College of Wisconsin
Milwaukee, WI
* *Stereotactic Radiosurgery and Radiotherapy for Temporal Bone Tumors*

Ravi N. Samy, MD
Assistant Professor, Department of Otolaryngology
University of Cincinnati College of Medicine
Cincinnati, OH
* *Surgery of the Facial Nerve*

Michael C. Schubert, PT, PhD
Assistant Professor, Department of Otolaryngology—Head and Neck Surgery
Johns Hopkins School of Medicine
Baltimore, MD
* *Vestibular Rehabilitation*

Robert V. Shannon, PhD
Scientist, Auditory Implant Research Laboratory
House Ear Institute
Research Professor of Biomedical Engineering / Neuroscience
University of Southern California
Los Angeles, CA
* *Auditory Brainstem Implant*

Michael J. Shinners, MD
Clinical Assistant Professor, Pritzker School of Medicine
University of Chicago
Evanston, IL
* *Intracranial Complications of Otitis Media*

Aristides Athanasiadis-Sismanis, MD, FACS
Professor of Otorhinolaryngology, Medical School of Athens University
Director, ORL Clinic
Ippokration Hospital
Athens, Greece
* *Tympanoplasty: Tympanic Membrane Repair*
* *Ossicular Chain Reconstruction*

Brad A. Stach, PhD
Director, Division of Audiology
Department of Otolaryngology—Head & Neck Surgery
Henry Ford Hospital
Detroit, MI
* *Audiologic Evaluation of Otologic/Neurotologic Disease*
* *Rehabilitation: Hearing Aids*

Veronika Starlinger, MD
Department of Otolaryngology—Head & Neck Surgery
Medical University of Vienna
Vienna, Austria
* *Auditory Physiology: Inner Ear*

Barry Strasnick, MD, FACS
Professor and Chairman, Department of Otolaryngology—Head & Neck Surgery
Eastern Virginia Medical School
Norfolk, VA
* *Diseases of Auricle, External Auditory Canal, Tympanic Membrane*

Elizabeth H. Toh, MD
Department of Otolaryngology, Lahey Clinic
Burlington, MA
* *Auditory Brainstem Implant*

Galdino E. Valvassori, MD
Professor, Department of Radiology
University of Illinois
Chicago, IL
* *Imaging of the Temporal Bone*

P. Ashley Wackym, MD, FACS, FAAP
Vice President of Research, Legacy Health
President, Ear and Skull Base Institute
Portland, OR
* *Stereotactic Radiosurgery and Radiotherapy for Temporal Bone Tumors*

D. Bradley Welling, MD, PhD, FACS
Professor and Chair, Otology and Neurotology
The Ohio State University College of Medicine
Department of Otolaryngology—Head & Neck Surgery
The Ohio State University Medical Center
Columbus, OH
* *Tumor Biology*
* *Vestibular Schwannoma*

Richard Wiet, MD, FACS
Professor of Clinical Otolaryngology and Neurosurgery
Northwestern University
Chicago, IL
Ear Institute of Chicago
Hinsdale, IL
* *Aural Complications of Otitis Media*

Justin Wittkopf, MD
Otology/Neurotology and Skull Base Surgery
Affiliated Ear Nose and Throat Physicians
Woodstock, IL
* *Canal-Wall-Up Mastoidectomy*

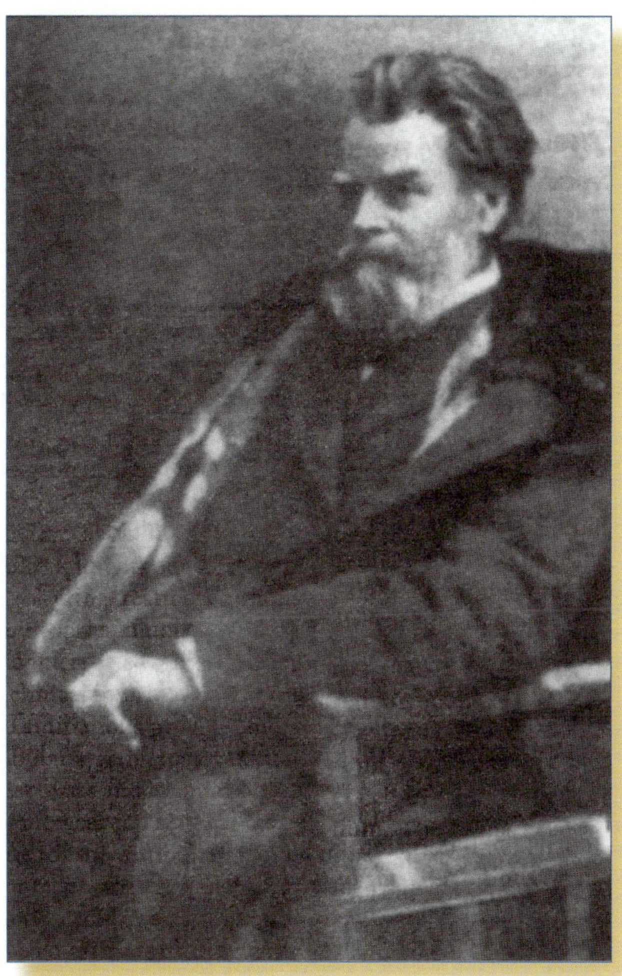

FRIEDRICH BEZOLD (1842-1908) • Clarified the differentiation by tuning fork tests of conductive and sensorineural hearing losses and the clinical diagnosis of otosclerosis. His clear and concise Textbook of Otology served as a model for Shambaugh as he wrote his Surgery of the Ear.

Scientific Foundations

1. Developmental Anatomy of the Temporal Bone and Skull Base
2. Anatomy of the Temporal Bone and Skull Base
3. Acoustics and Mechanics of the Middle Ear
4. Auditory Physiology: Inner Ear
5. Neurophysiology: The Central Auditory System
6. Vestibular Physiology and Disorders of the Labyrinth
7. Genetics in Otology and Neurotology
8. Tumor Biology

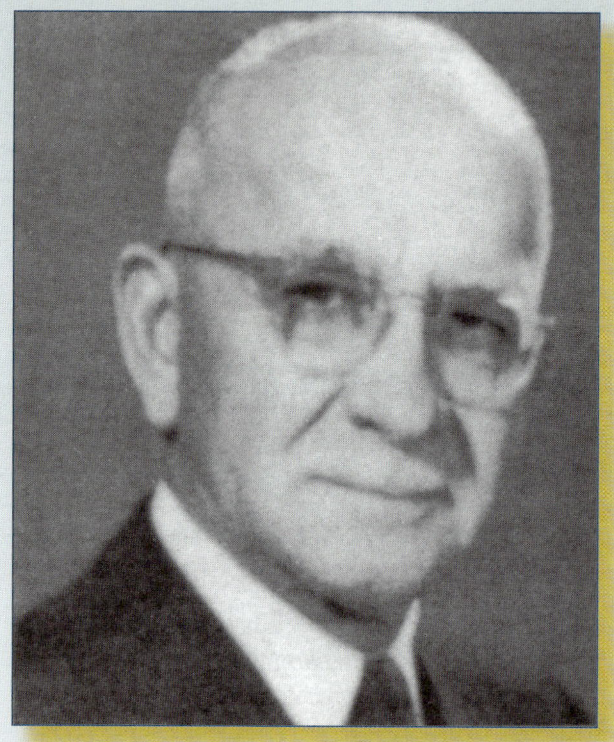

THEODORE H. BAST (1890–1959) • First described the utriculo-endolymphatic valve.

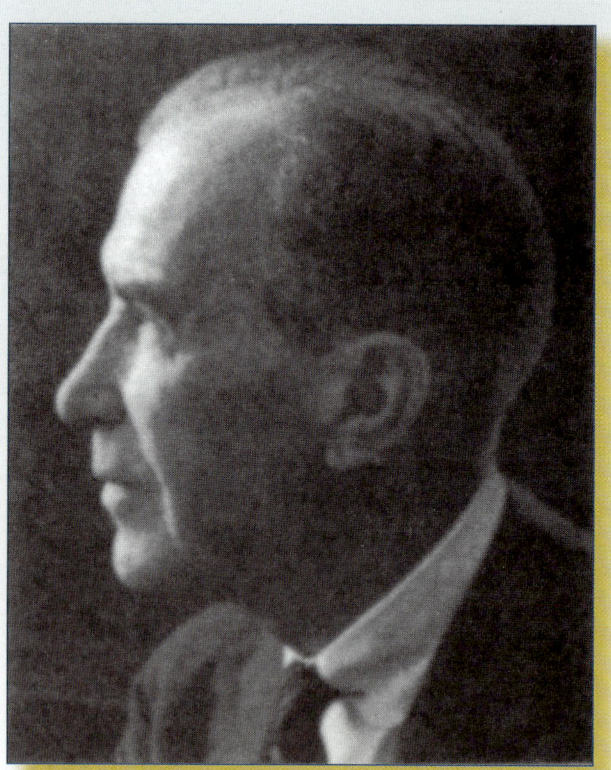

BARRY J. ANSON (1894–1974) • Student and investigator par excellence of the gross and microscopic anatomy of the temporal bone.

Developmental Anatomy of the Temporal Bone and Skull Base

1

Aina Julianna Gulya, MD, FACS

The complexity of nature's machinations is exemplified in the development of the ear, both in phylogenetic and ontogenetic terms. The labyrinth represents a parsimonious salvage and modification of the lateral line system of fish, whereas the ossicles originally participated in the masticatory apparatus of ancestral vertebrates.

As intriguing as the phylogeny of the ear is in an abstract sense, knowledge of its embryologic development is of crucial, concrete importance to the modern-day neurotologic surgeon. Management of major malformations of the ear, such as the manifestations of aural dysmorphogenesis, obviously demands such knowledge if a rational approach to the alleviation of associated hearing handicaps is to prevail. The surgeon who is able to anticipate more subtle irregularities of development, such as persistent stapedial arteries and high jugular bulbs, can confidently negotiate such potential hazards rather than fall prey to them.

This chapter presents a focused discussion of the development of the ear, emphasizing those features of particular surgical importance. The discussion begins with the most lateral structures of the temporal bone and progresses medially, just as a surgeon encounters these structures. The fetal ages are based on conversion of crown-rump measurements to postconceptual ages and thus may show some variations from figures based on alternative dating methods.

The reader interested in reviewing the pioneer works of Bast, Anson, Donaldson, Streeter, and Padget is referred to their referenced works. Comprehensive overviews of both phylogeny and anatomy are extant in such works as those by Gulya and Schuknecht,[1] Anson and Donaldson,[2] Pearson,[3] and Bast and Anson.[4]

DEVELOPMENT OF THE EXTERNAL EAR AND TEMPORAL BONE

External Ear

The development of the pinna commences at 4 weeks as tissue condensations of the mandibular and hyoid arches appear at the distal portion of the first branchial groove. Within 2 weeks, six ridges, known as the hillocks of His, arise from the tissue condensations (Figure 1–1). The significance of these hillocks varies, according to the investigator, from coincidental to integral to the development of the pinna. Accompanying these divergent views are studies that, on the one hand, suggest that the entire pinna except the tragus and anterior external auditory canal (of mandibular arch origin) arises from the hyoid (second branchial) arch.[5] Other studies demonstrate a balanced participation of both the first and second branchial arches in the development of the pinna.[3,6]

The hillocks fuse into an anterior fold of mandibular arch origin and a posterior fold of hyoid arch origin, oriented about the first branchial groove. The folds unite at the upper end of this groove (Figure 1–2).

Adult configuration (Figure 1–3) is achieved by the fifth month, independent of developmental progress in the middle

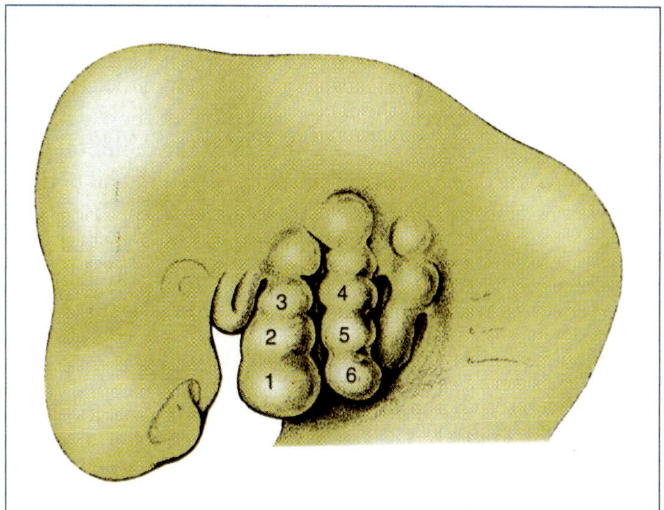

FIGURE 1-1 • The six hillocks of His at approximately 6 weeks. *After Levine.[6] Reproduced with permission from Gulya AJ. Gulya and Schuknecht's anatomy of the temporal bone with surgical implications. 3rd ed. New York: Informa Healthcare USA; 2007.*

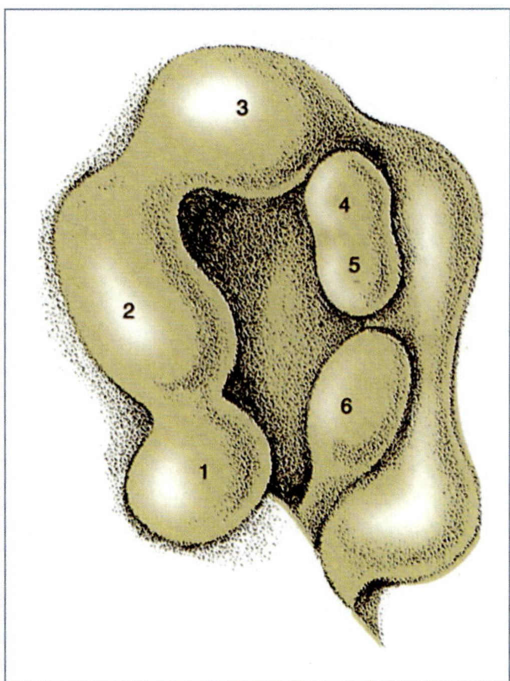

FIGURE 1–2 • At approximately 7 weeks, the six hillocks are fusing to form two folds, which will later fuse superiorly. *After Levine.*[6] *Reproduced with permission from Gulya AJ. Gulya and Schuknecht's anatomy of the temporal bone with surgical implications. 3rd ed. New York: Informa Healthcare USA; 2007.*

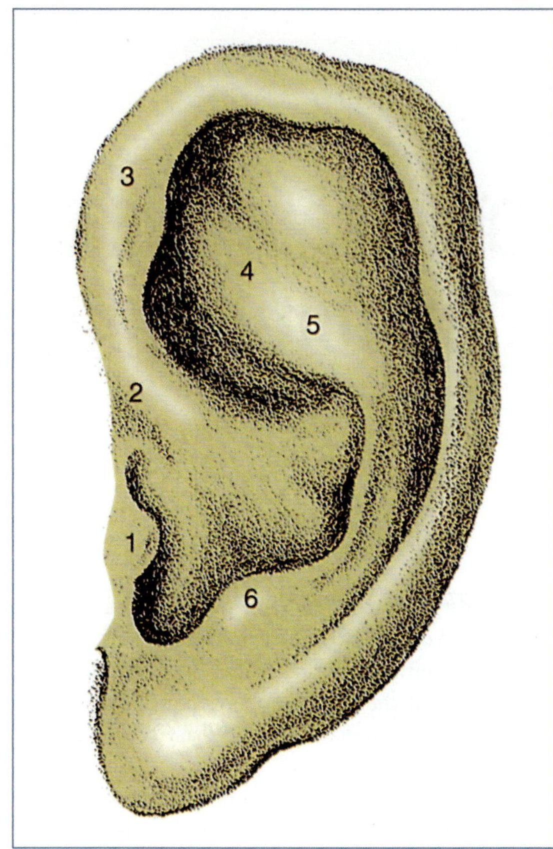

FIGURE 1–3 • The adult auricle with the derivatives of the six hillocks numbered. *After Levine.*[6] *Reproduced with permission from Gulya AJ. Gulya and Schuknecht's anatomy of the temporal bone with surgical implications. 3rd ed. New York: Informa Healthcare USA; 2007.*

and inner ears. The Darwinian tubercle, corresponding to the tip of the pinna in lower mammals, makes its appearance at roughly 6 months.

Temporal Bone, External Auditory Canal, Tympanic Ring, and Tympanic Membrane

The adult temporal bone is an amalgam of the squamous, petrous, mastoid, tympanic, and styloid bones. The close association of the external auditory canal, tympanic ring, and tympanic membrane justifies the inclusion of their developmental process in conjunction with that of the temporal bone as a whole. The development of the bony labyrinth and petrosa, however, because of its intricacy, warrants separate discussion. The following account of the development of the external auditory canal, tympanic ring, tympanic membrane, and temporal bone is derived from the works of Anson and associates[7] as well as Pearson.[3]

The dorsal part of the first branchial groove, which gives rise to the external auditory canal, progressively deepens during the second month. The ectoderm of the groove briefly abuts on the endoderm of the tubotympanic recess (first pharyngeal pouch), but during the sixth week, a mesodermal ingrowth breaks this contact. Beginning at 8 weeks, the inferior portion of the first branchial groove deepens again, forming the primary external auditory canal, which corresponds to the fibrocartilaginous canal of the adult. At the same time, development of the squama begins, marked by the appearance of a membranous bone ossification center. In the next week of development, a cord of epithelial cells at the depths of the primary external auditory canal grows medially into the mesenchyme to terminate in a solid (meatal) plate (Figure 1–4). The mesenchyme adjacent to the meatal plate gives rise to the lamina propria (fibrous layer) of the tympanic membrane and at 9 weeks is surrounded by the four membranous bone ossification centers of the tympanic ring. In addition to supporting the tympanic membrane, it has been theorized that the tympanic ring also functions to inhibit inward epithelial migration. Failure of this function may lead to cholesteatoma formation (ie, congenital cholesteatoma) at the junction of the first and second branchial arches.[8]

By the 10th week, the tympanic ring elements fuse except superiorly, where a defect remains, the notch of Rivinus. These elements then expand, accompanied by growth of the solid epithelial cord of cells. It is not until after the fifth month that the cord splits open, initially at its medial terminus, forming the bony external auditory canal by the seventh month. The cells remaining at the periphery form the epithelial lining of the bony external auditory canal, whereas those remaining medially form the superficial layer of the tympanic membrane. The medial layer of the tympanic membrane derives from the epithelial lining of the first pharyngeal pouch. These developmental changes in the external auditory canal occur at a time when the outer, middle, and inner ears are already well developed.

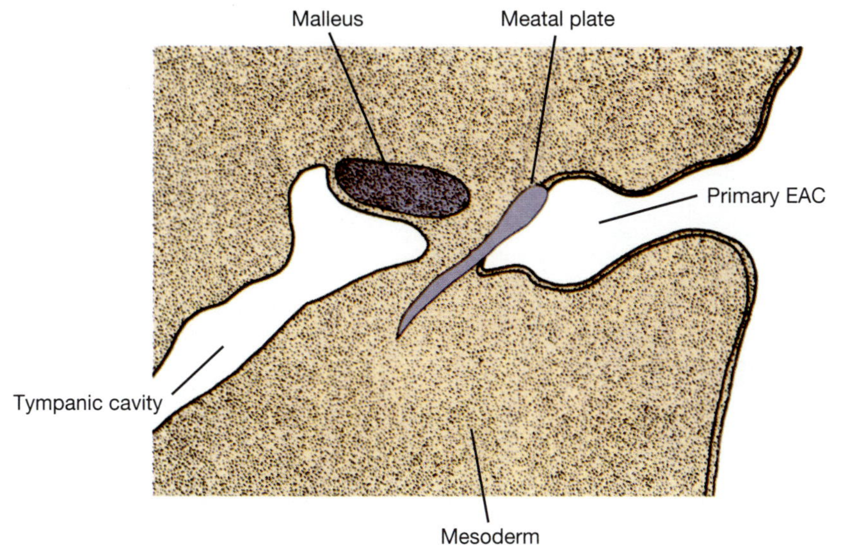

FIGURE 1–4 • The primary external auditory canal (EAC) is formed at 9 weeks with deepening of the first branchial groove. The meatal plate develops as epithelial cells grow medially toward the tympanic cavity. *After Anson and Donaldson.[2] Reproduced with permission from Gulya AJ. Gulya and Schuknecht's anatomy of the temporal bone with surgical implications. 3rd ed. New York: Informa Healthcare USA; 2007.*

Meanwhile, beginning at 4 months, the squama projects posterior to the tympanic ring, forming what will become the lateral (squamous) portion of the mastoid, roof of the external auditory canal, and lateral wall of the antrum. The medial (petrous) portion of the mastoid develops as air cells invade the periosteal layer of the bony labyrinth. The external petrosquamous fissure marks the junction of the petrosa with the squama and generally disappears by the second year of life.

The hypotympanum develops between 22 and 32 weeks as a tripartite bony amalgam[9] composed of the tympanic bone (membranous bone), the canalicular otic capsule (enchondral bone), and a petrosal ledge (periosteal bone). This variegated structure is thought to predispose this area to anomalous development, such as that which leaves bare the jugular bulb in the middle ear.

After the eighth month, the tympanic ring begins to fuse with the otic capsule, a process that is not completed until birth. Postnatally, lateral extensions of the tympanic ring and the squama (Figure 1–5) extend the external auditory canal and carry the tympanic membrane from the horizontal angulation of the neonate to the acute angulation of the adult (see Figure 1–5). The styloid process does not make its appearance until after birth, arising in an ossification center at the upper aspect of Reichert's cartilage.

Microtia, anotia, and aberrant positioning of the pinna derive from abnormal development of the first and second branchial arches. Developmental failure of the first branchial groove results in stenosis or atresia of the external auditory canal, based on either a lack of canalization of the meatal plate or a deficiency in epithelial ingrowth. The presence or absence of accompanying defects in the middle and inner ears depends on the time period at which development was disrupted.

Postnatal Development of the Temporal Bone

Although inner and middle ear structures have completed development long before birth, the mastoid and tympanic bones, in particular, manifest postnatal growth and development. Knowledge of these developmental changes is imperative for the otologic surgeon contemplating operative intervention in the very young pediatric patient or cochlear implantation in the profoundly deaf infant or child.

In the neonate, the squama is disproportionately large in comparison with that of the adult (Figure 1–6). The mastoid process is essentially nonexistent, and the tympanic bone is a relatively flat ring, rather than a cylinder. The relative position of the entire temporal bone in the neonate (see Figure 1–6) is inferolateral in comparison with the temporal bone in the adult and its more lateral orientation.

The facial nerve, in the absence of a mastoid process, exits the stylomastoid foramen to emerge on the lateral aspect of the skull and thus is especially vulnerable to injury if a standard postauricular incision is performed. After the first year of life, the mastoid process begins development both laterally and inferiorly, with the mastoid tip deriving from the petrous portion of the mastoid.[10] Similarly, the tympanic ring extends laterally, completing the formation of the bony external auditory canal, the sheath of the styloid process, and the nonarticular part of the glenoid fossa (see Figure 1–5). In the 1-year-old infant, opposing spurs of growing bone at the ventral aspect of the bony external auditory canal fuse, dividing the original external auditory canal into the adult external auditory canal and an inferior channel, known as the foramen of Huschke. The adult external auditory canal is cranial to, and larger than, the foramen of Huschke (see Figure 1–5). This secondary foramen closes in late childhood.[7] With these changes in the mastoid and tympanic bones, the lateral aspect of the temporal bone is vertically oriented, and the facial nerve is buried beneath the protective barrier of the mastoid process. The lateral growth of the tympanic ring, as mentioned previously, carries the tympanic membrane from the nearly horizontal orientation of the neonate to the adult angulation by age 4 or 5 years.

With a view toward cochlear implantation in the infant or young child, one study suggested that the dimensions that show

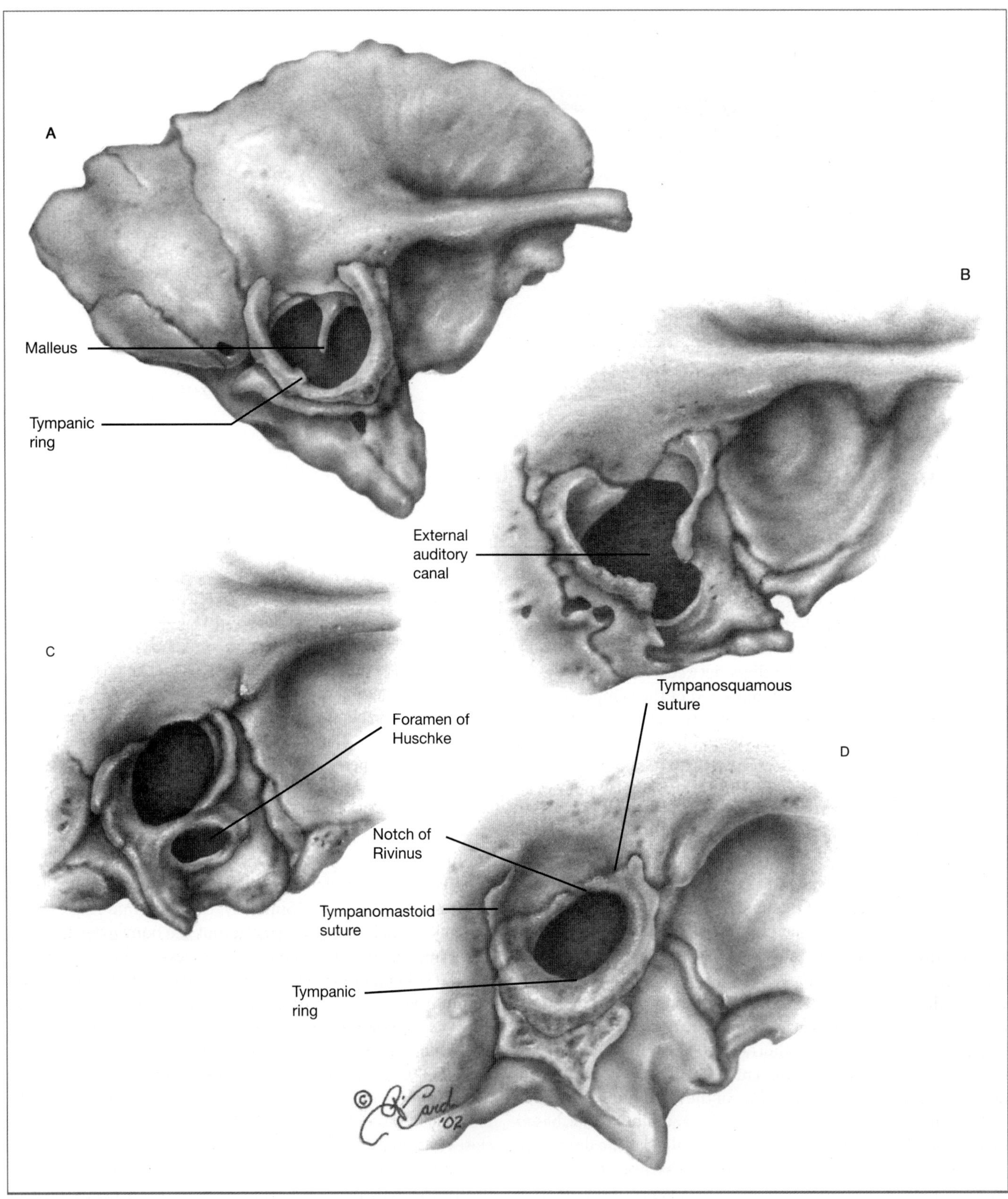

FIGURE 1–5 • Postnatal development of the tympanic portion of the temporal bone. *A*, Neonate. Note the flat tympanic ring and the exposed stylomastoid foramen. *B*, Infant, 11 months. The notch of Rivinus and the foramen of Huschke are becoming evident. *C*, Infant, 1 year. *D*, Adolescent. *After Anson BJ, Donaldson JA. Surgical anatomy of the temporal bone and ear. Philadelphia: WB Saunders; 1981.*

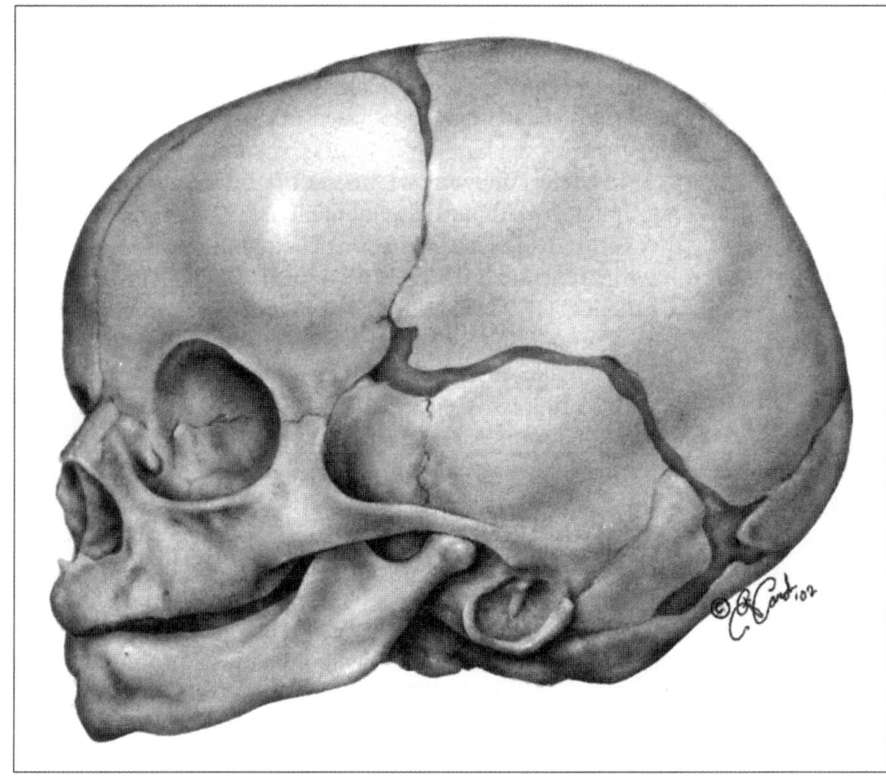

FIGURE 1–6 • The temporal bone of the infant, absent a mastoid process and laterally extending external auditory canal, is located more inferiorly on the skull than that of the adult.

significant growth, continuing into the teenage years, include the depth of the tympanic cavity (as measured by the distance between the tympanic membrane and the stapes footplate) and the length, width, and depth of the mastoid.[11] Cochlear wires, if reaching to the lateral skull, should be placed with approximately 2.5 cm of slack to accommodate anticipated growth. The facial recess, on the other hand, should be adult size at birth.[12]

DEVELOPMENT OF THE TYMPANOMASTOID COMPARTMENT AND EUSTACHIAN TUBE

The tympanomastoid compartment represents the phylogenetic salvage and functional adaptation of the aquatic gill apparatus, which transiently appears in the ontogeny of the human. As life forms evolved from a water environment to a terrestrial environment, a mechanism for matching the sound impedance of water with that of air became essential to auditory function. The middle ear and its contained ossicular chain serve this purpose. The first vestige of such an impedance-matching mechanism emerged as the spiracular diverticulum of the eusthenopteron (a crossopterygian fish).[13]

In the developing human, the tympanomastoid compartment appears at the 3-week stage as an outpouching of the first pharyngeal pouch known as the tubotympanic recess. The endodermal tissue of the dorsal end of this pouch eventually becomes the eustachian tube and tympanic cavity (Hammar, as cited in Proctor[14]). Expansion of the pouch begins at the inferior aspect of the definitive tympanic cavity and progresses by invasion of the adjacent mesenchyme, a loose, gelatinous derivative of mesoderm. By 7 weeks, concomitant growth of the second branchial arch constricts the midportion of the tubotympanic recess; according to Hammar (as cited in Proctor[14]), the primary tympanic cavity lies lateral and the primordial eustachian tube lies medial to this constriction. The terminal end of the first pharyngeal pouch buds into four sacci (anticus, posticus, superior, and medius[14]), which expand to progressively pneumatize the middle ear and the epitympanum. Expansion of the sacci envelops the ossicular chain and lines the tympanomastoid compartment, whereas the interface between two sacci gives rise to mesentery-like mucosal folds, transmitting blood vessels.

The further development of the eustachian tube is marked by its lengthening and narrowing, with mesodermal chondrification establishing the fibrocartilaginous eustachian tube. By the 21st week, pneumatization reaches the antrum. Although the tympanic cavity is essentially complete by 30 weeks, some configurational changes occur with finalization of the bony hypotympanum (see above).

Mastoid pneumatization is evident as early as 33 weeks and proceeds by well-established tracts.[15] Heredity, environment, nutrition, bacterial infection, and adequate ventilation provided by the eustachian tube are all thought to play a role in the interindividual variability of temporal bone pneumatization.[1]

By birth, the antrum approximates that of the adult. However, mesenchymal resolution may continue as late as 1 year postnatally,[16] or even later in some rare cases. Remnants of embryonic connective tissue in the adult are manifest as connective tissue strands draped over the oval and round windows.[10] Similarly, the mastoid continues to grow for up to 19 years after birth.[11]

Epitympanic fixation of the head of the malleus is a clinically encountered condition rooted in the incomplete pneumatization of the epitympanum.[17] Such bony fixation of the malleus is a normal occurrence in certain mammals.[18]

Alternative theories for the development of the middle ear have been proposed. Fraser (cited in Proctor[14]) suggested that the first, second, and third branchial arches, as well as the second branchial groove, give rise to the primitive tympanic cavity. Other workers suggested that the first pharyngeal pouch forms only the eustachian tube, whereas the remainder of the tympanomastoid compartment develops by the cavitation of mesenchyme.[19] In this scheme, mesenchymal derivatives, rather than the respiratory mucosa of the first pharyngeal pouch, form the lining of the middle ear.

DEVELOPMENT OF THE OSSICULAR CHAIN

The ossicular chain, a functional component of the middle ear impedance-matching mechanism, for the most part traces its phylogenetic roots to the branchial arch (gill slit) apparatus. In early vertebrates, the mesenchyme of branchial arches I (Meckel's cartilage, mandibular arch) and II (Reichert's cartilage, hyoid arch) was destined to become part of the masticatory apparatus. Evolutionary modifications that reduced the stresses on the jaw rendered certain of its components, namely, the articular and the quadrate, superfluous.[20] The malleus and the incus, respectively, are derived from these jaw components, whereas the origin of the stapes has been traced back to the columella auris of reptiles.

The first evidence of ossicular development in the human embryo occurs at approximately 4 weeks as an interbranchial bridge appears, connecting the upper end of that portion of the first branchial arch referred to as the mandibular visceral bar and the central region of the hyoid (second branchial arch) visceral bar. It is this condensed mesenchymal bridge, consisting of both first and second branchial arch elements, that through cartilaginous differentiation gives rise to the primordial malleus and incus.[21] All of the stapes blastema derives from the hyoid bar except for the medial surface of the footplate and its annular ligament, which are of otic capsular (lamina stapedialis) origin (Gradenigo, 1889, cited in Gulya and Schuknecht[1]) (Figure 1–7).

Over the following 11 weeks, the future ossicular chain continues growth and development as a cartilaginous model (see Figure 1–7); such formation of bone from a cartilage model is termed enchondral bone development (see "DEVELOPMENT OF THE OTIC CAPSULE"). The anterior process of the malleus is unique in that it develops as membranous bone without a cartilaginous model. Development of the stapes blastema involves progressive encirclement of the stapedial artery. The obturator foramen represents the completed ring left empty after the stapedial artery involutes (see "DEVELOPMENT OF THE ARTERIES"). Growth of the lamina stapedialis, an otic capsule structure, involves retrogressive changes in the cartilaginous rim of the oval window.

By 15 weeks, the ossicles have attained adult size, and ossification soon begins, first in the incus, then in the malleus, and finally in the stapes. As the footplate attains adult size, tissue at the oval window rim develops into the fibrous tissue of the annular ligament. During the same time frame, the tensor tympani and stapedius muscles develop from the mesenchyme of the first and second branchial arches, respectively. The ossicles assume their adult configuration by 20 weeks, although the megalithic stapes of the fetus continues to lose bulk well into the 32nd week. Otherwise, the endochondral bone of the ossicles, similar to that of the otic capsule, undergoes little change over the lifetime of the individual and demonstrates poor reparative capacity in response to trauma.

Meanwhile, pneumatization of the tympanic cavity extends into the epitympanum and antrum, and the ossicles are enveloped in the mucous membrane lining of the tubotympanic recess.

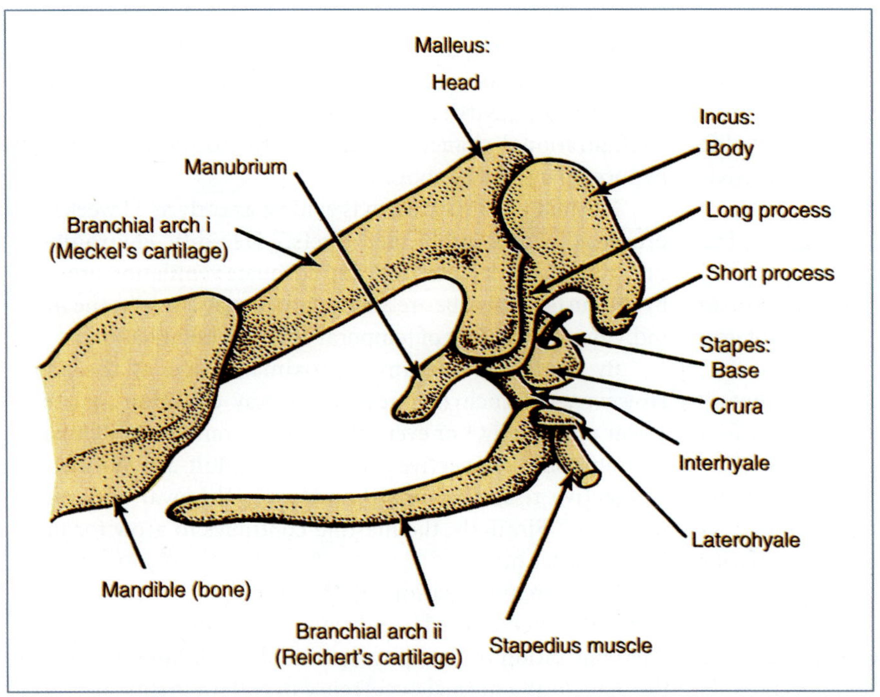

FIGURE 1–7 • The branchial arch origin of the ossicles at 8 to 9 weeks as seen in a left lateral view. The interhyale marks the site of development of attachment of the stapedius tendon, which is its derivative. The laterohyale, eventually migrating to lie posterior to the stapes, temporarily acts as part of the facial nerve canal. *After Hanson and colleagues.[21] Reproduced with permission from Gulya AJ. Gulya and Schuknecht's anatomy of the temporal bone with surgical implications. 3rd ed. New York: Informa Healthcare USA; 2007.*

DEVELOPMENT OF THE OTIC LABYRINTH

The precursor of the mammalian otic labyrinth is the cranial portion of the lateral line system of fish,[22] a water- motion detection system. This system of fluid-filled pits (ampullae) features epidermal placode derivation; innervation by cranial nerves VII, IX, and X; and a functional architecture consisting of hair cells, supporting cells, and surrounding fluid (sea water), recapitulated in the mammalian inner ear. Enclosure of the lateral line system, separating it from the ocean environment, is first seen in the hagfish (Myxinoidea) and results in the formation of the first true vestibular mechanism.[22] Ascending the vertebrate ladder, the vestibular mechanism becomes increasingly complex as it changes from a structure consisting of a utricle and two semicircular canals (the superior and posterior) by adding the endolymphatic duct passages; a third semicircular canal (the lateral), the saccule; and an outgrowth of the saccule, the lagena, which eventually gives rise to the cochlea. Endolymph replaced seawater as the surrounding fluid as the lateral line system evolved from use in aquatic to terrestrial organisms.

The development of the otic labyrinth in the human embryo faithfully follows much the same sequence as did the development of the mechanism in our vertebrate ancestors; hence, the phylogenetically older semicircular canals and utricle (pars superior) precede the development of the saccule and the cochlear duct (pars inferior). The phylogenetic seniority of the pars superior is thought to underlie its relative resistance to developmental malformations when contrasted with the newer pars superior.

The otic placode, a plaquelike thickening of surface ectoderm dorsal to the first branchial groove, appears at the end of the third week. Invagination into the underlying mesenchyme occurs within days, forming the auditory pit (Figure 1–8). The endolymphatic appendage appears at this stage, considerably in advance of the semicircular and cochlear ducts.[23] Expansion of the auditory pit and fusion of overlying tissue create the otocyst (otic vesicle), separated from the surface. The mesenchymal tissue that surrounds and differentiates in conjunction with the otocyst is the future otic capsule (bony labyrinth). By the fourth week, two flanges (the future semicircular ducts) arise from the otocyst. Development then involves elongation of the otocyst and the appearance of three deepening folds (I, II, and III), which demarcate the utricle with its three semicircular ducts, the endolymphatic duct and sac, and the saccule with its cochlear duct (Figure 1–9). The utriculoendolymphatic valve (of Bast) is a derivative of fold III, functionally separating the utricle and the dilated proximal aspect, or sinus, of the endolymphatic duct.[24]

In the 6-week embryo, the lumina of the semicircular ducts have formed, and the macula communis (the primordial macula at the medial wall of the otocyst) has divided into superior and inferior segments. The macula of the utricle and the ampullary crests of the superior and lateral semicircular ducts are derivatives of the superior segment, whereas the macula of the saccule and the ampullary crest of the posterior semicircular duct are derived from the inferior segment. At the same time, the cochlear duct has extended from the saccule, completing one turn during the course of the week.

As the semicircular ducts increase in both the radius of the arc of curvature and in luminal diameter (Figure 1–10), progressive deepening of the three folds (Figure 1–11) delineates the ductal connections of the utricle, saccule, and endolymphatic sac as well as of the cochlea and saccule. Meanwhile, the cochlear duct continues its spiraling growth, rapidly completing its 2½ turns by the eighth week (see Figure 1–8). A number of cochlear anomalies are recognized and are believed to reflect the stage at which normal development is disrupted.[25]

Between 8 and 16 weeks, the otic labyrinth approaches its adult configuration (Figure 1–12). The epithelium of the cristae ampullaries of the semicircular ducts differentiates to a sensory neuroepithelium with hair cells and gelatinous cupula as the semicircular ducts continue expansion. Similarly, the maculae of the otolithic organs (utricle and saccule) differentiate as hair

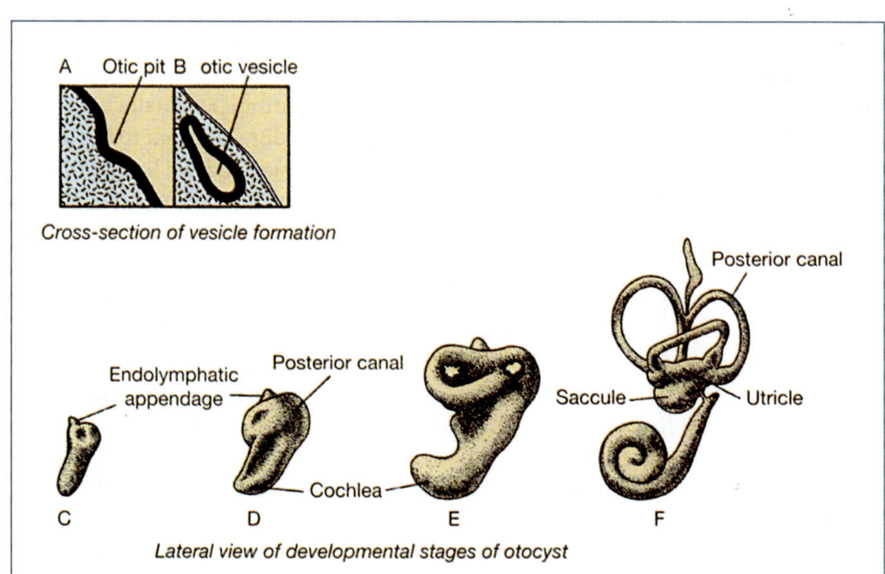

FIGURE 1–8 • The evolution of the endolymphatic (otic) labyrinth. *A*, 22 days, *B*, 4 weeks, *C*, 4½ weeks, *D*, 5½ weeks, *E*, 6 weeks, and *F*, 8+ weeks. *After Streeter.*[23] *Reproduced with permission from Gulya AJ. Gulya and Schuknecht's anatomy of the temporal bone with surgical implications. 3rd ed. New York: Informa Healthcare USA; 2007.*

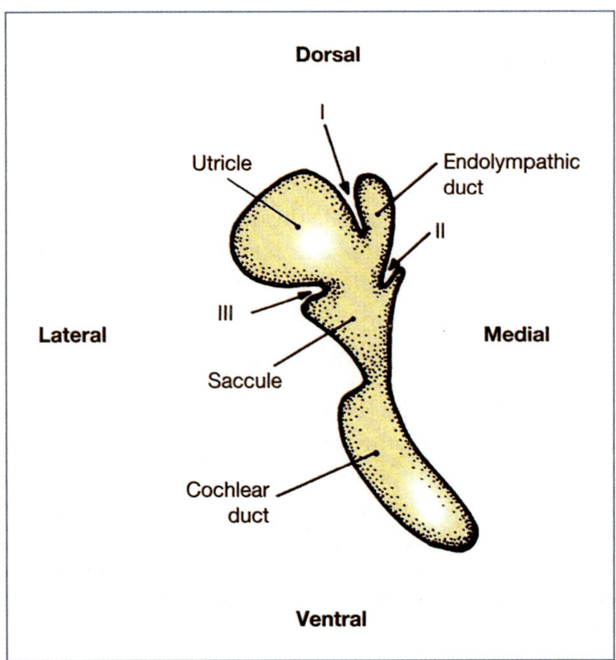

FIGURE 1–9 • The otic labyrinth at the 6- to 8-week stage. Folds I, II, and III begin to indent the otocyst. *After Bast and Anson.*[4] *Reproduced with permission from Gulya AJ. Gulya and Schuknecht's anatomy of the temporal bone with surgical implications. 3rd ed. New York: Informa Healthcare USA; 2007.*

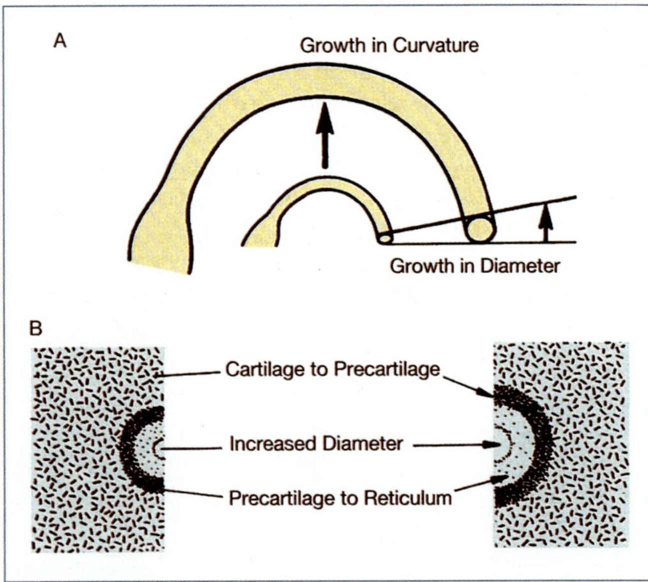

FIGURE 1–10 • Growth of the semicircular ducts involves retrogressive changes in the surrounding cartilage and precartilage. *After Pearson.*[3] *Reproduced with permission from Gulya AJ. Gulya and Schuknecht's anatomy of the temporal bone with surgical implications. 3rd ed. New York: Informa Healthcare USA; 2007.*

cells and otolithic membranes appear. The proximal endolymphatic sac begins to develop a rugose epithelium. The primitive circular cochlear duct assumes a more triangular outline as the neuroepithelium of the basal turn begins to differentiate into the organ of Corti (Figure 1–13).

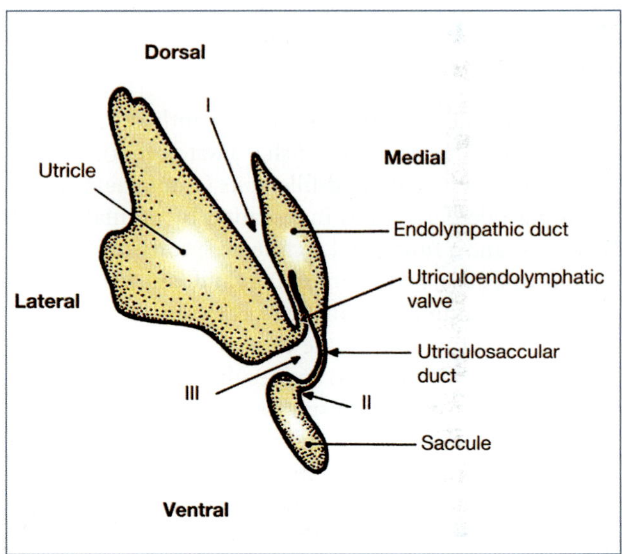

FIGURE 1–11 • The otic labyrinth at 9 weeks. Deepening of folds I, II, and III (compare with Figure 1–9) more clearly distinguishes the utricle, saccule, and endolymphatic duct. *After Bast and Anson.*[4] *Reproduced with permission from Gulya AJ. Gulya and Schuknecht's anatomy of the temporal bone with surgical implications. 3rd ed. New York: Informa Healthcare USA; 2007.*

At 20 weeks, the superior semicircular duct has reached adult size. In a phylogenetically determined sequence, the posterior and lateral ducts complete growth, and the cristae ampullares are completely differentiated. The endolymphatic duct, up to this stage, has followed a straight course, paralleling the crus commune to reach the endolymphatic sac; now the duct begins to develop a bend as it is dragged inferiorly and laterally along with the endolymphatic sac by the continuing growth of the sigmoid sinus and posterior fossa. The first part of the endolymphatic duct, then, is an anatomically constant structure in close relationship to the crus commune; the distal duct and sac, however, vary in position according to the degree of sigmoid sinus migration and posterior fossa development.[1] The sac continues to grow, with its size at term attaining quadruple that seen at midterm and with its lining further differentiating. The lining epithelium of the saccular, utricular, and endolymphatic ducts ranges from simple squamous to cuboidal. As demonstrated by Lundquist,[26] the proximal endolymphatic sac (Figure 1–14), located within the vestibular aqueduct, and the distal third, completely enveloped in dura adjacent to the lateral venous sinus, similarly possess a simple cuboidal lining. In contrast, the intermediate one-third, or rugose portion, which lies partly within the vestibular aqueduct and partly within folds of dura mater, has a highly differentiated epithelium. The tall, cylindrical cells of the epithelium possess microvilli and pinocytotic vesicles, are ruffled into papillae and crypts, and overlie a rich, subepithelial capillary network.

All of these features suggest resorptive and phagocytic functions, with the latter function providing for local immune defense.[27]

The organ of Corti is differentiated to such a degree by 20 weeks that the fetus can "hear" and respond to fluid-borne sounds.[28] The organ of Corti approximates the adult structure by 25 weeks.[3]

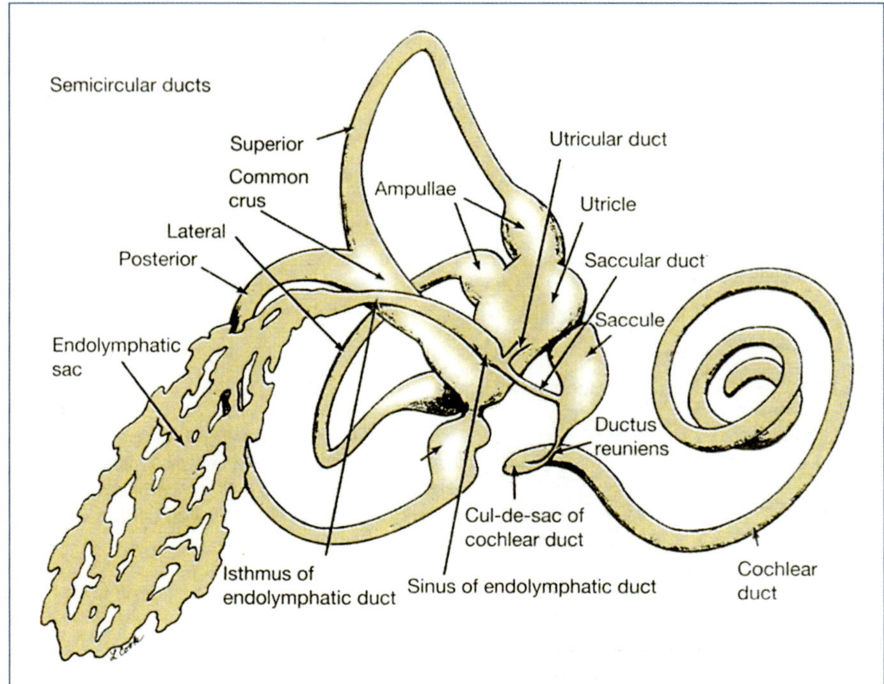

FIGURE 1–12 • The adult membranous labyrinth, medial aspect. The endolymphatic duct initially parallels the common crus and posterior semicircular duct but then diverges to the posterior cranial fossa location of the endolymphatic sac. *After Anson and Donaldson.[2] Reproduced with permission from Gulya AJ. Gulya and Schuknecht's anatomy of the temporal bone with surgical implications. 3rd ed. New York: Informa Healthcare USA; 2007.*

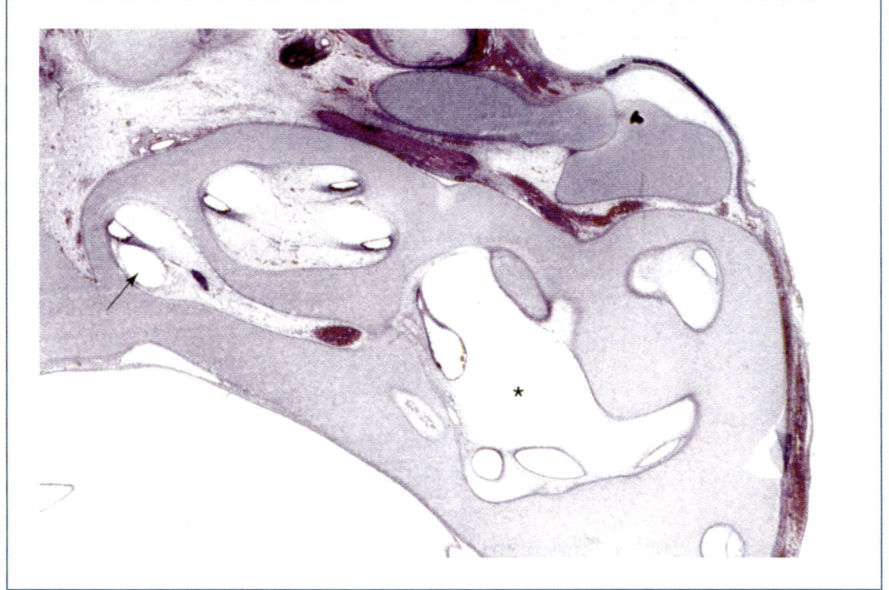

FIGURE 1–13 • In this 12-week fetus, the vestibule (asterisk) is advanced in development and the scala tympani (arrow) is evident in the basal turn of the cochlea. The cochlear duct of the basal turn assumes a more triangular configuration, whereas the apical turn still retains its circular outline. *Reproduced with permission from Gulya AJ. Gulya and Schuknecht's anatomy of the temporal bone with surgical implications. 3rd ed. New York: Informa Healthcare USA; 2007.*

DEVELOPMENT OF THE PERILYMPHATIC (PERIOTIC) LABYRINTH

The perilymphatic (periotic) labyrinth comprises the fluid-tissue space interposed between the membranous otic (or endolymphatic) labyrinth and its bony covering—the otic capsule. The perilymphatic cistern (of the vestibule), scala tympani, scala vestibuli, perilymphatic space of the semicircular canals, fissula ante fenestram, fossula post fenestram, and periotic duct are all considered part of the perilymphatic labyrinth.

It is not until the 8th week that the first sign of perilymphatic space formation is seen. Mesodermal tissue surrounding the membranous labyrinth (ie, the future otic capsule) retrogressively dedifferentiates from precartilage into a loose, vascular reticulum, initially around the ampullae of the semicircular ducts and in the region of the perilymphatic cistern of the vestibule. The scala tympani starts its emergence from precartilage as an area of retrogressive rarefaction in the precartilage just under the round window.

Rapidly changing over the next several weeks, the reticulum of the primordial perilymphatic labyrinth becomes highly vacuolated, its spaces traversed by supporting fibers for the walls of the saccule and the utricle and for the vascular and neural supplies of the inner ear.[3] The perilymphatic cistern of the vestibule, adjacent to the oval window, is the first recognizable space of the perilymphatic labyrinth, appearing late in the 12th week (see Figure 1–13). The scala tympani appears soon afterward, with the scala vestibuli appearing somewhat later as a diverticulum

FIGURE 1–14 • The osseous relationships of the endolymphatic duct and sac. *After Anson and Donaldson.*[2] *Reproduced with permission from Schuknecht HF. Pathology of the ear. Ontario: BC Decker; 1974.*

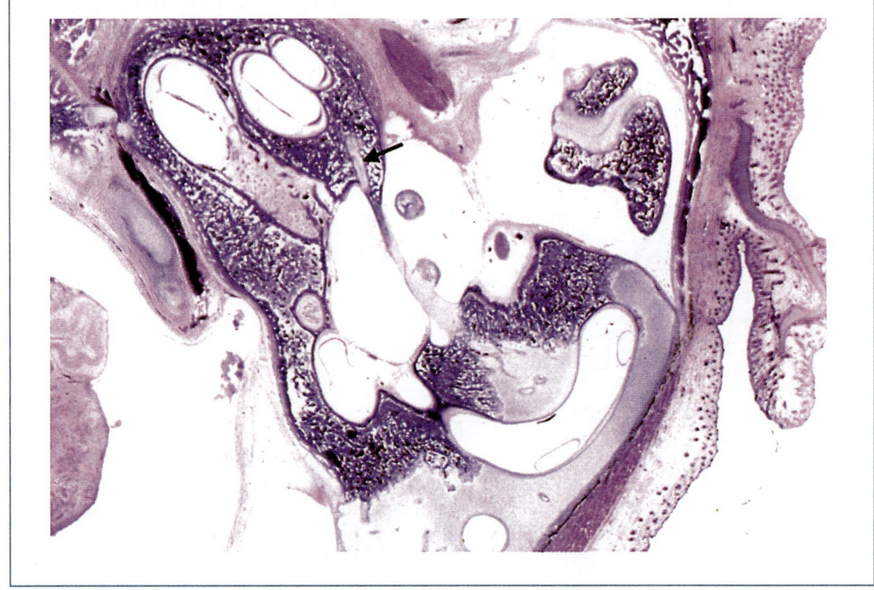

FIGURE 1–15 • This photomicrograph, from a 16-week specimen, shows the fissula ante fenestram (arrow). *Reproduced with permission from Gulya AJ. Gulya and Schuknecht's anatomy of the temporal bone with surgical implications. 3rd ed. New York: Informa Healthcare USA; 2007.*

of the perilymphatic cistern near the oval window. The expansion of both scalae is closely linked to that of the developing cochlear duct and cochlea. The canalicular portion of the perilymphatic labyrinth is relatively delayed in development. Only at 16 weeks does vacuolization begin; however, development is usually completed by 20 weeks.

Fissula Ante Fenestram

The fissula ante fenestram and the fossula post fenestram, although part of the perilymphatic labyrinth, undergo a different developmental sequence and hence merit separate discussion (Figure 1–15).

Apparently, the fissula ante fenestram is unique to humans, although Anson and Bast[10] detected a rudimentary, incomplete fissula in the rhesus monkey. The fissula is first apparent in the 9-week embryo as a strip of precartilage in the lateral wall of the cartilaginous otic capsule immediately anterior to the oval window (*ante* is Latin for "in front of," *fenestram* is Latin for "window"). In the course of the next 3 weeks, this extension of periotic tissue stretches as a connective tissue ribbon from the vestibule to the middle ear. Vertically, the ribbon extends from the scala vestibuli to the tympanic cavity, near the cochleariform process. The fissula continues to grow until midfetal life (about 21 weeks), at which time the ossification of the otic capsule is nearing completion.

Although the fissula is a constant tract in humans, it shows interindividual variation both in capacity and in form and undergoes alteration of its lining cartilage over the life of the individual. The cartilage border that separates the connective tissue of the fissula from the bone of the otic capsule is gradually replaced by intrachondral bone (see "Development of the Otic Capsule").[29]

Fossula Post Fenestram

The fossula post fenestram, an evagination of periotic tissue from the vestibule into the otic capsule (see Figure 1–15) posterior to the oval window, undergoes a developmental sequence similar to

FIGURE 1–16 • As seen in a 12-week fetus, the cochlear aqueduct (arrow) reaches from the posterior cranial fossa to the scala tympani of the basal turn. *Reproduced with permission from Gulya AJ. Gulya and Schuknecht's anatomy of the temporal bone with surgical implications. 3rd ed. New York: Informa Healthcare USA; 2007.*

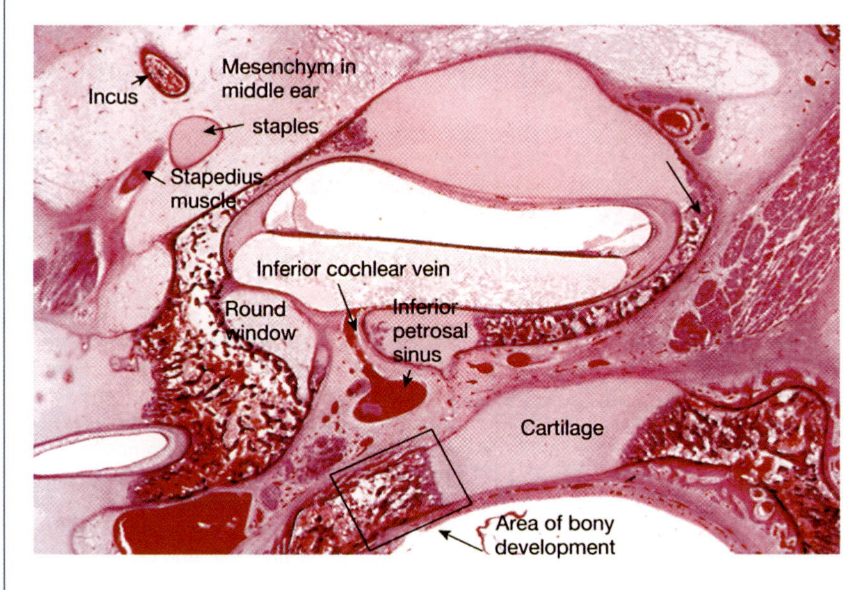

FIGURE 1–17 • The inferior cochlear vein occupies the primitive cochlear aqueduct, as seen in a fetus of approximately 17 weeks. The boxed area is enlarged in Figure 1–22. *Reproduced with permission from Gulya AJ. Gulya and Schuknecht's anatomy of the temporal bone with surgical implications. 3rd ed. New York: Informa Healthcare USA; 2007.*

that of the fissula ante fenestram. The fossula (*fossula* is Latin for "little ditch," *post* is Latin for "behind") is first seen in the fetus of 10½ weeks as an area of dedifferentiating precartilage. As early as 4½ weeks later, the fossula can be distinguished as a zone of connective tissue, which soon becomes surrounded by the bone of the otic capsule. Differing from the fissula, the fossula is an inconstantly occurring structure found in only 67% of all ears studied and extends through the otic capsule to the tympanic cavity in only 25% of those ears with a fossula.[4]

Although the fossula is an area of histologic instability for reasons similar to those for the fissula, cartilaginous and bony changes affect only 5% of all fossulae.[4]

Cochlear Aqueduct

The primordial (bony) cochlear aqueduct first appears at 7 weeks as a rarefaction of precartilage at the medial wall of the cochlear basal turn. The cochlear aqueduct extends from the area of the developing round window to the posterior cranial fossa. The reticulum of the primordial aqueduct links the loose mesenchyme of the round window niche with the connective tissue of the posterior cranial fossa dura, ninth cranial nerve, and inferior petrosal sinus (Figure 1–16).

By the 9th week, the inferior cochlear vein emerges from the syncytium of the cochlear aqueduct. Meanwhile, a cartilaginous bar, as it extends from the round window niche and ampulla of the posterior canal toward the opening of the cochlear aqueduct, gives rise to the floor and medial rim of the round window.

The development of the periotic duct and surroundings in the 16- to 40-week period has been detailed by Spector and associates.[30] In the 16- to 18-week stage (Figure 1–17), three structures are seen in the primitive cochlear aqueduct: the inferior cochlear vein (vein at the cochlear aqueduct), the tympanomeningeal hiatus (Hyrtl's fissure), and the periotic duct. There is still connective tissue continuity between the posterior cranial fossa

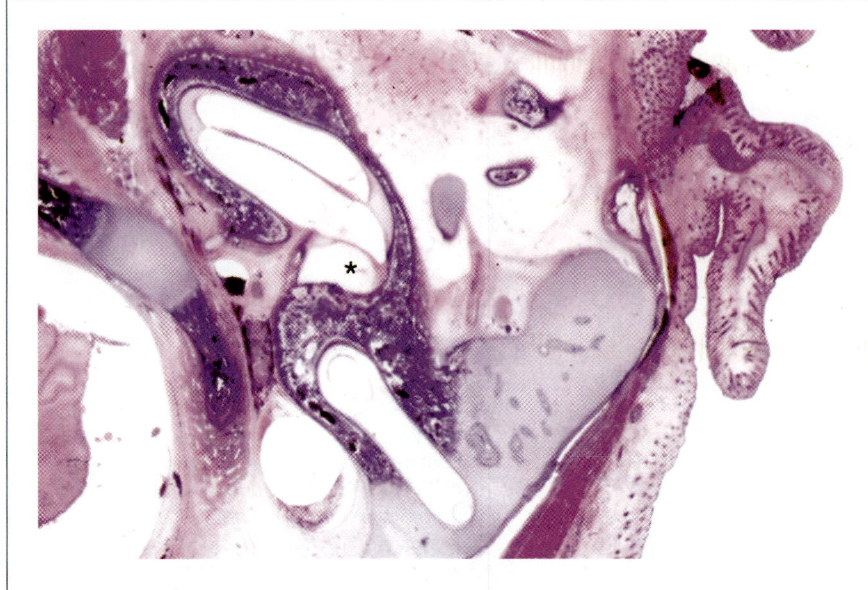

FIGURE 1–18 • Although younger than the fetus shown in Figure 1–17, this fetus shows more advanced ossification of the rim of the round window niche (asterisk) in particular, breaking the communication of the round window niche with the posterior cranial fossa (fetus, 16 weeks). *Reproduced with permission from Gulya AJ. Gulya and Schuknecht's anatomy of the temporal bone with surgical implications. 3rd ed. New York: Informa Healthcare USA; 2007.*

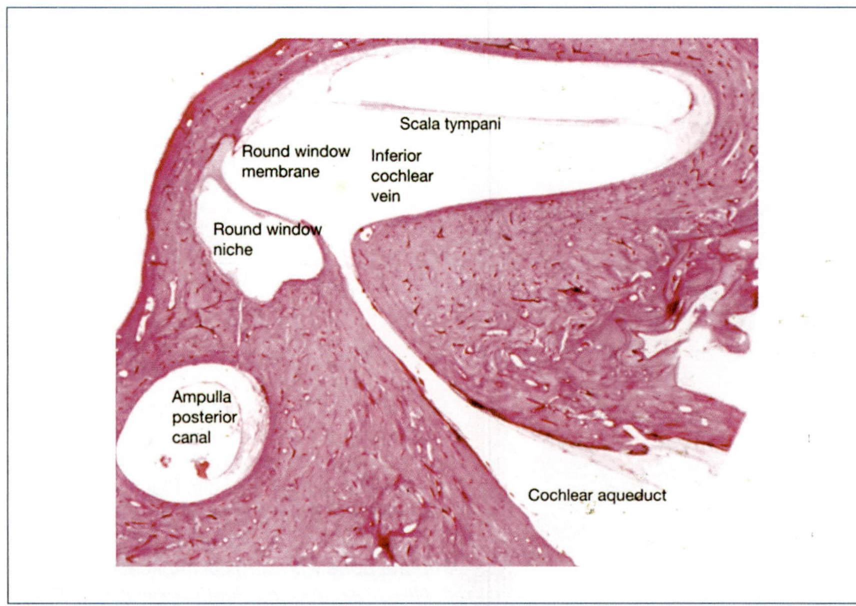

FIGURE 1–19 • The widely patent cochlear aqueduct is thought to underlie the "perilymph oozer" seen in stapes surgery (man, age 67 years). A microfissure is visible between the posterior semicircular canal ampulla and the round window niche. *Reproduced with permission from Schuknecht HF, Seifi AE. Experimental observations on the fluid physiology of the inner ear. Ann Otol Rhinol Laryngol 1963;72:687.*

and the tissue of the round window niche, especially through Hyrtl's fissure.

Ossification of the otic capsule, progressing to the round window by the 18- to 26-week stage (Figure 1–18), fuses the cochlear and canalicular segments of the otic capsule, caps Hyrtl's fissure, and relegates the round window niche to the tympanic cavity. The inferior cochlear vein is segregated into its own canal (of Cotugno) at 20 weeks through further growth and ossification of the otic capsule.

Completion of the cochlear aqueduct occurs between 32 and 40 weeks and entails elongation of the cochlear aqueduct with its contained periodic duct, widening of the cranial apertures of the cochlear aqueduct and periotic duct, and ingrowth of arachnoid tissue, which forms a lining membrane and meshwork. A widely patent cochlear aqueduct (Figure 1–19) is thought to underlie the "perilymph oozer"[1] occasionally encountered in stapes surgery. A persistent tympanomeningeal hiatus represents incomplete ossification. The hiatus extends from the depths of the round window niche to the posterior cranial fossa at the junction of the inferior petrosal sinus and jugular bulb (Figure 1–20).[1] The hiatus is a potential route that cerebrospinal fluid and brain tissue may follow to the middle ear.[30–33]

DEVELOPMENT OF THE OTIC CAPSULE

The otic capsule develops from the precartilage (compacted mesenchyme that is differentiating into embryonic cartilage) surrounding it. Eventually, the otic capsule becomes the petrous portion of the temporal bone.[4] The initial step in development of the otic capsule, as described by Bast and Anson,[4] occurs at the end of the 4th week as the cell density of the mesenchyme enveloping the otic capsule increases. By the 8th week, the

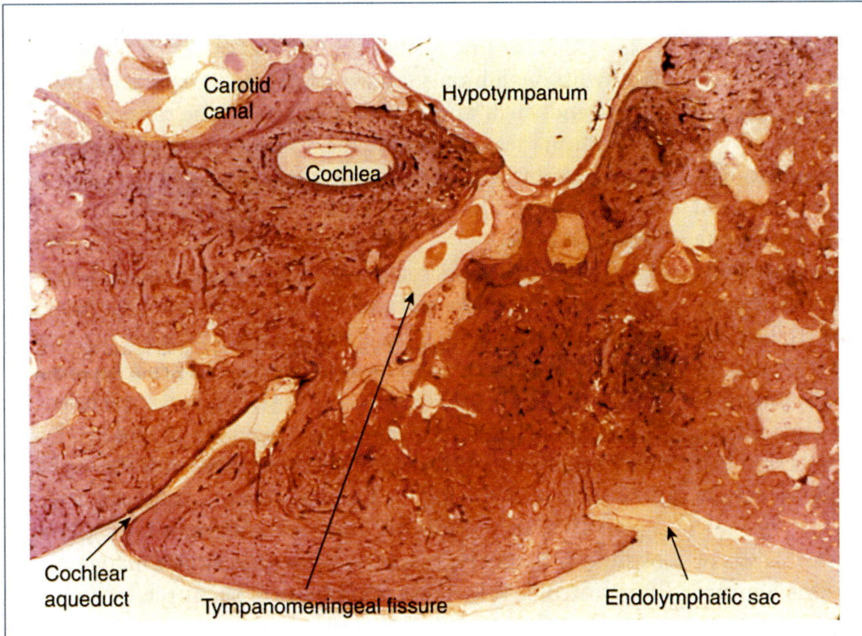

FIGURE 1–20 • The tympanomeningeal fissure (hiatus), occasionally persisting in the adult, is paralleled by the cochlear aqueduct (man, age 44 years). *Reproduced with permission from Gulya AJ. Gulya and Schuknecht's anatomy of the temporal bone with surgical implications. 3rd ed. New York: Informa Healthcare USA; 2007.*

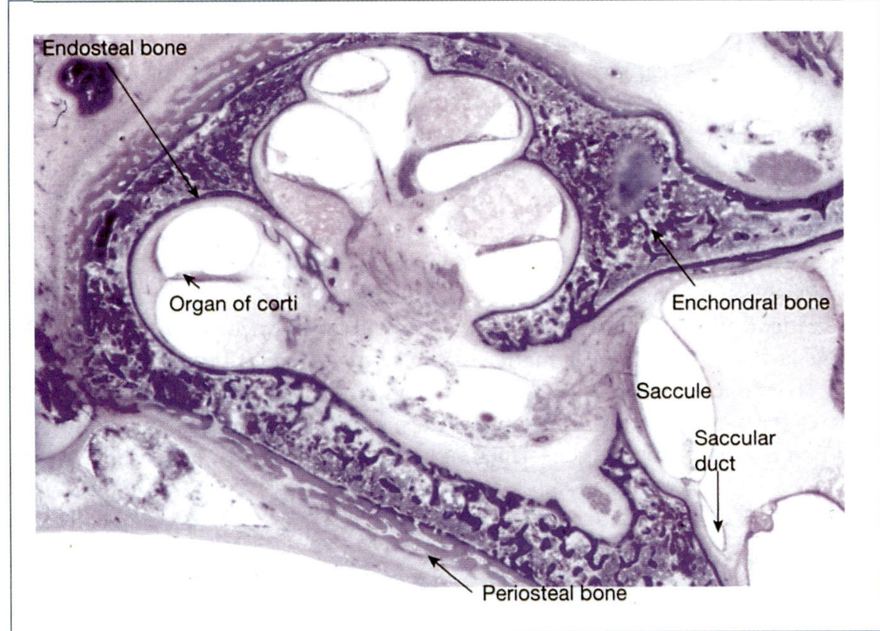

FIGURE 1–21 • With ossification of the otic capsule, three layers of bone are created (fetus, 16 weeks). *Reproduced with permission from Gulya AJ. Gulya and Schuknecht's anatomy of the temporal bone with surgical implications. 3rd ed. New York: Informa Healthcare USA; 2007.*

mesenchymal condensation has formed a cartilaginous model of the otic capsule. At this stage, although the membranous labyrinth, which the cartilaginous otic capsule surrounds, has attained adult configuration, it does not attain adult size until nearly midterm. Retrogressive dedifferentiation of otic capsular cartilage to a loose reticulum accommodates the expansion of the membranous labyrinth. Redifferentiation to cartilage occurs at the inner, trailing edge of the semicircular ducts (see Figure 1–10).

According to Bast and Anson,[4] the first ossification center of the otic capsule appears at the region of the cochlea only as the contained membranous labyrinth reaches adult size, usually by 16 weeks. A total of 14 centers eventually appear and fuse to complete the ossification of the otic capsule despite its small size. The last ossification center appears at 20 to 21 weeks in the posterolateral region of the posterior semicircular canal. The only areas that remain cartilaginous are those at the region of the fissula ante fenestram and an area that overlies part of the posterior and lateral semicircular ducts, where ossification does not begin until 2 weeks later.[4]

A detailed discussion of the ossification sequence of the otic capsule is beyond the scope of this chapter, and the interested reader is referred to Bast and Anson[4] and Gulya and Schuknecht[1] for a more detailed discussion. However, several unique features of the bone of the otic capsule are of clinical significance and are outlined below.

Three layers of bone emerge from the ossification of the cartilaginous otic capsule (Figure 1–21). The perichondrial membrane lining the external and the internal (facing the membranous labyrinth) surfaces of the otic capsule becomes a periosteal membrane as newly differentiated osteoblasts deposit calcium. The periosteal and endosteal bone layers are thus formed.

The endosteal layer does not significantly change throughout adult life, although in response to infection or trauma (including perhaps electrical stimulation), it may proliferate to such a degree as to obliterate the lumen of the labyrinth.[1] Alternatively, it has been proposed that undifferentiated mesenchymal cells, located around capillaries, are the true source of such obliterative, bony growths.[34] The periosteal layer, in contrast, does change, by lamellar addition of bone and by pneumatization, until early adult life.[10] This layer has the capability of good osteogenic repair in response to trauma and infection and remodels throughout life, similar to periosteal bone elsewhere in the body.

Sandwiched between the endosteal and periosteal layers of bone is the enchondral layer, consisting of both intrachondral (intrachondrial) and endochondral bone. Intrachondral bone (globuli interossei) comprises persistent islands of calcified hyaline cartilage, the lacunae of which are occupied by osteocytes and on which endochondral bone is deposited. Initial steps in the formation of intrachondral bone (Figure 1–22) are hypertrophy of cartilage cells in their lacunae, calcification of the cartilaginous matrix, and vascular bud invasion. Much of the calcified cartilage is removed, but scattered islands remain. Osteocytes repopulate the formerly cartilaginous lacunae and begin bone deposition.

Osteoblasts lining the surface of the calcified cartilage islands deposit layers of endochondral bone. This bone deposition nearly obliterates the vascular spaces and establishes the layer of very dense, poorly vascular bone characteristic of the petrous (rocklike) pyramid known as the enchondral layer.

The enchondral layer, similar to the endosteal layer, once formed in midfetal life undergoes little change save for conversion to increasingly dense bone.[10] Enchondral bone, also similar to endosteal bone, exhibits a minimal reparative response to insults, such as trauma and infection, at best healing by fibrous union. Because of the poor reparative capacity of the endosteal and enchondral layers, the ravages of stress and trauma leave indelible marks on the architecture of the bony labyrinth. Major trauma, sufficient to fracture the temporal bone, results in large fissures that may traverse the entire temporal bone.

The so-called microfissures are commonly encountered disruptions in the endosteal and enchondral layers of the bony labyrinth.[1] A microfissure found in all ears after the age of 6 years is located between the round window niche and the ampulla of the posterior canal (see Figure 1–19).[35] Additionally, microfissures can be found about the oval window region in 25% of ears examined, usually extending vertically above and below the oval window without involving the footplate, more commonly after the age of 40 years.[36] Typically, these microfissures are obstructed by fibrous tissue in association with an acellular matrix resembling osteoid. Why these microfissures occur remains unclear. It has been hypothesized that the microfissures represent stress fractures resulting from structural changes of the labyrinth[45] or from the transferred stresses of mastication.[37] Alternatively, the microfissures bridging the round window niche and the posterior canal ampulla may be related to an embryologic communication.[35] Although, by term, cartilage replaces the mesenchyme of this transient channel, this area may remain structurally weak and readily fractured.

The microfissures of the bony labyrinth have been thought to play a role in the contamination of the inner ear by inflammatory processes or ototoxic substances applied to the middle ear. Similarly, these microfissures have been theorized to give rise to spontaneous perilymph fistulae.

Attaching such clinical implications to microfissures remains a matter of conjecture. In an examination of 34 temporal bones, El Shazly and Linthicum were unable to find any relationship between the presence or absence of microfissures to sudden sensorineural hearing loss.[38]

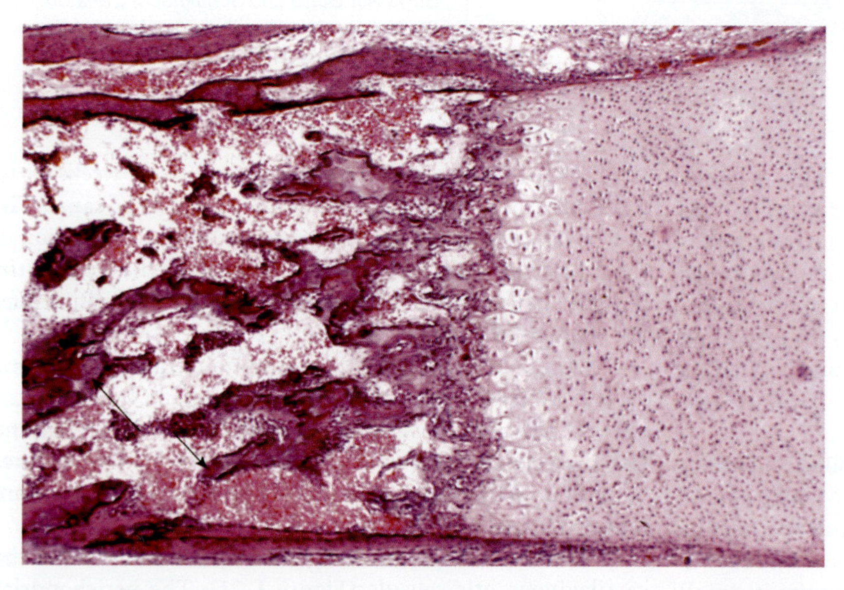

FIGURE 1–22 • This detailed view of the boxed area of Figure 1–17 illustrates the steps of enchondral bone formation. Going from right to left, cartilage cells multiply, enlarge, and are ossified. Globuli interossei (arrows) represent persisting islands of cartilage (fetus, age 17 weeks). *Reproduced with permission from Gulya AJ. Gulya and Schuknecht's anatomy of the temporal bone with surgical implications. 3rd ed. New York: Informa Healthcare USA; 2007.*

Distinct from and independent of the formation of the otic capsule from a cartilaginous model is the formation of the cochlear modiolus as membranous bone. The deposition of bone within the modiolus, housing the cochlear nerve, first occurs at 20 to 21 weeks in the region between the basal and second turns.[4] By 25 weeks, modiolar ossification is nearly complete.

Osseous extensions of the cochlear otic capsule, known as interscalar septa, serve to anchor the modiolus. The first septa appear in the 22nd week and within 5 weeks have stabilized the cochlear modiolus from base to apex. Following a similar time frame, the osseous spiral lamina begins ossification in the 23rd week and completes this process by the 25th.

Aberrations in the finer developmental steps of the cochlea may appear as structural anomalies that occasionally attain surgical importance. Partial absence of the interscalar septum (scala communis) is a relatively common developmental anomaly that does not interfere with normal cochlear function (Figure 1–23). Absence of the modiolus results in a wide communication between the subarachnoid space of the internal auditory canal and the scala vestibuli of the basal turn. This anomaly may represent the anatomic correlate of the "perilymph gusher," the voluminous outflow occasionally encountered in stapes surgery (Figure 1–24).

DEVELOPMENT OF THE ACOUSTIC NERVE AND GANGLION

The acoustic nerve, ganglion, and Schwann sheath cells begin development in the 4th week as cells of otic placode derivation begin to stream ventrally between the epithelium of the otocyst and its basement membrane. After penetrating the basement membrane, these cells reach the area at which the acoustic ganglion forms,[3,39] ventral and slightly medial to the otocyst.[40]

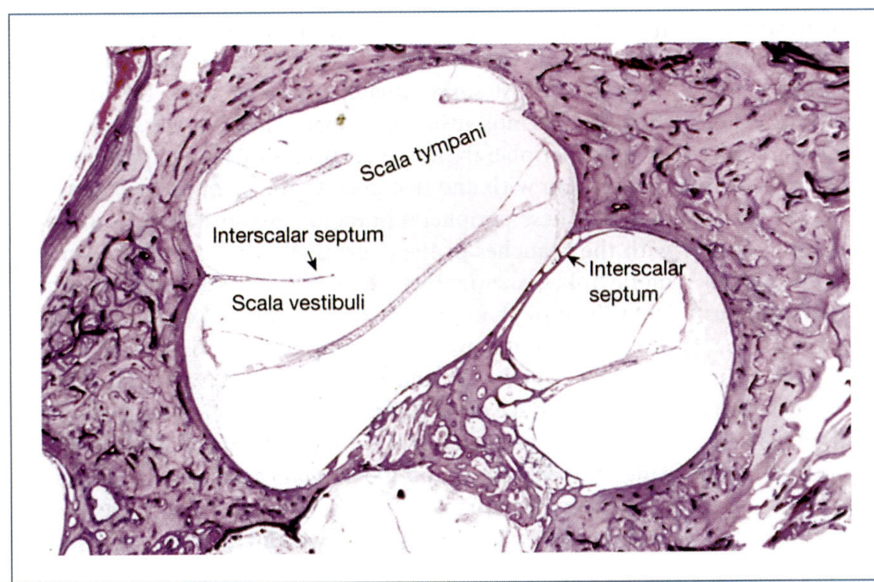

FIGURE 1–23 • Partial absence of the interscalar septum, as shown in this micrograph, is known as scala communis (woman, age 63 years). *Reproduced with permission from Gulya AJ. Gulya and Schuknecht's anatomy of the temporal bone with surgical implications. 3rd ed. New York: Informa Healthcare USA; 2007.*

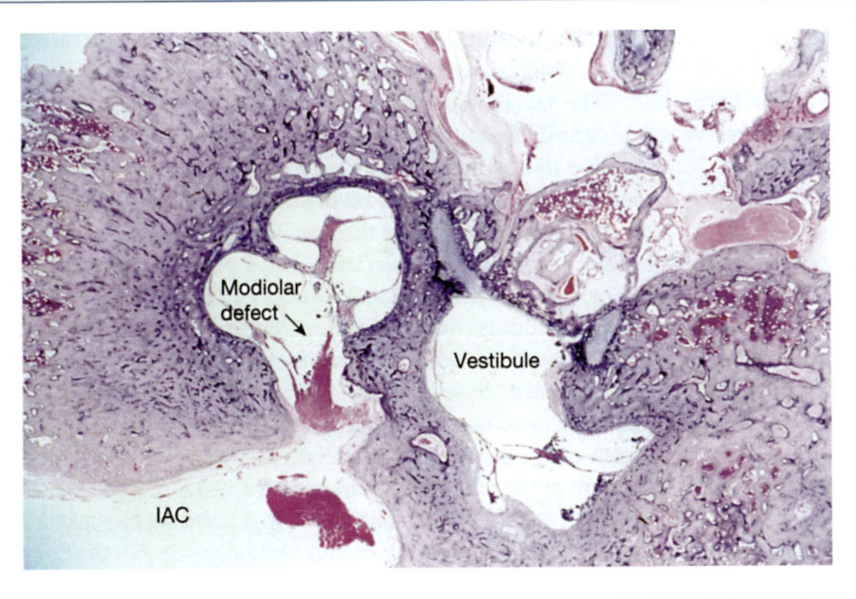

FIGURE 1–24 • The modiolar defect in the cochlea of this 2½-year-old child with a congenital conductive hearing loss results in a wide communication of the subarachnoid space of the internal auditory canal (IAC) with the scala vestibuli of the basal turn. Stapedectomy in such cases results in a "perilymph gusher." *Reproduced with permission from Shi S-R. Temporal bone findings in a case of otopalatodigital syndrome. Arch Otolaryngol 1985;111:120. Copyright 1985, American Medical Association.*

Over the remainder of the 4th and 5th weeks, the acoustic ganglion divides into superior and inferior segments.[23] The superior segment gives rise to the fibers that innervate the crista of the superior and lateral semicircular ducts as well as the utricular macula. Slightly later, the inferior segment divides into upper and lower portions. The upper portion supplies fibers to the saccular macula and to the crista of the posterior semicircular duct, whereas the lower portion innervates the organ of Corti.

By the end of 8 weeks, the acoustic nerve approaches full maturity. The ganglia of the vestibular division are spread along the nerve trunks, and its terminal branches, derived from the bipolar ganglion cells, develop as fairly long, discretely individual nerve fibers. The cochlear ganglion, in contrast, ends up at the distal terminus of the nerve trunk, and its terminal branches are short, anastomosing fibers.[23] Similarly, central connections (to the brainstem) are established, initially by the vestibular nerve and then later by the cochlear nerve fibers.[40] As soon as central connections (to the brainstem) are established, migration of glial cells from the brain tube begins to envelop the proximal portion of the acoustic nerve fibers, but it is only later in development that Schwann cells begin to migrate centrally. Thus, the central glial sheath extends for a considerable distance laterally along the acoustic nerve before Schwann cells migrate medially. Moreover, the distance covered by glial cells is greater on the vestibular nerve than on the cochlear nerve because of the earlier initiation of migration, the former when compared with the latter.[40] The junction of the Schwann cell and glial sheaths occurs variably about the region of the fundus of the internal auditory canal.

It is thought that the sensory neuroepithelium develops in those areas of the membranous labyrinth at which neural contact is established.[3] Such contact may not be required for neuroepithelial differentiation but may play a role in maintaining such specialization.[41,42]

DEVELOPMENT OF THE FACIAL NERVE AND GENICULATE GANGLION

At about 4 weeks, the facial nerve and its geniculate ganglion begin to develop from primordial tissue, arising from the rhombencephalon, which impinges on the deep aspect of the second branchial arch epibranchial placode,[43] a thickened area of surface ectoderm just caudal to the first branchial groove (Figures 1–25A and B, and 1–26A and B).

The later stages of facial nerve and geniculate ganglion development have been described by Gasser and colleagues.[43–45] Neuroblast differentiation in the region at which the primordial facial nerve tissue is in contiguity with the epibranchial placode results in a distinguishable geniculate ganglion by 6 weeks (Figures 1–25C and 1–26C). Meanwhile, the chorda tympani nerve, the first branch of the facial nerve to appear, is clearly evident. At approximately the same time, the facial motor nucleus appears in the future metencephalon; its intramedullary fibers are displaced by the abducens nucleus as the metencephalon grows, creating the internal genu of the facial nerve.

The chorda tympani nerve, at 6 weeks approximating the size of the facial nerve, dives into the mandibular arch to terminate in the same region as the lingual nerve ends and the submandibular ganglion develops.

The chorda tympani and lingual nerves clearly unite just proximal to the ganglion by the 7th week (Figures 1–25D and 1–26D). Also at approximately 6 weeks, the greater petrosal nerve, the second branch of the facial nerve to form, develops from the ventral aspect of the geniculate ganglion. The nervus intermedius (nerve of Wrisberg, the sensory fibers of the facial nerve) develops independently from the geniculate ganglion and extends to the brainstem bordered by the motor root of the facial nerve and the eighth cranial nerve. The main trunk of the facial nerve establishes its definitive intratemporal relationships within the cartilaginous otic capsule.

In sequence, the posterior auricular nerve and the fibers to the posterior belly of the digastric muscle appear. Branches of the posterior auricular nerve communicate with nerves of the second and third cervical ganglia, resulting in the formation of the transverse cervical and lesser occipital nerves.

At 7 weeks, a ventral offshoot from the geniculate ganglion reaches the glossopharyngeal ganglion. In the next week, the tympanic plexus and the lesser petrosal nerve form along this offshoot. At approximately the same time, the branch to the stapedius muscle has developed. The facial nerve grows and develops peripheral (muscular) branches, which appear in close conjunction with and just deep to the primitive facial muscle masses. These peripheral branches establish communications with the branches of the trigeminal nerve. Similarly, anastomotic linkages with other peripheral facial nerve fibers appear. With the growth of the facial nerve, the chorda tympani nerve diminishes in relative size (Figures 1–25E and 1–26E).

Between the 12th and 13th weeks, two twigs from the dorsomedial surface of the facial nerve (between the stapedius and the chorda tympani nerves) fuse and extend to the superior ganglia of the vagus and glossopharyngeal nerves. The nerve fiber emerging from this intermingling is Arnold's nerve (the auricular branch of the vagus), which traverses the primitive tympanomastoid fissure to innervate the subcutaneous tissue of the posterior aspect of the external auditory canal.

By 17 weeks, the definitive communications of the facial nerve, including those with the second and third cervical nerves, the three divisions of the trigeminal nerve, and the vagus and the glossopharyngeal nerves, are established.

The facial canal, originally a sulcus in the cartilaginous otic capsule, becomes a bony canal as it ossifies. Spector and Ge detailed the ossification of the tympanic segment of the fallopian canal, a process that involves two ossification centers: an anterior one developing at the apical cochlear ossification center at the end of 20 weeks gestation and a posterior one arising at the pyramidal eminence at 25 weeks gestation.[46] Each ossification center emits two bony projections that (ideally) encircle the facial nerve in its entirety. Each ossification center also extends from its point of origin, the anterior one posteriorly and the posterior one inferiorly, to envelop progressively more of the length of the facial nerve. By term, about 80% of the tympanic segment of the fallopian canal is present and is completely developed by roughly 3 months after birth. According to Spector and Ge, most of the surgically encountered dehiscences of the tympanic segment of the fallopian canal can be related to varying

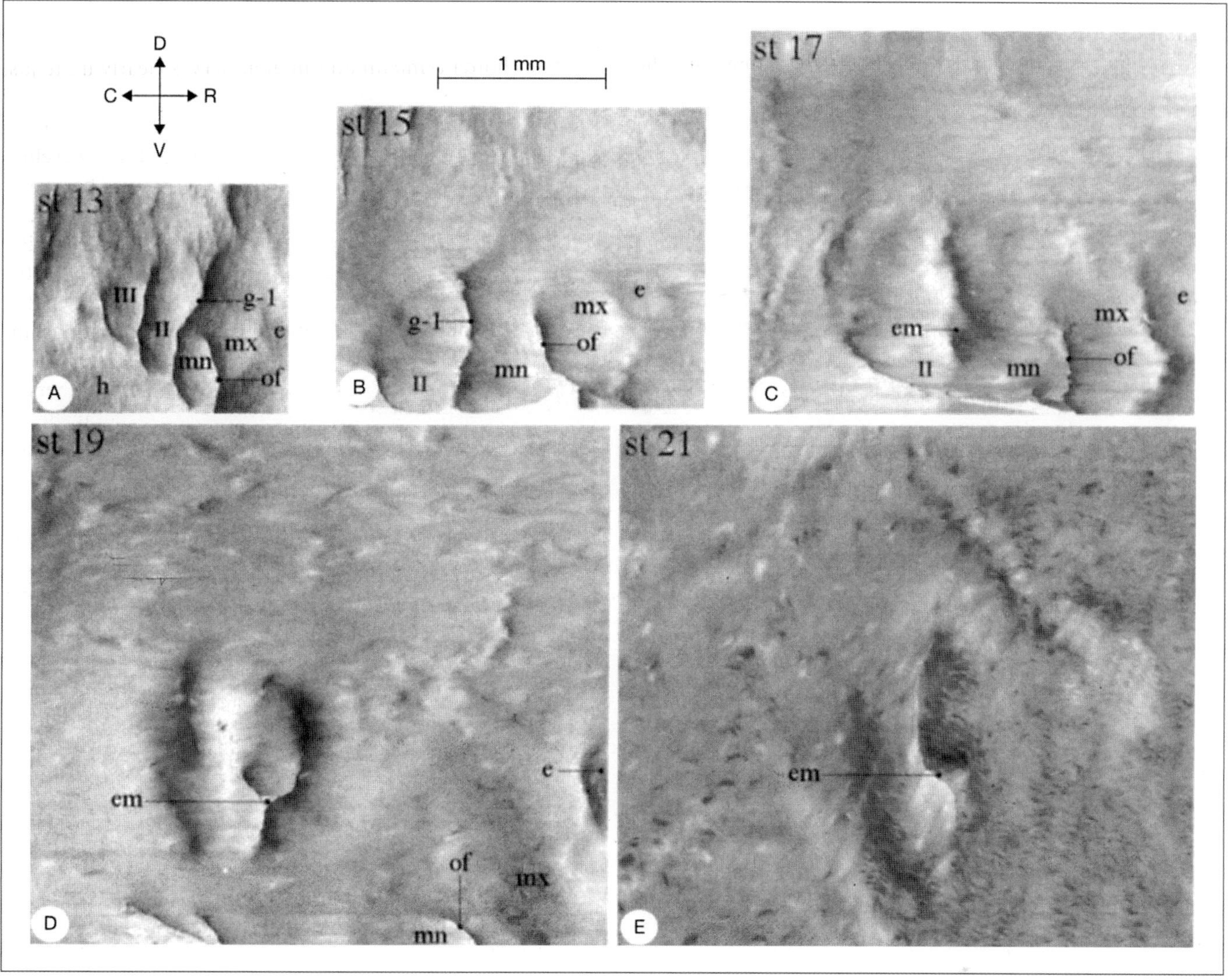

FIGURE 1–25 • Computer reconstructions of the ectoderm of the right external ear region at approximate ages 28 days (*A*), 33 days (*B*), 41 days (*C*), 48 days (*D*), and 52 days (*E*). Dorsal is superior, ventral is inferior, rostral is to the right, and caudal is to the left. This view, companion to Figure 1–26, reveals the structures anatomically related to the lateral aspect of the developing facial nerve. II, second arch; III, third arch; e, eye; em, external auditory meatus; g-1, first groove; h, heart; mn, mandibular part of first arch; mx, maxillary part of first arch; of, oral fissure. *Reproduced with permission from Gasser RF, Shigihara S, Shimada K. Three-dimensional development of the facial nerve path through the ear region in human embryos. Ann Otol Rhinol Laryngol 1994;103:395–403.*

degrees of failure of fusion of the two ossification centers and to failure of fusion of their bony projections.[46] Additionally, they report that the pattern of ossification of the tympanic segment is symmetric in 80% of the paired bones studied.

The mastoid process and tympanic ring grow postnatally, medially displacing and thus protecting the facial nerve.

DEVELOPMENT OF THE ARTERIES

The fetal circulatory system first appears in the 3rd week of development as mesenchymal vascular islands coalesce.[47] The primordial vascular supply to the brain derives from presegmental branches of the paired ("dorsal") aortae. A total of six aortic arches arise successively from the dilated region of the truncus arteriosus known as the aortic sac and course ventrally through their corresponding branchial arches into the ipsilateral dorsal aorta.[47] The primitive internal carotid artery is a branch of the first aortic arch. During this branchial phase of arterial development, there is a correspondence between each branchial arch and its aortic arch. However, not all of the aortic arch arteries exist at the same time. The first and second arch arteries disappear before the more caudal arch arteries develop. The following details of cranial arterial development are based on the comprehensive study of Padget.[48]

In the 4th week, as the first and second aortic arches begin to involute, they leave behind dorsal fragments, the mandibular and hyoid arteries, respectively, and the portion of the paired dorsal aortae extending anteriorly from the third arch artery becomes the adult internal carotid artery (Figure 1–27). In the hindbrain region, the bilateral longitudinal neural arteries

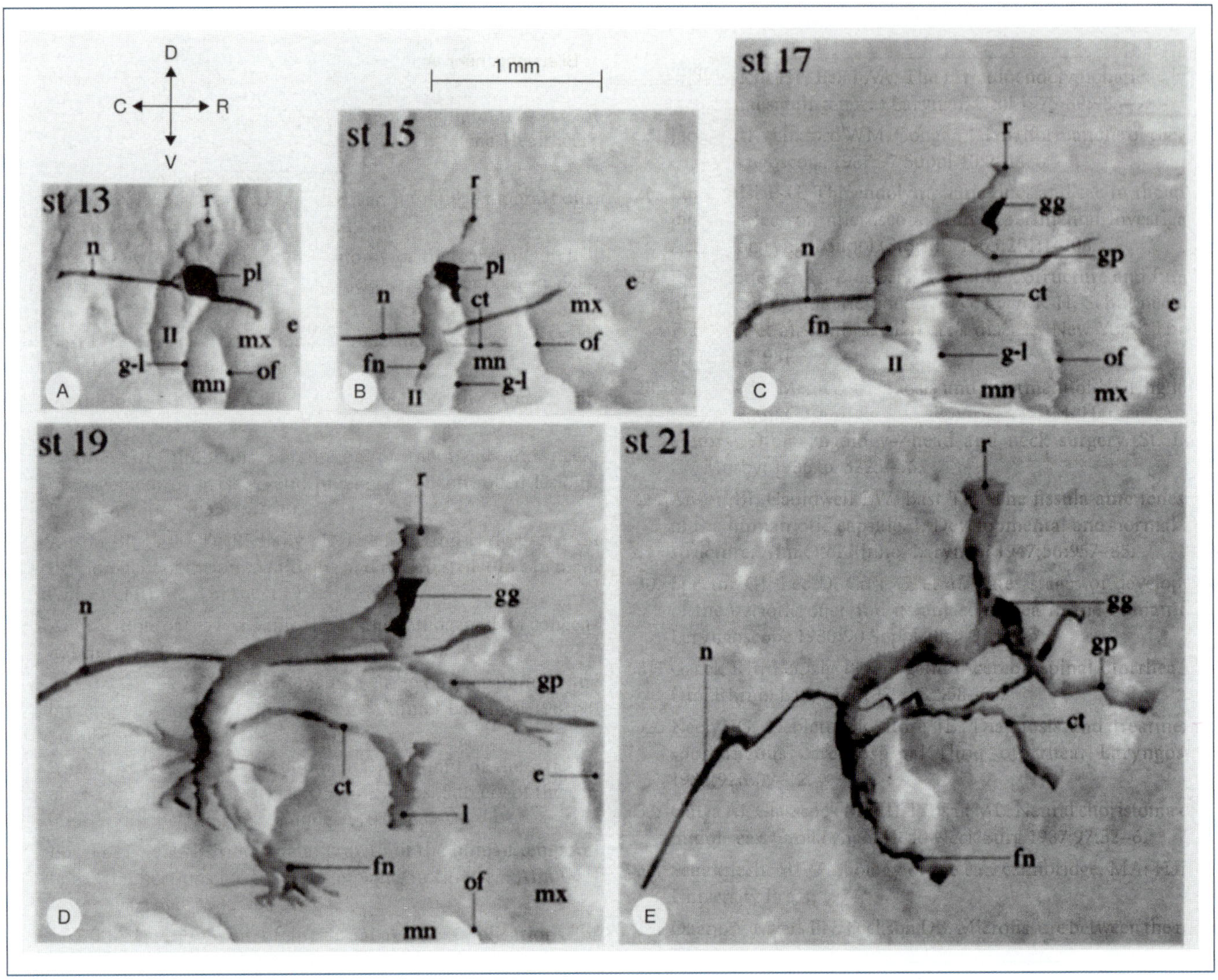

FIGURE 1–26 • Same specimens as Figure 1–25 but with computer reconstruction making the surface ectoderm relatively transparent, allowing visualization of the developing facial nerve. II, second arch; III, third arch; ct, chorda tympani nerve; e, eye; fn, facial nerve; g-1, first groove; gg, geniculate ganglion; gp, greater petrosal nerve; l, lingual nerve; mn, mandibular part of first arch; mx, maxillary part of first arch; of, oral fissure; pl, placode; n, notocord; r, facial nerve root. *Reproduced with permission from Gasser RF, Shigihara S, Shimada K. Three-dimensional development of the facial nerve path through the ear region in human embryos. Ann Otol Rhinol Laryngol 1994;103:395–403.*

emerge, supplied at the level of the otocyst and acoustic nerve by the primitive otic artery, a remnant of a presegmental branch of the paired aortae (see Figure 1–27).

In the 4- to 5-week stage, the ventral pharyngeal artery, which parallels the internal carotid artery, arises in the area formerly occupied by the ventral aspects of the first and second arch arteries. This artery supplies the bulk of the first two pharyngeal bars and subsequently is involved in the formation of the stapedial and external carotid arteries. At the same time, the bilateral longitudinal neural arteries fuse to form the basilar artery.

At 6 weeks, as the transition from branchial phase to postbranchial phase takes place, the stapedial artery appears as a small offshoot of the hyoid artery and passes through the stapes blastema to enter the mandibular bar; here the stapedial artery anastomoses with the distal remnant of the shrinking ventral pharyngeal artery. The maxillomandibular division of the stapedial artery is the result of this anastomosis, and it divides into maxillary and mandibular branches. The proximal remnant of the ventral pharyngeal artery evolves into the root of the external carotid artery, whereas the common carotid artery develops from the ventral union of the third and fourth arch arteries.

The development of the labyrinthine and anterior inferior cerebellar arteries during the 4th through 6th weeks passes through a ring configuration, with the abducens nerve in the center. Whether the labyrinthine artery arises from the anterior inferior cerebellar artery or from the basilar artery is determined by the point at which the vascular ring atrophies.

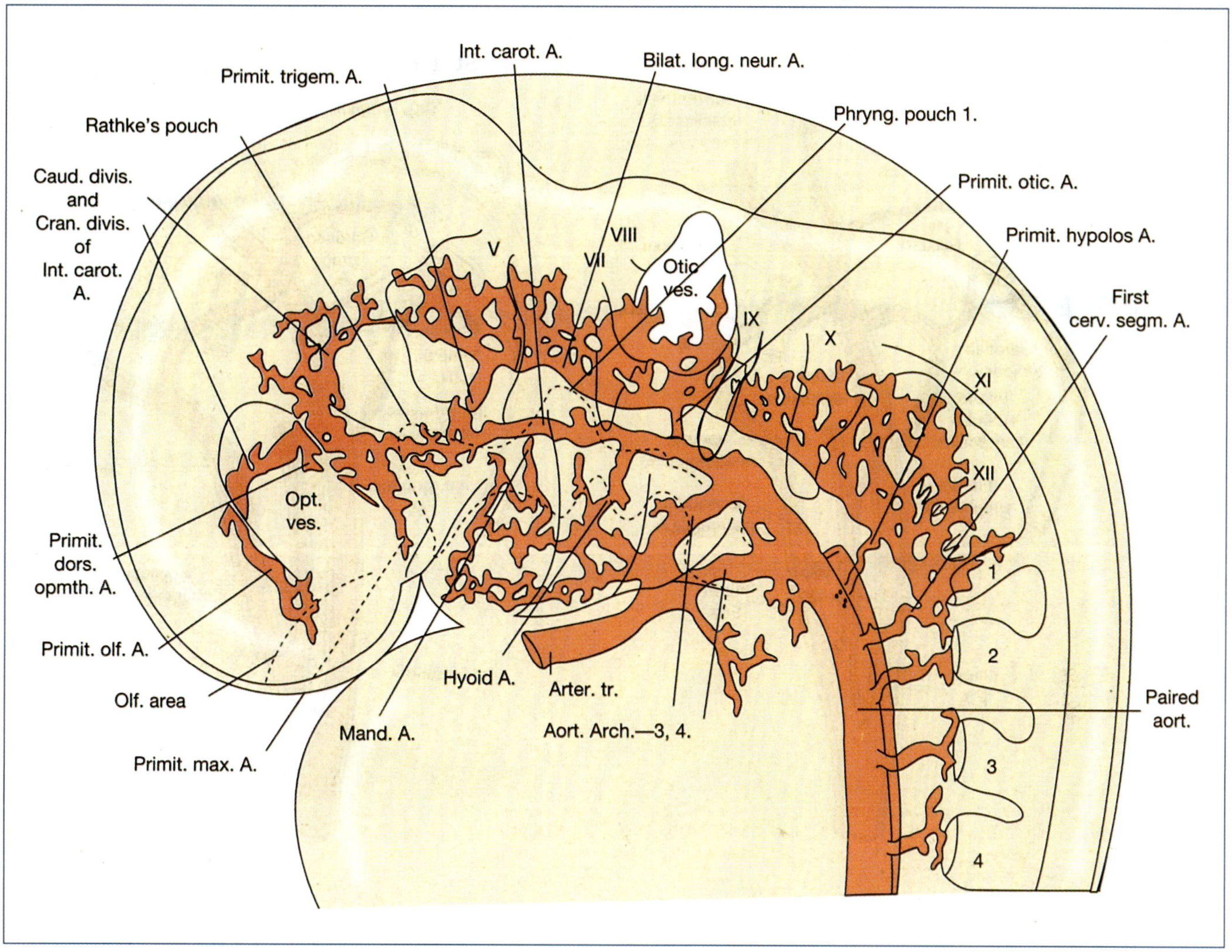

FIGURE 1–27 • Graphic reconstruction of the cranial arteries in a 4-week embryo. The mandibular and hyoid arteries are remnants of the first two aortic arches; the internal carotid artery originates from the third arch, and the bilateral neural arteries are starting to emerge. *Reproduced with permission from Padget DH. The development of the cranial arteries in the human embryo. Contrib Embryol 1948;32:205.*

The stapedial artery reaches the height of its development at 7 weeks (Figure 1–28A) and has two divisions, the maxillomandibular and the supraorbital; the latter division supplies the primitive orbit. Branches of the external carotid artery that can be identified now are the thyroid, lingual, occipital, and external maxillary arteries. Over the next week, the two major divisions of the stapedial artery are annexed by the internal maxillary artery of the external carotid artery and the ophthalmic artery, respectively. The trunk of the maxillomandibular division becomes the stem of the middle meningeal artery (Figure 1–28B). As the stapedialartery withers proximal to the stapes, its more distal stem becomes the superior tympanic branch of the adult middle meningeal artery. The hyoid artery, which originally gave rise to the stapedial artery, dwindles to a mere twig and is partially retained as a caroticotympanic branch of the adult internal carotid artery (Figure 1–28C). Remnants of the stapedial artery also are thought to play a role in the development of the caroticotympanic arteries, anterior tympanic artery, and superior petrosal artery (Tandler, as cited in Gulya and Schuknecht[1] and Altmann[49]).

The subarcuate artery, traversing the subarcuate fossa, develops as a branch of either the labyrinthine or anterior inferior cerebellar artery by the end of the eighth week and supplies part of the otic capsule and mastoid. The adult pattern of origin of all of the cranial arteries is visible by the ninth week.

The stapedial artery, usually a transient structure, may abnormally persist into adulthood, interfering with stapes operations especially (Figure 1–29). After passing through the stapes, the stapedial artery branches; bifurcation of the stapedial artery proximal to the stapes, with both branches penetrating the stapes blastema, may give rise to a three-legged stapes.[50] The stapedial artery, either directly or indirectly through a branch, may fix the developing internal carotid artery so as to pull it into the middle ear (Figure 1–30A and B) more posteriorly and laterally than it ordinarily would run.[50] Such aberrant internal

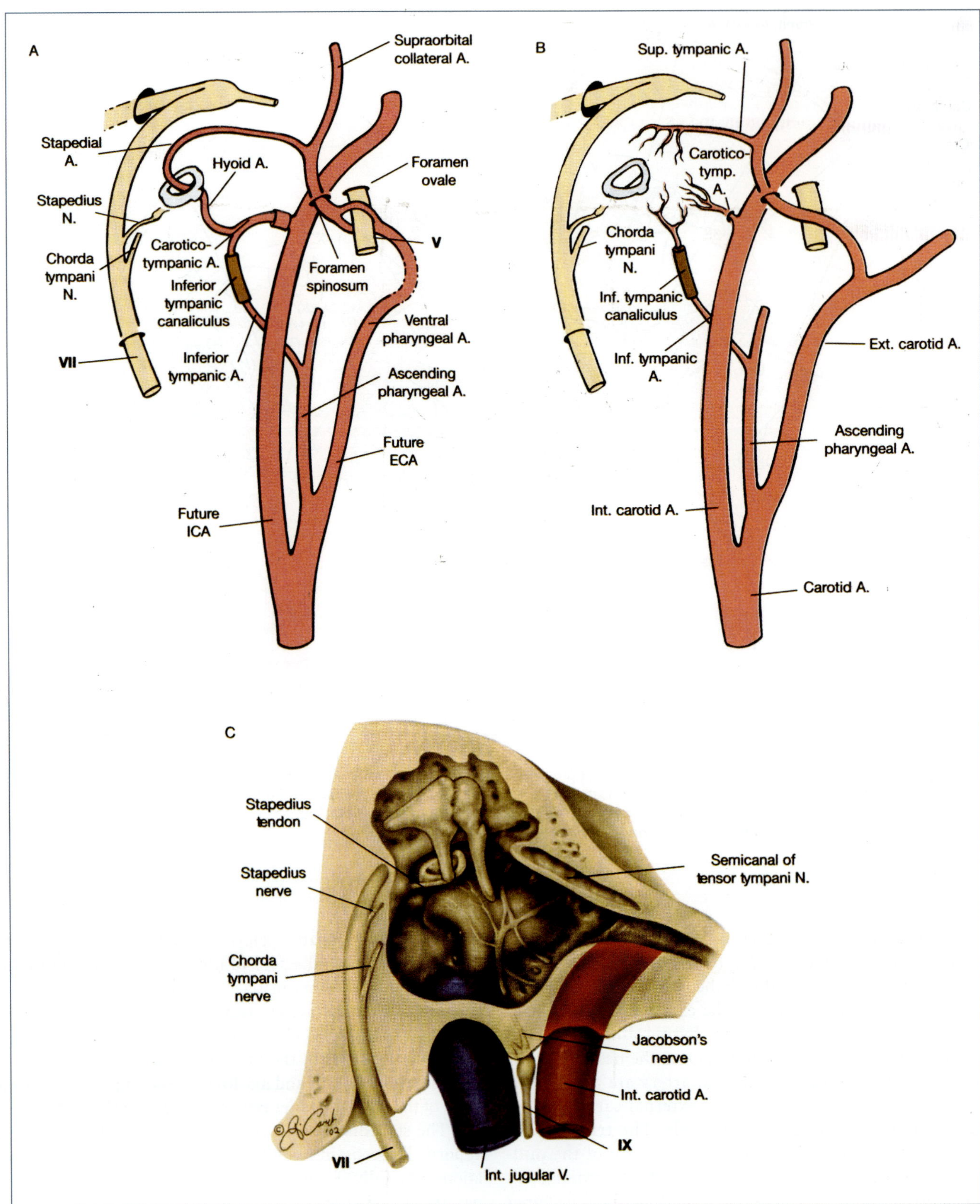

FIGURE 1–28 • Development of the cranial arteries. *A*, Approximately 7 weeks. *B*, Adult configuration. *C*, The internal carotid artery, internal jugular vein, and their interrelationships with the tympanomastoid compartment. *After Moret and colleagues. Abnormal vessels in the middle ear. J Neuroradiol 1982;9:227.*

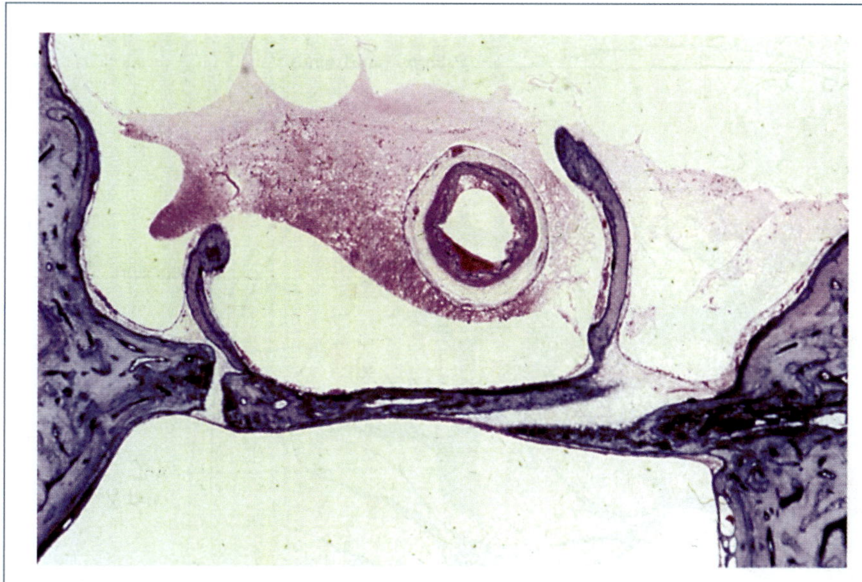

FIGURE 1–29 • The persistent stapedial artery traverses the obturator foramen (man, age 84 years). Reproduced with permission from Gulya AJ. Gulya and Schuknecht's anatomy of the temporal bone with surgical implications. 3rd ed. New York: Informa Healthcare USA; 2007.

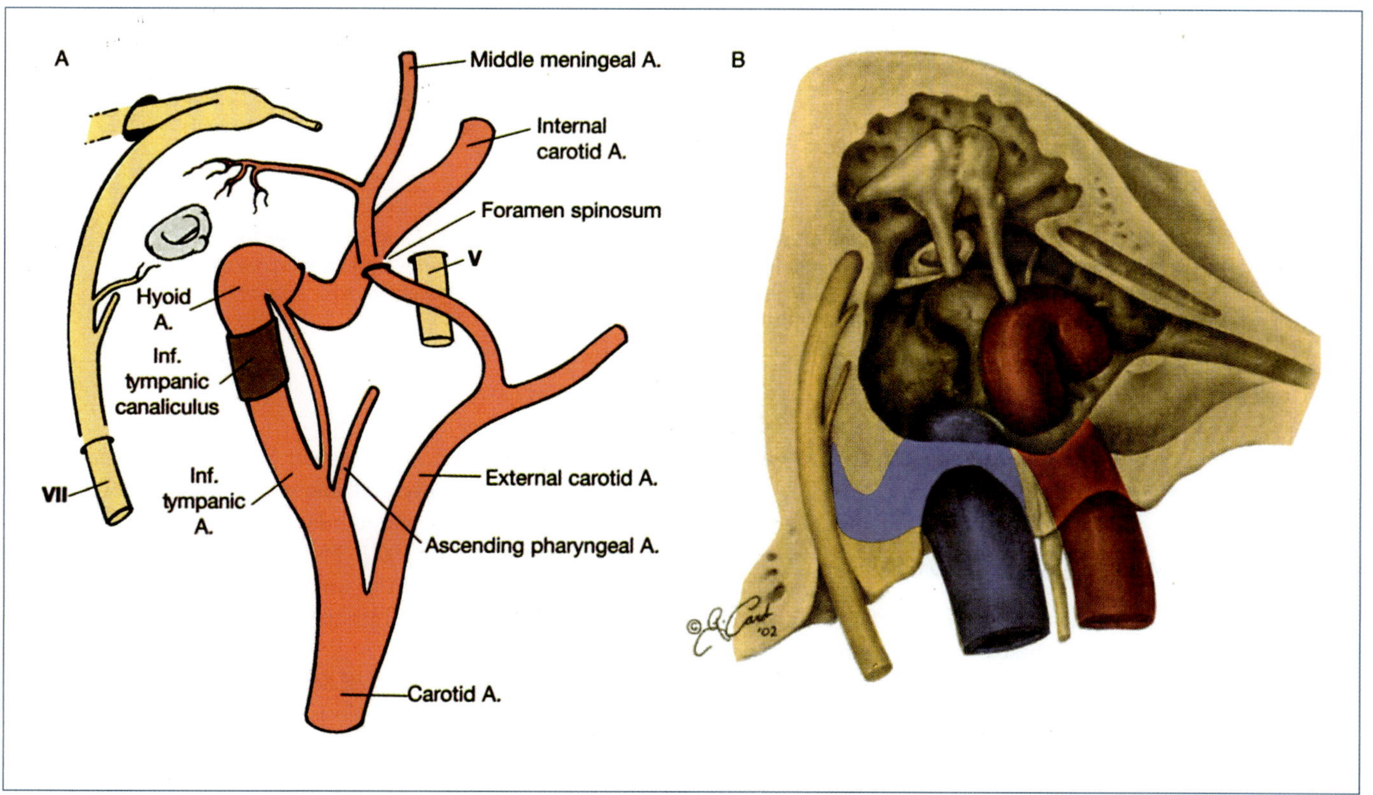

FIGURE 1–30 • *A,* The aberrant internal carotid artery, feeding into the horizontal portion of the intrapetrous internal carotid artery, is seen in association with the inferior tympanic artery and a persisting hyoid artery. *B*, The aberrant internal carotid artery is seen protruding into the tympanic cavity. *After Moret and colleagues. Abnormal vessels in the middle ear. J Neuroradiol 1982;9:227.*

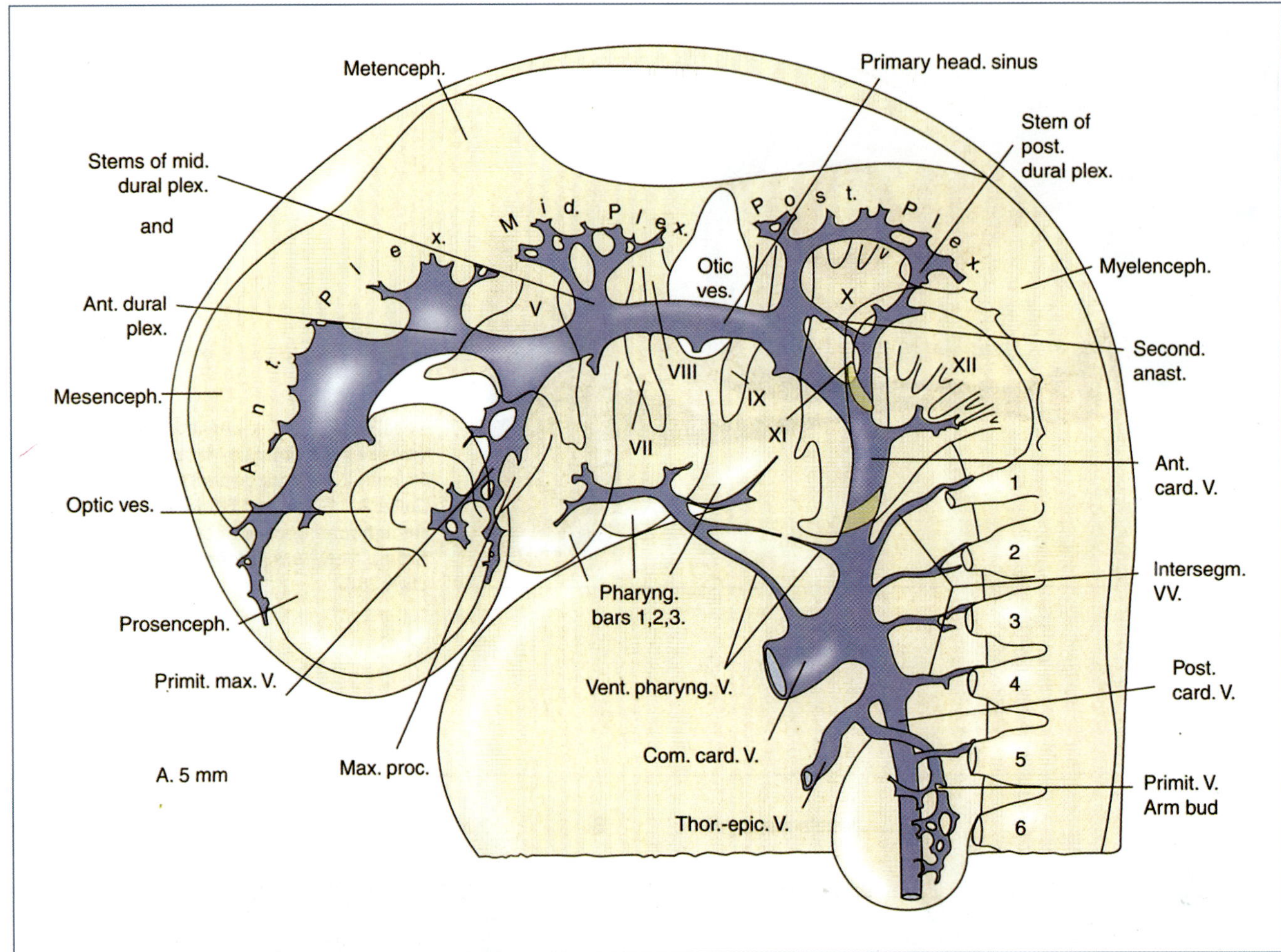

FIGURE 1–31 • The cranial venous system at approximately 4 weeks. Venous blood of the brain drains to the primary head sinus through three stems. The primary head sinus is in continuity with the anterior cardinal vein. *Reproduced with permission from Padget DH. Development of the cranial venous system in man, from the viewpoint of comparative anatomy. Contrib Embryol 1957;36:79.*

carotid arteries occasionally are encountered clinically as pulsatile middle ear masses.

DEVELOPMENT OF THE VEINS

The following account of the development of the venous circulation of the human is largely based on the exhaustive reviews of Padget.[51,52] In general, the venous system lags behind the arterial system in approaching adult configuration; in fact, adult configuration of the cranial venous system is not usually present at birth.[52]

In the developing human of 3 to 4 weeks, most of the neural tube is covered by a primitive capillary plexus, which drains dorsolaterally into a more superficial plexus. Through anterior, middle, and posterior venous stems, the superficial plexus drains into the primary head sinus (also known as the lateral capital vein), a channel that is medial to cranial nerves V and X and lateral to cranial nerves VII, VIII, and IX and the otocyst. The primary head sinus is the first true drainage channel of the craniocervical region and is present by 4 weeks (Figure 1–31). The primary head sinus is continuous with the anterior cardinal vein (the primitive internal jugular vein), which lies medial to cranial nerves X, XI, and XII. The anterior cardinal vein joins the posterior cardinal vein to form the common cardinal vein (duct of Cuvier), draining into the sinus venosus of the embryonic heart.

In the 5th and 6th weeks of development, the primary head sinus encircles and then completes its migration to lie lateral to the vagus nerve. The medial aspect of the ring around the vagus nerve forms the ventral myelencephalic vein. As the primary head sinus moves laterally, the posterior stem moves caudally, becoming continuous with the primitive internal jugular vein and thus constituting the caudal end of the definitive sigmoid sinus. The anterior cardinal (internal jugular) vein also moves to lie lateral to cranial nerves X, XI, and XII.

The jugular foramen, demarcating the internal jugular vein inferiorly and the sigmoid sinus superiorly, is completed by the 7th week. At the same time, a plexiform channel

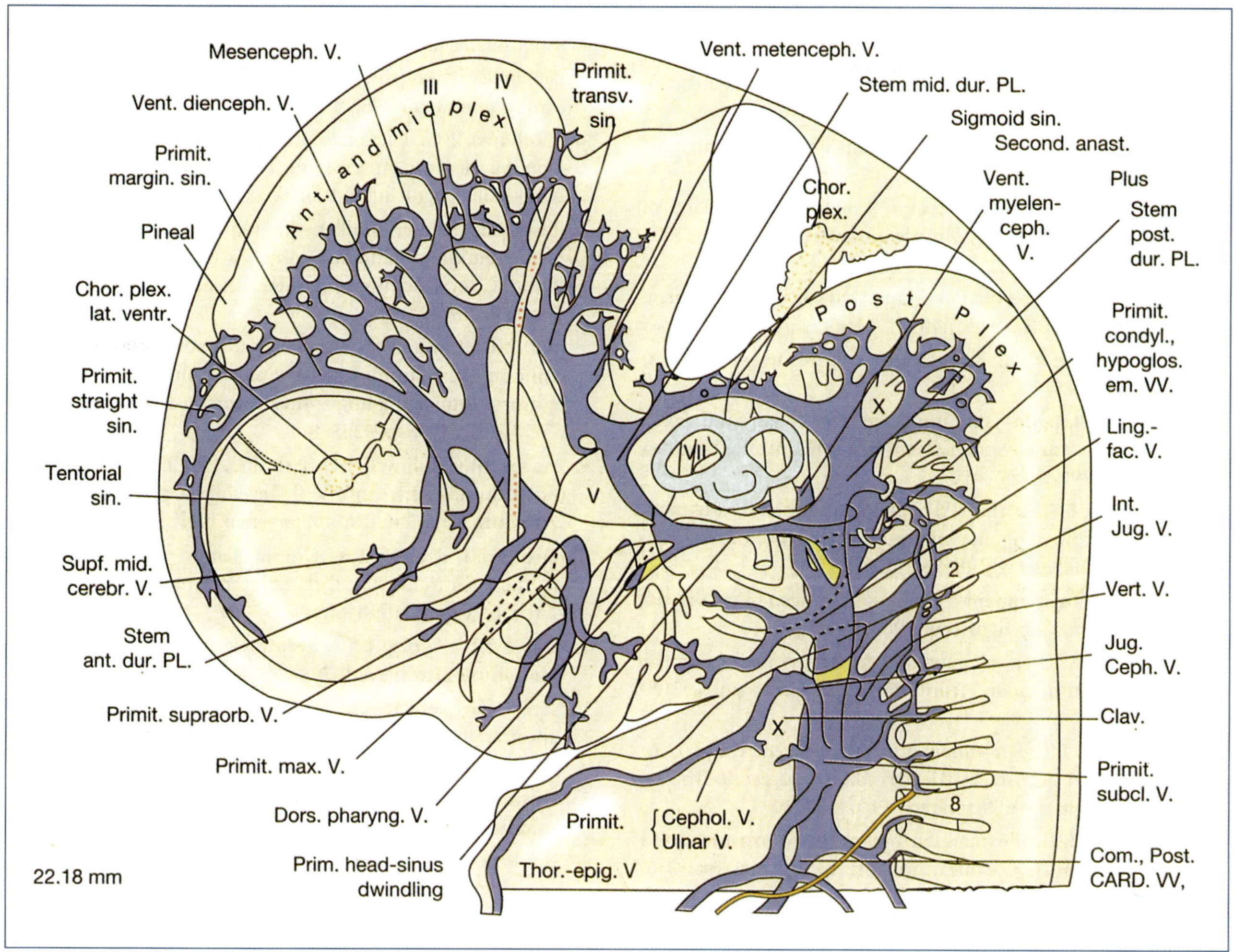

FIGURE 1–32 • The venous system at approximately 8 weeks shows the development of the sigmoid sinus from the anastomotic linkage of the middle and posterior dural plexuses. *Reproduced with permission from Padget DH. Development of the cranial venous system in man, from the viewpoint of comparative anatomy. Contrib Embryol 1957;36:79–140.*

develops, parallel and dorsal to the primary head sinus. This channel links the anterior, middle, and posterior stems and lies dorsal to the trigeminal nerve and the otocyst. Also during the 7th week, the primary head sinus begins to involute, being replaced by the dorsal channel, and the direction of flow reverses in the middle stem as it becomes the pro-otic sinus (Figure 1–32). The definitive sigmoid sinus is composed of the channel connecting the middle and posterior stems and the ventral remainder of the posterior stem. The transverse sinus develops from the anastomotic channel between the anterior and middle stems.

In embryos of approximately 8 weeks, the primary head sinus has essentially disappeared except for three remnants. The cranial remnant medial to the trigeminal nerve (part of the pro-otic sinus) becomes the lateral wing of the cavernous sinus. A caudal remnant contributes to the formation of the veins accompanying the superficial petrosal and stylomastoid arteries and draining the middle ear region, whereas yet another remnant of the primary head sinus accompanies the facial nerve extracranially, ventral to the otic capsule. Also at this stage, for the first time, the tendency of the venous drainage to pass more to the right than to the left is apparent and is accompanied by greater developmental maturity of the venous system of the right side when compared with that of the left side.

In the 9th and 10th weeks, the ventral myelencephalic vein receives the hypoglossal emissary and inferior cochlear veins. The inferior petrosal sinus is thus established.

By 12 weeks, cerebral expansion pushes the transverse sinus into its adult position. A medial tributary of the pro-otic sinus, the ventral metencephalic vein, becomes recognizable as the superior petrosal sinus.

After birth, anastomoses develop that add cavernous and inferior petrosal sinus drainage routes to the drainage of the cerebral and cerebellar veins into the junction of the transverse and sigmoid sinuses.[52]

References

1. Gulya AJ, Schuknecht H.F. Anatomy of the temporal bone with surgical implications. 3rd ed. New York: Informa Healthcare USA; 2007.
2. Anson BJ, Donaldson JA. Surgical anatomy of the temporal bone. 3rd ed. Philadelphia: WB Saunders; 1981.
3. Pearson AA. Developmental anatomy of the ear. In: English GM, editor. Otolaryngology. Philadelphia: Harper & Row; 1984. p. 1–68.
4. Bast TH, Anson BJ. The temporal bone and the ear. Springfield, IL: Charles C. Thomas; 1949.
5. Wood-Jones F, Wen I-C. The development of the external ear. J Anat 1934;68:525–33.
6. Levine H. Cutaneous carcinoma of the head and neck: Management of massive and previously uncontrolled lesions. Laryngoscope 1983;93:87–105.
7. Anson BJ, Bast TH, Richany SF. The fetal and early postnatal development of the tympanic ring and related structures in man. Ann Otol Rhinol Laryngol 1955;64:802–23.
8. Aimi K. Role of the tympanic ring in the pathogenesis of congenital cholesteatoma. Laryngoscope 1983;93:1140–6.
9. Spector GJ, Ge X-X. Development of the hypotympanum in the human fetus and neonate. Ann Otol Rhinol Laryngol 1981;90 Suppl 88:2–20.
10. Anson BJ, Bast TH. Developmental anatomy of the ear. In: Shambaugh GE Jr, Glasscock ME III, editors. Surgery of the ear. 3rd ed. Philadelphia: WB Saunders; 1980. p. 5–29.
11. Eby TL, Nadol JB Jr. Postnatal growth of the human temporal bone: Implications for cochlear implants in children. Ann Otol Rhinol Laryngol 1986;95:356–64.
12. Eby TL. Development of the facial recess: Implications for cochlear implantation. Laryngoscope 1996;106 Suppl 80:1–7.
13. van Bergeijk WA. Evolution of the sense of hearing in vertebrates. Am Zoologist 1966;6:371–7.
14. Proctor B. Embryology and anatomy of the eustachian tube. Arch Otolaryngol 1967;86:503–14.
15. Allam AF. Pneumatization of the temporal bone. Ann Otol Rhinol Laryngol 1969;78:49–64.
16. Takahara T, Sando I, Hashida Y, Shibahara Y. Mesenchyme remaining in human temporal bones. Otolaryngol Head Neck Surg 1986;95:349–57.
17. Davies DG. Malleus fixation. J Laryngol Otol 1968;82:331–51.
18. Pye A, Hinchcliffe R. Comparative anatomy of the ear. In: Hinchcliffe R, Harrison D, editors. Scientific foundations of otolaryngology. London: William Heinemann Medical Books; 1976.
19. Marovitz WF, Porubsky ES. The embryological development of the middle ear: A new concept. Ann Otol Rhinol Laryngol 1971;80:384–9.
20. Van de Water TR, Maderson PFA, Jaskoll TF. The morphogenesis of the middle and external ear. Birth Defects 1980;16:147–80.
21. Hanson JR, Anson BJ, Strickland EM. Branchial sources of the auditory ossicles in man. Part II: Observations of embryonic stages from 7 mm to 28 mm (CR length). Arch Otolaryngol 1962;76:200–15.
22. Guggenheim L. Phylogenesis of the ear. Culver City, CA: Murray and Gee; 1948.
23. Streeter GL. On the development of the membranous labyrinth and the acoustic and facial nerves in the human embryo. Am J Anat 1906;6:139–65.
24. Schuknecht HF, Belal AA. The utriculoendolymphatic valve: Its functional significance. J Laryngol Otol 1975;89:985–96.
25. Jackler RK, Luxford WM. Congenital malformations of the inner ear. Laryngoscope 1987;97 Suppl 40:2–14.
26. Lundquist P-G. The endolymphatic duct and sac in the guinea pig: An electron microscopic and experimental investigation. Acta Otolaryngol Suppl (Stockh) 1965;201:1–108.
27. Rask-Andersen H, Bredberg G, Stahle J. Structure and function of the endolymphatic duct. In: Vosteen K-H, Schuknecht HF, Pfaltz C, et al, editors. Meniere's disease. New York: Thieme-Stratton; 1981.
28. Smith RJH. Medical diagnosis and treatment of hearing loss in children. In: Cummings CW, Fredrickson JM, Harker LA, et al, editors. Otolaryngology—head and neck surgery. St. Louis: CV Mosby; 1986. p. 3225–46.
29. Anson BJ, Cauldwell EW, Bast TH. The fissula ante fenestram of the human otic capsule. I. Developmental and normal adult structure. Ann Otol Rhinol Laryngol 1947;56:957–85.
30. Spector GJ, Lee D, Carr C, et al. Later stages of development of the periotic duct and its adjacent area in the human fetus. Laryngoscope 1980;90 Suppl 20:1–31.
31. Gacek RR, Leipzig B. Congenital cerebrospinal otorrhea. Ann Otol Rhinol Laryngol 1979;88:358–65.
32. Neely JG, Neblett CR, Rose JE. Diagnosis and treatment of spontaneous cerebrospinal fluid otorrhea. Laryngoscope 1982;92:609–12.
33. Gulya AJ, Glasscock ME III, Pensak ML. Neural choristoma of the middle ear. Otolaryngol Head Neck Surg 1987;97:52–6.
34. Schuknecht HF. Pathology of the ear. Cambridge, MA: Harvard University Press; 1974.
35. Okano Y, Myers EN, Dickson DB. Microfissure between the round window niche and posterior canal ampulla. Ann Otol Rhinol Laryngol 1977;86:49–57.
36. Harada T, Sando I, Myers EN. Microfissure in the oval window area. Ann Otol Rhinol Laryngol 1981;90:174–80.
37. Proops DW, Hawke WM, Berger G. Microfractures of the otic capsule: The possible role of masticatory stress. J Laryngol Otol 1986;100:749–58.
38. El Shazly MAR, Linthicum FH Jr. Microfissures of the temporal bone: Do they have any clinical significance? Am J Otol 1991;12:169–71.
39. Batten EH. The origin of the acoustic ganglion in sheep. J Embryol Exp Morph 1958;6:597–615.
40. Skinner HA. The origin of acoustic nerve tumors. Br J Surg 1928–1929;16:440–63.
41. Van De Water TR, Ruben RJ. Organogenesis of the ear. In: Hinchcliffe R, Harrison D, editors. Scientific foundations of otolaryngology. London: William Heinemann Medical Books; 1976. p. 173–84.
42. Hilding DA. Electron microscopy of the developing hearing organ. Laryngoscope 1969;79:1691–704.
43. Gasser RF, Shigihara S, Shimada K. Three-dimensional development of the facial nerve path through the ear region in human embryos. Ann Otol Rhinol Laryngol 1994;103:395–403.
44. Gasser RF. The development of the facial nerve in man. Ann Otol Rhinol Laryngol 1967;6:37–56.
45. Gasser RF, May M. Embryonic development of the facial nerve. In: May M, editor. The facial nerve. New York: Thieme; 1986. p. 3–19.

46. Spector JG, Ge X. Ossification patterns of the tympanic facial canal in the human fetus and neonate. Laryngoscope 1993;103:1052–65.
47. Pansky B. Review of medical embryology. New York: Macmillan; 1982.
48. Padget DH. The development of the cranial arteries in the human embryo. Contrib Embryol 1948;32:205–61.
49. Altmann F. Anomalies of the internal carotid artery and its branches. Their embryological and comparative anatomical significance. Report of a new case of persistent stapedial artery in man. Laryngoscope 1947;57:313–39.
50. Steffen TN. Vascular anomalies of the middle ear. Laryngoscope 1968;78:171–97.
51. Padget DH. Development of the cranial venous system in man, from the viewpoint of comparative anatomy. Contrib Embryol 1957;36:79–140.
52. Padget DH. The cranial venous system in man in reference to development, adult configuration, and relation to the arteries. Am J Anat 1956;98:307–55.

Anatomy of the Temporal Bone and Skull Base

2

Aina Julianna Gulya, MD, FACS

The temporal bone is a fascinating, intricate, and complex structure, and developing a three-dimensional appreciation of the anatomic interrelationships of its components is an intellectually demanding task. To the otologic/neurotologic surgeon, such a three-dimensional grasp is critical to understanding the pathophysiology of, and skillfully diagnosing and managing, otologic disorders. This chapter presents a brief overview of those features of the anatomy of the temporal bone and its environs critical to the otologist; the interested reader is referred to *Anatomy of the Temporal Bone with Surgical Implications*[1] for detail beyond the scope of this chapter. In addition, since there is (as yet) no substitute for supplementing the acquisition of anatomic facts by careful dissection of a wide variety of temporal bone specimens, the reader is strongly encouraged to review the Appendix, "Surgical Anatomy of the Temporal Bone through Dissection," and to practice the described dissections.

PINNA AND EXTERNAL AUDITORY CANAL

Pinna

The pinna acts to focus and aid in the localization of sound. Its shape, showing considerable interindividual variability, reflects its multicomponent embryologic origin. Nonetheless, there are constant features.

The contour of the pinna is determined by the configuration of its elastic cartilage frame. The lateral surface of the pinna is dominated by concavities, in particular the concha (Figure 2–1). The skin of the lateral and medial surfaces of the pinna possesses hair and both sebaceous and sudoriferous glands; however, the attachment of the skin differs, being tightly bound down to the perichondrium on the lateral aspect and only loosely attached on the medial.

The pinna is securely attached to the tympanic bone by the continuity of its cartilage with that of the cartilaginous external auditory canal (EAC). Otherwise, the pinna loosely attaches to the skull by its skin, connective tissue, ligaments, and three extrinsic and six intrinsic muscles. A branch of the facial nerve, the posterior auricular nerve, innervates the intrinsic muscles, in general poorly developed in the human.

External Auditory Canal

The lateral one-third of the EAC comprises a continuation of the cartilage of the pinna and is deficient superiorly at the incisura terminalis (see Figure 2–1); the extracartilaginous endaural incision for access to the underlying temporal bone capitalizes on this gap. The two or three variably present perforations in the anterior aspect of the cartilaginous canal are the fissures of Santorini. The remaining medial two-thirds of the approximately 2.5-cm length of the canal are bony. The isthmus, the narrowest portion of the EAC, lies just medial to the junction of the bony and cartilaginous canals.

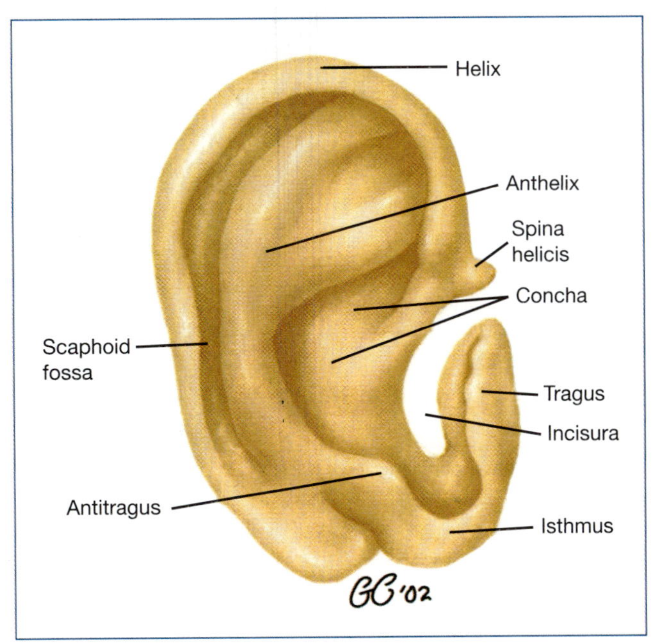

FIGURE 2–1 • Auricular cartilage.

The skin of the cartilaginous canal has a substantial subcutaneous layer, replete with hair follicles, sebaceous glands, and cerumen glands. The skin of the osseous canal, in contrast, is very thin and its subcutaneous layer is bereft of the usual adnexal structures. Accordingly, the absence of hair serves to distinguish the bony and cartilaginous canals.

Innervation

The auriculotemporal branch of the trigeminal nerve, greater auricular nerve (a branch of C3), lesser occipital nerve (of C2 and C3 derivation), auricular branch of the vagus nerve (Arnold's nerve), and twigs from the facial nerve all contribute to the sensory innervation of the pinna and EAC (Figures 2–2 and 2–3).

Effective local anesthesia can be obtained by 1 to 2% lidocaine infiltration of the postauricular region accompanied by infiltration of the cartilaginous canal in a four-quadrant (ie, at the 2, 4, 8, and 10 o'clock positions) fashion. Infiltration of the bony canal must be done gently to avoid troublesome bleb formation; if done properly, the anchoring of the skin of the bony EAC "outlines" the tympanomastoid and tympanosquamous sutures, which are the landmarks for the "vascular strip" incisions (see below). Inflammation, as with infection of the middle ear or external ear, reduces the efficacy of local anesthesia.

Vascular Supply

Two branches of the external carotid artery, the posterior auricular artery and the superficial temporal artery, are the sources of arterial blood supply to the pinna and EAC (see Figure 2–2). The posterior auricular artery, as it courses superiorly on the mastoid portion of the temporal bone, supplies the skin of the pinna and the skin and bone of the mastoid; its stylomastoid branch enters the fallopian canal to supply the inferior segment of the facial nerve. Anteriorly, a few twigs of the superficial temporal artery provide additional supply to the pinna and EAC. The veins accompanying the arteries drain into the internal jugular vein by either the facial or external jugular veins.

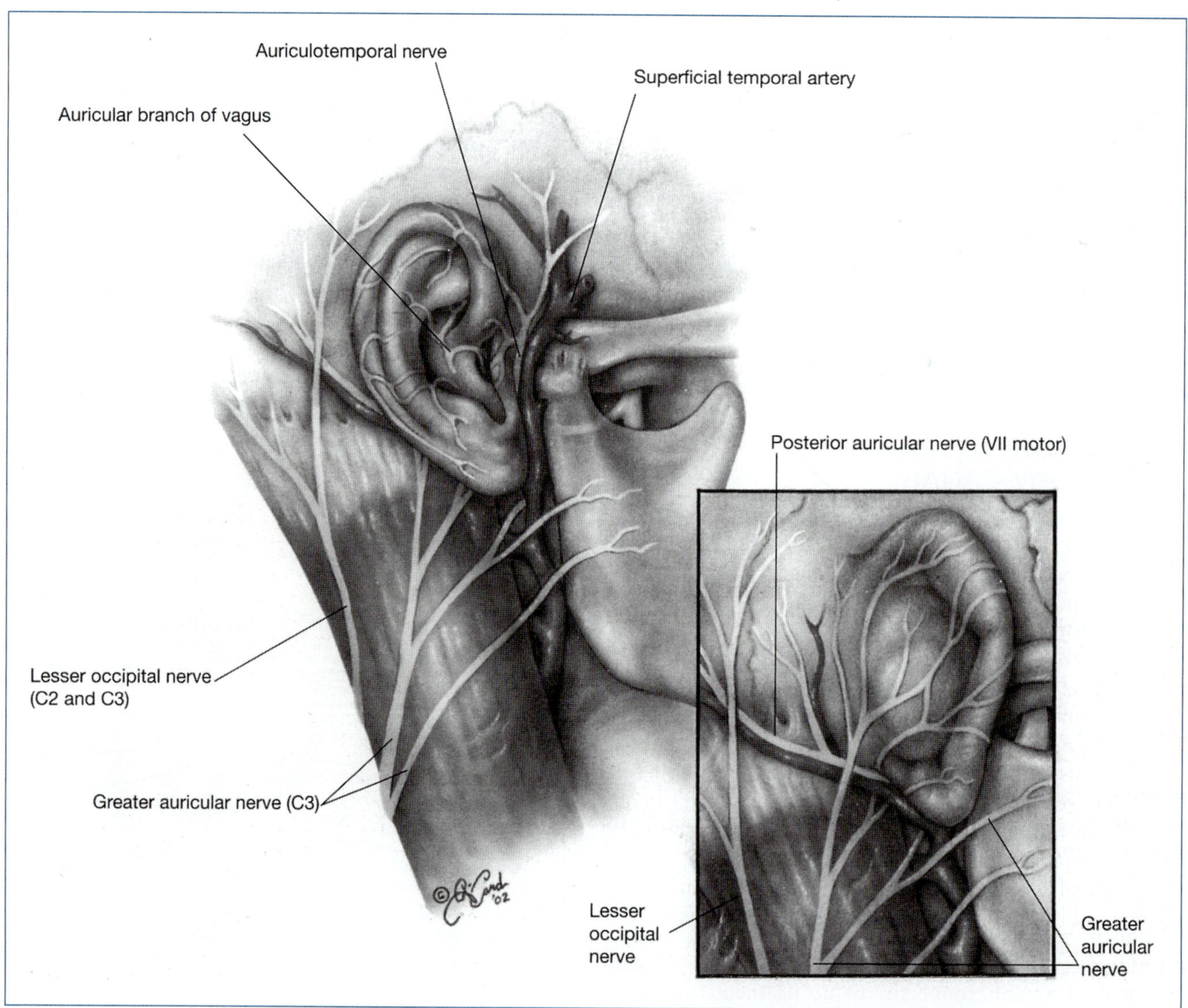

FIGURE 2–2 • Innervation of the external ear (lateral view). The inset shows the innervation of the posterior aspect of the pinna.

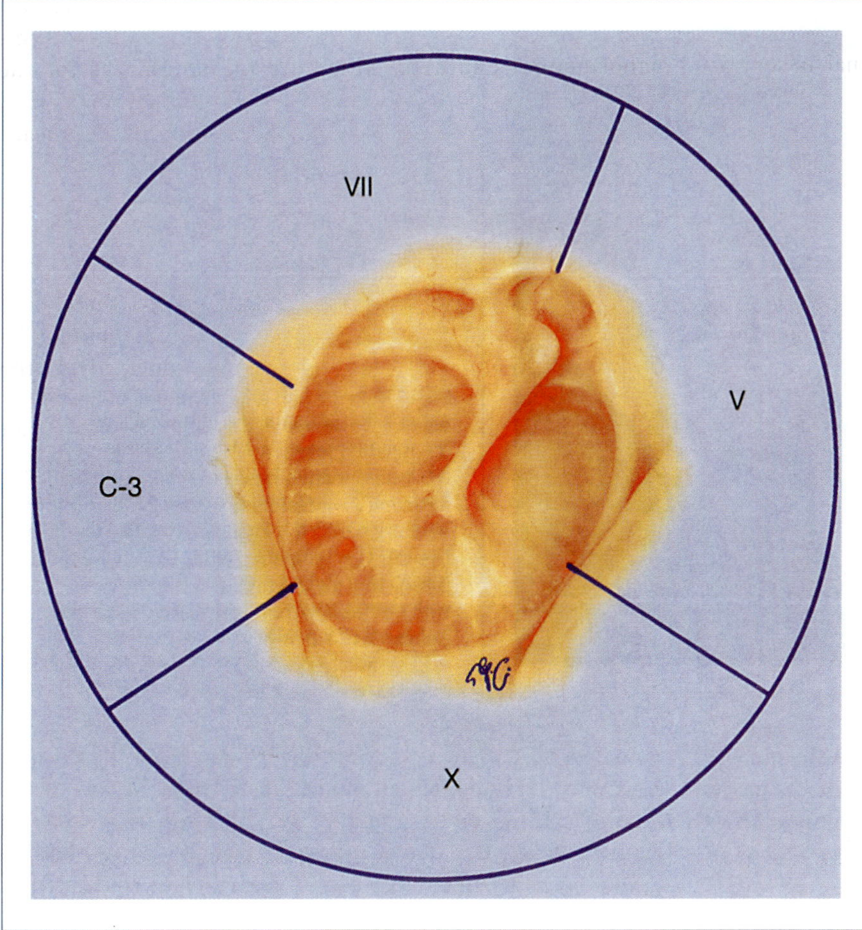

FIGURE 2–3 • The innervation of the external auditory canal.

TEMPORAL BONE, SKULL BASE, AND RELATED STRUCTURES

Temporal Bone and Skull Base

The temporal bone is a composite structure consisting of the tympanic bone, mastoid process, squama (also known as the squamous portion of the temporal bone), and petrosa (also known as the petrous portion of the temporal bone). Although the styloid process is closely related to the temporal bone, it is not considered a portion of it.

The tympanic, squamous, and mastoid portions of the temporal bone are evident on a lateral view (Figure 2–4). The tympanic bone forms the anterior, inferior, and parts of the posterior wall of the EAC. It interfaces with the squama at the tympanosquamous suture, the mastoid at the tympanomastoid suture, and the petrosa at the petrotympanic fissure and constitutes the posterior wall of the glenoid fossa for the temporomandibular joint (TMJ). The tympanomastoid suture is traversed by Arnold's nerve, whereas the chorda tympani nerve, anterior process of the malleus, and anterior tympanic artery traverse the petrotympanic fissure. Henle's spine is a projection of variable prominence at the posterosuperior aspect of the EAC. Inferiorly, the vaginal process, a projection of tympanic bone, forms the sheath of the styloid bone. Laterally, the tympanic bone borders the cartilaginous EAC, whereas medially it bears a circular groove, the annular sulcus. The annular sulcus houses the annulus of the tympanic membrane except superiorly, where it is deficient; at this point, known as the notch of Rivinus, the tympanic membrane attaches directly to the squama.

The tympanosquamous and tympanomastoid sutures are landmarks for the "vascular strip" incisions used in tympanomastoid surgery. The elevation of EAC skin and periosteum at these two sutures often requires sharp dissection to divide the contained periosteum, particularly at the tympanosquamous suture. Elevation of the tympanic membrane, as for a transcanal exploratory tympanotomy, typically commences just above the notch of Rivinus; the surgeon is thus able to identify and elevate the annulus in continuity with the tympanic membrane. The apparent size of the EAC may be diminished by excessive prominence of the bone at the tympanosquamous suture; access to the EAC in such cases can be improved by removal of the offending spur. Henle's spine marks the anterior limit of dissection in a canal wall up mastoidectomy. On occasion, posterior bulging of the anterior canal wall may obscure full visualization of the tympanic membrane. Anterior canalplasty can improve surgical visualization but if overzealous may result in prolapse of the TMJ into the EAC with, eg, opening the mouth. Temporomandibular joint dysfunction, as well as disease of the molar teeth, may manifest in referred otalgia, owing both to the proximity of the EAC and the shared innervation by the mandibular division of the trigeminal (fifth cranial) nerve.

The squamous portion of the temporal bone serves as the lateral wall of the middle cranial fossa and (see Figures 2–4

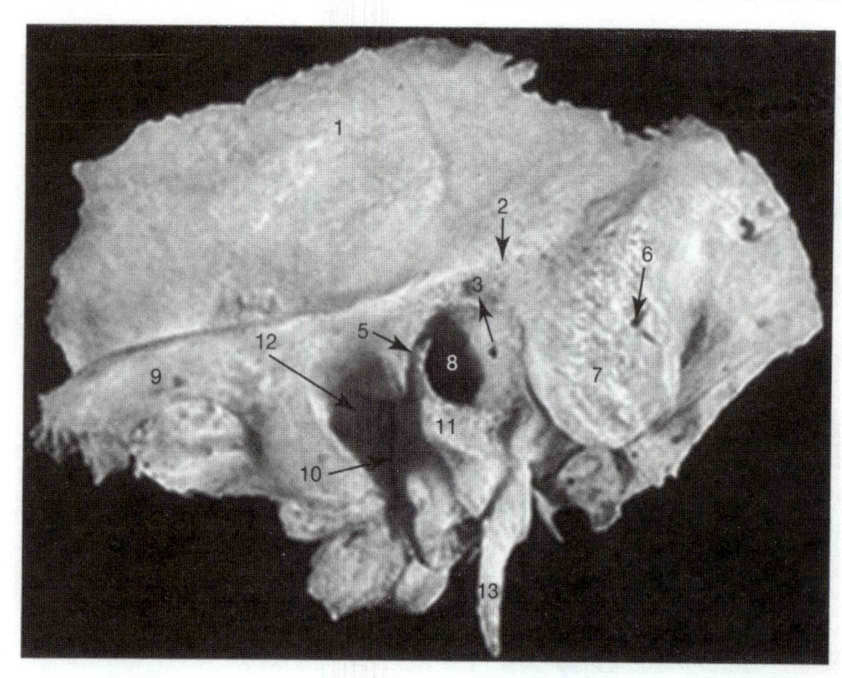

FIGURE 2–4 • Left adult temporal bone, lateral aspect. 1 = squama; 2 = temporal line; 3 = mastoid fossa; 4 = Henle's spine; 5 = tympanosquamous suture; 6 = mastoid foramen; 7 = mastoid process; 8 = external auditory canal; 9 = zygoma; 10 = petrotympanic fissure; 11 = tympanic bone; 12 = mandibular fossa; 13 = styloid process. *Reproduced with permission from Gulya, AJ. Gulya and Schuknecht's anatomy of the temporal bone with surgical implications. 3rd ed. New York: Informa Healthcare USA; 2007.*

and 2–5) interfaces with the parietal bone superiorly and with the zygomatic process and the sphenoid anteriorly. Its medial surface is grooved by a sulcus for the middle meningeal artery, whereas the middle temporal artery runs in a groove on its lateral aspect.

The mastoid portion of the temporal bone (see Figure 2–4) is the inferiorly extending projection seen on the lateral surface of the temporal bone. It is composed of a squamous portion (laterally) and a petrous portion (medially) separated by Körner's (petrosquamous) septum. The fossa mastoidea (Macewen's triangle) is defined by the linea temporalis (temporal line), a ridge of bone extending posteriorly from the zygomatic process (marking the lower margin of the temporalis muscle and approximating the inferior descent of the middle cranial fossa dura), the posterosuperior margin of the EAC, and a tangent to the posterior margin of the EAC. The fossa mastoidea, a cribrose (cribriform) area, is identified by its numerous, perforating small blood vessels.

The mastoid foramen, located posteriorly on the mastoid process, is traversed by the mastoid emissary vein and one or two mastoid arteries. Inferiorly, the sternocleidomastoid muscle attaches to the mastoid tip.

The linea temporalis is an avascular plane, a feature that makes it an ideal location for the superior limb of the "T" musculoperiosteal incision used in the postauricular approach to the tympanomastoid compartment. The fossa mastoidea is an important surgical landmark as it laterally overlies the mastoid antrum. The mastoid antrum, medial to the fossa mastoidea (Macewen's triangle), develops in the earliest stages of mastoid pneumatization and is ordinarily present in even the least pneumatized temporal bones. Therefore, the fossa mastoidea is the site at which mastoid drilling ordinarily commences.

The petrosa (see Figures 2–5, 2–6, and 2–7) is evident on superior, medial, and posterior views of the temporal bone; the term "petrous" (Greek for "rocklike") stems from the extreme density of its bone, which guards the sensory organs of the inner ear. Important landmarks seen on a superior view (see Figure 2–6) are the arcuate eminence (roughly corresponding to the superior semicircular canal), meatal plane (indicative of the internal auditory canal), foramen spinosum for the middle meningeal artery, and facial hiatus (marking the departure of the greater petrosal nerve from the anterior aspect of the geniculate ganglion). The lesser petrosal nerve, accompanied by the superior tympanic artery, occupies the superior tympanic canaliculus, lying lateral to and paralleling the path of the greater petrosal nerve to the petrous apex. The petrous apex points anteromedially and is marked by the transition of the intrapetrous to the intracranial internal carotid artery, orifice of the bony eustachian tube, and, anterolaterally, ganglion of the trigeminal nerve in Meckel's cave.

The medial view of the temporal bone (see Figure 2–5) features the porus of the internal auditory canal (IAC). The foramen seen at the petrous apex is the internal carotid foramen, by which the internal carotid artery exits the temporal bone. The sigmoid portion of the lateral venous sinus runs in the deep sulcus seen posteriorly, whereas the superior petrosal sinus runs in the sulcus located at the junction of the posterior and middle fossa faces of the temporal bone.

The vertically oriented posterior face of the petrosa dominates the posterior view of the temporal bone (see Figure 2–7) as it delimits the anterolateral aspect of the posterior cranial fossa and lies between the superior and inferior petrosal sinuses. The porus of the IAC, operculum, endolymphatic fossette cradling the endolymphatic sac, and subarcuate fossa are the key anatomic features on this surface.

The inferior surface of the temporal bone (Figure 2–8) figures prominently in skull base anatomy as it interfaces with the sphenoid and occipital bones. It provides attachment for the deep muscles of the neck and is perforated by a multitude

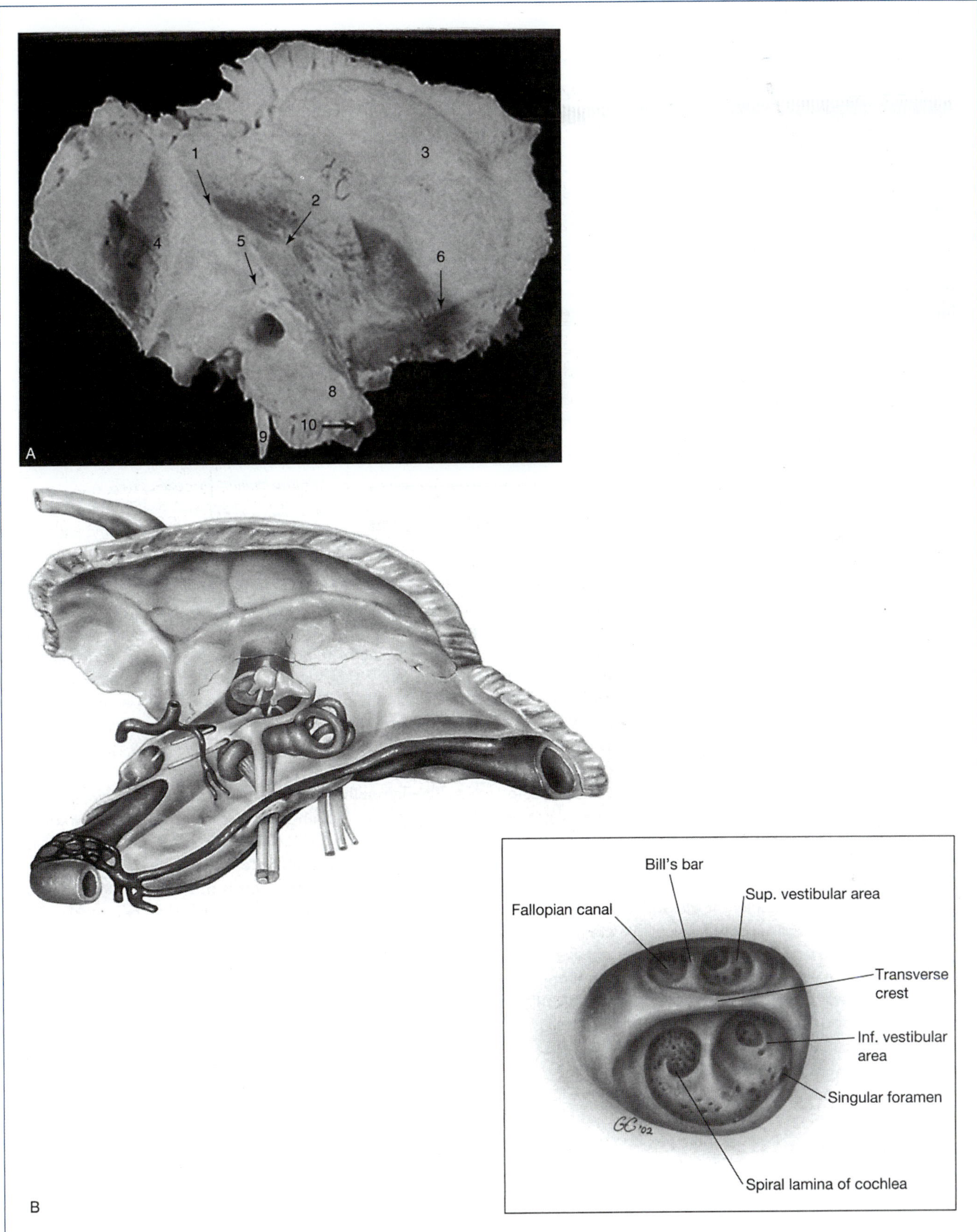

FIGURE 2–5 • *A*, Left adult temporal bone, medial aspect. 1 = superior petrosal sulcus; 2 = arcuate eminence; 3 = squama; 4 = sigmoid sulcus; 5 = petromastoid canal; 6 = middle meningeal artery sulcus; 7 = internal auditory canal; 8 = petrous apex; 9 = styloid process; 10 = internal carotid artery foramen. *Reproduced with permission from Gulya, AJ. Gulya and Schuknecht's anatomy of the temporal bone with surgical implications. 3rd ed. New York: Informa Healthcare USA; 2007. B*, Drawing indicating approximate anatomic relationships of the internal carotid artery, superior petrosal sinus, facial nerve, bony labyrinth, and ossicular chain (right temporal bone). Inset shows the anatomic interrelationships at the fundus of the internal auditory canal.

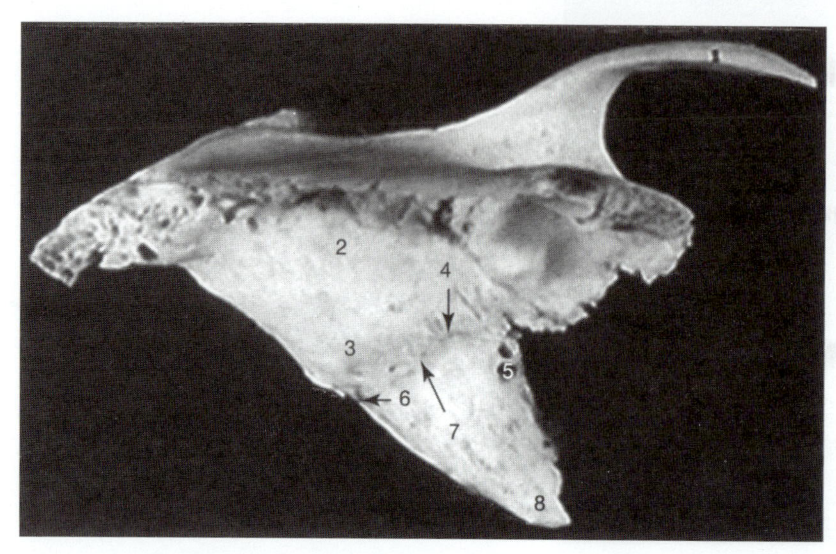

FIGURE 2–6 • Left adult temporal bone, superior aspect. 1 = zygoma; 2 = tegmen; 3 = arcuate eminence; 4 = lesser superficial petrosal canal; 5 = internal carotid artery foramen; 6 = internal audotory canal; 7 = facial hiatus; 8 = petrous apex. *Reproduced with permission from Gulya, AJ. Gulya and Schuknecht's anatomy of the temporal bone with surgical implications. 3rd ed. New York: Informa Healthcare USA; 2007.*

of foramina. The jugular fossa, housing the jugular bulb, is separated from the internal carotid artery by the jugulocarotid crest. The aperture of the inferior tympanic canaliculus, traversed by the inferior tympanic artery and the tympanic branch of the glossopharyngeal nerve (Jacobson's nerve), is sited in the jugulocarotid crest, whereas the cranial aperture of the cochlear aqueduct is located anteromedial to the jugular fossa. The groove for the inferior petrosal sinus can be seen near the petrous apex. The stylomastoid foramen of the facial nerve is located just posterior to the styloid process. The occipital artery and the digastric muscle occupy the temporal groove and the mastoid incisure, respectively, at the medial aspect of the tip.

The jugular foramen is of particular importance in skull base surgery as it is traversed by the glossopharyngeal (ninth), vagus (tenth), and spinal accessory (eleventh) cranial nerves as they exit the skull (Figures 2–9, 2–10, and 2–11). In the course of posterolateral skull base exposure, decortication and fibrous tissue dissection reveal the internal jugular vein, its bulb, and the internal carotid artery. Posterior retraction of the internal jugular vein and resection of the jugular bulb allow visualization of the lower cranial nerves exiting the skull (see Figure 2–11), the most anterior and lateral of which is cranial nerve IX, as it passes just posterior to the jugulocarotid crest.[2,3] Cranial nerves X and XI are located progressively more posterior (and medial) to cranial nerve IX. Cranial nerve XI is generally identified as it crosses over the internal jugular vein in the neck and the lateral process of the atlas; however, it is important to recognize that nearly as often cranial nerve XI can pass medial to the internal jugular vein.[4]

Contradictory reports exist in the literature regarding the bony/fibrous compartmentalization of the jugular foramen and the distribution of contained neurovascular structures; in the compartmentalized jugular foramen, cranial nerve IX is found in the anteromedial compartment, whereas cranial nerves X and XI and the jugular bulb are located posterolaterally. The contradiction appears particularly when contrasting neurosurgical studies, which use an intracranial approach to the jugular foramen, to neurotologic studies, in which a lateral approach predominates. One suggested resolution to the discrepancy is to consider the jugular foramen as a "short canal rather than a simple foramen"[4] in which a medially positioned bony/thick fibrous tissue septum thins as one approaches the lateral aspect of the foramen.

The hypoglossal canal, located in the anterior portion of the occipital condyle and anteroinferior to the jugular foramen, carries cranial nerve XII, which courses medial to cranial nerve X and inferior to the jugular foramen.[3]

The inferior petrosal sinus is in close anatomic relation to cranial nerves IX through XI as it drains, in two-thirds of cases via multiple openings, into the anterior aspect of the jugular bulb (see Figure 2–10). Most commonly, the inferior petrosal sinus runs inferior and medial to cranial nerve IX and superior and lateral to cranial nerves X and XI.[4] The condylar emissary vein, draining the suboccipital plexus, opens into the jugular bulb inferiorly and posteriorly, in proximity to cranial nerves X and XI.[4]

The cochlear aqueduct, carrying the periotic (or perilymphatic) duct, is an important landmark for the neuro-otologist. As the cochlear aqueduct runs from the medial aspect of the scala tympani of the basal cochlear turn to terminate anteromedial to the jugular bulb, it parallels, and lies inferior to, the IAC. From the transmastoid perspective, the aqueduct is encountered when drilling medial to the jugular bulb; opening the aqueduct results in the flow of cerebrospinal fluid into the mastoid, a useful maneuver in translabyrinthine cerebellopontine angle tumor surgery as it decompresses cerebrospinal fluid pressure. In addition, cranial nerve IX, the inferior petrosal sinus, and, in some cases, cranial nerves X and XI can be found immediately inferior to the lateral terminus of the cochlear aqueduct.[5]

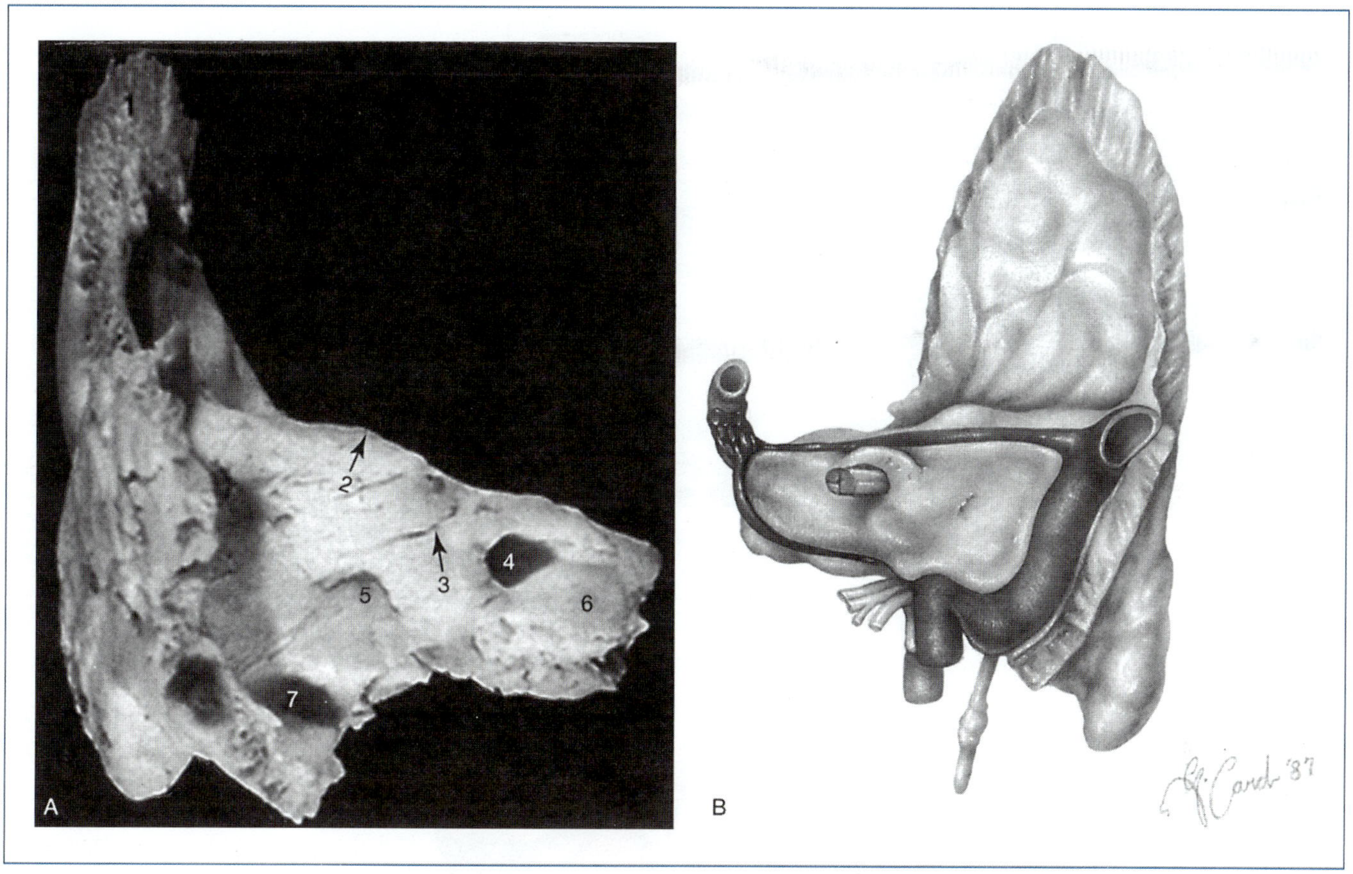

FIGURE 2–7 • *A*, Left adult temporal bone, posterior aspect. 1 = squama; 2 = arcuate eminence; 3 = petromastoid canal; 4 = internal auditory canal; 5 = endolymphatic fossette; 6 = petrous apex; 7 = sigmoid sulcus. *Reproduced with permission from Gulya, AJ. Gulya and Schuknecht's anatomy of the temporal bone with surgical implications. 3rd ed. New York: Informa Healthcare USA; 2007. B*, Artist's depiction of the posterior aspect of the right temporal bone, with neovascular structures.

Therefore, the cochlear aqueduct can be used as a guide to the lower limits of IAC dissection in, eg, the translabyrinthine approach as it allows full exposure of the IAC without risking the lower cranial nerves.

Related Structures

Tympanic Membrane

The tympanic membrane (see Figure 2–3) emulates an irregular cone, the apex of which is formed by the umbo (at the tip of the manubrium). The adult tympanic membrane is about 9 mm in diameter and subtends an acute angle with respect to the inferior wall of the EAC. The fibrous annulus of the tympanic membrane anchors it in the tympanic sulcus. In addition, the tympanic membrane firmly attaches to the malleus at the lateral process and at the umbo; between these two points, only a flimsy mucosal fold, the plica mallearis, connects the tympanic membrane to the malleus.

The tympanic membrane is separated into a superior pars flaccida (Shrapnell's membrane) and a pars inferior by the anterior and posterior tympanic stria, which run from the lateral process of the malleus to the anterior and posterior tympanic spines, respectively. Shrapnell's membrane serves as the lateral wall of Prussak's space (the superior recess of the tympanic membrane); the head and neck of the malleus, the lateral malleal ligament, and anterior and posterior malleal folds form the medial, anterosuperior, and inferior limits of Prussak's space.

The tympanic membrane is a trilaminar structure. The lateral surface is formed by squamous epithelium, whereas the medial layer is a continuation of the mucosal epithelium of the middle ear. Between these layers is a fibrous layer, known as the pars propria. The pars propria at the umbo splits to envelop the distal tip of the manubrium.

Ossicles

The ossicular chain (Figure 2–12), made up of the malleus, incus, and stapes, serves to conduct sound from the tympanic membrane to the cochlea.

The malleus, the most lateral of the ossicles, has a head (caput), manubrium (handle), neck, and anterior and lateral

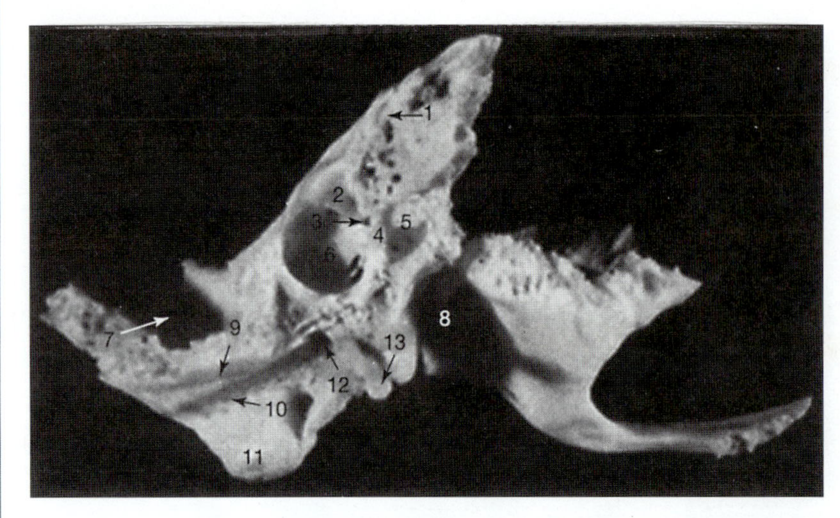

FIGURE 2–8 • Left adult temporal bone, inferior aspect. 1, inferior petrosal sulcus; 2, cochlear aqueduct; 3, inferior tympanic canaliculus; 4, jugulocarotid crest; 5, internal carotid artery formaen; 6, jugular fossa; 7, sigmoid sulcus; 8, mandibular fossa; 9, temporal groove; 10, mastoid incisure; 11, mastoid tip; 12, stylomastoid foramen; 13, styloid process. *Reproduced with permission from Gulya, AJ. Gulya and Schuknecht's anatomy of the temporal bone with surgical implications. 3rd ed. New York: Informa Healthcare USA; 2007.*

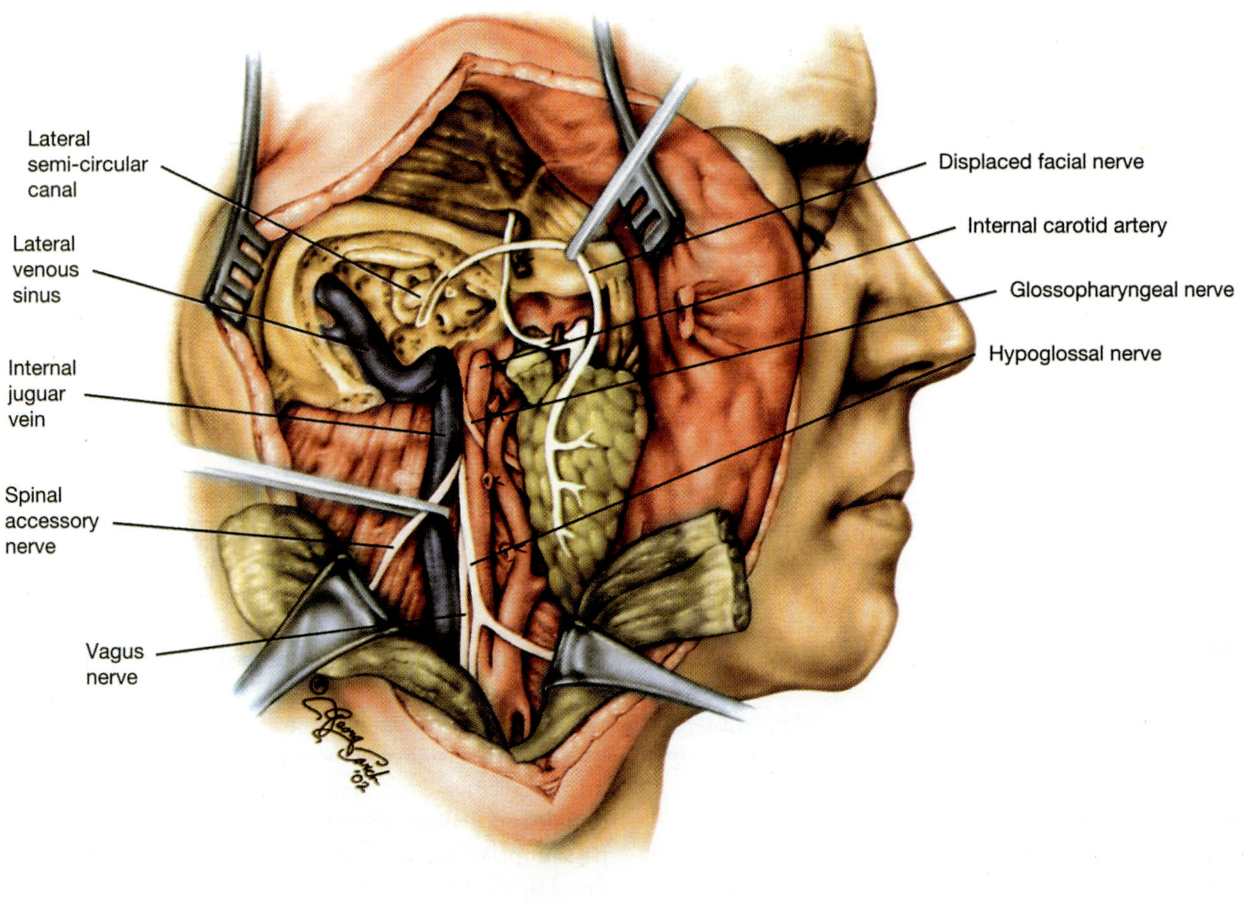

FIGURE 2–9 • Skull base dissection, right. A radical mastoidectomy and neck dissection have been done. The sigmoid sinus and internal carotid artery (ICA) have been decorticated, and the cochlea has been partially removed. The facial nerve has been rerouted anteriorly, and the lower cranial nerves are seen emerging from the crevice between the ICA and the internal jugular vein. *After Goldenberg RA. Surgeon's view of the skull base from the lateral approach. Laryngoscope 1984;94:1–21.*

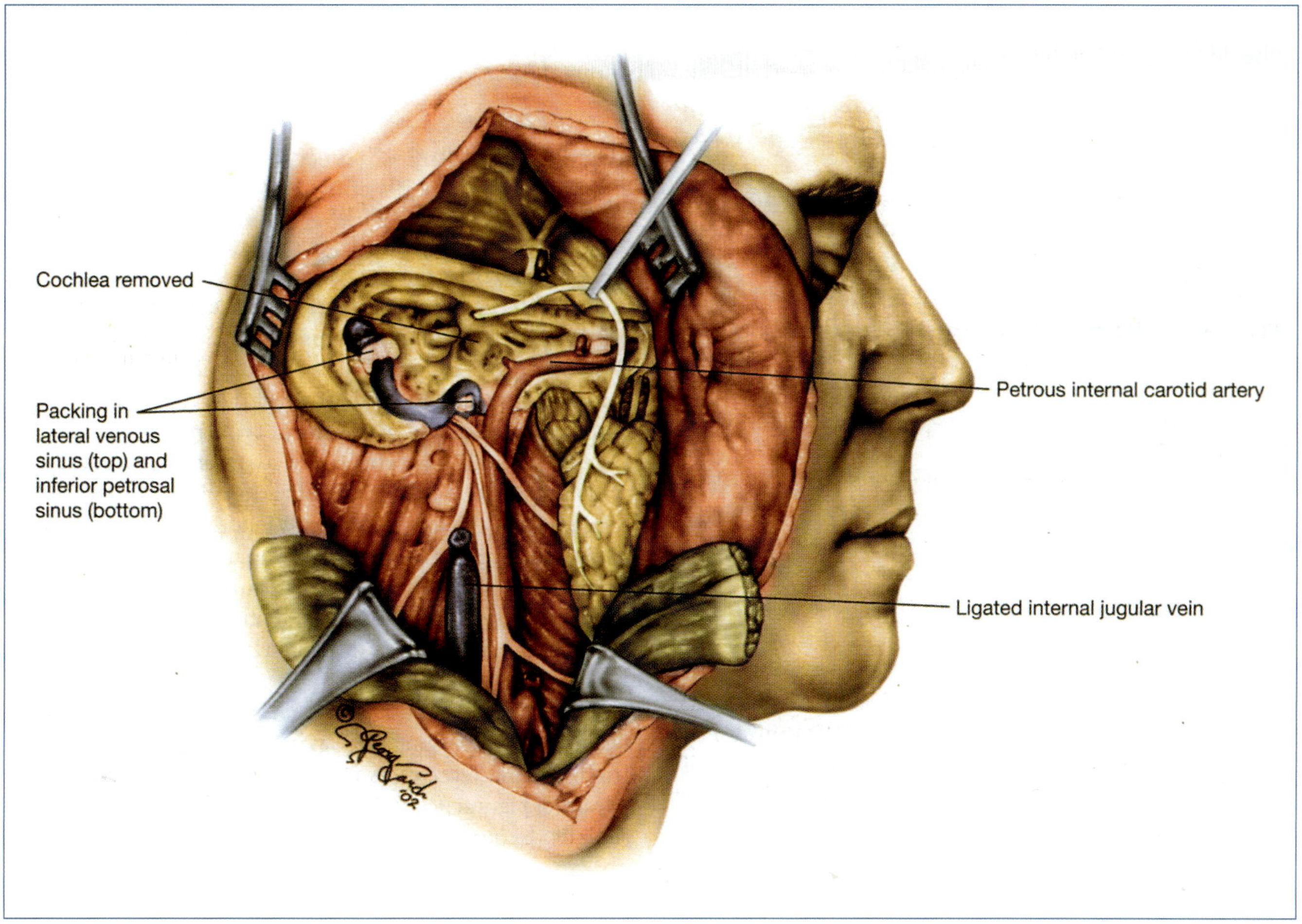

Cochlea removed

Packing in lateral venous sinus (top) and inferior petrosal sinus (bottom)

Petrous internal carotid artery

Ligated internal jugular vein

FIGURE 2–10 • With further dissection, the eustachian tube is removed, and the petrous internal carotid artery has been exposed. *After Goldenberg RA. Surgeon's view of the skull base from the lateral approach. Laryngoscope 1984;94:1–21.*

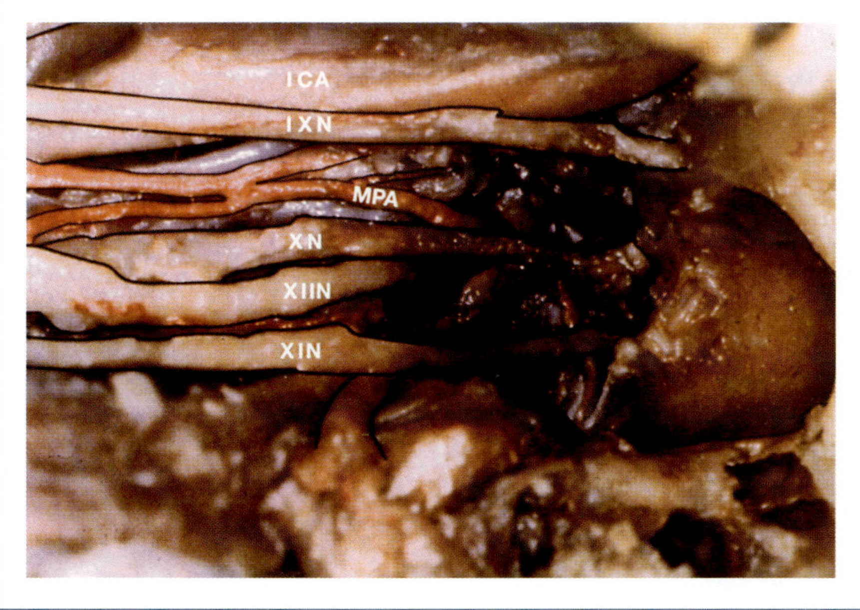

FIGURE 2–11 • Left skull base dissection. Removal of the internal jugular vein and the jugular bulb exposes the exit of the lower cranial nerves from the posterior fossa. (ICA, internal carotid artery; IXN, glossopharyngeal nerve; XN, vagus nerve; XIN, spinal accessory nerve; XIIN, hypoglosal nerve; MPA, posterior meningeal artery) Photo courtesy of John Kveton, MD; *reproduced with permission from Kveton JF. Anatomy of the jugular foramen: the neurotologic perspective. Op Tech ORL-HNS 1996;7:95–8.*

processes. The lateral process has a cartilaginous "cap" that imperceptibly merges with the pars propria of the tympanic membrane. The anterior ligament of the malleus, extending from the anterior process, passes through the petrotympanic fissure and, with the posterior incudal ligament, creates the axis of ossicular rotation.

The incus, the largest of the three ossicles, is immediately medial to the malleus. The incus has a body and three processes: a long, a short, and a lenticular. The body of the incus articulates with the head of the malleus in the epitympanum. The short process of the incus is anchored in the incudal fossa by the posterior incudal ligament. The long process extends inferiorly, roughly paralleling and lying posterior to the manubrium. The lenticular process, at the terminus of the long process, articulates with the stapes.

The stapes is the smallest and most medial of the ossicles. Its head articulates with the lenticular process of the incus, whereas its footplate sits in the oval window, surrounded by the stapediovestibular ligament. The arch of the stapes, composed of an anterior and a posterior crus, links the head and the footplate.

In the course of tympanic membrane elevation, as for instance in tympanoplasty, since the cartilaginous "cap" of the lateral process of the malleus blends into the pars propria of the drum, it is more expedient to sharply dissect it from the malleus rather than tediously attempting to dissect the drum from the "cap." The long process of the incus, perhaps owing to its tenuous blood supply, is particularly prone to osteitic resorption in the face of chronic otitis media. Although the ossicles are held in position by their ligaments and tendons, the force of injudicious surgical manipulation can easily overcome these restraints, resulting in subluxation or complete luxation. When dissecting disease from the stapes, one should parallel the plane of the stapedius tendon, in a posterior to an anterior direction, so that the tendon resists displacement of the stapes.

Middle Ear Muscles

The tensor tympani muscle, innervated by the trigeminal nerve, originates from the walls of its semicanal, greater wing of the sphenoid, and cartilage of the eustachian tube. The tendon of the tensor tympani muscle sweeps around the cochleariform process and across the tympanic cavity to attach to the medial aspect of the neck and manubrium of the malleus.

The medial pull of the tensor tympani muscle is ordinarily opposed by the intact tympanic membrane. In the case of a chronic, substantial perforation of the tympanic membrane, the unopposed action of the tensor tympani muscle can medialize the manubrium, effectively contracting the depth of the tympanic cavity. Forcible lateralization of the malleus, or even sectioning of the tensor tympani tendon, may be required to allow the surgeon to perform tympanic membrane grafting or ossiculoplasty. The cochleariform process is a landmark to the anterior aspect of the tympanic segment of the facial nerve as the nerve runs immediately superior to this process (Figure 2–13).

The stapedius muscle runs in a vertical sulcus in the posterior wall of the tympanic cavity adjacent to the facial nerve, from which it receives its innervation. Its tendon traverses the pyramidal eminence to attach to the posterior crus, and occasionally the head, of the stapes.

Middle Ear Spaces

The tympanic cavity is a sagittally oriented slit that lies immediately medial to the tympanic membrane. Its roof, or tegmen, also serves as part of the floor of the middle cranial fossa,

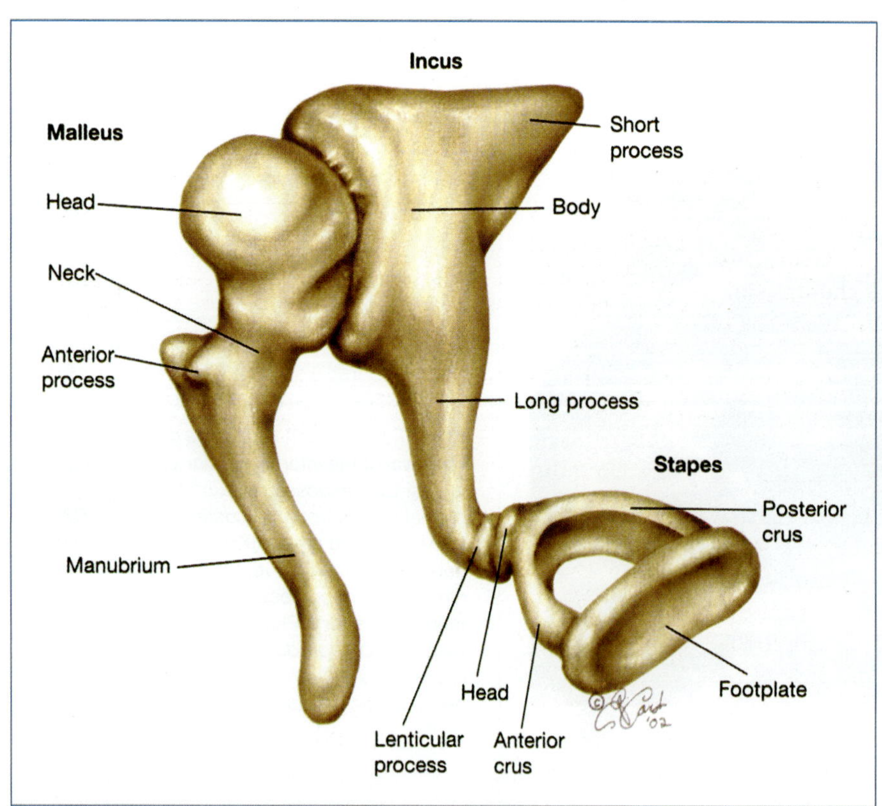

FIGURE 2–12 • The ossicular chain, medial aspect.

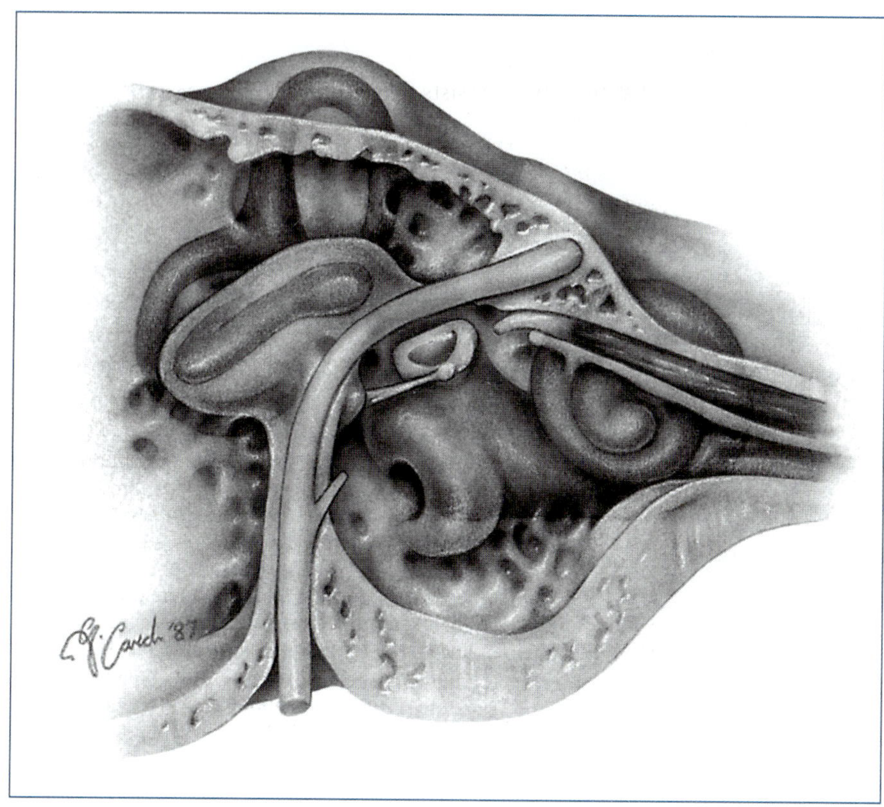

FIGURE 2–13 • The facial nerve is seen in its vertical and tympanic segments. Anterosuperiorly, the facial nerve passes superior to the tensor tympani tendon, which is seen sectioned just after it exits the cochleariform process.

whereas its irregularly contoured floor features the jugular bulb and, posteriorly, the root of the styloid process. The tympanic cavity is in continuity with the eustachian tube anteriorly and with the mastoid air cells via the aditus and antrum. It is traversed by the ossicular chain and is lined with a mucosal epithelium. Planes extended from the tympanic annulus subdivide the tympanic cavity into a mesotympanum, hypotympanum, protympanum, and posterior tympanic cavity. The epitympanum lies above the plane of the anterior and posterior tympanic spines.

Anteriorly, the mesotympanum is dominated by the bulge of the semicanal of the tensor tympani muscle; the tympanic orifice of the eustachian tube is immediately inferior to this bulge (Figure 2–14). Posteriorly, the key anatomic features are the pyramidal eminence and, lateral to it, the chordal eminence. The chordal eminence houses the iter chordae posterius by which the chorda tympani nerve enters the tympanic cavity.

The medial wall (the surgical "floor" of the middle ear) features three depressions: the sinus tympani, oval window niche, and round window niche (Figure 2–15). The sinus tympani is defined by the ponticulus superiorly, the subiculum inferiorly, the mastoid segment of the facial nerve laterally, and the posterior semicircular canal medially; there is substantial variability in the posterior extension (surgical "depth") of the sinus tympani, ranging from "shallow" to "deep." The oval window niche, occupied by the stapes footplate, is located anterosuperior to the ponticulus. The round window niche can be found posteroinferior to the promontory, the bulge created by the basal turn of the cochlea.

The sinus tympani evades direct surgical visualization, which is particularly worrisome in cholesteatoma surgery as it can harbor the nidus of recurrence. Inspection of this region has been somewhat improved by the advent of endoscopes appropriate for otologic surgery. The oval window niche may be the site of a perilymphatic fistula. Similarly, the round window niche may be implicated in perilymph leakage. In assessing the round window, it is important to realize that in the vast majority of cases, the true round window membrane is obscured by some kind of mucosal veil (Figure 2–16); most often, the veil is perforated, giving the false impression of seeing a defect in the round window membrane.[6]

Eustachian Tube

The eustachian tube extends approximately 35 mm from the anterior aspect of the tympanic cavity to the posterior aspect of the nasopharynx and serves to ventilate, clear, and protect the middle ear (see Figures 2–9 and 2–14). The lining mucosa of the tube has an abundance of mucociliary cells, important to its clearance function. The anteromedial two-thirds of the eustachian tube are fibrocartilaginous, whereas the remainder is bony. The tympanic orifice is in the anterior wall of the middle ear, a few millimeters above the floor. In its normal resting position, the tube is closed; opening of the tube is accomplished by the tensor veli palatini muscle, innervated by the trigeminal nerve. A body of fat, the lateral fat pad of Ostmann, abuts the lateral aspect of the fibrocartilaginous tube and aids in maintaining the resting closure of the tube.

Mucosa of the Tympanomastoid Compartment

The medial surface of the tympanic membrane, tympanic cavity, and mastoid air cells are all lined with a mucosal epithelium, reflecting their common heritage from the tubotympanic recess. The predominant cell type varies with location in the

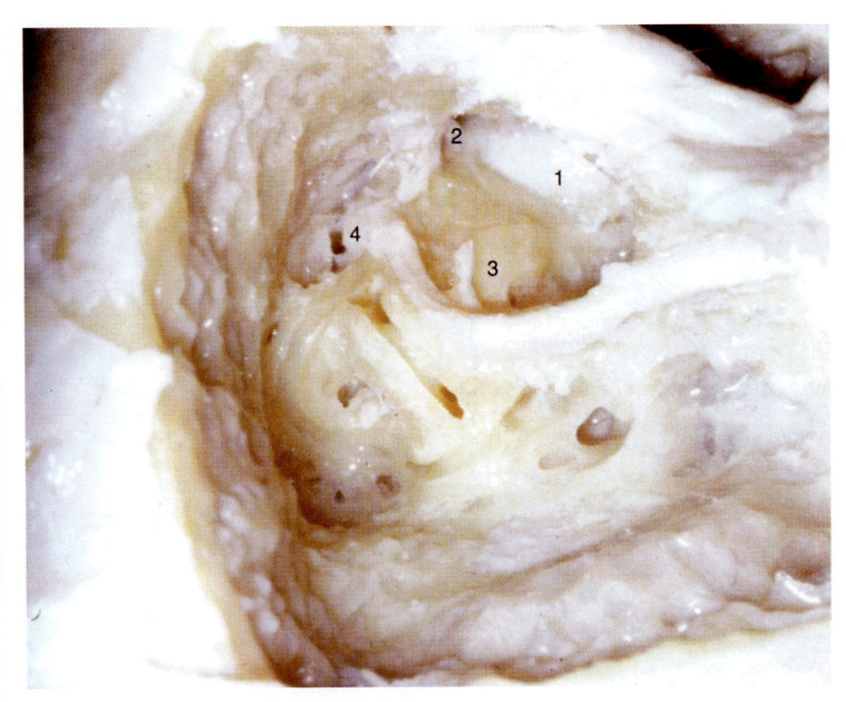

FIGURE 2–14 • Radical mastoid dissection view of a right temporal bone. The three semicircular canals have been opened. The anatomic interrelationships between the internal carotid artery (1), eustachian tube (2), promontory (3), and geniculate ganglion (4) are seen. *Reproduced with permission from Gulya AJ. Gulya and Schuknecht's anatomy of the temporal bone with surgical implications. 3rd ed. New York: Informa Healthcare USA; 2007.*

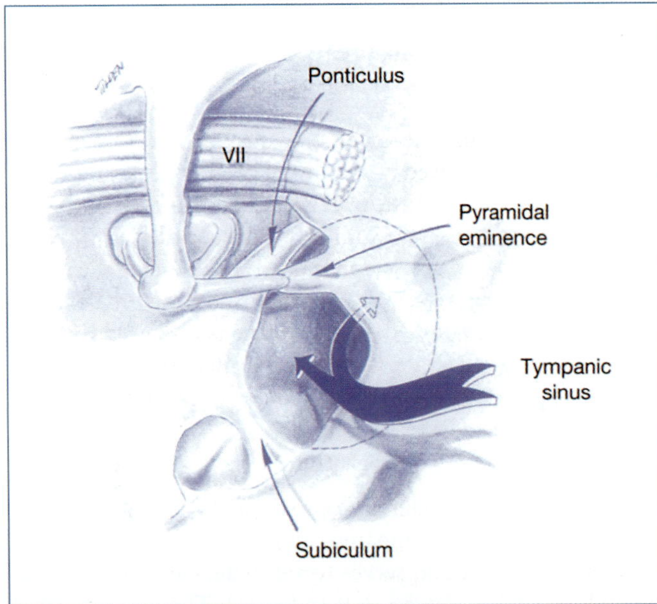

FIGURE 2–15 • The sinus tympani is bordered superiorly by the ponticulus and inferiorly by the subiculum. *Reproduced with permission from Schuknecht HF. Pathology of the ear. Ontario, Canada: Decker; 1974.*

tympanomastoid compartment. Ciliated cells intermingle with secretory cells on the promontory, in the hypotympanum, and in the epitympanum,[7] the mucociliary tracts thus formed act in concert with the mucociliary clearance system of the eustachian tube.

Pneumatization

The extent of pneumatization of the temporal bone varies according to heredity, environment, nutrition, infection, and eustachian tube function. There are five recognized regions of pneumatization: the middle ear, mastoid, perilabyrinthine, petrous apex, and accessory (Figure 2–17). The middle ear region, as described above, is divided into epitympanic, hypotympanic, mesotympanic, protympanic, and posterior tympanic areas. The mastoid region is subdivided into the mastoid antrum, central mastoid, and peripheral mastoid. The bony labyrinth divides the perilabyrinthine region into supralabyrinthine and infralabyrinthine areas. The apical area and the peritubal area comprise the petrous apex region. The accessory region encompasses the zygomatic, squamous, occipital, and styloid areas. There are five recognized air cell tracts. The posterosuperior tract runs at the juncture of the posterior and middle fossa aspects of the temporal bone. The posteromedial cell tract parallels and runs inferior to the posterosuperior tract. The subarcuate tract passes through the arch of the superior semicircular canal. The perilabyrinthine tracts run superior and inferior to the bony labyrinth, whereas the peritubal tract surrounds the eustachian tube.

The anterior petrous apex is pneumatized in only 10 to 15% of specimens studied.[8] Most often, it is diploic; in a small percentage of cases, it is sclerotic.

Troublesome cerebrospinal fluid leakage, persisting after translabyrinthine vestibular schwannoma resection despite apparently adequate tympanomastoid obliteration, has been linked to the presence of peritubal cells that open directly into the eustachian tube anterior to its tympanic orifice.[9]

Inner Ear

The bony labyrinth (see Figure 2–17) houses the sensory organs and soft tissue structures of the inner ear and consists of the cochlea, three semicircular canals, and vestibule. Its bone has three layers: an inner, or endosteal, layer; an outer, or periosteal, layer; and a middle layer consisting of enchondral and

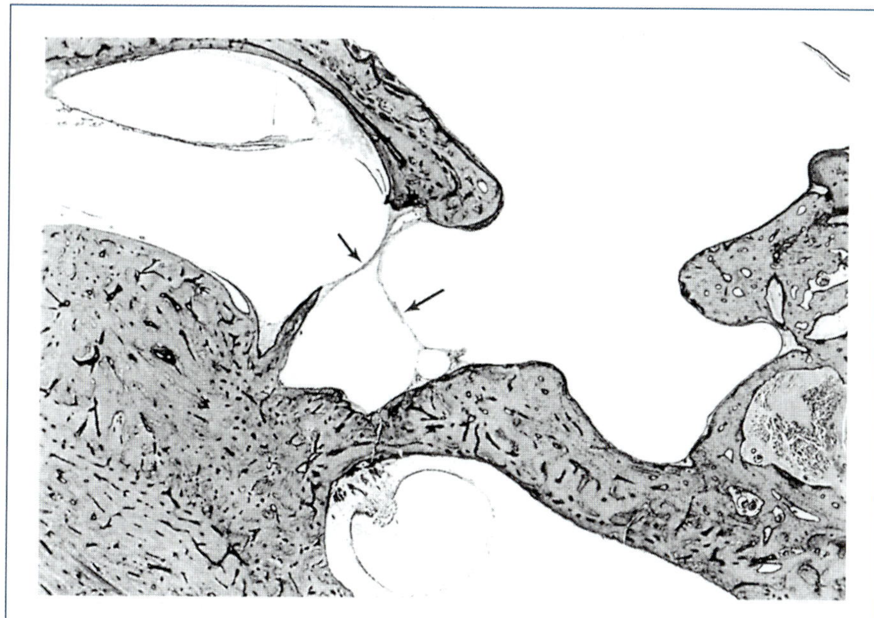

FIGURE 2–16 • The true round window membrane (left arrow) is covered by a veil of mucosa (right arrow). There is a microfissure extending from the medial aspect of the round window niche to the ampulla of the posterior semicircular canal. Right temporal bone; *reproduced with permission from Gulya AJ. Gulya and Schuknecht's anatomy of the temporal bone with surgical implications. 3rd ed. New York: Informa Healthcare USA; 2007.*

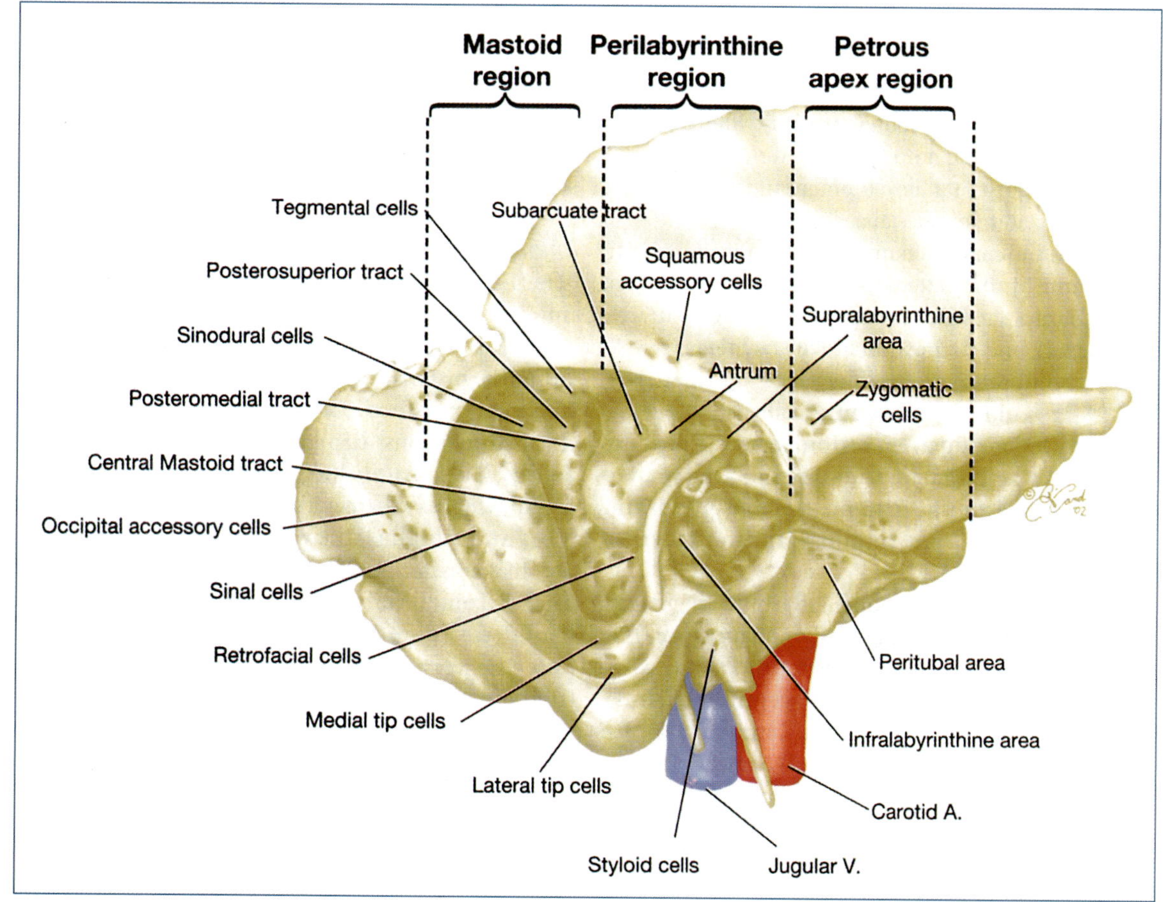

FIGURE 2–17 • Pneumatization of the temporal bone, with regions, areas, and tracts indicated. *After Nadol JB Jr, Schuknecht HF, editors. Surgery of the ear and temporal bone. New York: Raven Press; 1993.*

intrachondrial bone. Intrachondrial bone (globuli interossei) is characterized by cartilage islands, the lacunae of which have a thin bony layer owing to their invasion by osteoblasts.

The cochlea spirals 2½ turns about its central axis, the modiolus, and has a height of 5 mm. The base of the cochlea abuts the fundus of the IAC and is perforated (cribrose), allowing for the passage of cochlear nerve fibers. The apex lies medial to the tensor tympani muscle. The osseous spiral lamina winds about the modiolus and, along with the basilar membrane, separates the scala media (the cochlear duct) from the scala tympani. Adjacent turns of the cochlea are separated by an inter-scalar septum.

The three semicircular canals (see Figure 2–14) are the lateral (horizontal), superior (anterior vertical), and posterior (posterior vertical). The three canals are orthogonally related to one another and arc over a span of 240 degrees. Each canal has an ampullated limb, measuring 2 mm in diameter, and a nonampullated limb, which is 1 mm in diameter. The ampulla is cribrose for passage of nerve fibers. The nonampullated limbs of the posterior and superior canals fuse to form the crus commune. The ampullated and nonampullated limbs all open into the vestibule. The angle formed by the three semicircular canals is the solid angle, whereas the triangle bounded by the bony labyrinth, sigmoid sinus, and superior petrosal sinus is known as Trautmann's triangle.

Thinning, or frank dehiscence, of the bone of the superior semicircular canal is recognized as underlying some cases of sound- and/or pressure-induced vertigo.[10] Such dehiscence has been found in 0.5% of temporal bones studied, whereas thinning was encountered in 1.4%; both findings were "frequently" bilateral.[11] A failure in postnatal development of the bony labyrinth has been theorized to be the cause.[11]

The vestibule is the central chamber of the bony labyrinth and measures 4 mm in diameter. Its medial wall is marked by depressions for the saccule (the spherical recess), utricle (the elliptical recess), and cochlear duct (the cochlear recess). Cribrose areas accommodate nerve fiber access to their sensory organs. "Mike's dot" (the macula cribrosa superior) marks the passageway for superior vestibular nerve fibers to the cristae ampullares of the lateral and superior semicircular canals. As it corresponds to the extreme lateral aspect of the IAC, Mike's dot is an important landmark in translabyrinthine surgery.

There are three fissures of the bony labyrinth. The fissula ante fenestram is an evagination of the perilymphatic space that is invariably found extending anterosuperior to the oval window; in the adult, fibrous tissue and cartilage fill the fissula. The fossula post fenestram is a perilymphatic evagination that extends posterior to the oval window; it is a less constant feature of the temporal bone. Hyrtl's fissure (or the tympanomeningeal hiatus) is a remnant of embryologic development and is rarely present (see Chapter 1 for additional details).

There are two commonly encountered microfissures of the temporal bone. One extends between the round window niche and the ampulla of the posterior semicircular canal (see Figure 2–16). The other runs superior and inferior to the oval window. Both microfissures, or breaks in the endosteal and endochondral layers of the temporal bone, are filled with fibrous tissue and acellular matrix.

A persistent Hyrtl's fissure has been implicated as a route for cerebrospinal fluid leakage into the middle ear.[12] Although the oval and round window microfissures have been hypothesized to be the site of perilymph leakage, evidence refutes this theory.[13]

The membranous (endolymphatic) labyrinth housed within the bony labyrinth consists of the cochlear duct (scala media), the three semicircular ducts and their cristae ampullares, the otolithic organs (the utricle and the saccule), and the endolymphatic duct and sac. Generally interposed between the bony and membranous labyrinths are the connective tissue, blood vessels, and fluid of the perilymphatic space, including the scala tympani, scala vestibuli, perilymphatic cistern of the vestibule, perilymphatic duct, and perilymph spaces surrounding the semicircular ducts.

The endolymphatic duct originates in the medial wall of the vestibule. It first parallels the crus commune and then the posterior semicircular canal as it heads to the endolymphatic sac, anterior and medial to the sigmoid sinus. The endolymphatic sac lies approximately 10 mm inferior and lateral to the porus of the IAC; the sac has an intraosseous portion, which is covered by the operculum, and a more distal intradural portion (see Figure 1–14).

Donaldson's line, a surgical landmark in endolymphatic sac surgery, is derived by extending the plane of the lateral semicircular so that it bisects the posterior semicircular canal and contacts the posterior fossa dura (Figure 2–18); the endolymphatic sac lies inferior to this line. The precise position of the sac shows considerable variability.

Internal Auditory Canal

The IAC is the bony channel that shelters the superior and inferior vestibular, cochlear, facial, and intermediate nerves, as well as the labyrinthine artery and vein, as they course from the posterior cranial fossa to the labyrinth. On average, the canal measures 3.4 mm in diameter and 8 mm in length; these dimensions display considerable interindividual variability. The porus is the posterior cranial fossa opening of the canal, whereas the canal abuts the bony labyrinth at its fundus. At the fundus, the vestibular, facial, and cochlear nerves are in a constant anatomic relationship that is determined by the horizontal (falciform) crest and the vertical crest ("Bill's bar") (see Figure 2–5B). Progressing medially from the fundus, the nerves rotate, with fusion of the cochlear and vestibular nerves (Figure 2–19), so that the facial nerve assumes a location anterior to the cochleovestibular nerve bundle, whereas the cochlear nerve moves to lie inferior to the vestibular nerve.

Bill's bar is a useful landmark in translabyrinthine surgery of the cerebellopontine angle as it separates the superior vestibular nerve from the anteriorly located facial nerve. Although the medial anatomic relationships of the cochlear, vestibular, and facial nerves are useful in vestibular nerve section surgery, these relationships can undergo considerable distortion in the face of a cerebellopontine angle tumor.

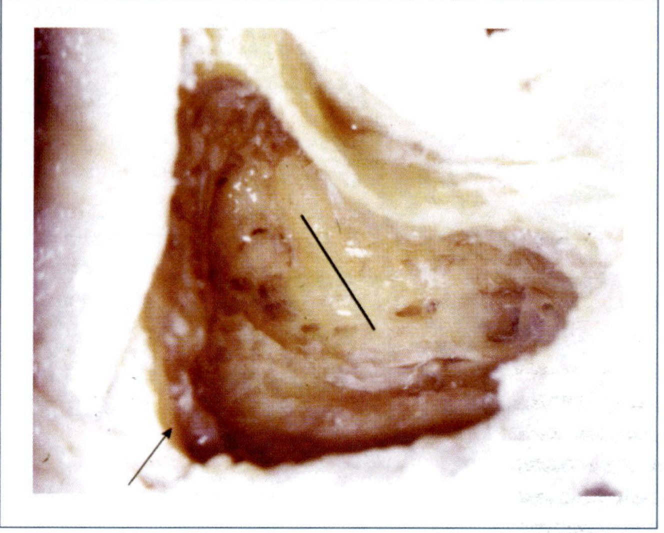

FIGURE 2–18 • Complete mastoidectomy view of a right temporal bone. The lateral and posterior semicircular canals form Donaldson's line (line). The angle of Citelli is indicated (arrow). *Reproduced with permission from Gulya AJ. Gulya and Schuknecht's anatomy of the temporal bone with surgical implications. 3rd ed. New York: Informa Healthcare USA; 2007.*

NEUROANATOMY

Trigeminal and Abducens Nerves

The gasserian ganglion of the trigeminal nerve occupies Meckel's cave on the middle cranial fossa face of the temporal bone, anterolateral to the petrous apex. The abducens (sixth cranial) nerve runs in Dorello's canal beneath the posterior petroclinoid (Gruber's) ligament. Petrous apicitis, with its attendant dural and venous inflammation, can manifest with purulent otorrhea, retro-orbital pain, and abducens palsy.

Facial Nerve

The facial nerve (the seventh cranial nerve) innervates structures derived from Reichert's cartilage. Three nuclei give rise to the fibers of the facial nerve: its motor nucleus in the caudal pons, the superior salivatory nucleus that is dorsal to the motor nucleus, and the nucleus of the solitary tract in the medulla oblongata. The superior aspect of the motor nucleus, innervating the frontalis and orbicularis oculi muscles, receives both crossed and uncrossed input from the motor cortex, whereas the inferior portion receives only ipsilateral input.

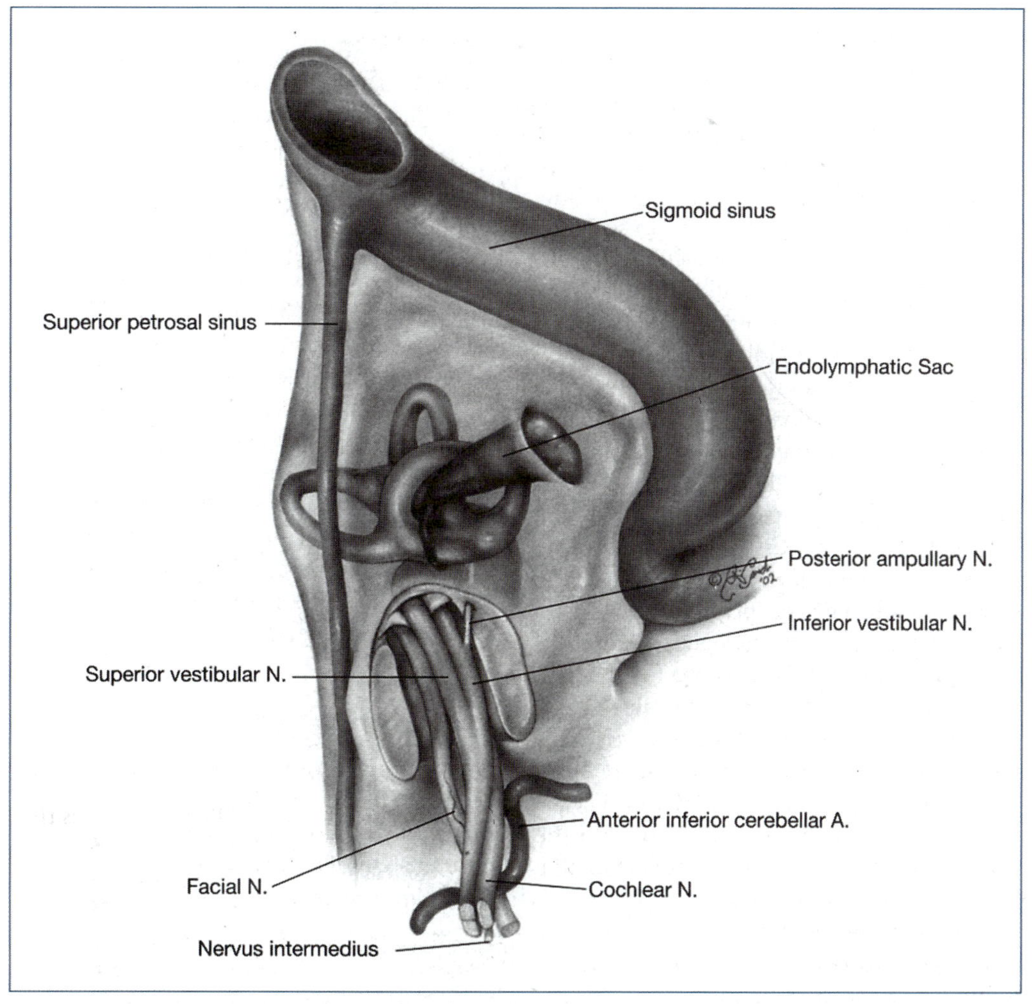

FIGURE 2–19 • The rotation of the facial, cochlear, and vestibular nerves as they traverse the internal auditory canal. *After Nadol JB Jr, Schuknecht HF, editors. Surgery of the ear and temporal bone. New York: Raven Press; 1993.*

Five fiber types make up the trunk of the facial nerve. Its special visceral efferent fibers supply the facial expression, stapedius, stylohyoid, and digastric (posterior belly) muscles. Its general visceral efferent fibers go to the lacrimal, nasal cavity seromucinous, sub-maxillary, and sublingual glands. The taste (sensory) fibers of the facial nerve derive from the anterior two-thirds of the tongue, tonsillar fossae, and posterior palate, whereas its somatic sensory fibers emanate from the EAC and concha. Visceral afferent fibers arise from the mucosa of the nose, pharynx, and palate.

The course of the facial nerve is divided into five segments. Its intracranial segment stretches 24 mm from the pons to the porus of the IAC. The intracanalicular segment traverses the IAC; at the fundus, it occupies the anterosuperior quadrant, where it is joined by the nervus intermedius. The shortest segment is the labyrinthine segment, running 4 mm from the beginning of the fallopian canal to the geniculate ganglion. The tympanic segment is roughly 13-mm long and courses in the medial wall of the tympanic cavity, superior to the cochleariform process and oval window. The mastoid segment spans the 20-mm distance from the second genu (at the lateral semicircular canal) to the stylomastoid foramen.

The facial nerve may follow an anomalous course. One such alternate path takes the tympanic segment of the facial nerve anterior and inferior to the oval window.[14] In another variant, the mastoid segment of the facial nerve bulges more posteriorly and laterally than usual as it runs inferior to the prominence of the lateral semicircular canal.[15] Rarely, the vertical segment of the facial nerve may be bipartite or even tripartite.

The fallopian canal has numerous gaps, or dehiscences, which render the facial nerve liable to injury. The tympanic segment over the oval window is the most likely site to be dehiscent; in one series, this site comprised 66% of dehiscences.[16] In approximately 75% of cases, the dehiscence at the oval window is bilateral.[17] On occasion, the facial nerve can protrude through the gap (Figure 2–20) to present as a middle ear mass.[18]

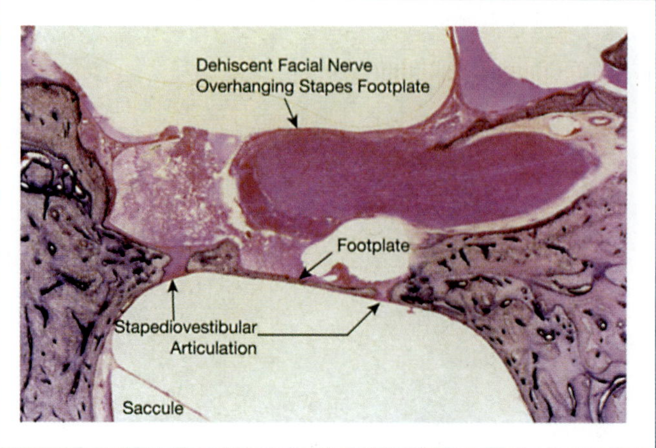

FIGURE 2–20 • The facial nerve is dehiscent at the oval window. *Reproduced with permission from Gulya AJ. Gulya and Schuknecht's anatomy of the temporal bone with surgical implications. 3rd ed. New York: Informa Healthcare USA; 2007.*

The subarachnoid space of the facial nerve usually extends no further than the junction of its labyrinthine and tympanic segments.[19] Occasionally, it extends into the geniculate ganglion and, rarely, onto the lateral aspect of the tympanic segment. Gacek theorized that the subarachnoid space extending onto the tympanic segment may spontaneously fistulize into the middle ear, resulting in cerebrospinal fluid otorrhea.[19] Alternatively, he suggested that it may gradually enlarge, presenting as a mass lesion with erosion or enlargement of the fallopian canal.

There are three intratemporal branches of the facial nerve: the greater petrosal nerve, nerve to the stapedius muscle, and chorda tympani nerve. The greater petrosal nerve arises from the anterior aspect of the geniculate ganglion (see Figure 2–14) and emerges onto the floor of the middle cranial fossa via the facial hiatus; in some cases, the geniculate ganglion and the greater petrosal nerve may lie exposed in the floor of the middle cranial fossa, lacking their usual bony covering. The nerve to the stapedius muscle arises from the mastoid segment of the facial nerve near the pyramidal eminence. The chorda tympani nerve, the sensory bundle making up some 10% of the cross-sectional area of the facial nerve, usually separates from the main trunk of the facial nerve approximately 4 mm proximal to the stylomastoid foramen (Figure 2–21); rarely, the chorda tympani and facial nerves separate extratemporally, and the chorda tympani re-enters the temporal bone via its own canal. Alternatively, the chorda may not separate from the facial nerve until it reaches the level of the lateral semicircular canal. After vertically ascending the temporal bone in a canal that lies lateral and anterior to the facial nerve, the chorda enters the tympanic cavity at the iter chordae posterius. It crosses lateral to the long process of the incus and medial to the malleus to exit the tympanic cavity via the iter chordae anterius (canal of Huguier) and the petrotympanic (glaserian) fissure. Rarely, the chorda may pass lateral to the malleus and the tympanic membrane.

The facial recess (see Figure 2–21) is a triangular area inferior to the incudal fossa, lateral to the facial nerve (vertical segment), and medial to the chorda tympani nerve; it is used in intact canal wall mastoidectomy to gain access to the middle ear.

The nervus intermedius (nerve of Wrisberg) carries the taste, secretory, and sensory fibers of the facial nerve. In the IAC, the nervus intermedius runs as a separate nerve between the facial and superior vestibular nerves. In the temporal bone, the nervus intermedius is within the facial nerve, occupying its dorsal aspect in the tympanic segment and its posterolateral aspect in the mastoid segment. The chorda tympani nerve represents the separation of the sensory fibers at the inferior mastoid segment.

Cochlear Nerve

The cochlear nerve arises from the spiral ganglion neurons. At the fundus of the IAC, the cochlear nerve is in the anteroinferior compartment. It rotates as it heads toward the porus and enters the brainstem a few millimeters caudal to the root entry zone of the trigeminal nerve.

Vestibular Nerves

The superior and inferior vestibular nerves occupy the posterior half of the IAC. The structures innervated by the superior vestibular nerve are the superior and lateral semicircular canals,

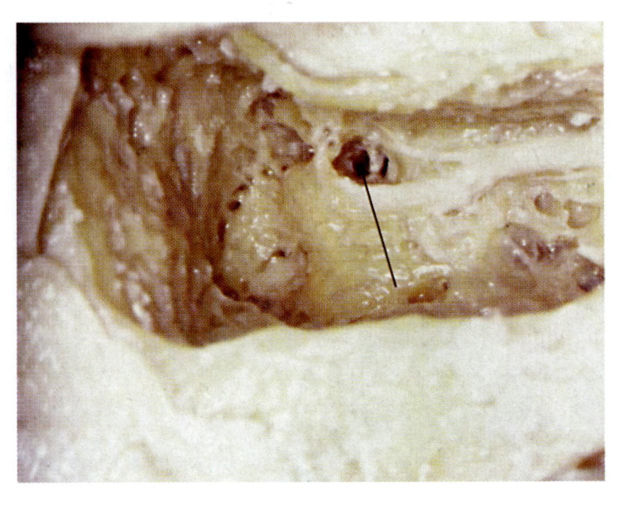

FIGURE 2–21 • The facial recess (arrow) lies between the facial and chorda tympani nerves. The incudostapedial joint is visible just to the right of the arrowhead. *Reproduced with permission from Gulya AJ. Gulya and Schuknecht's anatomy of the temporal bone with surgical implications. 3rd ed. New York: Informa Healthcare USA; 2007.*

utricular macula, and superior portion of the saccular macula. The inferior vestibular nerve innervates the inferior saccular macula and, by its posterior ampullary branch, the posterior semicircular canal. The posterior ampullary nerve separates from the main trunk of the inferior vestibular nerve a few millimeters from the porus of the IAC and traverses the singular canal to the posterior canal ampulla.

Sensory Nerves of the Tympanomastoid Compartment

Jacobson's nerve (the tympanic branch of cranial nerve IX) arises from the inferior (petrosal) ganglion of cranial nerve IX, which is located in the petrosal fossula of the jugulocarotid crest. It enters the tympanic cavity, accompanied by the inferior tympanic artery, through the inferior tympanic canaliculus. Subsequently, the nerve climbs the promontory and medial wall of the tympanic cavity to meet with the caroticotympanic nerves originating from the pericarotid plexus. The union of the preganglionic parasympathetic fibers of Jacobson's nerve and the postganglionic sympathetic caroticotympanic nerves at the tympanic plexus results in the formation of the lesser petrosal nerve. The lesser petrosal nerve heads to the floor of the middle cranial fossa adjacent to, or even within, the semicanal of the tensor tympani muscle. Jacobson's nerve mediates otalgia referred from the pharynx.

Arnold's nerve, the auricular branch of cranial nerve X, has fibers from the facial, glossopharyngeal, and vagus nerves. It originates in the jugular foramen, passes over the dome of the jugular bulb (via the mastoid canaliculus), and enters the fallopian canal. Arnold's nerve has been implicated in herpetic involvement of the EAC in herpes zoster oticus[20] and the cough reflex elicited by manipulation of the skin of the EAC.

VASCULAR ANATOMY

Temporal Bone Arteries

The internal carotid artery enters the temporal bone through the external carotid foramen, located just anteromedial to the styloid process. As it ascends in its intrapetrous segment, it passes first anterior to the tympanic cavity and cochlea and then bends (its "knee") to run medial to the eustachian tube and inferomedial to the semicanal of the tensor tympani muscle (see Figures 2–9 and 2–10). The artery climbs to exit the temporal bone at the internal carotid foramen. Accompanying the artery throughout its intrapetrous course are a venous and a neural (sympathetic) plexus. The bony shell protecting the artery is thin (often less than 0.5 mm thick) and can be dehiscent in 6% of cases.[21] In the course of surgery for chronic otitis media or cholesteatoma, the potential for injuring the internal carotid artery mandates gentle dissection in the medial wall of the eustachian tube.

Aberrant development of the carotid artery (see Chapter 1) can result in an artery that follows an anomalous course lateral and posterior to the vestibular line (a vertical line through the lateral aspect of the vestibule in the coronal plane).

The anterior inferior cerebellar artery (AICA) often extends a loop into the IAC. Its role of such a loop in the generation of symptoms such as tinnitus and vertigo is debatable.[22] Disruption of AICA causes hemorrhage in and infarction of the labyrinth and brainstem.

Temporal Bone Veins

The three dominant sinuses of the temporal bone are the sigmoid (portion of the lateral venous sinus), superior petrosal, and inferior petrosal (Figure 2–22). The lateral venous sinus occupies an S-shaped sulcus in the posterior mastoid—hence the term sigmoid—as it extends from the transverse sinus to the internal jugular vein. This drainage system on the right is larger than that on the left in 75% of cases.[23] The angle between the sigmoid sinus/posterior cranial fossa dura and the middle cranial fossa dura is known as the angle of Citelli (see Figure 2–18).

The superior petrosal sinus drains the cavernous sinus into the lateral venous sinus as it runs in the superior petrosal sulcus at the junction of the posterior and middle fossa dural plates. The inferior petrosal sinus courses in the petro-occipital suture line. It drains the cavernous sinus into the jugular bulb.

Arachnoid granulations (pacchionian bodies) are projections of pia-arachnoid into the venous sinuses and venous lacunae and are extensions of the subarachnoid space. Arachnoid granulations can also be found extending from the arachnoid of the middle and posterior cranial fossae into the adjacent mastoid air cells. Gacek has linked arachnoid granulations to adult-onset spontaneous cerebrospinal fluid otorrhea.[24,25]

The jugular bulb is interposed between the sigmoid sinus and internal jugular vein; in contrast to the thick wall of the sigmoid sinus, which quite readily contracts with bipolar cautery, the thin wall of the bulb does not and is prone to rupture with manipulation. The venous hemorrhage of a torn or incised sigmoid sinus can be controlled with pressure applied via a large square of gelatin sponge (Gelfoam®) surmounted by a neurosurgical cottonoid; several minutes after the bleeding has stopped,

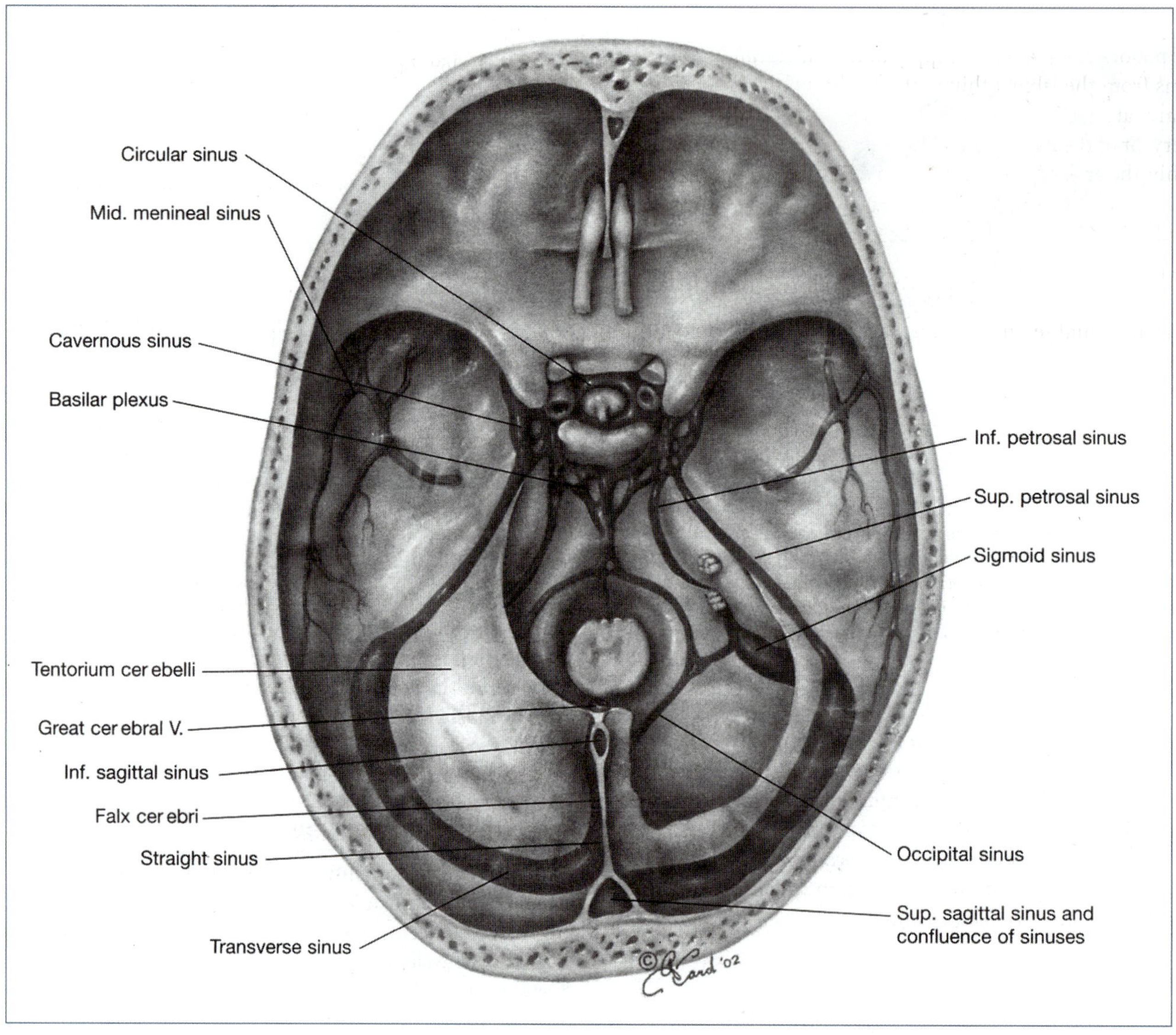

FIGURE 2–22 • The cranium has been opened and its contents removed to reveal the sinuses and related structures.

the cottonoid can be removed safely, and leaving the Gelfoam in place, surgery can be resumed.

The jugular bulb displays considerable variability in its position relative to the facial nerve and in its penetration into the tympanic cavity. A high-riding jugular bulb (one extending to or above the level of the inferior tympanic annulus) has been reported in 3.5 to 5% of temporal bone specimens studied[26,27] and may occur more frequently on the right side.[27] Its bony covering is very thin—only 0.1 to 0.3 mm. An alternate definition of the high-riding jugular bulb encompasses one encroaching to within 2 mm or less on the inferior aspect of the IAC.[28] Using this definition, one study reported that two-thirds of temporal bones from individuals older than 6 years housed a high-riding jugular bulb.[28] A jugular diverticulum is a "venous anomaly" and comprises an "irregular outpouching" of the jugular bulb.[29]

The high-riding jugular bulb may mimic a middle ear vascular mass, such as a glomus tympanicum, and may be the source of hemorrhage in tympanostomy tube insertion. Jugular bulbs reaching as high as the superior aspect of the IAC have been encountered in the course of posterior fossa vestibular schwannoma surgery,[23] rendering exposure of the IAC technically challenging. A jugular diverticulum has been implicated as the etiology of Meniere's disease–like symptoms.[29]

Middle Ear Blood Vessels

The inferior tympanic artery is a branch of the ascending pharyngeal artery (from the external carotid artery). It traverses the inferior tympanic canaliculus with Jacobson's nerve. The inferior tympanic artery is an important arterial feeder of tympanic paragangliomas.

A number of branches from the external carotid artery contribute to the anastomotic network of the tympanic cavity, including the anterior tympanic artery, deep auricular artery, mastoid artery, stylomastoid artery, superficial petrosal artery, and tubal artery.

Labyrinthine Vessels

The majority of the blood supply to the membranous labyrinth stems from the labyrinthine artery, a branch of the AICA. The subarcuate artery arises either as a branch of the labyrinthine artery, or of the AICA, or as multiple branches of both; it passes within the arch of the superior semicircular canal.

Facial Nerve Vessels

The facial nerve has both an intrinsic and an extrinsic vascular system. The extrinsic system consists of the AICA, supplying the intracranial segment of cranial nerve VII; the labyrinthine artery, supplying the intracanalicular segment; the superficial petrosal artery, which supplies the geniculate ganglion and the superior portion of the mastoid segment of the facial nerve; and the stylomastoid artery, which supplies the inferior mastoid segment of the nerve.

The intrinsic network, running within the nerve, is generally thought to be most poorly developed at its labyrinthine segment, in contrast to the tympanic and mastoid segments.[30]

References

1. Gulya AJ. Gulya and Schuknecht's anatomy of the temporal bone with surgical implications. 3rd edition. New York: Informa Healthcare USA; 2007.
2. Kveton JF, Cooper MH. Microsurgical anatomy of the jugular foramen region. Am J Otol 1988;9:109–12.
3. Kveton JF. Anatomy of the jugular foramen: The neurotologic perspective. Op Tech ORL-HNS 1996;7:95–8.
4. Saleh E, Naguib M, Aristegui M, Cokkeser Y, Sanna M. Lower skull base: Anatomic study with surgical implications. Ann Otol Rhinol Laryngol 1995;104:57–61.
5. Aslan A, Falcioni M, Balyan FR, et al. The cochlear aqueduct: An important landmark in lateral skull base surgery. Otolaryngol Head Neck Surg 1998;118:532–6.
6. Nomura Y. Otological significance of the round window. Adv Otorhinolaryngol 1984;33:1–162.
7. Lim DJ. Functional morphology of the lining membrane of the middle ear and eustachian tube. An overview. Ann Otol Rhinol Laryngol 1974;83 Suppl 11:5–22.
8. Lindsay JR. Suppuration in the petrous pyramid. Ann Otol Rhinol Laryngol 1938;47:3–36.
9. Saim L, McKenna MJ, Nadol JB Jr. Tubal and tympanic openings of the peritubal cells: Implications for cerebrospinal fluid otorrhea. Am J Otol 1996;17:335–9.
10. Minor LB, Solomon D, Zinreich JS, Zee DS. Sound- and/or pressure-induced vertigo due to bone dehiscence of the superior semicircular canal. Arch Otolaryngol Head Neck Surg 1998;124:249–58.
11. Carey JP, Minor LB, Nager GT. Dehiscence or thinning of bone overlying the superior semicircular canal in a temporal bone survey. Arch Otolaryngol Head Neck Surg 2000;126:137–47.
12. Gacek RR, Leipzig B. Congenital cerebrospinal fluid otorrhea. Ann Otol Rhinol Laryngol 1979;88:358–65.
13. El Shazly MAR, Linthicum FH Jr. Microfissures of the temporal bone: Do they have any clinical significance? Am J Otol 1991;12:169–71.
14. Hough JVD. Malformations and anatomical variations seen in the middle ear during the operation for mobilization of the stapes. Laryngoscope 1958;68:1337–79.
15. Procter B, Nager GT. The facial canal: Normal anatomy, variations and anomalies. Ann Otol Rhinol Laryngol 1982;91 Suppl 97:33–61.
16. Baxter A. Dehiscence of the fallopian canal: An anatomical study. J Laryngol Otol 1971;85:587–94.
17. Moreano EH, Paparella MM, Zelterman D, Goycoolea MV. Prevalence of facial canal dehiscence and of persistent stapedial artery in the human middle ear: A report of 1000 temporal bones. Laryngoscope 1994;104:309–20.
18. Johnsson L-G, Kingsley TC. Herniation of the facial nerve in the middle ear. Arch Otolaryngol 1970;91:598–602.
19. Gacek RR. Anatomy and significance of the subarachnoid space in the fallopian canal. Am J Otol 1998;19:358–64.
20. Eshraghi AA, Buchman C, Telischi FF. Facial nerve branch to the external auditory canal. American Neurotology Society 2001 Annual Meeting abstracts. http://itsa.ucsf.edu/~ajo/ANS/ANSspr21ab.html (accessed Mar 31, 2001).
21. Moreano EH, Paparella MM, Zelterman D, Goycoolea MV. Prevalence of carotid canal dehiscence in the human middle ear: A report of 1000 temporal bones. Laryngoscope 1994;104:612–18.
22. Makins AE, Nikolopoulus TP, Ludman C, O'Donoghue GM. Is there a correlation between vascular loops and unilateral auditory symptoms? Laryngoscope 1998;108:1739–42.
23. Kennedy DW, El-Sirsy HH, Nager GT. The jugular bulb in otologic surgery: Anatomic, clinical, and surgical considerations. Otolaryngol Head Neck Surg 1986;94:6–15.
24. Gacek RR. Arachnoid granulation cerebrospinal fluid otorrhea. Ann Otol Rhinol Laryngol 1990;99:854–62.
25. Gacek RR. Evaluation and management of temporal bone arachnoid granulations. Arch Otolaryngol Head Neck Surg 1992;118:327–32.
26. Overton SB, Ritter FN. A high placed jugular bulb in the middle ear: A clinical and temporal bone study. Laryngoscope 1973;83:1986–91.
27. Subotic R. The high position of the jugular bulb. Acta Otolaryngol (Stockh) 1979;87:340–4.
28. Rausch SD, Xu W-Z, Nadol JB Jr. High jugular bulb: Implications for posterior fossa neurotologic and cranial base surgery. Ann Otol Rhinol Laryngol 1993;102:100–7.
29. Jahrsdoerfer RA, Cain WS, Cantrell RW. Endolymphatic duct obstruction from a jugular bulb diverticulum. Ann Otol Rhinol Laryngol 1981;90:619–23.
30. Balkany T, Fradis M, Jafek BW, Rucker NC. Intrinsic vasculature of the labyrinthine segment of the facial nerve—Implications for site of lesion in Bell's palsy. Otolaryngol Head Neck Surg 1991;104:20–3.

Acoustics and Mechanics of the Middle Ear

3

Saumil N. Merchant MD / John J. Rosowski, PhD

Two of the primary tasks of the otologic surgeon include: *diagnosis*, the understanding of how pathological variations in external and middle-ear structure lead to hearing loss, and *surgical treatment* of external and middle ears ravaged by disease, such that the reconstructed ear has near-normal mechanical and acoustic function. The authors believe that a basic knowledge of physiology of the normal ear and pathophysiology of the diseased ear is necessary for proper diagnosis and surgical treatment of otologic disorders. This chapter provides a review of some fundamental principles of acoustics that are relevant to sound transmission in normal, diseased and reconstructed middle ears. The review concentrates on middle-ear mechanics and does not cover the physiological maintenance of middle-ear gases or static air pressures. The chapter is meant as a guide rather than an exhaustive treatise, and has been written with clinicians as its primary audience.

HISTORICAL ASPECTS

The histories of otology, audiology and acoustics have been documented by several authors.[1–5] The early events may be summarized as follows.[6]

Early Greek physicians (5th century BC) knew of the tympanic membrane and middle-ear space. The Greeks considered the middle-ear space to be the seat of hearing. Galen (AD 131 to 201) described the auditory nerve but suggested it originated in the middle ear. The Renaissance produced several great anatomists who described the ear in detail. Vesalius, in 1543, described the malleus and incus. In 1546, Ingrassia described the stapes and the oval and round windows. In 1561, Fallopius named the cochlea, the labyrinth, and the canal for the facial nerve. Eustachius described the auditory tube bearing his name in 1564.

These anatomic discoveries formed the basis for tracing the pathway of sound through the ear by Coiter in 1566, and the later more elaborate description of Durverney in 1683. Neither Coiter nor Duverney appreciated the impedance matching function of the middle ear because both thought the inner ear was filled with air. That the labyrinth contained fluid was established by Meckel, who, in 1777, demonstrated that frozen temporal bones were always filled with ice. The microscopic structures of the inner ear were first described by Corti in 1851, followed by Retzius's description of hair cells and their innervation by auditory nerve fibers in 1892.

Helmholtz, in 1868,[7] initiated the period of modern auditory physiology by defining the principles of impedance matching and how the middle ear served this function. Stating the problem of matching the transmission of sound in low-impedance air to the high impedance of the fluid-filled cochlea, Helmholtz conceived of three means by which this pressure transformation takes place: a lever action that resulted from the shape of the drumhead itself, a lever effect of the ossicular chain, and a hydraulic action of the large tympanic membrane acting upon the small stapes footplate.

In the 20th century, many investigators expanded, corrected, or quantified these basic concepts. Notable contributors to our knowledge of middle-ear mechanics include Nobel laureate Georg von Békésy, Ernst Glenn Wever, Merle Lawrence, Juergen Tonndorf, Shyam Khanna, William Peake, Richard Goode, Aage Møller, and Josef Zwislocki. Clinical observations and surgical advances that have stimulated physiologic investigations have included the question of altered sound conduction as a result of middle-ear diseases, and the restoration of hearing in pathologic middle ears through tympanoplasty and stapedectomy procedures.

SOUND AND ITS MEASUREMENT

Sound results when particles of a medium are set into vibration. For example, the vibrating tines of a struck tuning fork produce backward and forward motions of the air particles that surround the tines (Figure 3–1). The particles set in motion by the vibrating tines then push on adjacent air particles, where the push is proportional to the sound pressure, setting the next layer of particles into back and forth motion. The physical disturbance of sound pressure and particle motion, not the particles themselves, propagates through the medium, as succeeding layers of air particles are set into vibration. The *frequency* of the resulting

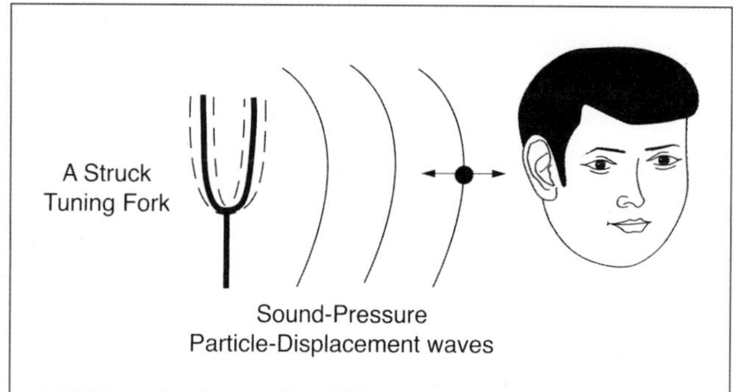

FIGURE 3–1 • The vibrating tines of a struck tuning fork set nearby air particles into motion with a frequency equal to the natural frequency of the fork. The air particles that are set in motion push on adjacent particles and so forth, resulting in a propagating physical disturbance that is perceived as sound. The black dot with the arrow is a hypothetical air particle set into back and forth motion, by the waves (curved lines) propagating from the struck fork.

sound is the number of cycles per second of the back and forth motion of the air particles. The unit of frequency is Hertz (Hz, with 1 Hz = 1 cycle per second). The amplitude of the propagating physical disturbance can be quantified either in terms of the sound pressure acting on the particles or the amplitude of the particle motion. In practice, it is easier to measure pressure variations than to measure motion of the particles; hence, sound pressure is the primary measure of sound.

Sound pressure refers to the magnitude of the temporal variations in pressure produced around ambient static pressure (Figure 3–2). A pressure is a force per area. The international unit of pressure is the pascal (Pa), where 1 Pa = one Newton of force per square meter of area. The quietest sounds heard by a human ear are of very low pressure; the change in pressure associated with sound at the threshold of hearing for a 1,000 Hz tone is about 20 μPa (or two-tenths of a billionth atmospheres). There are many ways to quantify sound pressure, the most common being in terms of the rms or the root of the mean squared deviation in pressure. For a sinusoidal pure tone like that in Figure 3–2A, the sound pressure can be quantified in terms of the peak, peak-to-peak or rms measures of amplitude. In the case of sinusoids, there is a fixed relationship between the three different measures, and for the tone shown in Figure 3–2A, these different measures yield values of 1, 2, or 0.71 Pa, respectively. The intensity or power within a complex sound waveform as illustrated in Figure 3–2B, is not readily quantified by peak measures but is well described by the rms value of the sound pressure. In fact, the rms sound pressure of this complex sound is 0.71 Pa, a value identical to that of the tonal sound pressure shown in Figure 3–2A. In general then, sound pressure measurements are usually quantified in terms of the rms pressure.

The human auditory system is sensitive to a wide range of sound pressures. Conversational speech is typically 100 to 500 times threshold, music often contains sound pressures that are 10,000 times threshold, while jet engines, guns, and fireworks can produce pressures that are more than 1 million times threshold. Because of the ear's sensitivity to pressures that vary by more than a million times, and because the human ear can discriminate fractional changes in pressure, it is common to use a logarithmic scale to grade sound pressures.[8] The decibel (dB, one-tenth of a Bell) is a logarithmic measure of relative energy where 10 dB (1 Bell) represents an increase over a given reference energy level of 1 order of magnitude (ie, 1 common log unit or a factor of 10). The reference level for sound pressure level (SPL) is 2×10^{-5} rms pascals (or Pa), and since energy is proportional to pressure squared:

$$\text{Sound level in dB SPL} = 10\log_{10}\left(\frac{X}{0.00002\,rms\,Pa}\right)^2$$

$$= 20\log_{10}\left(\frac{X}{0.00002\,rms\,Pa}\right)$$

where X is the sound pressure in rms pascals and 0.00002 rms Pa is the reference pressure. Different dB sound pressure scales use different reference pressures. For example, the dB Hearing Level scale (dB HL) of the clinical audiogram uses the average sound pressure threshold of the normal population at a given frequency as the reference pressure. The sound pressure level of both sounds shown in Figure 3–2 is 91 dB SPL, where 91 = 20 log10 (0.71/0.00002). The loudness of a sound is a monotonic function of the sound pressure; for mid-level sounds a 20 dB increase in sound pressure produces about a factor of six increase in loudness.[9] The sound pressures of various commonly experienced sounds are noted in terms of rms Pa and dB SPL in Table 3–1.

Sound is a variation in pressure with time. A pure tone, as in Figure 3–2A, is a sound in which the relationship between sound pressure and time can be described by a sine function, eg,

$$p(t) = A\cos(2\pi f t + \phi)$$

where we use the cosine function that is the common standard in engineering applications, $p(t)$ describes the variation in sound pressure with time, A describes the peak amplitude or *magnitude* of the pressure, f is the *frequency* of the sinusoid and ϕ is the *phase.* The phase ϕ determines the time when the pressure is maximum relative to some reference time zero. The relative phases of the sound pressure in the ear canal, and the mechanical and neural responses within the ear are useful in determining the physical and biological processes associated with hearing.[10,11] Also, the relative timing information in the phase is critical when waveforms are combined; two waves of the same frequency added together can sum constructively if they have similar phases, sum to near zero if the waves are out of phase and of identical amplitude, or somewhere in between for intermediate phases. Complex sounds (eg, Figure 3–2B) can be described by the addition of pure tones of different frequencies and different phases. A complex sound can be broken down into its individual components (individual sinusoids with magnitude and phase information) by using a Fourier analysis. While the ear is insensitive to the absolute phase of a single tone, a complex acoustic signal with a fixed number of frequency components of fixed magnitude can sound quite different depending on the relative phases of the components.

While the human ear can hear sound frequencies ranging from 20 to 20,000 Hz, the ear is differentially sensitive to sounds of different frequencies, and measurements of the

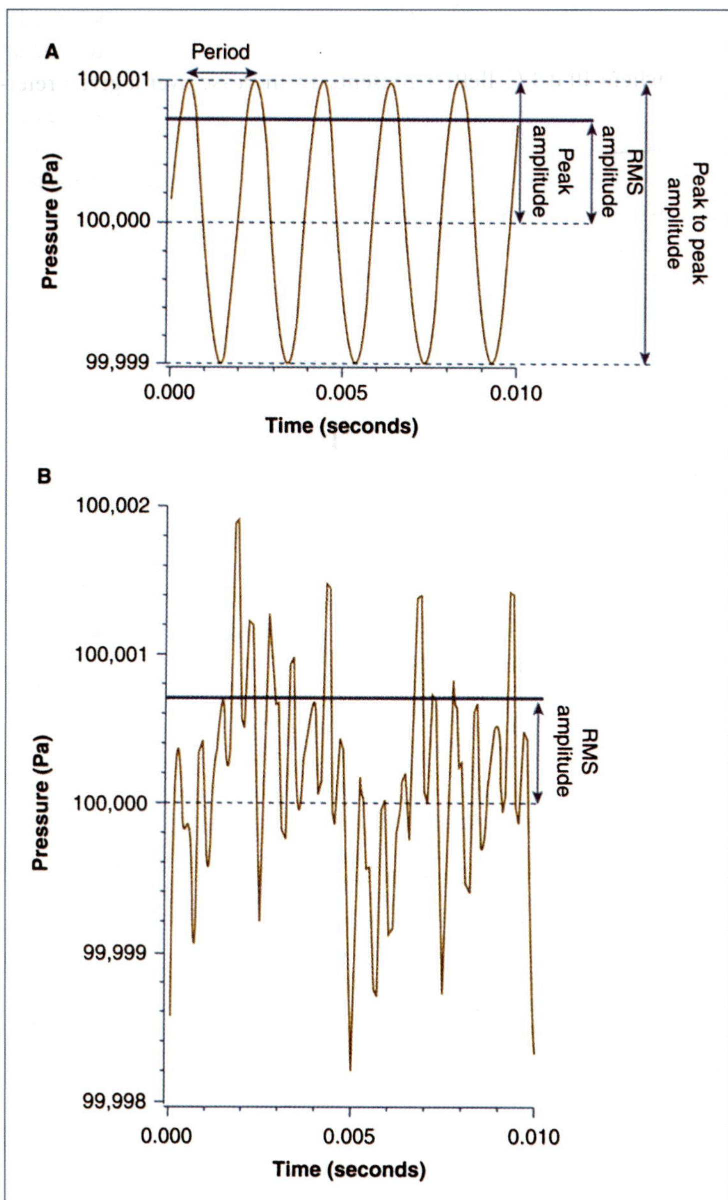

FIGURE 3–2 • Two patterns of temporal variations and air pressure produced by sounds. The schematic in *A,* depicts that produced by a 512-Hz pure tone, while *B,* depicts that produced by a complex sound. The absolute value of pressure is scaled in both plots, and, therefore, the sound-induced variations occur around a static value of 100,000 Pa = 1 atmosphere. The sound pressure corresponds to amplitude of variations around the static value. In both *A* and *B*, while the static atmospheric pressure is 100,000 Pa, the amplitude of the sound pressure is on the order of 1 Pa. *A*, The pressure variations are those of a 512-Hz pure tone. The pressure varies sinusoidally with a period of 1/512 = 0.00195 seconds. The amplitude of pressure variations around the static value can be quantified in terms of the peak-to-peak value of 2 Pa, the peak value of 1 Pa, or the rms (root mean square) value of 0.71 Pa. (The rms value is the square root of the mean of the squared pressure deviations from static values averaged over some time. In the case of a sinusoid, a convenient averaging time is an integral number of periods of the sine wave. With sinusoidal sound pressures, the rms value equals the peak amplitude/$\sqrt{2}$). *B*, The pressure variations are those of a complex sound with many irregular risings and fallings of the sound pressure. With this kind of sound, peak amplitude and peak-to-peak amplitude are poor indicators of the average sound level. However, rms is an excellent measure as long as one specifies an averaging time. In the case depicted, the rms sound pressure was computed over the 0.01 second time window. Note that the sound pressure in *B* has the same rms value as the sound pressure in *A*.

TABLE 3–1 Sound pressures of common sounds

APPROXIMATE SOUND LEVEL		
rms Pa	dB SPL	SOUND SOURCE
0.0001–0.0002	14–20	Just audible whisper
0.002–0.02	40–60	Conversational speech
0.02–0.6	60–90	Noisy room
0.6–20	90–120	Loud music
>20	>120	Gun fire

hearing threshold vary depending on how the sound stimulus is specified. Sound pressure thresholds (the lowest sound pressures that are audible) measured in normal young adults with pure tones of different frequencies under two different measurement conditions are shown in Figure 3–3. The lower curve depicts thresholds determined with subjects in an open space or free field,[12] where the sound pressure measurement was made at the location of the subject's head when the subject was not present. The upper curve is the ANSI (American National Standards Institute[13]) standard measurement of thresholds made under earphones, where the sound pressures are those generated by the earphones in a calibration coupler. The differences between these two curves can be explained by the effect of the human subject on the open sound field, sound gathering by the external ear, the effect of closing the ear canal by earphones and differences in calibration between the two circumstances.[14] Both curves clearly show that normal young adult humans are most sensitive to sound frequencies of 500 to 8,000 Hz. The best frequency differs depending on the measurement circumstance, being 1,500 Hz under earphones and 4,000 Hz in the free field. At higher and lower

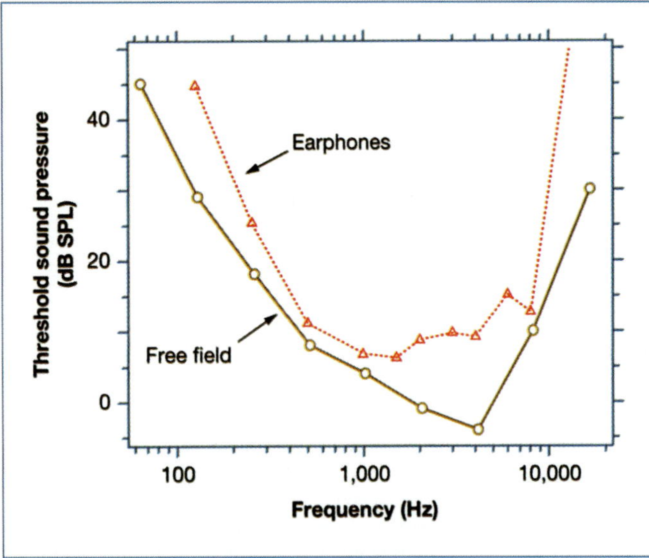

FIGURE 3–3 • Sensitivity of the ear to sounds of different frequencies. The figure depicts measurements of auditory threshold made under earphones (ANSI standards[13]) and those made in the free field (Sivian and White[12]). The mean normal threshold at 1,000 Hz under both measurement conditions is about zero dB SPL.

frequencies, more sound pressure is required to be audible, and the thresholds increase steeply below 500 Hz and above 8,000 Hz.

Clinicians are most interested in how an individual's hearing threshold differs from normal; in practice, normal is defined by the ANSI standard earphone measurements shown in Figure 3–3. A powerful graphical tool for comparing two different functions is to plot their difference. The *clinical audiogram* (Figure 3–4, discussed more in Chapter 8) uses this difference technique by plotting an individual's threshold relative to the ANSI standard normal hearing level. For example, a person whose hearing threshold at 1,000 Hz is 10 dB greater than the ANSI standard is assigned a hearing level of 10 dB at that frequency. In clinical audiograms, threshold sound pressure levels relative to the standard *Hearing Level* are quantified in dB relative to normal at frequencies of octave or half octave intervals. It is important to remember that the normal curve is based on mean hearing thresholds in normal subjects and that there is normal variation (plus or minus 20 dB) around the mean.

The *speed* or *propagation velocity* of sound through a medium determines the *sound wave length* for a given frequency, which is the distance it takes a propagating sound wave to repeat itself. Specifically, the wave length λ equals the propagation velocity divided by sound frequency. The wave length describes how a tone varies in space and the relative size of the wavelength and an object's dimensions determines how sound interacts with the object. If the wave length of a sound is at least five times larger than the largest dimension of an object, the object will have little effect on the sound, ie, as the sound propagates around the object, the sound pressure at the front and back side of the object will be very similar to the sound pressure measured when the object is not present. On the other hand, if the wave length is similar to or smaller than the dimensions of an object, variations in sound pressure will be introduced by the object. In general, as short wave length sound interacts with the object, the sound pressure along the front surface of the object will increase because of reflection of sound, and sound pressure along the back surface will be decreased because the object shields that location from the sound. A common analogy is between light and sound, where in the small wave length case, the object casts a sound shadow.

The size of body and ear structures relative to sound wave length plays a significant role in determining the interaction of the ear with sounds of different frequencies.[14] A 20 Hz sound wave (wave length of 17 m) is affected very little by the head or body. A 200 Hz sound (wave length of 1.7 m) can be effectively scattered by the head and torso so that there is a small gain in sound pressure at the ear. A 2,000 Hz tone (wave length of 17 cm) is diffracted by the head so that there is a doubling of sound pressure on the side of the head directed toward the sound source and a shadow on the opposite side of the head. A 4,000 Hz tone (8.5 cm wave length) is scattered by the pinna such that there is an increase in sound pressure for sound

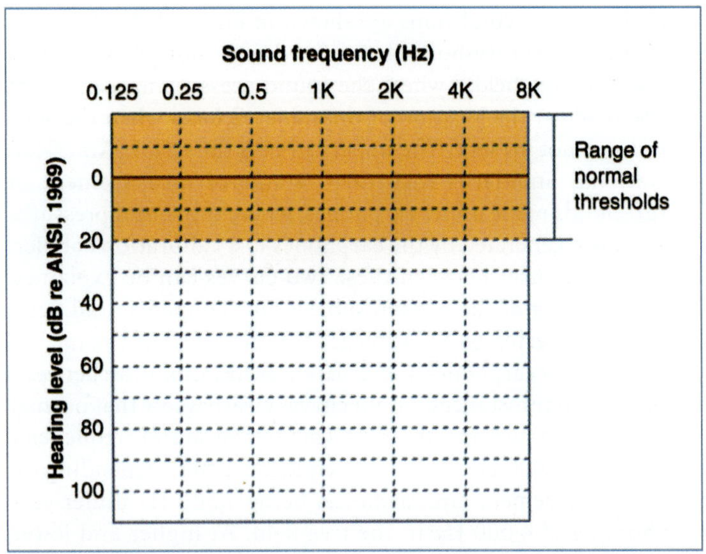

FIGURE 3–4 • Clinical audiogram, where an individual's hearing threshold relative to the ANSI standard normal hearing level is plotted versus frequency. The ordinate scale is inverted so that higher thresholds are plotted lower on the graph.

TABLE 3–2 Wavelengths of sound and body structures with which wave interactions are important

FREQUENCY (Hz)	WAVELENGTH	ANATOMICAL STRUCTURE	STRUCTURAL DIMENSIONS
340	1 m	Torso	0.5 m
2,000	17 cm	Head	10 cm
4,000	8.5 cm	Pinna Ear canal length	4 cm 2.5 cm
20,000	1.7 cm	Diameter of ear canal and tympanic membrane	0.8 cm

sources pointing directly at the meatus and decreases in sound pressure for other directions. Another kind of wave length interaction occurs in the external ear canal; resonances occur within the ear at frequencies where the length of the ear canal and depth of the concha are odd multiples of $\lambda/4$.[14] Table 3–2 lists some of the critical frequencies above which sound wave lengths allow interactions with various parts of the body and ear. In general, the interaction of the structures of the external ear and sound are restricted to sound frequencies of 1,000 Hz and above.

SOUND TRANSMISSION IN THE NORMAL EAR

The Problem of Transferring Air-Borne Sound Power to the Fluids of the Inner Ear: The Air-Fluid Impedance Mismatch

Acoustic signals are transmitted from the air of the external environment to the fluid-filled inner ear. The transmission of sound power at an air–fluid interface depends on the relative impedances of air and fluid. In the case of the inner ear, only about 0.1% of the intensity of an incident sound wave is transmitted to the fluid, and this is equivalent to a 30 dB loss. The external and middle ears act to better match the sound conducting properties of air and cochlear fluid by increasing the sound pressures that reach the inner ear at certain frequencies as described below. The discussion that follows is meant to be an overview, and readers seeking more detailed descriptions are referred to other sources.[15–17]

The External Ear

The external ear, along with the head and body, has a significant influence on the sounds that reach the middle ear. This acoustic function of the external ear, sometimes called the *external ear gain*, can be described by a frequency- and directionally-dependent alteration in the sound pressure at the tympanic membrane when compared to the sound pressure in the free field. As illustrated in Figure 3–5, when a sound source is positioned facing the ear, the external ear produces a gain of as much as 20 dB at 2,500 Hz, with less gain at lower and higher frequencies. As also illustrated in Figure 3–5, this gain results from the combination of sound scattering and diffraction around the head and torso, as well as the acoustic influence of the pinna, concha, ear canal, and middle-ear load impedance. The figure illustrates the frequency dependence of these different contributions and shows how the gains add (in dB terms) to define the total external-ear gain. Not shown in Figure 3–5 is how this external ear gain is directionally dependent for frequencies above 500 Hz. In fact, for sounds coming from the opposite side of the head, the sound pressure at the tympanic membrane can

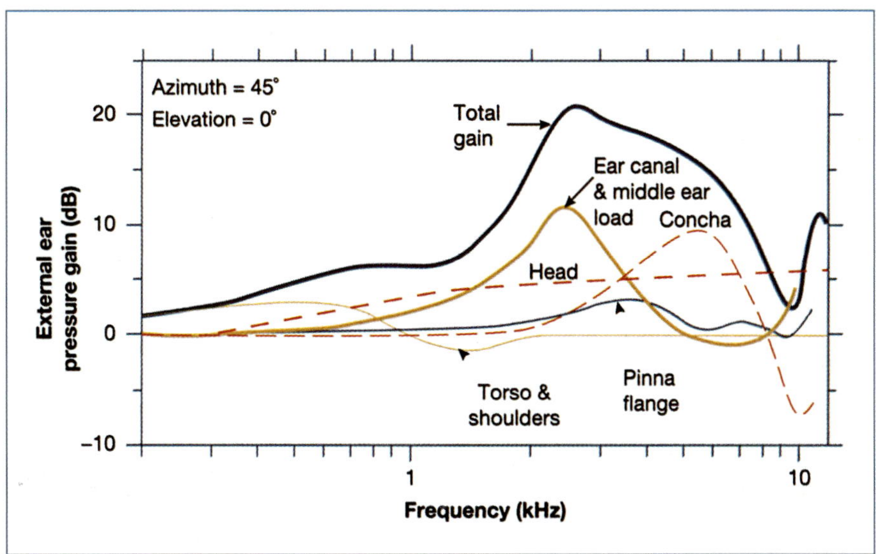

FIGURE 3–5 • Schematic representation of the external ear gain. The total gain and the gain of individual components in dB is plotted versus frequency. The plots describe the gains for a sound source that is positioned on the same horizontal plane as the interaural axis (elevation of 0 degrees) and which is 45 degrees off of the midline towards the ear that is measured (azimuth of 45 degrees). The gains of the different components are all multiplied (added in dB) together to achieve the total gain. *After Shaw.*[14]

be less than the sound pressure in the stimulus (ie, the external ear gain in dB is negative).

The Middle Ear

The middle ear couples sound signals from the ear canal to the cochlea primarily through the action of the tympanic membrane and the ossicular chain. Figure 3–6 is a schematic depicting the important structures in the *transformation* of sound power from the external ear to the inner ear. (Power is a product of pressure and volume velocity. Volume velocity refers to how much particle volume flows through a given area and is equal to the product of the average linear velocity across a surface and surface area. An acoustical transformer increases either pressure or volume velocity, while decreasing the other, thereby equalizing the sound power at the input and output). The middle ear acts as a transformer to increase sound pressure at the footplate relative to that at the tympanic membrane at the expense of a decrease in stapes volume velocity relative to the tympanic membrane volume velocity. The major transformer mechanism within the middle ear is the ratio of the tympanic membrane area to the stapes footplate area (*the area ratio*). The tympanic membrane gathers force over its entire surface and then couples the gathered force to the smaller footplate of the stapes. Since pressure is force per area, and the human tympanic has an area that is 20 times larger than the footplate,[2] if the transformer action of the area ratio is "ideal," the sound pressure applied to the inner ear by the stapes footplate should be 20 times or 26 dB larger than the sound pressure at the tympanic membrane. Another transformer within the middle ear is the ossicular lever: the lever action that results from the different lengths of the rotating malleus and incus arms around the axis of rotation of the ossicles. The axis of rotation is an imaginary line joining the anterior malleal ligament to the incudal ligament that anchors the short process of the incus. The malleus and incus lever arms in humans are nearly the same length. Hence, the ratio of these lengths, which is 1.3,[18] predicts only a small 2 dB increase in sound pressure applied by the stapes to the inner ear. Thus, if these transformers acted ideally, then the *theoretical middle-ear sound pressure gain* is about 28 dB (=26 dB area ratio + 2 dB ossicular lever).

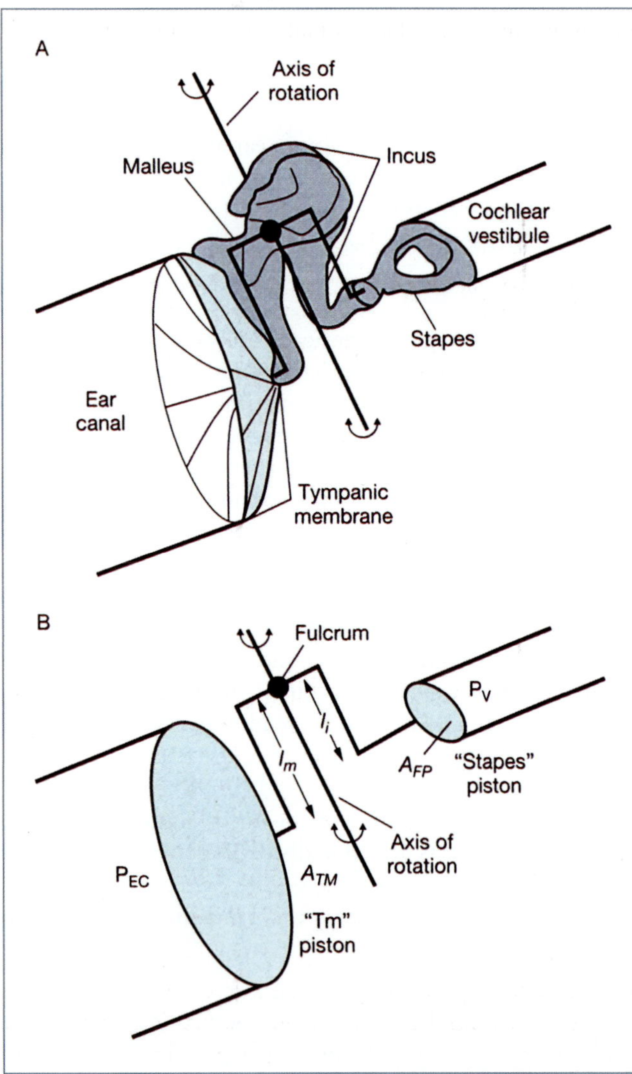

FIGURE 3–6 • Schematics of the tympano-ossicular system (*A*), and a mechanical analog (*B*), depicting important structures in the transformation of sound power from the middle ear to the inner ear. The key transformer within the middle ear is the ratio of the tympanic membrane area (*A*TM) to the area of the stapes footplate (*A*FP). Another transformer is the ossicular lever: this is the lever action due to differing lengths of the manubrium (*l*m) and long process of incus (*l*i) around the axis of rotation of the ossicles. This axis of rotation is an imaginary line joining the anterior malleal ligament to the incudal ligament that anchors the short process of the incus. The total middle-ear sound pressure gain, which is the result of the area ratio and the ossicular lever, can be quantified and measured using the ratio of sound pressure in the vestibule (P_V) to the sound pressure in the ear canal (P_{EC}). As described in the text, the theoretical (ideal) middle ear gain is 28 dB, whereas the actual (measured) middle-ear gain is only about 20 dB.

Measurements of the *actual middle-ear sound pressure gain* of the human middle ear performed in normal temporal bones under physiologic conditions[19] are illustrated in Figure 3–7. The data demonstrate that the pressure gain is frequency dependent, with a maximum gain of only about 20 dB near 1,000 Hz with lower gains at other frequencies. Similar findings have also been reported by other investigators.[20,21] Thus, the measured middle-ear gain is less than the 28 dB gain predicted by the ideal anatomical transformer model of Figure 3–6. The difference between the measured and theoretical gains is the result of several nonideal conditions within the middle ear: (1) The anatomical transformer model assumes that the entire tympanic membrane moves as a rigid body. However, measurements of tympanic membrane motion[22,23] show that portions of the membrane move differently than others. At low frequencies, the entire tympanic membrane moves with the same phase, but the magnitude varies. At frequencies above 1,000 Hz, the patterns of vibration become more complicated with the tympanic membrane breaking up into smaller vibrating portions that vibrate with different phases. This decreases the efficacy of the tympanic membrane as a coupler of sound pressure. (2) The simple transformer model does not account for the forces and pressures needed to stretch the tympanic membrane and ossicular ligaments and accelerate the mass of the middle-ear components. Part of the force generated by a sound pressure in the ear canal is used to move the tympanic membrane and ossicles themselves, and this force is lost before it

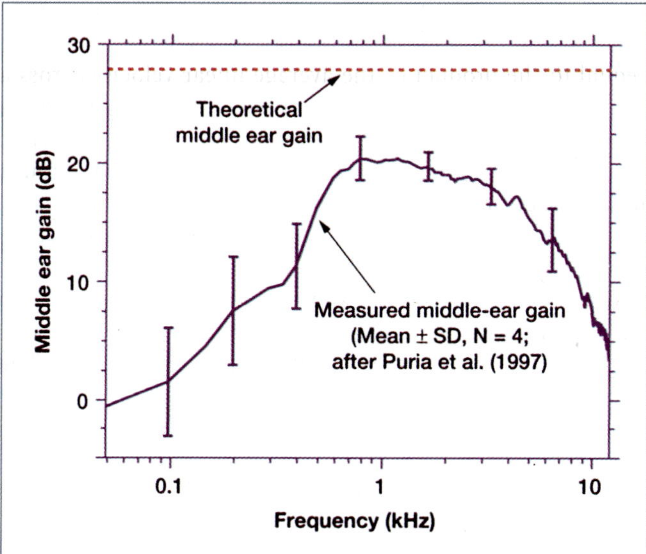

FIGURE 3–7 • Middle-ear sound pressure gain. The dashed line at the top shows the theoretical (ideal) transformer ratio produced by the tympanic membrane to footplate area ratio and the ossicular lever. The theoretical middle-ear gain, which is approximately 28 dB, is independent of frequency. The curve represents the mean ± standard deviation of measurements of middle-ear gain made in 4 normal temporal bones (Puria et al.[19]). The measurements consist of the increase in magnitude of the sound pressure in the cochlear vestibule over the sound pressure at the tympanic membrane. It is evident that the actual middle-ear gain is frequency dependent, and is only about 20 dB at best (around 1,000 Hz).

reaches the cochlea. (3) Other acoustical structures of the ear such as the middle-ear air spaces load the motion of the tympanic membrane and ossicles, and use up some of the pressure increase produced by the middle-ear transformer. (4) The anatomical transformer model implies that the ossicular system acts as a rigid body. In reality, there is slippage in the ossicular system particularly at frequencies above 1,000 to 2,000 Hz, which reduces the motion of the stapes relative to that of the manubrium. This slippage has been associated with translational movement in the rotational axis of the ossicles[24] or flexion in the ossicular joints.[10,25,26]

As will be discussed later, the effective stimulus to the inner ears is a difference in sound pressure between the oval and round windows. The middle ear maximizes this window pressure difference via two mechanisms.[27,28] First, as described above, the tympano-ossicular system preferentially increases the sound pressure at the oval window of the inner ear. At the same time, the intact tympanic membrane reduces the sound pressure in the tympanic cavity by 10 to 20 dB compared to the sound pressure in the ear canal,[29,30] thereby protecting or shielding the round window from the sound in the ear canal. A third function of the middle ear related to the protective function is that the presence of middle-ear air outside the round window permits the window to move freely when the inner ear is stimulated by motion of the footplate. These concepts of middle-ear sound pressure gain, round window protection and round window mobility have important practical implications for tympanoplasty.

The Inner Ear

The cochlea is a coiled tube made of three fluid-filled chambers. The fluid is essentially incompressible, so that any movement of the stapes footplate within the oval window must be accompanied by fluid motion elsewhere. Over the auditory frequency range, the small fluid-filled cochlear and vestibular aqueducts and other connections between the cochlea and cerebrospinal fluid space are effectively closed,[31] and it is the compliant membrane covering the round window that permits large motions of the footplate. When the stapes footplate moves in, the round window moves out. (The footplate and round window have approximately the same volume velocities, but move with opposite phase.) It is this coupling of the round and oval windows by the incompressible cochlear fluids that leads to the importance of the *difference* in sound pressure at the two cochlear windows in stimulating the inner ear.[32,33]

The cochlear partition within the inner ear includes the basilar membrane, the organ of Corti, scala media, and Reissner's membrane. The mechanical properties of the cochlear partition are heavily influenced by the mechanics of the basilar membrane; the latter is narrow, stiff and thick at the base, and it is wider, compliant and thin at the apex. Because the fluid is essentially incompressible, inward motion of the stapes causes a near instantaneous transfer of the motion through the cochlear fluids, resulting in outward motion of the round window. Associated with this displacement of the fluid is a nearly instantaneous pressure distribution across the cochlear partition. The reaction of the cochlear partition with its graded mechanical properties to this pressure distribution, results in a *traveling wave* of cochlear partition displacement.[34] The maximum displacement of this wave is tonotopically organized in a manner consistent with place-dependent differences in partition mechanics. High-frequency sounds produce displacement maxima near the stiff and thick base, while low-frequency sounds produce displacement maxima near the compliant and thin apex.

Because the wave appears to travel from the base towards the apex and also appears to stop just past the location of maximum displacement, there is an asymmetry in the motion of the cochlear partition. All sounds produce some motion of the basal portions of the cochlear partition, while only low-frequency sounds produce significant partition motion in the apex. This asymmetry has implications in our perception of complex sounds (where low-frequency sounds can interfere with our perception of high-frequency sounds, but not vice versa[35]), and has also been suggested to play a role in the sensitivity of the high-frequency base to noise trauma and in presbycusis.[36] Motion of the cochlear partition stimulates hair cells of the organ of Corti, where larger stimuli result from larger motions.

Phase Difference Between the Cochlear Windows

As stated earlier, the cochlea responds to the *difference* in sound pressure between the cochlear windows,[32,33] where the sound pressure at the oval window is a sum of the pressure produced by the tympano-ossicular system and the acoustic pressure within the middle-ear air space. It is important to understand how this difference (the essential stimulus to the inner ear), depends on the relative magnitude and phase of the individual sound pressures at the two windows. When there is a significant difference in magnitude between the oval- and round-window sound pressures (as in the normal ear and after successful tympanoplasty when the tympano-ossicular system amplifies the pressure acting at the oval window), *differences in phase have little effect* in determining the window-pressure difference.[37,38] The lack of importance of phase when the magnitudes differ is illustrated in Figure 3–8, which shows a hypothetical situation where the magnitude of the oval window sound pressure is ten times (20 dB) greater than the round window sound pressure. The range of possible window-pressure difference is shown by two curves, one with an amplitude of 9 representing the difference when the two window pressures are in-phase (0-degree phase difference) and the other curve with an amplitude of 11 representing the difference when the window pressures are completely out-of-phase (180-degree phase difference). Even with this maximum effect of varying the phase difference, the two curves shown in Figure 3–8 are similar in magnitude, within 2 dB of each other. With larger magnitude differences such as factors of 100 to 1,000 (40–60 dB) that occur in the normal ear and in ears that have undergone successful tympanoplasty, variations in phase have a negligible effect.

However, phase differences can become important under conditions when the magnitudes of the sound pressures at the oval and round windows are similar (eg, with an interrupted ossicular chain). When the individual window pressures are of similar magnitude and similar phase, they tend to cancel each other and produce only a small net window-pressure difference. On the other hand, if the individual window pressures are of similar magnitude but opposite phase, then they will add to each other, resulting in a window-pressure difference that is similar in magnitude to the applied pressures.

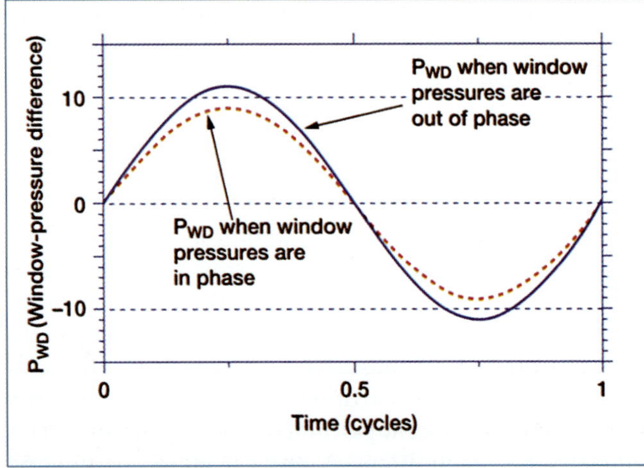

FIGURE 3–8 • Schematic showing that if there is a significant difference in magnitude between window pressures, then differences in phase are of little importance in determining the difference between the two sound pressures. In this specific case, the oval window sound pressure is 10 times (=20 dB) greater than the round window sound pressure. One cycle of the wave form of the window-pressure difference (P_{WD}) is plotted for two circumstances. The dashed line shows P_{WD} when the oval window and round window pressures are in-phase, and the result is a P_{WD} wave of peak amplitude 9 = 10 – 1. The solid line shows P_{WD} when the individual window pressures are completely out-of-phase, and the result is a P_{WD} wave of amplitude 11 = 10 – (– 1). Note that the two P_{WD} pressures differ by less than 2 dB ($20\log_{10}11/9 = 1.7$ dB), even though this phase variation produces the largest possible magnitude difference. Thus, in the normal ear and after successful tympanoplasty when the sound pressure at the oval window is large due to significant ossicular conduction of sound, differences in phase of sound pressures at the oval and round windows have little effect in determining the hearing outcome.

Multiple Pathways for Sound Stimulation of the Inner Ear

The contribution of the middle ear to the window-pressure difference that stimulates the inner ear can be split into several stimulus pathways. A previous section described how the tympano-ossicular system transforms sound pressure in the ear canal to sound pressure at the oval window. This pathway has been termed *ossicular coupling*.[39] There is another mechanism, called *acoustic coupling*,[39] through which the middle ear can stimulate the inner ear (Figure 3–9). Motion of the tympanic membrane in response to ear canal sound creates sound pressure in the middle ear cavity. Because the cochlear windows are separated by a few millimeters, the acoustic sound pressures at the oval and round windows respectively, are similar but *not* identical.[40] Small differences between the magnitudes and phases of the sound pressures outside the two windows result in a small but measurable difference in sound pressure between the two windows. In the normal ear, the magnitude of this acoustically-coupled window pressure difference is small, on the order of 60 dB less than ossicular coupling.[38,40] Hence, ossicular coupling dominates normal middle-ear function and one can

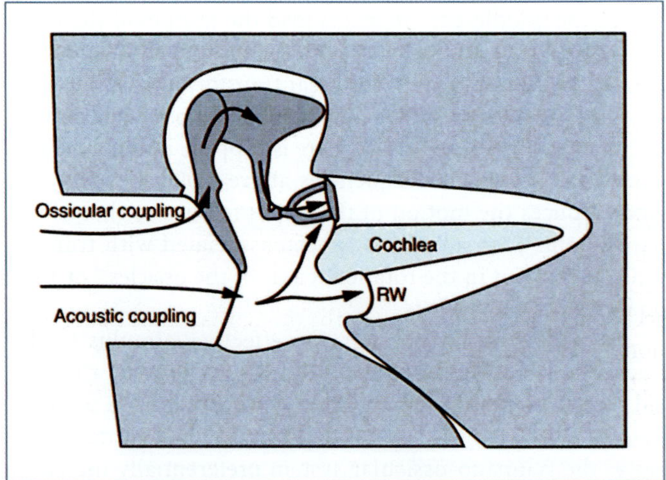

FIGURE 3–9 • Schematic showing the pathways of ossicular coupling and acoustic coupling. Ossicular coupling is produced by the coupled motion of the tympanic membrane, ossicles and stapes footplate. Acoustic coupling results from middle-ear sound pressure that is produced by ear canal sound pressure and motion of the tympanic membrane. Because the cochlear windows are spatially separated, the sound pressures within the middle ear cavity that act at the oval and round windows (RW), respectively, are *not* identical. The small differences between the magnitudes and phases of the two window pressures result in a small but measurable *difference* in sound pressure between the two windows. This difference is called acoustic coupling. In the normal ear, acoustic coupling is quite small and its magnitude is approximately 60 dB less than ossicular coupling.[38,39]

ignore acoustic coupling. However, as will be seen later, acoustic coupling can play an important role when ossicular coupling is compromised as in some diseased and reconstructed ears.

Environmental sound can also reach the inner ear by producing vibrations of the whole body and head, so-called whole body sound conduction.[41] This is a more general process than audiological *bone conduction* where a vibrator acts only on the mastoid portion of the skull. Sound-induced vibrations of the whole body and head can stimulate the inner ear by (1) generating external ear or middle-ear sound pressures via compressions of the ear canal and middle-ear walls, (2) producing relative motions between the ossicles and inner ear, and (3) direct compression of the inner ear and its contents by compression of the surrounding fluid and bone. Little is known about the contribution of *whole body sound conduction* to normal auditory function. However, measurements of hearing loss due to pathology such as congenital aural atresia suggest that the whole body route can provide a stimulus to the inner ear which is about 60 dB smaller than that provided by normal ossicular coupling.[41]

Audiological Bone Conduction

Sound energy transmitted to the skull by a bone vibrator (eg, a tuning fork or the electromagnetic vibrator of an audiometer) sets the basilar membrane in motion and is perceived as sound. Clinical bone conduction testing is used as a means to determine the functionality of the cochlea. The mechanisms by which a bone vibrator can stimulate the inner ear have been described by Tonndorf[42] and others[43,44] and are similar to those described earlier for whole-body sound transmission. It is important to realize that all of the hypothesized bone-conduction mechanisms involve relative motion between the ossicles and inner ear, and that bone-conduction hearing is influenced by pathologies in the external and middle ears. The so-called occlusion effect (easily demonstrated by occlusion of the external ear canal while talking, which results in increased loudness of sound heard in the occluded ear) occurs because vibrations of the ear canal wall produce significant sound pressures in the closed ear canal. Furthermore, a classic pattern in bone conduction audiometry known as the Carhart notch (see Chapter 10) is used to help identify cases of stapes footplate fixation.[45] The mechanical processes that underlie the Carhart notch phenomenon are not well understood. Therefore, the idea that vibrating the skull directly stimulates the cochlea in a manner that is independent of the middle ear is not strictly true.

Middle Ear Muscles

The stapedius and tensor tympani muscles contract under a variety of circumstances including loud sounds, before and during vocalization, tactile stimulation of the head or face, and fight or flight behavioral responses.[46] Such protective contractions reduce the transmission of low-frequency sound through the middle ear but have little effect on high-frequency sound.[2,47,48] Contraction of the stapedius muscle in response to sound is known as the *acoustic reflex*. The reflex is thought to help in speech discrimination (the reflex reduces masking by low-frequency sound of high-frequency stimuli[49,50]), and in protecting the inner ear from acoustic trauma of loud continuous sound.[51] Contractions of the tensor tympani have also been associated with opening of the eustachian tube where the inward motion of the tympanic membrane that results from the contraction produces an overpressure in the middle ear that helps open the tube.[52]

Middle Ear Joints

The incudomalleal and incudostapedial joints add flexibility to the ossicular system, which allows the middle ear to withstand large variations in the static pressure difference across the tympanic membrane without producing damage to the ear. Middle-ear static pressure variations that occur regularly in day-to-day activities (eg, those produced by sneezing and swallowing) generate millimeter-sized motions of the tympanic membrane; such large motions are not transmitted to the stapes due to the flexibility of the incudomalleal and incudostapedial joints.[53,54]

The ossicular joints also permit independent control of tympanic membrane and stapes motion by the middle-ear muscles. Large contractions of the stapedius muscle that cause 0.1 mm changes in position of the stapes head have been shown to have little effect on position of the other ossicles because of sliding in the incudostapedial joint.[55] Similarly, the tensor tympani can pull the malleus inwards by a millimeter or more but has little effect on the stapes because of the incudomalleal joint. There is some data from studies of ossicular motion in animals and human temporal bones to suggest that a consequence of the joint-induced flexibility is a decrease in the high-frequency response of the middle ear.[10,56] There is also evidence that flexion of the incudo-malleolar joint is a major component of the human ossicular response to sound at all frequencies.[25,57]

Investigation of Middle-Ear Mechanics

Broadly speaking, investigations of middle-ear mechanics have employed one or more of four approaches: behavioral and other assessments of hearing in normal and diseased ears, physiologic studies of the middle ears of animals, quantitative physics-based models, and acoustic measurements in cadaveric temporal bones.

The use of animal models to study the middle ear was pioneered by Wever and Lawrence in a series of studies of the effects of middle-ear modifications on cochlear potentials in cats.[2] Other landmark studies include: investigations of middle-ear impedance and ossicular motion,[10,58–61] investigations of the effect of middle-ear muscles,[62] and investigations of simulated pathologies on middle-ear transmission.[63–65] Animal studies continue to provide new insights into middle-ear function, including recent evidence that the ossicles are not completely rigid,[66] evidence of wave-motion in the tympanic membrane itself and within the ossicular chain[67–69] and new evidence of contractile elements within the support of the tympanic membrane.[70]

A "model" of the middle ear is essentially a set of mathematical equations that relate the physical structure of the ear to its acoustic function. The degree and complexity of the association of model elements with anatomic structures varies widely within models, ranging from simple "black-box" models of the ear,[71] through models where simple elements are associated with specific structures of the ear,[72] to complex three-dimensional finite-element models that include detailed depictions of middle-ear shape and approximations of the mechanical properties of the structural elements.[69,73,74] A wide variety of middle-ear models have been described, dealing with sound transmission in normal as well as in pathological ears. A discussion of such models is outside the scope of this review, and the reader is referred to other sources.[17]

Cadaveric temporal bones (the "temporal bone preparation") are also useful in studying middle-ear mechanics. It has been shown that the mechanical properties of the middle ear in carefully prepared temporal bones are indistinguishable from those measured in living human ears.[75–77] The temporal bones must be in a fresh state, kept moist and static pressure must not be allowed to build up within the middle ear. Besides its utility in studying normal middle-ear function, the temporal bone preparation allows one to make repeated measurements of acoustic and mechanical function after precise modifications that simulate specific pathologies or tympanoplasties. Measurements in such preparations have provided valuable insight into the mechanics of sound transmission in a variety of diseased and reconstructed ears.

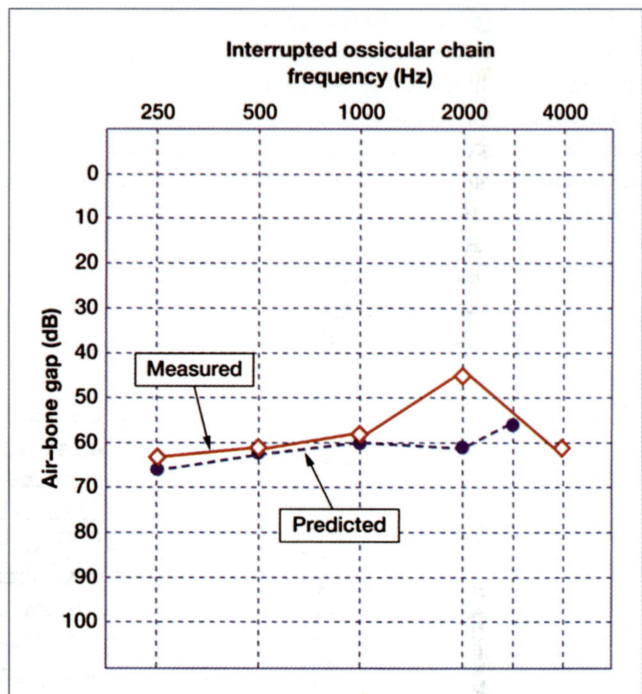

FIGURE 3–10 • Comparison of air–bone gaps measured in eight cases with surgically confirmed complete ossicular chain interruption with an intact tympanic membrane to air–bone gaps predicted on the basis of hearing resulting from acoustic coupling. In this pathological state, there is no ossicular coupling. Since acoustic coupling is about 60 dB smaller than ossicular coupling, the prediction is a 60 dB conductive hearing loss, which is consistent with the measured air–bone gaps. The standard deviation for each of the measured points is about ± 10 dB. *After Peake et al.*[39]

ACOUSTICS AND MECHANICS OF DISEASED MIDDLE EARS

The concepts discussed in the previous section help us to understand sound transmission in various pathological middle-ear conditions. In this review, we have chosen the "air–bone gap" as determined by standard clinical audiometry to describe the loss of middle-ear sound transmission in various pathological conditions. Our choice of the air–bone gap measure is a matter of ease and convenience, since the gap can be easily calculated from a clinical audiogram and it allows one to compare ears with disparate levels of sensorineural function. However, one must remember that the air–bone gap is not always an accurate measure of middle-ear sound transmission loss, because bone conduction thresholds can be influenced by middle-ear pathologies, as mentioned previously.

Ossicular Interruption With an Intact Tympanic Membrane

When there is ossicular interruption in the presence of an intact drum, ossicular coupling is lost and sound input to the cochlea via the middle ear occurs as a result of acoustic coupling.[39] Since acoustic coupling is about 60 dB smaller than ossicular coupling, one would predict that complete ossicular interruption would result in a 60 dB conductive hearing loss. This prediction is consistent with clinical observations as shown in Figure 3–10, where there is good agreement between the predicted and actual air–bone gap as measured in eight surgically confirmed cases of ossicular interruption with an intact tympanic membrane. Note that the consistency of the clinical results with the model of acoustic coupling suggests that stimuli reaching the inner ear through whole body or bone conduction mechanisms in this particular condition are small enough to be ignored.

A special type of ossicular interruption consists of resorption or a break in one of the ossicles and its replacement by connective tissue. An example is resorption of the long process of the incus and its replacement by a band of fibrous tissue in chronic otitis media. Such "partial ossicular interruption" is often associated with an air–bone gap that is greater at high versus low frequencies. It is one of the few types of middle-ear pathologies where the air–bone gap is greater at the high frequencies. The mechanism of hearing loss is probably related to a decrease in the rigidity within the ossicular chain. At low frequencies, a fibrous band seems to be tense enough to allow near-normal sound transmission; however, at higher frequencies, the fibrous band flexes such that motions of the tympanic membrane are not readily coupled to the stapes.

Loss of the Tympanic Membrane, Malleus, and Incus

In cases where the tympanic membrane, malleus, and incus are lost, the conductive hearing loss is on the order of 40 to 50 dB, ie, this condition results in hearing sensitivities that are 10 to 20 dB superior to cases with an intact tympanic membrane and complete ossicular interruption. The 40- to 50-dB loss can be explained by a loss of ossicular coupling together with an enhancement of acoustic coupling by about 10 to 20 dB, as compared to the normal ear.[39] The enhancement of acoustic coupling results from loss of the shielding effect of the tympanic membrane, which in the normal ear attenuates middle-ear sound pressure by 10 to 20 dB relative to ear canal sound pressure. The air–bone gap predicted by loss of ossicular coupling and enhanced acoustic coupling is similar to that measured in patients as shown in Figure 3–11. The increase in acoustic coupling due to loss of tympanic membrane shielding also explains why the hearing of a patient with an interrupted ossicular chain and an intact drum is improved by 10 to 20 dB when a perforation is created in the tympanic membrane.

Ossicular Fixation

Partial or complete fixation of the stapes footplate (eg, otosclerosis, tympanosclerosis, etc.) results in conductive hearing losses that range from 5 dB to 60 dB depending on the degree of fixation.[78] The losses are greater for the lower frequencies (Figure 3–12). Fixation of the footplate reduces ossicular coupling by hindering stapes motion, resulting in a conductive hearing loss. The amount of hearing loss depends upon the degree of decreased stapes motion. The primary effect of the otosclerotic lesion is an increase in the stiffness of the annular ligament that supports the stapes, where the normal ligament stiffness is a major constraint on the ossicular coupling route in the normal ear. Increases in ligament stiffness should first affect the low-frequency response of the ear, which is consistent with the observation that in early otosclerosis the hearing loss is mainly in the low frequencies.[78]

The conductive hearing loss resulting from fixation of the malleus is determined by the location, extent, and type of pathology causing the fixation.[79] Fixation at the level of the anterior malleal ligament (eg, calcification of the ligament) results in a hearing loss less than 10 dB. More commonly, fixation of the malleus is at the level of its head due to a bony spur that ankyloses the malleus head to the lateral epitympanic wall or to the tegmen tympani.[80] The resulting air–bone gap is small, usually in the range of 15 to 25 dB.[80,81] Malleus ankylosis can also be caused by extensive deposition of fibrous tissue and new bone in the epitympanum as the result of chronic otitis media.[80,82] In such a case, both the malleus and incus are usually fixed in the epitympanum, with an air–bone gap of 30 to 50 dB.[82] The differential effects of location, extent, and type of malleus fixation can be explained on the basis of the mechanics of rotation of the malleus (and incus) about an axis linking the anterior malleal and the posterior incudal ligaments.[79] In such a rotating system, the stiffening torque associated with malleus fixation is proportional to the distance between the fixation and the axis of rotation. When the fixation is at the axis of rotation (the anterior malleal ligament), the fixation-associated stiffening torque is small, whereas when a similar fixation is placed away from the axis of rotation at the malleus head (such as a bony spur), a much larger stiffening torque results.

Tympanic Membrane Perforation

Perforations of the tympanic membrane cause a conductive hearing loss that can range from negligible to 50 dB (Figure 3–13). The primary mechanism of conductive loss due to a perforation is a reduction in ossicular coupling caused by a loss in the sound-pressure difference across the tympanic membrane.[63,83–86] The sound–pressure difference across the tympanic membrane provides the primary drive to the motion of the drum and ossicles. Perforation-induced physical changes such as reduction in

FIGURE 3–11 • Comparison of air–bone gaps measured in 5 cases with missing tympanic membrane (TM), malleus and incus to air–bone gaps predicted on the basis of acoustic coupling. With loss of the tympanic membrane, there is enhancement of acoustic coupling by about 10 to 20 dB compared to the normal ear. The predicted and measured gaps are similar. *After Peake et al.*[39]

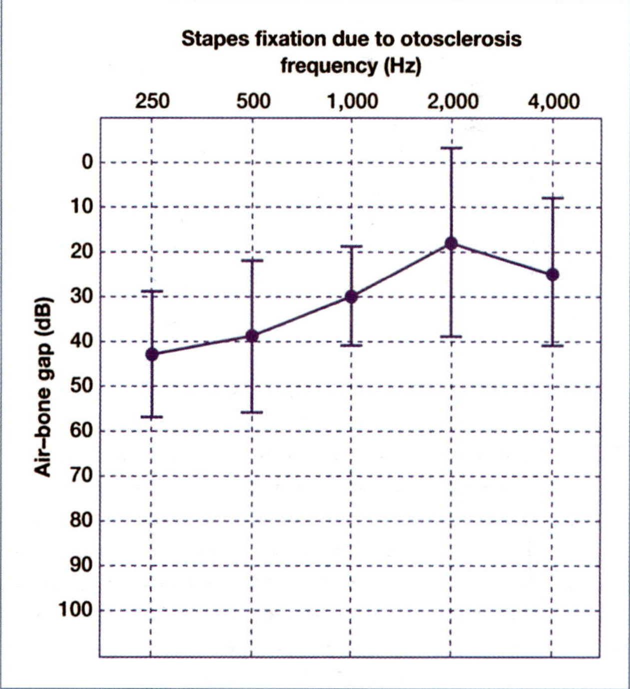

FIGURE 3–12 • Air–bone gaps measured in 75 cases of surgically confirmed stapes fixation of varying degrees due to otosclerosis. The mean ± 1 standard deviation of the air–bone gap at each frequency is shown. The conductive hearing loss is greater for the lower frequencies.

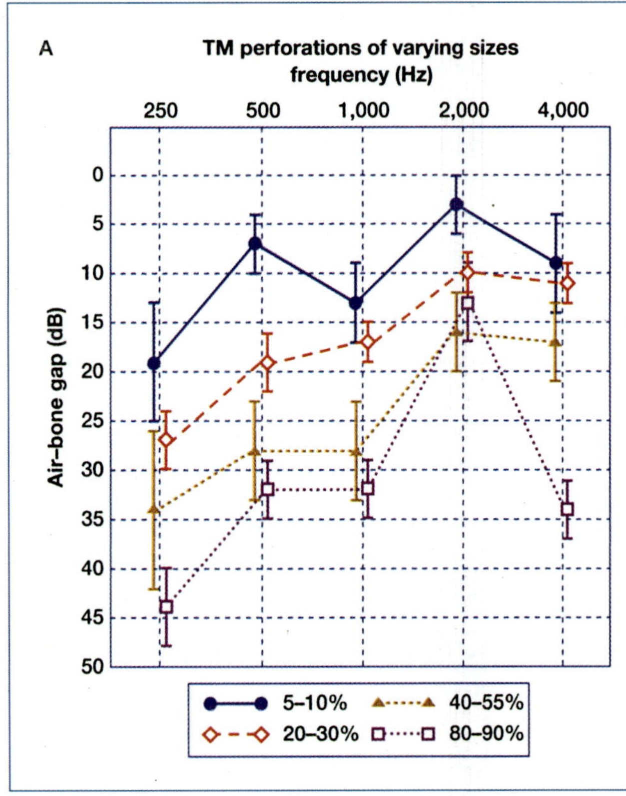

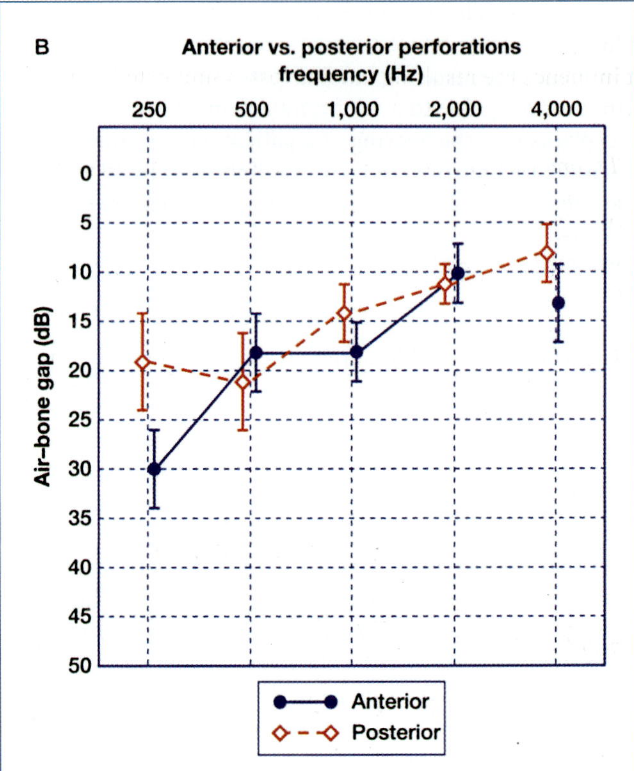

FIGURE 3–13 • Air–bone gaps measured in 42 ears with tympanic membrane perforations. In each case, the conductive hearing loss was caused solely by the perforation, because (1) the ossicular chain was found to be intact and mobile at subsequent tympanoplasty surgery done to repair the perforation, and (2) there was closure of the air–bone gap after the surgery. *A*, Air–bone gaps (mean ± one standard error of mean) are shown for perforations of varying sizes. Perforation size was estimated as a percentage of the area of the tympanic membrane. There were four groups of perforations, based on their size: 5 to 10% (5 ears), 20 to 30% (22 ears), 45 to 55% (6 ears), and 80 to 90 % (9 ears). Air–bone gaps are greater at the lower frequencies, and the gaps increase as the perforations get larger. The largest perforation-induced air–bone gaps are about 40 to 50 dB. *B*, Air–bone gaps (mean ± one standard error of mean) are shown for anterior versus posterior perforations of the same size. The ears of perforation size equal to 20 to 30% of tympanic membrane area from the dataset shown in *A*, were subdivided into anterior (11 ears), and posterior (8 ears) groups, based on location of the perforation with respect to the manubrium. There are no statistically significant differences between the two means at any frequency. (In 3 ears with 20 to 30% perforations, the perforation was directly inferior to the umbo, and they were excluded from the anterior versus posterior analysis.)

tympanic membrane area or changes in coupling of tympanic membrane motion to the malleus do not appear to contribute significantly to the hearing loss caused by a perforation.[84–86]

Perforations cause a loss that depends on frequency, perforation size, and middle-ear air space volume.[84–86] Perforation induced losses are greatest at the lowest frequencies and generally decrease as frequency increases. Perforation size is an important determinant of the loss; larger perforations result in larger hearing losses (Figure 3–13A). The volume of the middle-ear air space (combined tympanic cavity and mastoid air volume) is also an important parameter that determines the amount of hearing loss caused by a perforation; small middle-ear air space volumes result in larger air–bone gaps. Other things being equal, for a given sound pressure in the ear canal and a given perforation, the resulting sound pressure within the middle-ear cavity will vary inversely with middle-ear volume. Hence, the transtympanic membrane sound–pressure difference will be smaller (and the conductive loss correspondingly greater) with smaller middle-ear volumes.[84,87] Identical perforations in two different ears can have conductive losses that differ by up to 20 to 30 dB if the middle-ear air space volumes differ substantially (within normal ears, middle-ear air space volume can range from 2 to 20 cm^3).[88] Thus, a perforation will result in a larger air–bone gap when the mastoid is extremely sclerotic compared to one that is well pneumatized. The dependence of the hearing loss on the middle ear and mastoid air volume can explain the common clinical observation that seemingly identical perforations (in size and location) may produce significantly different degrees of hearing loss. It can also explain the clinical observation that an air–bone gap in a given perforation can vary from time to time in the same ear. For example, the air–bone gap is often smaller when the perforation is dry compared to when it is wet and draining. It is likely that in the infected situation, the volume of air in the middle ear and mastoid is reduced compared to the dry state.

The dependence of perforation-induced hearing loss on the transtympanic membrane sound–pressure difference also suggests that there should be *no* systematic differences in the air–bone gaps caused by perforations of identical size at different locations. The notion that location of a perforation should not influence the resulting hearing loss is supported by the following evidence-to-date:

1. *Theoretical calculations.* While it has been demonstrated that perforations of the tympanic membrane lead to increases in the sound pressure outside the cochlear windows, since the wave lengths of sound are generally larger than the middle-ear dimensions, the acoustically coupled window-pressure difference should not depend on perforation location.
2. *Experimental data.* Measurements in a temporal bone preparation have shown that the location of a perforation affects neither the resulting loss in sound transmission, nor the magnitude or phase of the sound pressures acting at the oval and round windows.[84–86]
3. *Clinical data.* Figure 3–13B compares air–bone gaps between same-sized perforations situated in anterior versus posterior locations, and there is no significant difference between the two groups. Mehta et al.,[87] in a study of 62 cases, found no significant differences in air–bone gaps at any frequency for perforations in the anterior versus posterior quadrants, after controlling for size of perforation and middle-ear air volumes. We speculate that the common clinical perception that perforations of similar size but different locations produce different hearing losses may result from inter-ear differences in the volume of the middle-ear and mastoid air space.[84–86]

Finally, measurements in temporal bones[40,84–86] demonstrate that tympanic membrane perforations lead to an increase in acoustic coupling by 10 to 20 dB due to loss of the shielding effect of the intact tympanic membrane. The increase in acoustic coupling allows one to predict that the maximum conductive loss following a perforation will be about 40 to 50 dB, which is consistent with clinical observations (Figure 3–13A).

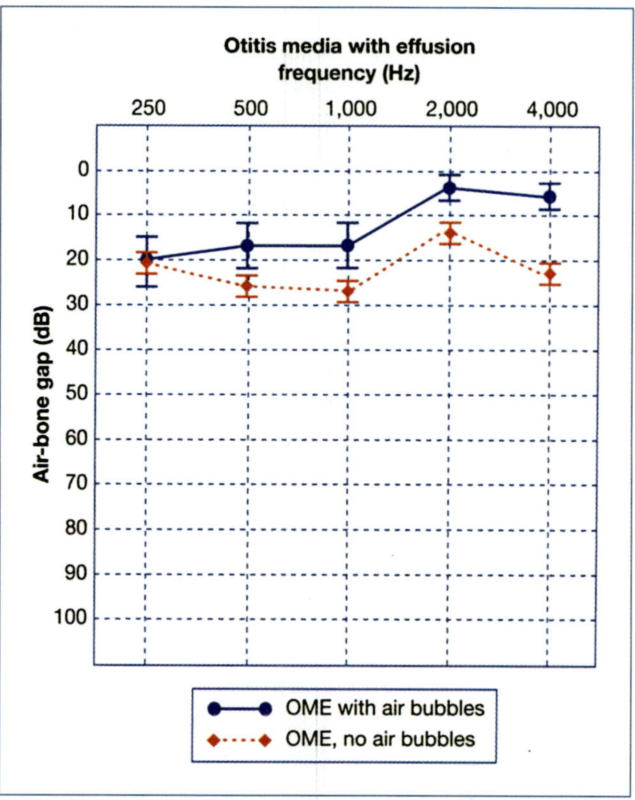

FIGURE 3–14 • Air–bone gaps (mean ± one standard error of mean) measured in 29 adult ears with otitis media with effusion (OME). In each case, the air–bone gap disappeared when the OME resolved, either spontaneously or after myringotomy. Two groups of ears are displayed, based on absence (N = 24) or presence (N = 5) of visible air bubbles behind the tympanic membrane at otoscopy, at the time the air–bone gaps were measured. Ears with air in the tympanic cavity show a smaller conductive loss than ears with no visible air bubbles. The differences between the two groups are statistically significant at the 5% level for 1,000, 2,000, and 4,000 Hz.

Middle Ear Effusion

Fluid in the middle ear, a primary feature of otitis media with effusion (OME), is associated with a conductive hearing loss of up to 30 to 35 dB,[89] though the degree and frequency dependence of individual losses vary (Figure 3–14). The conductive loss occurs because of a reduction in ossicular coupling due to several mechanisms.[90] At frequencies greater than 1,000 Hz, the loss is caused primarily by mass loading of the tympanic membrane by fluid, with decreases in sound transmission of up to 20 to 30 dB. The effect increases as more of the tympanic membrane surface area is covered with fluid. At frequencies below 1,000 Hz, the hearing loss is due to an increase in impedance of the middle-ear air space resulting from reduced middle-ear air volume, and possibly from negative middle-ear static pressure which is often associated with OME. Increasing the viscosity of the middle-ear fluid appears to have rather small effects (less than 5–10 dB) on the overall hearing loss.

Tympanic Membrane Atelectasis

Atelectasis of the tympanic membrane occurring without a tympanic membrane perforation (and in the presence of intact and mobile ossicles) can result in conductive hearing losses that vary in severity from negligible to 50 dB.[37] The conductive loss can be explained on the basis of a reduction in ossicular coupling due to the tympanic membrane abnormality. As long as the area outside the round window remains aerated and is shielded from the sound pressure in the ear canal by the tympanic membrane, the conductive hearing loss caused by the atelectasis should not exceed the amount of middle-ear sound pressure gain in normal ears, ie, air–bone gaps of up to 25 dB. If the atelectasis results in invagination of the tympanic membrane into the round window niche, the protective effect of the tympanic membrane and middle-ear air space on round window motion is lost, and larger 40 to 50 air–bone gaps should result. This prediction is consistent with the amount of acoustic coupling in cases where there is loss of the tympanic membrane, malleus, and incus.

Third Window Lesions of the Inner Ear

The majority of cases demonstrating an air–bone gap are the result of middle-ear pathology affecting the tympanic membrane or ossicular chain. However, there are a number of disorders affecting the inner ear that can result in an apparent conductive hearing loss in the absence of true middle-ear pathology. Their clinical presentation can mimic otosclerosis or other middle-ear disease. These disorders of the labyrinth produce an air–bone gap by creating a pathologic "third window' in the inner ear (in addition to the two normal windows, the oval and round windows).[91] The third window permits dissipation of air conducted sound energy away from the cochlea, thus resulting in a hearing loss by air conduction. At the same time, the third window improves thresholds for bone conducted sounds or leaves the bone thresholds unchanged. Thus, the net audiometric effect of the third window is a conductive hearing loss (air–bone gap).

The best characterized of these third window lesions is the syndrome of superior canal dehiscence.[92–95] The typical audiometric manifestation is an air–bone gap in the low and middle frequencies below 2,000 Hz, with no gap or only a small gap at higher frequencies. Low-frequency bone conduction thresholds may be at supra-normal levels of up to -20 dB or better.

Besides superior canal dehiscence, a number of disorders of the inner ear can result in pathologic third windows (Table 3–3).[96,97] Such lesions may be anatomically discrete or diffuse. Anatomically discrete lesions may be classified by location: semicircular canals (superior, lateral or, posterior canal dehiscence), bony vestibule (enlarged vestibular aqueduct, other inner ear malformations) or the cochlea (carotid–cochlea dehiscence, X-linked deafness with stapes gusher). An example of an anatomically diffuse lesion is Paget disease which may behave as a distributed third window.

The syndrome of superior canal dehiscence has been used as a prototype to investigate the mechanisms by which an air–bone gap rises in third window lesions. These investigations have included theoretical model analyses,[91,98] measurements in cadaveric human temporal bone preparations,[99] experiments in animal models of superior canal dehiscence,[100,101] and measures of middle-ear sound transmission in patients.[95,102] These studies have suggested the following conceptual mechanism causing the air–bone gap (Figure 3–15). In the normal ear, air conducted sound stimuli entered the vestibule through motion of the stapes. An inward motion of the stapes is accompanied by an equal but outward motion of the round window membrane. The fluid flow between the windows produces a pressure difference between the scala vestibuli and scala tympani, resulting in motion of the cochlear partition, activation of hair cells, and perception of sound. A pathologic third window on the vestibular side of the cochlear partition shunts a portion of the acoustic energy away from the cochlear partition, producing a decrease in sound pressure within the vestibule, thus resulting in a loss of hearing sensitivity to air-conducted sound. The effect of a third window on bone conduction thresholds is less intuitive but can be understood based on the compression of mechanism of bone conduction. In the normal ear, compression of inner-ear fluids by bone conducted sound results in a hearing percept because of an inequality in the impedance between the scala vestibuli side and the scala tympani side of the cochlear partition, which in turn, is due to a difference between the impedance of the oval and round windows, respectively. This inequality leads to a pressure difference across the cochlear partition, resulting in motion of the basilar membrane that leads to the perception of bone-conducted sound. A pathologic third window on the vestibular side of the cochlear partition increases the pressure difference between the two sides of the cochlear partition by lowering the impedance on the vestibuli side, thereby improving the cochlear response to bone conduction. Therefore, supra-normal thresholds for bone conduction may be evident. It should be noted that such improvements of bone conducted thresholds produced by the third window may be masked by an accompanying true sensorineural hearing loss.

It is important to note that the pathologic third window must be on the scala vestibuli side of the cochlear partition to produce an air–bone gap (ie, the window must be in the bony vestibule, in one of the semicircular canals, or in the bony wall of the scala vestibuli of the cochlea). A third window on the scala tympani side, such as an enlarged cochlear aqueduct, is not predicted to result in a conductive hearing loss and may even lead to an improvement in hearing function by increasing the sound pressure difference across the cochlear partition that results from air- and bone-conducted sound.

A number of audiometric clues and tests are available to the clinician for making an accurate diagnosis of an air–bone gap caused by a third window lesion as opposed to a pathological lesion within the middle ear.[93,94,97] A low-frequency air–bone gap with bone conduction thresholds that are better than 0 dB can be a clue. Therefore, it is important to accurately assess audiometric bone conduction thresholds to levels below 0 dB HL. Acoustic reflexes are typically absent in true middle-ear disease, but are generally present in third window lesions. Vestibular evoked myogenic responses are typically absent in patients with true middle-ear pathology but may be larger than normal and present at lower stimulus levels in third window lesions. Vestibular manifestations comprising sound- or pressure-induced vertigo and eye movements may be evident in third window lesions caused by canal dehiscences. When audiometric and other tests suggest that an inner ear

TABLE 3–3 Third-window lesions of the inner ear causing air-bone gaps

1. Anatomical third window
   a. Semicircular canal
      - Superior canal dehiscence
      - Posterior canal dehiscence
      - Lateral canal dehiscence
   b. Vestibule
      - Large vestibular aqueduct syndrome
      - Inner ear malformations causing a dehiscence between internal auditory canal and vestibule
   c. Cochlea
      - Dehiscence between carotid canal and scala vestibuli
      - Inner ear malformations causing a dehiscence between internal auditory canal and scala vestibuli, eg, DFN-3 (X-linked deafness with stapes gusher)
2. Diffuse or distributed third window
   a. Paget disease of the temporal bone

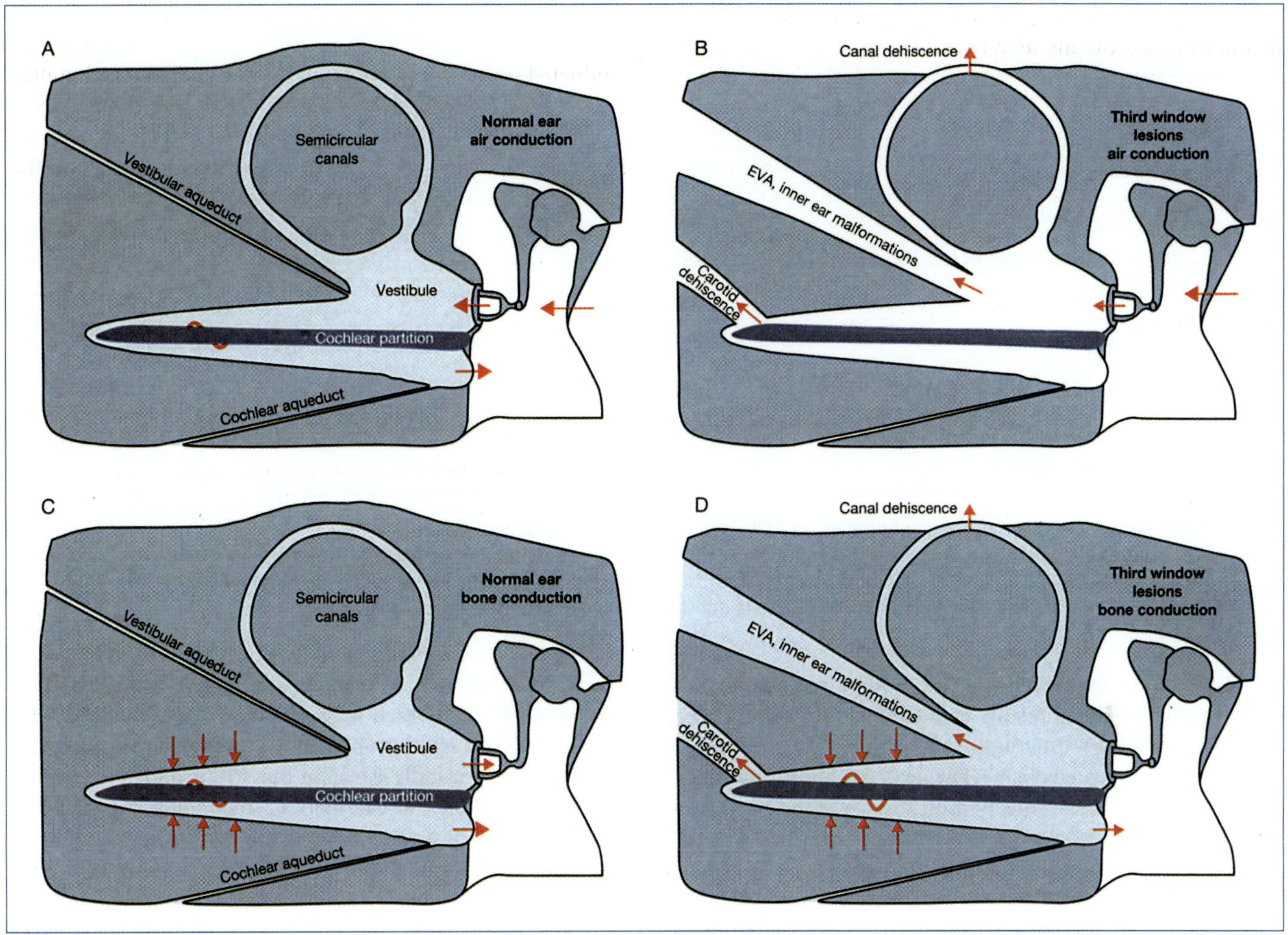

FIGURE 3–15 • Schematic representations of mechanism of air–bone gap in third window lesions. *A*, Normal ear, air conduction. Air-conducted sound stimuli enter the vestibule through motion of the stapes. There is a pressure difference between the scala vestibuli and the scala tympani, resulting in motion of the cochlear partition. The volume velocities of the oval and round windows are equal in magnitude but opposite in phase. *B*, Third-window lesion, air-conduction. It is hypothesized that a third window (in one of the canals, the vestibule or the scala vestibuli) allows a portion of the acoustic energy entering the vestibule through motion of the stapes to be shunted away from the cochlea. The shunting occurs primarily at low frequencies, resulting in a hearing loss by air-conduction. *C*, Normal ear, bone-conduction. Compression of inner ear fluid by bone-conducted sound results in a hearing percept because of an inequality in the impedance between the scala vestibuli side and the scala tympani side of the cochlear partition. This inequality is primarily due to a difference in the impedance between the oval and windows. As a result, there is a pressure difference across the cochlear partition, resulting in motion of the basilar membrane that leads to perception of bone-conducted sound. *D*, Third window lesion, bone-conduction. A third window increases the difference between the impedance on the scala vestibuli side and the scala tympani side of the cochlear partition by lowering the impedance on the vestibuli side, thereby improving the cochlear response to bone-conduction. In patients with healthy cochleae as in superior canal dehiscence, supranormal bone-conduction thresholds may be evident. In other patients with an accompanying true sensorineural hearing as in DFN-3, enlarged vestibular aqueduct (EVA), etc, the improved bone-conduction due to the third window mechanism may not be result in supranormal thresholds. *After Merchant and Rosowski.*[97]

lesion may be responsible for the conductive hearing loss, an appropriate imaging study such as a CT scan will help to make a definitive diagnosis.

ACOUSTICS AND MECHANICS OF RECONSTRUCTED MIDDLE EARS

Though tympanomastoid surgery for chronic otitis media is quite successful in controlling infection with reported success rates in excess of 80 to 90% (Chapter 28), it is well recognized that post-tympanoplasty hearing results are often unsatisfactory, especially with advanced lesions of the ossicular chain or when there is inadequate aeration of the middle ear. Table 3–4 is a summary of postsurgical hearing results from eight large clinical series[103–110] spanning the past three decades that demonstrates results are often less than satisfactory. When the ossicular chain has to be reconstructed, long term closure of the air–bone gap to ≤20 dB occurs in only 40 to 70% of cases when the stapes is intact, and only in 30 to 60% of cases when the stapes superstructure is missing.

TABLE 3–4 Hearing results after ossicular reconstruction: Cases (%) with postoperative air-bone gaps ≤ 20 dB

AUTHORS	NO. OF CASES	MINOR COLUMELLAS, INCLUDING PORPs	MAJOR COLUMELLAS, INCLUDING TORPs
1. Lee and Schuknecht, 1971[103]	936	40	—
2. Pennington, 1973[104]	216	70	—
3. Jackson, Glasscock et al., 1983[105]	417	64	43
4. Brackmann, Sheehy, and Luxford, 1984[106]	1,042	73	55
5. Lau and Tos, 1986[107]	229	54	40
6. Ragheb, Gantz, and McCabe, 1987[108]	455	52	37
7. Colletti et al., 1987[109]	832	48–80*	28–70*
8. Goldenberg, 1992[110]	262	57	58

PORP, partial ossicular replacement prosthesis; TORP, total ossicular replacement prosthesis.
Minor columella refers to an ossicular strut or prosthesis from the stapes head to the tympanic membrane/manubrium.
Major columella refers to an ossicular strut or prosthesis from the stapes footplate to the tympanic membrane/manubrium.
* Results varied with time interval after surgery: results got worse with increasing length of follow-up.

One factor responsible for the modest nature of post-tympanoplasty hearing results is lack of quantitative understanding of structure–function relationships in the mechanical response of reconstructed ears. The need for improved understanding of middle-ear mechanics is clearly shown by the clinical occurrence of many instances in which the structural differences between a good and poor hearing result are not apparent or where seemingly minor variations in structure are associated with large differences in function. For example, Liston et al.,[111] with the use of intraoperative monitoring by auditory evoked responses during ossiculoplasty, found that changes in prosthesis position of 0.5 to 1.0 mm had effects on hearing as large as 20 dB. It is also a common clinical observation that postsurgical ears, which seem identical in structure, can exhibit markedly different degrees of conductive hearing loss. Better quantitative understanding of the factors that determine the hearing response, eg, graft stiffness and tension, and the mechanical properties of the prosthesis, should permit us to understand what are the important structural differences that might account for these seemingly unexplainable results.

Other major factors contributing to unsatisfactory postsurgical hearing results are incomplete knowledge of the biology of chronic middle-ear disease (including pathology of middle-ear aeration and Eustachian tube function), and a lack of control over the histopathological and tissue responses of the middle ear to surgery. These factors are outside the scope of this chapter.

Reconstruction of the Sound Conduction Mechanisms

The goal of tympanoplasty is to restore sound pressure transformation at the oval window by coupling an intact tympanic membrane with a mobile stapes footplate via an intact or reconstructed ossicular chain, and to provide sound protection for the round window membrane by means of a closed, air-containing, mucosa-lined middle ear. As previously mentioned, the mean sound–pressure gain provided by the normal ear is only about 20 dB. Consequently, a mechanically mobile but suboptimal tympanoplasty, combined with adequate stapes mobility, adequate middle-ear aeration and round window sound protection, can result in no middle-ear gain but still produce a relatively good hearing result. For example, a tympanoplasty that gives a middle-ear gain of 5 dB but leaves the middle ear aerated and allows round window motion, will result in an air–bone gap of only 15 dB. (Of course, an immobile, rigid tympanoplasty graft will result in very little stapes motion and much larger hearing losses.) As previously discussed, the magnitude of the ossicularly coupled sound pressure at the oval window is significantly greater than the acoustically coupled sound pressure at the round window in the normal ear and we suspect a similar pressure gain after successful tympanoplasty. Under these circumstances, differences in phase of sound pressures at the oval and round windows have little effect in determining the hearing outcome. Therefore, the goal of a tympanoplasty should be to increase the magnitude of sound pressure at the oval window relative to the round window, *without* regard to phase.

The following subsections attempt to describe the structural parameters that are thought to be important to hearing results after middle-ear surgery.

Aeration of the Middle Ear

Aeration of the middle ear (including the round window) is *critical* to the success of any tympanoplasty procedure. Aeration allows the tympanic membrane, ossicles and round window to move. Clinical experience has shown that nonaerated ears often demonstrate 40-to 60-dB air–bone gaps.[38] The large gap in nonaerated ears occurs because (1) ossicular coupling is greatly reduced and (2) stapes motion is reduced because the round window membrane (which is coupled to the stapes by incompressible cochlear fluids) cannot move freely.

How much air is necessary behind the tympanic membrane (that is, within the middle ear and mastoid)? Model analyses of the effects of varying the volume of the middle ear and mastoid predict an increasing low frequency hearing loss as air volume is reduced[112] (Figure 3–16). The normal, average volume of the middle ear and mastoid is 6 cc; a combined middle ear and mastoid volume of 0.5 cc is predicted to result in a 10 dB conductive hearing loss. Volumes smaller than 0.5 cc should lead to progressively larger gaps, whereas increases in volume above about 1.0 cc should provide little additional acoustic benefit. Experimental studies[29,113] using a human temporal bone preparation where the middle ear and mastoid volume was reduced progressively show results consistent with the model prediction.

The above predictions of the effect of middle ear and mastoid air volume on the air–bone gap are applicable to those cases where the tympanic membrane is intact. Once there is a perforation of the tympanic membrane, then the volume of the middle ear and mastoid air space has an important bearing on the resulting air–bone gap, as discussed earlier.

Another parameter of the middle-ear air space that can influence middle-ear mechanics is the static air pressure within the space. Experiments in human perception dating back to the 19th century,[114] numerous animal studies[2,59] and measurements of ossicular motion in human temporal bones[115] have demonstrated that middle-ear static pressure can have different effects on sound transmission at different frequencies. Generally, transtympanic membrane static pressure differences produce decreases in sound transmission through the middle ear for frequencies less than 1,000 Hz, and have less effect at higher frequencies. Also, the effect of such static pressure differences are asymmetric with larger decreases observed when the middle-ear pressure is negative relative to that in the ear canal. The mechanisms by which pressure changes reduce middle-ear sound transmission are not well defined, and possible sites of pressure sensitivity include the tympanic membrane, annular ligament, incudo-malleal joint, and suspensory ligaments of the ossicles. Some of these structures are drastically altered as a result of tympanoplasty, and the acoustic effects of negative and positive middle-ear static pressure in reconstructed ears have not been characterized.

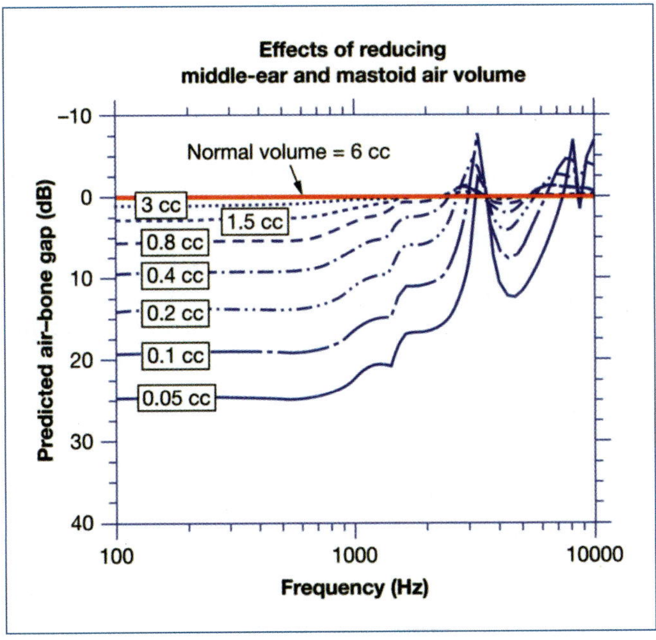

FIGURE 3–16 • Model predictions of the effects of reducing the volume of the middle ear and mastoid. The normal baseline volume is taken to be 6 cc. Note that reduction of the volume to 0.4 cc is predicted to result in an air–bone gap less than 10 dB. Volumes smaller than 0.4 cc are predicted to lead to progressively larger gaps. *After Rosowski and Merchant.*[112]

Tympanoplasty Techniques without Ossicular Linkage: Types IV and V

A type IV tympanoplasty[116] is a surgical option in cases where the tympanic membrane and ossicles are missing, the stapes footplate is mobile and there is a canal wall-down mastoid cavity. Incoming sound from the ear canal impinges directly on the stapes footplate while the round window is shielded from the sound in the ear canal by a tissue graft such as temporalis fascia (Figure 3–17). If the stapes footplate is ankylosed, it is removed and replaced by a fat graft and this arrangement constitutes a type V tympanoplasty.[117] In both type IV and type V procedures, there is no ossicular coupling and residual hearing depends on acoustic coupling.[39,118–120] The introduction of a tissue graft to shield the round window from sound enhances acoustic coupling by increasing the sound pressure difference between the oval and round windows. Model analyses of type IV reconstructions[118,119] suggest that an optimum reconstruction (defined by normal footplate mobility, a sufficiently stiff acoustic graft-shield, and adequate aeration of the round window) results in *maximum* acoustic coupling with a predicted residual conductive hearing loss of only 20 to 25 dB. This optimum result is consistent with the best type IV hearing results (Figure 3–18). These analyses also predict that decreased footplate mobility, inadequate acoustic shielding or inadequate round window aeration can lead to hearing losses as large as 60 dB.

Since the literature demonstrates that less than 50% of ears after type IV surgery have air–bone gaps less than 30 dB,[119] it is clear that many type IV reconstructions are nonoptimum.

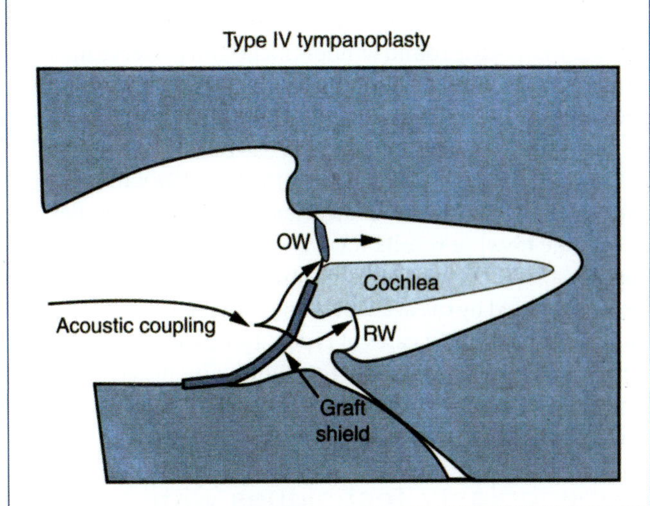

FIGURE 3–17 • Schematic of type IV tympanoplasty. Incoming sound from the ear canal impinges directly on a mobile stapes footplate within the oval window (OW), while the round window (RW) is acoustically protected by a graft-shield. With no ossicular coupling, cochlear stimulation depends on acoustic coupling.

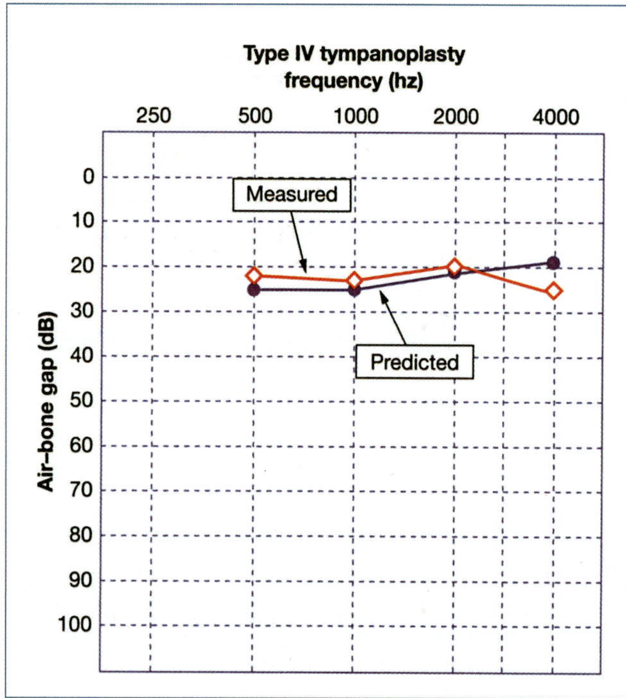

FIGURE 3–18 • Air–bone gaps after type IV tympanoplasty: the best surgical results are compared with a prediction based on "maximum" acoustic coupling. The predicted and measured results are similar, with an air–bone gap of approximately 20 dB. *After Peake et al.*[39]

The following surgical guidelines can be used to optimize the postoperative hearing results: (1) one should preserve normal stapes mobility by covering the footplate with a thin split-thickness skin graft and not a fascia graft (fascia is much thicker than skin and can increase footplate impedance), (2) one should reinforce the round window fascia graft-shield with cartilage or 1 mm thick Silastic™ (reinforcing the graft-shield in this manner increases its stiffness and improves its performance as an acoustic shield), and (3) one should create conditions that promote aeration of the round window niche and preserve mobility of the round window membrane (eg, by preserving all healthy mucosa in the protympanum and hypotympanum).

In a type V tympanoplasty, it is reasonable to assume that the mobility of the fat used to replace the footplate will be greater than that of the normal footplate. Hence, one would predict that the average hearing results for a type V would be better than those for a type IV, especially for low frequencies. This prediction is supported by the available clinical evidence. For example, in a clinical series of 64 cases of type V tympanoplasty[121] 86% of ears with conditions favorable for round window aeration had an air–bone gap smaller than the 20-dB gap that occurs with an optimum type IV.

Tympanoplasty Techniques with Reconstruction or Preservation of Ossicular Linkage: Types I, II, and III

Type I, II, and III tympanoplasty involve reconstruction of the tympanic membrane and/or the ossicular chain. Besides maintenance of middle-ear aeration and static pressure, the postoperative hearing result depends on the efficacies of the reconstructed eardrum and the reconstructed ossicular chain.

Tympanic Membrane Reconstruction

While the tympanic membrane is responsible for most of the middle-ear sound pressure gain, the details of how that gain is achieved are not well understood. Motion of the normal tympanic membrane is complex, especially at frequencies above 1,000 Hz.[22] Clinical observations suggest that surgical techniques that restore or preserve the normal anatomy of the tympanic membrane can lead to good hearing results.[37,38] However, more research is needed to define the optimum acoustic and mechanical properties of reconstructed tympanic membranes. For example: (1) Little is known of the mechanical significance of the arrangements of structural fibers in the tympanic membrane. (2) While it has been argued that the conical shape of the normal tympanic membrane plays an important role in middle-ear function,[7,22] the possible effects of changes in tympanic membrane shape on postoperative hearing results are not understood. (3) While many existing models of tympanic membrane function have been shown to fit some of the available data,[73] there are wide differences in the structure of these models, and little effort has been made to compare their significant differences and similarities. Further, these models generally have not been applied to reconstructed tympanic membranes. Better understanding of the features of tympanic membrane structure that are critical to its function should lead to improved methods for reconstructing the ear drum.

Ossicular Reconstruction

A wide variety of ossicular grafts and prostheses are in use. However, there are limited scientific data on the optimum acoustic and mechanical properties of ossicular prostheses. Factors that can influence the acoustic performance of an ossicular prosthesis include its *stiffness, mass,* and *position,* the *tension* imposed by the prosthesis on the drum and annular ligament, and mechanical features associated with *coupling* of the prosthesis to the drum and stapes.[37,38]

In general, the stiffness of a prosthesis will not be a significant factor as long as the stiffness is much greater than that of the stapes footplate-cochlear impedance. For clinical purposes, prostheses made of ossicles, cortical bone, and many synthetic materials generally meet this requirement.

Model analysis[112] and experimental data[122,123] suggest that an increase in ossicular mass does not cause significant detriment in middle-ear sound transmission. Shown in Figure 3–19 are model predictions of air–bone gaps resulting from increasing the mass of an ossicle strut, relative to the stapes mass, which is 3 mg. Increases up to 16 times are predicted to cause less than 10 dB conductive loss and only at frequencies greater than 1,000 Hz.

The positioning of the prosthesis appears to be important to its function. Measurements in human temporal bone preparations suggest that the angle between the stapes and a prosthesis should be less than 45 degrees for optimal sound transmission.[124,125] There is also evidence that some variations in positioning produce only small changes. For example, while it is ideal to attach a prosthesis to the manubrium, experimental data show that acceptable results can occur with a prosthesis placed against the posterior-superior quadrant of the tympanic

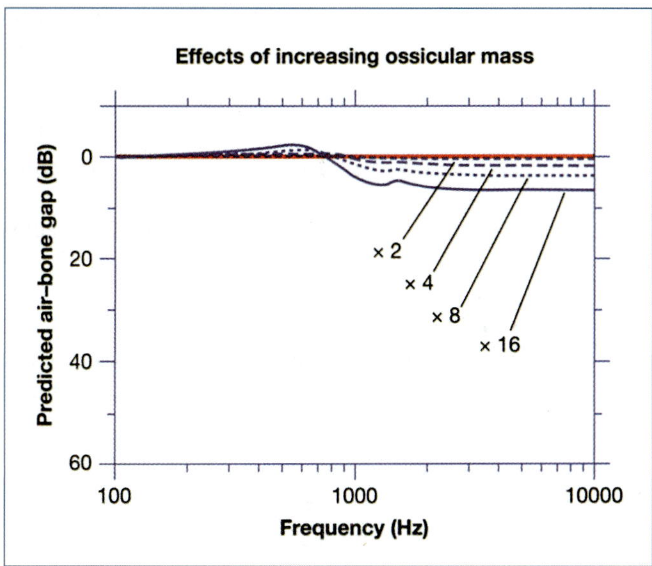

FIGURE 3–19 • Model prediction of the effects of increasing ossicular mass. The mass of an ossicular strut is increased as shown. These increases are relative to the stapes mass which is 3 mg. Increases up to 16 times are predicted to cause less than 10 dB conductive loss and only at frequencies greater than 1,000 Hz. *After Rosowski and Merchant.*[112]

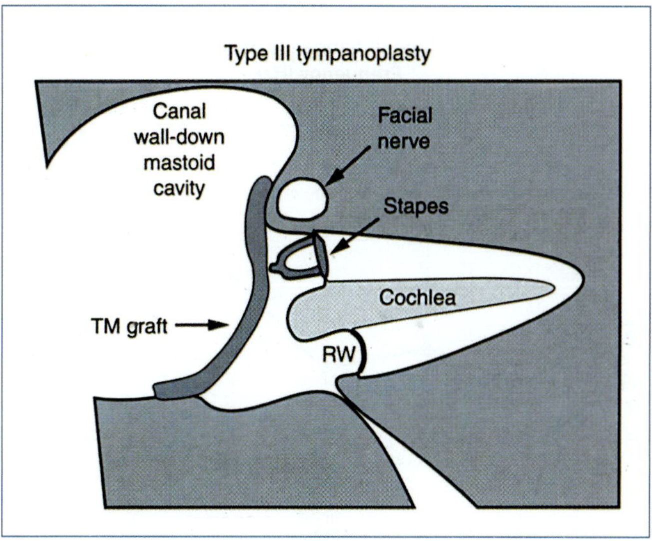

FIGURE 3–20 • Schematic of type III tympanoplasty, stapes columella. A tympanic membrane (TM) graft, usually temporalis fascia, is placed directly onto the stapes head. The procedure is typically performed in conjunction with a canal-wall-down mastoidectomy. RW, round window.

membrane as long as 3 to 4 mm of the prosthesis's diameter contacts the drum.[126]

The tension the prosthesis creates in the middle ear, which is generally a function of prosthesis length, appears critical in determining the hearing result.[127] The mechanical impedance of biological structures is inherently nonlinear, and measurements such as tympanometry have shown that the tympanic membrane and annular ligament act as linear elements only over the range of small motions (less than 10 micrometers) associated with physiological sound levels. Larger displacements of the ligament and membrane stiffen these structures. The large static displacements produced by a prosthesis that is too long would stretch the annular ligament and tympanic membrane, resulting in a stiffening of these structures, a reduction in tympano-ossicular motion and an air–bone gap. Currently, tension cannot be assessed intraoperatively in an objective fashion; a reliable objective test of this tension would be useful to the otosurgeon.

"Coupling" refers to how well a prosthesis adheres to the footplate or tympanic membrane, and the degree of coupling will determine whether or not there is slippage in sound transmission at the ends of a prosthesis. Thus, a prosthesis transmits sound effectively only if there is good coupling at both ends. Clinical observations indicate that it is rare to obtain a firm union between a prosthesis and the stapes footplate. Hence, inadequate coupling at the prosthesis-footplate joint may be an important cause of a persistent postoperative air–bone gap. The physical factors that control coupling have not been determined in a quantitative manner, and further study of this parameter is warranted.

Type III Tympanoplasty, Stapes Columella

A classical type III or stapes columella tympanoplasty (Figure 3–20) involves placement of a tympanic membrane graft such as temporalis fascia directly onto the stapes head,[116] ie, the ossicular chain is replaced by the single columella of the stapes. This tympanoplasty is typically performed in conjunction with a canal-wall-down mastoidectomy. The hearing results after this procedure vary widely with air–bone gaps ranging from 10 to 60 dB. Large air–bone gaps (40–60 dB) occur as a result of stapes fixation, nonaeration of the middle ear, or both (Figure 3–21). When the stapes is mobile and the middle ear is aerated, the average postoperative air–bone gap is on the order of 20 to 25 dB, suggesting that there is little middle-ear sound pressure gain occurring through the reconstruction. Experimental and clinical studies of the type III stapes columellar reconstruction have shown that interposing a thin disk of cartilage between the graft and the stapes head improves hearing in the lower frequencies by 5 to 10 dB.[128–130] We hypothesize that the cartilage acts to increase the "effective" area of the graft that is coupled to the stapes, which leads to an increase in the middle-ear gain of the reconstructed ear.

Canal Wall-Up Versus Canal Wall-Down Mastoidectomy

In a canal wall-down mastoidectomy, the bony tympanic annulus and much of the ear canal is removed, and the tympanic-membrane graft is placed onto the facial ridge and medial attic wall. This results in a significant reduction in the size of the residual middle-ear air space. However, as long as this air space is greater than or equal to 0.5 cc, the resultant loss of sound transmission should be less than 10 dB (see above). Since the average volume of the tympanic cavity is 0.5 to 1.0 cc,[88] a canal-wall-down procedure should create no significant acoustic detriment, so long as the middle ear is aerated. Indeed, clinical studies comparing the acoustic results of canal-wall-down versus canal-wall-up mastoidectomy have shown no significant differences in hearing between the two conditions.[106,109,130,131]

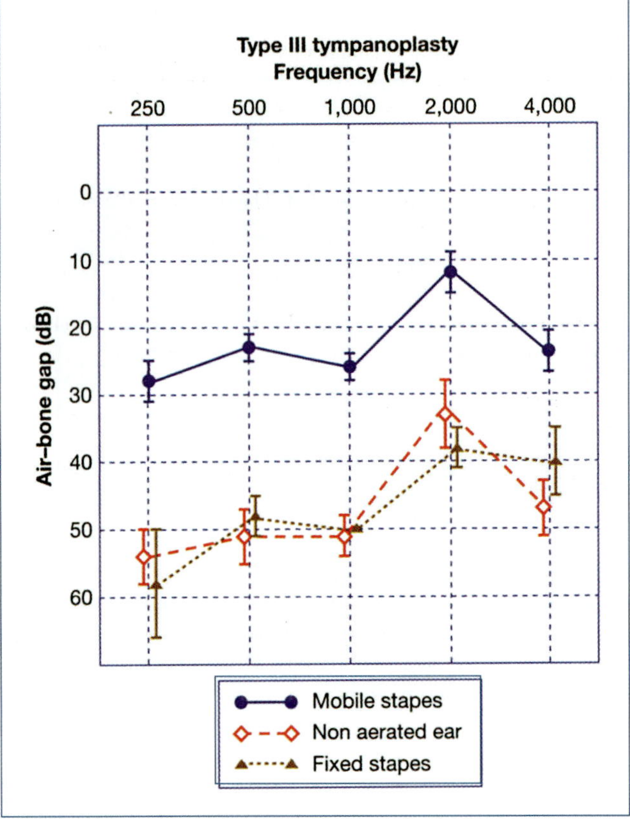

FIGURE 3–21 • Air–bone gaps (mean ± one standard error of mean) measured in 35 ears after canal-wall-down mastoidectomy and type III tympanoplasty with temporalis fascia graft onto stapes head. Results are displayed in three groups: (1) ears with a mobile stapes and an aerated middle ear after surgery, N = 23; (2) ears with a mobile stapes but no aeration of the middle ear postoperatively, N = 10; and (3) ears with an aerated middle ear postoperatively, but a fixed stapes footplate, N = 2. Mobility of the stapes was judged at time of surgery, and aeration of the middle ear was determined on the basis of postoperative CT scan assessments, pneumatic otoscopy and visible motion of the graft during a Valsalva maneuver. The best hearing results (air–bone gaps of 20 to 25 dB) are seen in those cases where the middle ear becomes aerated and the stapes is mobile. Large air–bone gaps of 40 to 60 dB occur as a result of stapes fixation, nonaeration of the middle ear or both.

A canal-wall-down procedure also results in the creation of a large air space lateral to the eardrum, ie, the air space within the mastoid bowl including the external auditory canal. This mastoid bowl and ear canal air space generates resonances which can influence middle-ear sound transmission favorably or unfavourably.[132] The structure-function relationships between the size and shape of the mastoid cavity, and cavity resonances have not been well defined. An improved understanding of this issue may help otosurgeons to configure mastoid cavities in ways that are acoustically beneficial.

Stapedotomy

The output of the middle ear can be quantified by the "volume velocity" of the stapes,[112] where volume velocity is the product of stapes linear velocity and the area of the stapes footplate. After a stapedotomy, the effective area of the footplate is reduced to the area of the prosthesis, thereby reducing the volume velocity produced by a given stapes linear velocity. The reduction in effective footplate area also reduces the area of the cochlear fluid over which the force generated by the stapes is applied. While the reduced footplate area leads to a local increase in pressure over the surface of the prosthesis, the average pressure at the cochlear entrance is reduced. The reduction in stapes volume velocity and cochlear sound pressure lead to a decrease in ossicular coupling and the development of an air–bone gap. The smaller the area of the stapes prosthesis, the greater the air–bone gap. Model predictions of the relationship between piston diameter and residual air–bone gap after stapedotomy were made using a simple lumped element model of the middle ear.[112] This analysis predicted the 0.8-mm piston diameter will produce 5 dB better hearing results than the 0.6-mm piston and 10 dB better results than the 0.4-mm piston. These predictions are in general agreement with (1) experimental temporal bone data,[133] (2) results of finite element modeling data,[134,135] and (3) clinical observations.[136–140] The predictions made in the simple lumped element model[112] assumed that the effective vibrating footplate surface area after a stapedotomy is no more than the area of the lower end of the prosthesis. In cases of partial or total stapedectomy with placement of a tissue graft and a stapes prosthesis, the effective vibrating surface may be greater than the area of the prosthesis alone, and the model predictions may overestimate the air–bone gap.

Conclusions Regarding the Contribution of Middle-Ear Mechanics to Otologic Practice

Till recently, the history of middle-ear surgery has generally progressed with minimal input from basic scientists and engineers who studied the acoustics, mechanics, and physiology of the middle ear. In this chapter, we have made a case for how knowledge of middle-ear mechanics can help the clinician to understand important aspects of present day otologic practice, and how close collaboration between clinicians and basic scientists can lead to improvements in an otologist's diagnostic and surgical capabilities. We have pointed out areas where recent work and new knowledge have produced new guidelines to optimize surgical results (eg, type III and IV tympanoplasty, stapedotomy, some aspects of ossiculoplasty), and also pointed out areas where our knowledge is incomplete and more research is needed (eg, tympanic membrane reconstruction, effect of static pressures, some aspects of ossicular reconstruction). Hopefully, some of these latter areas will be better understood by the time the next edition of this book is produced.

ACKNOWLEDGMENTS

We thank Joseph B. Nadol, Jr., MD, Michael J. McKenna, MD, Steven D. Rauch, MD, and William T. Peake, ScD, for advice and comments on previous versions of this chapter. The authors' efforts were supported by funding from the National Institute on Deafness and Other Communication Disorders of the National Institutes of Health, as well as by Mr. Axel Eliasen and Mr. Lakshmi Mittal.

References

1. Polizter A. Geschichte der Ohrenheilkunde. (2 volumes). Stuggart: F. Enke; 1907–13. (Reprinted, Hildesheim, 1967).
2. Wever EG, Lawrence M. Physiological acoustics. Princeton (NJ): Princeton University Press; 1954.
3. Leicher H, Mittermaier R, Theissing G, editors. Awanglose Abhandlungen aus dem Gebief der Hals-Nasen-Ohren-Heilkunde. Stuttgart: Georg Thieme Verlag; 1960. (English translation: A history of audiology: a comprehensive report and bibliography from the earliest beginnings to the present. Transactions of the Beltone Institute for Hearing Research, 1970.)
4. Hunt FV. Origins in acoustics: The science of sound from antiquity to the age of Newton. New Haven (CT): Yale University Press; 1978.
5. Pappas DG and Kent L. Otology's great moments. Birmingham (UK): Pappas; 2000.
6. Austin DF. Mechanics of hearing. In: Glasscock ME, Shambaugh GE, editors. Surgery of the ear. 4th ed. Philadelphia: WB Saunders; 1990. p. 297–8.
7. Helmholtz HLF. Die Mechanik der Gehörknöchelchen und des Trommelfells. Pflüg Arch ges Physiol 1868;1:1–60.
8. Yost WA. Fundamentals of hearing. New York: Academic Press; 1994.
9. Stevens SS, Davis H. Hearing. New York: Wiley; 1938.
10. Guinan JJ, Peake WT. Middle ear characteristics of anesthetized cats. J Acoust Soc Am 1967;41:1237–61.
11. Ruggero MA, Rich NC, Shivapuja BG, Temchin AN. Auditory-nerve responses to low-frequency tones: Intensity dependence. Auditory Neurosci 1996;2:159–85.
12. Sivian LJ, White SD. On minimum sound audible fields. J Acoust Soc Am 1933;4:288–321.
13. American National Standards Institute. American national standard specifications for audiometers. New York: ANSI; 1970. ANSI-S3.6-1969.
14. Shaw EAG. The external ear. In: Keidel WD, Neff WD, editors. Handbook of sensory physiology. Vol V, Part I: Auditory system. New York: Springer-Verlag; 1974. p. 455–90.
15. Dallos P. The auditory periphery. New York: Academic Press; 1973.
16. Zwislocki J. The role of the external and middle ear in sound transmission. In: Tower DB, editor. The nervous system. Vol 3: Human communication and its disorders. New York: Raven Press; 1975. p. 45–55.
17. Rosowski JJ. Models of external and middle ear function. In: Hawkins HS, McMullen TA, Popper AN, Fay RR, editors. The Springer handbook of auditory research. Vol 6: Auditory computation. New York: Springer-Verlag; 1996. p. 15–61.
18. Kirikae I. The structure and function of the middle ear. Tokyo: University of Tokyo Press; 1960.
19. Puria S, Peake WT, Rosowski JJ. Sound pressure measurements in the cochlear vestibule of human cadaver ears. J Acoust Soc Am 1997;101:2754–70.
20. Kurokawa G, Goode RL. Sound pressure gain produced by the human middle ear. Otolaryngol Head Neck Surg 1995;113:349–55.
21. Aibara R, Welsh J, Puria S, Goode R. Human middle-ear sound transfer function and cochlear input impedance. Hear Res 2001;152:100–9.
22. Tonndorf J, Khanna SM. Tympanic membrane vibrations in human cadaver ears studied by time-averaged holography. J Acoust Soc Am 1972;52:1221–33.
23. Decraemer WF, Khanna SM, Funnell WRJ. Interferometric measurement of the amplitude and phase of tympanic membrane vibrations in cat. Hear Res 1989;38:1–18.
24. Goode RL, Killion M, Nakamura K, Nishihara S. New knowledge about the function of the human middle ear: Development of an improved analog model. Am J Otol 1994;15:145–54.
25. Willi UB, Ferrazzini MA, Huber AM. The incudo-malleolar joint and sound transmission loss. Hear Res 2002;174:32–44.
26. Decraemer WF, Khanna S. Measurement, visualization and quantitative analysis of complete three-dimensional kinematical data sets of human and cat middle ear. In: K Gyo, H Wada, N Hato, T Koike,editors. Middle ear mchanics in research and otology. Singapore:World Scientific; 2004. p. 3–10.
27. Schmitt H. Über die bedeutung der Schalldrucktransformation und der Schallprotektion für die Hörschwelle. Acta Otolaryngol (Stock) 1958;49:71–80.
28. Terkildsen K. Pathologies and their effect on middle ear function. In: Feldman A, Wilber L, editors. Acoustic impedance and admittance: The measurement of middle-ear function. Baltimore: Williams & Wilkins; 1976. p. 78–102.
29. Whittemore KR, Merchant SN, Rosowski JJ. Acoustic mechanisms: Canal wall-up versus canal wall-down mastoidectomy. Otolaryngol Head, Neck Surg 1998;118:751–61.
30. Voss SE, Rosowski JJ, Merchant SN, Peake WT. Acoustic responses of the human middle ear. Hear Res 2000;150:43–69.
31. Gopen Q, Rosowski JJ, Merchant SN. Anatomy of the normal cochlear aqueduct with functional implications. Hear Res 1997;107:9–22.
32. Wever EG, Lawrence M. The acoustic pathway to the cochlea. J Acoust Soc Am 1950;22:460–7.
33. Voss SE, Rosowski JJ, Peake WT. Is the pressure difference between the oval and round windows the effective acoustic stimulus for the cochlea? J Acoust Soc Am 1996;100:1602–16.
34. Bekesy GV. Experiments in hearing. New York: McGraw Hill; 1960.
35. Wegel RL, Lane CE. The auditory masking of one pure tone by another and its probable relation to the dynamics of the inner ear. Physiol Rev 1924;23:266–85.
36. Rosen S, Bergman M, Plester D, El-Mofty A, Satti MH. Presbycusis study of a relatively noise-free population in the Sudan. Ann. Otol. Rhinol. Laryngol. 1962;71:727–43.
37. Merchant SN, Ravicz ME, Puria S, et al. Analysis of middle ear mechanics and application to diseased and reconstructed ears. Am J Otol 1997;18:139–54.
38. Merchant SN, Ravicz ME, Voss SE, Peake WT, Rosowski JJ. Toynbee Memorial Lecture 1997. Middle ear mechanics in normal, diseased and reconstructed ears. J Laryngol Otol 1998;112:715–31.
39. Peake WT, Rosowski JJ, Lynch TJ III. Middle ear transmission: Acoustic versus ossicular coupling in cat and human. Hear Res 1992;57:245–68.
40. Voss SE, Rosowski JJ, Merchant SN, Peake WT. Nonossicular signal transmission in human middle ears: Experimental assessment of the "acoustic route" with perforated tympanic membrane. J Acoust Soc Am. 2007;122:2154–73.
41. Rosowski JJ. Mechanisms of sound conduction in normal and diseased ears. In: Rosowski JJ, Merchant SN, editors. The function and mechanics of normal, diseased and reconstructed middle ears. The Hague, The Netherlands: Kugler; 2000. p. 137–45.

42. Tonndorf J. Bone conduction hearing. In: Keidel WD, Neff WD, editors. Handbook of sensory physiology. Vol V/Part III. Berlin: Springer-Verlag; 1974. p. 37–84.
43. Sohmer H, Freeman S, Geal-Dor M, Adelman C, Savion I. Bone conduction experiments in humans—A fluid pathway from bone to ear. Hear Res 2000;146:81–8.
44. Stenfelt S, Goode RL. Bone-conducted sound: Physiological and clinical aspects. Otol Neurotol 2005;26:1245–61.
45. Carhart R. The clinical application of bone conduction audiometry. Arch Otol 1950;51:798–808.
46. Carmel PW, Starr A. Acoustic and nonacoustic factors modifying middle ear muscle activity in waking cats. J. Neurophysiol 1963;26:598–616.
47. Borg E. A quantitative study of the effect of the acoustic stapedius reflex on sound transmission through the middle ear of man. Acta Otolaryngol (Stock) 1968;66:461–72.
48. Møller AR. The acoustic middle-ear muscle reflex. In: Keidel WD, Neff WD, editors. Handbook of sensory physiology: Auditory system. Vol V/Part I.Berlin: Springer-Verlag; 1974. p. 519–48.
49. Borg E, Zakrisson JE. Stapedius muscle and monaural masking. Acta Oto-Laryngol (Stockh) 1974;94:385–93.
50. Pang XD, Guinan JJ. Effects of stapedius-muscle contractions on the masking of auditory nerve responses. J Acoust Soc Am 1997;102:3576–86.
51. Borg E, Nilsson R, Engstrom B. Effect of the acoustic reflex on inner ear damage induced by industrial noise. Acta Otolaryngol (Stock) 1983;96:361–9.
52. Ingelstedt S, Jonson B. Mechanisms of gas exchange in the normal human middle ear. Acta Otolaryngol (Stock) 1966; Suppl 224: 452–61.
53. Marquet J. The incudo-malleal joint. J Laryngol Otol 1981;95:542–65.
54. Hüttenbrink KB. The mechanics of the middle-ear at static air pressures. Acta Otolaryngol (Stock) 1988; Suppl 451:1–35.
55. Pang XD, Peake WT. How do contractions of the stapedius muscle alter the acoustic properties of the middle ear? In: Allen JB, Hall JL, Hubbard A, Neely ST, Tubis A, editors. Peripheral auditory mechanisms. New York: Springer-Verlag; 1986. p. 36–43.
56. Gyo K, Aritomo H, Goode RL. Measurement of the ossicular vibration ratio in human temporal bones by use of a video measuring system. Acta Otolaryngol (Stock) 1987;103:87–95.
57. Nakajima HH, Ravicz ME, Merchant SN, Peake WT, Rosowski JJ. Experimental ossicular fixations and the middle-ear's response to sound: Evidence for a flexible ossicular chain. Hear Res 2005;204:60–77.
58. Zwislocki J. Analysis of the middle ear function. Part II. Guinea-pig ear. J Acoust Soc Amer 1963;35:1034–40.
59. Møller AR. Experimental study of the acoustic impedance of the middle ear and its transmission properties. Acta Otolaryngol (Stock) 1965;60:129–49.
60. Khanna SM, Tonndorf J. Tympanic membrane vibrations in cats studied by time-averaged holography. J Acoust Soc Am 1972;51:1904–20.
61. Nedzelnitsky V. Sound pressures in the basal turn of the cat cochlea. J Acoust Soc Am 1980;68:1676–89.
62. Nuttall AL. Tympanic muscle effects on middle-ear transfer characteristics. J Acoust Soc Am 1974;56:1239–47.
63. McArdle FE, Tonndorf J. Perforations of the tympanic membrane and their effects upon middle ear transmission. Arch Klin Exp Ohren Nasen Kehlkopfheilkd 1968;192:145–62.
64. Bigelow DC, Swanson PB, Saunders JC. The effect of tympanic membrane perforation size on umbo velocity in the rat. Laryngoscope 1996;106:71–6.
65. Wiederhold ML, Zajtchuk JT, Vap JG, Paggi RE. Hearing loss in relation to physical properties of middle ear effusions. Ann Otol Rhinol Laryngol 1980;89, Supp 68:185–89.
66. Decraemer WF, Khanna SM. Funnell WRJ. Bending of the manubrium in cat under normal sound stimulation. Prog in Biomedl Optics 1995;2329:74–84.
67. Puria S, Allen JB. Measurements and model of the cat middle ear: Evidence of tympanic membrane acoustic delay. J Acoust Soc Am 1998;104:3463–81.
68. Olson L. Observing middle and inner ear mechanics with novel intracochlear pressure sensors. J Acoust Soc Am 1998;103:3445–63.
69. Fay J, Puria S, Decraemer WF, Steele C. Three approaches for estimating the elastic modulus of the tympanic membrane. J Biomech 2005;38:1807–15.
70. Henson OW, Henson MM. The tympanic membrane: highly developed smooth muscle arrays in the annulus fibrosus of mustached bats. J Assoc Research Otolaryngol 2000;1:25–32.
71. Rosowski JJ, Carney LH, Lynch TJ, Peake WT. The effectiveness of external and middle ears in coupling acoustic power into the cochlea. In: Allen JB, Hall JL, Hubbard A, Neely ST, Tubis A,editors. Peripheral auditory mechanisms: proceedings of a conference held at Boston University, Boston, MA, August 13–16, 1985. New York: Springer-Verlag; 1986. p. 3–12.
72. Zwislocki, J. Analysis of the middle-ear function. Part I: Input impedance. J Acoust Soc Amer 1962;34:1514–23.
73. Funnell WRJ, Decraemer WM. On the incorporation of moiré shape measurements in finite-element models of the cat eardrum. J Acoust Soc Am 1996;100:925–32.
74. Gan R, Sun Q, Feng B, Wood MW. Acoustical-structural coupled finite element analysis for sound transmission in human ear pressure distributions. Med Engin Phys. 2006;28:395–404.
75. Rosowski JJ, Davis PJ, Merchant SN, Donahue KM, Coltrera MD. Cadaver middle ears as models for living ears: Comparisons of middle ear input immittance. Ann Otol Rhinol Laryngol 1990;99:403–12.
76. Goode RL, Ball G, Nishihara S, Nakamura K. Laser Doppler Vibrometer (LDV)—A new clinical tool for the otologist. Am J Otol 1996;17:813–22.
77. Chien W, Ravicz ME, Merchant SN, Rosowski JJ. The effect of methodological differences in the measurement of stapes motion in live and cadaver ears. Audiol Neurotol 2006;11:183–97.
78. Schuknecht HF. Stapedectomy. Boston: Little, Brown; 1972.
79. Nakajima HH, Ravicz ME, Rosowski JJ, Peake WT, Merchant SN. Experimental and clinical studies of malleus fixation. Laryngoscope 2005;115:147–54.
80. Schuknecht HF. Pathology of the ear. 2nd edition Philadelphia: Lea & Febiger; 1993.
81. Vincent R, Lopez A, Sperling NM. Malleus-ankylosis: A clinical, audiometric, histologic and surgical study of 123 cases. Am J Otology 1999;20:717–25.
82. Harris JP, Mehta RP, Nadol JB. Malleus fixation: Clinical and histopathologic findings. Ann Otol Rhinol Laryngol. 2002;111:246–54.
83. Kruger B, Tonndorf J. Middle ear transmission in cats with experimentally induced tympanic membrane perforations. J Acoust Soc Am 1977;61:126–32.

84. Voss SE, Rosowski JJ, Merchant SN, Peake WT. How do tympanic membrane perforations affect human middle-ear sound transmission? Acta Otolaryngol (Stockh) 2001;121:169–73.
85. Voss SE, Rosowski JJ, Merchant SN, Peake WT. Middle-ear function with tympanic membrane perforations I: Measurements and mechanisms. J Acoust Soc Am 2001;110:1432–44.
86. Voss SE, Rosowski JJ, Merchant SN, Peake WT. Middle-ear function with tympanic membrane perforations II: A simple model. J Acoust Soc Am 2001;110:1445–52.
87. Mehta RP, Rosowski JJ, Voss SE, O'Neil E, Merchant SN. Determinants of hearing loss in perforations of the tympanic membrane. Otol Neurotol 2006;27:136–43.
88. Molvaer O, Vallersnes F, Kringelbotn M. The size of the middle ear and the mastoid air cell. Acta Otolarygol (Stock) 1978;85:24–32.
89. Fria T, Cantekin E, Eichler J. Hearing acuity of children with otitis media. Arch Otolaryngol 1985;111:10–16.
90. Ravicz ME, Rosowski JJ, Merchant SN. Mechanisms of hearing loss resulting from middle ear fluid. Hear Res 2004;195: 103–1301.
91. Rosowski JJ, Songer JE, Nakajima HH, Brinsko KM, Merchant SN. Clinical, experimental and theoretical investigations of the effect of superior semicircular canal dehiscence on hearing mechanisms. Otol Neurotol 2004;25:323–32.
92. Minor LB, Solomon D, Zinreich JS, Zee DS. Sound- and/or pressure-induced vertigo due to bone dehiscence of the superior semicircular canal. Arch Otolaryngol Head Neck Surg. 1998;124:249–58.
93. Minor LB, Carey JP, Cremer PD, Lustig LR, Streubel SO, Ruckenstein MJ. Dehiscence of bone overlying the superior canal as a cause of apparent conductive hearing loss. Otol Neurotol 2003;24:270–8.
94. Halmagyi GM, Aw ST, McGarvie LA, et al. Superior semicircular canal dehiscence simulating otosclerosis. J Laryngol Otol 2003;117:553–7.
95. Mikulec AA, McKenna MJ, Ramsey MJ, et al. Superior semicircular canal dehiscence presenting as conductive hearing loss without vertigo. Otol Neurotol 2004; 25:121–29.
96. Merchant SN, Nakajima HH, Halpin C, et al. Clinical investigation and mechanism of air–bone gaps in large vestibular aqueduct syndrome. Annals Otol Rhinol Laryngol 2007;116:532–41.
97. Merchant SN, Rosowski JJ. Conductive hearing loss caused by third-window lesions of the inner ear. Otol Neurotol (in press).
98. Songer JE, Rosowski JJ. A mechano-acoustic model of the effect of superior canal dehiscence on hearing in chinchilla. J Acoust Soc Am 2007;122:943–51.
99. Chien W, Ravicz ME, Merchant SN, Rosowski JJ. Measurements of human middle- and inner-ear mechanics with dehiscence of the superior semicircular canal. Otol Neurotol 2007;28:250–57.
100. Songer JE, Rosowski JJ. The effect of superior canal dehiscence on cochlear potential in response to air-conducted stimuli in chinchilla. Hear Res 2005;210:53–62.
101. Songer JE, Rosowski JJ. The effect of superior-canal opening on middle-ear input admittance and air-conducted stapes velocity in chinchilla. J Acoust Soc Am 2006;120:258–69.
102. Rosowski JJ, Nakajima HH, Merchant SN. Clinical utility of laser-Doppler vibrometer measurements in live normal and pathologic human ears. Ear and Hearing 2008;29:3–19.
103. Lee K, Schuknecht HF. Results of tympanoplasty and mastoidectomy at the Massachusetts eye and ear infirmary. Laryngoscope 1971;81:529–43.
104. Pennington CL. Incus interposition techniques. Ann Otol 1973;82:518–31.
105. Jackson CG, Glasscock ME, Schwaber MK, Nissen AJ, Christiansen SG. Ossicular chain reconstruction: The TORP and PORP in chronic ear disease. Laryngoscope 1983;93:981–8.
106. Brackmann DE, Sheehy JL, Luxford WM. TORPS and PORPS in tympanoplasty: A review of 1042 operations. Otolaryngol Head Neck Surg 1984;92:32–7.
107. Lau T, Tos M. Long-term results of surgery for granulating otitis. Amer J Otolaryngol 1986;7:341–5.
108. Ragheb SM, Gantz BJ, McCabe BF. Hearing results after cholesteatoma surgery: The Iowa experience. Laryngoscope 1987;97:1254–63.
109. Colletti V, Fiorino FG, Sittoni V. Minisculptured ossicle grafts versus implants: Long term results. Am J Otol 1987;8: 553–59.
110. Goldenberg RA. Hydroxylapatite ossicular replacement prostheses: A four year experience. Otolaryngol-Head Neck Surg 1992;106:261–9.
111. Liston SL, Levine SC, Margolis RH, Yanz JL. Use of intraoperative auditory brainstem responses to guide prosthesis positioning. Laryngoscope 1991;101:1009–12.
112. Rosowski JJ, Merchant SN. Mechanical and acoustic analysis of middle-ear reconstruction. Am J Otol 1995;16:486–97.
113. Gyo K, Goode RL, Miller C. Effect of middle-ear modification on umbo vibration-human temporal bone experiments with a new vibration measuring system. Arch Otolaryngol Head Neck Surg 1986;112:1262–8.
114. Mach E, J Kessel. Die Function der Trommelhöhle und der Tuba Eustachii. Sitzungsber. Akad Wiss Wein math-nat Cl 1872;66:329–66.
115. Murakami S, Gyo K, Goode RL. Effect of middle ear pressure change on middle ear mechanics. Acta Otolaryngol (Stock) 1997;117:390–5.
116. Wullstein H. The restoration of the function of the middle ear, in chronic otitis media. Ann Otol Rhinol Laryngol 1956;65:1020–41.
117. Gacek RR. Symposium on tympanoplasty. Results of modified type V tympanoplasty. Laryngoscope 1973;83:437–47.
118. Rosowski JJ, Merchant SN, Ravicz ME. Middle ear mechanics of type IV and type V tympanoplasty. I. Model analysis and predictions. Am J Otol 1995;16:555–64.
119. Merchant SN, Rosowski JJ, Ravicz ME. Middle ear mechanics of type IV and type V tympanoplasty. II. Clinical analysis and surgical implications. Am J Otol 1995;16:565–75.
120. Merchant SN, Ravicz ME, Rosowski JJ. Experimental investigation of the mechanics of type IV tympanoplasty. Ann Otol Rhinol Laryngol 1997;106:49–60.
121. Montandon P, Chatelain C. Restoration of hearing with type V tympanoplasty. ORL J Otorhinolaryngol Relat Spec 1991;53:342–5.
122. Gan RZ, Dyer RK, Wood MW, Dormer KJ. Mass loading on the ossicles and middle ear function. Ann Otol Rhinol Laryngol 2001;110:478–85.
123. Bance M, Morris DP, Van Wijhe R. Effects of ossicular prosthesis mass and section of the stapes tendon on middle ear transmission. J Otolaryngol. 2007;36:113–9.
124. Vlaming MSMG, Feenstra L. Studies on the mechanics of the reconstructed human middle ear. Clin Otolaryngol 1986;11:411–22.

125. Nishihara S, Goode RL. Experimental study of the acoustic properties of incus replacement prostheses in a human temporal bone model. Am J Otol 1994;15:485–94.

126. Goode RL, Nishihara S. Experimental models of ossiculoplasty. In: Monsell E, editor. Ossiculoplasty. Otolaryngol Clin North Am 1994;27:663–75.

127. Morris DP, Bance M, van Wijhe RG, Kiefte M, Smith R. Optimum tension for partial ossicular replacement prosthesis reconstruction in the human middle ear. Laryngoscope. 2004;114:305–8.

128. Mehta RP, Ravicz ME, Rosowski JJ, Merchant SN. Middle-ear mechanics of type III tympanoplasty (stapes columella). I. Experimental studies. Otol Neurotol 2003;24:176–85.

129. Merchant SN, McKenna MJ, Mehta RP, Ravicz ME, Rosowski JJ. Middle-ear mechanics of type III tympanoplasty (stapes columella). II. Clinical studies. Otol Neurotol 2003;24:186–94.

130. Merchant SN, Rosowski JJ, McKenna MJ. Tympanoplasty: operative techniques. Otolaryngol Head Neck Surg 2003;14:224–36.

131. Toner JG, Smyth GD. Surgical treatment of cholesteatoma: a comparison of three techniques. Am J Otol. 1990;11:247–9.

132. Goode RL, Friedrichs R, Falk S. Effect on hearing thresholds of surgical modification of the external ear. Ann Otol Rhinol Laryngol 1977;86:441–51.

133. Honda N and Goode RL. The acoustic evaluation of stapedotomy using a temporal bone otosclerosis model. In Gyo K, Wada H, editors. Middle ear mechanics in research and otology. Singapore:World Scientific; 2004. p. 203–8.

134. Koike T, Wada H, Goode RL. Finite-element method analysis of transfer function of middle ear reconstructed using stapes prosthesis. In: Association for Research in Otolaryngology (ARO) Abstracts of the 24th Midwinter Meeting. Mt. Royal, (NJ): Association for Research in Otolaryngology; 2001. p. 221.

135. Bohnke F, Arnold W. Finite element model of the stapes-inner ear interface. Adv Otorhinolaryngol 2007;65:150–4.

136. Smyth GDL, Hassard TH. Eighteen years experience in stapedectomy. The case for the small fenestra operation. Ann Otol Rhinol Laryngol 1978;Suppl 49:3–36.

137. Schuknecht HF, Bentkover SH. Partial stapedectomy and piston prosthesis. In: Snow JB Jr., editor. Controversy in otolaryngology. Philadelphia: WB Saunders; 1980. p. 281–91.

138. Teig E and Lindeman HH. Stapedectomy piston diameter: is bigger better? Otorhinolaryngol Nova 1999; 9:252–6.

139. Sennaroglu L, Unal OF, Sennaroglu G, Gursel B, Belgin E. Effect of teflon piston diameter on hearing result after stapedotomy. Otolaryngol Head Neck Surg 2001;124:279–81.

140. Marchese MR, Cianfrone F, Passali GC, Paludetti G. Hearing results after stapedotomy: role of the prosthesis diameter. Audiol Neurootol 2007;12:221–5.

Auditory Physiology: Inner Ear

4

Veronika Starlinger, MD / Kinuko Masaki, PhD / Stefan Heller, PhD

INTRODUCTION

The cochlea, the mammalian auditory organ, is enclosed by the temporal bone and appears as a snail-shaped osseous structure (*cochlos* is Greek for "snail"). In humans, the cochlea is coiled for about $2^2/_3$ turns around a central axis, the modiolus. Within the bony cochlea (also known as the osseous labyrinth), three canals, or scalae, are formed by the membranous labyrinth: the central scala media, also known as the cochlear duct, is separated from the scala vestibuli by the Reissner's membrane and from the scala tympani by the basilar membrane (Figure 4–1). The connection of the scala vestibuli with the middle ear occurs via the oval window, which is attached to the stapes footplate. The round window links the scala tympani to the middle ear and is covered by the round window membrane. The scalae vestibuli and tympani merge at the cochlear apex (at the helicotrema); the scala media ends blindly. The scalae vestibuli and tympani are filled with perilymph, an extracellular fluid with high Na^+ and low K^+ concentration, whereas the scala media is filled with endolymph, which is defined by a unique ion composition of high K^+ and low Na^+ concentrations. Cochlear endolymph has a positive electrical potential of approximately +85 mV. This difference in ion composition between perilymph and endolymph and the electrical potential difference provide the energy required for the cochlea's work.

From a physiological viewpoint, three functional units within the cochlea can be distinguished: (1) The organ of Corti represents the "sensor" of the cochlea converting and amplifying mechanical sound stimuli into electrical signals (mechanoelectrical transduction). (2) The stria vascularis is the cochlea's "battery," generating the energy (endocochlear potential) necessary for mechanoelectrical transduction and influencing cochlear fluid homeostasis. (3) The spiral ganglion contains the neurons featuring axons ("electrical wires") that transport the electrical signals from the cochlea to the central nervous system. All three parts are essential for proper function of the cochlea and they will be discussed in detail in this chapter.

THE ORGAN OF CORTI

Overview

The organ of Corti is the auditory receptor organ of the mammalian cochlea. It is named after the 19th century Italian microscopist Alfonso Giacomo Gaspare Corti, who was the first to visualize and to describe this morphologically complex hearing organ.

The organ of Corti comprises two types of sensory receptors, the inner and outer hair cells. About 3,500 flask-shaped inner hair cells are lined up in a single row throughout the entire length of the human cochlear duct. Lateral to the inner hair cell row are three rows of outer hair cells that can be distinguished by their unique cylindrical shape (Figure 4–1B). Both hair cell types contain hair bundles that consist of highly organized actin-filled stereocilia that are graded in height with the most lateral row being the tallest and the most medial row being the shortest. The hair bundles of inner hair cells are organized as a smoothly curved line of two to three rows of stereocilia. Outer hair cell stereociliary bundles are arranged in a shallow V-shape (Figure 4–2). Hair bundles are the mechanosensitive organelles of hair cells. Every hair cell sits atop a phalangeal supporting cell, which for the outer hair cells are called Deiters cells. The inner and outer pillar cells delineate the area between inner and outer hair cells and frame the tunnel of Corti. Other supporting cells embrace the hair cell-bearing part of the organ of Corti. Medially, there are the inner marginal, and laterally, the Hensen's (outer marginal cells), Claudius, and Boettcher cells (Figure 4–1B). Along its entire length, the organ of Corti is covered by the tectorial membrane. This acellular structure is medially attached to the spiral limbus and connects to the hair bundles of outer hair cells.

The Basilar Membrane and Tonotopy

When sound strikes the eardrum, vibration is transmitted to the inner ear via the three middle ear ossicles. Movement of the stapes causes the displacement of the cochlear fluid in the scala

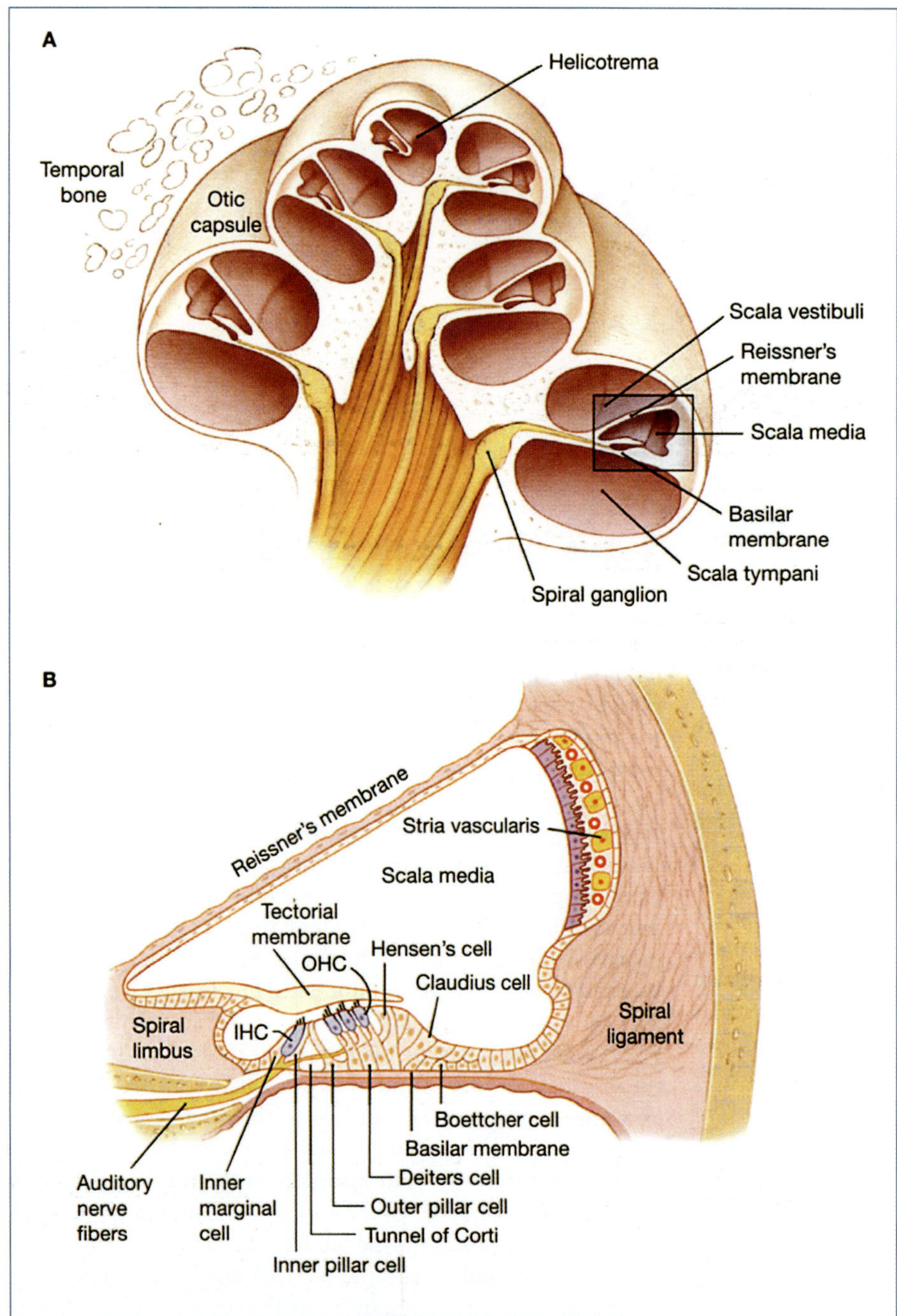

FIGURE 4–1 • Cross-section of the cochlea. *A*, schematic drawing of a cochlear cross-section. The rectangle delineates the area shown in *B*, illustrating a section of the scala media with surrounding structures such as the organ of Corti and the stria vascularis. IHC, inner hair cell; OHC, outer hair cell.

vestibuli. The incompressibility of perilymph causes a pressure gradient between the scala vestibuli and scala tympani, leading to movement of the basilar membrane and the organ of Corti. This displacement can be conceptualized as a travelling wave that moves from base to apex along the basilar membrane.[1] For a pure tone stimulus, the travelling wave reaches a maximum at a characteristic place along the basilar membrane and then decays. The precise location of this maximum depends on the frequency of the stimulus, which is the underlying principle of the tonotopic organization of the cochlea. Characteristic frequency at a specific basilar membrane location is governed by the properties of both the passive components such as extracellular, cellular, and molecular structures at that location (Figure 4–3), as well as the properties of the active system such as the cochlear amplifier (described below). The base of the cochlea is tuned for frequencies as high as 20 kHz in humans and at its apex the organ is sensitive to frequencies as low as 20 Hz. The tonotopic gradient is anatomically manifested not only in a continuous gradient in basilar membrane width but also in changes in hair cell height and the length of cellular structures such as the stereociliary hair bundles.

Inner Hair Cells and Mechanoelectrical Transduction

The cochlear inner hair cells are the linchpins in hearing as they are the sensory cells that convert mechanical stimulation into electrical signals and synaptic activity transmitted to the brain.

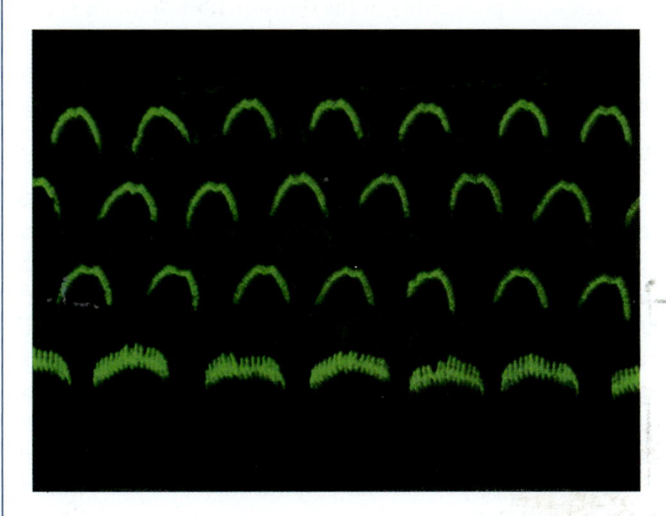

FIGURE 4–2 • Cochlear stereocilia. Shown is a view of the apical surface of a whole-mount preparation of a 150-μm long segment of the mouse organ of Corti. The stereociliary hair bundles are strongly labeled with fluorescein-conjugated phalloidin, which binds to filamentous actin. The curved hair bundles of inner hair cells are visible at the bottom as well as the three rows of V-shaped outer hair cell hair bundles at the top. *Image courtesy of Anthony W. Peng, Stanford University.*

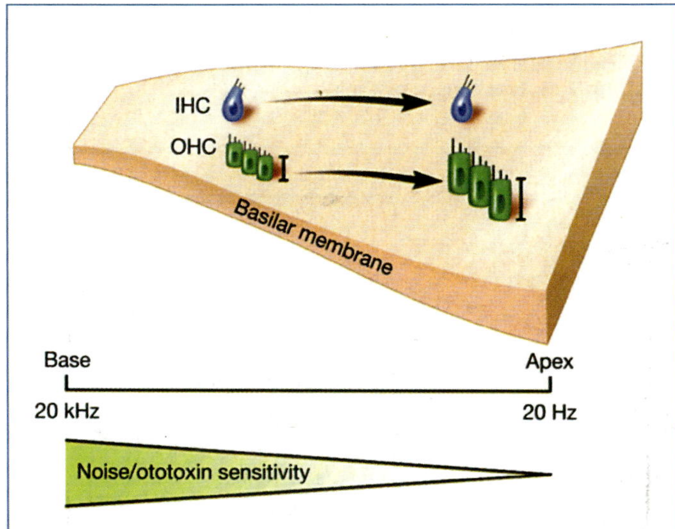

FIGURE 4–3 • Tonotopic organization of the organ of Corti. Schematic drawing of the anatomical changes along the length of the cochlea from base to apex, which include increasing width of the basilar membrane and size of the outer hair cells. These changes contribute to the frequency tuning of the organ of Corti. Likewise, sensitivity to ototoxic insults such as noise or aminoglycosides is highest at the cochlear base and decreases toward the apex.

At the core of this process is the mechanoelectrical transduction that occurs at or near the tips of the stereocilia. This mechanoelectrical transduction apparatus is present in all hair cells and consists of one or more mechanically gated cation channels, closely associated elastic structures, and a tip link that connects the tip of one stereocilium to the side of the next tallest stereocilium (Figure 4–4).[2–4]

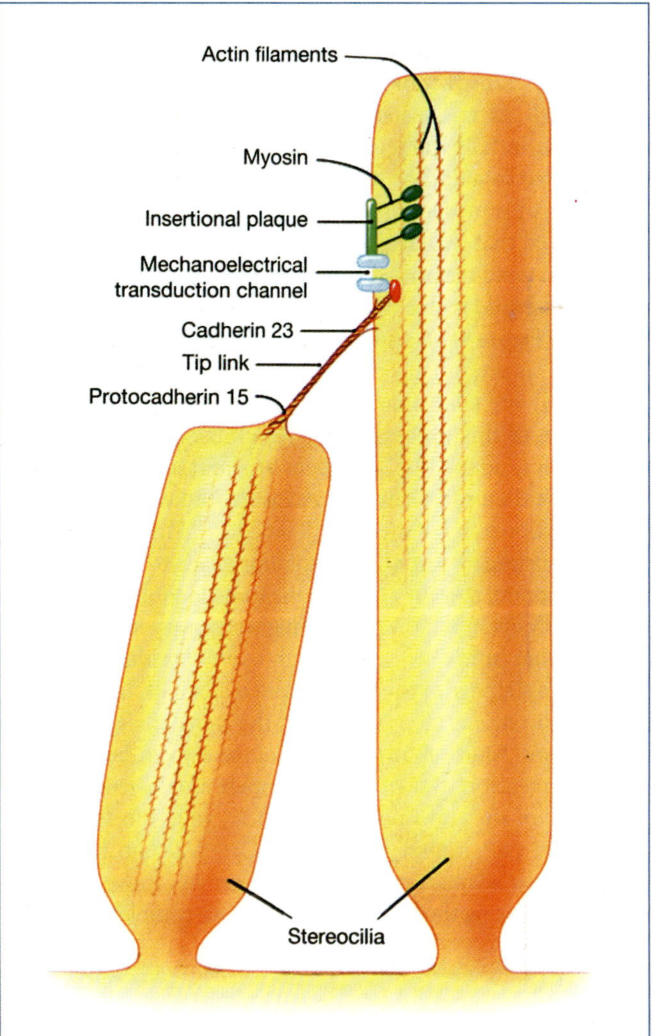

FIGURE 4–4 • Model of the stereociliary mechanoelectrical transduction apparatus. Known and proposed components of the mechanoelectrical transduction apparatus are shown.

Mechanical deflection of the hair cell's stereociliary bundle toward the tallest row of stereocilia leads to shearing motions between adjacent stereocilia.[4] The consequential increase of mechanical tension in the transduction apparatus leads to a conformational change in the transduction channel protein, leading to an increase in the channel open probability, which is about 40 to 50% at rest in the mammalian cochlea. Despite a few candidate proteins, none of the putative components of the hair cell transduction apparatus has been unequivocally linked functionally with the biophysical process of mechanotransduction. The most attractive candidates are cadherin 23 and protocadherin 15, which have been proposed as components of the tip link, and myosin 1c, which is essential for the adaptation process that controls the set point of mechanosensitivity (Figure 4–4). Mutations in the human genes encoding either cadherin 23 or protocadherin 15 cause Usher Syndrome (congenital hearing loss with progressive loss of vision from retinitis pigmentosa).

Upon mechanical stimulation toward the tallest row of stereocilia, K^+ and Ca^{2+} ions enter the hair cell through open mechanoelectrical transduction channels located near the stereociliary tips. This excitatory deflection leads to depolarization of the cell. When the stereocilia are deflected toward the shorter stereocilia, the transduction channels close, thereby hyperpolarizing the cell. After a sustained excitatory deflection of the hair bundle, the initially large transduction current adapts, which is manifested in a decline of the current that is correlated with the closure of transduction channels (Figure 4–5A). It has been hypothesized that two distinct processes are responsible for this adaptation: rapid reclosure of transduction channels and sliding of a myosin-based motor that is associated with the transduction apparatus (Figure 4–5B and C). Rapid channel reclosure or "fast adaptation" is presumably caused by Ca^{2+} binding to a proposed intracellular site near the channel's gate. The exact underlying mechanism of this process is not yet understood. The second process, "slow adaptation," happens at about a 10 times slower time course than rapid channel reclosure and occurs when the upper insertion point of the tip link slides down the stereocilium. During a sustained stimulus, adaptation leads to a resetting of the resting point, thereby allowing the transduction apparatus to continuously operate at the point of highest sensitivity. It has been proposed that influx of Ca^{2+} through open transduction channels leads to slippage of the myosin-based adaptation motor that continuously strives to crawl toward the stereociliary tip along the actin core (Figure 4–5B). Slippage of the myosin-based motor reduces the tension in the tip link complex and lowers the open probability of the transduction channels, which in turn shuts off the local Ca^{2+} influx. At low local Ca^{2+} concentrations, the myosins of the adaptation motor will effectively move upwards, thereby readjusting the tension in the tip link complex to a point where the open probability of the transduction channels is close to the open probability at rest. Myosin 1c has been put forward as a crucial component of the adaptation motor, which does not preclude the involvement of other myosins in this process.[5]

Outer Hair Cells and Amplification

The outer hair cells play a key role in the amplification of basilar membrane motion. Amplification is necessary for the detection of sounds at low sound pressure levels. The importance of the outer hair cells was illustrated when kanamycin, an ototoxic antibiotic, was used to selectively damage outer hair cells while keeping inner hair cells intact. Outer hair cell loss resulted in elimination of the auditory nerve's low threshold sensitivity and its sharp tuning while not affecting its high threshold characteristics.[6] This observation led to the hypothesis that the outer hair cells are mainly responsible for amplification and sharp tuning of the auditory system.

One mechanism for amplification is somatic electromotility.[7] Isolated outer hair cells have been shown to change their length by 3 to 5% in response to electrical stimulation. When depolarized, outer hair cells contract, whereas they elongate when hyperpolarized. As a result, outer hair cells exert mechanical force that feeds back into movements of the basilar membrane for stimuli up to a few kHz.

Upward stimulation of the basilar membrane, eg, moves the stereocilia in an excitatory direction and depolarizes the outer hair cells, which in turn shorten, further pulling the basilar membrane upward. In this way, outer hair cell electromotility amplifies basilar membrane motion caused by the traveling wave.

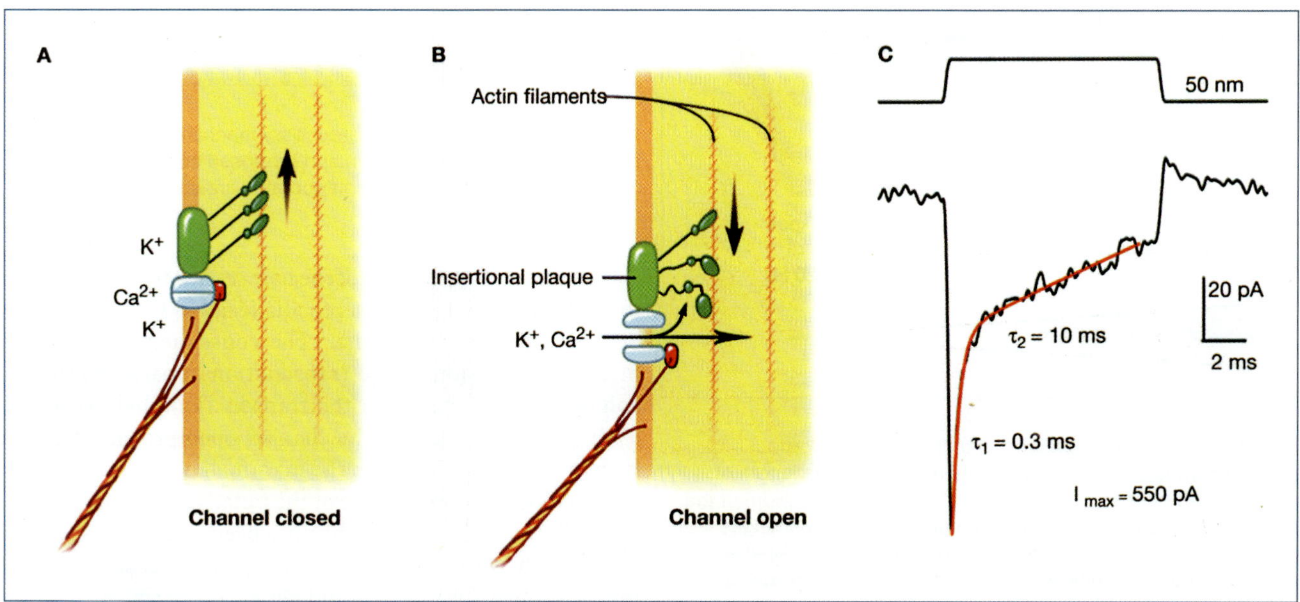

FIGURE 4–5 • Mechanoelectrical transduction. *A*, At rest, approximately 90% of the transduction channels are closed. Myosin-based molecular motors climb toward the stereociliary tips and adjust the tension in the tip link and associated structures to assure that the transduction apparatus operates at the highest sensitivity. *B*, Increased mechanical tension in the tip link and associated structures leads to opening of the transduction channels and incoming cations depolarize the cell. Local increase of the Ca^{2+} concentration affect the myosin motors and result in slippage of the transduction apparatus, thereby decreasing the mechanical tension and open probability of the transduction channels. *C*, Depolarization of a rat outer hair cell in response to a moderate mechanical deflection of 50 nm. Shown is the rapid rise of the receptor potential that is capable of reaching a maximum current of 550 pA in this specific cell, when fully stimulated. The current trace is labeled with the time courses of the fast (τ_1) and slow (τ_2) adaptation. *Data courtesy of Dr. Anthony Ricci, Stanford University.*

Prestin is thought to be the motor protein responsible for somatic electromotility in outer hair cells. Several lines of evidence support this fact.[8] First, cells transfected with prestin were found to be electromotile with magnitudes ranging up to 0.2 μm, showing that prestin is sufficient for motility. Second, prestin is located at the right place, namely in the lateral membrane of outer hair cells. And finally, mouse models with targeted deletion or modifications of prestin affect cochlear sensitivity and demonstrate that prestin is essential for outer hair cell electromotility. Prestin belongs to the SLC26 anion transporter superfamily whose members can mediate the electroneutral exchange of chloride and carbonate across the plasma membrane. The exact mechanism by which this motor works is still debated, but it is conceivable that a motor protein working on the principles of voltage displacement could operate much faster than the classical ATP-driven cellular motors.[9] A current working hypothesis suggests that intracellular anions act as voltage sensors that bind to prestin and trigger conformational changes. Hyperpolarization leads to anions binding to prestin, which causes the surface area of prestin to increase, leading to cell elongation. Depolarization, on the other hand, leads to dissociation of the anion and a decrease in the prestin surface area, leading to cell contraction. At rest, anions are usually bound to prestin; therefore, the protein assumes its longer conformation.

Another likely source of amplification is mediated by active hair bundle movements caused by interplay of mechanotransduction and adaptation. In cochleae of nonmammalian vertebrates, hair bundles are able to generate sustained oscillatory motion and similar net amplification rates as mammalian outer hair cells. Active stereocilia motion is an important amplification mechanism of nonmammalian vertebrates and it is likely that this process is also utilized for amplification or tuning in the mammalian organ of Corti, side-by-side with prestin-driven outer hair cell electromotility.

Tectorial Membrane

The tectorial membrane is an extracellular structure that overlies both the inner and outer hair cells. However, only the tallest stereocilia of the outer hair cells are directly embedded into the underside of the tectorial membrane. The tectorial membrane is attached on its inner edge to the spiral limbus and is loosely connected to the supporting cells such as the Hensen's cells by means of microscopically visible projections called trabeculae. The importance of the tectorial membrane is illustrated by the fact that mutations of tectorial membrane genes such as alpha- and beta-tectorin cause profound hearing loss both in humans and animal models.[10]

Based on anatomic observations, it was initially suggested that the tectorial membrane acts as a simple lever, shearing the hair bundles as the basilar membrane moves up and down. Other cochlear models treated it either as a simple mechanical load or as a resonant system consisting of a mass and spring. Recent findings suggest that the tectorial membrane is more like a resonant gel and is involved in enhancing the frequency selectivity of the cochlea. It is likely that all proposed functions of the tectorial membrane are relevant and because, like most structures in the organ of Corti, it changes its size from base to apex, the tectorial membrane may also contribute to the overall tonotopic organization of the cochlea.

THE STRIA VASCULARIS

Overview

The stria vascularis plays a pivotal role in cochlear homeostasis by generating the endocochlear potential and maintaining the unique ion composition of the endolymph.

The stria vascularis is a highly vascularized, multilayered tissue that is part of the lateral wall of the scala media (Figure 4–1 and 4–6). It is comprised of three distinct cell types: marginal,

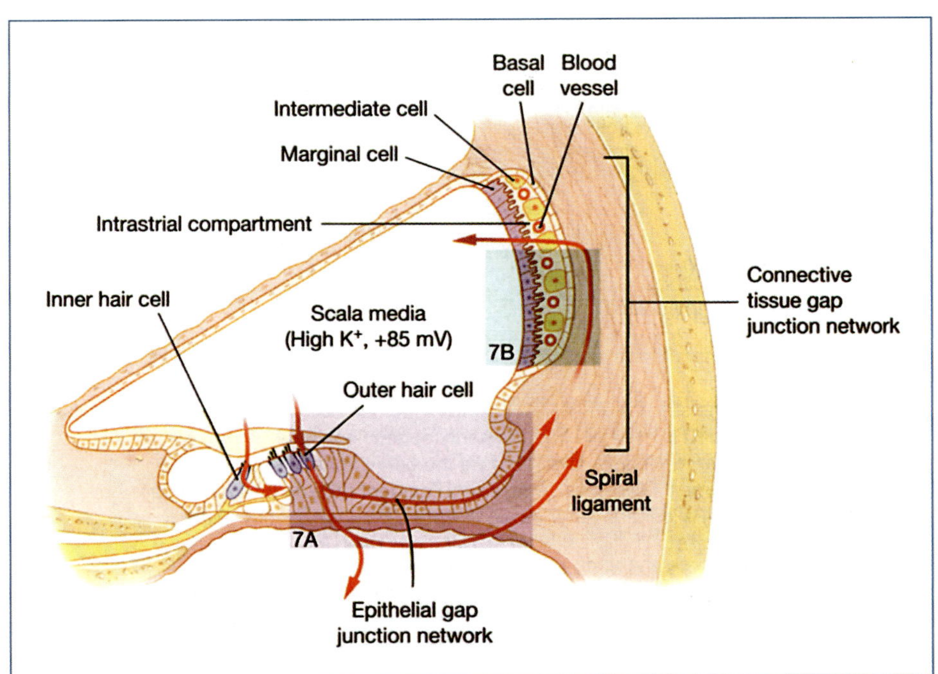

FIGURE 4–6 • Stria vascularis and K^+ circulation. Schematic drawing showing the flow of K^+ from the scala media through hair cells into the perilymphatic spaces as well as through the epithelial gap junction network into the spiral ligament. K^+ from the spiral ligament is transported via the stria vascularis into the scala media. Not shown are other pathways for K^+ out of the scala media, eg through outer sulcus cells and Reissner's membrane. The rectangles outline the areas shown in more detail in Figure 4–7.

intermediate, and basal cells, all of which are essential for its proper function. Tight junctions provide the ionic barriers that demarcate the strial tissue, one at the level of the marginal cells and the other at the level of the basal cells. The extracellular space in between these two barriers is called the intrastrial compartment.[11] As shown in Figure 4–7B, the marginal cells separate the endolymph-filled scala media from the intrastrial compartment that is filled with the intrastrial fluid, whereas the basal cells separate the intrastrial space from the perilymph that surrounds the fibrocytes of the spiral ligament. Intermediate cells as well as blood vessels are embedded in the intrastrial compartment. Gap junctions connect the basal cells with intermediate cells and with the fibrocytes of the spiral ligament, allowing electric coupling as well as exchange of ions and small molecules.[11,12] The regulation of cochlear fluid homeostasis also involves the endolymphatic sac, which responds to endolymph volume disturbances and probably disturbs homeostasis when it malfunctions.[13]

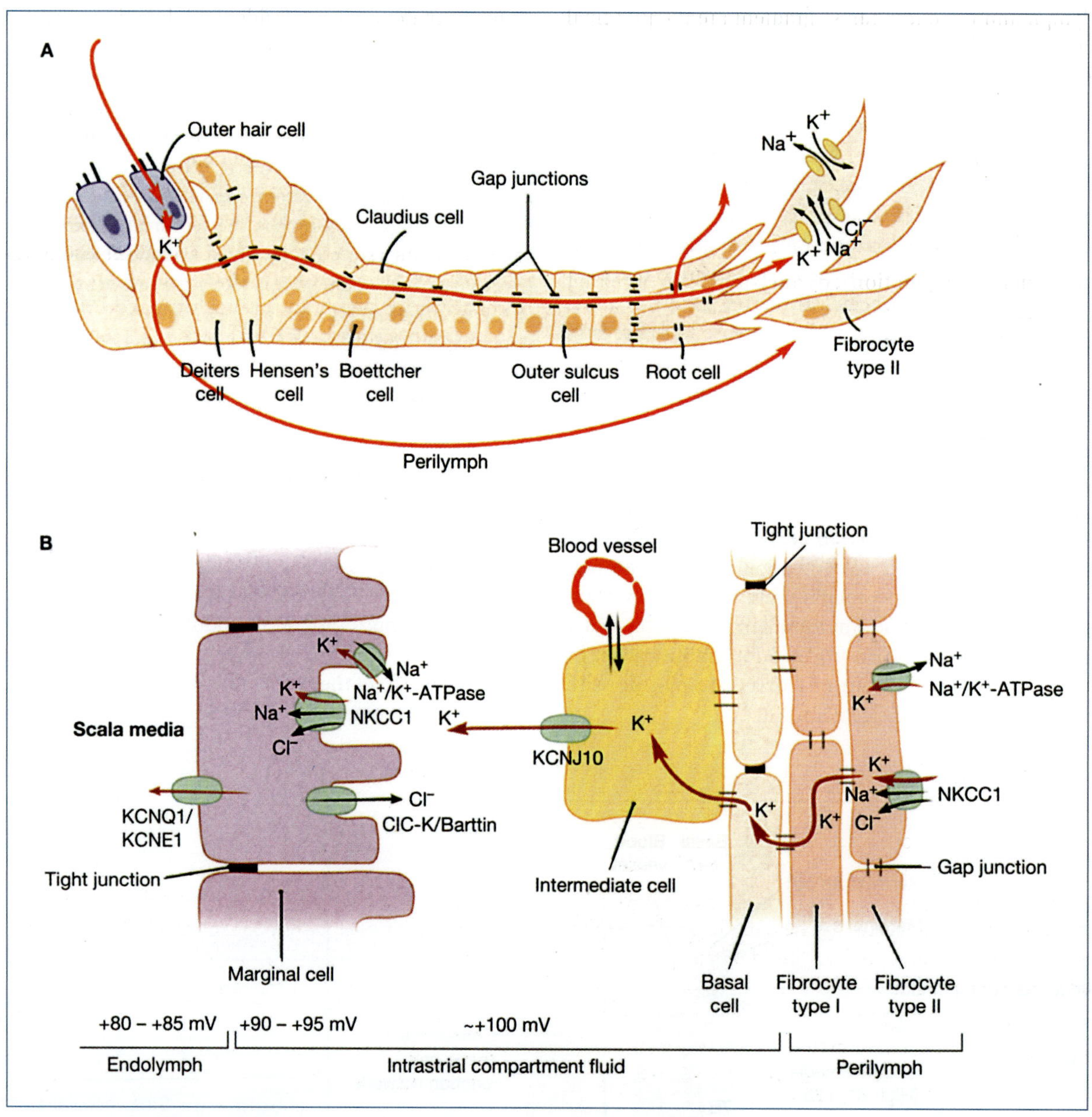

FIGURE 4–7 • K^+ flow through the organ of Corti and the stria vascularis. *A*, K^+ enters the hair cell via the mechanotransduction channels. On its basolateral side K^+ is released into the perilymphatic space via K^+ channels such as the KCNQ4 channel. K^+ can travel toward the spiral ligament via the perilymphatic space and, intracellularly, via the epithelial gap junction network. Type II fibrocytes in the spiral ligament take up K^+ and provide a path to the stria vascularis via the connective tissue gap junction network. *B*, K^+ enters basal and intermediate cells through gap junctions with type I and type II fibrocytes. The K^+ channel KCNJ10 has been identified as important for releasing K^+ into the intrastrial space. The gene encoding KCNJ10 is consequently essential for proper generation of the endocochlear potential. K^+ is efficiently removed from the intrastrial space by marginal cells, which actively take up K^+ via NKCC1 ($Na^+/K^+/2Cl^-$) cotransporters and by Na^+/K^+-ATPases. Finally, marginal cells secrete K^+ into the scala media via the KCNQ1/KCNE1 K^+ channel maintaining the high K^+ concentration of the endolymph essential for mechanoelectrical transduction.

Malfunctions in cochlear fluid homeostasis due to disruptions of the endocochlear potential, ionic composition, or its volume regulating mechanisms lead to various forms of hearing impairment in humans and animals.[11,12,14]

Endocochlear Potential and Potassium Homeostasis

Hair cell mechanoelectrical transduction works efficiently due to the large driving force for cations to enter the cell's cytoplasm from the scala media. The ≈ +85 mV endocochlear potential of the endolymph and the chemical K^+ gradient are the principal components of this driving force, which reaches about 130 mV when the hair cell's resting potential of –45 mV is taken into account.[4] Hearing threshold increases approximately 1 dB per mV loss of endocochlear potential.

K^+, the main cation of the endolymph, carries the majority of the electrical charge that generates the endocochlear potential. It is therefore important to understand how K^+ moves through the cochlea. K^+ can enter hair cells through mechanoelectrical transduction channels and it is released through the hair cells' basolateral membranes into the perilymphatic extracellular space (Figures 4–6 and 4–7A). It has been proposed that K^+ can enter supporting cells and move toward the spiral ligament by an extensive gap junction network. Alternatively, K^+ can diffuse extracellularly via the perilymphatic space. Spiral ligament type II and type I fibrocytes take up K^+ and provide an intracellular pathway into the basal and intermediate cells of the stria vascularis (Figures 4–6 and 4–7B). K^+ is released by intermediate cells via KCNJ10 channels into the intrastrial space from which it is actively pumped and cotransported into marginal cells. The marginal cells release K^+ into the scala media.[11,12] The overall K^+ circulation is probably not a true recycling as the perilymphatic and intrastrial spaces do not form an enclosed loop because these compartments are connected to other extracellular spaces as well as to the blood supply.

Malfunctions in several K^+ channels lead to perturbation of cochlear K^+ homeostasis, resulting in hearing impairment (Table 4–1). In mice, loss of the *KCNE1* gene that encodes a K^+ channel subunit expressed by marginal cells causes a phenotype highly similar to human Jervell and Lange–Nielsen syndrome, which is characterized by hearing loss and cardiac arrhythmia. This observation led to the identification of two human genes, *KCNE1* and *KCNQ1*, which both cause Jervell and Lange–Nielsen syndrome when mutated. It is conceivable that KCNQ1 and KCNE1 form the channel that allows secretion of K^+ from marginal cells into the scala media. Another member of the KCNQ family of potassium channels, KCNQ4, is likely involved in basolateral K^+ secretion by hair cells. Mutations in the human *KCNQ4* gene cause nonsyndromic deafness. Other known genetic dysfunctions involve ion transport proteins localized in the basolateral membrane of marginal cells (see below and Table 4–1). Probably the most well-known genes involved in cochlear K^+ homeostasis are the ones that encode connexin proteins. Connexins form the subunits of gap junction channels, which underlie the K^+ circulation networks described for the supporting cells of the organ of Corti, the spiral ligament, and stria vascularis. Mutations in genes encoding human connexins 26, 30, 31, and 43 are responsible for the majority of nonsyndromic hereditary hearing loss.[14]

Cochlear Fluid Homeostasis

Perilymph, endolymph, and intrastrial fluid are the three distinguishable fluids in the cochlea and can be seen as its metabolic support system. The proper ionic composition of these fluids is essential for generation and maintenance of the endocochlear potential. Perilymph and intrastrial fluid are characterized by a high Na^+ concentration and a low K^+ concentration, similar to other extracellular fluids. Endolymph not only has high K^+ and low Na^+ concentrations but also features an unusually low Ca^{2+} concentration compared to other extracellular fluids (Table 4–2).[15] Ca^{2+} ion homeostasis in the cochlea is controlled by ion channels and transporters located in the plasma membranes of its cells, as previously described for K^+.

In the stria vascularis, influx of Na^+ ions accompanies that of K^+ ions from the intrastrial compartment into the marginal cells. The cotransporter NKCC1 makes use of the strong Na^+ gradient to bring Na^+, K^+, and 2 Cl^- ions into the marginal cells. Na^+/K^+-ATPase is responsible for setting up this gradient by pumping Na^+ into the intrastrial space in exchange for K^+. Finally, K^+ leaves marginal cells into the endolymphatic space, driven by the high positive resting potential of marginal cells (Figure 4–7, B). This intricate process maintains a high Na^+ and low K^+ concentration of the intrastrial fluid that facilitates K^+ replenishment into the intrastrial space. Cl^- is transported back to the intrastrial space by ClC-K/Barttin channels. Inhibition of NKCC1 and the Na^+/K^+-ATPase by the loop diuretic furosemide and ouabain, respectively, leads to suppression of the endocochlear potential. Mutations of the Barttin gene, or the mutation of both the ClC-Ka and ClC-Kb subunits of the basolateral Cl^- channels, lead to Bartter's syndrome type 4, characterized by deafness and renal salt wasting (Table 4–1). Na^+ is reabsorbed from the endolymph by outer sulcus and Reissner's membrane cells, which play a role in maintaining the low Na^+ concentration in the scala media.[11,14]

Regulation of endolymphatic Ca^{2+} concentration is also of great importance. Hair cell physiology has revealed that tip links break at very low Ca^{2+} concentrations and that the mechanoelectrical transduction channels are blocked at high Ca^{2+} concentrations.[16,17] Furthermore, Ca^{2+} carries part of the transduction current and plays critical roles in adaptation and possibly in cochlear amplification.[18] Ca^{2+}-permeable channels, Ca^{2+}-ATPases, as well as Na^+/Ca^{2+}-exchangers are found in many cochlear cell types and could be involved in regulating Ca^{2+} efflux from and influx into the endolymph, but specific mechanisms have not been elucidated.

Cochlear fluid volume regulation is equally important for cochlear function and different mechanisms have been postulated.[13,19] Previously, longitudinal and radial flow patterns have been proposed as the underlying principle. Longitudinal flow of endolymph is described as its secretion along the membranous labyrinth with reabsorption in the endolymphatic duct and sac, whereas radial flow is based on local secretion and reabsorption, eg, via the stria vascularis. Under pathological conditions such as an increase or decrease of endolymph volume, longitudinal flow may be relevant. Experimental enlargement of

TABLE 4–1 Genes that alter cochlear K homeostasis when mutated

GENE	ENCODED PROTEIN	PROTEIN LOCALIZATION	PROTEIN FUNCTION	DISEASE
KCNE1	KCNE1	Marginal cells	K^+ channel	Jervell/Lange–Nielsen syndrome
KCNQ1	KCNQ1	Marginal cells	K^+ channel	Jervell/Lange–Nielsen syndrome
KCNQ4	KCNQ4	Outer and inner hair cells	K^+ channel	DFNA2
GJB2	Cx26	Fibrocytes in SL and SLi, epithelia on BM, intermediate and basal cells	Gap junction protein	DFNB1/DFNA3 Hereditary palmoplantar keratoderma with deafness
GJB6	Cx30	Fibrocytes in SL and SLi, supporting cells of the OoC	Gap junction protein	DFNA3
GJB3	Cx31	Fibrocytes in SL and SLi, epithelia on BM	Gap junction protein	DFNA2, AR-nonsyndromic deafness
GJB1	Cx32	Fibrocytes in SL and SLi, epithelia on BM	Gap junction protein	X-linked Charcot-Marie-Tooth and deafness
GJA1	Cx43	Fibrocytes in SL and SLi, epithelia on BM, intermediate and basal cells	Gap junction protein	AR-nonsyndromic deafness
BSND	Barttin	Marginal cells	Cl^- channel	Type 4 Bartter's syndrome

SL, spiral ligament; Sli, spiral limbus; BM, basilar membrane; OoC, Organ of Corti.

TABLE 4–2 Ionic composition of the endo- and perilymph

	COCHLEAR PERILYMPH (mM)	COCHLEAR ENDOLYMPH (mM)
Na^+	148	1.3
K^+	4.2	157
Cl^-	119	132
HCO_3^-	21	31
Ca^{2+}	1.3	0.023
pH	7.3	7.5

Adapted from Lang et al.[15]

the endolymph compartment was found to produce a longitudinal flow toward the base of the cochlea into the endolymphatic sac, decreasing both the volume of fluid and concentration of electrolytes within the cochlear duct. On the other hand, experimental decrease in endolymph compartment volume led to an apically directed flow, increasing fluid volume and electrolyte concentration. The radial flow theory has never been experimentally proven. Today, the prevailing thought is that there is no significant volume flow under physiological conditions. Experiments in animals have shown that markers iontophoresed into the endolymph without volume disturbance move solely by diffusion. The ions in the endolymph, therefore, turn over locally without concomitant volume flow. Similar regulatory mechanisms have been proposed for perilymph homeostasis. A low volume flow inside the cochlea has consequences for intracochlear drug applications where, under physiological conditions, diffusion of compounds inside the fluid-filled compartments appears to limit the equal dosing of potential drugs from base to apex.

On a cellular level, transmembraneous water movement largely depends on pore-like water-permeable channels such as aquaporins. Several aquaporins are found in the inner ear with only a few localized within the endolymph lining epithelium.[20] Lack of aquaporin 4 in mice results in hearing impairment. Other aquaporin knock-out mice either show no inner ear phenotype, are not available to date, or are embryonically lethal, such as aquaporin 2 knock-out mice. Nevertheless, aquaporin 2 is interesting as it is found in the endolymph-lining epithelium of the endolymphatic sac and is regulated by the hormone vasopressin. Animal models have shown that pathologically increased levels of vasopressin lead to a prominent endolymphatic hydrops, a morphological characteristic of Ménière's disease. Besides its potential relevance to the pathogenesis of Ménière's disease, this finding suggests a hormonal influence on inner ear volume regulation.[21] For example, vasopressin has not only been shown to influence the membrane expression of aquaporin 2 but also to increase the activity of epithelial Na^+ channels and the NKCC1 cotransporter found in strial marginal cells and type II fibrocytes of the spiral ligament.

Modulation of these channels could lead to increased K^+ secretion into the endolymph and consequently an osmotic volume movement, resulting in typical hydrops. Similar findings have been reported for another hormone, aldosterone, which increases activity of both epithelial Na^+ channels and Na^+/K^+-ATPase.[22] However, other hormones have an effect opposite to that of vasopression. Glucocorticoids, eg, have been shown to suppress the symptoms of Ménière's possibly due to a decrease of vasopressin production and modulation of the membrane expression of certain aquaporins.[23]

Cochlear fluid homeostasis, ion transport, and endocochlear potential are all required for proper cochlear function. Metabolic blockade or specific inhibitors of ion transport such as ouabain and furosemide rapidly affect this microenvironment and interfere with auditory function by disturbing the cochlea's battery, the endocochlear potential. It has been hypothesized that aging affects long-term maintenance of the endocochlear potential and that lowered metabolic rates of the stria vascularis could play a role in age-related hearing loss.

THE SPIRAL GANGLION

Overview

The spiral ganglion is located in Rosenthal's canal within the modiolus of the cochlea. It contains the cell bodies of afferent neurons, the dendrites of which are excited by neurotransmitters released by organ of Corti hair cells and the axons of which project centrally into the cochlear nucleus located in the brain stem. The majority (approximately 95%) of the afferent fibers are thick and myelinated and originate from type I ganglion neurons (Figure 4–8). These fibers exclusively innervate inner hair cells. The remaining afferent fibers are thin, unmyelinated, and emanate from type II ganglion neurons; these fibers contact outer hair cells. About a dozen type I ganglion neurons innervate each inner hair (converging innervation pattern), whereas the type II afferent nerve fibers divide into multiple branches and contact multiple outer hair cells (diverging innervation pattern). All auditory information is carried to the brain stem by the afferent system. The auditory and the vestibular nerves join each other to form the eighth cranial nerve (the vestibulocochlear nerve).

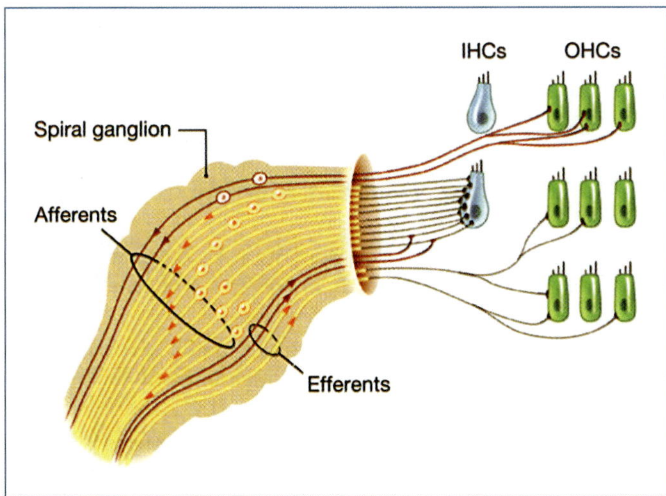

FIGURE 4–8 • Innervation of the organ of Corti. Schematic drawing of afferent and efferent innervation of inner and outer hair cells. Shown from top to bottom are unmyelinated type II afferent and myelinated type I afferent fibers, unmyelinated LOC efferent fibers, and myelinated MOC efferent fibers.

Efferent fibers originate in the brain stem from neurons located in the superior olivary complex and send information to the cochlea by synapsing with outer hair cells as well as with afferent fibers beneath inner hair cells. The efferent system allows the central nervous system to modulate the operation of the cochlea.[24]

The innervation pattern of the organ of Corti clearly underlines the functional differences of the two types of cochlear hair cells.

Neural Processing of Auditory Information and Inner Hair Cell Synapses

Afferent neurotransmitter release by inner hair cells is initiated at their 5 to 30 ribbon-type synapses where local influx of Ca^{2+} through voltage-gated Ca^{2+} channels leads to finely graded fusion of synaptic vesicles at presynaptic sites. The resulting exocytosis of neurotransmitters is, therefore, directly proportional to the presynaptic Ca^{2+} current, which in turn is dependent on voltage changes driven by mechanotransduction. Information coding at the afferent synapse is remarkably accurately, allowing high temporal precision as well as a considerable dynamic range of five orders of magnitude ranging from 0 dB to more than 100 dB.

Each ribbon synapse is composed of a presynaptic dense body (equivalent to the synaptic ribbon of photoreceptor cells) that is surrounded by vesicles containing neurotransmitters, a thickening of the underlying plasma membrane, a synaptic cleft, and the postsynaptic region containing the AMPA-type glutaminergic receptors of the afferent neurons. Glutamate, or a closely related compound, is thought to be the neurotransmitter of the inner hair cell afferents even though other yet unidentified transmitters may also be involved.

The tonotopic organization of the organ of Corti is maintained within the afferent system, where depolarization of inner hair cells at a specific location leads to the excitation of connected afferent spiral ganglion neurons. Each afferent fiber is characterized by a specific tuning curve (Figure 4–9), which describes the sound pressure level of the stimulus needed to elicit a response at a given frequency. An apparent feature of tuning curves is that they show the frequency at which the nerve fiber displays highest sensitivity, its characteristic frequency. Stimuli at higher or lower frequencies relative to the characteristic frequency can also evoke a response but only if presented at higher intensities. The sharpness and thresholds of afferent nerve fiber tuning curves depend on many factors including organ of Corti morphology and active processes associated with cochlear amplification. The activity of the efferent system plays an important role in modulating the afferent nerve characteristics (Figure 4–9). Loss of cochlear amplification, eg, as a result of outer hair cell loss, leads to a broadening of the tuning curve and an increase in the fibers' response thresholds.

The tonotopic organization of the cochlea is the basis for frequency coding in auditory nerve fibers (place coding).

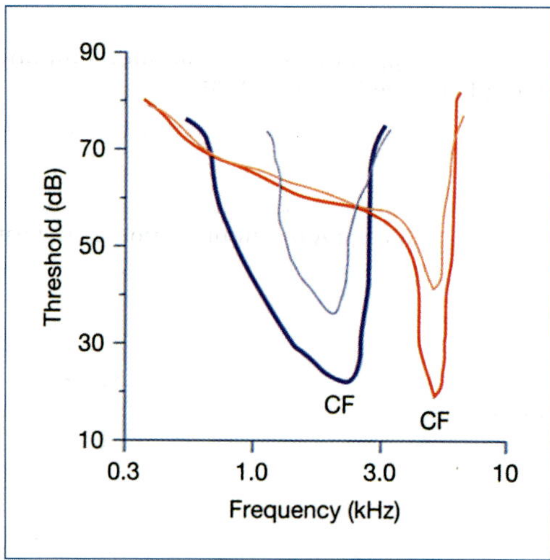

FIGURE 4–9 • Typical tuning curves of auditory nerve fibers. (Thick lines) Tuning curves of auditory nerve fibers with characteristic frequencies of ≈ 2 kHz (blue) and ≈ 5 kHz (red). (Thin lines) Substantial decrease of the auditory threshold in response to stimulation of the MOC system. Changes in the specific shapes of tuning curves depend on the characteristic frequencies (CF) of the individual fibers. *Adapted from Guinan.*[24]

Additionally, frequency is coded by the auditory nerve fibers' discharge characteristics known as phase locking. Here, an auditory nerve fiber fires at a particular phase of the stimulating frequency, which leads to a regular response pattern characterized by spacing of the nerve spikes in equals or multiples of the stimulus wavelength. Phase locking only happens at low frequencies. Above 5 kHz, spike responses of auditory nerve fibers occur at random intervals. Tonotopic organization and phase locking are both important for frequency discrimination. Discharge rates within the auditory nerve fibers are not only determined by the frequency but also by the intensity of the stimulus. As intensity increases, the discharge rate within a single auditory nerve fiber increases. Likewise, the number of auditory nerve fibers activated at a given characteristic frequency increases with intensifying stimuli. This recruitment of more fibers is due to the fact that auditory nerve fibers of the same characteristic frequency have different response thresholds. Furthermore, with increasing stimulus intensity, other afferent nerve fibers of nearby characteristic frequencies are also activated. These physiologically relevant features set some of the complex rules for cochlear implant design and application.

In summary, the frequency-dependent stimulation of cochlear hair cells leads to an increase in inner hair cell synaptic transmission at ribbon synapses. The ensuing excitatory postsynaptic currents in afferent nerve fibers lead to a timed discharge of action potentials in the auditory nerve. The acuity, temporal resolution, and dynamic range of the auditory system is unmatched by any other sensory system.

Efferent Innervation of the Cochlea

Two clearly distinguishable groups of efferent fibers originate in the brain stem.[24] First, myelinated medial olivocochlear (MOC) efferents arise from neurons located around the medial superior olivary nucleus. The MOC efferents project to the contralateral and ipsilateral cochleae, where they form cholinergic synapses with outer hair cells. The second group of fibers are the unmyelinated lateral olivocochlear (LOC) efferents that originate from neurons with small somata located in and around the lateral superior olivary nucleus. The LOC fibers project predominantly to the ipsilateral cochlea where they terminate on the dendrites of afferent type I neurons beneath inner hair cells. LOC efferent synapses are neurochemically complex and utilize cholinergic, GABAergic, and dopaminergic transmission as well as various neuropeptides.

The effects of stimulation of MOC fibers have been studied much more extensively than LOC fiber stimulation. In general, stimulation of the MOC system leads to increased thresholds, which is due to a decrease in the degree of cochlear amplification by outer hair cells (Figure 4–9). This sound-evoked feedback, therefore, decreases sensitivity of the hearing apparatus in situations when the metabolically expensive amplification mechanisms are not needed.

The function of the LOC efferent neurons appears to be more complex. Their direct input on the afferent neurons suggests that they regulate afferent activity, thereby affecting the dynamic range. Lesion studies support this view, where loss of specific neurotransmitters or destruction of cell bodies in the brainstem leads to either enhancement or suppression of auditory nerve response. These LOC feedback effects are slow and usually require minutes to become effective. An additional function of the LOC system is to perform slow integration and adjustment of binaural inputs needed for accurate binaural function and sound localization.[25]

Finally, activity of the MOC and the LOC efferent systems seem to have protective effects against acoustic injury and such a feedback could be important in loud noise environments.[26]

References

1. Raphael Y, Altschuler RA. Structure and innervation of the cochlea. Brain Res Bull 2003;60:397–422.
2. Pickles JO, Comis SD, Osborne MP. Cross-links between stereocilia in the guinea pig organ of Corti, and their possible relation to sensory transduction. Hear Res 1984;15:103–12.
3. Hudspeth AJ, Gillespie PG. Pulling springs to tune transduction: Adaptation by hair cells. Neuron 1994;12:1–9.
4. Hudspeth AJ. How the ear's works work: Mechanoelectrical transduction and amplification by hair cells. C R Biol 2005;328:155–62.
5. Holt JR, Gillespie SK, Provance DW, et al. A chemical-genetic strategy implicates myosin-1c in adaptation by hair cells. Cell 2002;108:371–81.
6. Kiang NY, Liberman MC, Levine RA. Auditory-nerve activity in cats exposed to ototoxic drugs and high-intensity sounds. Ann Otol Rhinol Laryngol 1976;85:752–68.
7. Brownell WE, Bader CR, Bertrand D, de Ribaupierre Y. Evoked mechanical responses of isolated cochlear outer hair cells. Science 1985;227:194–6.
8. Zheng J, Shen W, He DZ, Long KB, Madison LD, Dallos P. Prestin is the motor protein of cochlear outer hair cells. Nature 2000;405:149–55.
9. Ashmore J. Cochlear outer hair cell motility. Physiol Rev 2008;88:173–210.

10. Legan PK, Lukashkina VA, Goodyear RJ, Kossi M, Russell IJ, Richardson GP. A targeted deletion in alpha-tectorin reveals that the tectorial membrane is required for the gain and timing of cochlear feedback. Neuron 2000;28:273–85.
11. Wangemann P. Supporting sensory transduction: Cochlear fluid homeostasis and the endocochlear potential. J Physiol 2006;576:11–21.
12. Hibino H, Kurachi Y. Molecular and physiological bases of the K+ circulation in the mammalian inner ear. Physiol (Bethesda) 2006;21:336–45.
13. Salt AN. Regulation of endolymphatic fluid volume. Ann N Y Acad Sci 2001;942:306–12.
14. Heller S. Application of physiological genomics to the study of hearing disorders. J Physiol 2002;543:3–12.
15. Lang F, Vallon V, Knipper M, Wangemann P. Functional significance of channels and transporters expressed in the inner ear and kidney. Am J Physiol Cell Physiol 2007;293:C1187–208.
16. Assad JA, Shepherd GM, Corey DP. Tip-link integrity and mechanical transduction in vertebrate hair cells. Neuron 1991;7:985–94.
17. Farris HE, LeBlanc CL, Goswami J, Ricci AJ. Probing the pore of the auditory hair cell mechanotransducer channel in turtle. J Physiol 2004;558:769–92.
18. Mammano F, Bortolozzi M, Ortolano S, Anselmi F. Ca^{2+} signaling in the inner ear. Physiol (Bethesda) 2007;22:131–44.
19. Salt AN. Dynamics of inner ear fluids. In: Jahn AF, Santos-Sacchi J, editors. Physiology of the ear. 2nd ed. San Diego, CA: Singular Thompson Learning; 2001. p. 333–55.
20. Beitz E, Zenner HP, Schultz JE. Aquaporin-mediated fluid regulation in the inner ear. Cell Mol Neurobiol 2003;23:315–29.
21. Al-Mana D, Ceranic B, Djahanbakhch O, Luxon LM. Hormones and the auditory system: A review of physiology and pathophysiology. Neuroscience 2008;153:881–900.
22. Dunnebier EA, Segenhout JM, Wit HP, Albers FW. Two-phase endolymphatic hydrops: A new dynamic guinea pig model. Acta Otolaryngol 1997;117:13–9.
23. Fukushima M, Kitahara T, Uno Y, Fuse Y, Doi K, Kubo T. Effects of intratympanic injection of steroids on changes in rat inner ear aquaporin expression. Acta Otolaryngol 2002;122:600–6.
24. Guinan JJ. Physiology of olivocochlear efferents. In: Dallos P, Fay RR, Popper AN, editors. The cochlea. Springer handbook of auditory research. New-York: Springer; 1996. p. 435–502.
25. Darrow KN, Maison SF, Liberman MC. Cochlear efferent feedback balances interaural sensitivity. Nat Neurosci 2006;9:1474–6.
26. Maison SF, Luebke AE, Liberman MC, Zuo J. Efferent protection from acoustic injury is mediated via alpha 9 nicotinic acetylcholine receptors on outer hair cells. J Neurosci 2002;22:10838–46.

Neurophysiology: The Central Auditory System 5

Bradford J. May, PhD / Charles Limb, MD

Sounds are events inhabiting multidimensional space. The identity of each event is mapped by a listener in perceptual coordinates that include pitch, loudness, location, and time. The listener chooses to ignore or attend to the sound by weighing the biological context in which it occurs, where it originates, and what it means. Although this critical information is extracted in an instant without conscious effort, the act of listening requires the simultaneous analysis of multiple acoustic dimensions, and their interactions upon each other. Further increasing the demands of the listening task, the resulting auditory object must maintain a stable identity as it moves within the perceptual coordinate system, for example, by changing pitch or location. Natural auditory events rarely propagate under ideal listening conditions and therefore they also must be separated from environmental effects that are capable of distorting the original waveform with reflection or reverberation. Sounds seldom occur in isolation and therefore must be separated from competing stimuli that may mask or confuse the signal. This chapter will describe how neurons in the central nervous system are endowed with specialized sensitivities to meet the many challenges of auditory information processing and how this exquisitely tuned circuitry may break down after exposure to loud sounds, ototoxic agents, trauma, or the aging process.

A defining feature of the central auditory system is the elaborate neural network that governs sound representation. When sound-driven activity enters the brain by way of the auditory nerve, it is transformed by no less than 12 types of projection neurons in seven major processing centers before converging in the auditory thalamus. By contrast, visual information is conducted from the retina to thalamus without intermediate processing. In part, these differences in computational complexity may be traced back to the most elemental stage of sensory transduction. When light strikes the eye, its color, intensity, and location are unambiguously defined by the photoreceptors that it excites, the magnitude of the excitation, and their position on the retina. When sound propagates to the ear, auditory receptors are selectively excited by sound frequency. All other perceptual dimensions must be computed by integrating coincident activity across neural populations.

This review follows the central representation of sound information from cochlear nucleus to cerebral cortex (Figure 5–1). The descriptions of each of the major auditory nuclei summarize the anatomical pathways and physiological responses that give rise to the perceptual behaviors of normal and hearing impaired listeners. Each description begins with a brief summary of the essential functional characteristics of the processing center. Readers seeking the most general knowledge may quickly peruse this chapter by focusing their attention on this introductory material. Subsequent sections are intended to provide the reader with an understanding of basic concepts and

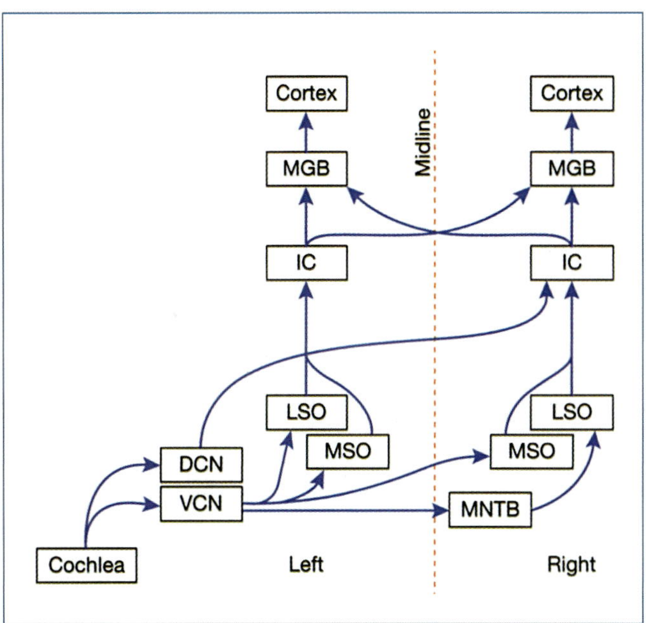

FIGURE 5–1 • Schematic diagram of the ascending pathways of the central auditory system. Principal connections between major nuclei are shown for the left ear. Symmetrical projections for the right ear are not shown. DCN, dorsal cochlear nucleus; IC, inferior colliculus; LSO, lateral superior olive; MGB, medial geniculate body; MNTB, medial nucleus of the trapezoid body; MSO, medial superior olive; VCN, ventral cochlear nucleus.

reference material to guide independent scholarship. Where it is possible, animal research is linked to clinical manifestations of processing disorders.

COCHLEAR NUCLEUS

As described in the accompanying chapter *Auditory Physiology: the Inner Ear,* a complex sound is broken apart into its constituent frequency components by the mechanical tuning of the cochlea. Because acoustic energy is tonotopically distributed along the length of cochlear partition, the discharge rates of individual auditory nerve fibers carry a single piece of the waveform puzzle. The complementary process of reconstructing the auditory signal from a dispersed peripheral representation begins in the cochlear nucleus where parallel streams of ascending information, each with a unique functional role, are established by the convergence patterns of auditory nerve fibers.[1]

The following discussion is organized around the broadest of functional dichotomies: the ventral and dorsal subdivisions of the cochlear nucleus complex. This parcellation was introduced by early anatomical descriptions of the auditory brainstem.[2] It endures because cellular morphology has proven to be an excellent predictor of function at the initial stages of central auditory processing.

VENTRAL COCHLEAR NUCLEUS

The ventral cochlear nucleus (VCN) serves as the primary input for afferent projections to the superior olive, lateral lemniscus, and inferior colliculus (ICC). Auditory information is channeled to each of these structures in discrete pathways that are optimized for the selective coding of local characteristics such as the phase and level of individual frequency components, or more global properties such as amplitude modulations of the stimulus envelope. This functional segregation is derived from striking differences in the synaptic structures, convergence patterns, and intrinsic electrical properties of VCN neurons.[3]

Anatomy

Approximately 30,000 auditory nerve fibers connect the human inner ear to the cochlear nucleus complex.[4] Upon entering the brainstem, the projections bifurcate into an ascending branch that proceeds to the anterior VCN and a descending branch that passes through the posterior VCN and dorsal cochlear nucleus (DCN). Although the systematic arrangement of the projections recapitulates the tonotopic organization of the cochlear partition, the one-dimensional frequency map is transformed into terminal fields. Within each two-dimensional frequency lamina, an orthogonal axis encodes other dimensions of sound.

The termination of the auditory nerve within the cochlear nucleus is obligatory. All sound information must be passed to higher centers by the discharge rates of cochlear nucleus neurons. There are approximately two VCN neurons for every auditory nerve fiber, suggesting a high degree of convergence within the nucleus.[5]

How VCN neurons integrate their multiple auditory nerve inputs is strongly influenced by the physical characteristics of cochlear nucleus synapses.[6] Two basic structures are observed. Neurons with wide-scale integration properties have profuse dendritic fields that are encrusted with the conventional bouton endings of large numbers of auditory nerve fibers. Neurons that faithfully preserve spike patterns in the auditory nerve are driven by large axosomatic endings, the endbulbs of Held.[7] These inputs are few in number but individually powerful enough to evoke postsynaptic activity.

The principal neuronal subtypes of the VCN are distinguished by three general cellular morphologies.[3] Bushy cells have stunted, shrub-shaped primary dendrites, globular or spherical cell bodies, and endbulb synapses. Like most neurons in the central nervous system, multipolar (or stellate) cells have long, relatively unbranched dendrites and bouton synapses. The integration properties of these cells are primarily determined by whether their dendritic fields lie within the plane of frequency laminae or radiate across them. Octopus cells have long, tufted dendrites that emanate from one side of the cell body creating the cephalopodal appearance for which they are named. These cells also receive highly convergent bouton inputs from the auditory nerve.

The cytoarchitecture of the VCN is regionally organized (Figure 5–2).[5] Spherical bushy cells are found in the most anterior subdivision, surrounding the entry point of the auditory nerve. Globular bushy cells occupy an intermediate location within the nucleus, while octopus cells are located in the

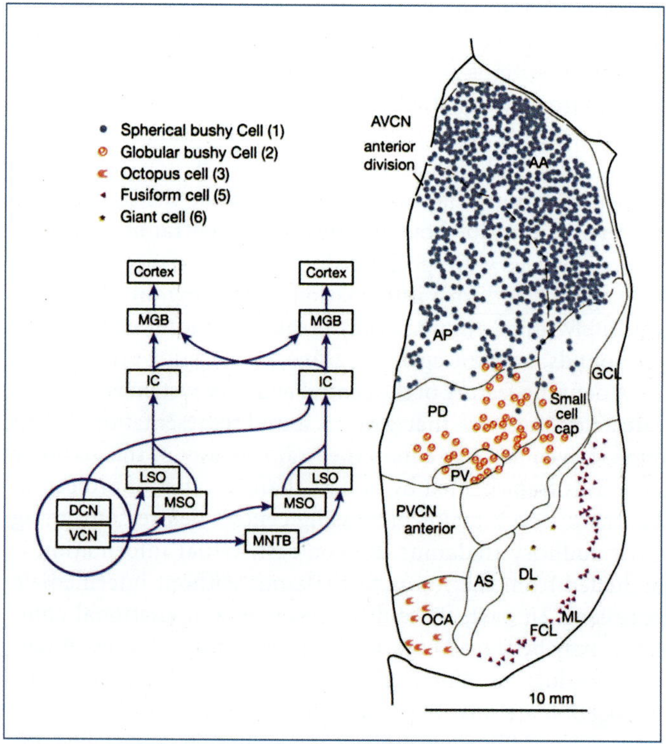

FIGURE 5–2 • Topographical clustering of morphological neuronal classes in the cochlear nucleus complex. See key for symbol identification. Inset shows relative position of the cochlear nucleus within the central auditory pathways. Abbreviations are explained in Figure 5–1. *Adapted with permission from Cant.*[3]

posterior subdivision. Multipolar cells, the most structurally diverse neurons, also show the most dispersed distribution.

Basic Physiological Properties

The regional separation of anatomically defined neuronal populations has allowed physiologists to relate the anatomical specializations of VCN neurons to their sound coding properties. Responses in the anterior nucleus are most likely recorded from bushy cells, while responses in the posterior nucleus are recorded from octopus cells. These inferences have been supported by intracellular experiments that have characterized the physiological properties of cochlear nucleus neurons before filling the cells with labeling material such as horseradish peroxidase (HRP) for later visualization.[8,9]

Single-unit electrophysiological activity in the VCN is typically classified by responses to short tone bursts at a neuron's best frequency (BF: the most sensitive frequency).[10,11] The timing of sound-driven action potentials, or spikes, is recorded and summed in temporal bins over many stimulus presentations to produce a peristimulus time histogram (PSTH). Six major response types can be identified by differences in PSTH shape (Figure 5–3).[1]

Primary-like neurons produce PSTHs that display an onset response that is robust but adapts rapidly to a lower sustained rate. Because primary-like units are found in the anterior subdivision of the VCN, they are assumed to be the functional counterpart of spherical bushy cells. As predicted by the high security endbulbs that bind bushy cells to auditory nerve fibers, the physiological characteristics of primary-like neurons are closely linked to their peripheral inputs.[12]

Primary-like with notch (PLN) neurons are found in regions containing large numbers of globular bushy cells.[13] Their PSTHs show a sharply peaked onset response that is followed by a brief period of inactivity. This "notch" reflects the neuron's refractory period after the onset spike. Primary-like with notch neurons display this property because modified endbulbs synchronize their responses to stimulus onsets.[14,15]

Onset neurons are named for their tendency to fire at stimulus onset and then show little activity for the remainder of the stimulus.[12] Onset-locker responses (onset-L) are typically recorded in the posterior subdivisions of the VCN and have been associated with octopus cell morphologies through intracellular labeling.[8] The precise onset response, broad frequency tuning, and wide dynamic range of onset neurons are consistent with the highly convergent afferent inputs of octopus cells.[16,17]

Onset chopper (onset-C) neurons show less variability than onset-L neurons. Because their spikes occur at regular intervals, onset-C neurons produce a "chopped" PSTH.[10] This response has been attributed to D stellate cells, which are large multipolar cells that send dorsally directed bilateral projections to the VCN.[18] The

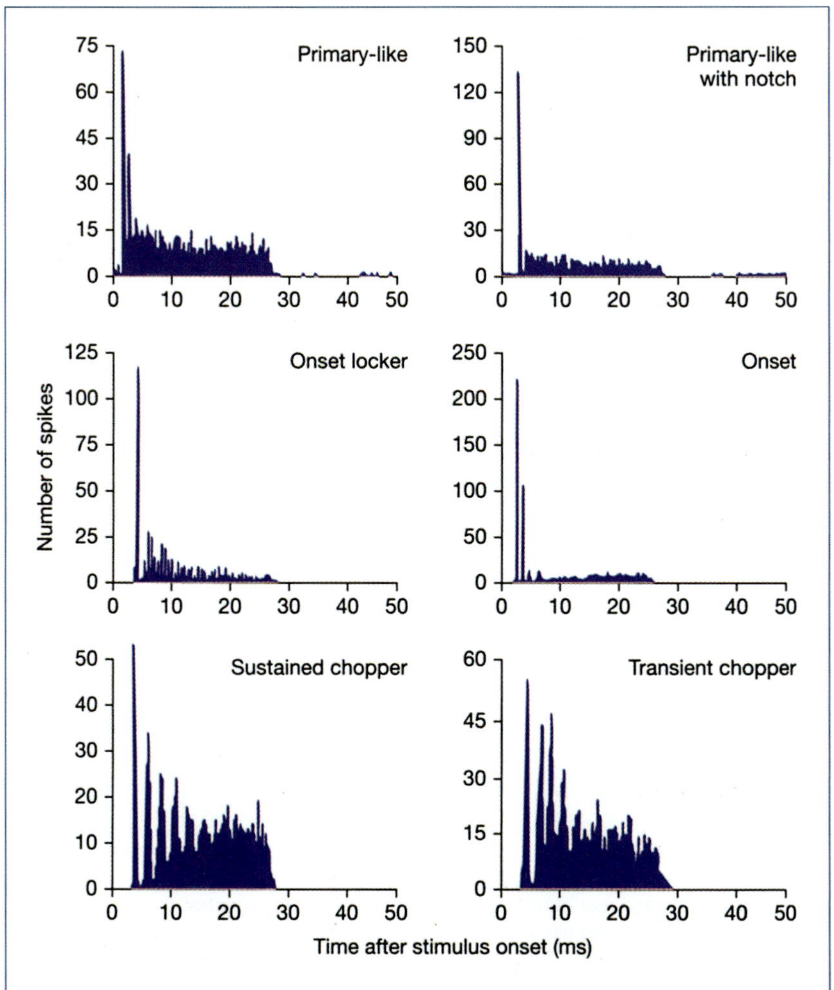

FIGURE 5–3 • Physiological response types in the ventral cochlear nucleus. Peristimulus time histograms for 30-millisecond tone bursts. *Adapted with permission from Rhode and Greenburg.*[1]

neurons have also been called "radiate" neurons because their dendritic fields fan out in three-dimensions integrating auditory nerve inputs across a wide frequency range.[19] They appear to be one source of the glycinergic inhibition that plays an important role in the sound coding properties of the cochlear nucleus.[18,20]

Chopper units are the physiological counterpart of T stellate cells.[1] These smaller multipolar cells project ventrally though the trapezoid body to the contralateral ICC.[3] The neurons are also referred to as "planar" neurons because their dendritic fields are oriented in the plane of frequency laminae.[19] In addition to sharp frequency tuning, chopper units display highly regular discharge rates and therefore produce "chopped" PSTH patterns. By integrating the responses of many auditory nerve fibers, chopper units produce signal representations that are robust across sound level and resistant to the degrading effects of background noise.[21]

Sound Coding in the Ventral Cochlear Nucleus

The diverse physiological patterns of cell populations in the VCN endow neurons with coding abilities that are selectively matched to the acoustic features of complex sounds.[22] With the exception of onset neurons, projection neurons tend to be sharply tuned in frequency. Consequently, as in the auditory nerve, complex spectra with multiple frequency components must be encoded by the discharge rates of many neurons with complementary tuning properties.[23,24]

From the perspective of human auditory experience, the veridical processing of complex spectral shapes is the foundation of speech perception. In the English language, the most rudimentary spectrum is a steady-state vowel. The perceptual identity of a vowel is defined by its formant frequencies,[25] which are high-energy bands within the stimulus. These information-bearing elements are encoded by hundreds of neurons in the auditory nerve and cochlear nucleus that combine to create a surprisingly straightforward representation in which discharge rates are linearly related to the amount of spectral energy within each neuron's range of frequency tuning.[21,26] The shape of the vowel emerges when vowel-driven activity is plotted at the BFs of the neural sample. For example, the vowel /e/, as in "bet," elicits high-discharge rates among neurons with BFs near 0.5 and 1.7 kHz, which are the frequency locations of its first and second formants (Figure 5–4).[25]

Sustained (Figure 5–4A) and transient chopper units (Figure 5–4B) provide excellent rate representations of vowel spectra across a wide range of sound levels.[21,27] It is hypothesized that this enhanced dynamic range reflects the dense convergence of auditory nerve fibers upon multipolar cells. Fibers with high spontaneous rates (SRs) tend to have low thresholds. Chopper units may accentuate these inputs at low sound levels. Conversely, fibers with low SRs have high thresholds, which may dominate chopper responses at high sound levels. A switching circuit for this "selective listening" has been proposed in which high SR inputs are located on distal dendrites and low SR inputs

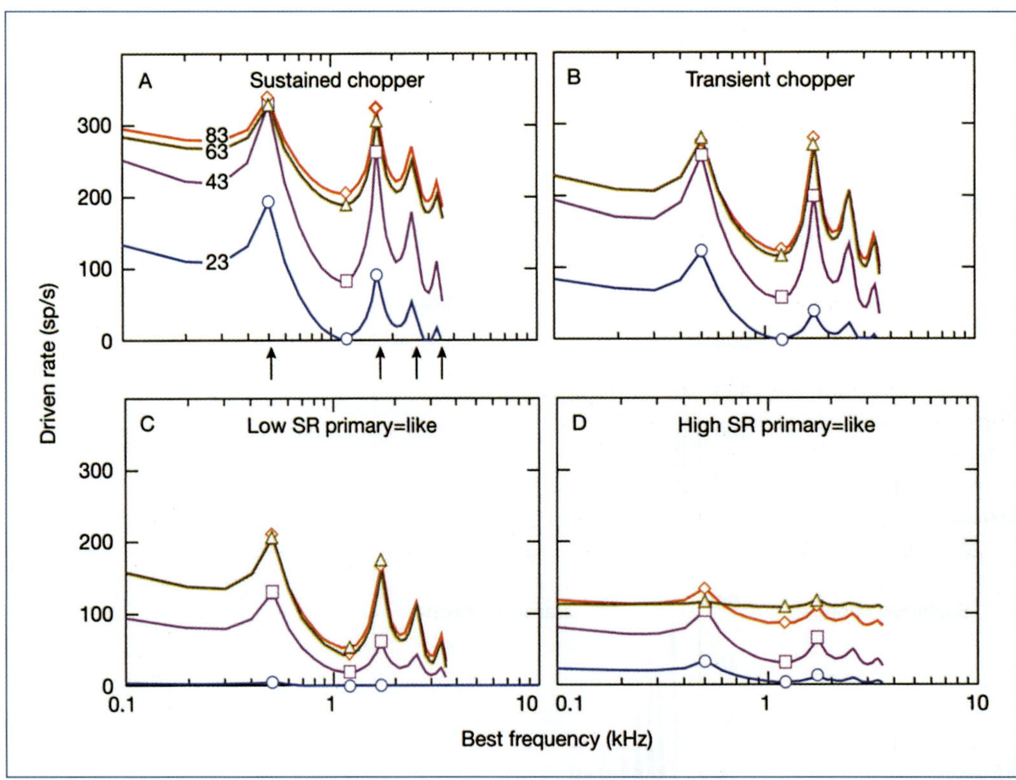

FIGURE 5–4 • Rate representation of the vowel /e/ by cochlear nucleus neurons. The formant frequencies of the vowel are indicated by arrows in *A*. Symbols indicate the average responses of actual neurons to three spectral features that define formant structure. Interpolated points are derived from the linear relationship between the level of those features and the discharge rates that they evoked. Numerical labels indicate the presentation level of the vowel stimuli. SR, spontaneous rates.

near the cell body of the chopper unit.[28] At high sound levels, the activation of intervening inhibitory inputs, possibly from radiate neurons, shunts the saturated high SR inputs away from the cell body. A reciprocal mechanism is not required for low SR inputs because their action is limited by threshold at low sound levels.

The vowel representations of VCN primary-like neurons manifest the dynamic range limitations of their auditory nerve inputs.[21,27] Primary-like neurons with low SRs (Figure 5–4C) provide a poor representation of formant structure at low sound levels because they are not effectively driven by the stimulus. The vowel's structure is apparent at suprathreshold sound levels because the highest discharge rates are restricted to formant-tuned neurons. Primary-like neurons with high SRs (Figure 5–4D) convey a good representation of formant structure at low levels but a featureless profile at high levels because the full complement of neurons responds at maximum driven rates. The threshold and saturation effects of primary-like neurons constrain their ability to encode spectral shapes in terms of discharge rates, but their responses are rich in temporal information.[12,27] In particular, the accurate timing of action potentials is critical for communicating the spatial location of auditory stimuli.

Many natural sounds are brief transients. Onset neurons respond vigorously to these stimuli and may participate in tightly coupled sensorimotor pathways that control acoustic startles and reflexive orientation movements.[29] A binaural comparison of stimulus onset time also exerts strong influences on spatial perception.[30,31] The event need not occur at the beginning of the stimulus. A sharp acoustic transition in the stimulus envelope will evoke similar responses. If the transients are repeated at a fixed rate, the responses of onset neurons will entrain to the period of stimulation. Periodicity is a fundamental characteristic of pitch perception and an essential cue for separating auditory signals from background noise.

Clinical Implications

The analysis of human neurological impairments has been essential for explaining the physiological foundations of higher cognitive function. Current understanding of the localization of speech and language in the human cortex can be traced back to the 19th century descriptions of aphasic patients by Broca[30] and Wernicke.[32] The clinical implications of damage within the pathways that bring information to the cortex have been largely determined by surgical manipulations of experimental animals.

Functional ablations of the VCN have been investigated by lesioning the projections that exit the nucleus by way of the trapezoid body.[33,34] The resulting deficits are as profound as those produced by removal of the cochlea or auditory nerve. If a trapezoid body lesion is made at the ventral midline of the brainstem, outputs from both cochlear nuclei are eliminated and the subject is rendered deaf. If a single lateralized lesion is made, outputs from one VCN are disrupted. Subjects maintain auditory function in one ear but they experience a pervasive loss of directional hearing because the brain is no longer about to make binaural comparisons of localization cues.

Temporary silencing of VCN inputs may have long-lasting clinical implications. During the early stages of development, sound-driven auditory nerve activity is needed to establish normal patterns of connectivity within the cochlear nucleus.[35] If the ear is silenced by conductive loss or sensorineural defects, the endbulbs of Held take on a hypertrophied appearance that is associated with temporal processing deficits. The synapses, and apparently higher cognitive function, may be rescued by swift interventions to restore input to the cochlear nucleus. These animal models may explain why cochlear implantation and hearing aid amplification is most effective when introduced at a young age.[36]

DORSAL COCHLEAR NUCLEUS

The DCN is a center for multisensory integration.[37] The principal output neurons are bipolar in shape and receive bouton endings on basal and apical dendritic arbors. Excitatory inputs from the cochlea are delivered to the basal dendrites. Mixed sources of excitation and inhibition contact the apical dendrites and cell body from the vestibular, cerebellar, and somatosensory nuclei.[38] Because these latter inputs are biased toward the head, neck, and outer ear, it is hypothesized that the cerebellar-like circuitry of the DCN may be involved in acousticomotor behaviors and pinna-based sound localization.[39]

Anatomy

In most mammalian species, the DCN is a three-layered structure (Figure 5–5).[3] The outer molecular layer contains descending inputs from outside the nucleus and their local target

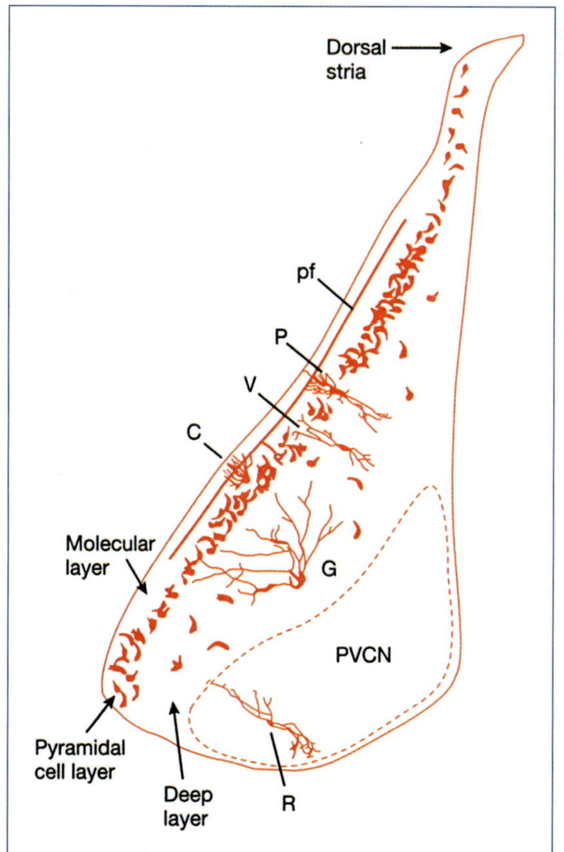

FIGURE 5–5 • Anatomical distribution of primary morphological classes within the layered structure of the dorsal cochlear nucleus. C, cartwheel cell; G, granule cell; P, pyramidal cell; pf, parallel fiber; PVCN, posteroventral cochlear nucleus; R, radiate cell; V, vertical cell. *Adapted with permission from Young and Davis.*[37]

neurons. The diverse sources of these "mossy fibers" have been determined by injecting HRP into the dorsal acoustic stria (DAS), where the fibers enter the nucleus.[38] After this procedure, heavy retrograde labeling is observed in the superior olivary complex because HRP is taken up by the axon collaterals of olivocochlear efferents. Extensive labeling of nonauditory cell groups is noted in the cerebellum and the vestibular nuclei. Retrograde labeling also is found in the lateral cuneate and sensory trigeminal nuclei. In combination, these structures carry proprioceptive information from the upper body, face, and ear.

The multisensory information conveyed to the DCN by mossy fibers is delivered to granule cells.[40] Granule cells are small cell bodies that are found scattered along the molecular layer and in the boundaries that separate the major subdivisions of the cochlear nucleus complex. The axons of granule cells form an array of parallel fibers that traverse the length of the nucleus. These fibers excite pyramidal cells through direct connections with apical dendrites or inhibit them through local interneurons, the cartwheel cells.

The pyramidal cell layer is occupied by the major projection neurons of the DCN.[5] Pyramidal cells, sometimes known as fusiform cells, are regularly arranged along the long axis of the nucleus. They send their apical dendrites into the complex neuropil of the molecular layer where they are contacted by granule and cartwheel cells. They project their basal dendrites into the deep layer where they receive inputs from auditory nerve fibers and additional sources of inhibition. The tonotopic map of the cochlea is transferred to the DCN by the systematic innervation of the dorsal branch of the auditory nerve.[41]

The deep layer of the DCN is inhabited by giant cells and vertical cells.[42] Giant cells are less frequently encountered projection neurons. Their basic physiological properties are similar to those of pyramidal cells, but their deeply located dendrites do not reach into the molecular layer to contact parallel fibers. Vertical cells are inhibitory interneurons. Their narrowband inhibitory influences reflect their alignment within DCN frequency lamina. Additional wideband glycinergic inhibition has been attributed to VCN radiate cells.[19]

Neural Coding of Spectral Cues for Sound Localization

The basic physiological properties of DCN projection neurons are shaped by complex interactions of their numerous excitatory and inhibitory inputs. Whereas VCN representations are linear, narrowly tuned, and distributed, DCN representations are nonlinear, broadly tuned, and integrative. Consequently, the discharge rates of individual pyramidal and giant cells are ideally suited for encoding the spectral shape of complex sounds.[37]

For the cat, which is the most developed animal model of DCN processing, biologically relevant spectral information is derived from the head-related transfer function (HRTF).[43,44] This filter shape describes the directional effects of the head and pinna on a free-field stimulus as it propagates to the ear drum. HRTF-based spectral cues are critical for the accurate localization of sound source elevation.

A prominent feature of the cat's HRTF is a single deep spectral notch, which is a sharp decrease in gain at frequencies between 5 and 20 kHz. When a broadband sound is passed through the transfer function, these frequencies are essentially filtered out of the stimulus. The frequency location of the notch changes systematically as a sound source moves in elevation or azimuth (Figure 5–6A). If these cues are removed from free-field sounds, cats make poorly directed orientation responses.[45]

The neural coding of spectral cues for sound localization has been examined by recording the HRTF-driven discharge rates of DCN projection neurons, which are known as type IV neurons. For best stimulus control, these experiments are performed with simulated spectral notches that are presented through headphones. The notch can be shifted in frequency with digital signal processing techniques to match the tuning of neurons that are encountered along the trajectory of the recording electrode.[46] The goal of these experiments is to mimic the movement of a sound source by manipulating the feature of interest relative to the inhibitory properties of the type IV neuron (Figure 5–6B). When the frequency of the notch is below the BF, the neuron is exclusively excited by the stimulus (Figure 5–6C, plots a and b). A similar response is produced when the notch is above BF (Figure 5–6D, plots d and e). These results are expected given the excitatory effects of broadband noise. However, when the notch coincides with BF, the neuron is strongly inhibited (Figure 5–6C and D, plot c).

The responses of type IV neurons to HRTF shapes are dictated by their nonlinear spectral integration properties.[47] Consequently, the neurons respond selectively to spectral shapes, and not merely the magnitude of individual frequency components. This feature-driven, level-tolerant representation is demonstrated by varying the presentation level of the HRTFs (Figure 5–6C and D). In contrast to the more generalized coding mechanisms of the VCN, major changes in spectral energy have little effect on the polarity of type IV responses to ON-BF and OFF-BF notches.

Clinical Implications

Perceptual abnormalities relating to DCN processing disorders have been investigated in the laboratory by sectioning the DAS (Figure 5–7A). This surgical manipulation eliminates the ascending axonal projections of pyramidal and giant cells en route to the ICC. Unlike lesions of the trapezoid body, lesions of the DAS have little effect on basic patterns of hearing. Absolute thresholds in quiet, and in background noise are not affected by the procedure.[34]

Significant deficits are observed when DAS lesioned cats are tested in localization paradigms that require the identification of sound source elevation.[48,49] Cats make reflexive head movements toward sudden, unexpected sounds. They also can be trained to perform these maneuvers repetitiously to gain access to food rewards. The cat is a natural predator, and the accuracy of these sound-guided responses approaches the limits of human directional hearing (Figure 5–7B).

When the output pathways of the DCN are bilaterally destroyed, cats exhibit clear deficits in localization behavior (Figure 5–7C).[49] Although performance is compromised in both horizontal and vertical dimensions, largest errors are observed in the determination of sound source elevation. These systematic errors confirm that the DCN is an important site for the auditory processing of spectral cues for sound localization. Cats

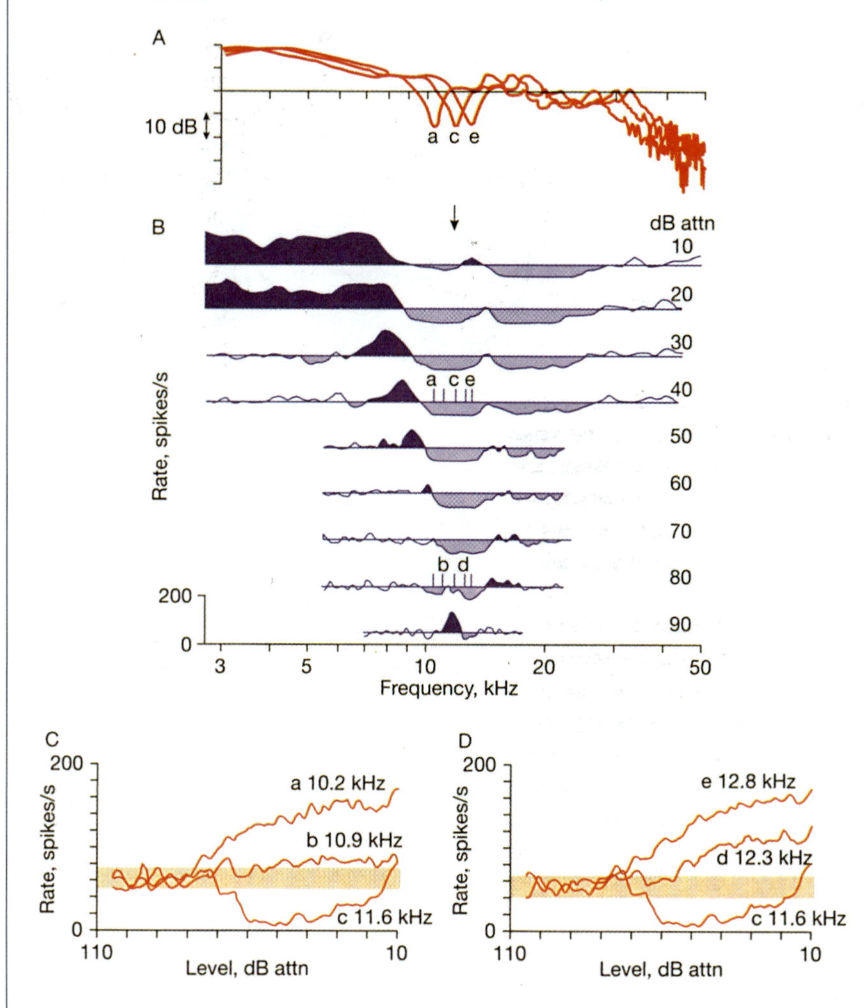

FIGURE 5–6 • Spectral coding in the dorsal cochlear nucleus. *A*, Generic head-related transfer functions of the cat. The biologically relevant spectral notch has been shifted in frequency by changing sampling rate during playback. *B*, The frequency response map of a DCN type IV unit. Letters relate the frequency location of the spectral notch at five sampling rates to the best frequency (BF) of the neuron. Excitatory responses (dark blue fill) are rates that exceed spontaneous activity. Inhibitory responses (light blue fill) are rates that fall below spontaneous activity. *C*, Rate-level functions obtained from the neuron when spectral notches were shifted to the unit's BF (c) or placed below BF (a,b). *D*, Rate-level functions for notches at BF (c) and above BF (d,e). The neuron's spontaneous rates are indicated by shading in *C* and *D*. *Adapted with permission from Young and Davis.*[37]

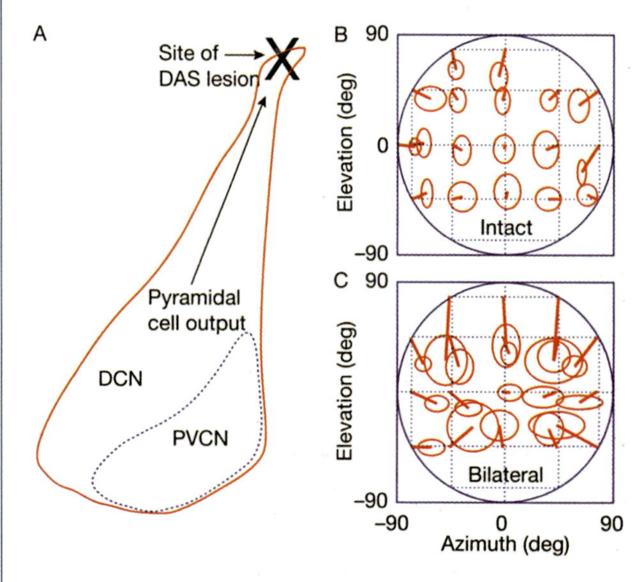

FIGURE 5–7 • Effects of dorsal acoustic stria (DAS) lesions on sound orientation behavior. *A*, Site of lesion. *B*, Accuracy of sound-evoked orientation responses in an intact cat. *C*, Accuracy after bilateral DAS lesions. Line segments connect actual source locations to average response locations. Ellipses indicate the standard deviation of responses in horizontal and vertical dimensions. *Adapted with permission from May.*[49]

with bilateral DAS lesions maintain directional hearing in the horizontal dimension by attending to binaural cues that are processed in the ventral pathways leading to the superior olivary complex.

The absolute silencing of DCN outputs by vascular accident or trauma is rare in human-patient populations. Tinnitus may reflect the less than complete disruption of this delicate circuitry.[50] If current physiological interpretations of tinnitus should prove to be correct, DCN processing deficits represent the most prevalent form of hearing disorder in industrial societies.

There is ample evidence that spontaneous discharge rates in the DCN increase when cochlear inputs are diminished by transient exposure to an intense sound or the long-term effects of aging. Because this hyperactivity mimics the normal auditory response to a physical stimulus, it creates the impression of phantom sound.[51,52]

The functional changes that accompany tinnitus have been extensively studied in animal models that allow controlled induction of the disorder and direct physiological evaluation of its consequences. This analysis has yet to reveal an unequivocal generator site and a unique pathology, but it is clear that candidate structures share common properties. The DCN, ICC, and auditory cortex have each been associated with tinnitus-like behavior.[53,54] These processing centers are key sites of multisensory integration where inputs from auditory and nonauditory nuclei converge to be acted upon by a constellation of excitatory and inhibitory neurotransmitters. Alterations of any component in this synaptic design have the potential to reorganize the resting and sound-driven properties of the neural circuit.

Neural hyperactivity remains the most influential physiological model of tinnitus. In part, the broad advocacy of this hypothetical mechanism lies in its intuitive simplicity. In addition, global changes in brain activity predict a metabolic signature that can be noninvasively imaged in human tinnitus patients.[55] While it is clear that some animal preparations respond to acoustic overexposure with generalized hyperactivity, important details of the proposed relationship between brain activity and sound perception remain unresolved. The effects may be specific to species, manner of induction, and methods of electrophysiological recording. A more comprehensive explanation of the underlying mechanisms of tinnitus may be gained from a more sophisticated statistical analysis of discharge patterns such as the regularity, synchronization, or long-term fluctuations of spontaneous activity.[56] These properties cannot be adequately described without direct electrophysiological recordings in animal preparations.

SUPERIOR OLIVARY COMPLEX

The superior olivary complex is situated in the ventral brainstem in close proximity to the trapezoid body. It consists of three primary auditory nuclei: the medial superior olive (MSO), lateral superior olive (LSO), and medial nucleus of the trapezoid body (MNTB). Ramon Y Cajal referred to the MSO and LSO as the accessory and superior olives in his classic Golgi studies.[57] These terms are occasionally encountered in modern texts. This central core is surrounded by a cluster of periolivary nuclei of which the lateral nucleus of the trapezoid body (LNTB) is the most prominent.

Ascending projections from both VCNs converge in the superior olivary complex to create binaural representations that are tuned to interaural disparities in time (interaural time differences, ITDs) and sound pressure level (interaural level differences, ILDs). Descending projections from the superior olive modulate cochlear sensitivity and cochlear nucleus inhibitory interactions through the action of olivocochlear efferent neurons.

Medial Superior Olive

The MSO performs a binaural comparison of the timing of sound-evoked discharge rates that reach the brain from the two ears. These temporal disparities are one of two essential cues for azimuthal (left–right) sound localization. The circuitry also plays an important role in spatial masking release, including the well-known "cocktail party effect." When competing auditory signals (eg, multiple talkers at a cocktail party) reach the listener's ear from different directions, spatial information facilitates their separation into distinct auditory objects. This process of "auditory streaming" may reduce the interference between signals by as much as 20 dB. Directional hearing relies heavily on binaural processes that are not available to individuals with unilateral hearing aids, which may explain why the devices perform poorly in complex listening environments.

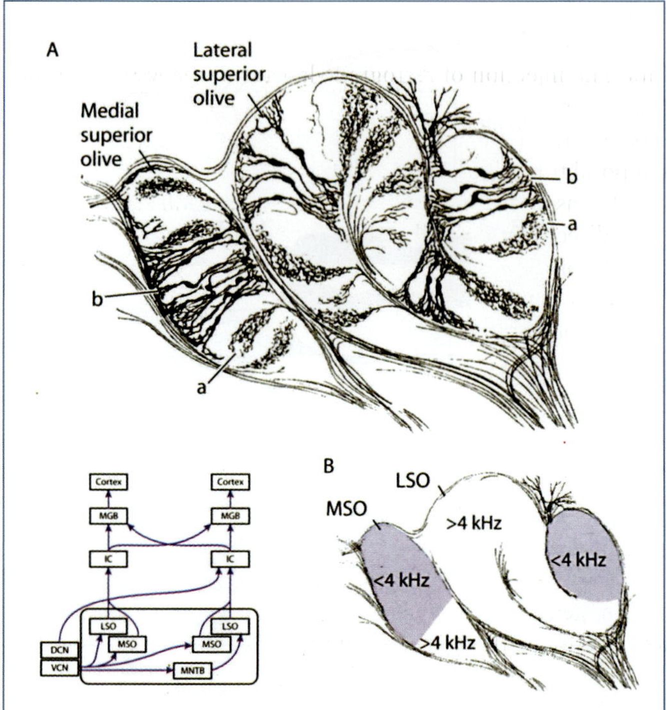

FIGURE 5–8 • The superior olivary complex. *A*, Golgi reconstructions of the lateral and medial superior olives showing bipolar neurons (a) and terminal axonal projections from the cochlear nucleus (b). *B*, Tonotopic map derived from electrophysiological recordings. Shaded regions indicate area devoted to frequencies below 4 kHz, the upper limits of temporal processing. Inset shows relative position of the superior olivary complex within the central auditory pathways. Abbreviations are explained in Figure 5–1. *Anatomical illustrations adapted from Scheibel and Scheibel[58] derived from Guinan et al.[59]*

Anatomy

In most mammals, the MSO is a two-dimensional sheet with bipolar dendritic fields (Figure 5–8A). The neurons receive afferent inputs from the ipsilateral VCN on lateral dendrites, and contralateral inputs medially. Because the inputs arise from spherical bushy cells,[60] high security endbulb synapses preserve the timing and frequency tuning of auditory nerve action potentials along their route to the MSO.[61]

The central cell region of the MSO is tonotopically organized along its dorsoventral axis (Figure 5–8B). Unlike the complete cochlear map that is found in the VCN, the MSO is biased toward low frequencies.[62] Although cats are capable of detecting frequencies above 64 kHz, the dorsal half of the feline nucleus is devoted to frequencies below 4 kHz. This frequency bias coincides with the upper limits of temporal coding by auditory neurons.[63]

Matching the delay sensitivity of auditory neurons to biologically relevant cues requires the interaction of a constellation of excitatory and inhibitory inputs, as well as the precisely timed delivery of each component. Results from immunocytochemical studies and intracellular recordings suggest that primary binaural inputs from the VCN are mediated by the excitatory amino acid glutamate through AMPA and NMDA receptors.[64] The MSO also shows a wide distribution of glycinergic receptors. The injection of retrograde label into the MSO indicates that the inhibitory inputs originate in the MNTB and LNTB.[65] Blocking the inhibition with strychnine compresses the range of temporal tuning shown by MSO neurons.[66]

The ascending projections of MSO neurons are almost exclusively directed ipsilaterally to low-frequency regions of the central nucleus of the ICC.[67] Injections of retrograde label into high-frequency regions has revealed few projections from the ventral subdivision of the MSO, where high-frequency neurons reside.[68]

Physiology

Neurons in the MSO are characterized by their monaural properties, binaural interactions, and ITD sensitivity. The sheet-like neuropil of MSO principal cells and the presence of powerful field potentials make isolation of single-unit activity in the nucleus difficult. Existing descriptions are typically founded on relatively small samples.

In general, MSO neurons show primary-like activity when tested with monaural stimuli. The discharge rates that are elicited by pure tones are irregularly timed, monotonically related to stimulus level, and narrowly tuned in frequency.[69] Responses to sounds in one ear cannot be considered in isolation because MSO neurons are excited by sounds in either ear. This excitatory-excitatory (EE) binaural interaction creates units with preferences for either contralateral or ipsilateral stimuli under monaural conditions.

The most influential model of binaural processing in the MSO is the Jeffress coincidence detector (Figure 5–9).[70] This anatomically based model was developed well before actual physiological recordings in the central auditory system. The key concept of coincidence is the existence of multiple delay lines in the afferent projections to MSO neurons. As a result, any acoustic delay in the interaural timing of a free-field sound is offset by a neural delay that is equal in magnitude but opposite in sign. The neuron with the appropriate delay line receives coincident inputs, which elicit maximum rates because of the EE binaural interaction. This pattern of excitatory ITD sensitivity is called a "peak-type" response. The neuron's delay sensitivity, therefore, represents a place code for the sound's location. It is interesting that, 50 years after the introduction of the Jeffress model, there is now anatomical evidence for coincidence detection circuits in the avian and mammalian MSO.[71,72]

Lateral Superior Olive

The LSO encodes the ILDs that signal the azimuth of high-frequency sounds. These cues are created by the "sound shadow" of the upper torso, head, and outer ear. Just as opaque objects block the path of light, acoustic reflections from the head produce interference patterns that reduce sound energy as it propagates to the two ears. A lateralized location will generate robust ILD cues because the interference is applied disproportionately to the far ear. The lower frequency limit of the shadowing effect is dictated by the geometry of the head. Larger animals are afforded lower frequency cues because their head attenuates longer acoustic wavelengths. Humans rely heavily on ILD cues at frequencies above 2 kHz.[73]

Anatomy

The LSO is arguably the most visually striking structure in the central auditory system. In cats, the LSO folds upon itself to take on an S-shaped conformation when viewed in transverse section (Figure 5–8A). The complexity and orientation of folding varies greatly in other species, depending on the biological significance of high-frequency sound localization.

The principal cells of the LSO have bipolar dendritic arbors that radiate across the hila of the nucleus. Axodendritic inputs arise from the same spherical bushy cell populations that project to the MSO; however, the inputs are confined to the ipsilateral cochlear nucleus.[3] The immunocytochemistry and morphological features of the synapses suggest that they evoke excitatory influences through the amino acid glutamate.[74]

Ascending inputs from the contralateral cochlear nucleus are relayed to the LSO by neurons in the MNTB. These indirect projections are the axonal tracts of globular bushy cells, which enter the trapezoid body and cross to the contralateral superior olivary complex.[60] Within the MNTB, the projections terminate in large calyceal synapses displaying glutamatergic pharmacological properties.[75] The postsynaptic targets of these projections label intensely for glycine.[76] Consequently, the excitatory input from the contralateral cochlear nucleus is reversed in sign before it reaches the LSO.

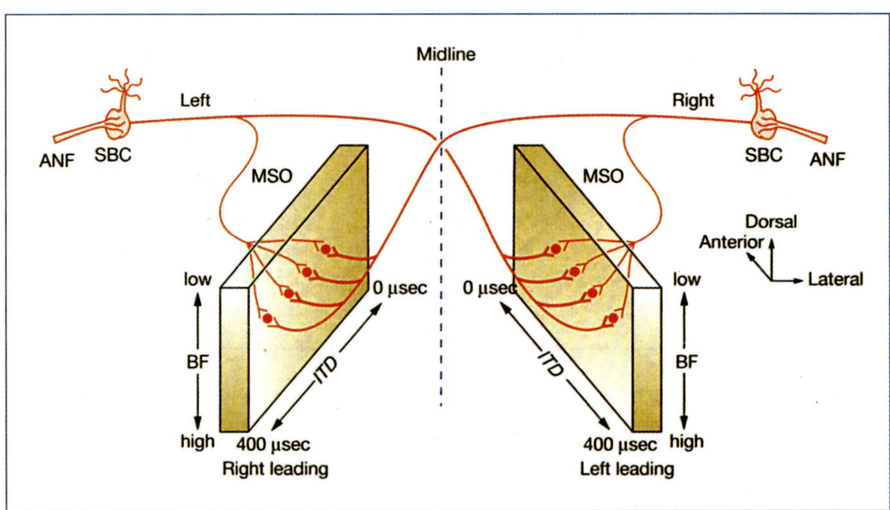

FIGURE 5–9 • The Jeffress coincidence detection model of sound localization. A single contralateral and ipsilateral input to the median superior olive (MSO) is shown. Neural delay lines are created by the arrayed termination pattern of the contralateral projections. ANF, auditory nerve fiber; BF, best frequency; ITD, interaural time difference; SBC, spherical bushy cell. *Adapted with permission from Yin.*[77]

The secure synaptic organization of MNTB principal cells preserves the timing and tuning of its cochlear nucleus inputs. Unlike the diffuse axosomatic endings of the monosynaptic excitatory input from the ipsilateral cochlear nucleus, disynaptic inhibitory inputs from the contralateral cochlear nucleus are delivered directly to the soma and proximal dendrites of LSO neurons.[78] This configuration aids a coincident binaural comparison by offsetting the synaptic delay that is introduced by additional transformations in the MNTB. Although many anatomical properties of the LSO are similar to those seen in the MSO, contralateral inhibition tunes its responses to the relative magnitude, and not timing of sound energy at the two ears.

Physiology

Single-unit recordings in the LSO reveal a tonotopic map with an exaggerated representation of high frequencies (Figure 5–8B). This bias corresponds favorably with the frequency domain of ILD information. Monaural responses to ipsilateral and contralateral stimuli show similar frequency tuning suggesting that underlying binaural comparisons are frequency specific. As expected, given the neurotransmitters of their ascending inputs, LSO neurons display IE binaural interactions. That is, they are inhibited by contralateral stimuli and excited by ipsilateral sounds. Because LSO neurons are maximally inhibited by coincident binaural inputs, they show minimum discharge rates. This inhibitory ITD sensitivity that is call a "trough-type" response.

Most LSO neurons exhibit monotonically increasing rate-level functions when ipsilateral tones are presented under closed-field conditions (Figure 5–10). This monaural response pattern recapitulates the coding of stimulus level by auditory nerve fibers and primary-like neurons in the anteroventral cochlear nucleus. Because monaural responses to contralateral tones are inhibitory, they simply suppress the neuron's spontaneous activity.

The effects of contralateral inhibition are better demonstrated under binaural conditions. To quantify the strength of inhibition, activity is evoked by an ipsilateral excitatory stimulus while a competing contralateral inhibitory stimulus is varied in level. This manipulation simulates the movement of a sound source from an ipsilateral location (lower contralateral levels) to a contralateral location (higher contralateral levels). The resulting rate changes show good agreement between LSO sensitivity and behavioral thresholds for ILD discrimination.[80]

The Acoustic Chiasm

The LSO sends bilateral projections through the lateral lemniscus to the central nucleus of the ICC. Approximately equal numbers of fibers ascend in an ipsilateral and contralateral direction. Tract tracing techniques have localized the source of ipsilateral projections to the lateral limb of the LSO. Contralateral projections originate in the medial limb. This sorting of output by physical location resembles the routing of optic nerve fibers through the optic chiasm. Because a tonotopic gradient is imposed on anatomical locations in the central auditory system, this "acoustic chiasm" separates high frequencies and routes them contralaterally, while low frequencies are sent ipsilaterally.[81]

The projection patterns and neurotransmitter systems of the superior olive enhance the contralateral representation of sound (Figure 5–11). A sound on the left side of the listener will produce bilateral activity in the anterior VCN, MNTB, and the MSO. Neural transmission in these pathways is mediated by excitatory amino acids. The ascending excitatory input carrying high-frequency information from the right LSO crosses to the left ICC.[82,83] Activity in the left LSO is silenced by MNTB inhibition. Both MSOs carry low-frequency information to the mid brain by ipsilateral excitatory projections but these inputs are inhibited in the right ICC by uncrossed glycinergic projections from the low-frequency LSO.[84] The net result of these reciprocal influences

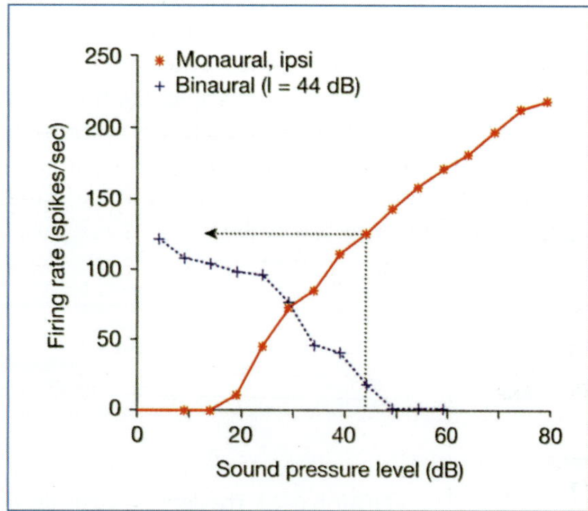

FIGURE 5–10 • Binaural interactions in the lateral super olive. Rate-level functions are compared for monaural ipsilateral tones and binaural tones. Dotted line indicates the firing rate evoked by a monaural ipsilateral tone at a presentation level of 44 dB SPL. This ipsilateral stimulus was fixed during binaural measures. Variations in contralateral tone levels during binaural testing are indicated on the abscissa. *Adapted with permission from Joris and Yin.*[79] SPL, sound pressure level.

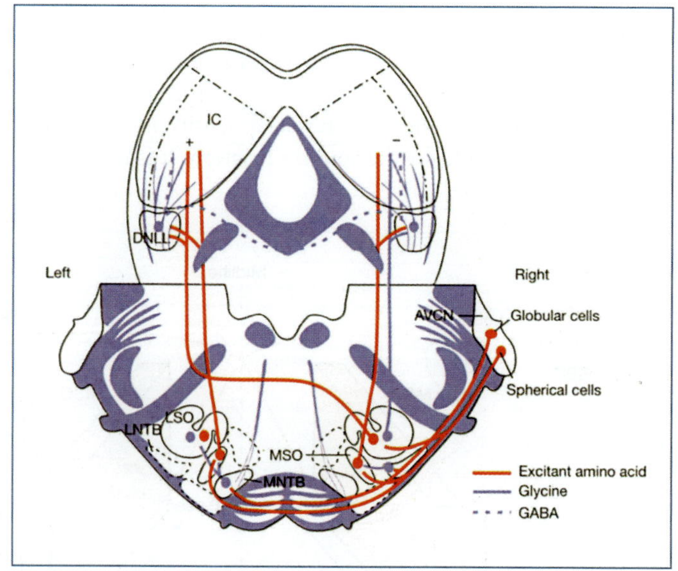

FIGURE 5–11 • The "acoustic chiasm" created by ascending projections from the superior olivary complex. Major connections are shown for the right ear. Putative neurotransmitters are indicated by line style. The strength of the input is represented by line width. *Adapted with permission from Helfert and Aschoff.*[85]

is a complete representation of low and high frequencies in the contralateral ICC. If a unilateral lesion is placed in the ICC or a higher structure in the central auditory system, sound localization deficits are restricted to the contralateral hemifield.[86]

Olivocochlear Efferent Pathway

Decades of research have probed the structure and function of the ascending auditory pathways. The reciprocal descending circuitry at present remains largely unexplored. The exception to this inattention is the olivocochlear efferent pathway, which is a mechanism that gives the brainstem control over the mechanical sensitivity of the auditory periphery. Olivocochlear feedback may play an important role in hearing protection, selective attention, and listening in noise.

Anatomy

Anatomical characteristics suggest that there are two separate olivocochlear systems (Figure 5–12).[87] The thin, unmyelinated axons of the more numerous lateral olivocochlear (LOC) neurons project from lateral regions of the superior olive to the distal processes of auditory nerve fibers. The innervation patterns of LOC fibers are heavily biased toward the ipsilateral cochlea. Medial olivocochlear (MOC) projections originate from cell bodies that are scattered in medial regions of the superior olivary complex. These neurons send thick myelinated axons to the inner ear, where they enter the organ of Corti through the habenulae perforatae, cross the tunnel of Corti, and terminate on the base of outer hair cells. The majority of the fibers project to the contralateral cochlea.

En route to the cochlea, MOC neurons send collateral projections to granule cell areas of the cochlear nucleus.[88] The projections target the dendritic fields of large multipolar cells that reside in the VCN. Because the target neurons are a source of inhibition, this feedback may compensate for efferent-based changes in the dynamic range properties of auditory nerve inputs to the cochlear nucleus. Any reduction in cochlear sensitivity by direct MOC influences may be offset by a reciprocal

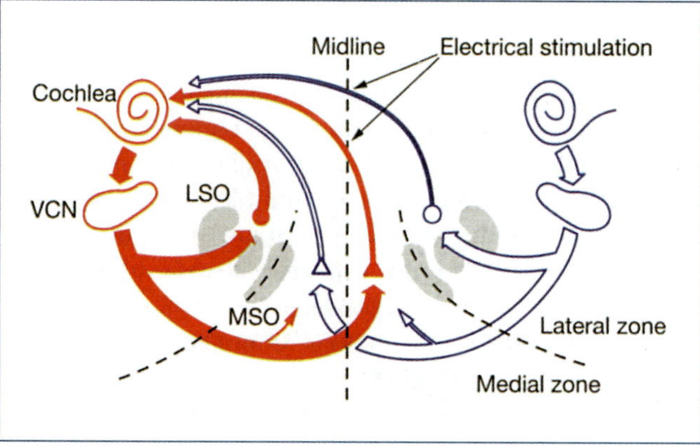

FIGURE 5–12 • The olivocochlear reflex arc. Inputs are shown from both ears, outputs to one ear. The cell bodies of medial olivocochlear efferents are located in the medial zones (triangles). Lateral olivocochlear efferents are located in the lateral zones (circles). The strength of input is indicated by line widths. LSO, lateral superior olive; MSO, medial superior olive; VCN, ventral cochlear nucleus. *Adapted with permission from Warr.*[89]

attenuation of cochlear nucleus inhibition. Consequently, the mechanical tuning of the cochlear partition can be tailored to the ongoing listening environment without a corruption of actual signal levels in higher processing centers.

Physiology

Classical physiological descriptions of olivocochlear function are performed by switching on the system with electrical shocks. The stimulating electrodes are placed on the midline of the IVth ventricle, where crossing fibers of the olivocochlear bundle (OCB) approach the dorsal surface of the medulla (Figure 5–12). This paradigm is assumed to selectively activate the medial efferent system. Electrical stimulation is less effective for the unmyelinated lateral efferent system. In addition, most LOC fibers project to the ipsilateral ear without approaching the site of stimulation.

The effects of olivocochlear feedback can be observed by comparing auditory nerve activity with and without OCB stimulation. The responses have been characterized in terms of compound action potentials (CAPs)[90] or direct single unit recording.[91] In both contexts, OCB stimulation reduces cochlear sensitivity.

Efferent-mediated changes in the dynamic range of the auditory nerve reflect alterations in the active mechanical properties of the cochlea.[92] Outer hair cells display the unique ability to move in response to depolarizing currents.[93] The force generated by this so-called electromotility amplifies and tunes the sound-generated movements of the cochlear partition. The release of acetylcholine by MOC neurons triggers an influx of calcium into the outer hair cells, which opens voltage-gated potassium channels in the cell membranes. The subsequent efflux of potassium hyperpolarizes the cells, making them less sensitive to depolarizing currents that enter through the stereocilia during movements of the basilar membrane. As a result, sound-generated deflections of the stereocilia bundle fail to elicit complementary electromechanical responses.

When sounds occur in the presence of background noise, a listening advantage may be gained by shifting the dynamic range of neural responses to higher levels.[94] Auditory nerve recordings have shown that a sensitive neuron may be driven to its maximum discharge rate by noise alone, leaving no additional response to encode the occurrence of a meaningful auditory event. When sensitivity is reduced by electrically stimulating the OCB, noise no longer saturates the neuron's response and coincident signals are able to evoke further rate increases.

Clinical Implications

Olivocochlear fibers enter the cochlea intermingled with the inferior vestibular nerve. Consequently, when the vestibular nerve is sectioned to alleviate intractable vertigo, the lesioned ear loses both vestibular and olivocochlear function.[95] What is most striking about these patients is the subtlety of their ensuing auditory deficits.[96] A battery of audiological assessments has identified one consistent abnormality. The loss of olivocochlear feedback reduces "selective listening." Under normal circumstances, this process allows an individual to listen to one channel of information while blocking out sounds in other competing channels. Auditory information channels are usually defined by frequency; that is, the subject focuses attention on one tone frequency at the expense of other frequencies. Because olivocochlear feedback is tuned in frequency, the listener may optimize performance by increasing cochlear sensitivity at the attended frequency and decreasing sensitivity at unattended frequencies. It is also possible to attend to auditory streams that are defined by their location, pitch, or temporal pattern. This ability is critical for separating important sounds from the acoustic clutter of real-world environments. Consequently, individuals with weak olivocochlear feedback tend to show deficits when listening in background noise.[97]

An important consideration for the audiological evaluation of vestibular neurectomy is that the patient populations upon which these studies have been performed are biased toward preexisting Meniere's disease with concomitant hearing loss. Such confounds are avoided in animal studies of olivocochlear function. The existing literature of controlled experimental manipulations has defined three roles for the efferent system: sound protection, listening in noise, and cochlear development. The ability of olivocochlear feedback to reduce acoustic trauma has received the greatest attention in the laboratory.[98]

Two qualities of the MOC pathways allow efferent feedback to be observed noninvasively in human listeners. First, olivocochlear activity may be induced by contralateral sound stimulation. Second, when the feedback is activated, there is a decrease in the magnitude of otoacoustic emissions, which depend on active cochlear processes. An intriguing aspect of these measures is the considerable variation in the strength of olivocochlear feedback among human subjects. Consequently, observers with weaker systems are less able to process sounds in noisy environments,[97] and may be more susceptible to acoustic trauma.[99]

INFERIOR COLLICULUS

The ICC may have the most elaborate neuronal connections of any auditory structure. It is comprised of a central core of sound processing neurons, the central nucleus, and a surrounding belt of polysensory nuclei with less robust sound-driven responses. The acoustic tuning of neurons in the central nucleus reflects the convergence of multiple parallel pathways that are created in the cochlear nucleus. Direct monaural projections originate in the ventral and dorsal subdivisions of the contralateral cochlear nucleus. Indirect binaural projections are routed through the superior olivary complex and nuclei of the lateral lemniscus. These ascending inputs are not simply relayed to higher structures. They are transformed into more selective representations of acoustic information and then delivered to higher processing centers in the auditory thalamus and cortex.

The sharp dichotomy of response patterns in the central and belt regions of the ICC has prompted the distinction of lemniscal pathways (the tonotopic core) versus extralemniscal pathways (the nontonotopic belt). Although auditory physiologists have focused on auditory activity in the lemniscal pathways, many clinicians have directed their attention to the extralemniscal system because disordered interactions of its multimodal inputs may serve as generator sites for audiogenic seizures, abnormal loudness perception, and certain types of tinnitus.[100]

Anatomy

The primary anatomical subdivision of the ICC is the central nucleus (Figure 5–13A).[101] The laminar structure of the ICC is created by incoming projections from the brainstem and the dendrites of disc-shaped principal cells. These fibrodendritic arrays are oriented in parallel creating isofrequency laminae. The cochlear tonotopic map is projected on the dorsal–ventral axis of the nucleus and preserved in its ascending outputs to the auditory thalamus.[102]

In addition to disc-shaped cells, stellate cells represent approximately 25% of the ICC cell population. They have ovoid or stellate dendritic fields that integrate synaptic inputs across isofrequency laminae. Immunostaining indicates that the ICC sends both excitatory and inhibitory projections to the medial geniculate body.[103] Because the number and size of cells that label positively for the inhibitory neurotransmitter gamma-amino butyric acid (GABA) match the characteristics of stellate cells, it is suspected that the neural population is an important source of thalamic inhibition.[104] It is not presently known if the broadband inhibitory influences of stellate cells are localized within particular processing pathways.

The ICC receives direct or indirect inputs from all of the major projection pathways of the cochlear nucleus. Within the ICC, there are regionalized differences in the topography of these inputs. The results of anterograde tracing studies suggest that excitatory inputs from ITD-sensitive MSO neurons and ILD-sensitive LSO neurons remain anatomically segregated (Figure 5–13B).[105] From a functional perspective, the discrete synaptic domains of these two binaural pathways mirror their separate roles in sound localization. Similarly, although the DCN and LSO both project to high-frequency regions, each lamina may be divided into a ventral portion that receives mixed inputs and a dorsal portion that is exclusively innervated by the DCN.[106] This pattern of input may establish functional modules that differ in their accentuation of binaural and monaural coding.

The belt regions of the ICC have been subdivided with varying degrees of complexity. Differences in existing maps of cellular anatomy reflect the histological methods used to identify cytoarchitectural features and connectivity. Most parcellations involve a dorsal cortex and paracentral nuclei of which the lateral or external nucleus is the most prominent.[107]

The dorsal cortex is the target of profuse descending inputs from multiple fields in auditory cortex[108] and commissural projections from the contralateral central nucleus.[109] Ascending auditory inputs are sparse. Incomplete regionalized innervation is received from the DCN and dorsal nucleus of the lateral lemniscus. Inputs from the MSO and LSO are conspicuously absent. The descending efferent projections of the dorsal cortex are directed bilaterally to the principal cell areas of the DCN.[110] This reciprocal circuitry suggests that the dorsal cortex may be specialized to enhance the analysis of monaural spectral cues for vertical sound localization.

The lateral nucleus receives somatosensory representations of the head from the dorsal column and trigeminal nuclei, as well as premotor inputs from components of the basal ganglia.[111] Auditory inputs are dominated by intracollicular projections from the ipsilateral central nucleus. Efferent projections of the lateral nucleus pass to the deep layers of the superior colliculus and cerebellum by way of the pontine nuclei where they may contribute to the integration of acoustically driven motor

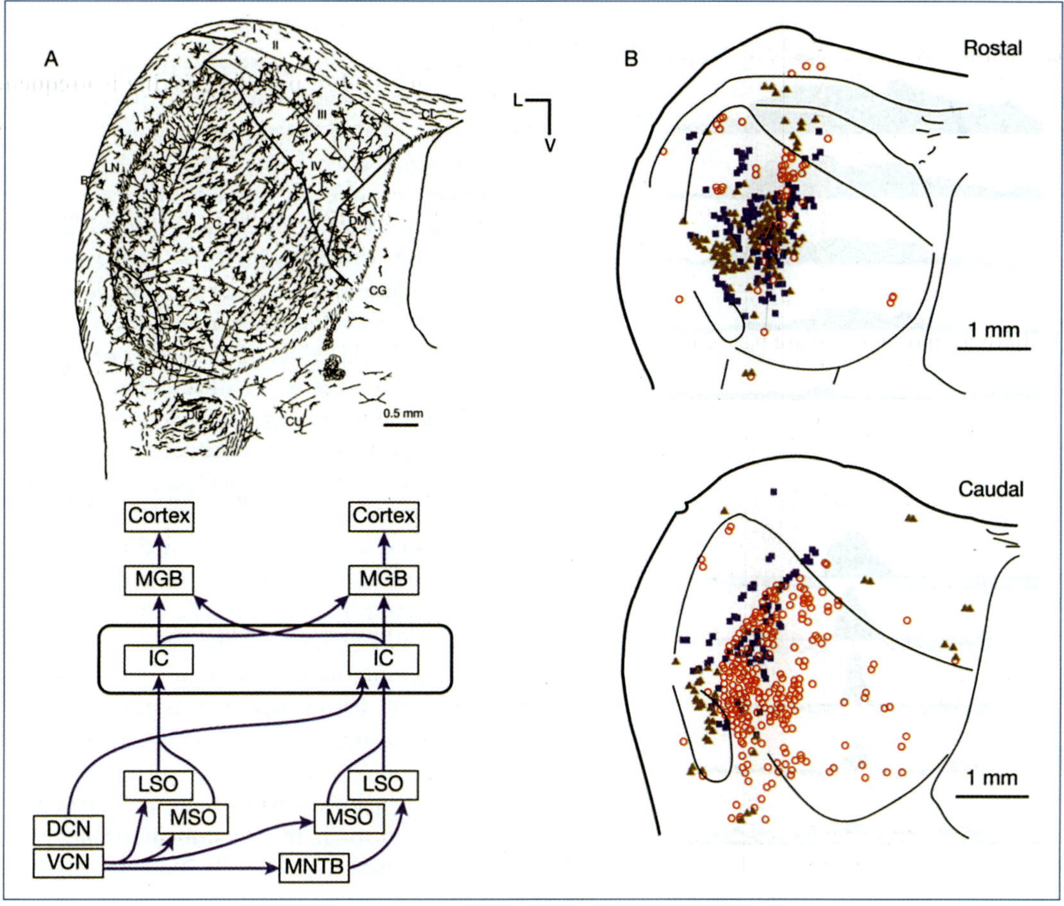

FIGURE 5–13 • Anatomical organization of the cat inferior colliculus. *A*, Laminar structure imposed by the trajectory of axonal projections and the dendritic fields of disc-shaped neurons. *B*, Terminal zones of projections from the superior olive. Excitatory projections from the contralateral LSO dominate rostral locations (filled triangles). Excitatory projections from the ipsilateral MSO are mostly found at caudal locations (open circles). Inhibitory inputs from the ipsilateral LSO are also shown (blue squares). Inset shows relative position of the inferior colliculus within the central auditory pathways. Abbreviations are explained in Figure 5–1. *Adapted with permission from Morest and Oliver[107] and Loftus et al.[105]*

behaviors such as startle responses, pinna reflexes, and sound target acquisitions by the head and eyes.[112]

Classification of Sound-Driven Activity in the Central Nucleus

The physiological properties of the central nucleus are strongly modified by barbiturate anesthesia. These influences may be avoided by recording single-unit activity in unanesthetized, decerebrate preparations. The subject's ability to initiate movements and experience pain is eliminated by transecting all fibers entering and exiting the cerebral cortex at the level of the thalamus. A limitation of this approach is that descending feedback systems from cortex are also removed from the neuronal circuitry of the auditory midbrain.

The principal cells of the ICC show three basic response patterns when frequency response maps (FRMs) are recorded in decerebrate cats (Figure 5–14).[113] The most common response has been designated the type-O unit because the neuron's excitatory receptive field is constrained to a small O-shaped island of frequencies near threshold. The remainder of the receptive field is dominated by inhibition. The neurons also tend to be insensitive to ITD cues.[114] These response patterns are reminiscent of monaural projection neurons in the DCN (type IV neurons). Type-O units are silenced when conduction is blocked in the DAS, further supporting a direct link between the DCN and the response type.[115] Type-O units are less commonly encountered in prey species (eg, guinea pigs, mice, gerbils),[116] which implies that they may play a specialized role in the predatory behaviors of the cat. The localization accuracy of cats is far superior to that of the prey upon which they feed.[117]

Type-I units are defined by a narrow I-shaped excitatory receptive field that is surrounded by lateral inhibition. The neurons tend to be tuned to higher frequencies and display trough-type ITD sensitivity. This cluster of physiological characteristics suggests that type-I units are the midbrain target of ascending excitatory projections from the contralateral LSO. Conversely, type-V units show an excitatory receptive field, low-frequency tuning, and peak-type ITD sensitivity. The controlling influences of these neurons are assumed to emanate from the ipsilateral MSO.

The FRM classification scheme is useful for interpreting the functional connections of the ICC. This simple conceptual framework reveals how physiologically defined pathways of the cochlear nucleus remain segregated en route to higher processing levels. It also provides a metric for evaluating

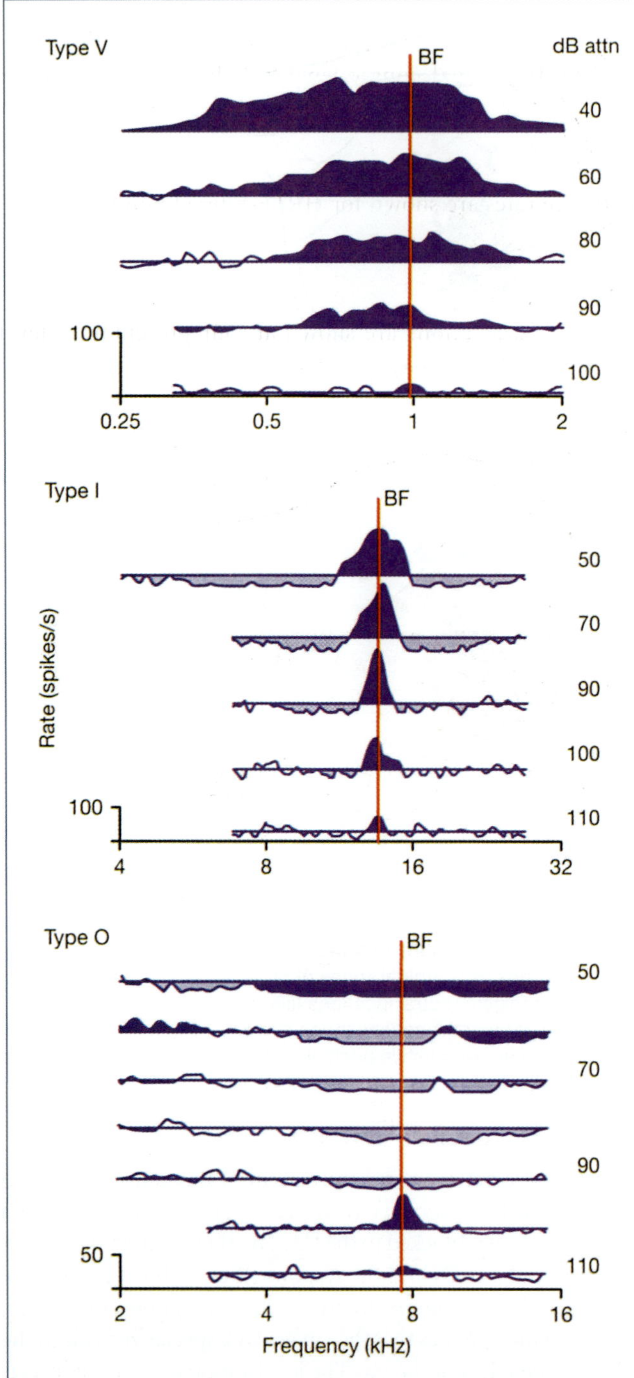

FIGURE 5–14 • Physiological properties of neurons in the central nucleus of the inferior colliculus. The responses were recorded in decerebrate cats. Frequency response maps plot sound-driven discharge rates as a function of pure tone frequency and level. Plotting conventions for frequency response maps are described in Figure 5–6. *Adapted with permission from Ramachandran et al.*[113]

how local transformations impact the quality of information coding. Nevertheless, it is clear from anatomical evidence that the central nucleus is the nexus of the auditory system; ie, the place where discrete representations from multiple input sources are bound together to form perceptual experience.[118]

Information Coding

Studies of information coding in the ICC have examined the representation of simple sound elements (amplitude, frequency, and timing), as well as the more complex constructs that support communication, localization, and perceptual grouping. A common theme in this research is the emergence of responses that are more selective than those observed in lower processing centers. Single-unit responses may be sharply tuned not only to frequency but also to sound pressure level[119] and temporal properties such as amplitude modulation (AM) or frequency modulation (FM).[120] Consequently, in contrast to the population codes of the auditory brainstem, the responses of individual neurons may signify critical biological information that lies in the spectral shape or dynamic patterns of natural sounds.

Temporal coding is founded on the ability of auditory neurons to entrain their discharge rates to time varying acoustic properties such as monaural AM and FM fluctuations as well as binaural temporal disparities. Modulation cues are important information-bearing elements of communication sounds and an essential reference for the segregation of auditory signals from background noise. Interaural time differences, as previously discussed, are the basis of azimuthal sound localization.

Amplitude and frequency modulations are encoded by the timing of action potentials in the auditory nerve and brainstem. At low tone frequencies, neurons fire at a particular phase of the stimulus waveform. In most mammals, the upper limit of phase-locking is reached around 5 kHz. Nevertheless, this mechanism remains in effect at much higher frequencies because discharge rates are synchronized to the envelope fluctuations of complex sounds.

Beyond the upper frequency limits of phase-locking and envelope following responses, temporal coding is constrained by the probabilistic nature of synaptic events. Each synapse adds error to the neural representation of time because of uncertainties in the release of neurotransmitter from the presynaptic neuron and the subsequent generation of action potentials in the postsynaptic neuron. The dedicated temporal pathways that project to the olivary complex minimize this "jitter" by integrating the inputs of multiple auditory nerve fibers and securely transmitting that information through powerful endbulb synapses.

Further synaptic degradation of temporal information may be avoided at high levels of auditory processing by transforming the temporal code into a rate code.[121] Neurons in the ICC are sharply tuned to specific modulation rates just as brainstem neurons are tuned in frequency. Consequently, the neuron acts as a "labeled line" signaling modulation frequency with its relative firing rates and not the temporal structure of its responses.

The ascending projections of the LSO and MSO endow neurons in the central nucleus with binaural temporal tuning. As in the brainstem, the majority of these neurons show peak-type or trough-type responses, which according to the Jeffress Model, may be explained by binaural excitatory and inhibitory interactions (see detailed descriptions in Superior Olivary Complex). A number of neurons, however, show intermediate-type ITD sensitivity.[122,123] The neurons may respond best to intermediate interaural phase disparities or show complex phase–frequency relationships. This temporal pattern is not compatible with the

Jeffress Model and probably reflects the convergence of olivary inputs with different ITD tuning.[124] It is likely that even ICC neurons with less complicated peak-type and trough-type responses integrate multiple inputs from the superior olive because the bandwidth of ITD tuning for both unit types is significantly sharper than their SOC counterparts.[125]

Spectral coding in the ICC is important for monaural sound localization and vocal communication.[126] The receptive fields of ICC neurons may span several octaves creating regions where spectral energy produces either excitatory or inhibitory effects. Sounds with energy at excitatory frequencies evoke strong responses; whereas, sounds with energy at inhibitory frequencies elicit weak responses. The response to a complex spectral shape, such as a broadband noise that has been filtered by the transfer function of the outer ear, is dictated by the balance of this excitation and inhibition.

The functional consequences of the template-matching process are summarized in Figure 5–15, which shows how the spatial tuning of an ICC neuron correlates with the frequency domain of its OFF-BF inhibition. In Figure 5–15A, the neuron's discharge rates are shown for HRTF-filtered noise bursts. The binaural stimuli were presented through headphones to simulate the acoustic effects of the two external ears at 99 different locations in the frontal sound field. Responses to these "virtual" sound locations are shown at four presentation levels. Each response is plotted according to the spectral energy in the contralateral (dominant) ear at the neuron's BF (~12 kHz). The distinguishing feature of the resulting rate-level function

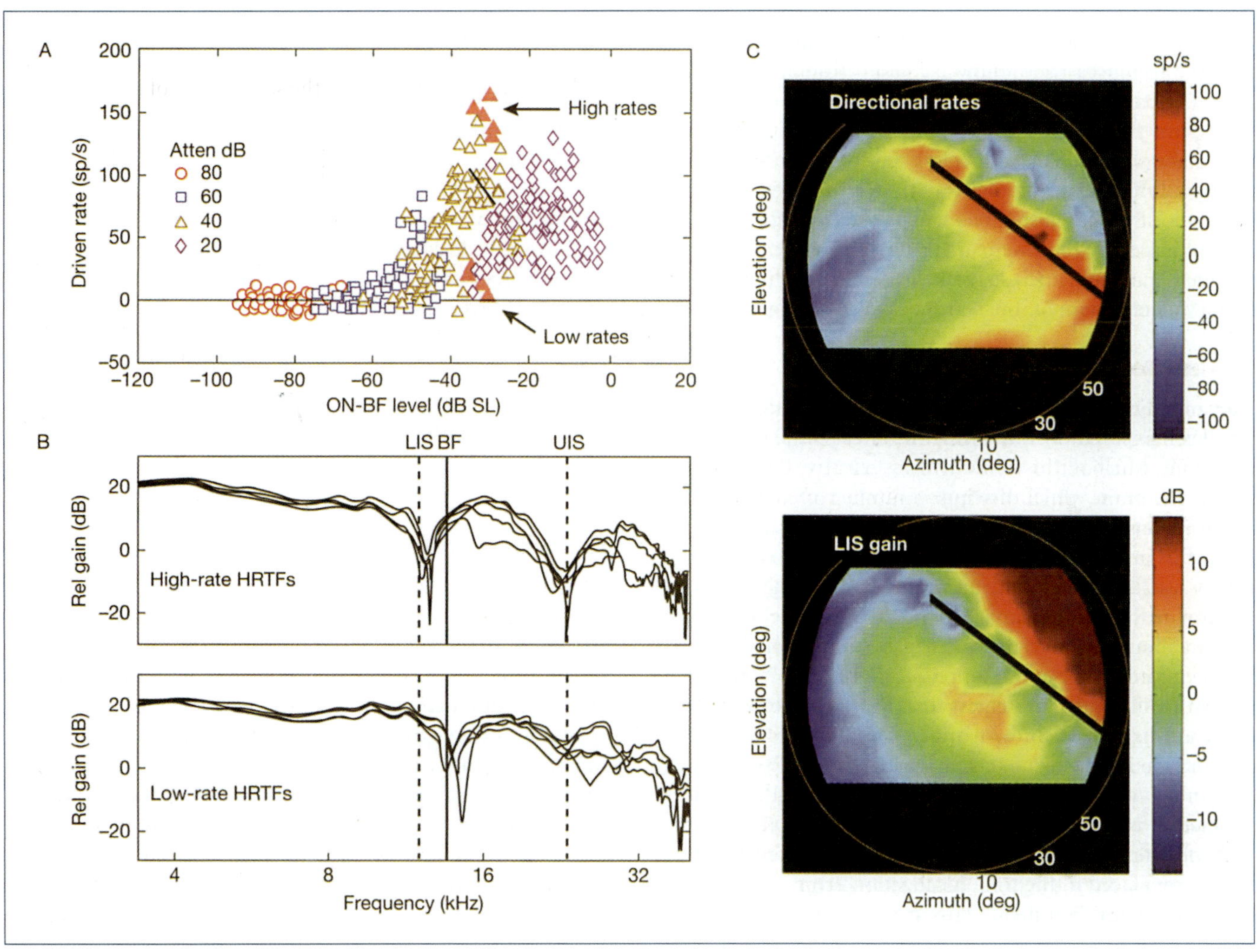

FIGURE 5–15 • Spatial tuning of a single-unit response in the inferior colliculus of a decerebrate cat. *A*, Discharge rates evoked by noise bursts that have been shaped by the cat's head-related transfer functions (HRTFs, see dorsal cochlear nucleus). Responses are shown for 99 locations in the frontal sound field at four presentation levels. Each data point is plotted in terms of spectrum level at the neuron's best frequency (BF). Filled symbols contrast HRTFs with similar ON-BF energy that elicited high versus low discharge rates. *B*, The spectral shapes of high- versus low-rate HRTFs. Vertical lines mark the relative gain of the functions at BF, and at a lower inhibitory sideband (LIS) and an upper inhibitory sideband (UIS). *C*, The role of sideband inhibition in the neuron's directional tuning. In the upper panel, the discharges rates in A are plotted in spatial coordinates. In the lower panel, the gain of the HRTFs at the LIS are plotted in spatial coordinates. Strongest responses (red) are observed where the transfer functions show the weakest gain at inhibitory frequencies. *Adapted with permission from May et al.*[126]

is the extreme variation in responses to HRTFs with similar ON-BF energy. These differences are observed because the neuron is sensitive to spectral features that exist at frequencies well beyond BF.

The HRTF shapes in Figure 5–15B are grouped by their ability to elicit high- or low-discharge rates from the IC neuron, as indicated by filled symbols in Figure 5–15A. Although the transfer functions have similar ON-BF energy, there are consistent differences in the frequency locations of their prominent spectral notches. High-rate HRTFs have notches that fall within lower and upper inhibitory sidebands (vertical dashed lines). Consequently, they produce relatively weak inhibitory responses. The low-rate HRTFs show the opposite polarity. Their spectral notches correspond to the central excitatory region surrounding the neuron's BF (vertical solid line).

The neuron's sensitivity to HRTF shapes is translated to spatial tuning in Figure 5–15C. The upper panel plots the discharge rates in Figure 5–15A, in spatial coordinates that indicate the virtual sound field location of the HRTF stimuli. The neuron's strongest responses (red) follow a contour from high ipsilateral to low contralateral elevations (superimposed line). The lower panel plots the relative gain of the HRTF stimuli in the same coordinate system. This gain refers selectively to the spectral energy falling within the neuron's powerful lower inhibitory sideband (LIS). The close agreement between locations with low gain (blue areas in the lower panel) and locations with high rates (red areas in upper panel) suggests that OFF-BF inhibition is the primary determinant of the neuron's spatial tuning.

Behavior/Ablation Studies

The contributions of the ICC to sound localization behavior have been explored by evaluating the effects of planned surgical lesions. Much of this work involves selective damage to one side of the brain, which disrupts a number of complex auditory functions without completely eliminating basic hearing.[118] When this procedure is performed on an experimental animal, there is a striking dichotomy between lesions of the lower commissural pathways and damage to the ICC. Unilateral lesions in the lower brainstem nuclei have a negative impact on directional hearing regardless of sound source location. [33,86,127,128] The pervasive nature of the deficit suggests that the foundations of localization are disrupted before a neural representation of directional information is fully formed. Damage to either side of the brain has global consequences because the timing and magnitude of binaural responses must be integrated to complete the first stage of directional processing. By contrast, when unilateral lesions are placed in the ICC, localization errors are limited to the contralateral hemifield. This spatial restriction implies a second-stage "distributive" process that biases the higher-order representation of auditory space toward contralateral source locations.[81,129] As previously noted, the acoustic chiasm is the proposed mechanism for the selective lateralized distribution of ascending olivary inputs to the central nucleus. Damage to the lateral lemniscus, therefore, produces similar deficits.

Behavior-ablation studies have relied heavily on free-field testing arenas to characterize the accuracy of directional hearing. In the classic two-alternative forced-choice paradigm, one of two goal boxes is unlocked to allow an animal access to a food reward. The left versus right location of the unlocked receptacle is signaled by the presentation of an auditory stimulus from an attached speaker. The limits of the subject's localization capabilities are measured by varying the angle of separation between the two goal box/speaker combinations. This is a true localization task that requires the subject to identify and approach the sound source for the food reward.

A review of this classic literature leads to the impression that destruction of the commissures of the ICC or cerebral cortex does not radically alter localization behavior.[33,128] Lesions of the trapezoid body may produce striking deficits, but these effects are only observed in some subjects and they tend to be transient.

Subsequent investigations have brought up the possibility that goal-box testing may be confounded by listening strategies that do not require directional hearing.[86] When two sound sources are located in the left and right hemifield of the testing arena, a subject with normal directional hearing may identify the active speaker by relying on binaural cues to distinguish *left* versus *right*. When spatial processing is distorted in one hemifield (eg, after a lesion of the left ICC disrupts localization in the right hemifield), the subject may continue to detect the food source by deciding whether the active goal box is *left* versus *not-left*. When the unilateral deficit is accompanied by hearing loss, the subject may respond *loud* versus *quiet*.

Covarying decision-criteria may be brought under stimulus control by increasing the number of sound sources in the testing arena, which requires the subject to select the active speaker from alternative locations in both hemifields. This procedural manipulation does not change the effects of trapezoid body lesions, but the behavioral consequences of higher-order lesions become more apparent.[86] Without the aid of nondirectional listening strategies, a complete and permanent disruption of sound localization is observed in the contralateral sound field.

Audiological Implications

The hallmark of auditory processing in the ICC is its delicate balance of excitation and inhibition. When these processes function normally, neurons show exquisite tuning to the many acoustic dimensions that give meaning to sound. Unfortunately, the mechanisms that shape the sound-driven activity of the auditory midbrain may spiral out of control in individuals who experience hearing loss, acoustic trauma, or aging. When excitatory inputs from the brainstem are reduced in number or strength, the ICC may grow silent. Conversely, a loss of tonic inhibition may produce abnormally responsive neurons. This hyperactivity has been implicated as a causal factor for audiogenic seizures, hyperacusis, loudness recruitment, and tinnitus.

Immunocytochemical studies[130] have demonstrated a substantial loss of the inhibitory neurotransmitter GABA in the central nucleus of aged rats. The loss is regionally selective. One-third fewer GABA-positive neurons are seen in the ventrolateral portion of the nucleus relative to young controls. Neurochemical analyses confirm that the potassium-evoked release of GABA by this tissue is significantly decreased, while the release of the excitatory neurotransmitter glutamate is up-regulated. These findings suggest that disordered GABAergic transmission in the ICC may contribute to a number of the audiological abnormalities that accompany neural presbycusis.[131] The effectiveness of GABAergic inhibition is also diminished by experimental manipulations that are known to induce tinnitus.[132,133]

The ICC has been proposed as a site for audiogenic seizures in animal models of epilepsy.[134] At the neural level, the induction of epileptiform activity is observed as a train of prolonged afterdischarges that follow sound stimulation. Insensitivity to endogenous GABA inhibition appears to lie at the core of these abnormal response patterns. When GABA is delivered to an ICC neuron by iontophoresis, the amount of neurotransmitter that is required to suppress activity in epilepsy-prone rats is significantly greater than in normal rats. A reduction of GABA-mediated inhibition also is indicated by the decreased efficacy of agonists such as benzodiazepine. Epileptiform activity may be induced in normal neurons by iontophoresis of bicuculline, a potent antagonist of GABA.

This same loss of central inhibition may lead to the perception of chronic tinnitus.[135] In addition to producing stronger, longer lasting responses to auditory stimuli, downregulation of GABA may increase spontaneous activity in the absence of sound. Because the hyperactivity mimics the sound-driven responses of auditory neurons, it is hypothesized that higher brain centers interpret the activity as sound even though no physical stimulus is present. The ICC may play a prominent role in the phenomenon because of the well-established physiological vulnerability of its inhibitory networks. Like the DCN, another putative generator site for tinnitus, the ICC receives converging inputs from both auditory and nonauditory pathways. One nonauditory function, the initiation of conditioned aversive responses, may be demonstrated with electrical or chemical stimulation of the auditory midbrain.[136] With reduction of central inhibition, these subsystems may potentiate the perceived severity of tinnitus, which often fails to correlate with objective loudness measures.[137]

The hypothesized role of GABA in tinnitus creates the opportunity to pursue pharmacological interventions. Because potentially toxic substances cannot be directly tested in human subjects, researchers must rely on animal models with experimentally induced tinnitus. This approach raises the conundrum, How do you characterize the subjective perception of phantom sound in an animal?[138] Although several behavioral testing procedures exist, the basic strategy is to train the subject to respond to the onset of a silent interval that is created by switching off a continuous background sound. After tinnitus is induced by exposure to a loud sound or a large dose of salicylate, the subject can no longer perform the task because it hears a phantom sound instead of silence. The success of a drug treatment is indicated by the restoration of normal behavioral performance. These paradigms are currently producing promising results with agents that modulate GABAergic transmission.[139]

THE AUDITORY THALAMUS

The auditory thalamus, or medial geniculate body (MGB), is an obligatory relay for the projections of the central nucleus of the ICC. Within the ventral division of the MGB, a rich intrinsic circuitry works in conjunction with descending feedback from cortex and the limbic systems to condition ascending auditory representations before they are passed on to the auditory cortex. In parallel to this tonotopic pathway, diffusely tuned and polysensory inputs from multiple brainstem nuclei converge within the dorsal and medial divisions. Each thalamic region maintains the separate functional identity of these diverse inputs by preferentially innervating distinct cortical areas.

Anatomy

Alternative anatomical parcellations of the MGB have been proposed based on cytoarchitectural structure and patterns of neural connectivity. Most recognize a tripartite scheme that divides the nucleus into a ventral principal cell area, a medial magnocellular area, and a structurally diverse dorsal area.[140,141] The ventral division alone shows robust sound-driven activity.

The major functional connections of the ventral division integrate ascending inputs from the ICC, local inhibitory neurons, and descending projections from the auditory cortex (Figure 5–16A). The thalamic targets of the predominately excitatory projections from the central nucleus of the ICC are large tufted cells that serve as the principal relay neurons, and small stellate cells that are inhibitory interneurons.[142] Because the dendritic fields of bushy cells are oriented in parallel to their afferent inputs, responses within the ventral division maintain the tonotopic organization and basic physiological characteristics of the midbrain. Excitatory outputs from the ventral division are mainly directed to cellular layer IV of A1.[143] The cortical region receiving these inputs sends reciprocal corticothalamic projections back to the ventral division.

As in other sensory relay nuclei of the thalamus, the inhibitory interneurons of the ventral division are organized in synaptic glomeruli (Figure 5–16B).[144] Excitatory inputs from the ICC form a triad synapse with the dendrites of interneurons and MGB principal cells. The synaptic complex is insulated from the surrounding neuropil by glial processes. When inputs from the ICC activate the triad, presynaptic terminals on the dendrites of the interneuron release GABA within the glomerulus.[145] The release of the inhibitory neurotransmitter is regulated by metabotrophic glutamate receptors, which require high input rates for activation and then maintain an active state for relatively long durations. Consequently, the transmission properties of the triad are ideal for modifying the long-term efficacy of midbrain inputs.

The MGB receives as many inputs from the cortex as it does from the ICC. Retrograde labeling suggests that corticothalamic feedback to the ventral MGB originates from small pyramidal cells in layer VI of area AI.[146] Synaptic morphology suggest that the descending projections are excitatory. En route to the dendritic fields of principal cells in the ventral division, the fibers send collaterals to the thalamic reticular nucleus (TRN), a large source of extrinsic GABAergic inhibition.[147] Therefore, cortical feedback has the potential to alter thalamic activity by direct action, or through its indirect influence on inhibitory networks. Additional inhibitory feedback is provided by the limbic system, particularly the mesencephalic reticular formation. This complex circuitry allows cognitive factors such as learning, attention, and state of arousal to activate a subset of thalamic neurons while suppressing others.[148]

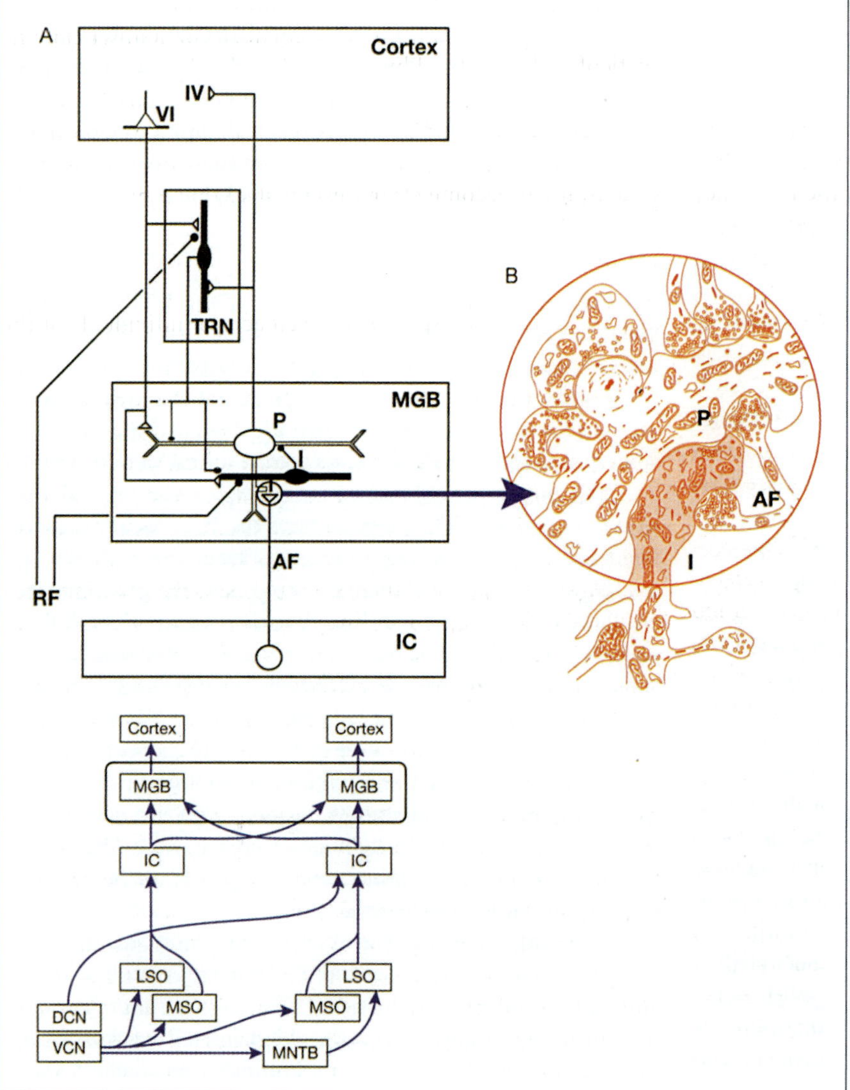

FIGURE 5–16 • Schematic diagram of the major inputs to principal cells in the ventral division of the auditory thalamus. *A*, Neural connections between the inferior colliculus (IC), medial geniculate body (MGB), and auditory cortex. Additional inputs are shown for the thalamic reticular nucleus (TRN) and mesencephalic reticular formation (RF). Cortical layers are identified by Roman numerals. Excitatory synapses are indicated by open triangles; inhibitory synapses, by filled circles. A synaptic glomerulus is encircled in the MGB. *Adapted from de Ribaupierre.*[149] *B*, Anatomical reconstruction of a synaptic glomerulus. The dendritic process of an inhibitory interneuron is shaded to facilitate visualization of triadic circuitry involving the dendrite of the interneuron (I), the dendrite of a thalamic principal cell (P), and an ascending axonal fiber from the inferior colliculus (AF). Inset shows relative position of the MGB within the central auditory pathways. Additional abbreviations are explained in Figure 5–1. *Adapted with permission from Morest.*[150]

Basic Physiology

Principal cells in the ventral division are organized in frequency laminae that reflect the tonotopic projections of the ICC. Within each laminae, the neurons form clusters of cells with similar binaural interactions and integration bandwidths.[151] These functional gradients suggest that parallel streams of information from the midbrain remain segregated in the auditory thalamus.

Detailed comparisons of the existing descriptions of sound-driven activity in the MGB and ICC are made difficult by procedural differences in subject species, testing parameters, and anesthetic state. Although there may be noteworthy changes in specific response patterns, the two structures appear to share fundamental coding properties. Like neurons in the central nucleus, many neurons in the ventral division are tuned in frequency, level, and time. They tend to be activated by sound presentations to either ear, but show a preference for one ear. Low-frequency neurons respond to ITD information in binaural sounds; whereas, high-frequency neurons are sensitive to ILD cues. It is clear that many of these properties are passed to the MGB from the brainstem. How these representations are transformed by local inhibitory networks and modulated by cortical feedback remains a subject of intense scientific interest.[148]

Adaptive Filtering of Biological Signals

The effects of corticofugal feedback on sound processing have been investigated by recording single-unit activity in the ventral division of the MGB during reversible cortical inactivation. When large areas of AI are silenced by cryogenic blockade in anesthetized cats, neurons in the ventral division show decreased spontaneous rates, increased signal-to-noise ratios, and changes in frequency tuning.[152] The selectivity of frequency tuning expands in some neurons and compresses in others. The diversity of the effects of cortical inactivation suggest that corticothalamic projections may operate through direct excitatory influences as well as by suppressing local inhibitory influences via projections from the TRN.

Adaptive filtering may enhance the auditory processing of biologically relevant sounds. For example, the MGB of the mustached bat displays an exaggerated neural representation of frequencies that are most important in the species' biosonar signals. These responses can be increased in magnitude and sharpened in their selectivity by stimulating matching frequency regions in auditory cortex. The effect is abolished by pharmacological blockade of cortical activity.[153]

Adaptive filtering is not only observed in specialized auditory systems, the magnitude of neural representations also may be modified by experience in more generalized listeners. When repeating tones are paired with noxious shocks, the frequency responses of central auditory neurons shift in frequency to produce an expanded reorganization of the fear-conditioned stimulus.[154] Pharmacological inactivation of auditory cortex abolishes the effect.[155]

Clinical Implication

Anatomical and functional abnormalities of the auditory thalamus have been implicated in language disorders that involve the inability to process rapidly changing speech sounds.[156] These temporal deficits have been related to aberrant thalamic anatomy by postmortem studies of dyslexic brains.[157] Although the MGB is bilaterally symmetrical in normal humans, the left MGB appears smaller in dyslexic brains because there are fewer large projection neurons. It is intriguing that the cortical target of the left MGB; ie, the left hemisphere of the cerebral cortex, is known to play a critical role in speech processing.[158]

Language impairments also have been linked to thalamic abnormalities by electrophysiological measures. Dyslexics show less mismatch negativity (MMN) when tested with rapid speech changes.[159] This electrical potential is evoked when the observer detects the presentation of a deviant stimulus in a repeating background. It is posited that dyslexics exhibit a reduced MMN because they cannot process the rapid change. Implanted electrodes in experimental animals have linked the MMN to activity in the extralemniscal divisions of the MGB.[160]

AUDITORY CORTEX

The auditory cortex receives all incoming sound representations from the thalamus. Whereas the separate subcortical structures are responsible for extracting specific features from acoustic stimuli, the auditory cortex must recombine these parallel information streams into integrated auditory percepts. These diverse perceptual behaviors include the discrimination of sound sources, localization of sound, recognition of voices, interpretation of sounds in a biological context, auditory memory, and training-induced plasticity. Much of our knowledge pertaining to the structure and function of the auditory cortex has been derived from studies in other species, with some of the most intriguing findings stemming from work in nonhuman primates. Given the limitations of experimental animals as a model system for the study of higher cognitive processes, our knowledge of human function has been significantly advanced by indirect measures of neural activity that can be applied to humans, particularly functional neuroimaging.

The technical difficulties of studying in vivo human auditory function are complicated by the broad heterogeneity of the auditory cortex, with its numerous areas and fields, each with their own distinctive anatomy and physiology. Many anatomical approaches have been utilized to define the subregions of the auditory cortex, including cytoarchitectonic and chemoarchitectonic methods, in addition to studies of fiber connectivity involved in thalamocortical, corticocortical, and corticofugal circuitry. Physiological studies based on receptive field properties, determination of BF (or characteristic frequencies), spectral bandwidth of target neurons, and temporal response qualities have also been utilized. As a result of these studies, it has become clearly established that a primary auditory field, often referred to as A1, exists in nearly all species, including humans. Beyond the A1, however, it has been difficult to establish uniform anatomical and functional criteria that are valid across species, or even across individuals of the same species.

Anatomy

The A1, constitutes the first stage of cortical processing for sound.[161] Much of what we know about the anatomy of A1 is based on work in primate models, especially monkeys, and therefore, some as of yet unidentified details may differ in humans. On a histological level, the A1 has several unique features of koniocortex, including densely packed small cells of layer 4, heavily myelinated fibers, and the presence of abundant cytochrome oxidase.[162] As stated earlier, it receives much of its input directly from the ventral subdivision of the thalamus.[163] Functionally, the neurons of the A1 tend to respond to pure tones well, with well-tuned BF ranges, and a tonotopic arrangement of isofrequency bands.[161]

Hackett and Kaas use the term *core* to describe primary or primary-like regions, which includes three areas (A1, rostral or R, and rostrotemporal or RT).[162] These areas appear to be activated in parallel, and each of these core subregions shows distinctive neural connections from other cortical areas. These three regions are organized caudo-rostrally along the plane of the lateral fissure, and have a tonotopic arrangement.[164] In humans, much of Heschl's gyrus (transverse temporal gyrus) consists of auditory core (Figure 5–17).

A cytoarchitecturally distinct *belt* of auditory cortex surrounds the centralized core. This region receives few inputs from the ventral thalamic nucleus (MGV), instead its main thalamic inputs originate in the dorsal (MGD) and medial (MGM) nuclei.[165–169] Neurons in the belt receive almost all of their auditory inputs from the core regions, and do not exhibit primary-like activity. A third *parabelt* region, just ventral to the belt, receives dense connections from the belt, but almost none from the core.[170] The parabelt receives thalamic inputs from the MGD and MGM, and cortical inputs from nonauditory regions adjacent to the superior temporal sulcus. This circuitry may play an important role in polysensory processing (audiovisual interactions). Additional prefrontal connections suggest a role in auditory memory and visuospatial representation.[164]

From the parabelt and belt regions, auditory signals are sent to a fourth level of neural processing within temporal, parietal, and frontal lobes. The implication of these relationships is that many areas of the brain, even those not strictly considered to be auditory processing centers, receive auditory inputs and are crucial for proper auditory processing. Polysensory interactions are critical here, and further work is needed to clarify the exact nature of the neural interactions between auditory and visual cortices. Furthermore, the role of homologous regions of the

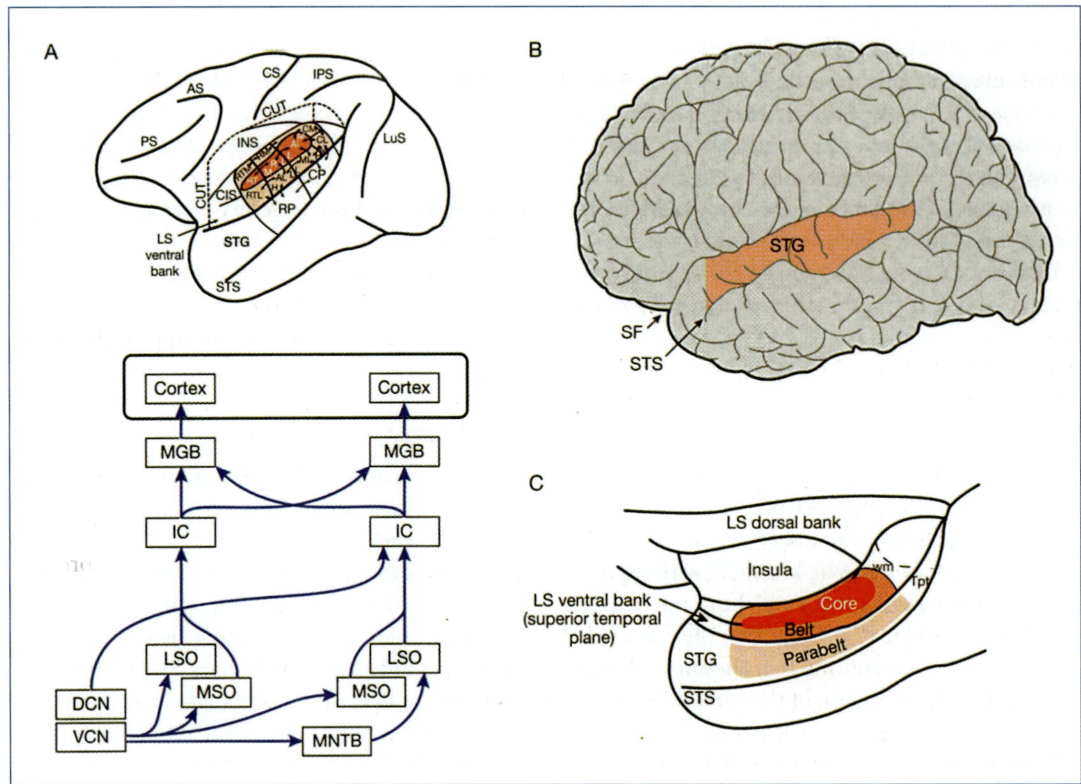

FIGURE 5–17 • *A*, Depiction of auditory cortical regions in the macaque monkey, showing the approximate locations of primary and secondary auditory regions along the left superior temporal plane. *B*, Schematic drawing of left lateral surface of the human brain, with the superior temporal gyrus outlined. The temporal lobe must be reflected laterally to see the contents that lie within the Sylvian fissure. *C*, Schematic drawing of the locations of core, belt and parabelt after reflection of the temporal lobe in primates. Inset shows relative position of the cortex within the central auditory pathways. Abbreviations are explained in Figure 5–1. *Adapted with permission from Hackett et al.,[162] Kaas and Hackett,[171] and Sweet et al.[172]*

brain connected by the corpus callosum is very poorly understood. In spite of these vagaries, it is the transfer of auditory information in this ascending fashion that ultimately allows humans to have conscious, cognitive perception of incoming auditory input.

Although the descriptions of auditory core, belt, and parabelt regions in monkeys are somewhat clear, our understanding of the human auditory system remains relatively poor, with recent functional imaging studies responsible for much of our current knowledge. In part, this limited understanding can be attributed to the difficulty of interpreting human lesion studies. It is clearly established that the human auditory cortex is concentrated along the superior temporal gyrus (Figure 5–18).

The superior temporal plane—which contains the planum polare, Heschl's gyrus, and planum temporale (from anterior to posterior)—appears to be the locus of the human auditory cortex. This region has notably high variation from person to person, and the parcellation of cortex into Brodmann areas may not apply very well. Within Brodmann's area 41, which corresponds to the anterior transverse temporal area (where A1 is located), a vertical columnar organization of auditory neurons appears to be present (referred to as Te1.1, Te1.0, and Te1.2 medial or posterior to lateral).[173]

As detailed in the first half of this chapter, a substantial amount of processing of auditory information takes place in the brainstem. Therefore, the auditory cortex receives "preprocessed" signals that are then further processed by the core, belt and parabelt regions. The A1 appears to be involved in auditory object identification, as well as integrating spectral and temporal qualities of sounds. Overall, our understanding of non-A1 is sparser in comparison to that of A1, in part due to the fact that most primate studies have utilized electrophysiologic techniques, while most human studies have utilized functional

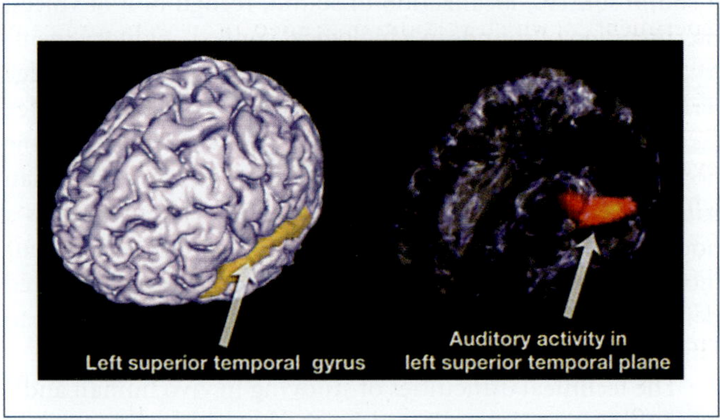

FIGURE 5–18 • Three-dimensional surface rendering of the human brain, showing the anatomical location of the left superior temporal gyrus (left side). Auditory activation within the left superior temporal plane revealed by functional MRI (right side).

neuroimaging methods. The latter approach has low temporal resolution and is complicated by the presence of loud scanner noise. For example, even establishing the exact parameters of the human tonotopic axis has been a challenge, since non-A1 responds weakly to pure tones, while A1 responds transiently. Studies using bandpass filtered stimuli with spectral variations strongly suggest that the human auditory cortex retains a tonotopic axis.[174–176]

The cortical processing of temporal information depends on the transmission rate of the information. In general, sounds can be subdivided into slow-rate (< 30 Hz) and fast-rate temporal structures (> 50 Hz). At slow rates, temporal information is coded directly by neural discharge rates. Both Heschl's gyrus and non-A1 are critical elements for the slow-rate modulations that are integral for processes such as speech envelope detection. At faster rates that outpace the frequency following capability of the neural response, other strategies must be used. Fast-rate (or fine) temporal structure occurs on the scale of milliseconds, and is relevant for issues such as ITDs (important for localization of sound) and important for perception of musical melodies. Several studies have examined how the brain responds to temporal variance of fast rates. Neural responses to regular-interval noise are stronger than for control noise, suggesting that high-frequency patterns trigger specific responses in the A1.[177,178]

It took until the latter half of the 19th century to reach consensus on the idea that sensorimotor functions could be localized to the cerebral cortex. In part, the reluctance to accept the idea of functional localization may have been a reaction to the misinformed theories of phrenologists, who localized sensorimotor function to the shape of the head. In 1861, a patient with expressive aphasia underwent a postmortem autopsy that revealed a left inferior frontal gyrus lesion in a region that has since been named Broca's area.[179] Damage to the posterior superior temporal gyrus in a region commonly referred to as Wernicke's area, leads to a receptive language deficit that is readily apparent clinically.[180] The concept of tonotopicity was identified in the mid 1900s,[181] and many early studies of the specific role of the auditory cortex for frequency discrimination were inconclusive. In 1975, it was discovered that bilateral auditory cortex lesions led to the loss of sound localization abilities.[33] Through a series of ablation experiments in which portions of the neocortex were surgically removed in macaque monkeys, it was determined that bilateral removal of the superior temporal gyrus led to immediate unresponsiveness to sound stimulation with delayed recovery after several months, while unilateral lesions led to contralateral deficits.[182–184] As described earlier, species-specific differences in auditory behavior and neural organization has impeded our understanding of auditory cortex. Critical questions concerning both normal and pathological mechanisms of hearing—remain unanswered.

The ultimate goal of neuroscience is to understand how the brain works. In relationship to the auditory system, the goal is to understand how the central and peripheral auditory systems are able to provide auditory cognition and accurate perception of auditory stimuli. To a certain extent, our current understanding has largely been shaped by approaches that subdivide the central nervous system into smaller subunits and examine the anatomy and physiology of each subunit. Consequently, we know a good deal more about each individual subunit than we do about how the numerous subunits interact with one another. Furthermore, we know relatively little about how the subunits of the auditory systems react with other sensory systems to provide an auditory percept that is correctly interpreted within a practical real-world context.

While it is undoubtedly helpful to break down the study of the auditory system into component features, such as A1 and secondary auditory cortex, this approach has intrinsic limitations that may never lead to a satisfying whole brain model of audition. The notion that auditory function can be specifically "localized" to a particular neuroanatomical region, as discussed briefly above, is likely to be a crude oversimplification. Yet, it is reasonable to consider the function of each subunit in order to be able to interpret how they function within an organic context. For these reasons, the utilization of broad methodologies is to be encouraged, and the development of whole brain mapping strategies, such as functional magnetic resonance imaging (fMRI), should provide important new information as to how auditory regions interact both to one another but perhaps more importantly, to nonauditory regions that ultimately place auditory information in a behavioral context. One of the clear benefits of fMRI is that information from diverse regions of the brain can be accrued simultaneously, allowing us to capture activity in regions of the brain for which we might not necessarily anticipate an obvious relationship to auditory perception. It is important to acknowledge that many classically "nonauditory" regions may play critical roles for the perception or production of complex sounds.

The "What" and "Where" Pathways

Based largely on the principles of parallel cortical processing streams present in the visual system, it has been suggested that auditory processing may possess a similar parallel structure. Specifically, an acoustic signal may be deconstructed during neural processing into separate components that can then be directed toward discrete neural substrates, thereby allowing for the parallel analysis of different aspects of the sound. These pathways have been described as the "what" and "where" pathways of sound, and have been proposed to relate to the identification of a sound's identity (what is it?) and localization of that sound (where is it?). Kraus and Nicol[185] argued that for spoken language, the identity of the speaker and the semantic meaning of the words contained in the spoken message could each be linked to separate brainstem responses that indicate the presence of a subcortical parcellation of information into separate streams akin to visual "what" and "where" processing. In the first behavioral study of the auditory "what" and "where" pathways, Lomber and Malhotra[186] applied the technique of reversible cooling deactivation to selective regions of the cat non-A1. In this study, they found that bilateral deactivation of the posterior auditory fields resulted in sound-localization deficits, while bilateral deactivation of the anterior auditory fields resulted in pattern-discrimination deficits only. These findings support the notion of parallel cortical processing streams within the auditory cortex.

Voice Recognition

In work that also stemmed from studies of facial recognition in the visual system, it has been demonstrated that the human voice is uniquely processed by the auditory system, and is in many ways comparable to an "auditory face" for which humans are specially geared to process and perceive. Given the critical importance of spoken language, these findings are not surprising, yet their demonstration over a series of elegant fMRI findings illustrates the power of these methods to study complex areas of human cognition. Belin et al.[187] reported the identification of voice-selective regions within bilateral STS of the auditory cortex (Figure 5–19). This study utilized fMRI during passive listening to vocal versus nonvocal environmental stimuli, and found greater activation of the STS during vocal stimulation. In addition, the central region of the STS displayed greater activation and selectivity for vocal sounds in comparison to scrambled voice or AM noise. In a follow-up study designed to explore affective/emotional components of vocal stimuli, referred to as paralinguistic vocal information, Belin et al.[188] used fMRI to examine differential responses to speech versus nonspeech vocalizations, and to explore the effect of frequency scrambling on cortical activation. They found that responses to speech versus nonspeech were greater throughout the auditory cortex (including A1) bilaterally, whereas A1 showed little attenuation when listening to frequency-scrambled stimuli as exhibited by the anterior STS. The authors also found that right anterior STS responses to nonspeech vocal sounds exceeded those in response to scrambled versions, suggesting that these regions might be responsible for perception of paralinguistic voice perception.

These human studies were recently confirmed in an fMRI study of monkeys by Petkov et al.,[189] which showed higher activation along the superior temporal plane during perception of species-specific vocalization than during non-species specific vocalizations, indicating that nonhuman primates also contain neural specializations for voice recognition. It should be emphasized that these specializations are different from (but related to) the nonauditory specializations that exist for language perception within the inferior frontal gyrus and inferior parietal lobule.

Nonprimary Pitch Centers

One of the basic elements of auditory processing is the ability to convert the fundamental frequency of a periodic signal into a subjective pitch. Pitch perception is an essential component of music and language perception, and several studies have recently identified the presence of neural centers devoted to the processing of pitch. In an fMRI study of individuals listening to pitches, melodies, and spectrally matched sounds without pitch, Patterson et al.[190] found that only the lateral portion of Heschl's gyrus was activated by pitch, and that the processing of melody recruited auditory neurons that were situated anterolaterally to Heschl's gyrus within the superior temporal gyrus and planum polare. A related study by Penagos et al.[191] utilized fMRI to assess brain activity in response to harmonic tone complexes where pitch varied, but not temporal regularity (ie, periodicity linked to pitch perception). The authors found that pitch information activated an area of non-A1 that overlapped the anterolateral end of Heschl's gyrus, These results suggest that pitch processing may be centered in non-A1.

Single-unit recordings of awake marmoset monkeys have described an area of auditory cortex near the anterolateral border of the A1 that exhibits a strong selectivity for the pitch of pure tones and harmonic tone complexes.[192] This finding extends the notion of a specialized pitch processing center residing outside the A1. Furthermore, the study demonstrates a high degree of congruence in the neural substrate for pitch processing among human and nonhuman primates.

Music Perception and Production

In many ways, the perception and production of music represents the pinnacle of auditory function. An enormously complex acoustic stimulus with an inherent abstractness of meaning is transformed into a unified auditory percept that provides an emotional experience for the listener. The mechanisms by which the brain is able to achieve this remarkable feat are far from understood, yet it is certainly reliant upon the basic auditory circuitry and processing mechanisms outlined throughout this chapter. Multimodal interactions between the brainstem, temporal lobe, and nonauditory centers transform sound into something that may be judged as beautiful or sublime.

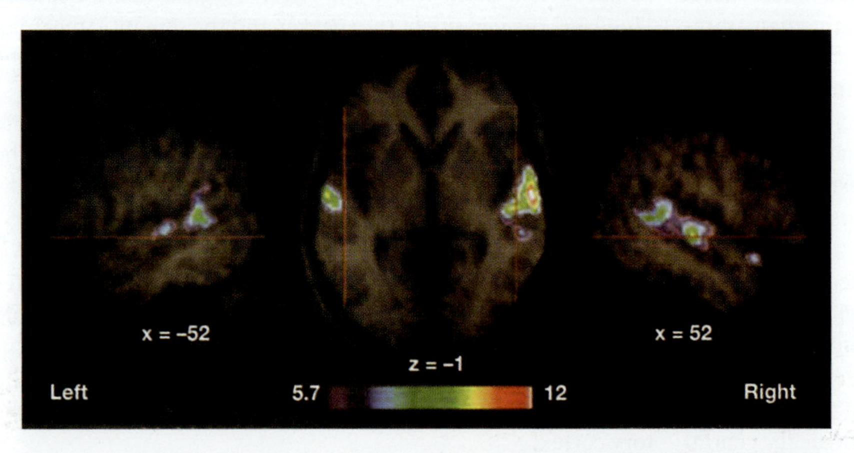

FIGURE 5–19 • Activation maps derived from functional MRI of volunteers listening to vocal stimuli. Activation clusters were identified by a contrast analysis of [Vocal] > [Nonvocal] stimuli. Significant activation along the upper bank of the superior temporal sulcus reveals voice-selective processing areas in human cortex. *Adapted with permission from Belin et al.*[187]

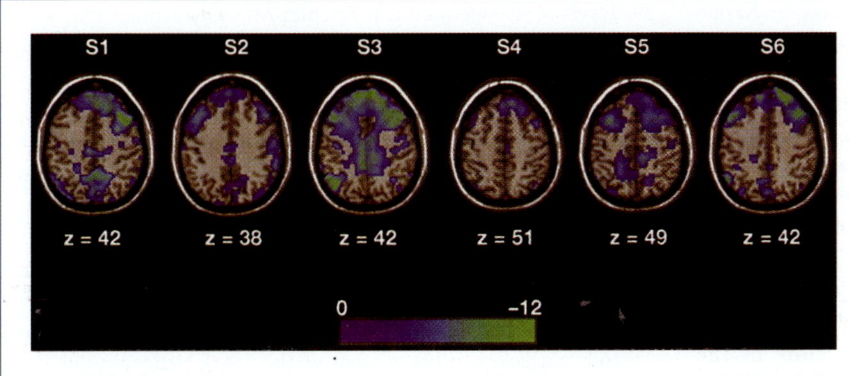

FIGURE 5–20 • Cortical deactivation within six pianists during spontaneous musical improvisation. All subjects show pronounced deactivation during improvisation in comparison to performance of memorized music. The broad region of deactivation is located within the prefrontal cortex, demonstrating the notion that complex auditory tasks show critical changes in nonauditory regions of the brain.

Music has persisted throughout all known historical epochs, and in all human cultures, even though it renders no clear survival benefit. It seems that the pleasure in producing and listening to music is sufficient justification for its persistence throughout history. By using music as a window into the brain, we can begin to understand numerous facets of brain function, under conditions as diverse as extended musical training (plasticity), instrumental performance (complex sensorimotor function), music induced emotion (limbic responses to sound), and spontaneous musical improvisation (neural mechanisms of creativity).

Over the past decade, it has become apparent that the human cortex is uniquely specialized for the processing of music. These observations vary from the hemispheric dominance of spectral versus temporal processing,[193] to links between language and music processing in Broca's area, and on to the detection of musical syntactic expectancies.[194,195] Music that is associated with strong emotional responses (described as "chills down the spine") elicits the same patterns of paralimbic activity that are commonly ascribed to the primitive substrates responsible for aversive or pleasurable reactions.[196] These observations underscore the fact that music, without additional sensory input, can induce changes in the extra-auditory regions that mediate the most basic of human impulses.

In a striking study of central auditory plasticity, Musacchia et al.[197] compared auditory brainstem responses of nonmusicians and highly trained musicians. Responses to speech and music suggest that musicians have earlier and more robust sound-evoked brain activity, superior phase-locking to periodic stimuli, and more sharply tuned temporal/frequency coding. This enhanced performance may be attributable to experience-based modifications of cortical processing that modify sound-driven activity in the brainstem by way of descending projections.

An fMRI study of jazz improvisation, a high level musical task of spontaneous creativity, has revealed unique patterns of brain activity in the prefrontal cortex of professional musicians (Figure 5–20).[198] Improvisation is associated with a focal increase in medial prefrontal activity, and a broad decrease in dorsolateral prefrontal activity. In addition, increased activity is seen in temporal cortices, where responses to simple auditory stimuli are not state dependent. These findings, which may reflect the neural signature of creativity, indicate that the whole brain is involved in the execution of multisensory processes that govern music perception and production.

Whitfield has suggested that the sensory cortices are a site for the formation of the concepts that facilitate the interpretation of external events.[199] In contrast to the auditory brainstem where features are extracted from complex sounds, the auditory cortex assembles these diverse streams of information into unified perceptual objects. The resulting higher-order transformations are shaped as much by a listener's experience, biological context, and behavioral state as they are by ascending sensory inputs. A challenge for future studies of the central auditory system is to move beyond neural representations of the physical dimensions of sound to explorations of the perceptual dimensions of human auditory experience. These questions may be best addressed by physiological approaches that define hearing as the global activity of the brain and not the isolated activity of its localized components.

References

1. Rhode WS, Greenburg S. Physiology of the cochlear nuclei. In: Popper AN, Fay RR, editors. The mammalian auditory pathway: Neurophysiology. New York: Springer-Verlag; 1992. p. 94–152.
2. Lorente de Nó R. The primary acoustic nuclei. New York: Raven Press; 1981.
3. Cant NB. The cochlear nucleus: Neuronal types and their synaptic organization. In: Webster DB, Popper AN, Fay RR, editors. The mammalian auditory pathway: Neuroanatomy. New York: Springer-Verlag; 1992. p. 66–116.
4. Rasmussen GL. Studies of the VIIIth cranial nerve of man. Laryngoscope 1940;50:67–83.
5. Osen KK. Cytoarchitecture of the cochlear nuclei in the cat. J Comp Neurol 1969;136:453–84.
6. Ryugo DK, Fekete DM. Morphology of primary axosomatic endings in the anteroventral cochlear nucleus of the cat: A study of the endbulbs of Held. J Comp Neurol 1982;210:239–57.
7. Held H. Die Cochlea der Säuger und der Vögel, ihre Entwicklung und ihr Bau. In: Bethe A, v Bergman G, Ellinger A, editors. Handbuch der Normalen und Pathologischen Physiologie. Berlin: Springer; 1926. p. 467–534.
8. Rhode WS, Oertel D, Smith PH. Physiological response properties of cells labeled intracellularly with horseradish peroxidase in cat ventral cochlear nucleus. J Comp Neurol 1983;213:448–63.
9. Rhode WS, Smith PH, Oertel D. Physiological response properties of cells labeled intracellularly with horseradish peroxidase in cat dorsal cochlear nucleus. J Comp Neurol 1983;213:426–47.

10. Pfeiffer RR. Classification of response patterns of spike discharges for units in the cochlear nucleus: Tone-burst stimulation. Exp Brain Res 1966;1:220–35.
11. Blackburn CC, Sachs MB. Classification of unit types in the anteroventral cochlear nucleus: PST histograms and regularity analysis. J Neurophysiol 1989;62:1303–29.
12. Rhode WS, Smith PH. Encoding timing and intensity in the ventral cochlear nucleus of the cat. J Neurophysiol 1986;56:261–86.
13. Smith PH, Joris PX, Carney LH, Yin TC. Projections of physiologically characterized globular bushy cell axons from the cochlear nucleus of the cat. J Comp Neurol 1991;304:387–407.
14. Tolbert LP, Morest DK. The neuronal architecture of the anteroventral cochlear nucleus of the cat in the region of the cochlear nerve root: Golgi and Nissl methods. Neuroscience 1982;7:3013–30.
15. Oertel D. Use of brain slices in the study of the auditory system: Spatial and temporal summation of synaptic inputs in cells in the anteroventral cochlear nucleus of the mouse. J Acoust Soc Am 1985;78:328–33.
16. Kane EC. Octopus cells in the cochlear nucleus of the cat: Heterotypic synapses upon homeotypic neurons. Int J Neurosci 1973;5:251–79.
17. Cant NB, Morest DK. The structural basis for stimulus coding in the cochlear nucleus of the cat. In: Berlin CI, editor. Hearing science. San Diego: College-Hill Press; 1984. p. 374–422.
18. Oertel D, Wu SH, Garb MW, Dizack C. Morphology and physiology of cells in slice preparations of the posteroventral cochlear nucleus of mice. J Comp Neurol 1990;295:136–54.
19. Doucet JR, Ryugo DK. Projections from the ventral cochlear nucleus to the dorsal cochlear nucleus in rats. J Comp Neurol 1997;385:245–64.
20. Doucet JR, Ross AT, Gillespie MB, Ryugo DK. Glycine immunoreactivity of multipolar neurons in the ventral cochlear nucleus which project to the dorsal cochlear nucleus. J Comp Neurol 1999;408:515–31.
21. May BJ, Prell GS, Sachs MB. Vowel representations in the ventral cochlear nucleus of the cat: Effects of level, background noise, and behavioral state. J Neurophysiol 1998;79:1755–67.
22. Young ED, Shofner WP, White JA, Robert J-M, Voigt HF. Response properties of cochlear nucleus neurons in relationship to physiological mechanisms. In: Edelman GM, Gall WE, Cowan WM, editors. Auditory function: neurobiological bases of hearing. New York: John Wiley & Sons; 1988. p. 277–312.
23. Kim DO, Molnar CE. A population study of cochlear nerve fibers: Comparison of spatial distributions of average-rate and phase-locking measures of responses to single tones. J Neurophysiol 1979;42:16–30.
24. Sachs MB, Young ED. Encoding of steady-state vowels in the auditory nerve: Representation in terms of discharge rate. J Acoust Soc Am 1979;66:470–9.
25. Peterson GE, Barney HL. Control methods used in the study of the vowels. J Acoust Soc Am 1952;24:175–84.
26. Le Prell GS, Sachs MB, May BJ. Representation of vowel-like spectra by discharge rate responses of individual auditory-nerve fibers. Aud Neurosci 1996;2:275–88.
27. Blackburn CC, Sachs MB. The representations of the steady-state vowel sound /e/ in the discharge patterns of cat anteroventral cochlear nucleus neurons. J Neurophysiol 1990;63:1191–212.
28. Wang X, Sachs MB. Transformation of temporal discharge patterns in a ventral cochlear nucleus stellate cell model: implications for physiological mechanisms. J Neurophysiol 1995;73:1600–16.
29. Davis M, Gendelman DS, Tischler MD, Gendelman PM. A primary acoustic startle circuit: Lesion and stimulation studies. J Neurosci 1982;2:791–805.
30. Berker EA, Berker AH, Smith A. Translation of Broca's 1865 report. Localization of speech in the third left frontal convolution. Arch Neurol 1986;43:1065–72.
31. Heil P. Neuronal coding of interaural transient envelope disparities. Eur J Neurosci 1998;10:2831–47.
32. Wernicke K. The aphasia symptom complex: A psychological study on an anatomical basis. The Hague: Mouton; 1874.
33. Casseday JH, Neff WD. Auditory localization: Role of auditory pathways in brain stem of the cat. J Neurophysiol 1975; 38:842–58.
34. Masterton RB, Granger EM, Glendenning KK. Role of acoustic striae in hearing: Mechanism for enhancement of sound detection in cats. Hear Res 1994;73:209–22.
35. Ryugo DK, Pongstaporn T, Huchton DM, Niparko JK. Ultrastructural analysis of primary endings in deaf white cats: Morphologic alterations in endbulbs of Held. J Comp Neurol 1997;385:230–44.
36. Ryugo DK, Kretzmer EA, Niparko JK. Restoration of auditory nerve synapses in cats by cochlear implants. Science 2005;310:1490–2.
37. Young ED, Davis KA. Circuitry and function of the dorsal cochlear nucleus. In: Oertel D, Fay RR, Popper AN, editors. Integrative functions in the mammalian auditory pathway. New York: Springer-Verlag; 2002. p. 160–206.
38. Adams JC, Warr WB. Origins of axons in the cat's acoustic striae determined by injection of horseradish peroxidase into severed tracts. J Comp Neurol 1976;170:107–21.
39. Kanold PO, Young ED. Proprioceptive information from the pinna provides somatosensory input to cat dorsal cochlear nucleus. J Neurosci 2001;21:7848–58.
40. Manis PB. Responses to parallel fiber stimulation in the guinea pig dorsal cochlear nucleus in vitro. J Neurophysiol 1989;61:149–61.
41. Spirou GA, May BJ, Wright DD, Ryugo DK. Frequency organization of the dorsal cochlear nucleus in cats. J Comp Neurol 1993;329:36–52.
42. Kane ES, Puglisi SG, Gordon BS. Neuronal types in the deep dorsal cochlear nucleus of the cat: I. Giant neurons. J Comp Neurol 1981;198:483–513.
43. Musicant AD, Chan JC, Hind JE. Direction-dependent spectral properties of cat external ear: New data and cross-species comparisons. J Acoust Soc Am 1990;87:757–81.
44. Rice JJ, May BJ, Spirou GA, Young ED. Pinna-based spectral cues for sound localization in cat. Hear Res 1992;58:132–52.
45. Huang AY, May BJ. Sound orientation behavior in cats. II. Mid-frequency spectral cues for sound localization. J Acoust Soc Am 1996;100:1070–80.
46. Young ED, Rice JJ, Spirou GA, Nelken I, Conley RA. Head-related transfer functions in cat: Neural representation and the effects of pinna movement. In: Gilkey RH, Anderson TR, editors. Binaural and spatial hearing in real and virtual environments. Mahwah, NJ: Lawrence Erlbaum Assoc; 1997. p. 475–98.
47. Yu JJ, Young ED. Linear and nonlinear pathways of spectral information transmission in the cochlear nucleus. Proc Natl Acad Sci U S A 2000;97:11780–6.
48. Sutherland DP, Masterton RB, Glendenning KK. Role of acoustic striae in hearing: Reflexive responses to elevated sound-sources. Behav Brain Res 1998;97:1–12.

49. May BJ. Role of the dorsal cochlear nucleus in the sound localization behavior of cats. Hear Res 2000;148:74–87.
50. Kaltenbach JA. Summary of evidence pointing to a role of the dorsal cochlear nucleus in the etiology of tinnitus. Acta Otolaryngol Suppl 2006;556:20–6.
51. Brozoski TJ, Bauer CA, Caspary DM. Elevated fusiform cell activity in the dorsal cochlear nucleus of chinchillas with psychophysical evidence of tinnitus. J Neurosci 2002;22:2383–90.
52. Kaltenbach JA, Afman CE. Hyperactivity in the dorsal cochlear nucleus after intense sound exposure and its resemblance to tone-evoked activity: A physiological model for tinnitus. Hear Res 2000;140:165–72.
53. Bartels H, Staal MJ, Albers FW. Tinnitus and neural plasticity of the brain. Otol Neurotol 2007;28:178–84.
54. Saunders JC. The role of central nervous system plasticity in tinnitus. J Commun Disord 2007;40:313–34.
55. Melcher JR, Sigalovsky IS, Guinan JJ Jr, Levine RA. Lateralized tinnitus studied with functional magnetic resonance imaging: abnormal inferior colliculus activation. J Neurophysiol 2000;83:1058–72.
56. Eggermont JJ. On the pathophysiology of tinnitus; a review and a peripheral model. Hear Res 1990;48:111–23.
57. Ramon Y Cajal S. English translation of new ideas on the structure of the nervous system in man and vetebrates, 1894. Cambridge, MA: The MIT Press; 1990.
58. Scheibel ME, Scheibel AB. Neuropil organization in the superior olive of the cat. Exp Neurol 1974;43:339–348.
59. Guinan JJ, Norris BE, Guinan SS. Single auditory units in the superior olivary complex. II: Locations of unit categories and tonotopic organization. Int J Neurosci 1972;4:147–166.
60. Cant NB, Casseday JH. Projections from the anteroventral cochlear nucleus to the lateral and medial superior olivary nuclei. J Comp Neurol 1986;247:457–76.
61. Smith PH, Joris PX, Yin TC. Projections of physiologically characterized spherical bushy cell axons from the cochlear nucleus of the cat: Evidence for delay lines to the medial superior olive. J Comp Neurol 1993;331:245–60.
62. Tsuchitani C, Boudreau JC. Single unit analysis of cat superior olive S segment with tonal stimuli. J Neurophysiol 1966;29:684–97.
63. Rose JE, Brugge JF, Anderson DJ, Hind JE. Phase-locked response to low-frequency tones in single auditory nerve fibers of the squirrel monkey. J Neurophysiol 1967;30:769–93.
64. Smith AJ, Owens S, Forsythe ID. Characterisation of inhibitory and excitatory postsynaptic currents of the rat medial superior olive. J Physiol 2000;529 (Pt 3):681–98.
65. Cant NB, Hyson RL. Projections from the lateral nucleus of the trapezoid body to the medial superior olivary nucleus in the gerbil. Hear Res 1992;58:26–34.
66. Pecka M, Brand A, Behrend O, Grothe B. Interaural time difference processing in the mammalian medial superior olive: The role of glycinergic inhibition. J Neurosci 2008;28:6914–25.
67. Aitkin L, Schuck D. Low frequency neurons in the lateral central nucleus of the cat inferior colliculus receive their input predominantly from the medial superior olive. Hear Res 1985;17:87–93.
68. Adams JC. Ascending projections to the inferior colliculus. J Comp Neurol 1979;183:519–38.
69. Goldberg JM, Brown PB. Response of binaural neurons of dog superior olivary complex to dichotic tonal stimuli: Some physiological mechanisms of sound localization. J Neurophysiol 1969;32:613–36.
70. Jeffress LA. A place theory of sound localization. J Comp Physiol Psychol 1941;41:35–9.
71. Carr CE, Konishi M. A circuit for detection of interaural time differences in the brain stem of the barn owl. J Neurosci 1990;10:3227–46.
72. Joris PX, Smith PH, Yin TC. Coincidence detection in the auditory system: 50 years after Jeffress. Neuron 1998;21:1235–8.
73. Mills AW. On the minimum audible angle. J Acoust Soc Am 1958;30:237–46.
74. Helfert RH, Juiz JM, Bledsoe SC Jr, Bonneau JM, Wenthold RJ, Altschuler RA. Patterns of glutamate, glycine, and GABA immunolabeling in four synaptic terminal classes in the lateral superior olive of the guinea pig. J Comp Neurol 1992;323:305–25.
75. Barnes-Davies M, Forsythe ID. Pre- and postsynaptic glutamate receptors at a giant excitatory synapse in rat auditory brainstem slices. J Physiol 1995;488 (Pt 2):387–406.
76. Helfert RH, Bonneau JM, Wenthold RJ, Altschuler RA. GABA and glycine immunoreactivity in the guinea pig superior olivary complex. Brain Res 1989;501:269–86.
77. Yin TCT. Neural mechanisms of encoding binaural localization cues in the auditory brainstem. In: Oertel D, Fay RR, Popper AN, editors. Integrative functions in the mammalian auditory pathway. New York: Springer; 2002. p. 99–159.
78. Spangler KM, Warr WB, Henkel CK. The projections of principal cells of the medial nucleus of the trapezoid body in the cat. J Comp Neurol 1985;238:249–62.
79. Joris PX, Yin TCT . Envelope coding in the lateral superior olive. I. Sensitivity to interaural time differences. J Neurophysiol 1995;73:1043–1062.
80. Tollin DJ, Koka K, Tsai JJ. Interaural level difference discrimination thresholds for single neurons in the lateral superior olive. J Neurosci 2008;28:4848–60.
81. Glendenning KK, Masterton RB. Acoustic chiasm: Efferent projections of the lateral superior olive. J Neurosci 1983;3:1521–37.
82. Oliver DL, Shneiderman A. An EM study of the dorsal nucleus of the lateral lemniscus: Inhibitory, commissural, synaptic connections between ascending auditory pathways. J Neurosci 1989;9:967–82.
83. Glendenning KK, Baker BN, Hutson KA, Masterton RB. Acoustic chiasm V: Inhibition and excitation in the ipsilateral and contralateral projections of LSO. J Comp Neurol 1992;319:100–22.
84. Saint Marie RL, Ostapoff EM, Morest DK, Wenthold RJ. Glycine-immunoreactive projection of the cat lateral superior olive: possible role in midbrain ear dominance. J Comp Neurol 1989;279:382–96.
85. Helfert RH, Aschoff A. Superior olivary complex and nuclei of the lateral lemniscus. In: Ehret G, Romand R, editors. The central auditory system. New York: Oxford University Press; 1997. p. 193–258.
86. Jenkins WM, Masterton RB. Sound localization: Effects of unilateral lesions in central auditory system. J Neurophysiol 1982;47:987–1016.
87. White JS, Warr WB. The dual origins of the olivocochlear bundle in the albino rat. J Comp Neurol 1983;219:203–14.
88. Brown MC, Liberman MC, Benson TE, Ryugo DK. Brainstem branches from olivocochlear axons in cats and rodents. J Comp Neurol 1988;278:591–603.
89. Warr WB. Organization of olivocochlear efferent systems in mammals. In: Webster WB, Popper AN, Fay RR, editors. The mammalian auditory pathway: Neuroanatomy. New York: Springer. p. 410–448.

90. Galambos R. Suppression of auditory nerve activity by stimulation of efferent fibers to cochlea. J Neurophysiol 1956;19:424–37.
91. Wiederhold ML, Kiang NY. Effects of electric stimulation of the crossed olivocochlear bundle on single auditory-nerve fibers in the cat. J Acoust Soc Am 1970;48:950–65.
92. Fuchs PA, Murrow BW. Cholinergic inhibition of short (outer) hair cells of the chick's cochlea. J Neurosci 1992;12:800–9.
93. Brownell WE, Bader CR, Bertrand D, de Ribaupierre Y. Evoked mechanical responses of isolated cochlear outer hair cells. Science 1985;227:194–6.
94. Winslow RL, Sachs MB. Effect of electrical stimulation of the crossed olivocochlear bundle on auditory nerve response to tones in noise. J Neurophysiol 1987;57:1002–21.
95. Chays A, Maison S, Robaglia-Schlupp A, Cau P, Broder L, Magnan J. [Are we sectioning the cochlear efferent system during vestibular neurotomy?] Rev Laryngol Otol Rhinol (Bord) 2003;124:53–8.
96. Scharf B, Magnan J, Chays A. On the role of the olivocochlear bundle in hearing: 16 case studies. Hear Res 1997;103:101–22.
97. Micheyl C, Collet L. Involvement of the olivocochlear bundle in the detection of tones in noise. J Acoust Soc Am 1996; 99:1604–10.
98. Rajan R. Effect of electrical stimulation of the crossed olivocochlear bundle on temporary threshold shifts in auditory sensitivity. II. Dependence on the level of temporary threshold shifts. J Neurophysiol 1988;60:569–79.
99. Maison SF, Liberman MC. Predicting vulnerability to acoustic injury with a noninvasive assay of olivocochlear reflex strength. J Neurosci 2000;20:4701–7.
100. Moller AR, Moller MB, Yokota M. Some forms of tinnitus may involve the extralemniscal auditory pathway. Laryngoscope 1992;102:1165–71.
101. Oliver DL, Morest DK. The central nucleus of the inferior colliculus in the cat. J Comp Neurol 1984;222:237–64.
102. Merzenich MM, Reid MD. Representation of the cochlea within the inferior colliculus of the cat. Brain Res 1974;77:397–415.
103. Winer JA, Saint Marie RL, Larue DT, Oliver DL. GABAergic feed-forward projections from the inferior colliculus to the medial geniculate body. Proc Natl Acad Sci U S A 1996;93:8005–10.
104. Oliver DL, Winer JA, Beckius GE, Saint Marie RL. Morphology of GABAergic neurons in the inferior colliculus of the cat. J Comp Neurol 1994;340:27–42.
105. Loftus WC, Bishop DC, Saint Marie RL, Oliver DL. Organization of binaural excitatory and inhibitory inputs to the inferior colliculus from the superior olive. J Comp Neurol 2004;472:330–44.
106. Oliver DL, Beckius GE, Bishop DC, Kuwada S. Simultaneous anterograde labeling of axonal layers from lateral superior olive and dorsal cochlear nucleus in the inferior colliculus of cat. J Comp Neurol 1997;382:215–29.
107. Morest DK, Oliver DL. The neuronal architecture of the inferior colliculus in the cat: Defining the functional anatomy of the auditory midbrain. J Comp Neurol 1984;222:209–36.
108. Andersen RA, Knight PL, Merzenich MM. The thalamocortical and corticothalamic connections of AI, AII, and the anterior auditory field (AAF) in the cat: Evidence for two largely segregated systems of connections. J Comp Neurol 1980;194:663–701.
109. Aitkin LM, Phillips SC. The interconnections of the inferior colliculi through their commissure. J Comp Neurol 1984;228:210–16.
110. Malmierca MS, Le Beau FE, Rees A. The topographical organization of descending projections from the central nucleus of the inferior colliculus in guinea pig. Hear Res 1996;93:167–80.
111. Aitkin LM, Kenyon CE, Philpott P. The representation of the auditory and somatosensory systems in the external nucleus of the cat inferior colliculus. J Comp Neurol 1981;196:25–40.
112. King AJ, Jiang ZD, Moore DR. Auditory brainstem projections to the ferret superior colliculus: Anatomical contribution to the neural coding of sound azimuth. J Comp Neurol 1998;390:342–65.
113. Ramachandran R, Davis KA, May BJ. Single-unit responses in the inferior colliculus of decerebrate cats. I. Classification based on frequency response maps. J Neurophysiol 1999;82:152–63.
114. Ramachandran R, May BJ. Functional segregation of ITD sensitivity in the inferior colliculus of decerebrate cats. J Neurophysiol 2002;88:2251–61.
115. Davis KA. Evidence of a functionally segregated pathway from dorsal cochlear nucleus to inferior colliculus. J Neurophysiol 2002;87:1824–35.
116. Le Beau FE, Rees A, Malmierca MS. Contribution of GABA- and glycine-mediated inhibition to the monaural temporal response properties of neurons in the inferior colliculus. J Neurophysiol 1996;75:902–19.
117. Heffner RS, Heffner HE. Sound localization in a predatory rodent, the northern grasshopper mouse (Onychomys leucogaster). J Comp Psychol 1988;102:66–71.
118. Aitkin L. The auditory midbrain: Structure and function in the central auditory pathway. Clifton, NJ: Humana Press; 1986.
119. Semple MN, Aitkin LM. Physiology of pathway from dorsal cochlear nucleus to inferior colliculus revealed by electrical and auditory stimulation. Exp Brain Res 1980;41:19–28.
120. Rees A, Moller AR. Responses of neurons in the inferior colliculus of the rat to AM and FM tones. Hear Res 1983;10:301–30.
121. Rees A, Moller AR. Stimulus properties influencing the responses of inferior colliculus neurons to amplitude-modulated sounds. Hear Res 1987;27:129–43.
122. Rose JE, Gross NB, Geisler CD, Hind JE. Some neural mechanisms in the inferior colliculus of the cat which may be relevant to localization of a sound source. J Neurophysiol 1966;29: 288–314.
123. Yin TC, Kuwada S. Binaural interaction in low-frequency neurons in inferior colliculus of the cat. III. Effects of changing frequency. J Neurophysiol 1983;50:1020–42.
124. McAlpine D, Jiang D, Shackleton TM, Palmer AR. Convergent input from brainstem coincidence detectors onto delay-sensitive neurons in the inferior colliculus. J Neurosci 1998;18: 6026–39.
125. Palmer AR, Kuwada S. Binaural and spatial coding in the inferior colliculus. In: Winer JA, Schreiner CE, editors. The inferior colliculus. New York: Springer; 2005. p. 377–410.
126. May BJ, Anderson M, Roos M. The role of broadband inhibition in the rate representation of spectral cues for sound localization in the inferior colliculus. Hear Res 2008;238:77–93.
127. Masterton RB, Jane JA, Diamond IT. Role of brainstem auditory structures in sound localization. I. Trapezoid body, superior olive, and lateral lemniscus. J Neurophysiol 1967;30:341–59.
128. Moore CN, Casseday JH, Neff WD. Sound localization: The role of the commissural pathways of the auditory system of the cat. Brain Res 1974;82:13–26.
129. Masterton RB. Neurobehavioral studies of the central auditory system. Ann Otol Rhinol Laryngol Suppl 1997;168:31–4.

130. Caspary DM, Milbrandt JC, Helfert RH. Central auditory aging: GABA changes in the inferior colliculus. Exp Gerontol 1995;30:349–60.
131. Caspary DM, Ling L, Turner JG, Hughes LF. Inhibitory neurotransmission, plasticity and aging in the mammalian central auditory system. J Exp Biol 2008;211:1781–91.
132. Bauer CA, Brozoski TJ, Holder TM, Caspary DM. Effects of chronic salicylate on GABAergic activity in rat inferior colliculus. Hear Res 2000;147:175–82.
133. Mossop JE, Wilson MJ, Caspary DM, Moore DR. Down-regulation of inhibition following unilateral deafening. Hear Res 2000;147:183–7.
134. Faingold CL. Role of GABA abnormalities in the inferior colliculus pathophysiology—audiogenic seizures. Hear Res 2002;168:223–37.
135. Bauer CA, Turner JG, Caspary DM, Myers KS, Brozoski TJ. Tinnitus and inferior colliculus activity in chinchillas related to three distinct patterns of cochlear trauma. J Neurosci Res 2008;86:2564–78.
136. Gerken GM. Central tinnitus and lateral inhibition: An auditory brainstem model. Hear Res 1996;97:75–83.
137. Meikle MB, Vernon J, Johnson RM. The perceived severity of tinnitus. Some observations concerning a large population of tinnitus clinic patients. Otolaryngol Head Neck Surg 1984;92:689–96.
138. Jastreboff PJ, Sasaki CT. An animal model of tinnitus: A decade of development. Am J Otol 1994;15:19–27.
139. Brozoski TJ, Spires TJ, Bauer CA. Vigabatrin, a GABA transaminase inhibitor, reversibly eliminates tinnitus in an animal model. J Assoc Res Otolaryngol 2007;8:105–18.
140. Rioch DM. Studies on the diencephalon of carnivora. Part 1. The nuclear configuration of the thalamus, epithalamus, and hypothalamus of the dog and cat. J Comp Neurol 1929;49:1–119.
141. Morest DK. The neuronal architecture of the medial geniculate body of the cat. J Anat 1964;98:611–30.
142. Andersen RA, Roth GL, Aitkin LM, Merzenich MM. The efferent projections of the central nucleus and the pericentral nucleus of the inferior colliculus in the cat. J Comp Neurol 1980;194: 649–62.
143. Winer JA, Diamond IT, Raczkowski D. Subdivisions of the auditory cortex of the cat: The retrograde transport of horseradish peroxidase to the medial geniculate body and posterior thalamic nuclei. J Comp Neurol 1977;176:387–417.
144. Jones EG, Rockel AJ. The synaptic organization in the medial geniculate body of afferent fibres ascending from the inferior colliculus. Z Zellforsch Mikrosk Anat 1971;113:44–66.
145. Schwarz DW, Tennigkeit F, Puil E. Metabotropic transmitter actions in auditory thalamus. Acta Otolaryngol 2000;120:251–4.
146. Rouiller EM, Colomb E, Capt M, De Ribaupierre F. Projections of the reticular complex of the thalamus onto physiologically characterized regions of the medial geniculate body. Neurosci Lett 1985;53:227–32.
147. Houser CR, Vaughn JE, Barber RP, Roberts E. GABA neurons are the major cell type of the nucleus reticularis thalami. Brain Res 1980;200:341–54.
148. Suga N, Zhang Y, Yan J. Sharpening of frequency tuning by inhibition in the thalamic auditory nucleus of the mustached bat. J Neurophysiol 1997;77:2098–114.
149. De Ribaupierre F. Acoustical information processing in the auditory thalamus and cerebral cortex. In: Ehret G, Romand R, editors. The central auditory system. New York: Oxford University Press; 1997. p. 317–397.
150. Morest DK. Synaptic relationships of Golgi type II cells in the medial geniculate body of the cat. J Comp Neurol 1975;162:157–193.
151. Rodrigues-Dagaeff C, Simm G, De Ribaupierre Y, Villa A, De Ribaupierre F, Rouiller EM. Functional organization of the ventral division of the medial geniculate body of the cat: Evidence for a rostro-caudal gradient of response properties and cortical projections. Hear Res 1989;39:103–25.
152. Villa AE, Rouiller EM, Simm GM, Zurita P, de Ribaupierre Y, de Ribaupierre F. Corticofugal modulation of the information processing in the auditory thalamus of the cat. Exp Brain Res 1991;86:506–17.
153. Zhang Y, Suga N. Modulation of responses and frequency tuning of thalamic and collicular neurons by cortical activation in mustached bats. J Neurophysiol 2000;84:325–33.
154. Gao E, Suga N. Experience-dependent corticofugal adjustment of midbrain frequency map in bat auditory system. Proc Natl Acad Sci U S A 1998;95:12663–70.
155. Gao E, Suga N. Experience-dependent plasticity in the auditory cortex and the inferior colliculus of bats: Role of the corticofugal system. Proc Natl Acad Sci U S A 2000;97:8081–6.
156. Tallal P. Auditory temporal perception, phonics, and reading disabilities in children. Brain Lang 1980;9:182–98.
157. Galaburda AM, Menard MT, Rosen GD. Evidence for aberrant auditory anatomy in developmental dyslexia. Proc Natl Acad Sci U S A 1994;91:8010–13.
158. Wada JA, Clarke R, Hamm A. Cerebral hemispheric asymmetry in humans. Cortical speech zones in 100 adults and 100 infant brains. Arch Neurol 1975;32:239–46.
159. Kraus N, McGee TJ, Carrell TD, Zecker SG, Nicol TG, Koch DB. Auditory neurophysiologic responses and discrimination deficits in children with learning problems. Science 1996;273:971–3.
160. Kraus N, McGee T, Littman T, Nicol T, King C. Nonprimary auditory thalamic representation of acoustic change. J Neurophysiol 1994;72:1270–7.
161. Luethke LE, Krubitzer LA, Kaas JH. Cortical connections of electrophysiologically and architectonically defined subdivisions of auditory cortex in squirrels. J Comp Neurol 1988;268: 181–203.
162. Hackett TA, Preuss TM, Kaas JH. Architectonic identification of the core region in auditory cortex of macaques, chimpanzees, and humans. J Comp Neurol 2001;441:197–222.
163. Kaas JH, Hackett TA, Tramo MJ. Auditory processing in primate cerebral cortex. Current opinion in neurobiology 1999;9:164–70.
164. Hackett TA, Stepniewska I, Kaas JH. Prefrontal connections of the parabelt auditory cortex in macaque monkeys. Brain Res 1999;817:45–58.
165. Imig TJ, Ruggero MA, Kitzes LM, Javel E, Brugge JF. Organization of auditory cortex in the owl monkey (Aotus trivirgatus). J Comp Neurol 1977;171:111–28.
166. Merzenich MM, Brugge JF. Representation of the cochlear partition of the superior temporal plane of the macaque monkey. Brain Res 1973;50:275–96.
167. Morel A, Garraghty PE, Kaas JH. Tonotopic organization, architectonic fields, and connections of auditory cortex in macaque monkeys. J Comp Neurol 1993;335:437–59.
168. Morel A, Kaas JH. Subdivisions and connections of auditory cortex in owl monkeys. J Comp Neurol 1992;318:27–63.

169. Rauschecker JP, Tian B, Hauser M. Processing of complex sounds in the macaque nonprimary auditory cortex. Science 1995;268:111–14.

170. Hackett TA, Stepniewska I, Kaas JH. Subdivisions of auditory cortex and ipsilateral cortical connections of the parabelt auditory cortex in macaque monkeys. J Comp Neurol 1998;394:475–95.

171. Kaas JH, Hackett TA. Subdivisions of auditory cortex and levels of processing in primates. Audiol Neurootol 1998;3:73–85.

172. Sweet RA, Dorph-Petersen KA, Lewis DA. Mapping auditory core, lateral belt, and parabelt cortices in the human superior temporal gyrus. J Comp Neurol 2005;491:270–289.

173. Morosan P, Rademacher J, Schleicher A, Amunts K, Schormann T, Zilles K. Human primary auditory cortex: cytoarchitectonic subdivisions and mapping into a spatial reference system. NeuroImage 2001;13:684–701.

174. Schonwiesner M, von Cramon DY, Rubsamen R. Is it tonotopy after all? Neuroimage 2002;17:1144–61.

175. Talavage TM, Ledden PJ, Benson RR, Rosen BR, Melcher JR. Frequency-dependent responses exhibited by multiple regions in human auditory cortex. Hear Res 2000;150:225–44.

176. Talavage TM, Sereno MI, Melcher JR, Ledden PJ, Rosen BR, Dale AM. Tonotopic organization in human auditory cortex revealed by progressions of frequency sensitivity. J Neurophysiol 2004;91:1282–96.

177. Griffiths TD, Buchel C, Frackowiak RS, Patterson RD. Analysis of temporal structure in sound by the human brain. Nat Neurosci 1998;1:422–7.

178. Griffiths TD, Uppenkamp S, Johnsrude I, Josephs O, Patterson RD. Encoding of the temporal regularity of sound in the human brainstem. Nat Neurosci 2001;4:633–7.

179. Broca P. Remarks on the seat of the faculty of articulate language, followed by an observation of aphema. Bulletin de la societe anatomique de Paris 1861;6:330–57.

180. James W. The principles of psychology. New York: Henry Holt; 1890.

181. Woolsey CN. Organization of cortical auditory system: A review and a synthesis. In: Rasmussen GL, Windle WF, editors. Neural mechanisms of the auditory and vestibular systems. Springfield, IL: Charles C. Thomas; 1960. p. 165–80.

182. Heffner HE, Heffner RS. Unilateral auditory cortex ablation in macaques results in a contralateral hearing loss. J Neurophysiol 1989;62:789–801.

183. Heffner HE, Heffner RS. Effect of restricted cortical lesions on absolute thresholds and aphasia-like deficits in Japanese macaques. Behav Neurosc 1989;103:158–69.

184. Heffner HE, Heffner RS. Cortical deafness cannot account for the inability of Japanese macaques to discriminate species-specific vocalizations. Brain Lang 1989;36:275–85.

185. Kraus N, Nicol T. Brainstem origins for cortical "what" and "where" pathways in the auditory system. Trends Neurosci 2005;28:176–81.

186. Lomber SG, Malhotra S. Double dissociation of "what" and "where" processing in auditory cortex. Nat Neurosci 2008;11:609–16.

187. Belin P, Zatorre RJ, Lafaille P, Ahad P, Pike B. Voice-selective areas in human auditory cortex. Nature 2000;403:309–12.

188. Belin P, Zatorre RJ, Ahad P. Human temporal-lobe response to vocal sounds. Brain Res 2002;13:17–26.

189. Petkov CI, Kayser C, Steudel T, Whittingstall K, Augath M, Logothetis NK. A voice region in the monkey brain. Nat Neurosci 2008;11:367–74.

190. Patterson RD, Uppenkamp S, Johnsrude IS, Griffiths TD. The processing of temporal pitch and melody information in auditory cortex. Neuron 2002;36:767–76.

191. Penagos H, Melcher JR, Oxenham AJ. A neural representation of pitch salience in nonprimary human auditory cortex revealed with functional magnetic resonance imaging. J Neurosci 2004;24:6810–15.

192. Bendor D, Wang X. The neuronal representation of pitch in primate auditory cortex. Nature 2005;436:1161–5.

193. Zatorre RJ, Belin P. Spectral and temporal processing in human auditory cortex. Cereb Cortex 2001;11:946–53.

194. Koelsch S. Significance of Broca's area and ventral premotor cortex for music-syntactic processing. Cortex 2006;42:518–20.

195. Maess B, Koelsch S, Gunter TC, Friederici AD. Musical syntax is processed in Broca's area: An MEG study. Nat Neurosci 2001;4:540–5.

196. Blood AJ, Zatorre RJ, Bermudez P, Evans AC. Emotional responses to pleasant and unpleasant music correlate with activity in paralimbic brain regions. Nat Neurosci 1999;2:382–7.

197. Musacchia G, Sams M, Skoe E, Kraus N. Musicians have enhanced subcortical auditory and audiovisual processing of speech and music. Proc Natl Acad Sci U S A 2007;104:15894–8.

198. Limb CJ, Braun AR. Neural substrates of spontaneous musical performance: An FMRI study of jazz improvisation. PLoS ONE 2008;3:e1679.

199. Whitfield IC. The object of the sensory cortex. Brain Behav Evol 1979;16:129–54.

Vestibular Physiology and Disorders of the Labyrinth

6

Timothy E. Hullar, MD, FACS / Nathan C. Page, MD / Lloyd B. Minor, MD, FACS

The vestibular system collects information about the position and motion of the head. Together with visual and proprioceptive signals, the brain uses this information to coordinate the eyes, head, and body during movement and to give a conscious perception of orientation and motion. Disturbances in this integrative process can lead to dizziness, which is the ninth most common cause of visits to primary care physicians and the most common among patients over 75 years.[1,2] Many of these patients are referred to otologists to determine if a vestibular abnormality accounts for their complaint and to develop a treatment plan. Knowledge of the anatomy and physiology of the vestibular system gives a rational basis for understanding the causes, diagnosis, and treatment of many types of dizziness.

ANATOMIC ORGANIZATION OF THE VESTIBULAR SYSTEM

Dividing the vestibular system into its peripheral and central parts helps to localize pathologies. The periphery is responsible for measuring accelerations of the head. All accelerations can be divided into six components: rotation around an axis lying in each of the three dimensions and linear motion along each of these axes. The periphery consists of the horizontal, superior (also known as anterior), and posterior semicircular canals, which measure rotation, and the utricle and saccule, which measure linear accelerations (Figure 6–1). Each semicircular canal has a synergistic canal in the opposite temporal bone lying approximately parallel to it. The horizontal canals act as a pair, while each superior canal is paired with the posterior canal on the opposite side (Figure 6–2). Linear forces can arise from translation of the head front to back, side to side, or up and down, as well as from the orientation of the head relative to the pull of gravity. The central vestibular system consists of the lateral, medial, superior, and inferior vestibular nuclei and their projections to the thalamus, cortex, cerebellum, descending spinal cord, and extraocular motor nuclei.

Each membranous semicircular canal is filled with endolymph, a potassium-rich extracellular fluid, and is bathed in perilymph, which has the approximate composition of cerebrospinal fluid. The ends of the canals open into the vestibule. Near one end of each membranous canal is a widening known as the ampulla, which contains the crista ampullaris and cupula. The crista ampullaris is a saddle-shaped gelatinous structure along one wall of the membranous canal that contains the sensory hair cells of the vestibular system. The cupula acts as a membranous diaphragm, stretching from the crista to the opposite walls of the canal (Figure 6–3). Because the membranous labyrinth is tethered to the skull, the crista and cupula accelerate with the head as it rotates, but the endolymph's inertia causes it to lag behind. The endolymph accumulates with higher pressure on one side of the cupula than the other, indenting it and bending the hair cells within the crista. When the head ceases to accelerate, the cupula and crista gradually return to their resting positions.

The utricle and saccule, together called the otolith organs, also contain hair cells that bend in response to acceleration of the head. Instead of cristae, however, the sensory epithelium of these organs is covered by flat, kidney-shaped sheets called maculae. One macula lies horizontally against the ceiling of the utricle, whereas the other hangs sagittally on the wall of the saccule. Each macula is a gelatinous matrix into which hair cells project and which is studded with tiny calcium carbonate granules called otoconia.

The maculae of the otolith organs are sensitive to linear accelerations because of the presence of otoconia on their surface. These increase the density of the maculae so that any time the head moves linearly, the heavy maculae lag behind, bending the hair cells embedded in them (Figure 6–4). The utricle primarily senses lateral tilt and translation of the head, whereas the saccule measures front-to-back tilt and translation as well as motion aligned with the pull of gravity.

Hair cells located in the sensory epithelia of the semicircular canals and otolith organs are responsible for coding head acceleration into a modulation in the discharge rate of vestibular afferent fibers. Each hair cell contains a bundle of 50 to 100 stereocilia and one long kinocilium at the edge of each bundle (Figure 6–5). The location of this kinocilium relative to the stereocilia gives each hair cell an intrinsic polarity. In the

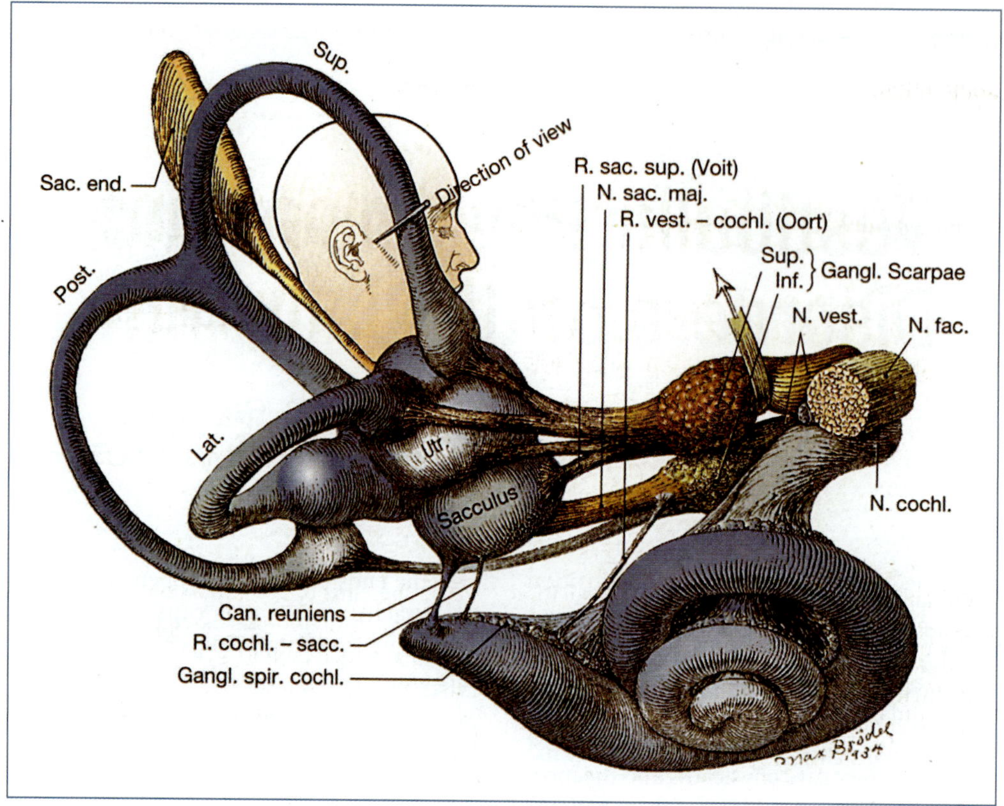

FIGURE 6–1 • Structures of the labyrinth. Structures shown include the utricle (utr.), sacculus, anterior or superior semicircular canal (sup.), posterior semicircular canal (post.), and horizontal or lateral semicircular canal (lat.). The superior vestibular nerve innervates the horizontal and anterior semicircular canals and the utricle. The inferior vestibular nerve innervates the posterior semicircular canal and the saccule. The cell bodies for the vestibular nerves are located in Scarpa's ganglion (Gangl. Scarpae). Drawing from the Brödel Archives, No. 933. *Reproduced with permission of the Department of Art as Applied to Medicine, Johns Hopkins University.*

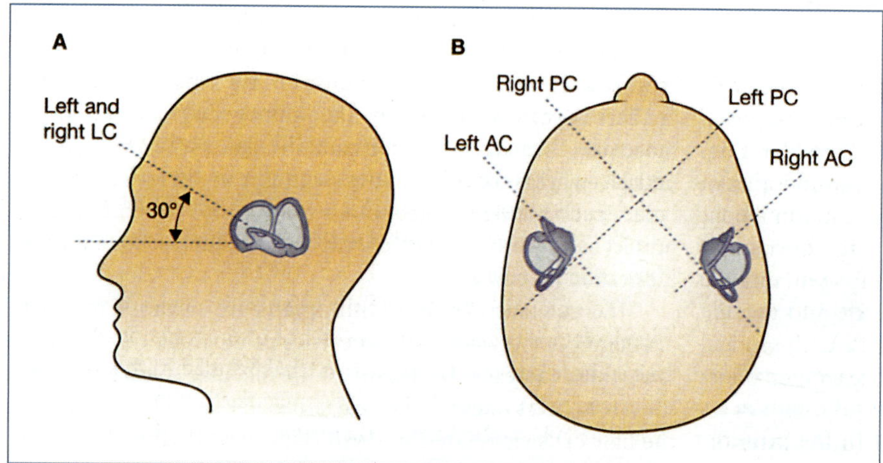

FIGURE 6–2 • Orientation of the semicircular canals. *A*, Horizontal (lateral) semicircular canals. *B*, Anterior (superior) and posterior canals. LC, lateral canal; AC, anterior canal; PC, posterior canal. Relative size of canals exaggerated for clarity. *Reproduced with permission from Barber H, Stockwell C. Textbook of electronystagmography. St. Louis: Mosby; 1976.*

horizontal canals, the kinocilium of every hair cell is located on the side of the ciliary bundle facing the utricle, whereas this arrangement is reversed in the superior and posterior canals. The hair cells of each otolith organ are arranged in two bands along a central stripe called the striola. The kinocilia of the hair bundles in the utricle are oriented toward the striola and those in the saccule face away.[3]

Displacement of a ciliary bundle toward its kinocilium opens potassium channels along the cilia and depolarizes the hair cell from its resting membrane potential of between −50 and −70 mV. The sensitivity of the hair cell can approach 20 mV of depolarization per micrometer of displacement. This depolarization leads to calcium influx at the basal end of the hair cells and increased flow of neurotransmitter into the synapse, whereas displacement in the opposite direction hyperpolarizes the cell and reduces neurotransmitter release.[4] The orientation of the kinocilia of the semicircular canals determines the excitatory direction of the canals. Each horizontal canal is maximally

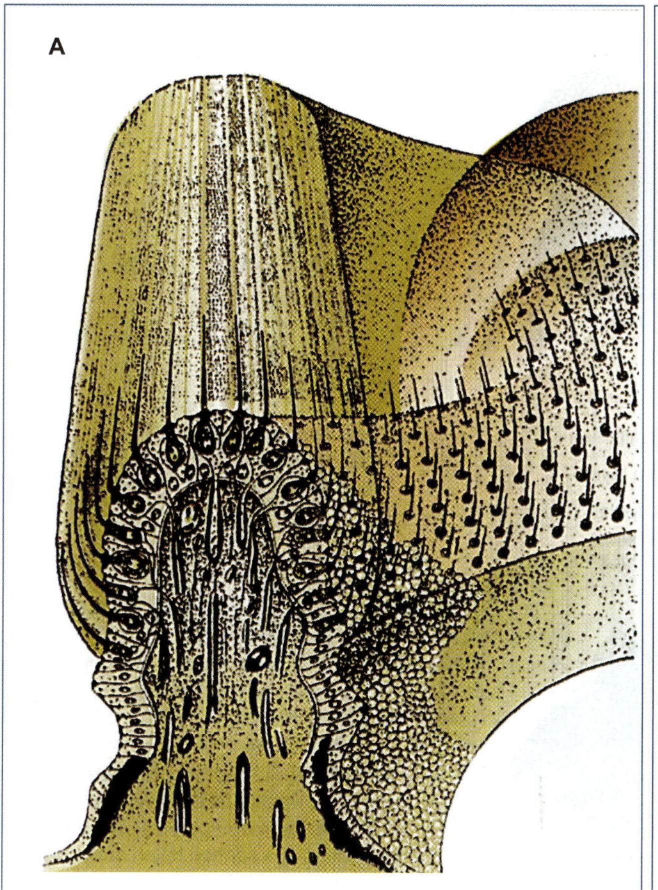

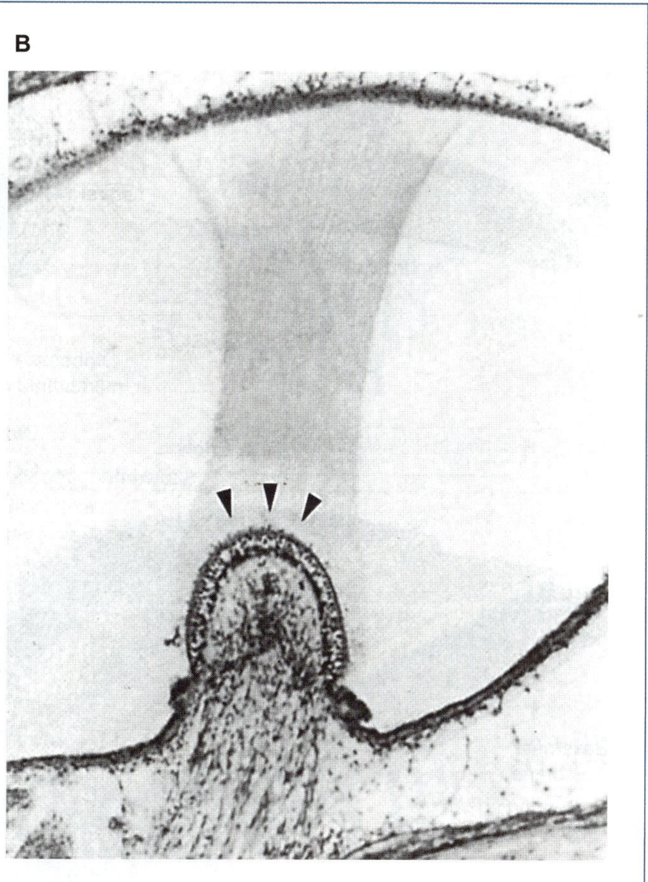

FIGURE 6–3 • Structure of the crista ampullaris and cupula. *A*, Artist's reconstruction of the crista ampullaris. *B*, Transverse section of the crista ampullaris of the monkey. The histologic techniques preserved the attachment of the cupula, which extends from the apex of the crista to the opposite wall of the membranous ampulla. Arrowheads indicate subcupular space. *A, Reproduced with permission from Wersäll J, Lundquist PG. In: Graybiel A, editor. Second Symposium on the Role of Vestibular Organs in Space Exploration, NASA SP-115. Washington DC: US Government Printing Office; 1966. B, Reproduced with permission from Igarashi M. In: Graybiel A, editor. Second Symposium on the Role of Vestibular Organs in Space Exploration, NASA SP-115. Washington DC: US Government Printing Office; 1966.*

excited by a rotation toward the side of the canal and inhibited by a rotation in the opposite direction. This results in an excitatory slow-phase movement toward the side opposite the canal and a resetting saccade toward the canal. The superior canal is excited by a rotation downward and to the side, in the plane of the canal. This results in a vertical–torsional nystagmus, with the slow phase of the vertical component upward and the resetting saccade downward. The posterior canal is excited by an upward rotation and to the side, in the plane of the canal, so that the slow phase is downward and the resetting phase upward.

Afferent nerve fibers in the superior vestibular nerve extend from sensory structures in the superior and horizontal canals and the utricle to the vestibular nuclei in the brain stem. The inferior vestibular nerve leads from the posterior semicircular canal and the saccule. In humans, each vestibular nerve is made up of about 25,000 neurons.[5] These neurons are bipolar, with cell bodies located in the vestibular nerve near the brain stem in Scarpa's ganglion. In addition to afferents, about 400 to 600 efferent nerves lead from the vestibular nuclei to hair cells and afferent nerves in each labyrinth. The precise role of these efferents in modulating the physiology of vestibular reflexes is unknown but may be related to adjusting the sensitivity of the vestibular system to an upcoming volitional movement.[6]

Almost all vestibular nerve afferents have a spontaneous or resting discharge rate, with some fibers firing up to approximately 100 spikes/sec.[7] This resting discharge rate enables each afferent to respond both to excitatory and inhibitory stimuli (Figure 6–6). Discharge regularity, measured by the spacing between action potentials of the afferent's discharge, has provided a useful marker for many important physiologic processes. Three groups of vestibular nerve afferents have been identified in mammals based on their responses to motion and their innervation profiles within the sensory epithelia of the labyrinth (Figure 6–7).[8] Bouton-only afferents have terminations exclusively onto type II hair cells in the peripheral zone of the cristae. These afferents are regularly discharging and have low rotational sensitivities. Dimorphic afferents have calyx endings terminating on type I hair cells and bouton endings terminating on type II hair cells. Their physiologic properties vary according to the location within the crista. Those dimorphic afferents

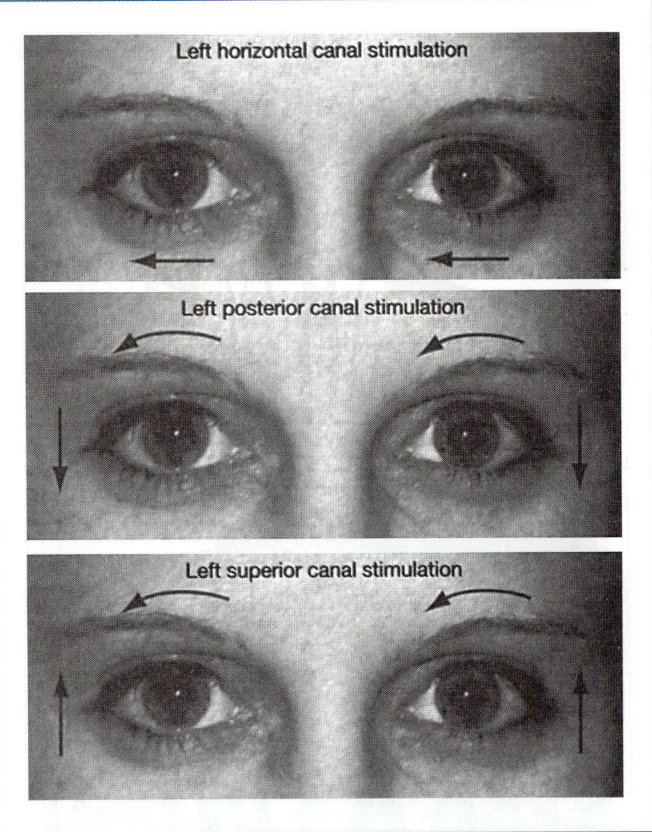

FIGURE 6–8 • Eye movements evoked by excitatory stimulation of individual semicircular canals. The arrows depict the motion of the slow-phase components of the nystagmus. Stimulation of the left horizontal canal results in a horizontal nystagmus with rightward slow phases. A vertical-torsional nystagmus is elicited by excitatory stimulation of either the superior or posterior canals. For the left superior canal, the slow-phase components are directed upward and clockwise with respect to the patient (superior poles of the eyes moving rightward with extorsion of the right eye and intorsion of the left eye). For the left posterior canal, the slow-phase components are the same for torsion but are directed downward in the vertical plane.

gaze during rapid head movements because it has a latency of 50 milliseconds or more. Deficits of the AVOR therefore lead to the symptom of oscillopsia (the apparent motion of objects that are known to be stationary) during rapid head movements. Patients with vestibular loss are less likely to have symptoms of oscillopsia during slower head movements because the visual system can stabilize gaze at lower head velocities.

The oculomotor system must also compensate for linear accelerations (tilt with respect to gravity and linear movements of the head). The linear vestibulo-ocular reflex (LVOR) is responsible for this compensation. Tilting the head side to side evokes ocular counterrolling, which is torsional movement of the eye about the line of sight that partially compensates for the effect of the rotation. Translational motion in which the head is moved laterally, however, requires the eyes to track with horizontal rotations. The otolith organs cannot distinguish between a tilt and a translational movement, so the system must use other information from the semicircular canals and other sensory inputs to decide how to move the eyes.

Several central processes are critical to understanding tests used to diagnose vestibular disorders. Velocity storage is the name given to the process that maintains the sense of rotation even after the rotation has stopped.[15] The neural source of this process is probably located in the vestibular commissure.[16] Signals from the semicircular canals decay away slowly, with a time constant (the time required for the response to decay to 37% of its initial value) of approximately 5 sec. However, the time constant of the AVOR (calculated from the time over which the slow-phase eye velocity declines after a rotation has stopped) in normal subjects is much longer, typically between 12 to 20 sec. The difference between these two values is due to the velocity storage mechanism. In patients with peripheral vestibular dysfunction, the velocity storage mechanism may cease to function. This causes rotation-induced nystagmus, and the conscious perception of rotation, to decay in a shorter period of time than normal.

A second central process whose function is important for measuring vestibular function is the *neural integrator*.[17] The neural integration circuit may be located in the medial vestibular and prepositus hypoglossi nuclei.[18] The neural integrator is the process that provides the signal to hold the eyes away from "primary position" facing straight ahead. When looking away from primary position, the extraocular muscles require a burst of activity to move the eyes to their eccentric position and then a sustained level of discharge that signals the muscles to hold the eye in an eccentric position. In patients with vestibular loss, this process may become dysfunctional and the eyes may drift inappropriately toward primary position.

BEDSIDE EVALUATION OF THE VESTIBULAR SYSTEM

History

A patient's history is often sufficient to identify a likely cause of his or her symptoms. Taking the history of a patient with a complaint related to dizziness should begin in an open-ended fashion, allowing the patient to describe the symptoms with minimal direction from the physician. The process can be facilitated by requesting the patient to complete a questionnaire that asks the patient to describe and respond to queries about symptoms before the first appointment.[19,20] Key elements of the history are described below.

The Nature of the Sensation

Dizziness is a term often used by patients to describe their symptoms in a general way, but categorizing their symptoms more precisely can help determine their cause more accurately. *Vertigo* is an illusory sense of motion when the patient is still. The patient may feel that the motion is internal or that objects in the surroundings are moving or tilting. The sense of motion can be rotatory, linear, or a change in orientation relative to the vertical. Vertigo often indicates a problem within the peripheral vestibular system. Horizontal rotatory movement of objects in the visual surround suggests dysfunction of the semicircular canals, while drop attacks or abnormal sensations of tilt suggest otolith dysfunction. Typical causes of vertigo include benign positional vertigo, viral labyrinthitis, or Ménière's disease, although

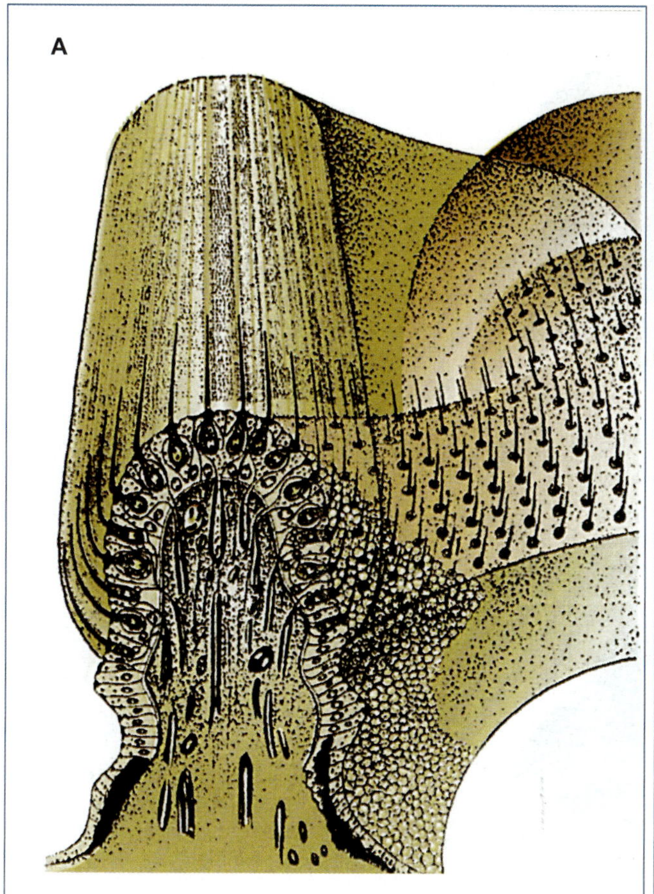

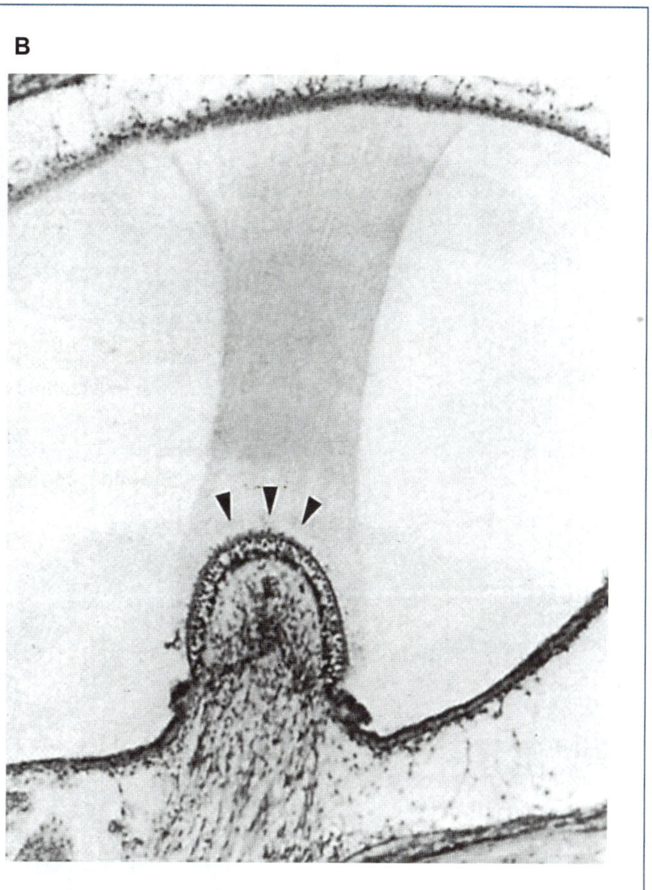

FIGURE 6–3 • Structure of the crista ampullaris and cupula. *A*, Artist's reconstruction of the crista ampullaris. *B*, Transverse section of the crista ampullaris of the monkey. The histologic techniques preserved the attachment of the cupula, which extends from the apex of the crista to the opposite wall of the membranous ampulla. Arrowheads indicate subcupular space. *A, Reproduced with permission from Wersäll J, Lundquist PG. In: Graybiel A, editor. Second Symposium on the Role of Vestibular Organs in Space Exploration, NASA SP-115. Washington DC: US Government Printing Office; 1966. B, Reproduced with permission from Igarashi M. In: Graybiel A, editor. Second Symposium on the Role of Vestibular Organs in Space Exploration, NASA SP-115. Washington DC: US Government Printing Office; 1966.*

excited by a rotation toward the side of the canal and inhibited by a rotation in the opposite direction. This results in an excitatory slow-phase movement toward the side opposite the canal and a resetting saccade toward the canal. The superior canal is excited by a rotation downward and to the side, in the plane of the canal. This results in a vertical–torsional nystagmus, with the slow phase of the vertical component upward and the resetting saccade downward. The posterior canal is excited by an upward rotation and to the side, in the plane of the canal, so that the slow phase is downward and the resetting phase upward.

Afferent nerve fibers in the superior vestibular nerve extend from sensory structures in the superior and horizontal canals and the utricle to the vestibular nuclei in the brain stem. The inferior vestibular nerve leads from the posterior semicircular canal and the saccule. In humans, each vestibular nerve is made up of about 25,000 neurons.[5] These neurons are bipolar, with cell bodies located in the vestibular nerve near the brain stem in Scarpa's ganglion. In addition to afferents, about 400 to 600 efferent nerves lead from the vestibular nuclei to hair cells and afferent nerves in each labyrinth. The precise role of these efferents in modulating the physiology of vestibular reflexes is unknown but may be related to adjusting the sensitivity of the vestibular system to an upcoming volitional movement.[6]

Almost all vestibular nerve afferents have a spontaneous or resting discharge rate, with some fibers firing up to approximately 100 spikes/sec.[7] This resting discharge rate enables each afferent to respond both to excitatory and inhibitory stimuli (Figure 6–6). Discharge regularity, measured by the spacing between action potentials of the afferent's discharge, has provided a useful marker for many important physiologic processes. Three groups of vestibular nerve afferents have been identified in mammals based on their responses to motion and their innervation profiles within the sensory epithelia of the labyrinth (Figure 6–7).[8] Bouton-only afferents have terminations exclusively onto type II hair cells in the peripheral zone of the cristae. These afferents are regularly discharging and have low rotational sensitivities. Dimorphic afferents have calyx endings terminating on type I hair cells and bouton endings terminating on type II hair cells. Their physiologic properties vary according to the location within the crista. Those dimorphic afferents

FIGURE 6–4 • Structure of the otolith organs. *A*, Sacculus. *B*, Utriculus. *C*, Composition of otoconial membrane of the saccus in a section taken at the level shown in *A*. *Reproduced with permission from Paparella MM, Shumrick DA, editors. Textbook of Otolaryngology. Vol 1. Philadelphia: WB Saunders; 1980.*

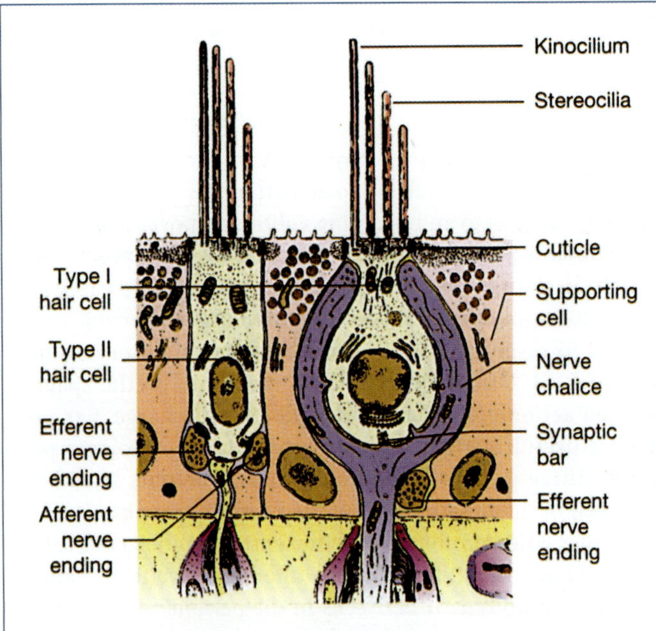

FIGURE 6–5 • Two types of sensory hair cells (types I and II) are found in the mammalian labyrinth. *Reproduced with permission from Wersäll J, Bagger-Sjöback D. In: Kornhuber HH, editor. Handbook of sensory physiology. New York: Springer-Verlag; 1974.*

terminating in the peripheral zone are regularly discharging, whereas those terminating near the central zone are irregularly discharging with higher rotational sensitivity. There is also a group of afferents that terminate exclusively with calyx endings onto type I hair cells in the central zone. The calyx-only afferents are irregularly discharging and have low rotational sensitivities at low stimulus frequencies and high sensitivities at higher frequencies.[9] The function of the different types of fibers may be related to the type of head motion each is coding.[10,11]

In work done over a century ago, Ewald identified two fundamental principles governing the relationship between the labyrinthine receptors and the vestibular reflexes that they mediate.[12] From experiments performed in pigeons, he noted that fenestration of a semicircular canal followed by mechanical stimulation of the membranous canal led to eye and head movements that were in the plane of that canal.

He also noted that excitatory stimuli led to larger amplitude responses than inhibitory stimuli. This is, at least in part, attributable to the resting discharge rate of vestibular nerve afferents and central vestibular neurons. These neurons can be excited up to a firing rate of at least 350 spikes/s but can be inhibited to only 0 spikes/s. Thus, there is a three- to fourfold higher range for excitation in comparison to inhibition. Many central vestibular neurons also have a resting discharge rate, suggesting that their

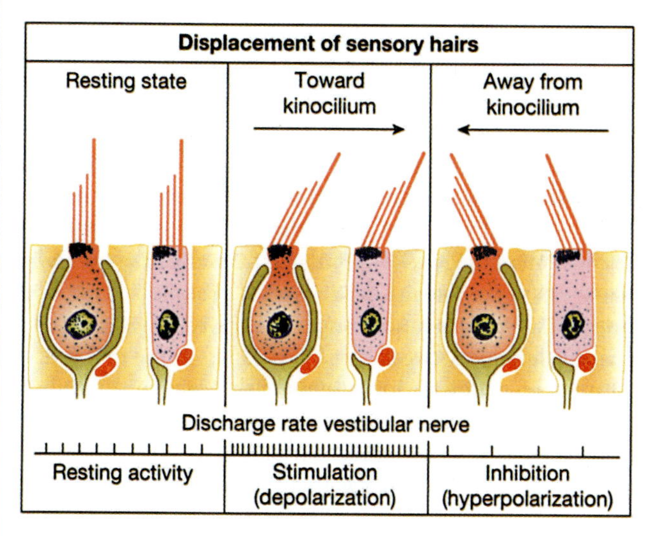

FIGURE 6–6 • Discharge rate of individual vestibular-nerve fibers as a function of the displacement of the cilia. The vestibular nerve afferents fire more frequently when the hair bundles are displaced toward the kinocilia; they fire more slowly when displaced in the opposite direction. *Reproduced with permission from Wersäll J, Lundquist P-G. In: Graybiel A, editor. Second Symposium on the Role of Vestibular Organs in Space Exploration, NASA SP-115. Washington DC: US Government Printing Office; 1966.*

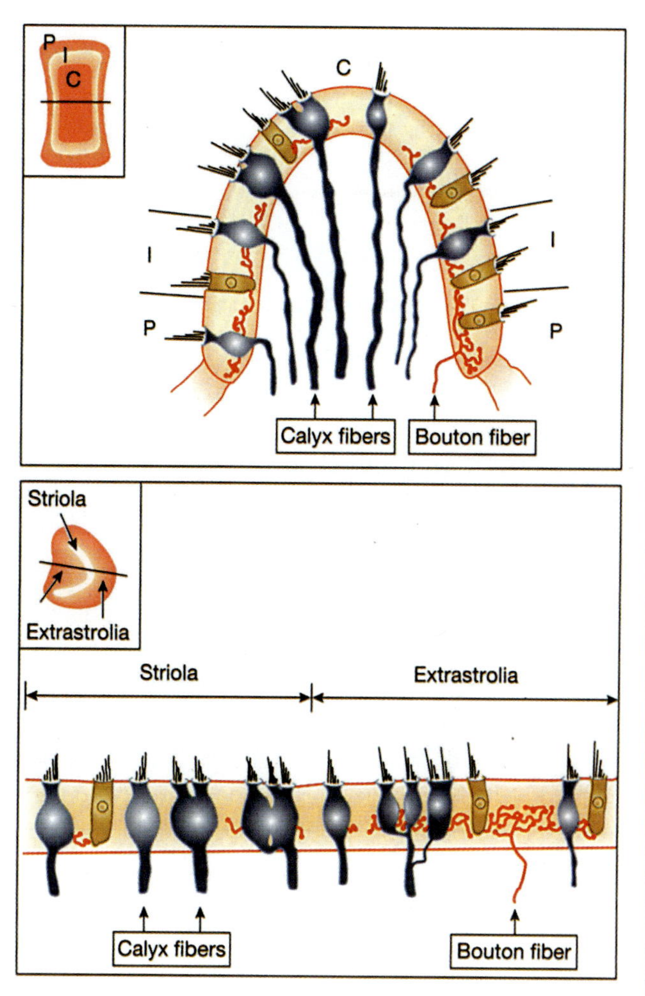

FIGURE 6–7 • Afferent innervation patterns in the mammalian vestibular end-organs. Top, The neuroepithelium of the cristae is divided into central (C), intermediate (I), and peripheral (P) zones, shown in plan in the inset and in cross-section in the main panel. Calyx fibers innervate the central zone, whereas bouton fibers innervate the peripheral zone. Dimorphic fibers are found throughout. Bottom, The macula is divided into the striola and the lateral and medial extrastriola (see inset). Calyx fibers are found in the striola, bouton fibers in the extrastriola, and dimorphs throughout. *Reproduced with permission from Goldberg JM. The vestibular end organs: morphological and physiological diversity of afferents. Curr Opin Neurobiol 1991;1:229–35.*

responses may also contribute to an asymmetry in responses. The first observation, motion of the eyes and head in the plane of the affected canal, is termed Ewald's first law (Figure 6–8). The second observation, excitatory responses are larger than inhibitory ones, is referred to as Ewald's second law. These relationships provide a basis for understanding many of the symptoms and signs that occur after injury to the labyrinth.

CENTRAL PROCESSES INVOLVED IN CONTROL OF VESTIBULAR REFLEXES

The central part of the vestibular system consists of the vestibular nuclei, which integrate information from vision, proprioception via spinal and cervical afferents, and vestibular signals from the labyrinth. These nuclei send projections that extend to the oculomotor system, where they help control eye movements; the muscles of the neck and spine, where they steady the head; and the thalamus and cortex. Central vestibular circuits also include parts of the cerebellum, which is involved in recalibrating the system when necessary.

Vestibular projections to the oculomotor nuclei reflexively maintain a steady image on the retina while the head is turning, tilted, or moving linearly in space. Quantification of these reflexes is the most common way of evaluating vestibular function. The angular vestibulo-ocular reflex (AVOR) is a three-neuron arc consisting of a vestibular afferent neuron, a vestibular interneuron, and an oculomotor neuron innervating the extraocular muscles. The brain interprets stimulation of a particular semicircular canal as motion of the head, and the eyes move reflexively in an equal but opposite amount to compensate. Turning the head to the left, for example, excites the left horizontal semicircular canal, and the eyes track to the right in response. This action leaves the angle of the target relative to the eye unchanged and its image steady on the retina. Similar relationships apply for the posterior and superior canals.

The AVOR is the fastest and one of the most exquisitely accurate reflexes in the body. It has a latency of about 7 milliseconds and produces eye movements that typically have <5% error with respect to rapid head movements.[13] This is critically important during rapid head movements, where even a small time delay might lead to instability of the visual image on the retina. Instability can occur when the image shifts even slightly, more than 2 to 3 degrees/s over the retina.[14] The visual system is unable to provide effective feedback to stabilize

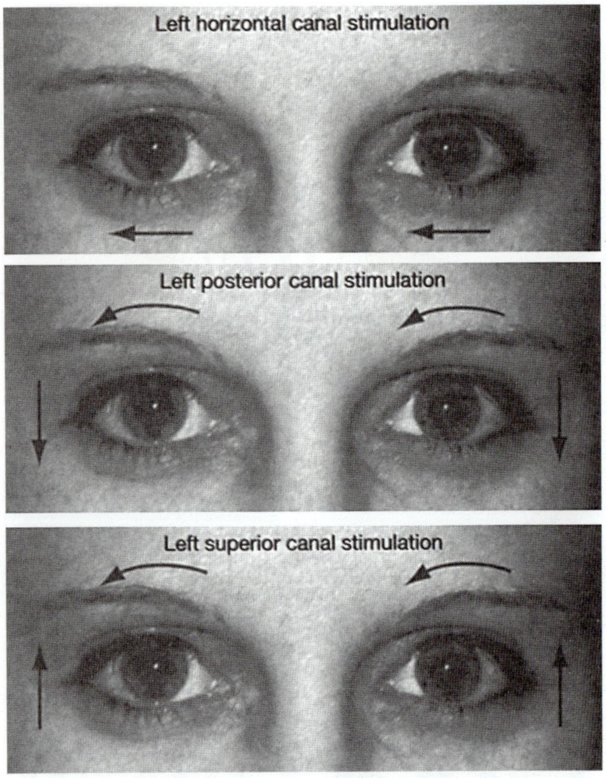

FIGURE 6–8 • Eye movements evoked by excitatory stimulation of individual semicircular canals. The arrows depict the motion of the slow-phase components of the nystagmus. Stimulation of the left horizontal canal results in a horizontal nystagmus with rightward slow phases. A vertical-torsional nystagmus is elicited by excitatory stimulation of either the superior or posterior canals. For the left superior canal, the slow-phase components are directed upward and clockwise with respect to the patient (superior poles of the eyes moving rightward with extorsion of the right eye and intorsion of the left eye). For the left posterior canal, the slow-phase components are the same for torsion but are directed downward in the vertical plane.

gaze during rapid head movements because it has a latency of 50 milliseconds or more. Deficits of the AVOR therefore lead to the symptom of oscillopsia (the apparent motion of objects that are known to be stationary) during rapid head movements. Patients with vestibular loss are less likely to have symptoms of oscillopsia during slower head movements because the visual system can stabilize gaze at lower head velocities.

The oculomotor system must also compensate for linear accelerations (tilt with respect to gravity and linear movements of the head). The linear vestibulo-ocular reflex (LVOR) is responsible for this compensation. Tilting the head side to side evokes ocular counterrolling, which is torsional movement of the eye about the line of sight that partially compensates for the effect of the rotation. Translational motion in which the head is moved laterally, however, requires the eyes to track with horizontal rotations. The otolith organs cannot distinguish between a tilt and a translational movement, so the system must use other information from the semicircular canals and other sensory inputs to decide how to move the eyes.

Several central processes are critical to understanding tests used to diagnose vestibular disorders. Velocity storage is the name given to the process that maintains the sense of rotation even after the rotation has stopped.[15] The neural source of this process is probably located in the vestibular commissure.[16] Signals from the semicircular canals decay away slowly, with a time constant (the time required for the response to decay to 37% of its initial value) of approximately 5 sec. However, the time constant of the AVOR (calculated from the time over which the slow-phase eye velocity declines after a rotation has stopped) in normal subjects is much longer, typically between 12 to 20 sec. The difference between these two values is due to the velocity storage mechanism. In patients with peripheral vestibular dysfunction, the velocity storage mechanism may cease to function. This causes rotation-induced nystagmus, and the conscious perception of rotation, to decay in a shorter period of time than normal.

A second central process whose function is important for measuring vestibular function is the *neural integrator*.[17] The neural integration circuit may be located in the medial vestibular and prepositus hypoglossi nuclei.[18] The neural integrator is the process that provides the signal to hold the eyes away from "primary position" facing straight ahead. When looking away from primary position, the extraocular muscles require a burst of activity to move the eyes to their eccentric position and then a sustained level of discharge that signals the muscles to hold the eye in an eccentric position. In patients with vestibular loss, this process may become dysfunctional and the eyes may drift inappropriately toward primary position.

BEDSIDE EVALUATION OF THE VESTIBULAR SYSTEM

History

A patient's history is often sufficient to identify a likely cause of his or her symptoms. Taking the history of a patient with a complaint related to dizziness should begin in an open-ended fashion, allowing the patient to describe the symptoms with minimal direction from the physician. The process can be facilitated by requesting the patient to complete a questionnaire that asks the patient to describe and respond to queries about symptoms before the first appointment.[19,20] Key elements of the history are described below.

The Nature of the Sensation

Dizziness is a term often used by patients to describe their symptoms in a general way, but categorizing their symptoms more precisely can help determine their cause more accurately. *Vertigo* is an illusory sense of motion when the patient is still. The patient may feel that the motion is internal or that objects in the surroundings are moving or tilting. The sense of motion can be rotatory, linear, or a change in orientation relative to the vertical. Vertigo often indicates a problem within the peripheral vestibular system. Horizontal rotatory movement of objects in the visual surround suggests dysfunction of the semicircular canals, while drop attacks or abnormal sensations of tilt suggest otolith dysfunction. Typical causes of vertigo include benign positional vertigo, viral labyrinthitis, or Ménière's disease, although other processes such as migraine-related vertigo may also be responsible. *Oscillopsia* is instability of the visual field caused by motion of the head. It is a common complaint in patients with unilateral or, more commonly, bilateral loss of peripheral vestibular function. *Disequilibrium* is the perception of unsteadiness, often with the sensation that a fall may be imminent. This may be related to dysfunction of the vestibular system, but may also be caused by faulty proprioception or other processes responsible for maintaining balance. Migraine-related vertigo, mal de debarquement, side effects of medication, or other conditions such as diabetes may be responsible. *Presyncope* may be related to anxiety, vascular disease, cardiac arrhythmia, or autonomic disorders.

Timing of the Initial Spell

Imbalance occurring shortly after a serious illness requiring hospitalization may be due to exposure to ototoxic antibiotics. Starting or stopping a new prescription or over-the-counter medicine, or changing the strength or dosing schedule of a medication, may lead to new symptoms of dizziness. An upper respiratory infection may precede the onset of symptoms of benign positional vertigo or vestibular neuritis. Trauma or infection can lead to symptoms of endolymphatic hydrops. Stapes surgery followed by episodic dizziness may reflect the development of a perilymphatic fistula. An initial spell of dizziness in a girl nearing menarche may indicate a hormonal influence on balance, often associated with migraine-related imbalance.

Frequency and Duration of Symptoms

Episodic imbalance may be divided into short-, medium-, or long-term events. Short-term symptoms, lasting seconds to minutes, may be caused by autonomic dysfunction or inner ear conditions such as benign positional vertigo, perilymphatic fistula, or semicircular canal dehiscence. Medium-length spells, typically up to 4/ h long, may be due to Ménière's disease. They may also be related to cardiac arrhythmias, transient ischemia, hypoglycemia, or seizure activity. Anxiety disorders may lead to medium-term vertigo. Longer spells, lasting up to days, are more likely to be related to migraine-associated vertigo. Chronic symptoms of dizziness indicate a stable level of dysfunction in any of the systems dedicated to maintaining balance. Unilateral or bilateral peripheral vestibular loss may cause chronic imbalance. It may also be due to dysfunction of other sensory symptoms, such as in patients with peripheral neuropathy. The elderly may suffer from chronic imbalance, as can patients with uncontrolled hypertension or other causes of widespread pathology of the central nervous system such as diffuse brain injury or syphilis. Semicircular canal dehiscence has recently been recognized as a cause of chronic imbalance.

Precipitating or Mitigating Factors

The diagnosis of certain vestibular disorders is strongly suggested from events, stimuli, or movements that trigger symptoms. Benign paroxysmal positional vertigo (BPPV) classically begins on rolling over in bed or tilting the head backward and toward the affected ear. Patients with superior canal dehiscence syndrome experience vertigo and oscillopsia with sound or pressure stimuli. Pressure sensitivity is also common in patients with perilymphatic fistula. Patients with migraine-related vertigo may have symptoms brought on by certain foods, changes in the weather, menses, significant motion stimuli, or exposure to lights or sounds. Seasonal relationships may suggest allergy, which has been linked to Ménière's disease. Migraine patients may benefit from sleep or rest in a darkened quiet room. Patients with BPPV tend to keep their heads as still as possible.

Associated Symptoms

Aural fullness and tinnitus can precede an attack of vertigo in patients with Ménière's disease, a correlation known as Lermoyez's syndrome.[21] Headache or visual symptoms sometimes accompany vestibular migraine. Dysarthria, diplopia, and paresthesias may accompany the vertigo seen in cases of vertebrobasilar insufficiency. Diplopia may be a sign of multiple sclerosis. Dysfunction of other cranial nerves, such as the fifth, seventh, or auditory nerve, may indicate a mass in the cerebellopontine angle or internal auditory canal. Ataxia suggests cerebellar dysfunction, sometimes related to a degenerative condition, but may also be due to the mass effect of a tumor in the cerebellopontine angle. More critically, it may be a manifestation of the lateral medullary syndrome due to brainstem infarct. Sweating, dyspnea, and palpitations often accompany panic attacks. Acute visual changes accompanying imbalance may be due to Cogan's syndrome, which is an otologic emergency affecting hearing, balance, and eyesight, or benign intracranial hypertension. Otosclerosis may cause hearing loss as well as imbalance. Temporomandibular joint disorder may cause headaches, subjective hearing loss, and tinnitus associated with imbalance.

Other Medical Conditions

Thyroid disease, diabetes mellitus, anemia, autoimmune diseases, and vascular or cardiac disease may cause imbalance. Hypoglycemia is a not uncommon cause of dizziness. Many medications, including those used to treat seizures, hypertension, cardiac arrhythmias, and hyperglycemia, can also produce symptoms that mimic peripheral or central vestibular disorders. Anxiety disorders, panic syndromes, and agoraphobia can lead to episodic vertigo that mimics a vestibulopathy. Previous ear surgery or otologic diseases such as cholesteatoma can lead to peripheral vestibular loss, sometimes through creation of a semicircular canal fistula.

Family History

Migraine, Ménière's disease, and otosclerosis can all be related to symptoms of imbalance and sometimes run in families.[22] Syndromic diseases, such as CHARGE syndrome and Usher's syndrome, may be accompanied by vestibular dysfunction. A mutation of the *CACNA1A* gene leads to autosomal-dominant episodic vertigo and ataxia type EA-2.[23]

Examination

The neurotologic examination evaluates components of vestibular and related oculomotor and postural function to identify abnormalities that are characteristic of pathologic entities. One such approach is presented below in an order that would correspond to the actual examination. Much of the examination of peripheral labyrinthine function is dedicated to evaluating semicircular canal function, but tests of otolith function are becoming more commonly used. In both cases, vestibular function is evaluated primarily by measuring eye movements. The general otolaryngologic examination is a part of the assessment but is not reviewed here.

Inspection for Spontaneous Nystagmus

Vestibulo-ocular reflexes are responsible for maintaining the stability of objects on the retina during head movements. Disorders in their physiology can result in nystagmus and impaired eye movements in response to head movements with consequent loss of visual acuity. Nystagmus is a to-and-fro beating of the eyes with slow and fast components. Spontaneous nystagmus is seen when there is an imbalance in the level of neural activity innervating the extraocular muscles. Vestibular-evoked nystagmus is termed "jerk nystagmus" and comprises a drifting slow phase followed by a rapid resetting motion. The direction of this type of nystagmus is typically named according to its fast phase because that is more obvious to the examiner, but is actually less diagnostically important than the slow phase, which is directly driven by afferent input from the vestibular end-organs. The amplitude of nystagmus is often reduced if a patient is able to fixate on a target. Examination for nystagmus should therefore take place with the patient wearing Frenzel goggles. These are high-diopter glasses, which allow the examiner to see the patient's eyes clearly but minimize the ability to fixate.

"Vestibular nystagmus" is a mixed horizontal-torsional motion of the eye that occurs with a recent vestibular loss. It occurs even if the head is held still and can be dampened by visual fixation. Afferent input to the brain stem is dominated by signal from the normal horizontal canal, which is interpreted by the brain as an ipsilateral turn. The AVOR compensates for this by moving the eye in a slow phase in the opposite direction, which is then reset by a fast phase toward the intact labyrinth. Torsional motion of the eye is provided by the sum of inputs from the intact superior and posterior canals. Because activity of the superior canal induces upward slow phases and the posterior canal induces downward slow phases, no net vertical motion of the eye is seen. Note that in some situations, nystagmus is caused by overstimulation of one labyrinth rather than loss of function of the other. This can occur following surgery on the inner ear or related to an attack of Ménière's disease.[24]

Vestibular nystagmus often changes its amplitude or direction with changes in the direction of gaze. Nystagmus seen in patients with benign positional vertigo related to canalithiasis of the posterior semicircular canal is more vertical when looking away from the involved side and more torsional when looking toward the involved side. This occurs because the eye is more in line with the plane of the posterior canal when looking away and more in line with the axis of the canal when looking toward the pathologic side. Nystagmus may also occur in normal subjects. "Convergence nystagmus" can be brought on voluntarily by focusing on a near target.[25] "Endpoint" nystagmus occurs when gaze is directed to the far limit of the range of motion of the eyes.[26] This may be accentuated in patients intoxicated with alcohol or using some medicines.

Alexander's law describes eye movements seen in patients with an acute unilateral vestibular loss (Figure 6–9). In these patients, the neural integrator is compromised and the eyes tend to drift back to their primary position. This motion combines with the slow phases of vestibular nystagmus caused by asymmetric input from the horizontal canals. The result accentuates the dominant vestibular nystagmus when gaze is directed toward the intact side and reduces it when gaze is directed toward the hypofunctional side.

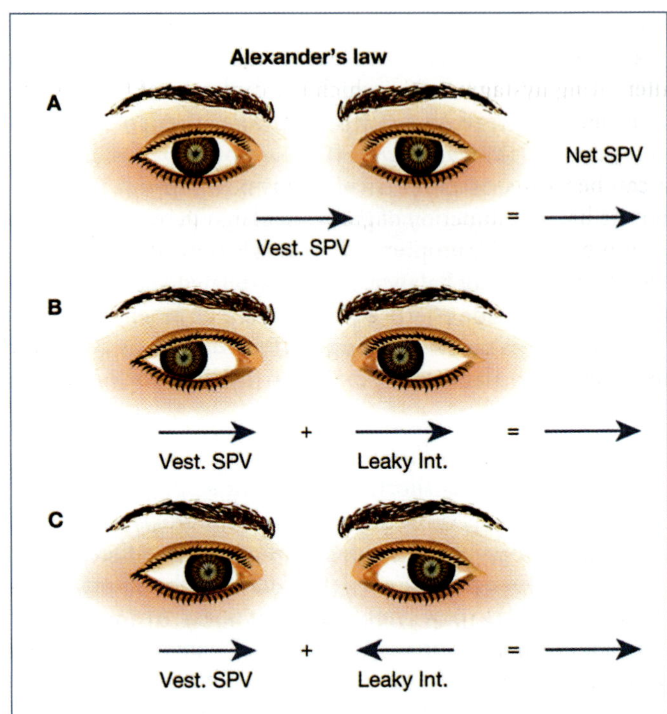

FIGURE 6–9 • Alexander's law. After unilateral vestibular loss, a central process (called the "leaky integrator") contributes to eye motion and nystagmus by allowing the eye to drift to center, regardless of its position. The interaction of this motion and the motion of the eye caused by the imbalance in vestibular activity between the two labyrinths cause nystagmus to be more pronounced when looking away from the lesion. In straight-ahead gaze *A*, the vestibular slow phase alone is manifest. When the eyes look to the direction of the fast phase (right, *B*), the leaky integrator causes the eye to drift to the left. This drift adds to the vestibular slow phase, and the net slow phase velocity (SPV) increases. When the eyes look to the direction of the slow phase (left, *C*), the leaky integrator causes the eye to drift to the right. This drift subtracts from the vestibular slow phase, and the net SPV decreases.

A related finding is seen in patients with Brun's nystagmus. This is seen in patients with a long-standing vestibular loss, such as due to an acoustic neuroma, in whom vestibular nystagmus is less pronounced due to central compensation. When looking toward the intact side, both the functional labyrinth and the loss of the neural integrator add to drive slow phases toward the hypofunctional side. However, when looking toward the hypofunctional side, the effect of the neural integrator letting the eyes drift toward the midline is actually stronger than the remaining, compensated vestibular signal driving their slow phases toward the hypofunctional side. The resulting slow phases are to the intact side and the fast phases beat toward the pathologic side.

Several types of nystagmus are caused by acute or chronic pathologies of the central nervous system. Upbeat or downbeat nystagmus can be caused by alcohol or medicine ingestion or disorders of the brain stem or cerebellum, including Chiari malformations. "Pendular nystagmus" consists only of slow phases and is often related to brainstem pathology. "Periodic alternating nystagmus," in which the direction of the nystagmus changes approximately every 2 min, is seen with brain stem and cerebellar disease including Chiari malformations. It can be treated with baclofen. "Congenital nystagmus" may appear like vestibular nystagmus, although patients may find a "null point" of gaze where the nystagmus is minimized and preferentially hold their eyes in that position in the orbit. Tourette's syndrome may cause ocular tics that mimic nystagmus. Other types of nystagmus are described in detail elsewhere.[27]

Ocular Tilt Reaction

The ocular tilt reaction is caused by an imbalance in tonic levels of activity along pathways mediating otolith-ocular reflexes. The ocular tilt reaction can occur with lesions anywhere along otolith-ocular pathways: labyrinth or vestibular nerve, vestibular nuclei, medial longitudinal fasciculus, or interstitial nucleus of Cajal. There are three components to the ocular tilt reaction arising from hypofunction of one labyrinth: head tilt toward the lesioned labyrinth, skew deviation with the lower eye being on the side of the lesion, and ocular counter-roll (torsional deviation of the superior poles of the eyes toward the side of the lesion). Patients with skew deviation often complain of vertical diplopia and sometimes torsional diplopia (one image tilted with respect to the other). The alternate cover test is used to detect skew deviation: the examiner covers one eye of the patient with a card and then moves the cover to the patient's other eye while looking for a vertical corrective movement as an index of a vertical misalignment.

Positional Testing

Benign paroxysmal positional vertigo (BPPV) is the most common cause of dizziness in patients who visit an otolaryngologist. It is usually caused by pathology in the posterior semicircular canal, but can affect the horizontal, superior, or multiple canals as well. Diagnosis of BPPV may be determined by the latency, direction, duration, and reversal properties of the nystagmus. The latency and duration of the perception of dizziness during positioning maneuvers, even without visible nystagmus, can also suggest the presence of BPPV. The Dix-Hallpike maneuver for identification of posterior canal BPPV is begun with the patient sitting upright on an examination table. For testing to detect the presence of right posterior canal BPPV, the head is turned 45 degrees, so the chin is toward the right shoulder. The patient is then brought straight back rapidly until the shoulders are flat on the bed and the neck is extended. This position is maintained for at least 30 sec.

Nystagmus due to BPPV typically begins after a latency of 2 to 10 sec, increases in amplitude over about 10 sec, and declines over the next 30 sec. This time course presumably reflects the sinking of the debris in the posterior canal. Posterior canal BPPV results in a vertical–torsional nystagmus with the slow-phase components of the nystagmus directed downward and toward the uppermost ear. The fast-phase vertical component of the nystagmus therefore is toward the forehead and the fast-phase torsional component directs the superior part of the eye toward the ground (Figure 6–8). Because of the orientation of pulling directions for the oblique and vertical recti muscles, the planar characteristics of the nystagmus change with the direction of gaze (when described with respect to an eye-fixed coordinate system): on looking to the dependent ear, it becomes more torsional; on looking to the higher ear, it becomes more vertical.

A horizontal canal (HC) variant of BPPV has also been described.[28] In these patients, a strong horizontal nystagmus builds up over the same time course as for posterior canal BPPV but persist much longer. The standard Dix-Hallpike maneuver may not elicit nystagmus in cases of HC BPPV. Nystagmus can instead be identified by bringing the patient backward into the supine position and then turning the head left or right ear down. The nystagmus seen with HC BPPV may last longer than that seen in posterior canal BPPV.

Nystagmus related to HC BPPV is exclusively horizontal and may beat either downward (geotropic) or upward (ageotropic) regardless of which direction the patient is facing. Geotropic nystagmus may reflect canalithiasis, while ageotropic nystagmus may indicate cupulolithiasis, where debris is stuck to the cupula and symptoms have a quicker onset and last longer following positioning. Geotropic nystagmus tends to be more vigorous than ageotropic nystagmus because geotropic nystagmus may be due to inhibition of the affected canal's afferents and ageotropic nystagmus may be due to their excitation. Anterior canal BPPV has been rarely described and is typified by vertical-torsional nystagmus with fast phases beating toward the patient's chin. This can be initiated with the patient in the standard Dix-Hallpike position, but in that case the involved canal is located in the upper ear.

Symptoms of positional vertigo with a minimal latent period suggest a central cause for dizziness. Sustained symptoms produced during testing for posterior canal BPPV may indicate a Chiari malformation or vertebrobasilar insufficiency worsened by neck extension. A central lesion is most likely when positional nystagmus is purely vertical or purely torsional or if there is a sustained unidirectional horizontal positional nystagmus of high enough intensity to be observed without Frenzel lenses. Multiple sclerosis can cause positional nystagmus, but limitations of eye movements due to internuclear ophthalmoplegia can sometimes mask its effects.[29] Brief symptoms on arising may be associated with orthostatic hypotension. A sustained, usually horizontal, positional nystagmus of low velocity is a common finding in patients with central or peripheral vestibular lesions and may also be present in asymptomatic human subjects.[30] Positional testing may also exacerbate a spontaneous nystagmus.[30] Alcohol intoxication is a common cause of positional nystagmus.[31]

Postheadshaking Nystagmus

Postheadshaking nystagmus (HSN) occurs in patients with imbalance in dynamic vestibular function. With Frenzel lenses in place, the patient is instructed to shake the head vigorously about 30 times side to side with the chin placed about 30 degrees downward to bring the horizontal canal into the plane of rotation. Head shaking is stopped abruptly, and the examiner looks for any nystagmus. Normal individuals usually have no or occasionally just a beat or two of post-HSN. With a unilateral loss of labyrinthine function, however, there is usually a vigorous nystagmus with slow-phase components initially directed toward the lesioned side.[32]

The initial phase of HSN arises because there is asymmetry of peripheral inputs during high-velocity head rotations: more activity is generated during rotation toward the intact side than toward the affected side. This asymmetry leads to an accumulation of activity within central velocity storage mechanisms during head shaking. Nystagmus following head shaking reflects discharge of that activity. The amplitude and duration of the initial phase of HSN are dependent on the state of the velocity storage mechanism. Because velocity storage is typically ineffective during the immediate period after an acute unilateral vestibular loss, the primary phase of HSN may be absent or attenuated in these circumstances.[33]

Head Thrust Test

The head thrust (or "head impulse") test allows examination of individual semicircular canals during vigorous motion. Brief, high-acceleration rotations of the head in the horizontal plane are applied while instructing the patient to look carefully at the examiner's nose. An AVOR of abnormally low amplitude will be evoked in response to head thrusts in the excitatory direction of a lesioned or hypoactive canal. For the horizontal canals, a rightward head thrust therefore tests the right horizontal canal and a leftward head thrust tests the left horizontal canal.[34] A corrective saccade, required to bring the eyes back to the intended point of fixation, is seen in such cases (Figure 6–10).[35] Corrective saccades observed in head thrust responses from patients with vestibular hypofunction can, with mechanisms of vestibular compensation, occur during the head movement and lead to an eye movement response that appears relatively normal on clinical examination. The sensitivity of the test can be improved by beginning each head movement with the patient's eyes in primary gaze position and moving the head at random intervals and order to the right and left. The test can also be used to detect dysfunction in each of the vertical canals by delivering the head thrusts in approximately the plane of the left anterior–right posterior or right anterior left posterior canals.[36]

Dynamic Visual Acuity

Vestibular dysfunction typically causes a pronounced loss of visual acuity during head movement. The patient reads a Snellen chart with the head stationary and visual acuity is recorded. Acuity is then checked during horizontal head oscillations at a frequency of about 2 Hz. Subjects with corrective lenses are instructed to wear their glasses or contact lenses during this testing. Subjects with normal vestibular function typically show no more than a one-line decline during head movement but those with vestibular hypofunction (particularly bilateral hypofunction) may show up to a five-line decline in acuity.[37] Predictive mechanisms during repetitive, sinusoidal oscillations of the head may augment performance during this test and obscure

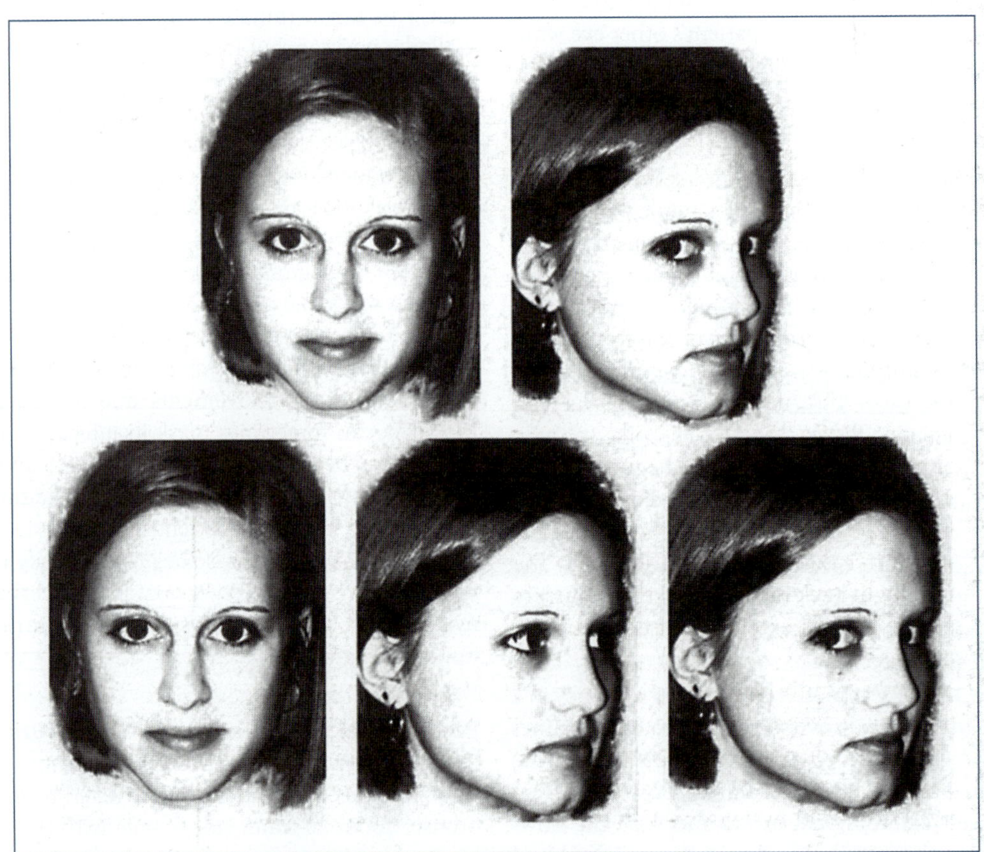

FIGURE 6–10 • Eye movements during head thrust test. Testing left horizontal canal by performing head thrust to subject's left. Top: normally functioning left horizontal canal drives eyes to right immediately following the thrust. Bottom: hypofunctional left horizontal canal fails to drive eyes to right. A catchup saccade brings them into position after a delay.

the identification of a deficit.[38] Computerized presentations of visual stimuli in a laboratory setting may avoid this problem.[39]

Other Bedside Tests of Vestibulo-Ocular Function

Changes in relative pressure between the middle and inner ears may induce nystagmus. A Valsalva maneuver with the glottis closed increases intracranial pressure, while a maneuver with the glottis open (blowing against a pinched nose) increases middle ear pressure. Nystagmus is best observed using Frenzel lenses or while examining small blood vessels on the sclera using an obliquely directed microscope. Similar symptoms may also be elicited by tragal compression or insufflation with a pneumatic otoscope or Siegle's speculum. Nystagmus induced during these maneuvers may reflect craniocervical junction anomalies such as Arnold–Chiari malformation, superior canal dehiscence syndrome, perilymph fistula, or compression of the vestibular nerve by tumor.[27]

Patients with pressure-induced eye movements may also have symptoms in response to sound. This may be evaluated by observing the eyes under Frenzel lenses when giving pure tones from 500 to 4,000 dB at intensities of 100 to 110 dB. Tullio's phenomenon is the occurrence of vestibular symptoms and eye movements with sound. Hennebert's sign is the occurrence of these symptoms and signs with motion of the tympanic membrane and ossicular chain. These signs have recently been documented in patients with superior canal dehiscence syndrome.[40, 41] The evoked eye movements in this syndrome align with the plane of the affected superior canal.(Figure 6–8).[42] Patients with superior canal dehiscence may also have eye movements induced by bone conducted vibrations. Otitic syphilis, Ménière's disease, and perilymph fistula have also been reported to cause these signs, although the specific features of their evoked eye movements have not been well characterized.

Hyperventilation may induce symptoms in patients with anxiety or phobic disorders but does not usually produce nystagmus. Patients with demyelinating lesions of the vestibular nerve (such as that caused by a vestibular schwannoma), or compression by a small blood vessel, or central lesions such as those related to multiple sclerosis may show hyperventilation-induced nystagmus.[43] Hyperventilation reduces pCO_2, which leads to an increase in serum and cerebrospinal fluid (CSF) pH. This relative alkalosis increases the binding of extracellular calcium to albumin and leads to an increase in the discharge rate and conduction in partially demyelinated axons.

Bedside Examination of Posture and Gait

Vestibulospinal reflexes maintain posture with respect to gravity and assist vestibulo-ocular reflexes by producing contraction of neck muscles that compensate for externally applied motion to the neck or body. Disorders of vestibulospinal reflexes can result in tilt of the head, abnormal posture, or ataxia. Other causes of similar symptoms may be dysfunctional proprioceptive inputs, visual inputs, or the inability to combine multiple sensory cues accurately. Static imbalance in vestibulospinal reflexes may be identified from a Romberg test, tandem walking, stepping tests, and evaluation of pastpointing. Romberg's test is used to assess sway with feet together and tandem, with eyes both open and closed. Falls during tandem walking or a positive Fukuda stepping test (turning while marching in place for 30 sec with eyes closed) are signs of vestibulospinal asymmetry due to vestibular lesions.[44] Pastpointing of the arms to previously seen targets with eyes closed may also be a sign of vestibulospinal imbalance. Dynamic vestibulospinal function is assessed by observing postural stability during rapid turns or in response to external perturbations imposed by the examiner (ie, a gentle shove forward, backward, or to the side).

Patients with vestibular dysfunction may rely largely on proprioceptive feedback for maintaining balance. Patients with this compensatory strategy often suffer from significantly increased sway when performing a Romberg test on a block of foam to reduce proprioceptive input from the feet and ankles. Patients with a compensatory strategy that depends on visual inputs may be unable to walk steadily with their eyes closed. The ability to combine multisensory cues can be tested at the bedside as part of the "Clinical Test of Sensory Integration and Balance," where both visual and proprioceptive cues are modified simultaneously similar to platform posturography.[45]

LABORATORY TESTES OF VESTIBULAR FUNCTION

Quantitative tests of physiologic processes under vestibular control can be an important adjunct to the history and clinical examination, but diagnoses are rarely made solely on their results. Laboratory tests are best used selectively to evaluate a patient suspected of particular conditions rather than applied to all patients. Many laboratory tests of vestibular function use electronystagmography (ENG) to record eye movements during various vestibular and oculomotor tests. The quantitative information from ENG enables the clinician to monitor progression of or recovery from disorders affecting vestibulo-ocular control. Three techniques can be used for recording eye movements: electro-oculography (EOG), infrared video image analysis, and magnetic search coil techniques.

Electro-oculography techniques are based on the corneoretinal potential (difference in electrical charge potential between the cornea and the retina). Movement of the eye relative to surface electrodes on the face produces an electrical signal corresponding to eye position. Horizontal eye movements can typically be resolved to an accuracy of 0.5 degrees, which is not as great as the sensitivity of direct visual inspection by a trained examiner (approximately 0.1 degrees). Examination of small-amplitude eye movements either directly or with the aid of Frenzel lenses or an ophthalmoscope is therefore important for identification of low-amplitude nystagmus. Torsional eye movements cannot be measured with EOG. Recently developed video imaging techniques are used instead of EOG in many clinical laboratories. In principle, infrared video recordings allow eye movements to be recorded in three dimensions and with an accuracy that is comparable to or greater than that achieved with EOG. Although algorithms and procedures are improving, there are still some patients for whom image fitting and analysis do not work properly.

The gold standard measurement of eye movements is the magnetic search coil technique.[46] This is based on the principle that changes in voltage are induced in a conductor moving relative to a magnetic field (Faraday's law). In humans, a minute wire is imbedded in a Silastic annulus that is inserted surrounding, but not actually touching, the cornea. Eye movements in three dimensions can be resolved to an accuracy of about 0.02 degrees. The main disadvantages of search coil recordings for general clinical use is the level of expertise required to set up the apparatus, conduct the recording sessions, and analyze the data. It can also be irritating to the eye and poses a hazard of corneal abrasion and is used only in specialized research laboratories.

Assessment of Spontaneous Nystagmus and Oculomotor Function

Eye movements are recorded with eyes closed and with eyes opened and while viewing a stationary visual target. Spontaneous nystagmus and the effects of visual fixation on this nystagmus are noted. The patient then looks to the left, right, up, and down so that a positional nystagmus can be detected.

Saccades are assessed by instructing the patient to fixate (eyes moving while keeping the head stationary) on a series of randomly displayed dots or lights at eccentricities of 5 to 30 degrees. The latency, velocity, and accuracy of saccades are analyzed. Defects in saccades may consist of prolonged latencies, abnormal velocities, and over- or under-shooting the target. These defects may be caused by muscular pathology such as myesthenia gravis, oculomotor paresis, multiple sclerosis, Huntington's disease, pathology in the brainstem or cerebellar vermis, or attentional lesions in the cerebellar hemispheres. Smooth pursuit eye movements are recorded while the patient is tracking a target that moves horizontally with a sinusoidal waveform at a low frequency (0.2–0.7 Hz) with a position amplitude of 20 degrees in each direction. Problems with smooth pursuit indicate a cerebellar pathology. Optokinetic testing is generally performed with the subject surrounded by a visual scene that moves in one direction at velocities of 30 to 60 degrees/sec. The optokinetic response is a nystagmus in the plane of motion of the visual scene. The slow-phase abnormalities on optokinetic tests parallel those detected with smooth pursuit testing, whereas abnormalities of the fast components of optokinetic nystagmus are correlated with those detected on saccade testing.

Caloric Testing

Evaluation of nystagmus induced by warm or cold water irrigation of the external canals has been used to measure vestibular function since the beginning of the twentieth century.[47] This test allows one labyrinth to be studied independently of the other. The stimuli can be applied relatively easily with techniques that are commonly available.

Bárány proposed that caloric nystagmus was the result of a convective movement of endolymph in the horizontal semicircular canal.[47] The convective flow mechanism is based on warm (44°C) or cold (30°C) water (or air) in the external auditory canal, creating a temperature gradient from one side of the horizontal canal to the other. This temperature gradient results in a density difference within the endolymph of the canal. When the horizontal canal is oriented in the plane of gravity (by elevating the head 30 degrees from the supine position or 60 degrees backward from the upright position), there is a flow of endolymph from the region with more dense fluid to the region with less dense fluid. This convective flow of endolymph leads to a deflection of the cupula and a change in the discharge rate of vestibular nerve afferents (Figure 6–11).

Endolymph will flow toward the ampulla of the horizontal canal (resulting in an increase in afferent discharge rate) for warm irrigations and away from the ampulla (resulting in a decrease in afferent discharge rate) for cold irrigations. This simple theory accounts for the dependence of the nystagmus direction on temperature and orientation of the head relative to gravity. Warm irrigations provoke a nystagmus with a slow phase away from the irrigated ear and a fast phase toward the irrigated ear, while nystagmus following irrigation with cold water is oriented in the opposite direction. Two lines of evidence support the existence of an additional, nonconvective component to the caloric response. First, caloric nystagmus can be elicited in the microgravity environment of orbital spaceflight under conditions in which there is no convection.[48] Second, caloric

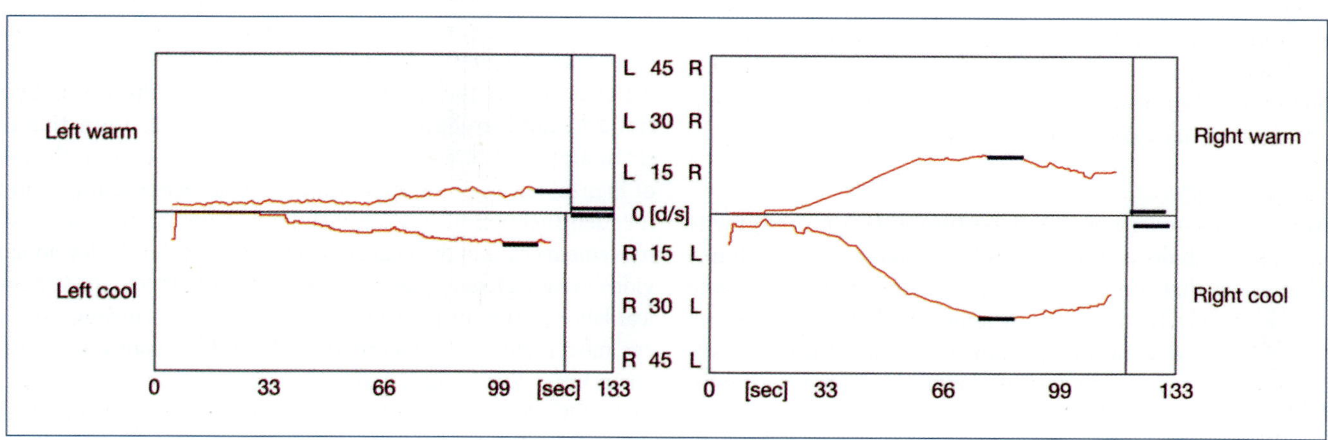

FIGURE 6–11• Caloric stimulation. Tracings represent slow-phase eye velocity following irrigation of a 49 year old female patient presenting with dizziness. Approximately 1 min is required to heat the inner ear enough to reach maximal stimulation. Both warm and cool responses on left are reduced. Jongkee's formulas reveal a 49% left weakness and a 17% left directional preponderance, with a total eye speed of 61 deg/sec. MRI suggested a meningioma in the cerebellopontine angle.

nystagmus can be elicited in animals whose canals are plugged, although the response is reduced to 30% of that obtained before plugging.[49] A direct effect of temperature on vestibular hair cells and/or afferent nerve fibers is the most likely source of the nonconvective component.

The conventional Fitzgerald-Hallpike technique for caloric stimuli consists of a single temperature irrigation for 60 to 90 sec.[50] Such stimuli result in a change in temperature in the temporal bone that lasts for 10 to 20 min. This prolonged warming or cooling of the temporal bone following a single-temperature irrigation makes it necessary to allow at least 10 minutes between successive irrigations. Biphasic caloric irrigations can be used to achieve roughly the same levels of eye velocity as noted with a single-temperature irrigation while substantially reducing the duration of the change in the temperature of the temporal bone.[51]

Responses to caloric tests are analyzed by calculating the velocity of each of the slow-phase components of the nystagmus. The maximum response for each irrigation is then determined based on the three to five slow-phase components with the highest velocity. Data are interpreted in terms of unilateral weakness (UW) and directional preponderance (DP) according to formulae described by Jongkees and colleagues, where R and L indicate right and left and W and C indicate warm and cold irrigations; values are velocity of slow-phase responses in degrees per second:[52]

$$\text{Unilateral weakness} = \frac{(RW + RC) - (LW + LC)}{(RW + RC + LW + LC)} \times 100\%$$

$$\text{Directional preponderance} = \frac{(RW + LC) - (LW + RC)}{(RW + LC + LW + RC)} \times 100\%$$

Normative values are established for each laboratory, with a UW greater than 20% and a DP of greater than 25% usually considered significant. Unilateral weakness is a sign of decreased responsiveness of the horizontal canal or the ampullary nerve that provides its innervation. In patients with reduced caloric responses, ice water may be used to elicit a response. This is a particularly provocative stimulus, however, and may cause nausea or vomiting in subjects with preserved function. Directional preponderance is commonly seen in patients with spontaneous nystagmus. Patients with minimal caloric responses may truly have bilaterally reduced vestibular function, but other possibilities such as cerumen impaction and variations in technique must also be considered. Caloric responses may also be affected by blink artifacts or blepharospasm. Rotational chair testing is advised for patients with bilaterally diminished calorics.

Rotatory Tests

Head rotation is the "natural" stimulus for the AVOR. Passive, whole-body rotations can be used to deliver consistent, reproducible rotational stimuli while eye movements are recorded. Standard clinical tests typically involve low-frequency sinusoidal rotations or rapid angular accelerations or decelerations ("steps" of head velocity) about an earth-vertical axis. Rotatory testing is particularly important in several situations. It can define the extent of disease in a patient with bilaterally reduced calorics. It can increase the sensitivity of caloric testing by identifying abnormalities in the vestibulo-ocular system of patients with imbalance but without abnormal caloric exams. Alternatively, caloric examination can sometimes pick up pathology that rotational chair misses, although this is sometimes a false-positive finding due to problems with head conduction as a result of the obstruction of the external ear or poor testing technique.

Rotational chair testing takes place in a darkened room. The head is held stationary on the body to prevent proprioceptive feedback from cervical receptors. The chair is moved sinusoidally at low frequencies, typically 0.01 Hz, up to higher frequencies, usually about 1 Hz as the eye velocity is recorded (Figure 6–12). Multiple cycles of each frequency are used. The results allow the gain, or sensitivity, of the vestibulo-ocular reflex to be quantified (in degrees/s of eye movement divided by degrees/s of head movement). The normal gain is approximately 0.4 at lower frequencies and rises to 0.6 at higher frequencies. Abnormally low gain may be due to unilateral or bilateral vestibular dysfunction but, especially when calorics are normal, may be due to the patient's loss of alertness. A patient's gain may be higher when turning in one direction than when turning in the other direction. The difference in gains is termed directional asymmetry. Directional asymmetry may reflect a weakness of one labyrinth (with a reduced gain when turning toward the dysfunctional side) or an asymmetric lesion in the central vestibular pathways. In cases of unilateral vestibular hypofunction, the stimulus velocity has to reach a peak velocity of 150 to 300 degrees/s to observe an asymmetry between responses for rotations toward in comparison with those away from the side of the lesion.[53]

Although the velocity profiles of the slow phases of the nystagmus follow the sinusoidal movements of the head, they do not correspond exactly in time. This phase shift between the head rotation and the eye response is due in part to the velocity storage mechanism. It is measured in degrees, with a perfectly compensatory AVOR (where the eyes move in perfect opposition to head movement) having a phase shift by convention of 0 degrees. If the eyes reach their maximum velocity slightly before the head does, the reflex shows a phase lead, typically of about 30 degrees at lower frequencies in normal subjects. This phase lead is related to the velocity storage mechanism. Patients with loss of vestibular function have a reduced time constant of the velocity storage mechanism, leading to an abnormally high phase lead at low frequencies.[54]

Another way to measure the gain and time constant of the vestibular system is to perform steps of velocity in the rotational chair (Figure 6–13). In these tests, the patient is accelerated to a steady speed, often of 60 degrees/s. After rotating long enough to have the sensation of rotation fade away (as the velocity storage system discharges), the chair is abruptly stopped and the patient has a sudden feeling of rotation (in the direction of the force used to decelerate the chair, opposite its original direction of rotation). The gain of the system is measured by the slow-phase eye velocity immediately after the chair stops and the time constant is measured by the time it takes for the eye velocity to drop to 37% of its initial value.

The AVOR can also be evaluated from eye movement responses to head-on-body rotations that are actively generated by the patient.[55] Recent evidence suggests that repetitive,

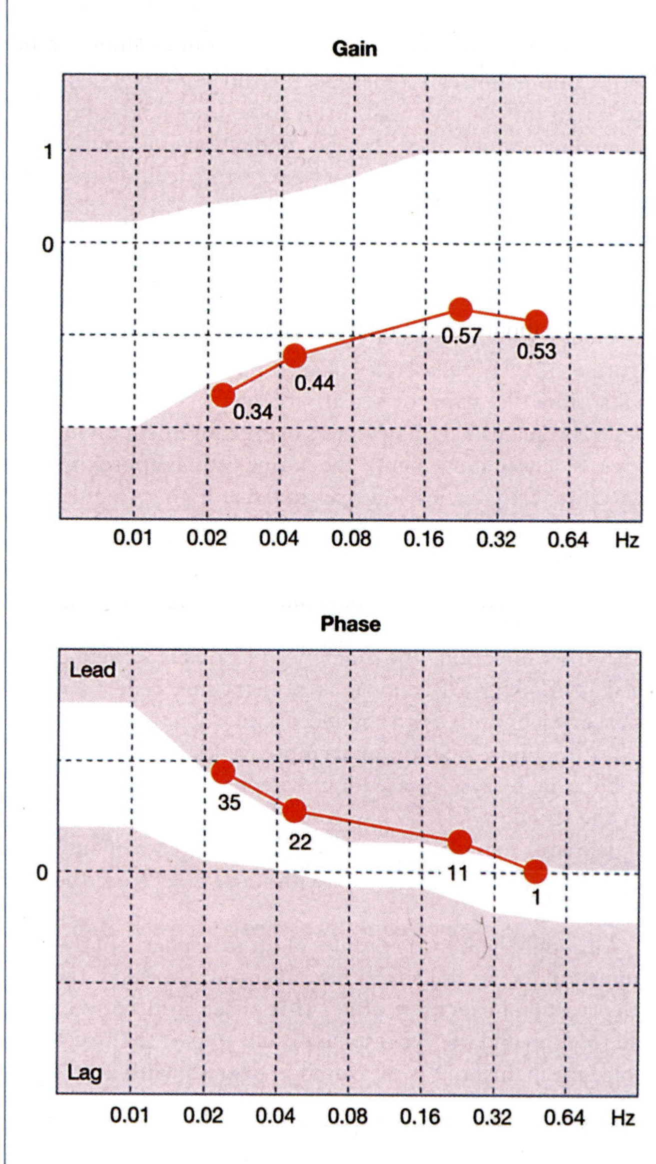

FIGURE 6–12 • Sinusoidal rotational velocity. Bilaterally deficient patient has decreased gain (falling below white band) and increased phase lead (falling above white band) at lower frequencies (0.01–0.04 Hz).

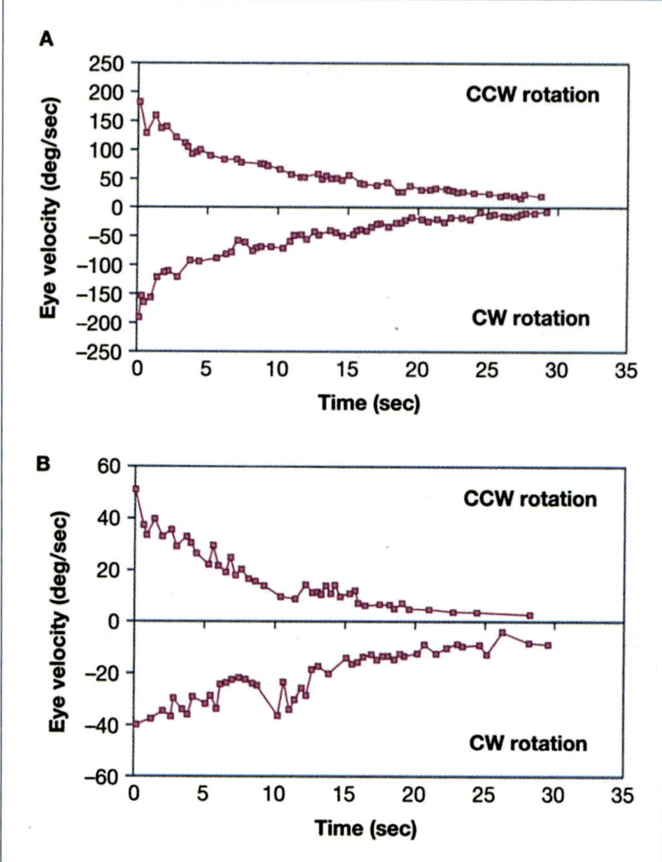

FIGURE 6–13 • Step of rotational velocity. Chair turning at 100 deg/s undergoes an abrupt stop. Normal responses shown in top panel, with a gain of 0.75 (measured as deg/s of eye velocity divided by deg/s of head velocity at the time the chair is stopped) and a time constant of 21 sec. Bilaterally deficient patient shown below, with gain of 0.4 and a time constant of 7 sec.

predictive rotational stimuli may lead to eye movement responses that arise from extralabyrinthine mechanisms (such as prediction or signals from neck proprioception).[56] Thus, the sensitivity of these tests in the identification of vestibular hypofunction may be lower than for those tests that use passive, unpredictable stimuli.

Posturography

Techniques for assessment of postural control in patients have developed in an attempt to provide quantitative measurements of processes that maintain upright stance under static and dynamic conditions.[57] These tests have conceptual appeal because they evaluate the major sensory systems (vestibular, visual, and somatosensory) that are important for maintaining balance.

The postural tests used most commonly include assessment of postural responses to platform movements and determination of effects of manipulations of visual and somatosensory information on balance while standing. The most commonly used posturography paradigm is termed the sensory organization test (SOT). This test includes six conditions selectively depriving the subject of modalities contributing to balance. The subject's balance is disrupted by blindfolding; allowing the platform to move "sway-referenced" along with the patient's center of gravity, reducing proprioceptive feedback; or moving the visual surround to remain fixed with respect to the patient as the center of gravity sways (sway-referenced vision). This last condition provides a conflicting stimulus, where vision indicates that no movement is occurring but vestibular and proprioceptive receptors indicating that it has (Figure 6–14).

The "equilibrium score" measures the patient's passive sway when standing upright in each of the six conditions. An "equilibrium score" of 100% indicates no sway and 0% indicates sway up to the theoretical limits of stability before falling. Normal equilibrium scores drop with increasing age. Patients who perform poorly on the "eyes closed, stable surface" condition may have loss of proprioceptive function; those who perform poorly on the "eyes open, sway-referenced surface" may have loss of

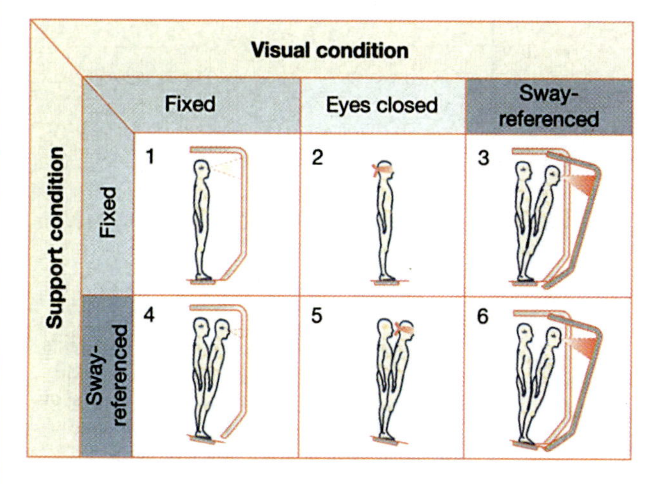

FIGURE 6–14 • Sensory organization test (SOT). Conditions 1–3 are on a stable surface; conditions 4–6 are sway-referenced. Conditions 1 and 4 are with a stable visual background, 2 and 5 are with no visual feedback, and 3 and 6 are with conflicting (sway-referenced) visual feedback.

visual contribution to balance; those who perform poorly on the "eyes closed, sway-referenced surface" may have vestibular problems, and those who perform better with their eyes closed than during "sway-referenced vision" conditions may have difficulty handling conflicting visual stimuli.

The SOT can also quantify the degree to which a subject relies on ankle motion versus hip motion to move the center of gravity to maintain balance. In normal subjects, small alignments are made by ankle movements and larger-amplitude alignments are made by hip movements. The degree to which a subject relies on each strategy is correlated with the shear force on the feet measured by the footplate. Hip dependence may occur with peripheral neuropathies that prevent the ankle joint from providing enough feedback to maintain balance. There are specifically defined clinical situations in which computerized postural assessment can have an effect on treatment outcome:[58] (1) planning a course of vestibular rehabilitation and monitoring response to this rehabilitation program in patients with vestibular hypofunction, central nervous system disorders that affect balance, or processes that require a procedure to ablate vestibular function in one ear; (2) determination of the need for procedures that remove CSF (eg, high-volume CSF drainage with lumbar punctures or a shunt) in patients with disequilibrium or gait disturbances caused by processes that result in abnormal CSF pressure dynamics; and (3) documentation of postural responses when there is suspected malingering, exaggeration of disability for compensation, or conversion disorder. Platform posturography may also be useful in evaluating a patient for proprioceptive loss and may allow cerebellar degeneration to be detected.

Evaluation of Otolith Function

Subjective Visual Vertical

The perception of the orientation of a laser-projected bar of light relative to the earth-vertical or earth-horizontal planes when subjects are in an otherwise dark room is dependent on vestibular function. The alignment of the subjective visual vertical and subjective visual horizontal has been shown to be tilted toward the lesioned side in cases of unilateral vestibular hypofunction.[59] In acute peripheral vestibular lesions, the tilt of the perception of verticality often initially measures 7 to 12 degrees. In cases of long-standing unilateral vestibular loss, the subjective visual vertical either returns to normal or remains tilted only by 2 to 3 degrees toward the side of the lesion.[60]

A modification of the test for subjective visual vertical allows the function of each ear to be tested independently. The patient is positioned in the rotational chair so that one labyrinth is on the axis of rotation and the other is slightly off-axis. In this position, centripetal force will activate the off-axis labyrinth but not the on-axis labyrinth. When the pathologic ear is off-axis, no change in the subjective vertical is elicited by rotation .[61]

Vestibular-Evoked Myogenic Potential Responses

Vestibular-evoked myogenic potential (VEMP) responses are short-latency responses measured from tonically contracting sternocleidomastoid muscles that relax in response to ipsilateral presentation of loud clicks (Figure 6–15).[62,63] These responses are thought to be of vestibular origin because they disappear after vestibular neurectomy and are still present in patients with absent hearing but intact vestibular function.[64,65] The inferior vestibular nerve has been implicated in the responses because all patients who developed posterior canal BPPV after vestibular neuritis had intact VEMP responses, whereas VEMP responses were absent in most patients after vestibular neuritis who did not develop similar symptoms of posterior canal BPPV.[66] Further work has indicated that VEMP responses probably originate in the sacculus. Vestibular-evoked myogenic potential responses can also be elicited from periocular sites, presumably related to electrical activity in the extraocular musclature in response to sound. These "oVEMP" responses have been shown to change their responsiveness in the case of superior canal dehiscence.[67] The threshold for eliciting a VEMP response is reduced in patients with superior canal dehiscence.[68] VEMP responses may be changed in patients with Ménière's disease.[69]

Audiometric Testing

Audiograms can be useful in diagnosing several causes of dizziness. Semicircular canal dehiscence often manifests with a supranormal bone-conduction line, particularly at low frequencies, with an air–bone gap.[70] Stapedial reflexes are normal. Similar findings are sometimes described in patients with enlarged vestibular aqueduct, who may become profoundly imbalanced following head trauma.[71] Patients with otosclerosis usually have conductive hearing loss with absent stapedial reflexes. Sensorineural loss is often found in patients with vestibular schwannoma. Hearing loss associated with Ménière's disease is typically low-frequency and typically varies over time. This finding can help distinguish Ménière's disease from vestibular migraine, conditions which often manifest with similar symptoms but whose treatments are generally distinct. However, migraine may also be related to hearing loss.[72] In later stages of the disease, the level of hearing loss tends to remain stable. Perilymphatic fistulas can also manifest with varying levels of hearing loss.

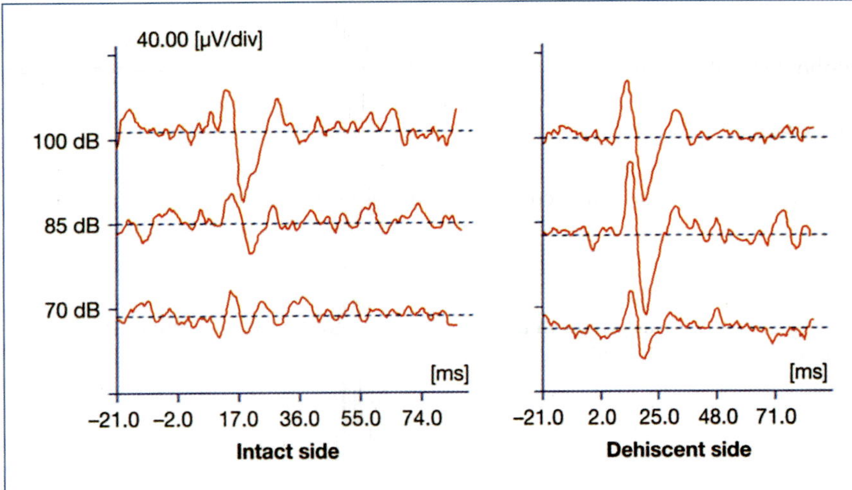

FIGURE 6–15 • Vestibular-evoked myogenic response. Both sides demonstrate a VEMP response to a click at a presentation level of 100 dB SPL. The dehiscent side remains sensitive even at lower amplitudes of stimulation.

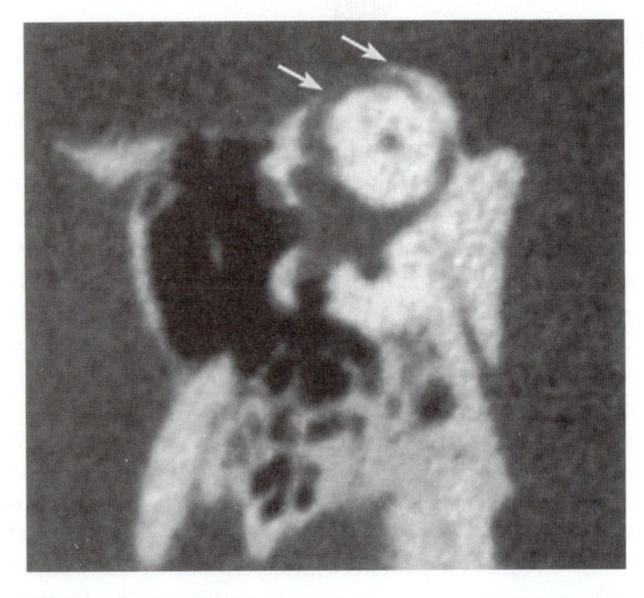

FIGURE 6–16 • Temporal bone CT scan from patient with superior canal dehiscence syndrome. Patient's responses shown in Figure 4–9. Projection of the CT image of the right temporal bone into the plane of the superior canal. A dehiscence measuring 3.7 mm in length is noted overlying the superior canal (arrows). *Reproduced with permission from Minor LB, Cremer PD, Carey JP, and colleagues. Symptoms and signs in superior canal dehiscence syndrome. Ann NY Acad Sci 2001;942: 259–273.*

Electrocochleography is an audiometric test that is sometimes used for diagnosing Ménière's disease. However, Ménière's is diagnosed based on clinical criteria, which are not closely matched by results of electrocochleography so its utility in identifying patients with Ménière's is limited.[73]

Radiologic and Serologic Tests

Computerized tomography is commonly used to evaluate patients with sound- or pressure-induced nystagmus. Dehiscence of the superior or posterior canals into the intracranial space as well as dehiscences of the horizontal canal into the middle ear (such as caused by cholesteatoma) may be visualized (Figure 6–16). Congenital dysplasia of the semicircular canals, enlarged vestibular aqueduct, and temporal bone fractures are also visualizable on CT scan.

MRI can be used to visualize tumors of the internal auditory canal, cerebellopontine angle, and brain. It can also indicate other central pathologies underlying symptoms of dizziness such as cerebellar degeneration, stroke, or multiple sclerosis. It may also indicate pathology of the temporal bone such as labyrinthine dysmorphisms and enlarged vestibular aqueduct or of the posterior fossa such as Arnold–Chiari malformation.

Serologic tests are of limited use for diagnosing patients with imbalance. Two notable exceptions are syphilis and Cogan's syndrome. In patients with episodic imbalance consistent with endolymphatic hydrops, or with a high likelihood of sexually transmitted disease, syphilis testing is appropriate.[74] In patients with abrupt onset of ocular symptoms with imbalance, testing for inflammatory markers of Cogan's syndrome is imperative as prompt initiation of treatment can be critical in controlling potentially life-threatening complications.[75]

DISORDERS AFFECTING VESTIBULAR FUNCTION

In this section, we review some of the more common vestibular disorders with an emphasis on their pathophysiology. This brief overview of labyrinthine abnormalities can be supplemented by other sources that address these and other peripheral and central vestibular disturbances in greater detail.

Benign Paroxysmal Positional Vertigo

Benign paroxysmal positional vertigo is the most common cause of vertigo arising from labyrinthine dysfunction.[76] It is characterized by rotatory vertigo brought on when the head is rolled to the side, as when turning over in bed, and backward with a sideways tilt, as when getting out of bed or walking up stairs. In order of frequency, known causes of BPPV include head trauma, middle ear infection, viral labyrinthitis, ear surgery, or bed rest. Half of occurrences have no clear precipitating event. BPPV occurs in children and in adults, although the incidence increases with age. Among those cases without a clear cause, the average age of onset was in the sixth decade, with females outnumbering males two to one.[77] Signs of BPPV may be present in up to 10% of the elderly, including those without specific complaints of imbalance.

Vertigo typically begins after a latent period—up to 20 sec after positioning the head—and continues for less than a minute before subsiding. It is provoked by the Dix-Hallpike maneuver, in which a patient is moved rapidly from a sitting to a supine position, head turned sharply to the side and shoulders hanging off the end of the examination table. Symptoms lessen if the head is repeatedly placed in the offending position. Knowledge of the anatomy and physiology of the labyrinth has allowed practitioners to develop a working theory for the cause of these symptoms and effective maneuvers to reverse them. Indeed, this sometimes crippling disease can often be completely cured in a single office visit.

In his original description of BPPV, Bárány[78] noted that if a patient's eyes were directed away from the affected ear, they tended to move with a vertical nystagmus (beating upward), whereas if they looked toward the affected ear, they moved with a torsional nystagmus (beating with the superior poles of the eyes directed toward the downward ear). These eye movements are identical to those expected from a stimulation of the posterior semicircular canal, leading this canal to be considered the source of pathology although it can affect the horizontal and superior canals as well.[79]

The actual mechanism of stimulation of the posterior semicircular canal has been confirmed with the observation of free-floating debris in the canal during surgery on a patient with BPPV, an occurrence that is now termed canalithiasis.[80] With the head tilted and hanging over the side of the table, free-floating debris in the posterior canal falls away from the cupula, drawing it away from the ampulla as the debris sinks.[81] The brain interprets that this deflection is caused by rotation of the head around the axis of the canal and creates a compensatory motion of the eyes—motion that is seen as nystagmus when a patient with BPPV is placed in the Dix-Hallpike position.

In addition to explaining the direction of nystagmus in BPPV, canalolithiasis also explains its time course: the sludgy debris in the posterior canal takes some time to begin sliding down the wall of the membranous canal after the head assumes a new position and requires about 1 min before coming to rest at the most dependent part of the canal and terminates the episode of vertigo. Repeated motion of the debris may allow some of it to escape through the open end of the canal, causing the signs and symptoms of posterior canal BPPV to wane with serial testing; this process may also explain the resolution of BPPV in some patients.

Current therapy for BPPV involves repositioning maneuvers that, in cases of canalolithiasis, use gravity to move canalith debris out of the affected semicircular canal and into the vestibule. For posterior canal BPPV, the maneuver developed by Epley[82] and later modified[83] is particularly effective. The maneuver begins with placement of the head into the Dix-Hallpike position that evokes vertigo. The posterior canal on the affected side is in the earth-vertical plane with the head in this position. After the initial nystagmus goes away, there is a 180-degree roll of the head (in two 90-degree increments, stopping in each position until any nystagmus resolves) to the position in which the offending ear is up (ie, the nose is pointed at a 45-degree angle toward the ground in this position). The patient is then brought to the sitting upright position (Figure 6–17). The maneuver is likely to be successful when nystagmus of the same direction continues to be elicited in each of the new positions (as the debris continues to move away from the cupula). The maneuver is repeated until no nystagmus is elicited. This treatment is typically effective in up to 90% of cases in eliminating BPPV.[84] The Semont maneuver moves the otoconial debris through the labyrinth in a manner similar to the Epley maneuver with similar efficacy.[85]

A horizontal canal variant of BPPV has also been identified.[86] The nystagmus typically has a longer duration than that noted with posterior canal BPPV. The direction may beat toward (geotropic) or away from (ageotropic) the downward ear. In cases that involve geotropic nystagmus, lying on one side with the affected ear up for about 12 h eliminates the disorder in most cases. Debris embedded in the cupula or in the canal relatively close to the ampulla may cause ageotropic nystagmus. A repositioning maneuver consisting of a "log roll" of the supine patient may sometimes be effective.[87] A superior canal variant of BPPV has also been described. It is very rare and difficult to treat successfully. Treatment with repositioning maneuvers for BPPV of any canal may direct otoconial debris into previously unaffected canals, necessitating a change in appropriate maneuvers.

Vestibular Migraine

Vestibular migraine is an increasingly recognized cause of episodic imbalance. Up to 25% of patients with migraine headaches have vertigo.[88] Vertigo may occur as an aura related to a migraine headache or may occur in isolation. Symptoms are typically brought on by strong visual or vestibular stimuli but may be provoked by other factors such as changes in the weather, menses,[89] or, quite commonly, particular foods, especially those containing caffeine. Symptoms typically last hours to days, which helps distinguish it from Ménière's disease whose symptoms generally resolve after a few hours.

Twenty-one percent of patients with vestibular migraine have reduced responses on vestibular testing.[90] Hearing loss may occur in patients with vestibular migraine.[91] It may occur in conjunction with BPPV[92] or in patients with symptoms of Ménière's.[93] Patients previously diagnosed with other conditions, in particular Ménière's disease, may in fact best be understood to have a migraine-related process. Children with paroxysmal vertigo of childhood, which typically occurs in patients 4 to 8 years old, may develop more typical symptoms of migraine as they age.[94,95] A positive family history is common in patients with migraine-like symptoms. Many patients who are now understood to have vestibular migraine carry a previous diagnosis of Ménière's disease.

Semicircular Canal Dehiscence Syndrome

A syndrome of vertigo and oscillopsia induced by loud noises or by stimuli that change middle ear or intracranial pressure has recently been defined in patients with a dehiscence of bone

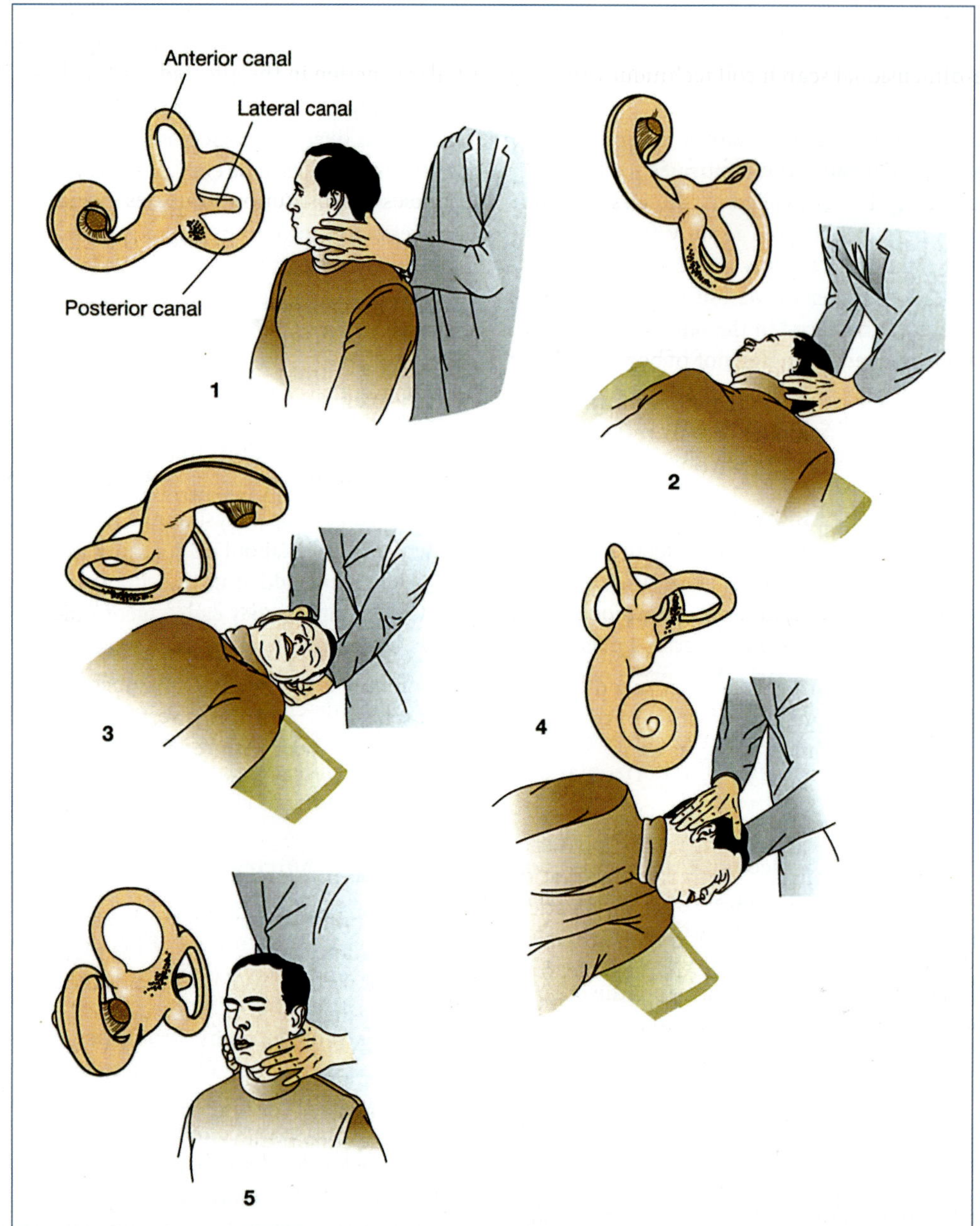

FIGURE 6–17 • Canalith repositioning maneuver for treatment of benign paroxysmal positional vertigo (BPPV) affecting the posterior canal. Panel 1 shows a patient with right posterior canal BPPV. The patient's head is turned to the right at the beginning of the canalith repositioning maneuver. The inset shows the location of the debris near the ampulla of the posterior canal. The diagram of the head in each inset shows the orientation from which the labyrinth is viewed. In panel 2, the patient is brought into the supine position with the head extended below the level of the bed. The debris falls toward the common crus as the head is moved backward. In panel 3, the head is moved approximately 180 degrees to the left while keeping the neck extended with the head below the level of the gurney. Debris enters the common crus as the head is turned toward the contralateral side. In panel 4, the patient's head is further rotated to the left by rolling onto the left side until the patient's head faces down. Debris begins to enter the vestibule. In panel 5, the patient is brought back to the upright position. Debris collects in the vestibule. *Illustration by David Rini.*

overlying the superior semicircular canal.[40,41] These patients may also experience chronic disequilibrium. The dehiscence creates a third mobile window into the inner ear, thereby allowing the superior canal to respond to sound and pressure stimuli. The evoked eye movements in this syndrome align with the affected superior canal (Ewald's first law).[42] Loud sounds, positive pressure in the external auditory canal, and Valsalva's maneuver against pinched nostrils stimulate the canal and produce a nystagmus that has slow-phase components that are directed upward with torsional motion of the superior pole of the eye away from the affected ear. Conversely, negative pressure in the external canal, Valsalva's maneuver against a closed glottis, and jugular venous compression can cause oppositely directed eye movements (slow-phase components directed downward with torsional motion of the superior pole of the eye toward the affected ear). These eye movement findings have been documented with three-dimensional search coil techniques and can be readily observed on clinical examination. Frenzel lenses should be used for this examination because visual fixation can lead to suppression of the evoked eye movements.

Patients with superior canal dehiscence syndrome have abnormally low thresholds for VEMP responses in the affected ear.[68] Patients often have supranormal bone line and a low-frequency conductive hearing loss with intact stapedial reflexes.[70,96] Temporal bone CT scans in patients with superior canal dehiscence syndrome reveal an absence of bone overlying the affected canal. It is important to remember, however, that a thin but intact layer of bone can appear as a dehiscence on a CT scan because of partial volume averaging. The specificity of temporal bone CT in the diagnosis of superior canal dehiscence syndrome can be improved with the use of reconstructed slice thickness of 0.5 mm or less and projection of images into the plane of the superior canal (Figure 6–11). The diagnosis of this syndrome depends on clinical symptoms and radiographic evidence of dehiscence. Similar symptoms may also be elicited in patients with a dehiscence in the posterior or horizontal canal.

Vestibular Neuritis

Vertigo associated with vestibular neuritis begins suddenly, may last for days with gradual resolution, and is frequently incapacitating early in its course. In support of an infectious etiology is the occurrence of cases around the same time within households or in association with upper respiratory infections. A vascular etiology has been suspected because the condition often spares the inferior division of the vestibular nerve, which is supplied by the posterior vestibular artery while the superior division of the vestibular nerve is supplied by the anterior vestibular artery.

Signs of unilateral vestibular hypofunction are readily apparent early in the course of the illness. These signs include a spontaneous nystagmus with horizontal and torsional slow components that are directed toward the ear with hypofunction and fast components directed oppositely. The horizontal eye velocity of this nystagmus frequently increases in amplitude when patients look in the direction of the fast component. It can be suppressed by looking at a stationary object, whereas the torsional eye velocity (rotation about the line of sight) of the nystagmus is not affected by this maneuver.

The vertigo and nystagmus in such a lesion of the cerebellum can be similar to that observed in vestibular neuritis.[97] It is important that these be distinguished, as a stroke involving the inferior cerebellum can lead to swelling, brain stem compression, and death unless there is prompt neurosurgical intervention. One key distinguishing feature is the degree of postural instability. Patients with cerebellar hemorrhage or infarction are typically unable to walk and are very unstable when standing. Patients with vestibular neuritis, in contrast, are likely to have an unsteady gait, but they can walk. Appropriate imaging such as a magnetic resonance imaging scan of the brain and posterior fossa should be obtained when there is suspicion that the symptoms may arise from an abnormality affecting the cerebellum or brain stem.

Recovery of balance reflexes following vestibular neuritis occurs through three mechanisms: spontaneous return of vestibular function in the affected ear (in about 50% of cases), vestibular adaptation, and substitution of other sensory or motor strategies. Vestibular adaptation involves recalibration of motor responses to diminished signals from a labyrinth. Some examples of substitution strategies include rapid eye movements in response to head movements toward the lesioned labyrinth and use of visual and proprioceptive information to maintain postural stability after loss of vestibular function.

Chemical Vestibulopathy

Vestibular neuritis leads to signs of an unequal level of activity between the two labyrinths, vestibular hypofunction resulting from chemical toxicity (often an aminoglycoside such as gentamicin administered intravenously) is commonly bilateral and symmetric.[98] Vestibulotoxicity is often noted without accompanying injury to the auditory system and can occur even when serum peak and trough levels are within appropriate ranges.[99] Patients typically do not experience vertigo, although oscillopsia with head movements and disequilibrium are commonly noted.

Ménière's Disease

Ménière's disease is characterized by episodic vertigo, tinnitus, fluctuating sensorineural hearing loss, and aural fullness (a pressure sensation deep within the ear). In contrast to the vertigo in BPPV, which typically lasts for only seconds during a single episode, the vertigo in an attack of Ménière's disease has a duration that varies from 30 min to several hours. It typically affects one ear, although bilateral involvement has been reported in 2 to 78% of cases.[100] Females are more often affected than males, and early middle age is a typical age of onset. An incidence of 15 per 100,000 and a prevalence of 218 per 100,000 have been reported.[101] Ménière's disease typically accounts for about 10% of the visits to clinics specializing in vestibular disorders.[76]

Abnormalities in the production and/or resorption of endolymph are thought to underlie the histopathologic changes that are seen in the cochlea and labyrinth of ears affected with Ménière's disease. Most cases are presumed to be idiopathic, although the clinical syndrome can follow infections affecting the inner ear such as mumps or measles, syphilis, or meningitis. Symptoms may also begin following head trauma. Antibodies to a 68-kDa protein (heat shock protein 70) have been noted in patients with Ménière's disease but the clinical utility of serologic testing for this marker is uncertain.[102]

Endolymphatic hydrops, the classic abnormality noted in Ménière's disease, is characterized by dilatation of the endolymphatic spaces with periodic rupture of the membranes that separate endolymphatic from perilymphatic compartments. Although endolymphatic hydrops is a consistent finding in the temporal bones of patients in whom a diagnosis of Ménière's disease had been made, it is not a specific finding as these pathologic changes have been noted in patients with no premorbid symptoms or signs suggestive of Ménière's disease.[103]

Attacks of vertigo are frequently the most disabling symptom in Ménière's disease. The vertigo may be rotatory, in which case semicircular canal dysfunction is suspected, or may consist of a precipitous sensation of being pulled toward one side, as might result from a sudden change in otolith activity. The nystagmus during an episode of vertigo may be "excitatory" with respect to the involved labyrinth (with slow components directed away from the affected ear), although clinical examination between episodes of vertigo may reveal signs of vestibular hypofunction. The hearing loss in Ménière's disease is commonly more severe for the low frequencies.

Low-salt diets and diuretics control episodes of vertigo in most patients. Intratympanic or oral steroids have also been shown to be useful.[104] Opening the endolymphatic sac on the affected side is used by some practitioners, although its effectiveness is in doubt. Refractory cases with unilateral involvement can be managed with procedures that ablate vestibular function in the affected ear. Selective sectioning of the vestibular nerve (when there is useful hearing remaining) and labyrinthectomy (when hearing is absent) have been the procedures of choice. More recent studies have demonstrated that vertigo can be controlled in most patients, with a low risk of hearing loss, by injecting gentamicin into the middle ear.[105] Recent studies have shown that a single intratympanic injection of gentamicin is effective in achieving control of vertigo in most cases.[106] Patients requiring cochlear implantation as a result of hearing loss due to Ménière's have been reported to have fewer attacks of vertigo following surgery.[107]

Vestibular Schwannoma

Vestibular schwannoma may present with imbalance, although typically the slow growth of the tumor allows compensation to occur and symptoms to be minimal. Frank vertigo affects a small percentage of patients, but vague imbalance is much more common. Vestibular schwannomas tend to occur on the superior vestibular nerve. Because this nerve carries fibers from the horizontal canal, standard caloric responses are often abnormal in patients. However, because VEMP responses are due to saccular reflexes carried by the inferior vestibular nerve, they may be preserved. Eye movements typical of posterior fossa mass lesions include Brun's nystagmus and nystagmus with lateral gaze that follows Alexander's law (Figure 6–9).

Vascular Disease

Both central and peripheral symptoms of imbalance may occur in patients with vertebrobasilar insufficiency. Sixty-two percent of patients with vertebrobasilar insufficiency have vertigo and 26% have paresis of the horizontal canal.[108] Transient ischemic attacks involving the posterior circulation may manifest as vertigo lasting for several minutes, with other neurologic symptoms appearing in more severe lesions. Patients with other types of vertigo are usually able to walk despite their symptoms, but those with serious brain stem lesions can be distinguished because they are often too ataxic to ambulate. Like patients with migraine, patients with vascular insufficiency may be more susceptible to BPPV. Several inflammatory conditions may affect the posterior circulation and cause dizziness, including Cogan's syndrome (which typically presents along with visual symptoms) and Susac's syndrome (which includes symptoms of encephalopathy).

References

1. Kroenke K, Arrington ME, Mangelsdorff AD. The prevalence of symptoms in medical outpatients and the adequacy of therapy. Arch Intern Med 1990;150:1685–89.
2. Kroenke K, Mangelsdorff AD. Common symptoms in ambulatory care: Incidence, evaluation, therapy, and outcome. Am J Med 1989;86:262–6.
3. Wersäll J, Bagger-Sjoback D. Morphology of the vestibular sense organ. In:. Vestibular system. part I: Basic mechanisms. Berlin: Springer; 1974. p. 123–70.
4. Precht W. Vestibular mechanisms. Annu Rev Neurosci 1979;2:265–89.
5. Park J, Tang Y, Lopez I, Ishiyama A. Age-related change in the number of neurons in the human vestibular ganglion. J Comp Neurol 2001;431:437–43.
6. Highstein SM, Baker R. Action of the efferent vestibular system on primary afferents in the toadfish. Opsanus tau. J Neurophysiol 1985;54:370–84.
7. Goldberg JM, Fernandez C. Physiology of peripheral neurons innervating semicircular canals of the squirrel monkey I. Resting discharge and response to constant angular accelerations. J Neurophysiol 1971;34:635–60.
8. Baird RA, Desmadryl G, Fernandez C, Goldberg JM. The vestibular nerve of the chinchilla. II. Relation between afferent response properties and peripheral innervation patterns in the semicircular canals. J Neurophysiol 1988;60:182–203.
9. Hullar TE, Della Santina CC, Hirvonen TP, et al. Responses of irregularly discharging chinchilla semicircular canal vestibular-nerve afferents during high-frequency head rotations. J Neurophysiol 2005;93:2777–86.
10. Hullar TE, Lasker DM, Carey JP, Minor LB. Responses of irregular vestibular nerve afferents to high-frequency rotations. J Vestib Res 2002;11:176.
11. Sadeghi SG, Chacron MJ, Taylor MC, Cullen KE. Neural variability, detection thresholds, and information transmission in the vestibular system. J Neurosci 2007;27:771–81.
12. Ewald JR. Physiologische Untersuchungen über das Endorgan des Nervus Octavus. Wiesbaden, Germany: Bergmann; 1892.
13. Tabak S, Collewijn H, Boumans LJJM, Van der Steen J. Gain and delay of human vestibulo-ocular reflexes to oscillation and steps of the head by a reactive torque helmet I. Normal subjects. Acta Otolaryngol 1997;117:785–95.
14. Burr DC, Ross J. Contrast sensitivity at high velocities. Vision Res 1982;22:479–84.
15. Raphan T, Matsuo V, Cohen B. Velocity storage in the vestibulo-ocular reflex arc (VOR). Exp Brain Res 1979;35:229–48.
16. Katz E, Vianney de Jong JMB, Buttner-Ennever JA, Cohen B. Effects of midline section on the velocity storage and the vestibulo-ocular reflex. Exp Brain Res 1991;87:505–29.
17. Arnold DB, Robinson DA. The oculomotor integrator: Testing of a neural network model. Exp Brain Res 1997;113:57–74.
18. Cannon SC, Robinson DA. Loss of the neural integrator of the oculomotor system from brain stem lesions in monkey. J Neurophysiol 1987;57:1383–409.
19. Zee DS, Fletcher WA. Bedside examination. In: Baloh RW, Halmagyi GM, editors. Disorders of the vestibular system. New York: Oxford University Press; 1996. p. 178–90.

20. Halmagyi GM, Cremer PD. Assessment and treatment of dizziness. J Neurol Neurosurg Psychiatry 2000;68:129–34.
21. Lermoyez M. Le vertige qui fait entendre (angiospasme labyrinthique). Presse Medicale 1919;27:1–3.
22. Cha YH, Kane MJ, Baloh RW. Familial clustering of migraine, episodic vertigo, and Ménière's disease. Otol Neurotol 2008;29:93–6.
23. Jen JC, Graves TD, Hess EJ, et al. Primary episodic ataxias: Diagnosis, pathogenesis and treatment. Brain 2007;130: 2484–93.
24. McClure JA, Copp JC, Lycett P. Recovery nystagmus in Ménière's disease. Laryngoscope 1981;91:1727–37.
25. Hotson JR. Convergence-initiated voluntary flutter: A normal intrinsic capability in man. Brain Res 1984;294:299–304.
26. Abel LA, Parker L, Daroff RB, Dell'Osso LF. End-point nystagmus. Invest Ophthalmol Vis Sci 1978;17:539–44.
27. Leigh R, Zee D. The neurology of eye movements. New York: Oxford University Press; 2006.
28. Baloh RW, Jacobson KJ, Honrubia V. Horizontal semicircular canal variant of benign positional vertigo. Neurology 1993;43:2542–49.
29. Katsarkas A. Positional nystagmus of the "central type" as an early sign of multiple sclerosis. J Otolaryngol 1982;11:91–3.
30. McAuley JR, Dickman JD, Mustain W, Anand VK. Positional nystagmus in asymptomatic human subjects. Otolaryngol Head Neck Surg 1996;114:545–53.
31. Fetter M, Haslwanter T, Bork M, Dichgans J. New insights into positional alcohol nystagmus using three-dimensional eye-movement analysis. Ann Neurol 1999;45:216–23.
32. Hain TC, Fetter M, Zee DS. Head-shaking nystagmus in patients with unilateral peripheral vestibular lesions. Am J Otolaryngol 1987;8:36–47.
33. Fetter M, Zee DS, Koenig E, Dichgans J. Head shaking nystagmus during vestibular compensation in humans and rhesus monkeys. Acta Otolaryngol 1990;110:175–81.
34. Halmagyi GM, Curthoys IS, Cremer PD, et al. The human horizontal vestibulo-ocular reflex in response to high-acceleration stimulation before and after unilateral vestibular neurectomy. Exp Brain Res 1990;81:479–90.
35. Tian J, Crane BT, Demer JL. Vestibular catch-up saccades in labyrinthine deficiency. Exp Brain Res 2000;131:448–57.
36. Cremer PD, Halmagyi GM, Aw ST, et al. Semicircular canal plane head impulses detect absent function of individual semicircular canals. Brain 1998;121:699–716.
37. Kasai T, Zee DS. Eye-head coordination in labyrinthine-defective human beings. Brain Res 1978;144:123–41.
38. Tian JR, Shubayev I, Demer JL. Dynamic visual acuity during transient and sinusoidal yaw rotation in normal and unilaterally vestibulopathic humans. Exp Brain Res 2001;137: 12–25.
39. Herdman SJ, Tusa RJ, Blatt P, et al. Computerized dynamic visual acuity test in the assessment of vestibular deficits. Am J Otol 1998;19:790–6.
40. Minor LB, Solomon D, Zinreich JS, Zee DS. Sound- and/or pressure-induced vertigo due to bone dehiscence of the superior semicircular canal. Arch Otolaryngol Head Neck Surg 1998;124:249–58.
41. Minor LB. Superior canal dehiscence syndrome. Am J Otol 2000;21:9–19.
42. Cremer PD, Minor LB, Carey JP, Della Santina CC. Eye movements in patients with superior canal dehiscence syndrome align with the abnormal canal. Neurology 2000;55:1833–41.
43. Minor LB, Haslwanter T, Straumann D, Zee DS. Hyperventilation-induced nystagmus in patients with vestibular schwannoma. Neurology 1999;53:2158–68.
44. Fukuda T. The stepping test: Two phases of the labyrinthine reflex. Acta Otolaryngol 1958;50:95–108.
45. Shumway-Cook A, Horak FB. Assessing the influence of sensory interaction of balance. Suggestion from the field. Phys Ther 1986;66:1548–50.
46. Robinson DA. A method of measuring eye movement using a scleral search coil in a magnetic field. IEEE Trans Biomed Eng 1963;10:137–45.
47. Bárány R. Untersuchungen über den vom Vestibularapparat des Ohres reflektorisch ausgelösten rythmischen Nystagmus und seine Begleiterscheinungen. Mschr Ohrenheilkd 1906;40: 193–297.
48. von Baumgarten R, Benson A, Berthoz A, et al. Effects of rectilinear acceleration and optokinetic and caloric stimulations in space. Science 1984;225:208–12.
49. Paige GD. Caloric responses after horizontal canal inactivation. Acta Otolaryngol 1985;100:321–7.
50. Fitzgerald G, Hallpike CS. Studies in human vestibular function: I. Observations on the directional preponderance ("Nystagmusbereitschaft") of caloric nystagmus resulting from cerebral lesions. Brain 1942;65:115–37.
51. Proctor LR, Dix RC. New approach to caloric stimulation of the vestibular receptor. Ann Otol Rhinol Laryngol 1975;84: 683–94.
52. Jongkees LBW, Maas JPM, Philipszoon AJ. Clinical nystagmography: A detailed study of electronystagmography in 341 patients with vertigo. Pract Otorhinolaryngol 1962;24:65–93.
53. Baloh RW, Jacobson KM, Beykirch K, Honrubia V. Horizontal vestibulo-ocular reflex after acute peripheral lesions. Acta Otolaryngol Suppl 1989;468:323–7.
54. Baloh RW, Honrubia V, Yee RD, Hess K. Changes in the human vestibulo-ocular reflex after loss of peripheral sensitivity. Ann Neurol 1997;16:222–28.
55. Hoffman DL, O'Leary DP, Munjack DJ. Autorotation test abnormalities of the horizontal and vertical vestibulo-ocular reflexes in panic disorder. Otolaryngol Head Neck Surg 1994;110:259–69.
56. Wiest G, Demer JL, Tian J, Crane BT, et al. Vestibular function in severe bilateral vestibulopathy. J Neurol Neurosurg Psychiatry 2001;71:53–7.
57. Nashner LM, Black FO, Wall III C. Adaptation to altered support and visual conditions during stance: patients with vestibular deficits. J Neurosci 1982;2:536–43.
58. Minor LB. Utility of posturography in management of selected conditions that cause dizziness. Am J Otol 1997;18:113–5.
59. Curthoys IS, Dai MJ, Halmagyi GM. Human ocular torsional position before and after unilateral vestibular neurectomy. Exp Brain Res 1991;85:218–25.
60. Tabak S, Collewijn H, Boumans LJJM. Deviation of the subjective vertical in long-standing unilateral vestibular loss. Acta Otolaryngol 1997;117:1–16.
61. Clarke AH, Schonfeld U, Hamann C, Scherer H. Measuring unilateral otolith function via the otolith-ocular response and the subjective visual vertical. Acta Otolaryngol Suppl 2001;545:84–7.

62. Colebatch JG, Halmagyi GM, Skuse NF. Myogenic potentials generated by a click-evoked vestibulocollic reflex. J Neurol Neurosurg Psychiatry 1994;57:190–7.
63. Ferber-Viart C, Dubreuil C, Duclaux R. Vestibular evoked myogenic potentials in humans: A review. Acta Otolaryngol 1999;119:6–15.
64. Colebatch JG, Halmagyi GM. Vestibular evoked potentials in human neck muscles before and after unilateral vestibular deafferentation. Neurology 1992;42:1635–6.
65. Matsuzaki M, Murofushi T, Mizuno M. Vestibular evoked myogenic potentials in acoustic tumor patients with normal auditory brainstem responses. Eur Arch Otorhinolaryngol 1999;256:1–4.
66. Murofushi T, Halmagyi GM, Yavor RA, Colebatch JG. Absent vestibular evoked myogenic potentials in vestibular neurolabyrinthitis. An indicator of inferior vestibular nerve involvement? Arch Otolaryngol Head Neck Surg 1996;122:845–8.
67. Todd NP, Rosengren SM, Aw ST, Colebatch JG. Ocular vestibular evoked myogenic potentials (OVEMPs) produced by air- and bone-conducted sound. Clin Neurophysiol 2007;118:381–90.
68. Streubel SO, Cremer PD, Carey JP, et al. Vestibular-evoked myogenic potentials in the diagnosis of superior canal dehiscence syndrome. Acta Otolaryngol Suppl 2001;545:41–9.
69. Timmer FC, Zhou G, Guinan JJ, Kujawa SG, et al. Vestibular evoked myogenic potential (VEMP) in patients with Ménière's disease with drop attacks. Laryngoscope 2006;116:776–9.
70. Mikulec AA, McKenna MJ, Ramsey MJ, Rosowski JJ, et al. Superior semicircular canal dehiscence presenting as conductive hearing loss without vertigo. Otol Neurotol 2004;25:121–9.
71. Merchant SN, Nakajima HH, Halpin C, Nadol JB, Jr., et al. Clinical investigation and mechanism of air–bone gaps in large vestibular aqueduct syndrome. Ann Otol Rhinol Laryngol 2007;116:532–41.
72. Bernard PA, Stenstrom RJ. Fluctuating hearing losses in children can be migraine equivalents. Int J Pediatr Otorhinolaryngol 1988;16:141–8.
73. Kim HH, Kumar A, Battista RA and Wiet RJ. Electrocochleography in patients with Ménière's disease. Am J Otolaryngol 2005;26:128–131.
74. Yimtae K, Srirompotong S, Lertsukprasert K. Otosyphilis: a review of 85 cases. Otolaryngol Head Neck Surg 2007;136:67–71.
75. Haynes BF, Kaiser-Kupfer MI, Mason P, Fauci AS. Cogan syndrome: Studies in thirteen patients, long-term follow-up, and a review of the literature. Medicine 1980;59:426–41.
76. Nedzelski JM, Barber HO, McIlmoyl L. Diagnosis in a dizziness unit. J Otolaryngol 1986;15:101–4.
77. Katsarkas A. Paroxysmal positional vertigo: an overview and the deposits repositioning maneuver. Am J Otol 1995;16:725–30.
78. Bárány R. Diagnose von Krankheitserscheinungen im Bereiche des Otolithenapparates. Acta Otolaryngol Suppl 1921;2:434–7.
79. Cohen B, Suzuki J-I, Bender MB. Eye movements from semicircular canal nerve stimulation in the cat. Ann Otol Rhinol Laryngol 1964;73:153–69.
80. Parnes LS, McClure JA. Free-floating endolymph particles: A new operative finding during posterior semicircular canal occlusion. Laryngoscope 1992;102:988–92.
81. Epley JM. New dimensions of benign paroxysmal positional vertigo. Otolaryngol Head Neck Surg 1980;88:599–605.
82. Epley JM. The canalith repositioning procedure: for treatment of benign paroxysmal positional vertigo. Otolaryngol Head Neck Surg 1992;107:399–404.
83. Herdman SJ, Tusa RJ, Zee DS, et al. Single treatment approaches to benign paroxysmal positional vertigo. Arch Otolaryngol Head Neck Surg 1993;119:450–4.
84. Lynn S, Pool A, Rose D, et al. Randomized trial of the canalith repositioning procedure. Otolaryngol Head Neck Surg 1995;113:712–20.
85. Semont A, Freyss G, Vitte E. Curing the BPPV with a liberatory maneuver. Adv Otorhinolaryngol 1988;42:290–3.
86. McClure JA. Horizontal canal BPV. J Otolaryngol 1985;14:30–5.
87. Fife T. Recognition and management of horizontal canal benign positional vertigo. Am J Otol 1998;19:345–51.
88. Kayan A, Hood J. Neuro-otological manifestations of migraine. Brain 1984;107:1123–42.
89. Grunfeld E, Price C, Goadsby P, Gresty M. Motion sickness, migraine, and menstruation in mariners. Lancet 1998;351:1106.
90. Cutrer FM, Baloh RW. Migraine-associated dizziness. Headache 1992;32:300–04.
91. Viirre ES, Baloh RW. Migraine as a cause of sudden hearing loss. Headache 1996;36:24–8.
92. Ishiyama A, Jacobson KM, Baloh RW. Migraine and benign positional vertigo. Ann Otol Rhinol Laryngol 2000;109:377–80.
93. Rassekh CH, Harker LA. The prevalence of migraine in Ménière's disease. Laryngoscope 1992;102:135–8.
94. Lanzi G, Balottin U, Fazzi E, et al. Benign paroxysmal vertigo of childhood: A long-term follow-up. Cephalgia 1999;14:458–60.
95. Basser L. Benign paroxysmal vertigo of childhood. Brain 1964;87:141–52.
96. Minor LB. Clinical manifestations of superior semicircular canal dehiscence. Laryngoscope 2005;115:1717–27.
97. Hotson JR, Baloh RW. Acute vestibular syndrome. N Engl J Med 1998;339:680–5.
98. Minor LB. Gentamicin-induced bilateral vestibular hypofunction. JAMA 1998;279:541–4.
99. Halmagyi GM, Fattore CM, Curthoys IS, Wade S. Gentamicin vestibulotoxicity. Otolaryngol Head Neck Surg 1994;111:571–4.
100. Balkany TJ, Sires B, Arenberg IK. Bilateral aspects of Ménière's disease: An underestimated clinical entity. Otolaryngol Clin North Am 1980;13:603–9.
101. Wladislavosky-Waserman P, Facer GW, Bahram M, Kurland LT. Ménière's disease: a 30-year epidemiologic and clinical study in Rochester, MN. 1951–1980. Laryngoscope 1984;94:1098–102.
102. Rauch SD, San Martin J, Moscicki RA, Bloch KJ. Serum antibodies against heat shock protein 70 in Ménière's disease. Am J Otol 1995;16:648–52.
103. Rauch SD, Merchant SN, Thedinger BA. Ménière's syndrome and endolymphatic hydrops: double-blind temporal bone study. Ann Otol Rhinol Laryngol 1989;98:873–83.

104. Boleas-Aguirre MS, Lin FR, Della Santina CC, et al. Longitudinal results with intratympanic dexamethasone in the treatment of Ménière's disease. Otol Neurotol 2008;29:33–8.
105. Minor LB. Intratympanic gentamicin for control of vertigo in Ménière's disease: Vestibular signs that specify completion of therapy. Am J Otol 1999;20:209–12.
106. Driscoll CLW, Kasperbauer JL, Facer GW, et al. Low-dose intratympanic gentamicin and the treatment of Ménière's disease: Preliminary results. Laryngoscope 1997;107:83–9.
107. Lustig LR, Yeagle J, Niparko JK, Minor LB. Cochlear implantation in patients with bilateral Ménière's syndrome. Otol Neurotol 2003;24:397–403.
108. Grad A, Baloh RW. Vertigo of vascular origin: Clinical and electronystagmographic features in 84 cases. Arch Neurol 1989;46:281–4.

Genetics in Otology and Neurotology

7

Anil K. Lalwani, MD / Anand N. Mhatre, PhD

The success of the human genome project in sequencing of the entire human genome has directly impacted our understanding of otologic and neurotologic disorders. Specifically, we have gained insights into the molecular mechanisms of hearing impairment, vestibular schwannomas, and glomus tumors. In this chapter, the principles of Mendelian genetics are reviewed and our understanding of the aforementioned diseases is summarized.[1]

PRINCIPLES OF MENDELIAN GENETICS

Autosomal Dominant Inheritance

In autosomal dominant disorders, the transmission of a rare allele of a gene by a single heterozygous parent is sufficient to generate an affected child (Figure 7–1A). A heterozygous parent can produce two types of gametes. One gamete carries the mutant form of the gene of interest and the other the normal form. Each of these gametes then has an equal chance of being used in the formation of a zygote. Thus, the chance that an offspring of an autosomal dominant affected parent will itself be affected is 50%. Equal numbers of affected males and females are expected for an autosomal dominant trait, and roughly half of the offspring of an affected individual will be affected. If male-to-male transmission of the trait is observed, the possibility that the trait is X-linked can be eliminated.

If the mutant phenotype is always expressed in individuals carrying the disease allele, then its penetrance is said to be complete; otherwise, it is incomplete. Where penetrance of the affected gene is complete, or 100%, the pattern of its inheritance may be discerned in a relatively straightforward manner. Complete penetrance of the dominant allele results in expression of the disease phenotype in all carriers of that allele without skipping generations. However, with incomplete penetrance of the affected gene, the inheritance pattern of the affected trait becomes relatively harder to discern, ie, one cannot easily distinguish between dominant inheritance with reduced penetrance and more complicated modes of inheritance. The failure of the gene to express itself may be owing to a variety of reasons. The most common rationale put forth to explain reduced penetrance is the effect of genetic background. Factors such as genetic redundancy, presence of more than one gene for the performance of a given function, and modifiers affect a variety of genes. Incomplete penetrance can also be seen in traits that are inherited in an autosomal recessive, X-linked recessive, and X-linked dominant manner.

Variable expression of different aspects of syndromes is common. Some aspects may be expressed in a range encompassing mild to severe forms and/or different combinations of associated symptoms may be expressed in different individuals carrying the same mutation within a single pedigree. An example of variable expressivity is seen in families transmitting autosomal dominant Waardenburg's syndrome. Within the same family, some affected members may have dystopia canthorum, white forelock, heterochromia irides, and hearing loss, whereas others with the same mutation may only have dystopia canthorum.

Autosomal Recessive Inheritance

An autosomal recessive trait is characterized by having two unaffected parents who are heterozygous carriers for mutant forms of the gene in question, but in whom the phenotypic expression of the mutant allele is masked by the normal allele. These heterozygous parents (A/a) can each generate two types of gametes, one carrying the mutant copy of the gene (a) and the other having a normal copy of the gene (A). Of the four possible combinations of these two gamete types from each of the parents, only the offspring that inherits both mutant copies (a/a) will exhibit the trait. Of the three remaining possibilities, all will have a normal hearing phenotype, but two of the three will be heterozygous carriers for the mutant form of the gene, similar to the carrier parents. A typical recessive pedigree with affected members in a single generation (horizontal pattern), showing a consanguineous mating between cousins, is depicted in Figure 7–1B.

X-Linked Inheritance

In humans, females have 22 pairs of autosomes and a pair of X chromosomes (46XX), and males have 22 autosomes, one X chromosome, and one Y chromosome (46XY). Accordingly,

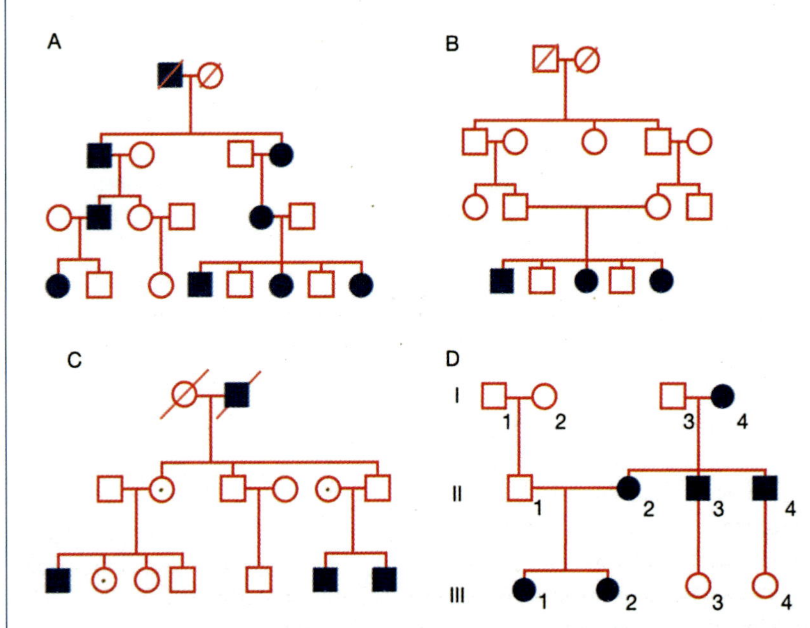

FIGURE 7–1 • Patterns of inheritance. Pedigrees showing autosomal dominant *A*, autosomal recessive *B*, X-linked *C*, and mitochondrial inheritance *D*. Autosomal dominant inheritance is characterized by vertical transmission in contrast to the horizontal pattern seen in recessive inheritance; transmission of recessive disease is more common in consanguineous mating depicted in the pedigree. In X-linked diseases, the unaffected carrier mothers (depicted as a *dot* in the center of the square or the circle) have affected and unaffected sons, whereas all daughters are unaffected. On the other hand, affected fathers only have unaffected children. Mitochondrial diseases can only be transmitted from the mother as mitochondrial DNA is present only in the egg.

males always receive their Y chromosome from their father and their X chromosome from their mother, whereas females receive one of their X chromosomes from each of their two parents. Because males have one copy of the X chromosome, they are hemizygous for genes on the X chromosome, and the X chromosome is active in all of their nucleated cells. In general, only one of the two X chromosomes carried by a female is active in any one cell, whereas the other is rendered inactive by a natural process known as lyonization. This random inactivation process makes all females who are heterozygous for X-linked traits mosaic at the tissue level, resulting in variable expression of the mutant gene. Diseases that are rarely expressed clinically in heterozygous females are called X-linked recessive. In female tissues, various proportions of cells may exist in which one or the other of two alleles for an X-linked locus is expressed. Occasionally, a carrier female may manifest some symptoms of an X-linked recessive disorder owing to this mosaicism if she, by chance, has an abundance of cells with the mutant allele being expressed. Transmission of an X-linked recessive trait in a pedigree is illustrated in Figure 7–1C.

VARIATIONS ON MENDELIAN PRINCIPLES

Mendel established the two fundamental principles of genetics: segregation of genes and their independent assortment. These principles refer to processes that occur in the formation of germ cells known as meiosis. Segregation refers to separation of homologous genes, representing the paternal and the maternal contribution to the individual's genotype, into two separate daughter cells. Thus, the diploid genome is reduced to the haploid state in the germ cells. The principle of independent assortment states that segregation of one gene occurs independently of other genes. These principles have served well for analysis and understanding of the inheritance of traits through a single locus. However, a number of variations on these principles do exist, some of which have already been stated implicitly above. These variations and their underlying principles have contributed toward increasing our understanding of the genetic etiology of disease.

Linkage and Recombination

Not all genes assort independently of each other. This variation of the Mendelian principle was initially identified by Thomas Morgan through analysis of transmission of selected traits in fruit flies. Experiments showed inheritance of specific pairs of alleles in a combination not present in the parental phenotype. This new combination of alleles was considered to result from crossing over and exchange of genetic material between two homologous chromosomes, known as homologous recombination, yielding the new combination of alleles not present in the original parental chromosomes. Analysis of recombination frequencies between two traits considered to be controlled by genes residing on the same linkage group, that is, the same chromosome, provided two essential concepts that led to the development of the genetic map: genes are arranged in a linear order and the frequency with which two alleles are inherited together is a function of the relative physical distance to each other. Thus, the closer the two genes, the greater the chance that they will remain linked post meiosis. The relative chromosomal positions of genes may be readily mapped through the application of these principles of linkage and recombination to generate genetic maps. The genetic distance between two linked genes as measured through the frequency of recombinants between the two alleles is measured in centiMorgans (cM); eg, two loci are one cM apart on the genetic map if there is a 1% chance of a recombination between them in meiosis. Thus, genes that are far apart on a chromosome will assort in an apparently independent manner, whereas genes that are close together will tend to remain linked postmeiosis.

Mitochondrial Inheritance

Not all genes are equally inherited from both parents. The extranuclear mitochondrial genome is inherited solely through the mother. Male mitochondria are not contributed to newly formed zygotes. This inheritance pattern gives rise to pedigrees in which all of the children of an affected mother may be affected and none of the children of an affected father will be affected (Figure 7–1D). In practice, the expression of mitochondrially inherited disorders is often variable and may be incompletely penetrant. If all of the mitochondria transmitted by the mother are of the same genotype, it is called homoplasmia; if there are genetic differences between them, it is called heteroplasmia.

Genomic Imprinting

The manifestation of some genetic diseases depends on the sex of the transmitting parent. This occurrence is considered to result from genomic imprinting. This phenomenon runs counter to the teachings of Mendelian genetics that emphasize equal contribution from paternal and maternal genes, with the obvious exception of genes on the sex chromosomes. Thus, in certain instances, despite the presence of both the paternal and maternal alleles, only one of the parental alleles is expressed. This differential expression of the parental alleles is detected in certain disease states when inheritance of that disorder is dependent on the sex of the parent who transmits the mutant gene. The gene-specific imprinting is presumed to be the consequence of reversible "epigenetic" modification of the parental allele during gametogenesis, leading to its differential expression. The precise mechanism of imprinting and its evolutionary significance remain unknown. Hypermethylation of the imprinted gene represents one possible mechanism.

Genomic imprinting at the level of a specific gene has been identified in familial cases of nonchromaffin paragangliomas (PGs; benign tumors of the paraganglionic cells, also known as glomus tumors). Although benign, their enlargement can cause deafness and/or facial palsy. Familial PGs have shown an autosomal dominant inheritance with genomic imprinting of the maternal allele. Thus, the transmission of the disease occurs via the affected paternal allele and not the maternal allele.

Multifactorial Inheritance

An expression of a phenotype, the outcome of which is determined by a single gene, is termed a Mendelian trait. Its pattern of transmission within a pedigree can be readily discerned in most cases, as described above. On the other hand, most common human diseases and traits show irregular inheritance patterns. These traits are considered to be determined from the action of multiple genes and/or nongenetic factors. A phenotype that is an outcome of both genetic and environmental factors is called a multifactorial, or complex, trait. The low proportion of Mendelian traits relative to the number of multifactorial traits in humans is better illustrated by considering the proportion of total number of Mendelian traits known (approximately 6,000 according to McKusick's Mendelian Inheritance in Man) to the total number of genes that are estimated to exist (approximately 30,000). It should be emphasized that classification of Mendelian traits as being "determined" by single genes is an oversimplification. As more Mendelian disorders are identified and their phenotypes investigated, their phenotypic variability and complexity are becoming increasingly clear, and, concomitantly, their distinction from complex or multifactorial traits is becoming increasingly blurred. Phenotype variability or variable expression seen in a single gene disorder such as Waardenburg's syndrome may reflect interaction of that major gene, such as PAX3, with "modifier" genes. Identification of these modifier genes has important implications for the understanding and treatment of Mendelian disorders with variable expressivity.

The relatively irregular mode of inheritance that characterizes a multifactorial trait is presumed to result from interaction of multiple genes (polygenic). This interaction is apparently distinct from that presumed for Mendelian traits. But this distinction may be at a quantitative rather than a qualitative level. For example, instead of a predominant influence or effect of one gene on expression of the phenotype, the multifactorial trait is characterized by a number of genes with equivalent influence or effect. The genetic component of multifactorial traits is referred to by terms such as increased risk, predisposition, or susceptibility. Because of their complexity, the factors that contribute to the multifactorial traits are poorly defined. Several well-studied diseases, such as cardiovascular conditions and diabetes, as well as distinct behavioral disorders, are classified as multifactorial. The influence of nongenetic factors, eg, environmental agents or stochastic processes during development, on a variety of traits is also clearly illustrated in the studies of identical twins.

GENETICS OF HERRING LOSS

Hearing loss is the most common form of sensory impairment in humans. Nearly 10% of the US population or 30 million Americans have significant auditory dysfunction. For some, the hearing loss is present at the beginning of life. The prevalence of permanent, moderate-to-severe sensorineural hearing loss (SNHL) is estimated to be between 1 and 3 per 1,000 live births.[2,3] Prelingual deafness, in contrast to late-onset hearing loss, can be devastating to the child. Significant delays in the acquisition of speech and language, as well as other developmental childhood milestones, can occur without adequate rehabilitation. The predominant etiology of hearing impairment in children has evolved with advances in medical knowledge and therapeutics. Historically, infectious disorders such as otitis media, maternal rubella infections, and bacterial meningitis, as well as environmental factors such as intrauterine teratogenic exposure or ototoxic insult, were the dominant causes of congenital and acquired hearing losses. The introduction of antibiotics, vaccines, and improved knowledge and enhanced awareness about teratogens has led to a decline in hearing loss resulting from infections and environmental agents. Currently, more than half of all childhood hearing impairment is thought to be hereditary. As a result of advances in clinical and basic medical research, significant progress has been made in understanding the causes of hereditary hearing impairment (HHI).

Classification

When SNHL occurs in isolation, it is called nonsyndromic.[4] On the other hand, hearing loss accompanied by other systemic disturbance is termed syndromic. Two-thirds of HHI is nonsyndromic, whereas the remaining one-third is syndromic. Over 1,100 syndromes are associated with otologic manifestations. Nonsyndromic HHI is further classified by the mode of inheritance. The majority of HHI is inherited in an autosomal recessive fashion (80%), with the autosomal dominant mode of inheritance being less common (15–18%).[5] Rare modes of transmission include X-linked and mitochondrial transmission, which account for the remaining 2% of hearing impairment.

Auditory Phenotype in HHI

Clinically, HHI can be described by several characteristics of the hearing loss: severity of hearing impairment, age of onset, type of hearing impairment, frequencies involved, unilateral/bilateral, stable/progressive, and syndromic/nonsyndromic. In general, recessive HHI tends to be more severe than dominantly inherited hearing impairment. Recessive HHI is predominantly congenital or prelingual in onset, whereas dominant HHI is delayed or postlingual. In contrast to the profound hearing loss associated with recessive deafness, autosomal dominant hearing loss is less severe and progresses with age. Many dominant hearing impairments progress at the rate of about 1 dB/year. Recessive deafness usually affects all frequencies equally. Although there are some types that have predominantly low-frequency or flat hearing loss, dominant hearing impairment more commonly affects the high frequencies, mimicking presbycusis. The frequencies involved in syndromic forms of hearing impairment are variable. Nonsyndromic hearing impairment is usually symmetric. In contrast, syndromic HHI can be unilateral or bilateral and symmetric or asymmetric.

Molecular Genetics of HHI

Rapid progress has been made in the identification of genes responsible for syndromic and nonsyndromic hereditary hearing impairment. In syndromic hearing impairment, more than 100 genes have been identified since 1990, showing a large heterogeneity even in the same type of syndromic hearing impairment. For example, Usher's syndrome type I has been associated with 11 different genetic loci; the genes responsible for nine of these loci have been identified (Table 7–1). In nonsyndromic hearing impairment, as of 2008, 57 autosomal dominant, 75 autosomal recessive, 6 X-linked, 2 mitochondrial loci, and 2 modified loci have been mapped on the human genome. In addition, the current count of nearly 50 nonsyndromic genes identified since 1994 will continue to rapidly increase (Table 7–2; Hereditary hearing loss homepage: http://webh01.ua.ac.be/hhh/).

The identified deafness genes play a variety of different roles in cellular physiology (see Tables 7–1 and 7–2). The responsible genes include cytoskeletal proteins important in maintaining cellular structure, division, and intracellular transport; transcription factors that regulate the expression of other genes; ion channels important in the transport of sodium, potassium, chloride, and iodine; developmental genes that regulate morphogenesis; and proteins involved in intercellular communications such as gap and tight junctions.

As a result of progress in the genetics of deafness (and genetics in general), several conventional notions have had to be modified. It is now clear that a single gene may cause syndromic or nonsyndromic forms of deafness or may be associated with autosomal dominant or autosomal recessive mode of inheritance. Identification of myosin 7A as the gene responsible for both syndromic and nonsyndromic deafness has led to the abandonment of the "one gene, one disease" dogma. In addition, pendrin mutations cause both Pendred's syndrome and isolated (nonsyndromic) large vestibular aqueduct (LVA). To muddle things further, different mutations in myosin 7A cause both dominant and recessive forms of nonsyndromic deafness. The same is true for connexin 26: it is associated with both a dominant and a recessive mode of transmission. In addition to the disease-causing gene, the patient's genetic background and the role of other modifier genes in determining the clinical severity is now better appreciated. For example, the severity of Waardenburg's syndrome in a given patient will be determined not only by the mutation in the PAX3 gene, but also by the nature of other genes present in the remaining genome.

Several of the genes and gene families are especially important in clinical otology including *GJB* (family of gap junction genes), *SLC26A4*, myosins, and mitochondrial gene 12S ribosomal ribonucleic acid (rRNA) and are discussed below.

GJB2

The apparent genetic heterogeneity of HHI is contrasted by the predominance of *GJB2* (encoding for connexin 26 gap junction protein) as a major cause of inherited and sporadic nonsyndromic deafness. Mutations of *GJB2* are responsible for both recessive (DFNB1—DFN for deafness, B for recessive) and dominant (DFNA3—DFN for deafness, A for dominant) forms of HHI; it is an important contributor to childhood hearing loss, accounting for nearly 50% of congenital recessive sensorineural hearing impairment. Connexin 26 (Cx26) is a member of a family of proteins that are involved in the formation of gap junctions. Connexins are transmembrane proteins that form channels allowing transport of ions or small molecules between adjacent cells. Each connexin subunit contains three intracellular domains and two extracellular domains, crossing the plasma membrane four times. The second intracellular domain contains the cytoplasmic loop. The other two intracellular domains consist of the N terminus and the C terminus.[6] Six connexin subunits join to form a connexon. A pair of connexons, one in each adjacent cell, comes together to form an intercellular channel. The family of connexin proteins plays an important role in normal hearing as mutations in several members of the family are associated with hearing impairment. To date, mutations in Cx26 (*GJB2*), Cx30 (*GJB6*), Cx31 (*GJB3*), Cx32 (*GJB1*), and Cx43 (*GJA1*) have been implicated in hearing loss (Connexin-deafness homepage: http://davinci.crg.es/deafness/). Its expression has been shown in the stria vascularis, basement membrane, limbus, and spiral prominence of the human cochlea.[7] One possible biochemical function of Cx26 has been suggested by studying rat cochlear gap junctions. The organization of gap junctions and information provided by other investigators suggest that

TABLE 7–1 Syndromic hereditary hearing impairment genes

SYNDROME/LOCUS	GENE	FUNCTION
Alport's	*COL4A3*	Cytoskeletal protein
	COL4A4	Cytoskeletal protein
	COL4A5	Cytoskeletal protein
Branchio-oto-renal	*EYA1*	Developmental gene
	SIX1	Developmental gene
Jervell and Lange-Nielsen	*KVLQT1*	Delayed rectifier potassium channel
	KCNE1	Delayed rectifier potassium channel
Norrie's	*NORRIN*	Cell-cell interactions?
Pendred's	*SLC26A4*	Chloride-iodide transporter
Stickler's	*COL2A1*	Cytoskeletal protein
	COL11A1	Cytoskeletal protein
	COL11A2	Cytoskeletal protein
Treacher Collins	*TCOF1*	Nucleolar-cytoplasmic transport
Usher's	*MYO7A*	Cytoskeletal protein
	USH1C	?
	CDH23	Intercellular adherence protein
	PCDH15	?
	SANS	Harmonin associated protein
	USH2A	Cell adhesion molecule
	VLGR1	G-protein coupled receptor
	WHRN	Calmodulin-dependent serine kinase
	USH3	?
	Others	
Waardenburg's type I, III	*PAX3*	Transcription factor
Waardenburg's type II	*MITF, SNAI2*	Transcription factor
Waardenburg's type IV	*EDNRB*	Endothelin-B receptor
	EDN3	Endothelin-B receptor ligand
	SOX10	Transcription factor

they serve as the structural basis for recycling of potassium ions back to the endolymph of the cochlear duct after stimulation of the sensory hair cells.[8,9]

Several studies have demonstrated the prevalence of Cx26 mutations in 50% of individuals with recessive deafness, with a carrier rate as high as 4%.[7,10–15] Currently, approximately 100 different mutations have been identified (Connexin-deafness homepage: http://davinci.crg.es/deafness/). Two single base pair deletions account for nearly half of all mutations in this gene: 35delG and 167delT. The 35delG mutation has been found to be common in several populations and accounts for up to 70% of Cx26 mutant alleles in families from the United Kingdom, France, Italy, Spain, Tunisia, Lebanon, Israel, Australia, Greece, United States, and New Zealand, as well as up to 40% of sporadic cases of congenital deafness in these countries.[12,13,16–20]

The 35delG mutation leads to frameshift, early termination of the nascent protein, and a nonfunctional intracellular domain in the protein.[12,16,21] Alternatively, this mutation may lead to an unstable RNA, leading to its early degradation or absence of its translation into protein. Clinically, homozygous patients with the 35delG mutation show a variable phenotype, ranging from mild to profound hearing impairment. However, most patients with the homozygous 35delG mutation show a severe to profound phenotype.

In contrast, the 35delG mutation may be less common in the Japanese populations in which 235delC is the prevalent

TABLE 7–2 Nonsyndromic hereditary hearing impairment genes

LOCUS	GENE	FUNCTION
Dominant loci		
Unnamed	*CRYM*	Thyroid hormone binding protein
DFNA1	*DIAPH1*	Cytoskeletal protein
DFNA2	*GJB3 (Cx31)*	Gap junctions
DFNA2	*KCNQ4*	Potassium channel
DFNA3	*GJB2 (Cx26)*	Gap junctions
DFNA3	*GJB6 (Cx30)*	Gap junctions
DFNA4	*MYH14*	Class II nonmuscle myosin
DFNA5	*DFNA5*	Unknown
DFNA6/14/38	*WFS1*	Endoplasmic reticulum protein
DFNA8/12	*TECTA*	Tectorial membrane protein
DFNA9	*COCH*	Unknown
DFNA10	*EYA4*	Developmental gene
DFNA11	*MYO7A*	Cytoskeletal protein
DFNA13	*COL11A2*	Cytoskeletal protein
DFNA15	*POU4F3*	Transcription factor
DFNA17	*MYH9*	Cytoskeletal protein
DFNA20/26	*ACTG1*	Cytoskeletal protein
DFNA22	*MYO6*	Unconventional myosin
DFNA28	*TFCP2L3*	Transcription factor
DFNA36	*TMC1*	Transmembrane protein
DFNA39	*DSPP*	Dentin phosphoprotein
DFNA44	*CCDC50*	Effector of EGF signaling
DFNA48	*MYO1A*	Unconventional myosin
Recessive Loci		
Unnamed	*SLC26A5 (prestin)*	Motor protein
DFNB1	*GJB2 (CX26)*	Gap junctions
DFNB2	*MYO7A*	Cytoskeletal protein
DFNB3	*MYO15*	Cytoskeletal protein
DFNB4	*PDS*	Chloride-iodide transporter
DFNB6	*TMIE*	Transmembrane protein
DFNB7/11	*TMC1*	Transmembrane protein
DFNB8/10	*TMPRSS3*	Transmembrane serine protease
DFNB9	*OTOF*	Trafficking of membrane vesicles
DFNB12	*CDH23*	Intercellular adherence protein
DFNB16	*STRC*	Stereocilia protein
DFNB18	*USH1C*	?

Continued

TABLE 7–2 Nonsyndromic hereditary hearing impairment genes (Continued)

LOCUS	GENE	FUNCTION
DFNB21	*TECTA*	Tectorial membrane protein
DFNB22	*OTOA*	Gel attachment to nonsensory cell
DFNB23	*PCDH15*	Morphogenesis and cohesion
DFNB24	*RDX*	Cross-link actin filaments
DFNB28	*TRIOBP*	Cytoskeletal-organizing protein
DFNB29	*CLDN14*	Tight junctions
DFNB30	*MYO3A*	Hybrid motor-signaling myosin
DFNB31	*WHRN*	PDZ domain-containing protein
DFNB36	*ESPN*	Calcium-insensitive actin-bundling protein
DFNB37	*MYO6*	Unconventional myosin
DFNB49	*MARVELD2*	Tight junction protein
DFNB53	*COL11A2*	Collagen protein
DFNB59	*PJVK*	Zinc binding protein
DFNB66/67	*LHFPL5*	Tetraspan membrane protein
X-linked Locus		
DFN3	*POU3F4*	Transcription factor

Cx26 mutation.[22–24] Likewise, in the Ashkenazi Jewish population, the 167delT mutation has been found to be more common than the 35delG mutation, with a carrier rate of 4%.[15]

Of the genes identified to date, Cx26, because of its small size, the single coding exon, frequency of involvement, and predominance of two mutations, lends itself to mutation screening. However, it is unlikely that screening for the two common mutations will be sufficient to identify the vast majority of Cx26 deafness. We screened 154 individuals with SNHL for mutations in Cx26by DNA sequencing and identified 34 patients with mutations for an overall incidence of 22% in the study population.[25] Of all Cx26 mutations, the 35delG mutation accounted for 26%. The 35delG mutation was present in a homozygous state in only four individuals (each of the two chromosomes harbored the 35delG mutation) and heterozygous in six individuals (only one chromosome had the 35delG mutation). Herein lies the fundamental problem with screening for only 35delG: only 4 of 34 individuals (12%) with Cx26 mutations, or 154 individuals in total (3%), had a homozygous mutation that would be required to clearly implicate Cx26 as the causative gene. The identification of a single copy of 35delG mutation does not implicate this gene in deafness and may simply reflect the high carrier rate that is present in the population. In this case, the rate of identifying the cause of childhood SNHL by genetic testing is significantly less than radiologic imaging. The predominance of the two common mutations in a heterozygous state (with a second uncommon Cx26 mutation) has been replicated by others.[26,27] Therefore, genetic testing for 35delG and 167delT mutations only, without sequencing the entire *GJB2* gene, is inadequate. *GJB2* testing is now readily available in many laboratories; its role in the management of children with hearing impairment remains to be determined.

SLC26A4 (Pendrin Protein)

Mutations in *SLC26A4* are associated with an isolated LVA (the most common radiologic abnormality associated with childhood deafness), as well as Pendred's syndrome. Vaughan Pendred, while he was working in the Ear, Nose, and Throat Department at Newcastle Royal Infirmary, observed the association between deaf-mutism and goiter in two sisters.[28,29] The first sister appeared to be profoundly deaf and developed goiter at the age of 13 years; the second sister was not completely deaf and also developed a notable thyroid mass at the age of 13. It has been estimated that as much as 10% of all HHI may be attributable to Pendred's syndrome, making it one of the most common syndromic HHI disorders.[30] Goiter may appear at birth, in childhood, or after puberty. The delay in onset, or sometimes absence of goiter can make clinical diagnosis of Pendred's syndrome difficult. Patients are usually euthyroid but can be hypothyroid. The elevation of thyrotropin-releasing hormone suggests a compensatory hypothyroidism.[31] The mild organification defect in Pendred's syndrome can be noted by the partial discharge of iodine in the perchlorate challenge test.[32] The perchlorate ion (ClO_4^-) is a competitor of iodine. When perchlorate is given orally or intravenously following radioactive iodine administration, the perchlorate blocks further uptake of iodine and releases unbound iodine in the thyroid follicular cells. In Pendred's syndrome, in which there is an intrinsic thyroid organification defect, the perchlorate displaces more iodine than in a normal thyroid gland, leading to a greater iodine "discharge" and a decrease in thyroid radioactivity over time. The hearing loss of Pendred's syndrome is usually congenital and profound. However, there are reports of milder or progressive hearing impairments. Hypoplasia of the cochlea and enlargement of the vestibular aqueduct can be associated with Pendred's syndrome as demonstrated by histologic and radiologic studies.[33,34]

Everett and colleagues identified mutations in the *SLC26A4* (formerly *PDS*) gene on chromosome 7q31 as the cause of Pendred's syndrome.[35] The gene contains 21 exons. The gene product pendrin encodes a 780-amino acid (86-kDa) protein that contains 11 transmembrane domains resembling sulfate transporters.[35] Evidence suggests that pendrin functions as a chloride–iodide anion transport protein.[36] In the mouse inner ear, pendrin localizes to the endolymphatic duct and sac, distinct areas in the utricle and saccule, and the external sulcus region within the cochlea, indicating a possible role in endolymph resorption. Van Hauwe and colleagues noted two particularly frequent missense mutations, L236P (707 T to C) and T416P (1246 A to C); subsequently, a third common mutation, E384G (1151 A to G), has also been identified.[37] Although the gene is too large for screening by direct sequencing, identification of common mutations opens the opportunity for screening for these isolated mutations.

SLC26A4 mutations are also responsible for nonsyndromic hearing loss associated with LVA. The isolated presence of an LVA is one of the most common forms of inner ear anomaly. Genetic studies of families with LVA disorder identified a recessive nonsyndromic locus, DFNB4, that also mapped to the same region as the *SLC26A4* gene.

This discovery led to the evaluation of the *SLC26A4* gene and the subsequent identification of seven pendrin mutations responsible for LVA with nonsyndromic HHI.[38] Like Pendred syndrome, different mutations, V480D, V653A, I490L and G497 S, have been found to be commonly associated with LVA. In a review of our experience, LVA was the most common imaging abnormality detected in children with nonsyndromic SNHL.[39] At least 40% of children with LVA will develop profound SNHL.[40] Patients with LVA are at risk for progressive hearing loss after minor head trauma. Identifying this anomaly influences parent counseling with respect to the dangers of incidental head trauma. In summary, the spectrum of *SLC26A4* mutations and the wide range of phenotypic manifestations show that pendrin is an important participant in ear structural development and in the normal functioning of the inner ear and thyroid. Screening for mutations may play an important role in the diagnosis and management of a child as well as their siblings with hearing impairment.

Myosins

The importance of myosins in inner ear function is manifest in the growing list of unconventional (nonclass II) myosin heavy chain genes pathogenically linked to HHI. These disease genes encode the heavy chains of myosin VI, VII, and XV. The expression of these unconventional myosins is not limited to the cells and the tissues of the inner ear. Yet the expression of their dysfunction is largely restricted to hearing impairment. In the mouse, myosin VI has been identified as the Snell's waltzer gene; the cochlear and vestibular neurosensory epithelium of Snell's waltzer mice degenerates soon after birth. The role of myosin VI in human deafness remains to be determined. Myosin VII has been linked to both rodent and human deafness. Mutations in the gene encoding myosin VIIA are responsible for mouse shaker 1, human Usher's syndrome type 1, and human nonsyndromic hearing impairment DFNB2 and DFNA11. Shaker 1 mice are deaf and have vestibular defects. Mice that are homozygous for mutant shaker 1 allele display disorganized stereocilia. Myosin XV is the largest of all myosin heavy chains, having a molecular weight of 395 kDa. Mutations in myosin XV have been pathogenically linked to DFNB3 in humans and the shaker 2 phenotype in mice.

The unconventional myosins are distributed throughout the mechanosensory hair cells. Moreover, histopathologic study of mouse models of myosin XV dysfunction has been valuable to understanding the consequences of myosin dysfunction on the sensory hair cells. Myosin VI is localized within the actin-rich cuticular plate, as well as in the rootlet actin filaments that descend from the stereocilia into the cuticular plate, suggesting a role in stabilizing the basal attachment of stereocilia.[41,42] Myosin VIIA is localized in the stereocilia and cell body of hair cells.[42] Postulated roles for myosin VIIA include maintaining stereocilia integrity and membrane trafficking in the inner hair cells. On histopathologic evaluation, the inner ears of mouse models of myosin XV dysfunction reveal significantly shortened stereocilia in the sensory hair cells, demonstrating the importance of myosin XV in the maintenance of hair cell structure and thereby its function.

A mutation in a conventional, or class II, myosin, MYH9, has been described. The class II myosins are broadly expressed in skeletal, cardiac, and smooth muscle, as well as nonmuscle tissue and consist of a pair of heavy chains, a pair of light chains, and a pair of regulatory light chains.[43] The N-terminal motor domain is the most highly conserved region of the myosin heavy chain and contains the adenosine triphosphate and actin-binding sites. The apparent molecular weight of the class II myosin heavy chain is 200 kDa. The myosin that mediates skeletal muscle contraction, also known as the sarcomeric myosin, represents the most well-characterized representative of the class II myosin family. Cardiac and smooth muscle cells also express isoforms of class II myosin, distinct from the sarcomeric myosin that mediates contraction in these muscle cells. Mutation in MYH9, a conventional nonmuscle myosin, was described in an American family with autosomal dominant nonsyndromic hereditary hearing impairment (DFNA17) associated with cochleosaccular degeneration.[44–46] The affected members of the DFNA17 family exhibit progressive, postlingual onset hearing loss, a pattern that is observed in the majority of nonsyndromic autosomal dominant HHI. The cosegregation of the mutant MYH9 with nonsyndromic hearing impairment illustrates a biologically significant role for MYH9 in hearing and an organ-specific pathology associated with the mutant allele.

Two other myosin genes have been predicted to have an important role in hearing. Myosin V is an abundant protein of afferent nerve fibers innervating both inner and outer hair cells.[47] Myosin Ip has been implicated as an effector of adaptation of the hair cell transduction apparatus.[48] The preponderance of myosins is not surprising given the diversity of actin filament systems in the inner ear.[49]

Aminoglycoside Ototoxicity

To date, there are 326 syndromes, disorders, or peculiar phenotypes associated with mutations in the mitochondrial genome.[50] Twenty-one of these disorders have some involvement with SNHL, indicating that the requirement for a healthy population of mitochondria is very important to the cells involved in normal hearing.[51–54] One of the most striking examples of a mitochondrially inherited trait whose expression is environmentally affected is the hearing loss caused by hypersensitivity to aminoglycosides.[51] The aminoglycoside hypersensitivity phenotype is the result of a single base transition of A to G at position 1555 in the mitochondrial 12S rRNA. This mutation causes a portion of the 12S rRNA transcript structure to closely resemble the binding site of aminoglycosides to bacterial rRNA. When an aminoglycoside such as streptomycin is administered to patients carrying this mutation, it binds to the mutant 12S rRNA and prevents it from functioning in the translation of mitochondrially transcribed genes, resulting in the loss of mitochondria in cells and perhaps cell death or impairment of normal function. Screening for this mutation prior to initiation of aminoglycoside therapy may reduce the incidence of ototoxicity.

GENETICS OF NEUROFIBROMATOSIS 2

Neurofibromatosis 2 (NF2) is much rarer than NF1, with an incidence estimated between 1 in 33,000 and 1 in 50,000.[55] Inheritance of NF2 is autosomal dominant, and gene penetrance is over 95%. Neurofibromatosis 2 most frequently presents in the second and third decades of life. The mean age of onset of symptoms from vestibular schwannomas in Kanter and colleagues's series was 20.4 years.[56] Vestibular schwannomas comprise approximately 8% of intracranial tumors and account for approximately 80% of cerebellopontine angle tumors.[57] The majority of vestibular schwannomas are sporadic in occurrence and unilateral, presenting in the fifth decade.

Patients with NF2 with bilateral vestibular schwannomas represent 2 to 4% of all vestibular schwannomas.[58,59]

Neurofibromatosis 2 has often been confused with NF1. The conclusive proof that NF1 and NF2 were distinct disease entities did not occur until 1987. Molecular biologic investigations by Barker and colleagues,[60] among others, showed that the gene responsible for NF1 was located near the proximal long arm of chromosome 17. At the same time, under separate investigation, the gene responsible for NF2 was located on chromosome 22 by Rouleau and colleagues.[61]

Neurofibromatosis 2 results from the inheritance of a mutation in the gene on chromosome 22. The incidence of mutation rate within the NF2 gene has been estimated at 6.5×10^{-6}.[55] In approximately 50% of cases, there is no family history, and these patients represent new germline mutations.[62] Chromosome 22 was first thought to be the likely source of the NF2 gene following cytogenetic studies of meningiomas in 1982.[63] The NF2 gene was subsequently mapped to chromosome 22 by both linkage studies and loss of heterozygosity analysis in 1986 and 1987, respectively.[61,64] In 1993, the NF2 gene, designated merlin or schwannomin, was isolated by two groups working independently.[65,66] The NF2 gene is spread over approximately 100 kb on chromosome 22q12.2 and contains 17 exons. The coding sequence of the messenger RNA is 1,785 bp in length and encodes a protein of 595 amino acids.[65,66] The gene product is similar in sequence to a family of proteins including moesin, ezrin, radixin, talin, and members of the protein 4.1 superfamily. These proteins are involved in linking cytoskeletal components with the plasma membrane and are located in actin-rich surface projections such as microvilli. The N-terminal region of the merlin protein is thought to interact with components of the plasma membrane and the C-terminal with the cytoskeleton.

Merlin or schwannomin is predominantly expressed in the cells of the nervous system and in the lens and is predominantly located in membrane ruffles and cellular protrusions.[67,68] It is currently believed that merlin protein overexpression can inhibit cell growth and that it induces cell surface protrusions and elongation of cells.[68,69] In 1994, Tikoo and colleagues[70] tested merlin's ability to function as a tumor suppressor gene. Following introduction of the NF2 protein into v-Ha-Ras-transformed NIH 3T3 cells, they were able to demonstrate the reversal of the malignant phenotype, thus confirming the tumor suppressor properties of merlin. Although the exact function of the NF2 protein is as yet unknown, the evidence available so far suggests that it is involved in cell–cell or cell–matrix interactions and that it is important for cell movement, cell shape, or communication. Loss of function of the merlin protein therefore could result in a loss of contact inhibition and consequently lead to tumorigenesis.

Mutations involving the NF2 gene have been observed in 22 to 59% of patients with sporadic vestibular schwannoma.[71] Welling and colleagues compared the rate of identification of genetic mutations in sporadic vestibular schwannoma versus patients with NF2 and found a significant difference, 66 to 33%, respectively, while noting that different mutational mechanisms may exist in tumorigenesis.[72] To date, more than 200 mutations of the NF2 gene have been identified, including single base substitutions, insertions, and deletions.[73,74] Most mutations lead to truncation of the C-terminal end of the protein; only 13 missense mutations have been identified.[74] NF2 gene defects have been detected in other malignancies including meningiomas, malignant mesotheliomas, melanomas, and breast carcinomas.[64,75–78]

Genotype–phenotype correlation studies suggest that mutations in the NF2 gene are associated with variable phenotypic expression. Ruttledge and colleagues found that mutations in the NF2 gene that result in protein truncation are associated with a more severe clinical presentation of NF2 (Wishart), whereas missense and splice site mutations are associated with a milder (Gardner) form of the disease.[79] Similarly, Parry and colleagues have reported that retinal abnormalities were associated with the more disruptive protein truncation mutations of the NF2 gene.[80] Both studies showed intrafamilial variability of phenotypic expression.

Although mutations in the NF2 gene play a dominant role in the biology of vestibular schwannoma, it is also possible that other genetic loci contribute to the development of vestibular schwannoma. In addition, NF2 gene mutations are not uniformly identified in patients with vestibular schwannoma, and published genotype–phenotype correlations are variable, which suggests that other genetic loci may contribute to the genesis of vestibular schwannoma and the ultimate phenotype of affected individuals.[79,80]

The identification of the gene responsible for NF2 has significantly advanced our understanding of the molecular pathology and factors responsible for the clinical heterogeneity among patients with NF2. Understanding the function of merlin in tumor formation will lead to the development of novel therapies, which may eventually alleviate the suffering associated with NF2.

GENETICS OF FAMILIAL PARAGANGLIOMAS (PG)

With the exception of the genes located on the sex chromosomes (X and Y), we inherit two copies of every gene. In most cases, both the maternal and the paternal copy of the gene are active. Therefore, when inheriting a disease that is transmitted in an autosomal dominant fashion, it usually does not matter which parent passes down the single mutated gene for the child to be affected. However, there are many genes in which only the paternal or maternal copy is active or functional and the inactive gene is said to be imprinted. Imprinted genes are normally involved in embryonic growth and behavioral development, but occasionally they also function inappropriately as oncogenes or tumor suppressor genes.

Familial PG is inherited in an autosomal-dominant manner with maternal imprinting. Therefore, when an individual inherits the PG gene from the mother (regardless of whether she herself is affected), that child is unaffected and becomes a silent carrier of the mutated gene. On the other hand, when a child inherits the PG gene from the father, the offspring will have PGs regardless of the affected status of the father. Subsequently, the affected/unaffected child harboring the abnormal PG gene will be able to pass the gene to his/her children; he/she will have affected children only if the transmitting parent is a father. This unusual form of incomplete genetic penetrance is caused by sex-specific gene modification during gametogenesis.[81]

Because of the unusual pattern of inheritance outlined above, it is difficult to determine whether every case of "sporadic" PGs is, in fact, sporadic or a hereditary tumor camouflaged as sporadic. In all likelihood, many sporadic tumors are probably familial and the incidence of hereditary tumors considerably higher than just 1 in 10 PGs. Similar to their familial counterparts, sporadic tumors also demonstrate loss of heterozygosity at PGL1 and PGL2. Bikhazi and colleagues demonstrated loss of heterozygosity to be present in 38% of sporadic cases of carotid body tumors and glomus tumors when tested with markers located at PGL1 and PGL2.[82] This indirectly suggests that one-third of sporadic tumors may indeed be inherited. Similar to NF2, sporadic and familial PGs likely have a common genetic etiology.

The quest for the identification of genes responsible for PG has been greatly aided by the human genome project and the availability of large families with inherited PG. This has led to the delineation of at least three different genes associated with PG.

The First Locus: PGL1

Genetic linkage analysis of a large Dutch family with hereditary PG mapped a gene called *PGL1* to the short arm of chromosome 11, 11q22-q23.[83,84] This finding was confirmed in North American families and further localized to 1 1q23.[85,86] Tumor cells from affected individuals with the PGL1 mutation revealed preferential loss of maternal DNA from chromosome 1 1q harboring the *PGL1* gene, providing genetic support for maternal imprinting. The phenomenon where DNA is deleted is termed a loss of heterozygosity.[85,87] This loss of heterozygosity associated with tumor formation strongly suggests that *PGL1* is a tumor suppressor gene. In the tumor suppressor hypothesis, tumor formation requires the loss of both functional copies of a tumor suppressor gene, since a single functioning copy of the tumor suppressor gene is sufficient to prevent tumors. The NF2 and retinoblastoma genes are examples of tumor suppressor genes. The loss of function of one tumor suppressor gene by inheritance of a mutated allele and a subsequent random mutation of the second allele results in tumorigenesis.[88] This phenomenon, described by Knudson,[88] is known as the "two-hit" hypothesis. In familial PG, like NF2, the inherited first "hit" predisposes the individual to multicentric tumors owing to multiple random second "hits."

The gene responsible for *PGL1* was cloned within the large chromosomal span of 11q23 by screening a candidate gene involved in oxygen metabolism located in this area.[89] This gene, known as *SDHD* (for succinate-ubiquinone oxidoreductase subunit D), encodes a small subunit of mitochrondrial cytochrome b (cybS) involved in Krebs cycle aerobic metabolism.[89] Using five families with hereditary PG, single base pair mutations leading to a loss of function of the *SDHD* gene product were identified. A nonsense mutation was found in two families leading to early truncation in the formation of the *SDHD* protein and consequently the loss of cybS production. The other three families showed evidence of missense mutations with change of a single amino acid, presumably dramatically altering cybS conformation, rendering it nonfunctional. Interestingly, typical postgametogenesis maternal imprinting was not found since biallelic expression of both the maternal and the paternal gene was found in somatic tissues. It appears that only when the normal maternal allele is later imprinted or lost that the mutated paternal allele encoding the mutated *SDHD* leads to tumor formation owing to a loss of tumor suppressor activity. The discovery of this gene will undoubtedly lead to more efficient efforts in screening family members at risk for heritable PG.

The Second Locus: PGL2

Mapping of another large, unrelated Dutch family with hereditary PGs has revealed a second locus, *PGL2*, found on the short arm of chromosome 11. This locus at chromosome 11 q13 harbors another gene for PG that by genetic mapping is clearly distinct from *PGL1*.[90,91]

The Third and Fourth Nonimprinted Loci: PGL3 and PGL4

A large German family with hereditary PG has revealed a third locus, PGL3.[92] Markers flanking the 11q23 and 11q13 loci associated with *PGL1* and *PGL2* excluded linkage to this area. Inheritance in this family was also autosomal-dominant, similar to *PGL1* and *PGL2,* but there was no evidence of maternal imprinting. This family was mapped to chromosome 1q21. Subsequently, as mutations in *SDHD* had been identified as the cause of type 1 PG, Niemann and Muller investigated *SDHC* in this family.[93] They found a G-to-A transition in exon 1 of *SDHC* in all affected members but not in unaffected members. The mutation destroyed the start codon ATG of the gene at nucleotide position 958. In mitochondrial complex II, *SDHA* and *SDHB* constitute the catalytic domains and are anchored in the inner mitochondrial membrane by subunits *SDHC* and *SDHD.* Screening for alterations within *SDHB* identified mutations associated with *PGL4*; mutations in *SDHB* are also associated with malignant pheochromocytoma. *PGL3* and *PGL4* are not maternally imprinted.

Genetic Screening

Rapid advances in molecular genetics and biology have allowed the practicing otolaryngologist insight into the etiology of a rare, yet well-described tumor of the head and neck. On evaluation of a patient with a PG, an extended family history should be elicited to identify additional members with evidence of head and neck tumors suspicious for PG. If hereditary PG is suspected, a detailed family pedigree should be obtained and the patient's family should be offered genetic screening. If the pedigree is sufficiently large, it could be determined by genetic linkage analysis if the family's PGs map to either *PGL1* or *PGL2.* Based on the genetic data, individuals harboring the affected chromosome and thus at risk for tumor formation could be identified. Individuals with a transmitted paternal allele who are at risk for PG should be aggressively followed both clinically and radiologically on a regular basis and offered genetic counseling. Those who have inherited the affected gene through maternal transmission should be advised of the clinically silent carrier state and be offered genetic counseling. Those with a noncarrier state can be advised that no increased risk for tumor development is present over the general population.[94]

Alternatively, the DNA extracted from the patient's blood could be directly tested for mutation in *SDHD* using polymerase chain reaction and direct DNA sequencing. If a mutation is identified, the family members could then be tested to see if they too harbor the mutation and therefore are at risk for tumor formation. It is hoped that genetic screening will lead to earlier identification of tumors to reduce the morbidity and mortality associated with its natural history and treatment. Ultimately, identification of the genetic alteration involved in both hereditary and sporadic PGs should lead to opportunities for genetic manipulation of tumor growth.

SUMMARY

A basic understanding of genetics is crucial to the practicing otologist and neuro-otologist. Genetic screening and genetic testing have already permeated into our daily practice. In the very near future, gene-based therapies too will dramatically change how we treat hearing loss and tumors of the temporal bone and cerebellopontine angle.

References

1. Lalwani AK, Lynch E, Mhatre AN. Molecular genetics: A brief overview. In: Lalwani A, Grundfast K, editors. Pediatric otology and neurotology. Philadelphia: Lippincot-Raven; 1998. p. 49–86.
2. Brookhouser P. Sensorineural hearing loss in children. Pediatr Clin North Am 1996;43:1195–216.
3. Mehl A, Thomson V. Newborn hearing screening: The great omission. Pediatrics 1998;101:e4.
4. Kheterpal U, Lalwani AK. Nonsyndromic hereditary hearing impairment. In: Lalwani A, Grundfast K, editors. Pediatric otology and neurotology. Philadelphia: Lippincott-Raven; 1998. p. 313–40.
5. Mhatre AN, Lalwani AK. Molecular genetics of deafness. Otolaryngol Clin North Am 1996;29:421–35.
6. Yaeger M, Nicholson BJ. Structural of gap junction intercellular channels. Curr Opin Struct Biol 1996;6:183–92.
7. Kelsell DP, Dunlop J, Stevens HP, et al. Connexin 26 mutations in hereditary non-syndromic sensorineural deafness. Nature 1997;387:80–3.
8. Kikuchi T, Adams JC, Paul DL, Kimura RS. Gap junction systems in the rat vestibular labyrinth: Immunohistochemical and ultrastructural analysis. Acta Otolaryngol (Stockh) 1994; 114:520–8.
9. Kikuchi T, Kimura RS, Paul DL, Adams JC. Gap junctions in the rat cochlea: Immunohistochemical and ultrastructural analysis. Anat Embryol 1995;191:101–18.
10. Guilford P, Ben Arab S, Blanchard S, et al. A non-syndromic form of neurosensory recessive deafness maps to the pericentromeric region of chromosome 13q. Nat Genet 1994;6:24–8.
11. Van Camp G, Willems PJ, Smith RJH. Nonsyndromic hearing impairment: Unparalleled heterogeneity. Am J Hum Genet 1997;60:758–64.
12. Zelante L, Gasparini P, Estivill X, et al. Connexin 26 mutations associated with the most common form of non-syndromic neurosensory autosomal recessive deafness (DFNB1) in Mediterraneans. Hum Mol Genet 1997;6:1605–9.
13. Kelley PM, Harris DJ, Comer BC, et al. Novel mutations in the connexin 26 gene (GJB2) that cause autosomal recessive (DFNB1) hearing loss. Am J Hum Genet 1998;62:792–9.
14. Cohn ES, Kelley PM. Clinical phenotype and mutations in connexin 26 (DFNB 1/GJB2), the most common cause of childhood hearing loss. Am J Med Genet 1999;89:130–6.
15. Morell RJ, Kim HJ, Hood LJ, et al. Mutations in the connexin 26 gene (GJB2) among Ashkenazi Jews with nonsyndromic recessive deafness. N Engl J Med 1998;339:1500–5.
16. Denoyelle F, Weil D, Maw MA, et al. Prelingual deafness: High prevalence of a 30delG mutation in the connexin 26 gene. Hum Mol Genet 1997;6:2173–7.
17. Estivill X, Fortina P, Surrey S, et al. Connexin 26 mutations in sporadic and inherited sensorineural deafness. Lancet 1998;351:394–8.
18. Lench N, Houseman M, Newton V, et al. Connexin 26 mutations in sporadic non-syndromal sensorineural deafness. Lancet 1998;351:415.

19. Antoniadi T, Rabionet R, Kroupis C, et al. High prevalence in the Greek population of the 35delG mutation in the connexin 26 gene causing prelingual deafness. Clin Genet 1999;55:381–2.
20. Sobe T, Vreugde S, Shahin H, et al. The prevalence and expression of inherited connexin 26 mutations associated with non-syndromic hearing loss in the Israeli population. Hum Genet 2000;106:50–7.
21. Carrasquillo MM, Zlotogora J, Barges S, Chakravarti A. Two different connexin 26 mutations in an inbred kindred segregating non-syndromic recessive deafness: Implications for genetic studies in isolated populations. Hum Mol Genet 1997;6: 2163–72.
22. Fuse Y, Doi K, Hasegawa T, et al. Three novel connexin 26 gene mutations in autosomal recessive non-syndromic deafness. Neuroreport 1999;10:1853–7.
23. Abe S, Usami S, Shinkawa H, et al. Prevalent connexin 26 (GJB2) mutations in Japanese. J Med Genet 2000;37:41–3.
24. Kudo T, Ikeda K, Kure S, et al. Novel mutations in the connexin 26 gene (GJB2) responsible for childhood deafness in the Japanese population. Am J Med Genet 2000;90:141–5.
25. Lin D, Goldstein JA, Mhatre AN, et al. Assessment of denaturing high-performance liquid chromatography (DHPLC) in screening for mutations in connexin 26. Hum Mutat 2001;18(1):42–51.
26. Denoyelle F, Marlin S, Weil D, et al. Clinical features of the prevalent form of childhood deafness, DFNB 1, due to a connexin-26 gene defect: Implications for genetic counselling. Lancet 1999;353:1298–303.
27. Marlin S, Garabedian EN, Roger G, et al. Connexin 26 gene mutations in congenitally deaf children: Pitfalls for genetic counseling. Arch Otolaryngol Head Neck Surg 2001;127:927–33.
28. Pendred V. Deaf mutism and goitre. Lancet 1896;11:532.
29. Smith RE. Pendred's syndrome. A historical note. Guys Hosp Rep 1969;118:519–21.
30. Batsakis JG, Nishiyama RH. Deafness with sporadic goiter: Pendred's syndrome. Arch Otolaryngol 1962;76:401–6.
31. Gomez-Pan A, Evered DC, Hall R. Pituitary-thyroid function in Pendred's syndrome. BMJ 1974;2:152–3.
32. Fraser GR, Morgans ME, Trotter WR. The syndrome of sporadic goiter and congenital deafness. Q J Med 1960;29:279–95.
33. Cremers CW, Admiraal RJ, Huygen PL, et al. Progressive hearing loss, hypoplasia of the cochlea and widened vestibular aqueducts are very common features in Pendred's syndrome. Int J Pediatr Otorhinolaryngol 1998;45:113–23.
34. Phelps PD, Coffey RA, Trembath RC, et al. Radiological malformations of the ear in Pendred's syndrome. Clin Radiol 1998;53:268–73.
35. Everett LA, Glaser B, Beck JC, et al. Pendred's syndrome is caused by mutations in a putative sulphate transporter gene (PDS). Nat Genet 1997;17:411–22.
36. Scott DA, Wang R, Kreman TM, et al. The Pendred's syndrome gene encodes a chloride-iodide transport protein. Nat Genet 1999;21:440–3.
37. Van Hauwe P, Everett LA, Coucke P, et al. Two frequent missense mutations in Pendred's syndrome. Hum Mol Genet 1998;7:1099–104.
38. Usami S, Abe S, Weston MD, et al. Non-syndromic hearing loss associated with enlarged vestibular aqueduct is caused by PDS mutations. Hum Genet 1999;104:188–92.
39. Scott DA, Wang R, Kreman TM, et al. Functional differences of the PDS gene product are associated with phenotypic variation in patients with Pendred's syndrome and non-syndromic hearing loss (DFNB4). Hum Mol Genet 2000;9:1709–15.
40. Mafong DD, Shin EJ, Lalwani AK. Utility of laboratory evaluation and radiologic imaging in the diagnostic evaluation of children with sensorineural hearing loss. Laryngoscope 2002;112:1–7.
41. Avraham KB, Hasson T, Sobe T, et al. Characterization of unconventional MYO6, the human homologue of the gene responsible for deafness in Snell's waltzer mice. Hum Mol Genet 1997;6:1225–31.
42. Hasson T, Walsh J, Cable J, et al. Effects of shaker-1 mutations on myosin-VIIa protein and mRNA expression. Cell Motil Cytoskeleton 1997;37:127–38.
43. Sellers JR. Myosins: a diverse superfamily. Biochim Biophys Acta 2000;1496:3–22.
44. Lalwani AK, Linthicum FH, Wilcox ER, et al. A three-generation family with late-onset, progressive hereditary hearing impairment and cochleosaccular degeneration. Audiol Neurootol 1997;2:139–54.
45. Lalwani AK, Luxford WM, Mhatre AN, et al. A new locus for nonsyndromic hereditary hearing impairment (DFNA17) maps to chromosome 22 and represents a gene for cochleosaccular degeneration. Am J Hum Genet 1999;64:318–23.
46. Lalwani AK, Goldstein JA, Kelley MJ, et al. Human nonsyndromic deafness DFNA17 is due to a mutation in nonmuscle myosin MYH9. Am J Hum Genet 2000;67:1121–8.
47. Coling DE, Espreafico EM, Kachar B. Cellular distribution of myosin-V in the guinea pig cochlea. J Neurocytol 1997;26:113–20.
48. Gillespie PG. Deaf and dizzy mice with mutated myosin motors. Nat Med 1996;2:27–9.
49. Tilney LG, Derosier DJ, Mulroy MJ. The organization of actin filaments in the stereocilia of cochlear hair cells. J Cell Biol 1980;86:244–59.
50. Wallace DC. Mitochondrial DNA mutations in diseases of energy metabolism. J Bioenerg Biomembr 1994;26:241–50.
51. Prezant TR, Agapian JV, Bohlman MC, et al. Mitochondrial ribosomal RNA mutation associated with both antibiotic-induced and non-syndromic deafness. Nat Genet 1993;4:289–94.
52. van den Ouweland JM, Lemkes HH, Trembath RC, et al. Maternally inherited diabetes and deafness is a distinct subtype of diabetes and associates with a single point mutation in the mitochondrial tRNA(Leu[UUR]) gene. Diabetes 1994;43:746–51.
53. Ballinger SW, Shoffner JM, Hedaya EV, et al. Maternally transmitted diabetes and deafness associated with a 10.4 kb mitochondrial DNA deletion. Nat Genet 1992;1:11–5.
54. Katagiri H, Asano T, Ishihara H, et al. Mitochondrial diabetes mellitus: Prevalence and clinical characterization of diabetes due to mitochondrial tRNA(Leu[UUR]) gene mutation in Japanese patients. Diabetologia 1994;37:504–10.
55. Evans DGR, Huson SM, Donnai D, et al. A genetic study of type 2 neurofibromatosis in the United Kingdom. 1. Prevalence, mutation rate, fitness and confirmation of maternal transmission effect on severity. J Med Genet 1992;29:841–6.
56. Kanter WR, Eldridge R, Fabricant R, et al. Central neurofibromatosis with bilateral acoustic neuroma: Genetic, clinical and

biochemical distinctions from peripheral neurofibromatosis. Neurology 1980;30:851–9.

57. King TT, Gibson WPR, Morrison AW. Tumors of the VIIIth cranial nerve. Br J Hosp Med 1976;16:259–72.
58. Abaza MM, Makariow EV, Armstrong M, Lalwani AK. Growth rate characteristics of acoustic neuromas associated with neurofibromatosis type 2. Laryngoscope 1996;106:694–9.
59. Lalwani AK, Abaza MM, Makariow EV, Armstrong M. Audiologic presentation of vestibular schwannomas in neurofibromatosis type 2. Am J Otol 1998;19:352–7.
60. Barker D, Wright E, Nguyen L, et al. Gene for von Recklinghausen neurofibromatosis is in the pericentromeric region of chromosome 17. Science 1987;236:1100–2.
61. Rouleau G, Seizinger VR, Ozelius LG, et al. Genetic linkage analysis of bilateral acoustic neurofibromatosis to a DNA marker on chromosome 22. Nature 1987;329:246–8.
62. Evans DG, Huson SM, Donnai D, et al. A genetic study of type 2 neurofibromatosis in the United Kingdom. II. Guidelines for genetic counselling. J Med Genet 1992;29:847–52.
63. Zang KD. Cytological and cytogenetics studies on human meningioma. Cancer Genet Cytogenet 1982;6:249–74.
64. Seizinger BR, Martuza RL, Gusella JF. Loss of genes on chromosome 22 in tumorigenesis of human acoustic neuroma. Nature 1986;322:644–7.
65. Rouleau GA, Merel P, Lutchman M, et al. Alteration in a new gene encoding a putative membrane-organizing protein causes neurofibromatosis type 2. Nature 1993;363:515–21.
66. Trofatter JA, MacCollin MM, Rutter JL, et al. A novel moesin-, ezrin-, radixin-like gene is a candidate for the neurofibromatosis 2 tumor suppressor. Cell 1993;72:791–800.
67. Gonzalez-Agosti C, Xu L, Pinney D, et al. The merlin tumor suppressor localises preferentially in membrane ruffles. Oncogene 1996;13:1239–47.
68. Vaheri A, Carpen O, Heiska L, et al. The ezrin protein family: membrane cytoskeleton interactions and disease associations. Curr Opin Cell Biol 1997;9:659–66.
69. Lutchman M, Rouleau GA. The neurofibromatosis type 2 gene product, schwannomin, suppresses growth of NIH 3T3 cells. Cancer Res 1995;55:2270–74.
70. Tikoo A, Varga M, Ramesh V, et al. An anti-RAS function of neurofibromatosis type 2 gene product. J Biol Chem 1994;269: 23389–90.
71. Irving RM, Moffat DA, Hardy DG, et al. Molecular genetic analysis of the mechanism of tumorigenesis in acoustic neuroma. Arch Otolaryngol Head Neck Surg 1993;119:1222–8.
72. Welling DB, Guida M, Goll F, et al. Mutational spectrum in the neurofibromatosis type 2 gene in sporadic and familial schwannomas. Hum Genet 1996;98:189–93.
73. Merel P, Hoang-Xuan K, Sanson M, et al. Predominant occurrence of somatic mutations of the NF2 gene in meningiomas and schwannomas. Genes Chromosomes Cancer 1995;13:211–6.
74. Kluwe L, Mautner VF. A missense mutation in the NF-2 gene results in moderate and mild clinical phenotypes of neurofibromatosis type 2. Hum Genet 1996;97:224–7.
75. Bianchi AB, Hara T, Ramesh V, et al. Mutations in transcript isoforms of the neurofibromatosis 2 gene in multiple human tumour types. Nat Genet 1994;6:185–92.
76. Bianchi AB, Mitsunaga SI, Cheng JQ, et al. High frequency of inactivating mutations in the neurofibromatosis type 2 gene (NF2) in primary malignant mesotheliomas. Proc Natl Acad Sci U S A 1995;92:10854–8.
77. Ruttledge MH, Sarrazin J, Rangaratnam S, et al. Evidence for the complete inactivation of the NF2 gene in the majority of sporadic meningiomas. Nat Genet 1994;6:180–4.
78. Sekido Y, Pass H, Bader S, et al. Neurofibromatosis type II (NF-2) gene is somatically mutated in mesothelioma but not in lung cancer. Cancer Res 1995;55:1227–31.
79. Ruttledge MH, Andermann AA, Phelan CM, et al. Type of mutation in the neurofibromatosis type 2 gene (NF2) frequently determines severity of disease. Am J Hum Genet 1996;59:331–42.
80. Parry DM, MacCollin MM, Kaiser-Kupfer MI, et al. Germ-like mutations in the neurofibromatosis 2 gene: correlation with disease severity and retinal abnormalities. Am J Hum Genet 1996; 59:529–39.
81. Hall JG. Genomic imprinting: review and relevance to human diseases. Am J Hum Genet 1990;46:857–73.
82. Bikhazi PH, Messina L, Mhatre AN, et al. Molecular pathogenesis in sporadic head and neck paraganglioma. Laryngoscope 2000;110:1346–8.
83. Heutink P, van der Mey AG, Sandkuijl LA, et al. A gene subject to genomic imprinting and responsible for hereditary paragangliomas maps to chromosome 1 1q23-qter. Hum Mol Genet 1992;1:7–10.
84. Heutink P, van Schothorst EM, van der Mey AG, et al. Further localization of the gene for hereditary paragangliomas and evidence for linkage in unrelated families. Eur J Hum Genet 1994;2:148–58.
85. Baysal BE, Farr JE, Rubinstein WS, et al. Fine mapping of an imprinted gene for familial nonchromaffin paragangliomas, on chromosome 11q23. Am J Hum Genet 1997;60:121–32.
86. Milunsky J, DeStefano AL, Huang XL, et al. Familial paragangliomas: linkage to chromosome 11q23 and clinical implications. Am J Med Genet 1997;72:66–70.
87. Devilee P, van Schothorst EM, Bardoel AF, et al. Allelotype of head and neck paragangliomas: allelic imbalance is confined to the long arm of chromosome 11, the site of the predisposing locus PGL. Genes Chromosomes Cancer 1994;11:71–8.
88. Knudson AG Jr. Genetics of human cancer. J Cell Physiol Suppl 1986;4:7–11.
89. Baysal BE, Ferrell RE, Willett-Brozick JE, et al. Mutations in SDHD, a mitochondrial complex II gene, in hereditary paraganglioma. Science 2000;287:848–51.
90. Mariman EC, van Beersum SE, Cremers CW, et al. Analysis of a second family with hereditary non-chromaffin paragangliomas locates the underlying gene at the proximal region of chromosome 1 1q. Hum Genet 1993;91:357–61.
91. Mariman EC, van Beersum SE, Cremers CW, et al. Fine mapping of a putatively imprinted gene for familial non-chromaffin paragangliomas to chromosome 11q13.1: evidence for genetic heterogeneity. Hum Genet 1995;95:56–62.
92. Niemann, S, Steinberger D, Muller U. PGL3, a third, not maternally imprinted locus in autosomal dominant paraganglioma. Neurogenetics 1999;2:167–70.
93. Niemann S, Muller U. Mutations in SDHC cause autosomal dominant paraganglioma, type 3. Nat Genet 2000;26:268–70.

94. Bikhazi PH, Roeder E, Attaie A, et al. Familial paragangliomas: The emerging impact of molecular genetics on evaluation and management. Am J Otol 1999;20:639–43.

Recent Review Articles of Interest

Kochhar A, Hildebrand MS, Smith RJ. Clinical aspects of hereditary hearing loss. Genet Med. 2007;9(7):393–408.

Brown SD, Hardisty-Hughes RE, Mburu P. Quiet as a mouse: Dissecting the molecular and genetic basis of hearing. Nat Rev Genet. 2008;9(4):277–90.

Welling DB, Packer MD, Chang LS. Molecular studies of vestibular schwannomas: A review. Curr Opin Otolaryngol Head Neck Surg. 2007;15(5):341–6.

Mittendorf EA, Evans DB, Lee JE, Perrier ND. Pheochromocytoma: Advances in genetics, diagnosis, localization, and treatment. Hematol Oncol Clin North Am 2007;21(3):509–25.

Tumor Biology 8

D. Bradley Welling, MD, PhD, FACS / Mark D. Packer, MD

INTRODUCTION

Recent advances in molecular biology have led to a better understanding of the etiology of many cranial base tumors. The development of new treatment options with improved outcomes and decreased morbidity by growth stabilization, or possible prevention is the goal of understanding the cellular mechanisms involved in the tumorigenesis. Indeed trials of several therapeutic agents targeting known pathways are underway.

As an example of the recent advances in this field, vestibular schwannomas (VS) will be highlighted. VS generally arise as sporadic unilateral tumors of the internal auditory canal (IAC) and the cerebellopontine angle (CPA); however, they are also found bilaterally as the hallmark of the inherited genetic disorder Neurofibromatosis 2 (NF2) [Online Mendelian Inheritance in Man (OMIM) #101000]. The NF2 syndrome is the autosomal-dominant manifestation of a biallelic mutation of the human chromosome 22, which gives rise to VS, as well as meningiomas, ependymomas, and presenile cataracts.

Fundamental understanding of the underlying molecular events leading to tumor formation began when the neurofibromatosis type 2 tumor suppressor gene (*NF2* gene) was identified and mutations confirmed in the VS or the germline.[1–3] The clinical characteristics of VS and NF2 syndromes have both been related to alterations in the *NF2* gene. The clinical manifestations of NF2 associated with various mutations have been described and signaling pathways affected by merlin, the product of the *NF2* gene, are becoming better understood.

For purposes of this chapter and elsewhere in the literature, abbreviations are as follows: "NF2" is used to indicate the human disease of neurofibromatosis type 2; the italicized "*NF2*" represents the human neurofibromatosis type 2 gene; and "*Nf2*" indicates the homolog or similar gene expressed in rodents. The mouse *Nf2* gene and the human *NF2* gene share greater than 98% amino acid homology, thus making the mouse a very relevant model for study. Interestingly, chickens have 94% and drosophila 50% human amino acid homology as well.[4]

The nomenclature $nf^{+/+}$ is wild type or normal nf gene. $nf^{-/-}$ refers to the absence of both alleles (homozygosity) and $nf^{+/-}$ refers to a heterozygosity or one allele only being nonfunctional.

Vestibular schwannomas can be grouped into unilateral sporadic solid VS or bilateral NF2-associated schwannomas. VS with true cysts or cystic schwannomas present a unique and aggressive phenotype, which may distinguish it from the more benign solid unilateral sporadic schwannoma. Mutations in the *NF2* gene have been identified in all three tumor types, but at the molecular level, the tumors are only beginning to be distinguished from each other.[5,6]

Schwannomas most commonly present as solitary tumors and constitute 95% of all VS. Sporadic unilateral VS occur in approximately 10 to 20 persons per million per year.[7,8] However, the true incidence may be higher, as highlighted by Anderson et al.[9] who demonstrated an incidence of 7 unsuspected schwannomas per 10,000 brain MRI studies (0.07%) or 70 per million. Sporadic tumors usually occur in the 4th and 5th decades with a mean presentation at about 50 years of age. Although histologically benign, schwannomas can compress the brain stem, leading to hydrocephalus, herniation, and death. Most commonly, however, they are associated with hearing loss, tinnitus, imbalance, facial paralysis, and facial paresthesias (see Figure 37–4).

NF2 [OMIM #101000] is clinically an autosomal-dominant disease that is highly penetrant.[10] NF2–associated tumors account for about 5% of all VS. Patients who inherit an abnormal copy of the *NF2* tumor suppressor gene have a 95% chance of developing bilateral VS (see Figure 37–2). However, about one half of patients have no family history of NF2, and thus as founders, they represent new germline mutations that were not inherited. Other disease features of NF2 include intracranial meningiomas, ependymomas, spinal schwannomas, and presenile lens opacities.[11–14] The onset of symptoms is usually between 11 and 30 years of age, but for some patients, the symptoms may present in their 5th or 6th decade. The incidence is estimated at between 1 in 33,000 and 1 in 40,000.[15,16] NF2 is not to be confused with neurofibromatosis type 1 (NF1) or von Recklinghausen's disease [OMIM #162200]. NF1, which is associated with multiple peripheral neurofibromas, is caused by a mutation in the *NF1* tumor suppressor gene on chromosome 17.

The spectrum of phenotypic expression in NF2 varies widely. In the past, the more severe clinical presentations were termed the Wishart type.[17] In addition to bilateral VS, patients often suffered from associated spinal tumors with a typical onset of symptoms in the late teens or early twenties. The less severe phenotypes have been termed the Gardner type with a later onset of bilateral schwannomas and fewer associated intracranial or spinal tumors.[18] In truth, the spectrum of disease does not always allow a clear distinction, but rather follows a continuum.

Occasionally segmental or mosaic categories of NF2 are also included to describe another classification of NF2.[19] The cause of segmental NF2 may be due to somatic mosaicism where a mutation occurs later in embryogenesis rather than in the germline DNA; therefore, only a portion of the patients' cells carry the mutation, and the disease is manifested in limited areas of the body.[20,21] In contrast, patients with familial NF2 inherit one mutation from a parent at conception and all cells carry one mutant allele. Kluwe et al.[21] estimated that mosaicism may account for 25% of the NF2 cases of any subtype among patients whose parents did not display the disease. Patients with somatic mosaicism can display bilateral VS if the postzygotic mutation occurred early in embryogenesis. However, they may also display an atypical presentation, or segmental NF2, in which the patient has a unilateral vestibular schwannoma and an ipsilateral, additional intracranial tumor, such as a meningioma, if the postzygotic mutation occurred later in development.[22] Unlike the traditional forms of NF2, the risk of passing NF2 caused by mosaicism to future offspring is low.

CYSTIC SCHWANNOMAS

Cystic VS are a particularly aggressive group of unilateral, sporadic schwannomas, which invade the surrounding cranial nerves, splaying them throughout the tumors. Cystic VS are associated with either intratumoral or extratumoral cysts, which develop in the loosely organized Antoni B tissues. In addition, a higher degree of nuclear atypia is seen in cystic tumors.[23,24] Careful distinction must be drawn between the truly cystic schwannomas and the very common heterogeneous schwannomas, which are not as aggressive in their clinical behavior. On magnetic resonance imaging (MRI), truly cystic regions of the tumors are hyperintense on T2-weighted images, and the cysts do not enhance with gadolinium administration. The noncystic component of the cystic tumors enhances with gadolinium in a manner similar to the unilateral and NF2-associated schwannomas (see Figure 37–5A and B). Cystic tumors may grow rapidly and are difficult to manage due to the high rate of hearing loss, facial nerve paralysis, and recurrence that occurs after surgical removal.[25] When compared to solid tumors of a similar size, the rate of complete facial nerve paralysis (House–Brachmann grade VI) with surgical removal of cystic tumors was 41%, as compared to 27% for that of solid unilateral schwannomas.[26] Cystic tumors are also more likely to have continued growth and facial nerve paralysis when treated with stereotactic radiation therapy than either the unilateral spontaneous or NF2-associated schwannomas.[27,28]

Although the effectiveness of treatment with current surgical and radiation treatments for VS are generally good, treatment-related morbidity continues to be problematic. A brief review of the recent discoveries and advances in the molecular biology of VS will follow.

The NF2 Gene

The *NF2* gene was localized to chromosome 22 band q12 through genetic and physical mapping (Figure 8–1A to C).[29,30] Positional cloning studies led to the discovery of the *NF2* gene in 1993 by two independent groups, Rouleau et al.[2] and Trofatter et al.[1] The gene was found to be frequently mutated in NF2-related VS. Since that time, mutations in the *NF2* gene have been found not only in NF2-associated tumors but also in sporadic unilateral schwannomas and cystic schwannomas.[3,31–37] Additionally, mutations within the *NF2* gene have been frequently identified in meningiomas and occasionally identified in other tumor types such as mesotheliomas.[35–43]

Human NF2 Mutations and Their Clinical Correlation

Specific *NF2* mutations in VS have been characterized in sporadic unilateral schwannomas and NF2-associated schwannomas.[3,32–36,38,44–58] The frequency, type, and distribution of *NF2* mutations were shown to be different between the sporadic and familial NF2 tumors.[3] Point mutations accounted for the majority of mutations identified in NF2 patients, whereas small deletions accounted for the majority of mutations found in the sporadic unilateral tumors.[46,47,55]

Two groups have recently published large data bases of NF2 mutations. Ahronowitz et al.[59] presented a meta-analysis of 1,070 small genetic changes detected primarily by exon scanning including 42 intragenic changes of 1 whole exon or larger, and 29 whole gene deletions and gross chromosomal rearrangements. Overall, somatic events detected by tumor analysis showed a significantly different genetic profile than constitutional events detected in the patients leukocytes. Over half of the mutations detected in tumors were frameshift mutations. The deletion of a single nucleotide (A < T < C < or G) from a gene can have a particularly disrupting affect because all of the codons downstream from the mutation are changed. In comparison constitutional or system wide inherited changes were primarily nonsense and splice site mutations (see Figure 8–2A to C).[60] Somatic events also differed markedly in meningiomas where most mutations were within the 5-prime four, ezrin, radixin, and moesin (FERM) domain of the transcript with a complete absence of mutations in exons 14 and 15. Less than 10% of small alterations were nontruncating or lesions, which would not completely destroy the protein. These changes were clustered in exons 2 and 3, suggesting that this region may be especially crucial to tumor suppressor activity in the protein. We and others have shown a frequent pattern of mutation changing arginine codons (CGA) to the thymine stop codon (TGA) (This type of "stop" codon not only terminates the transcription of mRNA, but often results in degradation of the mRNA already transcribed.) in both VS and meningiomas, causing a truncating lesion.[3,60] The chemical bonds associated with the configuration

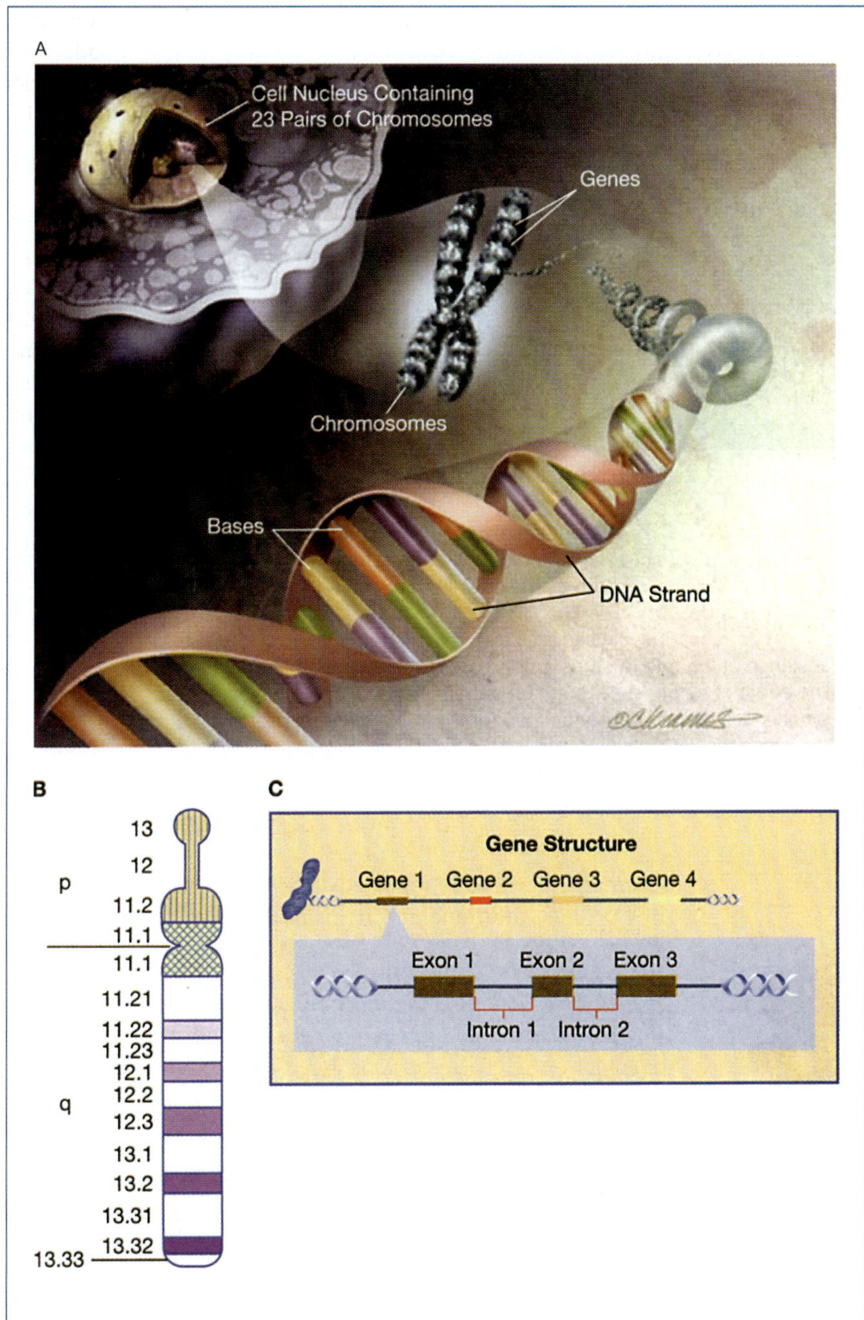

FIGURE 8–1 • *A*, Picture indicating the relationship of chromosomes, genes, and DNA nucleotide bases. *B*, Diagram of one arm of chromosome 22, depicting the p and q segments of the chromosome. *C*, A model of a human gene. The information contained in the gene and used for synthesis of the protein is split between exons (which code for the protein) and introns (noncoding sequences).

of these nucleotides make them less stable and more likely to undergo spontaneous mutation not only in NF2 but many other tumors as well. No mutations have been reported in exons 16 and 17, and few were noted in exon 9.

Studies to determine if genotype could be a predicator of disease severity showed that deletions that caused truncation of the NF2 protein have a more severe phenotype in NF2 pedigrees,[46,47,55] while missense mutations (see Figure 8–2) or small in-frame insertions in the *NF2*-coding region have been reported to associate with a mild phenotype.[3,35,36,54,56,57] However, exceptions are common as some missense mutations have been associated with severe phenotypes. It would appear that the location of the mutation within the gene may be important as missense mutations within the α-helical domain of the NF2 protein (see Figure 8–3) appear to associate with a less severe phenotype than those within the conserved ERM domain.[61] This lack of genotype–phenotype correlation was also seen for large deletions, which could give rise to mild phenotypes as well as the previously reported severe disease expression.[62] Clinical studies indicate that the phenotypic expression is more closely related within families than between families, but even within families, variability exists.[63] When statistically analyzed, the age of onset of NF2, the age at onset of hearing loss, and the number of intracranial meningiomas, were all found to have a significant intrafamilial correlation.[64] It is not known whether this variability occurs by chance, by epigenetic phenomena, or by modifying genes at other loci.[65] Epigenetic phenomena are not caused by a change in the coding sequence of the DNA but

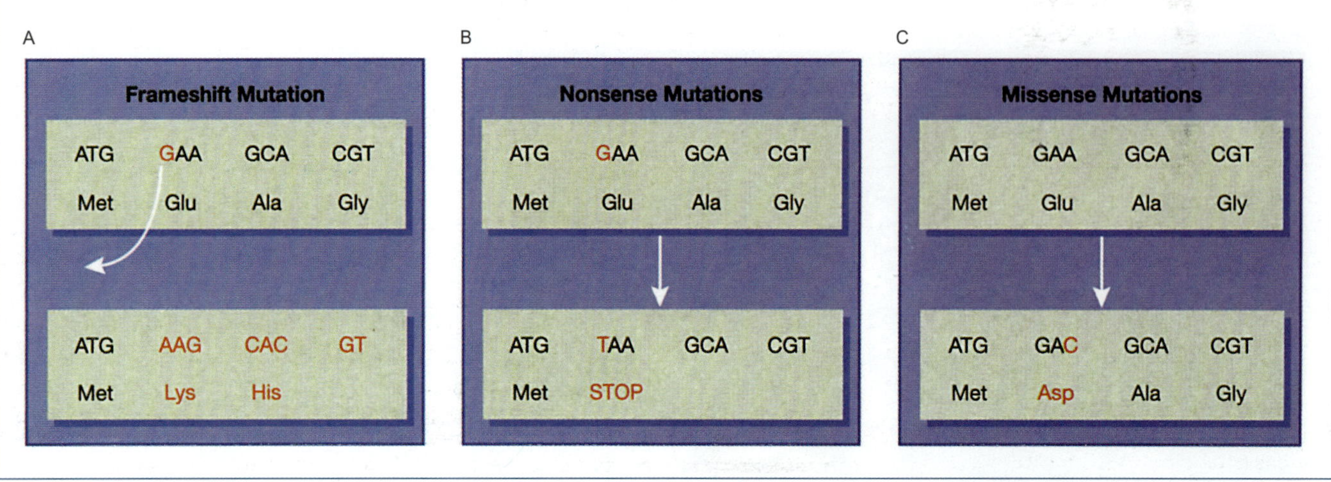

FIGURE 8–2 • *A*, The deletion of a single nucleotide (A, T, C, or G) from a gene can have a particularly disrupting affect on the gene because the deletion of one nucletide changes all of the codons downstream from the change, resulting in a frameshift mutation. The deletion of the "G" base changes the downstream coding such that instead of coding for…Glu-Ala-Gly, the mutated gene now codes for…Lys-His… downstream from the mutation. *B*, A nonsense mutation is one that converts a codon that specifies an amino acid into a termination codon. This results in a shortened protein, since the translation of the mRNA stops at this new termination codon and not the correct one which if further downstream. The effect of a nonsense mutation depends on how much of the protein is lost. *C*, A point mutation or change of a single nucleotide can change a codon so that a different protein is specified. This is called a missense mutation, since the wrong amino acid is specified. The protein coded by the gene therefore has a change to a single amino acid. This often has no significant effect on the protein, as most can tolerate a few amino acid changes without their biological function changing.

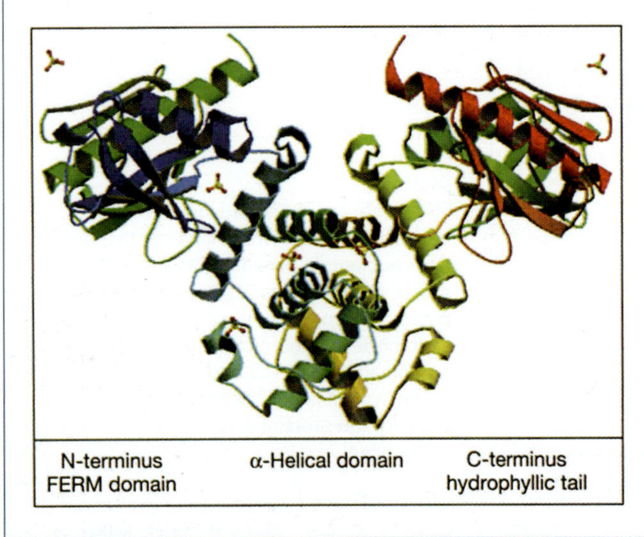

FIGURE 8–3 • The NF2 protein is divided into three general sections. The FERM domain is followed by an alpha-helical domain and a hydrophilic tail.[4] Merlin can dimerize with itself and heterodimerize with other ERM family proteins. *From Shimizu T, Seto A, Maita N, et al. (2002). Structural basis for neurofibromatosis type 2. Crystal structure of the merlin FERM domain. J. Biol. Chem. 277;(12):10332–6. doi:10.1074/jbc.M109979200. PMID 11756419*

rather alter the gene expression during gene development or cell proliferation. An example would be methylation of segments of the promoter region of the *NF2* gene, which suppress the expression of the gene. The *NF2*-coding region encompasses 17 exons spanning 90 kilo base-pairs (kBp) of DNA on chromosome 22.[1,2,66] By extensive screening of the entire *NF2* gene, Zucman-Rocci et al.[66] reported an 84% mutation detection rate in VS. Thus, additional mechanisms for inactivation of the *NF2* gene in some patients may exist. Mutation or methylation in the regulatory region of the *NF2* gene has been suggested (see Figure 8–4) as a possible mechanism of gene inactivation.[67–69] Posttranscriptional alternative splicing and differential polyadenylation may also be considered as possible means of inactivating the *NF2* gene.[68] Polyadenylation refers to the variable number of adenines that are attached at the 3′ end of the mRNA which may play a role in the way a gene is regulated. Alternative splicing refers to different patterns of splicing of exons which occurs, in this case the NF2 gene, resulting in differing isoforms of the gene. The two most common isoforms of NF2 have either exon 16 or exon 17 spliced out.

The NF2 Protein: Structure and Function

The *NF2* gene product is named merlin, for moesin-ezrin-radixin like protein, or *schwannomin*, a name derived from schwannoma.[1,2] For simplicity, the NF2 protein is referred to as "merlin" in this chapter. The *NF2* gene is transcribed into multiple RNA species by alternative splicing. Isoforms I and II are the two major RNA isoforms expressed in the cell. Isoform I encodes a 595-amino-acid protein and has exon 16 spliced out. Isoform II, containing all 17 exons, differs from isoform 1 only at the C-terminus. Insertion of exon 16 into the mRNA provides a new stop codon, resulting in a 590-amino-acid protein that is identical to isoform I over the first 579 residues. Intriguingly, only isoform I possess growth suppression activity.[70]

Merlin shares a high degree of homology to the erythrocyte protein 4.1-related superfamily of proteins, which act to

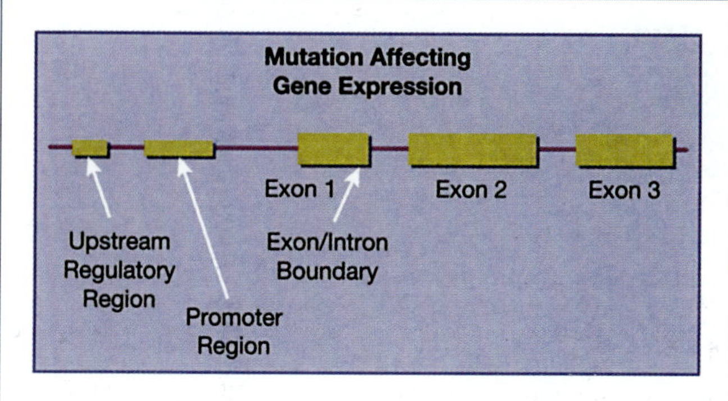

FIGURE 8–4 • Mutations can occur upstream of the gene itself in the promoter or regulatory regions or at the boundries between introns and exons (splice sites). Mutations in the promoter or regulatory regions may lead to over- or underexpression of the gene while mutations in the intron/exon boundaries may lead to aberrant splicing. Aberrant splicing might delete part of the resulting protein, add a new section of amino acids, or result in a frameshift.

link the actin cytoskeleton to the plasma membrane.[1,2] In particular, three proteins, ezrin, radixin, and moesin, referred to as the ERM family, share a great deal of structural similarity with merlin.[71,72] The proteins belonging to this family have a similar N-terminal globular domain, also known as the FERM domain, followed by an α-helical stretch, and finally a charged carboxyl-terminus.[72–74] The key functional domains of merlin may lie within the highly conserved FERM domains and the unique C-terminus of the protein. The ERM proteins have been shown to be involved in cellular remodeling involving the actin cytoskeleton.[75] These proteins bind actin filaments in the cytoskeleton via a conserved C-terminal domain and possibly via a second actin-binding site in the N-terminal half of the protein.[76,77]

Like the ERM proteins, merlin is expressed in a variety of cell types where it localizes to the areas of membrane remodeling, particularly membrane ruffles, although its precise distribution may differ from the ERM proteins expressed in the same cell.[78] Membrane ruffling is related to the interaction between the cytoskeleton with the cell body and the cell membrane. Schwannoma cells from NF2 tumors show dramatic alterations in the actin cytoskeleton and display abnormalities in cell spreading as well.[79] These results suggest that merlin may play an important role in regulating both the actin cytoskeleton-mediated processes and cell proliferation.[80] However, it should be noted that merlin has a growth suppression role, while other ERM-family members seem to facilitate cell growth.

Merlin Acts as a Tumor Suppressor

Overexpression of the *NF2* gene in mouse fibroblasts or rat schwannoma cells limits cell growth[57,81,82] and suppresses cell transformation by the ras oncogene.[83] Without the *NF2* gene overexpressed, transformation occurs when a cancer-causing protein, ras, allows the cellular proliferation machinery to become activated without proper regulatory mechanisms in place, causing malignant tumor growth. The growth control of certain Schwann cells and meningeal cells is lost in the absence of *NF2* function, suggesting that *NF2* mutations and merlin deficiency disrupt some aspect of intracellular signaling that leads to cellular transformation. Together, these findings demonstrate merlin's ability to act as a growth suppressor.

Nf2 knockout mouse models, which are either heterozygous or homozygous for the *Nf2* gene in the germline, have been created.[84,85] Heterozygous *Nf2* knockout mice go on to develop osteosarcomas, and less often, fibrosarcomas or hepatocellular carcinomas.[84] Metastatic disease is common in this model. Genetic analysis shows that nearly all of these malignant tumors are missing both *Nf2* alleles. Tumor growth in the absence of both *Nf2* alleles indicates that the *Nf2* gene possesses a classical tumor suppressor function. However, none of the heterozygous *Nf2* mice develop tumors or clinical manifestations associated with human NF2. The *Nf2* gene also plays an important role during early embryogenesis. Homozygous *Nf2* mutant mice, which are missing both *Nf2* alleles, die at approximately 7 days of gestation from a gastrulation defect or failure of inward migration of cells. Merlin is important in cell migration as we and others have shown during embryogenesis.[85,86]

By engineering mice whose Schwann cells have exon 2 excised from both *Nf2* alleles, conditional homozygous *Nf2* knockout mice have been produced, which display some characteristics of NF2 including schwannomas, Schwann cell hyperplasia, cataracts, and osseous metaplasia.[87] A conditional knockout model is engineered by inserting a regulatory mechanism into the gene, allowing the investigator to choose the time at which the desired gene (in this case *Nf2)* will be knocked out. Although these results are in favor of the argument that loss of merlin is sufficient for schwannoma formation in vivo, none of the tumors observed in these conditional knockout mice were found on the vestibular nerve. This is in contrast to those VS commonly found in patients with NF2.

Biallelic *NF2* inactivation is also frequently found in sporadic and in NF2-associated meningiomas. By engineering mice whose arachnoidal cells have exon 2 excised from both *Nf2* alleles, homozygous $Nf2^{-/-}$ mice show a range of meningioma subtypes histologically similar to the human tumors.[88] Taken together, these results demonstrate a tumor suppressor function for merlin in both Schwann cells and arachnoidal cells.

Merlin Signaling and Regulation

Merlin overexpression (see Figure 8–5), unlike the other members of the ERM protein family, causes growth suppression. In addition to the actin cytoskeleton, merlin has been shown to associate with cell membrane domains, which are highly enriched in signaling molecules that regulate cellular responses to proliferative and antiproliferative stimuli.[89] Vestibular schwannoma cells with *NF2* inactivation have dramatic alterations in cell spreading.[79] To date, several proteins that are likely to interact with merlin have been identified including the ERM proteins, CD44, F-actin, paxillin, microtubules, βII-spectrin, β1-integrin, β-fodrin, the regulatory cofactor of Na^+–H^+ exchanger (NHE-RF), SCHIP-1, hepatocyte growth factor-regulated tyrosine kinase substrate (HRS), p21-activated kinase 1 and 2 (Pak1 and Pak2), Rac1, the RIB subunit of protein kinase A, components of cadherin-mediated cell junctions, PIKE-L [phosphatidylinositol

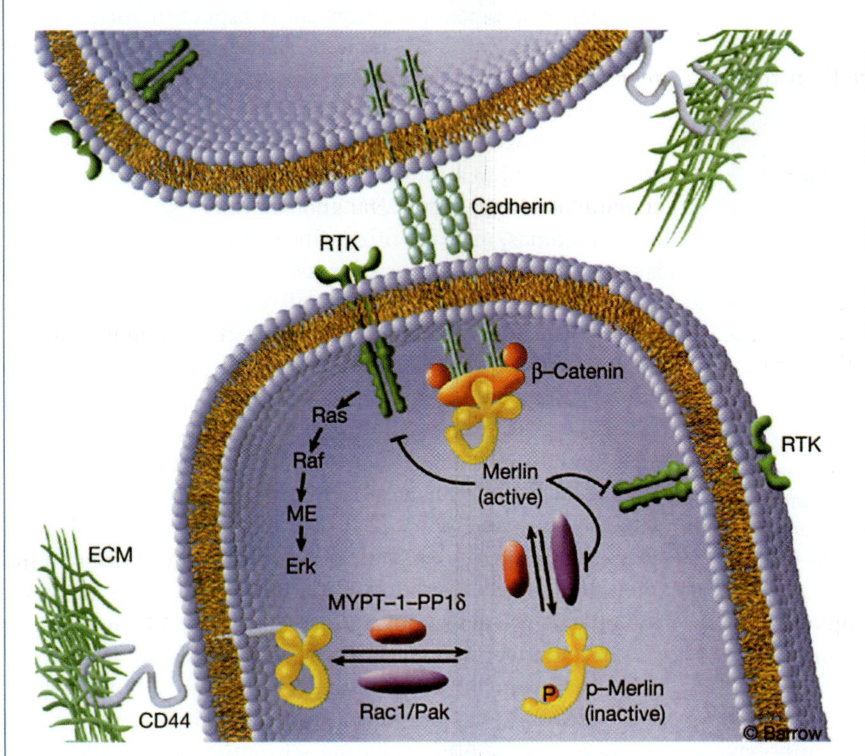

FIGURE 8–5 • Schematic diagram of merlin action. This diagram shows how Rac1 and Pak help convert the merlin protein from a closed conformation to an open conformation by phosphorylation of the protein. Consequently, merlin, in its open conformation, can interact with CD44 and facilitate linking the actin cytoskeleton to the cell membrane. p21-activated kinase 2 (Pak2) has been shown to phosphorylate merlin at serine 518 and inactivates its function. Merlin is activated by dephosphorylation by myosin phosphatase (MYPT-1-PP1δ).

3-kinase (PI3-kinase) enhancer], and erbin (erbB2-interacting protein).[82,90–107]

Presently, how all of these protein–protein interactions relate to the tumor suppressor activity of merlin is largely not understood. The association of merlin with CD44 and β1-integrin raises the possibility that merlin might function as a molecular switch in the signaling pathways. CD44 is a transmembrane hyaluronic acid receptor implicated in cell–cell adhesion, cell–matrix adhesion, cell motility, and metastasis.[90,101] Merlin mediates contact inhibition of cell growth through signals from the extracellular matrix. At high cell density, merlin becomes hypophosphorylated and inhibits cell growth in response to hyaluronate, a mucopolysaccharide that surrounds cells.[108] At low cell density, merlin is phosphorylated, growth permissive, and exists in a complex with ezrin, moesin, and CD44. These data indicate that merlin and CD44 form a molecular switch that specifies cell growth arrest or proliferation.

Lallemand et al.[105] showed that in *Nf2*$^{-/-}$ mouse embryo fibroblasts, *Nf2* deficiency led to piling-up of cells, hyperproliferation, and defective cadherin-mediated cell–cell interactions. When functioning normally, these interactions terminate proliferation by contact inhibition through specialized connections called adherens junctions. Furthermore, merlin colocalizes and interacts with and causes maturation of these adherens junction components in confluent or touching wild-type cells. Stated simply, when normal Schwann cells contact each other, special signaling through these junctions stops further growth. In the absence of merlin, the adherens junctions are immature and do not stop the schwannoma cells from terminating their growth when they contact each other. These results indicate that merlin functions as a tumor suppressor at least in part by controlling cadherin-mediated cell–cell contact.[109]

Merlin's function is regulated by phosphorylation.[106,110] Racl, a member of the RhoGTPase family, has been demonstrated to promote phosphorylation of merlin, thereby inactivating its growth suppressor mechanism.[111,112] Among the effectors of Racl and Cdc42 GTPases, members of the p21-activated kinase (PAK) family have demonstrated interactions with merlin. Specifically, (Pak2) has been shown to phosphorylate merlin at serine 518 and inactivate its function.[89,104,113,114] Kissil et al.[114] also reported an interaction between merlin and Pak1, and merlin could inhibit the activation dynamic of Pak1. Loss of merlin expression leads to the inappropriate activation of Pak1, while overexpression of merlin results in the inhibition of Pak1 activity. Conversely, Merlin is activated by dephosphorylation at serine 518, which occurs on serum withdrawal or on cell–cell or cell–matrix contact.[108] Although the members of the PAK family have been implicated in various cellular processes, such as cytoskeletal reorganization and apoptotic signaling, their exact roles and functions have not been clearly defined. Jin et al.[115] identified the myosin phosphatase (MYPT-1-PP1δ) as a merlin phosphatase. Interestingly, the cellular MYPT-1-PP1δ-specific inhibitor, CPI-17, could cause decreased merlin activity by merlin phosphorylation, Ras activation, and transformation. These results implicate MYPT-1-PP1δ and CPI-17 as important regulatory components in the merlin tumor suppressor pathway.

Merlin's Growth Regulatory Function Is Related to Its Conformation and Protein-Protein Interactions

The activities of the ERM proteins are controlled by self-association of the proteins' N-terminal and C-terminal regions.[116,117] The ERM proteins can exist in the "closed" conformation, where the N- and C-terminal regions undergo an intramolecular interaction, thus folding the protein to mask the conserved actin-binding site (Figure 8–3). The molecule can be converted to the "open" conformation in which the intramolecular interaction is disrupted by signals such as phosphorylation or treatment with phosphoinositides.[104,114,118]

Merlin's ability to function as a growth regulator is also related to its ability to form such intramolecular associations.[119] Two such interactions have been identified. The first interaction is between residues that fold the N-terminal end of the protein onto itself, while the second interaction folds the entire protein so that there is contact between N- and C-terminal ends of the protein.[82,119,120] In a fashion similar to the ERM proteins, merlin may cycle between the "open" and "closed" conformations that differentially determine whether it binds with the ERM proteins or other molecules to transduce merlin's growth inhibition signal.[121] In addition, the association between merlin and HRS, a substrate implicated in the signaling pathway initiated by hepatocyte growth factor (HGF) binding to the c-met receptor,[122] appears to be regulated by merlin folding.[120] These results suggest that the ability of merlin to cycle between the "open" and "closed" conformations may integrate CD44 and HGF signaling pathways. All of these findings are relevant to growth regulation. Also, merlin can exert its activity by inhibiting phophotidyl inositol 3-kinase (PI3-kinase) through binding to PIKE-L, a brain-specific GTPase that binds to PI3-kinase and stimulates its lipid kinase activity.[106] This finding suggests that PIKE-L is an important mediator of merlin growth suppression. Along this notion, we have found that the PI3-kinase/Akt pathway is activated in VS.[123]

The NF2 Gene Promoter

Characterization of the *NF2* regulatory regions is important for screening for mutations in both spontaneous and familial tumors in which no mutation was found in the *NF2*-coding region. We have shown that transcription of the *NF2* gene is initiated at multiple start sites and multiple regions in the *NF2* promoter are required for full *NF2* promoter activity.[68,124] Both positive and negative regulatory elements required for transcription of the *NF2* gene have been found in the 5′ flanking region of the promoter (see Figure 8–4). In particular, a sequence rich in guanine and cytosine nucleotide bases located in the proximal regulatory region, which can be bound by the Sp1 transcription factor, serves as a positive regulatory element.[68] This region is the area of the gene adjacent to 5′ of the coding region which regulates, either positively or negatively, the translation of the DNA into messenger RNA as we have described. Both the 5′ and 3′ flanking regions of the human *NF2* locus are G/C-rich and could serve as a target for gene methylation and inactivation as a form of therapy.[67,68]

We have also shown that a 2.4-kb human *NF2* promoter could direct where the NF2 gene expression would occur as early as embryonic day 5.5.[86] During early development, strong *NF2* promoter activity was detected in the developing brain and in sites containing migrating cells including the neural tube closure and branchial arches. (Figure 8–6). Interestingly, a transient change of *NF2* promoter activity during neural crest cell migration was noted. While little promoter activity was detected in premigratory neural crest cells at the dorsal ridge region of the neural fold, significant activity was seen in the neural crest cells already migrating away from the dorsal neural tube. In addition, we detected considerable *NF2* promoter activity in various NF2-affected tissues such as the acoustic and trigeminal ganglia, spinal ganglia, optic chiasma, the ependymal cell-containing tela choroidea, and the pigmented epithelium of the retina. The *NF2* promoter expression pattern during embryogenesis suggests a specific regulation of the *NF2* gene during neural crest cell migration and further supports the role of merlin in cell adhesion, motility, and proliferation during development.[86]

Alternatively Spliced NF2 mRNA Isoforms in Vestibular Schwannomas and Other Cell Types

The *NF2* gene undergoes alternative splicing in the coding exons.[38,47,68,125–130] Multiple alternatively spliced *NF2* transcripts have been identified in various human cells. The most common isoforms in these cells were isoforms II (containing all 17 exons) and isoform I (without exon 16). We have also examined the expression of alternatively spliced *NF2* mRNA isoforms in VS. Cloning and sequencing analysis showed that the expression pattern and relative frequency of the alternatively spliced *NF2* transcripts in VS appeared to be different from those detected in other human cell types. In addition to isoforms I and II, these schwannomas expressed a high percentage of the *NF2* isoform lacking exons 15 and 16. These alternatively spliced *NF2* transcripts could encode different protein products (unpublished data).

Presently, the role of alternative splicing of *NF2* mRNA is not well understood. It is possible that the functional contribution of the *NF2* tumor suppressor may require a balanced expression of various isoform proteins in Schwann cells and/or other cell lineages.[68,131] Alternative splicing may be another mechanism for Schwann cells to inactivate merlin function and/or to generate isoforms that have additional properties conducive to tumor formation.

Immunohistochemical Markers of Growth in Vestibular Schwannomas: Clinical Correlation

Attempts to correlate clinical parameters with immunohistologic evaluation of protein expression in VS have been performed. An increase in Ki-67, a protein, which is an index of nuclear proliferation, was shown to correlate with the growth of solid schwannomas on MRI.[132,133] Higher rates of tumor recurrence have also been suggested in tumors with an increased rate of nuclear proliferation and mitotic indexes, although the supporting data for this claim was not conclusive.[134] Positron emission tomography (PET) scanning has been conducted to assess the metabolic activity of VS preoperatively and to assess the metabolic activity with the proliferation index, Ki-67. However, no correlation was found. Additionally, there was no correlation between 18-fluorodeoxyglucose (FDG) uptake (indicator of metabolic activity in tissues) and Ki-67 expression measured by immunostaining.[135] This is most likely because VS are slow

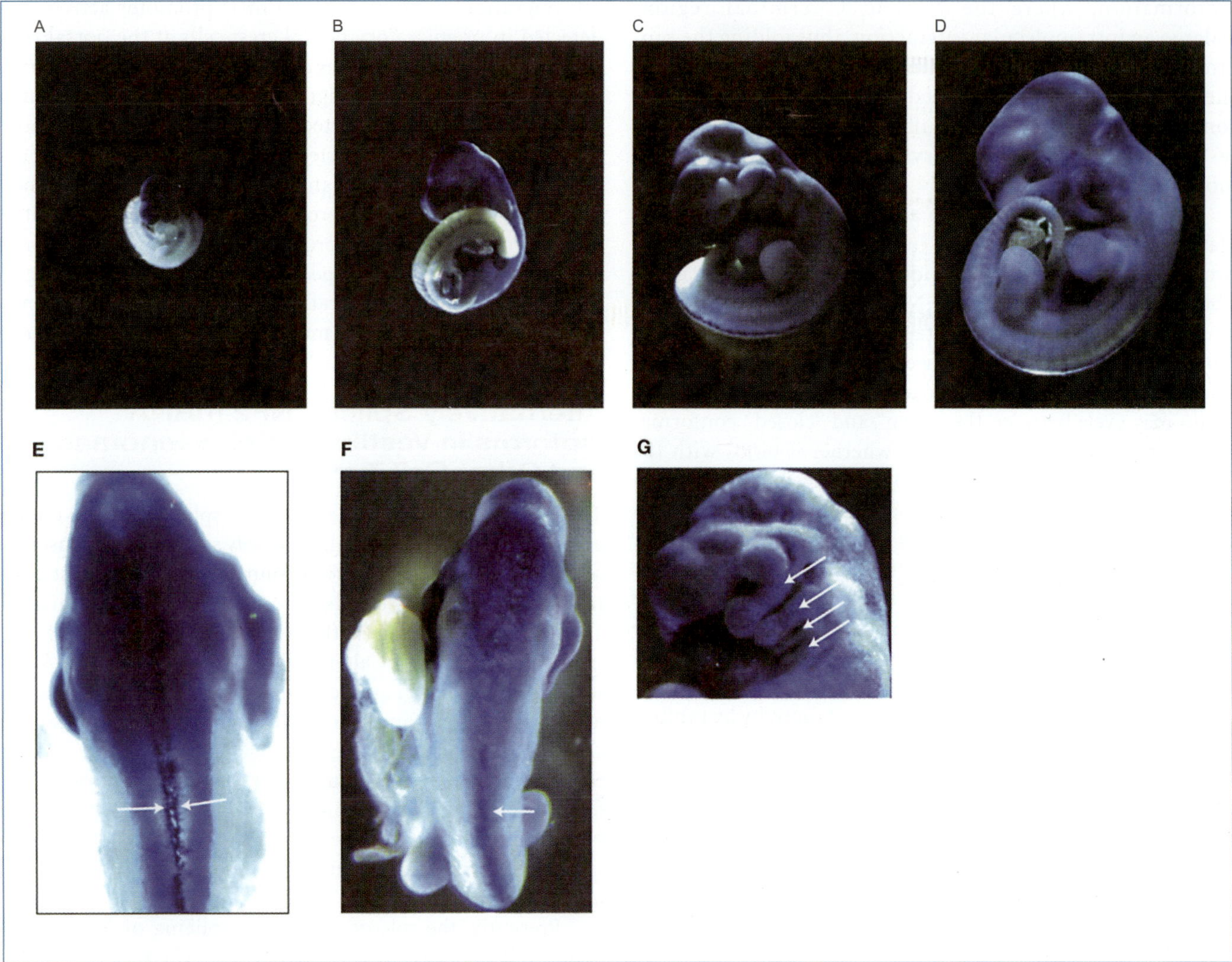

FIGURE 8–6 • *NF2* promoter expression in neural tube and neural crest. Lateral views of whole-mount X-gal-stained transgenic mouse embryos at various days p.c. *A*, E9.5, *B*, E10.5, *C*, E12.5, and *D*, E14.5. Scale bar 400 m. The most intense β-gal expression was detected along the dorsal closure (arrows) of neural tube in *E*, E9.5 and *F*, E10.5, transgenic embryos. Strong β-gal expression was also seen in the branchial arches I–IV (arrows) of the *G*, E10.5 embryo.

growing tumors with less than five percent of tumor cells being in S-phase or active division (Figure 8–7).[136]

Another possible marker for tumor growth is the transforming growth factor β1 (TGF-β1). Immunostaining for TGF-β1 was positive in 96% of blood vessels within schwannomas and in 84% of schwannoma tissue samples; however, no direct correlation with tumor growth was found.[137] Immunohistochemical association of β1-integrin with merlin has been demonstrated, but has not been related directly to tumor phenotypes.[95] Cystic schwannomas are associated with a 36-fold decrease in nuclear proliferation as measured with Ki-67 staining when compared to solid tumors, suggesting that the rapid clinical growth seen in cystic schwannomas is related to the accumulation of cyst formation but not by an actual increase in the growth rate of tumor cells.[138,139] Also, NF2-associated schwannomas have been shown to have an increased proliferation index by Ki-67 and proliferating cell nuclear antigen (PCNA) immunostaining, when compared to unilateral solid schwannomas.[140,141] PCNA is a proliferation index marker and is important in cell division.

Recently, we detected higher levels of cyclin D_3 expression, which is associated with G_1 cell-cycle progression, in 5 of 10 VS, compared to Schwann cells in adjacent normal vestibular nerve.[142] In contrast, expression of the cyclin D_1 protein, which controls Schwann cell differentiation, was not detected in any of the schwannomas examined. These results suggested a possible role for cyclin D_3 in the growth of some VS cells.

Taken together, these studies demonstrate relatively little correlation between clinical growth as assessed by MRI scans, historical data, and nuclear growth indexes in solid unilateral and *NF2*-associated schwannomas. Cystic tumor growth appears to occur via a different mechanism. Although the defective *NF2* gene is the underlying common denominator in tumor formation of all three tumor types, other differences at the molecular level likely account for the variable clinical presentations of these tumors.

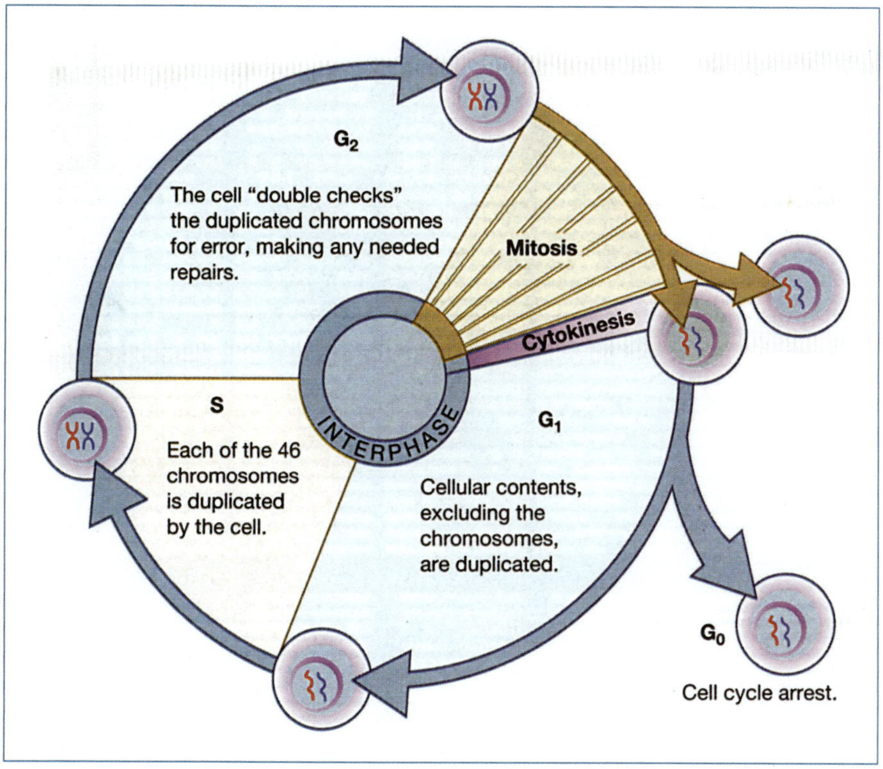

FIGURE 8–7 • Cell cycle revisited. During G1 phase, the cell grows. In S phase, the cell copies its chromosomes so that each chromosome now consist of two sister chromatids. During G2, the cell prepares for division and in M phase, the cell separates into two new cells (cytokinesis). www.le.ac.uk/ge/genie/vgec/sc/cellcycle.html. *From University of © Clinical Tools. Inc. Leicester.*

Identifying Deregulated Genes in Vestibular Schwannomas

To further elucidate the growth pathways in VS, the gene expression profiles have been studied. The study of large-scale gene expression profiles utilizing cDNA microarrays allows examination of the so-called transcriptome of a tissue, and gives a means of exploring a broad view of the basic biology of tumors.[143,144] cDNA is complimentary DNA, synthesized from a mature mRNA template. A microarray consists of thousands of "spots" of DNA attached to a solid surface, each containing a small amount of a specific DNA sequence corresponding to certain genes. A cDNA sample of interest is added to the microarray and allowed to hybridze. Hybridization of the sample and DNA on the array is detected and quantified using fluorescence. Using the technology of microarrays, gene expression profiles can be created in which the activity or expression of thousands of genes can be measured at once, creating a global picture of cellular function. By comparing gene expression profiles between the tumor and normal tissues, deregulated genes in the tumors tissues can be identified.[5,145] We studied gene regulation in VS using cDNA microarray analysis and found 42 genes, which were significantly upregulated including osteonectin, endoglin, and Rho B, when compared to normal vestibular nerve tissues.[5,145] Additionally, multiple genes were found to be significantly downregulated in the majority of VS examined. Of these genes, a putative tumor suppressor gene LUCA-15 was downregulated in 7 of 8 schwannomas studied (Figure 8–8).

Osteonectin is a secreted glycoprotein that interacts with extracellular matrix proteins to decrease adhesion of cells from the matrix, thereby inducing a biological state conducive to cell migration. Endoglin, a TGF-β receptor-binding protein was found to be significantly upregulated in all of the solid tumors but not in any of the cystic tumors examined. It is likely that the increased endoglin expression may induce downstream signaling proteins, somehow leading to an aggressive cystic phenotype.[5] An example of a deregulated signaling pathway suggested by the microarray data is the retinoblastoma protein (pRb)-cyclin dependent kinase (CDK) pathway.[145] Among genes involved in G_1-S progression (see Figure 8–7). CDK2 was found to be downregulated in 7 of 8 tumors. In addition, upregulation of transforming factor RhoB was found in all of the schwannomas examined.[5] Further examination of these deregulated genes as potential downstream targets of the *NF2* tumor suppressor should provide us with targets for pharmacotherapeutic interventions.

Environmental Exposures

There is evidence that radiation may be associated with the induction of vestibular schwannoma growth. While other sites and tumors also show propensity for growth in response to environmental exposures, the vestibular nerve appears to contain an increased sensitivity for tumor growth as compared to other regions within the central nervous system or elsewhere.

Evans and colleagues note an 18.8-fold increased relative risk of schwannoma induction and a 9.5-fold increased relative rate of meningioma induction following radiation doses of 2.5 Gy from the treatment of tinea capitis, adeno-tonsillar disease, and capillary hemangiomas.[146] The radiobiologic effect was dose-dependent similar to the tissue effect and tumor growth response observed in post-WWII Japan. Preston and

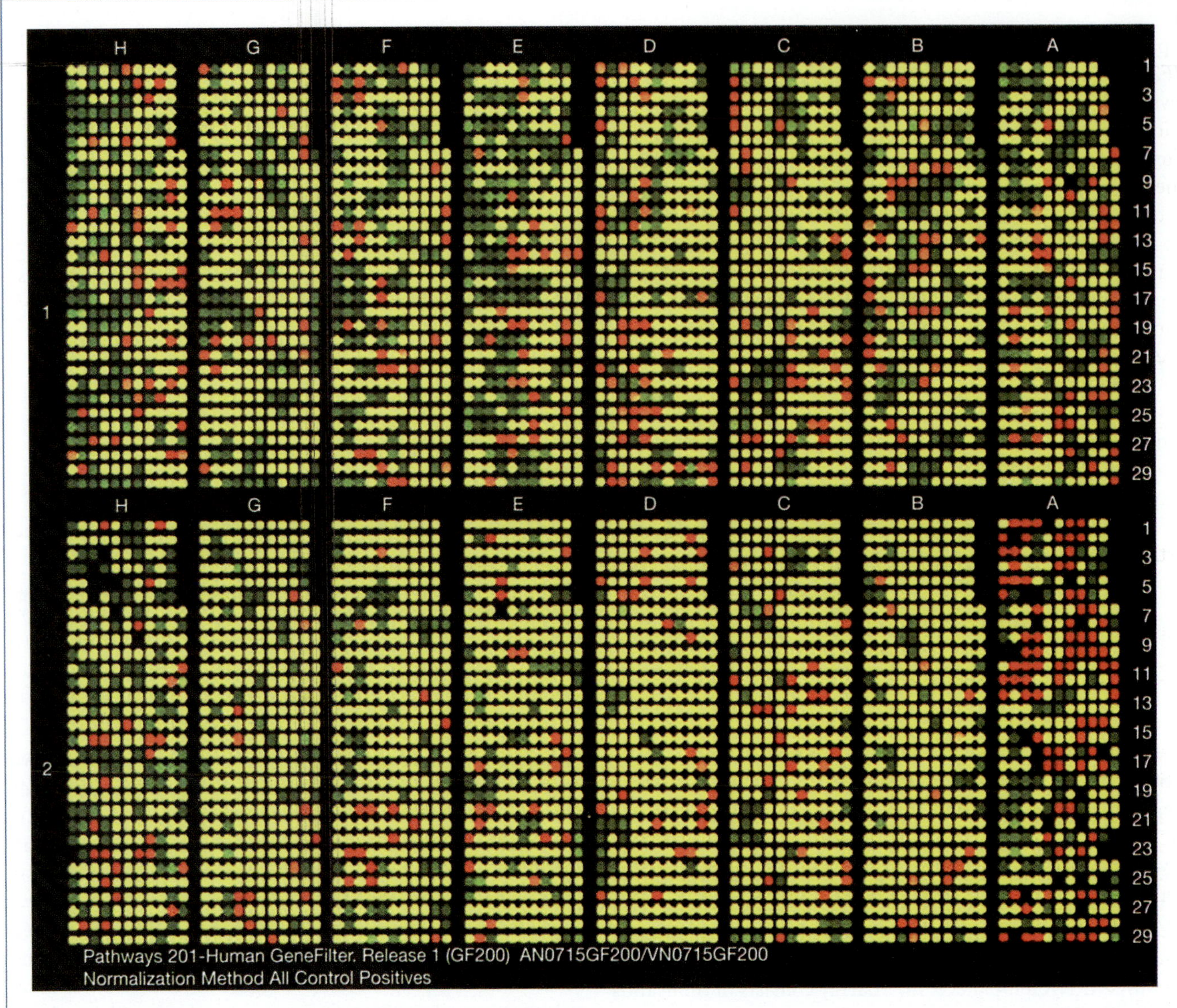

FIGURE 8–8 • cDNA microarray comparison of gene expression of a vestibular schwannoma and adjacent normal vestibular nerve (gene filter 200, Research Genetics, Huntsville, AL). The phosphor image shows red genes overexpressed in the tumor and green genes overexpressed in the vestibular nerve. Yellow images are genes that are nearly equally expressed in both tissues. *From Welling. Otol Neurotol, Volume 23(5).September 2002;736–748.*

colleagues[147] showed that VS were the most abundant intracranial tumors encountered, with a high propensity for Schwann cell mutation in response to radiation damage.

Overall, the risk of tumors induced by therapeutic radiation appears to be approximately 0.1 to 3% after 30 years.[146,148] In light of the 33 to 40% lifetime risk of malignancy in the general population, Evans[146] argues that the benefits of single-dose radiation treatment for VS may be justified for those with documented tumor growth that refuse surgery, or for the elderly or infirm. However, patients with NF2, in particular, are the disproportionate recipients of radiation-induced malignant tumors. Although only 7% of patients with VS have NF2, 50% of malignant changes induced by stereotactic irradiation of VS occur in NF2 patients. Evans strongly cautions the use of radiation treatment for benign tumors in childhood and in tumor-prone conditions such as neurofibromatosis. We concur.

Cellular Telephone Risk

Several studies addressed the risk of cellular telephone use and the formation of VS presumably secondary to electromagnetic radiation over a long exposure period. Hardell et al.[149] reviewed 13 case-controlled studies and found 9 case control studies to have reported patients with over 10 years of cellular telephone use. They concluded that the odds ratios for ipsilateral cellphone use and the development of VS was 2.4 (95% confidence interval 1.1–5.3). A consistent pattern emerges from the case-controlled studies of increased risk for vestibular schwannoma and also glioma with risk elevation greatest for high-grade gliomas associated with unilateral long-term exposure.[149,150]

Genetic Screening for NF2

A parent with NF2 has a 50% chance of passing the affected *NF2* allele along to their offspring if (1) their spouse does not have NF2 and if (2) they do not have a mosaic form of NF2. (Mosaicism occurs when a mutation in the NF2 gene occurs after an embryo has undergone several sets of cell division. Therefore only a portion of the child's cells carry a mutation in the NF2 gene.) A child who inherits an abnormal copy of the *NF2* tumor suppressor gene has a 95% chance of developing bilateral VS.

Because early intervention is very important in clinical outcome, genetic and clinical screening for at-risk patients is advocated. We feel that routine clinical and imaging examinations are mandatory for those who are at-risk to develop NF2. This includes anyone with a first-degree relative with NF2, patients under 30 years old with a unilateral VS, or any patient with multiple intracranial, spinal, or peripheral skin tumors that are associated with NF2. Any offspring of patients with NF2 should have annual ophthalmology examinations starting soon after birth since cataracts can begin at a very early age. Annual neurology examinations should be started at 7 years of age or earlier if neurologic deficits are noted. We recommend bi-annual audiograms and annual MRI evaluations beginning at age 7. Others have recommended starting a similar screening process at 10 years of age with an MRI every other year and annually once a tumor is found.[151]

Mutation screening for the first-degree relatives of NF2 patients is recommended when the probands' mutation has been identified either from a schwannoma or from leukocyte screening.[151,152] A proband is the person who is being studied in whom the disease is first clinically detected. Other family members at risk can be identified and screened for developing NF2 or receive appropriate genetic counseling. Patients who are first-degree relatives of NF2 patients where the mutation in the *NF2* gene has not been identified may have more ambiguity regarding the screening of their *NF2* gene for mutations if no mutation is localized. Appropriate audiometric testing and neural imaging needs to be carried out as false negatives in mutation screening can occur in up to 25% of patients. Taking this fact into consideration, we feel that annual MRI screening and biannual audiometric testing would still be needed for children older than 7 years of age who had a negative test. Additionally, if a mutation was detected during DNA sequencing, we would still recommend annual MRIs and biannual audiometric testing in order to detect the development of VS at the earliest possible stage. Early detection in NF2 does make a significant difference in the ability to successfully preserve hearing and facial nerve function.

When an *NF2* mutation has already been identified in an affected family member, screening additional first degree family members for the same mutation is considerably less costly and is recommended. The sensitivity of genetic testing in this circumstance is extremely high since the DNA being screened can be directly compared to the known mutation in the affected family member. In this case, knowing with near certainty that a child does not carry a *NF2* mutation can avoid the frequent MRI examinations that would otherwise be required.[44,153] Therefore, if a family has multiple members (more than two people) diagnosed with NF2 and mutation testing has not been performed, it may be worthwhile to identify the mutation in at least one family member so that future family members can be screened. This is most effectively done when tumor tissues are available for mutation screening. However, biopsy for genetic diagnosis alone is not suggested if tumor removal is otherwise not indicated as clinical screening protocols are also effective.

Potential Drug Treatments

As the understanding of merlin and its interacting partners is better understood, new means of targeting these pathways for intervention in schwannoma cells is occurring. Some treatments are aimed at restoring the wild-type merlin protein to the mutant cells, while other strategies attempt to block the proliferation of schwannoma cells by blocking its growth pathways or by increasing programmed cell death or apoptosis. For example, Messerli et al.[154] showed effective reduction of schwannoma growth in both a transgenic and a xenograft mouse model by injecting wild-type merlin packaged in an oncolytic recombinant herpes simplex virus vector in the tumor as noted in the text directly. The vehicle for delivery was a replication-competent herpes simplex virus, which has tumoricidal properties. There were no apparent toxicities with the injection of the oncolytic vector. A paradigm for the use of oncolytic vectors to reduce the volume of benign tumors when surgical resection may cause nerve damage is suggested.

Hansen et al.[155] and Doherty et al.[156] demonstrated cell surface human epidermal growth factor, also known as erythroblastic leukemia viral oncogene homolog 2 or ErbB2 receptors as possible targets for VS cell growth inhibition. Blocking the ligand or interacting proteins, which activates this receptor by treatment with blocking antineuregulin antibodies, also inhibited schwannoma cell proliferation. ErbB2 is a tyrosine kinase receptor, a common cellular switch, on the VS cell surface, which triggers the MAPK kinase cascade, a process that leads sequentially to nuclear activation of cell division. One of its ligands, neuregulin-1, is a growth factor produced by schwannoma cells, thus creating an autocrine feedback loop; the schwannomma cells cause further stimulation of schwannoma growth.

Plotkin et al. (Children's Tumor Foundation meeting, June 2008, Bonita Springs, FL) showed that epidermal growth factor receptor (EGFR) blockade with erlotanib HCl was tolerated and showed radiographic and audiometric response to treatment in a patient with NF2 in short follow-up. Although hepatotoxicity may limit this agent's use, other trials with EGFR and ErbB inhibitors are expected.

Several investigators demonstrated that intervention at the intracellular proliferation pathways, specifically the MAPK pathway and the phosphatidylinositol 3-kinase (PI3K) pathway, respectively, may also result in schwannoma growth suppression. Nakai et al.[112] showed that merlin is involved in suppression of Rac signaling, and cultured schwannoma cells contain elevated, GTP-bound, active Rac. Application of a Rac-specific inhibitor, the chemical compound NSC23766, to schwannoma cells restored neuronal interaction. The data support the significance of regulated Rac signaling in mediating Schwann cell–axon interaction and suggest controlling Rac activity as a possible therapy for schwannomas.

FIGURE 8–9 • PI3K/AKT signaling. Insulin and other growth factors activate cell surface tyrosine kinase receptors that stimulate PI3K activity. PI3K converts PIP2 to PIP3. PTEN is a negative regulator of the AKT pathway that catalyzes the conversion of PIP3 back to PIP2. PDK1 and PDK2 maximally activate AKT. Phosphorylation of downstream effectors of the AKT pathway inhibit these proteins. Existing as a complex, TSC1 and TSC2 normally inhibits mTOR activity. However, when TSC2 is phosphorylated by AKT, it dissociates from TSC1, and mTOR becomes active. Active GSK and FOXO function within the nucleus as transcriptional regulators that activate genes promoting apoptosis. Merlin, the NF2 gene product, can bind PIKE-L and inactivate PI3K. A small molecule PDK1 inhibitor can inhibit phosphorylation of AKT at the 308 site. PNAS 2004

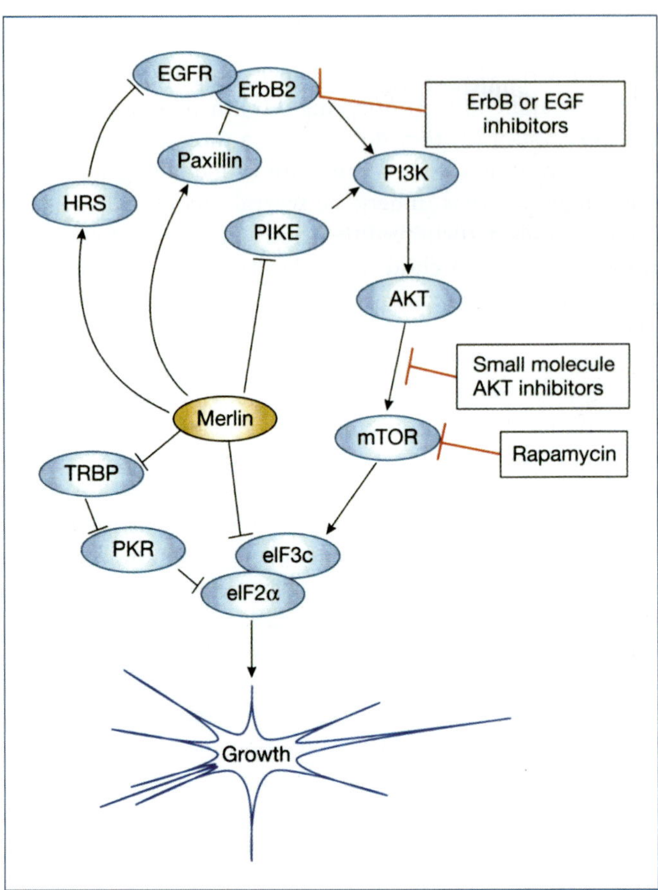

FIGURE 8–10 • Alternative pathways. In this schematic in a recent review by Dan Scoles, Merlin's interaction with the ErbB2—Paxillin complex, PIKE, and eIF3c, effect of NGB and merlin on cyclin D1 expression, and functional consequences of merlin loss on proliferation mediated by these interaction suggest that signaling in the ErbB2–PI3kinase–mTOR–eIF3c–cyclin D1 pathway may contribute to NF2 pathogenesis. PIKE-L is free to enhance PI3K which leads to complete phosphorylation and activation of PDK1 and PDK2, which in turn activate the cells mitotic machinery. Drugs targeting this pathway therefore may be useful for inhibition of NF2 tumors with overactive mTOR signaling, including trastuzumab (herceptin, LY294002, AKT inhibitors, UCN-01, Rad-001, CCI-779, and AP23573, and small molecule AKT pathway and histone deacetylase inhibitors. HSP90 inhibitor 17AAG (17-allylamino-17-desmethoxygeldanamycin) may affect Akt and C-Raf, Cdk4 and Cyclin D-1. (NexGenix)

Jacob et al.[123] demonstrated the activation of the PI3-kinase/AKT pathway in human schwannomas. It has been shown that merlin can inhibit PI3-kinase through its binding to the PI3-kinase enhancer-L (PIKE-L). PIKE-L is a GTPase which binds to and stimulates PI3K. (Figure 8–9) The suppression of PI3-kinase activity results from merlin disrupting the binding of PIKE-L to PI3-kinase. Our recent studies using cultured schwannoma cells further suggest that both an AKT pathway inhibitor as well as a histone deacetylase inhibitor could suppress schwannoma cell growth by blocking the PI3-kinase pathway. Utilizing a quantifiable xenograft model for VS we are currently testing the efficacy of these novel compounds.

Transduction of growth factor stimulation of the mammalian target of rapamycin (mTOR) signaling pathway ultimately results in stimulation of protein synthesis and entry into the G1 phase of the cell cycle. Decreased phosphatase and tensin homolog gene (PTEN), a human gene that acts as a tumor suppressor gene, manifests as AKT and mTOR activation stimulating growth. Additionally hypoxia inducible factors HIF-1 alpha, and HIF-2 alpha show increased expression and account for enhanced angiogenesis with mTOR activation. This may lead to the necessary blood vessel supply to schwannomas. AKT and mTOR activation have been noted in VS. The immunosuppressant, rapamycin, inhibits mTOR and induces G1 arrest and apoptosis. Newer mTOR inhibitors, such as temsirolimus, have shown good effect in the treatment of renal cell carcinoma alone and in combination with other agents. (Figure 8–10)

A novel treatment approach has been proposed and is being evaluated in benign tumors. Nonsense mutations account for up to 39% of NF2 related VS and 23% of mutations leading to unilateral sporadic tumors. These mutations are related to a dominant C to T transition, replacing arginine with a premature termination codon (PTC) within the developing protein molecule as mentioned earlier. PTC 124 is a low-molecular-weight compound that shows an ability to "read through" premature termination codons while still responding to true stops, allowing for synthesis of a full protein product (Figure 8–11). It is showing promise in phase II trials of nonsense mutations in

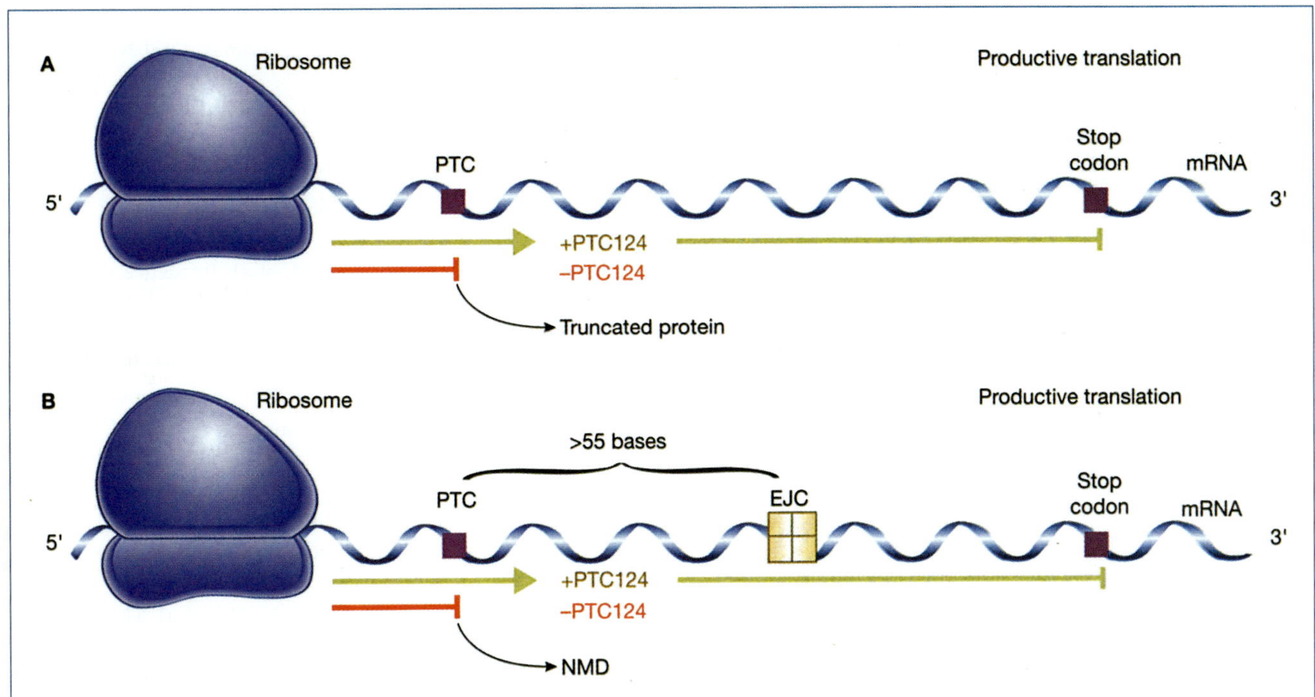

FIGURE 8–11 • Possible mechanisms of PTC124-enhanced translation. *A*, PTC124 could directly suppress termination of "productive" protein translation at a premature termination codon (PTC), leading to increased levels of functional full-length proteins. *B*, Alternatively, PTC124 might suppress the identification of PTCs in "pioneer" translation, thereby preventing nonsense-mediated mRNA decay (NMD), which is induced if a ribosome hits a stop codon more than 55 bases upstream of an exonjunction complex (EJC). This would lead to the stabilization of PTC-containing mRNAs, allowing their translation, presumably through the mechanism shown in View *A*. The work of Welch et al. supports the model depicted in View *A*.

genetically compatible patients with Duchenne's muscular dystrophy and cystic fibrosis.[157,158] Because PTC 124 is a genetically dependant therapeutic as opposed to a disease-specific agent, it holds promise for genetically screened patients displaying nonsense-related tumors.

Angiogenesis inhibitors such as Avastin (Bevacizumab) have been used alone or in combination for treatment of colorectal, and lung and prostate carcinomas.[159–162] It acts by inhibiting vascular endothelial growth factor (VEGF), and is used in several combination treatment protocols. Avastin has anecdotally shown temporary suppression of VS growth. Its temporary effect on tumor growth reduction, the potential side effects of leukopenia, and bleeding limit its use in surgical patients, and it is currently considered a temporizing agent. PTC 299 similarly blocks angiogenesis, but by inhibiting the production of VEGF. It has been shown to be effective against cancer cell lines including breast, cervical, colorectal, gastric, lung, ovarian, pancreatic, prostate, and renal cell carcinomas, fibrosarcoma, melanoma, and neuroblastoma. Animal studies have documented its efficacy in reducing VEGF in tumor and serum, decreasing blood vessel density in tumor, and substantially impeding tumor progression by itself and as a component of combined therapy with other antitumor agents or Avastin. Tolerance in phase I studies has been acceptable, and phase II trials in breast cancer are commencing (unpublished data).

The medical treatment of slow growing benign tumors must maintain efficacy over decades of potential treatment. Perhaps combined modality treatments might be considered. Two agents we are currently studying (a histone deacytelase inhibitor and an AKT pathway inhibitor) have shown capacity to modulate radiation response in an additive fashion. By sensitizing targeted tissues, radiation doses could be lowered to optimistically promote killing effect of tumor cells, reduce adverse effect on surrounding structures, preserve physiologic function, and decrease the risk of tumor promotion or malignant transformation.

Schwannomatosis (OMIM #162091), a recently defined form of neurofibromatosis, is characterized by multiple schwannomas but this condition distinctly lacks any VS. Patients with schwannomatosis frequently present with intractable pain rather than cranial nerve deficits. They do not develop other intracranial tumors or malignancies. MacCollin et al.[163] noted that about one-third of patients with schwannomatosis had tumors in an anatomically limited distribution, such as a single limb, several contiguous segments of spine, or one half of the body. Sporadic cases of schwannomatosis are as common as NF2, but few cases of familial schwannomatosis have been identified in contradistinction to NF1 and NF2, which are autosomal-dominant and highly penetrant. The underlying molecular disruption in schwannomatosis is a pattern of somatic *NF2* gene inactivation incompatible with NF1 or NF2, associated with alterations in the SMARCB1 (hSnf5/INI1) tumor suppressor gene in familial disease.[164,165]

Genetics of Paragangliomas

Paragangliomas of the head and neck are rare, mostly benign tumors. The hereditary paraganglioma syndromes are autosomal-dominant conditions with increased risk for multifocal tumors of the sympathetic and parasympathetic neuroendocrine systems. Approximately 30% of paraganglioma patients harbor a germline mutation, which is carried by all of the cells of the body (as opposed to a somatic mutation, which is only found in the tumor tissues). In more than a third of these patients, there is no prior family history thus representing new mutations.

Ten to 15% of paragangliomas are caused by mutations in the succinate dehydrogenase (SDH) genes or its anchoring subunits B, C, or D.[166] They may be hormone secreting. Malignant paragangliomas have been particularly associated with mutations in SDHB, but have also been reported in SDHD.[167] The succinate dehydrogenase genes provide a protein that is a small part of the cytochrome *b* complex in the mitochondrial complex II, one of the five protein assemblies or complexes that form the electron transport chain. By production of reactive oxygen molecules, this pathway is considered important in the signaling and detection of oxygen tension. The gene encoding SDHD consist of 4 exons and yields 159 amino acid polypeptides.[168]

Other mutations found to be associated with paragangliomas include the prolyl hydroxylase domain (PHD) proteins, which play a major role in regulating the hypoxia-inducible factor (HIF) that induces expression of genes involved in angiogenesis, erythropoiesis, and cell metabolism, proliferation, and survival. Mutations in the prolyl hydroxylase domain 2 gene (PHD2) have recently been described in a patient with erythrocytosis and recurrent paragangliomas.[169]

SUMMARY

The discovery of molecular mechanisms underlying VS formation is moving forward. Understanding merlin's function and its interactions with other proteins and signaling pathways, and regulation of the *NF2* gene will eventually lead to the development of novel treatments for VS. Ultimately, drug therapies will be designed to stop schwannoma progression. This will offer alternatives to the current options of untreated observation of tumor growth, stereotactic radiation, or surgical removal.

References

1. Trofatter JA, MacCollin MM, Rutter JL, et al. A novel moesin-, ezrin-, radixin-like gene is a candidate for the neurofibromatosis 2 tumor-suppressor. Cell 1993;72:791–800.
2. Rouleau GA, Merel P, Lutchman M, et al. Alteration in a new gene encoding a putative membrane-organizing protein causes neurofibromatosis type 2. Nature 1993;363:515–21.
3. Welling DB, Guida M, Goll F, et al. Mutational spectrums in the neurofibromatosis type 2 gene in sporadic and familial schwannomas. Hum Genet 1996;98:189–93.
4. Chen Y, Gutmann DH, Haipek CA, et al. Characterization of chicken Nf2/merlin indicates regulatory roles in cell proliferation and migration. Dev Dyn 2004;229:541–54.
5. Welling DB, Lasak JM, Akhmametyeva E, et al. cDNA microarray analysis of vestibular schwannomas. Otol Neurotol 2002 Sep;23(5):736–48.
6. Chang LS, Jacob A, Lorenz M, et al. Growth of benign and malignant schwannoma xenografts in severe combined immunodeficiency mice. Laryngoscope 2006 Nov;116(11):2018–26.
7. Tos M, Thomsen J, Charabi S. Incidence of acoustic neuromas. Ear Nose Throat J 1992;71:391–3.
8. Howitz MF, Johansen C, Tos M, et al. Incidence of vestibular schwannoma in denmark, 1977–95. Amer J Otol 2000;21:690–4.
9. Anderson TD, Loevner LA, Bigelow DC, Mirza N. Prevalence of unsuspected acoustic neuroma found by magnetic resonance imaging. Otolaryngol Head Neck Surg 2000;122:643–6.
10. Bull World Health Org. Prevention and control of neurofibromatosis: memorandum from a joint WHO/NNFF meeting. 1992;70:173–82.
11. Fontaine B, Rouleau GA, Seizinger BR, et al. Molecular genetics of neurofibromatosis 2 and related tumors (acoustic neuroma and meningioma). Ann NY Acad Sci 1991;615:338–43.
12. Kaiser-Kupfer M, Freidlin V, Datiles MB, et al. The association of posterior capsular lens opacities with bilateral acoustic neuromas in patients with neurofibromatosis type 2. Arch Ophthalmol 1989;107:541–4.
13. Kanter WR, Eldridge R, Fabricant R, et al. Central neurofibromatosis with bilateral acoustic neuroma: Genetic, clinical and biochemical distinctions from peripheral neurofibromatosis. Neurology 1980;30:851–9.
14. Martuza RL, Eldridge R. Neurofibromatosis 2 (bilateral acoustic neurofibromatosis). New Engl J Med 1988;318:684–8.
15. Evans DGR, Huson SM, Donnai D, et al. A clinical study of type 2 neurofibromatosis. Q J Med 1992;84:603–18.
16. Evans DGR, Huson SM, Donnai D, et al. A genetic study of type 2 neurofibromatosis in the united kingdom. I: prevalence, mutation rate, fitness, and confirmation of maternal transmission effect on severity. J Med Genet 1992;29:841–6.
17. Wishart JH. Case of tumors in skull, dura mater, and brain. Edinburgh Med Surg J 1822;18:393–7.
18. Gardner WJ, Frazier CH. Bilateral acoustic neurofibromatosis: a clinical study and field survey of a family of five generations with bilateral deafness in thirty-eight members. Arch Neurol Psychiatry 1930;23:266–302.
19. Evans DGR, Wallace AJ, Wu CL,et al. Somatic mosaicism: a common cause of classic disease in tumor-prone syndromes? Lessons from type 2 neurofibromatosis. Am J Hum Genet 1998;63:727–36.
20. Ruggieri M, Huson SM. The clinical and diagnostic implications of mosaicism in neurofibromatosis. Neurology 2001;56:1433–43.
21. Kluwe L, Mautner VF, Heinrich B, et al. Molecular study of frequency of mosaicism in neurofibromatosis 2 patients with bilateral vestibular schwannomas. J Med Genet 2003;40:109–14.
22. Moyhuddin A, Baser ME, Watson C, et al. Somatic mosaicism in neurofibromatosis 2: Prevalence and risk of disease transmission to offspring. J Med Genet 203;40:459–63.
23. Kameyama S, Tanaka R, Kawaguchi T, et al. Cystic acoustic neurinomas: studies of 14 cases. Acta Neurochir 1996;138: 695–9.
24. Charabi S, Tos M, Thomsen J, et al. Cystic vestibular schwannoma-clinical and experimental studies. Acta Otolaryngol (Suppl) 2000;543:11–3.

25. Charabi S, Tos M, Borgesen SE, Thomsen J. Cystic acoustic neuromas. Results of translabyrinthine surgery. Arch Otolaryngol Head Neck Surg 1994;120:1333–8.

26. Fundova P, Charabi S, Tos M,Thomsen J. Cystic vestibular schwannoma: surgical outcome. J Laryngol Otol 2000;114:935–9.

27. Pendl G, Ganz JC, Kitz K, Eustacchio S. Acoustic neuromas with macrocysts treated with gamma knife radiosurgery. Stereotact Funct Neurosurg 1995;66 (Suppl 1):103–11.

28. Shirato H, Sakamoto T, Takeichi N, et al. Fractionated stereotactic radiotherapy for vestibular schwannoma (VS): comparison between cystic-type and solid-type VS. Int J Radiat Oncol Biol Phys 2000;48:1395–401.

29. Rouleau GA, Wertelecki W, Haines JL, et al. Genetic linkage of bilateral acoustic neurofibromatosis to a DNA marker on chromosome 22. Nature 1987;329:246–8.

30. Wertelecki W, Rouleau GA, Superneau DW, et al. Neurofibromatosis 2: clinical and DNA linkage studies of a larger kindred. New Engl J Med 1988;319:278–83.

31. Welling DB. Clinical manifestations of mutations in the neurofibromatosis type 2 gene in vestibular schwannomas (acoustic neuromas). Laryngoscope 1998;108:178–89.

32. Jacoby LB, MacCollin MM, Barone R, et al. Frequency and distribution of NF2 mutations in schwannomas. Genes Chrom Cancer 1996;17:45–55.

33. Irving RM, Harada T, Moffat DA, et al. Somatic neurofibromatosis type 2 gene mutations and growth characteristics in vestibular schwannoma. Amer J Otol 1997;18:754–60.

34. Lekanne Deprez RH, Bianchi AB, Groen NA, et al. Frequent NF2 gene transcript mutations in sporadic meningiomas and vestibular schwannomas. Am J Hum Genet 1994;54:1022–9.

35. Merel P, Hoang-Xuan K, Sanson M, et al. Predominant occurrence of somatic mutations of the NF2 gene in meningiomas and schwannomas. Genes Chrom Cancer 1995;13:1211–6.

36. Merel P, Khe HX, Sanson M, et al. Screening for germ-line mutations in the NF2 gene. Genes Chrom Cancer 1995;12:117–27.

37. Lasota J, Fetsch JF, Wozniak A, et al. The neurofibromatosis type 2 gene is mutated in perineurial cell tumors: A molecular genetic study of eight cases. Am J Pathol 2001;158:1223–9.

38. Bianchi AB, Hara T, Ramesh V, et al. Mutations in transcript isoforms of the neurofibromatosis 2 gene in multiple human tumour types. Nat Genet 1994;6:185–92.

39. Bianchi AB, Mitsunnaga SI, Cheng JQ, et al. High frequency of inactivating mutations in the neurofibromatosis type 2 gene (NF2) in primary malignant mesotheliomas. Proc Natl Acad Sci USA 1995;92:10854–8.

40. Ruttledge MH, Sarrazin J, Rangaratnam S, et al. Evidence for the complete inactivation of the NF2 gene in the majority of sporadic meningiomas. Nat Genet 1994;6:180–4.

41. Sekido Y, Pass HI, Bader S, et al. Neurofibromatosis type 2 (NF2) gene is somatically mutated in mesothelioma but not in lung cancer. Cancer Res 1995;55:1227–31.

42. Deguen B, Goutebroze L, Giovannini M, et al. Heterogeneity of mesothelioma cell lines as defined by altered genomic structure and expression of the NF2 gene. Int J Cancer 1998;77:554–60.

43. Sanson M, Marineau C, Desmaze C, et al. Germline detection in a neurofibromatosis type 2 kindred inactivates the NF2 gene and a candidate meningioma locus. Hum Mol Genet 1993;2:1215–20.

44. MacCollin M, Mohney T, Trofatter JA, et al. DNA diagnosis of neurofibromatosis 2. altered coding sequence of the merlin tumor suppressor in an extended pedigree. JAMA 1993;270:2316–20.

45. MacCollin MM, Ramesh V, Jacoby LB, et al. Mutational anaylsis of patients with neurofibromatosis 2. Am J Hum Genet 1994;55:314–20.

46. Irving RM, Moffat DA, Hardy DG, et al. Somatic NF2 gene mutations in familial and non-familial vestibular schwannoma. Hum Mol Genet 1994;3:347–50.

47. Jacoby LB, MacCollin MM, Louis DN, et al. Exon scanning for mutation of the NF2 gene in schwannomas. Hum Mol Genet 1994;3:413–9.

48. Jacoby LB, Jones D, Davis K, et al. Molecular analysis of the NF2 tumor-suppressor gene in schwannomatosis. Am J Hum Genet 1997;61:1293–302.

49. Sainz J, Figueroa K, Baser ME, et al. High frequency of nonsense mutations in the NF2 gene caused by C to T transitions in five CGA codons. Hum Genet 1995;4:137–9.

50. Sainz J, Figueroa K, Baser ME, et al. Identification of three neurofibromatosis type 2 (NF2) gene mutations in vestibular schwannomas. Hum Mol Genet 1996;97:121–3.

51. Sainz J, Huynh DP, Figueroa K, et al. Mutations of the neurofibromatosis type 2 gene and lack of the gene product in vestibular schwannomas. Hum Mol Genet 1994;3:885–91.

52. Twist EC, Ruttledge MH, Rousseau M, et al. The neurofibromatosis type 2 gene is inactivated in schwannomas. Hum Mol Genet 1994;3:147–51.

53. Bourn D, Carter SA, Mason S, et al. Germline mutations in the neurofibromatosis type 2 tumour suppressor gene. Hum Mol Genet 1994;3:813–6.

54. Bourn D, Evans DGR, Mason S, et al. Eleven novel mutations in the NF2 tumour suppressor gene. Hum Genet 1995;95:572–4.

55. Parry DM, MacCollin MM, Kaiser-Kupfer M, et al. Germ-line mutations in the neurofibromatosis 2 gene: Correlation with disease severity and retinal abnormalities. Am J Hum Genet 1996;59:529–39.

56. Ruttledge MH, Andermann AA, Phelan CM, et al. Type of mutation in the neurofibromatosis type 2 gene (NF2) frequently determines severity of disease. Am J Hum Genet 1996;59:331–42.

57. Gutmann DH, Geist RT, Xu HM, et al. Defects in neurofibromatosis 2 protein function can arise at multiple levels. Hum Mol Genet 1998;7:335–45.

58. Stokowski RP, Cox DR. Functional analysis of the neurofibromatosis type 2 protein by means of disease-causing point mutations. Am J Hum Genet 2000;66:873–91.

59. Ahronowitz I, Xin W, Kiely R, et al. Mutational spectrum of the NF2 gene: A meta-analysis of 12 years of research and diagnostic laboratory findings. Hum Mutat 2007;28:1–12.

60. Baser ME, Contributors to the International NF2 Mutation Database. The distribution of constitutional and somatic mutations in the neurofibromatosis 2 gene. Hum Mutat 2006;27: 297–306.

61. Gutmann DH, Hirbe AC, Haipek CA. Functional analysis of neurofibromatosis 2 (NF2) missense mutations. Hum Mol Genet 2001;10:1519–29.

62. Bruder CE, Hirvela C, Tapia-Paez I, et al. High resolution deletion analysis of constitutional DNA from neurofibromatosis type 2 (NF2) patients using microarray-CGH. Hum Mol Genet 2001;10:271–82.

63. Mautner VF, Baser ME, Kluwe L. Phenotypic variability in two families with novel splice-site and frameshift NF2 mutations. Hum Genet 1996;98:203–6.

64. Zhao Y, Kumar RA, Bader S, et al. Intrafamilial correlation of clinical manifestations in neurofibromatosis 2 (NF2). Genet Epidemiol 2002;23:245–59.
65. Bruder CE, Ichimura K, Blennow E, et al. Severe phenotype of neurofibromatosis type 2 in a patient with a 7.4-MB constitutional deletion on chromosome 22: possible localization of a neurofibromatosis type 2 modifier gene? Genes Chrom Cancer 1999;25:184–90.
66. Zucman-Rossi J, Legoix P, et al. NF2 gene in neurofibromatosis type 2 patients. Hum Mol Genet 1999;7:2095–101.
67. Kino T, Takeshima H, Nakao M, et al. Identification of the cis-acting region in the NF2 gene promoter as a potential target for mutation and methylation-dependent silencing in schwannoma. Genes Cells 2001;6:441–54.
68. Chang LS, Akhmametyeva EM, Wu Y, et al. Multiple transcription initiation sites, alternative splicing, and differential polyadenylation contribute to the complexity of human neurofibromatosis 2 transcripts. Genomics 2002 Jan;79(1):63–76.
69. Gonzalez-Gomez P, Bello MJ, Alonso ME, et al. CpG island methylation in sporadic and neurofibromatosis type 2-associated schwannomas. Clin Cancer Res 2003;9:5601–6.
70. Gutmann DH, Sherman L, Seftor L, et al. Increased expression of the NF2 tumor suppressor gene product, merlin, impairs cell motility, adhesion, and spreading. Hum Mol Genet 1999;8:267–75.
71. Algrain M, Arpin M, Louvard D. Wizardry at the cell cortex. Current Biol 1993;3:451–4.
72. Golovnina K, Blinov A, Akhmametyeva EM, et al. Evolution and origin of merlin, the product of the *neurofibromatosis type 2* (NF2) tumor-suppressor gene. BMC Evol Biol 2005;5:69–86.
73. Chishti AH, Kim AC, Marfatia SM, et al. The FERM domain: a unique module involved in the linkage of cytoplasmic proteins to the membrane. TIBS 1998;23:281–2.
74. Shimizu T, Seto A, Maita N, et al. Structural basis for neurofibromatosis type 2 crystal structure of the merlin FERM domain. J Biol Chem 2002;277:10332–6.
75. Bretscher A, Chambers D, Nguyen R, et al. ERM-merlin and EBP50 protein families in plasma membrane organization and function. Ann Rev Cell Dev Biol 2000;16:113–43.
76. Turunen O, Wahlstrom T, Vaheri A. Ezrin has a COOH-terminal actin-binding site that is conserved in the ezrin protein family. J Cell Biol 1994;126:1445–53.
77. Roy C, Martin M, Mangeat P. A dual involvement of the amino-terminal domain of ezrin in F- and G-actin binding. J Biol Chem 1997;272:20088–95.
78. Gonzalez-Agosti C, Xu L, Pinney D, et al. The merlin tumor suppressor localizes preferentially in membrane ruffles. Oncogene 1996;13:1239–47.
79. Pelton PD, Sherman LS, Rizvi TA, et al. Ruffling membrane, stress fiber, cell spreading and proliferation abnormalities in human schwannoma cells. Oncogene 1998;17:2195–209.
80. Deguen B, Merel P, Goutebroze L, et al. Impaired interaction of naturally occurring mutant NF2 protein with actin-based cytoskeleton and membrane. Hum Mol Genet 1998;7:217–26.
81. Lutchman M, Rouleau GA. The neurofibromatosis type 2 gene product, schwannomin, suppresses growth of NIH 3T3 cells. Cancer Res 1995;55:2270–4.
82. Sherman L, Xu HM, Geist RT, et al. Interdomain binding mediates tumor growth suppression by the NF2 gene product. Oncogene 1997;15:2505–9.
83. Tikoo A, Varga M, Ramesh V, et al. An anti-ras function of neurofibromatosis type 2 gene product (NF2/merlin). J Biol Chem 1994;269:23387–90.
84. McClatchey AI, Saotome I, Mercer K, et al. Mice heterozygous for a mutation at the NF2 tumor suppressor locus develop a range of highly metastatic tumors. Genes Dev 1998;12:1121–33.
85. McClatchey AI, Saotome I, Ramesh V, et al. The NF2 tumor suppressor gene product is essential for extraembryonic development immediately prior to gastrulation. Genes Dev 1997;11:1253–65.
86. Akhmametyeva EM, Mihaylova MM, Luo H, et al. Regulation of the neurofibromatosis 2 gene promoter expression during embryonic development. Dev Dyn 2006 Oct;235(10):2771–85.
87. Giovannini M, Robanus-Maandag E, van der Valk M, et al. Conditional bialleic *Nf2* mutation in the mouse promotes manifestations of human neurofibromatosis type 2. Genes Dev 2000;14:1617–30.
88. Kalamarides M, Niwa-Kawakita M, Leblois H, et al. *Nf2* gene inactivation in arachnoidal cells is rate-limiting for meningioma development in the mouse. Genes Dev 2002;16:1060–5.
89. Shaw RJ, Paez JG, Curto M, et al. The NF2 tumor suppressor, merlin, functions in rac-dependent signaling. Dev Cell 2001;1:63–72.
90. Sherman L, Sleeman J, Herrlich P, et al. Hyaluronate receptors: key players in growth, differentiation, migration and tumor progression. Curr Opin Cell Biol 1994;6:726–33.
91. Takeshima H, Izawa I, Lee PS, et al. Detection of cellular proteins that interact with the NF2 tumor suppressor gene product. Oncogene 1994;9:2135–44.
92. Sainio M, Zhao F, Heiska L, et al. Neurofibromatosis 2 tumor suppressor protein colocalizes with ezrin and CD44 and associates with actin-containing cytoskeleton. J Cell Sci 1997;110:2249–60.
93. Huang L, Ichimaru E, Pestonjamasp K, et al. Merlin differs from moesin in binding to F-actin and in its intra- and intermolecular interactions. Biochim Biophys Res Comm 1998;248:548–53.
94. Murthy A, Gonzalez-Agosti C, Cordero E, et al. NHE-RF, a regulatory cofactor for na(+)-H+ exchange, is a common interactor for merlin and ERM (MERM) proteins. J Biol Chem 1998;273:1273–6.
95. Obremski VJ, Hall AM, Fernandez-Valle C. Merlin, the neurofibromatosis type 2 gene product, and b1 integrin associate in isolated and differentiating schwann cells. J Neurobiol 1998;37:487–501.
96. Scoles DR, Huynh DP, Morcos PA, et al. Neurofibromatosis 2 tumor suppressor schwannomin interacts with bII-spectrin. Nat Genet 1998;18:354–9.
97. Xu HM, Gutmann DH. Merlin differentially associates with the microtubule and actin cytoskeleton. J Neurosci Res 1998;51:403–15.
98. Fernandez-Valle C, Tang Y, Ricard J, et al. Paxillin binds schwannomin and regulates its density-dependent localization and effect on cell morphology. Nat Genet 2000;31:354–62.
99. Gonzalez-Agosti C, Wiederhold T, Herndon ME, et al. Interdomain interaction of merlin isoforms and its influence on intermolecular binding to NHE-RF. J Biol Chem 1999;274:34438–42.
100. Goutebroze L, Brault E, Muchardt C, et al. Cloning and characterization of SCHIP-1, a novel protein interacting specifically with spliced isoforms and naturally occurring mutant NF2 proteins. Mol Cell Biol 2000;20:1699–712.

101. Herrlich P, Morrison H, Sleeman J, et al. CD44 acts both as a growth and invasiveness-promoting molecule and as a tumor-suppressing cofactor. Ann NY Acad Sci 2000;910:106–18.

102. Scoles DR, Huynh DP, Chen MS, et al. The neurofibromatosis 2 tumor suppressor protein interacts with hepatocyte growth factor-regulated tyrosine kinase substrate. Hum Mol Genet 2000;9:1567–74.

103. Gronholm M, Vossebein L, Carlson CR, et al. Merlin links to the cAMP neuronal signaling pathway by anchoring the R1 beta subunit of protein kinase A. J Biol Chem 2003;278:41167–72.

104. Kissil JL, Wilker EW, Johnson KC, et al. Merlin, the product of the NF2 tumor suppressor gene, is an inhibitor of the p21-activated kinase, PAK1. Mol Cell 2003;12:841–9.

105. Lallemand D, Curto M, Saotome I, et al. NF2 deficiency promotes tumorigenesis and metastasis by destabilizing adherens junctions. Genes Dev 2003;17:1090–100.

106. Rong R, Tang X, Gutmann DH, et al. Neurofibromatosis 2 (NF2) tumor suppressor merlin inhibits phosphatidylinositol 3-kinase through binding to PIKE-L. Proc Natl Acad Sci USA 2004;101:18200–5.

107. Rangwala R, Banine F, Borg JP, Sherman LS. Erbin regulates mitogen-activated protein (MAP) kinase activation and MAP kinase-dependent interactions between merlin and adherens junction protein complexes in schwann cells. J Biol Chem 2005;280:11790–7.

108. Morrison H, Sherman LS, Legg J, et al. The NF2 tumor suppressor gene product, merlin, mediates contact inhibition of growth through interactions with CD44. Genes Dev 2001;15:968–80.

109. Flaiz C, Utermark T, Parkinson DB, et al. Impaired intercellular adhesion and immature adherens junctions in merlin-deficient human primary schwannoma cells. Glia 2008;56:506–15.

110. Surace EI, Haipek CA, Gutmann DH. Effect of merlin phosphorylation on neurofibromatosis 2 (NF2) gene function. Oncogene 2004;23:580–7.

111. Okada T, Lopez-Lago M, Giancotti FG. Merlin/NF-2 mediates contact inhibition of growth by suppressing recruitment of rac to the plasma membrane. J Cell Biol 2005;171:361–71.

112. Nakai Y, Zheng Y, MacCollin MM, Ratner N. Temporal control of rac in schwann cell–axon interaction is disrupted in NF2-mutant schwannoma cells. J Neurosci 2006;26:3390–5.

113. Xiao GH, Beeser A, Chernoff J, et al. P21-activated kinase links Rac/Cdc42 signaling to merlin. J Biol Chem 2002;277:883–6.

114. Kissil JL, Johnson KC, Eckman MS, et al. Merlin phosphorylation by p21-activated kinase 2 and effects of phosphorylation on merlin localization. J Biol Chem 2002;277:10394–9.

115. Jin H, Sperka T, Herrlich P, Morrison H. Tumorigenic transformation by CPI-17 through inhibition of a merlin phosphatase. Nature 2006;442:576–9.

116. Bretscher A, Reczek D, Berryman M. Ezrin: a protein requiring conformational activation to link microfilaments to the plasma membrane in the assembly of cell surface structures. J Cell Sci 1997;110:3011–8.

117. Tsukita S, Yonemura S, Tsukita S. ERM proteins: Head-to-tail regulation of actin-plasma membrane interaction. TIBS 1997;22:53–8.

118. Hirao M, Sato N, Kondo T, et al. Regulation mechanism of ERM (ezrin/radixin/moesin) protein/plasma membrane association: possible involvement of phosphatidylinositol turnover and rho-dependent signaling pathway. J Cell Biol 1996;135:37–51.

119. Gutmann DH, Haipek CA, Hoang Lu K. Neurofibromatosis 2 tumor suppressor protein, merlin, forms two functionally important intramolecular associations. J Neurosci Res 1999;58:706–16.

120. Gutmann DH, Haipek CA, Burke SP, et al. The *NF2* interactor, hepatocyte growth factor-regulated tyrosine kinase substrate (HRS), associates with merlin in the 'open' conformation and suppresses cell growth and motility. Hum Mol Genet 2001;10:825–34.

121. Pearson MA, Reczek D, Bretscher A, et al. Structure of the ERM protein moesin reveals the FERM domain fold masked by an extended actin binding tail domain. Cell 2000;101:259–70.

122. Komada M, Kitamura N. Growth factor-induced tyrosine phosphorylation of hrs, a novel 115-kilodalton protein with a structurally conserved putative zinc finger domain. Mol Cell Biol 1995;15:6213–21.

123. Jacob A, Lee TX, Neff BA, et al. Phosphatidylinositol 3 kinase/AKT pathway activation in human vestibular schwannoma. Otol Neurotol 2008;29:58–68.

124. Welling DB, Akhmametyeva EM, Daniels RL, et al. Analysis of the human neurofibromatosis type 2 gene promoter and its expression. Otolaryngol Head Neck Surg 2000 Oct;123(4):413–8.

125. Arakawa H, Hayashi N, Nagase H, et al. Alternative splicing of the NF2 gene and its mutation analysis of breast and colorectal cancers. Hum Mol Genet 1994;3:565–8.

126. Hitotsumatsu T, Kitamoto T, Iwaki T, et al. An exon 8-spliced out transcript of neurofibromatosis 2 gene is constitutively expressed in various human tissues. J Biochem 1994;116:1205–7.

127. Koga H, Araki N, Takeshima H, et al. Impairment of cell adhesion by expression of the mutant neurofibromatosis type 2 (NF2) gene which lacks exons in the ERM-homology domain. Oncogene 1998;17:801–10.

128. Nishi T, Takeshima H, Hamada K, et al. Neurofibromatosis 2 gene has novel alternative splicing which control intracellular protein binding. Int J Oncol 1997;10:1025–9.

129. Pykett MJ, Murphy M, Harnish PR, et al. The neurofibromatosis type 2 tumor suppressor gene encodes multiple alternatively spliced transcripts. Hum Mol Genet 1994;3(559):564.

130. Schmucker B, Tang Y, Kressel M. Novel alternatively spliced isoforms of the neurofibromatosis type 2 tumor suppressor are targeted to the nucleus and cytoplasmic granules. Hum Mol Genet 1999;8:1561–70.

131. Giovannini M, Robanus-Maandag E, Niwa-Kawakita M, et al. Schwann cell hyperplasia and tumors in transgenic mice expressing a naturally occurring mutant NF2 protein. Genes Dev 1999;13:978–86.

132. Labit-Bouvier C, Crebassa B, Bouvier C, et al. Clinicopathologic growth factors in vestibular schwannomas: A morphological and immunohistochemical study of 69 tumours. Acta Otolaryngol 2000;120:950–4.

133. Niemczyk K, Vaneecloo FN, Lecomte MH, et al. Correlation between ki-67 index and some clinical aspects of acoustic neuromas (vestibular schwannomas). Otolaryngol Head Neck Surg 2000;123:779–83.

134. Light JP, Roland JT, Jr, Fishman A, et al. Atypical and low-grade malignant vestibular schwannomas: Clinical implications of proliferative activity. Otol Neurotol 2001;22:922–7.

135. Chen JM, Houle S, Ang LC, et al. A study of vestibular schwannomas using positron emission tomography and monoclonal antibody ki-67. Am J Otol 1998;19:840–5.

136. Kesterson L, Shelton C, Dressler L, et al. Clinical behavior of acoustic tumors. A flow cytometric analysis. Arch Otolaryngol Head Neck Surg 1993;119:269–71.

137. Cardillo MR, Filipo R, Monini S, et al. Transforming growth factor-b1 expression in human acoustic neuroma. Am J Otol 1999;20:65–8.

138. Charabi S, Mantoni M, Tos M, et al. Cystic vestibular schwannomas: neuroimaging and growth rate. J Laryngol Otol 1994;108:375–9.

139. Charabi S, Klinken L, Tos M, Thomsen J. Histopathology and growth pattern of cystic acoustic neuromas. Laryngoscope 1994;104:1348–52.

140. Antinheimo J, Haapasalo H, Seppala M, et al. Proliferative potential of sporadic and neurofibromatosis 2-associated schwannomas as studied by MIB-1 (ki-67) and PCNA labeling. J Neuropathol Exp Neurol 1995;54:776–82.

141. Aguiar PH, Tatagiba M, Samii M, et al. The comparison between the growth fraction of bilateral vestibular schwannomas in neurofibromatosis 2 (NF2) and unilateral vestibular schwannomas using the monoclonal antibody MIB1. Acta Neurochir 1995;134:40–5.

142. Neff BA, Oberstien E, Lorenz M, et al. Cyclin D(1) and D(3) expression in vestibular schwannomas. Laryngoscope 2006 Mar;116(3):423–6.

143. Bassett DEJ, Eisen MB, Boguski MS. Gene expression informatics—it's all in your mind. Nat Genet 1999;21:51–5.

144. Lockhart DJ, Winzeler EA. Genomics, gene expression, and DNA arrays. Nature 2000;405:827–36.

145. Lasak JM, Welling DB, Akhmametyeva EM, et al. Retinoblastoma-cyclin-dependent kinase pathway deregulation in vestibular schwannomas. Laryngoscope 2002 Sep;112(9):1555–61.

146. Evans DGR, Birch JM, Ramsden RT, et al. Malignant transformation and new primary tumours after therapeutic radiation for benign disease: substantial risks in certain tumour prone syndromes. J Med Genet 2006;43:289–94.

147. Preston DL, Ron E, Yonehara S, et al. Tumors of the nervous system and pituitary gland associated with atomic bomb radiation exposure. J Natl Cancer Inst 2002;94:1555–63.

148. Schneider AB, Ron E, Lubin J, et al. Acoustic neuromas following childhood radiation treatment for benign conditions of the head and neck. Neuro Oncol 2008;10:73–8.

149. Hardell L, Carlberg M, Soderquist F, Mild KH. Meta-analysis of long-term mobile phone use and the association with brain tumors. Int J Oncol 2008;32:1097–103.

150. Hardell L, Carlberg M, Soderquist F, et al. Long-term use of cellular phones and brain tumours: Increased risk associated with use for > or = 10 years. Occup Environ Med 2007;64:626–32.

151. Evans DGR, Sainio M, Baser ME. Neurofibromatosis type 2. J Med Genet 2000;37:897–904.

152. Neff BA, Welling DB. Current concepts in the evaluation and treatment of neurofibromatosis type II. Otolaryngol Clin North Am 2005 Aug;38(4):671,684, ix.

153. Evans DG, Baser ME, O'Reilly B, et al. Management of the patient and family with neurofibromatosis 2: A consensus conference statement. Br J Neurosurg 2005;19:5–12.

154. Messerli SM, Prabhakar S, Tang Y, et al. Treatment of schwannomas with an oncolytic recombinant herpes simplex virus in murine models of neurofibromatosis type 2. Hum Gene Ther 2006;17:20–30.

155. Hansen MR, Roehm PC, Chatterjee P, Green SH. Constitutive neuregulin-1/ErbB signaling contributes to human vestibular schwannoma proliferation. Glia 2006;53:593–600.

156. Doherty JK, Ongekeko W, Crawley B, et al. ErbB and nrg potential targets for vestibular schwannoma pharmacotherapy. Otol Neurotol 2008;29:50–7.

157. Welch EM, Barton ER, Zhuo J, et al. PTC124 targets genetic disorders caused by nonsense mutations. Nature 2007;447:87–91.

158. Schmitz A, Famulok M. Chemical biology: ignore the nonsense. Nature 2007;447:42–3.

159. Pirker R, Filipits M. Targeted therapies in lung cancer. Curr Pharm Des 2009;15:188–206.

160. Aragon-Ching JB, Dahut WL. The role of angiogenesis inhibitors in prostate cancer. Cancer J 2008;14:20–5.

161. Ranieri G, Patruno R, Ruggieri E, et al. Vascular endothelial growth factor (VEGF) as a target of bevacizumab in cancer: from the biology to the clinic. Curr Med Chem 2006;13:1845–57.

162. Chase JL. Clinical use of anti-vascular endothelial growth factor monoclonal antibodies in metastatic colorectal cancer. Pharmacotherapy 2008;28:23S–30S.

163. MacCollin MM, Chiocca EA, Evans DGR, et al. Diagnostic criteria for schwannomatosis. Neurology 2005;18:38–45.

164. Boyd C, Smith MJ, Kluwe L, et al. Alterations in the SMARCB1 (INI1) tumor suppressor gene in familial schwannomatosis. Clin Genet 2008;74:358–66.

165. Sestini R, Bacci C, Provenzano A, et al. Evidence of a four-hit mechanism involving SMARCB1 and NF2 in schwannomatosis-associated schwannomas. Hum Mutat 2008;29:227–31.

166. Papaspyrou K, Rossmann H, Fottner C, et al. Malignant paraganglioma caused by a novel germline mutation of the succinate dehydrogenase D-gene: A case report. Head Neck 2008;30:964–9.

167. Marvin ML, Bradford CR, Sisson JC, Gruber SB. Diagnosis and management of hereditary paraganglioma syndrome due to the F933>X67 SDHD mutation. Head Neck 2009;31:689–94.

168. Mhatre AN, Lalwani AK. Molecular genetics in neurotology. In: Jackler RK, Brackmann DE, editors. Neurotology. Philadelphia, PA: Ellsevier Mosby; 2005.

169. Ladroue C, Carcenac R, Leporrier M, et al. PHD2 mutation and congenital erythrocystosis with paraganglioma. N Engl J Med 2008;359:2685–92.

II

Clinical Evaluation and Rehabilitation

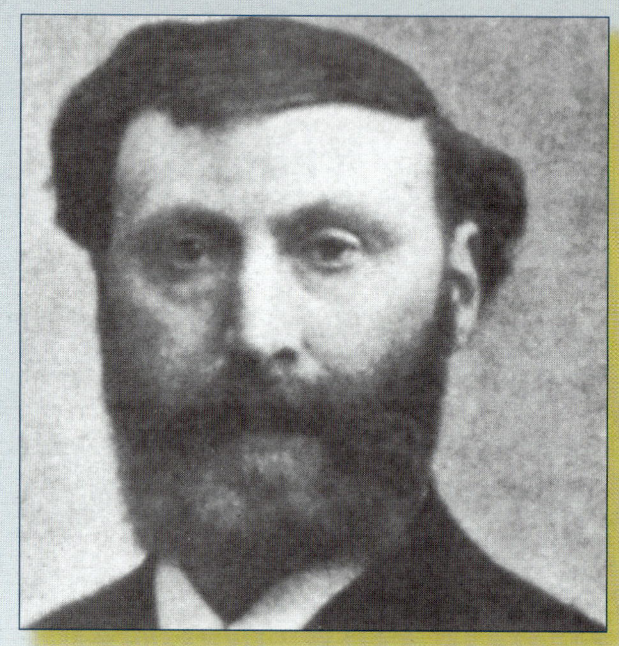

ADAM POLITZER (1835-1920) • Foremost teacher of otologic diagnosis and therapy of the Vienna school.

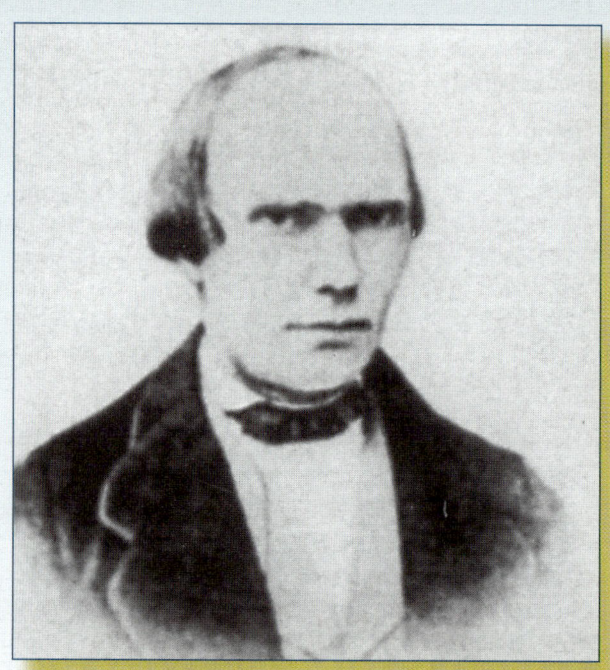

HEINRICH ADOLPH RINNE (1819-1868)• In 1855 described the tuning fork test, which is still the best method for diagnosis of conductive versus sensorineural hearing loss. *Reproduced with permission from Heck WE., Rinne A. Laryngoscope 1962;72:647.*

Clinical Diagnosis 9

Matthew R. O'Malley, MD / David S. Haynes, MD

Establishing a diagnosis in a patient with a hearing or balance disorder begins with a thorough history and physical examination. In particular, the history is of critical importance in ascertaining an accurate diagnosis, thereby allowing the physician to provide adequate counseling and institute appropriate therapy. This chapter addresses the basic neurotologic history and physical examination techniques that are important in the complete assessment of the patient with a hearing or balance complaint. This chapter also discusses the differential diagnosis of otologic and neurotologic diseases and provides a brief overview of common disorders.

HISTORY

General

As with any medical disorder, a thorough history and physical examination are essential in the evaluation of the patient with a neurotologic disorder.[1,2] As subsequent chapters will present, technological advancements over the past three decades have provided the clinician with incredibly powerful and accurate diagnostic imaging and testing techniques. Despite these advances, the mainstay of diagnosis is the history and physical examination, and it is the clinical evaluation that allows the practitioner to effectively and efficiently utilize ancillary testing.

When evaluating patients with disorders of hearing or balance, assessment forms (Figure 9–1) are commonly employed. Different forms may be designed for initial and follow-up visits. An otologic assessment form is advantageous for several reasons: (1) it allows the examination to be focused and directed, (2) it ensures that all critical information is obtained and not inadvertently omitted, and (3) it provides a precise, organized reference for follow-up examinations, surgery, research, or administrative purposes. Additionally, the American Academy of Otolaryngology—Head and Neck Surgery (AAO-HNS) Committee on Hearing and Equilibrium has advocated the documentation of certain elements of history in the evaluation of patients with specific balance disorders.[3]

A questionnaire completed by the patient is also very useful in the otologic evaluation. The questionnaire may be completed on arrival or may be mailed to the patient and completed prior to the office visit. The questionnaire should include all aspects of the patient history, including history of present illness, previous clinical evaluations, prior medical imaging, previous medical or surgical therapy, previous and current medication regimens, medication allergies, history of trauma, history of noise exposure, social history, family history, and review of systems. This history, recorded by the patient, does not supplant, but rather complements the standard history taken by the examiner. This questionnaire may also be useful because it is a history taken "by the patient" and can avoid discrepancies regarding onset of symptoms, previous evaluation, or previous surgery, which can be areas of significance in medical, legal cases. Further, it is encouraged that, when possible, the patients are asked to provide a list of their medical allergies in their own writing for reference in the chart.

The standard clinical encounter should begin with the chief complaint. When dealing with complaints pertaining to the ears, patients frequently have multiple complaints (eg, tinnitus and imbalance, drainage, and hearing loss). Spending a moment to allow the patient to prioritize their complaints can be enlightening to both the patient and the clinician. After establishing the patient's complaints, the history of present illness should be elucidated. Specific elements to be addressed include symptom onset, duration, frequency, associated symptoms, and exacerbating or relieving factors. In many instances, it is important to prompt the patient to report which ear (or ears) is causing the symptom being described, as it is not uncommon to have different complaints in each ear (eg, "... my right ear hurts, my left ear doesn't hear well, but both ears drain..."). The past medical history, past surgical history, review of symptoms, medications, allergies, previous therapy (including medications used and their efficacy or complications), history of trauma, history of noise exposure, social history, and family history are then systematically reviewed.

The history should not concentrate just on symptoms of hearing and balance but on the patient as a whole as many

Vanderbilt University Medical Center

OTOLARYNGOLOGY
Nashville, TN 37232-5555

OTOLOGY/NEUROTOLOGY ASSESSMENT FORM

Patient Name: Date:
DOB: AGE:
MR #
Referring Physician:
Dictation: Y N
Chief Complaint:

HPI:

HEARING	Right	Left	VERTIGO
Duration			Onset
Prog.			Frequency
Tinnitus			Duration
Fullness			Spinning
Otitis			Unsteadiness
Bet. Ear			Nausea
Fluctuation			Positional
Hearing Aid			MRI

Current Medications:

Allergies:

Trauma:

Family History

Noise Exposure:

Physical Exam:

Right		Left
	Normal	
	Perf w/ chol	
	Perf w/o chol	
	Serous OM	
	Acute OM	
AC>BC ; BC>AC	(W)	AC>BC ; BC>AC

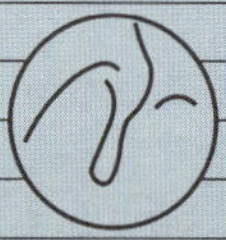

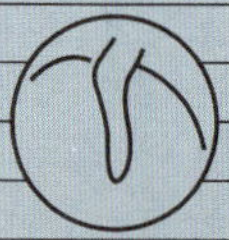

Neorotology Exam
Romberg
Cerebellar
Cranial Nerve
Nystagmus
Dix Hallpike

HEENT: Bruits:

IMPRESSION:

EVALUATION:

Imaging:	Lab Work	Vestibular Testing
CT	FTA	ENG
Temporal Bone	ESR	ECoG
Coronal Sinus	ANA	Rotary Chair
MRI head w/GAD	RF	Posturography
w/o GAD	Chol	Vestibular Rehab.
	SMA-20	

TREATMENT

Follow up

Audiogram

FIGURE 9–1 • Neurotologic assessment form. *Courtesy of Vanderbilt University Medical Center.*

systemic disorders can affect the vestibular or auditory system (Table 9–1).[4] Rheumatologic disorders, diabetes, multiple sclerosis, and thyroid disorders are just a few of the systemic disorders that can cause or exacerbate neurotologic symptoms. Occupational, recreational, and military noise exposure should be specifically documented[5] as should the influence of any type of potential trauma surrounding the complaint. As indicated previously, the use of an encounter form assists the clinician in assessing all of these points.

All current medications should be recorded as well as any past medications that have been employed to treat the patient's current symptoms. A list of potentially ototoxic medications is provided in Table 9–2.[6–9] Aminoglycoside antibiotics, salicylates, furosemide, hydrocodone, and other commonly used medications may be directly ototoxic. The prior use of ototoxic agents must be specifically asked for in most instances, as the patient with imbalance or hearing loss may not spontaneously report the prior use of medications to treat conditions elsewhere in the body, particularly if those conditions have resolved (eg, gentamicin used to treat an intra-abdominal infection 6 months prior to presentation). Other medications may lead to a sense of imbalance (antihypertensives, antidepressants) without being directly ototoxic. Somnolence is common with many medications (antihistamines, benzodiazepines) and can exacerbate symptoms of imbalance, especially among elderly patients.

The use of topical agents applied to the ear is of particular importance. Often these agents are used intermittently, and not spontaneously remembered by the patient on the day of the office visit. Many topical preparations carry a risk of ototoxicity, even when used appropriately, and in certain instances uncovering a history of use of these agents may aid in diagnosis and treatment.

The use of over-the-counter medications and supplements should be specifically addressed during the evaluation and on the patient questionnaire. These agents are often overlooked by patients and clinicians alike. The use of supplements is commonplace. The clinician is not infrequently confronted by a patient taking a supplement that is poorly characterized. Furthermore, some patients take "mega-doses" of vitamins or supplements; the physiologic ramifications of this practice are poorly understood in most instances. Many patients with imbalance may take or have taken over-the-counter meclizine preparations, which may impact their compensation abilities or interact with other prescribed agents. It seems safe to assume that the overwhelming

TABLE 9–1 Systemic disorders affecting the ear[4]

Granulomatous/infectious disease	Progressive systemic sclerosis
Langerhans' cell histiocytosis	Bone disease
Eosinophilic granuloma	Paget's disease
Hand-Schüller-Christian disease	Osteogenesis imperfecta
Letterer-Siwe disease	Fibrous dysplasia
Sarcoidosis	Osteopetrosis
Lyme disease	Osteitis fibrosa cystica
Fungal infections	Chronic osteomyelitis
Wegener's granulomatosis	Miscellaneous
Tuberculosis	Acquired immune deficiency syndrome (AIDS)
Autoimmune disease/collagen vascular disease	Mucopolysaccharidoses
Relapsing polychondritis	Polyarteritis nodosa
Systemic lupus erythematosus	Cogan's syndrome
Rheumatoid arthritis	Neoplastic disease
Giant cell arteritis	Leukemia
Sjögren's syndrome	Lymphoma
Polymyositis/dermatomyositis	Paraganglioma
Ankylosing spondylitis	Multiple myeloma
Vogt-Koyanagi-Harada syndrome	Metastatic disease/meningeal carcinomatosis
Behcet's syndrome	
Autoimmune inner ear disease	
Cardiac disorders (arrhythmias)	
Anemia	

TABLE 9–2 Agents and medications that can cause vestibular and auditory ototoxicity[6-9]

Antibiotics	Diuretics
Aminoglycoside antibiotics	Furosemide
Primarily cochleotoxic	Ethacrynic acid
Neomycin	Bumetanide
Kanamycin	Antiinflammatory agents
Tobramycin	Salicylates
Dihydrostreptomycin	Quinine
Amikacin	Nonsteroidal antiinflammatory agents
Primarily vestibulotoxic	Chloroquine
Gentamicin	Chelating agents
Streptomycin	Desferoxime
Other	Chemicals
Erythromycin	Mercury
Vancomycin	Gold
Antineoplastic agents	Lead arsenic aniline dyes
Cisplatin	
Carboplatin	
Nitrogen mustard	
Vincristine	
Vinblastine	

majority of adult patients have taken at least one drug or supplement in the 2 weeks prior to their office visit (eg, aspirin, Tylenol, or nonsteroidal antiinflammatory drugs (NSAIDS) for headache or cramps, vitamin E as an antioxidant, etc.), and it is recommended that the thorough clinician elicit such a history.

Certain elements of a patient's history are particularly pertinent to the surgeon, and should be reviewed and documented as a matter of routine, to avoid catastrophic omission. A personal history of anesthetic or bleeding complications with prior surgical procedures should be sought and documented, even if negative, as should a family history of bleeding disorders or inability to tolerate anesthetic. Asking about a history of any prior blood transfusions can sometimes prompt a patient to recall a forgotten surgical complication.

Auditory System

A history for the patient with hearing loss should include the following:

- Duration, age of onset
- Rate of progression (sudden or gradual)
- Stable or fluctuating
- Unilateral or bilateral
- Prior use of amplification
- Other associated symptoms (ie, tinnitus, vertigo, infections, fullness, otalgia, otorrhea)
- Previous ear surgery for hearing loss or other indications
- Family history of hearing loss, including ear surgery
- Better-hearing ear.

The patient should always be asked which ear is the better-hearing ear regardless of what the physical evaluation, tuning fork test, or audiogram reveals. In instances when the patient has reviewed an audiogram prior to the meeting with the physician, it is important to ascertain if the patient subjectively notices hearing loss that is discrepant with the audiometric testing.

In addition to the standard history, evaluation of a child for hearing loss also requires gestational, perinatal, postnatal, and detailed family histories. Inquiries should be made to explore possible syndromic associations (other systemic problems, neurological/developmental abnormalities, growth disturbances, craniofacial abnormalities, or disorders of renal, cardiac, hematologic, or metabolic systems.) Parental, other family members,' and teachers' concerns regarding hearing loss should be addressed. Parents may notice hearing difficulty in their children, but smaller losses may not actually be detected by family members. Particularly in the case of unilateral hearing loss or mid- or high-frequency hearing loss, the problem may go unrecognized until a screening audiogram is performed. Approximately 50% of congenital hearing impairment is hereditary, with 60 to 70% of these cases being of autosomal recessive mode of inheritance.[10] The majority of hereditary hearing losses are nonsyndromic and the most common genetic mutation identified to date is in Connexin 26, a protein important for ion homeostasis within the inner ear. Genetic testing is available to evaluate a child for a number of different mutations causing hereditary hearing loss, and its application is recommended in specific circumstances that are continually expanding.[11] The application of genetic testing in the evaluation of children with hearing loss is a rapidly changing field, not without controversy, and the clinician is encouraged to keep current with the literature on this subject. Regardless of testing, genetic counseling should be offered to any family who has a child with a suspected hereditary hearing loss.

A list of some of the causes of hearing loss is provided in Tables 9–3 and 9–4.[12–16] Congenital cytomegalovirus (CMV) infection has been shown to be an important cause of hearing loss.[17,18] In certain settings, it may soon be possible to establish congenital CMV infection as a possible etiology for hearing loss greater than a year after birth using heel blood cards collected at birth.[19]

Establishing a definitive etiology for congenital hearing loss may prove difficult. In one large series,[20] 31.9% of the children tested had no obvious etiology; establishing an etiology in unilateral cases was lower (50%) than in bilateral cases (75.4%). Despite the multiple diagnostic tests available, the history remains an important instrument in diagnosing childhood hearing loss.

Tinnitus is a symptom that is defined as any sound perceived by the patient when no external source of the sound exists. Tinnitus can be primarily divided into two categories, objective and subjective. Within each category, one can further classify tinnitus as pulsatile or nonpulsatile.

Objective tinnitus is infrequent and is audible to the examiner. Subjective tinnitus, much more common than objective

TABLE 9–3 Causes of sensorineural hearing loss[13-15]

Infectious disease	Autoimmune disorders
Acute otitis media	Vascular disease
Bacterial (suppurative) labyrinthitis	Neoplasms
Serous labyrinthitis	Meningeal carcinomatosis
Meningitis	Congenital disorders
Syphilis	Perinatal infections
Chronic osteomyelitis	Rubella
Lyme disease	Cytomegalovirus
Viral	Cochlear otosclerosis
Mumps	Migraine-associated hearing loss
Herpes zoster oticus	Metabolic disorders
Trauma	Diabetes
Noise-induced hearing loss	Renal failure
Occupational	Thyroid disorders
Recreational	Mucopolysaccharidoses
Basilar skull fracture	Hematologic disorders
Cochlear concussion	Psychogenic deafness
Barotrauma	Presbycusis
Perilymph fistula	Vasculitis
Drug toxicity	Paget's disease
Neurologic disorders	Multiple sclerosis
Systemic disease (see Table 9–4)	

tinnitus, is not audible to the examiner. Objective tinnitus may be caused by vascular, neurologic, or eustachian tube or palatal disorders. Vascular disorders may cause pulsatile tinnitus by generating turbulent flow in arterial or venous vessels in the neck, cranial vault, or temporal bone. Vascular disorders that may cause objective tinnitus include venous hums, arterial bruits, arteriovenous malformations and shunts, aneurysms, aberrant vessels, abnormalities in the lateral sinus (strictures, venous lakes) and vascular neoplasms. Neurologic disorders that cause objective tinnitus include palatal myoclonus and idiopathic stapedius and tensor tympani muscle spasm. Palatomyoclonus is an uncommon disorder characterized by regular or irregular, rapid, clicking sounds. Palatal myoclonus can be due to central nervous system pathology and neurotologic evaluation and imaging may be appropriate. The sounds are generated when the mucosa of the Eustachian tube snaps open or closed as the palatal muscles undergo myoclonic contractions. Middle ear muscle spasms (stapedius, tensor tympani) produce an intermittent, bothersome, fluttering sound in the ear as the muscles contract during spasm. External sounds may accentuate these spasms.

Subjective tinnitus is far more common than objective tinnitus and is generally associated with high-frequency sensorineural hearing loss, typically as a result of noise exposure or aging (presbycusis). Other causes are idiopathic, metabolic, genetic, cardiologic/vascular, neurologic, pharmacologic, dental, psychologic, and otologic factors. Tinnitus associated with symmetric sensorineural hearing loss may not necessitate evaluation beyond a complete audiologic and head and neck examination. Unilateral or pulsatile tinnitus and tinnitus associated with asymmetric sensorineural hearing loss or conductive hearing loss generally necessitate additional investigation by means of imaging or neurophysiologic testing.[2]

The presence or absence of otalgia should be reviewed in any ear of the patient who has presented for medical consultation. If otalgia is present, an evaluation of its severity should be made. The presence of otalgia is expected in patients with an acute infection of the external canal, tympanic membrane, middle ear, or mastoid. Though each individual's pain perception will vary, chronic infection of the middle ear is generally less painful than acute infection. As a general rule of thumb, a chronically draining ear with a tympanic membrane perforation should not be expected to produce severe pain. If severe otalgia (especially pain out of proportion for the clinical signs) is present in this condition, the clinicians should broaden their differential diagnosis to include causes other than isolated infection.

TABLE 9–4 Causes of conductive hearing loss[16,17]

Inflammatory or infectious causes	Neoplasia
Otitis externa	Paraganglioma
Eustachian tube dysfunction	Facial nerve neuroma
Adhesive middle ear disease	Rhabdomyosarcoma
Acute otitis media	Squamous cell carcinoma
Serous otitis media	Middle ear adenoma
Chronic otitis media	Neurofibroma
Malignant otitis externa	Hemangiopericytoma
Cholesteatoma	Lymphangioma
Tympanosclerosis	Lymphoma
Myringosclerosis	Leukemia
Tympanic membrane perforation	Multiple myeloma
Otomycosis	Pleomorphic adenoma
Aural tuberculosis	Adenoid cystic carcinoma
Syphilis	Hemangioma
Systemic disorders	Basal cell carcinoma
Sarcoidosis	Congenital abnormalities
Fibrous dysplasia	Microtia
Mucopolysaccharidosis	Atresia
Wegener's granulomatosis	Branchial cleft cyst
Histiocytosis/eosinophilic granuloma (Langerhans' cell histiocytosis)	Congenital ossicular fixation
Relapsing polychondritis	Otosclerosis
Polyarteritis nodosa	Osteogenesis imperfecta
Keratosis obturans	Treacher Collins syndrome
Cerumen	Pierre Robin syndrome
Trauma	Marfan syndrome
Barotrauma	Mohr syndrome
Basilar skull fracture/temporal bone fracture	Pyle's disease
Hemotympanum	Achondroplasia
Traumatic perforation	Paget's disease
External canal laceration/avulsion	Apert's disease
Miscellaneous	Goldenhar's syndrome
Cerebrospinal fluid effusion	Turner's syndrome
Keloid	Crouzon's disease
External canal osteoma	
External canal exostosis	
Osteopetrosis	

Disproportionate pain can be an indication of the development of complications. In an infected ear, pus under pressure and acute or subacute bone erosion generally cause pain. When the otoscopic examination is unremarkable, an evaluation of exacerbating and alleviating factors can sometimes reveal a source of otalgia. For instance, pain with chewing, at nighttime, or during stressful times in the day, may suggest temporomandibular joint (TMJ) dysfunction. A history of recent dental work or poorly fitting dentures may also suggest a cause for pain referred from the oral cavity. Head and neck muscle pain is commonly referred to the ear and can be the source of acute or chronic otalgia.

Otalgia without an obvious cause should alert the clinician to the possibility of malignancy. Malignancies arising in the upper aerodigestive tract (ie, nasopharynx, tonsil, base of tongue, oropharynx, hypopharynx, and larynx) can cause referred pain to the ear. Therefore in patients with otalgia and a normal otoscopic evaluation, elements of history designed to elicit symptoms of malignancy such as laryngitis, hoarseness, previous malignancy, or previous head and neck surgery, should be sought. Further, metastasis to the temporal bone from distant sites has been reported, and thus a history of malignancy elsewhere in the body should be reviewed.

Other elements of history pertinent to the evaluation of patients with otalgia include history of prior ear surgery or tympanostomy tube placement, a history of prior radiation treatment to the head or neck, a history of herpes zoster, a history of recurrent headaches or migraines, and/or a history of trauma.

If drainage is the primary complaint, the patient should be questioned regarding its characteristics, such as profuse or scant, purulent, clear, mucoid, bloody, or foul smelling. When otorrhea is present, knowledge of any prior surgical procedure is of undeniable importance. Multiple and bilateral procedures performed over many years and by multiple surgeons can obviously be confusing to patients and examiners. Occasionally, a patient may not remember having had ear surgery at all. Although the patient's reporting of previous procedures and even the medical records are not always entirely accurate, the information may be very important and it is imperative to document the type, approximate date, and side of the procedure. As with any complaint regarding hearing, the patient should always be asked which ear is the better-hearing ear regardless of what the physical evaluation, tuning fork test, or audiogram reveals. The presence of otorrhea without tympanic membrane perforation generally suggests either a dermatologic condition of the ear canal, or some variety of external ear infection.

Pruritis of the ear canal is encountered with some frequency. Isolated pruritis is rarely an indicator of a threatening disease process. Thus, the patient with an itchy ear should be questioned regarding associated symptoms (such as drainage, pain, hearing loss, etc.), which could suggest a more sinister cause. In cases of isolated pruritis, the clinician should consider asking about ear swabbing, ear canal manipulation, water exposure, cerumen build-up, and systemic or local dermatologic complaints.

Vestibular System

In the assessment of the patient with a balance complaint, the physical examination is often unrevealing, leaving the history as the most important diagnostic tool.[21] Dysequilibrium is a complex symptom that can result from aberrations of the vestibular system. Unsteadiness, drunkenness, giddiness, wooziness, vertigo, dizziness, a sensation of being off-balance, imbalance, light-headedness, heavy-headedness, wobbliness, and spinning are some of the terms used to describe vestibular symptoms. The distinction of vertigo from other varieties of disequilibrium is stressed in certain contexts. Some clinicians maintain that vertigo is to be defined strictly as the perception of movement when there is none. A survey of greater than 300 members of American Otological Society found that there is substantial variability in what clinicians term vertigo.[22]

In patients aged 75 years or older, dizziness is the most common complaint discussed with their physician.[23] Symptoms of vertigo should never be attributed to normal aging; a specific etiology should be identifiable in the majority of cases.[24] The clinician should address the following features of dysequilibrium in the evaluation of a balance complaint:

- Onset (date of first sense of imbalance, and gradual vs sudden)?
- How is the dysequilibrium described? (primarily differentiate between unsteadiness or true spinning)?
- Duration?
- Episodic or constant?
- If episodic, how long does each episode last? Are there symptoms between episodes? Frequency of episodes?
- Severity?
- Recovery from episodes—brief, prolonged, period of disability?
- Presence or absence of syncope?
- Progression (improving or worsening)?
- Conditions that can reliably cause symptoms (eg, head position, exercise, cough/sneeze/Valsalva maneuver, stress, diet/certain foods or sodium)?
- Exacerbating or alleviating factors?
- Are the vestibular symptoms associated with hearing loss, tinnitus, focal neurologic signs, migraine, or nausea and vomiting?
- Have there been past or present symptoms of migraine (visual hallucinations/scintillating scotomata, other transient neurological symptoms, photophobia or hyperacusis? (headache is not required!)
- Family history of migraine?
- Is there a history of head and neck trauma or barotrauma?
- Is there a history of chronic ear disease? Is there a history of otorrhea? Family history of chronic ear disease or other ear/hearing/balance problems?
- Is there a history of previous ear, head, neck, vascular, cardiac, or intracranial surgery?
- Is there a history of recurrent falling?
- Is the patient able to work, drive, or perform activities of daily living?
- Is the patient currently receiving, or seeking to receive, disability support (for dizziness or other causes)?

Determining whether the patient's symptoms are episodic or constant, and whether or not hearing loss is present, may be two of the more important points of the history for a patient with a balance complaint. In a prospective study, Kentala and Rauch found that 60% of patients with common otogenic causes of vertigo could be accurately diagnosed on the basis of these elements of history alone.[25]

To certain patients, the initial history taking may seem somewhat argumentative, as the clinician may frequently need to interject in order to clarify elements of the history. If the patient seems frustrated by the history taking, the clinician can often relieve some of the frustration by verbally acknowledging that providing a vertigo history can be difficult, but is important for effective diagnosis and treatment.

A history of syncope with dizziness attacks is a very important finding and should be sought out. Strictly speaking, otogenic vertigo should not cause syncope, though it may cause drop attacks. Drop attacks, or otolithic crises of Tumarkin, are characterized by a sudden, unexpected loss of vertical orientation in space that results in a drop straight downward, usually without the patient being able to react appropriately to protect themselves. Although dramatic, they are usually brief events that do not involve any loss of consciousness. Specifically differentiating syncope and drop attacks is therefore essential. A history of syncopal attacks should prompt a thorough evaluation for the cause of syncope, which may or may not be related to the cause of vertigo. Most often, the evaluation of a patient with syncope is coordinated with consultation and input from internists, cardiologists, neurologists, and other specialists. In very rare circumstances, true syncope can result from an extraordinarily severe vertigo spell in which there is a strong vaso-vagal response. Syncope from vertigo must be diagnosed by exclusion of medical and neurological causes and in association with a strong history, related the syncope to severe vertigo.

In most instances, inquiring about a patient's disability status is also useful. Patients who have already established disability likely represent a more severely affected group of patients, and may be less responsive to treatment. For those patients seeking to establish a disability claim, the clinician is frequently asked to complete lengthy forms requiring detailed information about the patient's capabilities, far beyond what may be traditionally asked in a purely clinical encounter. Knowing in advance that such information is required may allow the clinician to allot additional time for questioning, and collect additional information.

All too often the physical examination in the patient with vertigo is unrevealing and vestibular testing inconclusive, leaving the history the most important, if not the only instrument, that can be used to establish a clinical diagnosis. The importance of the history in correctly diagnosing these disorders cannot be overemphasized.

PHYSICAL EXAMINATION

This section will review the general examination of the patient with a hearing or balance disorder, which includes a general examination of the head and neck, ear, nose, and throat. The examination also includes a neurotologic examination in which cerebellar testing, cranial nerve evaluation, clinical balance testing, and a focused neurologic examination are done.

OTOLOGIC EXAMINATION

Auricle

The auricle is inspected for incisions, scarring, congenital abnormalities, trauma, infection, cellulitis, dermatitis, or neoplasia. Specific attention is to be paid to the postauricular/mastoid region. Scars in this area may indicate prior ear surgery, cosmetic surgery, or trauma. Erythema, swelling, and tenderness in this area suggest mastoiditis. Specific attention should also be paid to the tragal region, as scars here are likely the result of prior surgery. One may also specifically look for evidence of an endaural or preauricular incision.

A misshapen auricle, preauricular pits, or skin tags may be present and indicate faulty fusion of the auricular hillocks or other congenital abnormalities. Such abnormalities may create an opportunity for infection, or may alert the clinician to the possibility of other associated malformations. Following inspection, the auricle should be grasped and gently moved. Movement of the auricle often elicits tenderness when external otitis, cellulitis, or perichondritis is present. Tenderness elicited with movement of the auricle is less common in cases of otitis media and herpes zoster oticus.

External Auditory Canal

Although a handheld otoscope is useful as a screening tool, its use is limited by the absence of binocular, stereoscopic vision, and it offers limited magnification. The operating microscope (Figure 9–2) is a superior instrument to examine a pathologic condition of the external canal, tympanic membrane, and middle ear. Microscopic examination is particularly helpful in the preoperative evaluation. The patient may be reclined, and the head is positioned properly to compensate for the natural superiorly rising angle of the canal. As the head is turned slightly away from the examiner, the ear canal is straightened by gently pulling the auricle posteriorly and superiorly. Typically, the largest speculum that can be inserted comfortably into the ear canal is chosen to maximize light and exposure. The examiner may also pull the tragus slightly anteriorly to assist in inspection. Care is taken to insert the speculum only into the cartilaginous canal because deeper penetration near the bony canal can be painful. Both adults and children are informed in advance of the above steps. This simple forewarning facilitates the examination, avoids patient apprehension, and gains trust.

To truly examine the ear, cerumen, desquamated skin, and purulent debris must be removed with loops, alligator forceps, curettes, or suction until an unobstructed view is obtained. Cleaning the ear of even a small amount of cerumen or debris may be crucial for proper inspection and important in the avoidance of missing an otologic diagnosis on the basis of limited exposure. Video-otoscopic examination can be performed easily in the office and may assist in photo-documentation and patient counseling. With video monitors in the patient's direct view, the patient can better appreciate an existing abnormality such as a tympanic membrane perforation, retraction, or cholesteatoma. Most patients have never seen their tympanic membranes and appreciate seeing for themselves any abnormalities

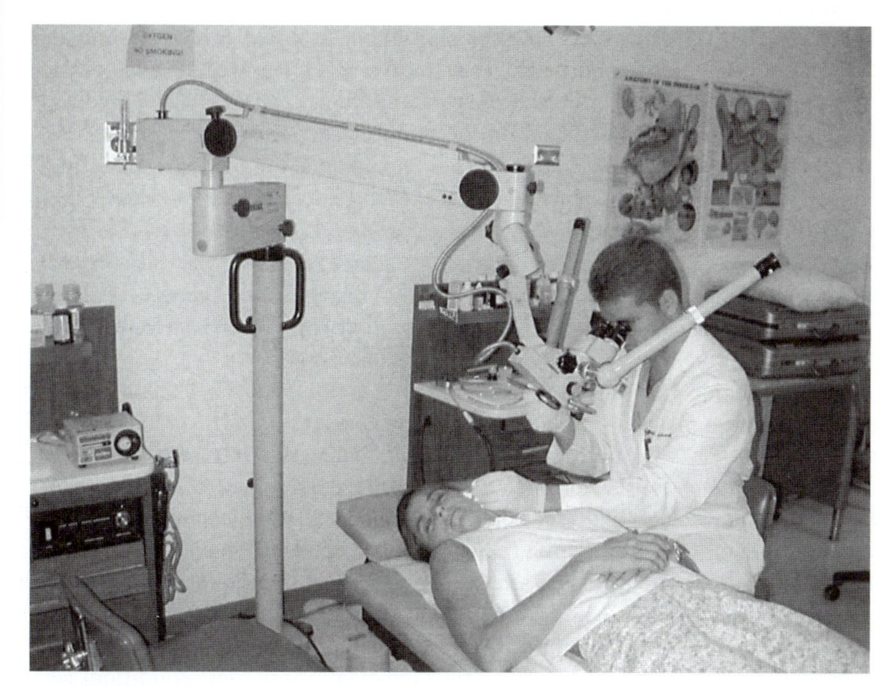

FIGURE 9–2 • Technique of otomicroscopy.

that may exist. Video-otoscopic examination can be performed with either an endoscope or with a microscope fitted with appropriate imaging equipment.

The external auditory canal is inspected for stenosis, cellulitis, furuncles, cysts, edema, dermatitis, exposed bone, osteomas, exostoses, and neoplastic changes. The presence of granulation tissue, purulent or mucoid discharge, or squamous debris is assessed. Bony osteomas or exostoses are confirmed to be hard by means of gentle, direct palpation. Aural polyps may be carefully manipulated to determine their site of origin. It is reasonable to differentiate polyps of external ear canal origin from those that arise from the middle ear or tympanic membrane, though this can sometimes be challenging in the office. Polyps protruding directly from the middle ear through a tympanic membrane perforation or, less commonly, directly from the tympanic membrane suggest chronic middle ear disease or cholesteatoma. Removal of aural polyps that protrude through the tympanic membrane as an office procedure is generally not recommended as these lesions indicate more significant disease not amenable to simple removal and may be intimately involved with vital structures such as the ossicular chain and facial nerve. Further, in rare instances, tumors, such as a facial nerve schwannoma or glomus tumor, may present with a mass that appears to be a simple aural polyp. In these cases, a seemingly minor office procedure can produce catastrophic results.

Tympanic Membrane

The otoscope or microscope is used to inspect the tympanic membrane for retraction, lateralization, perforation, effusion, myringitis, granulation tissue, cholesteatoma, or other pathologic process. A dimeric (formerly called "monomeric") area of the tympanic membrane should be differentiated from a true perforation, and this is generally possible using a microscope. The mobility of the tympanic membrane can be assessed with a handheld otoscope outfitted with a pneumatic bulb or by tympanometry. The most effective means for evaluating the mobility and character of the tympanic membrane is by pneumatic otoscopy using a Siegel lens and speculum, especially when combined with inspection under an operating microscope. Pneumatic otoscopy is especially useful in assessing middle ear fluid when the examination is inconclusive (ie, no air-fluid level, bubbles, or discoloration is evident). Pneumatic otoscopy is also useful in distinguishing tympanosclerosis from middle ear cholesteatoma and in evaluating atelectatic or retracted areas of the tympanic membrane. Adherent atelectasis or pockets represent a more advanced stage of chronic disease and may be more likely to require surgery than nonadherent defects in the tympanic membrane. A dehiscent jugular bulb or carotid artery, glomus tumor, facial neuroma (tympanic segment), middle ear adenoma or other tumor, and an aneurysm may appear as a vascular mass behind an intact tympanic membrane. Any mass in the middle ear with a vascular appearance (red, blue, violaceous, pulsatile) should be evaluated by imaging studies, preferably with contrast agents before any surgical exploration is considered. Computerized tomography (CT), angiography, or magnetic resonance imaging (MRI) angiography, may be indicated if the diagnosis remains uncertain after routine imaging. Biopsy of a vascular mass without preoperative imaging could result in injury to a major structure, such as an aberrant internal carotid artery, with disastrous consequences. A white mass visible medial to the tympanic membrane may represent purulent debris, congenital or acquired cholesteatoma, tympanosclerosis, or a middle ear mass such as a neuroma. Abnormal development of the ossicular chain may also manifest as a middle ear mass.

Occasionally, atelectasis, atrophy, or retraction of the tympanic membrane can be difficult to diagnose. Assessment is best performed with the binocular vision provided by the operating microscope. Pneumatic otoscopy may be of use in certain cases. Positive or negative pressure applied to the tympanic membrane may cause the retracted segment to move, allowing the examiner to assess the extent of retraction or atelectasis. Application of positive or negative pressure may also be useful to distinguish between a dimeric membrane and a tympanic membrane perforation. Serous fluid may be more evident with pneumatic otoscopy as the fluid may shift or may adhere to the tympanic membrane as the drum moves with applied pressure. The extent of retraction, presence of squamous debris or cholesteatoma, otorrhea, associated perforation, and, if possible, the status of the ossicular chain must be assessed to recommend proper therapy.

Examination of the patient who has undergone previous surgery is more difficult owing to altered anatomy and surgical scarring. Determining the type of surgical procedure(s) performed, such as canal wall down or intact canal wall mastoidectomy, can be more difficult in some ears than expected. Pathology particular to revision ears includes recurrent cholesteatoma, graft failure (perforation, lateralization, blunting, or retraction), and prosthesis extrusion. In canal wall down cavities, an assessment of meatal size, dependent or retracted areas, graft failure, inflammation, granulations, otorrhea, recurrent cholesteatoma, and height of the facial ridge is necessary.[26] The removal of debris from a canal wall down cavity is essential in an ear causing complaint. In some instances, the full removal of debris cannot be accomplished in the office, and such patients should be further evaluated with either imaging or examination or exploration in the operating room. The use of suction in the patient with a canal wall down cavity can cause vertigo, and thus patients should be suitably forewarned.

HEAD AND NECK EXAMINATION

Examination of the head and neck is an integral part of the neurotologic examination. The systematic examination of the skin, face, nose, nasal cavity, oral cavity, oropharynx, and neck should be performed in all patients presenting with a new otologic complaint. Though in most instances, this examination will be unrevealing, the routine inclusion of these elements of examination will facilitate diagnosis of less common etiologies. For example, the detection of a nasal septum lesion in a patient presenting with an effusion may allow the diagnosis of Wegener's granulomatosis with otologic involvement, a diagnosis that is less likely to be obtained had the septum not been examined.

The presence of otalgia may represent referred pain from the aerodigestive tract, thus the nasopharynx, oropharynx, hypopharynx, larynx and oral cavity should be examined for occult malignancy or other lesions in cases where the cause of the otalgia is not evident. Temporomandibular joint abnormalities may also cause otalgia, and the palpation of the joint during opening and closing of the mouth may alert the clinician to this possibility. The joint is examined for tenderness with deep palpation into the glenoid fossa along the posterior and superior aspects of the mandibular condyle. Intraoral examination for tenderness of the masseter and temporalis muscles along the anterior border of the mandibular ramus is often revealing for TMJ dysfunction, despite a negative history of jaw problems. The neck and parotid are palpated for masses, especially when signs of partial or total facial paralysis are evident. The suspected presence of a glomus jugulare tumor should alert the clinician to be vigilant when examining the neck in order to detect possible concomitant carotid body tumors. Further, an evaluation of laryngeal mobility may be helpful for the clinician when encountering a skull base lesion.

A funduscopic examination may be obtained either as part of the neurotologic examination or by consultation with an ophthalmologist when increased intracranial pressure is suspected. Pulsatile tinnitus may be a sign of benign intracranial hypertension. The presence of papilledema on funduscopic examination further supports the suspicion of elevated intracranial pressure and warrants referral to an ophthalmologist. It is important to note, however, that elevated intracranial pressure and benign intracranial hypertension can occur without papilledema,[27] and thus the diagnosis of these conditions generally cannot be ruled out without a measurement of cerebrospinal fluid pressure (CSF) (most commonly via lumbar puncture).

Auscultation of the head and neck is mandatory for all patients with pulsatile tinnitus. Bruits may be appreciable when turbulent blood flow is present. Auscultation is performed not only over the carotid bifurcation but also over the ear canal, the pre- and postauricular areas, and adjacent areas of the temporal bone. Vascular malformations or fistulae in the region of the occipital artery can be a cause of pulsatile tinnitus, and thus auscultation over these areas should be included when auscultating behind the ear. Auscultation of the ear canal may be performed with a Toynbee otoscope, modified electronic stethoscope, or standard stethoscope.

Venous flow abnormalities (venous hum) may occasionally be auscultated. They are most often described as a "swooshing type" of sound and are not necessarily pulsatile. The loudness is generally diminished by reducing venous blood flow with gentle compression of the jugular vein without compression of the carotid artery. Turning the head toward the uninvolved side, deep breathing, or Valsalva's maneuver may objectively or subjectively make the hum louder.

Tuning Fork Tests

A tuning fork examination comprises a part of the routine neurotologic examination and may be performed easily at the bedside or in the office. Even though most patients with otologic symptomatology are likely to undergo formal audiometric testing, tuning fork testing remains an important component of the neurotologic evaluation. It is particularly recommended to confirm audiometric findings before undertaking surgery for conductive hearing loss, especially stapedectomy.

To perform a Weber's test, a vibrating tuning fork (512 Hz) is placed on the midline of the patient (the forehead, nasal dorsum, central incisors of the maxilla, or mandibular symphysis) to conduct the tone directly to the cochlea. It is important to strike the tuning fork on a soft surface to prevent the development of high-frequency overtones, as may occur when striking the fork on a hard surface. A patient who hears the tone more clearly in one ear is said to have lateralized to that ear. If the sound does not lateralize, then the test is reported as midline or normal. As a rule, sound lateralizing to one ear implies either an ipsilateral conductive loss (typically 3 to 5 dB with a 512 Hz fork) or a contralateral sensorineural loss. Patients with a unilateral conductive hearing loss are sometimes hesitant to acknowledge hearing a tone louder in the "bad" ear. Although a Weber's test is a reliable and trusted test, its acoustic basis is unclear.

The Rinne test is performed, ideally with a 512-Hz tuning fork, by placing the vibrating fork against the mastoid process (bone conduction) and comparing its loudness with that of the tuning fork placed just outside the ear canal (air conduction). If the patient perceives the tone as being louder at the ear canal level, air conduction is said to be greater than bone conduction (AC > BC — a "positive" Rinne), consistent with either ipsilateral normal hearing or a sensorineural hearing loss. If the tone is louder when the tuning fork is placed on the mastoid tip, bone conduction is said to be greater than air conduction (BC > AC — a "negative" Rinne) and implies a conductive hearing loss in the tested ear. The positive/negative Rinne terminology is a frequent source of confusion as a positive test is a normal result. The authors prefer to describe the test results as AC > BC, AC = BC, or BC > AC. BC > AC (a negative Rinne) with a 512-Hz tuning fork suggests a conductive hearing loss of 20 dB or worse.

The importance of both the Weber's and Rinne tests in the bedside and office examinations cannot be overemphasized as they may confirm or refute audiometric test results; therefore, these tests are critical in otologic diagnosis.

Vestibular Evaluation

The vestibular system is located safely within the temporal bone, and in most instances cannot be directly examined. Thus, the physical examination of the vestibular system is typically inferred based on an examination of eye movements (either saccades or nystagmus) elicited by manipulation of the patient. The presence or absence of elicited ocular movements allows inferences to be made about the function of the peripheral vestibular system based on current understanding of the physiology of the vestibular and ocular systems. Most evaluations of the vestibular system are based on the presence of nystagmus.

Nystagmus is an involuntary rapid eye movement that may occur as a result of vestibular, optokinetic, or pursuit system dysfunction. A disturbance of one of these systems leads to a drift of the eyes during attempts at visual fixation (slow phase or slow component of nystagmus). A corrective phase of the eyes (quick phase or quick component) attempts to reset the drift. Constant velocity drifts create repetitive, quick corrective responses, resulting in nystagmus. A peripheral vestibular abnormality resulting in unilateral hypofunction leads to a drift of the eyes directed toward the side of the lesion, and the subsequent fast, corrective phase is directed contralaterally. By convention, the direction of the nystagmus is designated by the fast phase of nystagmus.

Nystagmus can be classified as either spontaneous or evoked. Nystagmus is described on physical examination in terms of direction (right-beating or left-beating, geotrophic-beating toward the ground or ageotrophic-beating away from the ground, plane (horizontal, rotary, or vertical), and intensity (first, second, or third degree). First-degree nystagmus is the least intense and occurs when gaze is in the direction of the fast component of nystagmus. Second-degree nystagmus occurs with gaze in the direction of the fast component as well as midline. Third-degree nystagmus occurs in all directions of gaze, including the slow phase, indicating the most severe form of nystagmus. Nystagmus may also be described as direction fixed (beating in the same direction despite different head positions) or direction changing (beating in different directions with associated different head positions).

Frenzel lenses are magnifying (20 diopter) lenses incorporated into glasses that are used to aid the examiner in observing nystagmus and to prevent the patient from visual fixation, which may lead to suppression of nystagmus. The evaluation of nystagmus can also be enhanced by using electronystagmographic (ENG) recording with surface electrodes or videonystagmography (VNG) recording with infrared goggles.

Fistula Test

The fistula test is performed by applying positive and negative pressure to the tympanic membrane using a pneumatic otoscope; nystagmus and vertigo with applied pressure constitute a positive fistula test. A positive fistula test may be reported as subjectively positive if the applied pressure produces vertigo without objective nystagmus. Examiner observation of nystagmus can be supplemented with Frenzel lenses, ENG or VNG recording, or the use of infrared goggles. Hennebert's sign is a positive fistula test in an ear with an intact tympanic membrane and without evidence of middle ear disease.[28,29] In the presence of a fistula, or vestibulofibrosis, the applied pressure causes deviation of the cupula, resulting in nystagmus and vertigo.[29] A positive fistula test can be seen in oval or round window fistulae, poststapedectomy perilymph leaks, horizontal canal fistulae, Ménière's disease, labyrinthitis, or syphilis.[28,29] Nystagmus that occurs with tragal compression over the external auditory meatus or a Valsalva's maneuver may be caused by superior semicircular canal dehiscence syndrome and a fistula test may produce characteristic vertical and torsional nystagmus in the plane of the affected semicircular canal.[30,31]

Dix-Hallpike Maneuver

The Dix-Hallpike maneuver (Hallpike testing, the Nylèn-Bárány maneuver) may be performed routinely on all patients complaining of vertigo, or may be limited to those patients who have positional vertigo, ie, vertigo provoked by certain head positions such as looking up or rolling over in bed. As for other aspects of the physical examination, the nature of this test and why it is being performed are briefly explained to the patient before the test is performed. The test is performed on a table or a chair capable of reclining completely flat, and begins with the patient sitting up and positioned so that when reclined, the head extends beyond the edge of the

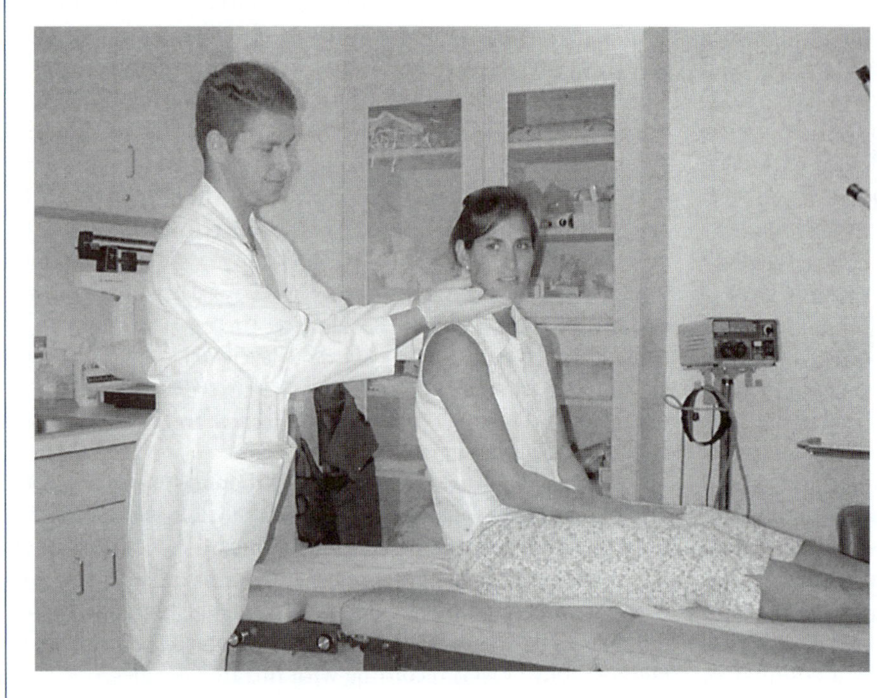

FIGURE 9–3 • Dix-Hallpike examination testing the right ear.

table (Figure 9–3). The patient is positioned with the head turned toward the suspected side, and then rapidly brought to the supine position, with the head turned and hanging slightly (Figure 9–4). The presence of nystagmus and subjective complaints of vertigo are noted. The patient is then gently returned to the sitting position, which may again provoke dizziness. Finally, the test may be repeated with the head turned to the opposite side. The abnormal ear is the one that, when placed in the "down" or lowermost position, elicits vertigo and nystagmus. Performing this test in patients who have limited mobility or neck extension, or those who are obese, can be challenging.

Head Shaking Nystagmus Testing

In this test, the patient's head, with the chin inclined down 30 degrees, is rotated rapidly to the right and left in the horizontal plane, either by the examiner or by the patient, and the patient is examined for nystagmus.[32] A normal response comprises no, or a few beats, of nystagmus. With a unilateral loss of labyrinthine function, nystagmus is seen with the fast phase initially directed toward the opposite (uninvolved) side and which then reverses and becomes directed toward the dysfunctional labyrinth.[32]

TESTS OF NEUROLOGIC FUNCTION

Cranial Nerve Examination

The neurotologic examination includes an evaluation of the cranial nerves. In general, tests of smell and visual acuity are not usually performed unless indicated clinically. Cranial nerves III through XII are assessed systematically as part of the routine neurotologic examination. The reader is referred elsewhere for a full description of the cranial nerve examination.[2,33]

Cerebellar Function

Cerebellar testing is included in the neurotologic examination when there is a complaint of vertigo or dysequilibrium. Cerebellar disease may manifest with ataxia, dysmetria, hyperdysmetria, or dysdiadochokinesia. Poor coordination with repetitive finger-to-nose testing or rapid alternating head movements (dysmetria) may be a sign of cerebellar dysfunction. Uncoordinated heel-to-toe testing or tandem gait (ataxia) is also a sign of cerebellar dysfunction. Patients tend to deviate toward the side of an uncompensated vestibular lesion during gait testing. When moving a limb against resistance, a patient should be able to compensate adequately when the resistance is suddenly removed. Failure to compensate adequately is termed hyperdysmetria. Fine motor control may be tested by having the patient flip his/her hands over, rapidly alternating the palm and the back of the hand side up. Failure to perform this test adequately is termed dysdiadochokinesia.

Romberg's test (Figure 9–5) is a test of vestibulospinal tract function. Romberg's test and gait assessment are measures of both central and peripheral input to the limb and spinal muscles. This test is performed with the patient standing erect with feet together both with eyes open and with eyes closed. Consistent falling to one side is an abnormal test; there is a tendency to fall to the side of an uncompensated, unilateral vestibular lesion. The sharpened Romberg's test (Figure 9–6), thought to be more sensitive than the standard Romberg's test, is performed by having the patient stand with the feet aligned in tandem and arms folded to the chest. The Fukuda stepping test is performed by having the patient march in place (30–50 steps) with eyes closed and arms extended anteriorly. The arms tend to deviate to, or the patient may turn excessively toward the side of, a vestibular lesion. Vestibulospinal testing depends on integration of

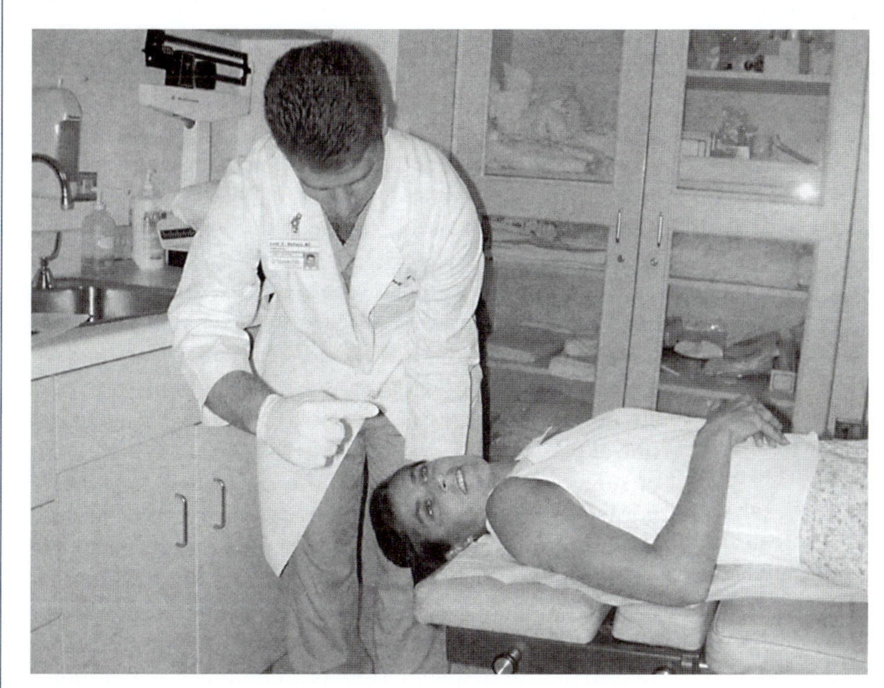

FIGURE 9–4 • Dix-Hallpike examination of the right ear.

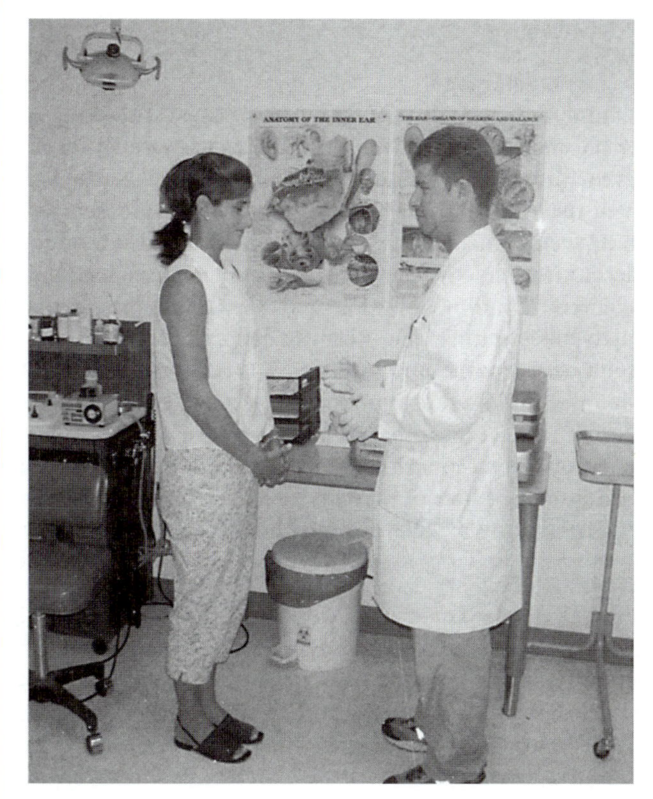

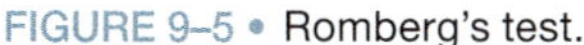

FIGURE 9–5 • Romberg's test.

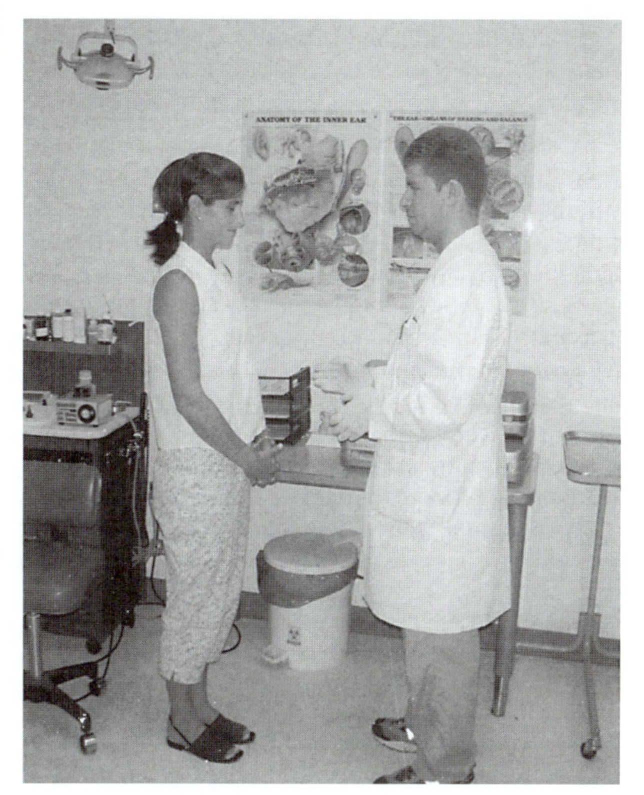

FIGURE 9–6 • Sharpened Romberg's test.

proprioceptive, visual, and vestibular inputs. Closing the eyes during Romberg's test eliminates visual input, and Romberg's test on a 6-inch foam mat reduces proprioceptive input, rendering the patient nearly solely dependent on vestibular input for orientation.[34]

DIAGNOSIS OF OTOLOGIC DISEASE

The previous section discussed the otologic/neurootologic history and physical examination and their importance in establishing a clinical diagnosis. A brief overview of common or important otologic and neurotologic diagnoses is presented in the following section.

Disorders of the Auditory and Vestibular System

Sensorineural Hearing Loss

There are a myriad of etiologies for sensorineural hearing loss.[13] Presbycusis and noise-induced hearing loss are by far the most common. Other causes of sensorineural hearing loss are listed in Tables 9–1 and 9–3. The diagnosis of both common and uncommon causes ultimately depends on a thorough history and physical examination.

Noise-Induced Hearing Loss

Hearing loss affects approximately 28 million people in the United States, with 10 million attributed at least in part to noise exposure. Sound loud enough to damage the inner ear can produce hearing loss not reversible by any known medical or surgical therapy. Sound levels of 75 dB or less, even after long exposure, are unlikely to cause any permanent hearing loss. Sound levels above 85 dB, with exposure of at least 8 h per day, will generally produce a permanent hearing loss.[5]

Conductive Hearing Loss

Twenty to thirty percent of the 28 million people with hearing loss in the United States are estimated to have conductive hearing loss.[15] Patients with conductive hearing losses are generally younger than patients with sensorineural loss and have no cognitive or other sensory deficits.[35] Etiologies of conductive hearing loss are listed in Table 9–4.

Sudden Sensorineural Hearing Loss

Sudden sensorineural hearing loss is defined as a loss of at least 30 dB in at least three contiguous frequencies occurring over a period of no more than 3 days.[36] Certain pathologies, such as vestibular schwannoma, are known to present with sudden sensorineural hearing loss. For the majority of patients with sudden sensorineural hearing loss, a definitive cause of hearing loss will not be identified. Thus, in some contexts, the term sudden sensorineural hearing refers only to the symptom of hearing loss, whereas in idiopathic cases, sudden sensorineural hearing loss is considered a diagnosis. Viral, vascular, and inflammatory processes have been proposed as possible etiologies for idiopathic sudden sensorineural hearing loss. Hearing loss is generally the presenting symptom, but some degree of vertigo, imbalance, aural fullness, and potentially even mild pain, may accompany the hearing loss. There are no formal guidelines to separate the diagnoses of sudden sensorineural hearing loss and labyrinthitis. Generally, the patient who presents with a complaint of sudden hearing loss and acknowledges imbalance on questioning is diagnosed with sudden sensorineural hearing loss, whereas the patient who presents with a complaint of sudden vertigo who acknowledges hearing loss is diagnosed with labyrinthitis. The management of sudden sensorineural hearing loss is currently an area of very active research. Reviews of this disorder are available.[37]

Labyrinthitis

Inflammation of the labyrinth is known as labyrinthitis. Bacterial (suppurative) labyrinthitis takes a more fulminant course than nonsuppurative, serous labyrinthitis and manifests in the sudden onset of profound hearing loss and fulminant vertigo that lasts several days and is usually associated with nausea and vomiting. It should be treated aggressively and promptly as the prognosis for hearing recovery is poor and there is an elevated risk of meningitis. Unsteadiness, as in vestibular neuritis, may last for several months. However, unlike vestibular neuritis, there are usually associated cochlear symptoms, eg, hearing loss, fullness, otalgia, and tinnitus. Serous labyrinthitis is an inflammatory process within the labyrinth without actual inner ear infection. A viral labyrinthitis may be suspected in a patient presenting with the acute onset of vertigo and sensorineural hearing loss in the absence of any other precipitating circumstance. Other causes of labyrinthitis include contamination of perilymph with bacterial or inflammatory toxins, blood, or surgery (eg, stapedectomy). The ear examination should be normal. Inner ear symptoms associated with acute otitis media, cholesteatoma, or chronic ear disease, must be assumed to be complications of the existing ear disease and treated promptly. Nystagmus may be present and should beat away from the affected ear. Nystagmus beating toward the affected ear indicates irritative nystagmus and is an ominous sign of inner ear injury. Nonotolaryngologists typically refer to a wide variety of otologic disorders that cause vertigo as labyrinthitis; otolaryngologists usually reserve the term for the specific entities as described above.

Vestibular Neuritis

Inflammation of the vestibular nerve confined within the bony internal auditory canal (IAC) and leading to dysfunction of the nerve with vertigo is termed vestibular neuritis.[38] Isolated atrophy of the vestibular nerve with little end-organ degeneration can be seen on histopathologic examination and is thought to reflect a viral etiology. The vertigo is abrupt in onset, is described as a severe, spinning sensation, and is usually accompanied by nausea and vomiting. Few other otologic symptoms are present except, occasionally, aural fullness. The acute phase lasts 48 to 72 h and is followed by a period of dysequilibrium and a sensation of unsteadiness that usually lasts 4 to 6 weeks but may persist for several months. The variability of time to recovery depends on the extent of the damage to the vestibular nerve and on compensation for the vestibular injury.[39]

Ménière's Disease

Ménière's disease is a clinical disorder classified as idiopathic endolymphatic hydrops. The diagnosis of Ménière's disease can only be made with certainty after death by demonstrating endolymphatic hydrops on temporal bone histopathologic examination. During life, the diagnosis is suggested by a low-tone, fluctuating sensorineural hearing loss, tinnitus, aural fullness, and episodic vertigo. The AAO-HNS Committee on Hearing and Equilibrium elaborated on the definition of Ménière's disease for the purposes of diagnosis and reporting.[3] The Committee delineated four levels of certainty in the diagnosis of Ménière's disease, which are reproduced in Table 9–5.

The vertigo of Ménière's disease is characteristically a true spinning vertigo; it can be incapacitating and severe and is often the most distressing symptom. Variants of Ménière's disease include Lermoyez[40] attacks, in which the hearing loss and

TABLE 9–5 AAO-HNS committee of hearing and equilibrium diagnosis of Ménière's disease

Certain Ménière's disease Definite Ménière's disease plus histologic confirmation
Definite Ménière's disease Two or more definitive spontaneous episodes of vertigo 20 minutes or longer Audiometrically documented hearing loss on at least one occasion Tinnitus or aural fullness in the treated ear Other causes excluded
Probable Ménière's disease One definitive episode of vertigo Audiometrically documented hearing loss on at least one occasion Tinnitus or aural fullness in the treated ear Other causes excluded
Possible Ménière's disease Episodic vertigo of the Ménière type without hearing loss, or
Sensorineural hearing loss, fluctuating or fixed, with dysequilibrium but without definitive episodes Other causes excluded

tinnitus improve with the attack of vertigo, and the otolithic crises of Tumarkin,[41] in which vestibular dysfunction manifests not as spinning vertigo but as a sudden, severe fall or "drop attack." The terms cochlear Ménière's disease (hearing loss, tinnitus, and aural fullness, without vertigo) and vestibular Ménière's disease (the vestibular symptoms of Ménière's with no auditory symptoms) are occasionally used to describe patients who do not have the full spectrum of symptoms of Ménière's disease. Although these terms remain in use clinically, The AAO-HNS Committee on Hearing and Equilibrium[42] has recommended abandoning these terms, in favor of the diagnostic criteria presented in Table 9–5.

Benign Paroxysmal Positional Vertigo

Benign paroxysmal positional vertigo (BPPV, also referred to as benign positional vertigo, or BPV) is a disorder frequently seen in otologic and neurotologic practice. In general, the symptoms of vertigo in this condition are thought to be caused by the movement of particulate matter, specifically otoconia, in the labyrinth. The most commonly involved location for such otoliths is in the posterior semicircular canal.

In its classical form, the presentation of BPPV should include a relatively consistent history and an appropriately positive physical examination. The patient should present with a history of intense vertiginous attacks that occur with a sudden onset. The attacks can be reproducibly brought on by assuming certain positions, most commonly by lying down and turning onto the affected side. The attacks of vertigo are generally not accompanied by sensations of aural fullness, tinnitus, or fluctuations in hearing. Typically attacks will last less than 1 min. Often patients will report that they have given up sleeping on the affected side in order to avoid the development of symptoms.

Dix-Hallpike testing (as described above) will be positive when the condition is active; establishing the diagnosis and revealing the involved side in posterior canal BPPV. The nystagmus of BPPV is pathognomonic: it has a several (2- to 10-) second latency, is geotropic (beating toward the ground) and horizontal-rotary, lasts no more than 30 sec before abating, and fatigues with repetition of the Hallpike maneuver.

Variants of BPPV have been described based on the presence of otoliths affecting the cupula versus the canal (ie, cupulolithiasis and canalolithiasis), and based on the presence of the otoliths in the horizontal or superior semicircular canals.[43–46] The presentation of these variants can be considerably different from the description offered above. A modified Hallpike maneuver is used to test for horizontal canal BPPV. In this test, the patient lies supine and the head is rapidly rotated to one side (without extension beyond the table edge); the head is returned to the supine position and is then turned to the contralateral ear. The evoked nystagmus is horizontal, geotrophic, or ageotrophic and is less likely to fatigue.[47]

Superior Semicircular Canal Dehiscence Syndrome

Sound- or pressure-induced vertigo caused by dehiscence of the superior semicircular canal has been described.[30,31,48] Patients with this disorder develop vertical-torsional eye movements aligned with the plane of the superior canal in response to loud sounds or maneuvers that change middle ear or intracranial pressure. The diagnosis is made by observing vertical-torsional nystagmus with the slow phase directed upward and away from the suspect ear following positive tragal pressure, Valsalva's maneuver, or a loud (110-dB) sound. Ultrahigh-resolution computed tomographic scanning of the temporal bones may demonstrate thinning or dehiscence of the bone of the superior canal.

Migraine-Related Vertigo

Migraine is a neurologic disorder characterized by headache and/or other neurologic symptoms that affects 6 to 18% of adults in the United States. Migraine is a frequent but often overlooked cause of episodic vertigo. In practices that treat patients with headaches, dysequilibrium or episodic vertigo has been reported in 33 to 72% of cases.[49,50] Both true vertigo and nonvertiginous dizziness can occur and the episodic nature of the symptoms can be easily mistaken for Ménière's disease or other vestibular system disorders. Interestingly, in the majority of patients, the vertigo is unassociated with their headache, and many patients have no headache history at all.[51]

Perilymph Fistula

Inner ear fistulae include labyrinthine fistulae, perilymph fistulae, and intramembranous communications. Although all are considered inner ear fistulae, each represents a distinct clinical entity. A perilymph fistula is a leak of perilymph fluid into the middle ear or mastoid, or a leak of air from the middle ear into the inner ear. Actual visual recognition of fluid, even with microscopic examination, is unusual. Precipitating insults include surgery, blunt trauma, penetrating trauma, barotrauma, infection, cholesteatoma, or sudden changes in CSF pressure as can occur with straining, sneezing, or Valsalva's maneuver. Congenital ear abnormalities may predispose to perilymph leaks. Spontaneous perilymph fistulae are believed to be infrequent.[52] The clinical picture of perilymph fistulae is variable, with symptoms ranging from mild to incapacitating. Vertigo, or more often unsteadiness, is the most common symptom. Hearing loss, tinnitus, or aural fullness may be present. A thorough history inquiring about activities such as trauma, scuba diving, flying, and straining is critical in the diagnosis of this disorder as the symptoms are vague and coincident with other vestibular disorders. A fistula test should be performed in a patient suspected of having a perilymph fistula (see above).

Another type of inner ear fistula is defined as an abnormal communication between the endolymphatic space and the perilymphatic space. This type of fistula is usually referred to as an intramembranous communication or a cochlear membrane tear and is theorized to be an etiology of (idiopathic) sudden sensorineural hearing loss.

The term labyrinthine fistula is used to describe an inner ear fistula that typically involves the semicircular canals. The usual etiologies are trauma and infection. Erosion of the horizontal canal (or less frequently the posterior or superior canals) from cholesteatoma or granulation tissue may lead to a labyrinthine fistula if the integrity of the bony labyrinth is violated. Inflammatory hypertrophy of the perilymphatic space endothelium usually prevents the flow of perilymph through the fistula, however, surgical disruption of the barrier precipitates the flow of perilymph. A patient known to have cholesteatoma in whom dysequilibrium develops is considered to have a labyrinthine fistula until proven otherwise.

Cerebellopontine Angle Tumors

Benign cerebellopontine angle tumors (eg, vestibular schwannomas and meningiomas) may underlie unilateral (or asymmetric) sensorineural hearing loss, tinnitus, and dysequilibrium. Even small tumors may cause considerable symptoms when they exert pressure on the seventh and eighth cranial nerves within the IAC. Other less common symptoms include facial weakness or paralysis, fifth cranial nerve involvement (facial numbness and decreased corneal reflex), sixth nerve symptoms of diplopia, ninth and tenth nerve problems with hoarseness or dysphagia, and pain or headache. Generally, the presence of clinically evident facial weakness in all but the largest tumors suggests the tumor originates from the facial nerve. Despite compression and destruction of the vestibular nerves, imbalance is a relatively uncommon presenting symptom; the gradual progression of vestibular dysfunction allows for compensation of the deficit. Dysequilibrium, if present, is usually mild; true spinning vertigo is rare. Large tumors may be associated with dysequilibrium, ataxia, nausea, vomiting, and headache, indicative of brain stem, cerebellar, or fourth ventricular compression or increased intracranial pressure. A list of disorders affecting the vestibular system is provided in Table 9–6.

Systemic Disorders Affecting the Ear and Temporal Bone

Systemic disorders (see Table 9–1) can directly or indirectly affect hearing and balance. These diagnoses may be elusive as many of the disorders are uncommon.[4] Also, some of the more common disorders (eg, diabetes mellitus) do not consistently affect hearing and balance.

TABLE 9–6 Disorders of the vestibular system

Benign paroxysmal positional vertigo
Labyrinthitis
Ménière's disease
Vestibular neuronitis
Drug toxicity (ototoxicity)
Cerebellopontine angle tumors
Metabolic disorders
Perilymph fistula
Trauma
Systemic disorders (see Table 9–1)
Autoimmune inner ear disease
Central disorders
Vertebral basilar insufficiency
Presyncope
Multiple sclerosis
Trauma
Familial ataxia
Arnold-Chiari malformation
Communicating hydrocephalus
Migraine Central nervous system lesion or tumor
Cerebellar degeneration
Parkinson's disease
Nutritional disorders (vitamin B_{12} deficiency)

Eustachian Tube Dysfunction

Eustachian tube dysfunction is a common disorder generally described as ear fullness or pressure, or sometimes creating an intermittent "popping sensation." The type of Eustachian tube dysfunction encountered most frequently entails inadequate tubal opening. Inflammatory processes, mucosal edema, allergic rhinitis, rhinosinusitis, and tumors of the nasopharynx can lead to Eustachian tube dysfunction. Disorders such as craniofacial anomalies, cleft palate, Down syndrome and neuromuscular diseases, with levator or tensor veli palatini muscle dysfunction, can cause Eustachian tube dysfunction. Hearing loss, mild aural fullness, and, rarely, tinnitus are associated symptoms. The fullness may be alleviated with Valsalva's maneuver. The physical examination in these patients varies depending on the disease process. In mild cases of dysfunction, the tympanic membrane may appear to be normal, however, tympanic membrane abnormalities ranging from atelectasis to retraction to cholesteatoma may be seen in more severely affected patients. In more chronic or severe cases of dysfunction, there may be an associated serous effusion.

Far less commonly encountered than inadequate Eustachian tube dilation, is a patulous (or open) Eustachian tube. A history of autophony (abnormal hearing of one's voice and breathing) in the problematic ear suggests a patulous Eustachian tube. Surprisingly, many of the symptoms of a blocked Eustachian tube and a patulous Eustachian tube are markedly similar, contributing to the difficulty of making the correct diagnosis. Aural fullness may be more bothersome in patients with patulous Eustachian tube than in those with dilatory dysfunction, and they generally do not have allergic rhinitis, sinusitis, or other historical risk factors associated with tubal obstruction. On examination, the tympanic membrane is normal, and the diagnosis is confirmed by observing lateral and medial excursions of the posterior eardrum with breathing through the ispilateral nostril during active symptoms. The symptoms of a patulous tube may be alleviated by maneuvers that close the tube, such as bending over, which, in effect, creates venous engorgement of the tissues of the tubal orifice.

Otosyphilis

Otosyphilis is mentioned here because this disease continues to present a diagnostic challenge.[53] The diagnosis is suggested in patients with cochleovestibular dysfunction and positive serologic testing (eg, fluorescent treponemal antibody absorption (FTA-Abs) or microhemagglutination-Treponema palladium [MHA-TP]). The manifestation(s) of syphilitic cochleovestibular dysfunction are extremely variable.[53,54] Hearing loss, which may be fluctuant, is the most common symptom (bilateral in 82% of the cases), followed by vertigo in 42%. Approximately one-fourth of patients with otosyphilis have symptoms consistent with endolymphatic hydrops.[55] The accurate diagnosis of otosyphilis remains challenging due to the variable symptomatology and the poor predictive value of serological testing in an otologic population.[56] A high index of suspicion is usually necessary to make the diagnosis in this condition that is known as, "the great mimicker."

CONCLUSION

Despite the wide array of electrophysiologic and imaging modalities that are used in the diagnosis of otologic disease, the history and physical examination remain the most important and most informative aspects of a thorough patient evaluation. Numerous conditions may be diagnosed on the basis of history alone, and a thorough history and complete physical examination promote efficient diagnosis and treatment of all otologic and neurotologic complaints, potentially minimizing expensive tests and unnecessary interventions. We have provided an extensive discussion of the key points of the history and physical examination for disorders of the ear, in addition to an overview of many of the pathologic conditions encountered in clinical practice.

References

1. Glasscock ME, Haynes DS, Storper IS, Bohrer P. Otology and neurotology. In: Adkins RB, Scott HW, editors. Surgical care of the elderly. 2nd ed. Philadelphia, PA: Lippincott-Raven; 1998. p. 193–200.
2. Strasnick B, Haynes DS. Otologic history and physical examination of the ear. In: Canalis RF, Lambert PR, editors. The ear: comprehensive otology. Philadelphia, PA: Lippincott Williams and Wilkins; 2000. p. 157–66.
3. Committee on Hearing and Equilibrium. Committee on Hearing and Equilibrium guidelines for the diagnosis and evaluation of therapy in Ménière's disease. Otolaryngol Head Neck Surg 1995;113:181–5.
4. Nadol JB, Merchant SN. Systemic disease manifestations in the middle ear and temporal bone. In: Cummings CW, Harker LA, Krause CJ, et al, editors. Otolaryngology-head and neck surgery. Vol 3. St. Louis, MO: Mosby; 1998. p. 3088–107.
5. Noise and hearing loss: consensus conference. JAMA 1990;263: 3185–90.
6. Roland JT, Cohen NL. Vestibular and auditory ototoxicity. In: Cummings CW, Harker LA, Krause CJ, et al, editors. Otolaryngology-head and neck surgery. Vol 3. St. Louis, MO: Mosby; 1998. p. 3186–95.
7. Van Der Hulst RJAM, Dreschler W, Urbanus NAM. High-frequency audiometry in prospective clinical research of ototoxicity due to platinum derivatives. Ann Otol Rhinol Laryngol 1988;97:133–7.
8. Rybak LP. Ototoxicity of loop diuretics. Otolaryngol Clin North Am 1993;26:829–43.
9. Jung TK, Rhee CK, Lee CS, et al. Ototoxicity of salicylate, non-steroidal anti-inflammatory drugs and quinine. Otolaryngol Clin North Am 1993;26:791–809.
10. Grundfast KM, Lalwani AK. Practical approach to diagnosis and management of hereditary hearing impairment (HHI). Ear Nose Throat J 1992;71:479–93.
11. Kochhar A, Hildebrand MS, Smith RJ. Clinical aspects of hereditary hearing loss. Genet Med 2007;9(7):393–408.
12. Bauer CA, Jenkins HA. Otologic symptoms and syndromes. In: Cummings CW, Harker LA, Krause CJ, et al, editors. Otolaryngology-head and neck surgery. Vol 3. St. Louis, MO: Mosby; 1998. p. 2547–58.
13. Arts A. Differential diagnosis of sensorineural hearing loss. In: Cummings CW, Harker LA, Krause CJ, et al, editors. Otolaryngology-head and neck surgery. Vol 3. St. Louis, MO: Mosby; 1998. p. 2908–28.
14. Okumura T, Takahashi H, Takagi A, Mitamura K. Sensorineural hearing loss in patients with large vestibular aqueduct. Laryngoscope 1995;105:289–93.
15. Backous D, Niparko J. Evaluation and surgical management of conductive hearing loss. In: Cummings CW, Harker LA, Krause CJ, et al, editors. Otolaryngology-head and neck surgery. Vol 3. St. Louis, MO: Mosby; 1998. p. 2894–907.
16. Scholtz AW, Fish JH, Kammen-Jolly K, et al. Goldenhar's syndrome: congenital hearing deficit of conductive or sensorineural origin? Temporal bone histopathologic study. Otol Neurootol 2001;22:501–5.
17. Fowler KB, Boppana SB. Congenital cytomegalovirus (CMV) infection and hearing deficit. J Clin Virol 2006;35(2):226–31.
18. Nance WE, Lim BG, Dodson KM. Importance of congenital cytomegalovirus infections as a cause for pre-lingual hearing loss. J Clin Virol 2006 Feb;35(2):221–5.
19. Walter S, Atkinson C, Sharland M, Rice P, Raglan E, Emery VC, Griffiths PD. Congenital cytomegalovirus: Association between dried blood spot viral load and hearing loss. Arch Dis Child Fetal Neonatal Ed. 2007 Nov 26.
20. Billings KR, Kenna MA. Causes of pediatric sensorineural hearing loss. Arch Otolaryngol Head Neck Surg 1999;125:517–21.
21. Bojrab DI, Bhansali SA. Objective evaluation of a patient with vertigo. In: Canalis RF, Lambert PR, editors. The ear: comprehensive

otology. Philadelphia, PA: Lippincott Williams and Wilkins; 2000. p. 181–96.

22. Blakley BW, Goebel J. The meaning of the word "vertigo". Otolaryngol Head Neck Surg 2001 Sep;125(3):147–50.
23. Kroenke K, Arrington ME, Manglesdorff AD. The prevalence of symptoms in medical outpatients and the adequacy of therapy. Arch Intern Med 1990;150:1685–9.
24. Sloane PD, Baloh RW, Honrubia V. The vestibular system in the elderly: clinical implications. Am J Otolaryngol 1989;10: 422–9.
25. Kentala E, Rauch SD. A practical assessment algorithm for diagnosis of dizziness. Otolaryngol Head Neck Surg 2003;128(1):54–9.
26. Jackson CG, Schall DG, Glasscock ME 3rd, et al. A surgical solution for the difficult chronic ear. Am J Otol 1996;17(1):7–14.
27. Marcelis J, Silberstein SD. Idiopathic intracranial hypertension without papilledema. Arch Neurol 1991;48(4):392–9.
28. Hennebert C. A new syndrome in hereditary syphilis of the labyrinth. Presse Med Belg Brux 1911;63:467.
29. Nadol JB. Positive Hennebert's sign in Ménière's disease. Arch Otolaryngol Head Neck Surg 1977;103:524–30.
30. Minor LB. The superior canal dehiscence syndrome. Am J Otolaryngol 2000;2:9–19.
31. Minor LB, Solomon D, Zinreich JS, Zee DS. Sound- and/or pressure-induced vertigo due to bone dehiscence of the superior semicircular canal. Arch Otolaryngol Head Neck Surg 1998;124:249–58.
32. Hain TC, Fetter M, Zee DS. Head-shaking nystagmus in patients with unilateral peripheral lesions. Am J Otolaryngol 1987;8:36–47.
33. Burton MJ, Niparko JK. Evaluation of the cranial nerves. In: Hughes GB, Pensak ML, editors. Clinical otology. New York: Thieme; 1997. p. 131–46.
34. Lambert PR. History and physical examination of a patient with dizziness. In: Canalis RF, Lambert PR, editors. The ear: comprehensive otology. Philadelphia, PA: Lippincott Williams and Wilkins; 2000. p. 167–79.
35. Stewart MG, Coker NJ, Jenkins HA, et al. Outcomes and quality of life in conductive hearing loss. Otolaryngol Head Neck Surg 2000;123:527–32.
36. National Institute on Deafness and Other Communication Disorders (NIDCD). Sudden deafness. Available at http://www.nicdc.nih.gov/health/hearing/sudden.asp Accessed August 02, 2008.
37. O'Malley MR, Haynes DS. Sudden hearing loss. Otolaryngol Clin North Am. 2008 Jun;41(3):633–49.
38. Schuknecht HF, Kitamura K. Vestibular neuritis. Ann Otol Rhinol Laryngol Suppl 1981;78:1–19.
39. Glasscock ME, Haynes DS. Evaluation and treatment of the patient with vertigo. Volta Rev 1998;99:129–40.
40. Lermoyez M. Le vertige qui fait entendre (angiospasme labyrinthique) Presse Med 1919;27:1.
41. Tumarkin A. The otolithic catastrophe: a new syndrome. BMJ 1936;2:175.
42. Pearson BW, Brackmann DE. Committee on Hearing and Equilibrium guidelines for reporting treatment results in Ménière's disease. Otolaryngol Head Neck Surg 1985;93:579.
43. Parnes LS, Agrawal SK, Atlas J. Diagnosis and management of benign paroxysmal positional vertigo (BPPV). CMAJ. 2003 Sep 30;169(7):681–93.
44. Furman JM, Cass SP. Benign paroxysmal positional vertigo. N Engl J Med. 1999 Nov 18;341(21):1590–6.
45. Jackson LE, Morgan B, Fletcher JC Jr, Krueger WW. Anterior canal benign paroxysmal positional vertigo: an underappreciated entity. Otol Neurotol. 2007 Feb;28(2):218–22
46. Choung YH, Shin YR, Kahng H, Park K, Choi SJ. 'Bow and lean test' to determine the affected ear of horizontal canal benign paroxysmal positional vertigo. Laryngoscope. 2006;116(10):1776–81.
47. Schessel DA, Minor LA, Nedzelski J. Ménières disease and other peripheral disorders. In: Cummings CW, Harker LA, Krause CJ, et al, editors. Otolaryngology-head and neck surgery. Vol 3. St. Louis, MO: Mosby; 1998. p. 2672–705.
48. Ostrowski VB, Byskosh A, Hain TC. Tullio phenomenon with dehiscence of the superior semicircular canal. Otol Neurotol 2001;22:61–5.
49. Selby G, Lance JW. Observations on 500 cases of migraine and allied vascular headache. J Neurol Neurosurg Psychiatry 1960; 23:23–32.
50. Kayan A, Hood JD. Neuro-otological manifestations of migraine. Brain 1984;107:1123–42.
51. Johnson GD. Medical management of migraine-related dizziness and vertigo. Laryngoscope 1998;108 Suppl:1–20.
52. Friedland DR, Wackym PA. A critical appraisal of spontaneous perilymphatic fistulas of the inner ear. Am J Otolaryngol 1999;20:261–79.
53. Gleich LL, Linstrom CJ, Kimmelman CP. Otosyphilis: a diagnostic and therapeutic dilemma. Laryngoscope 1992;102:1255–9.
54. Birdsall HH, Baughn RE, Jenkins HA. The diagnostic dilemma of otosyphilis. Arch Otolaryngol Head Neck Surg 1990;116:617–21.
55. Steckleberg JM, McDonald TJ. Otologic involvement in late syphyilis. Laryngoscope 1984;94:753–7.
56. Hughes GB, Rutherford I. Predictive value of serologic tests for syphilis in otology. Ann Otol Rhinol Laryngol. 1986 May–Jun;95(3 Pt 1):250–9.

Audiologic Evaluation of Otologic/Neurotologic Disease

10

Brad A. Stach, PhD

AUDIOLOGIC CONTRIBUTION TO DIAGNOSIS

The process and strategies used to evaluate hearing have their greatest utility in the audiologic diagnosis of communication disorder resulting from hearing loss. Nevertheless, results of the audiologic evaluation can be useful in the otologic/neurotologic diagnosis of ear disease. Patterns of results on measures of pure-tone audiometry, speech recognition, acoustic immittance, otoacoustic emissions (OAEs), and auditory evoked potentials may indicate the need for additional diagnostic testing or may serve to corroborate clinical otologic findings. They may also serve as a useful means of quantifying posttreatment outcomes.

Audiometric measures evaluate auditory system function. The extent to which a disease process interferes with function will dictate their usefulness in the diagnostic process. Should the condition not interfere measurably with function, the audiologic outcomes will be of little utility diagnostically. In contrast, if function is affected, results on these audiometric measures may serve a useful diagnostic purpose and may help to quantify the impact of the disorder.

The value of specific audiometric test results varies with the nature of the disorder. For example, a middle-ear disorder is readily identifiable with immittance measures and OAEs, whereas a brain-stem disorder might elude audiologic diagnosis if the influence on function is too subtle. The value of audiometric test results in the diagnostic process also depends on the sensitivity of other diagnostic measures. For example, the increased sensitivity of imaging techniques, capable of detecting ever-smaller lesions, has reduced the utility of the auditory brain-stem response (ABR) in the diagnosis of disorders of the eighth nerve and has relegated audiometric measures to the role of screening for, rather than identifying, specific lesions.

Regardless, the audiologic evaluation of otologic/neurotologic disease plays an important role in the diagnosis and management of patients. Whether for the purposes of corroboration, identification, or quantification, audiometric outcomes are often valuable components of the clinical evaluation. This chapter provides an overview of hearing disorders, audiometric measures and audiologic approaches, and anticipated measurement outcomes as a function of type of hearing disorder.

NATURE AND IMPACT OF HEARING DISORDERS

A hearing disorder is classified as (1) a hearing sensitivity loss, (2) a suprathreshold hearing disorder, or (3) a functional hearing loss. Hearing sensitivity loss is the most common form of hearing disorder. It is characterized by a reduction in the sensitivity of the auditory mechanism so that sounds need to be of higher intensity than normal before they are perceived. Suprathreshold disorders result in reduced ability to hear or perceive sounds properly at intensity levels above threshold. Functional hearing loss is the exaggeration or fabrication of a hearing loss.

Hearing Sensitivity Loss

Hearing sensitivity loss is caused by an abnormal reduction of sound being delivered to the brain by a disordered ear. This reduction of sound can result from any number of factors that affect the auditory mechanism. When sound is not conducted well through a disordered outer or middle ear, the result is a conductive hearing loss. When the sensory or neural mechanisms within the cochlea are absent or not functioning, the result is a sensorineural hearing loss. When structures of both the conductive mechanism and the cochlea are disordered, the result is referred to as a mixed hearing loss. A sensorineural hearing loss can also be caused by a disorder of the eighth nerve or auditory brain stem. Such disorders are usually referred to separately as retrocochlear disorders, because their diagnosis, treatment, and impact on hearing ability can differ substantially from a hearing loss of cochlear origin.

Conductive Hearing Loss

A conductive hearing loss is caused by an abnormal reduction or attenuation of sound as it travels through the conductive mechanisms of the outer and middle ear. A conductive hearing loss or the conductive component of a hearing loss is quantified by comparing the air- and bone-conduction thresholds on an audiogram. Air-conduction thresholds represent hearing sensitivity as measured through the outer, middle, and inner ears. Bone-conduction thresholds represent hearing sensitivity as measured primarily through the inner ear. Thus, if air-conduction thresholds are poorer than bone-conduction thresholds, it can be assumed that the attenuation of sound is occurring at the level of the outer or middle ears. The size of the conductive component is usually referred to as the air–bone gap. The audiometric configuration of a conductive hearing loss varies from low frequency to flat to high frequency, depending on the physical obstruction of the structures of the conductive mechanism. In general, any disorder that adds mass to the conductive system predominantly affects the higher audiometric frequencies. Any disorder that adds or reduces stiffness to the system predominantly affects the lower audiometric frequencies. Any disorder that changes both mass and stiffness affects a broad range of audiometric frequencies.

Because a conductive hearing loss acts primarily as an attenuator of sound, it has little or no impact on suprathreshold hearing. That is, once sound is of sufficient intensity, the ear acts as it normally would at suprathreshold intensities. Thus, perception and growth of loudness, ability to discriminate loudness and pitch changes, and speech-recognition ability are all normal once the conductive hearing loss is overcome by raising the intensity of the signal.

Although readily amenable to otologic treatment, there can be a more insidious effect of conductive hearing loss. Some children with chronic otitis media with effusion experience inconsistent auditory input during their formative years and do not develop appropriate suprathreshold auditory and listening skills.[1–4] Such children may be at risk for later learning and achievement problems.

Sensorineural Hearing Loss

A sensorineural hearing loss is caused by a failure in the cochlear transduction of sound from mechanical energy in the middle ear to neural impulses of the eighth nerve. When a structure of this sensorineural mechanism is in some way damaged, its ability to transduce mechanical energy into electrical energy is reduced, resulting in a number of changes in cochlear processing, including a reduction in the sensitivity of the cochlear receptor cells, in the frequency-resolving ability of the cochlea, and in the dynamic range of the hearing mechanism.

A sensorineural hearing loss is most often characterized clinically by its effect on cochlear sensitivity and, thus, the audiogram. If the outer and middle ears are functioning properly, then air-conduction thresholds accurately represent the sensitivity of the cochlea and are equal to bone-conduction thresholds. The audiometric configuration of a sensorineural hearing loss varies from low frequency to flat to high frequency depending on the location along the basilar membrane of hair cell loss or other damage.

A sensorineural hearing has at least three fundamentally important effects on hearing: a reduction in the cochlear sensitivity, in frequency resolution, and in the dynamic range of the hearing mechanism. In many ways, the reduction in hearing sensitivity can be thought of as having the same effect as a conductive hearing loss in terms of reducing the audibility of speech. That is, a conductive hearing loss and a sensorineural hearing loss of the same degree and configuration will have the same effect on audibility of speech sounds. The difference between the two types of hearing loss becomes manifest at suprathreshold levels.

One of the consequences of sensorineural hearing loss is recruitment (abnormal loudness growth). Loudness grows more rapidly than normal at intensity levels just above threshold in an ear with sensorineural hearing loss. This recruitment results in a reduced dynamic range from the threshold level to the discomfort level.

Reduction in frequency resolution and in dynamic range affects the perception of speech. In most sensorineural hearing losses, this effect on speech understanding is predictable from the audiogram and is poorer than would be expected from a conductive hearing loss of similar magnitude. In the extreme, the reduction in frequency resolution and dynamic range can severely limit the usefulness of residual hearing.

Mixed Hearing Loss

A hearing loss comprising both sensorineural and conductive components is termed a mixed hearing loss. A mixed hearing loss indicates that a disordered outer or middle ear attenuates the sound delivered to an impaired cochlea. Bone-conduction thresholds reflect the degree and configuration of the sensorineural component of the hearing loss. Air-conduction thresholds reflect both the sensorineural loss and the additional conductive component.

Retrocochlear Hearing Loss

A retrocochlear hearing loss is caused by a change in neural structure and function of some component of the peripheral or central auditory nervous system. As a rule of thumb, the more peripheral a lesion, the greater its impact will be on hearing sensitivity and on auditory function in general—sometimes referred to as the "bottleneck" principle. Conversely, the more central the lesion, the more subtle its impact. One might conceptualize this by thinking of the nervous system as a large tree. If one of its many branches were damaged, overall growth of the tree would be affected only subtly. Damage to its trunk, however, would affect the entire tree significantly. A well-placed tumor on the auditory nerve can substantially affect hearing, whereas a lesion in the mid brain is likely to have a more subtle effect.

Perhaps the best illustration of the bottleneck principle comes from reports of cases with lesions that effectively disconnect the cochlea from the brain stem. These cases manifest severe or profound hearing loss and very poor speech recognition despite normal cochlear function, as indicated by normal OAEs or eighth-nerve action potentials. In cases involving lesions of the cerebellopontine angle secondary to tumor,[5,6] multiple sclerosis,[7] and miliary tuberculosis,[8] the results have shown how a lesion strategically placed at the bottleneck can substantially affect hearing ability. The bottleneck in the case of the auditory system is, of course, the eighth nerve as it enters the auditory brain stem.

A retrocochlear lesion, then, may or may not affect auditory sensitivity, depending on many factors, including lesion size, location, and impact. A vestibular schwannoma on the eighth cranial nerve can cause a substantial sensorineural hearing loss, depending on how much pressure it places on the nerve or the damage that it causes to the nerve. A temporal-lobe tumor, however, is quite unlikely to result in any change in hearing sensitivity.

These influences of tumors and other retrocochlear lesions on function of the nervous system can be thought of as the primary effect of the neurologic disorder. Sometimes, however, a vestibular schwannoma can also cause cochlear dysfunction.[9] That is, the presence of a tumor on the eighth nerve can result in changes in the function of the cochlea, related to the presence of tumor-associated proteinaceous material in the cochlear space. Thus, although the primary site of the lesion may be the eighth nerve, its influence may be more peripheral. Clinical signs will vary from those consistent with retrocochlear disorder, when the influence of the tumor is primarily on nerve function, to those consistent with cochlear disorder, when the influence is primarily on the labyrinth. It may be that the clinical picture progresses from the former to the latter as the tumor persists.

If the bottleneck is unaffected, then lesions at higher levels will have effects on auditory processing ability that are more subtle. These effects tend to become increasingly subtle, as the lesions are located more centrally in the system. For example, whereas a lesion at the bottleneck can cause a substantial hearing sensitivity loss, a brain-stem lesion often results in only a mild low-frequency sensitivity loss[10], and a temporal-lobe lesion is unlikely to affect hearing sensitivity at all. Similarly speech recognition of words presented in quiet can be very poor in the case of a lesion at the periphery but will be unaffected by a lesion at the level of the temporal lobe.

Auditory Neuropathy and Hearing Loss

One specific type of auditory nervous system disorder is auditory neuropathy,[11,12] a term used originally to describe a condition in which cochlear function is normal and eighth nerve function is abnormal. As such, auditory neuropathy is a condition that exemplifies the consequences of a disorder at the level of the bottleneck. It is distinguishable from disorders due to space-occupying lesions in that imaging results of the nerve and brain stem are normal.

Auditory neuropathy was first described as a specific disorder of the auditory nerve that causes a loss of synchrony of neural firing.[11] Because of the nature of the disorder, it is also referred to as auditory dys-synchrony.[13] The cause of auditory neuropathy is often unknown, although it may be observed in cases of syndromic peripheral pathologies (eg, Freidreich's ataxia, Charcot-Marie-Tooth syndrome). The age of onset is usually before 10 years. Hearing sensitivity loss ranges from normal to profound and is most often flat or reverse-sloped in configuration. The hearing loss often fluctuates and is progressive in some patients. Speech perception is often substantially poorer that what would be expected from the audiogram.[14,15] Auditory neuropathy may not be as amenable to conventional amplification and implant treatment as disorders of sensory origin.

Auditory neuropathy, in its original form, is a neurogenic disorder, operationally defined based on a constellation of clinical findings that suggest normal functioning of some cochlear structures and abnormal functioning of the eighth nerve or brain stem. These clinical findings include absent ABR, poor speech perception, varying levels of hearing sensitivity loss, absence of acoustic reflexes, and preservation of some cochlear function as evidenced by the presence of OAEs and/or cochlear microphonics (CMs).

As increasing numbers of babies are being screened at birth, it appears that a substantial proportion of those with significant hearing loss have two of the clinical signs of auditory neuropathy—absent ABRs and present OAEs and/or CMs. Because of the early age of identification, measures of hearing sensitivity, acoustic reflex thresholds, and speech perception cannot be obtained. The label of auditory neuropathy has quickly become associated with these isolated findings in newborns.

It is becoming apparent that the term auditory neuropathy as it is defined clinically probably represents at least two fairly different disorders, one sensory and the other neural.[16,17] The auditory neuropathy (AN) of sensory origin—cochleogenic AN—is probably a sensory hearing disorder that represents a transduction problem, comprising a failure of the cochlea to transmit signals to the auditory nerve. The most likely origin of this transduction problem rests in the inner hair cells, a concept that has been reported both in patient populations[18,19] and in animal models.[20] Preservation of the OAEs and cochlear microphonics represents normal function of outer-hair cells. In cases of cochleogenic AN the absence of an ABR is a reflection of the sensitivity loss of the system and accurately predicts a substantial hearing loss. The hearing loss acts like any other sensitivity loss in terms of its influence on speech and language acquisition and its amenability to hearing aids and cochlear implants.

Auditory neuropathy of neural origin—or neurogenic AN—is probably accurately described as a specific disorder of the auditory nerve that interferes with the synchrony of neural firing. Hearing sensitivity loss is considerably more variable than in patients with cochleogenic AN, and other clinical signs are more consistent with retrocochlear disorder.

Suprathreshold Hearing Disorder

Although there is a tendency to think of hearing impairment as the sensitivity loss that can be measured on an audiogram, there is another type of hearing impairment that may or may not be accompanied by sensitivity loss. This other impairment results from disease, damage, or decline of the auditory nervous system in adults or delayed or disordered auditory nervous system development in children.

A disordered auditory nervous system, regardless of cause, will have functional consequences that can vary considerably in severity. When impairment is caused by active, measurable disease process, such as a tumor or other space-occupying lesion, or from damage due to trauma or stroke, it is often referred to as a retrocochlear disorder. When impairment is due to developmental disorder or delay or from diffuse changes such as aging, it is often referred to as an auditory processing disorder. The consequences of both types of disorder are often similar from an audiologic perspective, but the disorders are treated differently because of the consequences of diagnosis and the likelihood of a significant residual communication disorder.

Retrocochlear Disorder

In addition to possible hearing sensitivity loss, retrocochlear disease can cause more subtle hearing disorder that is often noted in measures of suprathreshold function such as speech-recognition ability. In general, hearing loss from retrocochlear disorder is distinguishable from cochlear or conductive hearing loss by the extent to which it can adversely affect speech perception. Conductive loss affects speech perception only by attenuating sound. Cochlear hearing loss adds distortion, but it is often minimal and predictable. A retrocochlear disorder can cause severe distortion of incoming speech signals in a manner that limits the usefulness of hearing.

In addition to speech-recognition deficits, other suprathreshold abnormalities can occur. Loudness growth can be abnormal in patients with retrocochlear disorder. Instead of the abnormally rapid growth of loudness characteristic of cochlear hearing loss, retrocochlear disorder can actually result in decruitment, an abnormally slow growth in loudness with increasing intensity. A retrocochlear disorder can also result in abnormal auditory adaptation. The normal auditory system tends to adapt to ongoing sound, especially at near-threshold levels, so that, as adaptation occurs, an audible signal becomes inaudible. At higher intensity levels, ongoing sound tends to remain audible without adaptation. However, in an ear with retrocochlear disorder, the audibility may diminish rapidly owing to excessive auditory adaptation, even at higher intensity levels.

The impact of retrocochlear disorder depends on the level in the auditory nervous system at which the disorder is exerting influence. If, for example, a vestibular schwannoma is having a retrograde influence on the cochlea, speech perception should be consistent with degree of sensitivity loss. A primary disorder of the eighth nerve itself, however, is likely to have a significant impact on hearing sensitivity and on speech perception. A disorder of the brain stem may spare hearing sensitivity and negatively influence only hearing of speech in noisy or other complex acoustic environments.

Auditory Processing Disorder

Auditory processing disorders are most common in children and in aging adults. These disorders are characterized by poor suprathreshold hearing. A primary sign of auditory processing disorder is hearing ability that seems to be disproportionate to the degree of hearing sensitivity loss. The most common symptom is difficulty extracting a signal of interest from a background of noise. Patients simply have difficulty hearing in noise. Another related symptom is difficulty with spatial hearing, such as localizing a sound source, especially in the presence of background noise. These symptoms are not unlike those of patients with peripheral hearing sensitivity loss, but they are usually out of proportion to what might be expected from the degree of loss. It should be no surprise that an auditory disorder, regardless of its locus, would result in similar perceived difficulties. Perhaps the distinguishing feature for patients with an auditory processing disorder is the inability to extract sounds of interest in noisy environments despite an ability to perceive the sounds with adequate loudness. These patients also exhibit difficulty on various tasks related to temporal processing.

Functional Hearing Loss

Functional hearing loss is the exaggeration or feigning of hearing impairment. Many terms have been used to describe this type of hearing "impairment," including nonorganic hearing loss, pseudohypacusis, malingering, factitious hearing loss, and so on. In many cases of functional hearing loss, particularly in adults, an organic hearing sensitivity loss exists but is willfully exaggerated.[21] In other cases, often secondary to trauma of some kind, the entire hearing loss will be willfully feigned. Because there may be some organicity to the hearing loss, it is probably best considered as an exaggerated hearing loss or a functional overlay to an organic loss. Functional hearing loss is the term most commonly used to describe such outcomes.

One way to understand functional hearing loss is to define it by a patient's motivation.[22] Motivation can be defined by two factors, the intent of the person in creating the symptoms and the nature of the gain that results. Thinking of functional hearing loss in this way results in a continuum that can be divided into at least three categories, malingering, factitious disorder, and conversion disorder.

Malingering occurs when an individual feigns a hearing loss, typically for financial gain. Malingering occurs mostly in adults. For example, an employee may apply for worker's compensation for hearing loss secondary to excessive sound exposure in the workplace; alternatively, an individual discharged from the military may seek compensation for hearing loss from excessive noise exposure. Although most patients have legitimate concerns and provide honest results, a small percentage tries to exaggerate the degree of hearing loss in the mistaken notion that they will receive greater compensation. There are also those who have had an accident or altercation and are involved in a lawsuit against an insurance company, for example. Occasionally, such a person will think that feigning a hearing loss will lead to a greater monetary award.

A factitious disorder is one in which the feigning of a hearing loss is done to assume a "sick" role, and the motivation is internal rather than external. Children with functional hearing loss are more likely to have a factitious disorder, using hearing impairment as an explanation for poor performance in school or to gain attention. The idea may have emerged from watching a classmate or sibling receive special treatment for having a hearing impairment. It may also be secondary to a bout of otitis media and the consequent parental attention paid to the episode.

A conversion disorder is a rare cause of functional hearing loss; here, the symptom of a hearing loss occurs unintentionally with little or no organic basis. A conversion disorder results following psychological distress of some nature.

AUDIOLOGIC ASSESSMENT TOOLS

Behavioral Measures

Pure-Tone Audiometry

Pure-tone audiometry is used to establish hearing sensitivity thresholds at discrete frequencies across a range important for human communication. Threshold levels are plotted on an audiogram to show how threshold sensitivity varies across the frequency range. The complete pure-tone audiogram consists of air-conduction and bone-conduction threshold curves for each ear.

The pure-tone audiogram is based on audiometric zero, or average normal hearing, across a defined frequency range. By definition, 0 dB hearing level (HL) is the average intensity level at which threshold of sensitivity is measured in normal-hearing individuals. For clinical purposes, the standard deviation is considered to be 5 dB, so that 99% of the normal population will have thresholds varying from –15 to +15 dB HL. Based on the pure-tone audiogram, then, hearing loss severity is often classified as minimal (15–25 dB), mild (25–40 dB), moderate (40–55 dB), moderately severe (55–70 dB), severe (70–90 dB), or profound (more than 90 dB). Although hearing loss in the minimal range may or may not result in impairment or handicap, it is incorrect to consider thresholds in this range to be within normal limits. The pure-tone audiogram is also used to describe the shape of loss or the audiometric contour or configuration. The audiogram also provides a measure of interaural symmetry, or the extent to which hearing sensitivity is the same in both ears or better in one than the other. In addition, the combination of air- and bone-conduction audiometry is used to determine type of hearing loss.

Pure-tone audiograms are readily established in cooperative older children and adults. In younger children, behavioral responses can be obtained, but may be more limited in accuracy and completeness.[23] In infants 0 to 6 months of age, behavioral observation audiometry is used to estimate binaural hearing thresholds. Behavioral observation audiometry involves controlled presentation of signals in the sound field and careful observation of the infant's response to those signals. Minimal response levels to signals across the frequency range can be determined with a fair degree of accuracy and reliability. In children aged 6 months to 2 years, visual reinforcement audiometry is used, in which a child's behavioral response to a sound, usually a head turn toward the sound source, is conditioned by reinforcement with some type of visual stimulus. If the child will wear earphones, thresholds can be estimated for both ears. In older children, conditioned play audiometry is used, in which the reinforcer is some form of play activity such as tossing blocks into a box.

Speech Audiometry

Speech audiometric measures are used routinely in an audiologic evaluation to measure threshold for speech, cross-check pure-tone sensitivity, quantify suprathreshold hearing, and assist in differential diagnosis.

For clinical purposes, speech audiometric measures fall into one of three categories, speech-recognition threshold, word-recognition score, and sensitized speech measures. In a typical clinical situation, a speech threshold (awareness or recognition) will be determined early as a cross-check for the validity of pure-tone thresholds.[24] Following completion of pure-tone audiometry, word-recognition scores will be obtained as estimates of suprathreshold speech understanding in quiet. Finally, either as part of a comprehensive audiological evaluation or as part of an expanded speech audiometric battery, sensitized speech measures will be obtained to assess processing at the level of the central auditory nervous system.

A speech threshold is the lowest level at which speech can be either detected or recognized. The threshold of detection is referred to as the speech detection threshold (SDT) or the speech awareness threshold. Although synonymous, the term SDT is probably more accurate to designate the lowest level at which speech is perceived. A SDT is used only in patients with limited language competence, such as young children. The threshold of recognition is referred to as the speech-recognition threshold, speech reception threshold, or spondee threshold. Historically, speech reception threshold was the more common term, though spondee threshold is the more accurate one. The term speech-recognition threshold (SRT) is now used to designate the lowest level at which spondee words can be identified.

The SRT is a measure of the threshold of sensitivity for identifying speech signals. The main purpose of obtaining a SRT is for comparison with pure-tone thresholds. The SRT should agree closely with the pure-tone thresholds averaged across 500, 1,000, and 2,000 Hz, differing by no more than ±6 dB. A larger discrepancy between the pure-tone average (PTA) and SRT usually indicates that pure-tone thresholds are inaccurate and may need to be remeasured.

The most common way to describe suprathreshold hearing ability is with word-recognition measures. Word-recognition testing, also referred to as speech discrimination, word discrimination, and phonetically balanced word testing is an assessment of a patient's ability to identify and repeat single-syllable words presented at some suprathreshold level. Speech-recognition ability is usually measured with monosyllabic word tests. A number of tests have been developed over the years.[25–27] Most use single-syllable words in lists of 25 or 50. Lists are usually developed to resemble, to some degree, the phonetic content of speech in a particular language. Word lists are presented to patients at suprathreshold levels, and the patients are instructed to repeat the words. Speech recognition is expressed as a percentage of correct identification of words presented.

The goal of word-recognition testing is to estimate the patient's maximum ability or score. To obtain a maximum score, lists of words or sentences are presented at several intensity levels, extending from just above the speech threshold to the upper level of comfortable listening. In this way, a performance versus intensity PI function is generated for each ear. The shape of this function often has important diagnostic significance. In most cases, the PI function rises systematically as speech intensity is increased, to an asymptotic level representing the best speech understanding that can be achieved in the test ear. In some cases, however, there is a paradoxical rollover effect, in which the function declines substantially as speech intensity increases beyond the level producing the maximal performance score. In other words, as speech intensity increases, performance rises to a maximum level, then declines or "rolls over" sharply as intensity continues to increase. This rollover effect is commonly observed when the site of the hearing loss is retrocochlear, in the auditory nerve or the auditory pathways in the brain stem.[28,29] The use of PI functions is a way of sensitizing speech by challenging the auditory system at high-intensity levels. Because of its ease of administration, many audiologists use it routinely as a screening measure for retrocochlear disorders. The most efficacious clinical strategy is to present a word list simply at the highest intensity level (usually 80 dB HL) and terminate testing if the score is sufficient to rule out rollover.

Interpretation of word-recognition measures is based on the predictable relation of maximum word-recognition scores to degree of hearing loss.[30,31] If the maximum score falls within a given range for a given degree of hearing loss, then the results are considered to be within expectation for a cochlea hearing loss. If the score is poorer than expected, then word-recognition ability is considered to be abnormal for the degree of hearing loss and consistent with retrocochlear disorder. Several approaches have been used to establish what is normal for a given hearing loss. One approach is to determine the lower limits of normal empirically from large data sets of patients with hearing loss. Tables have been generated that provide the lowest maximum score that 95% of individuals with cochlear hearing loss will obtain on a specified measure. Any score below this number for a given hearing loss is considered to be abnormal. Another approach is to establish a prediction for a given hearing loss based on the relationship of the sounds that are audible to the patient and the predicted score based on that audibility.[32]

Other techniques for measuring suprathreshold hearing involve sensitizing speech in some way to more effectively challenge the auditory system. Such measures include low-pass filtered speech,[33–35] time-compressed speech,[36,37] and the presentation of speech in noise or competition.[38] Another effective approach for assessing suprathreshold hearing is the use of dichotic tests.[39–43] In the dichotic paradigm, two different speech targets are presented simultaneously to the two ears. The patterns of results can reveal auditory processing deficits, especially those due to disorders of the temporal lobe and corpus callosum.

Speech audiometric measures can be useful in differentiating whether a hearing disorder is due to changes in the outer or middle ear, cochlea, or auditory peripheral or central nervous systems. A summary is presented in Table 10–1. In the cases of cochlear disorder, word-recognition ability is usually predictable from the degree and slope of the audiogram. Although there are some exceptions, such as hearing loss due to endolymphatic hydrops, word-recognition ability and performance on other forms of speech audiometric measures are highly correlated with degree of hearing impairment in certain frequency regions. When performance is poorer than expected, the likely culprit is a disorder of the eighth nerve or central auditory nervous system structures. Thus, unusually poor performance on speech audiometric tests lends a measure of suspicion about the site of the disorder causing the hearing impairment.

Speech audiometric tests are also used to measure auditory processing ability. As neural impulses travel from the cochlea through the eighth nerve to the auditory brain stem and cortex, the number and complexity of neural pathways expands progressively. The system, in its vastness of pathways, includes a certain level of redundancy or excess capacity of processing ability. Such redundancy serves many useful purposes, but it also makes the function of the auditory nervous system impervious to examination. For example, a patient can have a rather substantial lesion of the auditory brain stem or auditory cortex and still have normal hearing sensitivity and normal word recognition ability. Accordingly, sensitized speech audiometric measures must be used to assess nervous system function and dysfunction.

TABLE 10–1 Expected Patterns of abnormality on speech audiometric tests as a function of site of disorder

SITE	WRS MAX	WRS PI	SC MAX	SC PI	DICHOTIC
Cochlea	–	–	–	–	–
VIIIth nerve	++	++	++	++	–
Brain stem	–	+	++	++	–
Temporal lobe	–	–	+	+	++

Tests include maximum word-recognition scores presented in quiet (WRS max), performance-intensity function of word-recognition scores in quiet (WRS PI), maximum score on sentence identification in competition (SC max), performance intensity function of sentence identification in competition (SC PI), and score on a dichotic measur. Predicted performance on these measures would be (–) normal or predictable from the degree of hearing sensitivity loss, (+) sometimes abnormal, depending on the site, size, and extent of influence of the lesion or (++) usually abnormal.

Speech audiometric measures have been modified for use in pediatric assessment, although they are somewhat limited by the linguistic competence of younger children. Tests used with younger patients usually involve picture-pointing tasks in an effort to assess speech-recognition ability.

Other Behavioral Measures

A number of other behavioral measures can be used for various purposes in the audiologic evaluation. Some of the early strategies designed to differentiate cochlear from retrocochlear disorder were based primarily on measures of auditory adaptation and recruitment. They are seldom used in modern practice and will be described only briefly here.

One of the consequences of cochlear hearing loss is recruitment, or abnormal loudness growth. That is, loudness grows more rapidly than normal at intensity levels just above threshold in an ear with cochlear site of disorder. Clinically, this means that if recruitment is present, then the site of disorder is cochlear rather than retrocochlear. One effective way to measure recruitment is with the alternate binaural loudness balance (ABLB) test.[44] The ABLB was designed to be used in patients with unilateral hearing loss and was shown to be reasonably effective in identifying cochlear site.[45,46] Another strategy involved measuring the difference limen for intensity. An indirect method that was used clinically for a number of years is the short increment sensitivity index (SISI).[47–50] It too was shown to be effective in identifying cochlear hearing loss.

Another consequence of retrocochlear hearing loss is abnormal auditory adaptation. The normal auditory system tends to adapt to ongoing sound, especially at near-threshold levels, so that, as adaptation occurs, an audible signal becomes inaudible. At higher intensity levels, ongoing sound tends to remain audible without adaptation. However, in an ear with retrocochlear disorder, the audibility may diminish rapidly owing to excessive auditory adaptation even at higher intensity levels. Two popular behavioral measures of adaptation in the past were the tone decay test (TDT)[51–53] and diagnostic Békésy audiometry.[54,55] These tests were designed to assess a patient's ability to perceive sustained tones. Although popular for a time, the tests were not particularly sensitive to eighth-nerve disorder or specific to cochlear disorder.[56–59]

All of these measures, ABLB, SISI, TDT, and Békésy audiometry, were useful in the diagnosis of retrocochlear site in the days when tumors had to reach a substantial size before they could be diagnosed radiographically. As imaging and radiographic techniques improved, smaller lesions that had less functional impact on the auditory system could be visualized, and the utility of the classic test battery diminished. Today these measures are mostly of historic interest, although they can occasionally be useful in evaluating patients with severe hearing loss.

Another behavioral diagnostic measure that is sometimes useful is a measure of lower brain-stem function known as the masking level difference (MLD). Abnormal performance on the MLD is consistent with brain-stem disorder.[60–63] The MLD measures binaural release from masking owing to interaural phase relationships. The binaural auditory system is an exquisite detector of differences in timing of sound reaching the two ears and thus helps in localizing low-frequency sounds, which reach the ears at different points in time. The MLD is based on the concept of binaural release from masking, which occurs as a result of processing by the brain stem at the level of the superior olivary complex. The concept can be described as follows: if identical low-frequency tones are presented in-phase to both ears and noise is added to both ears to mask the tones, when the phase of the tone delivered to one earphone is reversed, the tone will becomes audible again.

The MLD test is designed to measure binaural release from masking. A 500-Hz interrupted tone is split and presented in-phase to both ears. Narrowband noise is also presented, at a fixed level of 60 dB HL. Using a tracking procedure, threshold for the in-phase tones is determined in the presence of the noise. Then the phase of one of the tones is reversed, and threshold is tracked again. The MLD is the difference in threshold between the in-phase and the out-of-phase conditions. For a 500-Hz tone, the MLD should be greater than 7 dB and is usually around 12 dB.

A number of behavioral measures are used to identify patients who are feigning hearing loss and to try to quantify the degree of any underlying organic disorder.[64] The two measures that have withstood the test of time are the Stenger and Lombard tests.

The Stenger test is designed to identify functional hearing loss in patients with unilateral or significantly asymmetric hearing loss. If the hearing loss is feigned or exaggerated, the Stenger test can detect the functional component. The test is based on the principle that tones presented to both ears will be perceived only in the ear in which the tone is louder if an ear difference exists. To carry out the test, either speech or pure-tone stimuli are presented simultaneously to both ears. Initially, the signal is presented to the good ear at a comfortable, audible level of about 20 dB sensation level and to the poorer ear at 20 dB below the level of the good ear. The patient will respond, because he/she will hear the signal presented to the good ear. Testing proceeds by increasing the intensity level of the signal presented to the poorer ear. If the loss in the poorer ear is organic, the patient will continue to respond to the signal being presented to the good ear (ie, a negative Stenger). If the loss is functional, the patient will stop responding when the loudness of the signal in the poorer ear exceeds that in the good ear because the signal will be heard only in the poorer ear owing to the Stenger principle. Because an audible signal is still being presented to the good ear, it becomes clear that the patient is not cooperating. This result is a positive Stenger, indicative of functional hearing loss.

The Lombard test is used in the case of suspected bilateral functional hearing loss. It is based on the principle that a patient's vocal effort will be raised in the presence of background noise. The test involves the sudden presentation of noise to a patient reading aloud, and an assessment of any change in vocal intensity. An increase in vocal intensity indicates the presence of functional hearing loss.

The audiologic goal in cases of functional hearing loss is to establish a valid and reliable behavioral audiogram that indicates the true extent of the hearing loss. Should behavioral measures fail, auditory evoked potentials are used to predict hearing sensitivity.

Pure-tone audiometry, speech audiometry, and these other procedures noted above constitute the basic behavioral measures available to quantify hearing impairment and determine the type and site of auditory disorder.

Electroacoustic and Electrophysiologic Measures

Immittance Measures

Immittance testing is one of the most powerful tools available for the evaluation of auditory disorder.[65] It serves at least three functions in audiologic assessment: (1) it is sensitive in detecting middle-ear disorder, (2) it can be useful in differentiating cochlear from retrocochlear disorder, and (3) it can be helpful in detecting the presence of peripheral hearing sensitivity loss and can be used as a cross-check to pure-tone audiometry in pediatric assessment. Because of its comprehensive value, immittance measurement is a routine component of the audiologic evaluation and is often the first assessment administered in the test battery.

Immittance is a physical characteristic of all mechanical vibratory systems. In very general terms, it is a measure of how readily a system can be set into vibration by a driving force. The ease with which energy will flow through the vibrating system is called its admittance. The reciprocal concept, the extent to which the system resists the flow of energy through it, is called its impedance. If a vibrating system can be forced into motion with little applied force, the admittance is high and the impedance is low. On the other hand, if the system resists being set into motion until the driving force is relatively high, then the admittance of the system is low and the impedance is high. Immittance is a term that is meant to encompass both of these concepts.

Immittance measurement can be thought of as a way to assess the manner in which energy flows through the outer and middle ears to the cochlea. If the middle-ear system is normal, energy will flow in a predictable way. If it is not, then energy will flow either too well (high admittance) or not well enough (high impedance).

Immittance is measured by delivering a pure-tone signal of a constant sound pressure level into the ear canal through a mechanical probe that is seated at the entrance of the ear canal. The signal, which is referred to by convention as the probe tone, is a 226-Hz pure-tone that is delivered at 85 dB SPL. The SPL of the probe tone is monitored by an immittance meter, and any change is noted as a change in energy flow through the middle-ear system.

Three immittance measures are generally used in the clinical assessment of middle-ear function: tympanometry, static immittance, and acoustic reflex thresholds.

Tympanometry measures how the acoustic immittance of the middle-ear vibratory system changes as air pressure is varied in the external ear canal. Transmission of sound through the middle-ear mechanism is maximal when air pressure is equal on both sides of the tympanic membrane. For a normal ear, maximum transmission occurs at, or near, atmospheric pressure. The clinical value of tympanometry is that a middle-ear disorder modifies the shape of the tympanogram in predictable ways. Various patterns of tympanometric shapes are related to various auditory disorders. The conventional classification system designates three tympanogram types, Types, A, B, and C.[66] The characteristically normal shape, with its peak at atmospheric pressure (0 daPa) is designated Type A.

If the middle-ear space is filled with fluid (eg, as in otitis media with effusion), then the tympanogram loses its sharp peak and become relatively flat or slightly rounded; this pattern is caused by the mass added to the ossicular chain by the fluid. This shape is designated Type B.

In eustachian tube dysfunction, air becomes trapped in the middle ear and is absorbed by the mucosal lining, resulting in a reduction of air pressure in the middle-ear space relative to the pressure in the external ear canal. This pressure differential draws the tympanic membrane medially. The effect on the tympanogram is to move the sharp peak away from 0 daPa and into the negative air pressure region, reflecting the fact that the maximum energy flow occurs when the pressure in the ear canal is negative, matching that in the middle-ear space. This tympanogram, which is normal in shape but peaks at a substantially negative air pressure, is designated Type C.

Anything that causes the ossicular chain to become stiffer than normal can result in a reduction in energy flow through the middle ear. The added stiffness simply attenuates the peak of the tympanogram. The shape will remain normal Type A, but the entire tympanogram will become shallower. Such a tympanogram is designated Type A_s to indicate that the shape is normal, with the peak at or near 0 daPa of air pressure but with significant reduction in the height at the peak. The subscript "s" denotes stiffness or shallowness. The disorder most commonly associated with a Type A_s tympanogram is otosclerosis.

Anything that causes the ossicular chain to lose stiffness can result in too much energy flow through the middle ear. For example, in ossicular discontinuity (essentially detaching the tympanic membrane from the cochlea), the tympanogram retains its normal shape, but the peak is much greater than normal. With the heavy load of the cochlear fluid system removed from the chain, the tympanic membrane responds more freely to forced vibration. The energy flow through the middle ear is greatly enhanced, resulting in a very deep tympanogram. This shape is designated A_d to indicate that the shape of the tympanogram is normal, with the peak at or near 0 daPa of air pressure, but the height is significantly increased. The subscript "d" denotes deep or discontinuity.

Classifying tympanograms based on descriptive types is a simple, effective approach to describing tympanometric outcomes. There are, however, other ways to analyze the tympanogram with more refinement. For example, a tympanogram can be described by its peak pressure, which is simply the number in daPa that corresponds to the peak of the tympanogram trace. Another way is to try to describe the actual shape of the tympanometric curve, which is done either by quantifying its gradient, which is the relationship of its height and width, or by measuring the tympanometric width. Tympanometric width is measured by calculating the daPa at the point corresponding to 50% of the static immittance value. This is a very effective way to describe a rounded tympanogram, and excessive widths are often found in ears with middle-ear effusion.[67]

A number of other strategies for tympanometric assessment have emerged over the years in an effort to more accurately and sensitively measure middle-ear function.[68,69] Measures of multifrequency tympanometry,[70] multicomponent analysis,[71] reflectance,[72,73] and other methods can be used for this purpose. The clinical challenge relating to these sensitive measures of function is one of understanding the relation of measurement outcome to active ear disease. Because they are so sensitive, such measures are prone to false-positive identification of meaningful otologic conditions.

The value of high-frequency tympanometry has become increasingly clear in the measurement of middle-ear function in infants. It is now common clinical practice to use a 1,000-Hz probe tone when testing newborns and young infants.[74–76] The reason is probably best demonstrated by the results shown in Figure 10–1. Tympanograms from a 7-week-old infant, measured with both 226- and 1,000-Hz probe tones, are shown. One ear of the child has middle-ear effusion, while the other does not, as judged by otoscopy. Results show fairly normal, peaked tympanograms in both ears with the 226-Hz probe but a clearly different picture with the 1,000-Hz probe. The use of higher frequency probe tones is an important consideration in infant testing.

In contrast to the dynamic measure of middle-ear function represented by the tympanogram, static immittance refers to the isolated contribution of the middle ear to the overall acoustic immittance of the auditory system. It can be thought of as simply the absolute height of the tympanogram at its peak. The

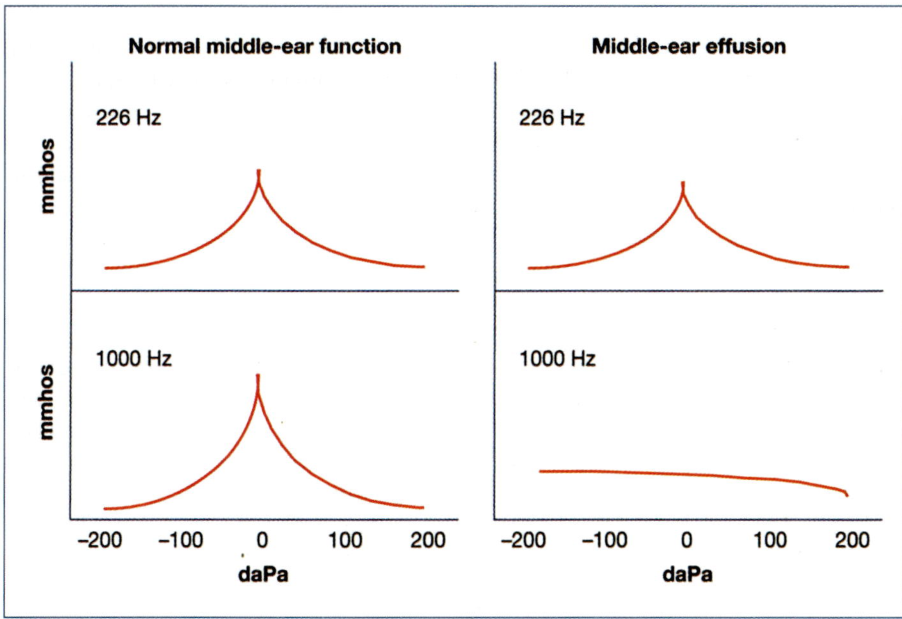

FIGURE 10–1 • 226-Hz and 1,000-Hz probe-tone tympanograms of a 7-week-old infant in whom one ear has normal middle-ear function and the other has middle-ear effusion.

static immittance is measured by comparing the probe-tone sound pressure level or immittance when the air pressure is at 0 daPa, or at the air pressure corresponding to the peak, with the immittance when the air pressure is raised to positive 200 daPa. Values lying below 0.3 cc or above 1.6 cc are strong evidence of middle-ear disorder. This information is useful in deciding whether a Type A tympanogram is normal, shallow, or deep. For example, if the tympanogram is Type A and the static immittance is 0.2, then the tympanogram can be considered shallow and indicative of increased stiffness of the middle-ear mechanism. Unfortunately, the range of normal static immittance is so large that many milder forms of middle-ear disorder will fall within the normal boundaries. Thus, the test lacks transitivity in that only one outcome is meaningful. That is, if the static immittance falls outside the normal range, it is safe to predict middle-ear disorder. But, values within the normal range do not necessarily exclude the possibility of middle-ear disorder.

The third measure of the typical immittance battery is the acoustic stapedial reflex. The stapedius muscle is attached, via its tendon, to the head of the stapes. When the muscle contracts, the tendon exerts tension on the stapes, stiffens the ossicular chain, and reduces low-frequency energy transmission through the middle ear. The result of this reduced energy transmission is an increase in probe-tone SPL in the external ear canal. Therefore, when the stapedius muscle contracts in response to high-intensity sound, a slight change in immittance can be detected by the circuitry of the immittance instrument.

Both stapedius muscles contract in response to sound delivered to one ear. Therefore, ipsilateral (uncrossed) and contralateral (crossed) reflexes are recorded with sound presented to each ear. For example, when a signal of sufficient magnitude is presented to the right ear, a stapedius reflex will occur in both the right (ipsilateral or uncrossed) and the left (contralateral or crossed) ears. These are called the right uncrossed and the right crossed reflexes, respectively. When a signal is presented to the left ear and a reflex is measured in that ear, it is referred to as a left uncrossed reflex. When a signal is presented to the left ear and a reflex is measured in the right ear, it is referred to as a left crossed reflex.

The threshold is the most common measure of the acoustic stapedial reflex and is defined as the lowest intensity level at which a middle-ear immittance change can be detected in response to sound. In patients with normal hearing and normal middle-ear function, reflex thresholds for pure tones will be reached at levels ranging from 70 to 100 dB HL. The average threshold level is approximately 85 dB. These levels are constant across the frequency range from 500 to 4,000 Hz. Threshold measures are useful for at least two purposes, screening for the presence of hearing sensitivity loss and differential assessment of auditory disorder.

Several methods have been developed for using acoustic reflex thresholds to predict whether hearing sensitivity loss exists. One example is the sensitivity prediction by the acoustic reflex (SPAR) test.[77,78] The SPAR test is based on the well-documented difference between acoustic reflex thresholds to pure tones versus broadband noise (BBN) and on the change in BBN thresholds, but not pure-tone thresholds, as a result of sensorineural hearing loss. That is, thresholds to BBN signals are lower than thresholds to pure-tone signals. However, sensorineural hearing loss has a differential effect on the two signals, raising the threshold to BBN signals, but not to pure-tone signals. The SPAR test capitalizes on this effect to provide a general prediction of the presence or absence of hearing loss.

To compute the SPAR value, the BBN threshold is subtracted from the average reflex threshold to pure-tones of 500, 1,000, and 2,000 Hz. The magnitude of this difference will vary according to the specific equipment used to carry out the measures. A correction factor is then applied to yield a SPAR value of 20 in normal-hearing subjects. If a patient's SPAR value is less than 15, there is a high probability of a sensorineural hearing loss.

Clinical application of such techniques based on acoustic reflex thresholds appears to be most effective when used to predict presence or absence of a sensorineural hearing loss.

Prediction of hearing sensitivity by acoustic reflex thresholds can be very valuable in testing a child on whom behavioral thresholds cannot be obtained and for sensitivity prediction is in the case of a patient who is feigning hearing loss.

Reflex threshold measurement has been valuable in both the assessment of middle-ear function and the differentiation of cochlear from retrocochlear disorder.[79–81] In terms of the latter, whereas reflex thresholds occur at reduced sensation levels in ears with cochlear hearing loss, they are typically elevated or absent in ears having eighth-nerve disorder. Similarly, reflex thresholds are often abnormal for patients with brain-stem disorder. Comparison of crossed and uncrossed thresholds has also been found to be helpful in differentiating eighth nerve from brain-stem disorders.[82]

Auditory Evoked Potentials

An auditory evoked potential is a waveform that reflects the electrophysiologic function of a certain portion of the central auditory nervous system in response to sound. For audiologic purposes, it is convenient to group the auditory evoked potentials into categories based loosely on the latency ranges over which the potentials are observed. The earliest of the evoked potentials, occurring within the first 5 milliseconds following signal presentation is the electrocochleogram (ECoG), which reflects activity of the cochlea and eighth nerve. The most frequently used evoked potential is the ABR, which occurs within the first 10 milliseconds following signal onset. The ABR reflects neural activity from the eighth nerve to the midbrain. The middle-latency response (MLR) occurs within the first 50 milliseconds following signal onset and reflects activity at or near the auditory cortex. The late-latency, or cortical, response (LLR) occurs within the first 250 milliseconds following signal onset and reflects activity of the primary auditory and association areas of the cerebral cortex.

These measures, the ECoG, ABR, MLR, and LLR are known as transient potentials in that they occur and are recorded in response to a single stimulus presentation. The response is allowed to end before the next signal is presented. The process is then repeated numerous times, and the responses are averaged. A different type of evoked potential, called the auditory steady-state response (ASSR), is measured by evaluating the ongoing activity of the brain in response to a modulation, or change, in an ongoing stimulus. The ASSR reflects activity from different portions of the brain, depending on the modulation rate used. Responses from slower rates emanate from more central structures of the brain, while responses from faster rates emanate from the more peripheral auditory nerve and brain-stem structures.

Diagnostic assessment is usually made with the ABR, MLR, and LLR. The ABR is highly sensitive to disorders of the eighth-nerve and auditory brain stem and is often used in conjunction with imaging and radiologic measures to assist in the diagnosis of acoustic tumors and brain-stem disorders.[83–88] Surgical monitoring of evoked potentials is usually carried out with ECoG, ABR, and/or direct-nerve recordings.[89,90] These evoked potentials are monitored during eighth-nerve tumor removal in an effort to preserve hearing. Threshold prediction is usually made with ABR and/or LLR in adults and ABR and ASSR in infants and young children.

The ECoG is a response composed mainly of the compound action potential (AP) that occurs at the distal portion of the eighth nerve. A click stimulus is used to elicit this response. The rapid onset of the click provides a stimulus that is sufficient to cause the fibers of the eighth nerve to respond in synchrony. This synchronous discharge of nerve fibers results in the action potential. There are two other, smaller components of the ECoG. One is referred to as the cochlear microphonic, which is a response from the cochlea that mimics the input stimulus. The other is the summating potential, which is a direct current response that reflects the envelope of the input stimulus.

The ECoG is best recorded as a near-field response, with an electrode close to the source. Unlike the ABR, MLR, and LLR, which can readily be recorded as far-field responses with remote electrodes, it is more difficult to record the ECoG from surface electrodes. Thus, the best recordings of the ECoG are made from an electrode that is placed through the tympanic membrane and onto the promontory of the temporal bone or from an electrode in the ear canal placed near the tympanic membrane.

The ABR occurs within the first 10 milliseconds following signal onset and consist of a series of five positive peaks or waves. The ABR has properties that make it very useful clinically. First, the response can be recorded from surface electrodes. Second, the waves are robust and can be recorded easily in patients with adequate hearing and normal auditory nervous system function. Third, the response is immune to the influences of the patient's state, so that it can be recorded in patients who are sleeping or sedated. Fourth, the latencies of the various waves are quite comparable within and across people so that they serve as a sensitive measure of brain-stem integrity. In addition, the time intervals between peaks are prolonged by auditory disorders central to the cochlea, which makes the ABR useful for differentiating cochlear from retrocochlear sites of disorder.

The ABR is generated by the auditory nerve and by structures in the auditory brain stem. Wave I originates in the distal or peripheral portion of the eighth nerve near the point at which the nerve fibers leave the cochlea. Wave II originates from the proximal portion of the nerve near the brain stem. Wave III has contribution from this proximal portion of the nerve and from the cochlear nucleus. Waves IV and V have contributions from the cochlear nucleus, superior olivary complex, and lateral lemniscus.

The "stacked" ABR is a modification of the conventional manner of ABR data collection. It is a strategy designed to enhance diagnostic effectiveness by assessing auditory system function across a broad frequency range rather than in the limited high-frequency region that responds to conventional click stimuli. Through a series of progressive band-pass filterings, ABRs are generated that correspond to frequency bands across the spectrum. The component wave Vs of the resultant ABRs are aligned in time and summed, and amplitudes are compared between ears and against normative data. Results have been encouraging in terms of sensitivity to small tumors of the eighth nerve.[91–93]

The MLR is characterized by two successive positive peaks: the first (P_a) at about 25 to 35 milliseconds and the second (P_b) at about 40 to 60 milliseconds following stimulus presentation.

The MLR is probably generated by some combination of projections to the primary auditory cortex and the cortical area itself. Although the MLR is the most difficult auditory evoked potential to record clinically, it is sometimes used diagnostically and as an aid to the identification of auditory processing disorder.

The LLR is characterized by a negative peak (N1) at a latency of about 90 milliseconds and a positive peak (P2) at about 180 milliseconds following stimulus presentation. This potential is greatly affected by subject state. It is best recorded when the patient is awake and carefully attending to the sounds being presented. There is an important developmental effect on the LLR during infancy and childhood. In older children or adults, however, it is robust and relatively easy to record. In children or adults with relatively normal-hearing sensitivity, abnormality or absence of the LLR is associated with auditory processing disorder. There are other late potentials, known as event-related potentials (ERPs), that can be recorded as well, including the mismatch negativity (MMN), late positive component, and object-related negativity, which seem to hold promise as objective measures of auditory nervous system function.[94,95]

The ASSR is used to predict hearing sensitivity.[96,97] The response itself is an evoked neural potential that follows the envelope of a complex stimulus. It is evoked by the periodic modulation of a tone. The neural response is a brain potential that closely follows the time course of the modulation. The response can be detected objectively at intensity levels close to behavioral threshold. The ASSR can yield a clinically acceptable, frequency-specific prediction of the behavioral audiogram. The ASSR is elicited by a tone. In clinical applications, the frequencies of 500, 1,000, 2,000, and 4,000 Hz are commonly used. The puretone is either modulated in the amplitude domain or modulated in both the amplitude and frequency domains. Brain electrical activity at the frequency corresponding to the modulation rate is measured. For example, when a tone of any frequency is modulated periodically at a rate of 90/s, the 90 Hz component of the brain electrical activity is measured. Measurement is made of the amplitude or variability of the phase of the electrical activity to determine if it is "following" the modulation envelope. When the modulated tone is at an intensity above threshold, the brain activity at the modulation rate is enhanced and time-locked to the modulation. If the tone is below a patient's threshold, brain activity is not enhanced and is random in relation to the modulation.

Otoacoustic Emissions

OAEs are low-intensity sounds that are generated by the cochlea and propogate through the middle ear into the ear canal[98,99]. OAEs are probably not essential to hearing, but rather are the by-product of active processing by the outer-hair cell system. Of clinical interest is that OAEs are present when outer-hair cells are healthy and absent when outer-hair cells are damaged. Thus, OAEs reveal, with considerable sensitivity, the integrity of outer-hair cell function.

There are two broad categories of OAEs: spontaneous and evoked. Spontaneous OAEs (SOAEs) are narrowband signals that occur in the ear canal without the introduction of an eliciting signal. Spontaneous emissions are present in over half of all normal-hearing ears and absent in all ears at frequencies where sensorineural hearing loss exceeds approximately 30 dB. It appears that SOAEs originate from outer-hair cells corresponding to that portion of the basilar membrane tuned to their frequency.

A sensitive, low-noise microphone housed in a probe is used to record SOAEs. The probe is secured in the external auditory canal with a flexible cuff. Signals detected by the microphone are routed to a spectrum analyzer, which provides frequency analysis of the signal. Usually the frequency range of interest is sampled several times, and the results are signal averaged to reduce background noise. SOAEs, when they occur, appear as peaks of energy along the frequency spectrum.

Because SOAEs are absent in many ears with normal hearing, clinical applications have not been forthcoming. Efforts to relate SOAEs to tinnitus have revealed a relationship in some, but not many subjects who have both.

Evoked OAEs are elicited by a stimulus and occur during and after signal presentation. Evoked OAEs bear a close resemblance to the eliciting signal. There are several classes of evoked OAEs, two of which have proven to be useful clinically: transient-evoked OAEs (TEOAEs) and distortion-product OAEs (DPOAEs).[100,101]

TEOAEs are elicited with transient signals or clicks. Series of click stimuli are presented, usually at an intensity level of about 80–85 dB SPL. Output from the microphone is signal averaged, usually within a time window of 20 milliseconds. In a typical clinical paradigm, alternating samples of the emission are placed into separate memory locations, so that the final result provides two traces of the response for comparison purposes.

TEOAEs occur about 4 milliseconds following stimulus presentation and continue for about 10 milliseconds. Because a click is a broad-spectrum signal, the response is similarly broad in spectrum as well. By convention, these waveforms are subjected to spectral analysis, the results of which are often shown in a graph depicting the amplitude-versus-frequency components of the emission. One important aspect of TEOAE analysis is the reproducibility of the response. This similarity or reproducibility of successive samples of a response is expressed as a percentage, with 100% being identical. If the magnitude of the emission exceeds the magnitude of the noise, and if the reproducibility of the emission exceeds a predetermined level, then the emission is said to be present. If an emission is present, it is likely that the outer-hair cells are functioning in the frequency region of the emission.

DPOAEs occur as a result of nonlinear processes in the cochlea. When two tones are presented to the cochlea, distortion occurs in the form of other tones that are not present in the two-tone eliciting signals. These distortions are combination tones, or harmonics, that are related to the eliciting tones in a predictable mathematical way. The two tones used to elicit the DPOAE are, by convention, designated f_1 and f_2. The most robust distortion product occurs at the frequency represented by the equation $2f_1–f_2$. As with TEOAEs, a probe is used to deliver the tone pairs and to record the response. Pairs of tones are presented across the frequency range to elicit distortion products from approximately 1,000 to 6,000 Hz. The tone pairs usually have a fixed frequency and intensity relationship. Typically, the pairs are presented from high frequency to low frequency. As each pair is presented, measurements are made at the $2f_1-f_2$ frequency to determine the amplitude of the DPOAE and also at a nearby frequency to provide an estimate of the noise floor at that moment in time.

DPOAEs are typically depicted as the amplitude of the distortion product ($2f_1-f_2$) as a function of frequency of the f_2 tone. If the amplitude exceeds the background noise, the emission is said to be present. If an emission is present, it is likely that the outer-hair cells are functioning in the frequency region of the f_2 tone.

Results of TEOAE and DPOAE testing provide a measure of the integrity of outer-hair cell function. Both approaches have been successfully applied clinically as objective indicators of cochlear function.

DIFFERENTIAL DIAGNOSIS AND MEASUREMENT OUTCOME

Functional outcomes of structural changes in the auditory system are reasonably predictable from the battery of assessment tools described. Table 10–2 summarizes the probable outcomes as a function of disorder sites.

Outer-and Middle-Ear Disorders

Audiologic outcomes vary depending on the consequence that a disorder has on the function of the outer- and middle-ear structures. For example, excessive cerumen in the ear canal may or may not impede the transduction of sound to the tympanic membrane. Similarly, tympanosclerosis may or may not reduce the functioning of the tympanic membrane. The first goal is to determine whether these structural changes result in a disorder in function.

The second goal of the evaluation is to determine whether and how much this disorder in function is causing a hearing loss. In some circumstances, a structural change in the outer and middle ear can result in outer or middle-ear disorder without causing a measurable loss of hearing. For example, a tympanic membrane can be perforated without causing a significant conductive hearing loss. On the other hand, a similar perforation located elsewhere on the tympanic membrane can result in a substantial conductive hearing loss. Similarly, eustachian tube dysfunction, causing significant negative pressure in the middle-ear space, may result in hearing loss in one case but not in another.

Immittance audiometry is used to evaluate outer and middle-ear function, and pure-tone audiometry is used to evaluate the degree of conductive component caused by the presence of middle-ear disorder. In most cases, rudimentary speech audiometry will be carried out as a cross-check of pure-tone thresholds and as a gross assessment of suprathreshold word-recognition ability.

In cases of outer and middle-ear disorder, the pure-tone audiogram will often be an important metric by which the outcome of the treatment is judged. That is, the pretreatment audiogram will be compared to the posttreatment audiogram to evaluate the success of the treatment.

Immittance Audiometry

The first step in the evaluation process is immittance audiometry. Because it is the most sensitive indicator of middle-ear function, a full battery of tympanometry, static immittance, and acoustic reflex thresholds is indicated. Results will provide information indicating whether a disorder is caused by

- an increase in the mass of the middle-ear mechanism,
- an increase or decrease in the stiffness of the middle-ear system,
- the presence of a perforation of the tympanic membrane, or
- significant negative pressure in the middle-ear space.

If all immittance results are normal, any hearing loss measured by pure-tone audiometry can be attributed to sensorineural hearing loss. If immittance results indicate the presence of a middle-ear disorder, pure-tone audiometry by air- and bone-conduction must be carried out to assess the degree of conductive component of the hearing loss attributable to the middle-ear disorder.

Immittance results vary with the nature of the disorder. The pattern of results consistent with an increase in the mass of the middle-ear system—from, eg, otitis media with effusion and cholesteatoma—comprises a Type B tympanogram, excessively low static immittance, and absent reflexes recorded in the disordered ear (in the case of right-ear

TABLE 10–2 Expected outcomes on audiometric measures as a function of site of disorder

MEASURE	COCHLEA	VIII NERVE	BRAIN STEM	TEMPORAL LOBE
Otoacoustic emissions	++	+	–	–
Pure-tone audiometry	++	+	+	–
Word-recognition scores	–	++	+	–
Acoustic reflexes	–	++	+	–
Auditory brain stem response	–	++	++	–
Dichotic speech measures	–	–	+	++

Predicted performance on these measures would be (-) normal or predictable from the degree of hearing sensitivity loss, (+) sometimes abnormal, depending on the site, size, and extent of influence of the lesion, or (++) usually abnormal.

disorder, right uncrossed and left crossed acoustic reflexes would be absent).

An increase in the stiffness of the middle-ear system (from, eg, otosclerosis) results in a pattern characterized by a Type A_s tympanogram, relatively low static immittance, and absent acoustic reflexes in the probe ear.

Excessive immittance of the middle-ear system, exemplified by ossicular disarticulation, manifests a pattern of results characterized by a Type A_d tympanogram, excessively high static immittance, and absent acoustic reflexes in the probe ear (if the left ear is affected, then the left uncrossed and right crossed will be absent).

A perforation of the tympanic membrane yields another pattern of immittance findings, characterized by an inability to measure a tympanogram, excessive volume, and unmeasurable acoustic reflexes from the affected probe ear (in the case of right-ear disorder, the right uncrossed and left crossed reflexes would be absent).

The pattern of results consistent with significant negative pressure in the middle-ear space, secondary to eustachian tube dysfunction, includes a Type C tympanograms (peak at ≤–200), normal static immittance, and absent acoustic reflexes in the probe ear.

Diagnosis of outer and middle-ear disorder in infants is not quite as straightforward. Because acoustic reflexes are not as readily identifiable in infants under 6 months of age, assessment is limited to tympanometric measures. Confounding the evaluation further is the need for use of higher frequency probe tones due primarily to physical ear canal size. Recent clinical finding suggest that the use of 1,000-Hz probe tones may permit classification of tympanograms for diagnostic purposes.[74] Wideband reflectance measures may also provide value in identifying infants with middle-ear effusion or other disorders.[102]

Pure-Tone Audiometry

Pure-tone audiometry is used to quantify the degree to which middle-ear disorder is contributing to a hearing sensitivity loss. If immittance audiometry shows any abnormality in outer or middle-ear function, then complete air- and bone-conduction audiometry is indicated for both ears to determine the degree of conductive hearing loss.

It is important to carry out both air- and bone-conduction to quantify the extent of the conductive component. It is important to test both ears because the presence of conductive hearing loss requires the use of masking in the nontest ear, and that ear cannot be properly masked without knowledge of its air- and bone-conduction thresholds.

Generally, a middle-ear disorder manifests as an air–bone gap on the audiogram. A disorder that adds mass to the system influences higher frequencies; a disorder that adds or subtracts stiffness affects the lower frequencies. Although the presence of middle-ear disorder is correlated with conductive hearing loss, the correlation is not perfect. The measurement of air- and bone-conduction thresholds is not as sensitive to middle-ear disorder as immittance audiometry or other measures. Consequently, a middle-ear disorder can exist without an air–bone gap. Nevertheless, a middle-ear disorder is likely to result in some degree of conductive hearing loss, and pure-tone audiometry can serve as a useful quantification of pre- and posttreatment function.

Speech Audiometry

In cases of outer and middle-ear disorder, the most important component of speech audiometry is determination of the speech-recognition threshold as a cross-check of the accuracy of pure-tone thresholds. A speech threshold is often established prior to pure-tone audiometry to establish a benchmark for the level at which pure-tone thresholds should occur. Although this is good practice in general, it is particularly useful in the assessment of young children. Speech thresholds can also be established by bone conduction, permitting the quantification of an air–bone gap to speech signals.

Assessment of word recognition is also often carried out, though more as a matter of routine than importance. Conductive hearing loss has a predictable influence on word-recognition scores, and if such testing is of value, it is usually only to confirm this expectation.

In conductive hearing loss caused by a middle-ear disorder, the effect on speech recognition will be negligible except to elevate the speech threshold by the degree of hearing loss in the ear with the disorder. Suprathreshold speech recognition is not affected by the hearing loss, except to shift the intensity level at which maximum performance is reached by the amount of the air–bone gap.

Auditory Evoked Potentials

Auditory evoked potentials are affected by conductive hearing loss only to the extent that attenuation of the eliciting signals influences waveform interpretation. For example, ABR waveform latencies become longer, and earlier waves become less identifiable, as intensity level is reduced. A 30-dB conductive hearing loss causes an ABR waveform elicited at 90 dB nHL to resemble a waveform elicited at 60 dB in an otherwise normal ear. Absolute latencies are delayed, but in a predictable manner. Inter-wave intervals are unaffected. So long as the amount of the air–bone gap is considered, interpretation of the ABR should not be affected.

The predictable delay in ABR latency actually helps in the identification of conductive disorders in infant assessment. Because a conductive component delays all component waves uniformly, assessment at higher intensity levels can reveal delays in both waves I and V, indicating that a predicted sensitivity loss is due primarily to conductive disorder. The conductive component can be confirmed with bone-conduction ABR, with the difference in thresholds predicted by air-conducted clicks and bone-conducted clicks revealing the extent of an air–bone gap.

Otoacoustic Emissions

OAEs are likely to be absent in cases of middle-ear disorder.[103–107] Their presence or absence depends both on an adequate signal reaching the cochlea and on the ability of the middle ear to transduce the emission into the ear canal. Thus, if the middle-ear disorder is causing a conductive hearing loss of a magnitude sufficient to block the elicitation of a measurable emission, no response will be recorded. Similarly, if the cochlea generates an emission but the middle-ear mechanism does not convey a sufficient response to the ear canal, no emission will be recorded. In routine clinical assessment, the distinction is probably unimportant. Efforts to elicit OAEs with bone-conduction stimulation may clarify the contributing factor in some cases, but the clinical relevance remains unclear.

As is usually the case with OAEs, their absence lends little to the diagnostic process other than corroboration of other findings. The presence of a response, however, may provide useful information about the severity of a disorder.

Cochlear Disorders

Audiologic contribution to the assessment of a cochlear disorder is directed at answering the following questions:

- Is there a hearing loss and what is its extent?
- Is the loss solely cochlear or is there also a conductive component?
- Is the loss truly cochlear or is it retrocochlear?
- Is the loss fluctuating or stable?
- Could the loss be attributed to a treatable condition such as endolymphatic hydrops?

The first step in the process is to determine whether a middle-ear disorder is contributing to the problem. The second is to determine the degree and type of hearing loss. The third is to scrutinize the audiologic findings for any evidence of retrocochlear disorder. Immittance audiometry is used to evaluate outer and middle-ear function, indicate the presence of cochlear hearing loss, and assess the integrity of eighth nerve and lower auditory brain-stem function. Pure-tone audiometry is used to evaluate the degree and type of hearing loss. Speech audiometry is used as a cross-check of pure-tone thresholds and as an estimate of suprathreshold word-recognition ability.

Immittance Audiometry

In cochlear hearing loss, the tympanogram is normal, static immittance is normal, and acoustic reflex thresholds are consistent with the degree of sensorineural hearing loss. If immittance audiometry suggests the presence of middle-ear disorder, then any cochlear loss is likely to have a superimposed conductive component that must be quantified by pure-tone audiometry. If immittance audiometry is consistent with normal middle-ear function but acoustic reflexes are elevated above what would be expected from the degree of sensorineural hearing loss, then suspicion is raised about the possibility of retrocochlear disorder.

Again, the typical immittance pattern associated with cochlear disorder includes a normal tympanogram, normal static immittance, and normal reflex thresholds.[108] Reflex thresholds are only normal, however, as long as the sensitivity loss by air-conduction does not exceed 50 dB HL. Above this level, the reflex threshold is usually elevated in proportion to the degree of loss. Once a behavioral threshold exceeds 70 dB, the absence of a reflex is an equivocal finding because it can be attributed to either the degree of peripheral hearing loss or a retrocochlear disorder.

In ears with cochlear hearing loss, acoustic reflex thresholds are present at reduced sensation levels.[108,109] In normal-hearing ears, behavioral thresholds to pure-tones are, by definition, at or around 0 dB HL. Acoustic reflex thresholds occur at or around 85 dB HL, or at a sensation level of 85 dB. In a patient with a sensorineural hearing loss of 40 dB, reflex thresholds still occur at around 85 dB HL, or at a sensation level of 45 dB. This reduced sensation level of the acoustic reflex threshold is characteristic of cochlear hearing loss.

Ears with cochlear hearing loss will also show reduced SPARs. That is, the sensitivity prediction by acoustic reflexes will be at or below 15 dB, indicative of the presence of cochlear hearing loss.[78]

Pure-Tone Audiometry

Pure-tone audiometry is used to quantify the degree of sensorineural hearing loss caused by the cochlear disorder. If all immittance measures are normal, then air-conduction testing must be completed on both ears. Bone conduction may not be necessary because outer and middle-ear functions are normal, and air-conducted signals can properly evaluate the sensitivity of the cochlea. If not all immittance measures are normal, then air- and bone-conduction thresholds must be obtained for both ears to assess the possibility of the presence of a mixed hearing loss. In either case, both ears must be tested, because the use of masking is likely to be necessary and cannot be properly carried out without knowledge of the air- and bone-conduction thresholds of the nontest ear.

Pure-tone audiometry is also an important measure for assessing the symmetry of the hearing loss. If a sensorineural hearing loss is asymmetric, in the absence of another explanation, suspicion is raised for the presence of retrocochlear disorder.

The hearing loss configuration may provide additional clinical evidence for the cause of the auditory disorder. Characteristic configurations are associated with noise-induced hearing loss, congenital hearing loss, and Ménière's disease, and provide some clinical insight as to the nature of the hearing loss.

Pure-tone audiometry can be useful in the otologic diagnosis of cochlear disorder in other ways. For those that are dynamic and may be treatable at various stages, the results of pure-tone audiometry can be used as both partial evidence of the presence of the disorder and as a means for assessing benefit from the treatment regimen.

Speech Audiometry

Speech audiometry is used in two ways in the assessment of cochlear disorder. First, speech reception thresholds are used as a cross-check of the validity of pure-tone thresholds in an effort to ensure the organicity of the disorder. Second, word-recognition and other suprathreshold measures are used to assess whether the cochlear hearing loss has the expected effect on speech recognition. That is, in most cases, suprathreshold speech-recognition ability is predictable from the degree and configuration of a sensorineural hearing loss if the loss is cochlear.[31] Therefore, if word-recognition scores are appropriate for the degree of hearing loss, then the results are consistent with a cochlear site of disorder. If scores are poorer than would be expected from the degree of hearing loss, then suspicion is aroused that the disorder may be retrocochlear.

If a sensorineural hearing loss is caused by a cochlear disorder, the speech threshold is elevated in that ear to a degree predictable by the pure-tone average of audiometric thresholds obtained at 500, 1,000, and 2,000 Hz. Suprathreshold word-recognition scores are predictable from the degree of hearing sensitivity loss.

Sensitized speech measures are normal or predictable from degree of loss, and dichotic measures are normal. One exception is in endolymphatic hydrops, where the cochlear disorder can cause so much distortion that word-recognition scores may be poorer than predicted from degree of hearing loss.[110]

Auditory Evoked Potentials

Auditory evoked potentials can be used for several purposes in the assessment of a cochlear disorder.

First, if there is suspicion that the disorder might be retrocochlear, the ABR can be used in an effort to differentiate a cochlear from a retrocochlear site. Cochlear hearing loss has a predictable influence on ABR waveform latency and morphology. Once that influence is accounted for, ABR results will be consistent with the degree and configuration of the cochlear hearing loss. If the high frequency pure-tone average of 1,000, 2,000, and 4,000 Hz exceeds 70 dB, the absence of a response is equivocal because it can be explained equally by the degree of cochlear hearing loss and by retrocochlear disorder.[111]

Second, ECoG measures have been used successfully to assist in the diagnosis of Ménière's disease,[112,113] as the ratio of the action potential to summating potential amplitudes can be abnormal in such cases. Recent modifications of this strategy have demonstrated that action potential latencies to condensation and rarefaction clicks are significantly different in patients with Ménière's disease when compared to the negligible polarity differences in patients with normal hearing or other forms of cochlear hearing loss.[114,115] In addition, a strategy similar to that used in deriving stacked ABRs may also prove to be useful in the differentiation of cochlear disorder due to Ménière's disease.[116]

Third, auditory evoked potentials can be used to predict or quantify the degree and configuration of cochlear hearing sensitivity loss. In infants and young children, the ABR and ASSR are often used alone or in combination to quantify thresholds. In adults, if there is suspicion that the hearing loss is exaggerated, evoked potentials can be used to estimate the degree of organic hearing loss. Typically, ABR thresholds to click stimuli are used to predict high-frequency hearing, and late-latency or other evoked potentials are used to predict lower frequency thresholds.[117]

Otoacoustic Emissions

OAEs can be used in the assessment of sensorineural hearing loss as a means of verifying that there is a cochlear component to the disorder. If the cochlea is disordered, OAEs are expected to be abnormal or absent.[118] Although this finding does not preclude the presence of retrocochlear disorder, it does implicate the cochlea. Conversely, if OAEs are normal in the presence of a sensorineural hearing loss, a retrocochlear site of disorder is implicated.[8,119]

Because of their sensitivity to sensorineural hearing loss, OAEs have been used to screen for significant hearing loss in infants. Although found to be a sensitive indicator of the presence of cochlear outer-hair cell loss, OAEs are confounded by two primary factors for screening purposes. First, OAE measurement is very sensitive to the presence of outer- and middle-ear disorder, resulting in unacceptable false-positive rates when screening for significant sensorineural hearing loss. Perhaps even more problematic, however, is that cochleogenic auditory neuropathy, due presumably to inner hair cell loss, will go undetected, resulting in unacceptable false-negative outcomes.

OAE measures have also been used effectively to monitor cochlear function, particularly for patients undergoing treatment with potentially ototoxic medications.[120–122] For example, it is not uncommon for DPOAEs to be used to monitor outer-hair cell function in an attempt to detect ototoxicity during chemotherapy. The sensitivity of DPOAEs to change in cochlear function across a focused frequency range enables detection of the onset of ototoxic effects before can be identified with the pure-tone audiogram.

Retrocochlear Disorders

Audiologic contribution to the assessment of retrocochlear disorder is directed at answering the following questions:

- Is there a hearing loss, and what is its extent?
- Is the loss unilateral or asymmetric?
- Is speech understanding asymmetric or poorer than predicted from the hearing loss?
- Are acoustic reflexes normal or elevated?
- Is there other evidence of a retrocochlear disorder?

One goal of the audiologic evaluation is to determine the degree and type of hearing loss. Another goal is to scrutinize the audiologic findings for any evidence of retrocochlear disorder. Often a third goal is to assess the integrity of the eighth nerve and auditory brain stem with electrophysiologic measures.

On most audiologic measures, there are indicators that can alert the otologist to the possibility of retrocochlear disorder. Acoustic reflex thresholds, symmetry of hearing sensitivity, configuration of hearing sensitivity, and measures of speech recognition all provide clues as to the nature of the disorder.

Prior to the advent of sophisticated imaging and radiographic techniques, specialized audiologic assessment was an integral part of the differential diagnosis of auditory nervous system disorders. Behavioral measures of differential sensitivity to loudness, loudness growth, and auditory adaptation were designed to assist in the diagnostic process. Then, for a number of years in the late 1970s and early 1980s, auditory evoked potentials were used as a very sensitive technique for assisting in the diagnosis of neurologic disorders.[84,85,88] For a time, these measures of neurologic function were thought to be even more sensitive than radiographic techniques in the detection of lesions. However, progress in imaging and radiographic assessment of structural changes has advanced to a point where functional measures such as the ABR have lost some of their utility and, thus, importance. That is, imaging studies have permitted the visualization of ever-smaller lesions in the brain. Sometimes the lesions are of a small enough size or are in such a location that they result in little or no measurable functional consequence. Thus, measures of function, such as behavioral measures and the ABR, may not detect their presence.[123–126] Regardless, auditory evoked potentials, particularly the ABR, remain valuable indicators of eighth nerve and auditory brain-stem function. Technique enhancement, such as the stacked ABR, should help to maintain the clinical value of such measures.[91] Although not as often as in the past, auditory evoked potentials are still used to assess neural function as a supplement to the assessment of structure provided by magnetic resonance imaging and other imaging studies.

The diagnostic use of OAEs has begun to reveal distinctions between primary influences of retrocochlear disease on auditory nervous system function and secondary influences of retrocochlear disease on cochlear function.[119,127,128] For example, in some vestibular schwannomas, audiologic outcomes reflect a primary effect on nerve function in a pattern of results that includes abnormal acoustic reflexes, abnormal auditory adaptation, disproportionately poor speech recognition, rollover of the speech function, abnormal ABR, and preserved OAEs. In other vestibular schwannomas, audiologic outcomes reflect what appears to be a secondary influence of the tumor on cochlear function. In such cases, the results may be more consistent with cochlear hearing loss than retrocochlear loss, including the absence of OAEs. The distinction is probably important in appreciating the relative value of audiologic measures in the diagnostic process.

Immittance audiometry is used to evaluate outer and middle-ear function and to assess the integrity of the seventh and eighth cranial nerves and lower auditory brain-stem function. Pure-tone audiometry is used to evaluate the extent of any hearing asymmetry. Speech audiometry is used (1) as a cross-check of pure-tone thresholds, (2) an estimate of suprathreshold speech-recognition ability, (3) a measure of hearing symmetry, and (4) an assessment of any abnormality of hearing under adverse listening conditions. Electroacoustic and electrophysiologic measures are used in an effort to assess integrity of the cochlea, eighth nerve, and auditory brain stem.

Immittance Measures

Acoustic reflex threshold or suprathreshold patterns can be helpful in differentiating cochlear from retrocochlear disorders. Immittance audiometry can also be important in assessing middle-ear function in cases of suspected retrocochlear disorder, because middle-ear disorder and any resultant conductive hearing loss can affect interpretation of other audiometric measures.

If the disorder is retrocochlear, the typical immittance pattern is characterized by normal tympanometry, normal static immittance, and abnormal elevation of reflex thresholds, or absence of reflex responses, whenever the reflex-eliciting signal is delivered to the suspect ear in either the crossed or the uncrossed mode.[81,82] For example, with a right-sided vestibular schwannoma, the tympanograms, and static immittance would be normal. Abnormal elevation of reflex thresholds would be observed for the right uncrossed and the right-to-left crossed reflex responses. A retrocochlear disorder can also result in acoustic reflex decay, reflecting abnormal auditory adaptation.[81,129–131] Abnormal decay occurs when a reflex contraction is not sustained to continuous stimulation at suprathreshold levels.

A key to differentiating elevated reflex thresholds from retrocochlear versus cochlear disorder is the audiometric level at the test frequency. As stated previously, in cochlear hearing loss, reflex thresholds are not elevated until the audiometric loss exceeds 50 dB HL, and even above this level the degree of elevation is proportional to the audiometric level. In the case of retrocochlear disorder, however, the elevation is more than would be predicted from the audiometric level. The reflex threshold may be elevated by 20 to 25 dB even though the audiometric level shows no more than a 5- or 10-dB loss. If the audiometric loss exceeds 70 to 75 dB, then the absence of the acoustic reflex is ambiguous. The abnormality could be attributed either to retrocochlear disorder or to cochlear loss.

For diagnostic interpretation, acoustic reflex measures are probably best understood if viewed in the context of a three-part reflex arc, (1) the sensory or input portion (afferent), (2) the central nervous system portion that transmits neural information (central), and (3) the motor or output portion (efferent).[132,133]

An afferent abnormality occurs as the result of a disordered sensory system in one ear. An example of a pure afferent effect is a profound unilateral cochlear hearing loss on the right or a vestibular schwannoma of the right eighth nerve. Both reflexes with signal presented to the right ear (right uncrossed and right-to-left crossed) would be absent.

An efferent abnormality occurs as the result of a disordered motor system or middle ear in one ear. An example of a pure efferent effect is a right facial nerve paralysis. Both reflexes measured by the probe in the right ear (right uncrossed and left-to-right crossed) would be absent.

A central pathway abnormality occurs as the result of brain-stem disorder. An example of a pure central effect is multiple sclerosis that affects the crossing fibers of the central auditory nervous system. In this situation, one or both of the crossed acoustic reflexes would be elevated or absent in the presence of normal uncrossed reflex thresholds.

Disorders of the eighth nerve, then, often result in afferent abnormalities.[82,130,133,134] Brain-stem disorders can result in afferent, efferent, or central pathway abnormalities,[133,135–137] depending on the effect of the lesion.

Pure-Tone Audiometry

Pure-tone audiometry is useful in assessing the symmetry of hearing loss. Asymmetric sensorineural hearing loss, in the absence of another explanation, raises suspicion for the presence of retrocochlear disorder.

Certain audiometric configurations have been attributed to various retrocochlear disorders. Although any configuration can occur, progressive asymmetric high-frequency hearing loss has been associated with eighth-nerve disorders.[138] Similarly, low-frequency hearing loss has been associated with brain-stem disorder.[10,139] Although hearing loss is usually insidious in neurologic disorders, it is not uncommon for a sudden hearing loss to be associated with a retrocochlear lesion.[140,141]

Although asymmetric hearing loss is a common finding in retrocochlear disorders, so is normal hearing.[141–145] As diagnosis has improved generally, reports have increased of normal-hearing sensitivity in patients with eighth-nerve disorder.

Speech Audiometry

Measurement of speech recognition is important in screening for a retrocochlear disorder. In most cochlear hearing losses, speech-recognition ability is predictable from the degree of loss and configuration of the audiogram. That is, given a hearing sensitivity loss of a known severity and configuration, the ability to recognize speech is roughly equivalent among individuals and nearly equivalent between ears within an individual.

Expectations of speech-recognition ability, then, lie within a certain predictable range for a given cochlear hearing loss. In many retrocochlear hearing losses, however, speech-recognition ability is poorer than would be expected from the audiogram. Thus, if performance on speech-recognition measures falls below that expected, suspicion is aroused that the hearing loss is caused by a retrocochlear rather than a cochlear disorder.[31]

If a sensorineural hearing loss is caused by an eighth-nerve disorder, the speech threshold is elevated in that ear to a degree predictable by the pure-tone average. Suprathreshold word-recognition ability is likely to be substantially affected.[58,146] Maximum scores are likely to be poorer than predicted from the degree of hearing loss, and rollover of the performance-intensity function is likely to occur.[28,29,147,148] Speech-in-competition measures are also likely to be depressed.[38,149,150] Abnormal results occur in the same, or ipsilateral, ear in which the lesion occurs. Dichotic measures are normal.

If a hearing disorder occurs as a result of a brain-stem lesion, the speech threshold is predictable from the pure-tone average. Suprathreshold word-recognition ability is likely to be affected substantially.[150,151] Word-recognition scores in quiet may be normal or depressed or show rollover. Speech-in-competition measures are likely to be depressed in the ear ipsilateral to the lesion. Dichotic measures are likely to be normal.

If a hearing disorder occurs as the result of a temporal-lobe lesion, hearing sensitivity is unlikely to be affected, and the speech threshold and word-recognition scores are likely to be normal. Sensitized speech measures may or may not be abnormal in the ear contralateral to the lesion.[33–35,37] Dichotic measures are the most likely of all to show a deficit because of the temporal-lobe lesion.[40,41,152,153]

Auditory Evoked Potentials

If a retrocochlear disorder is suspected, and if audiometric indicators heighten suspicion, it is customary to assess the integrity of the auditory nervous system directly with the ABR. The ABR is a sensitive indicator of the integrity of eighth nerve and auditory brain-stem function.[86,154,155] If it is abnormal, there is a very high likelihood of a retrocochlear disorder.

In recent years, imaging techniques have improved to the point that structural changes in the nervous system can sometimes be identified before those changes have a functional influence. Thus, the presence of a normal ABR does not rule out the presence of a neurologic disease process.[156] It simply indicates that the process is without apparent functional consequence. The presence of an abnormal ABR, however, remains a strong indicator of neurologic disorder and is useful in the diagnosis of retrocochlear disease.[92,124,157]

The ABR component waves, especially waves I, III, and V, are easily recordable and are very reliable in terms of their latency. As a general rule, wave I occurs at about 2 msec following signal presentation; wave III at 4 milliseconds; wave V at 6 milliseconds. Although these absolute numbers vary among clinical instrumentation, the latencies are quite stable across individuals. In most adults, the I–V interpeak interval is approximately 4 milliseconds, with a standard deviation of about 0.2 milliseconds. Thus, 99% of the adult population has *I–V* interpeak intervals of 4.6 or less. If the *I–V* interval exceeds this amount, it can be considered abnormal. These latency measures are reasonably consistent across the population. In newborns, they are prolonged compared to adult values, but in a predictable way. Once a child reaches 18 months, normal adult latency values can be expected and will continue throughout life. Because of the consistency of latencies within an individual over time and across individuals in the population, assessment of latency is relied on as an indicator of integrity of the VIII nerve and auditory brain stem.[158]

The decision about whether an ABR is normal is usually based on the following considerations:

- Interaural latency difference in *I–V* interpeak interval
- *I–V* interpeak interval
- Interaural difference in wave *V* latency
- Absolute latency of wave *V*
- Interaural differences in *V/I* amplitude ratio
- *V/I* amplitude ratio
- Selective loss of late waves
- Grossly degraded waveform morphology

Again, the ABR is used to assess the integrity of the eighth nerve and auditory brain stem in patients who are suspected of having vestibular schwannomas or other neurologic disorder. In interpreting ABRs, the consistency of the response across individuals is exploited to ask whether the measured latencies compare well between ears and with the population in general.

The MLR and LLR are less useful than the ABR in identifying discrete lesions.[159,160] Sometimes a vestibular schwannoma that affects the ABR will also affect the MLR. Also, sometimes a cerebral vascular accident or other discrete insult to the brain will result in an abnormality in the MLR.[161,162] However, these measures are probably more useful as indicators of generalized disorders of auditory processing ability rather than in the diagnosis of a specific disease process. For example, MLRs and LLRs have been found to be abnormal in patients with multiple sclerosis.[160,163] Although neither response has proven to be particularly useful in helping to diagnose this disorder, the fact that MLR and LLR abnormalities occur has proven to be valuable in describing the resultant auditory disorders. That is, patients with neurologic disorders often have auditory complaints that cannot be measured on an audiogram or with simple speech audiometric measures. The MLR and LLR are sometimes helpful in quantifying such auditory complaints.

Otoacoustic Emissions

OAEs can be used in the assessment of a retrocochlear disorder, although the results are often equivocal. If a hearing loss is caused by a retrocochlear disorder through an effect on eighth-nerve function, OAEs may be normal despite the hearing loss.[6,8] In such cases, outer-hair cell function is considered normal, and the hearing loss can be attributable to the neurologic diseases process. That is, the loss is caused by neural disorder, and the cochlea is functioning normally. However, in some cases, a retrocochlear disorder can affect cochlear function, resulting in a hearing loss and abnormality of OAEs.[119,127,128] Thus, in the presence of hearing loss and normal middle-ear function, the absence of OAEs indicates either a cochlear or a retrocochlear disorder. On the other hand, the preservation of OAEs in the presence of a hearing loss suggests that the disorder is retrocochlear.

One other aspect of OAEs that may be interesting from a diagnostic perspective is that the amplitude of a TEOAE is suppressed to a certain extent by stimulation of the contralateral ear. This contralateral suppression is a small but consistent effect that occurs when broad-spectrum noise is presented to one ear and transient emissions are recorded in the other.[164,165] The effect is mediated by the medial olivocochlear system, which is part of the auditory system's complex efferent mechanism. In some cases of peripheral and central auditory disorder, contralateral suppression is absent,[166] so that the TEOAE is unaffected by stimulation of the contralateral ear.

Suprathreshold Processing Disorders

Over the past three decades, techniques that were once used to assist in the diagnosis of neurologic disease have been adapted for use in the assessment of communication impairment that occurs as a result of auditory processing disorder. Sensitized speech audiometric measures are now commonly used to evaluate auditory processing ability. A typical battery of tests might include the following:

- The assessment of speech recognition across a range of signal intensities;
- The assessment of speech recognition in the presence of competing speech signals; and
- The measurement of dichotic listening—the ability to process two different signals presented simultaneously to both ears.

The results of such an assessment provide an estimate of auditory processing ability and a more complete profile of a patient's auditory abilities and impairments. Such information is often useful in providing guidance regarding appropriate amplification strategies or other rehabilitation approaches.

Many patients with an auditory processing disorder are elderly and consequently have some degree of cochlear hearing loss. Outcomes of assessment with immittance measures, pure-tone audiometry, and OAEs do not differ substantially in these patients from those found in patients with purely peripheral deficits. The differences that do exist are most readily identified by speech audiometry, and, to a lesser extent, auditory evoked potentials.

Immittance Measures

Immittance audiometry can be expected to show normal middle-ear function and reflex results consistent with normal-hearing sensitivity or cochlear hearing loss. Tympanograms, static immittance, and acoustic reflex thresholds are normal or consistent with the degree of sensorineural hearing loss.

Pure-Tone Audiometry

In the absence of middle-ear disorder, pure-tone audiometry demonstrates normal-hearing sensitivity or sensorineural hearing loss. There is some evidence of a low-frequency sensorineural component to the hearing loss in patients with auditory processing disorder.

Speech Audiometry

Speech audiometric deficits in patients with auditory processing disorders can be categorized as (1) deficits in hearing in noise (or competition), (2) difficulty processing in the temporal domain, (3) binaural hearing deficits, and (4) disordered spatial hearing.

One of the most common indicators of auditory processing disorder is an inability to extract signals of interest from a background of noise. This inability can be measured directly with a number of different speech audiometric techniques. The results show that patients with auditory processing disorders have considerable difficulty identifying speech in the presence of competition.[38,167–172] In general, the more meaningful or speech-like the competition, the more interfering will be its influence on perception.[173,174]

Much of the early work in this area focused on monaural perception of speech targets in a background of competition presented to the same ear. Other studies have shown deficits in patients with auditory processing disorders when competition is presented to the opposite ear or when both targets and competition are presented to both ears in a soundfield.[175]

Impairment in processing in the time domain is also a common sign in auditory processing disorders.[176–182] Temporal processing deficits have been identified on the basis of a number of measures, including time compression of speech, duration pattern discrimination, duration difference limens, and gap detection. Deficits in temporal processing are often considered the underlying cause of and primary contributor to many of the other measurable deficits associated with auditory processing disorders.

Most individuals with intact auditory nervous systems are able to identify different signals presented simultaneously to both ears and demonstrate a slight right-ear advantage in dichotic listening ability for linguistic signals. In a patient with an auditory processing disorder, particularly one caused by impairment of the corpus callosum and auditory cortex, a dichotic deficit, characterized by substantial reduction in left ear performance, is often seen.[39,183,184]

A stated earlier, the auditory system is exquisitely sensitive to differences in the timing of sound reaching the two ears. This sensitivity helps localize low-frequency sounds, which reach the ears at different points in time. One way of assessing how sensitive the ears are to these timing or phase, is by measuring binaural release from masking. Abnormal binaural release from masking is a sign of auditory processing disorder and occurs as a result of impairment in the lower auditory brain stem.[1,61,63]

A different kind of deficit in binaural processing is referred to as binaural interference. Normally, binaural hearing provides an advantage over monaural hearing. This "binaural advantage" has been noted in loudness judgments, speech recognition, and evoked potential amplitudes. In contrast, with binaural interference, binaural performance is actually poorer than the best monaural performance. In such cases, performance on a perceptual task with both ears can actually be poorer than performance on the better ear in cases of asymmetric perceptual ability.[185] It appears that the poorer ear actually reduces binaural performance below the better monaural performance. Binaural interference has been reported in elderly individuals, in patients with multiple sclerosis, and in children.[185–187]

The ability to locate acoustic stimuli in space generally requires auditory system integration of sound from both ears. Some patients with auditory disorders have difficulty locating the directional source of a sound. Disorders of the auditory nervous system have been associated with deficits in ability to localize the source of a sound in a soundfield or to lateralize the perception of a sound within the head.[180,188–191]

Auditory Evoked Potentials

In auditory processing disorders, the ABR may be abnormal if the disorder is secondary to nervous system disruption in the lower brain stem or in extreme cases of neuromaturational delay or disorder. More commonly, however, the ABR is normal. Recent evidence suggests that a speech-evoked ABR strategy may be helpful in identifying certain types of children with language processing disorders.[192]

Abnormal MLR and LVR have been associated with auditory processing disorders secondary to diffuse changes in brain function.[193] There is also evidence to suggest that event-related potentials may be useful in identifying patients with processing difficulty.[94,95] Although these conventionally measured evoked potentials are often normal, assessment with topographic brain mapping has revealed abnormalities in patients with auditory processing disorders.[194]

Otoacoustic Emissions

In an auditory processing disorder, OAEs are either normal or abnormal consistent with the degree on hearing sensitivity loss. However, in some cases of auditory processing disorder, contralateral suppression of OAEs is absent.

Illustrative Cases

Middle-Ear Disorder

Case 1 is a 28-year-old woman with bilateral otosclerosis, who developed hearing problems during pregnancy. She describes her problem as a muffling of other people's voices. She also reports bilateral tinnitus that bothers her at night. There is a family history of otosclerosis on her mother's side.

Results of immittance audiometry, as shown in Figure 10–2A, are consistent with middle-ear disorder, characterized by a Type A_s tympanogram, low static immittance, and bilaterally absent crossed and uncrossed acoustic reflexes. This pattern of results suggests an increase in the stiffness of the middle-ear mechanism and is often associated with fixation of the ossicular chain.

Pure-tone audiometric results are shown in Figure 10–2B. The patient has a moderate, bilaterally symmetric, conductive hearing loss. Typical for otosclerosis, the patient also has an apparent bone-conduction hearing loss at around 2,000 Hz in both ears—the so-called Carhart's notch. Carhart's notch actually reflects the elimination of the middle-ear contribution to bone-conducted hearing rather than a loss in cochlear sensitivity.[195]

Speech audiometric results show speech thresholds consistent with pure-tone thresholds. Suprathreshold speech-recognition ability is normal once the effect of the hearing loss is overcome by presenting speech at higher intensity levels. Word-recognition scores are 100% bilaterally.

Cochlear Disorder

Case 2 is a 60-year-old man with bilateral sensorineural hearing loss of cochlear origin, secondary to ototoxicity. The patient recently finished a round of chemotherapy that included cisplatin.

Immittance audiometry (Figure 10–3A) is consistent with normal middle-ear function bilaterally, characterized by Type A tympanograms, normal static immittance, and normal crossed and uncrossed acoustic reflex thresholds. The SPAR results (below 15 dB) predict a sensorineural hearing loss.

Pure-tone audiometry (Figure 10–3B) shows bilaterally symmetric, high-frequency sensorineural hearing loss, progressing from mild levels at 2,000 Hz to profound at 8,000 Hz. Further doses of chemotherapy would be expected to begin to affect the remaining high-frequency hearing and progress downward toward the low frequencies.

Speech audiometric results are consistent with the degree and configuration of cochlear hearing loss. Speech thresholds match the pure-tone thresholds, and word-recognition scores, although reduced, are consistent with this degree of hearing loss. Maximum word-recognition scores are 100% for the right ear and 92% for the left ear.

Case 3 is a 38-year-old man with unilateral sensorineural hearing loss secondary to endolymphatic hydrops. Two weeks prior to evaluation, the patient experienced fluctuating hearing loss, aural fullness, tinnitus, and an episode of severe vertigo. After multiple attacks, the hearing loss has persisted. A diagnosis of Ménière's disease was made following otologic examination.

Immittance audiometry is consistent with normal middle-ear function bilaterally, characterized by a Type A tympanograms, normal static immittance, and normal crossed and uncrossed reflex thresholds.

Pure-tone audiometry is shown in Figure 10–4. The results show a moderate, rising (upward sloping), sensorineural hearing loss on the left ear and normal-hearing sensitivity on the right.

Speech audiometric results are normal for the right ear. On the left, however, although speech thresholds agree with the pure-tone thresholds, suprathreshold speech-recognition scores are very poor. This performance is significantly reduced from what would normally be expected from a cochlear hearing loss. These results are atypical for cochlear hearing loss other than Ménière's disease.

Auditory brain-stem response results showed absolute and interpeak latencies that are normal and symmetric, supporting the diagnosis of cochlear disorder.

Case 4 is a 14-week-old girl who failed newborn hearing screening by automated ABR in the regular-care nursery shortly after birth. She had a maternal family history of congenital hearing loss. At a follow-up screening evaluation at 9-weeks of age, she again did not pass ABR screening in either ear.

Tympanometry, carried out with a 1,000-Hz probe tone, suggests normal tympanic membrane dynamics bilaterally, characterized by Type A tympanograms and normal static immittance.

Auditory brain-stem responses were used to predict hearing sensitivity. Result showed air-conducted click thresholds down to 40 dB nHL in the right ear and 35 dB nHL in the left. Unmasked bone-conducted ABRs were observed down to 35 dB nHL. These results are consistent with a mild high-frequency sensorineural hearing loss bilaterally.

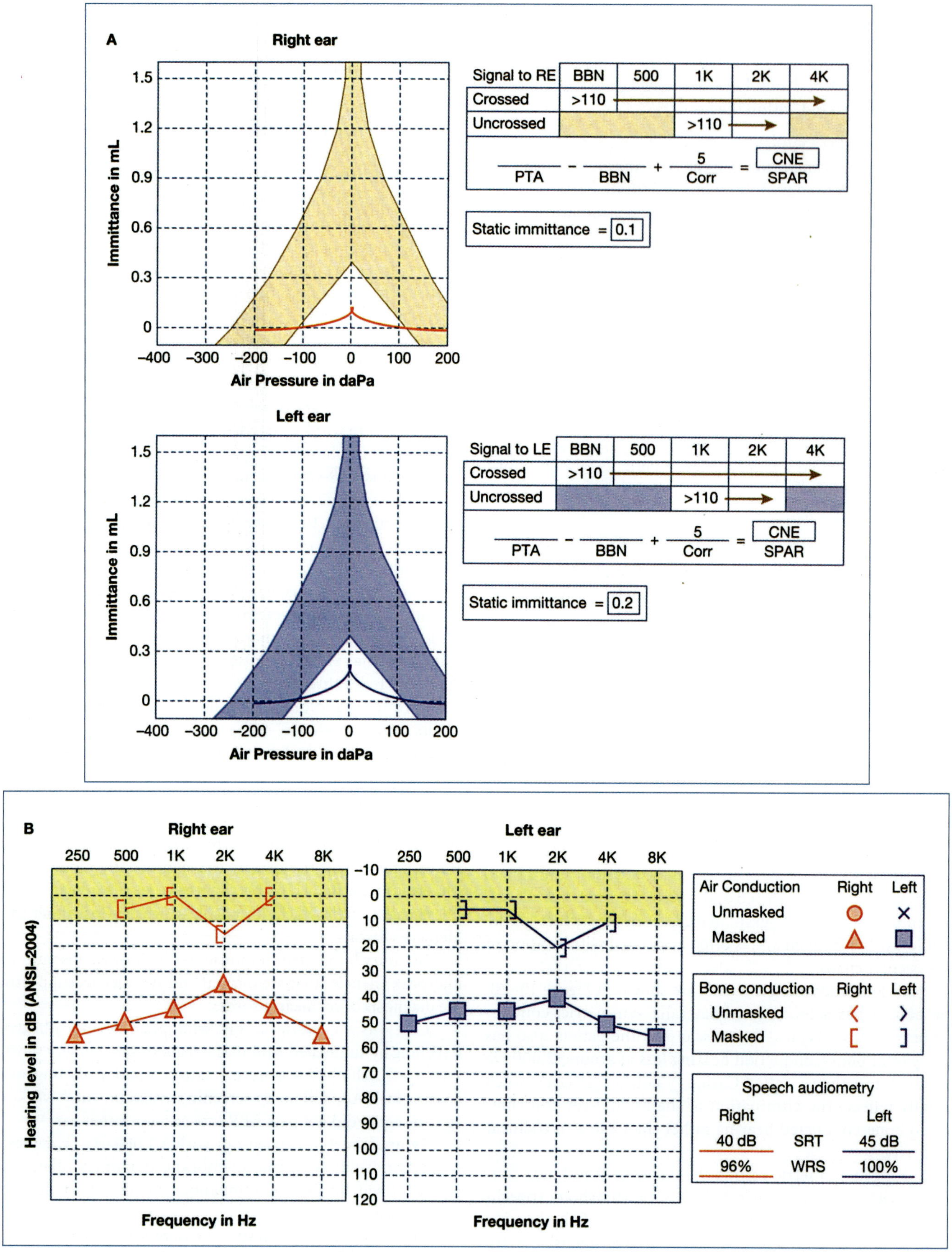

A

Right ear

Immittance in mL: 1.5, 1.2, 0.9, 0.6, 0.3, 0

Air Pressure in daPa: –400, –300, –200, –100, 0, 100, 200

Signal to RE	BBN	500	1K	2K	4K
Crossed	>110 →				
Uncrossed			>110 →		

PTA – BBN + 5 Corr = CNE SPAR

Static immittance = 0.1

Left ear

Immittance in mL: 1.5, 1.2, 0.9, 0.6, 0.3, 0

Air Pressure in daPa: –400, –300, –200, –100, 0, 100, 200

Signal to LE	BBN	500	1K	2K	4K
Crossed	>110 →				
Uncrossed			>110 →		

PTA – BBN + 5 Corr = CNE SPAR

Static immittance = 0.2

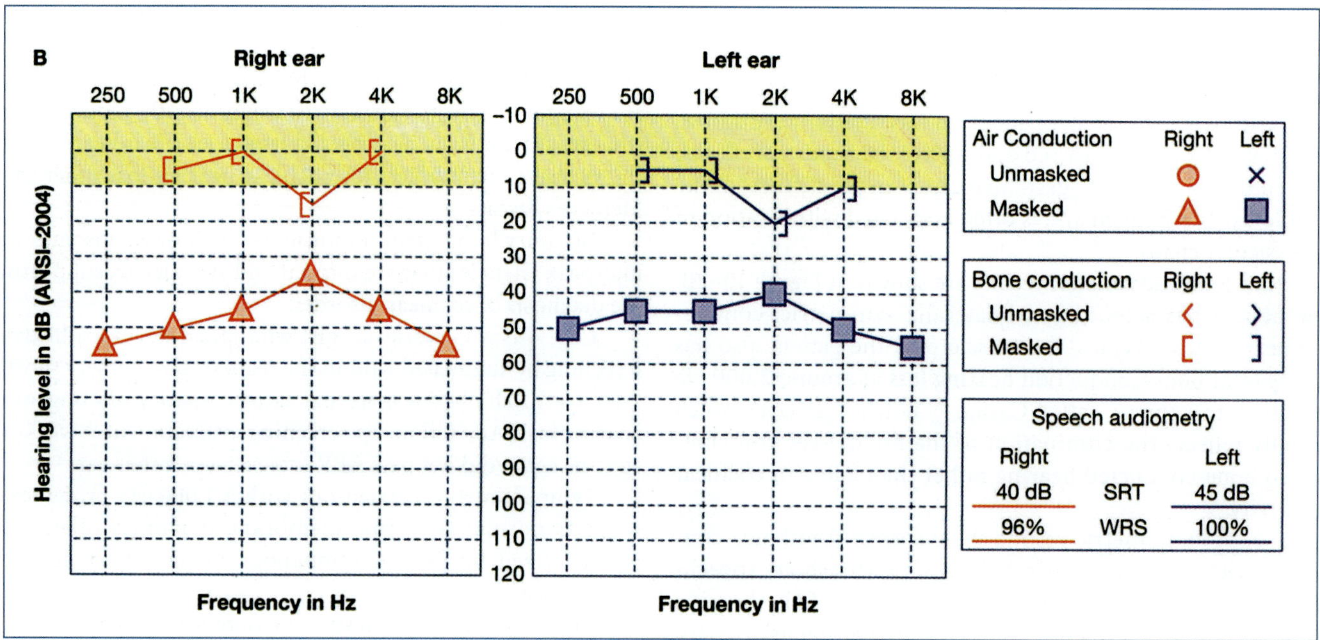

FIGURE 10–2 • Audiometric results in a 28-year-old female with otosclerosis. Immittance measures *A*, are consistent with an increase in the stiffness of the middle-ear mechanism. Pure-tone audiometric results *B*, show a moderate conductive hearing loss bilaterally. Speech-recognition thresholds (SRT) are consistent with pure-tone thresholds, and word-recognition scores (WRS) are consistent with conductive hearing loss.

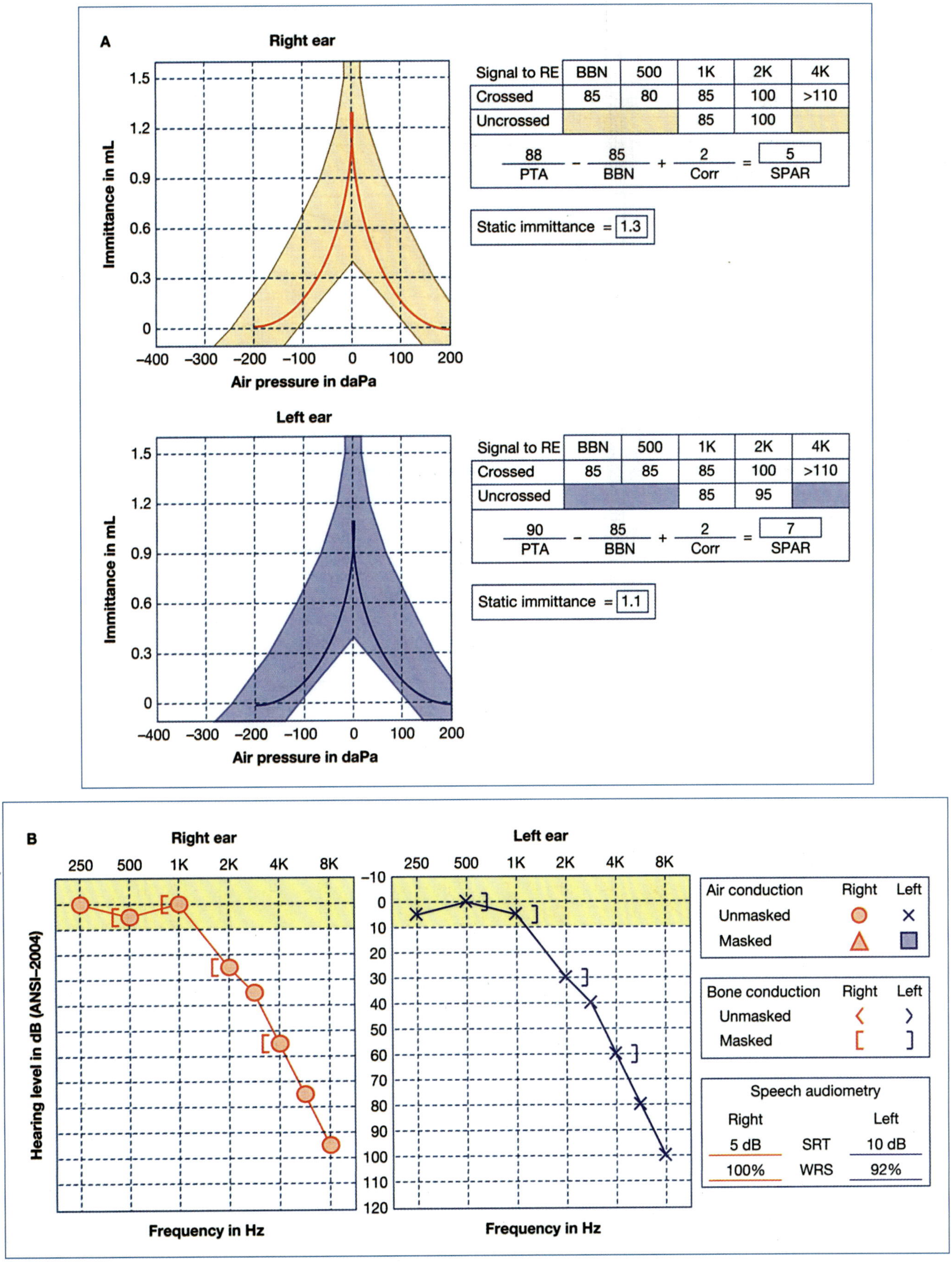

A

Right ear

Immittance in mL: 1.5, 1.2, 0.9, 0.6, 0.3, 0

Air pressure in daPa: –400, –300, –200, –100, 0, 100, 200

Signal to RE	BBN	500	1K	2K	4K
Crossed	85	80	85	100	>110
Uncrossed			85	100	

$$\frac{88}{\text{PTA}} - \frac{85}{\text{BBN}} + \frac{2}{\text{Corr}} = \frac{5}{\text{SPAR}}$$

Static immittance = 1.3

Left ear

Immittance in mL: 1.5, 1.2, 0.9, 0.6, 0.3, 0

Air pressure in daPa: –400, –300, –200, –100, 0, 100, 200

Signal to RE	BBN	500	1K	2K	4K
Crossed	85	85	85	100	>110
Uncrossed			85	95	

$$\frac{90}{\text{PTA}} - \frac{85}{\text{BBN}} + \frac{2}{\text{Corr}} = \frac{7}{\text{SPAR}}$$

Static immittance = 1.1

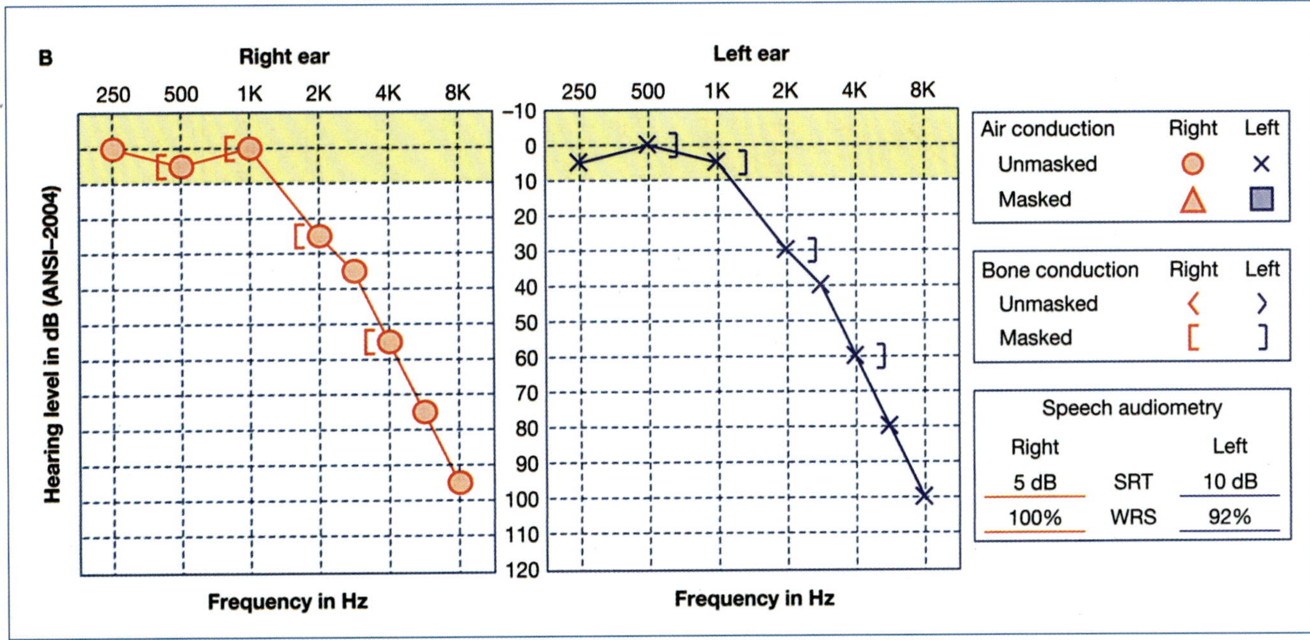

FIGURE 10–3 • Audiometric results in a 60-year-old male with cochlear hearing loss due to ototoxicity. Immittance measures *A*, are consistent with normal middle-ear function. SPARs predict the presence of hearing loss. Pure-tone audiometric results *B*, show a high-frequency sensorineural hearing loss bilaterally. Speech-recognition thresholds (SRT) are consistent with pure-tone thresholds, and word-recognition scores (WRS) are consistent with the degree and configuration of the cochlear hearing loss.

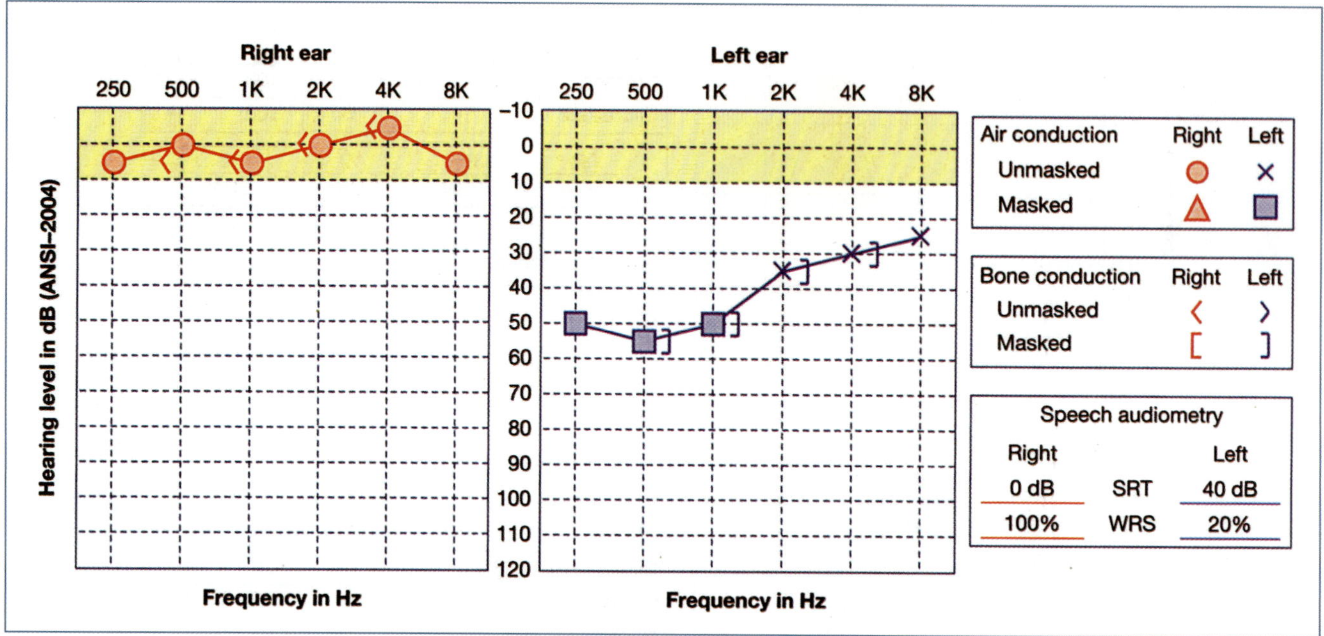

FIGURE 10–4 • Audiometric results in a 38-year-old male with cochlear hearing loss due to endolymphatic hydrops. Pure-tone audiometric results show normal hearing sensitivity on the right ear and a moderate, rising sensorineural hearing loss on the left. The word-recognition score (WRS) on the left ear is poorer than would be expected from the degree and configuration of the cochlear hearing loss.

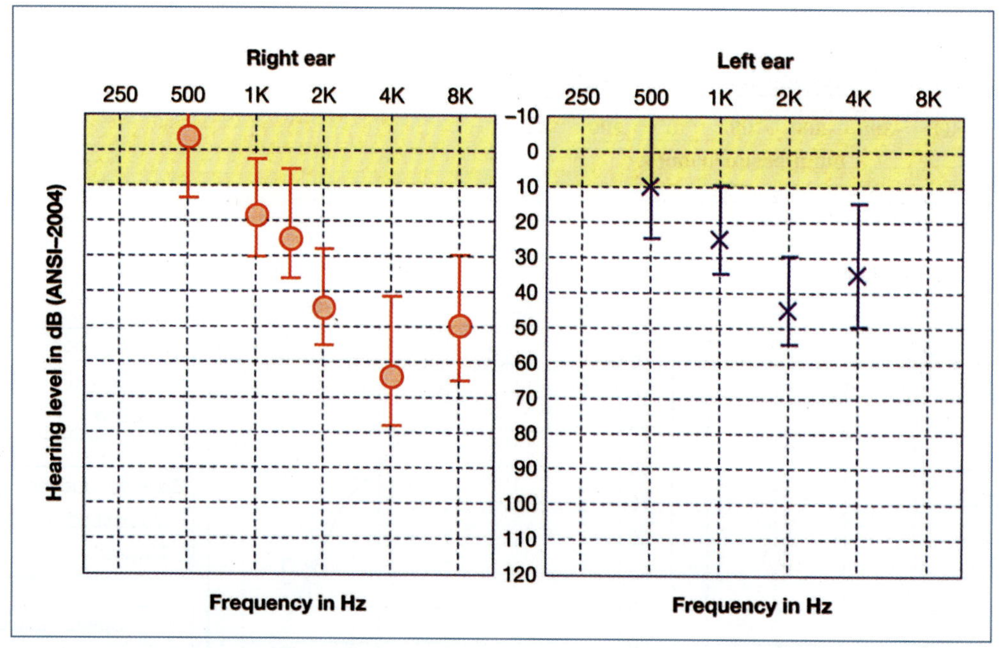

FIGURE 10–5 • Predicted audiogram based on ASSR thresholds in a 14-week-old girl with mild to moderate sensorineural hearing loss.

To evaluate the audiometric configuration of the hearing loss, auditory steady-state response measures were carried out. Tones at octave intervals across the audiometric frequency range were modulated at a rate of 90/s. Response detection was made by assessing the stability of the phase relationship of the modulation to the response. The predicted audiograms are shown in Figure 10–5, confirming the presence of mild to moderate high-frequency sensorineural hearing loss bilaterally.

Eighth-Nerve Disorder

Case 5 is a 54-year-old woman with a 4-month history of left tinnitus caused by a left vestibular schwannoma. Her health and hearing histories are otherwise unremarkable.

Immittance audiometry (Figure 10–6A) is consistent with normal middle-ear function bilaterally, characterized by a Type A tympanograms, normal static immittance, and normal right crossed and right uncrossed reflex thresholds. Left crossed and

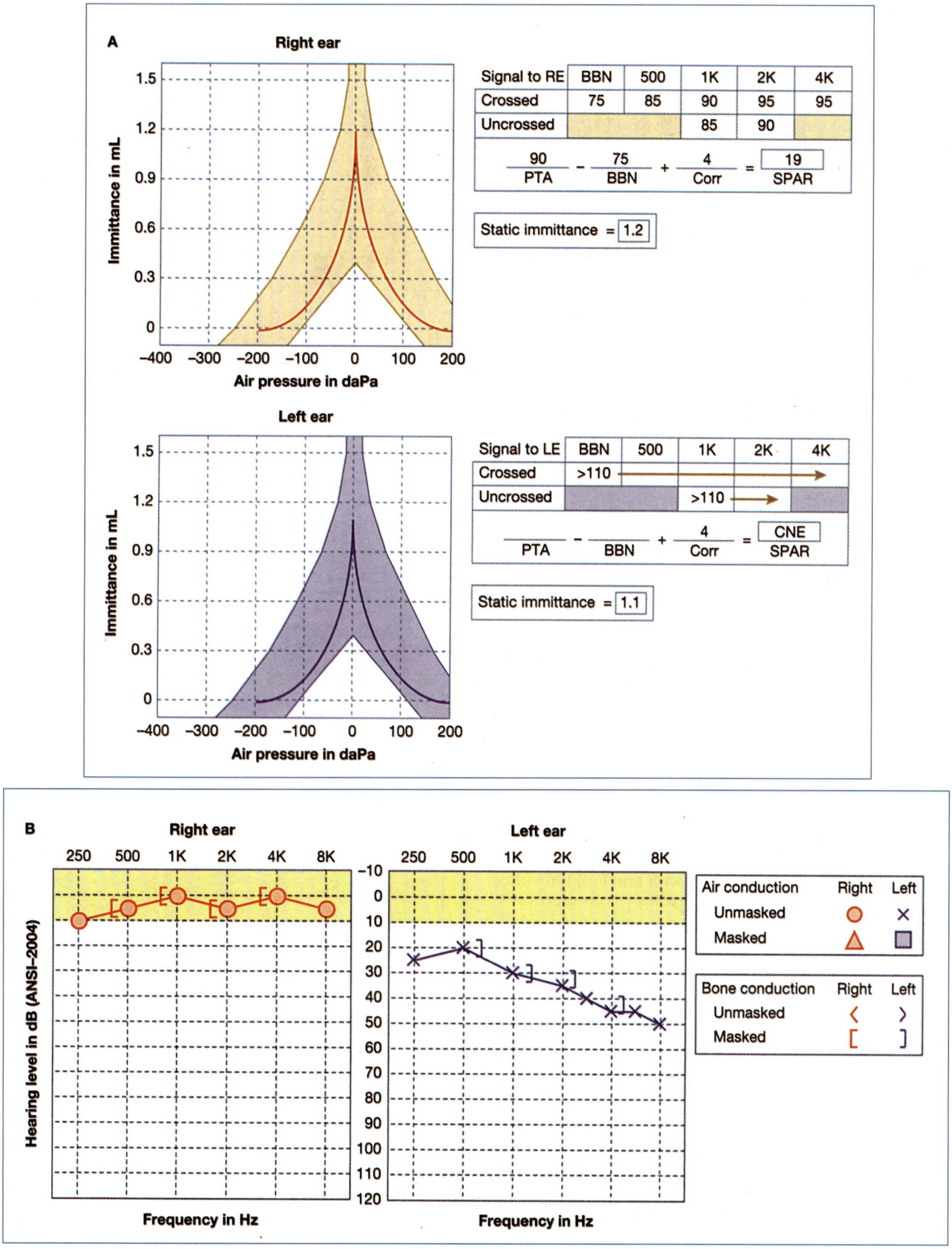

A
Right ear
Immittance in mL
1.5
1.2
0.9
0.6
0.3
0
−400 −300 −200 −100 0 100 200
Air pressure in daPa
Signal to RE | BBN | 500 | 1K | 2K | 4K
Crossed | 75 | 85 | 90 | 95 | 95
Uncrossed | | | 85 | 90 |
90 PTA − 75 BBN + 4 Corr = 19 SPAR
Static immittance = 1.2
Left ear
Immittance in mL
1.5
1.2
0.9
0.6
0.3
0
−400 −300 −200 −100 0 100 200
Air pressure in daPa
Signal to LE | BBN | 500 | 1K | 2K | 4K
Crossed | >110
Uncrossed | | | >110
PTA − BBN + 4 Corr = CNE SPAR
Static immittance = 1.1
B
Right ear
Left ear
250 500 1K 2K 4K 8K
−10 0 10 20 30 40 50 60 70 80 90 100 110 120
Hearing level in dB (ANSI–2004)
Frequency in Hz
Air conduction | Right | Left
Unmasked
Masked
Bone conduction | Right | Left
Unmasked
Masked

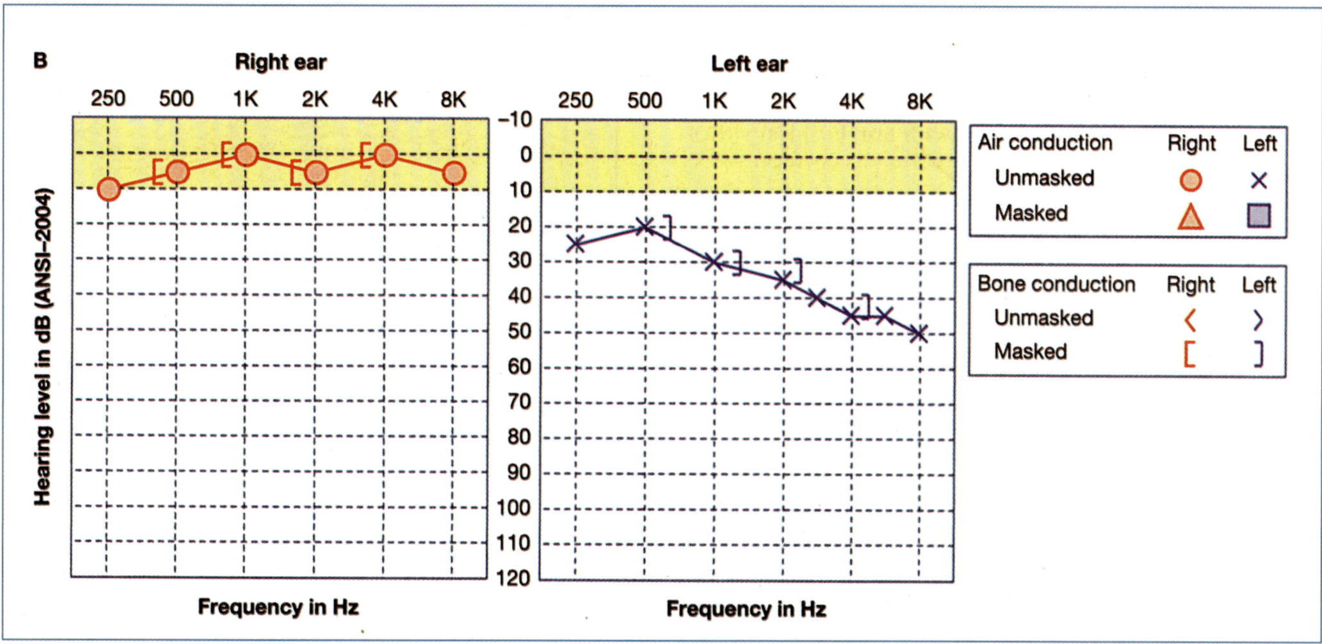

FIGURE 10–6 • Audiometric results in a 54-year-old male with a left VIII nerve tumor. Immittance measures *A*, are consistent with normal middle-ear function. Left crossed and left uncrossed reflexes are absent consistent with left afferent disorder. Pure-tone audiometric results *B*, show normal-hearing sensitivity on the right ear and a mild, relatively flat sensorineural hearing loss on the left.

Continued

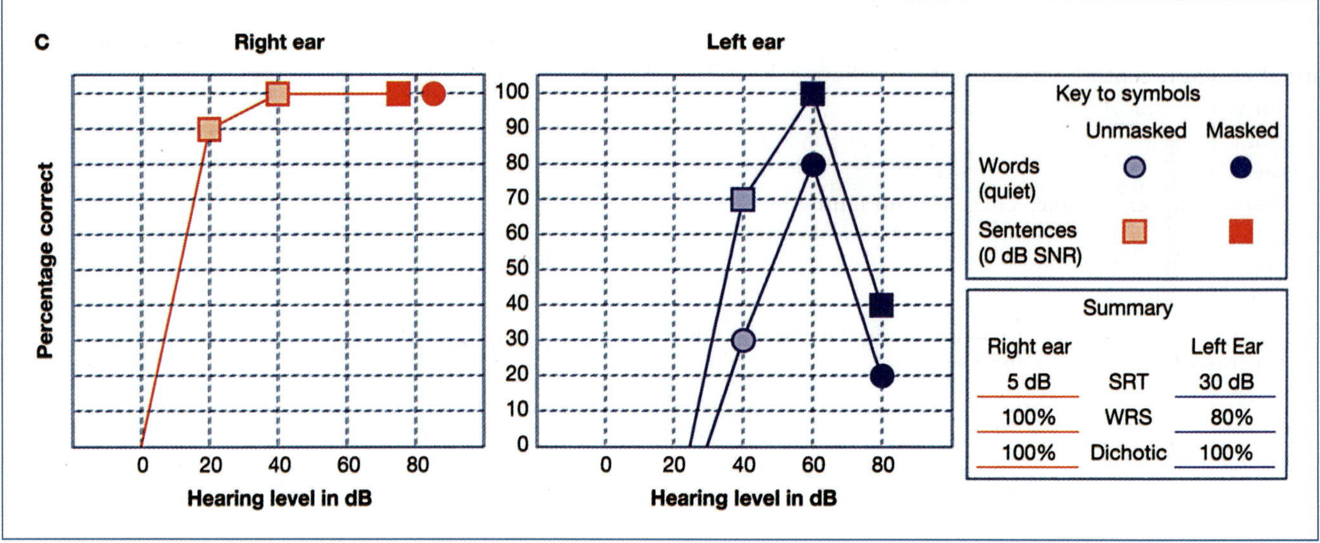

FIGURE 10–6 • *Continued.* Speech audiometric results C, show rollover of the performance intensity function on the left.

left uncrossed reflexes are absent, consistent with an afferent abnormality on the left—the vestibular schwannoma.

Pure-tone audiometric results are shown in Figure 10–6B. The patient has normal-hearing sensitivity on the right ear and a mild, relatively flat sensorineural hearing loss on the left.

Speech audiometric results, shown in Figure 10–6C, are normal on the right ear but abnormal on the left. Although maximum speech-recognition scores are normal at lower intensity levels, the PI function demonstrates significant rollover, or poorer performance at higher intensity levels, consistent with retrocochlear site of lesion.

The ABR results are normal on the right ear. Left ear results show delayed latency of wave *V* and prolonged interpeak intervals. These results are also consistent with retrocochlear site of disorder.

Case 6 is a 49-year-old man with a history of HIV infection. At the time of the evaluation, he was diagnosed as having cryptococcal meningitis. He had a long-standing history of profound sensorineural hearing loss in his left ear. He reported a sudden drop in right-ear hearing following the spinal tap done to confirm the meningitis diagnosis.

Immittance audiometry showed normal, Type A tympanograms and normal static immittance, although both crossed and uncrossed reflexes were absent to stimulation in both ears.

Pure-tone audiometry showed a profound sensitivity loss on the left ear and very inconsistent responses on the right. Speech-recognition thresholds are 25 dB for both air-and bone-conduction stimulation. Pure-tone thresholds could not be determined definitively, with responses ranging from 50 to 90 dB. Word-recognition scores could not be determined due to inconsistent responses. The initial diagnosis was sensorineural hearing loss on the left and functional or exaggerated hearing sensitivity loss on the right.

Despite considerable apparent hearing loss on the right, distortion product emissions are present across the frequency range.

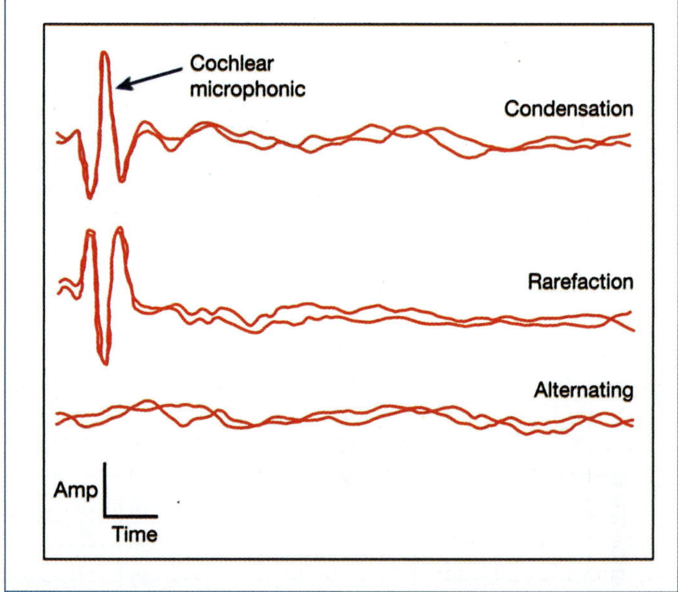

FIGURE 10–7 • ABR results from the right ear of a 49-year-old male with HIV infection and neurogenic auditory neuropathy. The only repeatable response is the cochlear microphonic to condensation and rarefaction clicks that are expectedly antiphasic and that cancel to alternating-polarity clicks.

ABR results (Figure 10–7) are consistent with auditory neuropathy on the right. Although a cochlear microphonic is clearly recordable, consistent with normal peripheral function, no repeatable synchronous ABR is observable beyond the microphonic. Although some of the clinical signs and symptoms are consistent with functional hearing loss, the combination of absent acoustic reflexes, absent ABR, poor speech recognition, variable thresholds, and present OAEs and cochlear microphonics is consistent with a diagnosis of neurogenic auditory neuropathy.

Cerebollopontine Angle Disorder

Case 7 is a 28-year-old female with a unilateral hearing loss of unusual etiology, central nervous system miliary tuberculosis.[8] Four weeks prior to evaluation, the patient noticed that she could not use the telephone with her left ear. She also reported "heaviness" on the left side of her head. Her hearing history was otherwise unremarkable. There was no family history of hearing loss or history of other risk factors for hearing loss. The results of a neurotologic evaluation, including otoscopic examination, were normal. She had no significant otologic history and no reported dizziness or tinnitus. Significantly, the patient had a long history of tuberculosis and had recently begun medical therapy for miliary tuberculosis involving her nervous system.

Immittance audiometry indicated normal middle-ear function bilaterally, characterized by Type A tympanograms, normal static immittance, and normal right crossed and right uncrossed reflex thresholds. However, crossed and uncrossed acoustic reflexes were absent when the eliciting signal was presented to the left ear. This reflex pattern is consistent with a left afferent abnormality, either a significant cochlear or retrocochlear disorder on that side.

Pure-tone results are shown in Figure 10–8A. Left ear results revealed a profound hearing loss. Hearing sensitivity could only be measured at 250 and 500 Hz at 105 and 110 dB HL, respectively. No responses were obtained at any other frequencies, and no responses were obtained to bone-conducted signals at equipment limits. The speech awareness threshold was 105 dB HL. Word-recognition ability could not be measured. Right-ear results showed normal-hearing sensitivity from 250 to 4,000 Hz and a minimal sensitivity loss at 6,000 and 8,000 Hz. The word-recognition score was 100% at 80 dB HL.

As a matter of routine clinical procedure in the evaluation of a unilateral hearing loss, a Stenger test was carried out to assess the organicity of the hearing loss. The result of a speech Stenger test was negative for functional hearing loss on the left. As a further indication of the organic nature of the loss, a shadow curve was noted on the left audiogram at expected levels for insert earphones when the right ear was not masked.

Distortion-product OAEs were measured to assess cochlear function. Distortion-product OAE amplitudes as a function of f_2 frequency are plotted in Figure 10–8B. The results showed substantive emissions across the frequency range for both the right and left ears. These results are consistent with normal cochlear outer-hair cell function in both ears and suggest that, despite the presence of a profound hearing sensitivity loss on the left, cochlear function, or at least outer-hair cell function, was normal.

Auditory brain-stem response results are shown in Figure 10–8C. Right-ear responses were well formed, with component peaks at normal absolute and interpeak latencies. Left ear results were abnormal. Only component Wave I was observable. The absolute latency of Wave I was 1.5 milliseconds in both ears. The presence of Wave I on the left is consistent with the OAE results, indicating near-normal cochlear function. The absence of later waves suggests a site of lesion at the proximal end of the eighth nerve or low auditory brain stem.

Audiologic and otologic findings were consistent with left retrocochlear disorder, characterized by a profound hearing sensitivity loss, absent acoustic reflexes, normal OAEs, and the presence of only Wave I of the auditory brain-stem response. Imaging studies revealed the presence of multiple punctate lesions, one of which was extra-axial and located in the left cerebellopontine angle.

Brain Stem Disorder

Case 8 is a 42-year-old woman with auditory complaints secondary to multiple sclerosis. Two years prior to her evaluation, she experienced an episode of diplopia, accompanied by tingling and weakness in her left leg. These symptoms gradually subsided, only to reappear in a slightly more severe form a year later. Ultimately, she was diagnosed as having multiple sclerosis. Among a variety of complaints, she had vague hearing difficulty, particularly in the presence of background noise.

Immittance audiometry is consistent with normal middle-ear function, characterized by a Type A tympanogram, normal static immittance, and normal right and left uncrossed reflex thresholds. However, crossed reflexes are absent bilaterally. This unusual pattern of results is consistent with a central pathway disorder of the lower brain stem.

Pure-tone audiometric results are shown in Figure 10–9A. The patient has a mild low-frequency sensorineural hearing loss bilaterally, a finding that is not uncommon in brain-stem disorder.[10,139]

Suprathreshold speech-recognition performance is abnormal in both ears. Although word-recognition scores are normal when presented in quiet, scores on sentence recognition in the presence of competition are abnormal, as shown in Figure 10–9B. Dichotic scores are normal. Auditory evoked potentials are also consistent with an abnormality in brainstem function. On the left, no waves were identifiable beyond component Wave II, and on the right, none were identifiable beyond Wave III.

Auditory Processing Disorder

Case 9 is a 72-year-old man with a long-standing, bilateral sensorineural hearing loss that has progressed slowly over the past 15 years. He has worn hearing aids for the past 10 years and has an annual audiologic reevaluation each year. His major complaints relate to communicating with his grandchildren and trying to hear in noisy restaurants. Although his hearing aids initially worked well, they no longer provide the benefits that they did 10 years ago.

The results of immittance audiometry are consistent with normal middle-ear function, characterized by a Type A tympanogram, normal static immittance, and normal crossed and uncrossed reflex thresholds bilaterally.

Pure-tone audiometric results are shown in Figure 10–10A. The patient has a moderate, bilaterally symmetric, sensorineural hearing loss. Hearing sensitivity is slightly better in the low frequencies than in the high frequencies.

Speech audiometric results are consistent with those found in older patients. Word-recognition scores are reduced, but not below the level predicted from the degree of hearing sensitivity loss. However, speech recognition in the presence of competition is substantially reduced, as shown in Figure 10–10B, consistent with the patient's age. Performance on a sentence-recognition task at an easy signal-to-noise ratio (SNR) was 100% bilaterally.

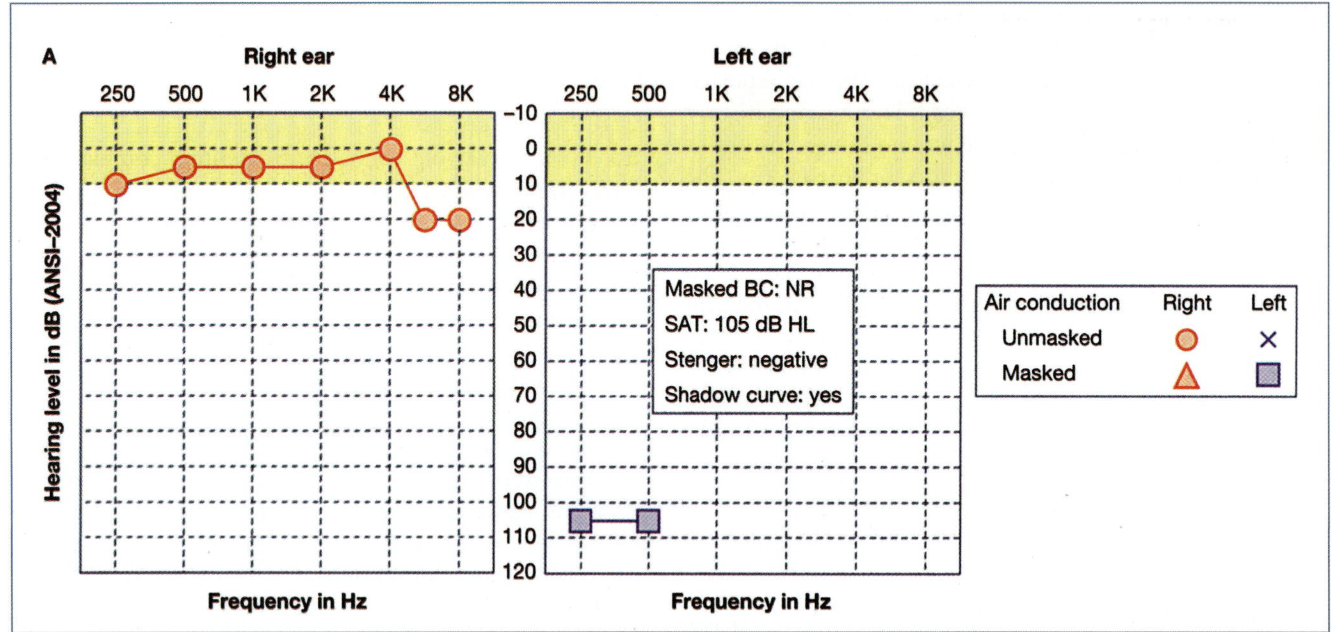

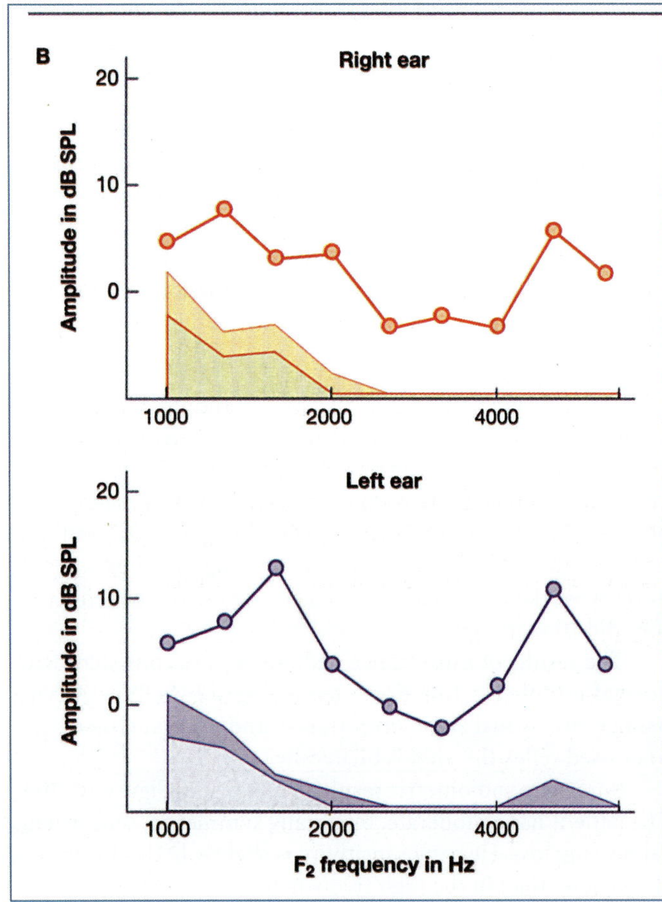

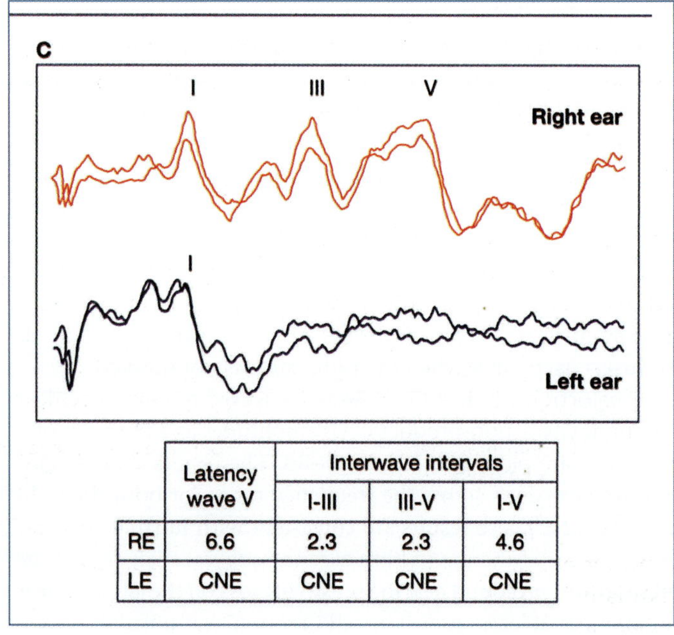

	Latency wave V	Interwave intervals		
		I-III	III-V	I-V
RE	6.6	2.3	2.3	4.6
LE	CNE	CNE	CNE	CNE

FIGURE 10–8 • Audiometric results in a 28-year-old female with central nervous system miliary tuberculosis. Pure-tone audiometric results *A* show normal-hearing sensitivity on the right ear and a profound sensorineural hearing loss on the left. Distortion product otoacoustic emissions *B* are consistent with normal cochlear function bilaterally. Auditory brain stem response results *C* are normal for the right ear but show only an observable Wave I on the left.

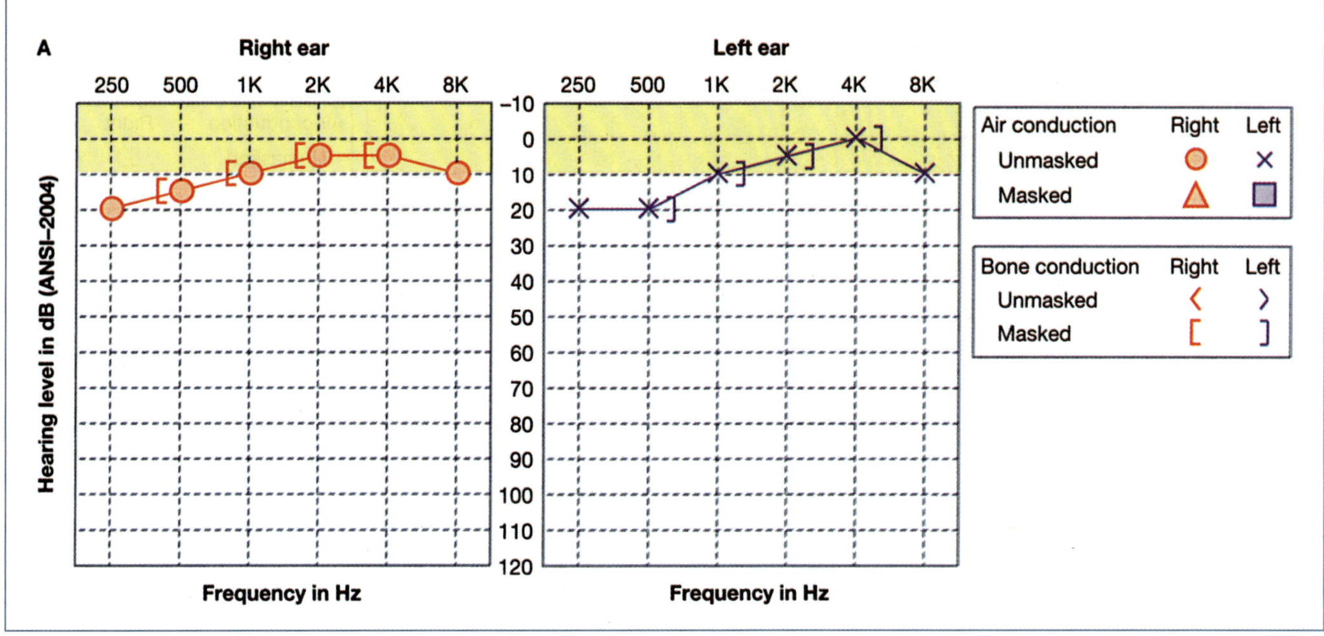

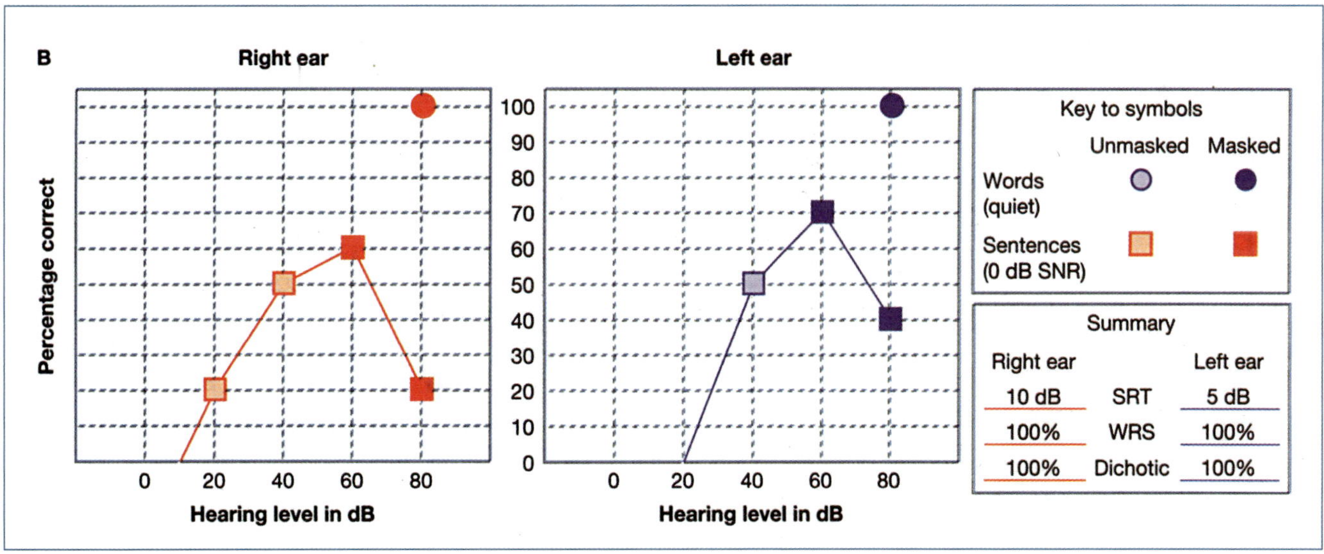

FIGURE 10–9 • Audiometric results in a 42-year-old female with multiple sclerosis. Pure-tone audiometric results *A* show mild low-frequency sensorineural hearing loss bilaterally. Speech audiometric results *B* show reduced maximum performance and rollover of the performance intensity function on a measure of sentence recognition in competition.

However, at a more difficult SNR (0 dB), performance was substantially reduced. In addition to these monotic deficits, the patient also shows evidence of a dichotic deficit, with reduced performance in the left ear.

SUMMARY: SOME DIAGNOSTIC LESSONS

By way of summary, following are some of the diagnostic lessons learned from the audiologic evaluation of patients with auditory disorder:

1. In eighth nerve tumors, size of the lesion matters generally, although location is critical. Size and location interact to dictate the extent to which a tumor will affect hearing function. A small tumor confined to the internal auditory canal can have a substantial impact on hearing, while a large tumor growing in the cerebellopontine angle can have a negligible effect on hearing.
2. There seem to be two influences of eighth nerve tumors on hearing; primary influences on the nerve function itself and secondary influences on cochlear function. Depending on the influence, audiologic outcomes might reflect retrocochlear patterns, cochlear patterns, or mixed patterns of results.
3. With immittance measures, tympanometry by itself is seldom useful unless it is abnormal. In combination with acoustic reflexes, immittance audiometry can be a powerful diagnostic tool.

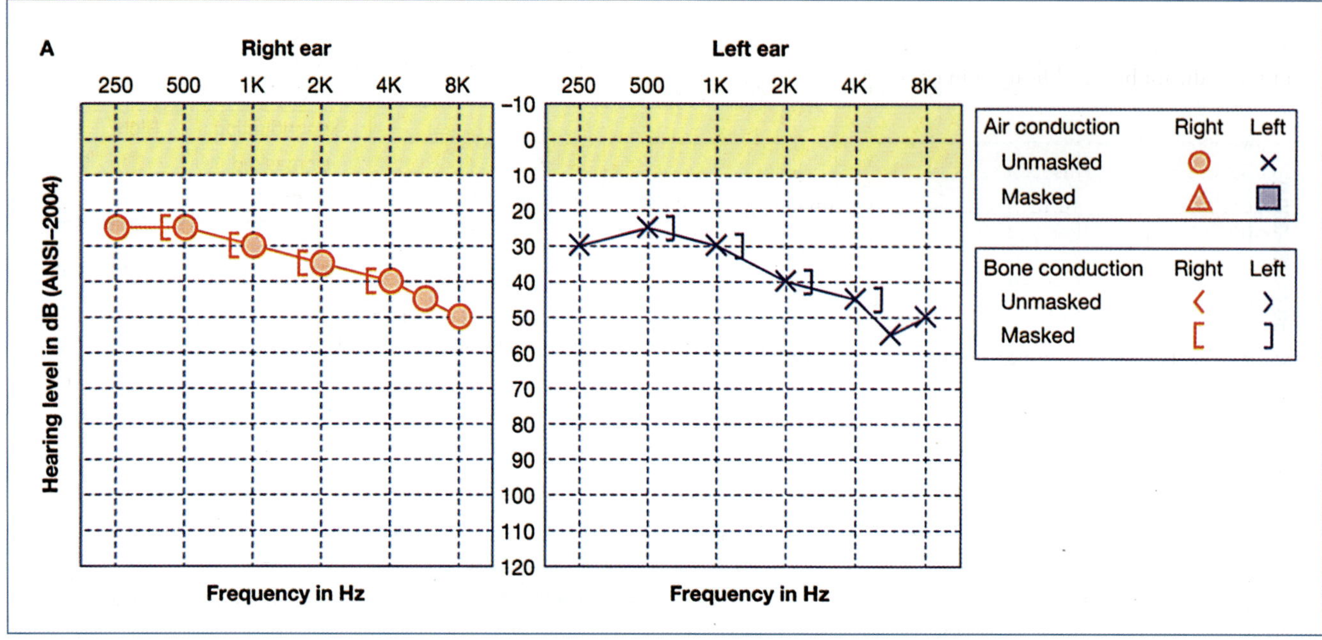

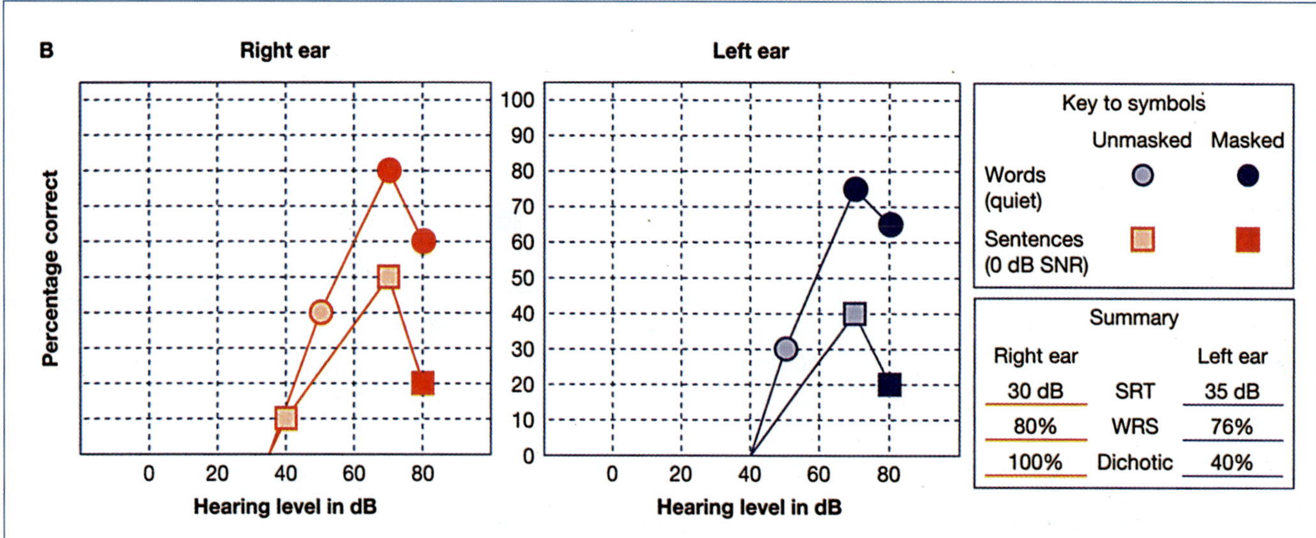

FIGURE 10–10 • Audiometric results in a 72-year-old male with sensorineural hearing loss and auditory processing disorder. Pure-tone audiometric results *A* show bilateral, symmetric, moderate sensorineural hearing loss. Speech audiometric results *B* show reduced word recognition in quiet, consistent with the degree and configuration of the cochlear hearing loss. Sentence recognition in competition and dichotic performance are substantially reduced.

4. Regarding acoustic reflexes, the patterns of ipsilateral and contralateral reflexes are critical to understanding the nature of a disorder. Reflexes correlate well with the integrity of ABR wave III and with results on the MLD.
5. In pure-tone audiometry, the more peripheral the retrocochlear disorder, the more likely is there to be a significant sensorineural hearing loss. The more central the disorder, the more likely is the influence on hearing to be subtle.
6. Disorders of the eighth nerve and lower brain stem are likely to show ipsilateral deficits on speech audiometric measures. The more peripheral the disorder, the more likely it is to affect word-recognition scores. The more peripheral the disorder, the less need there is for sensitized speech measures.
7. Disorders of the more central portions of the auditory nervous system are likely to show both ipsilateral and contralateral deficits on speech audiometric measures. Such disorders are unlikely to affect work recognition scores. The more central the disorder, the more need there is for sensitized speech measures to reveal its influence.
8. The ABR is correlated with other measures in peripheral nervous system disorder. The more central the disorder, generally the more normal the ABR.
9. Otoacoustic emissions are of limited value diagnostically if they are abnormal. In contrast, the presence of normal OAEs in an ear with sensorineural hearing loss is a powerful diagnostic indicator of retrocochlear disorder.

References

1. Hall JW, Grose JH, Pillsbury HC. Long-term effects of chronic otitis media on binaural hearing in children. Arch Otolaryngol 1995;121:847–52.
2. Brown DP. Speech recognition in recurrent otitis media: Results in a set of identical twins. J Am Acad Audiol 1994;5:1–6.
3. Jerger S, Jerger J, Alford BR, Abrams S. Development of speech intelligibility in children with recurrent otitis media. Ear Hear 1983;4:138–45.
4. Schilder AGM, Snik AFM, Straatman H, van den Broek P. The effect of otitis media with effusion at preschool age on some aspects of auditory perception at school age. Ear Hear 1994;15:224–31.
5. Cacace AT, Parnes SM, Lovely TJ, Kalathia A. The disconnected ear: Phenomenological effects of a large acoustic tumor. Ear Hear 1994;15:287–98.
6. Kileny PR, Edwards BM, Disher MJ, Telian SA. Hearing improvement after resection of cerebellopontine angle meningioma: Case study of the preoperative role of transient otoacoustic emissions. J Am Acad Audiol 1998;9:1–6.
7. Stach BA, Delgado-Vilches G. Sudden hearing loss in multiple sclerosis: Case report. J Am Acad Audiol 1993;4:370–5.
8. Stach BA, Westerberg BD, Roberson JB. Auditory disorder in central nervous system miliary tuberculosis: A case report. J Am Acad Audiol 1998;9:305–10.
9. Mahmud MR, Khan AM, Nadol JB. Histopathology of the inner ear in unoperated acoustic neuroma. Ann Otol Rhinol Laryngol 2003;112:979–86.
10. Jerger S, Jerger J. Low frequency hearing loss in central auditory disorders. Am J Otol 1980;2:1–4.
11. Starr A, Picton TW, Sininger Y, Hood LJ, Berlin CI. Auditory neuropathy. Brain 1996;119:741–53.
12. Starr A, Sininger Y, Winter M, et al. Transient deafness due to temperature-sensitive auditory neuropathy. Ear Hear 1998;19:169–79.
13. Berlin C, Hood L, Rose K. On renaming auditory neuropathy as auditory dys-synchrony. Audiol Today 2002;13:15–17.
14. Rance G, Beer D, Cone-Wesson B, et al. Clinical findings for a group of infants and young children with auditory neuropathy. Ear Hear 1999;20:238–52.
15. Sinninger Y, Oba S. Patients with auditory neuropathy: Who are they and what can they hear? . In: Sinninger Y, Starr A, editors. Auditory Neuropathy. San Diego: Singular Thomson Learning; 2001. p. 15–36.
16. Gibson W, Sanli H. Auditory neuropathy: An update. Ear Hear 2007;28:102S–6S.
17. Rapin I, Gravel JS. Auditory neuropathy: A biologically inappropriate label unless acoustic nerve involvement is documented. J Am Acad Audiol 2006;17:147–50.
18. Konradsson K. Bilaterally preserved otoacoustic emissions in four children with profound idiopathic unilateral sensorineural hearing loss. Audiology 1996;35:217–27.
19. Loundon N, Marcolla A, Roux I, et al. Auditory neuropathy or endocochlear hearing loss? Oto Neurotol 2005;26:748–54.
20. Harrison RV. An animal model of auditory neuropathy. Ear Hear 1998;19:355–61.
21. Gelfand SA, Silman S. Functional hearing loss and its relationship to resolved hearing levels. Ear Hear 1985;6:151–8.
22. Austen S, Lynch C. Non-organic hearing loss redefined: Understanding, categorizing and managing non-organic behaviour. Int J Audiol 2004;43:449–57.
23. Madell J, Flexer C. Pediatric audiology: Diagnosis, technology, and management. New York: Thieme; 2008.
24. Carhart R. Speech reception in relation to pattern of pure tone loss. J Speech Dis 1946;11:97–108.
25. Tillman TW, Carhart R. An expanded test for speech discrimination utilizing CNC monosyllabic words (Northwestern University Test No. 6). Technical Report, SAM-TR-66–55. In: Brooks Air Force Base, Texas: USAF School of Aerospace Medicine, Aerospace Medical Division (AFSC); 1966.
26. Egan JP. Articulation testing methods. Laryngoscope 1948;58:955–91.
27. Hirsh IJ, Davis H, Silverman SR, et al. Development of materials for speech audiometry. J Speech Hear Dis 1952;17:321–37.
28. Jerger J, Jerger S. Diagnostic significance of PB word functions. Arch Otolaryngol 1971;93:573–80.
29. Dirks DD, Kamm C, Bower D, Betsworth A. Use of performance-intensity functions for diagnosis. J Speech Hear Dis 1977;42:408–15.
30. Dubno JR, Lee FS, Klein AJ, Matthews LJ, Lam CF. Confidence limits for maximum word-recognition scores. J Speech Hear Res 1995;38:490–502.
31. Yellin MW, Jerger J, Fifer RC. Norms for disproportionate loss of speech intelligibility. Ear Hear 1989;10:231–4.
32. Gates GA, Feeney MP, Higdon RJ. Word recognition and the articulation index in older listeners with probable age-relate auditory neuropathy. J Am Acad Audiol 2003;14:574–81.
33. Lynn GW, Gilroy J. Evaluation of central auditory dysfunction in patients with neurological disorders. In: Keith RW, editor. Central Auditory dysfunction. New York: Grune & Stratton; 1977. p. 177–222.
34. Bocca E, Calearo C, Cassinari V. A new method for testing hearing in temporal lobe tumours. Acta Otolaryngol 1954;44:219–21.
35. Jerger J. Observations on auditory behavior in lesions of the central auditory pathways. Arch Otolaryngol 1960;71:797–806.
36. Calearo C, Antonelli AR. Audiometric findings in brain stem lesions. Acta Otolaryngol 1968;66:305–19.
37. Kurdziel S, Noffsinger D, Olsen W. Performance by cortical lesion patients on 40 and 60% time-compressed materials. J Am Audiol Soc 1976(2):3–7.
38. Jerger J, Hayes D. Diagnostic speech audiometry. Arch Otolaryngol 1977;103:216–222.
39. Jerger J, Chmiel R, Allen J, Wilson A. Effects of age and gender on dichotic sentence identification. Ear Hear 1994;15:274–86.
40. Musiek FE. Results of three dichotic speech tests on subjects with intracranial lesions. Ear Hear 1983;4:318–23.
41. Kimura D. Some effects of temporal lobe damage on auditory perception. Can J Psychol 1961;15:157–65.
42. Berlin CI, Lowe-Bell SS, Jannetta PJ, Kline DG. Central auditory deficits of temporal lobectomy. Arch Otolaryngol 1972;96:4–10.
43. Fifer RC, Jerger JF, Berlin CI, Tobey EA, Campbell JC. Development of a dichotic sentence identification test for hearing-impaired adults. Ear Hear 1983;4:300–305.

44. Fowler EP. A method for the early detection of otosclerosis: A study of sounds well above threshold. Arch Otolaryngol 1936;24:731–41.
45. Dix MR, Hallpike CS, Hood JD. Observations upon the loudness recruitment phenomenon, with especial reference to the differential diagnosis of disorders of the internal ear and VIII nerve. Proc R Soc Med 1948;41:516–26.
46. Jerger J. Recruitment and allied phenomena in differential diagnosis. J Aud Res 1961;2:145–51.
47. Lüscher E, Zwislocki J. A simple method for indirect monaural determination of the recruitment phenomenon (difference limen in intensity in different types of deafness). Acta Otolaryngol Suppl 1949;78:156–72.
48. Jerger J. A difference limen test and its diagnostic significance. Laryngoscope 1952;62:1316–32.
49. Jerger J, Shedd J, Harford E. On the detection of extremely small changes in sound intensity. Arch Otolaryngol 1959;69:200–11.
50. Thompson GA. Modified SISI technique for selected cases with suspected acoustic neurinoma. J Speech Hear Dis 1963;28:299–302.
51. Carhart R. Clinical determination of abnormal auditory adaptation. Arch Otolaryngol 1957;65:32–9.
52. Olsen WO, Noffsinger D. Comparison of one new and three old tests of auditory adaptation. Arch Otolaryngol 1974;96:231–47.
53. Jerger J, Jerger S. A simplified tone decay test. Arch Otolaryngol 1975;101:403–7.
54. Békésy G. A new audiometer. Acta Otolaryngol 1947;35: 411–22.
55. Jerger J. Bekesy audiometry in analysis of auditory disorders. J Speech Hear Res 1960;3:275–87.
56. Turner RG, Shepard NT, Frazer GJ. Clinical performance of audiological and related diagnostic tests. Ear Hear 1984;5:187–94.
57. Sanders JW, Josey AF, Glasscock ME. Audiologic evaluation in cochlear and eighth-nerve disorders. Arch Otolaryngol 1974;100:283–93.
58. Johnson EW. Auditory test results in 500 cases of acoustic neuroma. Arch Otolaryngol 1977;103:152–8.
59. Jerger S, Jerger J. Evaluation of diagnostic audiometric tests. Audiology 1983;22:144–61.
60. Lynn GE, Gilroy J, Taylor PC, Leiser RP. Binaural masking-level differences in neurological disorders. Arch Otolaryngol 1981;107:357–62.
61. Noffsinger D, Kurdziel S, Applebaum EL. Value of special auditory tests in the latero-medial inferior pontine syndrome. Ann Otol 1975;84:384–90.
62. Olsen WO, Noffsinger D. Masking level differences for cochlear and brain stem lesions. Ann Otol 1976;85:820–5.
63. Hannley M, Jerger JF, Rivera VM. Relationships among auditory brain stem responses, masking level differences and the acoustic reflex in multiple sclerosis. Audiology 1983;22:20–33.
64. Silman S, Silverman CA. Functional hearing impairment. In: Silman S, Silverman CA editors, Auditory diagnosis: principles and applications. San Diego: Singular; 1997. p. 137–57.
65. Stach BA, Jerger JF. Immittance measures in auditory disorders. In: Jacobson JT, Northern JL eds, Diagnostic audiology. Austin, Texas: Pro-Ed; 1990:113–40.
66. Jerger J. Clinical experience with impedance audiometry. Arch Otolaryngol 1970;92:311–24.
67. Koebsell C, Margolis RH. Tympanometric gradient measured from normal preschool children. Audiology 1986;25:149–57.
68. Shanks JE, Shelton C. Basic principles and clinical applications of tympanometry. Otolaryngol Clin North Am 1991;24:299–328.
69. Hunter LL, Margolis RH. Effects of tympanic membrane abnormalities on auditory function. J Am Acad Audiol 1997;8: 431–46.
70. Vanhuyse VJ, Creten WL, Van Camp KJ. On the W-notching of tympanograms. Scand Audiol 1975;4:45–50.
71. Shahnaz N, Polka L. Standard and multifrequency tympanometry in normal and otosclerotic ears. Ear Hear 1997;18:326–41.
72. Voss SE, Allen JB. Measurement of acoustic impedance and reflectance in the human ear canal. J Acoust Soc Am 1994;95:372–84.
73. Feeney MP, Grant I, Marryott L. Wideband energy reflectance measurements in adults with middle-ear disorders. J Speech Lang Hear Res 2003;46:901–11.
74. Alaerts J, Luts H, Wouters J. Evaluation of middle ear function in young children: Clinical guidelines for the use of 226- and 1,000-Hz tympanometry. Otol Neurotol 2007;28:727–32.
75. Baldwin M. Choice of probe tone and classification of trace patterns in tympanometry undertaken in early infancy. I J Audiol 2006;45:417–27.
76. Kei J, Mazlan R, Hickson L, Gavranich J, R. L. Measuring middle ear admittance in newborns using 1000 Hz tympanometry: a comparison of methodologies. J Am Acad Audiol 2007;18:739–48.
77. Niemeyer W, Sesterhenn G. Calculating the hearing threshold from the stapedius reflex threshold for different sound stimuli. Audiology 1974;13:421–7.
78. Jerger J, Burney P, Mauldin L. Predicting hearing loss from the acoustic reflex. J Speech Hear Dis 1974;39:11–22.
79. Mangham CA, Lindeman RC, Dawson WR. Stapedius reflex quantification in acoustic tumor patients. Laryngoscope 1980;90:242–50.
80. Anderson H, Barr B, Wedenberg E. Early diagnosis of Eighth-nerve tumours by acoustic reflex tests. Acta Otolaryngol 1970;262:232–37.
81. Jerger J, Harford E, Clemis J, Alford B. The acoustic reflex in eighth nerve disorder. Arch Otolaryngol 1974;99:409–13.
82. Jerger S, Jerger J. Diagnostic value of crossed vs. uncrossed acoustic reflexes. Eighth nerve and brainstem disorders. Arch Otolaryngol 1977;103:445–53.
83. Eggermont JJ, Don M, Brackmann DE. Electocochleography and auditory brainstem electric responses in patients with pontine angle tumors. Ann Otol Rhinol Laryngol Suppl 1980;75:1–19.
84. Stockard JJ, Stockard JE, Sharbrough FW. Detection and localization of occult lesions with brainstem auditory responses. Mayo Clinic Proc 1977;52:761–9.
85. Starr A, Achor J. Auditory brain stem responses in neurological disease. Arch Neurol 1975;32:761–8.
86. Selters WA, Brackmann DE. Acoustic tumor detection with brain stem electric response audiometry. Arch Otolaryngol 1977;103:181–7.
87. Clemis JD, McGee T. Brain stem electric response audiometry in the differential diagnosis of acoustic tumors. Laryngoscope 1979;89:31–42.
88. Musiek FE, Sach E, Geurkink NA, Weider DJ. Auditory brainstem response and eighth nerve lesions: A review and presentation of cases. Ear Hear 1980;1:297–301.

89. Grundy BI, Lina A, Procopio PT, Jannetta PJ. Reversible evoked potential changes with retraction of the eighth cranial nerve. Anesth Analg 1981;60:835–8.
90. Moller AR, Jannetta PJ. Monitoring auditory functions during the cranial nerve microvascular decompression operations by direct recording from the eighth nerve. J Neurosurg 1983;59:43–499.
91. Don M, Kwong B, Tanaka C, Brackmann DE, Nelson RA. The stacked ABR: A sensitive and specific screening tool for detecting small acoustic tumors. Audiol Neurootol 2005;10:274–90.
92. Don M, Masuda A, Nelson R, Brackmann D. Successful detection of small acoustic tumors using the stacked derived-band auditory brain stem response amplitude. Am J Otol 1997;18:608–21.
93. Philibert B, Durrant JD, Ferber-Viart C, et al. Stacked tone-burst-evoked auditory brainstem response (ABR): Preliminary findings. Int J Audiol 2003;42:71–81.
94. Alain C, Tremblay K. The role of event-related brain potentials in assessing central auditory processing. J Am Acad Audiol 2007;18:573–89.
95. Martin J, Jerger J, Mehta J. Divided-attention and directed-attention listening modes in children with dichotic deficits: An event-related potential study. J Am Acad Audiol 2007; 18:34–53.
96. Dimitrijevic A, John MS, Van Roon P, et al. Estimating the audiogram using multiple auditory steady-state responses. J Am Acad Audiol 2002;13:205–24.
97. Rance G, Rickards F. Prediction of hearing threshold in infants using auditory steady-state evoked potentials. J Am Acad Audiol 2002;13:236–45.
98. Kemp DT. Stimulated acoustic emissions from within the human auditory system. J Acoust Soc Amer 1978;64:1386–91.
99. Probst R. Otoacoustic emissions: An overview. Adv Otorhinolarygnol 1990;44:1–91.
100. Harris F, Probst R. Reporting click-evoked and distortion-product otoacoustic emission results with respect to the pure tone audiogram. Ear Hear 1991;12:399–405.
101. Probst R, Harris FP. Transiently evoked and distortion-product otoacoustic emissions: Comparison of results from normally hearing and hearing-impaired human ears. Otolaryngol Head Neck Surg 1993;119:858–60.
102. Vander Werff KR, Prieve BA, Georgantas LM. Test-retest reliability of wideband reflectance measures in infants under screening and diagnostic test conditions. Ear Hear 2007;28: 669–81.
103. Margolis RH, Trine MB. Influence of middle-ear disease on otoacoustic emissions. In: Robinette MS, Glattke TJ, editors. Otoacoustic emissions: Clinical applications. New York: Thieme Medical Publishers, Inc; 1997:130–50.
104. Lonsbury-Martin BL, Martin GK, McCoy MJ, Whitehead ML. Testing young children with otoacoustic emissions: Middle-ear influences. Am J Otol Suppl 1994;15:13–20.
105. Owens JJ, McCoy MJ, Lonsbury-Martin BL, Martin GK. Influence of otitis media on evoked otoacoustic emissions in children. Seminars Hear 1992;13:53–66.
106. Owens JJ, McCoy MJ, Lonsbury-Martin BL, Martin GK. Otoacoustic emissions in children with normal ears, middle-ear dysfunction, and ventilating tubes. Am J Otol 1993;14:34–40.
107. Trine MB, Hirsch JE, Marolis RH. The effect of middle ear pressure on transient evoked otoacoustic emissions. Ear Hear 1993;14:401–7.
108. Jerger J, Jerger S, Mauldin L. Studies in impedance audiometry. I. Normal and sensorineural ears. Arch Otolaryngol 1972;96:513–23.
109. Metz O. Threshold of reflex contractions of muscles of middle ear and recruitment of loudness. Arch Otolaryngol 1952;55:536–43.
110. Bess FH. Clinical assessment of speech recognition. In: Konkle DF, Rintelmann WF, editors. Principles of speech audiometry. Baltimore: University Park Press; 1983. p. 127–201.
111. Jerger J, Mauldin L. Prediction of sensorineural hearing level from the brainstem evoked response. Arch Otolaryngol 1978;104:456–61.
112. Portmann M, Aran JM. Electrocochleography. Laryngoscope 1971;81:899–910.
113. Gibson WR, Moffat DA, Ramsden RT. Clinical electrocochleography in the diagnosis and management of Meniere's disorder. Audiology 1977;16:389–401.
114. Margolis RH, Rieks D, Fournier EM, Levine SC. Tympanic electrocochleography for diagnosis of Meniere's disease. Arch Otolaryngol Head Neck Surg 1995;121:44–55.
115. Orchik DJ, Ge NN, Shea JJ. Action potential latency shift by rarefaction and condensation clicks in Meniere's disease. J Am Acad Audiol 1998;9:121–6.
116. Don M, Kwong B, Tanaka C. A diagnostic test for Ménière's disease and cochlear hydrops: Impaired high-pass noise masking of auditory brainstem responses. Otol Neurotol 2005;26:711–22.
117. Stach BA, Jerger J, Oliver TA. Auditory evoked potential testing strategies. In: Jacobson JT, editor. Principles and applications in auditory evoked potentials. Needham Heights, Mass achusetts: Allyn & Bacon; 1993. p. 541–60.
118. Probst R, Lonsbury-Martin BL, Martin GK, Coats AC. Otoacoustic emissions in ears with hearing loss. Am J Otol 1987;8:73–81.
119. Robinette MS. EOAE contributions in the evaluation of cochlear versus retrocochlear disorders. Seminars Hear 1999;20:13–28.
120. Ozturan O, Jerger J, Lew H, Lynch GR. Monitoring of cisplatin ototoxicity by distortion-product otoacoustic emissions. Auris Nasus Larynx 1996;23:147–51.
121. Balkany TJ, Telischi FF, Lonsbury-Martin BL, Martin GK. Otoacoustic emissions in clinical practice. Am J Otol Suppl 1 1994;;15:29–38.
122. Zorowka PG, Schmitt HJ, Gutjahr P. Evoked otoacoustic emissions and pure tone threshold audiometry in patients receiving cisplatinum therapy. Int J Ped Otorhinolaryngol 1993;25:73–80.
123. Ruckenstein MJ, Cueva RA, Morrison DH, Press G. A prospective study of ABR and MRI in the screening for vestibular schwannomas. Am J Otol 1996;17:317–20.
124. Chandrasekhar SS, Brackmann DE, Devgan KK. Utility of auditory brainstem response audiometry in diagnosis of acoustic neuromas. Am J Otol 1995;16:63–7.
125. Gordon ML, Cohen NL. Efficacy of auditory brainstem response as a screening test for small acoustic neuromas. Am J Otol 1995;16:136–9.
126. Cueva RA. Auditory brainstem response versus magnetic resonance imaging for the evaluation of asymmetric sensorineural hearing loss. Laryngoscope 2004;114:1686–92.
127. Telischi FF, Roth J, Stagner BB, Lonesbury-Martin BL, Balkany TJ. Patterns of evoked otoacoustic emissions associated with acoustic neuromas. Laryngoscope 1995;105:675–82.

128. Durrant JD, Kamerer DB, Chen D. Combined OAE and ABR studies in acoustic tumor patients. In: Hoehmann D, editor. ECoG, OAE and intraoperative monitoring. Amsterdam: Kugler; 1993. p. 231–9.
129. Olsen WO, Noffsinger D, Kurdziel S. Acoustic reflex and reflex decay. Occurrence in patients with cochlear and eighth nerve lesions. Arch Otolaryngol 1975;101:622–5.
130. Anderson H, Barr B, Wedenberg E. Intra-aural reflexes in retrocochlear lesions. In: Hamberger C, Wersall J, editor. Nobel Symposium 10: Disorders of the Skull Base Region. Stockholm: Almquist & Wiskell; 1969. p. 49–55.
131. Olsen WO, Stach BA, Kurdziel SA. Acoustic reflex decay in 10 seconds and in 5 seconds for Meniere's disease patients and for Eighth nerve patients. Ear Hear 1981;2:180–181.
132. Stach BA, Jerger JF. Acoustic reflex averaging. Ear Hear 1984;5:289–96.
133. Stach BA, Jerger JF. Acoustic reflex patterns in peripheral and central auditory system disease. Seminars Hear 1987;8:369–77.
134. Sanders JW, Josey AF, Glasscock ME, Jackson CG. The acoustic reflex test in cochlear and eighth nerve pathology ears. Laryngoscope 1981;91:787–93.
135. Greisen O, Rasmussen PE. Stapedius muscle reflexes and oto-neurological examinations in brain-stem tumors. Acta Otolaryngol 1970;70:366–70.
136. Bosatra A, Russolo M, Poli P. Modifications of the stapedius muscle reflex under spontaneous and experimental brain-stem impairment. Acta Otolaryngol 1975;80:61–6.
137. Jerger J, Oliver TA, Rivera V, Stach BA. Abnormalities of the acoustic reflex in multiple sclerosis. Am J Otolaryngol 1986;7:163–76.
138. Jerger S, Jerger J. Auditory disorders: A manual for clinical evaluation. Boston: Little, Brown; 1981.
139. Stach BA, Delgado-Vilches G, Smith-Farach S. Hearing loss in multiple sclerosis. Seminars Hear 1990;11:221–30.
140. Pensak ML, Glasscock ME, Josey AF, Jackson CG, Gulya AJ. Sudden hearing loss and cerebellopontine angle tumors. Laryngoscope 1985;95:1188–93.
141. Selesnick SH, Jackler RK. Atypical hearing loss in acoustic neuroma patients. Laryngoscope 1993;103:437–41.
142. Roland PS, Glasscock ME, Bojrab DI. Normal hearing in patients with acoustic neuromas. South Med J 1987;80:166–9.
143. Musiek FE, Josey AF, Glasscock ME. Auditory brain stem responses—interwave measurements in acoustic neuromas. Ear Hear 1986;7:100–5.
144. Saleh EA, Aristegui M, Naguib MB, et al. Normal hearing in acoustic neuroma patients: A critical evaluation. Am J Otol 1996;17:127–32.
145. Lustig LR, Rifkin S, Jackler RK, Pitts LH. Acoustic neuromas presenting with normal and symmetrical hearing: Factors associated with diagnosis and outcome. Am J Otol 1998;19:212–8.
146. Olsen WO, Noffsinger D, Kurdziel S. Speech discrimination in quiet and in white noise by patients with peripheral and central lesions. Acta Otolaryngol 1975;80:375–82.
147. Meyer DH, Mishler ET. Rollover measurements with the Auditec NU-6 word lists. J Speech Hear Dis 1985;50:356–60.
148. Bess FH, Josey AF, Humes LE. Performance intensity functions in cochlear and eighth nerve disorders. Am J Otol 1979;1: 27–31.
149. Russolo M, Poli P. Lateralization, impedance, auditory brain stem response and synthetic sentence audiometry in brain stem disorders. Audiology 1983;22:50–62.
150. Jerger J, Jerger S. Clinical validity of central auditory tests. Scand Audiol 1975;4:147–63.
151. Jerger JF, Jerger SW. Auditory findings in brainstem disorders. Arch Otolaryngol 1974;99:342–9.
152. Hurley R, Musiek FE. Effectiveness of three central auditory processing (CAP) tests in identifying cerebral lesions. J Am Acad Audiol 1997;8:257–62.
153. Sparks R, Goodglass H, Nickel B. Ipsilateral versus contralateral extinction in dichotic listening resulting from hemisphere lesions. Cortex 1970;6:249–60.
154. Josey AF, Glasscock ME, Musiek FE. Correlation of ABR and medical imaging in patients with cerebellopontine angle tumors. Am J Otol 1988;9:12–16.
155. Josey AF, Jackson CG, Glasscock ME. Brainstem evoked response audiometry in confirmed eighth nerve tumors. Am J Otolaryngol 1980;1:285–9.
156. Telian SA, Kileny PR, Niparko JK, Kemink JL, Graham MD. Normal auditory brainstem response in patients with acoustic neuroma. Laryngoscope 1989;99:10–14.
157. Stanton SG, Cashman MZ. Auditory brainstem response. A comparison of different interpretation strategies for detection of cerebellopontine angle tumors. Scand Audiol 1996;25:109–20.
158. Musiek FE, Lee WW. The auditory brain stem response in patients with brain stem or cochlear pathology. Ear Hear 1995;16:631–6.
159. Harker L, Backoff P. Middle latency electric auditory response in patients with acoustic neuroma. Otolaryngol Head Neck Surg 1981;89:131–6.
160. Stach BA, Hudson M. Middle and late auditory evoked potentials in multiple sclerosis. Seminars Hear 1990;11:265–75.
161. Kileny P, Paccioretti D, Wilson AF. Effects of cortical lesions on middle-latency auditory evoked responses (MLR). Electroencephalog Clin Neurophysiol 1987;66:108–20.
162. Kraus N, Özdamar Ö, Hier D, Stein L. Auditory middle latency responses (MLRs) in patients with cortical lesions. Electroencephalog Clin Neurophysiol 1982;54:275–87.
163. Robinson K, Rudge P. Abnormalities of the auditory evoked potentials in patients with multiple sclerosis. Brain 1977;100:19–40.
164. Collet L, Kemp DT, Veuillet E, et al. Effect of contralateral auditory stimuli on active cochlear micro-mechanical properties in human subjects. Hear Res 1990;43:251–62.
165. Berlin CI, Hood LJ, Wen H, et al. Contralateral suppression of non-linear click-evoked otoacoustic emissions. Hear Res 1993;71:1–11.
166. Berlin CI, Hood LJ, Hurley A, Wen H. Contralateral suppression of otoacoustic emissions: An index of the function of the medial olivocochlear system. Otolaryngol Head Neck Surg 1994;110:3–21.
167. Konig E. Audiological tests in presbycusis. Internat Audiol 1969;8:240–259.
168. Helfer KS, Wilber LA. Hearing loss, aging, and speech perception in reverberation and noise. J Speech Hear Res 1990;33:149–55.
169. Goetzinger C, Proud G, Dirks D, Embrey J. A study of hearing in advanced age. Arch Otolaryngol 1961;73:662–74.

170. Jerger J. Audiological findings in aging. Adv Oto-Rhino-Laryngol 1973;20:115–24.

171. Orchik D, Burgess J. Synthetic sentence identification as a function of age of the listener. J Am Audiol Soc 1977;3:42–6.

172. Wiley TL, Cruickshanks KJ, Nondahl DM, et al. Aging and word recognition in competing message. J Am Acad Audiol 1998;9:191–8.

173. Stuart A, Phillips DP. Word recognition in continuous and interrupted broadband noise by young normal-hearing, older normal-hearing, and presbyacusic listeners. Ear Hear 1996;17:478–89.

174. Sperry JL, Wiley TL, Chial MR. Word recognition performance in various background competitors. J Am Acad Audiol 1997;8:71–80.

175. Jerger J, Jordan C. Age-related asymmetry on a cued-listening task. Ear Hear 1992;4:272–7.

176. McCroskey R, Kasten R. Temporal factors and the aging auditory system. Ear Hear 1992;3:124–7.

177. Fitzgibbons PJ, Gordon-Salant S. Auditory temporal processing in elderly listeners. J Am Acad Audiol 1996;7:183–9.

178. Konkle D, Beasley D, Bess F. Intelligibility of time-altered speech in relation to chronological aging. J Speech Hear Res 1977;20:108–15.

179. Price PJ, Simon HJ. Perception of temporal differences in speech by "normal-hearing" adults: Effect of age and intensity. J Acoust Soc Am 1984;76:405–10.

180. Cranford JL, Romereim B. Precedence effect and speech understanding in elderly listeners. J Am Acad Audiol 1992;3:405–9.

181. Phillips SL, Gordon-Salant S, Fitzgibbons PJ, Yeni-Komshian GH. Auditory duration discrimination in young and elderly listeners with normal hearing. J Am Acad Audiol 1994;5:210–5.

182. Musiek FE, Shinn JB, Jirsa R, et al. GIN (Gaps in Noise) test performance in subjects with confirmed central auditory nervous system involvement. Ear Hear 2005;26:608–18.

183. Jerger J, Stach BA, Johnson K, Loiselle LH, Jerger S. Patterns of abnormality in dichotic listening in the elderly. In: Jensen JH, editor. Proceedings of the 14th Danavox Symposium on Presbyacusis and Other Age Relate Aspects. Odense, Denmark: Danavox; 1990:143–50.

184. Wilson RH, Jaffe MS. Interactions of age, ear, and stimulus complexity on dichotic digit recognition. J Am Acad Audiol 1996;7:358–64.

185. Jerger J, Silman S, Lew HL, Chmiel R. Case studies in binaural interference: Converging evidence from behavioral and electrophysiologic measures. J Am Acad Audiol 1993;4:122–31.

186. Silman S. Binaural interference in multiple sclerosis: Case study. J Am Acad Audiol 1995;6:193–6.

187. Schoepflin JR. Binaural interference in a child: a case study. J Am Acad Audiol 2007;18:515–21.

188. Cranford JL, Boose M, Moore CA. Tests of precedence effect in sound localization reveal abnormalities in multiple sclerosis. Ear Hear 1990;11:282–8.

189. Hausler R, Colburn S, Marr E. Sound localization in subjects with impaired hearing: Spacial-discrimination and interaural-discrimination tests. Acta Oto-Laryngol Suppl 1983;400:1–62.

190. Stephens SDG. Auditory temporal summation in patients with central nervous system lesions. In: Stephens SDG, editor. Disorders of auditory function. London: Academic Press; 1976:243–52.

191. Koehnke J, Besing JM. The effects of aging on binaural and spatial hearing. Seminars Hear 2001;22(3):241–54.

192. Johnson KL, Nicol TG, Kraus N. Brain stem response to speech: A biological marker of auditory processing. Ear Hear 2005;26:424–34.

193. Stach BA. Central auditory disorders. In: Lalwani AK, Grundfast KM, editors, Pediatric otology and neurotology. Philadelphia: Lippincott-Raven; 1998. p. 387–96.

194. Jerger J, B. A, Lew H, Rivera V, Chmiel R. Dichotic listening, event-related potentials, and interhemispheric transfer in the elderly. Ear Hear 1995;16:482–98.

195. Carhart R. Clinical application of bone conduction. Arch Otolaryngol 1950;51:798–807.

Vestibular Testing 11

Dennis I. Bojrab, MD / Sanjay A. Bhansali, MD, FACS /
Travis J. Pfannenstiel, MD / B. Maya Kato, MD

Vestibular testing is an important tool in the evaluation and management of the patient with dizziness. The bedside evaluation of the dizzy patient, with a careful history and a thorough neurotologic examination, is crucial in establishing an accurate clinical diagnosis. We do not believe that vestibular testing should be used as a solitary, one-time test for patients with dizziness. Vestibular testing may aid in establishing a diagnosis, determining the side or site of the lesion, staging of the illness, following the patient's condition with and without treatment over the course of the illness, and in selecting treatment options for the patient. We therefore advise a thorough understanding of how these tests are performed and interpreted, and how they are used in conjunction with other clinical information.

Although bedside and office examinations provide information about the status of the vestibular system, major limitations are the inability to quantify responses and to monitor the course of the illness or the results of medical and surgical management of the dizzy patient. The uses of the vestibular laboratory are cited in Table 11–1. Current technologies available for assessing the vestibular system include electronystagmography (ENG), rotation testing, computerized dynamic posturography (CDP), and vestibular-evoked myogenic potential (VEMP) testing. The first two modalities evaluate the vestibular system by testing vestibulo-ocular interactions or the vestibulo-ocular reflex (VOR). Dynamic posturography is a test of postural stability and reveals information about the vestibulospinal reflex (VSR). VEMP testing evaluates inner ear vestibular function through the VSR using auditory stimulation. We discuss how each of these tests is performed, what information each test provides, and provide guidelines for their use in various clinical situations.

ELECTRONYSTAGMOGRAPHY

Electronystagmography is the most commonly employed method of laboratory evaluation of the vestibular system. The examination consists of a battery of tests that are collectively referred to as the ENG. The vestibular and ocular systems are connected through the VOR; thus, patients with peripheral and/or central vestibular disorders often exhibit abnormal eye movements that can be measured and recorded. Electronystagmography assesses whether labyrinthine dysfunction is present, the degree of dysfunction, and provides specific information about each ear separately (ie, it lateralizes dysfunction).

There are a variety of methods currently available for recording eye movement: electric potentials (ENG or electro-oculography (EOG)), magnetic potentials (search coils), video cameras (video ENG or VNG), and infrared technology.

Corneoretinal Potential

The most commonly used technology (EOG) depends on the fact that there is a steady DC potential, termed the corneoretinal potential (CRP), between the cornea and the retina (Figure 11–1). These potentials create an electric field at the front of the head that rotates as the eyes rotate. The CRP is generated by the metabolic activity of the retinal pigment epithelium. The retina is negatively charged relative to the cornea; thus, an electrical potential can be measured between the two by means of skin surface electrodes. When the eyes are looking straight ahead (primary gaze), the average potential measured at the cornea is about 1 mV. As the eyes move, the potential changes, relative to the skin electrodes. Thus, differences in electric potential are measured and reflect movement of the eyes. Rotation of this electric field produces a roughly linear change in the voltage between electrodes attached to the skin on either side of the eyes. Horizontal eye position is monitored by electrodes placed on the temples; vertical eye position is monitored by electrodes placed above and below one eye. Of note, it is difficult to detect torsional nystagmus with traditional electro-oculography because rotation of the eye about the axis of the pupil does not effect a change in the CRP. The best methods for recording torsional eye movements are search coils or video/infrared methods.

ELECTRONYSTAGMOGRAPHIC TRACING

Electronystagmography results were previously recorded on a strip chart recorder in which time is plotted on the horizontal axis and eye movements are recorded on the vertical axis. The recordings are now done on computer. By convention, rightward

TABLE 11–1 Uses of vestibular laboratory

Aid in establishing diagnosis Location—central versus peripheral lesion Lateralization
Documentation
Assist in devising treatment plan Aid in long-term management

eye movement is recorded as an upward deflection, and leftward eye motion is shown as a downward deflection. When ENG testing was first developed, the data from the strip tracing were hand-calculated into meaningful results. The recent development of computerized ENG analysis has been a substantial enhancement and permits efficient storage and easy retrieval of eye movement data and eliminates the cutting and pasting of strip chart recordings. In addition, computerized ENG allows rapid and sophisticated analysis of saccade, tracking, and caloric tests—analyses that could not be done with strip chart recordings.

Video-oculography and Other Methods

Other techniques have been developed to record eye motion but are not available in all ENG laboratories. These alternative methods of evaluating eye movement include videonystagmography (VNG), magnetic scleral search coil devices, and infrared recording devices.

One current trend in many vestibular laboratories is toward the use of video-recorded nystagmography. Videonystagmography is a computer-based system for eye movement testing (Figure 11–2). This technique records eye movements with digital video technology using infrared illumination and a high-technology goggle. The images are then displayed on a computer monitor. The computer software records and analyzes the data. These images may then be recorded on videotape. The VNG technique determines eye position by locating the pupil and tracking its center; the internal computer program plots, measures, and analyzes the eye movement similar to traditional ENG.

The VNG technique permits visualization and recording of eye movements—helpful for later study and for teaching personnel and patients. This capacity is particularly useful in evaluating patients with benign paroxysmal positional vertigo (BPPV)—one of the most common vestibular abnormalities encountered. Videonystamographic tracings are clean with no drift, which improves the accuracy of analysis and interpretation. This technique is easier and quicker than using electrodes and only one calibration is necessary. There are limitations to the VNG that are noteworthy. Test equipment is more expensive, some patients with significant claustrophobia may not tolerate the sensation of confinement, and patients with ptosis, pupil-obscuring eyelashes, or other eye abnormalities may be difficult to test.

The magnetic search coil technique involves the patient sitting in a low-strength, alternating magnetic field. The patient wears a soft contact lens in which a wire coil is embedded. The

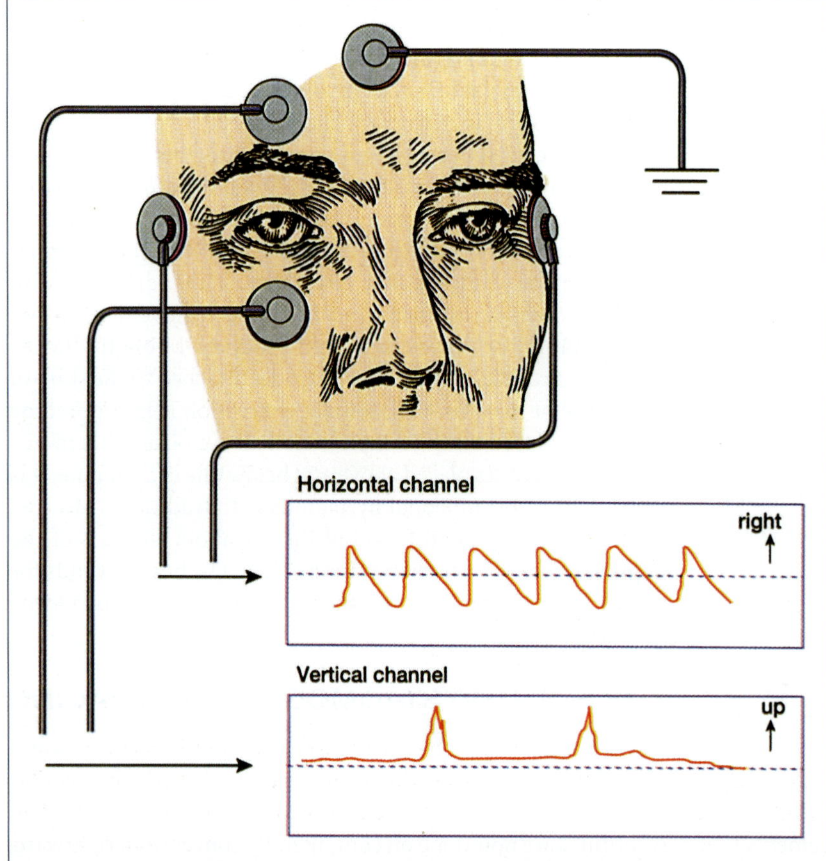

FIGURE 11–1 • Electro-oculography (EOG). The cornea is relatively positively charged in comparison to the retina; thus, an electric potential exists between the two. Electrodes are placed around the eyes, and rotation of the eye brings the cornea closer to one electrode and the negatively charged retina closer to the other. The relative voltage difference provides the basis for EOG. By convention, rightward movement of the eye is recorded as an upward deflection on the electronystagmographic tracing.

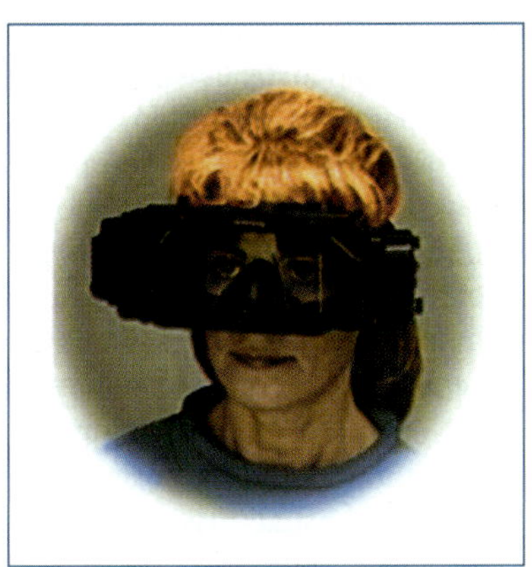

FIGURE 11–2 • Videonystagmography equipment. The goggles contain video cameras that allow the patient's eye movements to be recorded for later viewing and analysis. Direct visualization of the eyes allows for superior documentation of torsional nystagmus, when compared with traditional electro-oculography-based systems.

contact lens fits around but does not directly contact the cornea. Motion of the coil of wire in the alternating magnetic field induces a very small current in the wire (based on Faraday's law), and this signal can be used to obtain measurement of eye position. There are two major advantages of this method: it provides very precise determination of eye position in three dimensions and it allows eye position to be sampled and recorded very rapidly (500–1,000 times per sec). These features are responsible for the search coil technique providing the most accurate measurement of eye movements. The major disadvantage of the search coil technique is that it requires a sophisticated laboratory and highly experienced personnel. For these reasons, the search coil technique is usually limited to research laboratories.

Infrared oculography is based on the differing reflectance properties of the iris compared to the sclera and the fact that the photocells of the eye remain stationary while the edge of the iris moves with the eye. As a result, the light sensed by the photocells differs according to eye position. The advantage of this technique is that a direct estimate of the eye position as a function of time can be calculated. The disadvantages of this technique include the bulk of the equipment, which limits visual stimulation somewhat, and the interference with eyelid motion (eg, blink), which makes vertical recording difficult at times.[1]

ROUTINE COMPONENTS OF ELECTRONYSTAGMOGRAPHY

The ENG test battery usually consists of three groups of tests. By convention, the tests are performed in a systematic fashion to assess the oculomotor and vestibular systems and their corresponding interaction. Test procedures are designed to test each function and to detect the presence of pathologic (spontaneous, gaze, positional, and positioning) nystagmus.

The first group of tests investigates visual-oculomotor function and evaluates nonvestibular eye movements. The saccade test detects disorders of the saccadic control system. The tracking test and the optokinetic test both detect disorders of the pursuit control system.

The second group of tests looks for the presence of abnormal eye movements and whether they change with altered head position. The gaze test evaluates limitations of eye movement, gaze stability, ocular flutter, spontaneous nystagmus, and latent nystagmus. The positional test determines whether various head positions cause or modify nystagmus. The Dix-Hallpike maneuver looks for positioning nystagmus.

The third group assesses vestibulo-oculomotor function. The bithermal caloric test, involving four irrigations, is the most indispensable test of the ENG battery and primarily detects dysfunction of the labyrinth or vestibular nerve (ie, the peripheral vestibular system).

Tests of Visual-Oculomotor Function

Visual and vestibular inputs are both important in gaze stabilization during motion. A variety of oculomotor testing paradigms are used to test the central oculomotor control system. Three types of eye movements assessed as part of the ENG are saccades, smooth pursuit, and optokinetic eye movements. The oculomotor system interacts with vestibular reflexes to modulate visual input relevant to the task at hand. The saccade test detects disorders of the saccade control system, and the tracking test and the optokinetic test assess disorders of the pursuit control system.

Saccade (Calibration) Test

The saccade control system generates all voluntary and involuntary fast eye movements. The saccade test is performed at the beginning of the test while calibrating eye movements. The purpose of the saccade system is to rapidly capture interesting visual targets in the periphery of the visual field onto the fovea. This quick foveating eye movement is a saccade. It is the fastest type of eye movement, sometimes with peak velocities as high as 700 degrees/s and an average velocity of 200 degrees/s.

Horizontal eye movements are first calibrated by having the patient capture an image at a known distance that requires a 20-degree angle of visual excursion. Eye movements are calibrated in both the vertical and horizontal planes. Once calibrated, the patient's saccade function is tested; the testing paradigm may be performed differently in various laboratories. In one version of the test, the patient's horizontal eye movements are monitored with fixation on a computer-controlled visual target that jumps back and forth in the horizontal plane in random sequence. The complete sequence often consists of 80 target jumps (40 to the right and 40 to the left), with amplitudes ranging from 5 to 25 degrees. After testing, the computer calculates three values for each saccade: peak velocity, accuracy, and latency.

Abnormally slow-velocity saccades are seen in many degenerative and metabolic diseases of the central nervous system (CNS): internuclear ophthalmoplegia; disturbances in the cerebral hemispheres, the superior colliculus, the oculomotor nucleus, or the extraocular muscles; drug intoxication; or drowsy or inattentive patients. Abnormally fast-velocity saccades may occur with orbital tumors and myasthenia gravis.[2] The cerebellum plays an important role in determining the accuracy of saccadic movements. Inaccurate saccades, or ocular dysmetria, are classified as hypermetria (overshooting the target) or hypometria (undershooting) and may be seen with cerebellar disease or brainstem disorders. Saccadic latency abnormalities may be seen in patients with abnormal vision, Parkinson's disease, Huntington's chorea, Alzheimer's disease, and focal hemispheric lesions.[3]

Pursuit and Optokinetic Tests

Two tests of pursuit, the tracking test and the optokinetic test, are typically performed as part of the ENG. Pursuit tracking, or the smooth pursuit system, allows continuous tracking of moving objects and works with the saccade system to maintain images on the fovea when the target is moving. The smooth pursuit system is used to track targets at slower speeds and operates when the eyes move within the orbit and the head is still. The VOR is used to maintain the stability of images on the fovea when the head is moving. The VOR is particularly important in maintaining stable gaze during rapid head movements.

The smooth pursuit system has neural pathways from the fovea to several cortical and subcortical pathways. The pursuit tracking test (Figure 11–3) can be performed simply with a pendulum swinging back and forth, producing a sinusoidal moving target. In a computer-generated version of the test, the patient's horizontal eye movements are monitored while following a computer-controlled visual target that moves back and forth (at frequencies from 0.2–0.7 Hz) in the horizontal plane, following a sinusoidal waveform. After testing, the computer differentiates the eye position signal, calculates the gain of eye velocity with respect to target velocity separately for rightward and leftward tracking at each target frequency, and plots these data. Normal individuals are able to follow the target smoothly in both directions at all target frequencies. Deficits in smooth pursuit may result from age, medication, visual problems, attention deficit, or lesions of the brain stem, cerebellum, and occipitoparietal junction.

Optokinetic function is a phylogenetically older system that is also found in animals lacking well-developed foveae. The optokinetic pathways are subcortical, involving the accessory optic system. In humans, there is an overlap in function by neurons in the cortical and subcortical visual systems. The smooth pursuit system dominates the operation of the overall pursuit system. The optokinetic system differs from smooth pursuit in that optokinetic eye movements follow a moving object until the eye position becomes relatively eccentric. Optokinetic nystagmus consists of an involuntary pursuit of a repetitive image (slow phase) that is followed by a quick saccade that recenters the eyes (fast component). The specific methods and stimuli used in the optokinetic test vary according to testing laboratory. In one version, the patient's horizontal eye movements are monitored while following a series of visual targets that move to the right and then to the left. This stimulus evokes a nystagmus with the slow phase in the direction of target motion, periodically interrupted by fast phases in the opposite direction. The optokinetic test, like the tracking test, is a test of eye pursuit pathways, and the results of the tracking and optokinetic tests show concordance with tasks of similar difficulty. In normal individuals, the slow-phase eye velocities approximately match target velocities for both rightward- and leftward-moving targets. Figure 11–4 shows the results of the optokinetic test for a patient whose optokinetic nystagmus was defective for rightward-moving targets and normal for leftward-moving targets.

Abnormal Eye Movements

Gaze Test

This test is valuable in the detection of nystagmus that occurs without vestibular stimulation. It may reveal disorders, vestibular and nonvestibular, of CNS origin, congenital nystagmus, or a spontaneous nystagmus of peripheral vestibular origin. The test differentiates gaze-evoked, dysconjugate, rebound, and spontaneous nystagmus.

The gaze test is performed by recording eye movements first in the primary position and then while fixating on a target 30 degrees to the right, left, above, and below the center position. Each position should be held for at least 30 sec Some examiners

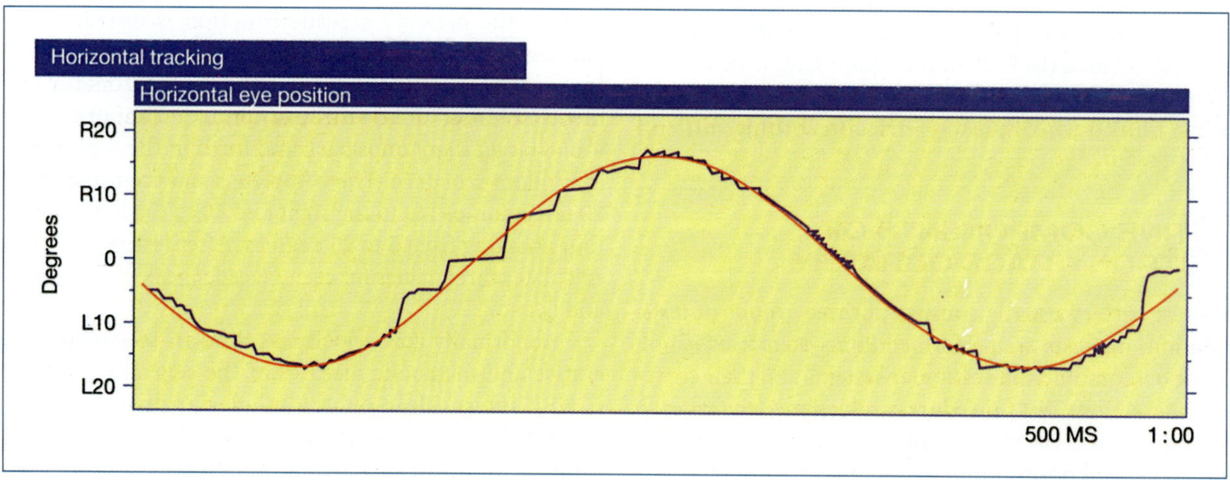

FIGURE 11–3 • The results of the tracking test in a patient with a unilateral pursuit defect. The patient was unable to follow the rightward-moving target smoothly and instead approximated its motion using successive saccades, producing a stair-step pattern on the eye movement tracing. Tracking of leftward-moving targets was normal. This patient's abnormality indicates an asymmetric central nervous system lesion involving the pursuit eye movement control system.

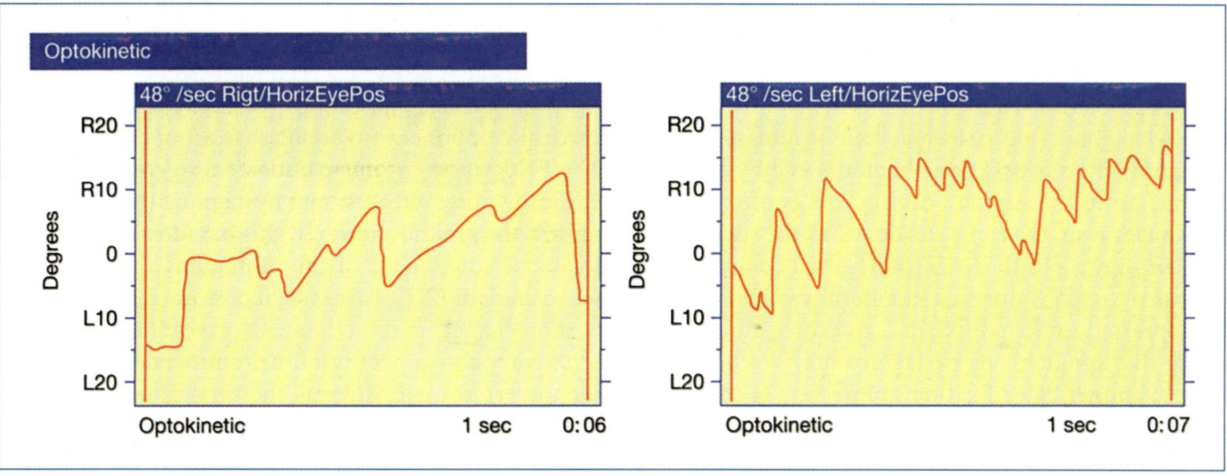

FIGURE 11–4 • Optokinetic test for a patient whose optokinetic system was defective for rightward-moving targets and normal for leftward-moving targets.

also attempt to monitor eye movements in these gaze positions (with visual fixation denied), but the tracing is often difficult to interpret. Young, normal individuals rarely have any nystagmus while fixating at any of these gaze positions, but many elderly individuals demonstrate end-gaze nystagmus. This nystagmus is usually subtle, with a centripetal slow phase, and generally is of equal intensity on right and left gaze.

Spontaneous vestibular nystagmus occurs when there is an imbalance in the tonic input from the labyrinth on the left and right sides. It is typically seen with unilateral vestibular lesions and usually beats away from the side of vestibular hypofunction. Frequently, it is better appreciated during the positional test with visual fixation prevented (in darkness or in light with the use of Frenzel lenses), and it manifests on ENG as a purely horizontal nystagmus because the ENG is insensitive to the torsional component; however, it is actually horizontal-torsional nystagmus. The intensity of spontaneous nystagmus may change with a change in the direction of the gaze, being stronger when looking toward the direction of the nystagmus (Alexander's law). Spontaneous nystagmus that is not diminished (or increases) with visual fixation (failure of fixation suppression) suggests a central lesion. Upbeat nystagmus usually is a result of medullary lesions that involve the vertical vestibular pathways. Other types of central nystagmus seen in the gaze test are described by Leigh and Zee,[4] and ENG tracings of many of these are illustrated by Barber and Stockwell.[5]

Gaze-evoked nystagmus (nystagmus exposed by directing gaze away from the primary position) may be a side effect of a variety of medications, including anticonvulsants, sedatives, and alcohol. It can also occur in such diverse conditions as myasthenia gravis, multiple sclerosis, and cerebellar atrophy. Dysconjugate gaze nystagmus is commonly present with medial longitudinal fasciculus lesions, such as internuclear ophthalmoplegia.

Positional Test

The purpose of the positional test is to determine if different head positions induce or modify vestibular nystagmus. Nystagmus induced by positional testing is referred to as positional nystagmus (or static positional nystagmus) to differentiate it from the paroxysmal or positioning nystagmus of the Dix-Hallpike maneuver. During the positional tests, the patient's eye movements are monitored while the head is in at least four positions: sitting, supine, head right (right ear down), and head left (left ear down). If nystagmus appears or is modified in either of the latter two positions, the patient is tested again while lying on that side to determine if the effect is caused by neck rotation. Eye movements are monitored in each position for about 20 sec, both with visual fixation (eyes open and fixating on a visual target at center gaze) and without visual fixation. Most examiners prevent fixation simply by asking patients to close their eyes, but eye closure may inhibit nystagmus. A better method is to monitor eye movements with eyes open in near total darkness. The examiner usually asks the patient to perform a mental task, such as arithmetic, while testing with visual fixation denied to stimulate mental alertness, thus avoiding suppression of nystagmus.

Positional nystagmus may be intermittent or persistent unlike positioning nystagmus that disappears over time after the head is brought into a new position. In both cases, the nystagmus induced by ampullopetal stimulation of the affected canal is greater than that induced by ampullofugal stimulation (Ewald's second law).[6] Persistent positional nystagmus is sustained as long as the head position is maintained and may reflect the effect of changing otolith influences on the central processes involved in control of the VOR. As with positioning nystagmus, the terms geotropic (beating toward the ground) and ageotropic may be used to describe the direction of the nystagmus. The nystagmus may be direction fixed (beating to the same direction in different head positions) or direction changing (changing direction with differing head positions). Both of these types of nystagmus occur most commonly with peripheral vestibular disorders, but they may also occur with central lesions. Peripheral vestibular nystagmus is eliminated or diminished with visual fixation. Thus, positional nystagmus is a valuable indicator of vestibular system dysfunction. Other signs and clinical data must be used to localize the lesion.

Spontaneous nystagmus has been defined as nystagmus that is unmodulated by changes in head position and has been distinguished from positional nystagmus, which is modulated by head position changes. The horizontal-torsional vestibular nystagmus that is seen acutely in unilateral vestibular hypofunction is occasionally modulated by a change from the sitting to the supine position and is often modulated by changes from the right-ear-down, to the supine, and to the left-ear-down positions. The horizontal component of spontaneous nystagmus due to a unilateral vestibular lesion may be suppressed by visual fixation, and often suppression is so strong that spontaneous nystagmus may not be identified by the examiner. Poor fixation suppression is an indication of CNS dysfunction in the pathways responsible for VOR cancellation.

When a persistent nystagmus is seen, it is important to extend the observation period to at least 2 min certain types of direction-changing nystagmus, eg, (acquired) periodic alternating nystagmus, reverse direction approximately every 2 min. Periodic alternating nystagmus is usually caused by a CNS lesion.[4]

Positioning Test

The most frequently employed test for positioning nystagmus is the Dix-Hallpike maneuver (Figure 11–5). In this test, the patient is subjected to two brisk movements, both beginning with the patient in the sitting position. The patient's head is first turned 45 degrees toward one side, and then the patient is briskly brought backward to assume the supine position with the head (still turned) hanging over the end of the examining table. The examiner holds the patient's head in position for at least 20 sec and looks for nystagmus. The duration and direction of any nystagmus are noted. Next the patient is returned to the sitting position and eye movements are observed for any nystagmus. The maneuver is then performed with the patient's head turned 45 degrees to the other side.

During the backward movement, the Dix-Hallpike maneuver normally induces a few beats of nystagmus, which is due to the VOR evoked by the head movement; however, after the head is in the hanging position, normal individuals do not have nystagmus. Patients with BPPV display a burst of intense nystagmus—paroxysmal positional nystagmus—the hallmark of the disorder. The nystagmus in BPPV typically begins after a latency of 10 to 20 sec following placement of the patient's head reaches in the Dix-Hallpike position and goes away about 15 to 45 sec after the onset. For this reason, BPPV is often referred to as a positioning nystagmus. Paroxysmal positional nystagmus can be readily appreciated by visual observation with the patient's eyes open or, better yet, with the patient wearing Frenzel lenses in a darkened room. In the case of BPPV affecting the posterior semicircular canal, the examiner sees a vertical-torsional nystagmus (up beating with torsional fast phases that involve motion of the superior pole of the eye toward the downward ear). Electronystagmography may be useful in documenting the response (Figure 11–6). It should be noted, however, that traditional methods of electro-oculography record only horizontal and vertical (and not torsional eye movements); thus, the findings noted with standard electro-oculography in BPPV may be difficult to interpret and misleading. The horizontal component of the nystagmus from posterior canal BPPV recorded with electro-oculography generally has the fast phase away from the undermost ear, and the vertical component invariably has an upbeating fast phase.[7] The ENG tracing seems paradoxical in comparison with the clinically observed torsional nystagmus that appears to beat toward the ground; however, this paradox occurs because the torsional component of the nystagmus cannot be recorded with standard ENG. Paroxysmal positional nystagmus appears to show changes in direction with respect to the patient's gaze.[8] The rotary component is more prominent during gaze toward the undermost ear, whereas the vertical component is more prominent during gaze toward the uppermost ear when the patient is in the Dix-Hallpike position. We are accustomed to describing eye movements with respect to an eye-fixed frame of reference, which explains why the direction of nystagmus appears to change with eye position. When described with respect to the canal planes, the nystagmus maintains the same alignment with the plane of the posterior canal regardless of eye position.

Positioning nystagmus has four distinctive features[9]:

1. It has a delayed onset. Usually, there is an interval of at least a few (2–20) seconds after the patient reaches the head-hanging position before the nystagmus begins.
2. It is always transient, ie, it rapidly builds in intensity (crescendos), slowly abates (decrescendos), and finally disappears (typically within 45 sec) as the head remains in position.
3. It is always accompanied by vertigo, usually intense, which follows the same time course as the nystagmus.
4. It is usually fatigable, ie, it progressively diminishes in intensity with repetition of the Dix-Hallpike maneuver. The disappearance of the response with repeated Dix-Hallpike maneuvers in many cases is due to the otoconial debris passing out of the posterior canal.

The Dix-Hallpike maneuver occasionally provokes other types of nystagmus, eg, downbeat nystagmus, which is exacerbated when the patient is moved to the head-hanging position. If downbeat nystagmus is mild, it may be missed during the gaze or positional tests and be observed for the first time with the Dix-Hallpike maneuver. It generally is not accompanied by vertigo. Rarely, other types of nystagmus, generally of CNS origin, are provoked by the Dix-Hallpike maneuver.

One limitation of the Dix-Hallpike maneuver is that it cannot be performed on patients with cervical spine disease that limits neck extension or back disorders that prohibit rapid positioning of the patient into the head-hanging position. In those patients, a sidelying Bojrab-Calvert maneuver may be employed. The senior author has been using this technique for over 14 years as his primary technique in elderly patients or patients with significant cervical neck disease. This maneuver allows the same positioning of the posterior semicircular canal as with the Dix-Hallpike maneuver, without the head hanging.

A

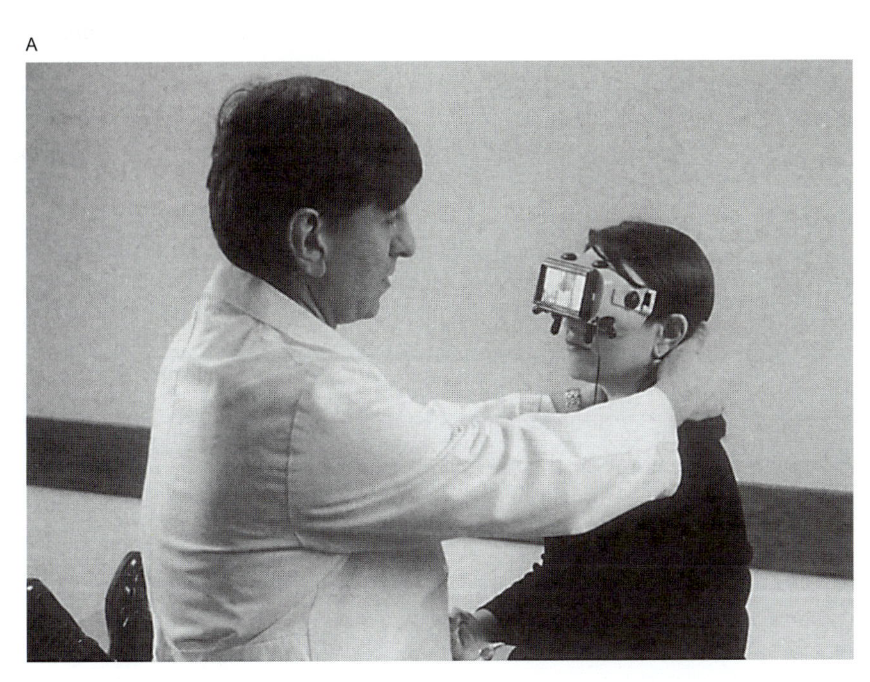

B

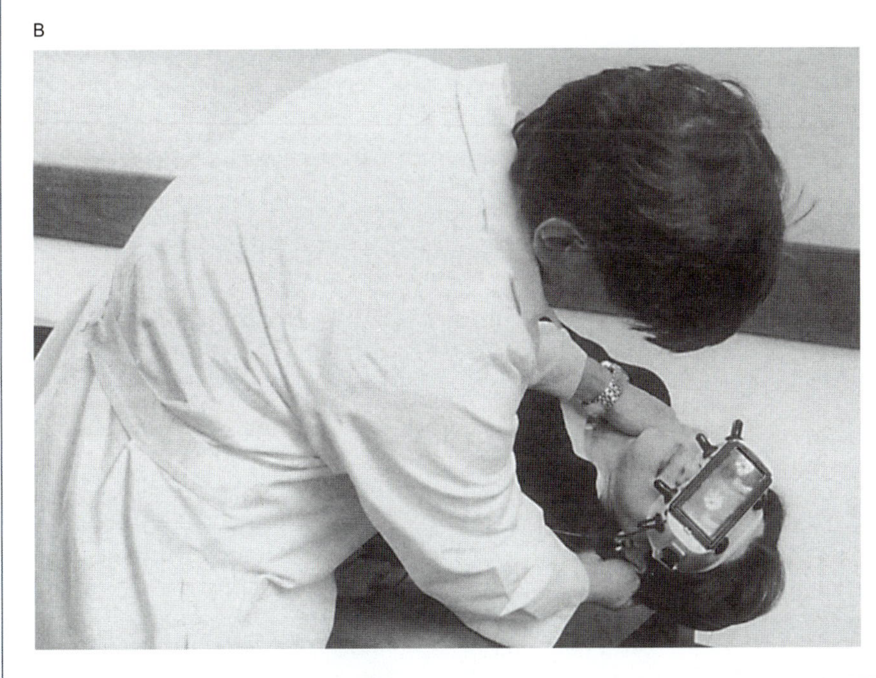

FIGURE 11–5 • Dix-Hallpike maneuver. The patient's head is first turned to the left. The patient is then rapidly brought into the head-hanging position. Patients with benign paroxysmal positional vertigo typically demonstrate a geotropic, torsional nystagmus with the affected ear down. Frenzel's lenses are used to prevent fixation-suppression. The test is repeated on the opposite side.

The Bojrab-Calvert maneuver (Figure 11–7) begins with the patient in the sitting position, facing the examiner. The head is turned 45 degrees to the right so that the pinna is perpendicular to the table surface. The examiner holds the head in that position as the patient is briskly lowered onto his/her shoulder with the head resting on the table. This position is held for at least 20 sec, while eye movements are monitored. The patient is then returned to the sitting position. If nystagmus was elicited, the examiner repeats the same maneuver to determine if the nystagmus is fatigable. The maneuver is performed with the contralateral side. As with the Dix-Hallpike maneuver, the ear that is dependent when nystagmus is elicited is thought to be the diseased side.

Lateral semicircular canal BPPV can often be detected with the Dix-Hallpike maneuver; however, a more effective maneuver involves placing the patient in the supine position, turning the head quickly to the right-ear-down position, and holding it there for at least 30 sec (or, if nystagmus is provoked, for up to several minutes). The patient's head is then returned slowly to the supine position; lastly, the head is turned quickly into the left-ear-down position and held there for at least 30 sec (or, if nystagmus is provoked, for up to several minutes). In patients

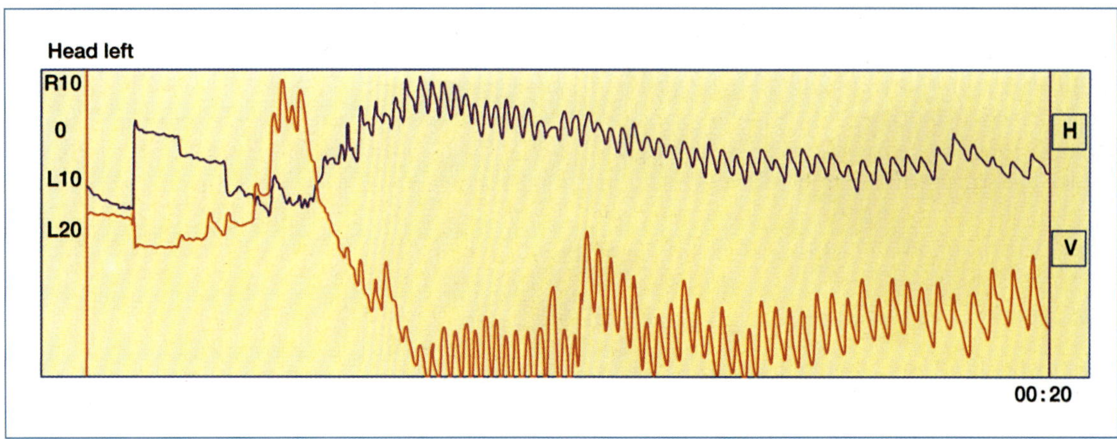

FIGURE 11–6 • Electronystagmographic tracing demonstrates horizontal and vertical components of the nystagmus seen in benign paroxysmal positional vertigo.

A

B

C

D

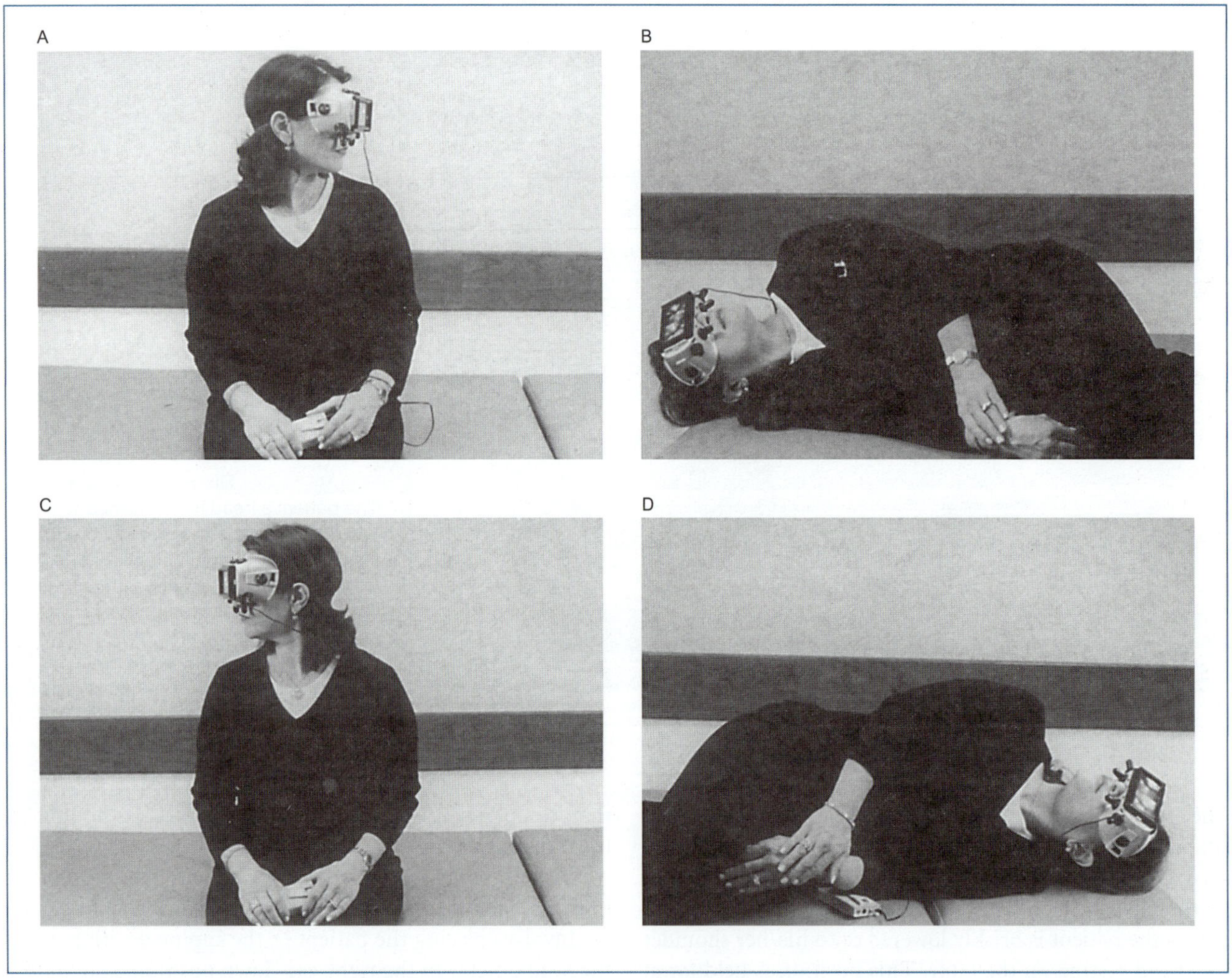

FIGURE 11–7 • Bojrab-Calvert maneuver for benign paroxysmal positional vertigo. This positioning maneuver is useful in assessing positioning nystagmus in elderly or other individuals who cannot tolerate the neck extension position used in the Dix-Hallpike maneuver.

with lateral canal BPPV, this maneuver provokes horizontal nystagmus, as described by Baloh and colleagues.[10] The nystagmus of lateral canal BPPV is (1) geotropic (right-beating in the right-ear-down position and left-beating in the left-ear-down position) and often followed by an ageotropic secondary nystagmus; (2) stronger when the ear presumed to be diseased is undermost; (3) transient (although more persistent than the response of posterior canal BPPV); (4) accompanied by vertigo, usually intense, which follows the same time course as the response; (5) not delayed in onset; and (6) not fatigable.

Tests of Vestibulo-Oculomotor Function

Bithermal Caloric Test

The bithermal caloric test has proven to be highly sensitive to unilateral lesions of the peripheral vestibular system because it allows the examiner to stimulate each ear separately. Other vestibular test procedures, such as rotation testing and posturography, stimulate both labyrinths simultaneously, thereby permitting the masking of abnormal responses from one labyrinth by normal responses from the opposite ear.

The bithermal (Hallpike) caloric tests evaluate the integrity of the lateral semicircular canals and their afferent pathways. The patient is placed in the supine position with the head elevated 30 degrees, thereby placing the lateral semicircular canal in the vertical plane (Figure 11–8). Testing is properly done with the patient wearing Frenzel goggles to prevent fixation-suppression. Asking the patient to engage in mental tasks can also be helpful in releasing the nystagmus.

Caloric testing uses a nonphysiologic stimulus (temperature) to induce fluid flow in the lateral semicircular canal. Each ear is irrigated twice: once with air (or water) at 7 degrees above body temperature and then with air (or water) at 7 degrees below body temperature. The caloric stimulus causes the endolymph to circulate, resulting, after a short latency period, in a brief (1–2 min) burst of nystagmus. In a healthy patient, irrigation with a warm stimulus provokes nystagmus with the fast phase directed toward the stimulated ear; irrigation with a cool stimulus evokes nystagmus with the fast phase directed away from the stimulated ear (cold, opposite; warm, the same).

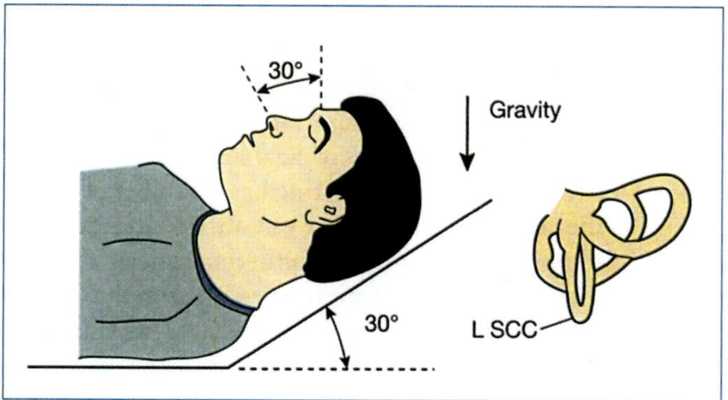

FIGURE 11–8 • Caloric testing may be performed with air or water. The correct position places the patient in the reclined position, 30 degrees elevated from the table, which places the horizontal canal in the vertical plane.

The caloric data are analyzed, and five characteristics of the calorically induced nystagmus are calculated: duration, latency, amplitude, frequency, and velocity. Of these parameters, the most important variable is the peak slow-phase eye velocity. In normal individuals, the slow-phase eye velocity should be equally strong in both directions. Comparing the peak slow-phase eye velocity of the cool and warm caloric responses of the right ear with those of the left ear allows the examiner to determine whether a unilateral vestibular weakness exists. To assess the function of each labyrinth, the caloric responses of the two ears are compared. Because both ears receive the same stimuli, they should demonstrate equal caloric responses.

Caloric stimuli are uncalibrated, ie, stimulus strength varies from person to person depending on the size and shape of the external ear canal and other uncontrollable variables. However, the basic assumption of the caloric test is that, for a given individual, the two ears receive equal caloric stimuli. If both ears are normal, they should produce responses of approximately equal intensity. Therefore, the intensity of the caloric responses of the two ears is compared by evaluating the peak slow-phase eye velocities using the following formula:

$$\frac{(RW + RC) - (LW + LC)}{RW + RC + LW + LC} \times 100\% = UW$$

where RW, RC, LW, and LC are peak slow-phase eye velocities of the responses to right warm, right cool, left warm, and left cool responses, respectively, and UW is unilateral weakness. In general, a unilateral caloric weakness (CW) of greater than 20% indicates peripheral vestibular dysfunction on the side of the weaker response.[11]

Patients with labyrinthine hypofunction may demonstrate reduced or absent caloric responses to the initial bithermal stimuli. In this case, the test is repeated with ice water (approximately 0°C) irrigations. However, one should keep in mind that the absence of a caloric response does not always imply absent peripheral function as the stimulus levels are below the level within which the VOR generally functions.[12]

Various patterns of ENG abnormalities can be seen with vestibular system dysfunction. For example, a patient with an acute, unilateral peripheral vestibular lesion often demonstrates spontaneous nystagmus and a unilateral caloric weakness (Figure 11–9).[13] The presence of spontaneous nystagmus may affect the results of the caloric test, creating a bias that resets the caloric baseline (Figure 11–10). Spontaneous nystagmus is not absolutely diagnostic of a recent peripheral vestibular lesion. Figure 11–11 shows data for a patient with spontaneous nystagmus but without caloric weakness. Such a finding is nonlocalizing as the nystagmus can be associated with numerous entities, including recovery from a previously compensated peripheral vestibular lesion or a central peripheral vestibular lesion.

Whereas the bithermal caloric test is highly sensitive to unilateral peripheral vestibular dysfunction, it is relatively insensitive to bilateral dysfunction because the caloric stimulus is uncalibrated. Even though the stimulus at the

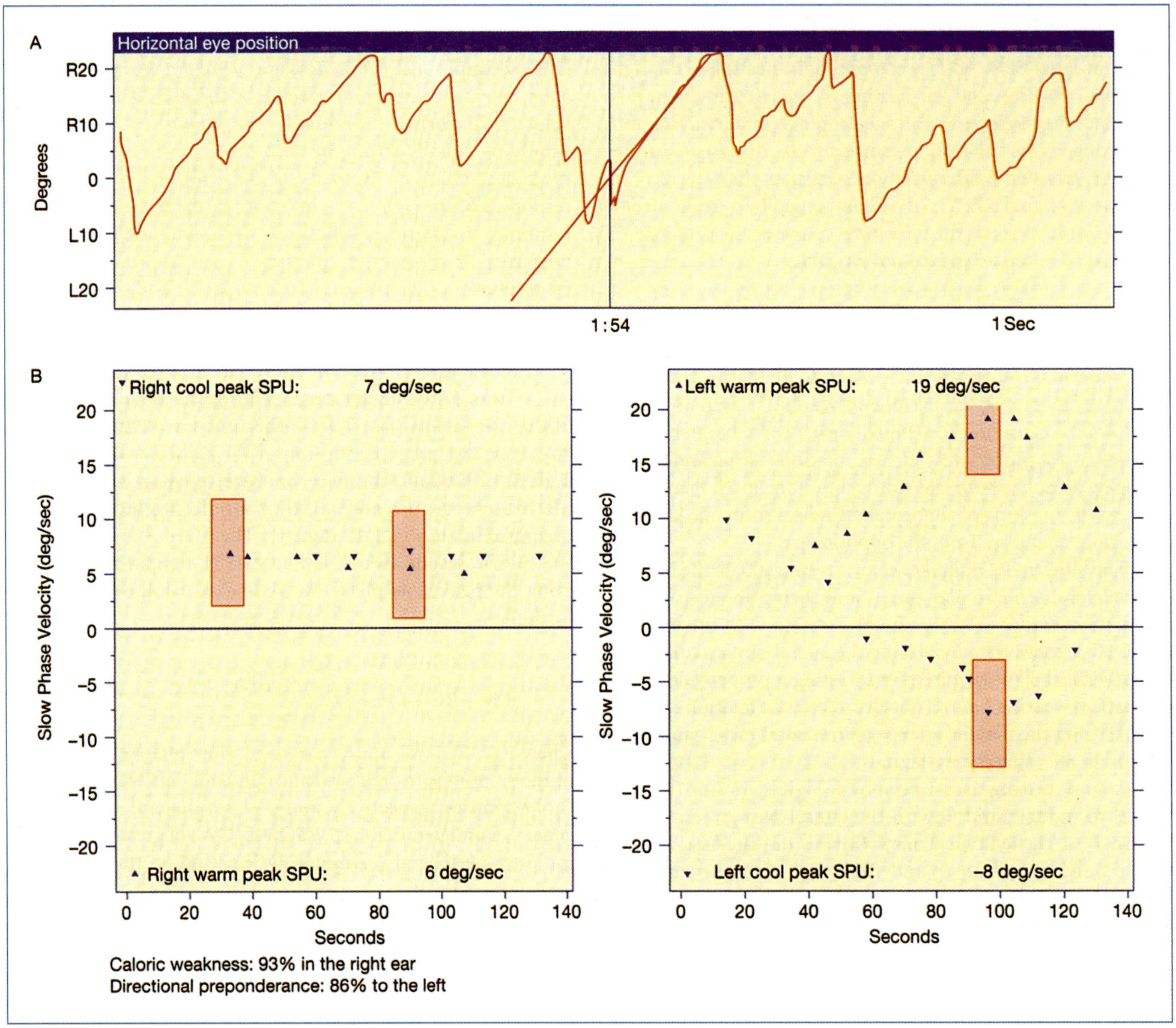

FIGURE 11–9 • Electronystagmographic data from a patient with an acute, left vestibular lesion. A reduction in the tonic resting input from the damaged ear causes a slow drift of the eyes toward the injured side, with a corrective saccade in the opposite direction. The caloric testing shows reduced responses to both warm and cold air in the left ear. *A*, ICE caloric: Right ear/prone; *B*, Bithernal caloric.

entrance to the external ear canal is the same for everyone, the stimulus reaching the inner ear shows great interindividual variability owing to differences in the size and shape of the ear canal and the status of the middle ear. Therefore, the range of normal absolute response intensities is extremely wide, and bilateral caloric weaknesses must be severe to fall below them. The usual rule of thumb is that a bilateral weakness exists if the caloric responses (warm response plus cool response) of both ears fall below 12 degrees/s, per side. A bilateral weakness usually indicates bilateral peripheral vestibular dysfunction.[5] Bilateral weaknesses can be of CNS origin but are usually accompanied by other signs of CNS dysfunction.

Although ENG has correlates with many portions of the physical examination, it is an important part of the evaluation of many patients with complaints of dizziness or balance disturbance. Electronystagmographic testing has a number of advantages: (1) the results of the test are quantified, and there are well-defined normal limits; (2) the bithermal caloric test cannot be done as accurately without the precise stimulus control and response quantification provided by ENG; (3) because ENG provides accurate documentation of results, it can be used to follow the patient with known vestibular disease; (4) standardized documentation is helpful in medical-legal and workers' compensation cases; and (5) it is the only test that assesses each ear separately and can give side-of-lesion localizing information.

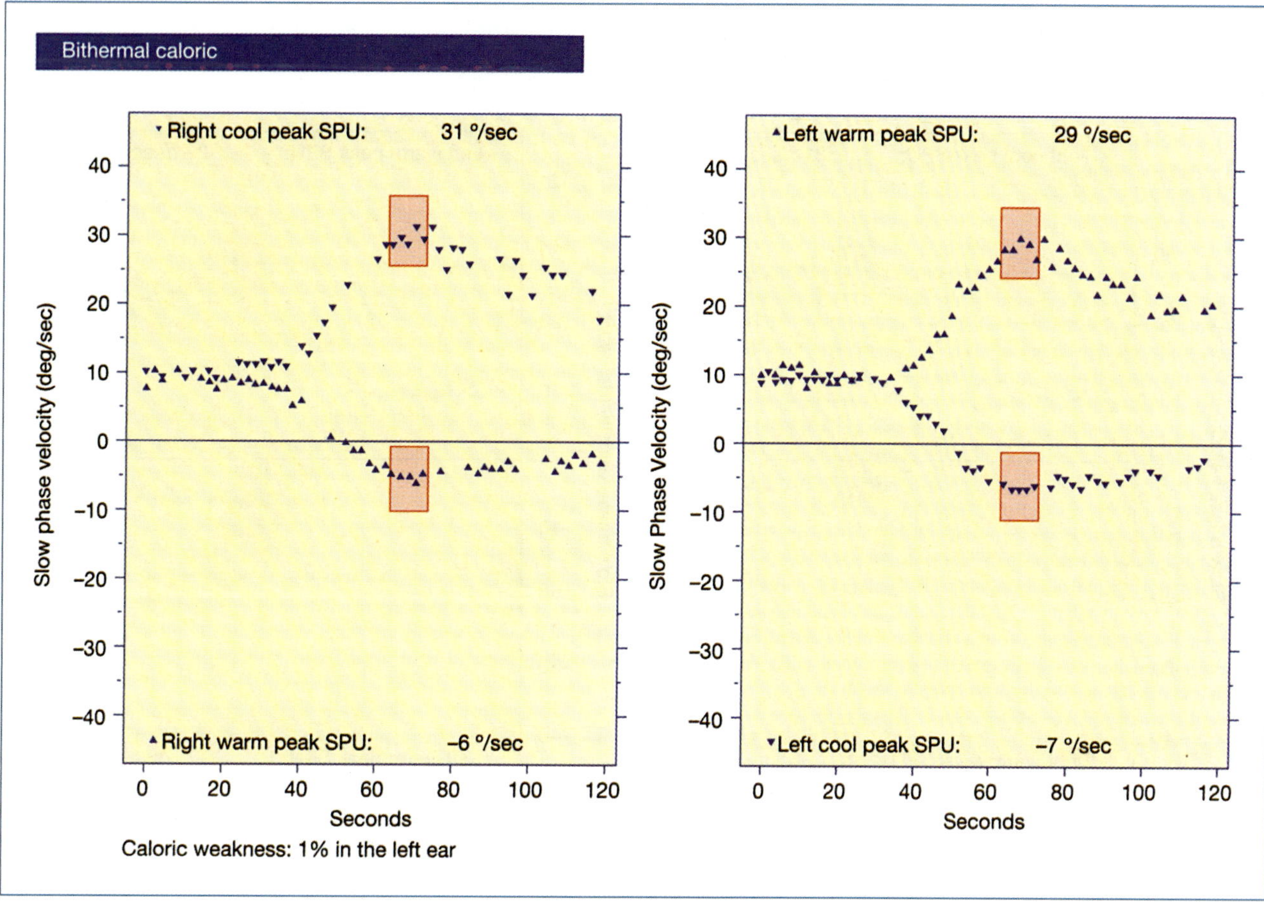

FIGURE 11–10 • Electronystagmographic data 3 days after an acute unilateral vestibular lesion. The patient has spontaneous nystagmus that creates a bias; caloric responses were symmetric about a new baseline corresponding to the slow-phase velocity of this nystagmus. It would be difficult to distinguish between the effects of this bias and a unilateral caloric weakness on the basis of peak slow-phase velocities if only one irrigation temperature were used in the test. When both warm and cool irrigations are used, responses are elicited in both directions, and the sum of the two peak responses is used as the measure of response strength of a particular ear. This cancels the effect of the bias and allows a valid comparison to be made between the two ears.

Limitations

Electronystagmography testing has its limitations. It is important to recognize that ENG tests only the lateral semicircular canal and provides little information about the status of the posterior or superior semicircular canals, utricle, or saccule. Traditional ENG testing using electro-oculography is also relatively insensitive to torsional nystagmus because rotational movement of the eye about the axis of the pupil does not move the cornea with respect to any of the skin electrodes. However, this limitation is easily overcome using VNG.

The results of ENG testing may fluctuate in concordance with the patient's disease process. Two of the more common illnesses seen in our patients are BPPV and Meniere's disease. Both illnesses can be associated with a normal ENG despite "classic" symptomatology. For example, on the day of testing a patient with complaints consistent with BPPV, the response may have been fatigued or the disease may have gone into remission. For that patient, the test results may be normal or indicate a unilateral vestibular weakness on the suspected side. Nevertheless, we maintain clinical suspicion of BPPV and ask the patient to return for retesting on a particularly "dizzy day." Similarly, the patient suspected of having Meniere's disease may have a normal ENG early in the course of the illness, and only later, on a particularly "dizzy day," will the caloric evaluation demonstrate a unilateral peripheral weakness, gaze-evoked nystagmus, or even spontaneous nystagmus. It is best to have patients abstain from vestibular suppressant medications (eg, diazepam) for at least 48 to 72 h prior to ENG testing as they can also cause a "false-negative" test or show abnormal central vestibular function.

Some patients may present with dizziness not related to vestibular system dysfunction, eg, syncope or presyncope, vertebral-basilar insufficiency, migraine-associated dizziness, multiple sclerosis, ocular dizziness, motion sickness syndrome, or cardiovascular disease. In these patients, a unilateral weakness found on ENG does not necessarily implicate vestibular dysfunction as the cause of their symptoms. The ENG finding may be incidental and must be considered in light of the clinical history and physical examination.

Summary

Electronystagmography testing is an important tool in the management of the patient with dizziness. It is by no means a substitute for a thorough neurotologic history and physical examination, and the results should be interpreted in light of

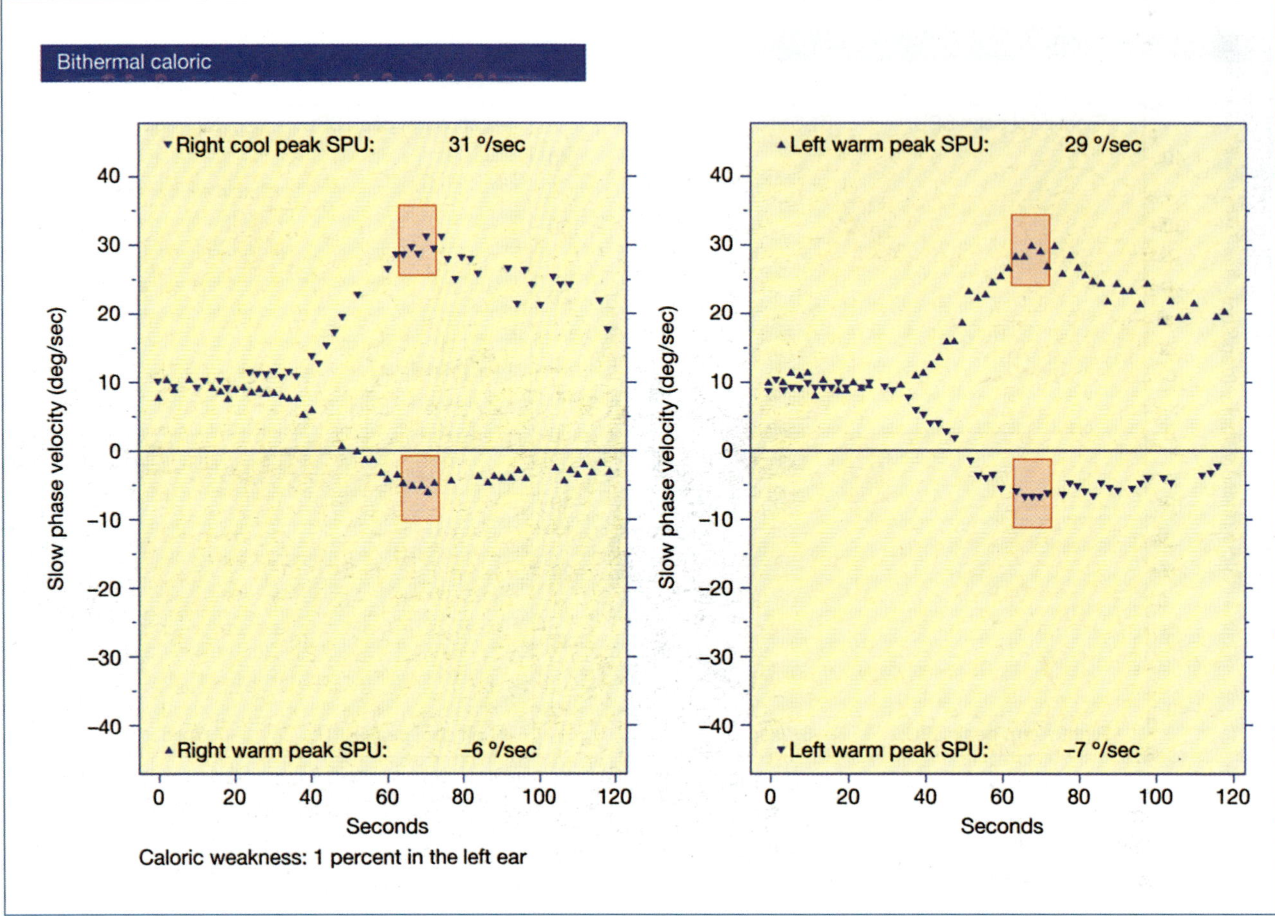

FIGURE 11–11 • Electronystagmographic data for a patient with spontaneous, left-beating nystagmus but no caloric weakness. The spontaneous nystagmus creates a new baseline on which the caloric responses are superimposed. The spontaneous nystagmus cannot be attributed to a recent vestibular lesion since the caloric responses of the two ears are equal. It could have been caused by a lesion within the central vestibular pathways, but other explanations, such as recovery of a previously compensated peripheral lesion, are also possible. Therefore, spontaneous nystagmus that cannot be attributed to a recent vestibular lesion must be regarded as nonlocalizing.

the clinical evaluation. Those who use ENG testing should have a thorough understanding of how the test is performed, what its components are, and the significance of the results. Electronystagmographic test reports should always be evaluated by the clinician with a critical eye. When used properly, ENG is the single most valuable test currently available in the vestibular laboratory.

ROTATIONAL TESTS

Rotational tests have been used to evaluate vestibular function for nearly a century. They provide another method of testing for vestibular disorders that affect the VOR. Rotational tests can be classified as either passive rotational tests, in which the patient's body is rotated without any movement between the head and body, or as active rotational tests, in which the patient rotates his or her own head back and forth while the body remains stationary.

Rotary Chair Test

The rotary chair test (RCT) has proven to be the most useful of the rotational tests.[14,15] It is a passive rotational test in which the patient is seated in a chair so that the axis of rotation is vertical and passes through the center of the head, thus stimulating only the lateral semicircular canals. The base of the chair is bolted to a computer-controlled servomotor that determines the frequency of chair rotation. The patient's head is positioned so that the lateral semicircular canals are in the plane of rotation and is firmly restrained so that it exactly follows body and chair motion (Figure 11–12). Horizontal eye movements are monitored using electro-oculography as in ENG testing.

Testing Paradigms

Rotary chair testing can be performed using various testing paradigms, but the one typically employed is slow harmonic acceleration. In this paradigm, the patient is oscillated in a sinusoidal fashion about a vertical axis at various test frequencies (ranging from 0.01–01.28 Hz). The exact test protocol varies somewhat among laboratories, but oscillation frequencies of 0.01, 0.02, 0.04, 0.08, 0.16, 0.32, and 0.64 Hz, with peak angular velocities of 50 degrees/s at each frequency, are usually used. The patient undergoes multiple cycles of oscillation at each frequency; the oscillations are gradually increased, and the chair is rotated in a

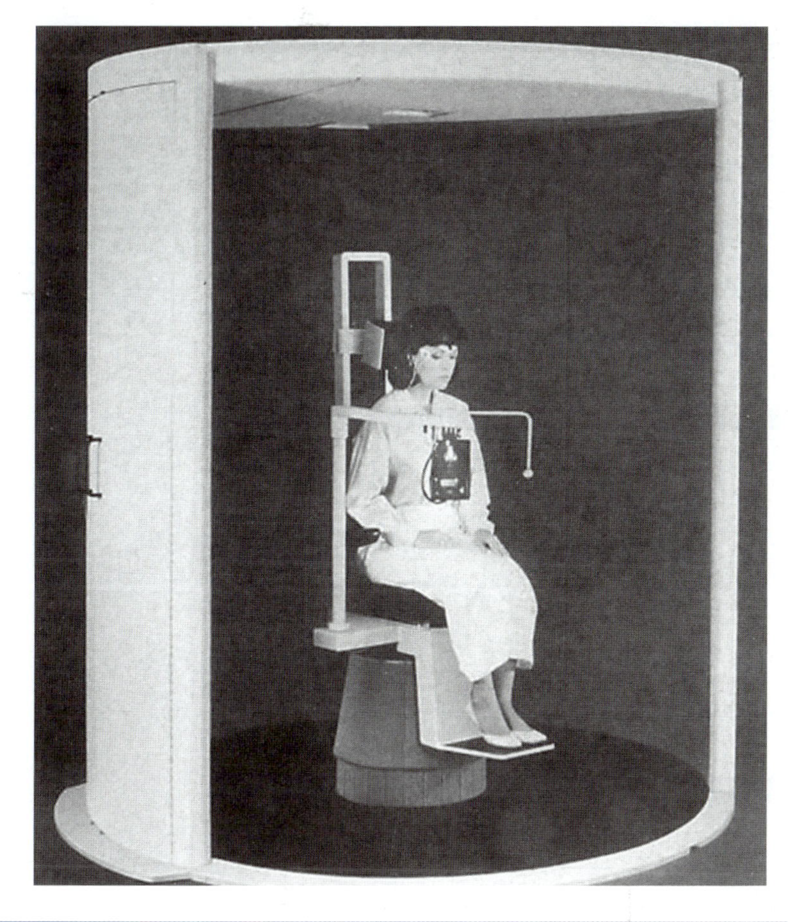

FIGURE 11–12 • Rotational chair testing equipment. The patient is seated in a chair so that the horizontal semicircular canals are in the plane of rotation. Electro-oculography is used to monitor eye movements.

sinusoidal harmonic acceleration paradigm. The stimulus level delivered by the rotary chair is much greater than that delivered in caloric testing, which delivers a stimulus equivalent only to frequencies between 0.002 and 0.004 Hz.

Components of Rotary Chair Testing

Rotary chair testing stimulation generates right-beating nystagmus when the patient is moving rightward and left-beating nystagmus when moving to the left. After testing, the computer differentiates the eye position signal and removes the fast phase of nystagmus, yielding the slow-phase eye velocity. The computer then compares the head velocity and slow-phase eye velocity and calculates three measurements, phase, gain, and symmetry, for each of the test frequencies.

Gain

Gain is defined as the slow eye velocity divided by the head velocity. It is used as an indicator of overall responsiveness of the system. Clinically, a reduction in gain is used to help determine the overall level of function reduction in patients with bilateral vestibular disease.

Phase Angle

The phase angle measures the temporal relationship between eye and head velocities and is measured in degrees. Of the three parameters, phase angle often has the greatest clinical significance. In normal individuals, through the function of the vestibulo-ocular reflex, movement of the head to the right results in deviation of the eyes to the left. If the patient is rotated at a low frequency for a prolonged period of time, eye movement actually precedes the head movement. Increased phase lead implies peripheral vestibular system dysfunction, whereas decreased phase lead may suggest a cerebellar lesion.

Symmetry

Symmetry is the ratio of rightward to leftward slow-phase eye velocity. This parameter gives information as to whether any bias is present in the system, favoring one direction over the other. Asymmetry may result from a peripheral vestibular weakness on the side of the larger slow-phase component or an excitatory lesion of the contralateral labyrinth.

The relationship between head and eye movement during several cycles of sinusoidal oscillation for a normal individual is shown in Figure 11–13. The purpose of the VOR is to produce eye movements that compensate for head movements, and the eye velocity is approximately 180 degrees out of phase with head velocity. When a normal individual is oscillated at low frequencies, slow-phase eye velocities exhibit progressively lower gains and are no longer exactly opposite in phase.[16] Instead, they display progressively larger phase leads, ie, changes in slow-phase eye velocity occur more and more in advance of head velocity. Figure 11–14 shows graphic plots of phase, gain, and symmetry data for a normal individual over the entire range of test frequencies.

The slow harmonic acceleration test shows abnormalities primarily at the lowest and at the highest oscillation frequencies.

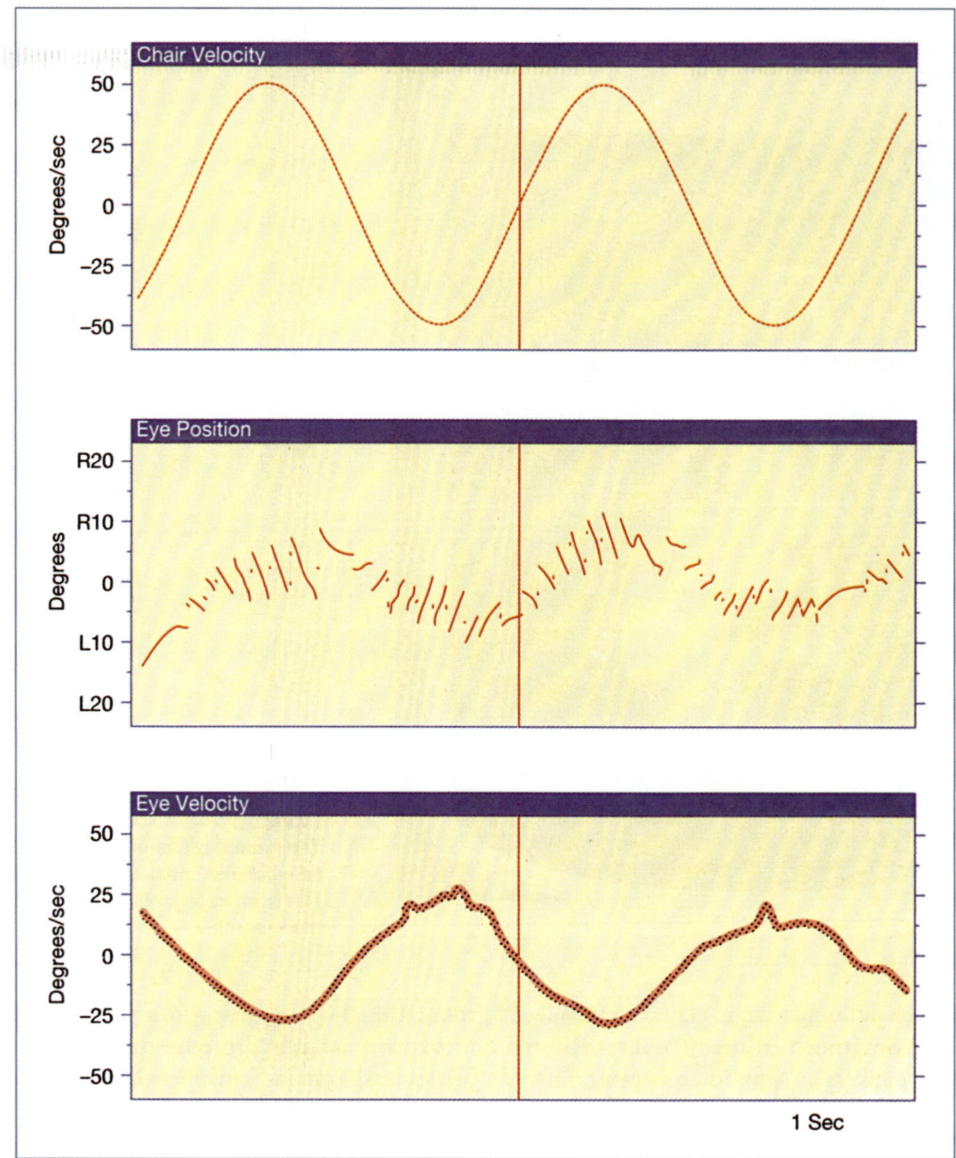

FIGURE 11–13 • Rotary chair test data from a normal individual. The oscillation frequency in this example was 0.16 Hz, near the middle of the test frequency range. Eye movements are 180 degrees out of phase with head movement. The patient had nystagmus with leftward slow phases when their head was moving rightward and nystagmus with rightward slow phases when their head was moving leftward.

Low frequencies reveal abnormal phase leads and gain reductions. High frequencies reveal asymmetries.

In our experience, abnormalities seen on RCT can be classified into four categories: (1) vestibular habituation and asymmetry, (2) vestibular habituation, (3) vestibular deficit, and (4) vestibular asymmetry.

Vestibular habituation and asymmetry—abnormal low-frequency phase leads and high-frequency asymmetry (with the asymmetry always toward the side of the lesion)—is most often seen in patients with acute unilateral peripheral dysfunction. These patients demonstrate the most severe abnormalities. Figure 11–15 shows test results in a patient who underwent the slow harmonic acceleration test shortly after the sudden onset of severe vertigo. Electronystagmography, performed at the same time as RCT, showed left-beating spontaneous nystagmus as well as right reduced caloric responses.

At the lower oscillation frequencies, this patient displayed progressively greater than normal phase leads, which are thought to be caused by a loss of velocity storage normally provided by the central vestibular system to enhance the low-frequency response of the vestibulo-ocular system.[17,18] Loss of velocity storage seems to represent habituation to the strong tonic asymmetry produced by the unilateral peripheral vestibular lesion.[18] Loss of velocity storage is not an exclusive feature of unilateral peripheral vestibular lesions as it is also seen in a variety of vestibular disorders, both peripheral and central, and has also been observed in normal individuals who have undergone prolonged rotation.[19]

This patient also had a rightward asymmetry, ie, nystagmus with rightward slow phases was stronger than nystagmus with leftward slow phases. At low oscillation frequencies, the asymmetry was about equal to the slow-phase velocities of the

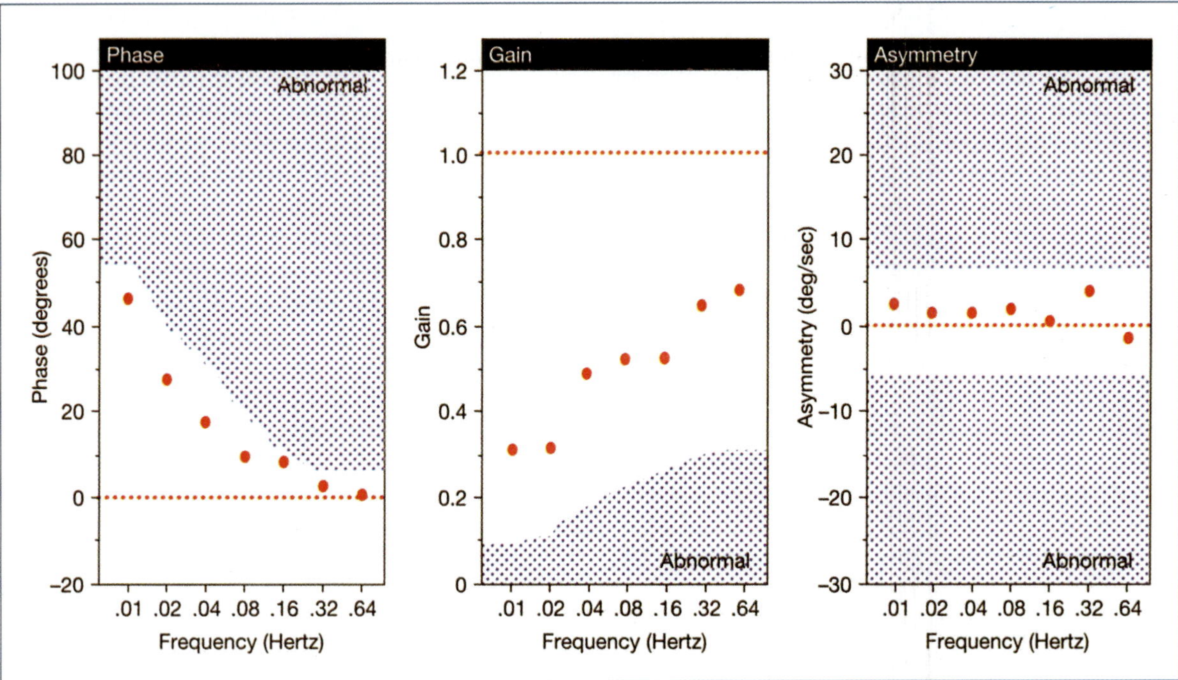

FIGURE 11–14 • Phase, gain, and asymmetry values in relation to oscillation frequency from a normal individual. Note that eye velocity signal is inverted during the analysis so that a phase angle of 180 degrees is expressed as a phase angle of 0 degrees. Phase leads become progressively larger and gains become progressively lower as oscillation frequency decreases. Symmetry values are approximately zero at all frequencies.

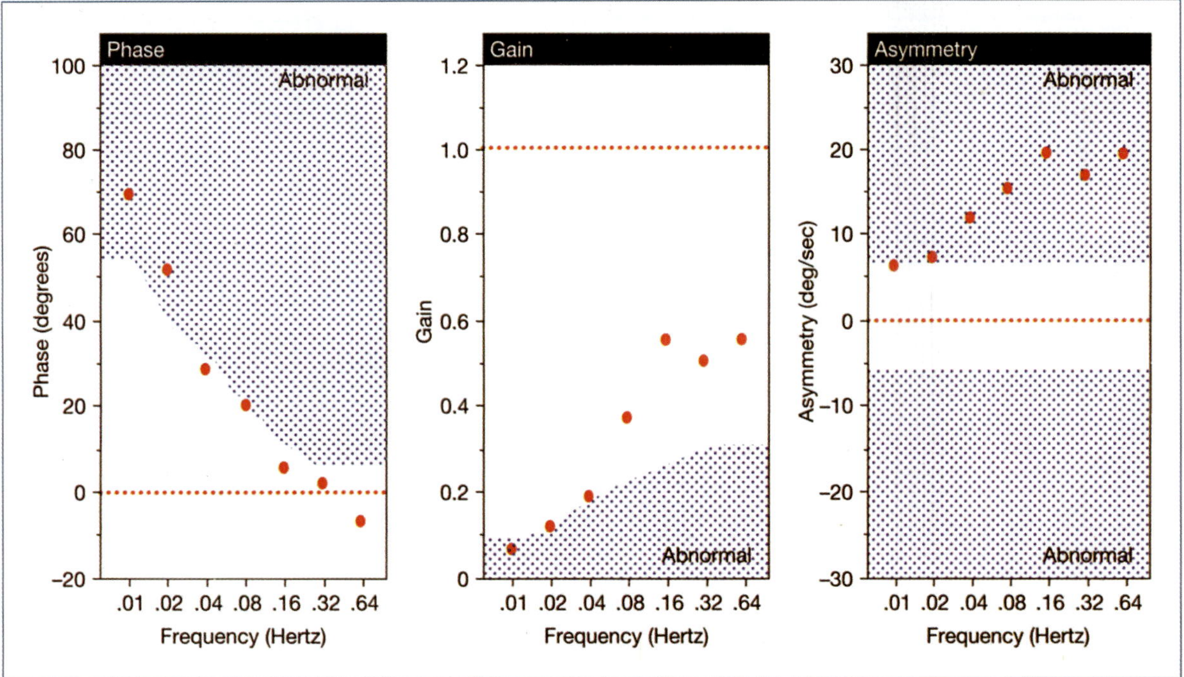

FIGURE 11–15 • Phase, gain, and asymmetry values in relation to oscillation frequency for a patient with an acute right peripheral vestibular lesion. At lower oscillation frequencies, this patient shows progressively greater than normal phase leads. The patient also has a rightward asymmetry. This response pattern—abnormal low-frequency phase leads and high-frequency asymmetry—is routinely observed in patients with acute unilateral vestibular loss. The asymmetry is always toward the side of the loss.

patient's spontaneous nystagmus with eyes closed, but at higher frequencies, the asymmetry was greater than could be accounted for by this bias. This additional asymmetry is thought to be attributable to either saturation of inhibitory responses of the intact labyrinth during rotation toward the side of the lesion or an asymmetric loss of velocity storage.[20]

Vestibular habituation is the most common abnormality found on RCT and consists solely of abnormally large phase leads at the lower oscillation frequencies. This abnormality is often seen in patients with a chronic, unilateral peripheral vestibular lesion. An example is seen in Figure 11–16 from a patient with a right vestibular schwannoma.

This response pattern—abnormal low-frequency phase leads—is by far the most common abnormality seen in the slow sinusoidal rotation test. Stockwell reported abnormal low-frequency phase leads as the sole abnormality on the slow harmonic acceleration test in 109 of 305 patients with dizziness.[21] Twenty-seven of these patients (eight with a diagnosis of unilateral Meniere's disease and the rest with a variety of diagnoses) showed no abnormality on ENG. Fifty-five of the 305 patients showed evidence of a chronic unilateral peripheral vestibular lesion, ie, a significant unilateral caloric weakness without significant spontaneous nystagmus, and most were diagnosed as having either Meniere's disease or a vestibular schwannoma. The reduction in vestibular caloric response in these patients was nearly always greater than 50%. Patients with a unilateral caloric weakness of less than 50% generally did not have abnormal phase leads. The remaining 27 patients showed a variety of abnormalities on ENG, mostly consistent with either CNS dysfunction or a combination of abnormalities.

The third abnormality, vestibular deficit, is relatively uncommon. The slow harmonic acceleration test reveals abnormalities in patients with bilateral loss of vestibular function. RCT has particular significance in cases of bilateral reduced or absent caloric responses. If rotatory chair responses are also diminished in these patients, then the findings provide a strong indication of bilateral vestibular hypofunction An example is shown in Figure 11–17 of a patient with bilateral absence of caloric response of unknown origin. Rotary chair testing confirmed the bilateral caloric loss. The patient failed to show a definite nystagmus response at any oscillation frequency. Some patients with bilaterally absent caloric responses show absent or reduced response gains at the lower oscillation frequencies but normal gains at the highest frequencies. An example is shown in Figure 11–18 of a patient who developed unsteadiness following a course of gentamicin therapy and showed a bilateral absence of caloric response. Baloh and colleagues reported that randomized controlled trial (RCT) often demonstrates normal vestibular function at high frequencies even when ice water irrigations have failed to provoke a response from either ear.[22] In these cases, the results of caloric and rotation tests are not contradictory because the caloric response is a response to a low-frequency stimulus and therefore should be similar to responses to low-frequency rotational stimuli. However, in

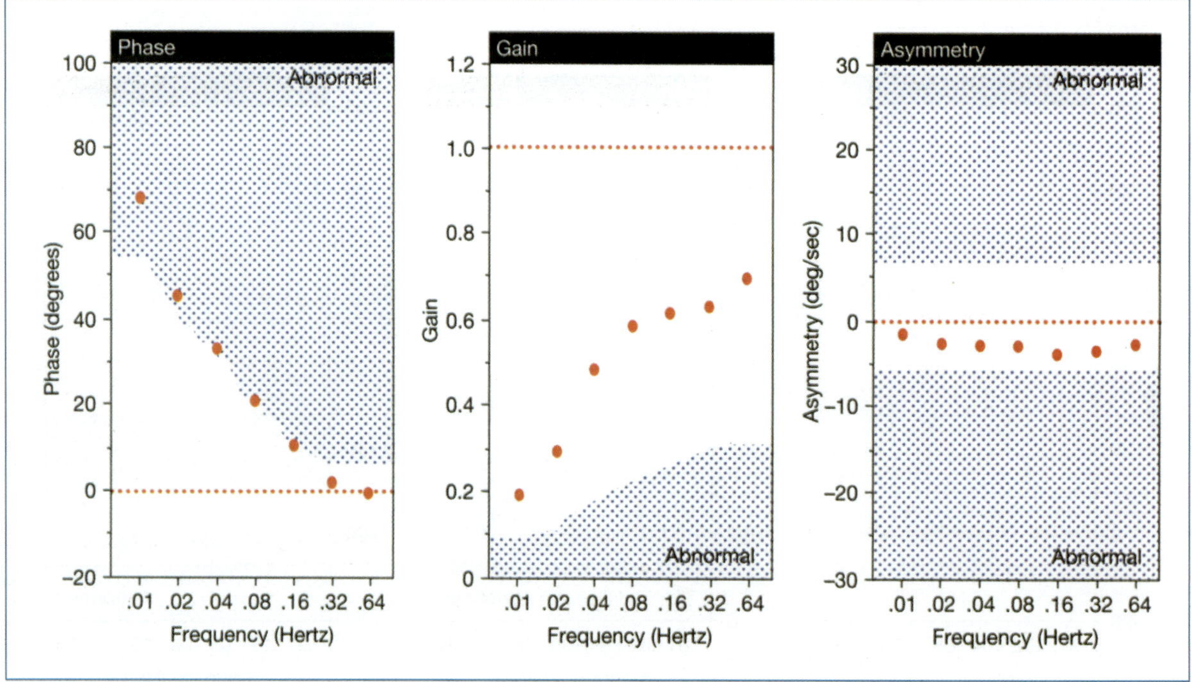

FIGURE 11–16 • Phase, gain, and asymmetry values in relation to oscillation frequency for a patient with a chronic left peripheral vestibular lesion (vestibular schwannoma). Electronystagmography showed a severe right caloric weakness. The rotational chair test shows greater than normal phase leads at lower test frequencies, reflecting a loss of velocity storage. This loss can be persistent, remaining for years following vestibular malfunction, although there is nearly always some recovery. The absence of tonic asymmetry in this individual illustrates the effect of vestibular compensation. If a peripheral vestibular lesion develops slowly, compensation is able to gradually rebalance the asymmetric input, preventing the vertigo and spontaneous nystagmus that would otherwise occur. Even when lesions develop suddenly, compensation quickly rebalances the tonic asymmetry over a period of days.

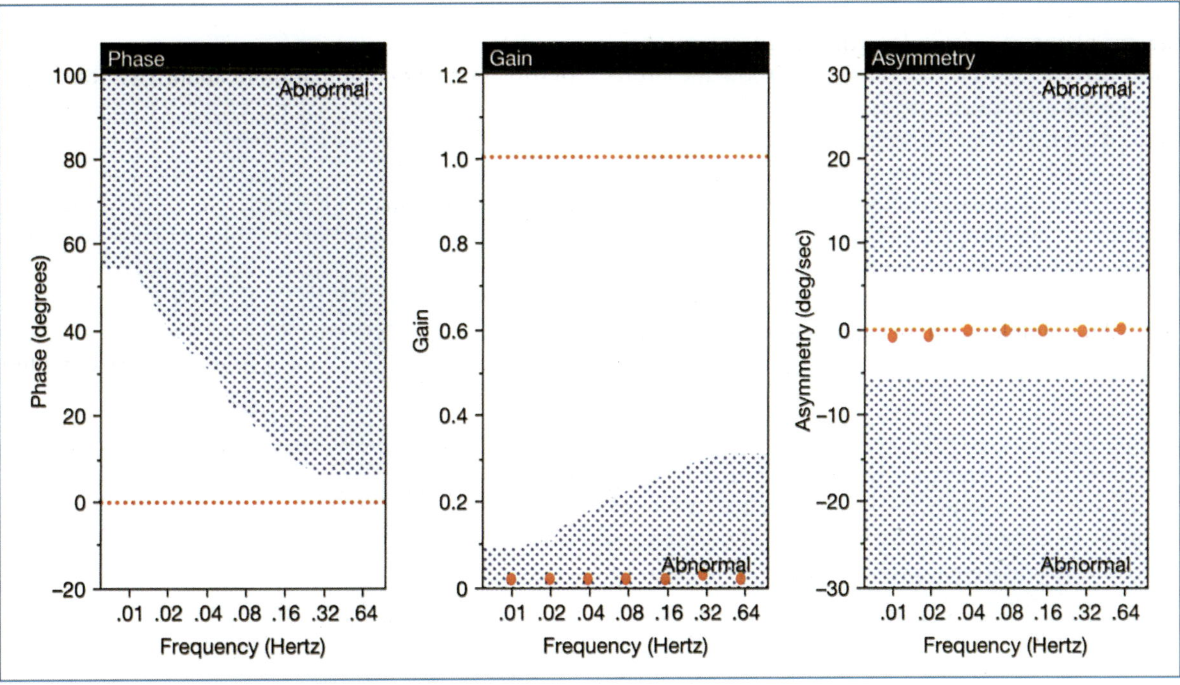

FIGURE 11–17 • Phase, gain, and asymmetry values in relation to oscillation frequency for a patient with bilateral absence of caloric responses, showing absent responses at all oscillation frequencies. Phase values were not plotted owing to low response gains.

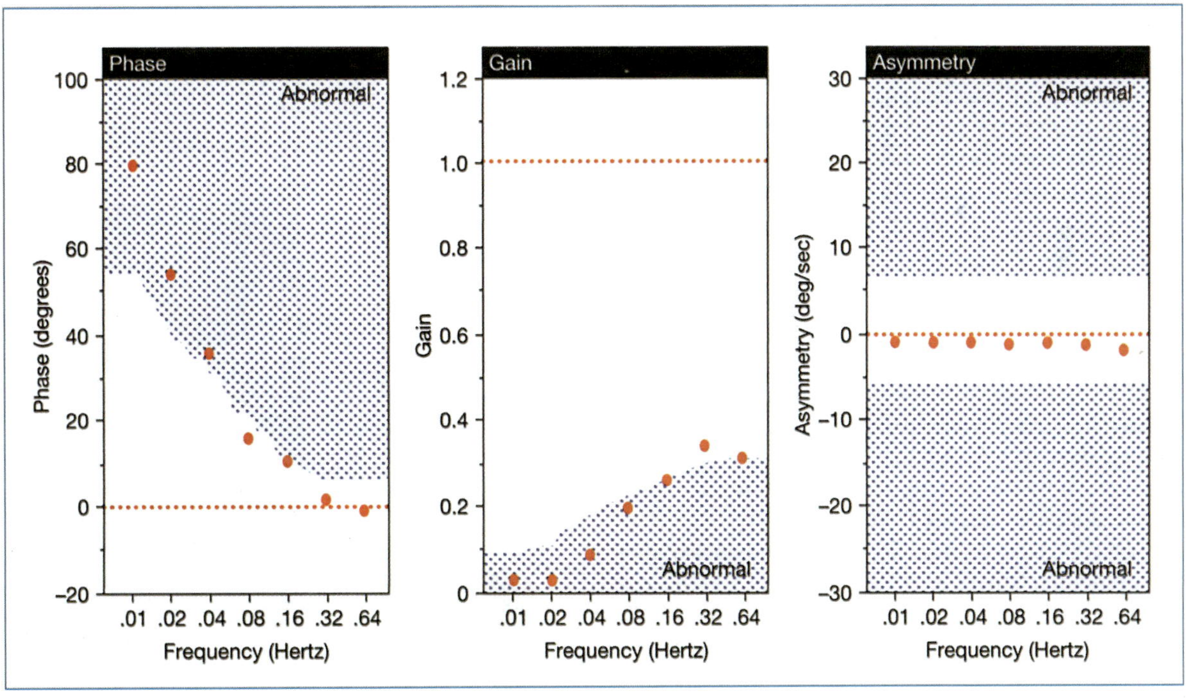

FIGURE 11–18 • Phase, gain, and asymmetry values in relation to oscillation frequencies for a patient with bilateral absence of caloric responses, showing normal response gains at the higher frequencies.

other cases, RCT shows normal response gains at all frequencies, despite absent caloric responses, indicating a false-positive caloric test result.[23] Clearly, the slow harmonic acceleration test is the procedure of choice in evaluating patients suspected of having bilateral loss of vestibular function because the caloric test, even with ice water, does not define the extent of the loss and sometimes yields false-positive results.

The final abnormality is vestibular asymmetry, which is characterized by an asymmetry at high frequencies. It is similar to the high-frequency asymmetry seen in patients with acute unilateral peripheral lesions, which we have attributed to low firing rates of central vestibular neurons. However, these patients have chronic complaints and do not show the spontaneous nystagmus and low-frequency phase leads of patients with acute peripheral lesions. We suspect that vestibular asymmetry reflects a central vestibular disorder because several patients have shown clear concomitant evidence of CNS dysfunction, but we do not have enough numbers to justify making a firm statement regarding the clinical significance of this finding.

Clinical Indications for Rotational Chair Testing

Rotational chair testing stimulates both peripheral vestibular systems simultaneously; however, it may be helpful in determining the site of lesion in certain disorders. Shepard makes some suggestions as to when chair testing may be helpful in patient evaluation.[24] First, when the ENG is normal and oculomotor results are either normal or observed abnormalities would not invalidate rotational chair results, RCT is used to expand the assessment of peripheral system dysfunction and status of compensation. Second, when the ENG suggests a well-compensated state, despite the presence of a clinically significant unilateral caloric weakness and active symptomatology, RCT is used to expand the investigation of compensation in a patient with a known lesion site and complaints suggesting poor compensation. Third, when the caloric irrigations are below 12 degrees/s bilaterally, when caloric irrigations cannot be performed, or when results in the two ears may not be compared reliably because of anatomic variability, RCT is used to verify the presence, and define the extent, of a bilateral weakness or to investigate further the relative responsiveness of the peripheral vestibular apparatus in each ear when caloric studies are unreliable or unavailable. Lastly, RCT may be beneficial when a baseline measure is needed to follow the natural history of the patient's disorder (eg, possible early Meniere's disease) or to assess the effectiveness of a particular treatment (such as chemical ablation).

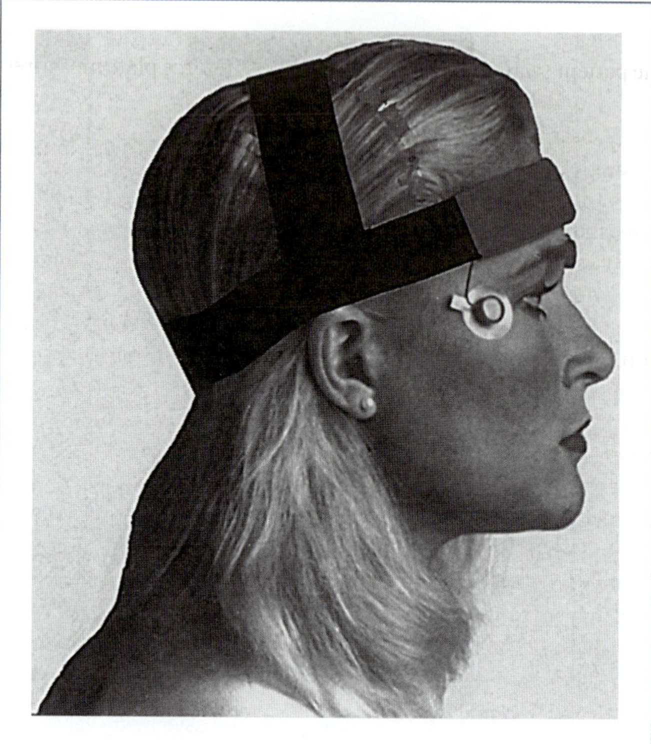

FIGURE 11–19 • Vestibular autorotational equipment. A portable computer is connected to an instrumented head strap containing a head velocity sensor. Active head oscillations are performed by the subject at frequencies from 2 to 6 Hz.

Vestibular Autorotational Testing

Vestibular autorotational testing is an active rotation test in which the patient actively shakes his/her head from side to side with increasing frequency. An angular sensor is fixed to a headband which is worn by the patient, and the eyes are evaluated with electro-oculography (Figure 11–19).

Advantages of VAT over the other tests include portability of testing equipment, relatively brief (18 sec) duration of the test, and ability to test high-frequency (2–6 kHz) oscillations (when the VOR is active).

POSTUROGRAPHY

Posturography is a quantitative balance test that assesses standing balance function under a variety of conditions. It is often performed on a computerized testing device, called the Equitest™ (manufactured by Neurocom International, Inc, Portland, Oregon) (Figure 11–20). This device consists of a platform that is capable of moving back and forth and tilting in the pitch plane about an axis colinear with the patient's ankle joints. During the test, the patient stands independently on the

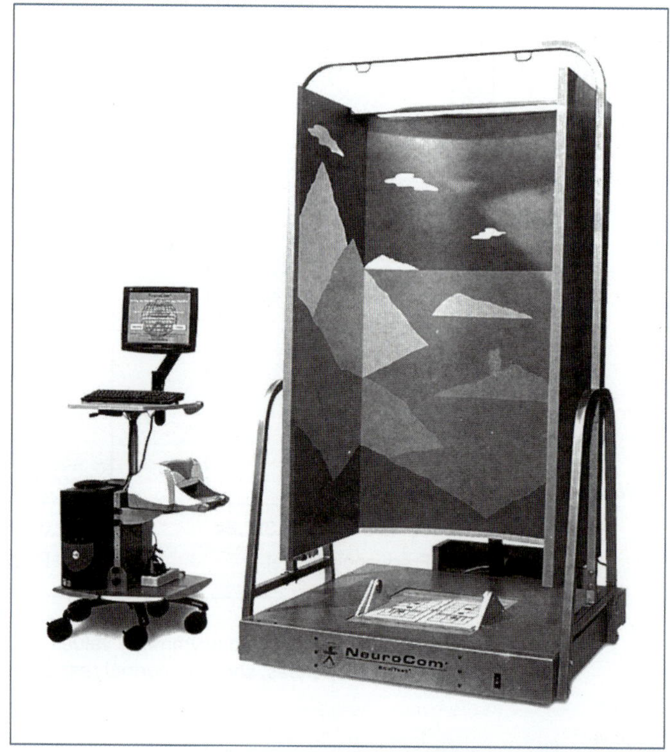

FIGURE 11–20 • Computerized dynamic posturography equipment. The subject stands on a computer-driven platform containing a force plate. Various testing paradigms are performed in which the platform and/or the visual surround can be either stationary or moved. A safety harness is worn at all times.

platform, wearing a harness for safety and facing a visual screen that is capable of tilting about the same axis as the platform. As the patient sways on the platform, a built-in force plate measures the changes in the position of the patient's center of gravity. These data are transmitted to the computer, which calculates the angle of the body sway in the pitch plane.

Computerized Dynamic Posturography with the Equitest™ consists of two tests: the sensory organization test and the movement coordination test. Of the two, the sensory organization test is the more useful in the evaluation of patients with dizziness because it is designed primarily to test vestibular function. In the sensory organization test, the patient's postural stability is evaluated under six conditions in which either visual or proprioceptive cues (or both) are denied. Normally, individuals maintain their balance by integrating visual and somatosensory cues. The visual cues can be disrupted in one of two ways: visual input can be denied (by blindfolding) or visual cues can be disrupted by sway-referencing the surroundings. Normal subjects ignore inaccurate sway-referenced visual input, relying on other information to maintain balance.[25,26]

The six test conditions in the sensory organization test are as follows:

1. Support fixed, eyes open, visual fixed
2. Support fixed, eyes closed, visual fixed
3. Support fixed, eyes open, visual sway-referenced
4. Support swayed, eyes open, visual fixed
5. Support swayed, eyes closed, visual fixed
6. Support swayed, eyes open, visual sway-referenced

The patient is subjected to each test condition three times, and an equilibrium score is calculated for each condition. The equilibrium score compares the patient's sway in the anteroposterior direction, compared to the theoretical limits of anteroposterior sway. A score of 100% implies little sway, and lower scores correspond to greater amounts of sway. The differences in scores for the six conditions are then analyzed to determine the specific nature of the patient's balance disorder. Of particular interest is the vestibular ratio, which compares conditions 1 and 5 and delineates the reduction in stability when visual and somatosensory inputs are disrupted. Although healthy subjects sway a little in condition 5, those with vestibular disease score poorer than average. An example of such a posturography test is shown in Figure 11–21.

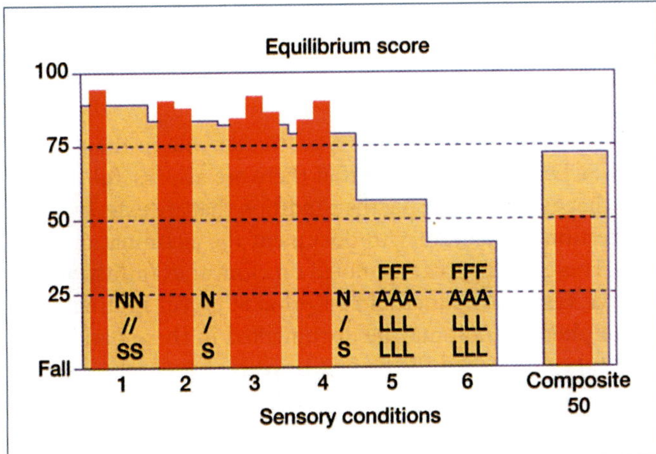

FIGURE 11–21 • Posturography test of a patient with total bilateral loss of vestibular function owing to ototoxicity. He has normal postural stability when tested under conditions 1 through 4 but marked instability on conditions 5 and 6, in which he had to rely solely on vestibular cues. This type of result may be seen in patients with acute unilateral peripheral vestibular lesions. Only rarely is it seen in patients with chronic unilateral vestibular dysfunction.

Posturography may be helpful in evaluating patients with balance disorders in whom the history and physical examination do not suggest any apparent etiology. In this regard, it is occasionally ordered for patients with vague symptoms of dizziness and unsteadiness, without vertigo. It can also be used to detect malingerers, who will tend to exaggerate their symptoms, thus producing results that are inconsistent with those seen in patients with true vestibular dysfunction. More than a diagnostic tool, it can also be used to evaluate how patients with known balance problems are progressing in terms of compensation and return to health.

VESTIBULAR EVOKED MYOGENIC POTENTIAL TESTING

Vestibular evoked myogenic potential (VEMP) testing is the newest method of assessing the vestibular system. It has only recently become available for clinical use and requires that each laboratory establish normative data. It can be very useful in testing a portion of the vestibular system that no other test measures. VEMP testing is the only commonly used electrophysiological test of the inferior vestibular nerve. The VEMP test uses an intense sound stimulus to stimulate the sacculus, one of the otolith organs in the inner ear, which evokes a response via the inferior vestibular nerve. A vestibulospinal response with relaxation in the ipsilateral sternocleidomastoid muscle is measured as a change in activity recorded on the electromyogram (EMG). The VEMP response provides information by comparing the left side to the right side, or by a change in certain parameters of the response (latency, stimulus threshold). The most commonly employed muscle in VEMP testing today is the sternocleidomastoid (SCM) muscle because the response at this muscle is robust and reliable using skin surface EMG electrode technology currently available.

The presence of the VEMP recording is dependent on the contraction of the muscle being monitored, so the test is performed by having the patient contract the muscle first, and then a loud (90–100 dB) repeating click or tone burst is delivered for 30 sec to the ear being tested. In our laboratory we primarily use a head lift protocol, in which patients are in the supine position, lying flat, and are instructed to lift the head 2 inches off the examination table and keep it lifted without sitting up or lifting the shoulders, thereby activating the SCM muscles bilaterally (Figure 11–22). If a patient is unable to perform a head lift maneuver, a head turn protocol is used (Figure 11–23). In this case, the patient is seated and instructed to turn the head sharply to the one side and keep turning the head without moving the trunk, thereby

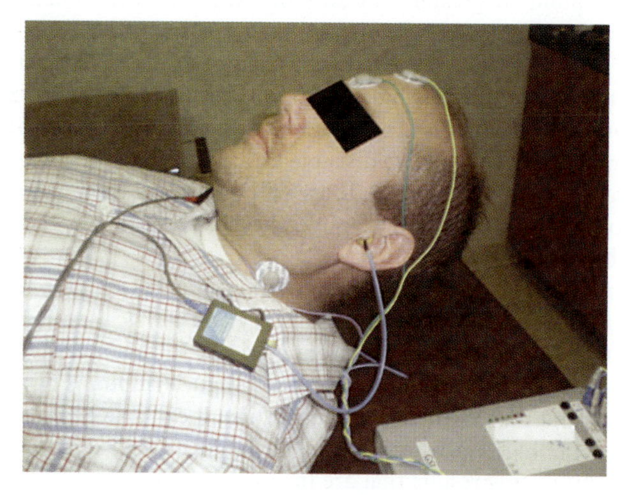

FIGURE 11–22 • VEMP testing is performed by having the patient elevate his or her head by about 30 degrees up from the examination table. Elevation of the head places the sternocleidomastoid muscle under contraction, thereby enabling the relaxation potentials associated with the VEMP response to be recorded.

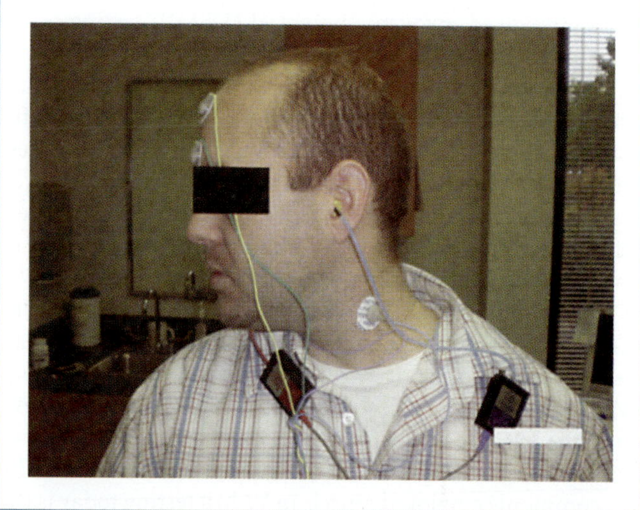

FIGURE 11–23 • In patients who are unable to maintain elevation of their head during VEMP testing, the head can be turned away from the ear being tested.

activating the SCM muscle on the opposite side to the direction of the head turn.

After the sound is presented, the EMG tracing shows a sharp biphasic deflection in its baseline tracing, reflecting a modulation of the EMG activity. An example of a normal VEMP tracing is shown in Figure 11–24. The first peak created by this wave is labeled P_1 (positive deflection) and the next peak is called N_1 (negative deflection). The peaks occur at predictable latencies in the normal patient: P_1 at 12 to 16 milliseconds and N_1 at 22 to 24 milliseconds. Latency and amplitude of the wave are the most commonly used parameters today. The threshold is more time-consuming and laborious to determine, but it can be very useful in identifying certain disorders. The amplitude of the wave (P_1 to N_1) generated by left ear stimulation is compared to the amplitude generated by right ear stimulation because the absolute amplitude varies significantly between individuals, but within subject asymmetry is minimal in the normal condition. An interaural asymmetry ratio (AR) is calculated and this determines whether one side is abnormally weak. The ratio is calculated by dividing the difference of the averages (usually two recordings are done per side and are averaged) of each side by the sum of the averages from both sides: $AR = (A_L - A_R) / (A_L + A_R) \times 100$. This formula is analogous to Jongkee's formula, which used to calculate unilateral weakness in ENG caloric testing. Since there is no standard AR that establishes abnormal, laboratories should establish normative data and consider using two standard deviations above and below as abnormal. In our laboratory, we consider a 30% difference significant. Figure 11–25 shows a unilateral weak response that can be clearly seen by the difference in amplitudes between left and right sides.

A significantly decreased amplitude on one side (AR > Amplitude ± 2SD), has been correlated with peripheral vestibular dysfunction from paretic lesions such as vestibular neuronitis, Meniere's disease, acoustic neuroma, and intratympanic gentamicin therapy.[27] An increased amplitude is seen in peripheral vestibular dysfunction from irritative lesions such as Meniere's disease (recovery phase) and superior canal dehiscence syndrome (SCDS).[28] The VEMP test is particularly useful in the diagnosis of SCDS. Patients with SCDS typically have a lower than normal VEMP threshold and elevated amplitude of VEMP responses in the affected ear. Increased latency of P_1 and N_1 has been associated with central vestibular dysfunction. Once again, the absolute value of what constitutes an increased latency should be established by each laboratory based on normative data. In our laboratory, we consider a latency of P_1 greater than 17 milliseconds abnormal and suggestive of central vestibular dysfunction. Although the VEMP test is new, it shows promise and provides an important window into inner ear function in the normal and abnormal state.

Since the VEMP test has a particular role in the diagnosis of SCDS, we should note that there are also useful bedside tests that aid in diagnosing the condition that are extended into the vestibular laboratory to document the examination findings. These findings can be noted on clinical examination and tests of vestibular function can provide useful findings. The Tullio phenomenon may be documented in these patients on physical exam (when the patient is wearing Frenzel goggles to prevent fixation) as well as with VNG recording. When a loud tone (using an audiometer) is presented to the patient, nystagmus may be recorded (Figure 11–26). Patients with SCDS will demonstrate a vertical-torsional nystagmus as long as the tone sounds. The plane of the eye movement in this nystagmus aligns with the plane of the affected superior canal. These patients may also display Hennebert's sign, vertigo, and nystagmus with motion of the tympanic membrane, and Valsalva-induced vestibular symptoms and nystagmus.

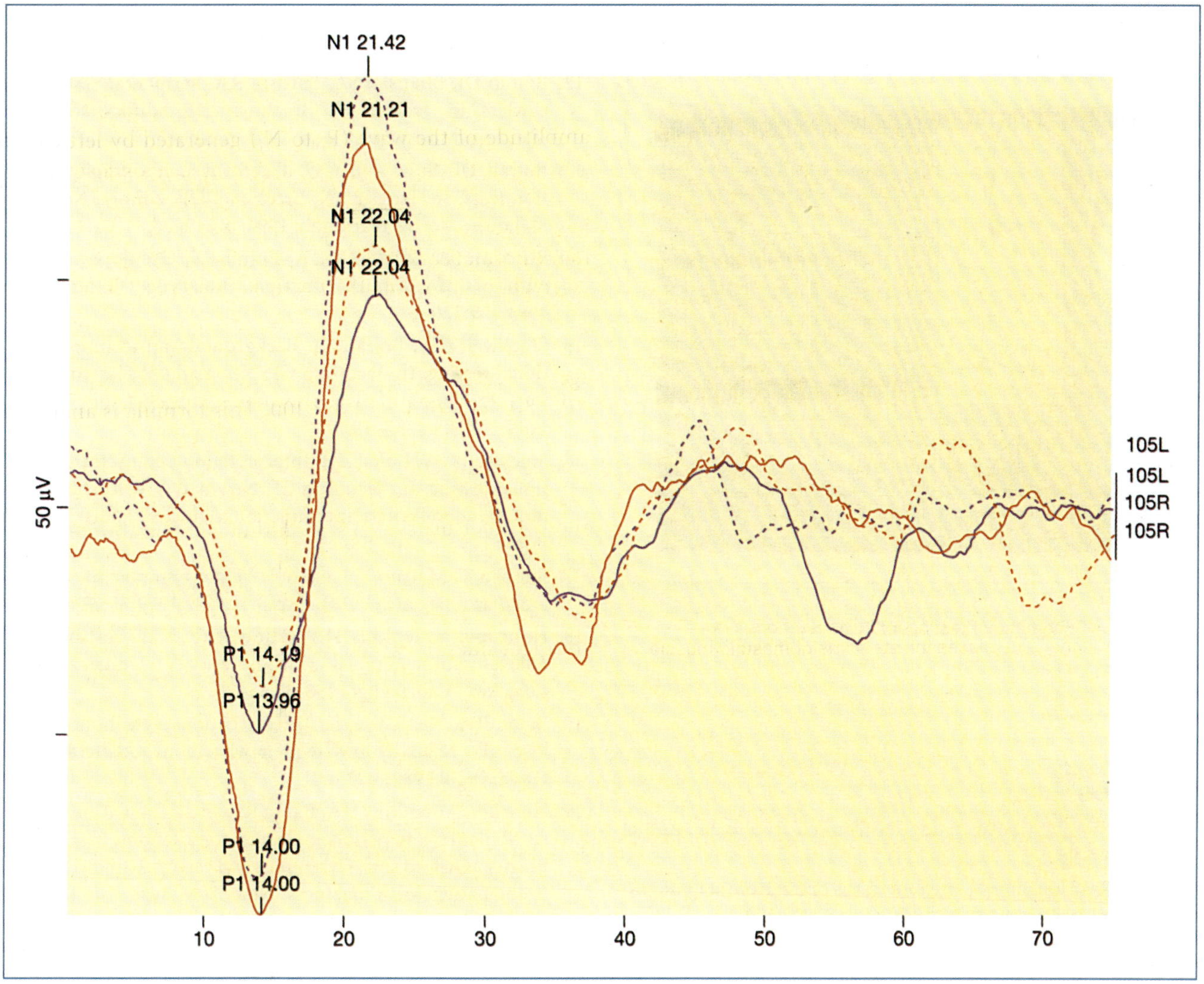

FIGURE 11–24 • A normal VEMP response consists of a biphasic waveform with the first wave (P1) reaching a peak approximately 13 to 14 milliseconds after the onset of the tone stimulus and the second peak (N1) reaching a peak approximately 21 to 23 milliseconds after the onset of the tone.

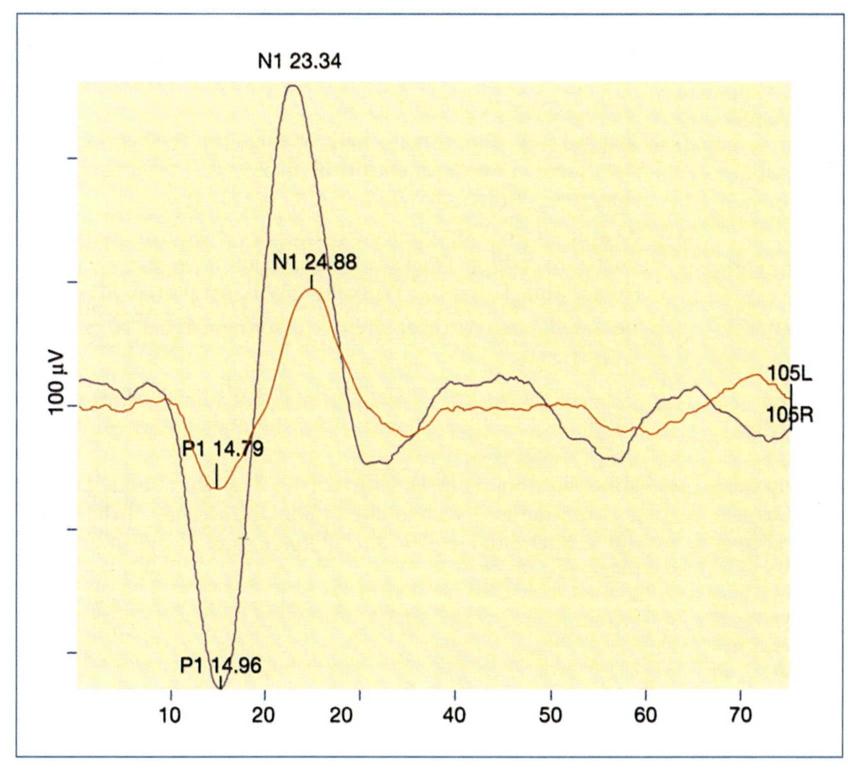

FIGURE 11–25 • Unilateral weakness for responses to the right VEMP stimulus is demonstrated in this figure.

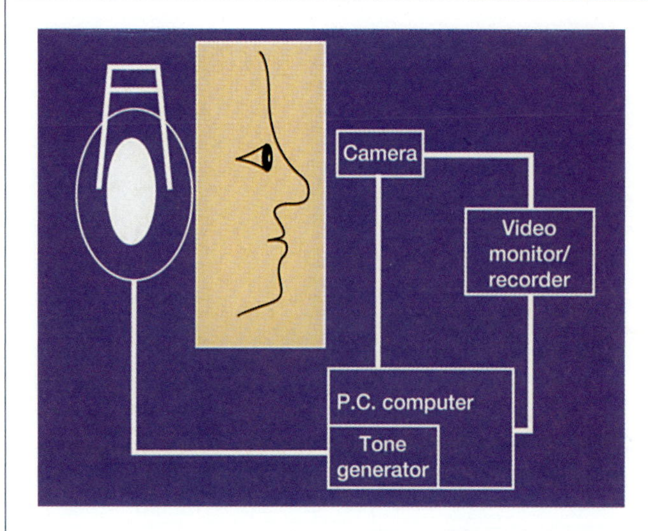

FIGURE 11–26 • Schematic of testing for Tullio phenomenon.

References

1. Stockwell CW. Vestibular testing: Past, present, future. Br J Audiol 1997;31:387–98.
2. Bhansali SA, Honrubia V. Current status of electronystagmography testing. Otolaryngol Head Neck Surg 1999;120:419–26.
3. Baloh RW, Honrubia V. Clinical neurophysiology of the vestibular system. Philadelphia: FA Davis; 1990.
4. Leigh RJ, Zee DS. The neurology of eye movements. Philadelphia: FA Davis; 1991.
5. Barber HO, Stockwell CW. Manual of electronystagmography. 2nd ed. St. Louis: CV Mosby; 1980.
6. Baloh RW, Honrubia V, Konrad HR. Ewald's second law reevaluated. Acta Otolaryngol (Stockh) 1977;83:474–9.
7. Baloh RW, Honrubia V, Jacobson K. Benign positional vertigo: Clinical and oculographic features in 240 cases. Neurology 1987;37:371–8.
8. Baloh RW, Yue O, Jacobson KM, Honrubia V. Persistent direction-changing positional nystagmus: Another variant of benign positional nystagmus? Neurology 1995;45:1297–301.
9. Bojrab DI, Bhansali SA. Objective evaluation of a patient with dizziness. In: Canalis RF, Lambert PR, editors. The ear—Comprehensive otology. Philadelphia: Lippincott, Williams & Wilkins; 2000. p. 181–96.
10. Baloh RW, Jacobson K, Honrubia V. Horizontal semicircular canal variant of benign positional vertigo. Neurology 1993;43:2542–9.
11. Jacobson GP, Newman CW, Peterson EL. Interpretation and usefulness of caloric testing. In: Jacobson GP, Newman CW, Kartush JM, editors. Handbook of balance function testing. San Diego: Singular; 1997. p. 193–234.
12. Bojrab DI, Bhansali SA, Battista RA. Peripheral vestibular discorders. In: Jackler RK, Brackman DE, editors. Neurotology. St. Louis: Mosby-Year Book; 1994. p. 629–50.
13. Bojrab DI, Stockwell CW. Electronystagmography and rotation tests. In: Jackler RK, Brackman DE, editors. Neurotology. St. Louis: Mosby-Year Book; 1994. p. 219–28.
14. Bhansali SA, Stockwell CW, Bojrab DI. Oscillopsia in patients with loss of vestibular function. Otolaryngol Head Neck Surg 1993;109:120–5.
15. Stockwell CW, Bojrab DI. Background and technique of rotational testing. In: Jacobson GP, Newman CW, Kartush JM, editors. Handbook of balance function testing. St. Louis: Mosby-Year Book; 1993. p. 237–48.
16. Stockwell CW, Bojrab DI. Interpretation and usefulness of rotational testing. In: Jacobson GP, Newman CW, Kartush JM, editors. Handbook of balance function testing. St. Louis: Mosby-Year Book; 1993. p. 249–58.
17. Raphan T, Matsuo V, Cohen B. Velocity storage in the vestibuloocular reflex arc (VOR). Exp Brain Res 1979;35:229–48.
18. Honrubia V, Jenkins HA, Balon RW, et al. Vestibulo-ocular reflexes in peripheral labyrinthine lesions: I. Unilateral dysfunction. Am J Otolaryngol 1984;5:15–26.
19. Baloh RW, Henn V, Jager J. Habituation of the human vestibulo-ocular reflex by low frequency harmonic acceleration. Am J Otolaryngol 1982;3:235–41.
20. Honrubia V, Jenkins HA, Balon RW, et al. Evaluation of rotatory vestibular tests in peripheral labyrinthine lesions. In: Honrubia V, Brazier MAB, editors. Nystagmus and vertigo. Clinical approaches to the patient with dizziness. New York: Academic Press; 1982. p. 57–78.
21. Stockwell CW. Vestibular function testing: 4-year update. In: Cummings CW, Harker, Kralee, et al, editors. Otolaryngology-head and neck surgery: Update II. St. Louis: Mosby-Year Book; 1989. p. 39–53.
22. Baloh RW, Honrubia V, Yee RD, et al. Changes in the human vestibulo-ocular reflex after loss of peripheral sensitivity. Ann Neurol 1984;16:222–8.
23. Baloh RW, Sills AW, Honrubia V. Impulsive and sinusoidal rotatory testing: A comparison with results of caloric testing. Laryngoscope 1979;89:646–54.
24. Shepard NT. Rotational chair testing. In: Goebel JA, editor. Practical management of the dizzy patient. Philadelphia: Lippincott Williams & Wilkins; 2001. p. 129–41.
25. Nashner LM. Computerized dynamic posturography. In: Goebel JA, editor. Practical management of the dizzy patient. Philadelphia: Lippincott Williams & Wilkins; 2001. p. 143–70.
26. Stockwell CW. Posturography. Otolaryngol Head Neck Surg 1981;89:333–5.
27. Welgampola MS, Colebatch JG. Characteristics and clinical applications of vestibular-evoked myogenic potentials. Neurology 2005;64:1682–88.
28. Minor LB, Solomon D, Zinreich JS, Zee DS. Sound- and/or pressure-induced vertigo due to bone dehiscence of the superior semicircular canal. Arch Otolaryngol Head Neck Surg 1998;124:249–58.

Endoscopic Diagnosis and Surgery of Eustachian Tube Dysfunction 12

Dennis S. Poe, MD, FACS / Quinton Gopen, MD

The Eustachian tube is a dynamic conduit connecting the middle ear with the nasopharynx. It performs the critical roles of aeration and drainage of the middle ear space and protects the middle ear from reflux of sound and material from the nasopharynx. Proper function of this tubular organ's secretory, ciliary, and dilatory actions is required for optimal conduction of sound through the middle ear cavity. This chapter will review the anatomy, physiology of dilation, and pathophysiology of the Eustachian tube and present updates in the medical and surgical treatments of dysfunctional and patulous conditions.

HISTORY

The Eustachian tube was first mentioned by Alcmaeon of Sparta in 400 BC,[1] but Bartolomeus Eustachius is credited with its discovery in 1562 when he published a detailed description of its anatomy and physiologic function.[2] Valsalva later described the Eustachian tube as having cartilaginous and osseous parts and was the first to recognize the importance of the tensor veli palatini muscle in opening the Eustachian tube.[3] He also described the Valsalva maneuver, which remains clinically relevant to this day. Toynbee furthered our understanding of the Eustachian tube through extensive investigations of the peritubal muscles[4] and Politzer made important contributions in connecting the role of the Eustachian tube in middle ear pathology.[1]

ANATOMY

The Eustachian tube in the normal adult measures approximately 31 to 38 mm in length.[5] It contains a physiological valve that is closed in the passive resting position and is dilated open by active muscular exertion. There is no generally accepted definition for Eustachian tube dysfunction but it is commonly taken to imply an inadequate ability to open the tubal valve. When the valve fails to function properly, numerous consequences may occur within the middle ear with the most common of these being otitis media.[1]

Since the direction of mucociliary clearance within the Eustachian tube flows from the ear to the nasopharyngeal orifice, the anatomy will be described with "proximal" referring to the middle ear end and "distal" referring toward the nasopharyngeal orifice. When viewing a cross-section of the tubal lumen, there are superior and inferior halves and anterolateral and posteromedial halves.

The proximal one-third is, in effect, a bony funnel-shaped extension of the middle ear, which becomes narrowest at the isthmus, the smallest aperture in the entire tube. The bony portion is lined with a thin layer of cuboidal respiratory epithelium[6] and is a fixed conduit and is normally patent.[7]

The distal two-third of the Eustachian tube is called the pharyngeal portion and is composed of a cartilaginous skeleton to which is attached a complex arrangement of peritubal muscles capable of a wide range of dynamic movements. The lumen is lined by respiratory epithelium that is taller, more columnar, and more ciliated inferiorly than the cuboidal epithelium in the superior one-half. A submucosal layer of lymphatics and fat adds to the lining's thickness within the tubal lumen. The cartilaginous portion is normally closed in the resting state due to apposition of the mucosal walls. The closure occurs over a variable length (5–10 mm segment) just a few millimeters distal to the bony isthmus where the cartilaginous skeleton becomes flexible. This portion that intermittently dilates to an open position is termed the "valve."

There are four peritubular muscles, the levator veli palatini, the salpingopharyngeus, the tensor tympani, and the tensor veli palatine. The TVP is thought to be the principal dilator of the tubal lumen.[1]

The levator veli palatini muscle (LVP) is a round-bellied muscle that looks like a sling running from the base of the temporal bone at the bony Eustachian tube and passing under a groove in the inferior aspect of the medial cartilaginous lamina and membranous floor of the Eustachian tube to insert into the palatal musculature. Contraction of the LVP raises the soft palate and medially rotates the medial cartilaginous lamina.

The tensor veli palatini muscle (TVP) is a flat, fan-shaped muscle with broad origins from the basisphenoid and includes dilator tubae muscle fibers originating from the membranous anterolateral wall of the Eustachian tube. It courses longitudinally along the length of the cartilaginous Eustachian tube and tapers to run under the hamulus of the palatal bone and then insert into the soft palate. The relaxed bulk of the TVP contributes to the anterolateral wall bulge into the lumen of the Eustachian tube and aids in closure of the lumen. Contraction of the TVP tenses the anterolateral membranous wall to dilate the tubal valve into the open position.

PHYSIOLOGY OF TUBAL DILATION

Intermittent brief tubal dilation is probably the principal mechanism for equilibration of middle ear pressure with the ambient atmosphere. Involuntary dilation of the Eustachian tube occurs throughout the day, usually through a swallow or yawn, but it does not accompany every swallow or yawn. Barometric and chemical receptors within the middle ear are thought to provide autonomic nervous system feedback to influence the frequency of involuntary tubal opening.[8,9] Tubal dilation occurs in normal subjects approximately 1.4 times per minute during the daytime with the duration of opening averaging 0.4 seconds.[10] During sleep, the frequency of tubal opening is substantially reduced.

Muscular contractions initiate rotational movements of the cartilaginous framework and create tension with effacement and lateral rounding of the anterolateral wall to produce active dilation of the lumen and transient opening. It is believed that intermittent brief dilation of the tube is the principal mechanism for equilibration of middle ear pressure with the ambient atmosphere.[11] Middle ear and mastoid gas exchange is an ongoing process that continually generates a net absorption of gases, resulting in an increasingly negative pressure between tubal dilations. Failure to dilate for an extended period of time can lead to pathologically severe negative pressure and consequences of tympanic membrane retraction, atelectasis, and otitis media with effusion (OME). Surfactants are produced within the tubal mucosa and probably aid in reducing the surface tension of the lumen and reduce the work required to dilate the tube.[12]

Fluid and secretions in the middle ear are cleared by a combination of muscular pumping action associated with the tubal closing process[6] and by mucociliary activity.[13] Reflux of nasopharyngeal secretions into the middle ear is limited or prevented by the closed position of the resting pharyngeal Eustachian tube and by the trapped volume of gas in the middle ear and mastoid bone which creates a "gas cushion." Reflux of the sounds of breathing and vocalization are also blocked by the closed resting position of the pharyngeal Eustachian tube.[13]

EUSTACHIAN TUBE ENDOSCOPY

Endoscopy of the human Eustachian tube has substantially increased our understanding of the functional processes in normal and pathological tubes. Initial work done by the insertion of microfiber-optic instruments into the tubal lumen yielded only limited information since the bony isthmus is only about 1.0 to 1.5 mm in horizontal diameter and 2 to 3 mm in vertical diameter.[14] In order to pass through the narrow isthmus, endoscope diameters must be restricted to 1 mm or less, which compromises image resolution that gross structures within the middle ear, such as ossicles, may be seen but fine details of movements cannot be appreciated. Direct contact of the endoscope lens with secretions and mucosal folds sufficiently obscures inspection within the lumen such that most reports have only been able to describe gross observations such as the presence of lesions or degree of patency.[15–18]

Larger diameter (=3–4 mm) fiber-optic nasopharyngoscopes or rigid Hopkins rod endoscopes have been used for more detailed studies of the tubal lumen. The endoscope should be carefully positioned in the nasopharyngeal orifice with the view directed superiorly and laterally into the lumen, allowing for observation of most of the pharyngeal portion of the tube as it rotates into the dilated position during the opening sequence. Careful observation of tubal dynamics has become possible with high-resolution optics. Avoidance of direct contact with the mucosa prevents interference with the dilating mechanism and limits problems with fogging of the lens. Video recordings can be made and replayed in slow motion for meticulous analysis of the dilation process and study of normal physiology and pathophysiology.[19,20]

Eustachian tube endoscopy generally yields views proximally well into the valve area during the time of maximal active dilation. The opening process can be seen endoscopically as the tube progressively dilates from the nasopharyngeal orifice up toward the isthmus, generally moving the lumen into full view of the endoscope. We have studied normal subjects and patients with tubal dysfunction using these techniques to establish some observed patterns of normal dynamic physiology and pathophysiology.

TECHNIQUE OF EUSTACHIAN TUBE VIDEO ENDOSCOPY

Patients are examined in the sitting position in an office setting. Topical spray anesthetic and decongestant, lidocaine (4%) topical mixed with equal parts of phenylepherine HCl 0.5% solution, is applied to both nasal cavities while the patient sniffs. Endoscopes are introduced into the nasal cavity and advanced up to the nasopharyngeal orifice of the Eustachian tube, just posterior to the inferior turbinate and identified by the torus torbaris. It is easy to pass by the torus and examine the fossa of Rosenmüller, believing it to be the Eustachian tube orifice.

The initial endoscopic exam is done with a 4 mm diameter steerable flexible fiber-optic nasopharyngoscope EMF-P3 (Olympus, Tokyo, Japan). Careful inspection of the nasal cavity, nasopharynx, hypopharynx, and larynx is done to look for mucosal inflammation or lesions, especially if there is any evidence for laryngo-pharyngeal reflux (LPR) or allergic disease. If the adenoid is enlarged, its proximity to the posterior cushion of the Eustachian tube is noted. Lastly, the Eustachian tube is closely examined. The optimal fiber-optic view is most commonly obtained introducing the endoscope along the floor of the contralateral nasal cavity and passing the tip behind the vomer. This brings the tip into the proper angle to view up the long axis of the Eustachian tube when it dilates. Occasionally, the lumen may be successfully viewed with a fiber-optic scope from the ipsilateral nasal cavity.

For a more detailed examination or if slow-motion recording is desired, rigid endoscopes are preferred, generally using a 4-mm diameter, 30 or 45 degree view angle, Hopkins rod rigid sinus surgery endoscope (Karl Storz, Culver City, CA). The rod endoscopes have high-resolution images but the fiber-optic endoscopes are easier to pass and can be steered deeper into the Eustachian tube lumen if desired.

The 30-degree rigid endoscope is introduced with the view angle looking directly laterally and passed along the nasal floor, following the inferior turbinate. After passing the posterior aspect of the inferior turbinate, the next landmark encountered is the anterior cushion of the Eustachian tube's nasopharyngeal orifice. Once at the orifice, the endoscope is rotated slightly to look superiorly toward the long axis of the tubal lumen.

The rigid endoscope is used with a charge coupled device (CCD) camera in place and images are viewed on a video monitor. Video recordings are made with a s-VHS video or DVD recorder.

The patient is initially asked to vocalize "K" "K" "K" repeatedly to view the isolated action of the LVP. The "Ks" stimulate palatal elevation and medial rotation of the posterior cushion and posteromedial wall of the Eustachian tube. Swallows are done to induce normal physiological tubal dilations, and forced yawns are performed to cause maximal sustained dilation. The Eustachian tube is not expected to open with every swallow and yawn and patients are coached to feel the muscular contractions in the back of their throats to generate some dilatory efforts. The procedure is repeated for the contralateral Eustachian tube orifice.

The video of tubal dilations is then reviewed and analyzed in normal time, slow motion, and even stepping through single frames that are captured at a rate of 30 frames per second.

ENDOSCOPY OF THE NORMAL EUSTACHIAN TUBE

The normal dilation process was initially studied endoscopically in 30 normal subjects.[19] Normal dilation and opening were observed to have four consistent sequential phases during a normal swallow (Figure 12–1A to C):

1. The soft palate elevated with simultaneous medial rotation of the posterior cushion and posteromedial wall. The lateral pharyngeal wall also medialized, causing transient constriction of the nasopharyngeal orifice despite the medial rotation of the posterior cushion and posteromedial wall. One hypothesis for this contrary movement could be to provide momentary protection of the Eustachian tube against reflux at the initiation of swallow.
2. The palate remained elevated, and the posteromedial wall remained medially rotated as the lateral pharyngeal wall displaced laterally to begin the dilation of the nasopharyngeal orifice.
3. The TVP began to contract causing dilation of the lumen to propagate from the nasopharynx proximally toward the bony isthmus. The dilation occurred by displacement of the anterolateral tubal wall laterally against the already contracted and medially rotated posteromedial wall.
4. Tubal opening occurred as the functional valve of the cartilaginous tube dilated into a roughly rounded aperture. The convex bulge seen in the resting anterolateral valve wall became visibly flattened or concave to produce the final opening.

Closure of the tube began with closure of the valve area and propagated distally toward the nasopharyngeal orifice. This proximal to distal closure has been hypothesized to have a pumping action that may protect against reflux.[6] Relaxation of the posteromedial wall, lateral pharyngeal wall, and palate occurred in variable order or even simultaneously.

The thin mucosa and subcutaneous tissues of the normal Eustachian tubes permitted viewing of the muscular contractions of the LVP and TVP. Even the ripples of distinct individual fiber contractions were often appreciated.

ENDOSCOPY OF THE DYSFUNCTIONAL EUSTACHIAN TUBE

Eustachian tube dysfunction is defined as inadequate dilatory function causing secondary ear pathology. It may result from anatomical obstruction or physiologic failure due to: (1) hereditary factors as seen in strong family histories of ear disease, (2) mucosal inflammation with functional obstruction or failure of dilation, (3) muscular problems causing dilatory dynamic dysfunction, and lastly (4) true anatomical obstruction due to

A

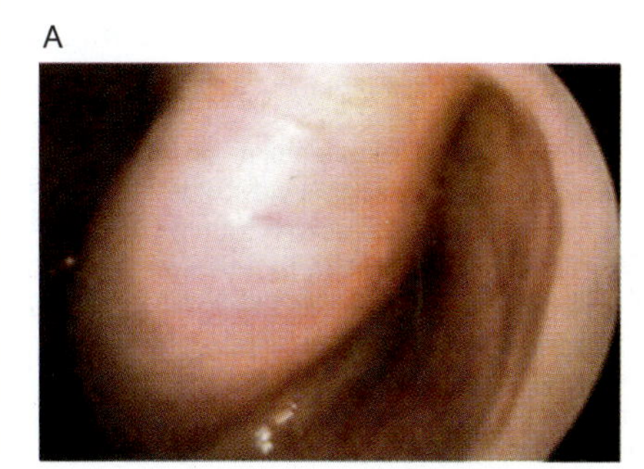

B

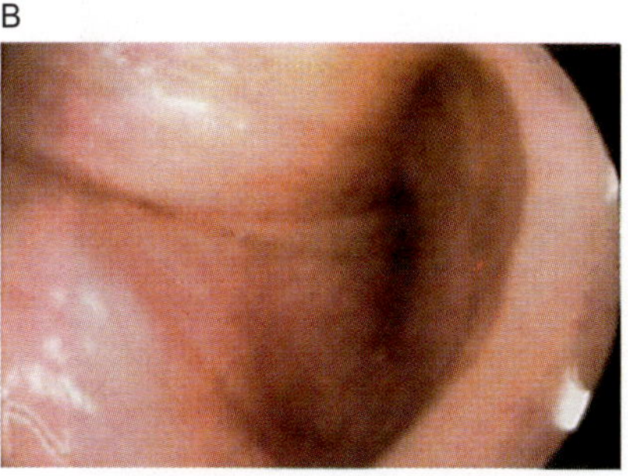

C

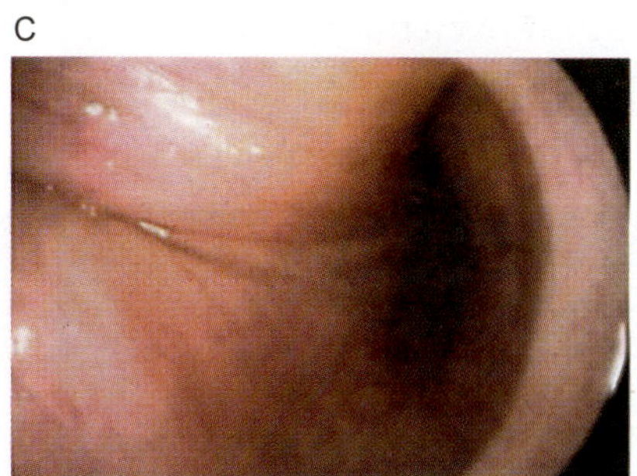

FIGURE 12–1 • Transnasal, 4-mm, 45-degree Hopkins rod endoscopic view of left normal Eustachian tube orifice: *A*, Resting position (valve closed). *B*, Initiation of swallow. Levator veli palatini muscle has elevated the palate and medially rotated the posterior cushion. *C*, Tensor veli palatini has contracted, dilating the valve to open position.

TABLE 12–1 Pathological findings in the 58 clinically dysfunctional Eustachian tubes

Mucosal edema—48 (83%)
Reduced lateral wall motion—43 (74%)
Obstructive mucosal disease—15 (26%)

neoplasms or other mass lesions, the least common cause. The etiologies of tubal dilatory failure can be separated into obstructive and dynamic dysfunctions. Most obstructive problems are not true anatomical blockage; rather, they are due to functional failures to dilate the tube sufficiently or often enough to adequately aerate the middle ear.

There is increasing evidence that Eustachian tube dysfunction results from pathology within the cartilaginous portion. Slow-motion video analysis was done on 58 ears (of 40 adult patients) with pathology suggestive of tubal dysfunction.[20] All subjects had significant pathology and compromise of tubal dilation within the cartilaginous portion compared to 4/30 (13%) of normal subjects who had only mild inflammatory changes. The pathological findings are summarized in Table 12–1. All 58 tubes had significantly compromised dilation, which was judged to be moderate opening ability—26 (45%); minimal opening—21 (36%); and no opening—11 (19%).

The components of the pharyngeal Eustachian tube can be classified as the cartilaginous skeleton, tubal muscles, submucosa, and epithelium of the lumen and defects were observed in each of the different components. Edema of the mucosa and submucosa were most often responsible for decreased luminal diameter and decreased ability to dilate the tube (Figure 12–2A–D).

Actual muscular dysfunction (dynamic dysfunction) as the primary problem was seen in 8%. Examples of hypofunction, hyperfunction, or lack of coordination of either the TVP, LVP, or both muscles were seen. Most commonly, reduced TVP muscle action with decreased excursion of the anterolateral wall was observed. Hypercontraction of either muscle could result in a bulky mass effect that could block the lumen. Several cases of LVP muscle dysfunction were also identified.[20]

In some cases the TVP showed weakness, disorganized fasciculations, or absence of the usual dilatory wave that should progress from the nasopharyngeal orifice toward the isthmus. Two cases demonstrated excessively strong contractions of the TVP with prominent ripples producing longitudinal ridges that paradoxically reduced the lumen diameter instead of dilating it. (Figure 12–3A and B). There were three Eustachian tubes in which a good dilatory effort was seen in the distal half of the tube but there was reduced dilatory effort or failure to open the valve area. Two cases demonstrated an unusual double contraction of the LVP muscle and palate that blocked the lumen while the TVP attempted to dilate the tube. In another case, the LVP paradoxically relaxed just at the time that the TVP began to contract. These three cases demonstrated a failure of coordination between the levator and tensor muscles that resulted in failure of dilation of the tube. LVP may serve a function of maintaining a "scaffold" that the TVP requires for effective dilation.

Typically mucosal edema within the tube was uniformly distributed along the length of Eustachian tube and tended to be most prominent in the inferior half of the cross-sectional diameter of the tube. Mucosal swelling was sometimes accompanied by erythema, mucoid secretions, or purulent drainage. There were several tubes that demonstrated severe edema with bulbous projections into the lumen resembling polyps. These tubes generally were unable to dilate open at all.

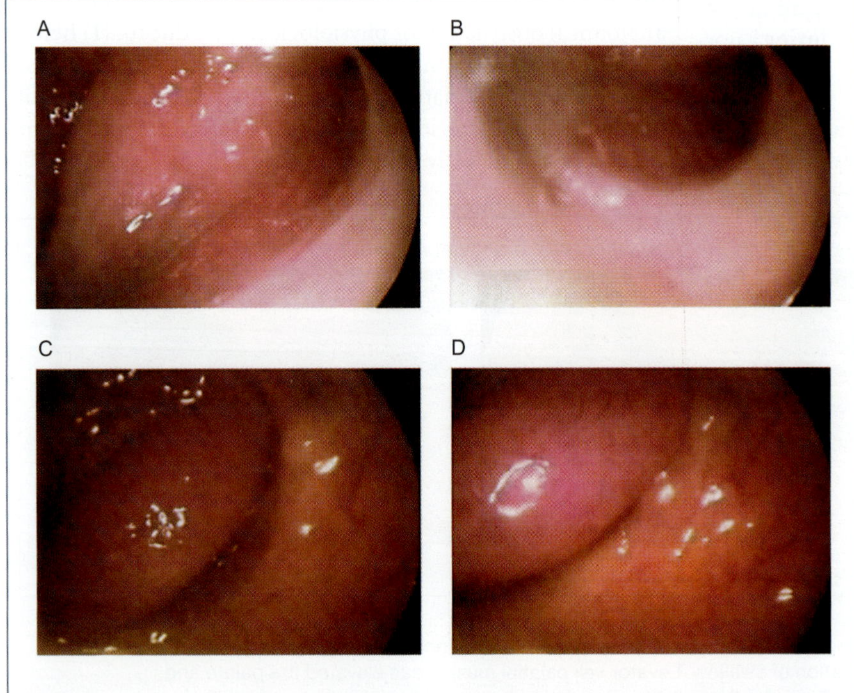

FIGURE 12–2 • Transnasal, 4-mm, 45-degree Hopkins rod endoscopic view of left inflamed and edematous Eustachian tube orifices *A*, Mildly inflamed posterior cushion in resting position (valve closed); *B*, Mildly inflamed posterior cushion in dilated position (same case as *A*); *C*, Severely inflamed posterior cushion in resting position (valve closed); *D*, Severely inflamed posterior cushion in dilated position. Posterior cushion is so edematous that pharyngeal constrictors and adenoids have forced the posterior cushion anteriorly during swallow completely preventing dilation (same case as *C*).

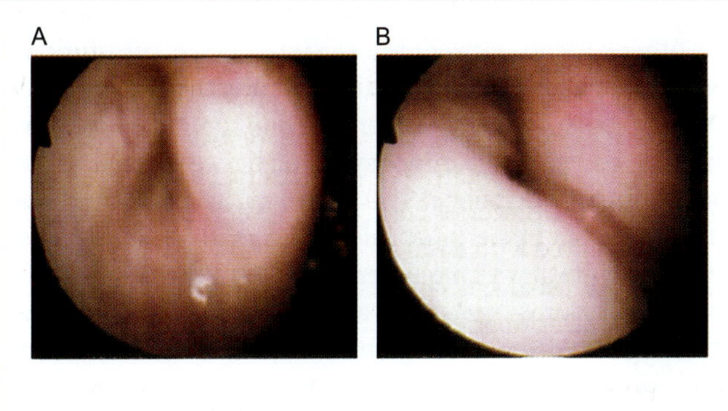

FIGURE 12–3 • Transnasal, 3.7-mm, fiber-optic endoscopic view of right Eustachian tube orifice with paradoxical blockage of the valve during dilation phase. *A*, Resting closed position; *B*, Bulging of the anterlateral wall that blocks valve opening during dilation phase.

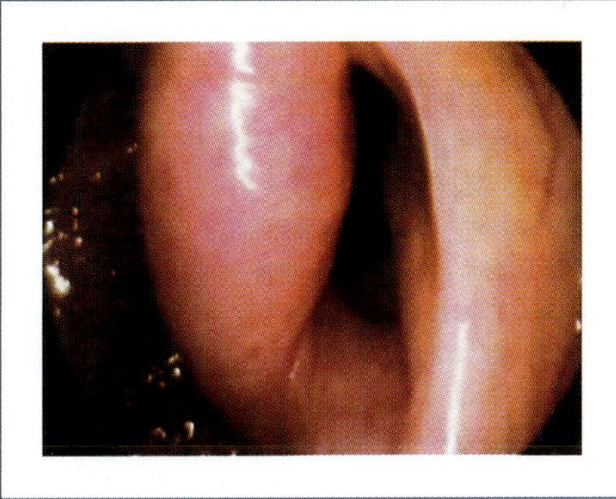

FIGURE 12–4 • Transnasal, 4-mm, 45-degree Hopkins rod endoscopic view of orifice of a left patulous Eustachian tube. Note concavity of antero-lateral wall extending through valve.

There was one patient who had adenoid hypertrophy that was not obstructing the nasopharyngeal orifice at rest. During swallowing, however, the adenoid was pressed into the tubal orifice that forced the posterior cushion (posteromedial wall) to completely cover and paradoxically obstruct the nasopharyngeal orifice at the time when it should be dilating. This type of bulbous posterior cushion with coverage of the tubal orifice during swallow has been repeatedly seen in subsequent clinical experience, especially in patients with severe allergic or LPR disease. Mucosal atrophy with observation of the underlying yellow Ostmann's fat was seen in 11 (19%) tubes.

There was a correlation between mucosal inflammation and LPR findings on nasopharynogoscopy or laryngoscopy. There was no correlation between the severity of middle ear pathology and the severity or type of Eustachian tube pathology. It appeared that changes in the tympanic membrane and middle ear took on an independent pathophysiological process once Eustachian tube dysfunction had passed some critical point.

There were six patulous tubes and all of them demonstrated a consistent concavity in the superior cross-sectional half of the anterolateral wall, within the valve area. Normal tubes have a convexity in this location that flattens during the final stage of dilation process. This absence of tissue in the superior anterolateral wall has been a consistent finding in patulous Eustachian tubes that have been subsequently studied including 14 cases of patulous tube surgical reconstructions. The defect is commonly a deficiency in the lateral cartilaginous lamina, thin mucosa/submucosa, reduced Ostmann's fat pad, and thin TVP muscle. Any of these abnormalities can contribute to reduction of the anterolateral wall bulge that comprises the valve and makes it incompetent[21] (Figure 12–4).

MEDICAL TREATMENT OF EUSTACHIAN TUBE DYSFUNCTION

Tubal dysfunction is predominantly due to mucosal inflammatory disease, similar to chronic sinusitis, and can be managed in most cases with medical treatment. Identification of the underlying etiology is critical for success. LPR should be treated with dietary management, daily or twice daily proton pump inhibitors, and H2 blockers at bedtime as indicated. Refractory cases may be treated by sleeping on an inclined bed, and ultimately, fundoplication if necessary.

Symptoms and signs of allergic disease should be thoroughly investigated, doing testing and dietary elimination trials as indicated. Avoidance of the offending allergen, oral second generation antihistamines, leukotriene inhibitors, nasal antihistamines or mast cell stabilizers, nasal steroid sprays; and immunotherapy should be pursued as required.

Careful consideration for other underlying pathology should be done. Recurrent infections should raise the suspicion for underlying nasal or sinus disease, immunosuppression or immunodeficiency, or primary mucosal disorders (eg, Samter's triad, Wegener's and other granulomatous disease). Etiologies for chronic tubal dysfunction are summarized in Table 12–2.

Anatomical obstruction due to neoplasm should be ruled out, especially in cases of unilateral persistent effusion. Contrast-enhanced imaging studies are often necessary to recognized nasopharyngeal carcinoma and other malignancies. Functional obstruction due to hypertrophic adenoid tissue contacting the posterior cushion can be excised.

TABLE 12–2 Differential diagnosis for etiology of chronic Eustachian tube dysfunction
Allergic disease
Laryngo-pharyngeal reflux (LPR)
Hypertrophied adenoid contacting posterior cushions
Chronic sinusitis
Tubal dynamic dysfunction
Pneumonia or chronic pulmonary disease
Primary mucosal disease
—Immune deficient/suppressed —Samter's (aspirin sensitivity, asthma, nasal polyps) triad —Wegener's or other granulomatous disease —Other middle ear or nasopharyngeal inflammation
Anatomical obstruction with neoplasm or other lesion

TABLE 12–3 Differential diagnosis with Minor's (semicircular canal dehiscence) syndrome

Symptoms/signs of Minor's syndrome (MS) may mimic:
• Otosclerosis—LF conductive HL – MS: Intact stapedius reflex, BC<0 dB HL
• Eustachian tube dysfunction—Persistant ear blockage – MS: Normal TM/tympanogram, no relief with tympanostomy
• Patulous Eustachian tube—Persistant ear blockage, autophony of voice, relief supine/valsalva – MS: Autophony of breathing, no TM excursions with breathing
• Ménière's disease/PLF—Persistant ear blockage, intermittent vertigo, tullio, positive fistula test, LF HL, hearing distortion/hyperacusis – MS: LF CHL, torsional nystagmus
• TMJ dysfunction—Persistant ear blockage/pain – MS: Tenderness in TMJ

Chronic fullness in the ear associated with a normal appearing mobile tympanic membrane, absence of any retraction or effusion, and a normal tympanogram should not be interpreted as Eustachian tube dysfunction, especially if myringotomy fails to relieve the symptoms. Instead, a search for other causes of fullness, blockage, or otalgia is indicated and should include evaluation of the temporomandibular joint as the most common cause followed by semicircular canal dehiscence (Minor's) syndrome and endolymphatic hydrops. Table 12–3 summarizes some of the differential diagnostic characteristics of Minor's syndrome.

Eustachian Tuboplasty for Tubal Dysfunction

Persistent tubal dysfunction with OME or atelectasis has been successfully managed in most cases with tympanostomy tubes with excellent long-term outcomes. Some patients, however, recur with effusion or atelectasis and require multiple tympanostomy tubes over many years. Eustachian tuboplasty (ETP) has been used in recent years to ablate mucosa and submucosa from within the tubal lumen on the posterolateral wall to widen the lumen and facilitate the dilatory process. Healing occurs with fibrosis and mucosa along the posterior cushion and posterior wall that is thinner and with reduced inflammation compared to preoperatively.[22,23] Results remain preliminary with small series to date, but the data is encouraging for patients in whom the underlying pathology has been controlled. If there are ongoing uncontrolled mucosal disease processes such as allergies or LPR, postoperative improvement may only be temporary and tubal dysfunction may recur. In patients with ongoing mucosal inflammation, symptoms and signs may fluctuate depending on how well the patient is managing the condition at the time. Cessation of antihistamines, or proton pump inhibitors, or resumption of allergen exposure may cause a relapse of tubal dysfunction.

In the senior author's two-year follow-up study of ETP using an otologic Argon or KTP laser for tissue ablation, 37% of 13 adults with refractory long-term OME and multiple prior tympanostomy tubes had remission of their effusion. There were three other patients with continuing intermittent effusions who considered themselves substantially improved. Failure correlated with LPR or allergic disease. There were no significant complications. One patient had a minor synechia between the nasal septum and inferior turbinate. Two patients had a small persistent granuloma in the posterior cushion for several weeks postoperatively that resolved with nasal steroid sprays. There were no cases of bleeding, or tubal synechiae, and no patient was made worse by the surgery. Postoperative pain was minimal and was less than the throat discomfort from the endotrachial intubation.

A trial of ETP using a microdebrider for tissue ablation was done in 20 patients with chronic OME and sinus disease along with their endoscopic sinus surgery; 14/20 (70%) improved subjectively and by improvement in tympanogram and or pure-tone averages. Failure correlated with higher preoperative CT sinus disease stage and with higher eosinophil counts in the biopsy specimens.

Indications for Surgery

All patients are investigated for possible underlying etiology and treated appropriately. Patients who have had maximal medical therapy for their underlying pathology, yet still have irreversible mucosal disease and persistent atelectasis, difficulty with airplane flights, or intermittent or persistent OME, may be candidates for ETP. Patients should have been helped with tympanostomy tubes but problems have continued to recur after two or more tubes. Slow-motion video endoscopy has demonstrated mucosal disease, causing obstructive dysfunction with inadequate dilation of the lumen.

Contraindications for Surgery

Primary middle ear disease that is not secondary to tubal dysfunction, such as recurrent thick proteinaceous "glue" ear that repeatedly occluded tympanostomy tubes, is a contraindication to surgery. Other contraindications include radiation therapy for nasopharyngeal cancer and extensive nasal or nasopharyngeal mucosal disease due to an underlying, uncontrolled inflammatory process.

Preoperative Management

Patients are treated with 6 weeks of nasal steroid sprays daily to see if any resolution of their ear or Eustachian tube pathology occurs. Other underlying etiologies are appropriately treated during this time.

Preoperative Planning

High-resolution computed tomography (CT) scanning is obtained of the nasopharynx and temporal bones to rule out concomitant sinus disease and other disorders in the nasopharynx, Eustachian tube, or ear. Contrast enhancement is used in cases with a unilateral effusion to reveal any associated neoplasm.

Video endoscopy is reviewed to determine the extent of Eustachian tube, nasal, sinus, and nasopharyngeal disease. Cases observed to date have had obstructive disorders and the results for dynamic disorders remains unknown. More extensive disease warrants more aggressive removal of soft tissue or even some of the medial cartilaginous lamina.

Operative Technique for Laser Eustachian Tuboplasty

Patients are operated in the supine position and maintained under general anesthesia with endotrachial intubation. A myringotomy with or without temporary tube insertion may be done to aspirate effusion. The patient is draped for nasal endoscopic surgery. Nasal decongestant spray is applied to both nasal cavities. A tonsil mouth gag is placed and the mouth opened moderately. The Eustachian tube is viewed with a 30-degree, 4 mm nasal endoscope, and the operation is performed watching a surgical video monitor using a CCD camera (Karl Storz, Culver City, CA) attached to the endoscope lens. Local infiltration with lidocaine 1% solution with 1 to 100,000 epinephrine is performed in the nasopharyngeal orifice of the Eustachian tube with a curved endosinus needle passed through the oral cavity. The Eustachian tube orifice may be dilated with a 2 mm wide sliver of Merocel™ (Medtronic Xomed, Inc., Jacksonville, Florida) compressed sponge-soaked in epinephrine solution (1–50,000) and delivered into the tubal lumen. After 5 minutes, the Merocel™ pack is removed and the medial cartilaginous lamina within the posterior cushion is palpated. A fiber-delivered diode pumped KTP laser (Iridex Corporation, Mountain View, California), with the handpiece manually gently bent into a 60-degree arc, is passed through the mouth to perform the tissue ablation. Settings of 2,500 mW, and 1 second continuous mode pulse duration are used. Laser cauterization of tissue begins on the mucosa overlying the leading edge of the medial cartilaginous lamina within the posterior cushion. From the leading edge, all mucosa and submucosa is ablated down to the exposed cartilage making a triangular defect that extends along the cartilage proximally up to the valve. The posterior cushion may be medially rotated using an olive tip maxillary antral suction. In cases with more advanced obstructive disease, ablation is continued into the valve, always taking great care to avoid injury to the contralateral wall of the tubal lumen that may cause synechiae and exacerbate the obstruction. No more than 40% of the circumference of the lumen is ablated. For ablation deep into the valve, the overlying mucosa may be preserved and ablation can be done of the underlying submucosa. Cases of severe obstructive disease or dynamic dysfunction may additionally be treated by some resection of the cartilage to thin it and weaken the spring of the cartilage. Cauterization for hemostasis is occasionally required. A pledget of Merogel™ (Medtronic Xomed, Inc., Jacksonville, Florida) soaked in sulfacetamide/prednisolone ophthalmic drops is applied to the surgical defect at the end of the procedure (Figure 12–5A to E).

Postoperative Management

Patients are discharged home from surgery on the same day and they are restricted to light activities for ten days. They are instructed to use saline sprays at least three times daily for two weeks. Patients suspected of LPR are put on daily proton pump inhibitors for at least 6 weeks, or longer if they remain with ongoing reflux. Patients with allergic disease continue with nasal steroid sprays for 6 weeks, or longer if indicated. Antihistamines and other measures are continued as needed. Follow-up examinations are done at 1, 6, 12, 24, and 36 months. An example of pre and post operative results is shown in Figure 12–6.

Complications and Pitfalls

The mucosa of the anterolateral wall, opposite of the surgical site, must be treated gently at all times to avoid any injury that could result in synechiae and worsening of the dysfunction. The Eustachian tube must be correctly identified as the first prominent

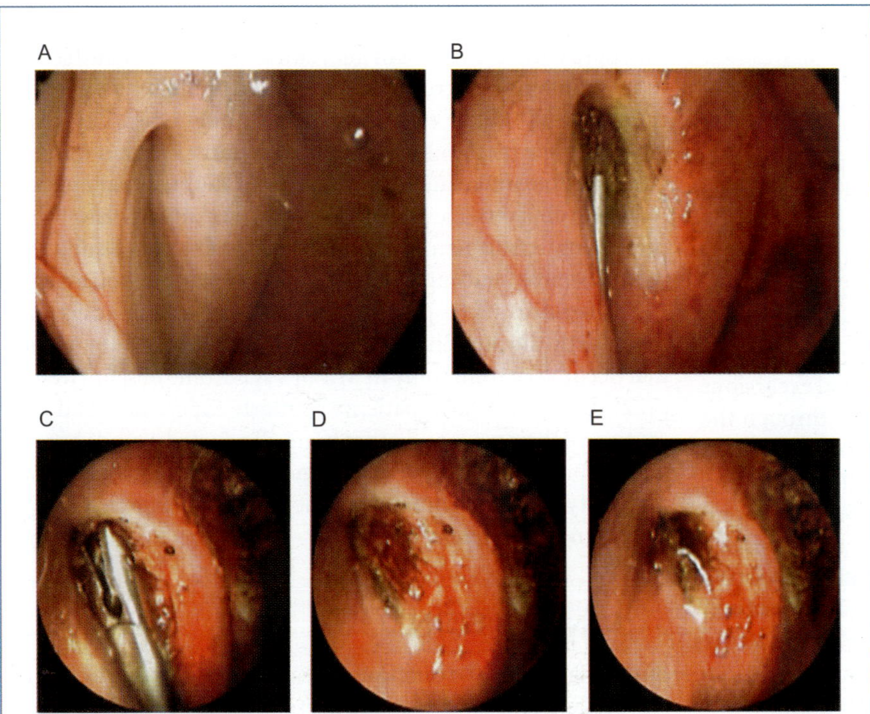

FIGURE 12–5 • Right Eustachian tuboplasty. Transnasal, 4-mm, 45-degree Hopkins rod endoscopic intraoperative views. *A*, Initial view of tubal orifice. Note edematous bulging of posterior cushion; *B*, Laser debulking of intraluminal mucosa and submucosa overlying medial cartilaginous lamina within the posterior cushion. Mucosa is left intact within the valve proper; *C*, Cup forceps resection of cartilage bulge protruding into valve lumen; *D*, Completed resection of tissue; *E*, Lumen of tubal valve packed with absorbable Merogel soaked in Sulfacetamide–Prednisolone ophthalmologic solution.

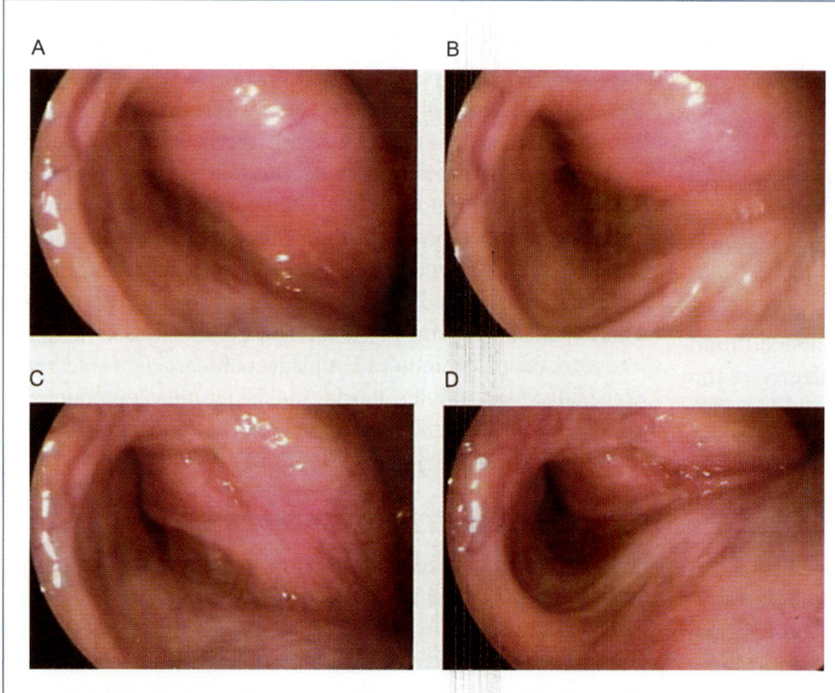

FIGURE 12–6 • Transnasal, 4-mm, 45-degree Hopkins rod endoscopic view of orifice of right Eustachian tube orifice pre and post op for Eustachian tuboplasty. *A*, Preop resting closed position; *B*, Preop dilated position; *C*, Six-month postop resting closed position. Note enlarged orifice and valve lumen; *D*, Six-month postop dilated postion.

structure immediately posterior to the inferior turbinate. If the tube is missed, the Fossa of Rosenmüller can appear like a tubal orifice and lies immediately posterior to the Eustachian tube. The internal carotid artery lies just deep to the apex of the fossa. A thorough knowledge of Eustachian tube surgical anatomy is essential. The medial cartilaginous lamina is the most important landmark and will not only lead the surgeon into the lumen up to the valve, but serves to protect the internal carotid artery. As long as the dissection remains along the luminal side of the cartilage, the artery is not in jeopardy. Care must be taken not to puncture through the cartilage and risk carotid injury that could result in life-threatening bleeding and brain complications.

Treatment of the Patulous Eustachian Tube

In the author's experience, the patulous Eustachian tube is associated with significant weight loss in approximately one-third of the cases, with rheumatologic or similar chronic conditions in one-third, and uncertain etiology in the remaining one-third. There is often a previous history of prior Eustachian tube dysfunction with multiple Valsalva maneuvers and sniffing, LPR, or allergic disease. The diagnosis can be most definitively confirmed by otoscopic observation of lateral and medial excursions of the tympanic membrane as the patient breathes through the nose. The excursions can be enhanced by having the patient occlude the opposite nostril. The excursions will only be seen if the patient is simultaneously experiencing their symptom of autophony during the nasal breathing. If there is an absence of tympanic membrane excursions despite the patient's reporting of concurrent active autophony, another cause of the autophony should be investigated and Minor's syndrome (semicircular canal dehiscence syndrome) should be suspected.

Medical treatment consists of good hydration and treatment of any underlying conditions. Nasal irrigations with saline or saline drops may be helpful. Nasal steroid sprays, decongestants, and antihistamines may exacerbate the condition.

SSKI is occasionally helpful in thickening mucous secretions. Temporary improvement may be gained by using estrogen nasal topical drops such as Premarin® or estradiol, which are not FDA approved for this use. Nasal irritant drops such as those containing chlorine are being investigated and their efficacy has not yet been established. Ventilating tubes may be helpful in alleviating the sensation of tympanic membrane excursions with breathing but are rarely helpful in alleviating autophony.

Obstruction of the Eustachian tube by transnasal or middle ear approaches is effective in alleviating the patulous Eustachian tube symptoms, but creates long-term Eustachian tube dysfunction that will usually require tympanostomy tubes. The senior author is now performing functional reconstruction of the convexity of the anterolateral wall with intraluminal submucosal cartilage implants. The procedure closes the patulous defect while preserving Eustachian tube function. Short-term results have been favorable, but long-term outcomes are not yet available.

Diagnosis of the patulous Eustachian tube is often confused with the autophony of voice, but not breathing sounds that occur very commonly in Minor's syndrome of semicircular canal dehiscence. Such patients similarly experience loud perception of their voice and other bone-conducted sounds but not of their breathing noises. They do not have patulous excursions of their tympanic membranes coincident with experiencing the symptom of autophony.

CONCLUSION

Eustachian tube dysfunction appears to result from failure of any of the components of the cartilaginous pharyngeal tube. Mucosal edema may be caused by inflammatory disease, infection, allergy, or reflux from the nasopharynx (including LPR). Medical treatment should be directed toward the underlying etiology of edema whenever possible and middle ear ventilation with tympanostomy tubes is generally recommended when medical treatment is inadequate. The persistence of mucosal edema despite maximal medical treatment and dissatisfaction with tympanostomy tubes may be considered an indication for tubal surgery. Primary muscular disorders including weakness or lack of coordination between LVP and TVP may benefit from medical treatment or speech therapy Eustachian tube exercises. Intratubal surgery may help some patients failing these conservative measures. Primary anatomical obstruction is less common but such cases should be studied individually to determine what medical or surgical interventions may be needed.

Endoscopic intraluminal surgery of the Eustachian tube is now being performed and developed. The principle of the surgery is to debulk the irreversibly injured swollen tissue in the posteromedial wall to allow for easier dilation of the tube as the TVP contracts. Cases involving muscular dysfunction may also have a portion of the medial cartilaginous lamina debulked to weaken the spring of the cartilaginous skeleton and facilitate LVP and TVP contraction.

References

1. Bluestone CD. Introduction. In: Bluestone MB, editor. Eustachian tube structure, function, role in otitis media. London: BC Decker Inc; 2005. p. 1–9.
2. Eustachius B. Epistola de auditus organis. Arch Otolaryngol 1944;20:123.
3. Canalis R. Valsalva's contribution to otology. Am J Otolaryngol 1990;11:420–7.
4. Toynbee J. On the muscles that open the Eustachian tube. Proc R Soc Med 1853;6:286–91.
5. Proctor B. Anatomy of the Eustachian tube. Arch Otolaryngol 1973;97:2.
6. Honjo I, Hayashi M, Ito S, et al. Pumping and clearance function of the Eustachian tube. Am J Otolaryngol 1985;6:241.
7. Hopf J, Linnarz M, Gundlach P, et al. Die Mikroendoskopie der Eustachischen Rohre und des Mittelhres. Indikationen und klinischer Einsatzpunkt. Laryngorhinootologie. 1991;70:391–4.
8. Eden A, Gannon P. Neural control of middle ear aeration. Arch Otolaryngol Head Neck Surg 1987;113:133–7.
9. Rockley T, Hawke W. The middle ear as a baroreceptor. Acta Otolaryngol (Stockh) 1992;112:816–23.
10. Mondain M, Vidal D, Bouhanna S, Uziel A. Monitoring eustachian tube opening: Preliminary results in normal subjects. Laryngoscope 1997;107(10):1414–19.
11. Honjo I. Eustachian tube and middle ear diseases. Tokyo: Springer-Verlag, 1988.
12. Chandrasekhar SS, Mautone AJ. Otitis media: Treatment with intranasal aerosolized surfactants. Laryngoscope 2004;114:472–85.
13. Bluestone CD, Klein JO. Otitis Media, atelectatis, and Eustachian tube dysfunction. In: Bluestone CD, Stool SE, Kenna MA (eds). Pediatric otolaryngology. 3rd ed. Philadelphia: WB Saunders 1996.
14. Schuknecht HF, Gulya AJ. Anatomy of the temporal bone with surgical implications. Philadelphia: Lea & Febiger, 1986.
15. Chays A, Cohen JM, Magnan J. La microfibroendoscopie tubotympanique. Technique Chirurgicale. 1995; 24:773–4.
16. Kimura H, Yamaguchi H, Cheng SS, et al. Direct observation of the tympanic cavity by the superfine fiberscope. Nippon Jibiinkoka Gakkai Kaiho, 1989;92:233–8.
17. Takahashi H, Honjo I, Fujita A. Endoscopic findings at the pharyngeal orifice of the Eustachian tube in otitis media with effusion. Eur Arch Otorhinolaryngol. 1996;253(1–2):42–4.
18. Klug C, Fabinyi B, Tschabitscher M. Endoscopy of the middle ear through the Eustachian tube: Anatomic possiblilites and limitations. Am J Otol 1999;20:299–303.
19. Poe DS, Pyykko I, Valtonen H, Silvola J. Analysis of Eustachian tube function by video endoscopy. Am J Otol, 2000;21:602–7.
20. Poe DS, Abou-Halawa A, Abdel-Razek O. Analysis of the Dysfunctional Eustachian tube by video endoscopy. Otol Neurotol 2001;22:590–5.
21. Poe DS, Diagnosis and surgery for the patulous Eustachian tube. Otol Neurotol. 2007;28(5):668–77.
22. Poe DS, Metson RB, Kujawski O. Laser eustachian tuboplasty-A preliminary study. Laryngoscope 2003;113:583–91.
23. Poe DS, Grimmer, JF, Metson RB. Laser Eustachian tuboplasty: Two-year results. Laryngoscope 2007;117:231–7.

Imaging of the Temporal Bone 13

Galdino E. Valvassori, MD / Masoud Hemmati, MD

The role of imaging in the assessment of temporal bone pathology has been enhanced by the refinement of the diagnostic equipment and new techniques. At present, three modalities are applied to study the temporal bone and central auditory-vestibular pathways: computed tomography (CT), magnetic resonance imaging (MRI), and angiography. Conventional radiography is no longer used except in a few cases for the evaluation of mastoid pneumatization and assessment of the position and integrity of cochlear implant electrodes.

COMPUTED TOMOGRAPHY

CT is a radiographic technique that allows the measurement of small absorption differentials not recognizable by direct recording on x-ray films. The digital signal produced by CT is a measure of the amount of ionizing radiation (x-rays) absorbed by each pixel of tissue. The scan is initiated at a chosen level and the x-ray tube, collimated to a pencil-thin beam, rotates around the patient. The nonabsorbed portion of radiation is picked up by detectors, as many as 64, arranged along the circumference of the tube trajectory and is converted into digital signals. Today the helical (or spiral) CT allows for continuous rotation of the gantry and thus a continuous acquisition of images. A block of ultrathin sections (0.35 mm thick) covering the entire temporal bone can be acquired in less than 1 min.

Acquisition of volumetric data is usually done in the axial plane since it is the easiest to obtain and the most comfortable for the patient. Since pixels are isotropic, reformatting the images is then performed in the *X*, *Y*, *Z*, as well as oblique planes without distortion. The CT images provide exquisite bony detail (Figure 13–1) and excellent demonstration of soft tissue density within the air spaces of the mastoid, external auditory canal, and the middle ear,[1] but very limited identification of the type of substance producing the abnormal density. For instance, the density of cholesteatoma is identical to that of a tumor or granulation tissue and even of fluid. The study is often repeated after intravenous infusion or bolus injection of contrast material, which produces an increased density or enhancement of several anatomic structures and pathologic processes. An enhanced study is mandatory whenever a vascular anomaly, a tumor, or an otogenic abscess is suspected.

MAGNETIC RESONANCE IMAGING

MRI is capable of producing cross-sectional images of the human body in any plane without exposing the patient to ionizing radiation. MR images are obtained by the interaction of hydrogen nuclei or protons of the human body, high magnetic field, and radiofrequency pulses. The strength of the MR signal to be converted into imaging data depends on the concentration of the hydrogen nuclei and two magnetic relaxation times, T1 and T2, which are tissue-specific.

MRI techniques have undergone several changes and refinement to increase definition of the images and to decrease acquisition time. First, the use of surface coils placed adjacent to the area of interest has increased the signal-to-noise ratio, consequently improving image quality. Faster acquisitions have been obtained by shortening the time between successive pulses (repetition time or TR), using pulses with flip angles smaller than 90 degrees (gradient echo imaging), by reducing the number of phase-encoded steps, and by increasing the data collected per excitation. The latter technique, known as fast spin echo (FSE), uses multiple echos (4 to 16 for excitation), thereby reducing the number of excitations necessary to create an image.

MR examination of the temporal bones is performed with the patient in the supine position so that a line drawn from the tragus to the inferior orbital rim is perpendicular to the tabletop. Different projections are obtained by changing the orientation of the magnetic field gradients without moving the patient's head. Because cortical or nondiploic bone and air emit a very weak signal, the normal mastoid, external auditory canal, and middle ear appear in the MR images as dark areas without any pattern or structure. The petrous pyramids are equally dark except for the signal received from the fluid within

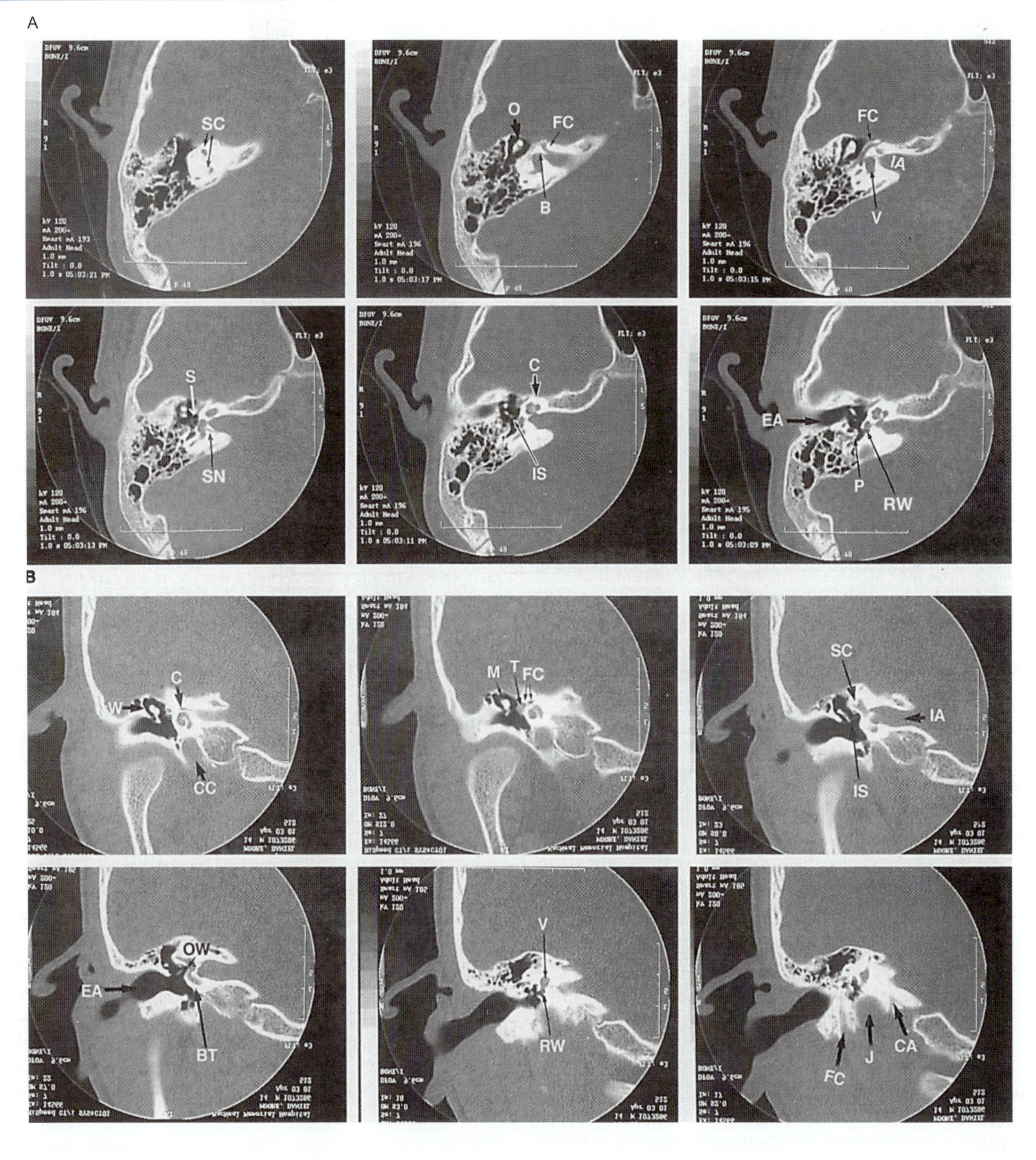

FIGURE 13–1 • Computed tomography sections of a normal right ear. *A*, axial. *B*, coronal. BT, basal turn cochlea; C, cochlea; CA, cochlear aqueduct; CC, carotid canal; CR, common crus; EA, external auditory canal; FC, facial canal; HS, horizontal semicircular canal; IA, internal auditory canal; IS, incudostapedial joint; J, jugular fossa; M, malleus; O, ossicles; OW, oval window; PE, pyramidal eminence; PS, posterior semicircular canal; RW, round window; S, stapes; SC, superior semicircular canal; SN, singular nerve canal; T, tensor tympani canal; V, vestibule; VA, vestibular aqueduct; W, lateral wall attic.

Continued

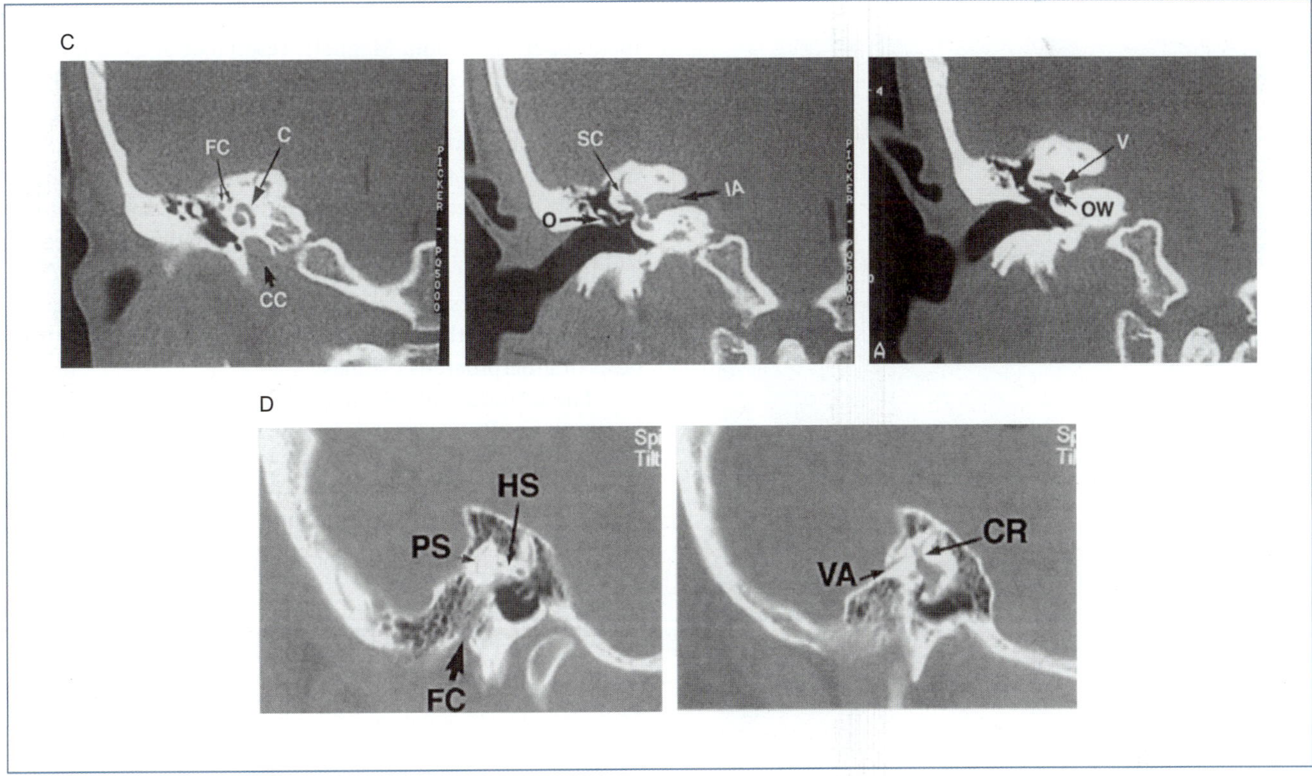

FIGURE 13–1 • *Continued.* Computed tomography sections of a normal right ear. *C,* 20 degrees coronal oblique. *D,* sagittal. BT, basal turn cochlea; C, cochlea; CA, cochlear aqueduct; CC, carotid canal; CR, common crus; EA, external auditory canal; FC, facial canal; HS, horizontal semicircular canal; IA, internal auditory canal; IS, incudostapedial joint; J, jugular fossa; M, malleus; O, ossicles; OW, oval window; PE, pyramidal eminence; PS, posterior semicircular canal; RW, round window; S, stapes; SC, superior semicircular canal; SN, singular nerve canal; T, tensor tympani canal; V, vestibule; VA, vestibular aqueduct; W, lateral wall attic.

the internal auditory canal, cochlea, vestibule, and semicircular canals. A white cast of these structures is therefore visible within the dark areas of the pyramids in T2-weighted sequences (Figure 13–2).[17]

Tissue and fluid caused by trauma or infection, and tumors within the mastoid, external auditory canal, and middle ear are readily identified by MR images as areas of abnormally high signal intensity in T2 and T1 postcontrast infusion sequences. MR imaging is more sensitive than CT scanning in the early identification of pathologic changes in the temporal bone. However, the exact location, extent, and involvement of structures, such as the ossicles, scutum, and labyrinthine capsule, cannot be determined by MR imaging because all of the landmarks within the temporal bone are absent, except for the lumen of the inner ear structures. For this reason, CT remains the study of choice for the assessment of middle ear pathology. If the lesion extends outside the confines of the temporal bone, both intracranially and extracranially, MRI defines involvement more precisely than CT scanning, particularly true for glomus tumors because involvement of the jugular vein and carotid artery may be demonstrated, thus avoiding the need for more invasive vascular studies.

The images shown in this chapter were obtained with a superconducting magnet and a magnetic field of 15,000 gauss (1.5 Tesla) or 30,000 gauss (3 Tesla). The stronger the magnetic field, the higher the signal-to-noise ratio. Therefore, it allows imaging of the smaller structures and thinner sections.

Pathologic processes are demonstrated by MRI whenever the hydrogen density and relaxation times of the pathologic tissues are different from those of the normal tissues.

The intravenous injection of ferromagnetic contrast agents has improved the recognition and differentiation of pathologic processes. Because the contrast material does not penetrate the intact blood–brain barrier, normal brain does not enhance except for structures, such as the pituitary gland and several cranial nerves that lack a complete blood–brain barrier. Enhancement of brain lesions occurs whenever the blood–brain barrier is disrupted, provided that there is sufficient blood flow to the lesions. Extra-axial lesions, such as meningiomas and schwannomas, lack a blood–brain barrier and therefore demonstrate strong enhancement.

ANGIOGRAPHY

Angiography is seldom required for the diagnosis of vascular tumors or anomalies within or adjacent to the temporal bone. Angiography, however, is mandatory for identifying the feeding vessels of a vascular lesion, usually a glomus, whenever embolization or surgical ligation is contemplated. Subtraction techniques are necessary to delineate the vascular mass and feeding vessels, which are otherwise obscured by the density of the surrounding temporal bone. The injection should be performed in the common carotid artery to visualize both internal and external carotid circulation. A vertebral arteriogram may also be performed.

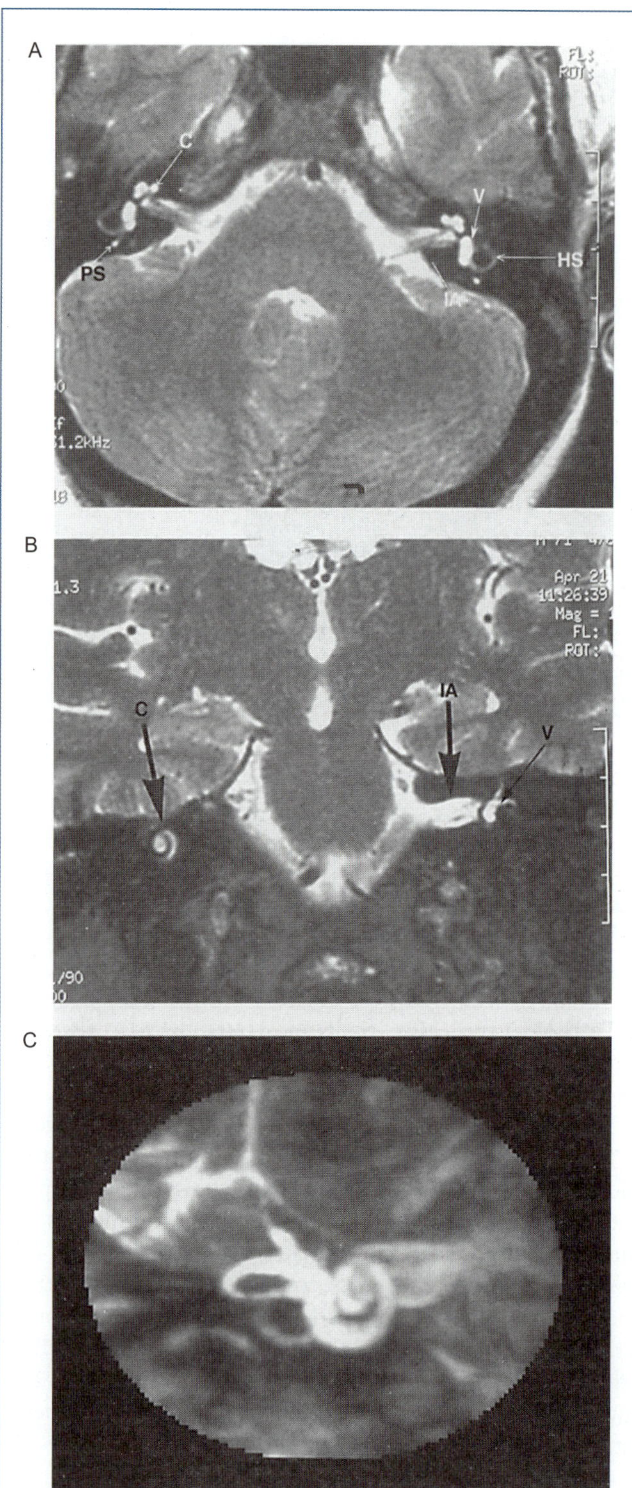

FIGURE 13–2 • Magnetic resonance images of the normal temporal bone. *A*, Fast spin-echo (FSE) axial. *B*, FSE coronal. *C*, Three-dimensional reconstruction of the inner ear structures. C, cochlea; HS, horizontal semicircular canal; IA, internal auditory canal; PS, posterior semicircular canal; V, vestibule.

Gradient echo techniques and flow-encoded gradients have enabled the development of magnetic resonance angiography.

The axial slices, after electronic removal of bone and soft tissues, are reconstructed into three-dimensional images, which can be rotated in different planes to separate vessels and eliminate superimposition. Magnetic resonance angiography of the intracranial vasculature has been particularly useful in the demonstration of aneurysms in the region of the circle of Willis, arteriovenous malformations (AVMs; particularly small dural AVMs that cannot be visualized on routine spin echo images), and vaso-occlusive pathology, including dural sinus thrombosis. MR angiography of the extracranial circulation provides excellent information regarding the patency of the carotid and vertebral arteries. These vessels may be compressed or displaced by neck masses and their lumens stenosed or obstructed by thrombosis or atheromatous plaques.[4]

The introduction of the ultrafast CT has made it possible to obtain excellent angiographic images. In CT angiography, the continuous acquisition of images allows following the rapidly injected intravenous bolus of contrast through the arteries and veins of the areas under investigation. The reconstructed images can be rotated in the plane that best demonstrates the vessels.

DEVELOPMENTAL VARIATIONS

Anatomical variations in the size and position of several components of the temporal bone are quite common. These variations should be recognized by the radiologist rather than mistaken for pathologic processes but, above all, should be known to the otologists as they develop their surgical plans.[7]

Mastoid

The development of the mastoid varies from person to person, as well as from side to side of the same individual. In some mastoids, pneumatization is limited to a single antral cell; in others, it may extend into the mastoid tip and squamosa of the temporal bone and even invade the adjacent zygoma and occipital bone. The nonpneumatized mastoid may be made up of solid bone or contain spongy diploic spaces filled with fatty marrow. The fatty marrow produces a high signal in the T1 sequence that decreases in the T2 sequence, and should not be confused with fluid or other pathologic processes that usually have a high signal in the T2 sequence.

Lateral Sinus

The lateral, or "sigmoid," sinus forms a shallow indentation on the posterior aspect of the mastoid. Occasionally, the sinus courses more anteriorly and produces a deep groove in the mastoid, best seen in the axial sections. In some cases, only a thin bony plate separates the sinus from the external auditory canal (Figure 13–3).

Tegmen

The tegmen of the mastoid and the attic is usually oriented in the horizontal plane, slightly lower than the arcuate eminence, which is formed by the top of the superior semicircular canal. A depression of the tegmental plate is not unusual, particularly in a patient with congenital atresia. As best seen in the coronal sections, the floor of the middle cranial fossa deepens to form a groove lateral to the attic and labyrinth (Figure 13–4). Low-lying dura may cover the roof of the external auditory canal and, when the canal is not developed, dip laterally to the mesotympanum.

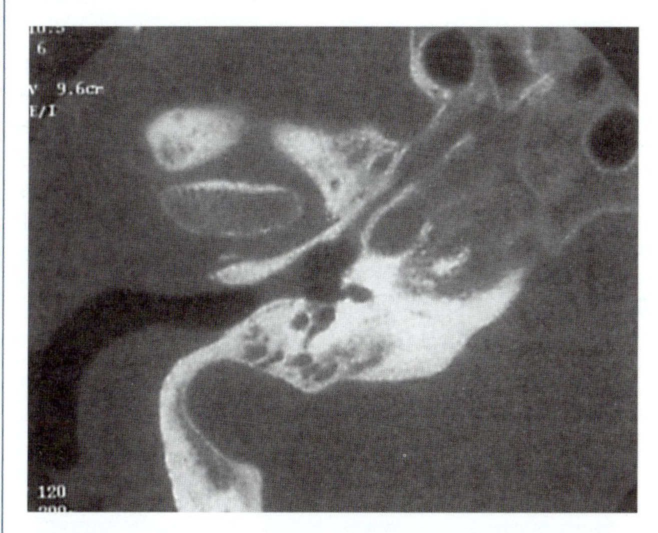

FIGURE 13–3 • Anterior lateral sinus: axial computed tomography of right ear.

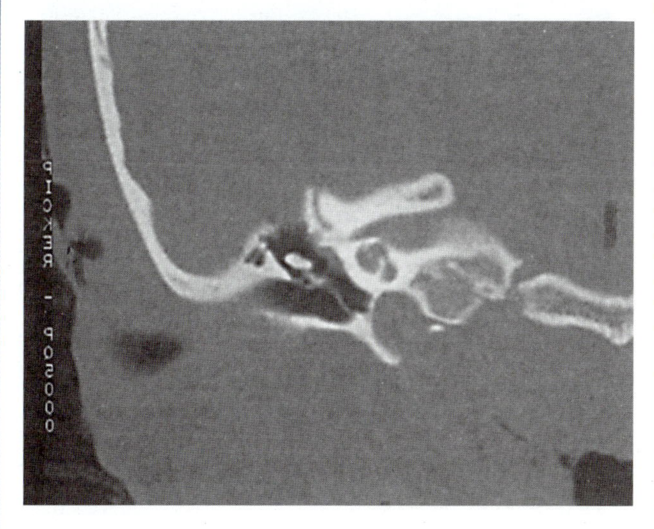

FIGURE 13–4 • Low dura: coronal computed tomography scan of right ear.

Jugular Fossa

There is tremendous variation in the size of the jugular fossa and jugular bulb. The variation occurs not only from patient to patient but also from side to side in the same patient. The size of the jugular fossa is not a criterion for any pathologic process. A normal jugular fossa may produce only a slight indentation on the undersurface of the petrous bone or may extend superiorly as high as the superior petrous ridge posterior to the labyrinth and internal auditory canal (Figure 13–5A and B). In these instances, the jugular bulb projects so high that it blocks access to the internal auditory canal by the translabyrinthine route in acoustic neuroma surgery. Often the high venous structure is not the jugular bulb itself but rather a diverticulum arising from the jugular bulb. At times, the jugular bulb projects into the hypo- and mesotympanum. There may be a bony cover over the jugular bulb, or the vein may lie exposed in the middle ear in contact with the medial surface of the tympanic membrane. Such a high jugular bulb appears otoscopically as a blue mass that can be misdiagnosed as a glomus tumor.

A

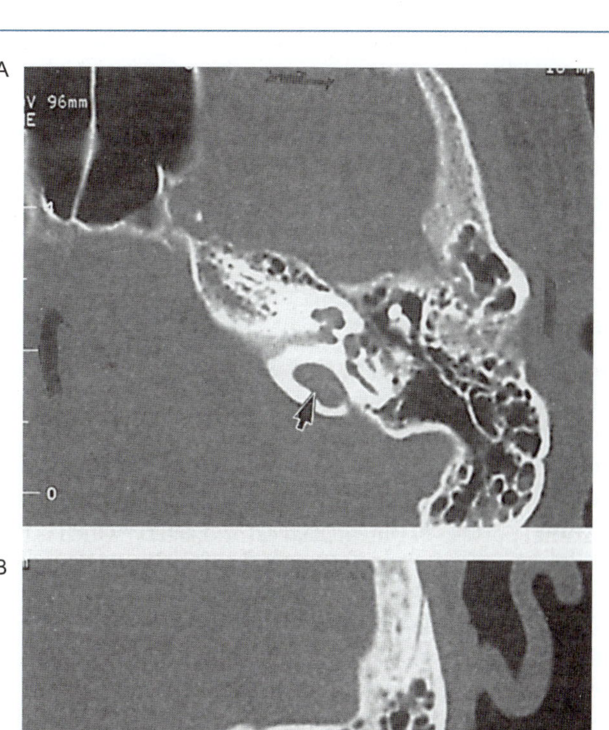

B

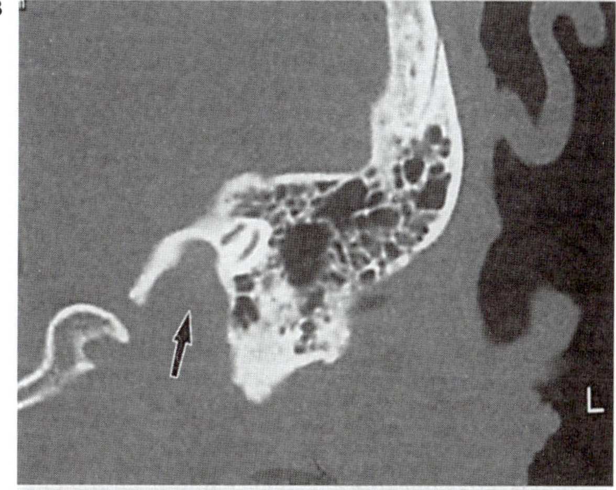

C

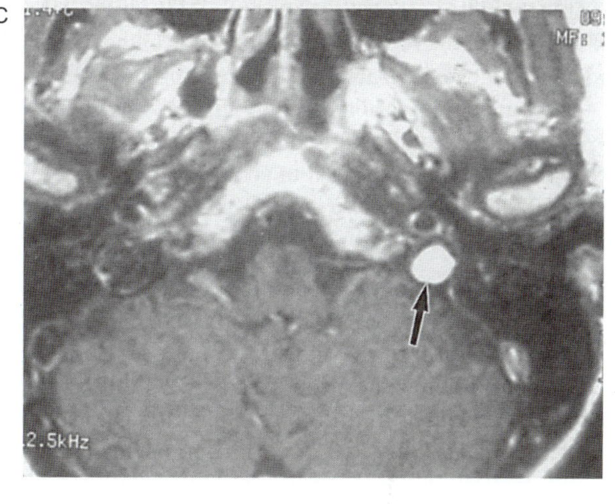

FIGURE 13–5 • High jugular bulb (*arrows*). *A*, Axial. and *B*, Coronal computed tomography sections. *C*, Magnetic resonance T1 image postcontrast.

The MRI appearance of a high jugular bulb may be misread as a glomus tumor because of the area of mixed signal within the bulb produced by turbulent flow. However, whereas a glomus tumor contains multiple dots of signal void within a mass of medium or high signal, with a high jugular bulb, linear streaks of high and low signal are seen within the lumen of the bulb, usually paralleling its walls due to variations in flow velocity (Figure13–5C).

Carotid Artery

Minor variations in the intratemporal course of the internal carotid artery are not uncommon but are of no clinical significance. In some cases, the internal carotid artery may take an ectopic course through the middle ear. This anomaly should be recognized prior to surgery to avoid tragic consequences. The proximal portion of the internal carotid artery, which is always seen in the coronal sections below the cochlea, is absent. The anomalous internal carotid artery enters the temporal bone through an enlarged tympanic canaliculus or via an opening in the floor of the posterior aspect of the hypotympanum. The artery extends through the entire length of the middle ear cavity and then passes through a defect in the anterior wall of the middle ear to regain its normal position in the petrous apex (Figure 13–6A and B).

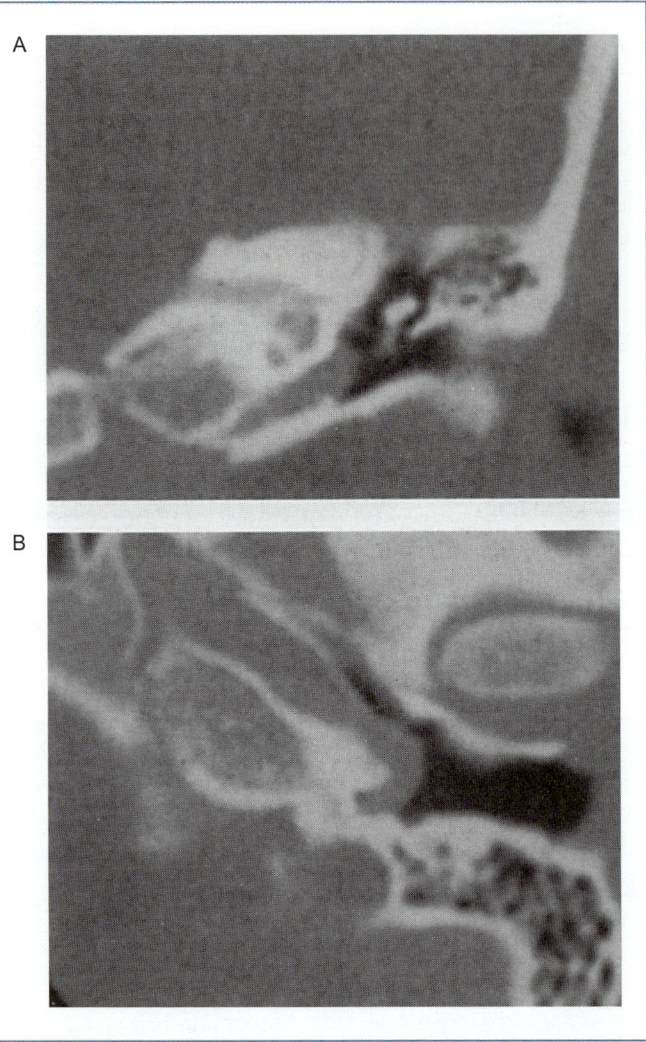

FIGURE 13–6 • Ectopic carotid, CT. *A*, Coronal. *B*, Axial sections.

Arachnoid Granulations

Arachnoid granulations are villous structures that herniate through small defects in the dura and drain cerebrospinal fluid from the subarachnoid space into the venous system.

A variable number of arachnoid granulations do not reach their venous target but come in contact with the intracranial surface of the middle ear and, less frequently, of the posterior surface of the temporal bone. Over time, the pulsation of the cerebrospinal fluid may produce small areas of bony resorption and erosion.

Arachnoid granulations become clinically significant when they open into the adjacent air spaces (attic, mastoid air cells) as they may lead to a spontaneous cerebrospinal otorrhea. If the mastoid and middle ear cavity are infected, intracranial complications such as abcess formation may develop.

Petrous Apex

The petrous apex may be significantly pneumatized or be made up of compact or diploic bone. In the MR study, the signal intensity of the apex varies with its bony texture: high or bright in the T1 images when diploic, low or dark when highly pneumatized or compact. Often the bony texture of the two petrous apices of the same person is different, resulting in one apex being brighter than the other (Figure13–7).

PATHOLOGIC CONDITIONS

The major categories of pathologic conditions that may involve the temporal bone and adjacent base of the skull are congenital malformations, traumatic effects, inflammatory processes, neoplastic conditions, and otodystrophies. The otolaryngologist should learn as much as possible about the nature and extent of the pathologic process before deciding how to treat the patient and, if surgery is indicated, how to approach the lesion.

Congenital Anomalies of the Temporal Bone

A proper imaging assessment is essential in all patients with congenital anomalies of the temporal bone. Otoscopy is of little value in atresia and aplasia of the external auditory canal. Audiometry is often unreliable in young children. Imaging should demonstrate the status of the anatomic structures of the ear, the development and course of the facial nerve canal, the position of the sigmoid sinus and jugular bulb, and the course of the carotid canal. Such information is of value for the otologist in determining the proper treatment for conductive and sensorineural hearing losses.

Anomalies of the Sound Conducting System

A good CT study provides the surgeon with the following basic information, which is needed in making decisions about the feasibility of corrective surgery and in determining which type of surgery is indicated:

1. The degree and type of abnormality of the tympanic bone. These abnormalities range from a relatively minor deformity to complete agenesis of the external auditory canal (Figures 13–8 and 13–9A and B).

A

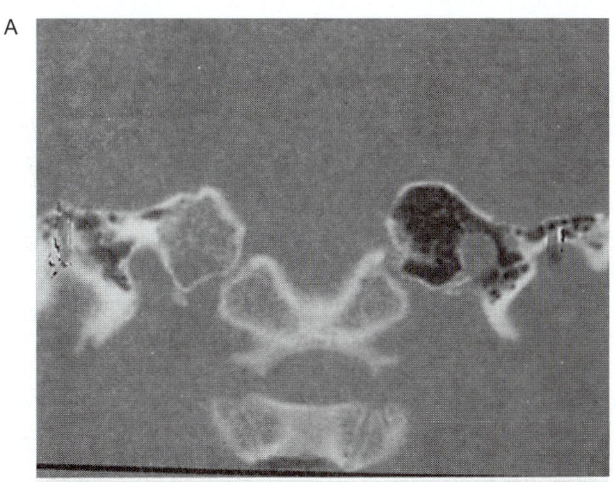

B

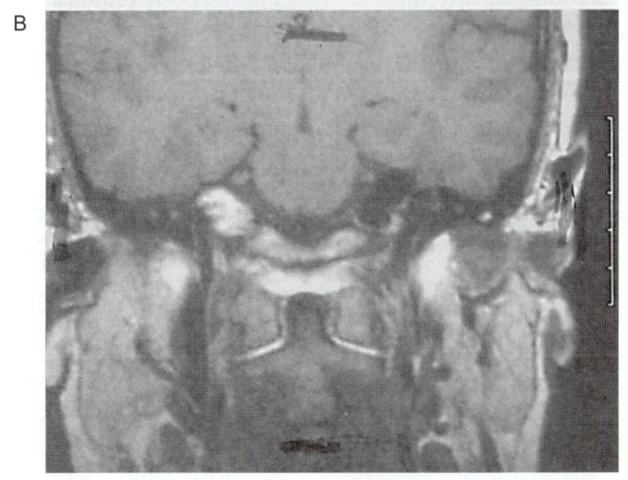

FIGURE 13–7 • Asymmetric pneumatization of the petrous apices. *A*, Coronal computed tomography scan. *B*, Magnetic resonance coronal T1 image.

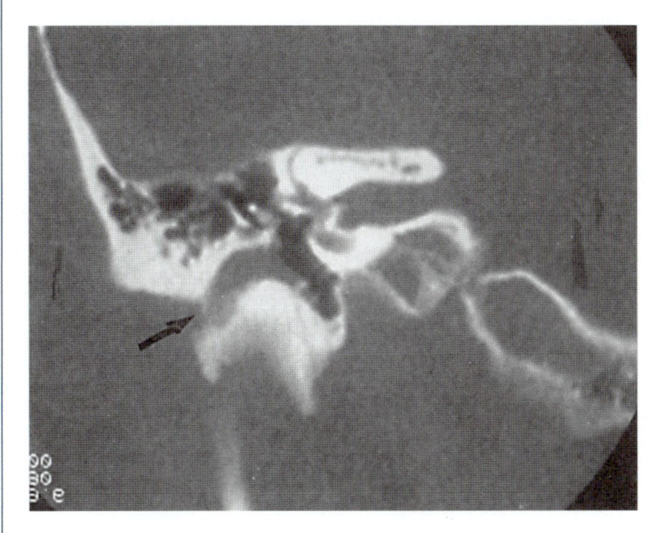

FIGURE 13–8 • Atresia of the external auditory canal: coronal CT scan. The external auditory canal is stenotic and closed at its lateral end by a thin bony plate (*arrow*). The middle ear cavity is aerated and normal in size, but the incus is deformed, with a short and stubby long process.

2. The degree and position of the pneumatization of the mastoid air cells and mastoid antrum.
3. The development and aeration of the middle ear cavity.
4. The status of the ossicular chain, the size and shape of the ossicles, and the presence of fusion or fixation (see Figures 13–8 and 13–9A and B).
5. The patency of the labyrinthine windows.
6. The course of the facial nerve canal.
7. The development of the inner ear structures. Defects in the otic capsule, including the modiolus and spiral lamina, are visualized by high-definition spiral CT.
8. The relationship of the meninges to the mastoid tegmen and superior petrous ridge. The middle cranial fossa often forms a deep groove lateral to the labyrinth, which results in a low-lying dura over the mastoid and external auditory canal.

Anomalies of the Ear

With advances in cochlear implantation for profound sensorineural deafness, the assessment of the inner ear structures has become essential. Only defects in the otic capsule are visible by

A

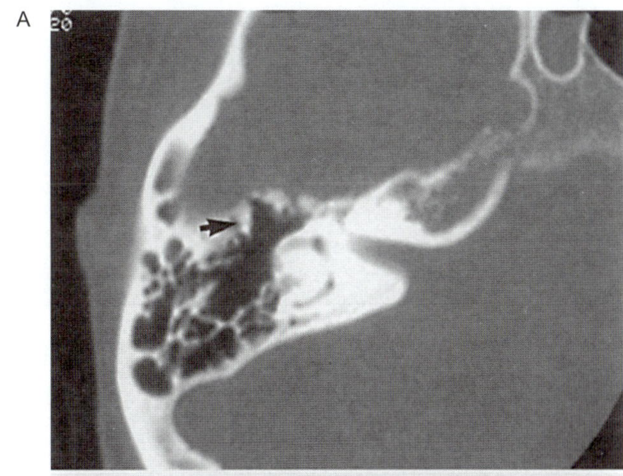

B

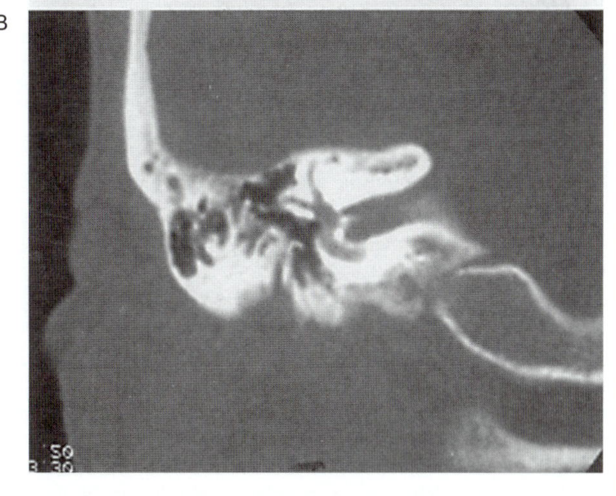

FIGURE 13–9 • Agenesis of the external auditory canal. *A*, axial. *B*, Coronal computed tomography scans. The external auditory canal is not developed; the middle ear cavity is aerated but smaller than normal. The malleus and incus are hypoplastic and fixed to the lateral attic wall (*short arrow*). The course of the facial canal, inner ear structures, and oval window are normal.

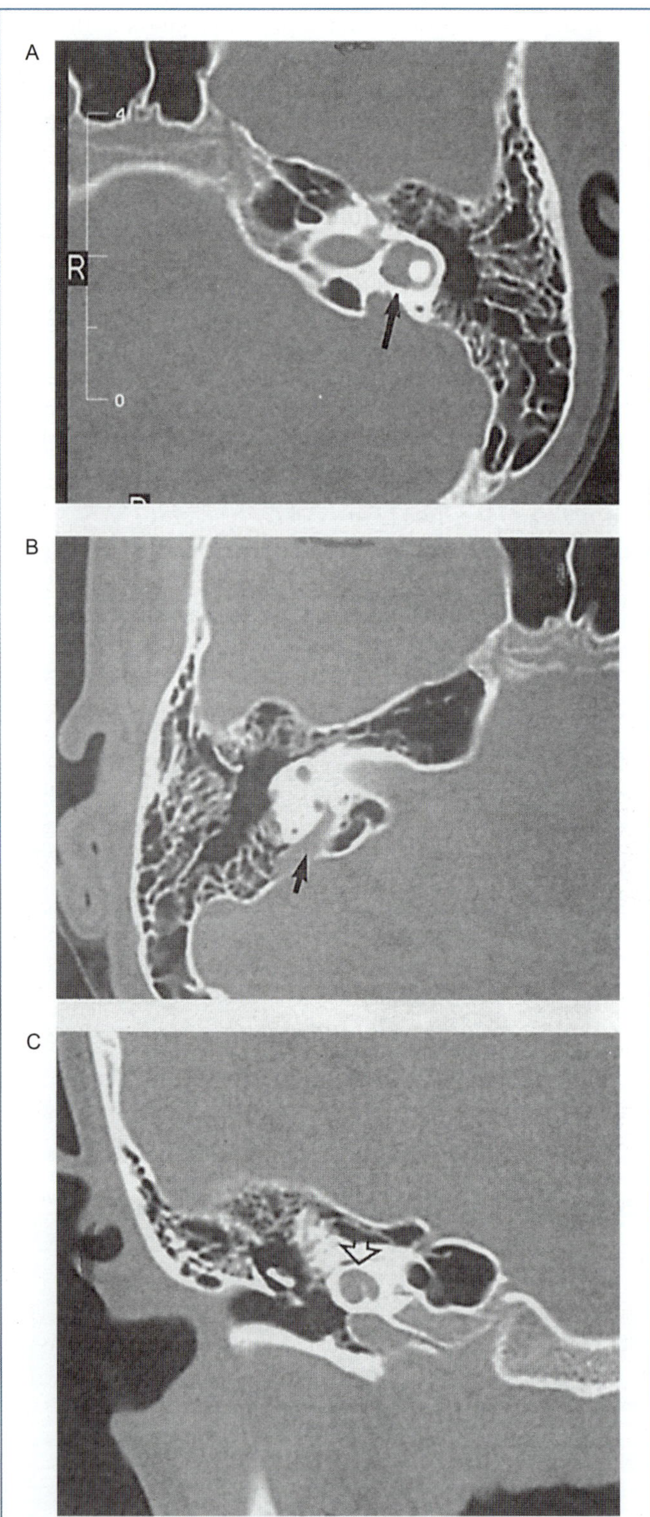

FIGURE 13–10 • Mondini defect. *A* and *B*, Axial. *C*, Coronal computed tomography scans. The cochlea (*open arrow*) is normal in size, but the bony partition between the cochlea coils is absent or hypoplastic. The vestibular aqueduct (*short arrow*) is enlarged and the vestibule (*long arrow*) is dilated.

imaging. Abnormal development of the membranous labyrinth is not detectable by the present imaging techniques. Anomalies of the otic capsule involve a single structure or the entire capsule and may range from a minor hypoplasia of a single structure to complete agenesis of the inner ear structures (Michel's anomaly). A common deformity of the labyrinthine capsule is Mondini's type, which is characterized by an abnormal development of the cochlea associated with dilatation of the vestibular aqueduct[18] and vestibule (Figure 13–10A to C). The semicircular canals are often malformed and usually hypoplastic.[8–14]

Imaging Assessment for Cochlear Implantation

Candidates for cochlear implantation require an imaging study to determine the feasibility of the procedure. The otologic surgeon must know if the mastoid and middle ear are large enough to gain access to the promontory and round window. If an intracochlear implant is contemplated, the surgeon should know if there is a patent round window and cochlear lumen. If the cochlea is obliterated by bone, the cochlea must be drilled or an extracochlear device used. Marked hypoplasia of the cochlea and internal auditory canal (Figure 13–11A and B) is often indicative of a lack of development of the acoustic nerve, which will make an implant infeasible. MR is indicated to establish the presence and status of the cochlear nerve, to rule out fibrous obliteration of the

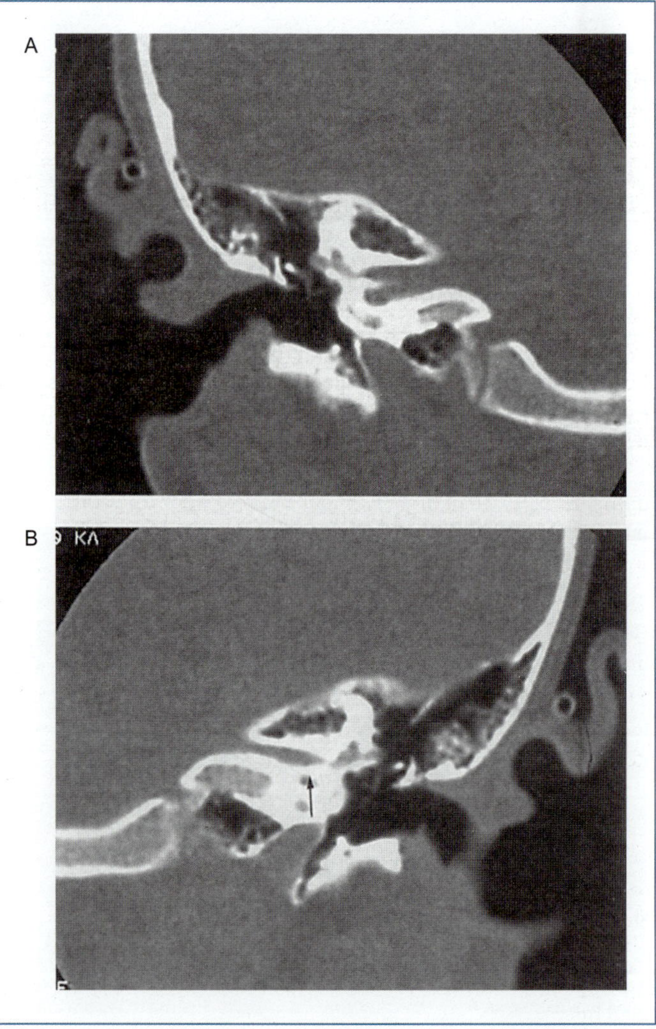

FIGURE 13–11 • Hypoplasia of the internal auditory canal: coronal computed tomography scans. *A*, Right; *B*, Left. The upper compartment of the left internal auditory canal is normal, but the lower compartment is absent or markedly hypoplastic as shown by the position of the falciform crest (*arrow*). Compare with the normal right side.

cochlear lumen that cannot be seen by the CT, and exclude the presence of central pathology affecting the auditory pathways. A postoperative transorbital or Schüller view should be obtained to determine the position of the electrodes and the integrity of the implanted wires. A more precise assessment is obtained by three-dimensional reconstruction of the CT data.

Anomalies of the Facial Nerve

Anomalies of the facial canal involve the size and course of the canal. There may be complete or partial agenesis of the facial nerve with total paralysis. Occasionally, the facial nerve canal may be unusually narrow and the nerve hypoplastic. In these cases, intermittent episodes of facial paresis may occur. The horizontal segment of the facial canal is at times displaced inferiorly to cover the oval window. Anomalies in the course of the mastoid segment are common in congenital atresia of the external auditory canal. The facial canal is usually rotated laterally. The rotation varies from a minor obliquity to a true horizontal course.

Temporal Bone Trauma

Imaging studies of the temporal bone following head trauma are indicated when there is cerebrospinal fluid otorrhea or rhinorrhea, hearing loss, or facial nerve paralysis.

The CT study should always include axial, coronal, and sagittal sections. In patients with unconsciousness or neurologic findings, the CT study should be extended to the entire brain to rule out the possibility of intracranial hemorrhage. In addition, a series of scans obtained after intrathecal injection of iodinated contrast material is often useful in demonstration of the site of leak in patients with cerebrospinal fluid rhinorrhea or otorrhea.[13]

Temporal bone fractures are divided into longitudinal and transverse types, depending on the direction of the fracture line. Longitudinal fractures occur more frequently than transverse fractures in a ratio of 5 to 1. This classification, however, is somewhat arbitrary because most fractures follow a serpiginous tract in the temporal bone.

The typical longitudinal fracture involves the temporal squama and extends into the mastoid. The fracture usually reaches the external auditory canal and passes medially into the epitympanum, where it produces a disruption of the ossicular chain. From the epitympanum, the fracture extends into the petrosa and follows an intralabyrinthine or extralabyrinthine course. An intralabyrinthine course of the fracture is rare because the otic capsule is quite resistant to trauma. Extralabyrinthine extension occurs either anterior or posterior to the labyrinth. Anterior extension is more common (Figure 13–12A and B).

A transverse fracture of the temporal bone typically crosses the petrous pyramid perpendicular to the long axis of the pyramid. The fracture usually follows the line of least resistance and runs from the dome of the jugular fossa through the labyrinth to the superior petrous ridge (Figure 13–13A and B).

The fracture line may disappear at certain levels only to reappear a few millimeters distant. This apparent gap is not caused by interruption of the fracture but rather by the fact that the plane of the fracture line changes course and becomes invisible in some sections.

Longitudinal fractures are best demonstrated in the axial and sagittal sections and transverse fractures are best seen in the axial and coronal sections.

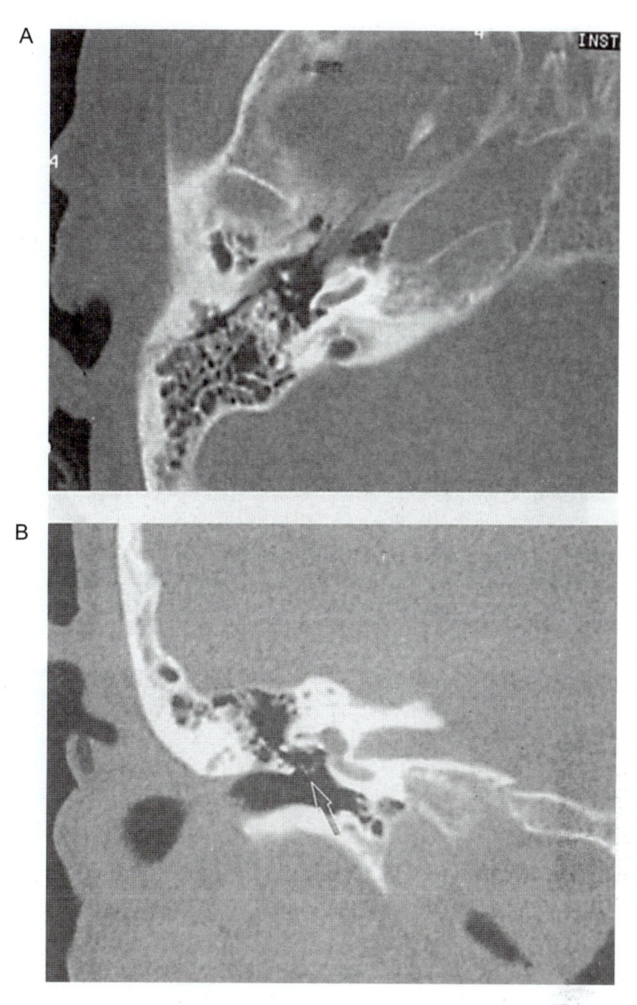

FIGURE 13–12 • Longitudinal fracture of the right temporal bone. *A*, Axial. *B*, Coronal computed tomography scans. The mastoid fracture extends to the superior canal wall and to the lateral wall of the attic. The ossicular chain is disrupted at the incudostapedial joint (*arrow*).

Traumatic disruption of the ossicular chain is most common in patients with longitudinal fractures but may occur even in the absence of an actual fracture. Dislocation of the malleus is rare because of its firm attachment to the tympanic membrane and the strong anterior malleal ligament. The incus is most commonly dislocated because its attachment to the malleus and stapes is easily torn (Figure 13–14). Fractures and dislocations of the footplate of the stapes are seldom recognizable but may be identified by the presence of air within the vestibule.

Labyrinthine Concussion and Bleeding

Bleeding within the lumen of inner ear structures may occur after trauma (Figure 13–15). If a fracture line traverses the inner ear, the detection of blood is of academic value since the patient has an irreversible total deafness, vestibular paralysis, or both. If bleeding occurs by concussion without actual fracture, MRI may be indicated to confirm the diagnosis. The study should be performed at least two days after the injury to allow the transformation of deoxyhemoglobin into methemoglobin, which has a bright signal in both T1 and T2 images. Intracranial bleeding in

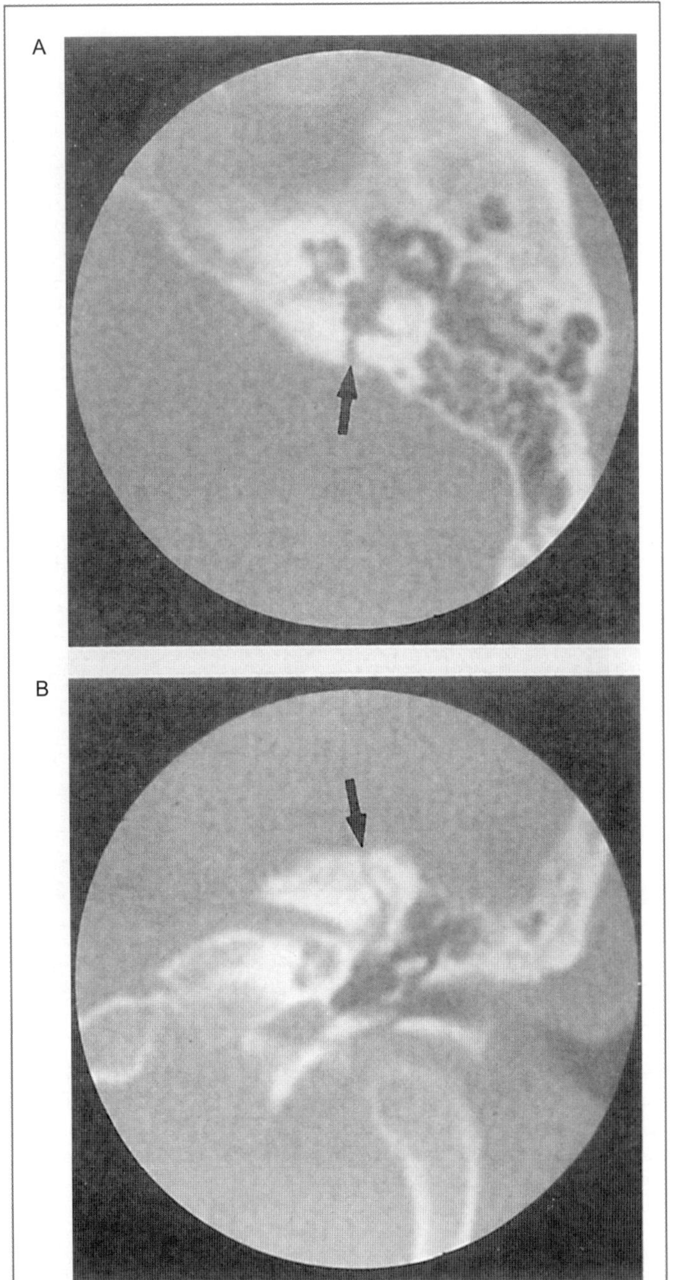

FIGURE 13–13 • Transverse fracture with facial paralysis. *A*, Axial. *B*, Coronal computed tomography scans. The fracture splits the vestibule and involves the facial canal anterior to the oval window (*arrow*).

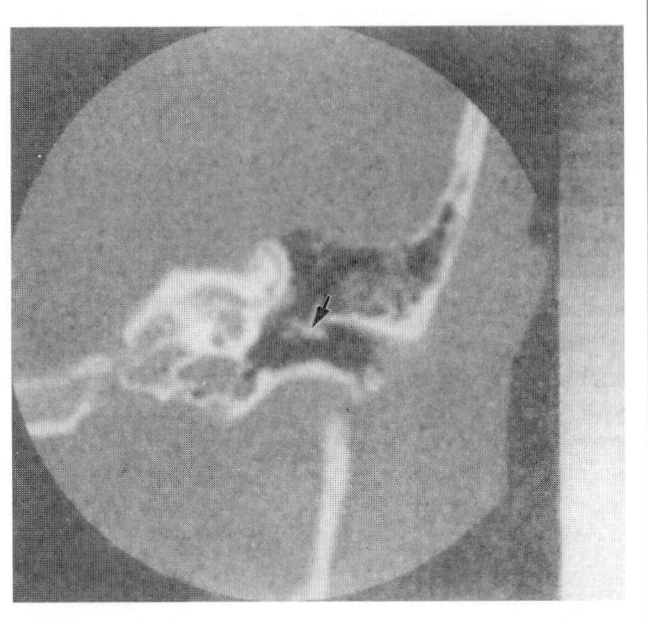

FIGURE 13–14 • Traumatic dislocation of the incus: coronal computed tomography scan. The body of the incus is displaced into the external auditory canal (*arrow*).

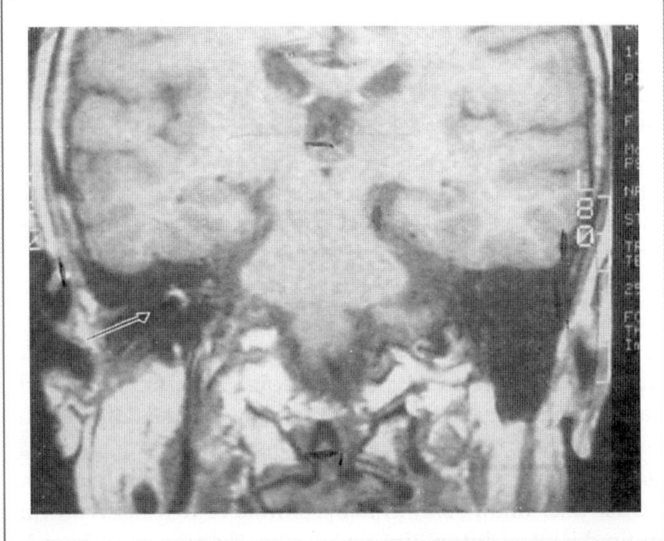

FIGURE 13–15 • Labyrinthine concussion with bleeding: magnetic resonance coronal T1 image; no contrast. Note the high signal within the vestibule and semicircular canals produced by blood (*arrow*).

the region of the cochlear nuclei and auditory pathway may also cause transient or irreversible deafness. Spontaneous intralabyrinthine hemorrhage has also been observed in patients with sickle cell disease owing to vaso-occlusive crisis.

Traumatic Facial Paralysis

Facial paralysis occurs immediately or after a period of a few hours or days following trauma. Immediate-onset facial paralysis is the result of transection of the facial nerve by the fracture. Delayed facial paralysis is caused by fracture of the facial canal and post-traumatic edema of the nerve. Facial paralysis occurs in approximately 25% of longitudinal fractures and is delayed, and often transient, in 50% of the cases. Facial paralysis is observed in 50% of transverse fractures and is almost always immediate and permanent (see Figure 13–13). In some cases, the site of involvement of the facial canal cannot be visualized in the CT sections. However, by evaluation of the course of the fracture line, the site of the lesion can be determined.

Meningocele and Meningoencephalocele

Meningocele and meningoencephalocele are usually post-traumatic owing to a tegmental fracture, or iatrogenic following mastoid surgery, and are rarely spontaneous. The brain and

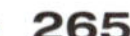

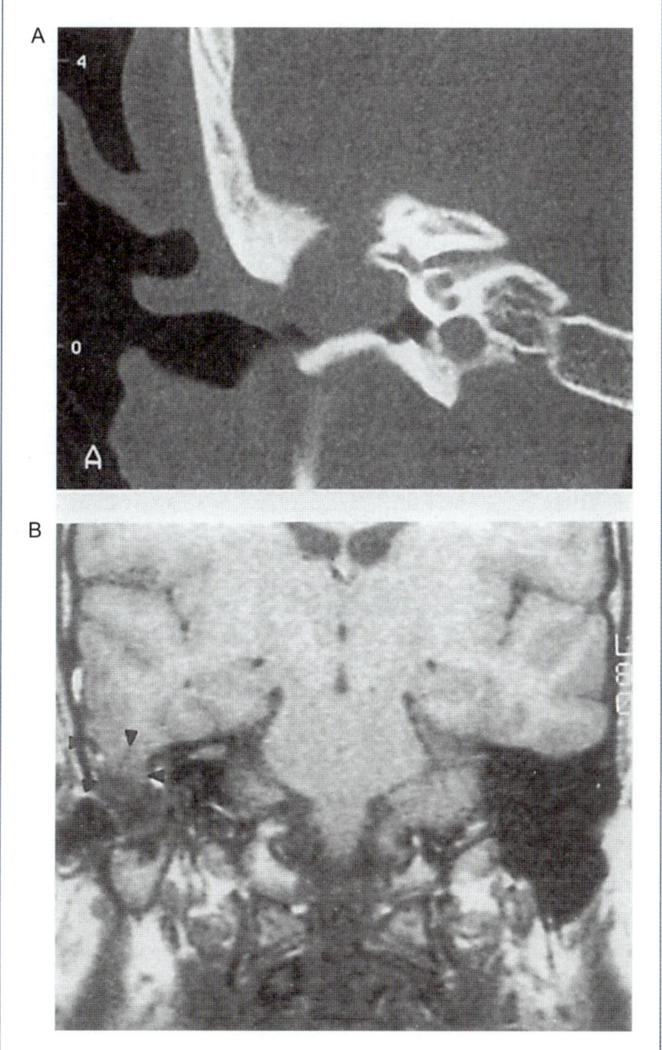

FIGURE 13–16 • Meningoencephalocele: *A*, Coronal computed tomography scan. *B*, Magnetic resonance (MR) T1 image. A large well-defined soft tissue mass protrudes into the right external auditory canal through a wide defect in the tegmen. The MR image confirms that the mass is a meningoencephalocele (*arrowheads*).

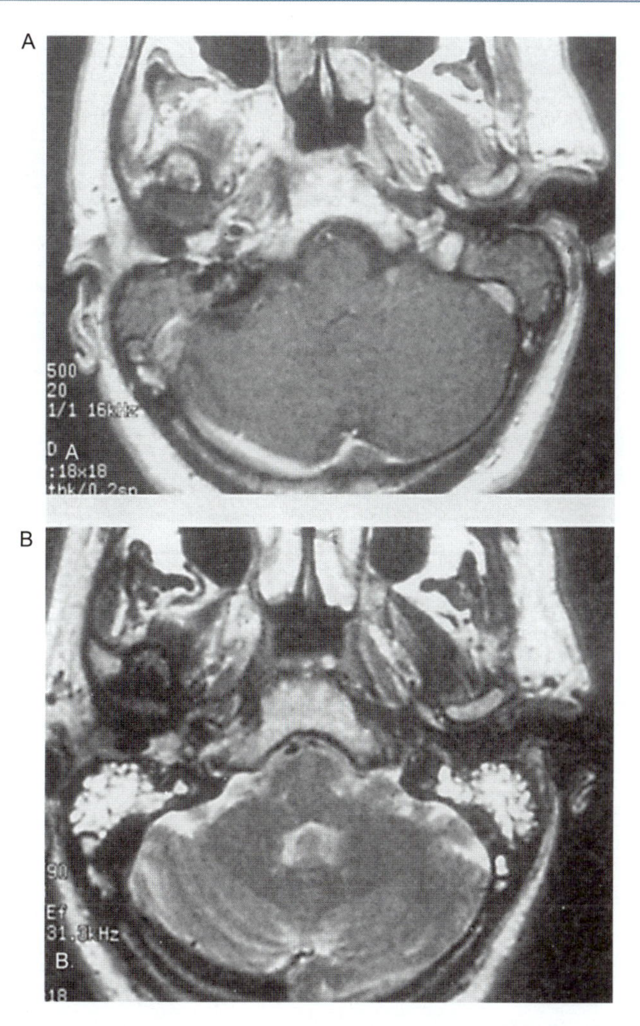

FIGURE 13–17 • Acute otomastoiditis: magnetic resonance images. *A*, T1; *B*, T2. In the T1 image, the mastoid air cells are filled by a medium (pus) of higher signal intensity than clear fluid, which becomes bright in T2.

meninges herniate through the defect in the tegmen into the mastoid antrum or attic. The constant pulsation of cerebrospinal fluid is transmitted through the walls of the meningocele, causing gradual resorption of the surrounding bony walls. CT scanning demonstrates the defect in the tegmen and the adjacent soft tissue mass (Figure 13–16A). An MR study is performed whenever the nature of the soft tissue mass is unclear. On MR examination, a meningocele has a signal identical to cerebrospinal fluid; the signal of an encephalocele is identical to that of brain (Figure 13–16B).

Inflammatory Process and Cholesteatomas

Acute Otomastoiditis

Acute otitis media with mastoiditis is a clinical diagnosis. Initially, the process is characterized by a nonspecific diffuse and homogenous opacification of the middle ear and mastoid air cells (Figure 13–17). If the infection is not arrested by proper treatment, necrosis of the cell walls occurs, which leads to the formation of areas of coalescence and abscesses. The coalescent infection may perforate the mastoid cortex and produce a variety of subperiosteal abscesses. If the tegmen or sinus plate is dehiscent or eroded, intracranial complications develop, such as epidural and brain abscesses, sigmoid sinus thrombosis, and perisinus abscesses (Figure 13–18).[12]

Whenever an intracranial complication is suspected, a CT or MR study of the brain with contrast should be obtained to confirm the intracranial involvement and demonstrate the site and extent of the process (Figure 13–19).

Chronic Otomastoiditis

Two types of chronic ear diseases are recognizable: chronic infection and tubotympanic disease. Chronic infection is the result of an infection by a low-virulence organism or of an acute infection with incomplete resolution. The typical radiographic findings consist of thickening of the mastoid trabeculae, inhomogeneous opacification of the air cells, and, if no perforation is present, inhomogeneous opacification of the middle ear cavity.

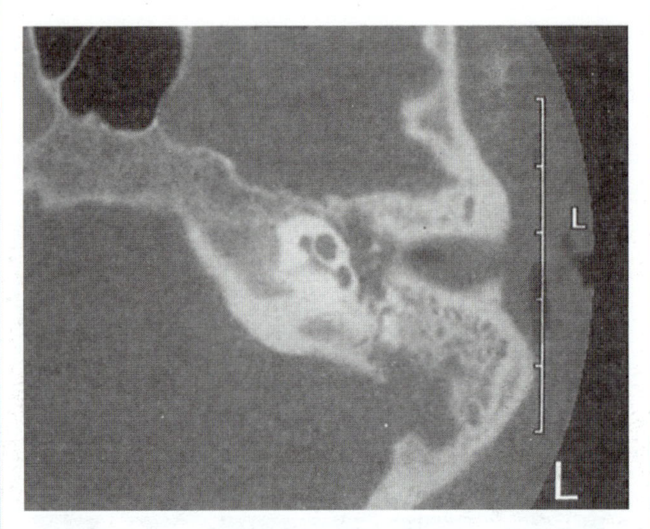

FIGURE 13–18 • Acute mastoiditis with perisinus abscess and sigmoid sinus thrombosis. The axial computed tomography scan shows a coalescent cavity in the left mastoid with erosion of the sinus plate. Note the clouding of the left middle ear cavity and swelling of the external auditory canal skin. L, left.

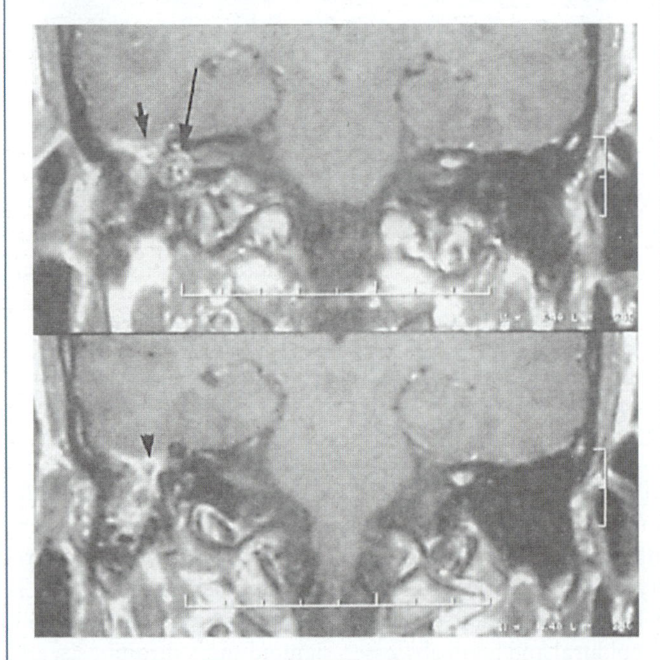

FIGURE 13–19 • Subacute mastoiditis with complications: magnetic resonance coronal T1 image postcontrast. Enhancing granulation tissue and an abscess fill the right mastoid. The tegmen is partially eroded with formation of an epidural abscess (*arrowhead*). Note the thickening and enhancement of the adjacent meninges (*short arrow*) and the enhancement of the inner ear structures caused by an acute labyrinthitis (*long arrow*).

The involved air cells become constricted at first and later are completely obliterated. The residual air cells, antrum, and middle ear are usually filled with granulation tissue and fluid. Erosion of the long process of the incus may occur.

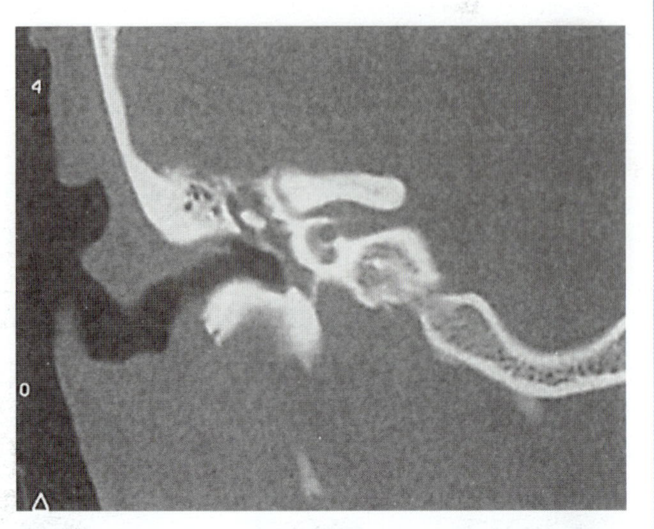

FIGURE 13–20 • Chronic otitis media: coronal computed tomography scan. The middle ear cavity is opacified, and the tympanic membrane is thickened and retracted.

Tubotympanic disease is the result of faulty aeration of the middle ear caused by eustachian tube malfunction or obstruction by mucositis. CT sections demonstrate opacification of the middle ear and mastoid and contraction of the middle ear space (Figure 13–20), caused by retraction of the tympanic membrane to the promontory. Tympanosclerotic plaques are not uncommon and, if large enough, appear as linear calcifications in the tympanic membrane and mucosa over the promontory, or as partially calcified masses in the attic, often surrounding and fixing the ossicles.

Malignant Necrotizing External Otitis

Malignant external otisis is an acute osteomyelitis of the temporal bone that occurs in diabetic and immunosuppressed patients and is caused by the *Pseudomonas* bacterium. The infection begins as an external otitis but spreads to involve the walls of the external canal (Figure 13–21A and B). The process often extends into the middle ear and mastoid. The infection usually breaks through the floor of the external canal at the bony–cartilaginous junction and spreads along the undersurface of the temporal bone to involve the facial nerve at the stylomastoid foramen. Further medial extension involves the jugular fossa and cranial nerves IX, X, XI, and XII. Anterior spread of the infection affects the temporomandibular joint (Figure 13–21). CT scanning is excellent for demonstrating involvement of the external auditory canal, middle ear, and petrous pyramid, but MRI becomes the study of choice when the infection spreads to the facial nerve or beyond the confines of the temporal bone.

Acute Labyrinthitis

Enhancement within the lumen of the bony labyrinth is often observed in MR images obtained after infusion of contrast material in patients with acute bacterial and viral labyrinthitis and sudden deafness (see Figures 13–19 and 13–22). The enhancement of inner structures is presumably caused by damage of the capillary endothelium, which leads to a disruption of the labyrinth–blood barrier.[3–11]

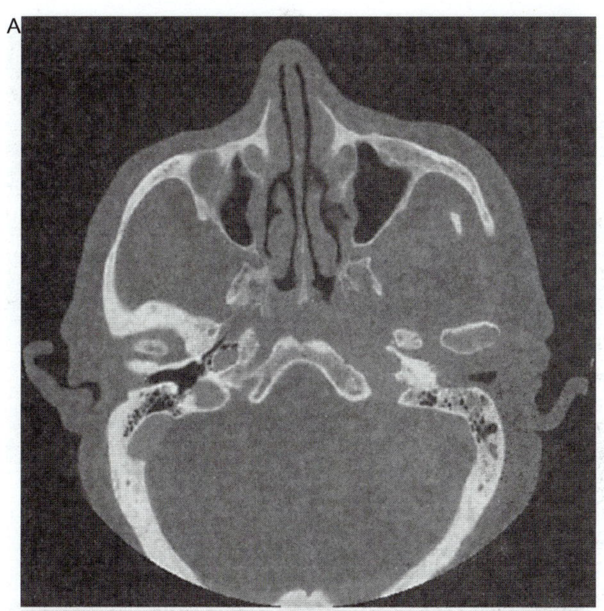

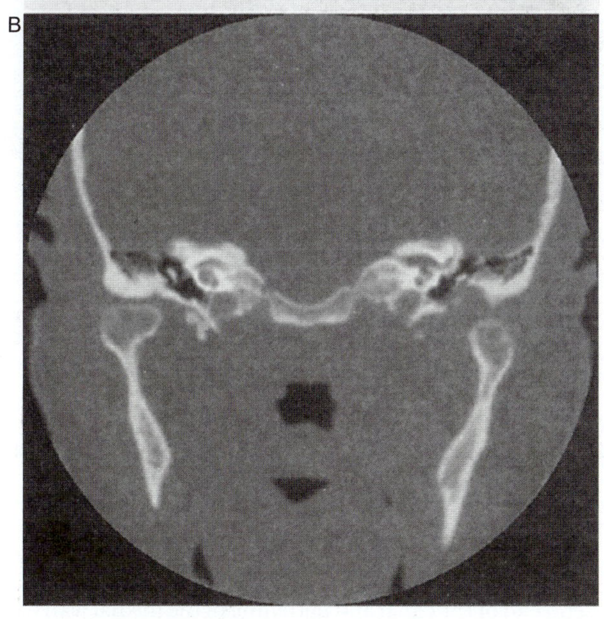

FIGURE 13–21 • Necrotizing otitis extreme. *A*, Axial. *B*, Coronal sections. The floor and anterior wall of the external auditory canal are destroyed with extension of the infection to the undersurface of the temporal bone and to the temporal mandibular joint.

Chronic Labyrinthitis

Chronic labyrinthitis varies from a localized reaction caused by a fistula of the bony labyrinth to a diffuse process. The lumen of the inner ear is partially or totally filled with granulation and fibrous tissue. Osteitis of the bony labyrinth occurs, which leads to a partial or complete bony obliteration of the lumen. Whereas bony obliteration of the inner ear is readily identified by CT scanning, fibrous obliteration is recognizable only by MR imaging. In the T2 sequence, the high signal seen within the normal inner ear structures is absent, making the involved structures no longer recognizable.

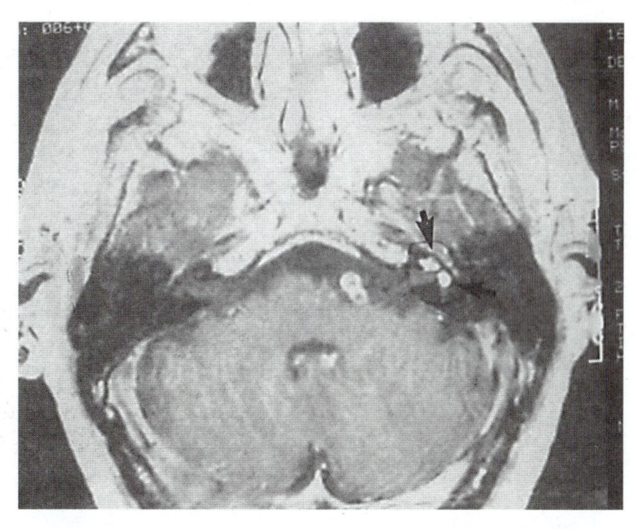

FIGURE 13–22 • Acute labyrinthitis: axial magnetic resonance T1 image postcontrast showing prominent enhancement of the left cochlea and vestibule (*arrow*).

Facial Neuritis

Moderate bilateral enhancement of the normal facial nerve, particularly in the region of anterior genu, is often observed in MR studies obtained after injection of contract material.

Asymmetric enhancement of the facial nerve, more prominent on the paralyzed side, is common in patients with Bell's palsy and Ramsey Hunt syndrome. The enhancement varies in intensity with the stage of the process. It is usually more prominent early in the course of the disease and gradually decreases whether or not the paralysis has resolved. In Bell's palsy, the involvement is segmental and usually confined to the anterior genu and adjacent labyrinthine and tympanic segments. Involvement of the mastoid segment is rare. In Ramsey Hunt syndrome, the involvement by the *Herpes zoster* virus is more diffuse and very often involves the nerve in the internal auditory canal (Figure 13–23A and B).

Cholesteatoma

Cholesteatomas are congenital or acquired epidermoid cysts. Congenital cholesteatomas arise from epithelial tissue rests within or adjacent to the temporal bone. Acquired cholesteatomas originate in the middle ear from the stratified squamous epithelium of the tympanic membrane or metaplasia of the middle ear mucosa. Another distinct form of cholesteatoma arises in the external auditory canal. CT scanning is the study of choice for the diagnosis and the extent of the cholesteatoma.

Acquired Cholesteatoma

Cholesteatomas appear as soft tissue masses in the maesotympanum or epitympanum. If the middle ear is aerated, the entire soft tissue mass is well outlined. When fluid or inflammatory tissue fills the middle ear, the contour of the cholesteatoma is obscured, and it may be difficult to determine its actual size. Characteristic bone changes occur in cholesteatomas that help in diagnosing the lesion and in establishing the site of origin and extension of the process.

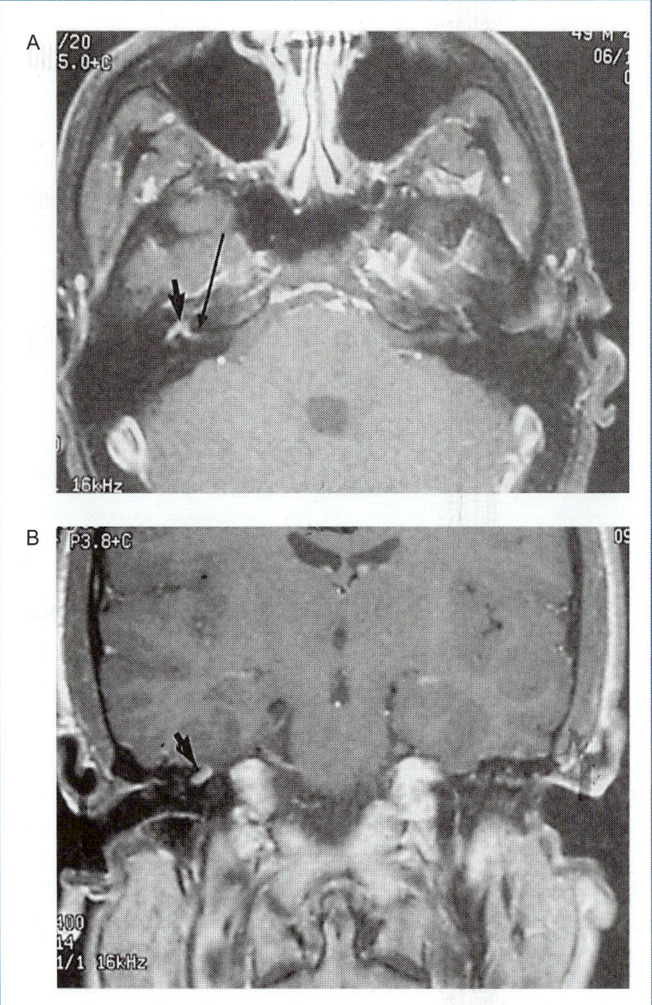

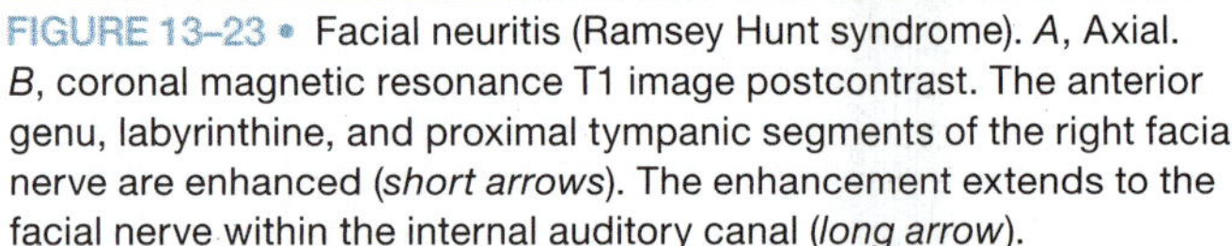
FIGURE 13–23 • Facial neuritis (Ramsey Hunt syndrome). *A*, Axial. *B*, coronal magnetic resonance T1 image postcontrast. The anterior genu, labyrinthine, and proximal tympanic segments of the right facial nerve are enhanced (*short arrows*). The enhancement extends to the facial nerve within the internal auditory canal (*long arrow*).

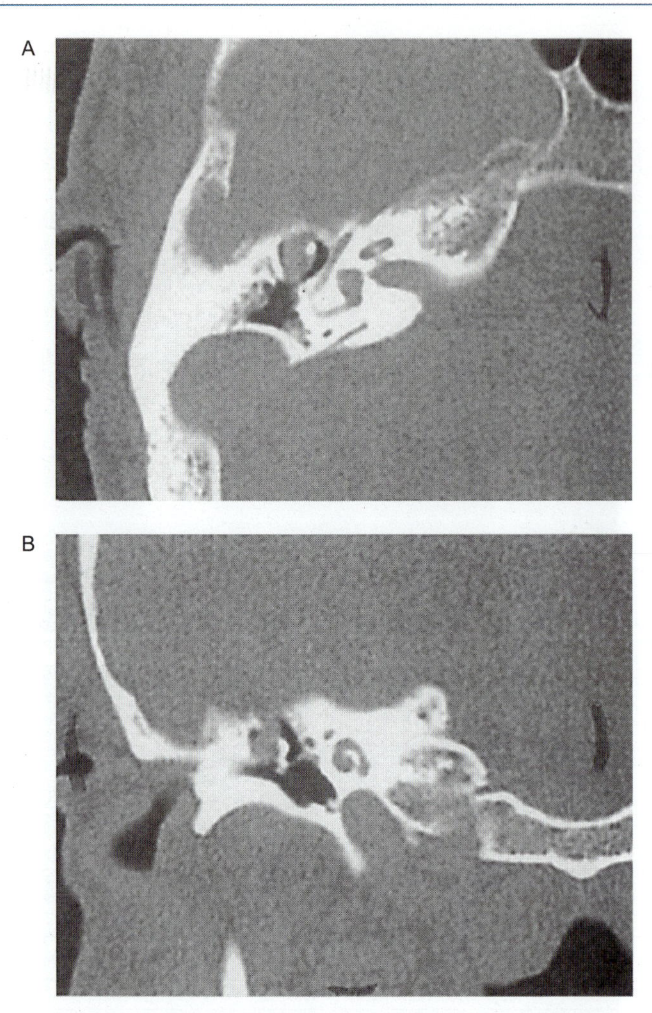

FIGURE 13–24 • Attic cholesteatoma (pars flaccida perforation). *A*, Axial. *B*, Coronal computed tomography scans. The anterior portion of the lateral wall of the attic is eroded by a soft tissue mass extending into the attic lateral to the ossicles, which appear partially eroded and displaced medialward.

Cholesteatomas associated with a perforation of the pars flaccida of the tympanic membrane produce erosion of the anterior portion of the lateral wall of the attic (Figure 13–24A and B) and of the anterior tympanic spine. The lesion extends lateral to the ossicles, which may be displaced medially. Cholesteatomas associated with perforation (usually a posterosuperior marginal perforation) of the pars tensa erode the posterior portion of the lateral wall of the attic and the adjacent posterosuperior wall of the external auditory canal. These lesions extend medial to the ossicles, which are often displaced laterally. The long process of the incus and the stapes superstructure are usually eroded. Further growth of the cholesteatoma produces enlargement of the attic, aditus, and mastoid antrum (see Figure 13–25A and B) and formation of a cavity in the mastoid as a result of erosion of the cell walls. Involvement of the medial wall of the middle ear cavity leads to the formation of a labyrinthine fistula (Figure 13–26A and B). The ampullated limb of the horizontal semicircular canal is the most common site of a fistula. Horizontal and coronal oblique sections show thinning or absence of the bone covering the lateral end of the canal and flattening of the medial wall of the epitympanic recess caused by erosion of the normal protuberance of the horizontal semicircular canal.

Congenital Cholesteatoma

Congenital cholesteatomas are epidermoid tumors originating from embryonic epidermoid rests located anywhere in the temporal bone or adjacent epidural and meningeal spaces.

The clinical symptoms of congenital cholesteatoma depend on the site and size of the lesion. Middle ear congenital cholesteatoma appear as whitish globular masses lying medial to an intact tympanic membrane. There is usually no history of antecedent inflammatory ear disease. Occasionally, there is an associated serous otitis media.

CT examination shows a well-defined soft tissue mass within the middle ear (Figure 13–27). If the cholesteatoma involves the entire middle ear space or if there is accompanying serous otitis media, the entire tympanic cavity is opacified, and the tympanic membrane bulges laterally. In these cases MR may be helpful in identifying the presence and size of the

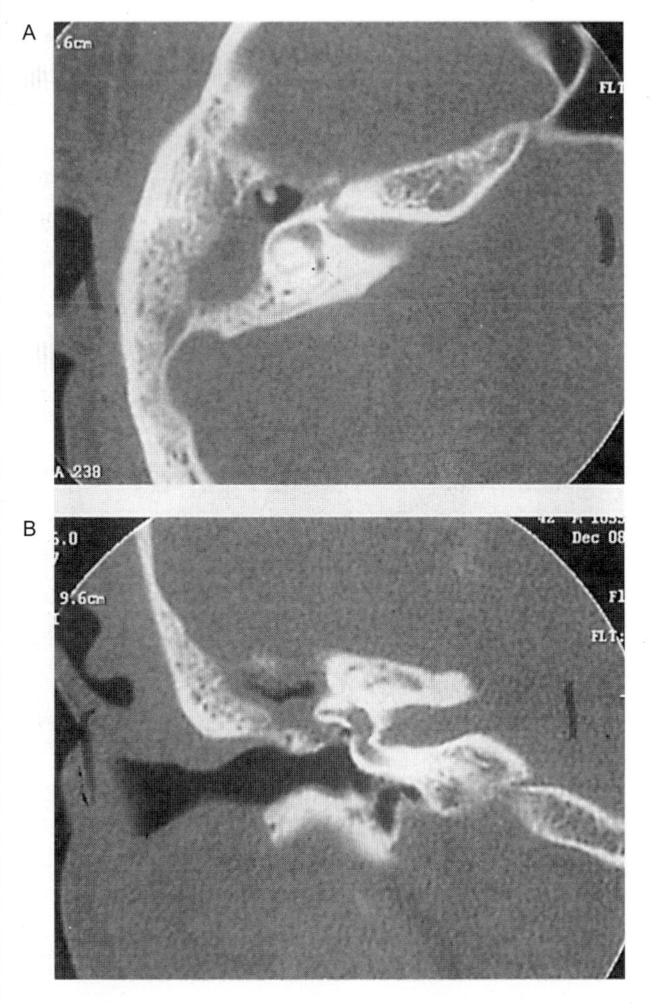

FIGURE 13–25 • Cholesteatoma, pars tensa perforation type. *A*, Axial. *B*, Coronal computed tomography scans. The posterior portion of the lateral wall of the attic is eroded by a soft tissue mass filling the posterosuperior quadrant of the middle ear cavity and the posterior portion of the attic. The cholesteatoma widens the aditus and passes into the mastoid antrum, which appears enlarged because of erosion of the periantral air cells.

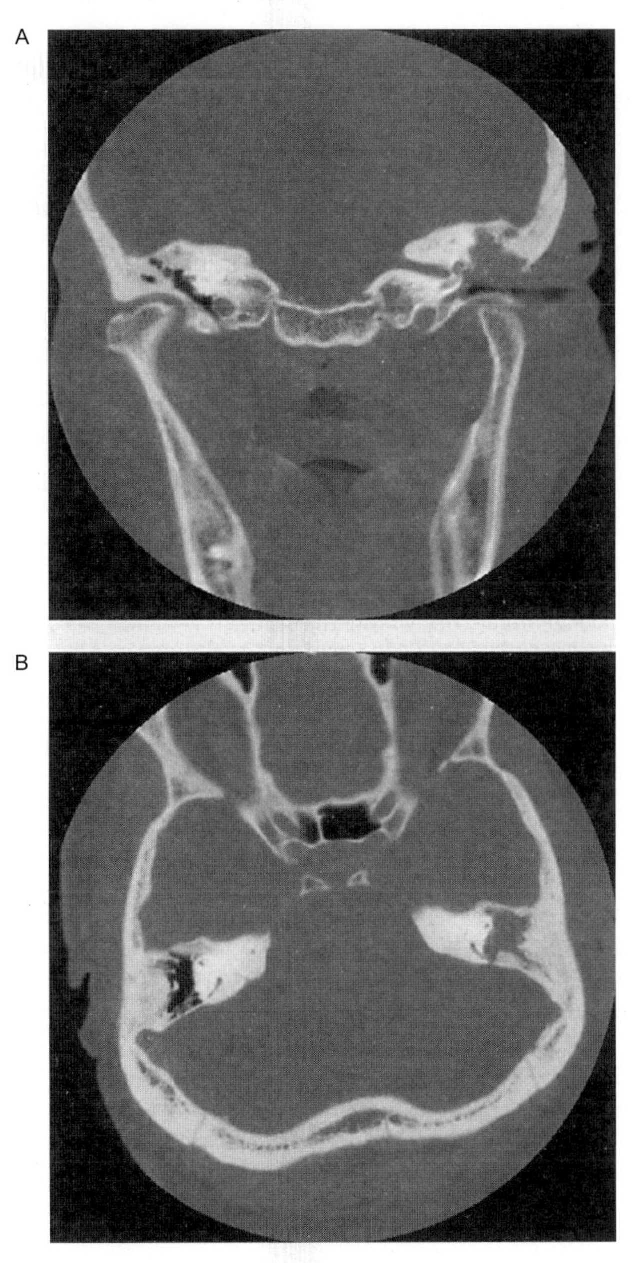

FIGURE 13–26 • *A*, Coronal. *B*, Axial computed tomography scans. A Large cholesteotoma with fistulas. This large cholesteotoma filling the entire middle ear and mastoid has eroded the labyrinthine wall of the middle ear including the capsule of the horizontal (coronal) and posterior semicircular canals (axial).

cholesteatoma. The cholesteatoma mass may erode portions of the ossicular chain.

The inferior margin of the lateral epitympanic wall, which is typically eroded in acquired cholesteatoma, is intact in congenital lesions. However, the lateral epitympanic wall is often eroded from within when the congenital lesion extends into the epitympanum.

Epidermoid Cyst or Congenital Cholesteatoma of the Petrous Pyramid

The findings depend on whether the cholesteatoma arises from within the petrous apex or from the adjacent epidural or meningeal spaces.

When the cholesteatoma arises from within the petrous apex, CT scanning reveals an expansile, cystic lesion in the apex. The involved area of the pyramid is expanded, and the superior petrous ridge is usually elevated and thinned. As the lesion expands, the internal auditory canal and the labyrinth are eroded. Large cholesterol granuloma cysts in the petrous pyramid have often been misdiagnosed as epidermoid cysts because they produce similar CT findings. The two lesions can be differentiated by MRI. Epidermoid cysts appear as areas of fairly low signal intensity in the T1 images and of high intensity in the T2 images. Cholesterol granuloma cysts are bright in both sequences because of short T1 and long T2 relaxation times (Figure 13–28A to C). Dark areas, produced by deposits of hemosiderin, are often observed within the bright mass.

Cholesteatomas arising from the epidural or meningeal spaces on the superior aspect of the petrous pyramid create a scooped-out defect of the adjacent aspect of the pyramid. The defect is caused by erosion of the pyramid from without, and

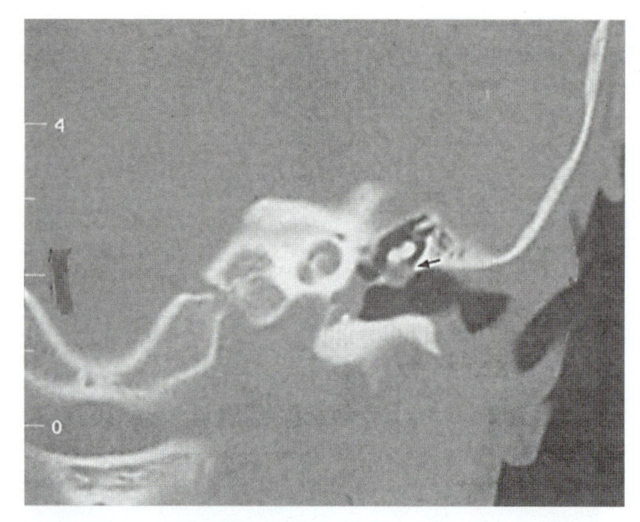

FIGURE 13-27 • Congenital cholesteatoma: coronal computed tomography scan. The tympanic membrane is intact, but two soft tissue masses are seen in the middle ear cavity: a larger in the inferior mesotympanum and a smaller (*arrow*) lateral to the malleus neck.

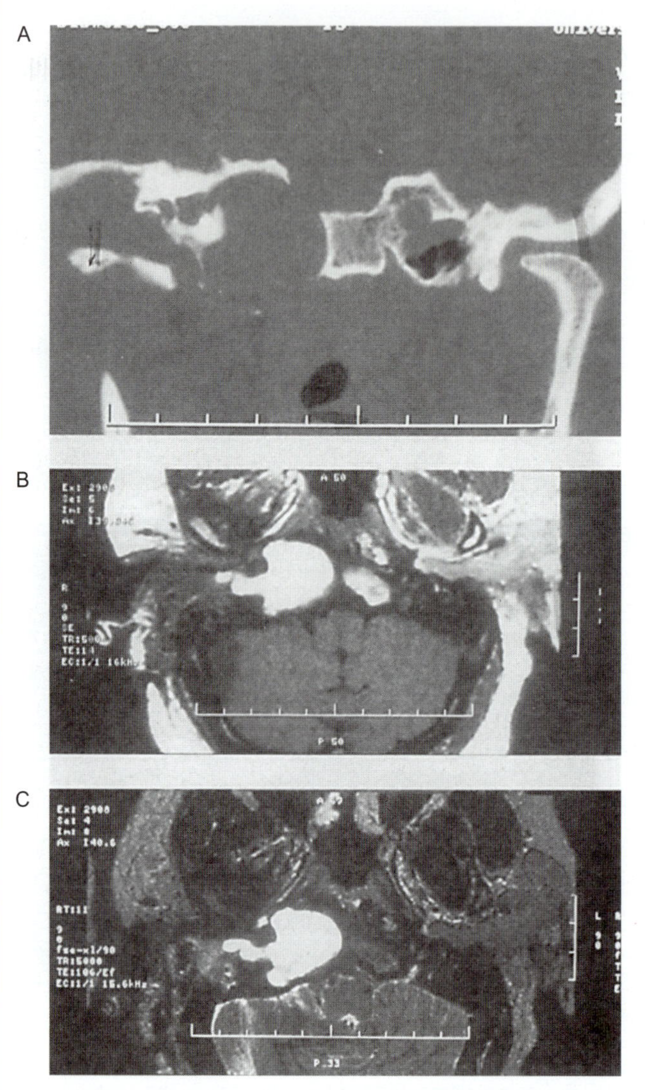

FIGURE 13-28 • Recurrent cholesterol granuloma. *A*, Coronal computed tomography scan. *B*, T1; *C*, T2 axial magnetic resonance image. An expansile lesion involves the right petrous apex and extends into the internal auditory canal. The mass has a characteristic high signal in both T1 and T2 sequences.

there is no bony rim, as in lesions that arise from within the pyramid.

Keratosis Obturans and Cholesteatomas of the External Auditory Canal

Keratosis obturans is caused by osteomas, stenosis of the canal, or hard masses of cerumen. Blockage of the external canal for a long period of time permits epithelial debris to accumulate in the canal and expand the bony contour of the external auditory canal (Figure 13–29A and B).

Cholesteatomas of the external auditory canal are a form of invasive keratitis characterized by accumulation of desquamated debris in the wall of the canal (Figure 13–30A). Removal of the debris reveals deep, localized erosion and exposed necrotic bone. As the lesion enlarges the entire circumference of the canal becomes involved. Large scooped-out defects of the bony canal wall are formed and a soft tissue mass containing small bony sequestra may fill the lumen of the canal (Figure 13–30B).

Neoplastic Conditions

Neoplastic conditions involving the temporal bone can be divided into five major groups, as follows:

1. Histologically benign tumors with a benign course.
2. Histologically benign tumors with a possible malignant clinical course due to extensive destruction of the base of the skull and intracranial extension by the tumor mass.
3. Primary malignant processes.
4. Malignant tumors arising in structures adjacent to the petrous bone and involving it by direct extension.
5. Metastatic lesions.

The first group includes conditions usually involving the external auditory canal, such as osteomas (Figure 13–31), fibromas, and lipomas. The second group includes neuromas (arising from the seventh through the twelfth cranial nerves), glomus tumors, and meningiomas. These lesions deserve special attention not only because of their relatively frequent occurrence, but above all because of the fundamental role imaging plays in their diagnosis. Carcinomas are the most common primary malignant tumors of the temporal bone. Carcinomas usually arise in the external auditory canal, where they produce a partial or total destruction of the canal walls. They may spread into the mastoid, involving the facial canal, or extend into the middle ear cavity, from there involving the jugular fossa and petrous pyramid. Owing to their tendency to infiltrate rather than destroy, carcinomas produce a typical mottled or moth-eaten appearance of the involved bone. Sarcomas usually occur in young children and manifest as destructive lesions of the petrous pyramid. Sarcomas may arise in the eustachian tube and spread by retrograde extension to the ear.

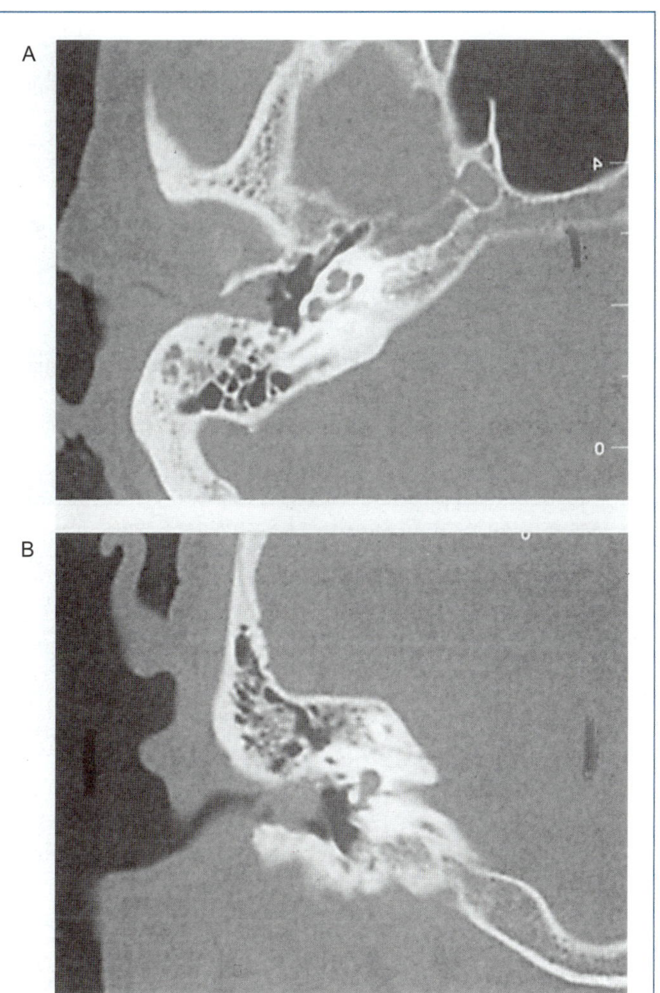

FIGURE 13-29 • External auditory canal cholesteatoma. *A*, Axial. *B*, Coronal computed tomography scans. The canal is stenotic in the region of the isthmus, and a moderately expansile soft tissue mass fills the lumen of the bony segment of the canal.

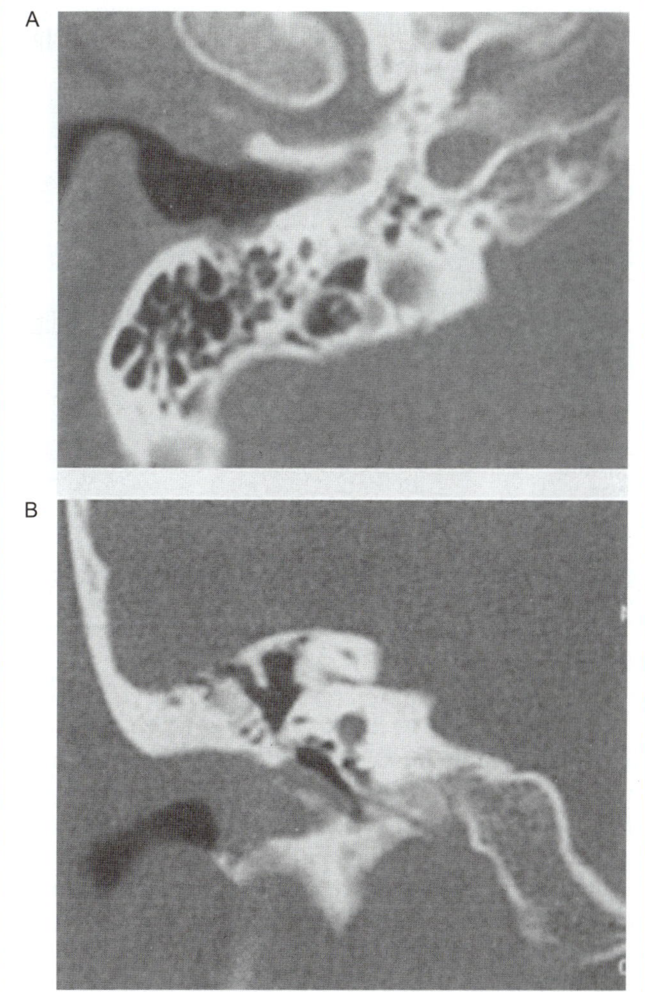

FIGURE 13-30 • External auditory canal cholesteotoma. *A*, Axial CT: incipient lesion of the posterior wall of the canal covered by desquamated debris. *B*, Coronal CT: a large soft tissue mass fills the canal and erodes its floor. Bony sequestra are seen within the mass.

Metastatic lesions to the temporal bone have been observed in carcinomas of the breast, prostate, lungs, and in melanomas. (Figure 13–32).

Glomus Tumors or Chemodectomas

Chemodectomas (or paragangliomas) arise from paraganglionic glomus tissues (chemoreceptors). The four common sites are the jugular fossa (glomus jugulare tumors), middle ear (glomus tympanicum tumors), carotid artery bifurcation (carotid body tumors), and inferior ganglion (ganglion nodosum) of the vagus nerve (glomus vagale). Only the first two are considered in this chapter.

Glomus Tympanicum Tumors

Glomus tympanicum tumors arise in the middle ear cavity over the promontory from glomus tissue located in the adventitia of vessels along the tympanic branch (Jacobson's nerve) of the glossopharyngeal nerve and auricular branch (Arnold's nerve) of the vagus nerve. Axial and coronal CT sections demonstrate a well-defined and enhancing soft tissue mass of variable size in the lower portion of the middle ear cavity and

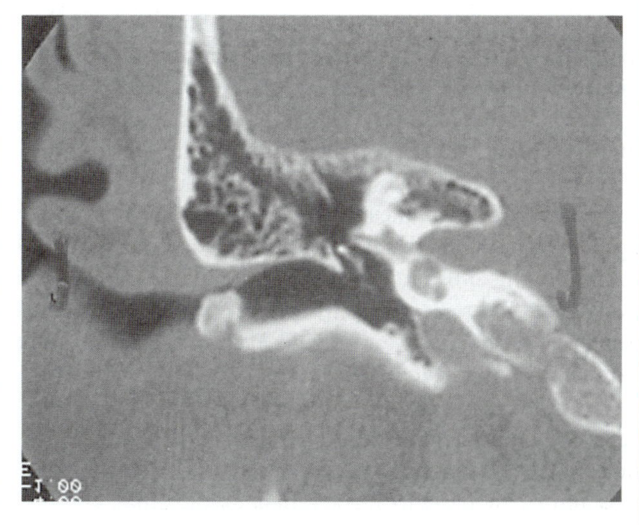

FIGURE 13-31 • Osteoma: coronal computed tomography scan. A bony mass obstructs the right external auditory canal at the isthmus.

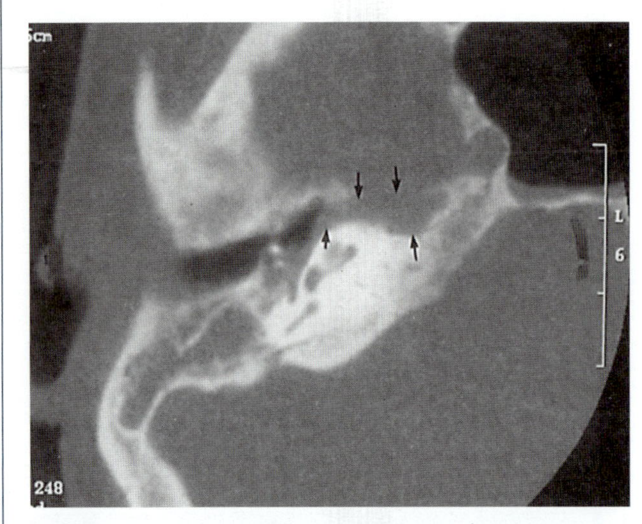

FIGURE 13-32 • Metastatic lesion from carcinoma of the breast: axial computed tomography scan showing a destructive lesion involving the anterior aspect of the right petrous pyramid and extending into the middle ear cavity (*arrows*).

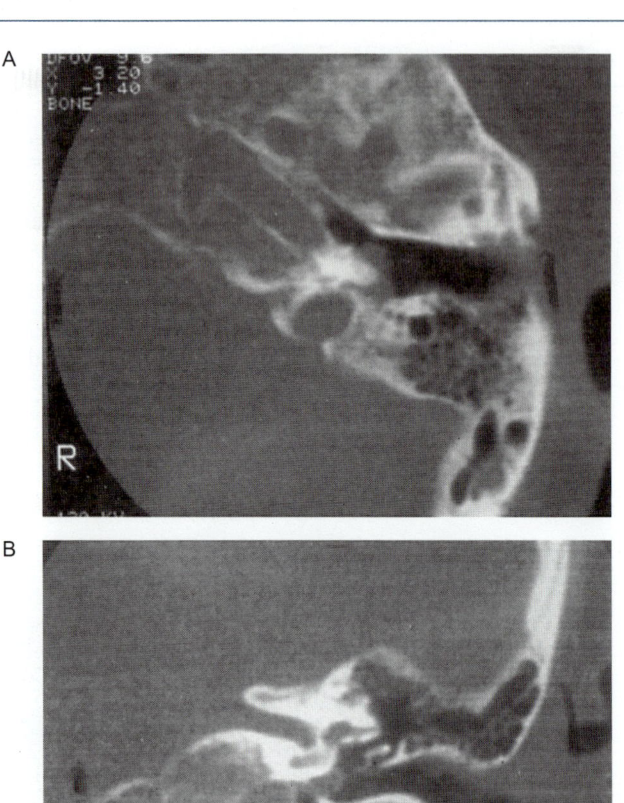

FIGURE 13-33 • Glomus tympanicum. *A*, Axial. *B*, Coronal computed tomography scan. A well-defined soft tissue mass is seen in the lower portion of the middle ear cavity adjacent to the promontory.

adjacent to the promontory (Figure 13–33A and B). The hypotympanic floor and jugular fossa are usually intact. As the tumor enlarges, it may fill the entire middle ear cavity, causing a lateral bulge of the tympanic membrane, and a smooth indentation of the promontory, and it may extend posteriorly into the mastoid and inferiorly into the hypotympanic air cells and jugular fossa.

Glomus Jugulare Tumors

Glomus jugulare tumors arise from paraganglions located in the jugular fossa and jugular bulb. The jugular fossa is usually enlarged, with erosion of its cortical outline (Figure 13–34A) and of the bony septum separating it from the external aperture of the carotid canal. Asymmetry of the jugular fossa and a large jugular bulb without cortical erosion are common anatomic variations of no clinical significance. As the floor of the hypotympanum is eroded, the tumor extends into the middle ear cavity and from there into the external auditory canal. Lateral extension of the lesion into the mastoid often leads to erosion of the facial canal and involvement of the facial nerve. Medial extension first produces undermining of the posteroinferior aspect of the petrous pyramid and then actual destruction of the perilabyrinthine bone and petrous apex. The resistant otic capsule is seldom involved, although the cochlea is often skeletonized by the erosion of the surrounding bone. Intracranial involvement is often observed in large tumors, although the lesion usually remains extradural. Extracranial extension occurs within and along the jugular vein.

CT scanning is ideal for the detection of the bony changes typical of glomus jugulare tumors. However, MRI is the study of choice since it is more precise in defining the size of the tumor mass and particularly its intracranial, extracranial, and intravascular extent.

The tumor appears as a mass of medium signal intensity in the T1 sequence that becomes brighter in T2 and enhances after infusion of contrast. Multiple punctated areas of signal void produced by blood vessels are observed within the tumor mass (Figure 13–34B and C). Involvement of the jugular vein and carotid artery is readily demonstrated because these vascular structures are clearly visible in the MR images, thus avoiding the need for more invasive vascular studies.

Vestibular Schwannomas

Vestibular schwannomas (acoustic neuromas) account for approximately 10% of cases of unilateral sensorineural hearing and vestibular loss of unknown origin. Most of the tumors arise from the vestibular nerve within the internal auditory canal. MR, at present, is the study of choice for the assessment of the cerebellopontine angle. The format of the examination varies with the clinical symptomatology.[9]

A limited study of the internal auditory canals is performed whenever the patient is referred for evaluation of unilateral sensorineural hearing loss, either sudden or progressive. The examination consists of 2-mm contiguous axial and coronal, T1 and T2 FSE images of the internal auditory canals obtained prior to the infusion of contrast. If a tumor is clearly outlined

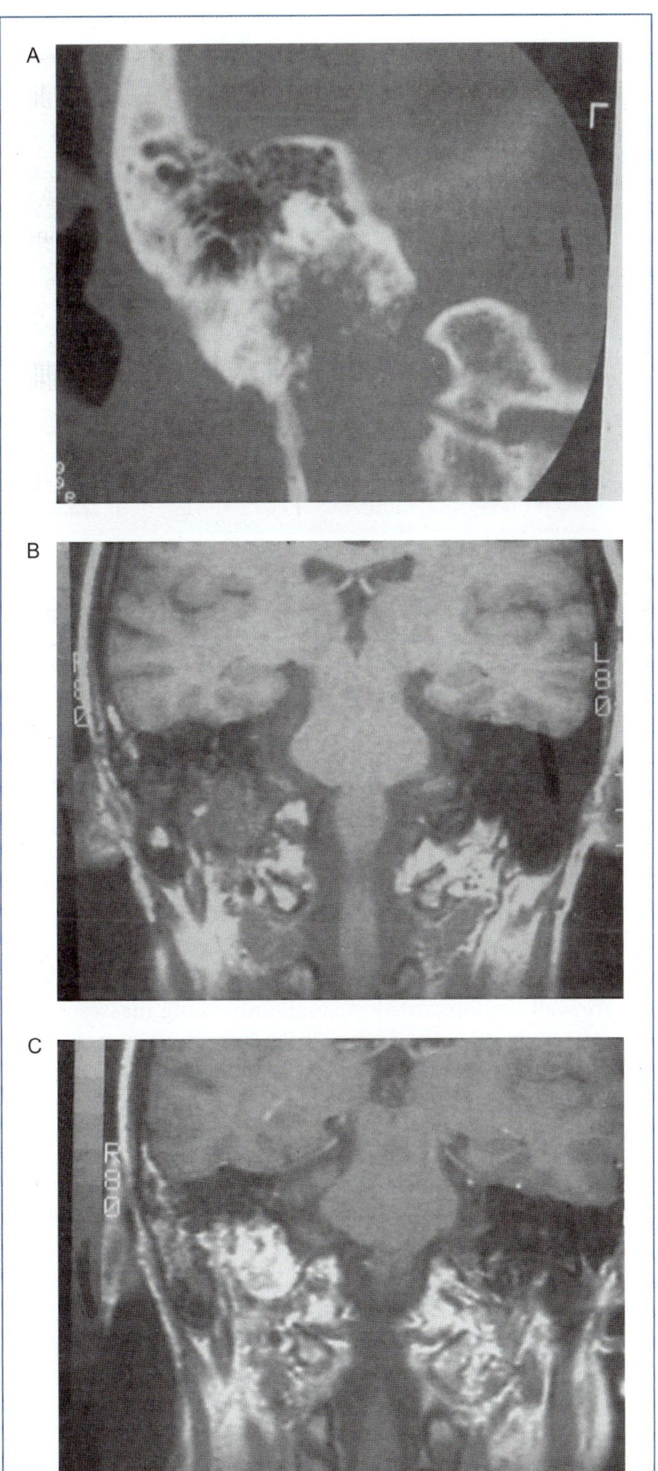

FIGURE 13–34 • Glomus jugulare. *A*, Coronal computed tomography scan. *B* and *C*, Coronal magnetic resonance (MR) T1 image prior to and after injection of contrast. The right jugular fossa appears enlarged and its contour eroded. The MR images demonstrate a mass of medium intensity, which enhances with contrast. Note the areas of signal void within the mass produced by blood vessels.

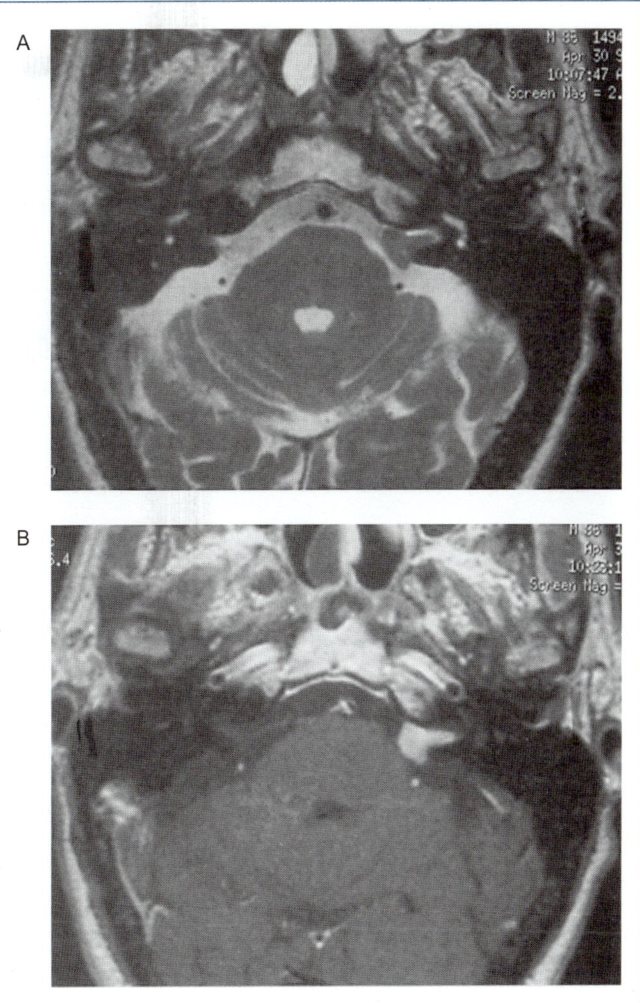

FIGURE 13–35 • Vestibular schwannoma; magnetic resonance images. *A*, Fast spin echo (FSE). *B*, T1 postcontrast. *A*, The tumor mass is well seen in the FSE image as a filling defect within the bright cerebrospinal fluid. *B*, The size of the tumor mass is more clearly defined in the postcontrast image.

in the FSE images, as a filling defect within the brightness of the cerebrospinal fluid (Figure 13–35A), the study is terminated.[16] Otherwise, contrast is infused, and T1 images are obtained in the axial and coronal planes with fat suppression, revealing tumors as small as 2 mm (Figure 13–35B).[15] Vestibular schwannomas should be differentiated from facial neuromas arising within the internal auditory canal, which usually extend into the fallopian canal (Figure 13–36).[6]

A complete study of the internal auditory canals and brain is performed in patients with bilateral sensorineural hearing loss to rule out neurofibromatosis, as well as in patients with vertigo. Before the infusion of contrast, this examination includes 2-mm FSE axial images of the posterior cranial fossa and internal auditory canals, 2-mm T1 coronal sections of the internal auditory canals, and 5-mm fluid-attenuated inversion recovery (flair) axial sections of the brain, which are particularly useful in ruling out a demyelinating process. After infusion of contrast, 2-mm T1 coronal images of the internal auditory canals and 5-mm axial sections of the brain are obtained.

Fat suppression images should always be obtained after infusion of contrast if the patient has previously had surgery for the removal of an acoustic tumor since that fat-containing graft used to fill the surgical defect may obscure the enhancing residual or recurrent tumor mass.

A

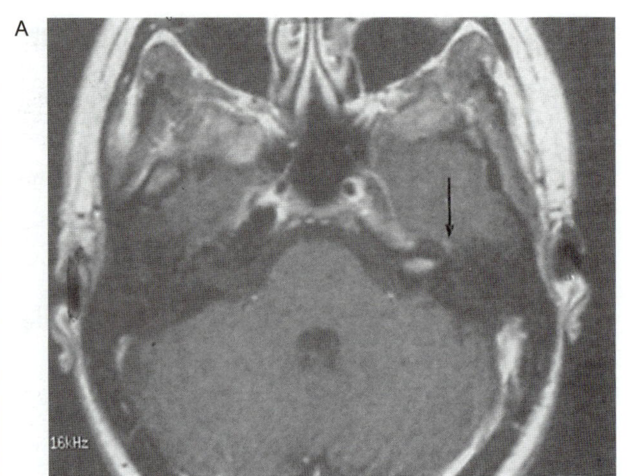

B

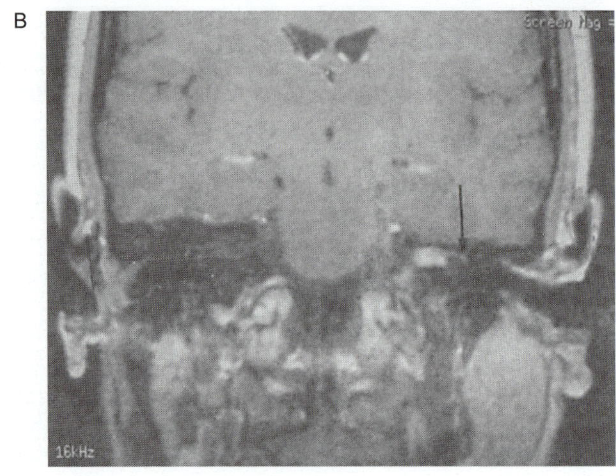

FIGURE 13–36 • Facial schwannoma; magnetic resonance images. *A*, Axial. *B*, Coronal T1 after contrast. The tumor fills the left internal auditory canal and extends into the facial canal (*arrow*).

A CT study should be performed only if MRI is not available or if the patient cannot undergo an MRI study because of an implanted medical device, such as a pacemaker.

CT scanning allows a precise assessment of the internal auditory canals. Because the internal auditory canals in the normal individual vary in size from 2 to 12 mm, whereas the two canals of any person are almost identical, both sides should always be examined for comparison purposes. Enlargement of 2 mm or more and shortening of the posterior canal wall by at least 3 mm in comparison with the canal of the normal-hearing side are usually indicative of a space-occupying lesion. Enlargement of 1 to 2 mm and shortening of the posterior wall by 2 mm are only suggestive of a lesion. Intravenous infusion of contrast material is then performed. The contrast study allows the detection of extracanalicular tumors as small as 5 mm. If the infusion study is negative, a spinal puncture is immediately performed, and 3 cc of air or gas (CO_2 or O_2) are injected into the subarachnoid space. By proper positioning, the gas is then moved into the cerebellopontine cistern under examination. When a tumor is present, the gas outlines the medial contour of the mass and reveals a complete or partial block of the internal auditory canal (Figure 13–37). By this technique, intracanalicular tumors, as small as 2 to 3 mm, are clearly identified.

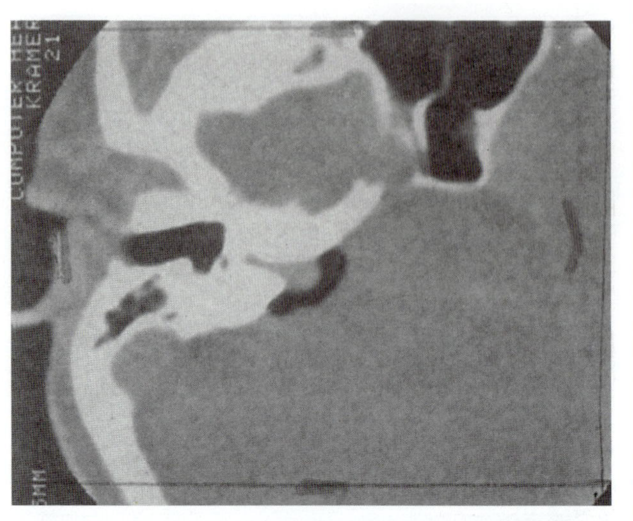

FIGURE 13–37 • Right vestibular schwannoma: computed tomography pneumocisternogram. The air outlines the convex medial aspect of the tumor, which protrudes from the internal auditory canal into the adjacent cerebellopontine cistern.

Labyrinthine Schwannomas

In the past, small schwannomas have been found within the vestibule and cochlea during postmortem dissection of the temporal bone. These lesions are usually not recognizable by CT but are well demonstrated as small enhancing masses in MR examinations performed after infusion of contrast material (Figure 13–38).[5]

Meningiomas

Meningiomas are the second most common tumor of the cerebellopontine angle and usually arise outside the internal auditory canal, although they may extend into the medial portion of the canal. Meningiomas limited to the internal auditory canal are rare and mimic vestibular schwannomas, both clinically and on imaging. Meningiomas grow as a solid mass or en plaque and may cause hyperostosis or erosion of the adjacent bony structures. Magnetic resonance images obtained after infusion of contrast show enhancement of the tumor and in 10% of cases small areas of signal void caused by calcifications within the mass (Figure 13–39).

En plaque lesions appear as focal areas of enhancing, thickened meninges. The meningeal involvement often extends from actual tumor mass, producing the so-called tail sign, which is helpful but not specific for meningiomas (Figure 13–39).

Hemangiomas

Small hemangiomas or AVMs limited to the lumen of the internal auditory canal are rare. They appear in precontrast MR images as an area of high signal intensity caused by slow flow, which becomes larger following the administration of contrast. The mass has a nonhomogeneous intensity and may contain

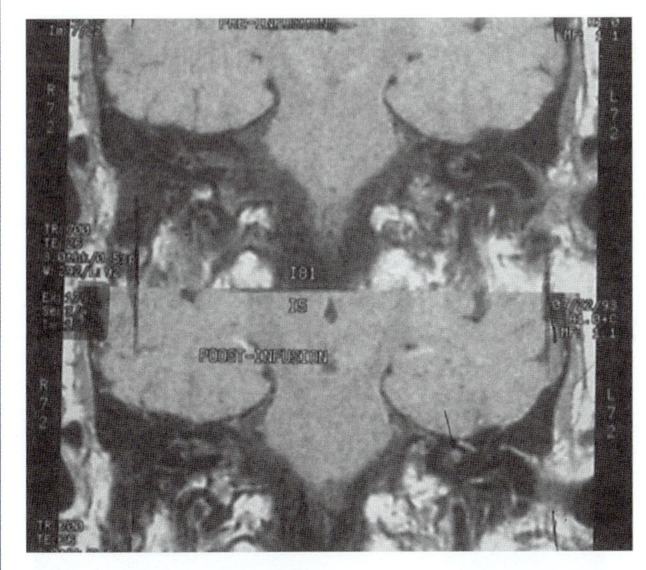

FIGURE 13–38 • Cochlear schwannoma: magnetic resonance image coronal T1, before (*top*) and after (*bottom*) contrast. A 2-mm enhancing mass is seen within the cochlea (*arrow*). The internal auditory canal is normal.

signal void areas caused by calcifications. A large hemangioma may involve the petrous pyramid and extend into the internal auditory canal. It is characterized by a mass of medium intensity in the T1 precontrast images, which contains multiple areas of signal void caused by bony spicules. The tumor becomes bright after infusion of contrast but maintains the same nonhomogeneous intensity (Figure 13–40).

Lipomas

Lipomas may occur within the cerebellopontine cistern or the internal auditory canal. In the five cases the senior author has seen, the lipoma was located at the fundus of the internal auditory canal. The diagnosis is made by obtaining T1 and T2 precontrast images or by fat suppression images whenever a bright mass is seen on postcontrast T1-weighted images (Figure 13–41).

Epidermoid Cysts

Epidermoid cysts usually occur in the cerebellopontine angle cistern and rarely within the internal auditory canal. The MR study shows a nonenhancing mass of low signal in the T1 images that becomes bright in the T2-weighted images.

Epidermoid cysts can be differentiated from arachnoid cysts since, contrary to the latter, they show absent or incomplete attenuation in the FLAIR sequence and restricted diffusion (high signal) in diffusion weighted images.

Aneurysm

An aneurysm within the internal auditory canal is extremely rare. The lesion appears on T1- and T2-weighted MR images as a small mass of high signal presumably caused by thrombosis or slow flow. Following the infusion of contrast, the lesion becomes slightly larger. Aneurysms within the cerebellopontine cistern

A

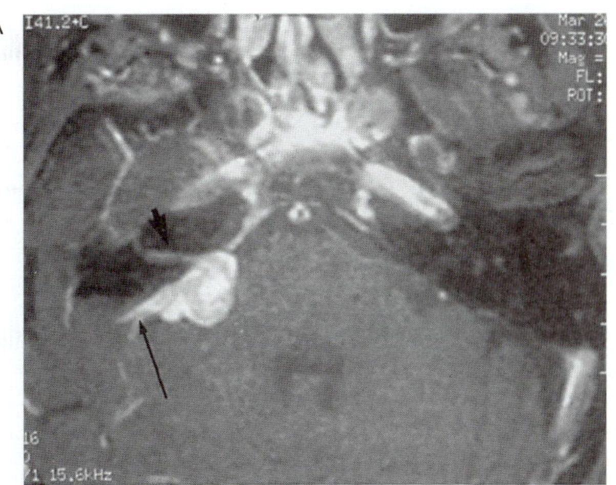

B

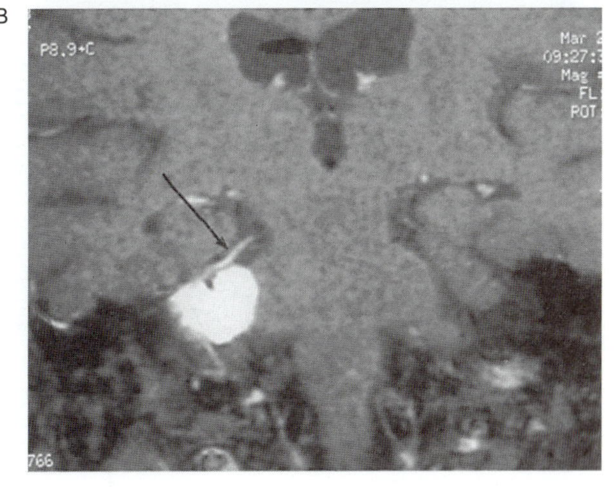

FIGURE 13–39 • Meningioma right cerebellopontine cistern. An unevenly enhancing mass is seen in the right cerebellopontine cistern. The tumor extends into but does not fill the internal auditory canal (*short arrow*). Note the extension of the tumor en plaque (*long arrow*). *A*, Axial. *B*, Coronal T1 images, after contrast.

may compress the acoustic or facial nerves causing symptoms similar to those of a vestibular schwannoma (Figure 13–42A and B). MR images reveal a mass of nonhomogeneous high signal intensity produced by the clot. If the lumen of the aneurysm is partially patent, the flowing blood will appear as an area of signal void (Figure 13–42A). An MR angiogram should be performed to confirm the diagnosis and to reveal from which vessel the aneurysm is arising.[4]

Endolymphatic Sac Tumors

Endolymphatic sac tumors are locally aggressive papillary adenomatous tumors. They are often associated with von Hippel-Lindau disease, a genetic multisystem neoplastic disorder. At first, endolymphatic sac tumors involve the adjacent dura and endolymphatic duct. From there, the lesion extends to the vestibule, semicircular canals, mastoid, and middle ear cavity, where it appears through an intact tympanic membrane as a bluish mass, often confused with a glomus tumor. Continued growth leads to complete replacement by tumor of the mastoid and petrous pyramid. Axial CT images initially

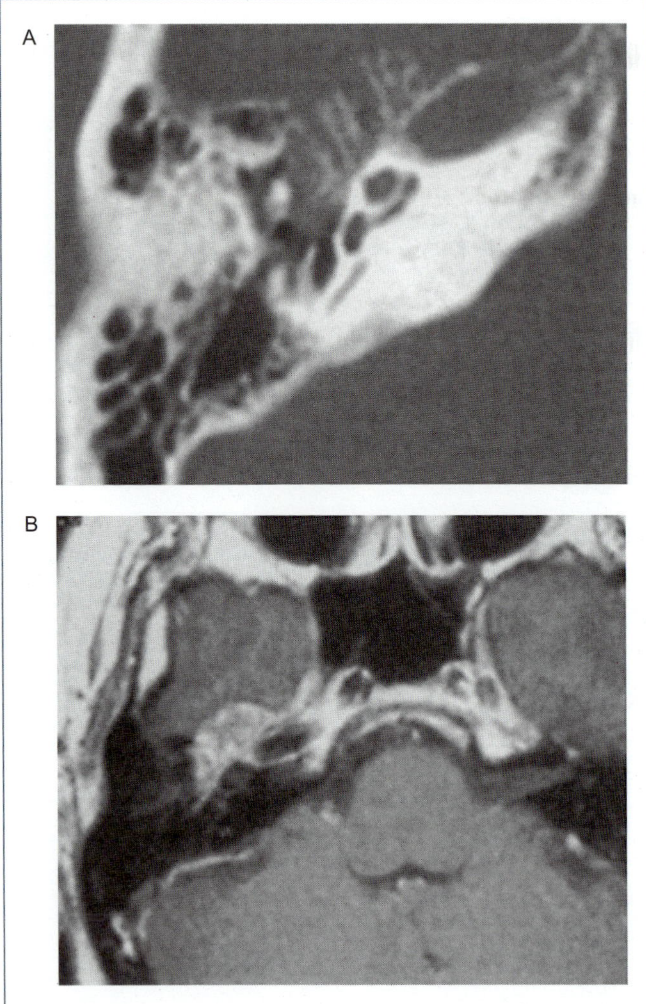

FIGURE 13–40 • Hemangioma. *A*, Axial CT: a mass containing multiple bony spicules erodes the anterior aspect of the petrous pyramid and extends into the attic lateral to the ossieles. *B*, MR axial T1 post contrast: the mass shows a nonhomogeneous enhancement.

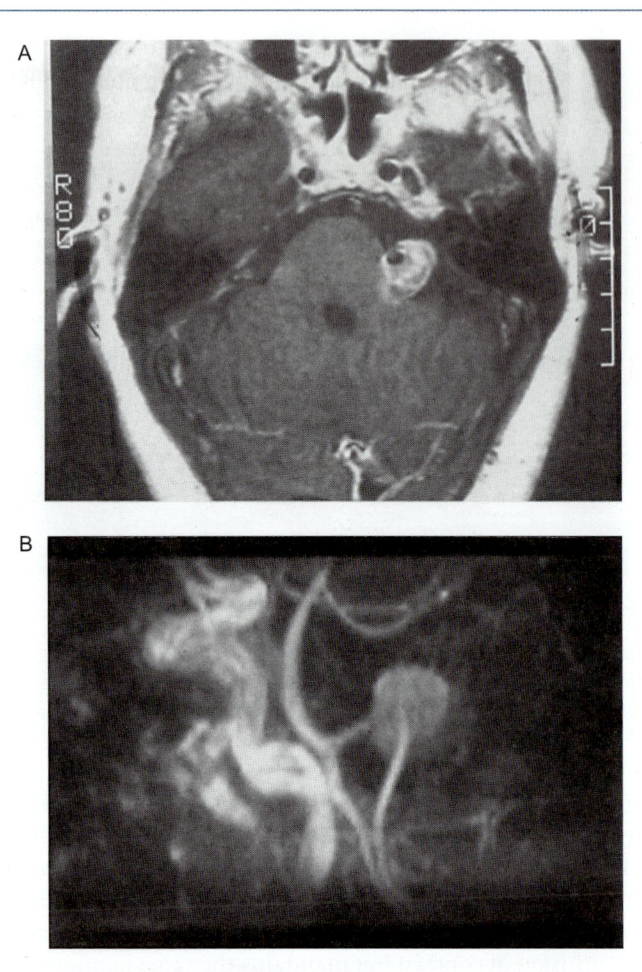

FIGURE 13–42 • Cerebellopontine cistern aneurysm. In the axial magnetic resonance (MR) T1 image obtained after contrast *A*, the clotted aneurysm appears as a mass of nonhomogeneous high signal. The area of signal void within it is the patent lumen. *B*, The MR angiogram confirms the presence of an aneurysm arising from the left vertebral artery.

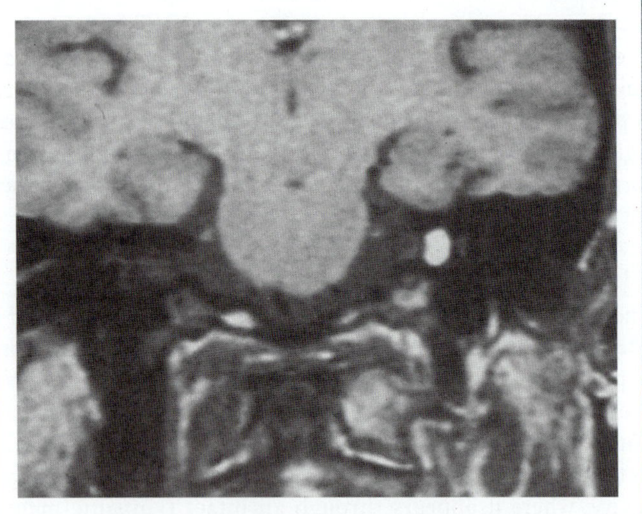

FIGURE 13–41 • Lipoma 1AC: MR T1 coronal precontrast shows a bright mass filling and expanding the left IAC.

show a localized area of erosion of the posterior aspect of the petrous pyramid in the region of the endolymphatic sac (Figure 13–43A). As the lesion enlarges, destruction of the petrous pyramid is observed with involvement of the inner ear structures. In T1-weighted MR images, the tumor has a heterogeneous appearance, with areas of high signal caused by cysts filled with blood or high proteinaceous fluid and multiple small areas of signal void caused by calcifications and blood vessels (Figure 13–43B). Following administration of contrast, the solid portion of the mass undergoes a nonhomogeneous enhancement (Figure 13–43C).[10]

Otodystrophies

Otosclerosis

The diagnosis of fenestral otosclerosis is usually suspected by the otologist on the basis of the clinical history and audiometric tests. A CT study may be performed in these cases to confirm the diagnosis and rule out other possible causes of conductive hearing impairment. The examination consists of axial and

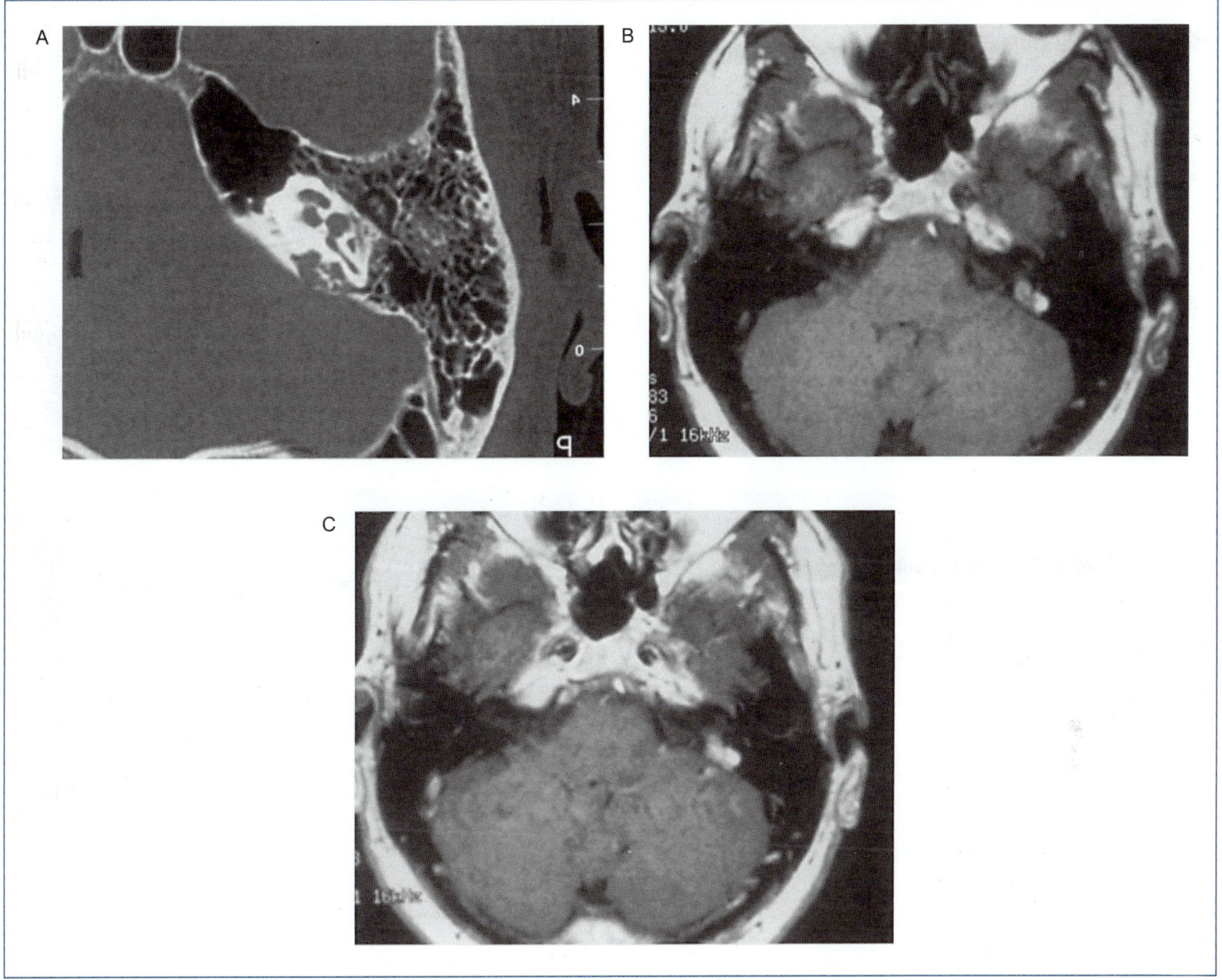

FIGURE 13–43 • Endolymphatic sac tumor. *A*, Axial computed tomography scan. *B* and *C*, Axial magnetic resonance image before and after contrast. The posterior aspect of the left petrous pyramid is eroded in the region of the endolymphatic sac. *B*, The tumor mass has a heterogeneous appearance before contrast. *C*, The solid portion of the tumor enhances with contrast.

20-degree coronal oblique sections at 1-mm increments. The CT findings vary from loss of definition of the margin of the oval window (owing to demineralization) to narrowing and finally complete obliteration of the oval window opening and niche (Figure 13–44A and C). CT is extremely helpful in evaluating postsurgical cases in which an initial hearing improvement is subsequently lost and in determining the cause of poststapedectomy vertigo. The CT study may disclose protrusion of the prosthesis into the vestibule, separation of the lateral end of the strut from the incus, dislocation of the medial end of the prosthesis, and reobliteration of the oval window with fixation of the strut (Figure 13–45).

Cochlear otosclerosis occurs by progressive enlargement of the perifenestral foci or as single or multiple foci in other locations of the cochlear and labyrinthine capsules. The diagnosis of cochlear otosclerosis is suspected by the otologist on the basis of the audiometric configuration, clinical history, and clinical findings, such as Schwartze's sign (blush at the promontory seen at the otoscopy) but further confirmation by a proper imaging study is required. The CT examination consists of axial and coronal oblique sections at 1-mm increments. The normal cochlear capsule, which appears as a sharply defined, homogeneously dense, bony shell outlining the lumen of the cochlea, becomes disrupted in cochlear otosclerosis. Otosclerotic changes range from small and isolated foci of decreased density to diffuse demineralization of a large area of the capsule with complete dissolution of its contour.

A typical sign of cochlear otosclerosis is the formation of a band of demineralization surrounding the cochlear canal (double-ring effect) caused by confluent spongiotic foci. The band of intracapsular demineralization is in some cases limited to a segment of the capsule, but in the others it follows almost the entire contour of the cochlea. A more precise and quantitative assessment of the involvement is accomplished by CT densitometric readings. Using the smallest cursor, the contour of the cochlear capsule is scanned, and 31 densitometric readings are obtained. A profile of the density of the capsule is obtained by plotting the densitometric values versus the 31 points where

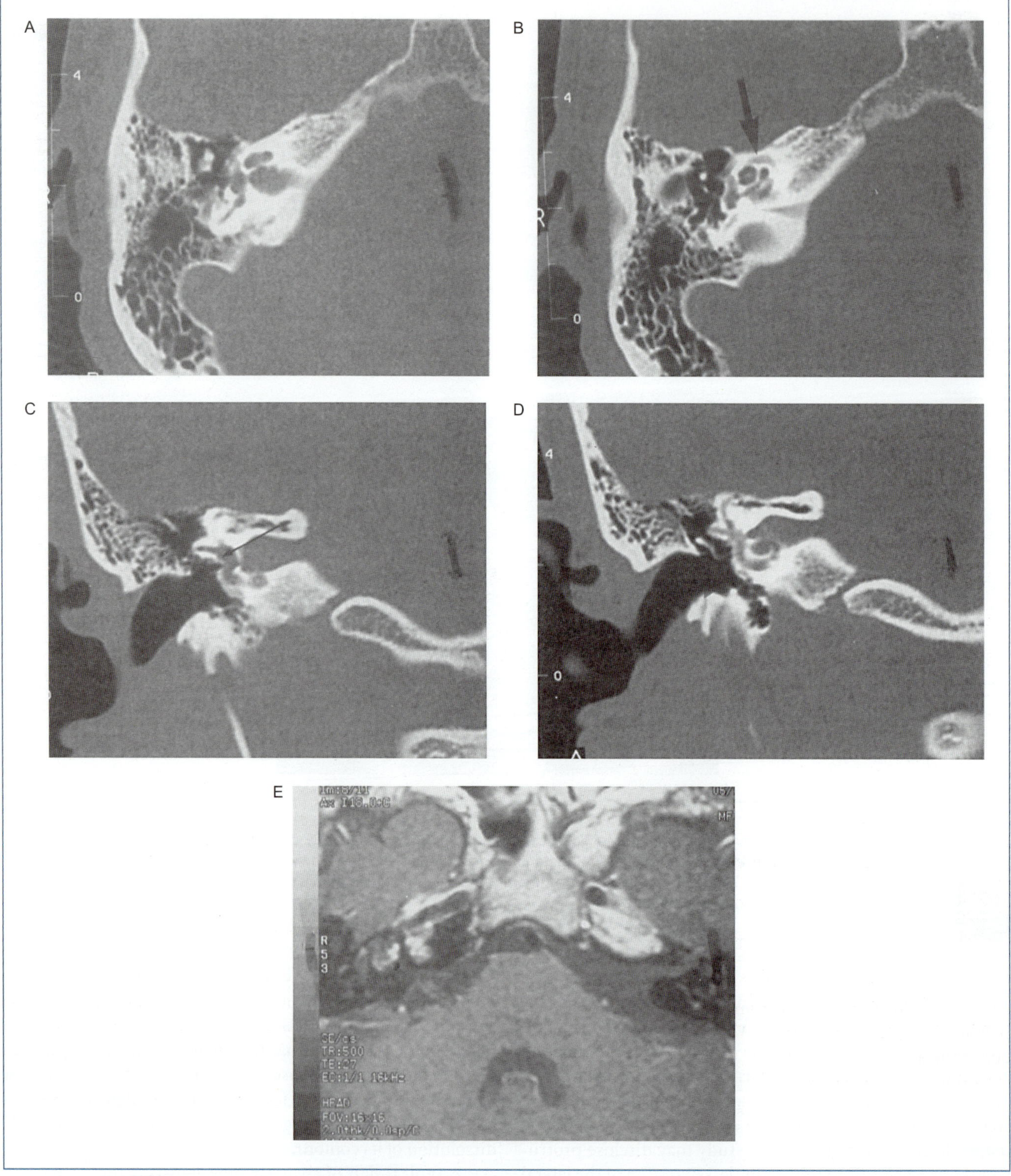

FIGURE 13–44 • Stapedial and cochlear otosclerosis. *A* and *B*, Axial. *C* and *D*, Coronal computed tomography. *E*, axial magnetic resonance (MR) T1 image after contrast. The footplate of the right stapes is thickened (*A* and *C*, *arrows*). Severe spongiotic changes are present throughout the cochlear capsule (*B* and *D*, *arrows*). The MR image reveals enhancement of the active and vascular foci of otosclerosis.

the reading are made. The obtained densitometric curve is then compared to the densitometric profile of the normal capsule that was previously determined.[2]

In several patients with a positive Schwartze's sign and severe spongiotic changes in the CT study, MR images obtained after infusion of contrast show enhancement within the demineralized foci (see Figure 13–44E). Presumably, the blushing is produced by pooling of contrast within the numerous blood vessels and lacunae found in active spongiotic foci.

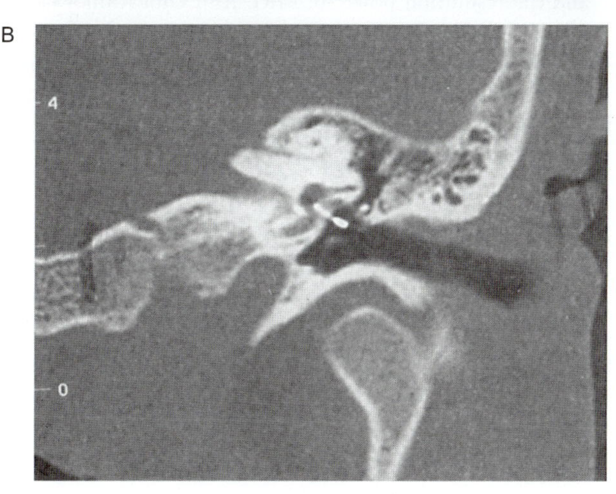

FIGURE 13–45 • Recurrent fenestral otosclerosis after stapedectomy. *A*, Axial. *B*, Coronal computed tomography scan. A metallic piston extends from the long process of the incus to the oval window, which appears reclosed. The medial end of the piston is in a good position but is fixed by the large focus obliterating the oval window niche (*arrow*). Otospongiotic changes are noted in the cochlear capsule.

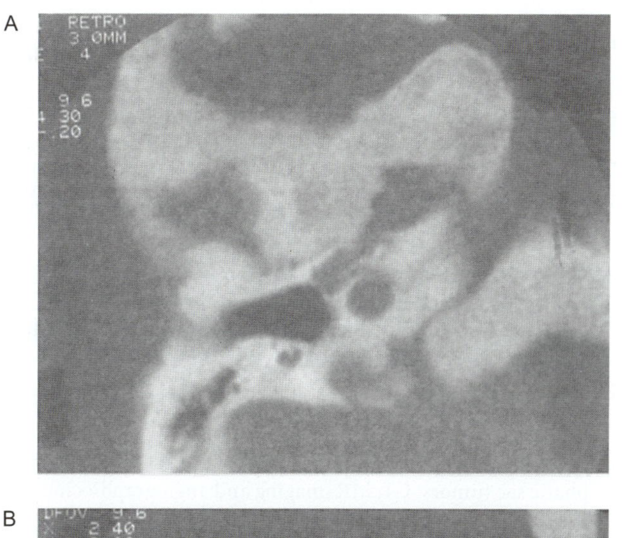

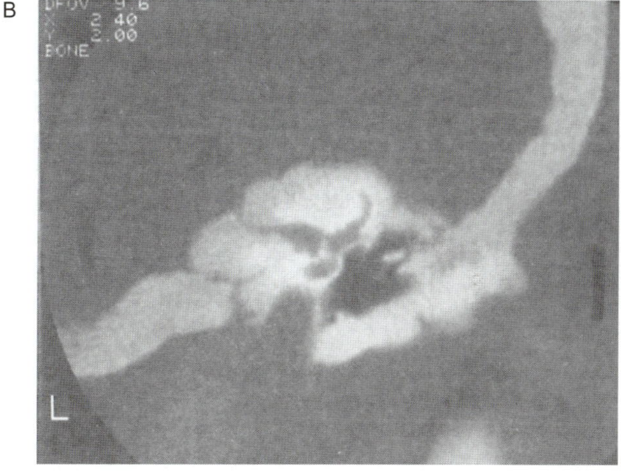

FIGURE 13–46 • Fibrous dysplasia. *A*, Axial. *B*, Coronal computed tomography. There is diffuse thickening and sclerosis of the temporal bone with narrowing of the external and internal auditory canals.

Paget's Disease

Paget's disease can affect the calvarium and the base of the skull, including the petrous pyramids. When the disease process extends into the otic capsule it will cause a progressive, mixed or sensorineural hearing loss.

The haversian bone of the petrosa is affected first, with spread of the disease from the apex laterally. At first, because of severe demineralization of the petrosa, the labyrinthine capsule becomes more prominent than normal. Involvement of the otic capsule begins at the periosteal surface. Slow demineralization occurs that at first produces thinning and finally complete dissolution of the capsule. The result is a washed-out appearance of the entire petrous bone characteristic of Paget's disease.

Fibrous Dysplasia

Fibrous dysplasia is the abnormal proliferation of fibrous tissue intermixed with trabeculae of woven bone within the medullary cavity, and causes increased density and thickening of affected areas. Involvement by fibrous dysplasia is usually unilateral, which leads to asymmetry. In the temporal bone, the squama becomes thickened and the pneumatized spaces are obliterated. The external auditory canal often is stenosed by new bone formation (Figure 13–46A). As the density of the petrous pyramid increases, the outline of the labyrinthine capsule becomes less distinguishable from the surrounding bone. Further progression may lead to narrowing of the internal auditory canal (Figure 13–46B) and obliteration of the lumen of the labyrinth.

References

1. Valvassori GE, Buckingham RA. Tomography and cross sections of the ear. Philadelphia: Georg Thieme Verlag; 1975.
2. Valvassori GE, Dobben GD. CT densitometry of the cochlear capsule in otosclerosis. AJNR Am J Neuroradiol 1985;6:661–7.
3. Seltzer S, Mark AS. Contrast enhancement of the labyrinth on MR scans in patients with sudden hearing loss and vertigo: Evidence of labyrinthine disease. AJNR Am J Neuroradiol 1991;12:13–6.
4. Rodgers GK, Applegate L, De La Cruz A, et al. Magnetic resonance angiography: Analysis of vascular lesions of the temporal bone and skull base. Am J Otol 1993;14:56–62.

5. Casselman JW, Kuhweide R, Ampe W, et al. Pathology of the membranous labyrinth: Comparison of T1-and T2-weighted and gadolinium-enhanced spin-echo and 3DFT-CIS imaging. AJNR Am J Neuroradiol 1993;14:59–69.
6. Casselman JW, Kuhweide R, Deimling M, et al. Constructive interference in steady state-3DFT-MR imaging of the inner ear and cerebellopontine angle. AJNR Am J Neuroradiol 1993;14:47–57.
7. Mafee MF, Valvassori GE, Becker M. Imaging of the head and neck. New York: Thieme Verlag; 2005.
8. Harnsberger HR, Dahlen RT, Shelton C, et al. Advanced techniques in magnetic resonance imaging in the evaluation of the large endolymphatic duct and sac syndrome. Laryngoscope 1995;105;1037–42.
9. Valvassori GE. The internal auditory canal revisited. Otolaryngol Clin North Am 1995;28:431–51.
10. Mukherji SK, Albernaz VS, Lo WW, et al. Papillary endolymphatic sac tumors: CT, MR imaging and angiographic findings in 20 patients. Radiology 1997;202:801–8.
11. Fitzgerald DC, Mark AS. Sudden hearing loss: Frequency of abnormal findings on contrast-enhanced MRI studies. AJNR Am J Neuroradial 1998;19:1433–6.
12. Antonelli PJ, Garside JA, Mancusso AA, et al. Computed tomography and the diagnosis of coalescent mastoiditis. Otolaryngol Head Neck Surg 1999;120:350–4.
13. Stone JA, Castillo M, Neelon B, Mukherji SK. Evaluation of CSF leaks: high resolution CT compared with contrast-enhanced CT and radionuclide cisternography. AJNR Am J Neuroradial 1999;20:706–12.
14. Bamiou DE, Phelps P, Sirimanna T. Temporal bone computed tomography findings in bilateral sensorineural hearing loss. Arch Dis Child 2000;82:257–60.
15. Dubrulle F, Ernst O, Vincent C, et al. Cochlear fossa enhancement at MR evaluation of vestibular schwannoma: Correlation with success at hearing preservation surgery. Radiology 2000; 215:458–62.
16. Schmalbrock P, Chakeres DW, Monroe W, et al. Assessment of internal auditory canal tumors: A comparison of contrast-enhanced T1 weighted and steady-state T2 weighted gradient echo MR imaging. AJNR Am J Neroradiol 1999;20:1207–13.
17. Buckingham RA, Valvassori GE. Inner ear fluid volumes and the resolution power of MRI. Ann Otol Rhinol Laryngol 2001;110(2):113–7.
18. Boston M, Halstead M, Meinzen-Derr J, et al. The large vestibular aqueduct: A new definition based on audiologic and computed tomography correlation. Otolaryngology-Head and Neck Surgery 2007;136:972–7.

Hearing Aids 14

Brad A. Stach, PhD / Virginia Ramachandran, AuD

Hearing aids are sufficiently robust and flexible in design and signal processing capability to be adapted to fit nearly any hearing loss that causes a communication disorder. Indeed, for the vast majority of individuals with hearing loss, hearing aids are currently the best and most appropriate solution available to minimize the impact of the disorder on communication. Although the essential components of all hearing aids remain the microphone, amplifier, and receiver, rapid advancement in component technology has increased the effectiveness of hearing aids and improved outcomes for treatment of hearing loss.[1] This chapter will review the current state of hearing aid technology including candidacy, selection, fitting and verification, and management.

THE DEVELOPMENT OF MODERN HEARING AIDS

Major changes have occurred in the design of hearing instruments in the recent past. As a consequence, both the range of patient candidacy and benefit from hearing instruments have increased substantially.

Electronic hearing aids were first developed in the early 1900s. They used carbon-granule technology and became widely available in the 1920s and 1930s. The first major step forward in technological development comprised vacuum-tube amplifiers, leading to the first vacuum-tube hearing aid in the late 1930s. The devices required a rather large battery pack as the power supply but were small enough that they could be worn on the body. In the early 1950s, the transistor was developed, which, along with the development of smaller batteries, led to the first behind-the-ear (BTE) hearing aids. Eyeglass hearing aids were developed in the 1960s, followed by in-the-ear (ITE) hearing aids in the 1970s and finally digital hearing aids in the late 1980s.

The modern era of hearing aids has been influenced by several significant trends. One important trend was the miniaturization of hearing instruments, resulting ultimately in hearing instruments that fit completely in the ear canal. Perhaps the most important change was the transformation from analog to digital processing platforms for hearing instruments. Digital processing permits sophisticated control of the acoustic signal without the space and power constraints imposed by analog circuitry. Digital signal processing (DSP) has many advantages, including fine-grain adjustment of amplification parameters, sophisticated noise and feedback reduction paradigms, and enhancements of directional microphones. The most recent trend in hearing aid development is that of wireless connectivity. This feature permits hearing aids from both ears to communicate with each other and with external sound sources, creating a direct link with other modern communication and entertainment technologies.

HEARING AID CANDIDACY

Fundamentals of Candidacy

The first question often asked by patients pursuing an audiologic evaluation is "Do I need a hearing aid?" In asking this question, the patient is trying to ascertain whether the provider believes that the degree of hearing loss warrants amplification. This is not necessarily an easy question to answer.

There are degrees of hearing loss that suggest candidacy for hearing instruments and those that do not. Fitting ranges are available for hearing instruments that indicate whether a particular hearing instrument will provide appropriate amplification for a hearing loss with a given degree and configuration as determined by audiometric evaluation. However, the audiogram offers only one piece of information needed to answer the patient's question.

The answer really lies with the patient's perspective on whether the hearing loss is causing a communication problem. Patients with impaired hearing often report that they perceive no difficulty with communication. Such patients use communication strategies effectively, including speech reading, manipulation of the environment, and cognitive skills to minimize the impact of the hearing loss. Other patients, with the same degree of sensitivity loss, perceive the loss and associated communication difficulties as significant problems and are anxious to quantify the hearing loss for the purpose of obtaining hearing aids. In all cases, counseling regarding expectations from hearing aid use is essential, and the use of an assessment of communication needs should be considered to determine candidacy and promote successful use of the hearing aid.[2]

For a small group of patients, hearing instrument use may be contraindicated. A more likely scenario is that certain patient and hearing-loss characteristics may result in communication outcomes that are less than ideal.

Patient motivation is a key factor in predicting success with hearing instruments. Often, an unwilling patient succumbs to the requests of a spouse or other family members to obtain hearing instruments. Individuals who have a negative attitude toward hearing aid use often have poorer outcomes and limited use of the instruments.[3]

In some ears, speech perception is poorer than expected for a given hearing loss and, if severe enough, may preclude successful use. Word recognition scores can be useful in providing an initial prognosis for success with amplification. When word recognition is poor, the prognosis is reduced for benefit from, and satisfaction with, hearing aid use.

Limited cognitive ability can also be a barrier to successful hearing aid use. Modern hearing aids have multiple programs, memory buttons, and volume controls to provide better audibility. Due to poor memory and other constraints, inappropriate use can work against the patient by causing poor audibility.[4]

When a patient has a progressive or fluctuating hearing loss, hearing instruments must be sufficiently flexible to allow for alterations in programming to accommodate the fluctuating hearing.

Occasionally, patients may have an absent, small, or misshapen pinna that precludes fitting with a traditional custom hearing aid or earmold, or BTE hearing instrument. More commonly, the size of the ear canal of a patient may sometimes limit the use of certain ITE hearing instruments, due to space limitations.

Trends in Candidacy

Candidacy for hearing aid use depends on the degree and configuration of hearing loss and patient factors that may impact success with hearing aid fitting. Recent trends in hearing instrument technology have led to an expansion of the hearing loss criteria appropriate for hearing aid use. The use of DSP in hearing aids and the use of open-fit and receiver-in-the-canal (RIC) technology are examples of these recent trends.

Advances in hearing aid sound-processing strategies have expanded candidacy for hearing aid benefit. The nearly universal change from analog processing to DSP circuits in hearing aids permits significantly greater flexibility to manipulate the auditory signal in a way that is appropriate for most patients with hearing loss.[5,6] In the past, a specific hearing aid was chosen to closely match the characteristics of the hearing loss. The current use of digital amplifiers permits programmable control in the frequency, amplitude, and time domains to better fit an individual's specific hearing loss and ability. The response of the hearing aid is based upon a prescriptive target for a given hearing-loss degree and configuration, with additional programming changes made to adapt to patient-specific characteristics. Although there are still some hearing losses for which hearing aids are less than optimal, such as rising configurations and losses that are too severe, the use of digital processing allows for greater flexibility in hearing-aid-response characteristics and, thus, for more patients to benefit from hearing aids.

Introduction of newer hearing aid designs also has contributed to increased patient candidacy. The "open-fit" design is one example. Here, amplified high-frequency signals are delivered to the ear canal via thin tubing, leaving the ear canal relatively open for natural hearing of lower-frequency sounds. This approach permits the fitting of ears with relatively normal low-frequency hearing.

The increasing flexibility offered by modern DSP technology and the benefits accrued for specific populations through the use of different sound delivery designs have led to greater range of candidacy for hearing aid use. Indications for successful use generally relate more to a given patient's communication needs rather than to the specific characteristics of the patient's hearing loss. In other words, in light of the expanded technology, candidacy is now based more upon whether the patients perceive they are struggling to communicate, rather than on the specific audiometric outcomes found on the audiogram.

Another overall trend in hearing aid candidacy is the use of binaural amplification when hearing loss is present in both ears. Binaural amplification offers several advantages over monaural fitting that can greatly increase positive communication outcomes for a patient.[7–9] Advantages include binaural summation, wherein the loudness of sound is increased when perceived from both ears rather than one, resulting in better hearing sensitivity, and binaural squelch, wherein the signal-to-noise ratio is effectively increased by greater elimination of background sounds.[10] In addition, listeners perceive a more natural and balanced sound quality with two hearing instruments. The benefits expected of many of the newer technology trends, including directional microphones and certain types of wireless connectivity, are predicated on an assumption of binaural hearing aid use.

The use of two hearing aids is also important because of the potential for monaural auditory deprivation in cases where only one hearing aid is fitted on a patient with bilateral hearing loss.[11] It appears likely that in a subset of patients with bilateral hearing loss, the fitting of a hearing aid on one ear will result in progressive deterioration of suprathreshold hearing in the unaided ear. Although these deprivation effects are reversible in some patients with the completion of binaural fitting, in others the effect may be permanent.[12]

In some rare circumstances, significantly asymmetric speech perception may actually contraindicate binaural use. In a case where one ear has significant distortion or poor processing ability, amplification of the distorted signal may actually serve to decrease overall speech perception below that of the better ear.[13,14] Examination of binaural speech-recognition performance can assist in determining whether a poorly functioning ear is actually undermining speech-perception performance of both ears.

HEARING AID SELECTION

Selection of hearing aids is based on determination of an amplification system that will effectively deliver sound to a patient's ear. Effectiveness is determined by the interaction of the electroacoustic response of the device, the design style for delivery of the amplified sound, and the device features necessary to optimize that sound delivery.

Electroacoustic Characteristics

Fundamental Signal Processing

Every hearing aid has a characteristic acoustic output, defined by its frequency gain, input–output, and output limiting. The gain of a hearing aid is the amount that the input signal is increased by the hearing aid amplifier. The frequency-gain characteristic of a hearing aid describes the gain as a function of frequency for a given input intensity level. In addition to varying with frequency, the gain of a hearing aid can also vary as a function of input intensity level. The input–output response describes the relationship between input intensity and output intensity for a given frequency.

There are two general classes of input–output functions for hearing aids, linear and nonlinear. Early forms of modern hearing instruments used a linear amplification approach, in which all sound inputs were amplified equally. Because most sensorineural hearing losses are nonlinear at near-threshold levels, the application of a linear solution proved inadequate. The solution was the use of compression circuits that allow a signal to be amplified differentially depending on the intensity of the input sound. Typically, lower intensity inputs are amplified to a greater extent than higher intensity inputs. The use of compression circuits allows the auditory signal to be "shrunk" to fit in the dynamic range of the listener, reducing distortion of the signal.[15,16]

In linear hearing aids the output of the aid was limited by a method known as "peak-clipping," in which energy output that exceeded a defined level was abruptly attenuated. This simple approach of linear amplification and peak clipping was an effective approach for fitting conductive hearing loss but proved to be wholly unsatisfactory for fitting ears with sensorineural hearing loss. Peak clipping also proved to be an unsatisfactory approach to output limiting because it caused substantial distortion of the acoustic signal. Compression-limiting strategies were implemented in analog circuits to reduce the distortion.

The fundamental way to specify a starting point for determining the response of a hearing aid is to prescribe frequency-gain characteristics based on audiometric measures.[17] A number of prescriptive rules have been developed. Some are based on hearing thresholds alone and attempt to specify gain that will amplify average conversational speech to a comfortable or preferred listening level. Simple gain rules, such as the half-gain rule, prescribe gain equal to one-half the amount of the hearing loss; the third-gain rule to gain equal to one-third the amount of the hearing loss. Most prescriptive rules use this simple approach as a basis and then adjust individual frequencies based on empirically determined correction factors. One popular early threshold-based procedure, which still serves as the basis for some current approaches is that of the National Acoustic Laboratory (NAL).[18]

Another approach has been to prescribe frequency-gain characteristics based on threshold and discomfort levels.[17] One such method is the desired sensation level (DSL) method.[19] The DSL was originally designed for fitting hearing aids in children, and it prescribed gain based on both thresholds and predicted discomfort levels.

Other considerations for determining targets include the type of hearing loss and whether one or both ears are being fitted. When there is a conductive component to the hearing loss, target gain is usually increased by approximately 25% of the air–bone gap at a given frequency. When the hearing aid fitting is binaural, the target gain for each ear should be reduced by 3 to 6 dB for binaural summation.[17,20]

Trends in Signal Processing

The change to DSP has had a dramatic impact on the flexibility of hearing aid selection. In the past, a specific hearing aid was chosen to closely match the electroacoustic characteristics of the hearing aid with the hearing sensitivity of the patient. That is, the patient's audiogram was used to determine a prescription for gain. Circuit matrices were then scrutinized to find one that would match the target gain, and a hearing aid was chosen with the selected circuit. Today, because of the flexibility of digital amplifiers, hearing aids have a broad fitting range, and the electroacoustic characteristics can be adjusted to match a wide range of prescriptive gains. Selection, then, is less a matter of gain issues and more a matter of design style and features. Enhancements in signal processing will be covered in greater detail under feature selection.

The advancements in nonlinear-amplifier characteristics have reduced the effectiveness of threshold-based prescriptive methods for specifying target gains. Newer alternative prescriptive procedures have been developed in response to these wide-dynamic-range compression amplifiers to determine targets for soft, moderate, and loud sound.[21] More recent procedures combine the linear approach of the early threshold-based prescription methods with different prescription requirements for soft and loud sounds.[17,22]

Hearing Aid Design

The placement of a hearing aid into the ear has consequences to the hearing in that ear and consequences to the functioning of the device. Merely placing an object such as a hearing aid or earmold into the ear causes a loss of hearing due to the attenuating effect of the object, a consequence known as insertion loss. This additional loss must be accounted for in selecting devices and specifying amplification characteristics. Insertion of the device into the ear canal also causes the "occlusion effect," wherein low-frequency components of an auditory signal are enhanced, including those of the patient's voice. This commonly results in a complaint of sounds being too loud, booming, or echoing.

Another important consequence of hearing aid use is displacement of the microphone away from the ear's natural sound enhancement of the pinna and ear canal. That is, the ear's natural microphone is the tympanic membrane, which benefits from resonant amplification of important speech frequencies from the ear canal and concha. The tympanic membrane also receives acoustic cues that are important for spatial localization. When a hearing device is added to the system, and the microphone is moved away from the tympanic membrane, these cues are altered. The further the microphone is from the ear canal, the greater is the loss of this important information. The loss of spatial cues and resonant peaks must also be accounted for in selecting devices and especially in considering technology features of the device.

An alternative to moving the microphone away from the tympanic membrane is to place it as deep in the ear canal as possible. Doing so, however, puts the microphone in proximity to the receiver or loudspeaker, which enhances the likelihood of acoustic feedback and decreases the amount of usable gain. Many of the technology features in hearing aids are designed to overcome the issues created by placement of the device in the first place.

As a result of these influences, there are a number of factors to consider when determining the best hearing-instrument design for a patient.[23] One of the most important factors is the degree and configuration of hearing sensitivity loss. Other factors that influence the design decision include feedback, venting, device size, durability, microphone location, and patient preference.

Design Fundamentals

Hearing instruments can be categorized generally as BTE or ITE styles. As a class, BTE instruments house the majority of the components outside the ear canal and auricle (Figure 14–1A). This type of hearing instrument is coupled to the ear via an earmold and tubing. Traditional BTE instruments have a custom earmold.

ITE hearing instruments vary in size from a full-shell hearing instrument, which fills up the entire bowl and helix of the auricle, to the smallest completely-in-the-canal hearing instruments that fit deeply in the ear canal (Figure 14–1B to D).

As mentioned previously, acoustic feedback occurs when the amplified sound emanating from a receiver is directed back into the microphone of the same amplifier system. The best method to eliminate feedback is to separate the microphone and receiver in space. Although advanced signal processing strategies have been developed to provide automatic feedback cancellation,[24] the physical elimination of feedback remains the most effective approach. Thus, for a patient with considerable sensitivity loss, for which a large amount of gain is required, selection of a device that permits physical separation, such as a BTE, is the preferred approach to feedback reduction.

One of the most effective ways of reducing the occlusion effect of hearing aid or earmold insertion is the use of venting. A small bore, called a vent, can be made through an earmold or hearing-instrument casing.[25] The vent allows exchange of air in the ear canal and the escape of low-frequency sound. In most cases, this reduction in low-frequency sound is desirable, as amplification of low frequencies can cause a patient's own voice to be "hollow" or "echoing." However, in cases where large amounts of gain are needed, the presence of a vent increases the opportunity for feedback as sound escapes through the vent.[25–27]

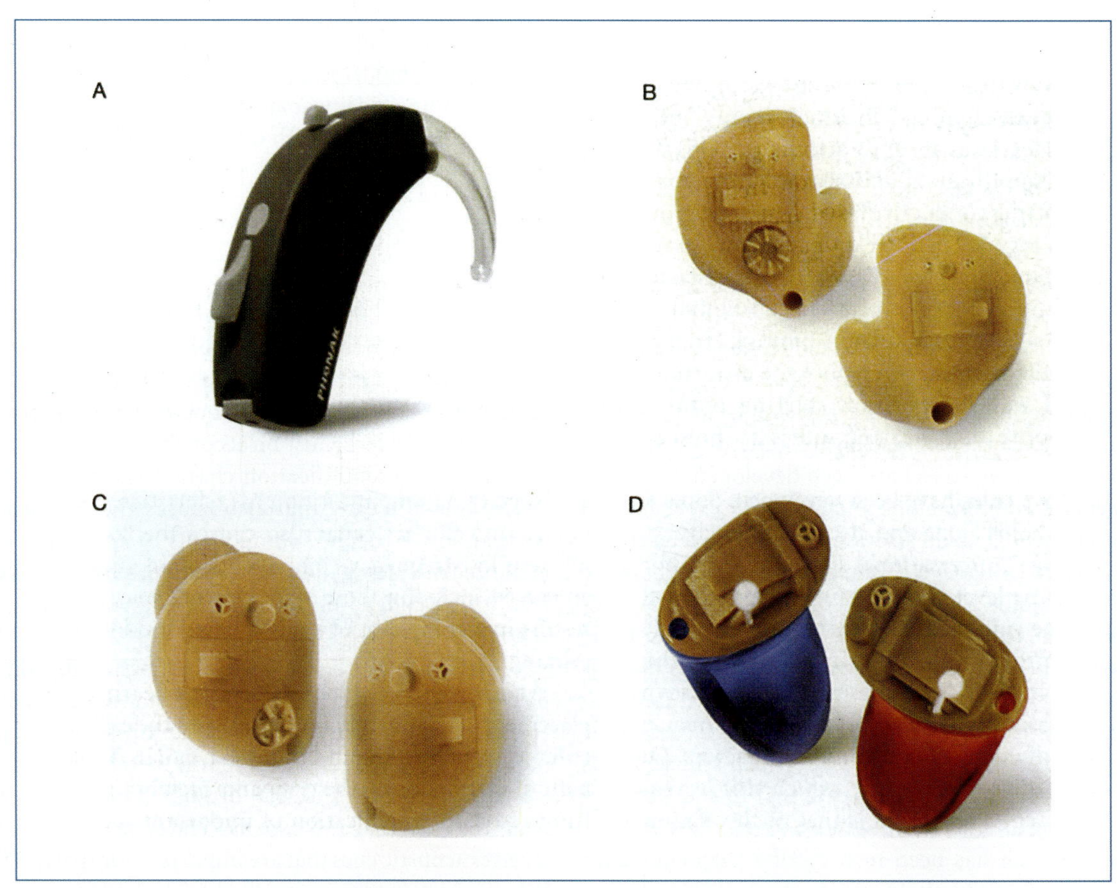

FIGURE 14–1 • Photographs of hearing instrument design styles. *A*, Behind-the-ear aid. *B*, In-the-ear full-shell aid. *C*, In-the-canal aid. *D*, Completely-in-the-canal aid. *Courtesy of Phonak.*

Another important consideration in the selection of hearing aids is the overall size of the device. As a general rule, the smaller a hearing instrument, the greater is the potential for feedback to occur, due to the necessarily closer proximity of the microphone and receiver. Device size also dictates what controls are available to the patient, as smaller hearing instruments have less physical space for the actual switches. In the case of completely-in-the-canal hearing instruments, directional microphone technology and telecoils are not available due to space limitations. Battery size is also limited in smaller hearing instruments. This may be an important factor when fitting a patient with limited manual dexterity or visual acuity. These patient needs and characteristics must be taken into account when determining appropriate device size.[28,29]

Hearing instruments are routinely subjected to conditions that are unfavorable for electronic devices. Moisture and cerumen in the ear canal are generally incompatible with electronic instruments. As such, hearing aids with the electronic components of the device behind the ear are generally found to be more durable than hearing instruments where these components are located in the ear.

Selection decisions about hearing aid styles represent a trade-off of all of these factors to arrive at a choice that balances the various physical constraints of the hearing aid design. Confounding the decision further, however, is the important consideration of patient preference. It is often patient preference for a particular style of hearing instrument that presents the greatest fitting challenge.

Design Trends

A general trend in hearing aid development is the miniaturization of hearing aids, for both ITE and BTE designs. The use of DSP has reduced the need for external controls on hearing aids, allowing the aids to be smaller and more streamlined in appearance. This change appeals to the cosmetic and comfort concerns of many potential hearing aid users.

A recent trend in hearing aid fittings is the use of open-fit and RIC hearing aids (Figure 14–2). The term "open-fit" refers to hearing aid fittings that leave the ear canal relatively unoccluded. Open-fit BTE (also called over-the-ear) hearing aids direct sound to the ear canal via thin tubing that rests in the ear canal or terminates in a non-custom flexible dome that fits in the ear canal. The earmold piece can also be customized for better device retention.

RIC technology refers to a style of aid wherein the microphone and amplifier are housed behind- or over-the-ear, typically in a miniaturized BTE style aid, while the receiver is located in the ear canal. The electrical signal is transmitted to the receiver via a thin wire. The receiver is coupled to the ear canal via a pliable dome, as with most open-fit styles, or via a custom earmold. There are two primary advantages to the RIC approach. First, the separation of the receiver from the microphone and amplifier permits the delivery of more amplification gain without feedback. Second, because the microphone/amplifier package does not include the receiver, space needs are reduced, permitting smaller size or more components within the BTE itself.

The use of open-fit and RIC technology has led to expanded hearing aid candidacy for precipitously sloping hearing losses and mild losses where the higher frequencies must be amplified, without occluding the ear in such a way to block off the relatively normal low-frequency hearing.[30]

Technology Features

Once a hearing aid style has been selected, determination is made of the electroacoustic and component features to be included in the device.

Fundamentals

Hearing instruments consist of three main components: a microphone that transduces acoustic energy to electrical energy; an amplifier that increases the strength of the electrical signal; and a receiver that transduces electrical energy back to acoustic energy (Figure 14–3). Additionally, hearing instruments require a power source in the form of a battery. Controls on a hearing instrument for volume or program manipulation are also commonly included on devices.

Most hearing aids include some form of input as an alternative to the microphone. Conventionally, hearing aids can be equipped with a telecoil (or t-coil) for electromagnetic coupling to a telephone or other induction-loop transducer. Many hearing aids can also receive direct audio input via a plug-in cord or can be fitted with a plug-in frequency modulation (FM) receiver.

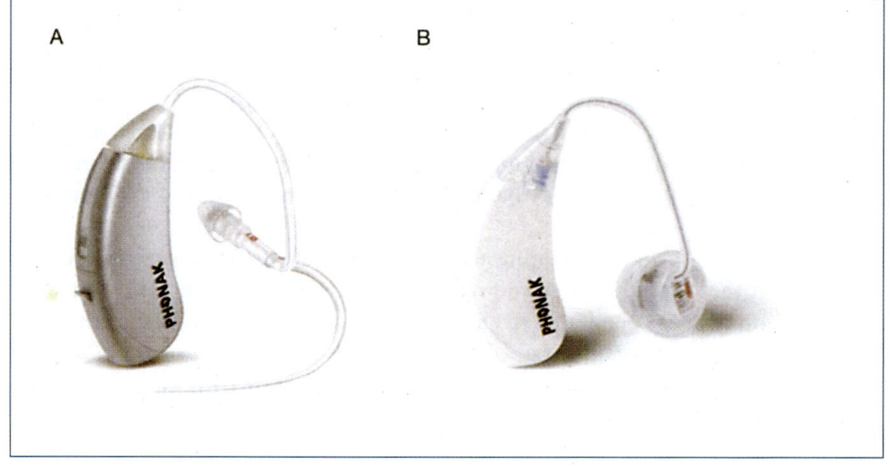

FIGURE 14–2 • Photograph of (A) open-fit slim tube hearing aid and receiver-in-the-canal hearing aid (B). *Courtesy of Phonak.*

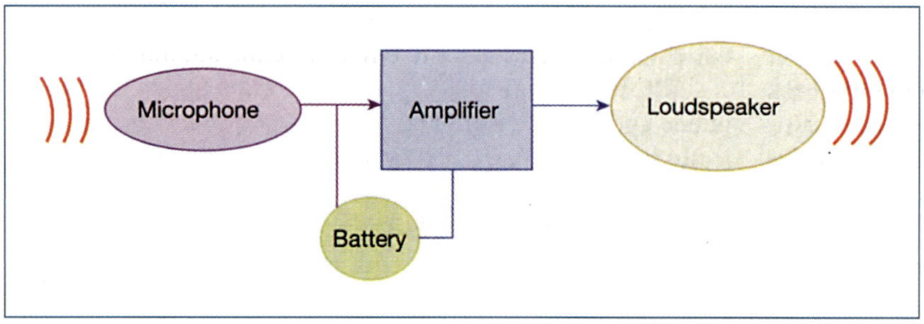

Microphone
Amplifier
Loudspeaker
Battery

FIGURE 14–3 • Schematic representation of the components of a hearing aid.

When a traditional BTE style of hearing instrument is selected, an earmold must be made to couple the instrument to the ear canal. There are many styles of earmolds, from a full-shell, which fills the auricle, to canal earmolds that fill the ear canal only. There are also several choices for earmold materials.[25] Acrylic, the hardest material, is typically the easiest to insert and remove. Silicone, the softest material, provides the best acoustic seal in the ear to prevent feedback. This softer silicone material is used most often with pediatric patients for safety reasons. Vinyl, an intermediate material, can provide a compromise among these factors. Nonallergenic materials are available as well.

Trends in Technology Features

DSP capability in hearings aids permits the flexibility to include a number of hearing aid features that can be of substantial benefit to hearing aid users. These features include adaptable directionality, multiple programs, digital noise reduction, digital feedback suppression, data logging, trainability, wireless connectivity, and the ability of the hearing aid to automatically control most of these features. The value and availability of these various features are determined by the type, degree, and configuration of the hearing loss, which in turn determines the style and type of signal processing indicated. Patient characteristics and communication needs are also factors in choosing appropriate hearing aid features.

A common feature in hearing aids is directionality. Most devices have an omnidirectional microphone, which is essentially unfocused in terms of direction of sound transduction, and some form of directionality, wherein the hearing aid is more sensitive to sound from a specified direction while not amplifying sounds originating from other directions. This feature enhances sound in front of the patient, where a presumed speaker would be, while reducing background noise.[31] The effect of directional microphone use is to increase the signal-to-noise ratio, thereby enhancing speech understanding in noise. Directional microphones are available in various configurations. In the simplest form the microphone can be switched from omnidirectional to directional. In more advanced forms, the amount of directionality can be varied over a continuum. In addition, some systems are automatic and adaptive, so that the amount of directionality varies automatically as a function of the amount of detected background noise.

Another feature of hearing aids is the availability of multiple programs or memories. The use of multiple programs allows the hearing aid to have several different responses available for different listening situations. For example, one hearing aid program may be appropriate for quiet situations, with an omnidirectional-microphone mode, while another hearing aid program may be appropriate for noisy situations, with a directional-microphone mode and a frequency-gain response that de-emphasizes low-frequency sounds. Other hearing aid programs may be most appropriate for telephone use, for listening to music, or for any particular listening environment that might require a specific hearing aid response. Programmatic control can be manual or can be changed automatically and adaptively by the hearing aid.

Reduced user control over hearing aid response is a current trend in hearing aids, with elimination of volume controls and manual program buttons or remote controls in favor of adaptive control by the hearing aid itself. Many hearing aids have the capability to continuously sample the acoustic environment and to make preprogrammed adjustments to the hearing aid response as the environment changes.

Noise-reduction circuitry is a feature available in most digital hearing aids. The goal of noise reduction is to reduce unwanted, ongoing background noises in an effort to enhance speech perception and listening comfort. Sophisticated processing algorithms allow the hearing aid to differentiate between noise sources and other signals based on their frequency, intensity, and temporal characteristics.[32] When an unwanted noise source is identified, the amplification characteristics are automatically adjusted accordingly.

As noted previously, acoustic feedback occurs when an amplified signal is redirected into the microphone of an amplification instrument. The most common and effective method of feedback suppression in hearing aids remains adequate physical separation of the microphone and receiver. However, DSP has allowed for additional feedback suppression mechanisms; as in the case of noise, feedback is recognized based on its frequency, intensity, and temporal characteristics. When the hearing instrument recognizes acoustic feedback it can be suppressed in most cases by reduction of gain in the offending frequency band, or by phase cancellation of the feedback signal.[24,33]

Data logging is a hearing aid feature that tracks and records user settings and usage patterns of the hearing aid. Statistics are generated to characterize use, which can be viewed via the programming software of the hearing aid. Information that is commonly utilized includes overall time of hearing aid use, use of automatic or manually controlled hearing aid programs and features, and in some cases, the classification of the listening environment in which the hearing aid was used. Data logging is helpful in troubleshooting patient complaints and in making changes to baseline programming to reflect the user's preferred settings. The process can even be automated to provide suggested changes based on listener preferences and experiences.[34] An example of a data logging screen is shown in Figure 14–4.

Trainability of hearing aids is an extension of data logging. In some cases, data logging may be used to automatically change programming based on user preferences. For certain hearing aids, changes may be made when the user initiates training via a manual control. For example, a patient may adjust the hearing aid volume and program characteristics to preferential settings for a particular environment. The user then initiates hearing aid training so that the aid will approximate these settings in the future in similar listening environments.[35]

Another feature available in certain hearing aid styles is self-diagnostic testing of the integrity of the hearing aid. For certain commonly encountered problems, the hearing aid is capable of determining malfunction, and voice indicators are used to direct the patient for basic hearing aid troubleshooting.

Wireless connectivity is a growing trend in hearing aids. This allows for convenient communication from hearing aids to electronic devices and signal sources, such as remote microphones. Other signal sources include mobile phones and personal music players. Newer technology also allows binaural hearing aids to communicate with each other, permitting synchronization of responses to environmental sounds.[36]

HEARING AID FITTING AND VERIFICATION

Fitting and Verification Fundamentals

Once a hearing aid has been selected, it is programmed with a prescriptive formula derived from audiometric data. Most DSP hearing aid programming software will predict a "best-fit" prescription, based on the proprietary nuances of the signal processing, which sets parameters for frequency gain, input–output, and maximum output levels. The algorithms used for prescriptive gain are based on the physical characteristics of an average ear. Because the specific characteristics of an individual patient's ear canal and pinna modify sound in a unique way, adjustments must be made to the acoustic response of the hearing aid to accommodate these individual variations.

Probe-microphone measurements are used for this purpose. These measurements are made by insertion of a small tube in the ear canal, close to the tympanic membrane. The external portion of the tube is attached to a microphone that is capable of recording sounds from inside the ear canal. Loudspeakers placed near the ear of the patient deliver various signals of different intensities.

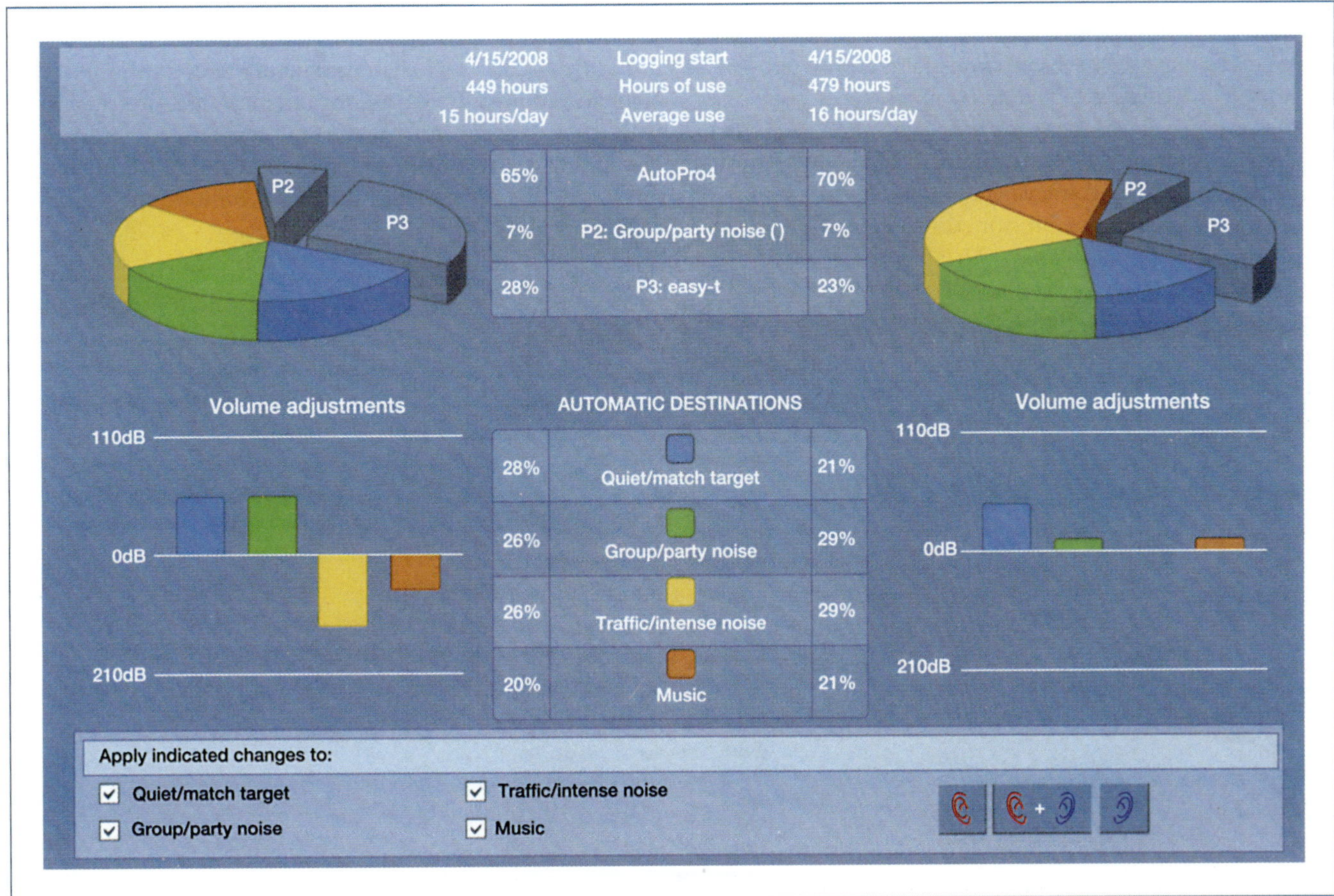

FIGURE 14–4 • Image of data logging screen from hearing aid programming software. *Courtesy of Unitron.*

With the probe-tube in the open ear canal, sounds are presented to determine the real-ear unaided response or gain. Then, with the hearing aid in place, the real-ear aided response or gain is determined by presentation of the same sounds. The difference between the recorded sounds, with and without the hearing aid in place, describes the real-ear insertion gain (REIG) provided by the hearing aid. The output of the hearing aid can be adjusted as needed so that the REIG approximates the desired output targets.[37–40]

Verification of the hearing aid response is a necessary component of fitting hearing aids. Traditionally this had been accomplished through the use of aided-response testing. Perceptual verification of hearing aid performance is accomplished with subjective quality judgments and functional measures including functional gain (how much hearing sensitivity improves with the hearing aid in situ) and speech recognition measures with the hearing aid in place. Such testing is often still used today following initial fitting to verify the benefit provided by hearing aids.

Trends in Hearing Aid Fitting and Verification

Real-ear measurement strategies have advanced in sophistication to accommodate changes in signal processing complexity. For example, simple tonal stimuli used in the past for real-ear measurement are now often eliminated by sophisticated noise-reduction paradigms, rendering them unacceptable for evaluating the functioning of the device. More complex signals, such as speech or speech-like noise, are now used to provide a more realistic assessment of the electroacoustic response of a device over time to varying levels of complex input.

One example of this type of approach is called speech mapping. In speech mapping, recorded speech is presented through a loudspeaker at various intensity levels while the response of the hearing aid is measured in situ via probe-microphone. An example is shown in Figure 14–5. In addition, live speech, such as that of a family member, can be used to examine the response of the hearing aid to realistic and highly relevant speech stimuli. The acoustic response of the hearing aid can be adjusted so that low-intensity speech becomes audible, medium-intensity speech is comfortable, and high-intensity speech is perceived as loud but not uncomfortable.[41]

Another advance in real-ear measurement is the integration of the probe-microphone into the hearing aid itself. Thus, built-in features of the hearing aid are used to provide real-ear measures, rather than an external probe-microphone.

As in all areas of healthcare, outcome measures are a common strategy for evaluating the impact of hearing aid use on communication ability. A variety of self-assessment scales exist that can be administered prior to and following amplification use to determine hearing aid benefit.[42] Scales that measure patient perceptions of hearing ability and the impact of communication disorder resulting from hearing loss include the Hearing Handicap Inventory for the Elderly (HHIE)[2], the Abbreviated Profile of Hearing Aid Benefit (APHAB),[43] and the Client Oriented Scale of Improvement (COSI).[44] Other measures, such as the Glasgow Hearing Aid Benefit Profile (GHABP)[45] and the International Outcome Inventory—Hearing Aids (IOI-HA)[46] provide quality-of-life measures related to hearing aid use. There are also evaluations, such as the HHIE, which can be administered to spouses and other family members to provide additional input regarding patients' experiences with hearing loss and hearing aid use. The Speech-Hearing, Spatial-Hearing and Qualities of Hearing (SSQ) Scale,[47] is a measure designed to evaluate not only a patient's ability to understand speech, but other factors such as sound quality and naturalness of all acoustic sounds. This type of outcome measure may prove particularly useful for the current generation of hearing aid technology, wherein the emphasis has shifted to include not only audibility of speech, but patient comfort and acceptance of hearing aids.

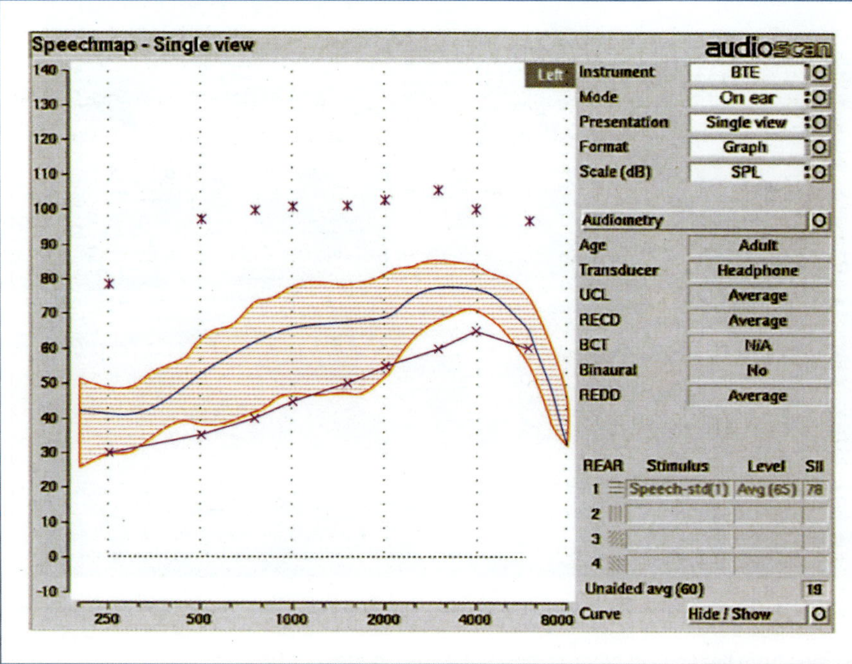

FIGURE 14–5 • Image of a real-ear speech mapping screen. *Courtesy of Audioscan.*

HEARING AIDS ONLY THE FIRST STEP

Orientation and Follow-Up

At the time a hearing aid is dispensed, the patient is oriented to the basic working of the instrument.[48,49] Instructions and training are provided in cleaning and care of the hearing instrument, including changing batteries. The patient is also counseled on insertion and removal of the hearing instruments, often the most challenging aspect of the fitting.

Follow-up appointments are typically made with new users of hearing instruments to ensure that the patient is acclimating to, and is correctly using, the hearing instruments. Often, due to the extent of information covered in the initial fitting appointment, the patient has additional questions or concerns. In addition, fine-tuning adjustments can be made to the hearing instrument programming as needed.

A number of problems occur related to fitting of hearing instruments that require sophistication in counseling, first to define the problem and then to manage it. In many cases, the complaints of hearing instrument users are ambiguous, as patients struggle to describe the often transient sensations which occur with hearing instrument use. Once a complaint is identified, there are often a number of possible causes, which must be systematically ruled out before a solution is found. In some cases, the solution lies in helping the patient to develop appropriate expectations for hearing instrument use.

Hearing Assistive Technology

Assistive technologies other than hearing aids are available for situation-specific hearing issues. Assistive technologies include assistive listening devices (ALDs), alerting and signaling devices, and telephone amplifiers. ALDs include personal amplifiers, FM systems, and television listeners. These devices are designed to enhance an acoustic signal over background noise by the use of a remote microphone. The use of a remote microphone allows the signal to be received by the listener without the degrading effects of distance and reverberation.[50]

Other assistive technologies are available to provide solutions for specific listening situations, such as telephone amplifiers and closed captioning of television shows. Alerting devices, such as alarm clocks, fire alarms, and doorbells are designed to flash a light or vibrate a bed when activated.

A recent trend with hearing assistive technology is the ability to wirelessly connect such devices to hearing aids. Through the use of wireless connectivity, such as Bluetooth, many hearing aids can be connected to a telephone, FM receiver, MP3 player, or other audio-input device. The audio input is typically connected or paired to a device that is worn around the neck and which transmits a signal to the hearing aids. Such technology allows users to hear the input signal acoustically modified by the hearing aid, and to hear this signal in both ears. In addition, it eliminates problems of feedback commonly encountered when using devices such as headphones or telephones with hearing aids.

Aural Rehabilitation

In addition to fitting patients with amplification and orienting them to optimal use of the hearing instruments, some patients receive benefit from structured auditory-rehabilitation programs. One aspect of auditory rehabilitation involves patient education regarding approaches to optimizing understanding of speech in challenging listening situations. Communication strategies may include behavior modifications such as rephrasing or asking for repetition, use of speechreading to enhance understanding of the auditory signal, and environmental modifications to reduce potentially interfering background sounds and barriers to audibility.

Another aspect of auditory rehabilitation involves the use of structured auditory- or listening-training programs. These programs include formal presentation of stimuli designed to train listeners to use the auditory signal more effectively. In order to provide more cost and time-effective means of administering such programs, computer-based rehabilitation models have been developed. One example is the Listening and Auditory Communication Enhancement (LACE) training program, which is available for patient use on a personal computer so that auditory training can occur in the patient's home environment.[51]

Counseling patients about reasonable expectations for hearing aid use begins at the time of hearing aid selection and continues throughout the rehabilitation process. Patients will benefit most and adjust more readily to hearing instruments if they are informed and knowledgeable regarding expectations for hearing instrument use.[52,53] Just as for listeners with normal hearing, patients will experience greater benefit in quiet than in noise, and when the face of the speaker can be clearly seen. Environmental sounds will be louder than previously experienced, but should not be uncomfortably loud. Listeners should expect hearing instruments to be visible to a certain degree, and while they may feel the hearing instruments, they should be physically comfortable. Patients will also benefit from prior understanding of how hearing instruments should be used to obtain maximum benefit. A key to success with hearing instruments is consistent use. Some patients have the expectation that hearing instruments will be used only in challenging listening situations. However, it is important for patients to understand that inconsistent use of hearing instruments typically leads to poorer results.[54] In addition, patients should be counseled that they will use their hearing instruments only during waking hours and not in situations where the hearing instruments would be exposed to excessive moisture.

References

1. Sammeth CA, Levitt H. Hearing aid selection and fitting in adults: History and evolution. In: Valente M, Hosford-Dunn H, Roeser RJ, editors. Audiology treatment. New York: Thieme Medical Publishers, Inc.; 2000. p. 213–59.
2. Ventry I, Weinstein B. The hearing handicap inventory for the elderly: A new tool. Ear Hear 1982;3:128–34.
3. Wilson C, Stephens D. Reasons for referral and attitudes toward hearing aids: Do they affect outcome? Clin Otolaryngol Allied Sci 2003;28:81–4.
4. Kricos PB. Audiologic management of older adults with hearing loss and compromised cognitive/psychoacoustic auditory processing capabilities. Trends Amplif 2006;10:1–28.
5. Levitt H. A historical perspective on digital hearing aids: How digital technology has changed modern hearing aids. Trends Amplif 2007;11:7–24.

6. Niklaus M. Flexible DSP circuits have put advances in hearing aid technology on a fast track. Hear J 2007;60:22–4.
7. Balfour PB, Hawkins DB. A comparison of sound quality judgments for monaural and binaural hearing aid processed stimuli. Ear Hear 1992;13:331–9.
8. Byrne D, Noble W, LePage B. Effects of long-term bilateral and unilateral fitting of different hearing aid types on the ability to locate sounds. J Am Acad Audiol 1992;3:369–82.
9. Day GA, Browning GG, Gatehouse S. Benefit from binaural hearing aids in individuals with a severe hearing impairment. Br J Audiol 1998;22:273–7.
10. Gelfand SA. Hearing: An introduction to psychological and physiological acoustics. 4th ed. New York: Mercal Dekker; 2004.
11. Silman S, Gelfand SA, Silverman CA. Late onset auditory deprivation: Effects of monaural versus binaural hearing aids. J Acoust Soc Am 1984;76:1357–62.
12. Silverman CA, Silman S. Apparent auditory deprivation from monaural amplification and recovery with binaural amplification. J Am Acad Audiol 1990;1:175–80.
13. Jerger J, Silman S, Lew HL, Chmiel R. Case studies in binaural interference: Converging evidence from behavioral and electrophysiologic measures. J Am Acad Audiol 1993;4:122–31.
14. Schoepflin JR. Binaural interference in a child: A case study. J Am Acad Audiol 2007;18:515–21.
15. Hickson LMH. Compression amplification in hearing aids. Am J Audiol 1994;3:51–65.
16. Venema TH. Compression for clinicians. San Diego, CA: Singular Publishing Group; 1998.
17. Palmer C, Lindley GA. Overview and rationale for prescriptive formulas for linear and nonlinear hearing aids. In: Valente M, editor. Strategies for selecting and verifying hearing aid fittings. 2nd ed. New York: Thieme Medical Publishers, Inc.; 1996. p. 1–22.
18. Byrne D, Dillon H. New procedure for selecting gain and frequency response of a hearing aid: The National Acoustics Laboratory (NAL) formula. Ear Hear 1986;7:257–65.
19. Seewald RC. The desired sensation level method for fitting children: Version 3.0. Hear J 1992;45:36–41.
20. Mueller HG, Hawkins DB. Three important considerations in hearing aid selection. In: Sandlin RE, editor. Handbook of hearing aid amplification, volume II: Clinical considerations and fitting practices. Boston, MA: College Hill Press; 1990. p. 31–60.
21. Van Vliet D. A comprehensive hearing aid fitting protocol. Audiol Today 1995;7:11–3.
22. Byrne D, Dillon H, Ching T, Katsch R, Keidser G. NAL-NL1 procedure for fitting nonlinear hearing aids: Characteristics and comparisons with other procedures. J Am Acad Audiol 2001;12:37–51.
23. May AE, Upfold LJ, Battaglia JA. The advantages and disadvantages of ITC, ITE and BTE hearing aids: Diary and interview reports from elderly users. Br J Audiol 1990;24:301–9.
24. Parsa V. Acoustic feedback and its reduction through digital signal processing. Hear J 2006;59:16–23.
25. Valente M, Valente M, Potts LG, Lybarger EH. Earhooks, tubing, earmolds, and shells. In: Valente M, Hosford-Dunn H, Roeser RJ, editors. Audiology treatment. New York: Thieme Medical Publishers, Inc.; 2000. p. 59–104.
26. Mueller HG, Bright KE, Northern JL. Studies of the hearing aid occlusion effect. Semin Hear 1996;17:21–32.
27. Kuk FK. Perceptual consequences of vents in hearing aids. Br J Audiol 1991;25:163–9.
28. Upfold L, May A, Battaglia J. Hearing aid manipulation skills in an elderly population: A comparison of ITE, BTE and ITC aids. Br J Audiol 1990;24:311–18.
29. Stephens SD, Meredith R. Physical handling of hearing aids by the elderly. Acta Otolaryngol Suppl 1990;476:281–5.
30. Mueller HG. Open is in. Hear J 2006;59:11–14.
31. Ricketts TA, Hornsby BWY, Johnson EE. Adaptive directional benefit in the near field: Competing sound angle and level effects. Semin Hear 2005;26:59–69.
32. Kates JM. Digital hearing aids. San Diego, CA: Plural Publishing, Inc.; 2008.
33. Greenberg JE, Zurek PM, Brantley M. Evaluation of feedback reduction algorithms for hearing aids. J Acoust Soc Am 2000;108:2366–76.
34. Mueller HG. Data logging: It's popular, but how can this feature be used to help patients? Hear J 2007;60:19–26.
35. Hayes D. Empowering the hearing aid wearer through logging plus learning. Hear J 2007;60:20–5.
36. Sandrock C, Schum DJ. Wireless transmission of speech and data to, from, and between hearing aids. Hear J 2007;60:12–16.
37. Hawkins DB. Clinical ear canal probe tube measurements. Ear Hear 1987;8(suppl 5):74S–81S.
38. Mueller HG, Hawkins DB, Northern JL. Probe-microphone measurements: Hearing aid selection and assessment. San Diego, CA: Singular Press; 1992.
39. Preves DA, Curran JR. Hearing aid instrumentation and procedures for electroacoustic testing. In: Valente M, Hosford-Dunn H, Roeser RJ, editors. Audiology treatment. New York: Thieme Medical Publishers, Inc.; 2000. p. 1–58.
40. Revit LJ. Real-ear measures. In: Valente M, Hosford-Dunn H, Roeser RJ, editors. Audiology treatment. New York: Thieme Medical Publishers, Inc.; 2000. p. 105–45.
41. Moore BCJ. Speech mapping is a valuable tool for fitting and counseling patients. Hear J 2006;59:26–30.
42. Johnson CE, Danhauer JL. Handbook of outcome measures in audiology. Albany, NY: Thomson Delmar; 2002.
43. Cox R, Alexander G. The abbreviated profile of hearing aid benefit (APHAB). Ear Hear 1995;16:176–86.
44. Dillon H, James A, Ginis J. The client oriented scale of improvement (COSI) and its relationship to several other measures of benefit and satisfaction provided by hearing aids. J Am Acad Audiol 1997;8:27–43.
45. Gatehouse S. Glasgow hearing aid benefit profile: Derivation and validation of a client-centered outcome measure for hearing aid services. J Am Acad Audiol 1999;10:80–103.
46. Cox R, Alexander G. The international outcome inventory for hearing aids (IOI-HA): Psychometric properties of the English version. Int J Audiol 2002;41:30–5.
47. Gatehouse S, Noble W. The speech, spatial and qualities of hearing scale (SSQ). Int J Audiol 2004;43:85–99.
48. Sinks B, Duddy D. Hearing aid orientation and counseling. In: Valente M, editor. Strategies for selecting and verifying hearing aid fittings. 2nd ed. New York: Thieme Medical Publishers; 2002. p. 345–68.

49. Mormer E, Palmer C. A systematic program for hearing aid orientation and adjustment. In: Sweetow R, editor. Counseling for hearing aid fittings. San Diego, CA: Singular Publishing; 1999. p. 165–207.
50. Martin RL. For severe losses, FM technology can add great value to a hearing aid fitting. Hear J 2004;57:64.
51. Sabes JH, Sweetow RW. Variables predicting outcomes on listening and communication enhancement (LACE™) training. Int J Audiol 2007;46:374–83.
52. Kricos PB, Lesner SA, Sandridge SA. Expectations of older adults regarding the use of hearing aids. J Am Acad Audiol 1991;2:129–33.
53. Kochkin S. Reducing hearing instrument returns with consumer education. Hear Rev 1999;6:18–20.
54. Nabelek AK, Tucker FM, Letowski TR. Toleration of background noises: Relationship with patterns of hearing aid use by elderly persons. J Speech Hear Res 1991;34:679–85.

Tinnitus 15

Elina Kari, MD / Douglas E. Mattox, MD /
Pawel J. Jastreboff, PhD, ScD, MBA

Tinnitus, "ringing in the ears," is one of the most common problems encountered in everyday otolaryngology or audiology practice. Fortunately, the majority of people with tinnitus are not bothered by it, or their level of annoyance is mild. For some, it can be debilitating problem. In spite of a long history of tinnitus research and a rapid increase in the understanding of the auditory system, tinnitus remains a mystery. A relatively recent shift toward recognizing that tinnitus is a phantom auditory perception and the importance of various structures and systems in the brain have yielded substantial progress in the understanding and treatment of tinnitus. Last, but not least, the development of valid animal models of tinnitus has expanded research into this challenging phenomenon from purely the clinical arena to the laboratory. Many treatments have been proposed during last 30 years and the effectiveness of these treatments has increased considerably during this time.

HISTORY

The word "tinnitus" is derived from Latin, meaning a "jingling, clink." Tinnitus is the sensation of noises in the ear(s) that have been described as any number of sounds—ringing, whistling, blowing, booming, sizzling, etc.

Attempts to treat tinnitus can be found in millennia past. For "the bewitched ear," ancient Egyptians would administer "oil, frankincense, tree sap, herbs, and soil" via the external ear. Hippocrates and Aristotle later introduced the idea of masking to diminish the perception of tinnitus. During the Middle Ages, the Welsh placed hot loaves of bread onto each ear, thinking that the subsequent perspiration and "help of God" would cure the tinnitus. During the Renaissance, surgery was introduced as a potential cure. Trephination of the mastoid was performed to release air thought to be trapped in the ear and causing tinnitus. Jean Marie Gaspard of France was credited for advancing the field of tinnitus management during the 19th century. Also known for his work with deaf-mutes, he gave the earliest descriptions of so-called objective versus subjective tinnitus.[1,2]

EPIDEMIOLOGY

The prevalence of tinnitus has been estimated to be as high as 30% in the adult population, with approximately 8% of this population reporting bothersome tinnitus.[3,4] The severity of tinnitus can range from trivial to completely disabling. Tinnitus patients sometimes are driven to extremely high levels of anxiety and some commit suicide. However, a systematic study showed that the prevalence of suicide is statistically the same in tinnitus sufferers and the general population. An Internet search (Google) for "tinnitus" revealed over 4,300,000 sites, including countless self-help Web sites, information blogs, and nonprofit organizations devoted to a tinnitus "cure."

Tinnitus presents a difficult clinical problem as it can be the result of any number of medical reasons and in many cases, a definitive cause cannot be identified. Various approaches to the classification of tinnitus have been proposed.

Classification and Etiology

It is hoped that the classification of tinnitus can aid in its diagnosis and management. Consensus holds that subjective tinnitus is a phantom auditory perception and that objective tinnitus is called a somatosound. Tinnitus is perceived only by the patient; somatosounds are generated either by structures within or adjacent to the ear, or by structures that transmit sound to the ear (eg, clicking associated with artificial heart valves). Theoretically, an examiner may be able to detect a somatosound, such as a carotid bruit, but all the factors that can cause such sounds are not often easily clinically discernible.

Auditory imagery (a.k.a. musical hallucinations) is the phantom perception of well-known musical tunes or of voices without any understandable speech.[5–8] This perception is much less frequent than other forms of tinnitus; nevertheless, it is well documented and occurs primarily in older people with hearing loss. It is presumably a central type of tinnitus involving reverberatory activity within neural loops at a high level in the auditory cortex.[5–8]

Somatosounds can be either pulsatile or nonpulsatile. Pulsatile somatosounds are usually secondary to vascular (e.g., arteriovenous fistulas or malformations, paragangliomas, carotid artery stenosis, atherosclerotic disease, arterial dissection, persistent stapedial artery, intratympanic carotid artery, vascular compression of the eighth cranial nerve, increased cardiac output, pseudotumor cerebri, venous hum, jugular bulb anomalies) or nonvascular causes (palatal myoclonus, tensor tympani or stapedius muscle myoclonus, vascular neoplasms of the skull base).[2]

Tinnitus can be secondary to a number of medical conditions but often exists in the absence of an identifiable cause. This form of tinnitus is by far the most common. Furthermore, there is significant variation in the degree of severity with which tinnitus affects an individual—ranging from benign to devastating—with associated affective disorders such as hyperacusis, misophonia, and depression. Notably, there is no correlation between tinnitus severity and its psychoacoustical characterization (i.e., pitch and loudness match, minimal masking level).[9]

Pathophysiology

Risk Factors

Epidemiological studies have implicated many risk factors associated with the development of tinnitus. Specifically, age, cardiovascular or cerebrovascular disease, drugs, ear infections/inflammation, head or neck trauma, thyroid abnormalities, loud noise exposure, Ménière's disease, otosclerosis, sudden deafness, vestibular schwannoma, anxiety, depression, familial inheritance, health status, body mass index, education, socioeconomic status, and cigarette use have all been associated with tinnitus.[4] The same data indicate that alcohol, in moderation, can actually be beneficial.

The Norway Hearing Study (1996–1998)[4] reported that people who consumed 1–14 alcoholic beverages over the preceding 2 weeks were less likely to report bothersome tinnitus than those who reported having no alcoholic beverages during the same time frame. A statistically significant relationship between tinnitus and alcohol for those individuals consuming more than 14 alcoholic beverages, however, could not be identified.

The same study, as well as the United States National Health Information Survey, Disability Supplement,[4] demonstrated that individuals with hearing loss were much more likely to report bothersome and chronic tinnitus. In addition, the more the severe the hearing loss, the more likely individuals were to report chronic or bothersome tinnitus. Noise exposure, even in the absence of hearing loss or other auditory conditions, has been associated with tinnitus. Ototoxic agents and numerous drugs have also been found to be likely culprits.[2,10] There have been a number of case reports of specific agents that have appeared to cause tinnitus, but there are specific agents that have been consistently reported, such as cisplatin[11] or quinine.

THE STUDY OF TINNITUS

While many disorders have been associated with tinnitus, the exact pathophysiology of tinnitus is unclear. Tinnitus is believed to originate from deterioration in, or damage, or alteration to the inner ear hair cells, and/or peripheral or central nervous system auditory pathways. The pathophysiological mechanisms and pathway that lead to such a deterioration or alteration are myriad, complex, and in many cases, unclear. Even in cases of well-defined dysfunction of the inner ear (eg, hearing loss) there are a variety of proposed mechanisms, but as of yet none have been definitely proven.

The study of tinnitus in humans is challenging. A common goal has been to identify differences between the cochlear and brain functions of tinnitus sufferers and those who do not suffer from tinnitus. The tests available, such as positron emission tomography (PET), functional magnetic resonance imaging (fMRI), otoacoustic emissions, and evoked potentials, can vary considerably based on patient's age, sex, and degree of hearing loss,[12] and provide a limited amount of useful information.

A number of animal models have evolved over the last 20 years and have greatly added to our understanding of the neuropathophysiology of tinnitus. In 1988, Jastreboff et al.[13] described a rat model of tinnitus using a conditioned suppression procedure. The animals were trained to associate silence with a shock that subsequently evoked fear (Pavlovian suppression training). Jastreboff used water deprivation to motivate the animals to lick from a waterspout. Fear induces a decrease in drinking that has been used to assess the extent of fear. When tinnitus was induced in animals trained to be afraid of silence, they were not as afraid when external background noise was switched off as they did not perceive silence, but tinnitus. Consequently, suppression of drinking was smaller and extinction of learned fear of silence occurred faster. When, on the other hand, animals were trained to be afraid of tinnitus rather than silence (by inducing tinnitus before Pavlovian suppression training), suppression was stronger and extinction of trained fear occurred slower.

Other models have evolved since Jastreboff's work that have also used conditioned responses to reflect tinnitus, such as pole jumping avoidance,[14] conditioned lick reward,[15] conditioned polydipsia avoidance,[16] conditioned two-choice (left/right responses),[17] and gap detection reflexes.[18,19]

The Discordant Dysfunction Theory

The discordant dysfunction theory[20–22] postulates that tinnitus can result from an imbalance that results from damaged or dysfunctional outer hair cells (OHCs) and relatively better functioning inner hair cells (IHCs). It is postulated that increased neuronal activity in the dorsal cochlear nucleus (DCN) is generated in response to the decreased or absent signal from type II auditory nerve fibers (originating from OHCs) due to neuronal disinhibition in the DCN. This increased neuronal activity is thought to be the signal source for tinnitus that is perceived at a high cortical level.[22]

Kaltenbach and colleagues' work with cisplatin and hamsters has supported the theory that loss of OHC function may be a trigger of tinnitus-related hyperactivity in the DCN.[11] His group demonstrated that cisplatin-treated animals showed DCN hyperactivity and that the degree of hyperactivity correlated with degree of OHC loss/damage. Furthermore, the portion of the DCN exhibiting hyperactivity represented the higher frequency half of the animals' audiometric range and corresponded to the OHC loss in the (mainly basal half) cochlea. Their work also demonstrated that increases in DCN activity were not related to degree of IHC damage. Their data, in fact, suggested that damage to IHCs may offset the condition of hyperactivity triggered by OHC loss, as predicted by the discordant damage theory.

Hyperactivity of the spontaneous activity of the central auditory system has also been observed at the inferior colliculus (IC) and auditory cortex (AC) in patients with tinnitus.[23] The DCN receives direct innervation from the auditory nerve and its output is relayed to higher order auditory centers. Kaltenbach presented several lines of evidence for the role of the DCN contributing to tinnitus.[23] His work, however, has been criticized. Namely, the finding that the DCN is involved in the network involved in tinnitus does not prove that DCN stimulation causes tinnitus. Also, note should be made that the time course of noise-induced hyperactivity in the DCN is completely different from the time course of noise-induced tinnitus. Finally, his data do not present reasonable proof that observed effects are not due simply to hearing loss that was induced simultaneously.

Work involving the ototoxic effects of salicylate has been done in the hope of elucidating the mechanisms of tinnitus. The use of high doses of salicylate analgesics has been consistently associated with acute tinnitus dating back to 1877 in the reports by Sée and Müller.[24,25] In fact, the dosage of salicylate for the treatment of rheumatoid arthritis was used to titrate the dose of salicylate by increasing the dose until tinnitus appeared and then decreasing the dose a little.[26] Cazals' review discusses many reports and studies of the ototoxic effects of salicylate.[26] Symptoms include alteration in sound perception, loss of absolute acoustic sensitivity, and vertigo. Data have suggested that this toxicity is, in fact, reversible.[27,28] Tinnitus has been consistently reported after ingestion of ≥3 g of salicylate.[24,27,28] Cazals reviewed the data of numerous studies that showed that tinnitus "loudness" increased in linear proportion to the plasma salicylate levels and that spontaneous otoacoustic emissions (OAEs) were greatly reduced or eliminated after salicylate ingestion. Further work on isolated outer hair cells and cochlear mechanics suggests that salicylate can interfere with baseline electromechanical properties, but these in vitro studies have employed levels of salicylate that are well beyond the usual therapeutic range. Others, however, have shown similar findings using levels of salicylate that are closer to or within physiologic levels.[29,30] Salicylate use has also been shown to increase the spontaneous auditory neural activity. Cazals' review also examined studies that argued that salicylate does not cause significant changes in the electrocochlear potential, cochlear microphonic, or summating potential.[26]

While salicylate is a useful tool in establishing animal models of tinnitus, it is argued that this type of tinnitus, which has no practical clinical significance, does not represent clinically relevant tinnitus and its mechanisms may be different. Therefore, in current animal models, overexposure of noise is used to evoke tinnitus. As this procedure typically induces hearing loss as well, it is paramount to have data that allow discrimination of the effects of hearing loss from the effects of tinnitus. Currently, the work with salicylate-induced tinnitus is limited to establishing new animal models of tinnitus.

Neural Plasticity

Neural plasticity is important in understanding both the generation of tinnitus and explaining the suffering caused by tinnitus. While many individuals will report experiencing tinnitus at some point in their lives, only a small proportion of them find their tinnitus to be sufficiently bothersome to seek intervention or medical treatment. Several studies have indicated that the severe tinnitus that causes suffering is related to changes in the function of nuclei in the ascending auditory pathways or by the redirection of information to regions of the central nervous system (CNS) that do not normally receive auditory input.[31–33] Møller has described the nonclassical auditory pathway and its role in crossmodulation between the auditory and somatosensory systems.[34]

The nonclassical auditory pathways, also known as the extralemniscal pathways, ascend in parallel to the classical pathways. The classical pathways involve the central nucleus of the medial geniculate body and projections from there that connect to the auditory cortex. The nonclassical auditory pathways, however, start from the DCN and involve parts of subsequent higher-level nuclei. Of particular interest is the connection between the thalamus (via the extralemniscal part of the medial geniculate body) and the limbic system (via the lateral nucleus of the amygdala). The nonclassical pathways also receive input from organs subserving other sensory modalities, such as the somatosensory and the visual systems.[31,34,35]

The involvement of the limbic and autonomic nervous systems can cause increased arousal, anxiety, panic, and awareness of tinnitus, and can enhance the perception of the tinnitus signal, helping to explain how perceived loudness can be related to stress, anxiety and emotional status.[22] Notably, there is a direct connection from amygdala to the inferior colliculus, allowing control by the limbic system of processing information within the auditory system. This interconnection between the auditory, and the limbic and autonomic nervous systems provides a basis for creating a series of conditioned reflexes with tinnitus as the conditioned stimulus and overactivation of the limbic and sympathetic parts of autonomic nervous systems as the response, in turn, leading to a set of emotional and psychological reactions that result in patient suffering (Figure 15–1).[22]

Neural plasticity is necessary for creating new functional connections, which are responsible for reactions evoked by tinnitus as well as in extinguishing them (by retraining the brain). Neural plasticity can consist of changes in synaptic efficacy, the creation or elimination of synapses, the elimination or creation of new connections, or alteration in the protein synthesis of nerve cells.[31,37] Animal experiments have shown that deprivation of auditory input caused by hearing loss and exposure to loud sounds can cause hyperactivity in the nuclei of the auditory pathways.[38–40] The unmasking of dormant synapses can cause redirection of information, which has been thought to not only cause tinnitus, but the subjective symptoms of suffering such as hyperacusis and affective disorders.[31]

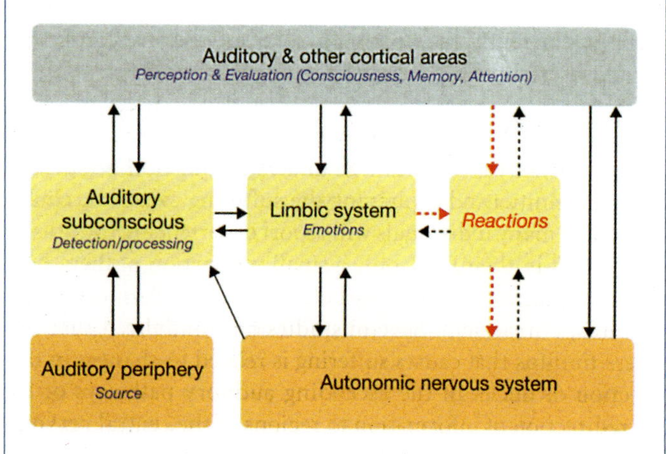

FIGURE 15–1 • The neurophysiological model of tinnitus. Block diagram outlining structures and connections involved in clinically significant tinnitus. The tinnitus signal, typically generated at the periphery of the auditory system, is detected and processed in subconscious pathways of the auditory system and finally perceived in the auditory cortex. If tinnitus is classified as an important negative stimulus, self-enhancing loops, governed by principles of conditioned reflexes, develop. Note the existence of two loops: high, involving consciousness, and low, the subconscious loop.[36]

Chronic Pain, Depression, and Psychological Aspects of Tinnitus

Similar neurologic changes have been observed in both chronic neuropathic pain and tinnitus sufferers that support proposals of similar mechanisms underlying these phenomena. Both lack physical signs and objective tests to confirm or characterize the disorders and are characterized by altered perceptions of physical stimuli. Similarly, both are often accompanied by affective disorders.[33,41–44]

Other researchers have also looked at the role of personality and psychological characteristics that may contribute to tinnitus severity. The strong placebo effect that is often seen in tinnitus treatment highlights the importance of psychological factors.[45] Langguth et al.[46] identified "the big five personality traits" that affected scores on two standard tinnitus grading instruments. They evaluated 72 individuals with chronic tinnitus by administering the tinnitus questionnaire (TQ),[47,48] the tinnitus handicap inventory (THI),[49] the Beck depression inventory (BDI),[50] and the NEO-Five factor inventory (NEO-FFI).[51] The five personality traits examined were neuroticism, extraversion, openness, agreeableness, and conscientiousness. A low "agreeableness" score is thought to correlate to people who are "highly competitive, self-centered, and more susceptible to anger."[52] A high "neuroticism" score is thought to correlate to people who "experience more anxiety, fear, sadness, embarrassment, and guilt."[46] They found that tinnitus severity correlated with low "agreeableness" and high "neuroticism" and that the degree of correlation depended on which measure of severity was used. They also found that "neuroticism" correlated strongly to female gender and younger age, independent of tinnitus. In addition, the authors found that 20.8% of subjects exhibited moderate to severe depression, 34.7% exhibited mild depression, and that tinnitus severity significantly correlated to depression.

Another study by McKenna et al. found that 45% of patients presenting with tinnitus for treatment had "significant levels of psychological distress."[53] Reynolds et al. examined the prevalence of psychological comorbidities in patients undergoing treatment for tinnitus in the United Kingdom. They found that both depression and anxiety affected patients with tinnitus and that anxiety, which was identified as the main psychological problem, affected 28% of the reported sample.[54]

The effect of depression and/or anxiety cannot be underestimated in evaluating and treating patients with tinnitus.[55] These psychological disorders can precede tinnitus, complicate treatment efforts, play a critical role in the maintenance of tinnitus symptoms, and subsequently become worse themselves as tinnitus symptoms continue.[46,47,54] A report on patients with tinnitus compared to a control group of patients presenting hearing loss revealed that 60% of the tinnitus patients met criteria for a major depressive disorder, or MDD, versus 7% of control patients. They also had higher lifetime prevalence of ever having had a MDD (73% vs 21%).[56] Psychological disorders, however, may be evoked by tinnitus and many patients experience depression and anxiety only after developing tinnitus. Therefore, the question remains open as to what extent tinnitus is facilitated by prior depression, anxiety, etc., versus causing these problems.

Diagnostic Techniques

History and Physical Examination

The evaluation of tinnitus should begin with a complete but focused history and physical examination. The physician should inquire into the duration, onset, severity, sound quality and intensity, trigger factors, mitigating factors, and laterality of the tinnitus. It is also important to inquire as to whether the sound is constant or intermittent, if the quality changes, if it worsens with additional noise or silence, and if the patient experiences decreased sound tolerance.

A complete review of a patient's past medical and surgical histories is helpful, paying particular attention to otologic or neurologic surgery, depression, anxiety, and family history, especially of ear disease or hearing loss.

A thorough review of the patient's medications, consumption of herbal or dietary supplements, over-the-counter agents, and recreational substances is also sometimes useful to identify agents that have been reported to cause tinnitus.

It is crucial to assess the degree of distress or handicap that tinnitus causes in the patient. Newman et al have described a patient-completed Tinnitus Handicap Inventory (THI) to aid in this assessment (see Appendix).[49] Other inventories have also been developed—the Tinnitus Effects Questionnaire, the Tinnitus Handicap Questionnaire, the Tinnitus Severity Scale, and the Tinnitus Coping Style Questionnaire.[57,58] Recently, a new questionnaire, the Tinnitus Functional Index, developed as the result of an extensive, 3-year project, has been presented,[59] but is not yet in the public domain.

The physical examination should include a full head and neck examination. Microscopic examination of the ears, pneumatic otoscopy, tuning fork examination, and cranial nerve testing should be included. If the patient is complaining of pulsatile tinnitus (or somatosounds), one should auscultate for vascular bruits over the ear canal, periauricular region (circumferentially around the ear), and over the neck. Similarly, compression of the internal jugular vein can cause an increase or decrease in tinnitus perception in some vascular causes of tinnitus, depending on the etiology.

Audiometry

Evaluation should always include pure-tone (air and bone conduction), Loudness discomfort levels and speech discrimination (word recognition) testing to assess the extent and functional impact of hearing loss. Tinnitus pitch, loudness match, and minimal masking levels are typically evaluated as well even though they do not provide insight into the diagnosis or proposed treatment. High-frequency-resolution distortion product otoacoustic emission (DPOAE) testing is very useful for counseling purposes, particularly in light of the discordant dysfunction theory of tinnitus. The frequency range of all measurements can be extended into the higher frequencies, i.e., 12.5 kHz for audiometry and 10 kHz for DPOAE.

Imaging

Additional diagnostic testing, such as imaging, should ultimately be guided by data garnered from the history and physical examination. A gadolinium-enhanced magnetic resonance imaging study is recommended in cases strongly suggestive of the presence of a vestibular schwannoma, eg, obvious asymmetry on audiogram, impaired speech discrimination, rollover in speech discrimination, or acoustic reflex decay.[2] Note that tinnitus alone is not a good indicator of a vestibular schwannoma, but the possibility should be considered in cases of significant unilateral tinnitus. In patients with very significantly reduced sound tolerance, it may be advisable not to perform acoustic reflex evaluation, and furthermore to use a "wait and monitor" approach using treatment aimed first at alleviating/ending the reduced sound tolerance prior to proceeding to an MRI study, which is inherently noisy.

Treatment

Physician Counseling and Reassurance

One of the most important aspects of treating tinnitus is the dialog that should take place between the patient and the physician. Most patients arriving in an otolaryngology clinic have already been evaluated by many other health professionals and often arrive frustrated and discouraged, having been told to, "Just learn to live with it" and that, "There is nothing I can do for you." Also crucial is the reassurance that the tinnitus is not a sign of another, more serious health malady, such as a brain tumor or severe illness.

Negative counseling plays a large role in how patients develop problems with their tinnitus. Our practice has had the experience of encountering many patients whose tinnitus has caused them much greater distress after they have been told there are no cures. Additionally, it is crucial to emphasize the benign implications of tinnitus. It should be made clear to the patient that tinnitus is not a predictor or harbinger of hearing loss or deafness, brain tumor, aneurysm, stroke, psychiatric problems or other serious medical illness.

While there is no cure for tinnitus, there are many management options that have shown variable degrees of success.

As previously noted, most cases of tinnitus do not have an easily identifiable cause. The following review of medical, surgical, and other modalities of management is meant to specifically address tinnitus treatment. Note that medication or surgical management offers some improvement for tinnitus in probably less than 1% of cases.

In cases in which the patient's evaluation has led to the identification of an offending drug or agent that can cause tinnitus, efforts should be made to eliminate this agent. For example, benzodiazepine withdrawal is a known cause of tinnitus.[60]

What follows is a review of many of the strategies and agents that have been examined in the treatment of tinnitus. We have grouped these into hearing aid/masking therapy, tinnitus retraining therapy (TRT), psychologic, pharmacologic, surgical, and other. The success of these therapies varies widely and the data that support them also vary significantly in their quality. Therapies directed at causes of somatosounds (typically pulsatile) are beyond the scope of this chapter. Note, that TRT is an effective method for treating somatosounds as well.

Hearing Aids and Masking Therapy

The use of hearing aids and masking therapy for tinnitus dates back to the work of Goodhill,[61] and Saltzman and Ersner.[62] The principle is, "... by amplification, much outside sound is enabled to reach the cochlea, crowding out and masking the patient's head noises."[62] Some work has described the concept of residual inhibition, in which tinnitus perception is reduced or eliminated by employing masking sound designed to precisely match various sounds to a person's tinnitus.[63] In spite of high expectations, after over 30 years of investigation, residual inhibition has never reached clinical usefulness, as it typically lasts only seconds to a minute. Vernon[64] discussed the utility of hearing aids in tinnitus sufferers with high-frequency hearing loss. He had highlighted that hearing aids will likely not be successful in patients in whom the tinnitus is so high-pitched that it is above the frequency capability of the hearing aid. Others, however, have shown this to be not true. Classical experiments of Feldman have shown that suppression of tinnitus perception is based on the neuronal suppression of the tinnitus signal and is not based on acoustic masking (due to interaction of two traveling waves at the basilar membrane of the cochlea).[65] Specifically, he has shown that there is no phenomenon of critical band, there is no "V"-shaped dependence of intensity of masker around pitch of tinnitus and that it is equally easy to suppress tinnitus perception by sounds of a wide range of frequencies. Sometimes contralateral suppression is even easier than ispilateral. Unfortunately, the label "masking," became associated with tinnitus suppression, creating the incorrect opinion that it is easier to suppress tinnitus perception by sounds covering the tinnitus pitch.

Vernon reported that tinnitus was "maskable in 95% of tinnitus patients."[66] These findings, however, have not been confirmed by other groups, including reports showing that masking is not better than placebo.[67] Others have found that the masking therapy only resulted in short-term benefit in a small group of patients.[13,68,69] The fact that continuous use of "maskers" after

6 months has been used as a criterion of success in Vernon's and some other authors' papers hindered validity of these reports.

Jastreboff and Jastreboff[70] highlighted some of the limitations of masking therapy. There have been cases in which hearing aids have worsened tinnitus, mostly in cases involving occlusive hearing aids that act as earplugs.

Folmer[71] reported the efficacy of ear-level devices (hearing aids or sounds generators) in 150 patients. According to a mailed questionnaire, 50 patients used hearing aids, 50 used in-ear sound generators, and 50 did not use ear-level devices. Follow-up was assessed 6 to 48 months subsequently. They found significant reduction in the Tinnitus Severity Index in all groups, but more improvement was seen in the groups that used hearing aids or ear-level devices.

Studies have also examined the role of "pink noise," a variety of artificial sounds, mimicking sounds of flowing water or air. Various compact discs and noise machines have been marketed and studied, but the efficacy of these have not yet been proven or confirmed with independent studies.[69]

Neuromonics® Tinnitus Treatment uses a device with headphones that patients wear for a prescribed period of time each day. According to the manufacturer, this device plays "music [that] is spectrally modified and customized with an embedded neural stimulus based upon the patient's audiological and tinnitus profile." It is available by prescription only but is often not covered by major insurance carriers. Subsequently, the cost (~$5000) can be prohibitive for many patients. It is not clear, however, if this approach is substantially better than using an iPod with high-quality earphones playing music for a few hours a day. There have been only two published studies that reported success with this program, but the researchers were shareholders of the Neuromonics company, and one of the studies did not include a control group.[72,73]

Tinnitus Retraining Therapy

Tinnitus retraining therapy (TRT) is aimed at "habituation of reactions evoked by tinnitus, and subsequently habituation of the tinnitus perception."[74] It incorporates two components that follow the principles of the neurophysiological model of tinnitus as described by Jastreboff (Figure 15–1).[20] These two components are (1) counseling, aimed at the "reclassification of tinnitus to a category of neutral signals" and (2) sound therapy, aimed at "weakening tinnitus-related neuronal activity."[74] Both components are strictly based on the neurophysiological model of tinnitus. The therapy attempts to achieve extinction of the abnormal conditioned reflex arc between the tinnitus signal within the auditory pathways and the emotional and physiological responses involving the limbic and sympathetic part of the autonomic nervous systems. The primary goal is to habituate tinnitus-evoked reactions. The final goal is to reach a stage at which tinnitus does not interfere with the patients' lives.

In an evaluation of 303 patients, Jastreboff found that 82% of patients showed a statistically significant decrease in THI scores at 12 months of treatment.[74] Other researchers have reported similar success with both short- and long-term follow-up.[75,76] The most interesting study so far was reported by Henry et al. (2006).[77] In a randomized, systematic study, Henry compared relief therapy, which he labeled "masking therapy" (any sound that provided immediate decrease of tinnitus), with TRT. Results showed superiority of and a high level of effectiveness for TRT.

In a prospective, nonrandomized, unblinded study of 152 patients with tinnitus, Herraiz et al.[76] found that 82% of patients had significant improvement in their tinnitus with TRT when compared with patients who received no intervention and were on a waiting list to be seen in the authors' clinic, in addition to patients who were partially treated but refused the recommended prostheses. Herraiz et al.[78] went on to report that certain prognostic factors could help predict success with TRT. Specifically, they found that more severe cases of tinnitus tended to have superior results. In addition, they found that patients who use the recommended sound-generating instrumentation also tended to have better results.

Wilson et al[79] reported a critical analysis of TRT in 1998. They identified problems with the "distinction between directive counseling and cognitive therapy, the adequacy of the cognitive therapy components, the nature of the outcome data which have been presented to date, the theoretical basis for the treatment, and the conceptual clarity of terms such as perception, attention and coping." They also highlighted the need for more controlled studies with no treatment or placebo arms, and in which the efficacy of the counseling and white noise components could be clearly isolated. Many of these critical points have been clarified in subsequent studies, such as those mentioned above.

Psychological Treatment

Although not widely employed in the United States, psychologically based therapy has been used as the sole mode of therapy for tinnitus in other countries, particularly Germany and Sweden. Cognitive-behavior therapy is a psychotherapeutic approach that aims to influence problematic and dysfunctional emotions, behaviors, and cognitions through a goal-oriented, systematic procedure based on behavioristic learning theory and cognitive psychology. It has been described as an approach to help patients better cope with tinnitus.[80] Others have reported on their success in treating the discomfort associated with tinnitus, but they had less success in decreasing depression, irritation, and tinnitus loudness.[81]

Pharmacologic Therapy

There is no proven medication for the treatment of tinnitus. The review that follows discusses some of the data that have reported success, but much of the data is confounded by the lack of rigorous research standards (ie, double-blinded, randomized control trials) or they demonstrated a benefit over a placebo effect, which itself was quite high (40% in some series). At this time, it is the position of the authors of this chapter that medical therapy is not generally effective, deleterious in some cases, and should not be considered first-line therapy in the treatment of tinnitus.

Antidepressants

The significant link between psychiatric disorders such as depression and anxiety with tinnitus has led researchers to treat tinnitus with various antidepressants. In 1993 Dobie et al.[45] reported the use of nortriptyline for tinnitus treatment in a double-blinded, randomized clinical trial in 92 patients with and without depression. Tinnitus, depression, and anxiety were assessed using the Iowa Tinnitus Handicap Questionnaire,

Beck Depression Inventory, and Hamilton Anxiety Rating scale, respectively. Their results indicated that 67% of patients stated that the drug "helped them," versus 40% of placebo. However, tinnitus severity was not significantly different between the placebo and nortriptyline groups, although both improved throughout the study.[55,82] Their work has also highlighted the importance of the placebo effect and that the regular contact with health care teams may not be inconsequential.[45]

Zöger et al.[83] reported in a double-blind, placebo-controlled study involving 76 patients with severe tinnitus that the use of sertraline was more effective than placebo in decreasing tinnitus severity, decreasing perceived tinnitus loudness, and improving symptoms of anxiety and depression. Tinnitus severity was assessed with the Tinnitus Severity Questionnaire (TSQ) and with a visual analog scale (VAS) for tinnitus loudness and annoyance. The Hamilton Anxiety Rating Scale and Hamilton Depression Rating Scale were used in the assessment of depression and anxiety. Psychiatric assessments were also performed by an experienced psychiatrist. Thirteen participants dropped out of the study; however, these individuals did not differ significantly in age, sex, or duration of tinnitus or scores for depression and anxiety from the remaining participants. At the conclusion of 16 weeks, the TSQ scores for the placebo group decreased from 22.68 to 19.99, whereas they had decreased from 21.96 to 17.28 in the treatment group. There were similar statistically significant decreases in depression in anxiety scores in the treatment group. While these differences were found to be statistically significant, they also highlighted the placebo effect.

Other studies have been published and reviewed with regard to the use of other selective serotonin reuptake inhibitors (SSRIs) and antidepressants, and overall found them to be more helpful in patients with coexisting depression and anxiety.[84,85] In all these studies, improvement in depression was shown, but there was no clear indication that these drugs have direct beneficial effect on tinnitus.

Antiepileptics: Gabapentin

The relationship between chronic pain and tinnitus has been suggested and reviewed in the references noted above. A case report by Zapp[86] in 2001 discussed a patient with chronic pain and a 10-month history of tinnitus. He was prescribed a 2-week course of gabapentin and was found to have significant improvement in his tinnitus symptoms, which persisted with continued therapy. Other researchers have attempted to reproduce these findings with randomized clinical studies without success. Piccirillo[87] reported in a double-blind, randomized clinical study involving 135 patients that gabapentin was no more effective than placebo in relieving tinnitus (11.3 vs. 11.0 point-reduction in the Tinnitus Handicap Inventory score, respectively).

Witsell[88] reported similar findings in a randomized double-blind, clinical trial. Seventy-six patients with tinnitus were treated either with placebo or gabapentin (1800 mg daily) for 5 weeks. Outcomes were assessed with the Tinnitus Handicap Inventory, Profile of Mood States rating scale, and subjective tinnitus severity. At the conclusion of the study, no significant differences could be identified between the two groups. In fact, as in the Piccirillo data, there were similar reductions in THI in both groups.

Bauer and Brozoski,[89] however, postulated that gabapentin would be beneficial in patients whose tinnitus is associated with acoustic trauma (as evidenced by an increased threshold, or "notch," between 3 and 6 Hz on audiometry) when compared to patients with tinnitus that is not associated with acoustic trauma. In a placebo-controlled, single-blind trial of 39 patients, they demonstrated a statistically significant improvement in tinnitus annoyance, and 20% or better improvement in subjective loudness in 6 out of 20 acoustic trauma patients and 4 out of 19 nontrauma patients. However, other subjective assessments, such as the Tinnitus Handicap Questionnaire (THQ), which are much better assessments of efficacy in the treatment of tinnitus, did not significantly differ between treatment and placebo groups.

Benzodiazepines

Anecdotally, some practitioners rely on benzodiazepines for the treatment of tinnitus. However, there are few well-designed studies showing that benzodiazepines are effective at controlling tinnitus and improving the suffering associated with tinnitus.[90] In a double-blind, randomized clinical trial using alprazolam for a 12-week period, researchers found that 76% of those taking alprazolam reported reduction of their tinnitus loudness, compared to only 5% of the placebo group.[91] However, this study did not evaluate the effect on tinnitus severity, quality of life, or the consequences of discontinuing therapy and problems related to dependence. The study has been criticized in subsequent publications as not being truly blinded as subjects were able to determine whether they were on placebo or active substance by side effects. Others have advocated the use of benzodiazepines in the treatment of tinnitus and hyperacusis,[66] largely based on anecdotal experience rather than data from randomized controlled trials.

It is important to recognize that upon discontinuation of therapy, patients note a return of their tinnitus symptoms, and in some cases, their symptoms worsened.[92,93] In a report by Busto,[94] three patients developed new-onset tinnitus after cessation of long-term diazepam therapy. One patient had resolution of symptoms after 6 months, another persisted with symptoms after 1 year, and the third patient resumed diazepam therapy to control the tinnitus.

Much attention has been drawn to the dependence that can develop with the use of benzodiazepines.[60] There are significant side effects from the use of benzodiazepines, such as tachycardia, hypotension, dizziness, sedation, and headache. Furthermore, some have argued that benzodiazepine dependence can limit an individual's ability to habituate to tinnitus symptoms, thereby worsening long-term management.[95] Furthermore, it has been documented that infusion of benzodiazepines into the amygdala blocks, even very basic learning (Pavlovian conditioning pairing tone with electrical shock) showing that benzodiazeines impair neural plasticity. They are, therefore, counterproductive in any treatment aimed at achieving modification of connections in the brain such as TRT or psychological therapies.

Alternative Therapies

A number of nontraditional pharmacologic, over-the-counter, and herbal remedies for tinnitus have been examined. A detailed examination into all of the agents available on the market would be beyond the scope of this chapter. We will, however, highlight some of the therapies examined. As with pharmacologic therapy, there are no agents that have been shown to be effective in double-blinded, randomized controlled studies.

Piccirillo,[96] in a literature review of melatonin, found that it may help patients with tinnitus and concomitant sleep disturbance, but that it did not seem to modify the severity or frequency of tinnitus.

Hilton[97] performed a systematic review of the literature available on gingko biloba and identified only three studies that met inclusion criteria. These studies revealed no evidence that tinnitus improved with ginko therapy.

Savastano[98] reported a nonrandomized trial with no placebo arm in which 31 patients with tinnitus were treated with antioxidant vitamins. They observed that patients reported "great improvement in the reduction of tinnitus." However, in light of previous placebo-controlled studies, the placebo effect cannot be excluded in this study.

Furthermore, in a review of various antioxidants, minerals, vitamins, and herbal remedies, Enrico[99] found many of these studies to be fraught with insubstantial scientific evidence, significant placebo effects, and potential harm from these substances.

Park[100] reviewed acupuncture therapy for tinnitus and identified six randomized clinical trials. Two of these were unblinded and showed improvement in tinnitus, whereas the four that were blinded showed no difference.

Transtympanic Therapy

Transtympanic therapy falls into four classes: (1) anesthetic agents (lidocaine), (2) ototoxic agents (gentamicin), (3) corticosteroids, and, (4) neuroactive agents (eg, antioxidants).[101] The tinnitus-reducing effects of lidocaine were discovered accidentally in 1935[102] and later led to use of anesthetic agents (intravenously) in the treatment of tinnitus.[103] The beneficial effects of lidocaine, both transtympanic and intravenous, have proven to be short-term.

Interest in transtympanic gentamicin for tinnitus has grown with its success in the treatment of Ménière's disease. Hoffer et al.[101] have reported their results with the use of transtympanic gentamicin in the treatment of Ménière's disease and transtympanic corticosteroids in the treatment of tinnitus in two nonrandomized, unblinded studies without placebo controls. In the Ménière's disease study, 65% of patients reported a reduction in their tinnitus.[104] Another group also reported success in treating Ménière's disease as well as Ménière's disease-related tinnitus in two small prospective trials that were also nonrandomized, unblinded studies without placebo controls.[105,106] Given that most tinnitus sufferers do not have Ménière's disease, the use of transtympanic gentamicin may actually be deleterious to a patient's hearing and vestibular function.

In a study examining transtympanic corticosteroids[101], 3 of 10 patients had almost complete resolution of their tinnitus and 3 of 10 experienced a significant reduction in their tinnitus. Of note, those patients with sudden sensorineural hearing loss were those that achieved complete tinnitus resolution with transtympanic corticosteroids. The three patients with significant reduction in tinnitus had noise-induced hearing loss. Sixty percent of the 10 patients "had a reduction or elimination of their hearing loss," so it is unclear if tinnitus improvement was a direct effect of treatment or secondary to hearing improvement.

Two other reports have reported similar findings.[107,108]

Surgical Intervention

The management of tinnitus is, overall, nonsurgical. However, a handful of surgical procedures have been identified as beneficial in some groups of tinnitus sufferers. Each of these, however, has specific inclusion criteria that most tinnitus sufferers would likely not meet.

Cochlear Implantation

As tinnitus is often associated with hearing loss, the implementation of cochlear implants for hearing rehabilitation has led to the examination of how cochlear implantation affects tinnitus. Various studies have been performed on cochlear implant patients and evaluated their subjective rating of their tinnitus pre and postimplantation.[109–113] In a comprehensive review, Baguley and Atlas[114] examined over 18 studies and found that the response to cochlear implantation was variable. The tinnitus prevalence varied from 35 to 100% of study subjects and tinnitus severity often was not quantified in a comparable manner across the studies. Success rates have overall been positive for tinnitus elimination or reduction (40%, up to 92% in some series), but some reports have indicated worsening of tinnitus in 2 to 15% of implanted patients studied.[114]

In order to qualify for cochlear implantation, it is recommended that adults have an audiogram that documents a PTA exceeding 70 dB bilaterally. If the patient can detect speech with best-fit hearing aids in place, a speech-recognition test in a sound field of 55 dB HL (hearing level) is performed. Current US Food and Drug Administration (FDA) guidelines permit implantation in patients whose open-set sentence recognition (e.g., HINT) is 60% or less in the best-aided condition. Criteria may vary depending on the third-party payer.[115]

Microvascular Decompression

It has been postulated that vascular compression of cranial nerves can cause or are associated with hyperactive disorders, such as trigeminal neuralgia, hemifacial spasm, and tinnitus.[116,117] Microvascular decompression (MVD) surgery involves moving the blood vessel off of the intracranial portion of the nerve involved.[116,118] In a study of 72 patients,[116] inclusion criteria were severe tinnitus and signs of change in the conduction properties of the auditory nerve as measured by narrow dips in the pure-tone audiogram and poorer speech discrimination. Thirteen patients, or 18.2%, had significant improvement, 22.2% had marked improvement, 11.1% had slight improvement, 45.8% had no improvement, and 2.8% became worse. The authors found that better results were observed in patients who had had tinnitus for less than 3 years and in those with unilateral tinnitus.

In another series by Brookes,[117] vascular compression was assessed with the use of air computed tomographic cisternography, and subsequently with MRI. Microvascular decompression surgery was performed in nine patients with severe tinnitus, resulting in complete abolition of symptoms in three (33%)

patients, significant reduction in five patients, and no change in two patients.

These data suggest that MVD could be considered in a very highly selected group of patients with tinnitus, but the data are limited to small series of patients and were not overwhelming in their success. Given the risks inherent to the procedure described, we would not consider this first-line therapy.

Cochlear Nerve Section

Other authors have discussed severing the cochlear nerve in order to alleviate tinnitus. This decision would clearly eliminate all hearing on that side. Others would argue that this surgery may make no difference given that individuals who are already deaf still experience tinnitus. Pulec[119] published data in a series of 151 patients in whom tinnitus was determined to originate within the cochlea. The cochlear nerve was severed medial to the spiral ganglion and resulted in 101 patients with complete resolution postoperatively, 43 who had improvement, seven who had no improvement. The length of follow-up was not clear, however. Given the elimination of all hearing coupled with the possibility that tinnitus could persist or worsen, the authors of this chapter do not recommend this line of therapy.

Other

Transcranial Magnetic Stimulation

Positron emission tomographic (PET) scans have provided researchers with data that may indicate that tinnitus is associated with cortical areas involved in the perception and processing of sounds and speech.[120,121] Regional cerebral blood flow was assessed in patients with tinnitus during tinnitus perception and after tinnitus reduction by lidocaine injection.[120,122] Based on these findings, Plewnia 2006[123] investigated the use of PET-navigated repetitive transcranial magnetic stimulation (TMS) with the objective being to interfere with the neuronal activity in the affected areas. While short-term results were promising,[124] all but one of the six patients in their study returned to their baseline level of tinnitus after 2 weeks of therapy. Other studies have examined TMS using various cortical targets, stimulation frequencies, and control groups. Kleinjung et al.[125] reviewed 11 clinical trials and the results varied considerably with regard to short- and long-term control. At this time, the data do not seem to indicate that this modality of therapy is widely effective.

Transcutaneous Electrical Stimulation

Tinnitus suppression via transcutaneous electrical stimulation was initially in the 1890s.[126–128] Although success rates of up to 66% have been reported, relief is often transient.[129] A more recent study by Steenerson and Cronin[126] reported data on transcutaneous electrical stimulation in 500 patients. A hand-held probe was used to deliver electrical stimulation to approximately 20 arbitrarily selected points on the external pinna and tragus of each ear. Patients were simultaneously guided through tinnitus-reduction activities, such as relaxation, breathing exercises, or biofeedback. Of the 500 patients, 53% received significant benefit as measured by subjective tinnitus intensity scores. The study did not, however, employ a validated questionnaire and 13 patients reported worsening tinnitus after therapy that returned to pretreatment levels in 11 of these patients. Furthermore, as the patients were treated simultaneously with other methods, one cannot conclude that the benefits were due to transcutaneous electrical stimulation.

Electrical Suppression with High-Rate Pulse Trains

The work of Rubinstein et al.[130] is predicated on the hypothesis that tinnitus is the result of the loss or alteration of normal spontaneous activity in certain regions of the cochlea or auditory nerve. In a prospective, nonrandomized trial without a control group, 11 subjects with tinnitus were treated with myringotomy and placement of a temporary round window electrode. High-rate pulse train stimuli (close to 5 kHz) were presented at various intensities. Five of the 11 subjects (45%) experienced substantial or complete temporal resolution of their tinnitus. Three subjects showed tinnitus suppression only in association with the perception of the stimulus and three showed no effect. At this time, however, there has only been this study and more work needs to be performed demonstrating the efficacy of this therapy prior to being recommended for widespread use.

Sound Therapy

A wide variety of sound therapies have been promoted over the years (eg, pink noise therapy dynamic tinnitus mitigation system, phase shift tinnitus reduction, auditory integration training). There are no results clearly showing effectiveness. It is generally recognized that sound enrichment can be helpful and proper utilization of sound is important for a number of therapies, such as music therapies, Neuromonics, relief therapy, and TRT.

CONCLUSIONS

The mechanism(s) of tinnitus are still under debate and there is no cure that removes tinnitus perception. A number of treatments, however, offer a possibility of substantial improvement. Of crucial importance is avoiding negative counseling (eg, "nothing can be done; you will have to live up to end of your life with tinnitus; tinnitus may get worse with aging and worsening of hearing"). Negative counseling can enhance preexisting tinnitus, annoyance and anxiety level, and turn a subject who is just experiencing tinnitus into a patient who is suffering from it.

While there is no drug that is consistently recommended for tinnitus, there are ongoing studies with the hope of finding a medication that will at least partially attenuate tinnitus. Notably, some drugs (eg, benzodiazepines) may make treatment more difficult, in addition to creating considerable side effects. No surgical procedure can consistently be recommended at this time.

There is a consensus that sound enrichment of the auditory background can be helpful and avoiding silence is of paramount importance. Most effective therapies combine counseling with sound therapy. It appears that therapies aimed at habituation of tinnitus, such as TRT, at the moment, offer advantages over other approaches.

APPENDIX: TNNITUS HANDICAP INVENTORY[49]

This questionnaire includes 25 items evaluating functional (F), emotional (E) and catastrophic (C) side effects, The patient is asked to respond with Yes (equaling 4 points), Sometimes (equaling 2 points), or No (equaling 0 points). Scoring is from 0 to 100 with 100 demonstrating extremely severe tinnitus handicap.

1 (F) Because of your tinnitus is it difficult for you to concentrate?
2 (F) Does the loudness of your tinnitus make it difficult for you to hear people?
3 (E) Does your tinnitus make you angry?
4 (F) Does your tinnitus make you feel confused?
5 (C) Because of your tinnitus do you feel desperate?
6 (E) Do you complain a great deal about your tinnitus?
7 (F) Because of your tinnitus do you have trouble falling asleep at night?
8 (C) Do you feel as though you cannot escape your tinnitus?
9 (F) Does your tinnitus interfere with your ability to enjoy social activities (such as going out to dinner, to the movies)?
10 (E) Because of your tinnitus, do you feel frustrated?
11 (C) Because of your tinnitus do you feel that you have a terrible disease?
12 (F) Does your tinnitus make it difficult for you to enjoy life?
13 (F) Does your tinnitus interfere with your job or household responsibilities?
14 (F) Because of your tinnitus do you find that you are often irritable?
15 (F) Because of your tinnitus is it difficult for you to read?
16 (E) Does your tinnitus make you upset?
17 (E) Do you feel that your tinnitus problem has placed stress on your relationship with members of your family and friends?
18 (F) Do you find it difficult to focus your attention away from your tinnitus and on other things?
19 (C) Do you feel that you have no control over your tinnitus?
20 (F) Because of your tinnitus do you often feel tired?
21 (E) Because of your tinnitus do you feel depressed?
22 (E) Does your tinnitus make you feel anxious?
23 (C) Do you feel that you can no longer cope with your tinnitus?
24 (F) Does your tinnitus get worse when you are under stress?
25 (E) Does your tinnitus make you feel insecure?

References

1. Willingham E. Tinnitus. Bobby D. Alford Department of Otolaryngology-Head and Neck Surgery Grand Rounds, Baylor College of Medicine; 2004.
2. Shiley SG, Folmer RL, McMenomey SO. Tinnitus and Hyperacusis. In: Cummings CW, Flint PW, Haughey BH, Robbins KT, Thomas JR, Harker LA, editors. Otolaryngology: Head and Neck Surgery. Philadelphia: Elsevier Mosby; 2005. p. 2832–47.
3. Heller AJ. Classification and epidemiology of tinnitus. Otolaryngol Clin North Am. 2003;36:239–48.
4. Hoffman HJ, Reed GW. Chapter 3: Epidemiology of Tinnitus. In: Snow JB, editor. Tinnitus: Theory and Management. London: BC Decker; 2004. p. 16–41.
5. Goodwin PE. Tinnitus and auditory imagery. Am J Otol. 1980;2:5–9.
6. Berrios GE. Musical hallucinations: A statistical analysis of 46 cases. Psychopathology 1991;24:356–60.
7. Berrios GE, Rose GS. Psychiatry of subjective tinnitus: Conceptual, historical and clinical aspects. Neurology, Psychiatry and Brain Research 1992;1:76–82.
8. Musiek F, Ballingham TM, Liu B, et al. Auditory Hallucinations: An audiological perspective. The Hearing Journal 2007;60:32–52.
9. Moller AR. Pathophysiology of tinnitus. Otolaryngol Clin North Am 2003;36:249–66.
10. Jastreboff PJJ, *Jastreboff* M.M. Chapter 31: Tinnitus and decreased sound tolerance. In: Snow JB, Wackym PA, editors. Bellinger's Otorhinolaryngology. 17th Edition. New York: 2009.
11. Kaltenbach JA, Rachel JD, Mathog TA, Zhang J, Falzarano PR, Lewandowski M. Cisplatin-induced hyperactivity in the dorsal cochlear nucleus and its relation to outer hair cell loss: Relevance to tinnitus. J Neurophysiol 2002;88:699–714.
12. Eggermont JJ. Pathophysiology of tinnitus. Prog Brain Res 2007;166:19–35.
13. Jastreboff PJ, Brennan JF, Coleman JK, Sasaki CT. Phantom Auditory Sensation in Rats: An Animal Model for Tinnitus. 1988:811–22.
14. Guitton MJ, Caston J, Ruel J, Johnson RM, Pujol R, Puel JL. Salicylate induces tinnitus through activation of cochlear NMDA receptors. J Neurosci 2003;23:3944–52.
15. Ruttiger L, Ciuffani J, Zenner HP, Knipper M. A behavioral paradigm to judge acute sodium salicylate-induced sound experience in rats: A new approach for an animal model on tinnitus. Hear Res 2003;180:3950.
16. Lobarinas E, Sun W, Cushing R, Salvi R. A novel behavioral paradigm for assessing tinnitus using schedule-induced polydipsia avoidance conditioning (SIP-AC). Hear Res 2004;190:109–14.
17. Heffner HE, Koay G. Tinnitus and hearing loss in hamsters (Mesocricetus auratus) exposed to loud sound. Behav Neurosci 2005;119:734–42.
18. Turner JG, Brozoski TJ, Bauer CA, et al. Gap detection deficits in rats with tinnitus: A potential novel screening tool. Behav Neurosci 2006;120:188–95.
19. Turner JG. Behavioral measures of tinnitus in laboratory animals. Prog Brain Res 2007;166:147–56.
20. Jastreboff PJ. Phantom auditory perception (tinnitus): Mechanisms of generation and perception. Neurosci Res. 1990;8:221–54.
21. Jastreboff PJ. Tinnitus as a phantom perception theory and clinical implications. In: Vernon JA, Moller AR, editors. Mechanisms of tinnitus. Boston: Allyn and Bacon, 1995. p. 73–93.
22. Jastreboff PJ. Chapter 8: The Neurophysiological model of tinnitus. In: Snow JB, editor. Tinnitus: Theory and management. London: BC Decker, 2004. p. 96–106.
23. Kaltenbach JA. The dorsal cochlear nucleus as a contributor to tinnitus: Mechanisms underlying the induction of hyperactivity. Prog Brain Res 2007;166:89–106.
24. Sée G. Etudes sur L'acide salicylique et les salicylates: traitement du rhumatisme aigu et chronique de la goutte, et de diverses affections du syste nerveux sensitif par les salicylates. Bulletin de l'Academie Nationale de Medecine 1877;26:689–706.
25. Müller G. Beitrag zur wirking der salicylasuren natrons beim diabetes mellus. Ber. Clin. Wochensch 1877;14:29–31.
26. Cazals Y. Auditory sensori-neural alterations induced by salicylate. Prog Neurobiol 2000;62:583–631.

27. Myers EN, Bernstein JM. Salicylate ototoxicity; a clinical and experimental study. Arch Otolaryngol 1965;82:483–93.
28. McCabe PA, Dey FL. The effect of aspirin upon auditory sensitivity. Ann Otol Rhinol Laryngol 1965;74:312–25.
29. Shehata WE, Brownell WE, Dieler R. Effects of salicylate on shape, electromotility and membrane characteristics of isolated outer hair cells from guinea pig cochlea. Acta Otolaryngol (Stockh) 1991;111:707–18.
30. Lue AJ, Brownell WE. Salicylate induced changes in outer hair cell lateral wall stiffness. Hear Res 1999;135:163–8.
31. Møller AR. Pathophysiology of tinnitus. Otolaryngol Clin North Am 2003;36:249–66.
32. Lockwood AH, Salvi RJ, Coad ML, Towsley ML, Wack DS, Murphy BW. The functional neuroanatomy of tinnitus: Evidence for limbic system links and neural plasticity [see comment]. Neurology 1998;50:114–20.
33. Møller AR. Similarities between severe tinnitus and chronic pain. J Am Acad Audiol 2000;11:115–24.
34. Møller AR, Møller MB, Yokota M. Some forms of tinnitus may involve the extralemniscal auditory pathway. Laryngoscope 1992;102:1165–71.
35. Møller AR, Rollins PR. The non-classical auditory pathways are involved in hearing in children but not in adults. Neuroscience Letters 2002;319:41.
36. Jastreboff PJ. Tinnitus. In: Adelman G, Smith B, editors. The New Encyclopedia of Neuroscience (NRSC): Elsevier; 2008.
37. Møller AR. The role of neural plasticity in tinnitus. Prog Brain Res 2007;166:37–45.
38. Gerken GM, Saunders SS, Paul RE. Hypersensitivity to electrical stimulation of auditory nuclei follows hearing loss in cats. Hear Res 1984;13:249.
39. Kaltenbach JA, Afman CE. Hyperactivity in the dorsal cochlear nucleus after intense sound exposure and its resemblance to tone-evoked activity: A physiological model for tinnitus. Hear Res 2000;140:165–72.
40. Szczepaniak WS, Møller AR. Evidence of decreased GABAergic influence on temporal integration in the inferior colliculus following acute noise exposure: A study of evoked potentials in the rat. Neuroscience Letters 1995;196:77–80.
41. Tonndorf J. The analogy between tinnitus and pain: A suggestion for a physiological basis of chronic tinnitus. Hear Res 1987;28:271–5.
42. Møller AR. Similarities between chronic pain and tinnitus. Am J Otol 1997;18:577–85.
43. Møller AR. Tinnitus and pain. Prog Brain Res 2007;166:47–53.
44. Price DD. Psychological and neural mechanisms of the affective dimension of pain. Science. 2000;288:1769–72.
45. Dobie RA, Sakai CS, Sullivan MD, Katon WJ, Russo J. Antidepressant treatment of tinnitus patients: Report of a randomized clinical trial and clinical prediction of benefit. Am J Otol 1993;14:18–23.
46. Langguth B, Kleinjung T, Fischer B, Hajak G, Eichhammer P, Sand PG. Tinnitus severity, depression, and the big five personality traits. Prog Brain Res 2007;166:221–5.
47. Hallam RS, Jakes SC, Hinchcliffe R. Cognitive variables in tinnitus annoyance. Br J Clin Psychol 1988;27:213–22.
48. Goebel G, Hiller W. [The tinnitus questionnaire. A standard instrument for grading the degree of tinnitus. Results of a multicenter study with the tinnitus questionnaire] Hno. 1994;42:166–72.
49. Newman CW, Jacobson GP, Spitzer JB. Development of the tinnitus handicap inventory. Arch Otolaryngol Head Neck Surg 1996;122:143–8.
50. Beck AT, Steer RA, Carbin MG. Psychometric properties of the Beck depression inventory: Twenty-five years of evaluation. Clinical Psychology Review 1988;8:77.
51. Costa P, McCrae R. The NEO personality inventory. In: Resources PA, editor. Manual Form S and Form R. Odessa: Psychological Assessment Resources, 1985.
52. Meier BP, Robinson MD. Does quick to blame mean quick to anger? The role of agreeableness in dissociating blame and anger. Personality & Social Psychology Bulletin 2004;30:856–7.
53. McKenna L, Hallam RS, Hinchcliffe R. The prevalence of psychological disturbance in neurotology outpatients. Clin Otolaryngol Allied Sci 1991;16:452–6.
54. Reynolds P, Gardner D, Lee R. Tinnitus and psychological morbidity: A cross-sectional study to investigate psychological morbidity in tinnitus patients and its relationship with severity of symptoms and illness perceptions. Clin Otolaryngol Allied Sci 2004;29:628–34.
55. Dobie RA. Depression and tinnitus. Otolaryngol Clin North Am 2003;36:383–8.
56. Sullivan MD, Katon W, Dobie R, Sakai C, Russo J, Harrop-Griffiths J. Disabling tinnitus. Association with affective disorder. Gen Hosp Psychiatry 1988;10:285–91.
57. Kuk FK, Tyler RS, Russell D, Jordan H. The psychometric properties of a tinnitus handicap questionnaire. Ear Hear 1990;11:434–45.
58. Budd RJ, Pugh R. Tinnitus coping style and its relationship to tinnitus severity and emotional distress. J Psychosom Res 1996;41:327–35.
59. Meikle M, Stewart BJ, Griest S, et al. Development of the tinnitus functional index (TFI): Part 2. Final dimensions, reliability and validity in a new clinical sample. Association for Research in Otolaryngology, 2008.
60. Ashton H. Benzodiazepine withdrawal: An unfinished story. Br Med J (Clin Res Ed). 1984;288:1135–40.
61. Goodhill V. Tinnitus: Otologic aspects. Trans. Am. Ophthalmol Otolaryngol 1954;44:67–77.
62. Saltzman M, Ersner M. A hearing aid for the relief of tinnitus aurium. Laryngoscope 1947;57:358–66.
63. Sockalingam R, Dunphy L, Nam KE, Gulliver M. Effectiveness of frequency-matched masking and residual inhibition in tinnitus therapy: A preliminary study. Audiological Medicine 2007;5:92–102.
64. Vernon J. Attemps to relieve tinnitus. J Am Audiol Soc 1977;2:124–31.
65. Feldmann H. Homolateral and contralateral masking of tinnitus by noise-bands and by pure tones. Audiology 1971;10:138–44.
66. Vernon JA, Meikle MB. Masking devices and alprazolam treatment for tinnitus. Otolaryngol Clin North Am 2003;36:307–20.
67. Erlandsson S, Ringdahl A, Hutchins T, Carlsson SG. Treatment of tinnitus: A controlled comparison of masking and placebo. Br J Audiol 1987;21:37–44.
68. Terry AM, Jones DM, Davis BR, Slater R. Parametric studies of tinnitus masking and residual inhibition. Br J Audiol 1983;17:245–56.
69. Jastreboff MM. Chapter 42: Sound therapies for tinnitus management. In: Langgtuh H, Kleinjung, Cacace and Moller, editors. Progress in brain research. Elsevier BV; 2007. p. 449–455.

70. Sheldrake JBJ, M.M. Chapter 22: Role of hearing aids in management of tinnitus. In: Snow JB, editor. Tinnitus: Theory and management. London: BC Decker; 2004. p. 310–3.
71. Folmer RL, Carroll JR. Long-term effectiveness of ear-level devices for tinnitus. Otolaryngology—Head and Neck Surgery 2006;134:131–137.
72. Davis PB, Paki B, Hanley PJ. Neuromonics tinnitus treatment: Third clinical trial. Ear Hear 2007;28:242–59.
73. Davis PB, Wilde RA, Steed LG, Hanley PJ. Treatment of tinnitus with a customized acoustic neural stimulus: A controlled clinical study. Ear Nose Throat J 2008;87:330–9.
74. Jastreboff PJ. Tinnitus retraining therapy. Prog Brain Res 2007;166:415–23.
75. Mazurek B, Fischer F, Haupt H, Georgiewa P, Reisshauer A, Klapp BF. A modified version of tinnitus retraining therapy: Observing long-term outcome and predictors. Audiol Neurootol 2006;11:276–86.
76. Herraiz C, Hernandez FJ, Plaza G, de los Santos G. Long-term clinical trial of tinnitus tetraining therapy. Otolaryngology—Head and Neck Surgery 2005;133:774.
77. Henry JA, Schechter MA, Zaugg TL, et al. Outcomes of clinical trial: Tinnitus masking versus tinnitus retraining therapy. J Am Acad Audiol 2006;17:104–32.
78. Herraiz C, Hernandez FJ, Toledano A, Aparicio JM. Tinnitus retraining therapy: prognosis factors. Am J Otolaryngol. 2007;28:225–9.
79. Wilson PH, Henry JL, Andersson G, Hallam RS, Lindberg P. A critical analysis of directive counselling as a component of tinnitus retraining therapy.[see comment]. Br J Audiol 1998;32:273–86.
80. Wilson PH. Classical conditioning as the basis for the effective treatment of tinnitus-related distress. ORL J Otorhinolaryngol Relat Spec 2006;68:6–11; discussion 11–13.
81. Lindberg P, Scott B, Melin L, Lyttkens L. Long-term effects of psychological treatment of tinnitus. Scand Audiol 1987;16:167–72.
82. Dobie RA, Sullivan MD, Katon WJ, Sakai CS, Russo J. Antidepressant treatment of tinnitus patients. Interim report of a randomized clinical trial. Acta Otolaryngol (Stockh) 1992;112:242–7.
83. Zoger S, Svedlund J, Holgers KM. The effects of sertraline on severe tinnitus suffering—a randomized, double-blind, placebo-controlled study. J Clin Psychopharmacol 2006;26:32–9.
84. Robinson SK, Viirre ES, Stein MB. Antidepressant therapy in tinnitus. Hear Res 2007;226:221–31.
85. Robinson S. Antidepressants for treatment of tinnitus. Prog Brain Res 2007;166:263–71.
86. Zapp JJ. Gabapentin for the treatment of tinnitus: A case report. Ear Nose Throat J 2001;80:114–6.
87. Piccirillo JF, Finnell J, Vlahiotis A, Chole RA, Spitznagel E, Jr. Relief of idiopathic subjective tinnitus: Is gabapentin effective? Arch Otolaryngol Head Neck Surg 2007;133:390–7.
88. Witsell DL, Hannley MT, Stinnet S, Tucci DL. Treatment of tinnitus with gabapentin: A pilot study. Otol Neurotol 2007;28:11–5.
89. Bauer CA, Brozoski TJ. Effect of gabapentin on the sensation and impact of tinnitus. Laryngoscope 2006;116:675–81.
90. Shulman A, Strashun AM, Goldstein BA. GABAA-benzodiazepine-chloride receptor-targeted therapy for tinnitus control: Preliminary report. Int Tinnitus J 2002;8:30–6.
91. Johnson RM, Brummett R, Schleuning A. Use of alprazolam for relief of tinnitus. A double-blind study. Arch Otolaryngol Head Neck Surg 1993;119:842–5.
92. Dobie RA. A review of randomized clinical trials in tinnitus. Laryngoscope 1999;109:1202–11.
93. Lechtenberg R, Shulman A. Benzodiazepines in the treatment of tinnitus. Archives of Neurology 1984;41:718–24.
94. Busto U, Fornazzari L, Naranjo CA. Protracted tinnitus after discontinuation of long-term therapeutic use of benzodiazepines. J Clin Psychopharmacol 1988;8:359–62.
95. Jastreboff MM, Mattox DE, Payne L, Jastreboff PJ. Medications used by tinnitus patients and their impact on treatment. Association for Research in Otolaryngology, 2004.
96. Piccirillo JF. Melatonin. Prog Brain Res 2007;166:331–3.
97. Hilton M, Stuart E. Ginkgo biloba for tinnitus. Cochrane Database Syst Rev. 2004:CD003852.
98. Savastano M, Brescia G, Marioni G. Antioxidant therapy in idiopathic tinnitus: Preliminary outcomes. Arch Med Res 2007;38:456–9.
99. Enrico P, Sirca D, Mereu M. Antioxidants, minerals, vitamins, and herbal remedies in tinnitus therapy. Prog Brain Res 2007;166:323–30.
100. Park J, White AR, Ernst E. Efficacy of acupuncture as a treatment for tinnitus: A Systematic Review. Arch Otolaryngol Head Neck Surg 2000;126:489–92.
101. Hoffer ME, Wester D, Kopke RD, Weisskopf P, Gottshall K. Transtympanic management of tinnitus. Otolaryngol Clin North Am 2003;36:353–8.
102. Barany R. Die Beeinflussung des Ohrensausens durch iv Injizierte Lokalanaesthetica. Acta Otolaryngol. 1935;23.
103. Baguley DM, Jones S, Wilkins I, Axon PR, Moffat DA. The inhibitory effect of intravenous lidocaine infusion on tinnitus after translabyrinthine removal of vestibular schwannoma: A double-blind, placebo-controlled, crossover study.[erratum appears in Otol Neurotol. 2005 Nov;26(6):1264]. Otol Neurotol 2005;26:169–76.
104. Hoffer ME, Kopke RD, Weisskopf P, et al. Use of the round window microcatheter in the treatment of Meniere's disease. Laryngoscope 2001;111:2046–49.
105. Kasemsuwan L, Jariengprasert C, Chaturapatranont S. Transtympanic gentamicin treatment in Meniere's disease: A preliminary report. J Med Assoc Thai 2006;89:979–85.
106. Kasemsuwan L, Jariengprasert C, Ruencharopen S, Orathai P. Low dose transtympanic gentamicin treatment for intractable Meniere's disease: A prospective study. J Med Assoc Thai 2007;90:327–34.
107. Shulman A, Goldstein B. Intratympanic drug therapy with steroids for tinnitus control: A preliminary report. Int Tinnitus J 2000;6:10–20.
108. Sakata E, Itoh A, Itoh Y. Treatment of cochlear tinnitus with dexamethasone infusion into the tympanic cavity. Int Tinnitus J 1996;2:129–35.
109. Miyamoto RT, Wynne MK, McKnight C, Bichey BG. Electrical suppression of tinnitus via cochlear implants. Int Tinnitus J 1997;3:35–8.
110. Ito J. Tinnitus suppression in cochlear implant patients. Otolaryngol Head Neck Surg 1997;117:701–3.
111. Dauman R, Tyler RS. Tinnitus suppression in cochlear implant users. Adv Otorhinolaryngol 1993;48:168–73.

112. Souliere CR, Jr., Kileny PR, Zwolan TA, Kemink JL. Tinnitus suppression following cochlear implantation. A multifactorial investigation. Arch Otolaryngol Head Neck Surg. 1992;118:1291–7.

113. Ruckenstein MJ, Hedgepeth C, Rafter KO, Montes ML, Bigelow DC. Tinnitus suppression in patients with cochlear implants. Otol Neurotol 2001;22:200–4.

114. Baguley DM, Atlas MD. Cochlear implants and tinnitus. Prog Brain Res 2007;166:347–55.

115. Isaacson B. Cochlear Implants, Indications eMedicine. WebMD; 2008.

116. Møller MB, Møller AR, Jannetta PJ, Jho HD. Vascular decompression surgery for severe tinnitus: Selection criteria and results. Laryngoscope 1993;103:421–7.

117. Brookes GB. Vascular-decompression surgery for severe tinnitus. Am J Otol 1996;17:569–76.

118. Møller AR, Møller MB. Microvascular decompression operations. Prog Brain Res 2007;166:397–400.

119. Pulec JL. Cochlear nerve section for intractable tinnitus. ENT: Ear, Nose & Throat Journal 1995;74:468.

120. Mirz F, Pedersen B, Ishizu K, et al. Positron emission tomography of cortical centers of tinnitus. Hear Res 1999;134:133–44.

121. Giraud AL, Chery-Croze S, Fischer G, et al. A selective imaging of tinnitus. Neuroreport 1999;10:1–5.

122. Reyes SA, Salvi RJ, Burkard RF, et al. Brain imaging of the effects of lidocaine on tinnitus. Hear Res 2002;171:43–50.

123. Plewnia C, Reimold M, Najib A, Reischl G, Plontke SK, Gerloff C. Moderate therapeutic efficacy of positron emission tomography-navigated repetitive transcranial magnetic stimulation for chronic tinnitus: A randomised, controlled pilot study.[see comment]. J Neurol Neurosurg Psychiatry 2007;78:152–6.

124. Plewnia C, Bartels M, Gerloff C. Transient suppression of tinnitus by transcranial magnetic stimulation. Ann Neurol 2003;53:263–6.

125. Kleinjung T, Steffens T, Londero A, Langguth B. Transcranial magnetic stimulation (TMS) for treatment of chronic tinnitus: Clinical effects. Prog Brain Res 2007;166:359–67.

126. Steenerson RL, Cronin GW. Tinnitus reduction using transcutaneous electrical stimulation. Otolaryngol Clin North Am 2003;36:337–44.

127. Graham JM, Hazell JW. Electrical stimulation of the human cochlea using a transtympanic electrode. Br J Audiol 1977;11:59–62.

128. Cazals Y, Negrevergne M, Aran JM. Electrical stimulation of the cochlea in man: Hearing induction and tinnitus suppression. J Am Audiol Soc 1978;3:209–13.

129. Portmann M, Negrevergne M, Aran JM, Cazals Y. Electrical stimulation of the ear: Clinical applications. Ann Otol Rhinol Laryngol 1983;92:621–2.

130. Rubinstein JT, Tyler RS, Johnson A, Brown CJ. Electrical suppression of tinnitus with high-rate pulse trains. Otol Neurotol 2003;24:478–85.

Vestibular Rehabilitation 16

Michael C. Schubert, PT, PhD

The vestibular system is responsible for sensing motion of the head in order to maintain postural control and stability of images on the fovea of the retina during that motion. When functioning normally, the vestibular receptors in the inner ear provide amazing precision in the representation of head motion in three dimensions. This information is then used by the central vestibular pathways to control reflexes and perceptions that are mediated by the vestibular system. Disorders of vestibular function result in abnormalities in these reflexes and lead to sensations that reflect abnormal information about motion from the vestibular receptors.

Normal activities of daily life (such as running) can have head velocities of up to 550 degrees/sec, head accelerations of up to 6,000 degrees/sec^2, and frequency content of head motion from 1 to 20 Hz.[1,2] Only the vestibular system can detect head motion over this range of velocity, acceleration, and frequency.[3] Additionally, the latency of the vestibulo-ocular reflex (VOR) has been reported to be as short as 5 to 7 milliseconds.[4] As a result, the vestibular system remains essential not only for detection of head motion, but generation of the appropriate motor signal to represent that head motion.

Physical therapists are likely to encounter patients with vestibular disorders regardless of clinical setting. It is estimated that the incidence of dizziness in the United States is 5.5%, or greater than 15 million people per year develop the symptom.[5] The reported prevalence of dizziness as a medical complaint in community-dwelling adults varies based on subjects' age, gender, and definition of the complaint (1–35%).[6–8] In multiple studies, it is clear that dizziness is one of the most common complaints adults report to their physicians, and its prevalence increases with age.[9] For patients older than 75 years, dizziness is the most common reason to see a physician.[10] Patients who experience dizziness report a significant disability that reduces their quality of life.[11] Furthermore, it has been reported that more than 70% of patients with initial complaints of dizziness will not have a resolution of symptoms at a 2-week follow up.

HISTORY

Cawthorne and Cooksey were the first clinicians to advocate exercises for persons suffering from dizziness and vertigo.[12,13] Years later, Harold Schuknecht proposed the cupulolithiasis theory, ie, otoconial debris attached to the cupula, which was later recognized as one of the two mechanisms responsible for the most common cause of vertigo, benign paroxysmal positional vertigo (BPPV).[14] In 1991, John Epley revolutionized treatment for BPPV, based on evidence that otoconia may also be free floating in the semicircular canals, known as the canalithiasis theory.[15,16] Overwhelmingly, these two forms of BPPV are successfully treated using physical maneuvers that remove the otoconia from their irritative location.

Recent studies have verified exercise incorporating visual targets and head motion as an effective means to reduce symptoms as well as improve function associated with vestibular impairment.[17] Therefore, it has only been within the last three or four decades that our knowledge of vestibular function and related disorders has profoundly changed, improving the rehabilitation approaches for individuals whose disorder pathology affects the vestibular system.

DIFFERENTIAL DIAGNOSIS

Clinicians treating patients who report dizziness and imbalance have the difficult task of distinguishing between vestibular and nonvestibular causes of dizziness. Ascertaining a thorough patient history is a critical component of the assessment. Many patients and clinicians use the imprecise term "dizziness" to describe a vague sensation of light-headedness or a feeling they have of a tendency to fall. The imprecision of the term may complicate clinical management decisions. Generally, most complaints of being "dizzy" can be categorized as light-headedness, disequilibrium, vertigo, or oscillopsia.

Light-headedness is often defined as a feeling that fainting is about to occur and can be caused by nonvestibular factors such as hypotension, hypoglycemia, or anxiety.[18] *Disequilibrium*

TABLE 16–1 Possible causes of vestibular and nonvestibular symptoms

	VESTIBULAR	NONVESTIBULAR
Symptoms	Oscillopsia with head movement, vertigo, imbalance	Light-headedness, disequilibrium
Causes	Unilateral vestibular hypofunction, bilateral vestibular hypofunction, benign paroxysmal positional vertigo, central lesion affecting the vestibular nuclei	Orthostatic hypotension, hypoglycemia, anxiety, panic disorder, lower-extremity somatosensory deficit, upper brain stem and motor pathway lesions

is defined as the sensation of being off balance. Often, disequilibrium is associated with nonvestibular problems such as decreased somatosensation or weakness in the lower extremities. *Vertigo* is defined as an illusion of movement. Vertigo tends to be episodic and often indicates pathology within the vestibular periphery or along the vestibular pathways. Vertigo is common during the acute stage of a unilateral vestibular lesion, but also may manifest itself through displaced otoconia (BPPV) or acute brain stem lesions affecting the root entry zone of the peripheral vestibular neurons or the vestibular nuclei.[18] *Oscillopsia* is the experience that objects in the visual environment that are known to be stationary are in motion. Oscillopsia can occur in association with head movements in patients with vestibular hypofunction because the vestibular system is not generating an adequate compensatory eye velocity during a head rotation.[19] A deficit in the VOR often results in motion of images on the fovea during head rotation with a resultant decline in visual acuity. The reduction of visual acuity during head motion, however, varies among people with vestibular hypofunction.[20] Listed in Table 16–1 are some of the more common symptoms and causes associated with vestibular and nonvestibular etiologies.

DIAGNOSTIC TECHNIQUES

The assessment of a patient with possible vestibular dysfunction begins with a careful history. The clinical examination then includes an assessment of eye movements, posture, and gait. Because of the direct relationship between vestibular receptors in the inner ear and eye movements produced by the VOR, the bedside examination of eye movements is of primary importance in defining and localizing vestibular pathology. Clinical evaluation of the vestibulo-ocular system takes advantage of two physiological principles: the high resting firing rate and the inequality in firing rates within the central vestibular neurons for excitation and inhibition. The presence of a high resting firing rate means each vestibular system can detect head motion through excitation or inhibition. During angular head rotations, ipsilateral vestibular afferents can be excited up to 400 spikes sec.[21] Such head movements also result in inhibition of peripheral afferents and of many central vestibular neurons receiving innervation from the labyrinth opposite the rotation. Because the resting discharge rate of these afferents and central vestibular neurons averages 70 to 100 spikes sec, inhibitory cutoff is more likely to occur than is excitation saturation.

Head Impulse Test

The head impulse test (HIT) is a widely accepted clinical tool that is used to assess semicircular canal function.[22] The head is flexed 30 degrees (to ensure cupular stimulation primarily in the tested lateral SCC). Patients are asked to keep their eyes focused on a target while their head is manually rotated in an unpredictable direction using a small-amplitude (5–15 degrees), high-acceleration (3,000–4,000 degrees/sec^2) angular impulse. When the VOR is functioning normally, the eyes move in the direction opposite to the head movement and through the exact angle required to keep images stable on the fovea. In the case of vestibular hypofunction, the eyes move less than the required amount. At the end of the head movement, the eyes are not looking at the intended target and images have shifted on the fovea. A rapid, corrective saccade is made to bring the target back on the fovea. The appearance of these corrective saccades indicates vestibular hypofunction as evaluated by the HIT (see Video 16–1). The HIT provides a sensitive indication of vestibular hypofunction in patients with complete loss of function in the affected labyrinth that occurs following ablative surgical procedures, such as labyrinthectomy.[23] The test is less sensitive in detecting hypofunction in patients with incomplete loss of function.[24]

Head-Shaking-Induced Nystagmus

Nystagmus is an involuntary back-and-forth motion of both eyes. Any nystagmus due to vestibular stimulation or pathology is composed of slow and fast eye movements. The slow component (slow eye velocity) is produced by the intact ear, which generates a normal VOR as a result of the asymmetry between the discharge rates of central vestibular neurons on each side. The fast component is a resetting eye movement that brings the eyes close to the center of the oculomotor range.[25] The head-shaking-induced nystagmus (HSN) test is a useful aid in the diagnosis of people with asymmetry of peripheral vestibular input to central vestibular regions. Patients undergoing the HSN test must have their vision blocked because fixation on a visual target can suppress nystagmus. Similar to the HIT, the head should initially be flexed 30 degrees. Next, the head is oscillated horizontally for 20 cycles at a frequency of two repetitions per second (2 Hz). Upon stopping the oscillation, people with symmetric peripheral vestibular input will not have HSN. Typically, a person with a unilateral loss of peripheral vestibular function will manifest a horizontal HSN; with the quick phases of the nystagmus directed toward the healthy ear and the slow phases directed toward the lesioned ear (see Video 16–2). Not all patients with a unilateral vestibular loss will have HSN. Patients with a complete loss of vestibular function bilaterally will not have HSN because neither system is functioning and there is no asymmetry between the tonic firing rates.

Positional Testing

Positional testing is commonly used to identify whether otoconia have been displaced into the SCC BPPV. The Dix-Hallpike test is commonly used to verify displaced otoconia (see Figure 16–1). The presence of otoconia in endolymph makes the semicircular canals sensitive to changes in head position. The abnormal signal results in nystagmus and vertigo, nausea with or without vomiting, and disequilibrium. Once the patients are in the provoking position, the resultant nystagmus indicates which semicircular canal is involved. Table 16–2 lists the pattern of nystagmus associated with the affected semicircular canal for both cupulolithiasis and canalithiasis. Please see Video 16–3 for an example of the nystagmus pattern generated from otoconia in the most common location for BPPV, the posterior semicircular canal.

Dynamic Visual Acuity

Dynamic visual acuity (DVA) is the measurement of visual acuity during self-generated horizontal motion of the head. A "bedside" and computerized form of the test can be used to identify the functional significance of the vestibular hypofunction.[26,27] Head velocities need to be greater than 100 degrees/sec at the time DVA is measured in order to ensure that the vestibular afferents from the semicircular canals on the contralateral side are driven into inhibition and the letters are not identified with a smooth pursuit eye movement. In people without vestibular problems, head movement results in little or no change of visual acuity, compared with the head still. For patients with vestibular hypofunction, the VOR will not keep the eyes stable in space during the rapid head movements, leading to decreased visual acuity during head motion, compared with the head still. DVA has been shown to correctly identify an individual semicircular canal lesion when tested with unpredictable head rotations, as produced from the surgical plugging of a dehiscent superior semicircular canal.[28]

Posture and Balance Testing

The assessment of gait and balance problems is important for determination of a patient's functional status. Testing should consist of a range of assessments including static balance, weight shifting, automatic postural responses, and ambulation. The balance tests cannot uniquely identify pathology within the vestibular system. Table 16–3 includes some common balance tests and expected results.

Physical Therapy Intervention

Vestibular rehabilitation refers to interventions such as repositioning techniques, vestibular adaptation exercises, habituation exercises, and general exercise to improve muscle force, gait, or balance. The beneficial effect of vestibular rehabilitation to improve gait and imbalance due to vestibular hypofunction is well documented.[29] In addition, controlled studies have been used to demonstrate improvements in DVA and to reduce complaints of oscillopsia as well as to reduce VOR gain asymmetry.[17,30,31]

Benign Paroxysmal Positional Vertigo

Nystagmus is generated when SCC with displaced otoconia are placed into gravity-dependent positions, as in the Dix-Hallpike test. Each SCC generates a unique eye rotation and directs the clinician to choose an appropriate treatment approach (Table 16–2). Three different treatment approaches have been developed, each based on pathophysiologic theories of this disorder. The techniques include the canalith repositioning maneuver, the liberatory (Semont) maneuver, and Brandt-Daroff exercises.

The canalith repositioning maneuver (CRM) is based on the canalithiasis theory of free-floating debris in the SCC.[16] The patient's head is moved into different positions in a sequence that will move the debris out of the involved SCC and into the vestibule. Once the debris is in the vestibule, the signs and symptoms should resolve. The positions used in the treatment of posterior and anterior SCC canalithiasis are the same. Figure 16–2 illustrates the CRM as applied to either the right posterior or right

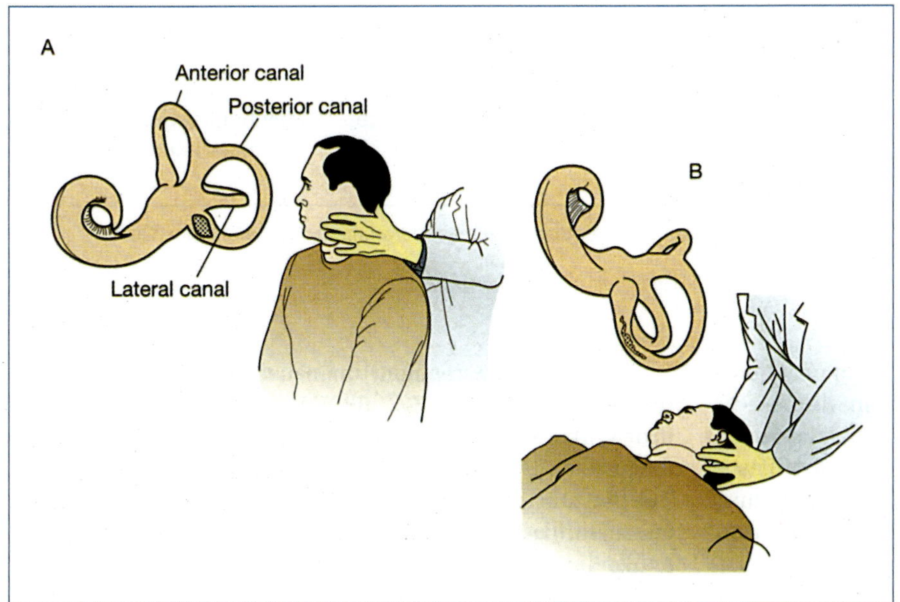

FIGURE 16–1 • Canalith repositioning maneuver for treatment of benign paroxysmal positional vertigo. Dix-Hallpike test for affecting the right ear. *A*, A patient with right posterior canal BPPV. The patient's head is turned to the right at the beginning of the canalith repositioning maneuver. The *inset* shows the location of the debris near the ampulla of the posterior canal. The diagram of the head in each inset shows the orientation from which the laybrinth is viewed. *B*, The patient is brought into the supine position with the head extended below the level of the gumey. The debris falls toward the common crus as the head is moved backward.

TABLE 16–2 Type of nystagmus on SCC location and mechanism of BPPV

AFFECTED SCC[a]	MECHANISM	NYSTAGMUS[b]
Right posterior	Cupololithiasis Canalithiasis	Persistent UBN and right torsion[c] Transient UBN and right torsion
Left posterior	Cupololithiasis Canalithiasis	Persistent UBN and left torsion Transient UBN and left torsion
Right anterior	Cupololithiasis Canalithiasis	Persistent DBN and right torsion Persistent DBN and right torsion
Left anterior	Cupololithiasis Canalithiasis	Persistent DBN and left torsion Persistent DBN and left torsion
Horizontal[d]	Cupololithiasis Canalithiasis	Persistent apogeotropic Transient geotropic

[a] Testing for BPPV in the SCC assumes the patient is in the appropriate positional test
[b] Nystagmus is labeled by the direction of the fast component (UBN means the fast component of the nystagmus is beating upwards; DBN, down beat nystagmus)
[c] The torsional rotation is noted as it relates to the superior poles of the eyes, from the perspective of the examiner
[d] When BPPV occurs in the horizontal SCC, nystagmus will be present when the head is positioned to the either side.
Apogeotropic nystagmus, fast component beats away from the earth; geotropic nystagmus, fast component beats towards the earth.

TABLE 16–3 Common balance and expected results related to specific diagnosis

TEST	BPPV	UVH	BVH	CENTRAL LESION
Romberg	Negative	Acute: positive Chronic: negative	Acute: positive Chronic: positive or negative	Often negative
Tandem Romberg	Negative	Positive, eyes closed	Positive	Positive
Single-legged stance	Negative	May be positive	Acute: positive Chronic: positive or negative	May be unable to perform
Gait	Normal or mildly ataxic	Acute: wide-based, slow, decreased arm swing and trunk rotation Compensated: normal	Acute: wide-based, slow, decreased arm swing and trunk rotation Compensated: mild gait deviation	May have pronounced ataxia
Turn head while walking	May produce slight ataxia	Acute: may not keep balance Compensated: normal	Ataxia, slows cadence to perform	May not keep balance, increased ataxia

BPPV, benign paroxysmal postural vertigo; UVH, unilateral vestibular hypofunction; BVH, bilateral vestibular hypofunction; Central lesion—lesion affecting central vestibular pathway.

anterior SCC. After the treatment, the patient may be cautioned to avoid vertical head movements that may again dislodge the otoconia. It is important to instruct the patient that horizontal movement of the head should be performed to prevent stiff neck muscles. CRM has also been adapted for application to the horizontal SCC.[31] BPPV is much less common in either the horizontal or anterior SCC and recurrence of BPPV is low.[32,33]

The liberatory (Semont) maneuver was first offered as a treatment for posterior SCC BPPV based on the cupulolithiasis theory.[34] It involves rapidly moving the patient through positions designed to dislodge the debris from the cupula (Figure 16–3). The liberatory maneuver is effective as an alternative treatment for canalithiasis, though it may be more difficult for the patient to tolerate.

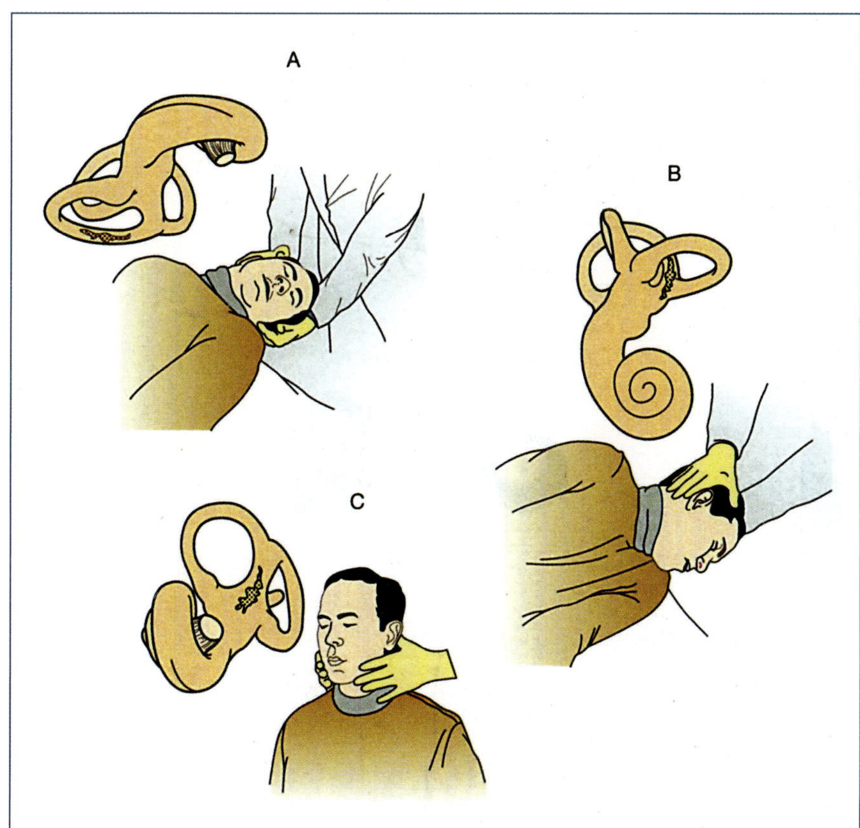

FIGURE 16–2 • Canalith repositioning maneuver for treatment of benign paroxysmal positional vertigo. *A*, The head is moved approximately 180 degrees to the left while keeping the neck extended with the head below the level of the gurney. Debris enters the common crus as the head is turned toward the contralateral side. *B*, The patient's head is further rotated to the left by rolling onto the left side until the patient's head faces down. Debris begins to enter the vestibule. *C*, The patient is brought back to the upright position. Debris collects in the vestibule.

Brandt-Daroff exercises were originally designed to habituate the CNS to the provoking position.[35] They may also act to dislodge debris from the cupula or by causing debris to move out of the canal. This exercise is illustrated in Figure 16–4. The exercise should be performed in 5 to 10 repetitions, three times a day until the patient has no vertigo for two consecutive days. If the patient has severe vertigo or complaints of nausea, decreasing the number of repetitions to three, performed three times a day, may render the exercises more tolerable. It is important to explain to the patient that the movements of the body toward the bed should be done rapidly and that this will probably provoke the patient's vertigo. Patients should also be made aware that some residual symptoms of dysequilibrium and nausea upon completing the exercise are common. Any residual symptoms are usually temporary.

The physical therapy goal of performing CRM and Liberatory procedures is to return the otoconia into the vestibule. The Brandt-Daroff exercises, although originally designed to habituate the peripheral vestibular response, have also led to a complete remission of symptoms, sometimes after the first exercise session.[35] Physical therapy should also include teaching the patient how to use the appropriate techniques at home, in the case of recurrence. See Table 16–4 for suggested guidelines for use of the CRM, the Liberatory maneuver, or Brandt-Daroff exercises.

Unilateral Vestibular Hypofunction

Patients with unilateral vestibular hypofunction (UVH) should be informed that recovery time upon initiating vestibular rehabilitation averages 6 to 8 weeks. To ensure compliance with the vestibular rehabilitation exercises, patients should be encouraged frequently and informed of the outcomes and goals. The primary focus of this type of rehabilitation is gaze and gait stability exercises. Vestibular adaptation exercises are a type of gaze stability exercise designed to expose patients to retinal slip. Retinal slip occurs when the visual image of an object moves off the fovea of the retina, resulting in visual blurring/motion. Retinal slip is necessary as this is the signal used to improve the response of the residual vestibular system. However, the brain can tolerate small amounts of retinal slip, yet see a target clearly.[36] The patient should be directed to keep the target in focus. Otherwise, head motion that is too rapid will result in excessive retinal slip. The purpose of these exercises is to improve the VOR and recruit other oculomotor systems that may assist gaze stability during the head motion. The two primary paradigms of vestibular adaptation are X1 (times 1) and X2 (times 2) exercises.[37] In the X1 exercise, the patient is asked to move the head horizontally (and vertically if appropriate) as quickly as possible while maintaining focus on a stable target. The patient must learn to slow the head movement if the target becomes blurred. A good target to use is a business card, asking the patient to focus on a word or a letter within a word. The starting target distance should be an arm's length away. The X2 paradigm requires the patient to move the head and target in opposite directions. Both paradigms should be made increasingly more difficult as the patient improves. Examples of increasing difficulty include the use of a distracting background while the patient attempts to read the letter or word (checkerboard, venetian blinds), varying the distance from which the patient performs the exercises, moving the head more rapidly, and performing the exercise while standing or walking.

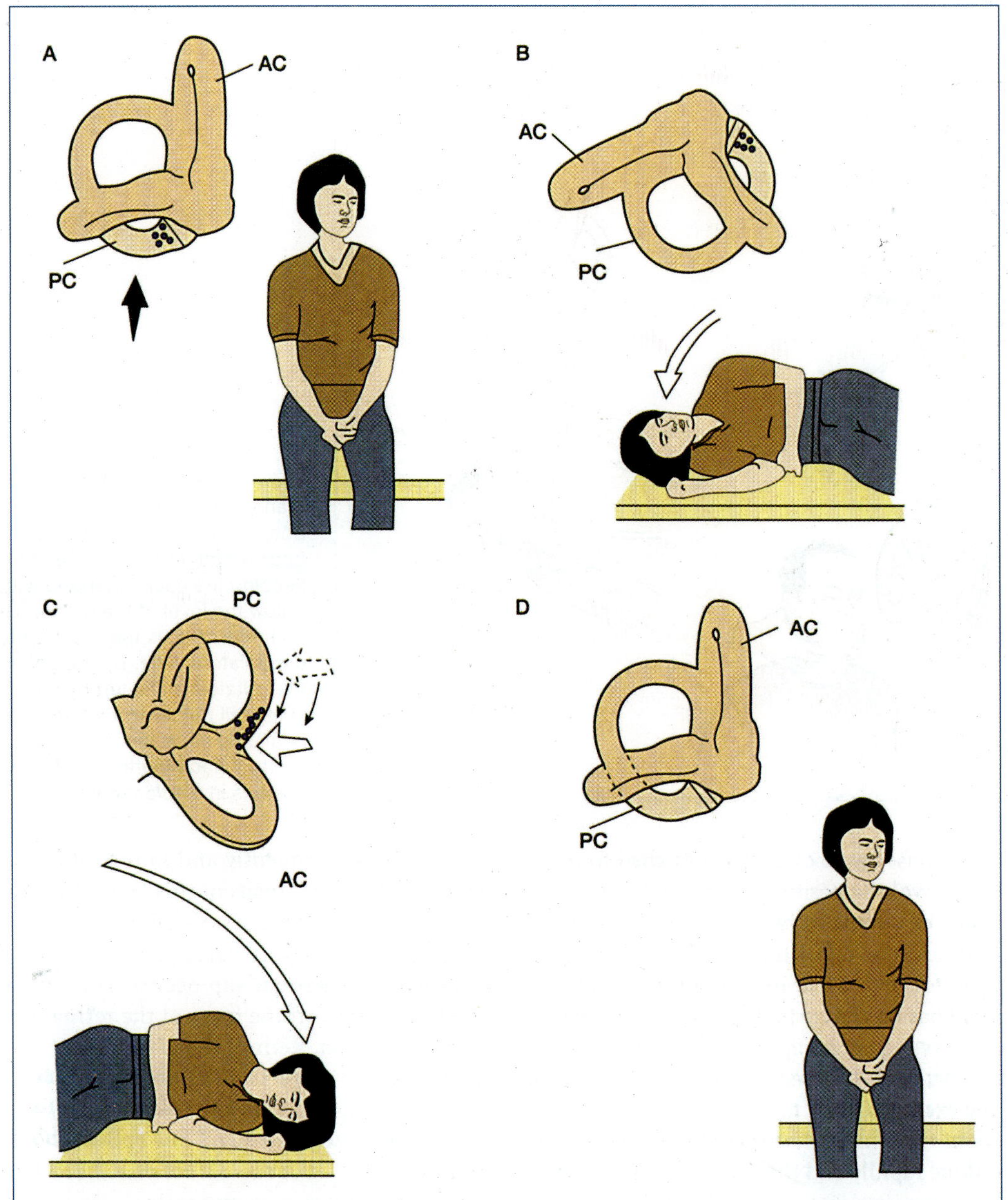

FIGURE 16–3 • Liberatory (Semont) maneuver for right posterior SCC BPPV. The clinician should assist the patient through this positioning procedure. Note the otoconia adherent to the cupula in A and B. *A*, The head is rotated 45 degrees to the left side. *B*, With assistance, the patient is moved from sitting to right sidelying and stays in this position for 1 min. *C*, The patient is then rapidly moved 180 degrees, from right sidelying to left sidelying. The head should be in the original starting position, left rotated (nose down in final position) in this example. Note the otoconia have been dislodged from the cupula. After 1 min in this position, *D*, the patient returns to sitting. AC, anterior SCC; PC, posterior SCC; HC, horizontal SCC. *Adapted from O'Sullivan and Schmitz, editors, Physical Rehabilitation, 5th edition, FA Davis, 2006.*

Postural stability exercises are designed to improve balance by encouraging the development of balance strategies within the limitations of the patient, be they somatosensory, visual, or vestibular. The exercises should challenge the patient and be safe enough to perform independently. Exercises must be updated and progressed to incorporate more challenges. It is important to incorporate head movement into the exercises because many patients with vestibular loss tend to decrease their head movement.

Motion sensitivity is a common complaint experienced by individuals with vestibular hypofunction. Habituation training is warranted when a patient with a UVH has continual complaints of motion sensitivity or dizziness. Habituation is defined as the reduction in response to a repeatedly performed movement. These exercises were the first successful methods used to treat persons with vestibular disorders.[12,13,38,39] To determine which habituation exercises to prescribe, the physical therapist must determine provoking positions first. When a position

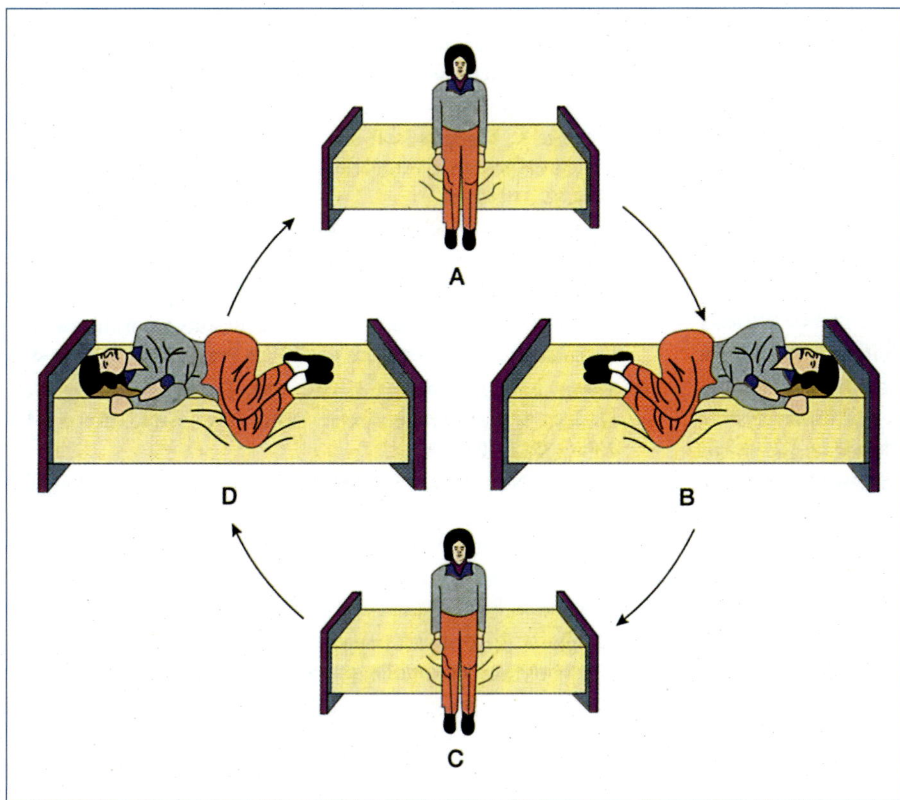

FIGURE 16–4 • Brandt–Daroff exercises for BPPV. Instructions to the patients include *A*, *Sit* on the edge of the bed and turn your head 45° to the right. *B*, Quickly lie down on your left side and wait 15 sec before sitting up. *C*, Sit up and wait another 15 sec with your head turned the entire time. *D*, Now turn your head to the left and lie down quickly on your right side. Wait 15 sec and then sit up, wait for 15 sec. Keep your head turned the entire time. The entire sequence is repeated 5 times and is performed 3 times a day. *From Arch Otolaryngol Head Neck Surg. 2005;131:344–348.*

TABLE 16–4 Benign paroxysmal positional vertigo treatment techniques

TREATMENT	DIAGNOSIS
CRM	BPPV due to canalithiasis
Liberatory maneuver	BPPV due to cupulolithiasis
Brandt-Daroff exercises	Persistent BPPV unresolved with CRM/Liberatory Residual vertigo without nystagmus May be useful for the patient who cannot tolerate CRM

CRM, canalith repositioning maneuver; BPPV, benign paroxysmal positional vertigo.

elicits a mild to moderate amount of dizziness, the patient remains in the provoking position for 30 sec or until the symptoms abate, whichever comes first.[40] The patient is provided with a home exercise program (HEP) based on the results of the positional evaluation. The provoking exercises are performed 3 to 5 times each, 2 to 3 times a day.

Bilateral Vestibular Hypofunction

Treatment of patients with a BVH is designed to address the primary complaints of gaze instability during head motion, dysequilibrium, and gait ataxia. Recovery from a lesion involving both vestibular systems takes much longer than a unilateral lesion. For this reason, patient education emphasizing daily activity is a high priority.

Gaze stability exercises can be similar to the X1 paradigm described in treatment for UVH. Use of the X2 paradigm may not be useful for a patient with a BVH because this exercise may cause excessive retinal slip. Instead, exercises that incorporate sequenced eye and head movements and the use of imaginary targets may improve gaze stability by enhancing central preprogramming of eye movements.[17] Patients with BVH depend on somatosensation and/or vision to maintain postural stability. Balance exercises should enhance the use of these cues. Care must be taken that the exercises are performed safely because people with BVH are more likely to fall.[41] It is imperative to begin the patient on a walking program, daily if tolerated. This can be progressed to ambulating on different surfaces (grass, gravel, sand) and in different environments (grocery store, mall). Daily activity must continue beyond the course of vestibular rehabilitation. Other recommended activities include exercises in a pool and Tai Chi. The pool provides the benefit of buoyancy, reducing the dangers of gravity, which allows the patient to move safely without the risk of falling quickly to the ground. Tai Chi incorporates slow, controlled motions used to improve balance, flexibility, and increase strength.[42] In most cases, a person with a BVH will incur a permanent functional disability. Certain activities may always be limited, such as walking in the dark, night driving, or sports involving quick movements of the head.[43] Older patients may have to use an assistive device such as a cane for safe ambulation at night or on uneven surfaces. Habituation exercises do not work for the patient with a bilateral vestibular loss.[44]

Central Vestibular Lesion

Once an accurate diagnosis of central vestibular pathology is made, the physical therapist must be careful in choosing rehabilitation strategies. Expectations for recovery should be described initially to the patient. Generally, the time to recover will be 6 months or more, and may be incomplete.[45] Many of the adaptive mechanisms thought responsible for recovery of the vestibular system are central processes that may have been damaged in the initial central lesion. Physical therapists treating patients with traumatic brain injury (TBI) must be careful not to be too aggressive thereby greatly exacerbating patient symptoms. Though vestibular rehabilitation offers promise for treating persons with TBI,[46] it may not always be the treatment of choice due to its irritating nature.

The physical therapy intervention for central vestibular lesions at the level of the brain stem (vestibular nuclei) likely will be similar to a UVH, with the same expectations for recovery. Vestibular cortical lesions may also recover, similar to the process by which recovery for cerebral vascular accident happens. Additionally, gait and balance exercises designed to incorporate somatosensory, visual, and vestibular contributions are also effective means with this patient population.

Nonvestibular Dizziness

Many patients with complaints of dizziness or imbalance will have a normal clinical vestibular exam (negative BPPV, hHSN, HIT), yet will have abnormal balance or will complain of motion sensitivity. These patients can be successfully treated with vestibular rehabilitation techniques similar to those patients with true vestibular pathology.

CONCLUSION

The vestibular system requires movement to recover from most lesions. The vestibular system will not improve to the greatest potential without head motion. This basic tenet should be thoroughly discussed when educating patients about returning to daily activity, exercising independently at home, and as a general guideline for their recovery. The challenge for the clinician is determining the amount of exertion the patient can tolerate in order to create an effective vestibular rehabilitation strategy without causing deleterious effects.

References

1. Grossman GE, Leigh RJ, Abel LA, et al. Frequency and velocity of rotational head perturbations during locomotion. Exp Brain Res 1988;70:470–6.
2. Das VE, Zivotofsky AZ, DiScenna AO, Leigh RJ. Head perturbations during walking while viewing a head-fixed target. Aviat Space Environ Med 1995;66:728–32.
3. Waespe W, Henn V. Gaze stabilization in the primate: The interaction of the vestibulo-ocular reflex, optokinetic nystagmus, and smooth pursuit. Rev Physiol Biochem Pharmacol 1987;106:37–125.
4. Minor LB, Lasker DM, Backous DD, Hullar TE. Horizontal vestibuloocular reflex evoked by high-acceleration rotations in the squirrel monkey, I: Normal responses. J Neurophysiol 999;82:1254–70.
5. Kroenke K, Mangelsdorff AD. Common symptoms in ambulatory care: Incidence, evaluation, therapy, and outcome. Am J Med 1989;86(3):262–6.
6. Yardley L, Owen N, Nazareth I, Luxon L. Prevalence and presentation of dizziness in a general practice community sample of working age people. Br J Gen Pract 1998;48(429):1131–5.
7. Sloane PD. Dizziness in primary care. Results from the national ambulatory medical care survey. J Fam Pract 1989;29(1):33–8.
8. Tinetti ME, Williams CS, Gill TM. Dizziness among older adults: A possible geriatric syndrome. Ann Intern Med 2000;132(5):337–44.
9. Colledge NR, Wilson JA, Macintyre CC, MacLennan WJ. The prevalence and characteristics of dizziness in an elderly community. Age Ageing 1994;23(2):117–20.
10. Sloane P, Blazer D, George LK. Dizziness in a community elderly population. J Am Geriatr Soc 1989;37(2):101–8.
11. Grimby A, Rosenhall U. Health related quality of life and dizziness in old age. Gerontology. 1995;41:286–98.
12. Cawthorne, T. The physiological basis for head exercises. J Chart Soc Physiother. 1944;30:106.
13. Cooksey FS. Rehabilitation in vestibular injuries. Proc R Soc Med 1946;39:273.
14. Schuknecht HF. Cupulolithiasis. Arch Otolaryngol 1969;90(6):765–78.
15. Epley JM. The canalith repositioning procedure: For treatment of benign paroxysmal positional vertigo. Otolaryngol Head Neck Surg. 1992;107:399.
16. Hall SF, Ruby RR, McClure JA. The mechanics of benign paroxysmal vertigo. J Otolaryngol. 1979;8(2):151–8.
17. Schubert MC, Migliaccio AA, Clendaniel RA, Allak A, Carey JP. Mechanism of dynamic visual acuity recovery with vestibular rehabilitation. Arch Phys Med Rehab 2008;89(3):500-7.
18. Baloh RW. Dizziness: Neurological emergencies. Neurol Clin 1998;16:305–21.
19. Gillespie MB, Minor LB. Prognosis in bilateral vestibular hypofunction. Laryngoscope. 1999;109:35–41.
20. Bhansali SA, Stockwell CW, Bojrab DI. Oscillopsia in patients with loss of vestibular function. Otolaryngol Head Neck Surg 1993;109:120–5.
21. Fernandez C, Goldberg JM. Physiology of peripheral neurons innervating semicircular canals of the squirrel monkey, II: Response to sinusoidal stimulation and dynamics of peripheral vestibular system. J Neurophysiol 1971;34:661–75.
22. Halmagyi GM, Curthoys IS. A clinical sign of canal paresis. Arch Neurol 1988;45:737–9.
23. Halmagyi GM, Curthoys IS, Cremer PD, et al. The human horizontal vestibulo-ocular reflex in response to high-acceleration stimulation before and after unilateral vestibular neurectomy. Exp Brain Res 1990;81:479–90.
24. Schubert MC, Tusa RJ, Grine LE, Herdman SJ. Optimizing the sensitivity of the head thrust test for identifying vestibular hypofunction. Phys Ther 2004;84(2):151–8.
25. Hain TC, Fetter M, Zee DS. Head-shaking nystagmus in patients with unilateral peripheral vestibular lesions. Am J Otolaryngol 1987;8:36–47.

26. Longridge NS, Mallinson AI. The dynamic illegible E (DIE) test: A simple technique for assessing the ability of the vestibulo-ocular reflex to overcome vestibular pathology. J Otolaryngol 1987;16:97–103.

27. Herdman SJ, Tusa RJ, Blatt P, et al. Computerized dynamic visual acuity test in the assessment of vestibular deficits. Am J Otol 1998;19:790–6.

28. Schubert MC, Migliaccio AA, Della Santina CC. Dynamic visual acuity during passive head thrusts in canal planes. J Assoc Res Otolaryngol 2006;7(4):329–38.

29. Hall CD, Schubert MC, Herdman SJ. Prediction of fall risk reduction as measured by dynamic gait index in individuals with unilateral vestibular hypofunction. Otol Neurotol 2004;25(5):746–51.

30. Szturm T, Ireland DJ, Lessing-Turner M. Comparison of different exercise programs in the rehabilitation of patients with chronic peripheral vestibular dysfunction. J Vestib Res 1994;4(6):461–79.

31. Baloh RW, Jacobson K, Honrubia V. Horizontal semicircular canal variant of benign positional vertigo. Neurology 1993;43(12):2542–9.

32. Simhadri S, Panda N, Raghunathan M. Efficacy of particle repositioning maneuver in BPPV: A prospective study. Am J Otolaryngol 2003;24(6):355–60.

33. Sakaida M, Takeuchi K, Ishinaga H, Adachi M, Majima Y. Long-term outcome of benign paroxysmal positional vertigo. Neurology 2003;60(9):1532–4.

34. Semont A, Freyss G, Vitte E. Curing the BPPV with a liberatory maneuver. Adv Oto-Rhino-Laryngol 1988;42:290.

35. Brandt T, Daroff RB. Physical therapy for benign paroxysmal positional vertigo. Arch Otolaryngol 1980;106:484.

36. Demer JL, Honrubia V, Baloh RW. Dynamic visual acuity: A test for oscillopsia and vestibulo-ocular reflex function. Am J Otol 1994;15(3):340–7.

37. Schubert MC, Das V, Tusa RJ, Herdman SJ. Cervico-ocular reflex in normal subjects and patients with unilateral vestibular hypofunction. Otol Neurotol 2004;25(1):65–71.

38. Norre, ME, DeWeerdt, W. Treatment of vertigo based on habituation. J Laryngol Otol 1980;94:971.

39. Dix, MR. The rationale and technique of head exercises in the treatment of vertigo. Acta Otorhinolaryngol Belg 1979;33:370.

40. Shumway-Cook A, Horak FB. Vestibular rehabilitation: An exercise approach to managing symptoms of vestibular dysfunction. Seminars in Hearing 1989;10:196.

41. Herdman SJ, Blatt P, Schubert MC, Tusa RJ. Falls in patients with vestibular deficits. Am J Otol 2000;21(6):847–51.

42. Wolf SL, Barnhart HX, Kutner NG, McNeely E, Coogler C, Xu T. Atlanta FICSIT Group. Reducing frailty and falls in older persons: An investigation of Tai Chi and computerized balance training. J Am Geriatr Soc. 2003;51(12):1794–803.

43. Cohen HS, Wells J, Kimball KT, Owsley C. Driving disability and dizziness. J Safety Res 2003;34(4):361–9.

44. Smith-Wheelock M, Shepard NT, Telian SA. Physical therapy program for vestibular rehabilitation. Am J Otol 1991;12(3):218–25.

45. Shepard NT, Telian SA, Smith-Wheelock M, Raj A. Vestibular and balance rehabilitation therapy. Ann Otol Rhinol Laryngol 1993;102(3 Pt 1):198–205.

46. Gurr B, Moffat N. Psychological consequences of vertigo and the effectiveness of vestibular rehabilitation for brain injury patients. Brain Inj 2001;15(5):387–400.

Fundamentals of Otologic and Neurotologic Surgery

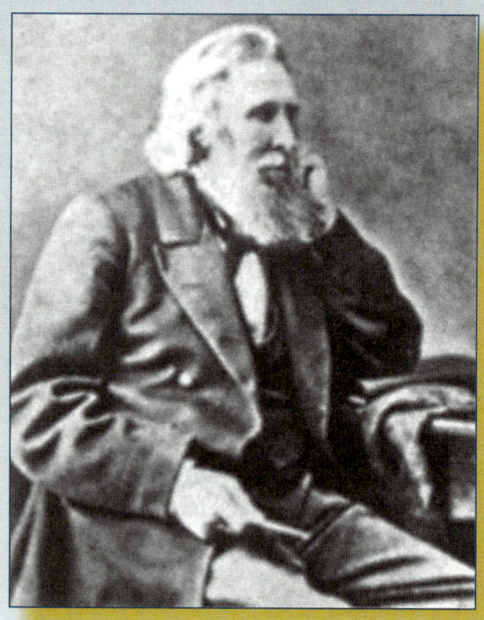

SIR WILLIAM WILDE (1815-1876) •
Described the postauricular incision for the management of acute subperiosteal mastoid abscess.

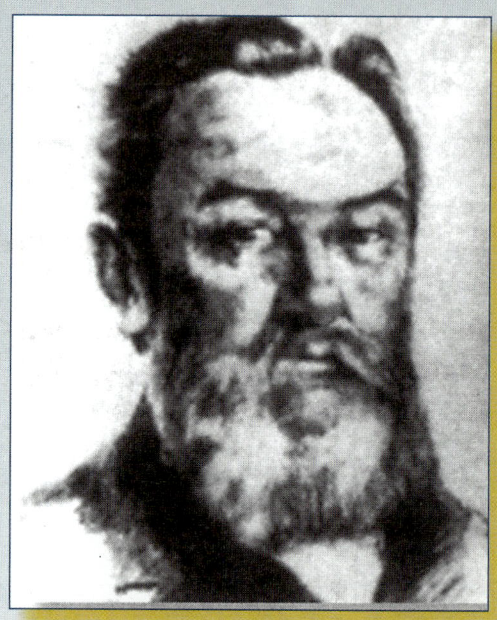

JOHANNES KESSEL (1837-1907) •
First performed endaural radical mastoidectomy, described by his chief resident in 1892. In 1878 performed the first stapes mobilization and in 1879 described sound protection for the round window.

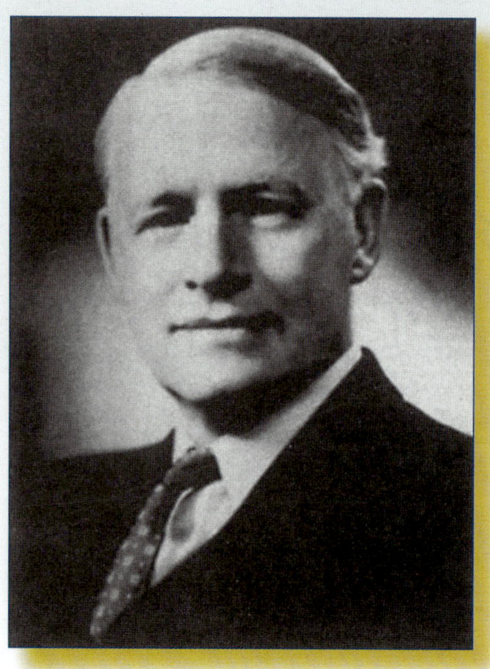

CARL OLAF NYLÉN (1892-1978) •
In 1921 introduced the (monocular) otomicroscope for ear surgery.

Principles of Temporal Bone and Skull Base Surgery 17

Roberto A. Cueva, MD, FACS / C. Gary Jackson, MD, FACS

INTRODUCTION

The goal of this chapter is to cover general issues related to temporal bone and skull base surgery. Specifics regarding surgical approaches and diseases will be covered in their respective chapters. Adherence to the fundamentals of appropriate anesthesia, hemostasis, exposure, illumination, magnification, knowledge of anatomy, and meticulous surgical technique (common to all surgery) leads to successful outcomes for the patient and the surgeon. Proper preparation and education of the patient for the surgical event creates appropriate expectations, reduces perioperative risk, and fosters a positive patient–physician rapport thereby reducing anxiety. Finally, postoperative care will be discussed for both otologic and skull base surgery.

PREOPERATIVE ASSESSMENT

In a tertiary care setting, patients will often be referred for surgery with all the appropriate tests and workup completed. However, both tertiary care specialists and general otolaryngologists alike must ensure that the workup is complete before embarking on performing the surgery. There are two aspects of preoperative assessment; the evaluation of the disease process leading to the consideration for surgery and evaluation of the patient's suitability to undergo surgery/anesthesia.

General Health

First, an integral part of any specialist's consultation is not only a thorough history of the presenting illness/disease process, but also a detailed review of the patient's general health status. Depending on the findings of this inquiry, more extensive medical evaluation may be required before surgery may be safely undertaken, or the consideration of surgery may be abandoned entirely and other management options recommended. A patient's suitability to undergo surgery/anesthesia depends on numerous factors including: type of anesthetic to be used, nature and duration of the surgical procedure, hemodynamic challenges of the operation (either from blood loss or fluid shifts), anticipated morbidity of the surgery, typical recovery, and the patient's health status as it relates to the aforementioned factors. Ever-increasing life expectancy, along with successful treatment of chronic illnesses, has resulted in a greater number of older patients with complex medical histories being considered for surgical management of temporal bone/skull base diseases. Proactive involvement of appropriate medical specialists in the perioperative management of patient's chronic illnesses is necessary to reduce risks associated with surgery. In certain situations consultation with an anesthesiologist, in advance of the morning of surgery, may be required to assess suitability to undergo general anesthesia or to avoid anesthetic complications.

Healthy patients, taking no daily medication, typically do not require any preoperative blood tests. Patients with chronic medical illness or patients who are on daily medication may require blood tests as indicated by their circumstances. Otherwise asymptomatic men over the age of 40 and women over the age of 50 should have an electrocardiogram. Patients with complex medical histories may require formal consultation with an internist or other specialist (eg, cardiologist). Medications that inhibit proper blood clotting (anticoagulants, aspirin, nonsteroidal anti-inflammatory drugs [NSAIDs], ginkgo biloba extract, vitamin E, etc.) should be stopped approximately 10 days before the planned procedure.

Disease Specific Evaluation

In addition to a thorough head and neck examination, including cranial nerve testing, patients considered for temporal bone/skull base surgery require specific examinations and testing appropriate to their diagnosis.

Otologic Surgery

Patients considered for surgery of the middle ear, tympanic membrane, and/or mastoid should all undergo microscopic otoscopy. Such careful examination reduces the likelihood that the operating surgeon will be surprised in the operating room and have to extend the operation beyond what was planned. Particularly important is the careful removal of any crusts covering the pars flaccida region that may hide the neck of a cholesteatoma. Furthermore, in patients requiring revision surgery following a previous intact canal wall mastoidectomy, careful inspection of the postero-lateral ear canal is important as a canal mastoid fistula may be present if the previous surgeon unnecessarily reduced the height of the posterior canal bone. The opening to such a fistula may be easily missed if attention is solely focused on the tympanic membrane.

Preoperative audiometric testing of both ears is mandatory. Operating on the only hearing ear should be approached with the utmost of caution as a potential complication is complete deafness. The preoperative audiogram not only serves as a baseline for postoperative comparison, but also allows the surgeon to counsel the patient regarding the potential for hearing improvement related to the planned surgery. Electronystagmography (ENG) should be performed on all patients prior to surgery targeting the vestibular system. Correlation of ENG findings with the audiogram and clinical symptoms when planning endolymphatic shunt decompression, semicircular canal occlusion, or labyrinthectomy is important. Although rare, a patient may have one ear symptomatic for hearing fluctuation, tinnitus, and aural pressure, while the opposite ear is the cause of vertigo. Performing surgery on the incorrect ear in this setting will not help patients and likely leave them worse.

The role of computed tomography (CT) scanning prior to middle-ear/mastoid surgery is dependent on the surgeon's judgment and disease process in question. An adult suspected of having otosclerosis with a normal microscopic otoscopy does not need a CT scan of the temporal bones. The opposite is true for a patient with two previous surgeries, recurrent cholesteatoma, and a history of transient facial weakness following the last surgery. Other indications for preoperative temporal-bone CT scanning include: ear canal atresia/hypoplasia; suspected middle-ear/mastoid/jugular foramen tumor; suspected cerebral spinal fluid (CSF) otorrhea; suspected fracture; suspected X-linked conductive hearing loss; preoperative cochlear assessment prior to cochlear implantation; and sensorineural hearing loss/vertigo/facial weakness in the setting of chronic otitis media and/or cholesteatoma.

Neurotologic/Skull Base Surgery

Patients being prepared for neurotologic/skull base surgery not only require the evaluation process described above, but also require a more extensive neurological examination. Skull base tumors often negatively impact the central nervous system in addition to regional cranial nerves. Sensory and motor function of the extremities, deep tendon reflexes, Hoffman's sign, pronator drift, cerebellar testing (Romberg—normal and tandem, heel to shin, finger to nose, rapid alternating movements), and gait should all be assessed. Consultation with a neurosurgeon is typically sought as such cases are managed in a team setting. In practice settings with sufficient patient volume a highly efficient multidisciplinary clinic can be established in which the neurotologist and neurosurgeon see the patient simultaneously. Such a "skull base clinic" promotes greater exchange of information between specialties, facilitates discussion of management options and approach selection, as well as other aspects of perioperative planning. Consultation with a plastic/reconstructive surgeon is recommended when complex reconstruction is anticipated following tumor extirpation.

Patients with skull base lesions commonly require preoperative audiologic and neurophysiologic testing. The results of the audiogram will help in determining whether a hearing preservation type approach should be employed and help predict potential for hearing preservation or loss. Auditory brain stem response (ABR) testing may help prognosticate chances of hearing preservation in vestibular schwannoma cases. The absence of ABR waveforms does not preclude attempted hearing preservation as intraoperative direct eighth nerve monitoring (DENM) routinely detects cochlear nerve action potentials when ABR is absent.[1,2] Postoperative testing of hearing demonstrates whether hearing was preserved and the quality of hearing if still present. Electronystagmography (ENG) has historically been used to try and predict the nerve branch of origin for vestibular schwannomas, but is unreliable and therefore of limited utility. Vestibular evoked myogenic potentials (VEMP) should be tested in all patients suspected of superior semicircular canal dehiscence to correlate with their CT findings.

Radiological studies are always required for patients undergoing neurotologic/skull base surgery. For most lesions magnetic resonance imaging (MRI), with and without gadolinium contrast, is the study of choice. Axial and coronal images help the surgeon form a three-dimensional picture of the tumor's relationship to the patient's anatomy. Lesions in the region of the sella turcica (ie, pituitary macroadenomas, craniopharyngiomas, and chordomas) warrant contrast-enhanced sagittal views as well. For epidermoid cysts/tumors of the central nervous system, which can mimic arachnoid cysts, diffusion-weighted images are optimal for establishing the diagnosis and delineating extent of disease.[3]

In cases where tumor embolization is not required, the use of magnetic resonance angiography (MRA) and magnetic resonance venography (MRV) may be used to assess a tumor's relationship to major vascular structures such as the internal carotid artery and jugular bulb/vein. When tumor embolization is anticipated, formal cerebral angiography, with its attendant risks, is necessary. Angiography with embolization is scheduled approximately 48 h prior to the planned tumor surgery to maximize tumor vessel occlusion without allowing excess time for dense fibrosis to occur within the tumor. Octreotide scanning can be useful for finding metachronous lesions in patients with neuroendocrine tumors such as paragangliomas, if cranial MRI does not include the neck down to the carotid bifurcation. CT scanning may be indicated to better define the bony anatomy of the skull base in lesions causing deformity, erosion, or destruction of the temporal bone or skull base.

Specific diseases require blood or urine testing for diagnosis and prevention of perioperative complications. Paragangliomas require 24-h urine collection testing for vanillylmandelic acid (VMA) and metanephrines. Patients with glomus tumors that secrete epinephrine/norepinephrine should have preoperative alpha and beta blockade to prevent potentially dangerous intraoperative hypertension. Such blockade should be in place at the time of angiography with embolization, as release of these vasoactive hormones can also occur related to embolization.

PREOPERATIVE PATIENT PREPARATION

Once the patient and the disease process have been appropriately evaluated and the decision made to proceed with surgery (after fully discussing the other management options), the patient must be prepared for the event.

Patient Education

This preparation includes educating the patient about the disease process, the planned surgical procedure, type of anesthesia, associated risks/complications, expected outcome of surgery, anticipated recovery time, postoperative care, and follow-up plans. The discussion about the surgical procedure should be detailed including: location and size of incisions, amount of hair to be clipped (if any), basic steps of the procedure, method of wound closure, and dressing(s). The description of the risks/complications and expected outcomes will occasionally overlap. The expected outcome in many temporal bone procedures involves improvement or preservation of function. However, in some procedures the expected outcome may involve a decline in function (hearing loss, cranial nerve dysfunction, altered cosmesis, etc.), which should not be considered as a complication. Complications are unplanned adverse events that may occur within a recognized statistical range. This difference should be made clear in settings when the expected outcome involves such an anticipated decrement of function. Whenever possible the quoted likelihood of success and/or risk of developing a complication should be based on the individual surgeon's practice experience. Surgeons early in their practice should rely on published statistical data.

Choice of anesthetic is dependent on the planned procedure, the temperament of the patient, and the surgeon's preference. Most transcanal middle-ear surgery is readily accomplished with local anesthetic and sedation. This allows intraoperative testing of hearing and more speedy recovery. Postauricular otologic procedures including tympanoplasty with or without mastoidectomy may also be done under local anesthesia with sedation, but proper patient selection is important. Additionally, the surgeon must reliably be able to complete the planned procedure within 2 to 3 h. Of course, all otologic procedures may also be done under general anesthetic. Skull base procedures are done under general anesthesia.

Anticipated course of recovery and timing for return to work/activities should be discussed. If hospitalization is required, duration of hospital stay will vary and should be determined by the patient's postoperative functional status. At the Skull Base Surgery Center for Southern California Permanente Medical Group, patients are advised that they will be able to leave the hospital when they are maintaining oral alimentation, ambulating with little or no assistance, pain relief is provided by oral medications, and that there are no signs of complications. This focuses the issue of hospital discharge on achieving appropriate functional level rather than a specific number of days. Using this simple algorithm over the past decade, length of stay for acoustic tumor patients has averaged less than 3 days. Reassuring the patient that he or she will not be discharged until they have achieved a suitable level of function is achieved relieves anxiety about readiness to go home. Identifying the functional goals required for discharge also motivates patients to achieve those goals. Creating the proper expectation regarding discharge criteria during the preoperative discussion is critical to optimizing duration of hospitalization. Hospitalization beyond what is medically or functionally indicated increases the risk of nosocomial infection, deep vein thrombosis, and other hospitalization related complications.

The patient and family should be informed about proper postoperative care following discharge. Topics to address are: proper wound care, symptoms or changes to watch for, eye care (if facial nerve weakness is present), medication schedule, activity level, and physician contact information should problems arise. Providing this information in written form is helpful as patients are often overwhelmed by the volume of information during this stressful time. Once home, patients are encouraged to pursue an appropriate level of activity to reduce the risk of deep venous thrombosis, as well as, maintain mobility and stamina. Exertion requiring a Valsalva maneuver, particularly in patients at risk for CSF leak, is discouraged for 1 month following surgery. The number, timing, and purpose of postoperative visits should be well delineated. Neurotologic/skull base lesions commonly require long-term radiological monitoring. The type and timing of imaging to be done should be discussed in advance as well as postoperatively. Establishing a system for tracking patients needing scans at recommended intervals is necessary to avoid losing a patient to follow-up.

To reduce confusion and anxiety on the day of surgery, patients should be given directions to the surgery center and/or hospital before arrival, and if possible visit the facility to preregister for their admission. Doing so will help familiarize them with the check-in process and the physical plant. Patients traveling to a distant tertiary care center should be provided a list of lodging resources close to the facility.

Medical Preparation

A brief discussion between surgeon and anesthesiologist regarding the surgery can help optimize the patient's surgical experience and avoid complications. Review of the anesthetic choice, anticipated duration of surgery, use/nonuse of neurophysiological monitoring, concerns regarding intracranial pressure, intraoperative fluid management, hyperventilation to lower Pco_2, and patient-specific health issues are examples of topics worthy of review. In centers where otologic/neurotologic surgery is common, the discussion may be more abbreviated as the anesthesia team will likely be familiar with the surgeon's preferences. The surgeon (or surrogate) should visit the patient in the preoperative area and confirm the site for surgery; mark it personally.

The topic of intraoperative fluid management during skull base surgeries merits specific attention. From the perspective of the anesthesiologist, the patient arrives in the preoperative area in a dehydrated state having foregone oral hydration for at least 8 h. The anesthesiologist will commonly want to "make up" the patient's fluid deficit using intravenous fluids. The first author and his neurosurgical colleague have instructed their anesthesia team to resist this impulse. Our instructions regarding fluid balance are to match the volume of intravenous fluids given to the quantity of urine output and blood loss during the course of the surgery. This avoids overhydration and possible brain edema. We have experienced situations in which the anesthetic team did not follow this request, giving patients as much as three liters of fluids during the course of an uncomplicated 3-hour surgery, causing the patients to develop cerebellar edema a few hours later requiring emergent measures. Excessive dehydration is to be avoided as well since it increases the risk of venous thrombosis.

Anxiolysis is typically provided by the anesthesiologist in the preoperative area depending on patient need. To reduce nausea related to otologic procedures, 4 to 8 mg of dexamethasone (Decadron) and 4 mg of ondansetron (Zofran) given intravenously at the start of surgery are a useful combination. Perioperative antibiotics for clean otologic procedures (intact tympanic membrane or dry perforation) are not employed as the infection rate is in the range of 1%.[4,5] Actively draining ears have a higher rate of postoperative infection compared to non-draining ears. The administration of a single dose of preoperative (within 1 h of incision) cephalosporin, in draining ears, has been shown to reduce early (within the first week) postoperative infection rates three-fold. However, this protective effect disappears in the second postoperative week.[5] As such, there is no compelling indication for the use of perioperative antibiotics for otologic surgery. Patients with diabetes have their blood glucose level checked and if necessary treated to prevent hyperglycemia, which has been associated with surgical site infection (SSI).[6] Neurotologic and skull base procedures require medications aimed at brain protection and infection control. For the purpose of brain protection, preoperative intravenous Mannitol 0.5 to 1 g/kg (usually 75 g) and dexamethasone 10 mg are given intravenously. In contrast to otological surgery, prophylactic antibiotics are routinely used for skull base procedures. The antibiotic of choice should be effective against *Staph. aureus* as this is the most commonly cultured organism from neurosurgical SSIs. Either oxacillin 1 g, or a cefazolin 1 g, is given intravenously within 1 h of incision. If the patient is allergic to both penicillin and cephalosporins, then vancomycin is employed in dose appropriate to the patient's weight. If the procedure is lengthy, intraoperative doses of antibiotics should be given at appropriate intervals. Prophylactic intravenous antibiotics are discontinued 24 h postoperatively.[6–8]

Transition to the Operating Room

As the patient is brought into the operating room, the staff present should introduce themselves to the patient and identify their role. If music is playing, it should be soothing and at a low volume to avoid affecting conversation. The patient is then assisted in transferring onto the operating table. The patient's head should be at the end of the bed with the most space underneath to accommodate the surgeon's legs while seated. While the patient is still awake, identity is confirmed and the planned procedure and site is reconfirmed with all staff participating in this "time out" check.

Once the patient is sedated or under general anesthetic, positioning for the planned surgery is undertaken. For all otologic and neurotologic surgeries the anesthetist is at the patient's feet. In addition to providing appropriate sedation/anesthesia, the anesthetist is charged with managing the bed controls to adjust side-to-side tilt and height. Attention is paid to protecting the patient's airway when moving the head during patient positioning. Stabilization of the endotracheal tube, once the patient is positioned, should be done in such a way so that movement of the head during dressing placement at the conclusion of surgery does not inadvertently extubate the patient. The patient then is secured to the operating table with adjustable straps to prevent patient movement when the bed is tilted side to side. The patient's head is placed on a "donut" pillow with the head turned to place the operative site "up." Additional elevation of the head may be needed in patients with large shoulders. Often slight neck flexion will help the surgeon gain access to the temporal bone in robustly proportioned patients. Pin fixation of the head is used in retrosigmoid craniotomy and most supratentorial craniotomy cases. Clipping of hair and skin cleansing with isopropyl alcohol is undertaken before incision marking is done. Injection of local anesthetic with epinephrine along the incision site is done for hemostasis. Electrophysiological monitoring set up is then undertaken as appropriate for the planned procedure.

The scrub technician/nurse (scrub) is positioned directly opposite the surgeon in most cases. In cases where the surgeon is positioned at the top of the patient's head then the scrub is positioned on the side of the surgeon's dominant hand to facilitate instrument transfers. A video monitor is positioned such that the scrub can see it, follow the course of surgery, and anticipate instrument changes. Some surgeons prefer that the scrub operate the foot pedals of all devices such as bipolar cautery and drills. Other surgeons control such foot pedals themselves as there is an inherent delay in starting and stopping the devices, since the surgeon must vocalize a command and the scrub then reacts to it. Figures 17–1 to 17–4 demonstrate idealized operating room organization of patient, equipment, and staff for different surgical site examples. Each surgeon's operating room size and configuration will dictate specifics of personnel and equipment positioning.

More important than the physical organization of the operating room are the personnel that make up the operative team. It is optimal to have a consistent crew of scrub technicians, circulating nurse, anesthesia team, and neurophysiologist working with the surgeon's team. By repetition and experience this consistent team will increase the quality of care as well as improve safety for the patient and for each other. Familiarity with the types of procedures, disease processes, surgeon preferences, and routines will decrease inadvertent errors and foster excellence from all participants.

Surgical Site Preparation

Preparation of the surgical site(s) is designed for the purpose of limiting colonization of the wound by normal skin flora. Adequate clipping of hair to accommodate the anticipated incision(s) and extent of surgery should be done. Shaving of hair with a razor has been associated with higher wound infection rates and clipping with an electric clipper is now recommended.[6] Cleansing of the skin with isopropyl alcohol helps to further reduce the bacterial count as well as remove skin oils in preparation for incision marking, application of gum resin adhesive, and adhesive plastic drapes. For otologic

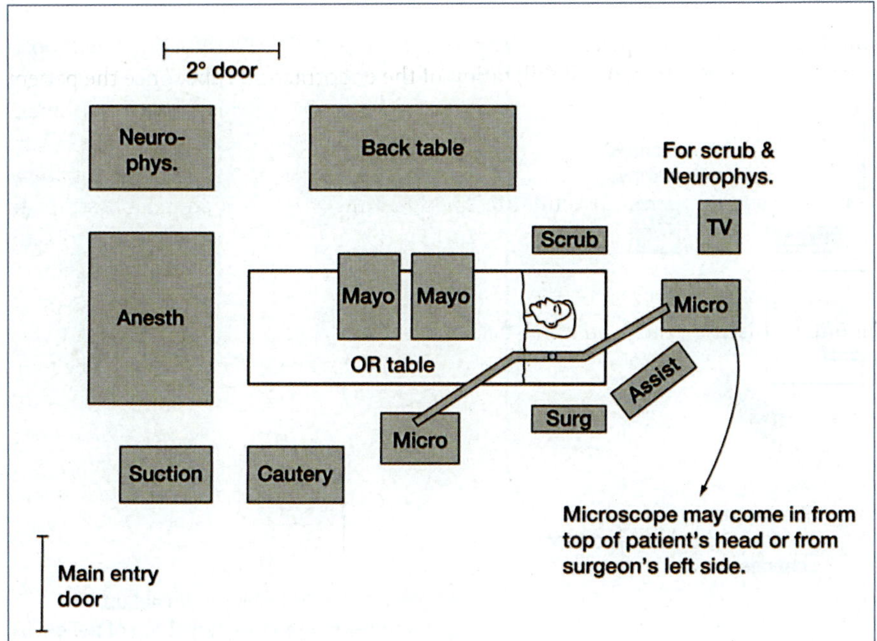

FIGURE 17–1 • Operating room set up for left-sided posterior fossa/temporal bone lesion.

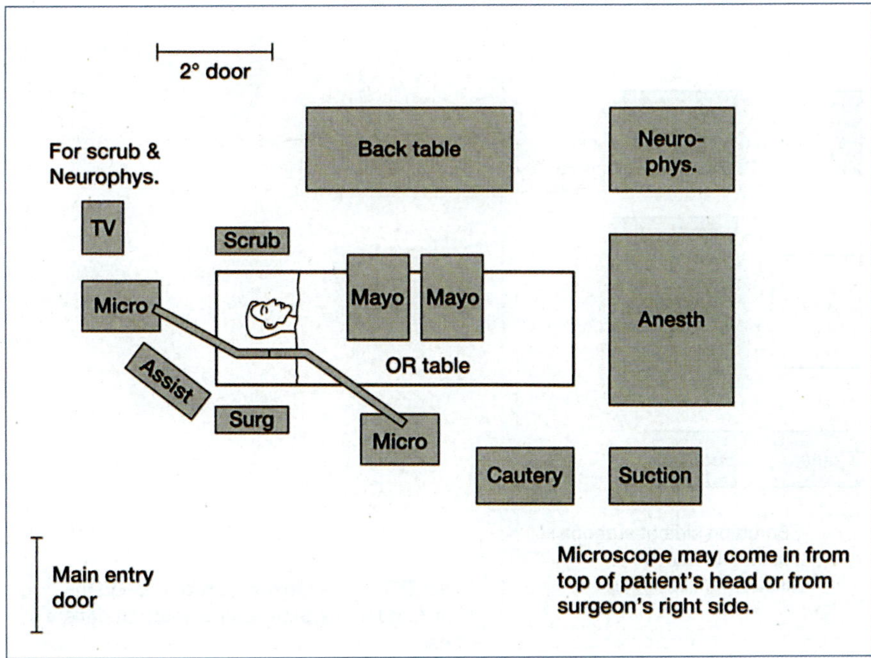

FIGURE 17–2 • Operating room set up for right-sided posterior fossa/temporal bone lesion.

surgery povidone-iodine (Betadine) soap is used for the prep. In neurotologic procedures alcohol-based iodine or chlorhexidine adhesive prep solutions (Duraprep or Chloraprep) are utilized. The sterile drapes used are nonabsorbent, self-adhering barrier drapes. In otologic cases there is a precut aperture through which the auricle protrudes. For neurotologic/skull base procedures a wide-field adhesive drape is employed and the drape cut as dictated by incision position. Attached pouches with suction are desirable to collect irrigation runoff. The latter is important as a pouch heavy with collected runoff may cause the drape to pull away from the skin creating an avenue for wound contamination. Stapling the drape in place along the posterior edge of the field can help prevent undesirable detachment of the drape from the skin. Aseptic technique is an absolute necessity. No amount of antibiotics will protect the patient from infection if aseptic technique is carelessly executed.

SURGICAL TECHNIQUE

This section will focus on basic principles. Specifics related to incisions, degree of bone removal, etc. for particular approaches/diseases will be covered in their respective chapters. Proper handling of tissues throughout the procedure will maximize tissue vitality and consequently proper healing. Tissue that is crushed, devascularized, or allowed to desiccate will not heal well and will be more susceptible to infection and necrosis.

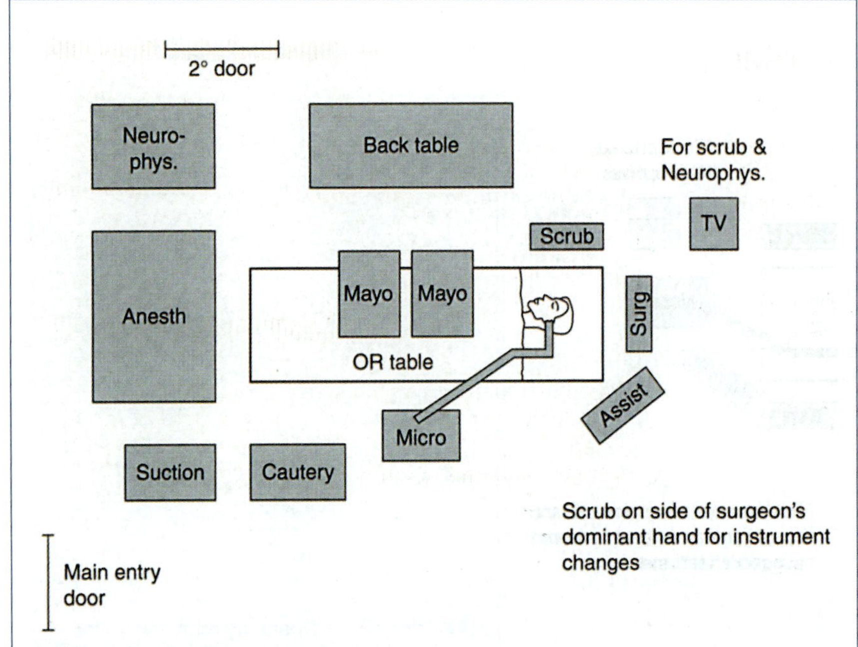

FIGURE 17–3 • Operating room set up for right-handed surgeon seated at top of patient's head.

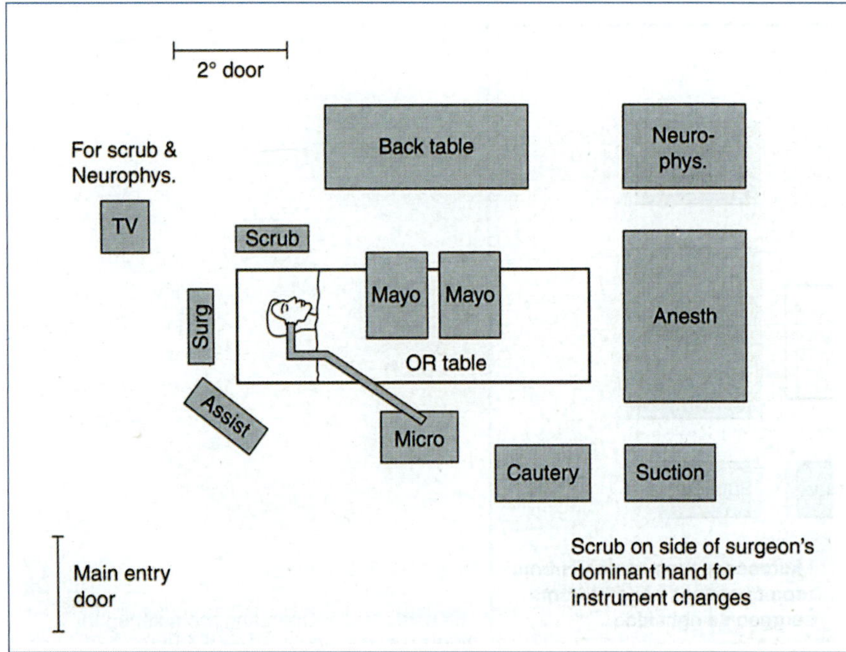

FIGURE 17–4 • Operating room set up for left-handed surgeon seated at top of patient's head.

Maintaining hemostasis and optimal exposure are critical elements contributing to successful otologic/neurotologic surgery. Proper bone dissection technique is critical for maximizing speed and safety during this phase of temporal bone/skull base surgery. Identification of vital structures away from involvement by pathology makes for safer disease removal. Finally, meticulous multilayered wound closure will provide better cosmesis and lower risk of complications such as CSF leak.

Hemostasis

The demand for hemostasis in microsurgery surpasses that required during more typical procedures in the head and neck. To achieve the degree of hemostasis required for microsurgery special tactics must be mastered. Injection of local anesthetic with epinephrine is the first step of both providing comfort for the patient and vasoconstriction of vessels in the surgical field. For otologic surgeries done under local anesthetic with sedation, the pattern of injections will differ based on the specific procedure. For transcanal procedures, injections of 2% xylocaine with 1:100,000 epinephrine (total volume usually 2–3 mL) are placed in the tragus (Figure 17–5), the incisura (cleft between the tragus and root of helix; Figure 17–6), the floor and posterior aspect of the lateral portion of the canal (Figures 17–7 and 17–8). Deeper canal injections can be made with 2% xylocaine with 1:50,000 epinephrine (usually less than 1 mL) starting in the vascular strip, then two anterior canal injections, and the last injection along the floor of the canal. These deeper injections start in the more mobile, hair bearing, portion of the canal

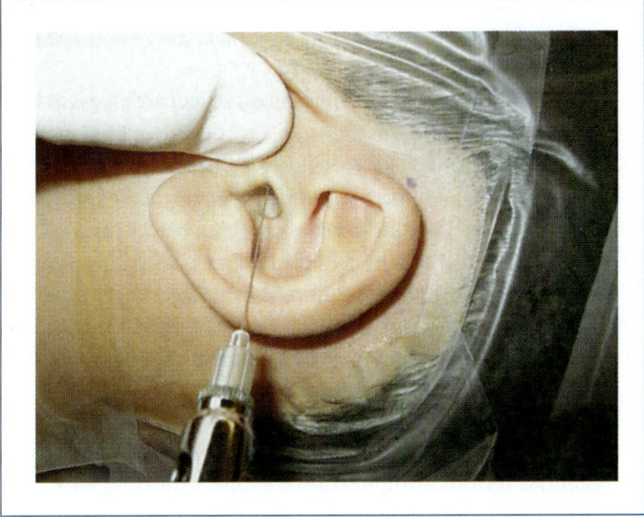

FIGURE 17–5 • Tragal injection of local anesthetic with epinephrine.

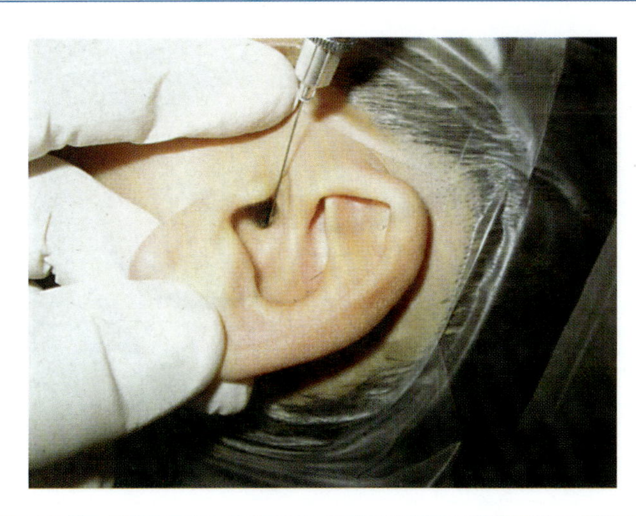

FIGURE 17–8 • Posterior ear canal injection.

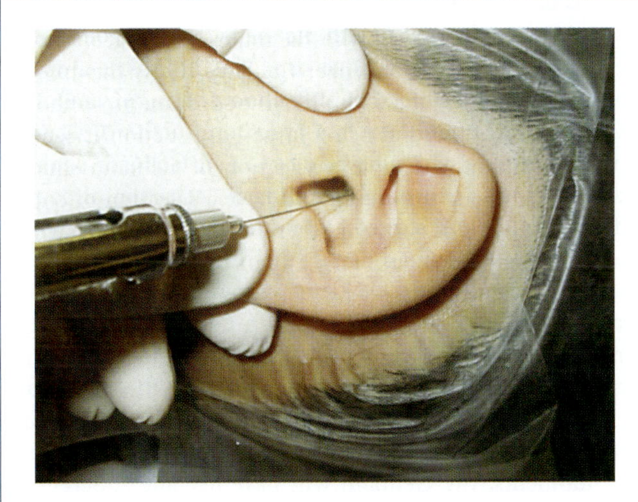

FIGURE 17–6 • Local anesthetic injection in incisura.

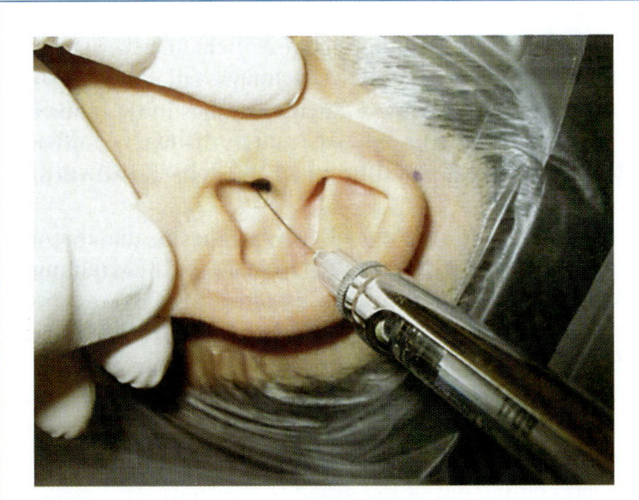

FIGURE 17–7 • Floor of lateral ear canal injection.

skin with the needle tip contacting the bone of the medial-ear canal. Gentle injection pressure must be used to prevent a bleb in the deep canal skin.

For postauricular procedures, the canal injections are the same, but are preceded first by placement of a greater auricular nerve block (Figure 17–9). This is followed by injection of the postauricular tissues along the anticipated incision line (Figure 17–10). The tissues from dermis to periosteum are injected with 2% xylocaine with 1:100,000 epinephrine. The areas of the zygomatic root, superior and posterior to the incision line receive additional injection for a total volume of 5 to 6 mL. If mastoidectomy is anticipated, these latter areas are augmented with 0.5% marcaine with 1:200,000 epinephrine (total of 3–5 mL). To better control the rate of injection, the authors favor the use of dental syringes with commercially available carpules of xylocaine/marcaine and epinephrine in the concentrations noted above. Additionally the carpules are labeled and reduce the likelihood of a medication error. The needle used is a 27-gauge, one and one-quarter inch long dental needle. Total volume and concentration of the injected local anesthetic is announced to the anesthetist and nurse, to be recorded. For procedures performed under general anesthetic the same pattern of injections is used (with the elimination of the greater auricular nerve block and marcaine injections) as a carrier for the epinephrine. The injections are administered prior to the surgeon scrubbing as this gives adequate time for optimal vasoconstriction to occur. Infiltration of the intended incision sites for neurotologic procedures with xylocaine/epinephrine is also undertaken for hemostasis.

Electrocautery is an indispensable tool for achieving hemostasis. Use of monopolar electrocautery is limited to the soft tissues of skin and muscles. Bipolar cautery, specifically micro bipolar cautery (usually irrigating), is most helpful once the microscope is being used. With bipolar cautery the strength of current required for hemostasis and the related current spread is reduced resulting in a lower risk of adjacent tissue damage. Bipolar cautery is most useful for achieving hemostasis on

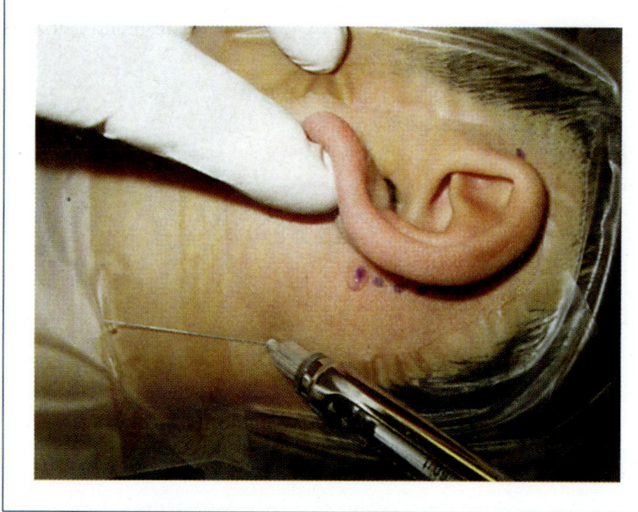

FIGURE 17–9 • Demonstration of entry point and subcutaneous course of needle for greater auricular nerve block.

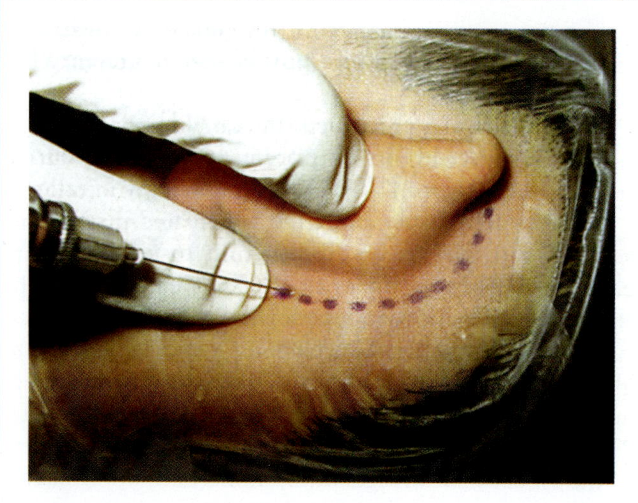

FIGURE 17–10 • Injection of postauricular tissues. The index finger palpates the mastoid tip.

exposed dura, the exposed sigmoid sinus, adjacent to the facial nerve, middle-ear mucosa, ear canal skin flaps, and the internal auditory canal. The surgeon's experience and familiarity with his equipment will guide the current level suitable for specific sites, but if questions arise, the current level may be tested on exposed muscle or other soft tissue in the surgical field.

Topical application of concentrated epinephrine is a valuable tool for achieving hemostasis in the middle ear and mastoid. Specific circumstances in which application of topical epinephrine are most helpful are: prior to tympanic membrane graft placement, prior to stapes manipulation, and when dissecting diseased middle-ear mucosa or granulation tissue. The authors employ absorbable gelatin sponge (Gelfoam) soaked in 1:1,000 epinephrine as the topical applicator. The gelfoam is placed in the area requiring hemostasis and left in place for a few minutes. Work is undertaken elsewhere and then when the surgeon removes the Gelfoam, remarkably good hemostasis is usually encountered. It is rare to have even minimal change in heart rate or blood pressure with the topical use of epinephrine as described.

Bone bleeding can sometimes be managed with topical epinephrine, but commonly bone wax is needed to achieve hemostasis. A piece of bone wax is delivered on an instrument then packed and smoothed into position with a cotton pledget. Bone wax should be considered a foreign body and used judiciously in infected fields. Drilling with a diamond bur is useful for achieving hemostasis in bone. The diamond bur works by pushing bone dust into vascular channels in the bone rather that generating heat to cauterize the bone. This maneuver should be done with copious irrigation to avoid thermal damage to adjacent vital structures.

Injury to the sigmoid sinus can result in startling bleeding and potential serious complications. Properly dealing with this event is necessary to reduce the risk of complication and to maximize the chance of maintaining vessel patency. Since the sigmoid sinuses are the main avenue for venous return from the brain "packing it off" should remain a last resort. Should the sinus be violated, rather than place suction at the opening while getting ready to deal with the injury, the surgeon should occlude the defect with a finger tip. This limits the amount of blood lost and reduces the likelihood of an air embolus. Next the scrub should attach a large-bore suction/irrigation tip to the tubing, assemble a selection of Gelfoam squares soaked in saline or thrombin, and have a selection of cotton pledgets ready. The surgeon then selects, with a bayonet forceps, a Gelfoam square larger than the size of the defect. The finger occluding the defect is removed and the Gelfoam square placed over the defect. Next a cotton pledget larger than the Gelfoam square is picked up using the suction and placed over the Gelfoam. Compression with the large-bore suction and bayonet forceps on this "Gelfoam patch" is maintained with irrigation turned on and off intermittently. Within a few moments, the Gelfoam will have become adherent to the exposed dura of the sinus effectively sealing the defect without occluding the vessel. Slight elevation of the patient's head done by placing the table in reverse Trendelenberg position will reduce venous pressure and can assist in achieving hemostasis but must be used with caution lest an air embolus occur. Defects in the sinus, as large as 1 cm, may be "patched" with this technique. Should this technique fail, suture repair of the sinus may be employed. Small openings in the sinus may be "welded" shut using bipolar cautery if there is sufficient mobility of the sinus wall to pinch the hole closed with the bipolar forceps.

Should all other options fail then packing the sinus becomes necessary. Proximal flow can often be managed by extraluminal packing. The dura of the sinus is dissected from its bony covering near the sinodural angle. Then absorbable oxidized regenerated cellulose (Surgicel) is packed between the bone and dura to extraluminally compress the sinus. The same technique may be used with the distal portion of the sinus. Should intraluminal packing be needed, longer strips of Surgicel should be used with a tail left coming out of the defect in the sinus. This prevents embolization of the packing material into the central venous circulation. Panic is to be avoided as the medial wall of the sinus may be breached and the intracranial contents compressed by overzealous packing.

Exposure

The key to all surgery, and in particular otologic/neurotologic surgery, is adequate exposure. One simply must see what one is doing in the anatomically complex temporal bone. Developing a sequential pattern of bone dissection for various temporal bone procedures will ensure that the optimal exposure is achieved for the task at hand. One must resist the temptation to reach the deeper structure of interest prior to achieving the desired degree of lateral exposure first. Creating a narrow, deep corridor can yield disorientation from a lack of orienting landmarks and result in injury to vital structures. While the details of specific incisions and bone removal will be left to other chapters, the principle of adequate exposure must be upheld. Incision and bone-removal planning should allow appropriate visualization and access (distal and proximal control) to the neurovascular structures traversing the intended surgical field. Furthermore, contingencies must be made should the exposure need extension to deal with intraoperative complications.

The authors recommend use of the operating microscope for all aspects of temporal bone and skull base surgery with the exception of initial soft tissue work. The microscope should possess the following characteristics: high-quality optics, variable magnification, objectives with appropriate focal distances, adjustable eye pieces, mounted camera for photo/video documentation, and finally a suitable stand, which may be finely balanced. The microscope must be prepared by the surgeon prior to draping. The surgeon should check the diopter settings and ensure that the observer and operating oculars are par focal. The microscope should be balanced to allow full range of motion with minimal effort. During surgery the surgeon should be in an ergonomically sound sitting position using a chair, which provides good back support during microscope use. This will reduce fatigue and avoid back and neck problems related to improper sitting position. Starting temporal bone drilling under microscopic magnification provides better illumination, a better view of the anatomy, and protection against bone dust and irrigation, which may carry potentially lethal viruses (Hepatitis C, HIV, prions). By using the lowest magnification suitable for each step in the surgery maximizes field of view and depth of field.

An intimate knowledge of the three-dimensional anatomic relationships (and their variations) within the temporal bone, especially the course of the facial nerve, is mandatory for efficient and safe bone removal. The temporal bone lab is where a beginning temporal bone surgeon should explore the complex temporal-bone anatomy. Likewise, the lab is where a practicing surgeon can rehearse an uncommonly done procedure. Learning the anatomic "pointers" to the facial nerve: the digastric ridge, chorda tympani, the lateral and posterior semicircular canals, the incus/fossa incudus, the cochleariform process, the "cog," the pyramidal process, the oval window, Jacobson's nerve, greater and lesser superficial petrosal nerves, Bill's bar, and the eighth cranial nerve are crucial to becoming an accomplished temporal bone surgeon.[9] This knowledge provides the surgeon a number of options for finding the nerve in a location away from where it is affected by pathology. The facial nerve should then be traced into the area of pathology. As the facial nerve is dissected, should direct exposure of the sheath be required, the bone overlying the nerve is thinned to an "eggshell," and then this thin layer of bone is carefully dissected from the sheath. This sequence of dissection will reduce the likelihood of facial nerve injury. The facial nerve should be viewed as a welcome landmark, routinely sought out during all manner of temporal bone procedures. Use of electromyographic facial nerve monitoring (covered more completely in Chapter 19) is a useful tool for informing the surgeon during dissection directly on the sheath or nerve itself. Such monitoring is no substitute for knowledge of anatomy or proper technique when seeking out the nerve during bone dissection.

Fearing the facial nerve and avoiding its identification makes inadvertent injury more likely. The same is true of the internal carotid artery in complex skull base surgeries. Identifying this important vessel away from the area of disease involvement and achieving proximal and distal control are prerequisites for embarking on tumor dissection along its course. The potential for morbidity/mortality is greatest in those tumors that intimately involve the internal carotid artery. The modern skull-base surgeon should be prepared to manage injury to this vessel themselves or by having appropriate team members assembled for such cases.

Bone Dissection

Next in importance is the use of drilling technique that allows rapid bone removal while sequentially identifying and delineating anatomic landmarks, which then help lead the surgeon to subsequent structures. Modern high-speed, high-torque drills (both pneumatic and electric) should rightfully be called bone dissection tools. These tools allow for rapid bone removal with minimal force needed from the surgeon's hand. This combination of attributes allows a sense of feel with the drill similar to that of a scalpel on tissue. Just as a surgeon would not use a dull scalpel, brand new burs should be used with every case. Dull burs require more pressure to remove bone, reduce sense of feel, and escalate the risk of injury.

Just as it takes time and experience to develop the "feel" required for soft tissue surgery, the same is true of bone dissection. The novice temporal bone surgeon will commonly use a very light pressure stroke with rapid side-to-side motion of the drill, which results in very little bone removal and sets up a dangerous rhythm that may be difficult to stop when a vital structure is encountered (Video 17–1). Additionally the irrigation component of the suction irrigator is commonly poorly aimed and either kept too wet or too dry. The safest and most efficient technique of bone dissection is similar to that of a computer numerical control (CNC) milling machine. In a CNC machine, the computer has a shape three-dimensionally programmed as numerical coordinates. The computer then drives a milling tool to create the programmed shape out of a block of solid material. The temporal bone surgeon should have in mind the idealized temporal bone anatomy as that programmed three-dimensional shape. Different from a CNC machine, the surgeon is able to see the temporal bone structures as they are approached and modify the bone dissection to follow the contours of the structures encountered. In this way the anatomy of the neurovascular structures that traverse the temporal bone are "liberated" from their bony encasement.

When drilling with well-applied suction irrigation, the bone is kept moist and does not develop significant, opaque, white dusting. Wet bone remains translucent. If one cannot see an anatomic structure through the wet bone to be drilled, it is likely to be at least 2 to 3 mm thick. That much bone can be safely removed in a single, measured stroke with a cutting bur; the pressure exerted to remove bone should be measured, not maximal. If maximal pressure is used there is greater risk of loss of control and therefore injury. The hands should be supported against the patient's head for optimal stability. Using the side of the bur achieves the most effective bone removal. Use of the tip should be avoided. The largest bur suitable for the task should be used as it will expose structures in a broader fashion. Inappropriately small burs tend to penetrate structures and cause injury. Expose and delineate the lateral anatomy developing a sequence of anatomic landmarks that lead to deeper structures. Broad, saucerized-lateral exposure eliminates ledges or overhangs that may obscure structures, reduce illumination, and inadvertently catch the flute of a cutting bur causing it to jump. Keep the field clear of bone dust as it can hide vital structures making them susceptible to injury. Furthermore, bone dust is prone to osteo-neogenesis and if left in the middle ear may contribute to conductive hearing loss.

The depth of bone removal should be predetermined by the surgeon and modified by feedback from one's senses. The senses of sight, touch, and hearing should be employed while drilling. The sound generated by drilling will change to a high-pitched tone when approaching areas of thin bone overlying the dura. The structures to be identified through thin bone will have different colors and characteristic locations through the temporal bone. Differences in bone density can be discerned by the degree of pressure required for bone removal while drilling. When the edge of a landmark is approached pressure is reduced to avoid the drill flipping past the edge or injuring the structure. When the bone over a structure is thinned, it may be visible through 0.5 to 1 mm of wet bone. The different bur types are used for different purposes. The cutting burs are aggressively fluted and used for rapid bone removal. The diamond bur is used for finer, more gradual bone removal when approaching a vital structure. However, care must be taken to use adequate irrigation as the diamond bur can generate significant heat that can burn bone and cause thermal injury to vital structures such as the facial nerve. Video 17–2 is an example of bone dissection technique employed in the early stages of a translabyrinthine approach in a right ear.

Integral to all surgery is the closure. While important in otologic surgery, attention to detail during wound closure in skull base surgery is essential. CSF leak remains one of the most commonly reported complications of skull base surgery.[10] Attention to approach design and meticulous, multilayer closure techniques can reduce the incidence to 1% or 2%.[11,12] Complex closures, more frequently seen in revision surgeries, may require regional or free-flap reconstructions.[13]

To close this section on operative technique, one must emphasize that part of doing the best possible job for the patient includes knowing when one has reached their own (or the team's) limit of expertise, encountered a problem they are unprepared to manage, or have become disoriented in the surgical field. In such circumstances often the best service rendered to the patient means "backing out." By persisting under the aforementioned conditions one greatly increases the risk of injuring the patient. Remember, "*Primum non nocere.*" Reassessment may allow reoperation in better circumstances or may prompt referral to a helpful colleague.

POSTOPERATIVE CARE

Patients following otologic/neurotologic surgery should be transferred from the operating room to a postanesthesia care unit (PACU). The PACU staff should be trained to recognize facial nerve, cranial nerve, and other neurological dysfunction related to these surgeries. Patients are closely monitored until they are sufficiently recovered to go home or be transferred to their hospital room (intensive care unit [ICU] or medical/surgical unit). Patients undergoing otologic surgery are routinely discharged to home the day of surgery itself. Should severe nausea persist then they are admitted overnight for hydration and control of nausea. This latter circumstance is most commonly seen in procedures, which open the labyrinth.

Following transcanal procedures, the patient is instructed to change the conchal cotton ball twice daily starting the morning after surgery. The ear canal is to be kept dry until instructed by the surgeon that it may get wet. For patients with postauricular incisions, the compressive mastoid dressing may be removed the day after surgery around mid-day. The authors favor a "Glasscock" ear dressing. Patients are readily able to remove the dressing at home and begin cleansing the postauricular incision (closed with subcuticular sutures) with rubbing alcohol and replace the conchal cotton ball twice daily. The ear canal must remain dry, but the postauricular incision is allowed to get wet 4 days after surgery. The first postoperative visit is 3 weeks later when the ear canal is cleared of crusts and ointment. Ear drops are not used unless an ear canal wick was placed at the time of surgery (ie, following ear canal atresia reconstruction).

Patients undergoing craniotomy are observed in the ICU overnight with hourly checks of the vital signs and neurological functions. The following day, if they are in suitable condition then they may be transferred to a medical/surgical unit for the remainder of their hospital stay. Prevention of perioperative deep venous thrombosis is important.[14] Routine use of sequential compression stockings is initiated in the operating room as part of the patient positioning. Subcutaneous heparin injections of 5,000 units twice daily are started the morning following surgery. Rapid mobilization of the patient further reduces the risk of thrombus formation in the lower extremities. As permitted by the presence or absence of postoperative vertigo, patients are encouraged to be out of bed the day following surgery. Physical therapy consultation is obtained on the first postoperative day to assess and assist in ambulating patients at least three times daily.

Following surgery for tumors affecting the lower cranial nerves patients may have significant problems with swallowing function and airway protection and are kept NPO. Early consultation with speech/swallowing therapists is critical before starting oral intake to reduce the likelihood of aspiration pneumonia.

Older patients have more difficulty compensating for these problems than do younger patients and rehabilitation can be a lengthy process. Procedures for temporary vocal cord medialization are suitable for patients in whom recovery of nerve function is expected. Otherwise more permanent vocal cord medialization may be needed. Though uncommon, tracheotomy and gastrostomy may be necessary temporary measures for such patients. For patients without lower cranial nerve involvement, a clear liquid diet is ordered postoperatively with advance as tolerated.

As previously mentioned, prophylactic antibiotics following skull base surgeries are continued for only 24 h postoperatively. The use of postoperative Dexamethasone (4 mg every 6 h) for 48 h after neurotologic cases is to prevent/reduce any brain or nerve edema. Patients with tumors causing significant preoperative brainstem/pontine compression are at risk for symptomatic re-expansion edema. Re-expansion edema can be so severe that it can cause cytotoxic changes in brain tissue resulting in permanent dysfunction. In such cases low-dose mannitol (25 g every 6 h for 2–3 days) may be prophylactically employed to mitigate the re-expansion edema and reduce the likelihood of cytotoxic damage. Urine and serum osmolality are monitored during the period of Mannitol use. Care must be taken not to excessively dehydrate the patient as this increases the risk for venous thrombosis.

Patients with facial nerve weakness following surgery require special attention to maintaining corneal lubrication. These issues are discussed preoperatively with patients in whom the facial nerve is in peril. Use of lubricating eye drops at least hourly during the day is recommended. Moisturizing ophthalmologic ointment is used at night. A moisture chamber may also be used. Ongoing monitoring of corneal status by an ophthalmologist is recommended in patients with significant facial weakness and poor eye closure. Consultation with an oculoplastic surgeon may be necessary if more aggressive measures (gold weight, lateral tarsorrhaphy, etc.) are required to protect the cornea.

Skin staple removal occurs 10 to 14 days following skull base surgery. At this visit the patient's recovery progress is assessed. Encouragement is given and instructions are reinforced regarding activity level and, if appropriate, eye care. For patients experiencing vertigo following their surgery Cawthorne exercises are given at this time. For patients not recovering well with Cawthorne exercises after 1 month, referral to physical therapy for balance rehabilitation is initiated. Most patients are able to return to work within 4 to 6 weeks following neurotologic surgery. If the patient is recovering well and there is no facial nerve dysfunction then radiological follow-up is arranged with telephonic visits arranged to review results and plan future studies. If facial nerve or other neurological dysfunction is present then follow up visits every 3 to 4 months, to monitor pace of recovery, are planned.

SUMMARY

Temporal bone and skull base surgery requires precision planning and execution to achieve the best results for patient and surgeon alike. The level of expectation for favorable outcome is very high and while we strive to achieve perfection, the disease process will often thwart our efforts. Proper patient education and preparation will help align expectation with the anticipated results. Every surgeon should constantly strive for excellence and routinely pursue self-critique to find opportunities for improvement in all aspects of care. Rigorous application of the principles discussed in this chapter will assist the temporal bone/skull base surgeon reach the highest levels of achievement possible.

References

1. Roberson JB, Jackson LE, McAuley JR. Acoustic neuroma surgery: Absent auditory brainstem response does not contraindicate attempted hearing preservation. Laryngoscope 1999;109:904–10.
2. Danner C, Mastrodimos B, Cueva RA. A comparison of direct eighth nerve monitoring and auditory brainstem response in hearing preservation surgery for vestibular schwannoma. Otol Neurotol 2004;25(5):826–32.
3. Doll A, Abu EM, Kehrli P, et al. Aspects of FLAIR sequences, 3D-CISS and diffusion-weighted MR imaging of intracranial epidermoid cysts. J Neuroradiol 2000;27(2):101–6.
4. Jackson CG. Antimicrobial prophylaxis in ear surgery. Laryngoscope 1988;98(10):1116–23.
5. Govaerts PJ, Raemaekers J, Verlinden M, et al. Use of antibiotic prophylaxis in ear surgery. Laryngoscope 1998;108(1):107–10.
6. Mangram AJ, Horan TC, Pearson ML, et al. Guideline for prevention of surgical site infection. Infect Control Hosp Epidemiol 1999;20(4):247–78.
7. Korinek AM, Golmard JL, Eicheick A, et al. Risk factors for neurosurgical site infections after craniotomy: A critical reappraisal of antibiotic prophylaxis in 4,578 patients. Br J Neurosurg 2005;19(2):155–62.
8. Barker FG. Efficacy of prophylactic antibiotics against meningitis after craniotomy: A meta-analysis. Neurosurgery 2007;60(5):887–94.
9. Sanna M, Khrais T, Mancini F, Russo A, Taibah A. The facial nerve in temporal bone and lateral skull base microsurgery. New York: Thieme Medical Publishers; 2006.
10. Selesnick SH, Liu JC, Jen A, Newman, J. The incidence of cerebrospinal fluid leak after vestibular schwannoma surgery. Otol Neurotol 2004;25:387–93.
11. Cueva RA, Mastrodimos B. Approach design and closure techniques to minimize cerebrospinal fluid lead after cerebellopontine angle tumor surgery. Otol Neurotol 2005;26(6):1176–81.
12. Sanna M, Taibah A, Russo A, et al. Perioperative complications in acoustic neuroma (vestibular schwannoma) surgery. Otol Neurotol 2004;25(3):379–86.
13. Jackson CG, Netterville JL, Glasscock ME, et al. Reconstruction and cerebrospinal fluid management in neurotologic skull base tumors with intracranial extension. Laryngoscope 1992;102(11):1205–14.
14. Epstein NE. A review of the risks and benefits of differing prophylaxis regimes for the treatment of deep venous thrombosis and pulmonary embolus in neurosurgery. Surg Neurol 2005;64(4):295–301.

Lasers in Otology 18

S. George Lesinski, MD

INTRODUCTION

Over the past two decades, four lasers have received the *Food and Drug Administration* (FDA) approval for otologic surgery in the United States—two lasers in the visible light spectrum—argon (514 nm) and potassium titanyl phosphate (KTP) (532 nm), and two in the infrared (IR)—carbon dioxide (CO_2) (10,600 nm) and erbium yttrium aluminum garnet (YAG) (2,960 nm). These lasers have increased surgical precision while reducing mechanical trauma to the inner ear and facial nerve. Otologic lasers have now been widely accepted for otosclerosis surgery. Many studies have demonstrated improved clinical results for primary and, in particular, revision otosclerosis surgery compared to standard nonlaser techniques. Otologic lasers have been used successfully for vaporizing glomus tumors, acoustic neuromas, small arteriovenous (AV) malformations, and in chronic ear surgery, for vaporizing granulation tissue and cholesteatomas, particularly on a mobile stapes. Recently, lasers have warmed nitinol prostheses—attaching these "metals with memory" to the incus without mechanical crimping. All four lasers have proven clinical efficacy and safety for these applications, provided the surgeon employs appropriate energy guidelines and microsurgical techniques.

Which laser is best for which otologic procedure? Is the laser's wavelength important? What potential future applications do lasers offer for otologic surgery? Understanding the biophysical effects resulting from the laser's electromagnetic (EM) energy being absorbed by the EM fields of the atoms in the target tissue provides the scientific foundation to answer these questions. This submicroscopic world is composed of powerful EM fields, a world that is very different than the world we experience through our senses. It is governed by rules of physics (quantum mechanics) that are counterintuitive to our daily experience and often seem to contradict the laws of Newtonian physics, the physics that most of us studied in college.

This chapter will first focus on a few essential principles of quantum mechanics that explain the interaction of light and matter. Then, results from relevant laboratory experiments that compare different lasers effects on water, bone, and collagen will be cited. Medical lasers approved for otologic surgery and their safe energy parameters will be detailed. Next, specific laser surgical procedures are discussed.

INTERACTION OF LIGHT AND MATTER—QUANTUM THEORY

To understand how the EM energy fields of light interact with the EM fields of atoms and molecules, we must examine the submicroscopic structure of matter at dimensions unfamiliar to our senses (smaller than 10^{-10} m).

To journey into this submicroscopic realm we will leave our familiar world of solid, stable matter, and enter the violent world of charged particles vibrating, spinning, and orbiting at unimaginable speeds, creating powerful EM forces and containing kinetic energy beyond our imagination.[1] "This is where the action is" when light interacts with matter.

Atoms and molecules are in constant motion (kinetic energy). There are five levels of kinetic energy within each molecule:

1. Nuclear
2. Electron "orbits"
3. Vibration of atoms relative to "core atom" in molecule
4. Rotation of entire molecule
5. Translational motion—Brownian movement

To maintain stability within the molecule, it can exist only in specific, quantized energy levels at each of the first four kinetic energy levels. The laws of quantum mechanics predict these energy levels. Charged particles in motion produce EM fields. When a specific kinetic energy state (eg, electron orbits) moves to a lower allowable energy level, the molecule emits photons of EM energy that precisely equals the lost energy. Conversely, each molecule can absorb only those photons that contain the precise amount of EM energy that will move the lower energy state to a higher "allowable" quantized level. Thus each molecule can absorb only specific photons (wave lengths or frequencies)—absorption of laser EM energy is wave length dependent.

Laser energy interacts with four of the five kinetic energy levels within a molecule:

1. *Nuclear kinetic energy.* The powerful kinetic energy fields of protons, neutrons and the strong nuclear force are far beyond the quanta of laser energy and therefore lasers cannot affect the nucleus.
2. *Electron orbits (EM force).* Electrons are attracted by positively charged protons into specific "quantized orbits." There are relatively few orbits allowed. Thus laser wavelengths (eg, ultraviolet [UV] and visible) that interact with electron orbits will be specific for the target atoms and molecules.
3. *Vibrational kinetic energy.* Atoms are bound into molecules by sharing their outer orbital electrons. These covalent and ionic bonds are "elastic" and all atoms vibrate in relationship to the central core of the molecule. Molecules can exist in a large number of closely spaced vibration energy levels and thus lasers interacting with these levels (eg, mid-IR) are absorbed by most molecules.
4. *Rotational kinetic energy.* The entire molecule rotates as a unit. The allowable rotational frequencies are numerous and closely spaced. Far-IR and microwave EM energy interacts with this level of kinetic energy.
5. *Translational kinetic energy.* The three-dimensional motion of an entire molecule in relationship to its neighboring molecules (Brownian movement) results from the total amount of kinetic energy contained within the molecule. The average amount of translational energy within a system is termed "heat." The more Brownian movement, the hotter it is. The amount of translational energy determines whether that group of molecules will exist as a solid (lowest), liquid, or gas (highest). Using the photothermal effect of lasers, we raise the kinetic energy level of the target molecules by adding the laser's EM energy to the electron orbits (UV and visible), vibrational (near- and mid-IR) or rotational (microwaves) kinetic energy states. Thus we heat the target molecules to a gas (vaporize) or a liquid (coagulate).

TABLE 18–1 Site of electromagnetic photon absorption

KINETIC ENERGY	ELECTROMAGNETIC PHOTON
Nucleus	None
Electrons (orbital)	Ultraviolet, visible, and near-infrared
Atoms (vibrational)	Infrared
Kinetic energy molecule (rotational)	Microwave

Table 18–1 indicates the four levels of kinetic energy stored within a molecule and the types of EM photons that each kinetic energy level will emit or absorb.

Light is a form of EM energy field made of photons—quantized units of energy. One photon equals one complete wavelength of EM. The amount of energy within a photon is proportional to its frequency and inversely proportional to its wavelength. The EM spectrum is represented in Figure 18–1, which shows wavelengths in meters and frequencies in hertz. The lowest energy frequencies (longer wavelength radio waves) are on the left. As we move across the graph to the right, the amount of energy contained within each photon increases as its frequency increases and its wavelength shortens.

The laws of quantum mechanics dictate the selective absorption of laser photons by molecules. Higher energy laser photons (eg, UV and visible) have limited absorption because they can be absorbed only by those molecules capable of adding the precise quantum of laser EM to raise its electron orbits to

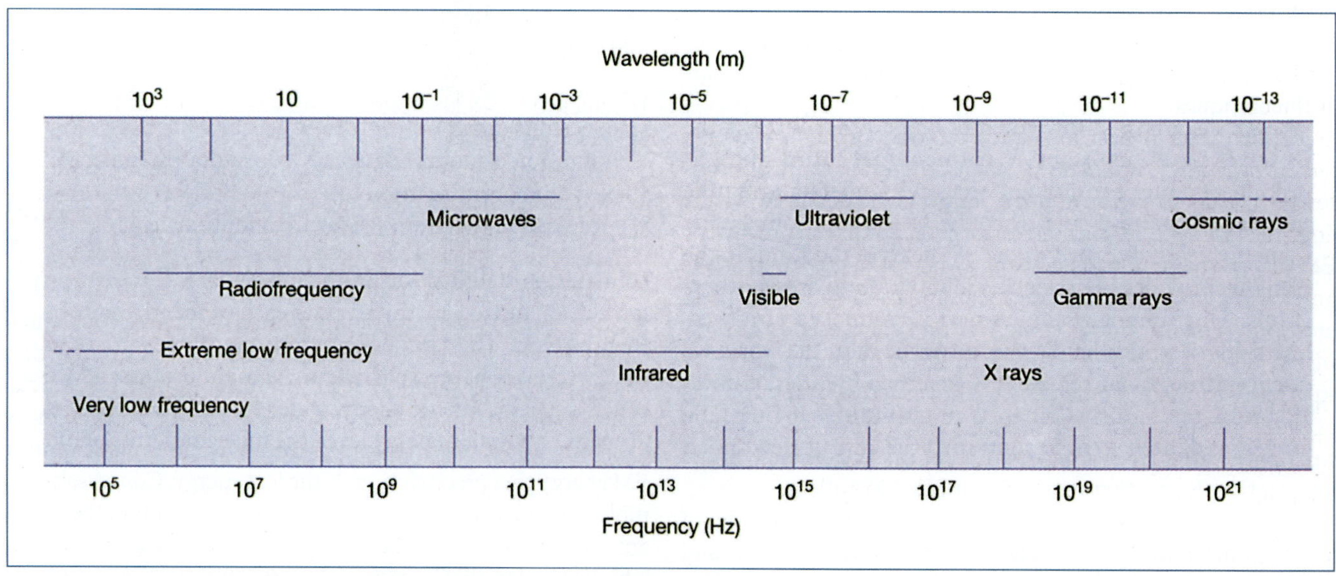

FIGURE 18–1 • Electromagnetic spectrum showing wavelengths (meters) and frequencies (hertz). Photon energy is proportional to frequency. Low-energy photons (low frequency, long wavelength) are on the left and high energy (high frequency, short wavelength) on the right.

one of the few allowable higher energy states. Conversely, lower energy laser photons (eg, mid-IR) are added to the many closely spaced atomic vibrational kinetic energy levels and thus are absorbed by most molecules.

Microwaves

The lower energy photons of microwaves (10^{-1}–10^{-3} M) are emitted and absorbed by the molecular rotation kinetic energy state. Though molecules can rotate at a large number of closely spaced frequencies, there are ideal "resonating" frequencies at which the molecule's EM fields are balanced. The ideal rotational kinetic energy state of water is 2,450 MHz—the frequency of an 11.8-cm microwave. Microwave ovens emit an 11.8-cm microwave because water selectively absorbs this EM wavelength and thus, more of the EM energy will heat the water of our coffee rather than its container.

Infrared

The IR wavelengths include far-IR (1,000–50 μ), mid-IR (50–2.5 μ), and near-IR (2.5–0.76 μ). Far-IR photons are emitted and absorbed by the translational motion and the molecular rotation of molecules. Every object warmer than its environment emits far-IR waves. "Night vision" optical instruments have photoelectric cells that detect this far-IR spectrum. There are no far-IR lasers.

Carbon dioxide (10.6 μ) and erbium YAG (2.9 μ) are in the mid-IR range. Atomic vibration kinetic energy states emit and absorb the mid-IR spectrum. Atoms are allowed to vibrate at many closely spaced frequencies but depending on its molecular bond, there are specific resonating frequencies whose quantum states are ideal. The hydrogen atoms of water ideally resonate at approximately 10^{14} Hz, the frequency of erbium YAG (2.9 μ); thus, erbium YAG is the EM photon best absorbed by water. Mid-IR lasers are absorbed by most molecules and until recently could not be transmitted by optical fibers. In 2007, OmniGuide® introduced a flexible fiber for delivery of CO_2 energy. The first generation product for ear surgery had a 0.9-mm outside diameter.

The near-IR photons are absorbed by outer electron orbits and by some atomic vibrational levels. Holmium YAG (2.1 μ) and neodynium YAG (1.06 μ) can be delivered efficiently by optical fibers. These lasers are used by several medical specialties including obstetrics/gynecology (OB/GYN), orthopedics, and cardiology. Because they possess higher energies and fewer molecules can absorb them, these lasers can be passed through optical fibers but tend to penetrate tissue deeply and scatter more readily than mid-IR lasers.

Visible Light

The visible spectrum (380–760 nm) is defined by those photons that are absorbed and activate photochemoreceptors in the human eye. Visible light photons are absorbed or emitted by the outer electron orbits of the atoms as these electron orbits rise and fall to specific allowable energy levels. Enhanced studies of visible spectra are important means of spectroscopically analyzing the electron structure of atoms and molecules. The blue-green argon (488 and 514 nm) laser photons are not absorbed by water molecules and readily pass through most of the molecules of our atmosphere. Red hemoglobin selectively absorbs these blue-green wavelengths. An object appears "red" in visible light because it reflects the red portion of the spectrum while absorbing the remainder of visible light photons.

Ultraviolet

The UV spectrum (1–380 nm) results from large transitions between allowable outer electron orbits. Ultraviolet photons contain higher energy than visible light and thus, are particularly useful for photodissociation of specific molecular bonds without heating molecules. The carbon-carbon double bond of collagen can specifically absorb 193 nm photons (argon fluoride [ArF]—excimer laser). This laser has been enormously successful in dividing collagen and reshaping the cornea without heating tissue (laser-assisted in situ keratomileusis [LASIK] procedure). Ultraviolet photons can also impart enough energy to cause an electron to escape the EM attraction of its original nucleus; thus, "ionizing" the atom. DNA and RNA are particularly sensitive to 248 and 312 nm. These UV wavelengths are potentially carcinogenic because they are capable of chemically altering the DNA and RNA sequences within cells. In our upper atmosphere, ozone absorbs most of the UV spectrum protecting us from the potentially harmful photons.

Lasers are unique forms of EM energy in that they are monochromatic (one wavelength), coherent (phase locked), and collimated (parallel waves). Depending on the laser's wavelength, the photons will interact with the molecules of the target tissue to produce:

1. Photothermal effects (eg, "heating" for coagulation or vaporization)
2. Photodissociation (eg, excimer laser for LASIK surgery)
3. Photoacoustic effects (eg, aluminum garnet laser for lithotripsy)
4. Photochemical effects (eg, UV lasers for photodynamic therapy)

Lasers have been employed in otology for their photothermal effects to vaporize bone (stapedotomy), collagen (stapedectomy revision), tumors (acoustic neuroma, glomus tympanicum, cholesteatoma, granulation tissue), or to coagulate blood vessels. The EM laser energy is absorbed by the EM fields, thus raising the molecular translational energy of electron orbits, atom vibrations, or molecular rotations. As the molecule's translational motion increases, the physical state of those molecules will change from solid to liquid to gas. Coagulation of blood vessels occurs when the collagen translational energy is raised enough to liquefy the collagen and then as it cools, it congeals into a solid mass—obliterating its lumen. Vaporization occurs when the molecule's translational energy is increased sufficiently enough to convert its physical state from solid to gas.

LASER TISSUE INTERACTION—LABORATORY STUDIES

Early applications for otologic lasers focused on otosclerosis—laser stapedotomy and laser stapedectomy revision. Four requirements are essential to safely apply laser energy to the stapes footplate (stapedotomy) or to the collagen sealing the oval

TABLE 18–2 Lasers for otosclerosis safety requirements
Optics
Bone and collagen absorption
No heating of perilymph
No damage to inner ear or facial nerve

window (stapedectomy revision) without damaging the inner ear or facial nerve (Table 18–2):

1. Precise optics
2. Efficient absorption by the bone and collagen
3. Minimal heating of perilymph
4. No damage to inner ear structures from photons transmitted through the perilymph

In the early 1980s, the use of argon and KTP lasers to perform stapedotomies became increasingly popular.[2–4] Until 1985, these were the only lasers that had satisfactory optical precision for microscopic ear surgery. Though little laboratory work had been done to establish their safety, clinical studies of visible laser stapedotomy demonstrated that they were safe and effective for vaporizing stapes bone. Could argon lasers be used for stapedectomy revision to improve our clinical results? If the oval window collagen neomembrane could gradually be vaporized without damage to the inner ear, the precise cause for the conductive hearing loss could be identified, the old prosthesis safely removed, and a new prosthesis stabilized in the center of the oval window. Argon lasers were being used by ophthalmologists to coagulate retinal blood vessels, specifically because they were not absorbed by the collagen of the cornea, lens, or ocular fluid.

THERMOCOUPLE EXPERIMENTS

By 1985, Sharplan had developed its first microscope delivery system that provided optical precision satisfactory for ear surgery. In the laboratories of the Midwest Ear Foundation (MEF), a series of thermocouple experiments were performed to evaluate the relative merits of each of argon, KTP, and CO_2 surgical lasers and to establish safe energy parameters for both stapedotomy and stapedectomy revision (Figure 18–2).[5–6] The 0.6-mm stapedotomies were vaporized in fresh human stapes footplates with appropriate energy settings using 0.2-mm "rosettes" for argon and KTP lasers, and a 0.6-mm-diameter pulsed CO_2 beam. Thin allograft collagen was then placed in an open oval window was then vaporized to simulate stapedectomy revision. Finally, all of the lasers were focused on surface perilymph to evaluate heating versus transmission effects.

These thermocouple experiments were designed to test all four requirements for safely using a laser to perform stapedotomy and stapedectomy revision (Table 18–2). Following data analysis, the author drew the following conclusions:

1. Provided safe energy parameters were used, argon, KTP, and CO_2 lasers could be used safely for laser stapedotomy.
2. The focused argon and KTP beams are not well absorbed by collagen, readily pass through the perilymph without absorption, and potentially could damage the inner ear. Therefore, the author recommended using a pulsed CO_2 beam for stapedectomy revision.

Many otologists who were successfully using argon and KTP lasers for stapedotomy challenged the experimental design of these thermocouple experiments claiming that the black thermocouple did not measure perilymph temperature change. This is true. However, the experiment was designed to measure all the EM energy that passed through the stapes, both those photons that were absorbed by perilymph (heating it) and those that passed through the perilymph that could potentially damage the inner ear. A second criticism was that only a focused argon and KTP laser beam was used for stapedotomy. This also was true. A KTP 200-μ fiber did not deliver enough energy to consistently vaporize a rosette into the footplate. The Gherini/Horn EndoOtoprobe® had not yet been invented for argon laser.

Several years later, Gherini redesigned the thermocouple experiments and performed argon stapedotomy with the HGM EndoOtoprobe®.[7] He used a silver thermocouple positioned in the vestibule but away from the stapes bone. He stated that he found "no significant change in perilymph temperature," concluding that the argon EndoOtoprobe® is safe because of the rapid dilution

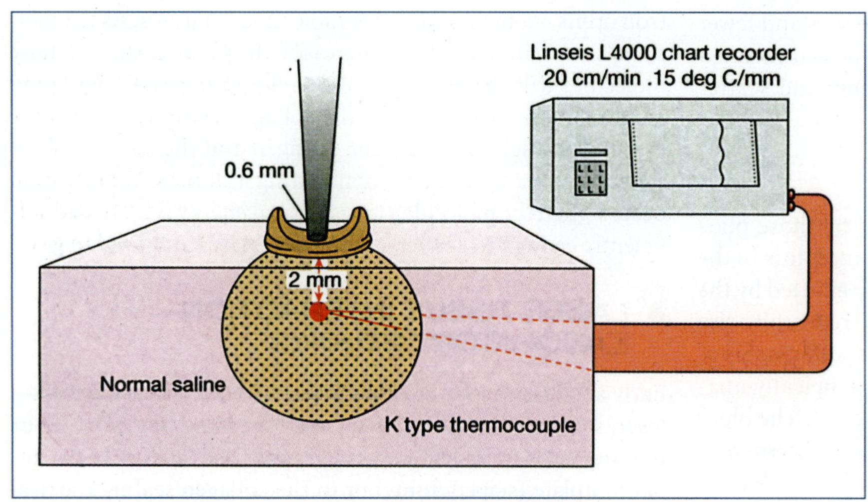

FIGURE 18–2 • Laser stapedotomy performed with argon, KTP, and CO_2 lasers. Ultrasensitive thermocouple in vestibule measure EM energy transmitted through stapes footplate (Midwest Ear Foundation—1984).

of energy caused by the 14-degree tip diffusion angle of the EndoOtoprobe®. Gherini, indeed, was measuring only perilymph temperature change. He was not measuring the argon EM energy that was being transmitted into the inner ear for three reasons:

1. Argon photons are not absorbed by perilymph and will not heat it.
2. The silver thermocouple will reflect argon photons and not measure them.
3. The silver thermocouple was positioned outside the diameter of the laser beam. Argon energy would pass directly into the inner ear without contacting the thermocouple.

There are many otologists who have reported the safe use of argon and KTP lasers for stapedotomy (both focused and fiber optic).[8,9,10] The author, however, continues to warn the surgeon to avoid applying visible lasers directly into the open vestibule.[11,12] Safe laser use is enhanced when the surgeon understands laser tissue interaction. Isolated cases of laser-induced postoperative nerve deafness, facial paralysis, and dizziness have occurred, particularly following laser stapedectomy revision. After confidentially discussing specific cases of complications with the involved surgeon, it became evident that the inner ear or facial nerve damage was indeed caused by inappropriate use of the CO_2 or visible laser. The most common error with the CO_2 laser was using the wrong energy parameter setting (average power for pulsed lasers is very misleading—see below). The common error was using a visible laser for revision techniques that were designed to be safe only with the CO_2 laser. This chapter was written to help otologic laser surgeons avoid such complications in the future.

The controversy between visible and IR otologic lasers continues to this day. It can be resolved by understanding how EM energy interacts with tissue. The EM wavelength is the single most important factor that determines its absorption by water, collagen, or bone. The spectral characteristics of water have been known for over a century. Many spectroscopy and fluence threshold experiments have studied the absorption characteristics of bone and collagen from UV through the IR spectrum.

Bone

Mechanism of Bone Vaporization

Izatt et al. vaporized bone with a dozen different lasers in the UV, visible, and IR spectrums.[13] Vaporization occurs when the molecules composing a solid or liquid absorb enough EM energy to raise their translational energy levels (heat) to the boiling point at which time the physical state of the molecule changes to a gas. Table 18–3 lists the chemical composition of bone and the respective boiling points of these components.

TABLE 18–3 Bone vaporization boiling temperature

COMPOSITION OF BONE	BOILING POINT
Hydroxylapatite 75%	~1,500°C
Collagen 20%	~300°C
Water 5%	100°C

The Laser Biomedical Research Center at Massachusetts Institute of Technology (MIT) in Boston has studied the wavelength dependency of bone vaporization. High-speed photography documented what occurred during laser vaporization of bone (Figure 18–3). Because the boiling point of hydroxyapatite is so high (1,500°C), both water (100°C) and collagen (300°C) are vaporized first carrying the free hydroxyapatite crystals into the air. Therefore, to ablate bone, the ideal laser wavelength should be absorbed readily by water and collagen. This fact is particularly fortunate for choosing the ideal wavelength for otosclerosis surgery because the same wavelength would be ideal for laser stapedotomy (bone) and laser stapedectomy revision (collagen), while the surface perilymph will protect the inner ear.

Fluence Thresholds

Izatt then performed fluence threshold experiments measuring the lowest energy levels (mJ/mm²) required for each laser to begin to vaporize surface bone molecules.[13] The lower the fluence threshold, the more efficiently the target bone absorbs that photon. Table 18–4 lists the mean fluence thresholds determined by Izatt's experiments for the wavelengths relevant to otologic surgery.

Transmission Spectroscopy—Stapes Bone

To evaluate which photons are best absorbed by the stapes bone, the Biomedical Laser Research Laboratories performed transmission spectroscopy in the UV through far-IR range (research supported by MEF).[14] Figures 18–4 to 18–7 graphically illustrate

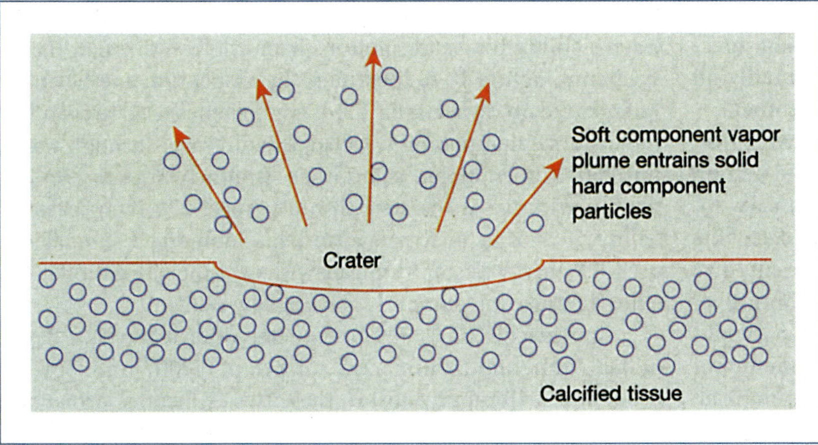

FIGURE 18–3 • Bone vaporization with laser. With sufficient fluence, photothermal effect of laser boils water and collagen. Hydroxyapatite particles are entrained in the vapor flume.

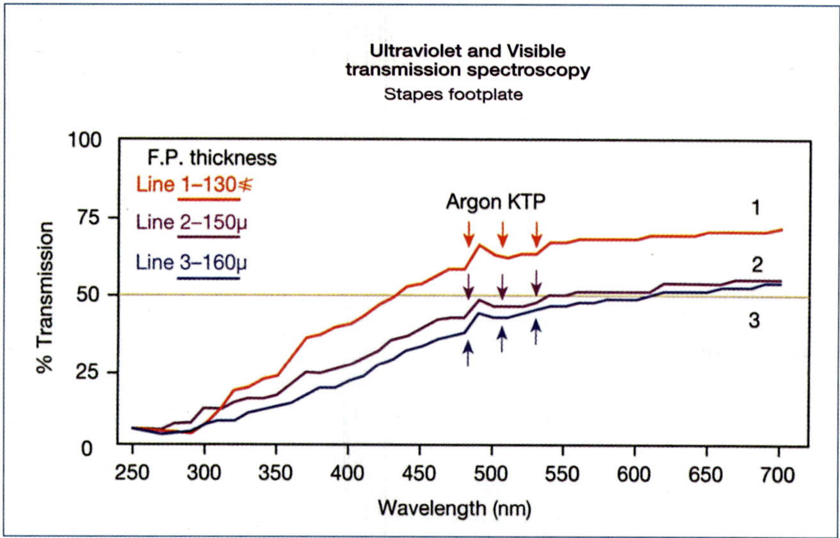

FIGURE 18–4 • Wavelength dependency of stapes footplate absorption—UV and visible wavelengths 250nm–300 nm (excimer lasers) are well absorbed. Visible photons around 500 nm (argon and KTP lasers—arrows) are not very well absorbed with approximately 50% of this wavelength passing through a footplate of average thickness (150 μ).

TABLE 18–4 Bone vaporization fluence thresholds

LASES	WAVELENGTH (μ)	BONE ABLATION FLUENCE THRESHOLDS (mJ/mm²)
XeCl	0.308	12
ErbYAG	2.9	12
CO_2	10.6	15
Ar	0.488 and 0.514	150
KTP	0.532	155

Ar, argon; CO_2, carbon dioxide; ErbYAG, erbium yttrium aluminum garnet; KTP, potassium titanyl phosphate; XeCl, xenon chloride.

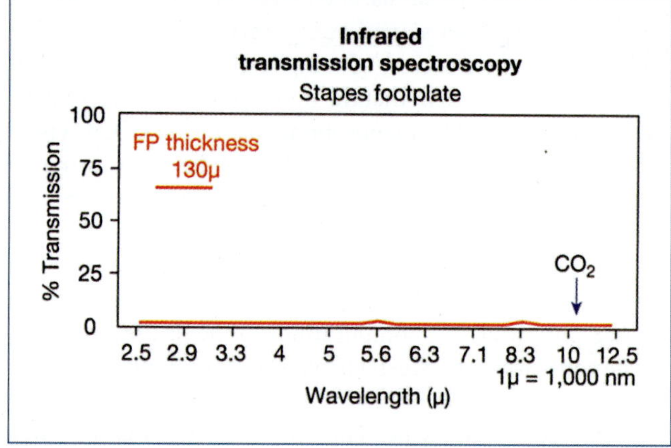

FIGURE 18–5 • Wavelength dependency of stapes footplate absorption—IR. The IR spectrum from 2.5–12.5 μ is completely absorbed by even the thinnest stapes footplate (130 μ).

the results. Figure 18–4 graphs the percentage of UV and visible light that was transmitted through the center of three different fresh stapes footplates that varied in thickness from 130 to 160 μ. The energy that was not transmitted was absorbed by the footplate bone (reflection and scatter is negligible). The stapes footplate selectively absorbs nearly all the energy in the 250 to 300 nm wavelengths (UV) and little is transmitted through even the thinnest footplate. The wavelengths of argon (488 and 512 nm) and KTP (532 nm) are highlighted with arrows. Absorption of these photons by the stapes footplate is only fair and an average of 50% of argon and KTP EM energy is transmitted through the footplate. Figure 18–5 illustrates the IR transmission spectroscopy on the thinnest stapes footplate (130 μ). Essentially, all the IR photons from 2.5 to 12.5 μ were completely absorbed.

To obtain a more sensitive evaluation of the IR wavelengths, the stapes footplate was then sectioned into a 10-μ thin section and the IR transmission spectroscopy repeated (Figure 18–6). Three-micron photons are completely absorbed within 10 μ of the stapes bone (the domain of the erbium YAG laser). Seventy-five percent of CO_2 laser photons (10.6 μ) were absorbed within 10 μ. Therefore, 100% of CO_2 laser energy would be absorbed at a depth of 50 μ in the stapes bone. Figure 18–7 illustrates the amount of EM energy that is transmitted through an average stapes footplate (150 μ) during vaporization with argon, KTP, and CO_2 lasers.

Water

Transmission Spectroscopy—Water

Most soft tissues in the human body contain 50–75% intracellular water. Laser ablation of soft tissue occurs when the intracellular water is heated to boiling—exploding the cell. The wavelength dependency of laser tissue interaction becomes readily apparent because there is an enormous variability in water's ability to absorb photons from the UV through the IR spectrum. Figure 18–8 illustrates the absorption coefficient of water based on wavelength.[15] This coefficient is used to calculate the distance that photon wavelength will travel through water, until 50% of irradiance is absorbed. In practical terms, an EM photon with 0.5-μ wavelength must travel 229 ft in seawater before 50% of its energy is absorbed. Submerged submarines use KTP energy to communicate with orbiting navigational satellites because it is so poorly absorbed by water.

Conversely, CO_2 is 50% attenuated after it travels a depth of 0.007 mm and erbium YAG a depth of 0.0007 mm. Surface perilymph will rapidly absorb these two IR beams, protecting the inner ear. However, these beams must be pulsed in brief microsecond bursts to prevent thermal spread from the surface of the perilymph to deeper layers in the vestibule.

Collagen

Transmission Spectroscopy—Collagen

Yannas performed transmission spectroscopy in the UV through far-IR wavelengths on powdered bovine collagen and hot cast gelatin to determine which EM wavelengths collagen best absorbs.[16]

Though various thicknesses of collagen were used for UV, visible, and IR light, the author has extrapolated the data for a 10-μ thick section of collagen in Table 18–5. This table lists the efficiency of absorption by collagen for the photons of the otologic lasers. Collagen absorbs erbium YAG the best and KTP the worst.

TABLE 18–5 Transmission spectroscopy

LASER	ABSORPTION
Erbium yttrium aluminum garnet (2.9 μ)	93%
Carbon dioxide (10.6 μ)	61%
Argon (0.488 and 0.512 μ)	28%
Potassium titanyl phosphate (0.532 μ)	18%

Histologic Studies—Laser Stapedotomy

A wide range of surgical lasers were used to perform stapedotomy on both human and animal bones and then evaluated histologically with both light and electron microscopy.[17–21] These studies were performed to evaluate the relative merits of various lasers' wavelength for creating "a clean laser crater" with little damage to the surrounding tissue. In addition, the ideal energy parameters were determined.[21]

As one reviews the details of these histologic studies, a consistent theme resonates through all of these studies. The cleanest and safest stapedotomies were produced by those wavelengths that were best absorbed by the stapes bone. Because these wavelengths required less energy to vaporize the bone and because there was less photon scatter, laser energy was precisely

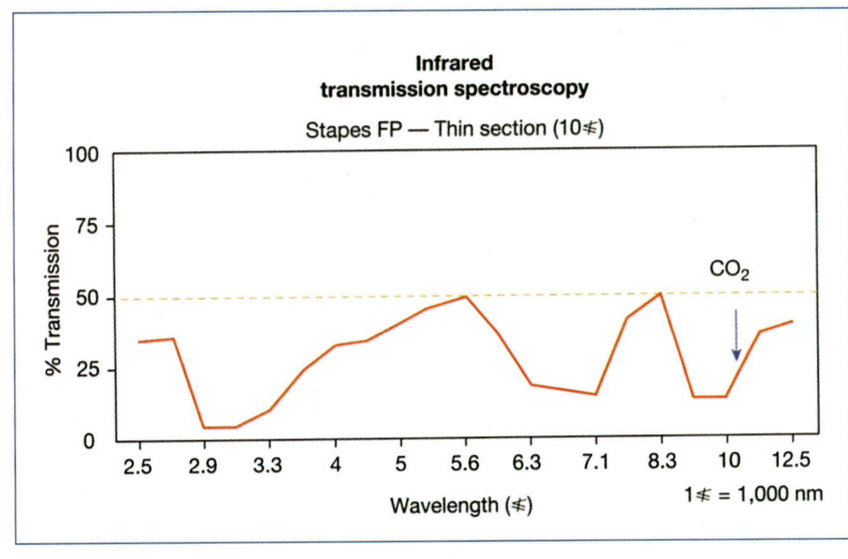

FIGURE 18–6 • Selective IR absorption by ultrathin (10 μ) stapes footplate. Photons with wavelengths 2.9–3.1 μ (erbium YAG 2.94 μ) are completely absorbed by the stapes footplate within 10 μ. Seventy-five percent of CO_2 laser photons (10.2 μ) are absorbed in the first 10 μ of stapes footplate thickness.

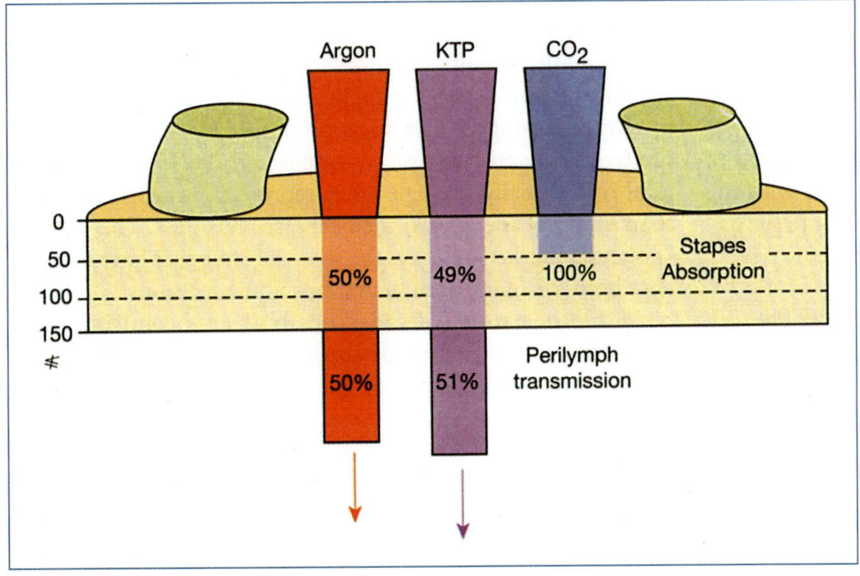

FIGURE 18–7 • Summary of transmission spectroscopy of human stapes footplate for argon, KTP, and CO_2 lasers.

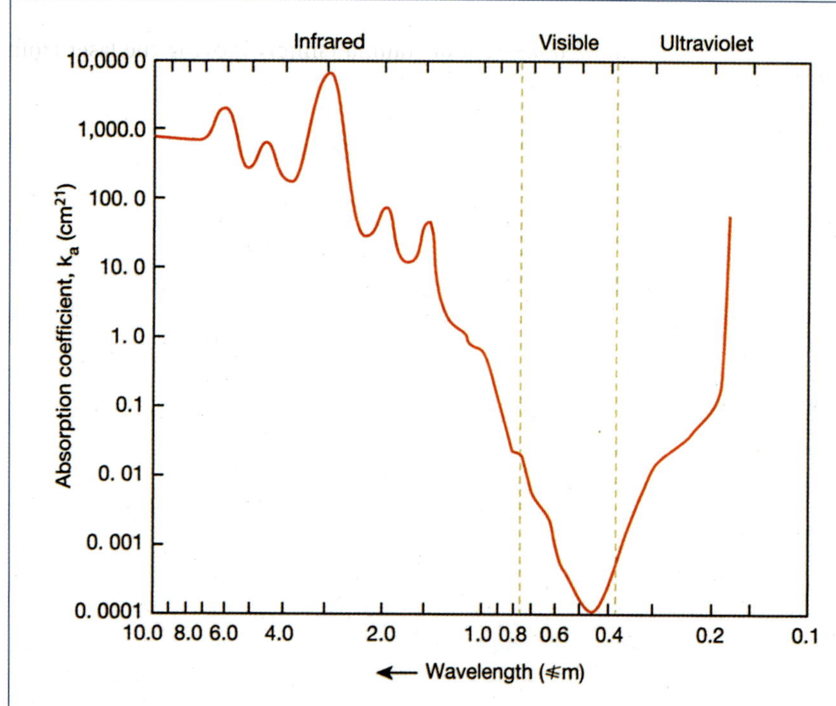

FIGURE 18–8 • Attenuation of seawater as a function of wavelength. EM wavelengths at 0.5 μ (argon and KTP) will travel 229 ft before half of the energy is absorbed. Fifty percent attenuation of irradiance occurs within 0.0007 mm for erbium YAG (2.94 μ) and 0.007 mm for CO_2 (10.6 μ). *Reproduced with permission from The Infrared Handbook, Office of Naval Research, pp. 3–107.*

converted to heating the tissue beneath the laser beam. Damage to the margins of the crater is further reduced by pulsing the laser in tiny microsecond bursts, limiting thermal spread by conduction through the tissue.

Summary

Quantum theory predicts that each molecule can absorb or emit only specific wavelength photons—those photons whose quanta of energy specifically equals the quanta of EM energy that has been gained or lost as the molecule moves among the various allowable energy levels in its four kinetic energy states. The laboratory studies confirm that laser tissue interaction is dependent on the laser's wavelength. To produce photothermal effects (vaporize or coagulate), those wavelengths that are best absorbed by the target tissue are the safest to use because there is less energy transmission and scatter through the tissue and because lower power densities can be used. For the well-absorbed photon, thermal conductivity through the tissue should be limited by pulsing the laser beam.

There was remarkable consistency between the date compiled with thermocouple studies, spectroscopy of the stapes bone, collagen and water, and histologic studies. As applied to otosclerosis surgery, these laboratory tests combined with the clinical experience of many surgeons lead this author to the following conclusions:

1. Provided safe energy parameters and surgical techniques are followed, argon, KTP, erbium YAG, and CO_2 lasers can be used safely for stapedotomy.
2. Because visible laser photons are poorly absorbed by both collagen and water, focused (microscope delivered) argon and KTP energy should not be aimed directly into the vestibule.
3. Infrared laser energy should be pulsed in microsecond bursts to minimize thermal spread to the inner ear.
4. The defocused argon EndoOtoprobe® beam is the safest visible laser to use for ear surgery.
5. The surgical techniques described for CO_2 laser stapedectomy revision can also be performed with the erbium YAG laser but should not be attempted with argon or KTP.

OTOLOGIC SURGICAL LASERS

The medical laser industry is a rapidly changing, highly competitive business. New surgical applications for lasers are occurring in every specialty at a very rapid rate, often requiring unique laser delivery systems and energy parameters. Acceptance of these new procedures occurs at a more gradual pace, when clinical studies confirm the advantage of a new laser technique over nonlaser alternatives.

Laser companies are pressured to produce lasers with a great deal of versatility so that a particular surgical laser can be used by many surgical specialties. With dwindling resources, hospitals' laser committees will usually only approve the purchase of a new laser if it has multispecialty applications. These laser committees usually require special certification training by the surgeon and the technical assistant because of perceived additional medical legal risks. Finally, otologic lasers represent a tiny fraction (less than 0.1%) of the overall medical laser business. This limited "potential market" restricts the leverage otologists have to influence both the manufacturer and hospitals' decisions.

Over the past two decades, nearly 20 laser companies producing otologic lasers have disappeared (merger or bankruptcy). In December, 2007, only four laser companies were producing otologic lasers:

1. HGM (argon): HGM Medical Laser Systems
3959 West 1820 South
Salt Lake City, Utah 84104

2. Laserscope (KTP): Laserscope
   3070 Orchard Dr.
   San Jose, California, 95134-2011
3. Zeiss (erbium YAG): Carl Zeiss
   D-73446
   Oberkochen, Germany
4. Lumenis (CO_2): Merger between Coherent and ESC Sharplan
   2400 Condensa St.
   Santa Clara, California, 95051

Visible Lasers

In 1980, Perkins reported a small series of 11 successful laser stapedotomies performed with a microscope-mounted focused argon beam.[2] He concluded that the lasers reduced mechanical trauma and increased surgical precision, should improve hearing results, and should reduce postoperative dysequilibrium compared to nonlaser stapedotomy. In 1983, McGee published a series of 100 consecutive argon laser stapedotomies.[3] Hearing results were similar between McGee's laser and nonlaser patients, but the laser patients were less dizzy postoperatively. These argon lasers had originally been designed for ophthalmology by Coherent. The continuous mode argon energy was carried by a fiber-optic cable to a microscope-mounted "micromanipulator" that then delivered a focused argon beam to the operative field. At a 250-mm focal length, the spot size could be focused down to 0.05 mm.

The HGM argon EndoOtoprobe® developed under the guidance of Gherini and Horn was introduced to otologists in the late 1980s.[7] This handheld probe conveniently delivers an argon beam with a spot size of 200 µ. The 14-degree diffusion angle rapidly increased the spot size as the distance from the probe tip increased.

The KTP laser developed by Laserscope™ under the direction of Perkins is still the only 532-nm laser available for otologic surgery.[4] Its laser energy is delivered via microscope-mounted micromanipulator. Laserscope™ has developed several fiber-optic handheld probes. They do not deliver sufficient power density to vaporize stapes bone.

These two visible lasers have ideal optical properties. The laser can be conveniently delivered to the microscope-mounted micromanipulator or a handheld probe through a fiber-optic cable. The micromanipulator can focus the visible beam down to 0.05 mm spot size at 250 mm focal length. Because argon and KTP are visible, the laser beam is used at a lower power for the "aiming" beam. Therefore, the laser will always hit the tissue exactly where it was aimed and with the same spot size of energy (parfocal and coaxial). Until 1985, these two visible lasers were the only lasers that were optically precise enough to use for otologic surgery.

Infrared CO_2 Lasers

Though CO_2 lasers are the most widely used medical lasers for tissue coagulation and vaporization, the inherent optical properties of the IR CO_2 laser made the early models too imprecise for the rigid demands of microscopic surgery. Optical fibers will not transmit CO_2 laser; therefore, the beam was delivered from the lasing console to a microscope-mounted micromanipulator by a series of 13 mirrors and lenses called the "flexible arm." A minimal amount of trauma (simply moving the laser from room to room) could misalign one or more of these mirrors. A second visible laser beam (helium-neon [HeNe]—632 nm) is required to aim the invisible CO_2 laser beam. This introduces another optical problem—chromatic aberration. When light passes through a lens, it is refracted inversely proportional to its wavelength. As both beams pass through the same focusing lens, the visible HeNe beam is refracted (bent) to a much greater degree than the longer CO_2 beam. It was nearly impossible to keep the HeNe beam and CO_2 beams parfocal and coaxial and the separation worsened with optical misalignment of the mirrors and lenses. Finally, because of its long wavelength, at 250 mm focal length, the early CO_2 beams could only be focused to a 2-mm spot size.

In the mid-1980s, researchers at Sharplan were experimenting with CO_2 laser reanastomosis of small blood vessels. This application required much greater optical precision. Their engineers developed a microscope-mounted micromanipulator that could focus the CO_2 beam down to 0.5 mm. This prototype model was used by the author for the stapes thermocouple experiments performed in the MEF laboratories and later was the first CO_2 laser used in the operating room for stapedotomy and stapedectomy revision.[5,6]

The early CO_2 lasers were less convenient to use in the operating room than the visible lasers. Each time the flexible arm was attached or detached from the micromanipulator, the operating microscope had to be rebalanced. To ensure proper alignment, the CO_2 laser was test-fired preoperatively. A technician routinely realigned the CO_2 and HeNe beams every few months. In the early models, the alignment of the HeNe beam and CO_2 beam could not be adjusted by the surgeon.

Since the mid-1980s, Sharplan has continued to refine the optical precision and reliability of its flexible arm—stabilizing the reflecting mirrors and permitting quick readjustment should misalignment ever occur. Its micromanipulator also has been improved. The initial "Microslad®" allowed focusing the beam size down to 0.2 mm. In the mid-1990s, the "Accuspot®" could reliably focus the spot size to 0.05 mm at 275 mm focal length. Recently, Sharplan introduced "Accublade®," a computer-driven vibrating mirror that distributes a 0.05-mm CO_2 beam homogeneously throughout the area of a target whose shape and size is determined by the surgeon. "Accublade®" vaporizes bone and collagen with remarkable precision and minimal thermal spread.

Finally, the convenience of CO_2 lasers for otologic microsurgery has also been improved. The laser cabinet can be mounted on the base of an operating microscope. The flexible arm parallels the microscope arm, no longer limiting the freedom of motion of the microscope. The laser can now remain attached to the microscope at all times. Preoperative test-firing and microscope counterbalancing are no longer required.

In 2007, OmniGuide introduced an otologic fiber that, for the first time, delivers CO_2 laser energy with a handheld probe. The first-generation OmniGuide fiber for otology had an outside diameter of 0.9 mm and is satisfactory for most otologic applications including stapedotomy and stapedectomy

TABLE 18–6 Energy parameters of visible (nonpulsed) and infrared (pulsed) lasers

ENERGY PARAMETERS—VISIBLE (NONPULSED) LASERS

	M.D. SETTINGS				ENERGY DELIVERED	
LASER	AVERAGE POWER (W)	MODE	PULSE DURATION (sec)	SPOT SIZE (mm)	PEAK POWER (W)	TOTAL FLUENCE (mJ/mm^2)
Argon (Endo-Otoprobe®)	2	Continuous	0.1	0.2	2	6,451
KTP (Laserscope®)	2	Q-switched (Quasi-continuous)	0.1	0.05	6 (30% duty cycle)	103,216
	2		0.1	0.2		6,450

ENERGY PARAMETERS—INFRARED (PULSED) LASERS

	M.D. SETTINGS				MICROPULSE ENERGY				
LASER	AVERAGE POWER (W)	MODE	PULSE DURATION (sec)	SPOT SIZE (mm)	PEAK POWER (W)	PULSE WIDTH (millisec)	MJ/ PULSE	NO. OF PULSES	TOTAL FLUENCE (mJ/mm^2)
Sharplan CO_2									
734	3.6	Superpulse	0.1	0.5	36	0.6	21.6	8	400
1040	2	Superpulse	0.1	0.5	280	0.09	25.2	2	117
1100A	Flexilase© #7	Chopped	0.1	0.5	130	0.075	9.75	20	450
Coherent CO_2									
5000C	Ultrapulse© #10	Chopped	0.1	0.5	120	0.08	10	20	465
Luxar Novapulse with OmniGuide OTO-S Fiber	6	Superpulse	0.1	0.3	65	0.1	16	16	229
Erbium YAG Zeiss OPMI ®TwinER	(20 mJ)	Pulsed	0.2	200	0.1	20	1	639	
	(70 mJ)	Continuous	0.6	350	0.2	70	1	240	

revision. The spot size at the tip is 0.25 mm (0.3–1 mm from the tip) the laser energy at the tip of the fiber is 50% reduced. The surgeon should double the laser settings to maintain effective and safe energy parameters (see Table 18–6).

OmniGuide has developed adaptors for Luxar Novapulse (Lumenis) CO_2 laser. Adaptors for various other CO_2 laser models were refined and have been available from 2008. In 2008, OmniGuide introduced the beampath OTO-S Fiber (0.5 mm outside diameter) specifically for more precise requirements of otosclerosis surgery. The advantage of a CO_2 handheld probe is its convenience and reliability. It eliminates the misalignment of the microscope-mounted CO_2 laser and its HeNe aiming beam that can occur when the flexible arm is roughly handled.

Infrared Erbium Yttrium Aluminum Garnet

In the late 1990s, Zeiss perfected a microscope-mounted erbium YAG laser designed specifically for ear surgery (OPMI®TwinER). As described earlier, spectroscopy studies on water, collagen, and bone and histologic experiments on both human and animal stapes suggested that this laser wavelength would be the most ideal for bone and collagen vaporization for otologic surgery. After extensive animal experiments and clinical human trials, the OPMI®TwinER was approved for otosclerosis surgery in Europe in 1997 and in the United States in early 1999.[22] As predicted, it vaporizes a precise stapedotomy with little lateral spread of energy (no charring and no significant heating of perilymph).

However, this efficient photon absorption introduces two disadvantages:

1. Hemostasis is poor because the lack of lateral thermal spread prevents the coagulation of blood vessels at the periphery of the laser crater.
2. A photoacoustic wave is produced and theoretically, if large enough, could damage hair cells.[21]

SAFE ENERGY PARAMETERS

Besides the laser's wavelength, two additional factors determine its effect upon tissue:

1. Power density (W/mm^2)
2. Fluence (mJ/mm^2)—the time that the power density is applied to the tissue.

Power density is determined by the watts of power delivered divided by its spot size. The power density will vary inversely to the area of the spot size. Therefore, reducing the diameter of the spot size in half increases the power density fourfold.

Fluence (mJ/mm^2) is calculated by multiplying power density (W/mm^2) times the total time that power density is striking the tissue. Fluence calculations for visible lasers are straightforward because these beams are delivered in a continuous mode (KTP—"quasi-continuous"). Infrared lasers are pulsed. When the surgeon sets a Sharplan 1100 or a Coherent 500C laser on *superpulse mode* and then adjusts the power to 5 W (*average power*) and 0.1 sec pulse duration, he is actually delivering a single micropulse with a peak power of 600 W and a micropulse width of 0.075 milliseconds. This micropulse is too powerful for vaporizing the stapes.

Table 18–6 tabulates the safe energy parameters for stapedotomy that were established by thermocouple experiments in the MEF laboratories for each of these lasers (except erbium YAG). The first four columns (average power, mode, pulse duration, spot size) are the variables that the surgeon adjusts. One column (peak power) is required for defining how the laser energy is being delivered for the continuous or quasi-continuous visible lasers. To determine energy characteristics of the pulsed IR laser the four characteristics of each micropulse must be known—peak power (W), pulse width (millisecond), work (mJ/micropulse), and number of micropulses. The final column compares the fluence levels (mJ/mm^2) actually being delivered to the tissue.

Visible Lasers

Two Watts of argon laser are delivered in a continuous mode by a 200-μ EndoOtoprobe® (Figure 18–9). Spot size at the probe tip is 0.2 mm and rapidly enlarges as the distance from the probe tip increases.

KTP lasers (Laserscope) are focused on the operative field by a microscope-mounted micromanipulator. Because KTP lasers are q-switched, an average power setting of 2 W actually delivers 780 micropulses in 0.1 sec (Figure 18–10). Each micropulse contains 6 W of peak power. Q-switching behaves like a continuous beam (quasi-continuous) because there is not enough time interval between each micropulse to allow for tissue cooling. Therefore, average power (30% duty cycle × 6 W peak power = 2 W) can be used to define the laser/tissue effect.

Because these two wavelengths are particularly well absorbed by hemoglobin, argon and KTP can be used to efficiently vaporize small amounts of vascular tissue, such as granulation tissue, small glomus, or small fragments of acoustic neuroma. Stapes bone vaporization can be enhanced by placing a small droplet of blood on the footplate (chromophore) or by overlapping rosettes (char). Because of poor absorption by water, visible lasers are inefficient for vaporizing most soft tissues and should not be aimed directly into the vestibule since the perilymph will not protect the inner ear.

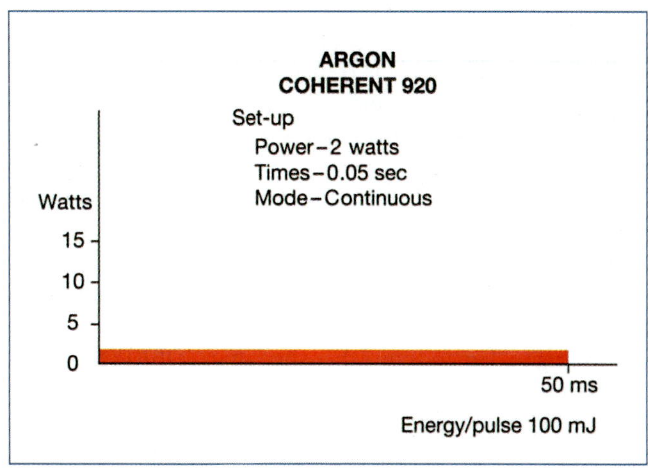

FIGURE 18–9 • Argon lasers are generated in continuous mode. With 2 W of average power—100 mJ of work are delivered to the operative field in 0.05 sec.

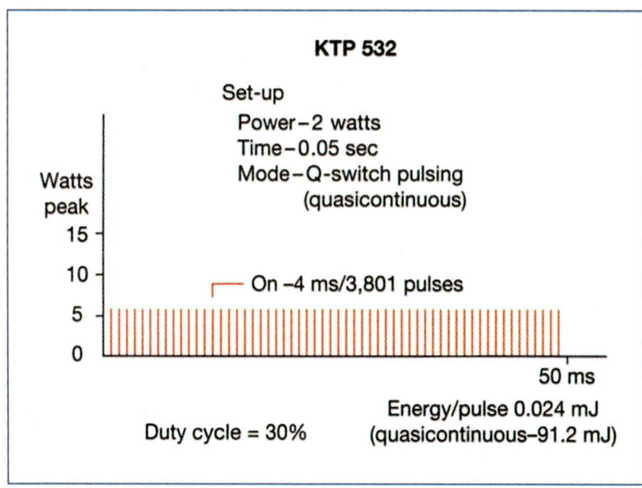

FIGURE 18–10 • KTP lasers are q-switched in a rapid succession of microsecond pulses. Because the micropulse interval is extremely short (8 μsec), there is little time for tissue cooling. Therefore, tissue response is similar to continuous beam (quasi-continuous). At 2-W average power, the surgeon delivers 91.2 mJ of work in 0.05 sec.

Infrared Lasers

Focused CO_2 laser energy is transmitted to the operative field by microscope-mounted micromanipulators. The energy can be delivered in one of three modes: continuous, chopped, or superpulsed.

When vaporizing tissue, efficiency is improved and thermal spread reduced by pulsing the energy in a series of micropulses with high peak power (W) that are on for a fraction of a millisecond. Figure 18–11 illustrates the pulsing parameters of Sharplan 734, the first CO_2 laser used by the author in 1985. Responding to demands by other specialties (OB/GYN, neurosurgery, general surgery) for more efficient tissue vaporization, Sharplan began progressively increasing the peak power of each micropulse while reducing its pulse width. Within a decade, Sharplan had raised its superpulse from 36 W (model #734) to 600 W (model #1100). Average power setting did not change this peak power but merely changed the number of 600-W micropulses that were being delivered. At its lowest setting (5 W average power) the 1100 was actually delivering 600 W of power, which was much too powerful for the delicate requirements for stapedotomy. This progression in pulsing power is analogous to bombarding the target with B-B's (small packets of energy) using the sharplan #734 versus a 70-mm machine gun (large packets of energy) with the sharplan #1100.

The ideal energy parameters for laser stapes vaporization were established in the MEF laboratory. Each micropulse should contain between 10–20 mJ of energy (peak W × micropulse width). Greater than 25 mJ/micropulse caused "flaring"—a literal microscopic explosion where a microflame could be seen rising toward the facial nerve.

By the mid-1990s, the two largest CO_2 laser companies (Sharplan and Coherent) were producing pulsed CO_2 lasers whose micropulses were delivering 500–600 W of peak power. The problem was that average power was adjusted not by changing peak power but by changing the number of micropulses being delivered per second. New software programs were developed in the late 1990s to accommodate the needs of otologic microsurgery. Sharplan developed Flexilase© for its 1100A, 1041S, and 1055S—a chopped mode that delivers 130 W of peak power and 9.75 mJ/micropip (Figure 18–12). Coherent 5,000C followed suit with an ultrapulse setting. Ultrapulse© at 10 mJ setting delivers 120 W peak power and 10 mJ/micropulse.

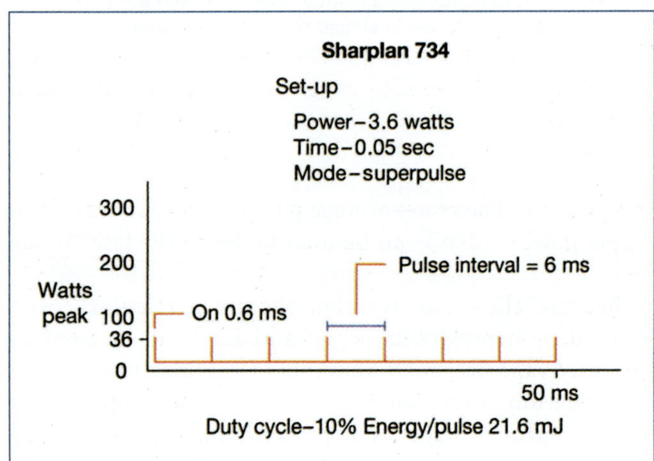

FIGURE 18–11 • CO_2 laser for tissue vaporization are delivered in superpulse mode. This early Sharplan laser had ideal energy characteristics for laser stapedotomy. Each micropulse contained 21.6 mJ of energy and a total of 173 mJ were delivered to operative field within 0.05 sec at a setting of 3.6 W average power.

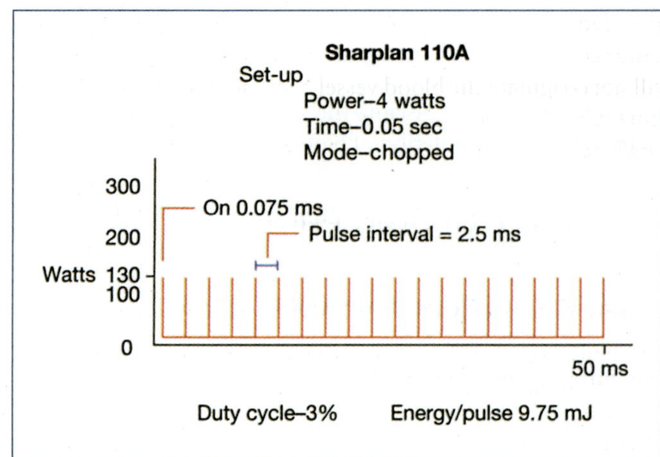

FIGURE 18–12 • Chopped mode for newer Sharplan and Coherent lasers. In superpulse mode, nearly all CO_2 surgical lasers developed by Sharplan and Coherent after 1988 generated 500–600 W of peak power—much too powerful for delicate otologic surgery. Sharplan adapted these lasers for ear surgery by adding Flexilase©—a chopped mode that delivers 130 W of peak power and 9.75 mJ per micropip (model #1100A, 1041S, and 1055S).

A word of caution. Several instances of thermal injury to the inner ear or facial nerve have been reported to me by surgeons who performed laser stapedotomy with Coherent and Sharplan CO_2 lasers in the superpulse mode. Guided by average power settings of 2 to 3 W, they performed laser stapedotomy, but were actually delivering 300 to 600 W of peak power (0.70 mm machine gun bullets). When laser energy is pulsed, the average power setting is very misleading. Both laser companies have now stopped using the average power setting.

Because of its ideal tissue characteristics, vaporization of soft tissue and bone can be efficiently performed with the CO_2 laser pulsed in brief microsecond pulses to minimize thermal spread. Slight thermal spread around the margins of the crater induces good hemostasis. To coagulate blood vessels, the CO_2 laser should be used on low power (2–3 W) in a continuous mode for 0.1 to 0.2 sec with a spot size of 0.5 to 1 mm.

Erbium Yttrium Aluminum Garnet

Zeiss' OPMI®TwinER was designed specifically for otologic surgery. The surgeon can adjust only the millijoules of the laser pulses (10–100 mJ) and the number that are delivered (frequency 1–3 per sec). The computer adapts the energy (mJ/pulse) by adjusting both the peak power (200–500 W) and the pulse width (0.05–0.2 milliseconds). In Europe, stapedotomies are performed by vaporizing 0.2 mm rosettes at a 20-mJ setting. I have been performing stapedotomies with a 0.6 mm spot size and a 70-mJ setting.

Erbium YAG is an ideal laser for vaporizing bone. Soft tissue vaporization is too efficient. Because of lack of thermal spread to the periphery of the target spot, blood vessels are not coagulated and therefore, hemostasis is poor when vaporizing tumor cells. When aimed directly at a blood vessel, erbium YAG will not coagulate the blood vessel because its pulse width is too short. Coagulation (raising collagen to 65 degrees) requires a continuous mode for hemostasis.

LASER OTOLOGIC PROCEDURES

Laser Stapedectomy Revision

Stapedectomy revision is presented first because in no other area of otology have lasers demonstrated such a profound advantage over nonlaser techniques. Nonlaser revision stapedectomies produce inconsistent hearing results and often damage the inner ear (3–20% surgical risk of significant postoperative nerve damage). Lasers improve our ability to safely identify and repair the conductive hearing losses encountered and have reduced the risk of postoperative nerve damage to 0.5%.[23,24] Hundreds of patients who had undergone one to three unsuccessful nonlaser attempts at revision have had their hearing restored with laser techniques.

Figure 18–13 illustrates the revising surgeon's dilemma. After elevating the tympanotomy flap, the surgeon must identify the margins and depths of the oval window, any residual stapes footplate, and the relationship of the prosthesis to the vestibule. Palpations of the prosthesis and neomembrane can be misleading because the oval window collagen usually has contracted and lateralized above the level of the vestibule. The prosthesis is often eccentric, not reaching the vestibule or migrated against the fixed otic capsule bone. A fixed footplate may be present 2 to 3 mm below the lateralized neomembrane.

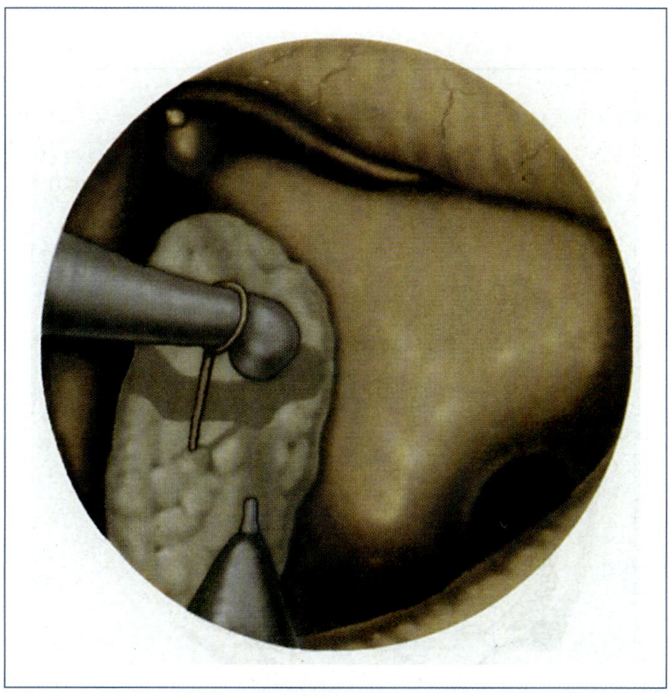

FIGURE 18–13 • Stapedectomy revision: a surgical dilemma (right ear). The surgeon must identify the margins and depth of the oval window, any residual stapes footplate, and the relationship of the prosthesis to the vestibule. The dilemma, surgical manipulation of the obliterating soft tissue or the prosthesis may produce significant dizziness and nerve deafness.

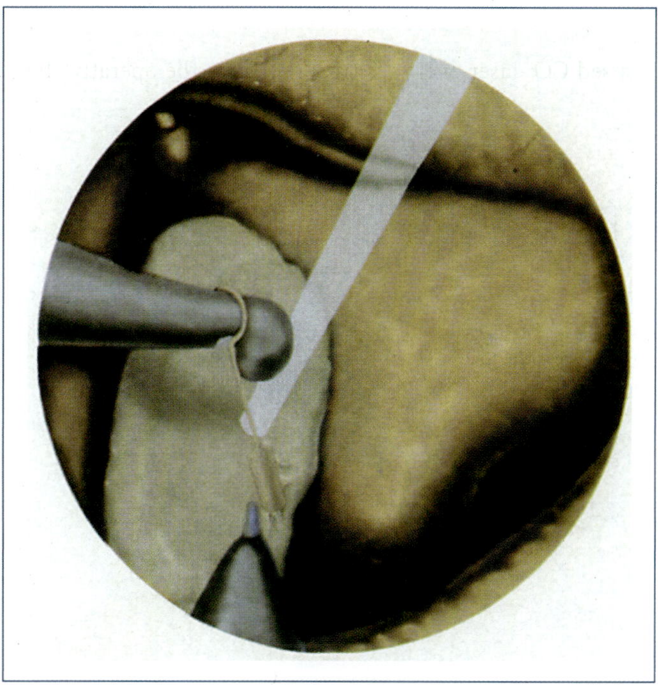

FIGURE 18–14 • Laser stapedectomy revision—the solution. CO_2 laser vaporizes (thins) collagen until margins and depth of oval window can be identified. Laser vaporization of soft tissue attachments of the distal end of the prosthesis permits removal of the prosthesis without mechanical trauma to the inner ear.

With appropriate energy settings, the CO_2 laser progressively vaporizes (thins) the collagen neomembrane until the margins of the oval window can be precisely identified (Figure 18–14). The relationship of the prosthesis to the oval window can now be established. Next, tissue surrounding the prosthesis is vaporized, and the prosthesis is removed. Depending on the status of the incus, a 0.6- or 1-mm "stapedotomy" is vaporized through the center of the oval window neomembrane (Figure 18–15), in order to

1. Identify residual fixed stapes footplate
2. Determine the exact length required for the new prosthesis
3. Stabilize the new prosthesis in the center of the oval window

When the incus is intact, a 0.6-mm stapedotomy is used. A teflon-piston, platinum-ribbon stapedotomy prosthesis (0.25 mm longer than the distance between the entrance into the vestibule and undersurface of the incus) is inserted into the stapedotomy opening and crimped to the neck of the incus. Clotted blood is then used to seal the oval window.

If the incus is eroded, a 1-mm stapedotomy opening is vaporized into the center of the oval window. Thin tragal perichondrium (2 × 3 mm) is then layered over the oval window neomembrane and depressed into enlarged stapedotomy opening. If 1 mm of the incus extends below the level of the facial ridge, a Lippy Moon Robinson offset stapes prosthesis is attached to the shortened incus (Figure 18–16). If the incus is

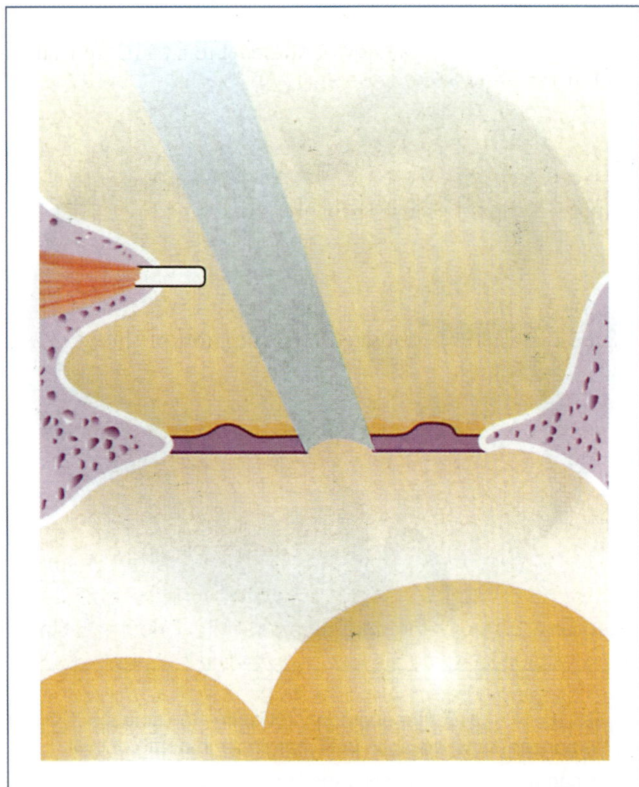

FIGURE 18–15 • A stapedotomy is vaporized in the center of the oval window, through the sealing neomembrane, until perilymph of the vestibule is encountered. Note: Fixed stapes footplate is found in 13%.

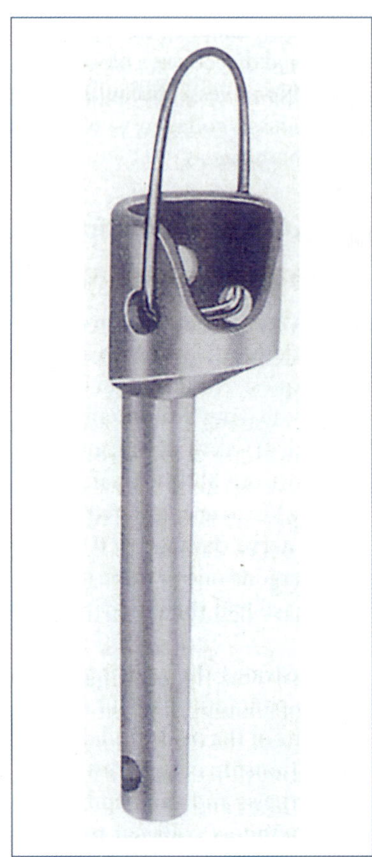

FIGURE 18–16 • Lippy Moon Robinson offset stapes prosthesis (Xomed/Medtronics #11–33009) for eroded incus when incus extends 1 mm or more below the facial ridge.

absent or too short, a Lesinski malleus to oval window prosthesis is employed (Figure 18–17). More recently, the new titanium *aerial* prosthesis from Kurz has been used (Figure 18–18). A sterile allograft collagen membrane (MEF) is placed between the tympanic membrane and the titanium prosthesis. The prosthesis is stabilized in the posterior superior quadrant by extending the allograft collagen below the malleus, over the prosthesis, and then under the lip of the bony canal.

If the malleus and incus are normal, postoperative hearing results approach that of primary stapedotomy. When the incus is eroded, 83% of the patients can expect to close the air–bone gap within 15 dB.[24] In a recent series of 300 consecutive CO_2 laser stapedectomy revisions, two patients (0.7%) developed a mild (less than 25 dB) drop in the bone level (mean 500 Hz, 1 KHz, 2 KHz, 3 KHz).[25] No patient exhibited a greater loss.

A word of caution. The safe energy parameter used for CO_2 laser revision techniques was established in the laboratory with human temporal bone thermocouple experiments, prior to its use in the operating room. Understanding the absorption tissue characteristics of argon and KTP lasers for water, bone, and collagen, the focused visible lasers should not be employed in the manner described above. Focused argon and KTP laser energy (microscope-mounted) can easily penetrate perilymph, traveling into the inner ear with enough fluence to potentially damage inner ear structures. The argon EndoOtoprobe® offers a greater degree of safety by rapidly diluting the power density but still should be used with caution since collagen does not absorb this wavelength very well.

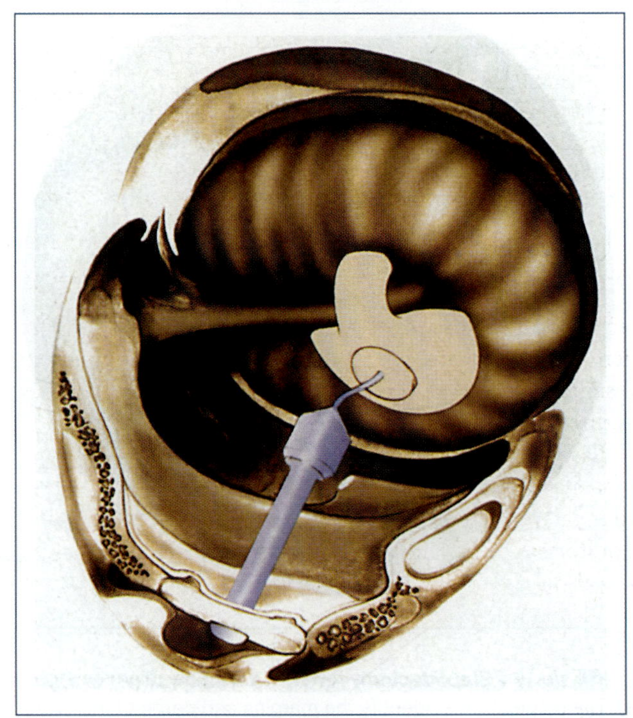

FIGURE 18–17 • Conductive repair when incus is significantly eroded using Lesinski malleus to oval window prosthesis (Xomed/Medtronics #0320). Note: Perichondrial graft sealing 1 mm stapedotomy and supporting prosthesis.

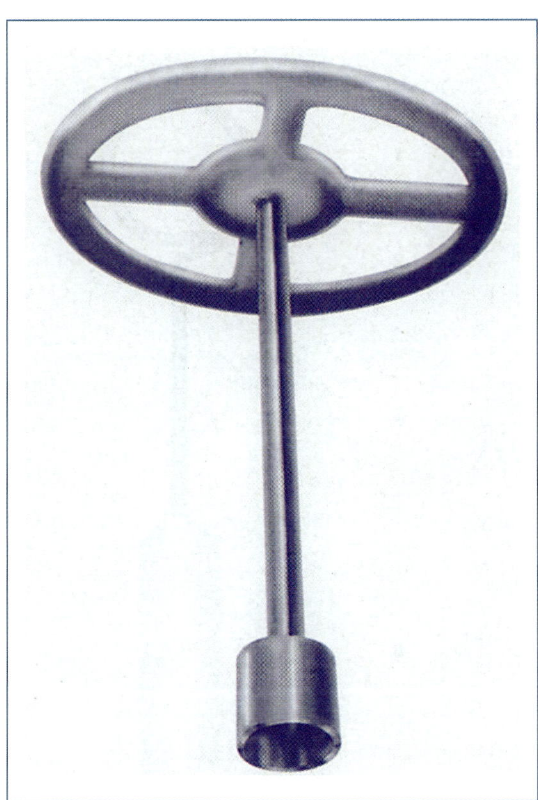

FIGURE 18–18 • Titanium AERIAL™ prosthesis (Kurz #1101–1113). Allograft collagen membrane (MEF) is placed under the malleus, over the prothesis, and under the posterior canal bony lip and then tympanotomy flap returned to anatomic position.

Laser Stapedotomy

The clinical advantages of stapedotomy versus stapedectomy include:[26–28]

1. Stabilization of the prosthesis in the center of the oval window
2. Reduced trauma to the inner ear (less postoperative sensorineural loss and dizziness)
3. Less mechanical trauma to the middle ear (reduced adhesions and less risk to facial nerve)

Mechanical stapedotomy techniques (trocar or low frequency microdrill) do not consistently produce a round symmetrical stapedotomy because the footplate frequently mobilizes or fractures.

Laser vaporization of the stapes footplate offers a nonmechanical solution. Safe energy parameters for argon, KTP, CO_2, and most recently, erbium YAG lasers have been established by laboratory experiments and confirmed by scores of successful clinical studies.

Visible lasers require vaporizing a series of tiny rosettes (0.05–0.2 mm) in the center of the stapes footplate. The 200-μ EndoOtoprobe® is the most popular mode of delivery. The result of this rosette technique is an irregular, scalloped stapedotomy whose precise diameter is difficult to control. Surgeons usually seal the visible laser stapedotomy with a vein or perichondrium.

For the past 21 years the author has been identifying and tabulating the precise causes for stapedectomy failure that are found at the time of revision surgery. Analysis from the data on 279 consecutive patients with conductive hearing loss following stapedectomy was presented to the American Otologic Society in May 2001. Eighty-one percent of those patients had a conductive failure because their prosthesis had migrated out of the oval window fenestration. Collagen contracture lifted the prosthesis out of a stapedotomy opening allowing the prosthesis to migrate onto the fixed footplate. Following stapedectomy, collagen contracture produced lateralization of the oval window neomembrane, allowing the prosthesis to migrate onto the fixed otic capsule bone (Figure 18–19). As the incus continued to vibrate against the fixed prosthesis, erosion occurred on the undersurface of the incus neck. Despite its inconvenience, the author prefers using a CO_2 laser. A round symmetrical stapedotomy, precisely the size of a prosthesis piston (0.6 mm), can be reliably produced in the footplate. Because the stapedotomy is precisely the size of the prosthesis piston, no collagen tissue seal is required and the oval window can be safely sealed with clotted blood. By avoiding a postoperative collagen contracture, prosthesis migration is minimized, and long-term hearing results are improved (Figure 18–20).[28]

Carbon dioxide laser stapedotomies are produced with a few "hits" of a pulsed CO_2 laser beam focused to a 0.6-mm

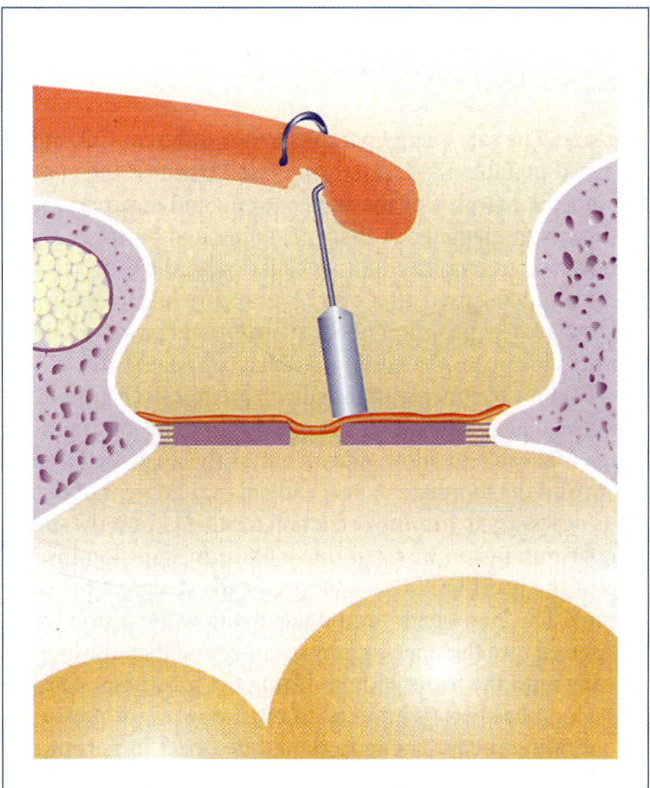

FIGURE 18–19 • The most common cause for conductive hearing loss following stapedotomy is prosthesis migration out of stapedotomy and onto solid fixed stapes footplate. Collagen contracture initiates the migration by lifting prosthesis out of the fenestration. Note: Incus erosion occurs as incus continues to vibrate against fixed prosthesis.

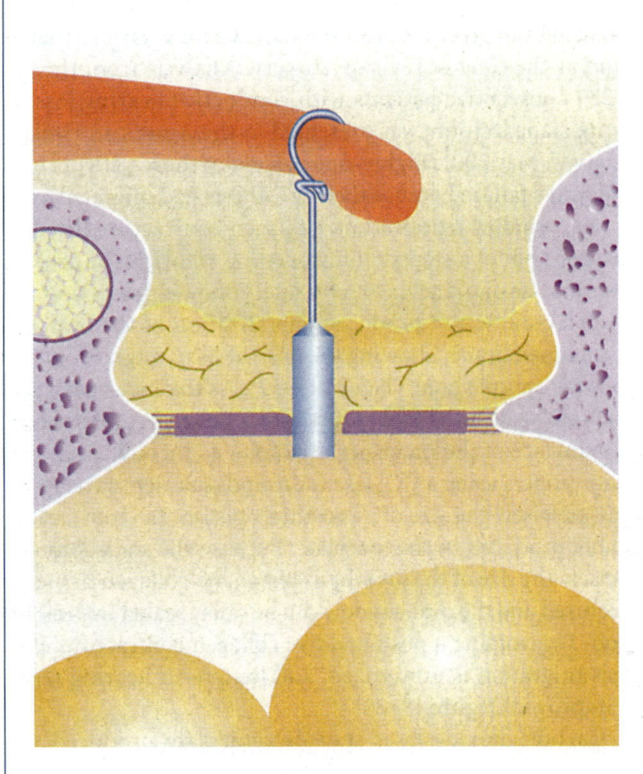

FIGURE 18–20 • CO_2 laser produces round symmetrical 0.6-mm stapedotomy opening. Clotted blood effectively seals the oval window. Collagen tissue seal is avoided eliminating collagen contracture and reducing the risk of postoperative prosthesis migration.

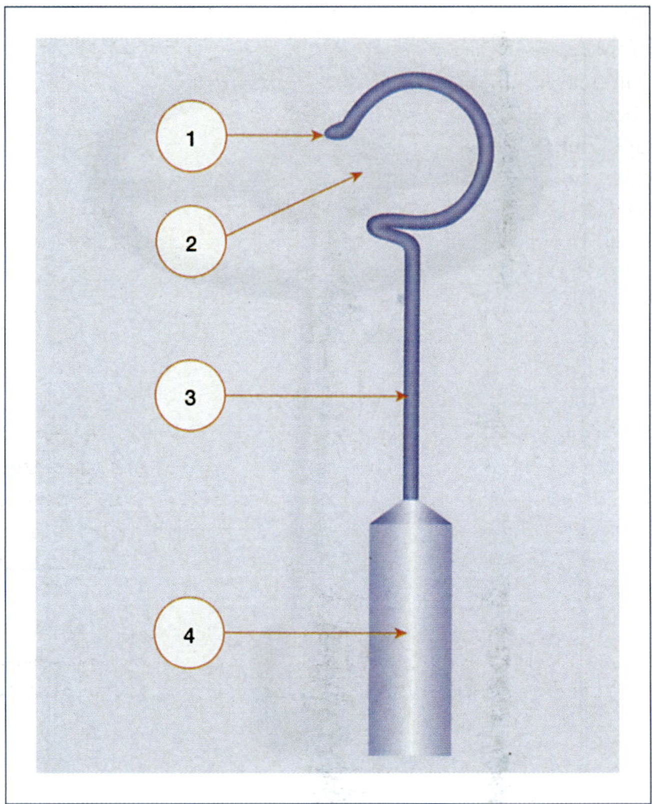

FIGURE 18–21 • Improved stapedotomy prosthesis (Xomed/Medtronics #385): 1. = Offset shepherd's crook; 2. = Lateral opening; 3. = Malleable platinum shaft is reinforced at the neck; 4. = Teflon piston (0.6 mm diameter).

spot size. The safe energy parameters for different CO_2 models are listed in Table 18–6. A 0.6-mm Fisch trocar is then used to smooth the margins of the stapedotomy and ensure symmetrical 0.6 mm diameter. A thick or obliterated footplate can be fenestrated but requires multiple "hits" with the CO_2 laser. The trocar should be used after every four or five hits to remove the crater char. The precision of the stapedotomy produced in this manner eliminates the need for a collagen tissue seal.

A Teflon-piston, platinum-ribbon prosthesis (Figure 18–21) was designed specifically for stapedotomy. The platinum ribbon is malleable to allow adjustment of the angle between the piston and the footplate. A perpendicular alignment of the piston is necessary to minimize friction resulting from the snug fit of a 0.6-mm piston inserted into a 0.6-mm stapedotomy. The loop of the prosthesis also was specifically designed for stapedotomy. The loop opens on the side to allow the piston to first be inserted into the stapedotomy opening and then the loop slid laterally onto the incus without lifting the prosthesis. The base of the loop has been reinforced to resist downward pressure of the vibrating incus. The loop should be offset to permit snug crimping. The stapedotomy prosthesis should measure 0.25 mm longer than the distance between the undersurface of the incus and the footplate. Generally, a 4.5-mm and occasionally a 4.75-mm prosthesis are required. This longer prosthesis resists displacement out of the stapedotomy opening during Valsalva's maneuvers or head trauma.

No collagen tissue seal is used. The surgeon can now directly observe the position length and mobility of the prosthesis in relation to the stapedotomy. Postoperative contracture of the collagen neomembrane can lift the prosthesis out of the stapedotomy and is the most common cause for stapedotomy failures. A drop of clotted blood reliably seals the oval window.

There are three instances when a thin tissue seal (vein or perichondrium) is recommended:

1. "Perilymph gusher"
2. Footplate fracture or mobilization
3. Stapedotomy that is too large for the prosthesis.

If a collagen tissue seal is used, the author prefers a Lippy Robinson bucket handle prosthesis because of its increased rigidity and stability. The platinum ribbon prosthesis is too malleable for the increased impedance of the collagen tissue seal.

Employing laser stapedotomy techniques, the surgeon can expect that 90% of his patients will close the air–bone gap to within 10 dB and 96% within 15 dB.[14] Lasers reduce inner ear trauma as evidence by less postoperative dizziness and sensorineural hearing loss. Finally, provided the surgeon employs appropriate laser energy parameters and techniques, the risk to the facial nerve is nearly eliminated.

Lasers for Tympanoplasty/Mastoidectomy

Otologic lasers can assist the surgeon in several situations where standard techniques are inadequate or potentially dangerous. Hemostasis can be obtained by coagulating blood vessels that are inaccessible to bipolar electrocautery. Frequently, the chronic ear surgeon encounters an oval window obliterated by cholesteatoma, granulation tissue, hyperplastic mucosa, and adhesions. In a chronically infected middle ear, dislocating the stapes bone potentially exposes the inner ear to bacterial contamination (bacterial labyrinthitis and meningitis). Visible or CO_2 lasers are used to meticulously vaporize the abnormal soft tissue. In addition, to facilitate complete tumor removal, the arches of a mobile stapes can be safely vaporized with a laser, providing free access to the footplate.

If the stapes head is eroded but the arches are intact, hearing reconstruction presents a challenge. Most prostheses designed for attachment to the stapes require an intact stapes head for stability. Optimal hearing results can be obtained by vaporizing the arches and centering a total ossicular replacement prosthesis (TORP) on the mobile stapes footplate. Mechanically crushing the arches (Wehr's or Fisch crura crusher) works well when the stapes footplate is fixed but will frequently dislocate a mobile footplate.

With appropriate laser energy settings, vaporization and coagulation of granulation tissue and hyperplastic mucosa can also be safely done in delicate areas such as the round window niche or overlying a dehiscent facial nerve.

Tumor Ablation

In the late 1980s, there was considerable enthusiasm for employing both visible and CO_2 lasers to vaporize acoustic neuroma, glomus tumors, and other base of skull tumors. The slow rate of laser tumor ablation coupled with the risk of adjacent tissue damage from thermal spread or a misdirected laser beam limited its advantages. Just as for middle ear surgery there are instances when the argon EndoOtoprobe® or the CO_2 lasers can be helpful (eg, vaporization and coagulation of small bits of acoustic neuroma still adherent to the facial nerve). The blood vessels feeding smaller glomus or acoustic neuroma tumors can be coagulated.

With carefully controlled energy parameters, the author has used CO_2 lasers to vaporize epidermoid carcinoma off the adventia of the carotid artery and benign tumors off a dehiscent facial nerve. Stage I epidermoid carcinomas and papillomas of the external ear canal can be vaporized without extensive surgical dissection though histologic evaluation of crater margins is required to ensure complete removal of the cancer cells. When the tumor is near the facial nerve, intraoperative electrical monitoring of the nerve is recommended.

THE FUTURE OF OTOLOGIC LASERS

Laser techniques are accepted by the otologic community only when the laser procedure offers significant clinical advantages over nonlaser techniques. When the first stapedotomy procedure was presented 20 years ago, many of the otologists in the audience were skeptical of the potential clinical advantages that lasers afforded. Ten years later, approximately half of the otologists were using lasers in the operating room; the other half, maintaining "my results are just as good without the laser." Today, nearly every otologist employs a laser for specific otologic surgical circumstances when the precision and lack of mechanical trauma offers a safer alternative.

Until now, lasers have been employed to vaporize or coagulate soft tissue or bone or warm nitinol prostheses. Besides its photothermal effects, EM energy could be used for many nonheating medical applications. Listed below are a few of the potential areas being explored in laser laboratories.

1. *Emission Spectroscopy.* The electron orbits of molecules within tissue are excited with UV lasers. As their electron orbits decay, each molecule emits the exact photon (wavelength) of EM energy it loses. Molecules are identified by their spectral patterns. Cancer cells contain unique molecules (eg, primitive amino acids). Therefore, cancer cells potentially could be identified through emission spectroscopy with a great degree of accuracy.[29] Emission spectroscopy is presently being performed on many different types of tumors and being compared with histologic sections to determine its diagnostic potential.
2. *Inner Ear Endoscopy and Spectroscopy.* Perhaps someday in the future, surgeons will cannulate the inner ear with tiny optical fibers and perform emission spectroscopy at various sites in the vestibular and cochlear partitions. Cupulolithiasis could be identified and ablated with UV or photoacoustic laser effects.

Do the dark cells have enough unique biochemistry that they could be partially ablated with appropriate UV lasers—reducing the production of endolymph in Ménière's patients? Is peripheral tinnitus caused by excitable hair cells or neurons whose critical firing potentials have been biochemically altered? Could we biochemically re-engineer these aberrant molecules using the photodissection effect of EM energy?

Over the past 50 years, ear surgery has traveled from completely macroscopic techniques to exclusively microscopic. Perhaps in the next 50 years, otology will journey into the submicroscopic world. Surgeons will operate with EM energy upon atoms and molecules—restructuring intracellular molecules to alter cell function. The road is well lit by the laws of quantum mechanics. Molecular physicists and biophysicists will guide us. Our ultimate destination is limited by our imagination.

References

1. Pollock S. Particle physics for nonphyscists—The Teaching Company. 2003. p. 20–4.
2. Perkins R. Laser stapedotomy for otosclerosis. Laryngoscope 1980;90:228–41.
3. McGee T. The argon laser in surgery for chronic ear disease and otosclerosis. Laryngoscope 1983;93:1177–82.
4. Perkins R. New instruments—The KTP/532 laser. Presented at the American Academy of Otolaryngology Head and Neck Surgery, Sept. 1984.
5. Lesinski SG. Lasers for otosclerosis: CO_2 vs. argon and KTP 532. Laryngoscope 1989;99:1–8.
6. Lesinski SG. CO_2 laser for otosclerosis: Safe energy parameters. Laryngoscope 1989;99:9–12.
7. Gherini S, Horn KL, Causse JP, et al. Fiberoptic argon laser stapedotomy: Is it safe? Am J Otol 1993;14(3):283–9.
8. Bartels L. KTP laser stapedotomy: Is it safe? Otolaryngol Head Neck Surg 1990;103:685–92.

9. McGee TM, Diaz-Ordaz EA, Kartus J, et al. The role of KTP laser in revision stapedectomy. Otolaryngol Head Neck Surg 1993;109:839–43.
10. Vernick DM. A comparison of the results of KTP and CO_2 laser stapedotomy. Am J Otol 1996;17(2):221–4.
11. Lesinski SG. Lasers in revision stapes surgery. Oper Tech in Otolaryngol Head Neck Surg 1992;3:21–31.
12. Lesinski SG. Lasers for otosclerosis—Which one and why? Lasers Surg Med 1990;10:448–57.
13. Izatt JA, Albagli D, Britton M, et al. Wavelength dependence of pulsed laser ablation of calcified tissue. Lasers Surg Med 1991;11:238–49.
14. Lesinski SG, Newrock R. CO_2 lasers for otosclerosis. Otolaryngol Clin North Am 1993;26(3):417–42.
15. Wolfe WL, Zissis GJ. The infrared handbook. Washington, DC: Office of Naval Research; 1978. p.#;3–107.
16. Yannas I. Collagen and gelatin in the solid state. J Macromol Chem C7 1972;1:49–104.
17. Pfalz R, Hibst N. Suitability of different lasers for operations ranging from the tympanic membrane to the base of stapes. Adv Otorhinolaryngol 1995;49:87–94.
18. Nuss R, Fabian R, Sarkar R, et al. Infrared laser bone ablation. Lasers Surg Med 1998;8:381–91.
19. Hibst R. Mechanical effects of erbium YAG laser bone ablation. Lasers Surg Med 1992;12:125–30.
20. Stubig IM, Reder PA, Facer GW, et al. Holmium YAG laser stapedotomy: Preliminary evaluation. Proc SPIE 1993;1876:10–19.
21. Jovanovic S, Schonfeld U, Prapavat V, et al. Effects of pulsed laser systems on stapes footplate. Lasers Surg Med 1997;21(4): 341–50.
22. Lenarz T, Heermann R, Brandis A, et al. Middle ear mechanics in research and otosurgery. In: Huttenbrink KB, editor. Erbium YAG laser in middle ear surgery. 1997. p. 233–37.
23. Haberkamp TJ, Harvey SA. Revision stapedectomy with and without the CO_2 laser: An analysis of results. Am J Otol 1996;17(2):225–9.
24. Lesinski SG. Revision surgery for otosclerosis—1998 perspective. Oper Tech in Otolaryngol Head Neck Surg 1998;9(2):72–81.
25. Lesinski SG, Newrock R. Carbon dioxide lasers for otoclerosis. Otolaryngol Clin North Am 1993;26(3):417–41.
26. Fisch U. Stapedotomy vs. stapedectomy. Am J Otol 1982;4:112–7.
27. Kursten R, Schneider B, Zrunek M, et al. Long term results after stapedectomy versus stapedotomy. Am J Otol 1994;15(6): 804–6.
28. Marquet J. Stapedotomy technique and results. J Otol 1985; 6:63–7.
29. Richards-Kortum R. Fluorescence spectroscopy as a technique for diagnosis [PhD thesis]. Massachusetts Institute of Technology; 1990.

Neurophysiologic Monitoring in Otologic/Neurotologic Surgery

19

Roberto A. Cueva, MD, FACS / Gayle E. Hicks, PhD, DABNM

Whereas surgical experimentation with facial nerve electrical stimulation during cerebellopontine angle (CPA) surgery dates back to the late 19th century,[1] the modern era of neurophysiologic monitoring during otologic/neurotologic surgery begins in 1979, when Delgado et al. reported on their experience with intraoperative electromyographic (EMG) monitoring of the facial nerve during intracranial surgery.[2] Historically, various methods for detecting facial nerve irritation/trauma during surgery have been employed, varying from an observer watching the face during dissection to the suturing of sterilized cat collar bells to specific locations on the face to signal facial movement by their ringing.[3,4] But it was Delgado et al., along with the efforts of Møller and Jannetta,[5] Gantz,[6] Harner et al.,[7] Prass and Luders,[8] and others, using neurophysiologic equipment to monitor and record facial nerve activity, who ushered us into the modern era.

Soon after, in the early 1980s, Møller and Jannetta and others began to report their success in monitoring and recording cochlear nerve function during CPA surgery.[9] Facial nerve monitoring quickly became the standard of care during surgery for acoustic neuromas and other CPA pathology as studies indicated improved facial nerve function related to the use of monitoring.[10] Auditory monitoring, although initially reported using direct eighth nerve monitoring (DENM), came to be widely employed using auditory brainstem responses (ABRs).[11] Difficulties with maintaining electrode position and signal degradation in cerebrospinal fluid hampered successful DENM, but advances in electrode design have largely overcome these problems.[12] More recently, DENM is receiving increasing attention by surgeons and authors as it provides the most rapid feedback to the surgeons on the status of auditory function during CPA surgery.

The techniques of EMG and direct nerve monitoring are being applied to monitor other cranial nerves in an effort to reduce patient morbidity following neurotologic surgery. Specifically, monitoring of the vagus, spinal accessory, and hypoglossal nerves is frequently done in skull base surgical cases.[13] Oculomotor and trigeminal nerve monitoring is becoming more common.

As a whole, neurophysiologic monitoring during surgery continues to grow in routine use and advance in technological sophistication. The driving motivation for its application and ongoing development is the desire to keep morbidity related to complex neurotologic surgery to an absolute minimum. Clearly, monitoring the facial nerve during CPA surgery has had a positive effect on functional outcome. The impact of facial nerve monitoring during routine otologic surgery remains less well defined. Auditory monitoring with DENM has been demonstrated as superior to ABR in facilitating hearing preservation during CPA surgery.[14] Future advances in application and technology hold the promise of better surgical outcomes.

FACIAL NERVE MONITORING

Neurophysiologic monitoring of the facial nerve most commonly involves EMG. Equipment for monitoring gross facial muscle contraction via strain gauges has been used in the past, but the technique has fallen into disuse as it is not as sensitive as EMG at detecting facial nerve irritation. Likewise, video monitoring of the face during surgery has fallen by the wayside as it is likely to miss subclinical muscular contractions. EMG voltages less than 100 μV are typically not visible as facial movement but are easily recorded using modern technology. Current artifact created during electrocautery effectively prevents EMG monitoring so care must be taken when cauterizing adjacent to the facial nerve.

As a consequence of EMG's reliance on the neuromuscular junction, paralytic agents must not be used during surgery in which motor nerve monitoring is being performed. A short-acting neuromuscular blocker may be used during anesthetic induction, but motor nerve activity should be allowed to return to normal during the course of the surgical procedure. If significant facial nerve manipulation is anticipated, testing to ensure reversal of the anesthetic induction neuromuscular blockade should be done prior to beginning facial nerve dissection.

EMG data may be recorded using three separate or simultaneous acquisition formats: continuous or free-run EMG (FEMG), triggered EMG (TEMG), and stimulated EMG (SEMG). Free-run EMG is recorded in real time, typically employing sweep durations of 200 milliseconds to 5 sec. Triggered EMG allows the capture of spontaneous responses that exceed a preset voltage. Many commercial systems provide an audible warning when the EMG activity exceeds the preset voltage. Stimulated EMG records responses to a stimulus source such as a hand-held probe designed specifically for cranial nerve stimulation. Figure 19–1 shows simultaneous recordings of FEMG and TEMG. Figure 19–2 demonstrates simultaneous recordings of FEMG and SEMG. Depending on the manufacturer, commercially available systems may employ one or a combination of the three acquisition formats.

Generally, two configurations may be employed for monitoring EMG from the face and other cranial nerves, monopolar and bipolar. In a monopolar and bipolar electrode configuration, the amplifier records the difference in activity between two strategically placed electrodes. Monopolar recordings use active electrodes placed in the desired myotomes (eg, orbicularis oculi muscle for the facial [VII] nerve and the masseter muscle for the trigeminal [V] nerve) and a reference electrode neutrally placed (eg, lateral forehead on the opposite side of the head from the active electrodes). Bipolar recordings are obtained by placing both the active and reference electrodes in the muscle. Both methods are acceptable and use a differential amplifier common to most current recording systems. True referential recorders may be used only with amplifiers specifically designed to provide this type of recording methodology. A referential amplifier subtracts the activity of the reference electrode from the activity of the active electrode or electrodes. This results in greater specificity, reduced noise, and the convenience of using fewer electrodes.

The most common EMG recording method employs paired subdermal needle electrodes in a bipolar configuration. Two subdermal needle electrodes are placed under the skin over the muscles or myotomes of the associated cranial nerve. Their distance is determined by the desired specificity. The closer the pair of electrodes are placed to each other, the fewer the muscle fibers represented in the EMG response. Electrode placement should take into consideration the size of the muscle group of interest as well as that of the surrounding muscles. For instance, the orbicularis oculi is in proximity to the frontalis and temporalis muscles. When placing electrodes to represent seventh nerve activity, the temporalis muscle should be avoided. Since the seventh nerve innervates the frontalis, activity from this muscle would be acceptable when the facial nerve is at risk. Thus, the recommended electrode placement for the orbicularis oculi muscle should be more centrally located over the orbit to avoid interference from temporalis electrodes reacting to inadvertent stimulation of the fifth nerve (Figure 19–3). In small tumors, overlap of activity from different cranial nerves is

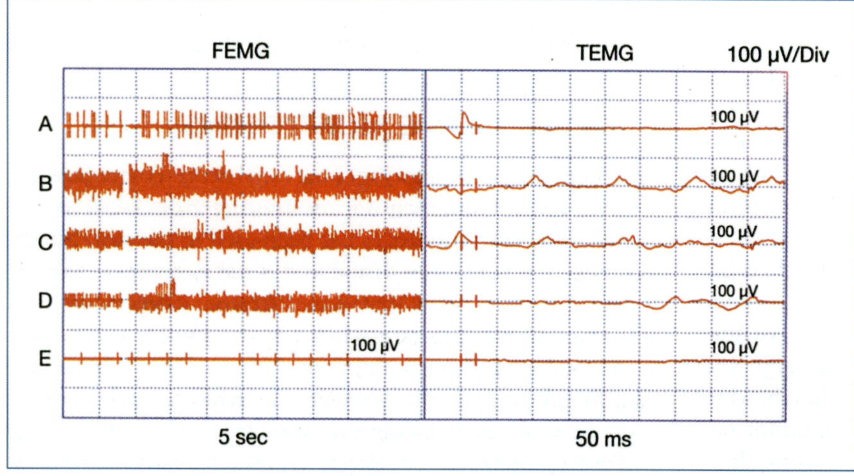

FIGURE 19–1 • Simultaneous recordings of free-run electromyography (FEMG) and triggered EMG (TEMG) acquired during acoustic neuroma surgery are shown. Traces *A* through *E* reflect EMG from the orbicularis oculi *A*, orbicularis oris *B*, mentalis *C*, masseter *D*, and trapezius *E* muscles for both the FEMG and TEMG recordings. The five channels of FEMG to the left were recorded with a 5-sec sweep window. All of the muscles, except the trapezius, exhibit spontaneous activity secondary to inadvertent stimulation of their respective nerves during tumor manipulation. The corresponding TEMG, to the right, is a 50-millisecond capture of the simultaneously recorded FEMG. In this recording, the trigger voltage was set at 50 µV. Any activity in the EMG exceeding 50 µV would trigger the capture.

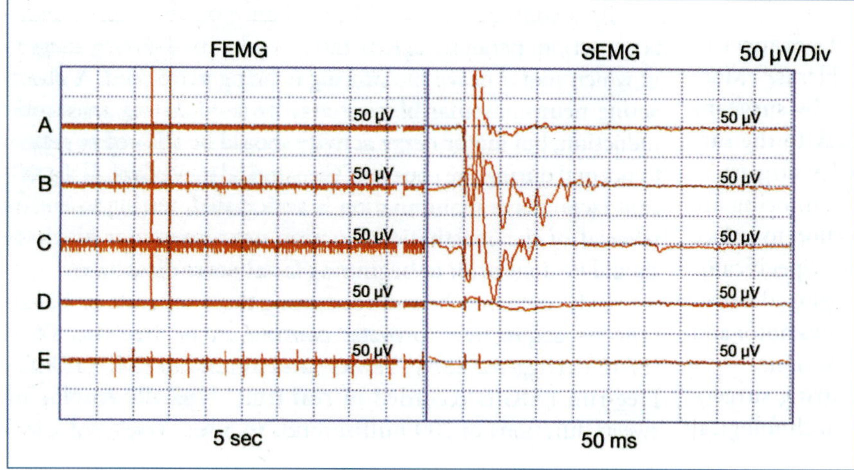

FIGURE 19–2 • Simultaneous recordings of free-run electromyography (FEMG) and stimulated EMG (SEMG) acquired during acoustic neuroma surgery are shown. As in Figure 14–1, traces *A* through *E* reflect EMG from the orbicularis oculi *A*, orbicularis oris *B*, mentalis *C*, masseter *D*, and trapezius *E* muscles. The FEMG, to the left, is a second sweep of continuous EMG. Evident in traces B and E are regularly spaced artifacts from the probe stimulator. Two larger events are seen at the same intervals as the stimuli artifacts and reflect responses from the facial muscles to the probe stimuli. These responses are more clearly seen in a 50-millisecond sweep of SEMG to the right. In this recording, the probe stimuli triggered the capture.

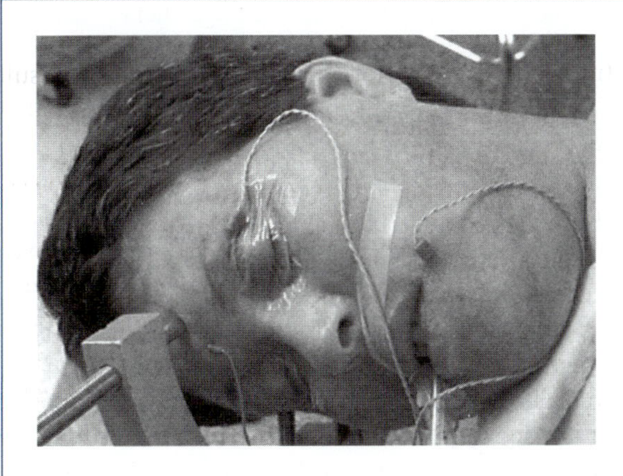

FIGURE 19–3 • Subdermal bipolar needle electrodes are placed in the superior portion of the orbicularis oculi muscle away from the temporalis and masseter muscles to avoid bleed-over of electromyographic activity.

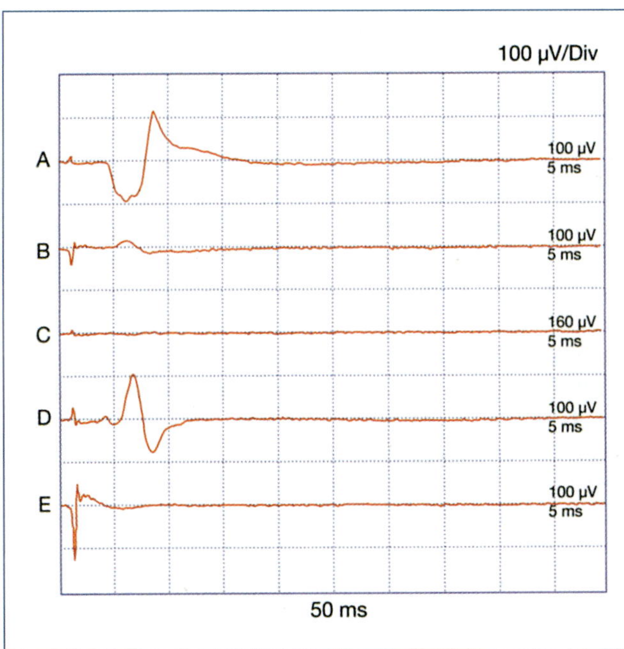

FIGURE 19–4 • Recordings of stimulated electromyography (EMG) to probe stimulation of the motor branch (V3) of the fifth nerve are shown. Traces *A* through *E* reflect EMG from the orbicularis oculi *A*, orbicularis oris *B*, mentalis *C*, masseter *D*, and trapezius *E* muscles. Note the large biphasic responses from the orbicularis oculi and masseter muscles. The response exhibited in trace *A* reflects temporalis activity in the orbicularis oculi channel. These muscles are in such close proximity that electrode placement near the lateral orbital rim results in activity to stimulation of either nerve (V or VII).

not usually a problem. However, for large tumors in which the anatomy may be significantly distorted, this overlap could be a critical issue. Figure 19–4 demonstrates a masseter response to fifth nerve stimulation and a "bleed-over" from the temporalis muscle to electrodes placed in the orbicularis oculi muscle. Note that these SEMG responses exhibit a simple biphasic waveform compared with typical multiphasic SEMG responses from the

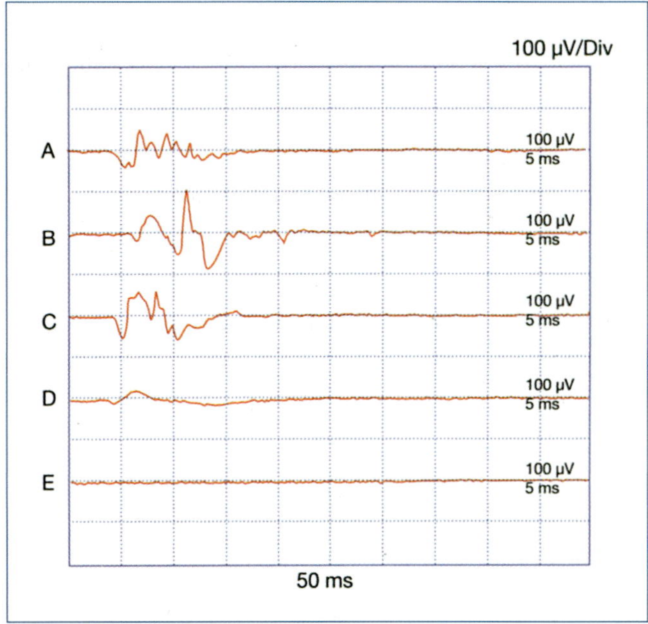

FIGURE 19–5 • Recordings of stimulated electromyography (EMG) to probe stimulation of the seventh nerve during the same surgery as those acquired in Figure 14–3 are shown. Traces *A* through *E* reflect EMG from the orbicularis oculi *A*, orbicularis oris *B*, mentalis *C*, masseter *D*, and trapezius *E* muscles. Note the complexity of the responses compared with those seen in Figure 14–3. The multiphasic and longer duration activity are typical of EMG responses to probe stimulation of the seventh nerve.

orbicularis oculi to stimulation of the seventh nerve, as demonstrated in Figure 19–5.

In most surgical conditions, two channels of facial nerve EMG are adequate. However, in large tumors in which the seventh nerve may be splayed over the tumor, three or four channels of EMG representing additional branches of the facial nerve provide greater sensitivity. Figure 19–6 shows EMG activity recorded continuously from four facial muscles. EMG activity limited to the mentalis muscle in response to tumor manipulation is evident.

Ephaptic Responses

The condition of hemifacial spasm (HFS) is caused by irritative arterial compression of the facial nerve near its root entry zone at the brain stem. Electrophysiological studies indicate that this vascular contact creates a physiologically active bridge between fibers, allowing crossover of antidromic impulses. These crossed impulses then travel distally through other branches to activate the facial muscles. The abnormal muscle response generated by nonsynaptic axonal activation (ephapse) may be recorded during EMG as the ephaptic response (ER).[15] Monitoring the facial nerve for ER during microvascular decompression (MVD) for HFS helps the surgeon identify the offending vessel.

Figure 19–7 demonstrates the stimulus and acquisition electrode positions for EMG with ER. Stimulating current, usually between 7 and 20 mA, is passed via the stimulus electrodes, resulting in antidromic crossover motor activity recorded on EMG. Examples of ER are shown in Figure 19–8. As the surgeon

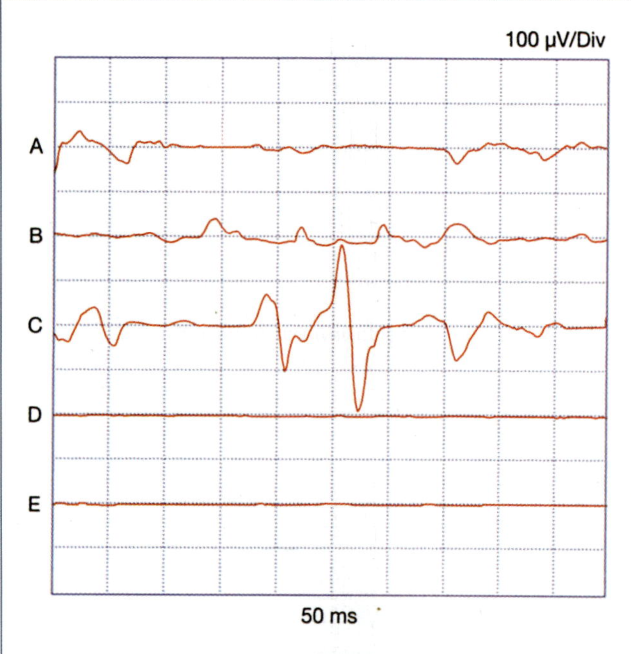

FIGURE 19–6 • Triggered electromyographic activity showing responses captured to a 100-μV trigger. Traces *A* through *E* reflect activity from the orbicularis oculi *A*, orbicularis oris *B*, mentalis *C*, masseter *D*, and trapezius *E* muscles. Note that the activity from the orbicularis oculi and oris muscles (traces *A* and *B*) did not reach an amplitude great enough to trigger a capture. Only the activity from the mentalis (trace *C*) reached adequate amplitude for a capture or an audible alert.

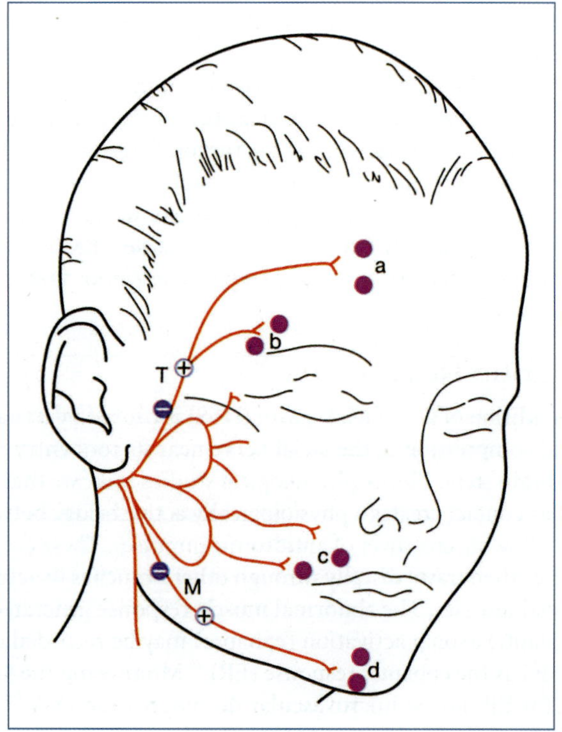

FIGURE 19–7 • The stimulus and acquisition sites are displayed. For stimulation of the temporal (T) and mandibular (M) branches of the seventh nerve the anode is typically placed proximally to enhance the antidromic conduction of the action potential. A bipolar recording montage is recommended for each muscle: (a) frontalis, (b) orbicularis oculi, (c) orbicularis oris, and (d) mentalis.

explores the root entry zone of the facial nerve, the ER will immediately extinguish when the compressing vessel is moved away from the nerve. Using ER to identify the vessel causing the HFS is felt to result in improved cure rates for MVD.

If the surgeon is very familiar with a particular, dedicated, motor nerve monitoring device and is able to differentiate true motor responses from artifact signals, then he/she may be comfortable interpreting the output of the monitoring equipment himself/herself. Otherwise, the use of personnel trained and qualified to perform neurophysiologic monitoring is strongly recommended. Using more sophisticated equipment and trained personnel has distinct advantages. As noted above, multichannel monitoring equipment allows monitoring of other motor nerves and helps differentiate true facial nerve stimulation from artifact or other cranial nerve stimulation. Additionally, a diffuse increase in EMG activity in multiple muscle groups may indicate reduced depth of anesthesia, which can be disastrous during posterior cranial fossa surgery. Furthermore, use of monitoring personnel allows the surgeon to concentrate on performing the surgery rather than having to divert attention to interpret the EMG feedback. Finally, for monitoring to be successful, the surgeon must respond appropriately to the feedback provided and alter activities to reduce or eliminate facial nerve irritation.

Stimulation of the nerve with electric current should be done at the lowest possible level. Pulse duration and the voltage or current determine the strength of the stimulus. Most commercial systems use a pulse width of 0.05 or 0.10 μsec and provide intensity integrals of 0.05 or 0.10 mA. During initial stages of tumor resection, when the location of the seventh nerve may not be obvious, spontaneous EMG activity would suggest close proximity to the nerve. In this instance, a slightly higher pulse intensity (0.10–0.20 mA) is useful when searching for the nerve in a field in which anatomy is distorted. At the conclusion of surgery, the functional integrity of the facial nerve may be estimated by determining the lowest current level required for facial nerve stimulation. If robust amplitude motor responses are obtained from the facial nerve at its exit from the brain stem with stimulation at 0.05 to 0.10 mA, then good facial function is expected.

Facial nerve monitoring during otologic surgery may be helpful in reducing the risk of facial nerve injury during cases in which the facial nerve may be exposed by disease (cholesteatoma, granulation tissue) or congenital variation of anatomy. Because of the fibrous sheath surrounding the nerve in the temporal bone, higher current levels, in the 0.20- to 0.50-mA range, are required to stimulate EMG responses. If attempts to stimulate the nerve are being performed through a thin bony layer, higher current levels, 0.50 to 1.0 mA, are required.

There is no substitute for an intimate and thorough knowledge of facial nerve anatomy and its variations within the temporal bone. For the experienced surgeon, facial nerve monitoring may reduce the risk of facial nerve injury during dissection of cholesteatoma or granulation tissue from an exposed nerve. It should not serve as a crutch for finding the nerve during otherwise routine otologic surgery. Clearly, any patient who has had facial nerve symptoms related to cholesteatoma or ear infection or as a consequence of previous otologic surgery

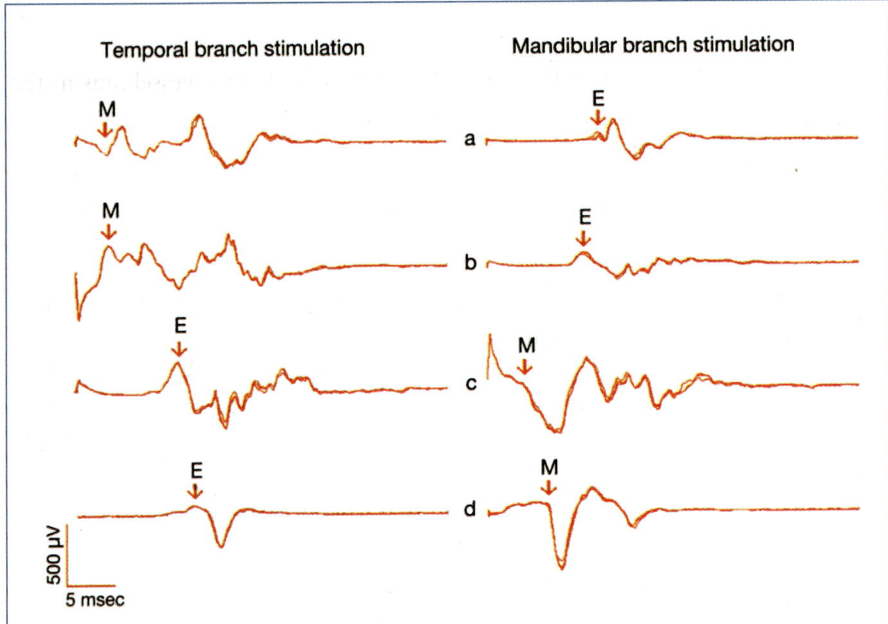

FIGURE 19–8 • Three superimposed trials are shown for the two stimulation conditions for each muscle; (a) frontalis, (b) orbicularis oculi, (c) orbicularis oris, and (d) mentalis. The downward arrows indicate the onset of a muscle response. The M wave (M) represents the compound muscle action potential to orthodromic conduction of the stimulus. The E wave (E) represents the Ephaptic response produced by antidromic conduction of the stimulus. The M wave is evident only in those muscles innervated by the peripheral nerve stimulated whereas the E wave is most clearly observed from the noninnervated muscles and exhibits a much later onset.

warrants facial nerve monitoring during surgery. These symptoms warn the surgeon of the high likelihood that the nerve is dehiscent and directly affected by the disease process, increasing surgical risk.

Routine facial nerve monitoring for otologic surgery remains somewhat controversial as there is disagreement regarding whether it provides significant, protective benefit to the nerve. Some authors express concern that routine use of facial nerve monitoring is no substitute for thorough knowledge of anatomy and may create a false sense of confidence for the inexperienced surgeon. For the experienced surgeon, medico-legal concerns may drive the decision regarding routine facial nerve monitoring during uncomplicated otologic cases. Although the senior author favors selective use of facial nerve monitoring for otologic surgery in his own practice, each surgeon must decide this issue for himself/herself.

AUDITORY MONITORING

Møller and Jannetta first reported recording compound action potentials from the auditory nerve in humans in 1981. This report focused on the correlation of anatomic locations and the different waveforms seen on ABR testing.[11] The year 1982 saw the first reports describing ABR, initially developed in the mid-1970s as a diagnostic tool, used for intraoperative monitoring during acoustic tumor surgery.[16,17] Although DENM provides much larger amplitude responses and faster feedback than ABR, difficulties maintaining electrode position hampered its widespread use. As a result, ABR came to be the preferred method for monitoring auditory function during CPA surgery throughout the 1980s and 1990s.[18,19]

The late-1990s saw a resurgence of interest in DENM.[20,21] With the traditional morbidities of CPA surgery greatly reduced owing to advances in surgical technique and motor nerve monitoring, increasing focus is being placed on improving rates of hearing preservation. The best way to improve hearing preservation rates, apart from earlier diagnosis of smaller tumors, is to obtain the most rapid intraoperative feedback possible regarding the functional status of the cochlear nerve. DENM provides the nearest thing to real-time auditory function during CPA surgery and has been shown to be superior to ABR in facilitating hearing preservation. [14,21] Recent reports on the use of DENM during resection of acoustic neuromas 10 mm and smaller demonstrate hearing preservation rates in the range of 80–85%.[22]

Scalp-recorded ABR is obtained by arranging surface or subdermal needle electrodes at opposing ends of the dipole or direction of the neuroelectric activity of the auditory neural pathway. Several hundred to several thousand click stimuli generated by a 100 μV square wave pulse are delivered to the ear via cushion or insert earphones. The small click-evoked responses (usually < 1.0 μV) are computer averaged and appear within 10 millisecond of stimulus onset as a series of five to seven waves originally labeled with Roman numerals by Jewett and colleagues.[23] In the normal ABR (Figure 19–9, right ear) the poststimulus latency of wave I evoked by a suprathreshold (60–80 dB nHL [normal hearing level]) click occurs at or before 2 millisecond. Subsequent waves exhibit latencies at approximately 1 millisecond intervals. Eighth nerve activity is reflected in waves I and II—the former near the cochlea and the latter near the brain stem.[24,25] The remaining waves are generated by brainstem structures rostral to the pontomedullary junction. Patients with eighth nerve or brain-stem lesions rarely exhibit normal ABRs on the affected side and require interpretation by an experienced clinician or technologist. Figure 19–10 shows a series of ABR tracings obtained during resection of an acoustic neuroma.

While recording the ABR during surgery, subdermal needle electrodes are preferred because of their impedance stability over long periods of time. An active electrode is placed at or near the vertex and a reference electrode on the mastoid, earlobe, or neck. Since the scalp-recorded ABR is a far-field response,

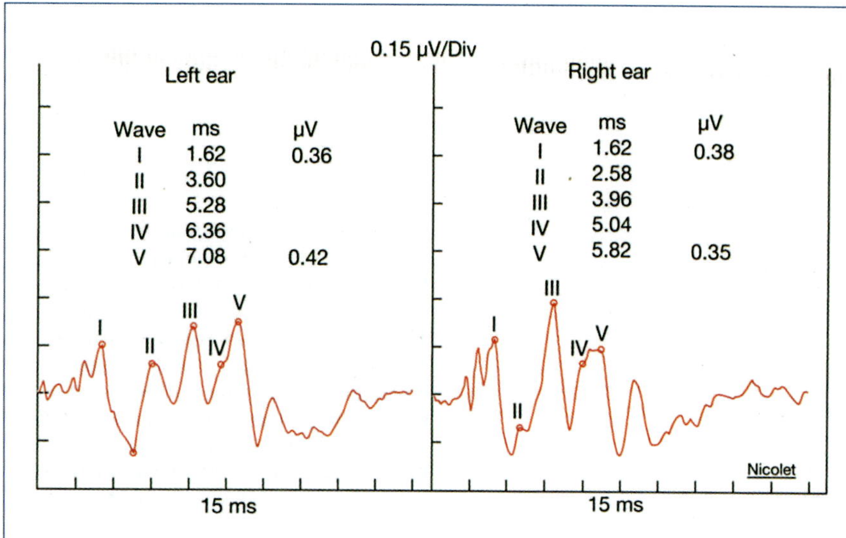

FIGURE 19–9 • Scalp-recorded auditory brainstem response (ABR) traces for the left and right ears of a patient with a left-sided cerebellopontine angle lesion are shown. The left ear ABR exhibits relatively normal morphology. Wave I latency is normal, but the remaining peaks exhibit abnormal absolute and interpeak latencies. The right ear ABR exhibits normal morphology and normal absolute and interpeak latencies.

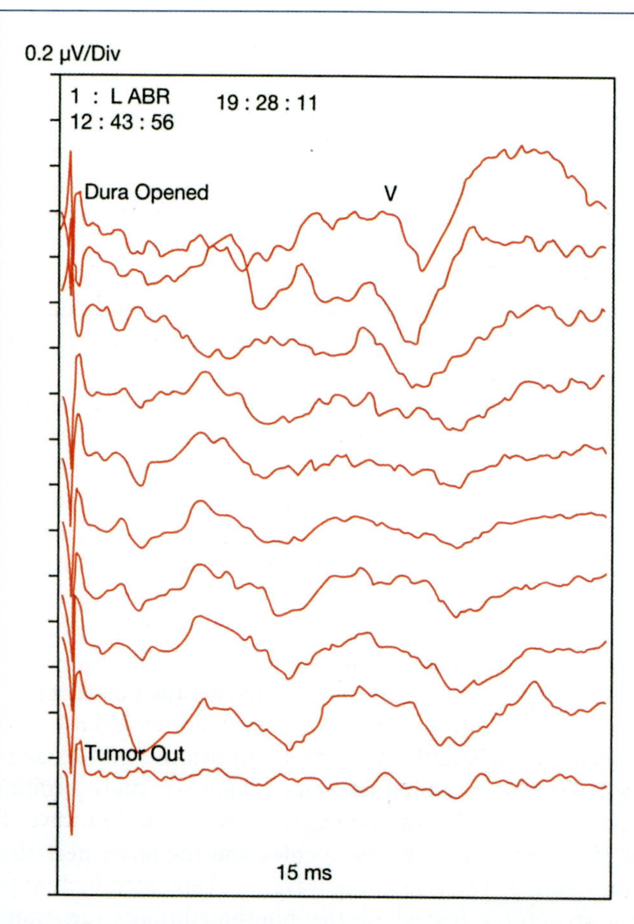

FIGURE 19–10 • Serial recordings of scalp-recorded auditory brainstem responses acquired during resection of a 2.5-cm acoustic neuroma. The top trace was acquired just subsequent to opening the dura and was used as a baseline trace by which all subsequent traces were compared. Only wave V was clearly identified in the baseline trace. Subsequent traces exhibited even greater morphologic abnormality.

slight variations in placing the vertex electrode are not critical. To optimize wave I, the reference electrode is placed on the mastoid or earlobe ipsilateral to the stimulated ear. However, this placement may be inconvenient for surgeries of the ear in which the surgical field lies close to the mastoid and/or earlobe. In such cases, placement of the reference electrode at the base of the skull or high cervical spine will yield a wave I comparable to the mastoid/earlobe placement.

Insert earphones with tube extensions deliver the acoustic click to the ear. The tube extension is secured in the ear with a flexible universal earmold (eg, Doc's Promold®) or a foam earmold. The universal mold is preferred to the foam earmold since it creates a more secure fit in the ear. However, the foam tip can be effective when secured in the ear with surgical bone wax. To avoid collection of preparatory or other fluids in the canal of the surgical ear, seal the earmold and tubing with a small adhesive drape (eg, Tegaderm®). A click of slow to moderate rate (7–27/sec) should be delivered with sufficient loudness to evoke the three most prominent waves (I, III, and V). Avoid click rates near or at multiples of 60 Hz that can result in cyclic interference from electrical lines and fields. Depending on the degree of hearing loss, 70 to 90 dB nHL is an adequate click intensity. Most patients who require monitoring of auditory function during surgery exhibit preoperative and intraoperative ABR abnormalities; a recording time window of 15 to 20 millisecond will account for any abnormally prolonged latencies. In an anesthetized patient, a reliable ABR can be identified within a few hundred averaged stimuli. Most difficulties in recording ABRs in the operating room are the result of technical conditions. A preoperative ABR study is recommended to determine the reliability of the ABR for the operative ear and will help avoid any questions regarding technical mishaps that can occur in the operating room. Additionally, occasional recording from the nonsurgical ear provides a control condition accounting for temperature and other nonpathologic events that can affect the ABR during surgery.

The operating room and surgical environment can create unpredictable events that can affect the reliability of the ABR. Continuous recording of the ABR during each stage of the surgery can help identify and troubleshoot these events. Although DENM recordings may be a more desirable method of monitoring during tumor resection, the scalp-recorded ABR is initially necessary to ensure technical reliability since the recording methodologies are similar, with the exception of the intracranial electrode. Additionally, brain retraction applied during initial exposure can alter eighth nerve function, and the scalp-recorded ABR can help identify this situation.

Technically, recording the cochlear nerve action potential (CNAP) is similar to recording the ABR, with some exceptions, including the placement of the reference electrode on or near the eighth nerve and the gain settings. The senior author has a long-standing interest in DENM and prefers an electrode of his own design (available through AD-Tech Medical Instrument Corporation, Racine, Wisconsin), which provides consistent but gentle positioning on the cochlear nerve.[12,14] This electrode (Figure 19–11) partially encircles the cochlear nerve but allows atraumatic escape of the nerve should the electrode be accidentally displaced. When the electrode is mounted on the applicator, the opening in the C-shaped ring is opened widely, allowing for atraumatic insinuation of the electrode around the cochlear nerve. Simple digital pressure on the finger pad of the applicator allows closure of the ring, securing it gently on the nerve. The electrode wire is then disengaged from the proximal yoke of the applicator and the applicator is carefully withdrawn, leaving the electrode on the cochlear nerve as seen in Figure 19–12.

The amplitude of the CNAP is anywhere from 10 to 100 times larger than that of the scalp-recorded ABR since the impedance of the head significantly reduces the voltage of the ABR generators to an amplitude range of 0.50 to 1.0 μV. Because of the proximity of the intracranial electrode, the CNAP can be as large as 50 μV, depending on the extent of eighth nerve compromise and

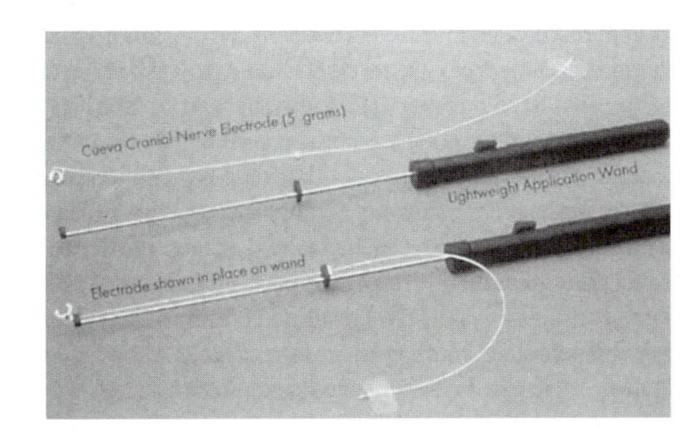

FIGURE 19–11 • The Cueva cranial nerve electrode is shown with its application wand. When mounted on the wand, tension along the lead wire opens the C-shaped ring, allowing atraumatic placement on the cochlear nerve.

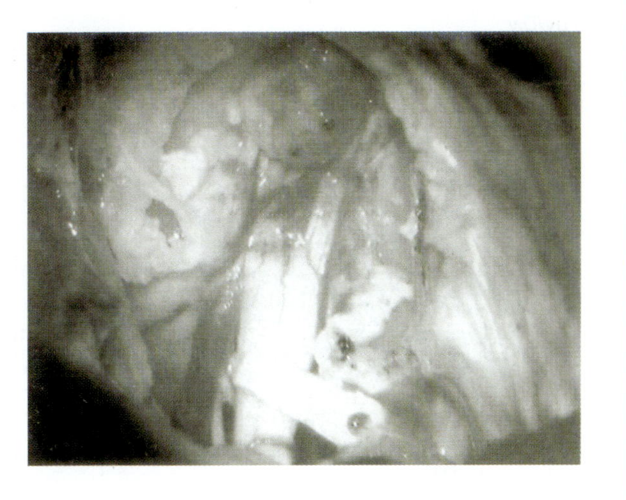

FIGURE 19–12 • The electrode is in place on the cochlear nerve during retrosigmoid craniotomy for removal of a right, intracanalicular acoustic neuroma. The tumor arose from the superior vestibular nerve. Postoperative pure-tone levels were maintained within 5 dB of preoperative levels, and speech discrimination remained at 96%.

electrode location. Additionally, the voltage of the CNAP provides an improved signal-to-noise ratio, requiring fewer averaged responses to yield a reliable waveform. In the surgical environment, the scalp-recorded ABR may require 1 to 2 min to yield a reliable tracing, whereas the CNAP may be obtained in as little as six-tenths of a second. Figure 19–13 demonstrates a scalp-recorded ABR and a DENM from a patient undergoing surgery for an acoustic neuroma. The DENM electrode was placed at the cochlear nerve root entry to the brain stem. The amplitude of the scalp-recorded ABR was less than 0.5 μV, whereas the DENM response exceeded 45.0 μV. Serially recorded DENM tracings acquired during removal of an acoustic neuroma are shown in Figure 19–14. The final tracing was recorded at the completion of tumor removal. Although the DENM response exhibited a decline, there was still evidence of cochlear nerve continuity and function at the conclusion of surgery.

It is not unusual to observe a significant decline in the scalp-recorded ABR during tumor resection, and, in many cases, the ABR may be absent despite neural continuity. Authors have reported hearing preservation in a substantial percentage of surgical patients in whom the scalp-recorded ABR disappeared during surgical removal of the CPA tumor.[24] In such cases, the CNAP can provide valuable information to the surgeon regarding the condition of the eighth nerve. Roberson et al reported their findings in a series of patients undergoing surgery for an acoustic neuroma in whom the ABR was absent, yet all had a detectable CNAP.[26] Figure 19–15 demonstrates the recordings from a patient in whom the ABR was absent, but a reliable CNAP was recorded using DENM.

Although the ABR will always be a part of auditory monitoring for CPA surgery, it has distinct disadvantages compared

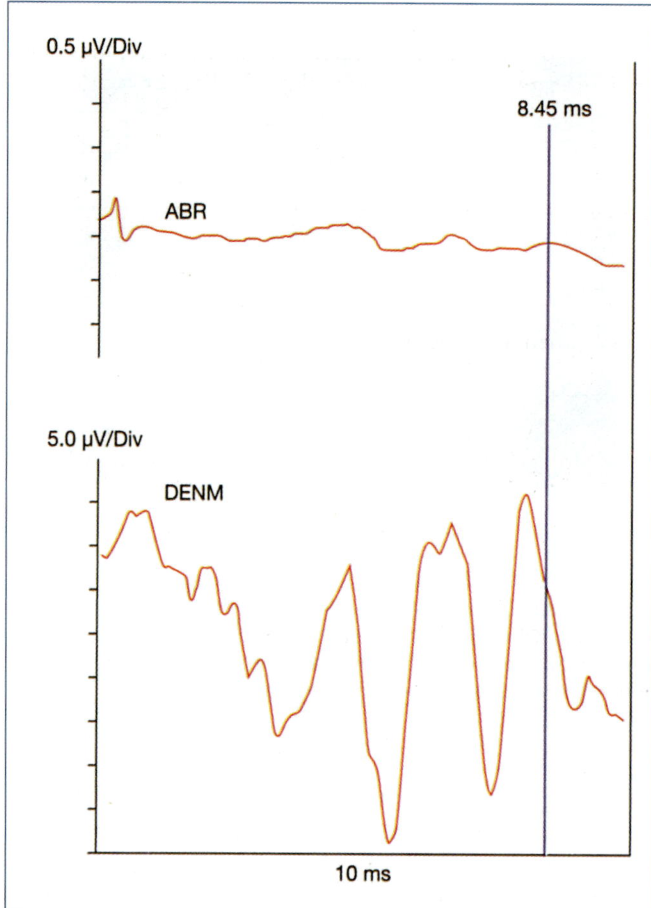

FIGURE 19–13 • Scalp-recorded auditory brainstem response (ABR) and direct eighth nerve monitoring (DENM) traces recorded from the same patient undergoing craniotomy for acoustic neuroma removal are shown. The DENM electrode was placed at the eighth nerve entry zone at the brain stem. The ABR is the averaged response to 300 stimuli, and the DENM is the averaged response to 20 stimuli. Both were acquired with the same click rate (17.1/sec) and click intensity (90 dB nHL), resulting in acquisition times of approximately 15 seconds and 1 sec, respectively. Both traces are displayed with a 10-millisecond time window for comparison. A cursor is placed at wave V of the ABR (8.45 millisecond) and corresponds closely to the latest peak seen in the DENM. The amplitudes of the DENM waveforms exceed the ABR by nearly 100 times.

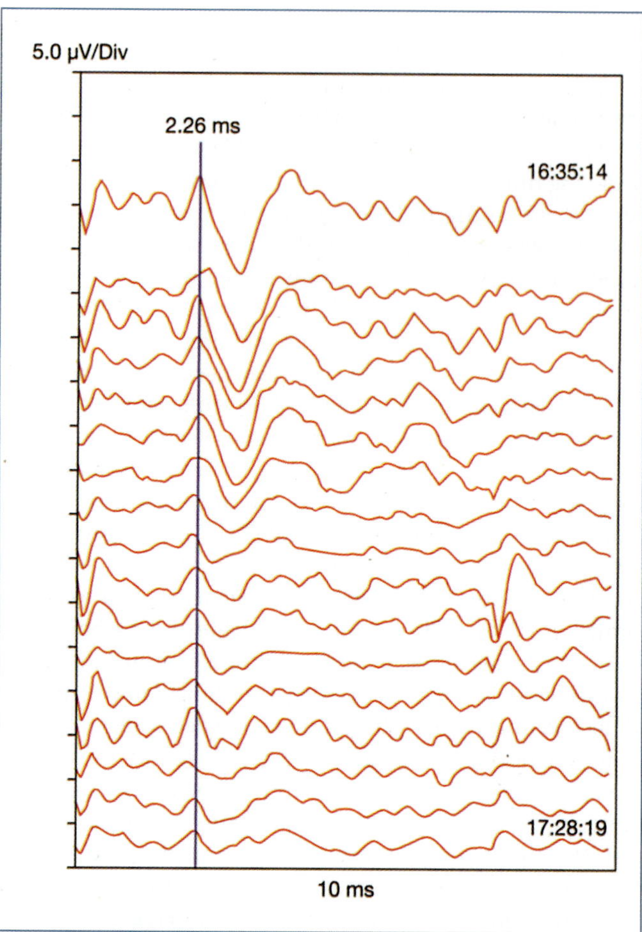

FIGURE 19–14 • Serially recorded direct eighth nerve monitoring (DENM) traces acquired during tumor removal are shown. The first trace was recorded at 16:35:14 and the last trace at 17:28:19, just following removal of the remaining sections of the tumor. Although the last trace shows a decline in the DENM, evidence of activity consistent with neural continuity is evident.

to DENM. The monitoring of cochlear nerve action potentials gives more rapid feedback with robust amplitudes. The CNAP can often identify neural integrity when ABR is no longer recordable. Hence, in their striving for optimal patient outcomes, an ever-increasing number of centers are using DENM as a routine part of CPA surgery.

OTHER CRANIAL NERVE MONITORING

Electromyography is widely used to monitor other motor cranial nerves during neurotologic surgery. The motor branch of the trigeminal nerve, the vagus nerve, the spinal accessory nerve, and the hypoglossal nerve are commonly monitored using EMG.[13] These nerves have been monitored primarily in patients undergoing surgery for tumors affecting the CPA, jugular foramen, and Meckel's cave.

Monitoring of the other motor cranial nerves involves placing either needle or surface electrodes in or near the muscles innervated by the nerve of interest. In the case of the trigeminal nerve, the masseter or temporalis muscle may be used. Needle electrode placement into the trapezius and tongue muscles for monitoring the spinal accessory and hypoglossal nerves, respectively, is readily accomplished. Monitoring the vagus nerve is more challenging and requires either direct laryngoscopy for needle electrode placement into the vocalis muscles of the true vocal cords or use of a specially designed endotracheal tube that incorporates surface electrodes on its surface. As with facial nerve monitoring using EMG, neuromuscular paralysis must be avoided during the course of surgery.

Direct nerve monitoring of motor nerves has not been previously reported, but the senior author has used this technique with good results in surgery for tumors of the jugular foramen, low CPA, and foramen magnum. The same electrode used to monitor the cochlear nerve in the CPA is secured around the vagus, spinal accessory, and hypoglossal nerves in the neck. To ensure stable positioning, the open part of the C-shaped electrode is sutured with fine (4-0 or 5-0) silk to create a ring. The

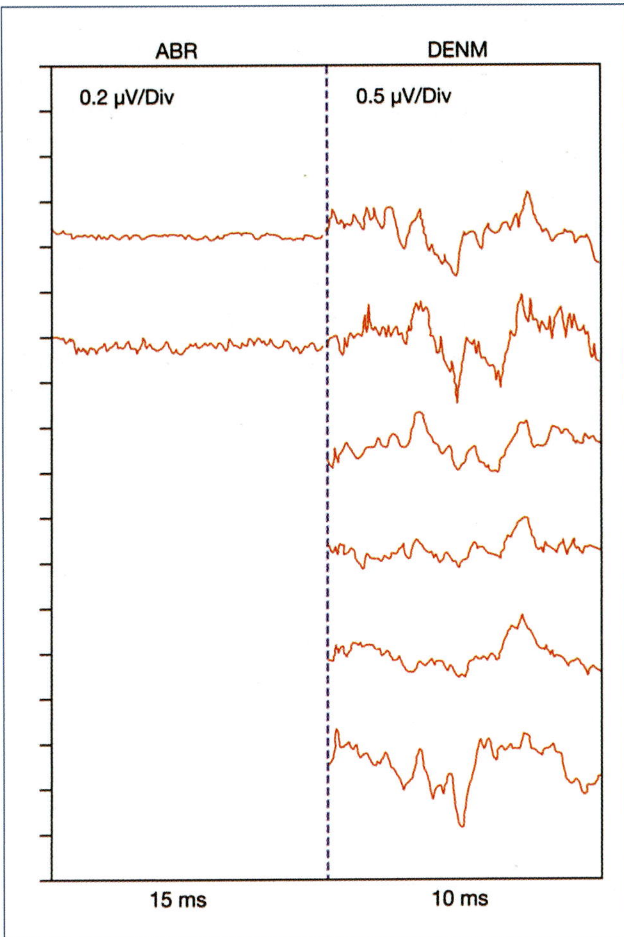

FIGURE 19–15 • Simultaneous recordings of the auditory brainstem response (ABR) and direct eighth nerve monitoring (DENM) are shown. No response peaks were observed in the ABR recordings. Although the peaks seen in the DENM traces are abnormally reduced in amplitude (approximately 1.0 μV), they could be reliably recorded during tumor removal. The last DENM trace was acquired subsequent to tumor removal.

suture needle is passed through the soft silicone of the electrode at the edges of the opening.

Direct motor nerve monitoring does not rely on the neuromuscular junction and therefore allows ongoing neuromuscular blockade, thereby simplifying the administration of anesthesia, which can be very helpful if use of the bipolar cautery is causing jerking muscular activity even from mild current spread. However, because the nerves of the jugular foramen are in direct contact with each other as they pass into the pars nervosa, electrical stimulation of one of the nerves intracranially often results in firing of all of the nerves. Mechanical stimulation of one of the nerves results in a compound action potential limited to that nerve; hence, the technique remains helpful during tumor dissection.

SUMMARY

Ever-growing numbers of surgeons are using neurophysiologic monitoring to help achieve optimal surgical outcomes for their patients undergoing neurotologic surgery. In fact, for many neurotologic and skull base surgeries, using monitoring is considered the standard of care. The last three decades have seen significant advances in technology facilitating routine use of these valuable monitoring methods. Future advances such as wireless connections between the monitoring head box/amplifiers and the averaging computer may reduce the impact of 60-cycle electrical interference in the operating room. The reader is encouraged to employ monitoring where judged appropriate in practice. In the final analysis, if the patient will likely have a better outcome because neurophysiologic monitoring was used, then it should be used.

References

1. Krause F. Surgery of the brain and spinal cord. Vol II. New York: Rebman Company; 1912.
2. Delgado TE, Buchheit WA, Rosenholtz HR, et al. Intraoperative monitoring of facial muscle evoked responses obtained by intracranial stimulation of the facial nerve: a more accurate technique for facial nerve dissection. Neurosurgery 1979;4:418–21.
3. Givre A, Olivecrona H. Surgical experiences with acoustic neuroma. J Neurosurg 1949;6:396–407.
4. Williams JD, Lehman R. Bells against palsy. Am J Otol 1988; 9: 81–2.
5. Møller AG, Jannetta PJ. Preservation of facial function during removal of acoustic neuromas. J Neurosurg 1984;61:757–60.
6. Gantz BJ. Intraoperative facial nerve monitoring. Am J Otol 1985;Nov. Suppl:58–61.
7. Harner SG, Daube JR, Ebersold MJ. Electrophysiologic monitoring of facial nerve during temporal bone surgery. Laryngoscope 1986;96:65–9.
8. Prass RL, Luders H. Evoked electromyographic activity during acoustic neuroma resection. Neurosurgery 1986;19:392–400.
9. Møller AG, Jannetta PJ. Compound action potentials recorded intracranially from the auditory nerve in man. Exp Neurol 1981;74:862–74.
10. Harner SG, Daube JR, Ebersold MJ, et al. Improved preservation of facial nerve function with use of electrical monitoring during removal of acoustic neuromas. Mayo Clin Proc 1987;62:92–102.
11. Ojemann RG, Levine RA, Montgomery WM. Use of intraoperative auditory evoked potentials to preserve hearing in unilateral acoustic neuroma removal. J Neurosurg 1984;61:938–48.
12. Cueva RA, Morris GF, Prioleau GR. Direct cochlear nerve monitoring: first report on a new atraumatic, self-retaining electrode. Am J Otol 1998;19:202–7.
13. Romstock J, Strauss C, Fahlbusch R. Continuous electromyography monitoring of motor cranial nerves during cerebellopontine angle surgery. J Neurosurg 2000;93:586–93.
14. Danner C, Mastrodimos B, Cueva RA. A comparison of direct eighth nerve monitoring and auditory brainstem response in hearing preservation surgery for vestibular schwannoma. Otol Neurotol 2004;25(5):826–32.
15. Nielsen VK. Pathophysiology of hemifacial spasm: I. Ephaptic transmission and ectopic excitation. Neurology 1984;34: 418–26.
16. Rausdzens PA, Shetter AG. Intraoperative monitoring of brainstem auditory evoked potentials. J Neurosurg 1982;57:341–8.
17. Grundy BL, Jannetta PJ, Procoio PT, et al. Intraoperative monitoring of brain stem auditory evoked potentials. J Neurosurg 1982;57:674–81.

18. Abramson M, Stein BM, Pedley TA, et al. Intraoperative BAER monitoring and hearing preservation in the treatment of acoustic neuromas. Laryngoscope 1985;95:1318–22.
19. Schramm J, Mokrusch T, Fahlbusch R, et al. Detailed analysis of intraoperative changes monitoring brain stem acoustic evoked potentials. Neurosurgery 1988;22:694–702.
20. Nedzelski JM, Chiong CM, Cashman MZ, et al. Hearing preservation in acoustic neuroma surgery: Value of monitoring cochlear nerve action potentials. Otolaryngol Head Neck Surg 1994;111:703–9.
21. Jackson LE, Roberson JB. Acoustic neuroma surgery: Use of cochlear nerve action potential monitoring for hearing preservation. Am J Otol 2000;21:249–59.
22. Meyer TA, Canty PA, Wilkinson EP, Hansen MR Rubinstein JT, Gantz BJ. Small acoustic neuromas: Surgical outcomes versus observation or radiation. Otol Neurotol 2006;27(3):380–92
23. Jewett DL, Romano MN, Williston JS. Human auditory evoked potentials: Possible brain stem components detected on the scalp. Science 1970;167:1517–8.
24. Levine RA, Ronner SF, Ojemann RG. Auditory evoked potential and other neurophysiologic monitoring techniques during tumor surgery in the cerebellopontine angle. In: Loftus CM, Traynelis VC, editors. Intraoperative monitoring techniques in neurosurgery. New York: McGraw-Hill; 1994:175–91.
25. Martin WH, Pratt H, Schwegler JW. The origin of the human auditory brainstem response wave II. Electroencephalogr Clin Neurophysiol 1995;96:357–70.
26. Roberson JB, Jackson LE, McAuley JR. Acoustic neuroma surgery: Absent auditory brainstem response does not contraindicate attempted hearing preservation. Laryngoscope 1999;109: 904–10.

Endoscope-Assisted Ear Surgery 20

Dennis S. Poe, MD, FACS

The introduction of endoscopy into the middle ear has opened up new opportunities for minimally invasive temporal bone surgery. The use of the surgical microscope brought revolutionary advances into the field of otologic surgery because its new technology expanded the ability of surgeons to see in limited confines of the temporal bone. Similarly, endoscopic imaging provides dramatic new vistas to the otologist, and we are just in the early exciting phases of developing the appropriate applications and supporting instrumentation. The endoscope lens brings the surgeon's view into the depths of the operative field and can provide a wide field of view with perspectives not possible through a surgical microscope.

The operating microscope provides magnified images in a straight line extending from the objective lens. Many deep recesses within the temporal bone cannot be directly seen without the surgeon taking measures to expand the operative exposure. Endoscopes have an immediate advantage with an inherently wide field of view that extends from the tip of the instrument's lens. Additional angulation of view is accomplished by placing prisms into the tip. Endoscopes, therefore, offer the surgeon the capability of wide fields of view with minimal exposure, looking behind the obstructions or overhangs, and peering into recesses with much less requirement for surgical exposure than demanded by conventional techniques. Surgical morbidity and operating time can be substantially reduced.

Clinically, there are many current applications of endoscopes in temporal bone surgery. The present chapter will focus on surgery of the middle ear and mastoid with endoscopic assistance. Endoscopy of the middle ear itself may be done through a myringotomy, offering immediately available, spectacular in vivo examinations free of the artifacts of blood, tissue transudates, and injected local anesthetic agents. Accordingly, endoscopy may be useful for various diagnostic purposes, such as perilymphatic fistula explorations. Endoscopes also improve the ability to inspect the entire middle ear after cholesteatoma removal. Examination of the undersurfaces of the ossicles and tympanic membrane and the deep recesses of the mastoid cavity can reduce cholesteatoma residual rates.

BRIEF HISTORY

The first published description of imaging of the middle ear by endoscopy was by Mer and colleagues in 1967.[1] They passed a fiberoptic instrument through existing tympanic membrane perforations in two patients, but the image resolution of their instruments was quite limited. Eichner obtained much improved images using 2.7-mm-diameter rigid endoscopes, however, the much larger diameter significantly restricted the endoscope's utility within the small spaces of the temporal bone.[2] Nomura introduced the concept of middle ear exploration by passing a rigid endoscope through a myringotomy in an otherwise intact tympanic membrane.[3]

Rapid advances were subsequently made in fiberoptic resolution by reducing the size of individual fibers and packing more of them within the same outer diameter. Kimura and colleagues,[4] Chays and colleagues,[5] and Hopf and colleagues[6] passed high-resolution fibers through the nasal cavity to inspect the lumen of the eustachian tube, sometimes passing fibers all the way into the middle ear cavity for a limited view of its contents. Takahashi and colleagues inspected the bony eustachian tube orifices of children with 1.7-mm rigid endoscopes passed through an anterior myringotomy, prior to the placement of ventilation tubes.[7] Poe and colleagues described the use of 1.9-mm rigid endoscopes through a myringotomy to aid in the diagnosis of perilymphatic fistulae.[8] Thomassin and colleagues developed successful rigid endoscopic techniques as an adjunct to conventional cholesteatoma surgery, dramatically reducing the residual rates of disease.[9] McKennan used minimally invasive endoscopic techniques to perform second-look operations to rule out residual cholesteatoma.[10] Magnan and colleagues[11] and O'Donoghue and O'Flynn[12] began to popularize the use of rigid endoscopes in cerebellopontine angle surgery.

EQUIPMENT

Rigid Hopkins rod endoscopes and fiberoptic endoscopes are both commonly available for use in the office setting and in temporal bone surgery. Generally, the rigid endoscopes are preferred because of their superior resolution. Fiberoptic instruments are continually improving, allowing for ever-increasing numbers of individual light-carrying fibers to be packed into small (outer) diameter endoscopes. Each light fiber carries a portion of the image representing a single pixel, and increasing the number of pixels increases the resolution of the overall image. There is a finite amount of cladding and cement between fibers that creates a visible "chicken wire fence appearance" when images are sharply focused. Rod lens endoscopes avoid this problem, yielding images with superior clarity and resolution. Fiberoptic endoscopes can be constructed with smaller diameters than most rigid endoscopes, but the resulting fiber-transmitted image is generally considered to be impractical for surgical purposes owing to the consequent reduction in resolution. Newer generation rigid endoscopes, using gradient index (GRIN) of refraction lenses, are becoming ever smaller, and are closing the gap with fiber technology.[8] GRIN microendoscopes are now being evaluated for intralabyrinthine imaging. The miniaturization of charge-coupled device (CCD) camera microchips has progressed sufficiently that they can be placed on the distal end of a flexible endoscope ("chip-tip" endoscope) of diameter as small as 3.1 mm and eliminating the need for fiberoptic or long lens systems entirely. These cameras have image resolution comparable to a rigid Hopkins rod endoscope without requiring any fiber or rigid optical elements other than the camera chip and covering lens. As these endoscopes become smaller, they will play an increasingly important role in endoscopic surgery because of their steerability and exceptional optics.

Endoscopic images have the disadvantage of spherical distortion ("fisheye views") and cannot ordinarily provide the three-dimensional view afforded with the binocular-operating microscope. Endoscopic magnification increases steeply as an object comes into close proximity to the lens and can approach the powers achieved with the operating microscope. Endoscopic surgeons learn to compensate for the variable magnification and two-dimensional views by watching how a structure and its surroundings change as the endoscope is moved in and out of proximity to it. The three-dimensionality of an image is re-created by these changes with motion of the endoscope.

Endoscopes intended to pass through the tympanic membrane must be 1.9 mm in diameter or less. Operating room exposures permit the use of larger endoscopes, such as 2.3 to 4.0 mm, which are preferred since they yield larger images with improved brightness and clarity. Endoscopes typically have 0-, 30-, and 70-degree view angles.

Endoscopic illumination is provided by a halogen or xenon fiberoptic light source, generally using 150 to 300 W. Images may be viewed directly through the endoscope lens, or, more commonly, a CCD camera is attached to the endoscope's proximal lens to deliver the images to a monitor. Computer interfaces, digital or video recording devices, and printing systems are optional.

ENDOSCOPY OF THE EXTERNAL AUDITORY CANAL AND TYMPANIC MEMBRANE

Endoscopes may be used in the office for inspecting areas of the ear that are inaccessible to the operating microscope and for photodocumentation. The panoramic view achieved with a 2.7- or 4-mm endoscope makes for excellent otologic photography. The endoscopes may be used to inspect the tympanic membrane or the medial external auditory canal when the microscopic view is limited by a canal stenosis or other obstruction. Bony canal defects or recesses and the depths of limited mastoid cavities may be easily seen. Tympanic membrane retraction pockets may be inspected to determine their depth and the presence or absence of cholesteatoma. Surgeons may benefit from such information when considering whether a patient should undergo cholesteatoma surgery and determining the optimal approach.

TRANSTYMPANIC ENDOSCOPY

An endoscope may be passed through an existing perforation or myringotomy in the tympanic membrane to perform a limited middle ear exploration. The procedure may be performed in the office or operating room and is commonly done using Hopkins rod endoscopes with outside diameters of 1.7 or 1.9 mm. The 1.7-mm-diameter endoscope is often preferred as it passes more readily through the tympanic membrane. Indications for transtympanic endoscopy are listed in Table 20–1.

Technique for Office Transtympanic Endoscopy

The patient is reclined to the supine position in the office examination chair. The tympanic membrane is initially inspected with the operating microscope, and the location of the incision is planned to overlie the area of anticipated pathology. Working through an ear speculum, the tympanic membrane is anesthetized with topical phenol solution (USP) applied by dipping a 20-gauge suction tip into the solution and touching the adherent bead of solution to the tympanic membrane over the incision site only. Phenol is the preferred anesthetic because of its rapid onset of action and local cautery effect that provides a dry, bloodless field. A radial myringotomy is carried out from

TABLE 20–1 Indication for transtympanic endoscopy

N = 119 PATIENTS IN OFFICE	
DIAGNOSIS	NO. OF PATIENTS
Vertigo to rule out perilymphatic fistula	59
RW exam before IT gentamicin	37
Conductive hearing loss	7
Middle ear mass	9
TM granulations, suspected cholesteatoma	2
Exam RW for failed IT gentamicin	2
Vertigo, rule out recurrent cholesteatoma	1
Hyperacusis, rule out absent stapedius	1
Exam perilymph fistula site after repair	1

IT, intratympanic administration; RW, round window; TM, tympanic membrane.

the umbo to the annulus, creating an opening sufficiently large to readily admit the endoscope without tearing the tympanic membrane. The incision for exploration of a possible perilymphatic fistula is made halfway between the shadow of the round window niche and the distal end of the long process of the incus seen through the tympanic membrane.

Defogger is applied to the endoscope lens at the tip. A drop of defogger is blotted with a cotton sponge, taking care to avoid contact with the lens, which would smear the solution and thus obscure the image.

Initial inspection of the middle ear is done with a 0-degree endoscope, which provides a good overall view of the middle ear. The 30-degree endoscope is usually required to obtain a definitive close-up view of areas with suspected pathology. The angled endoscope is more difficult to use, to a certain extent, because of its off-center view, and it requires some practice for atraumatic insertion through a myringotomy.

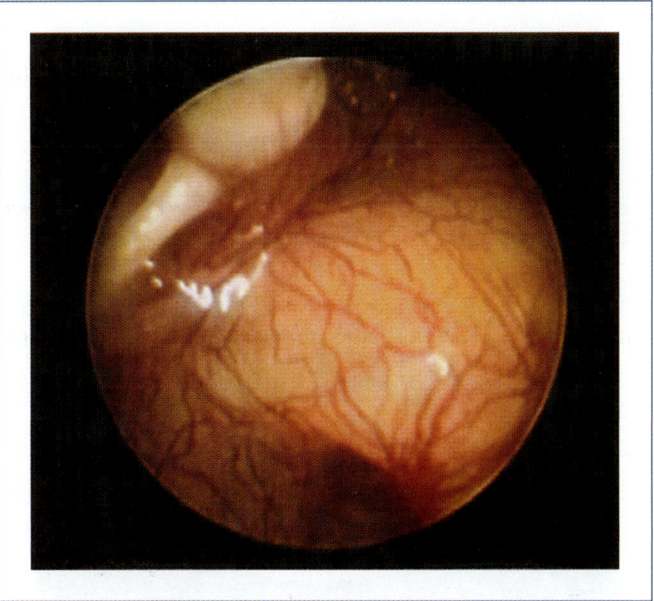

FIGURE 20–1 • Transtympanic endoscopic view of the middle ear: 1.9-mm, 0-degree angled Hopkins rod endoscope.

MIDDLE EAR ENDOSCOPIC SURGERY

Surgeons with little endoscopic experience would be well advised to introduce the endoscope through the tympanic membrane perforation while looking directly through the eyepiece. Although the image appears quite small to the eye, it allows for an adequate examination and it is easier to maintain control of the endoscope within the ear. Adding a CCD camera can cause disorientation by forcing the surgeon to look at a video monitor remote from the surgical field. Any rotation of the camera produces errors in hand–eye-coordinated movements. The camera also adds additional weight to the endoscope system. With practice, most endoscopists eventually prefer video images, which are considerably enlarged and offer more detail of the surgical field.

Endoscopes are passed through a handheld ear speculum slightly smaller than one that would ordinarily be used with a microscope. The smaller speculum extends deeper into the external auditory canal and helps protect the sensitive canal skin from inadvertent contact with the endoscope shaft that could produce pain or bleeding. The speculum and endoscope shaft are supported by the surgeon's nondominant hand, and fine fingertip movements are used to guide the endoscope tip atraumatically through the myringotomy. The dominant hand is used to hold the eyepiece and camera, helping to guide the endoscope tip and allowing for some minimal rotation of the field of view as desired. With the endoscope fully passed through the tympanic membrane, a wide view of the middle ear can be appreciated (Figure 20–1). Close-up, angled views, especially beneath overhangs, are best achieved with a 30-degree endoscope, which is introduced by rotating the view angle to the appropriate direction prior to insertion into the middle ear (Figures 20–2 and 20–3). When viewing on the video monitor, it is especially important to ensure that the camera is properly oriented to avoid trauma to the ear from inadvertent movements. The endoscope is generally withdrawn and reinserted whenever a significant change in the direction of view angle is desired.

Patients may experience a heat-induced caloric effect with vertigo when using the 300-W light source if the endoscope remains in situ more than 45 to 60 sec. Withdrawal of the endoscope relieves the symptoms, and the examination may proceed, either with reduced brightness or by removing the endoscope periodically. The author has had no cases of thermal injury, but elevations of temperature, up to 50 degrees, have been produced in dry temporal bones exposed for 2 min or more.[13] Vertigo has not occurred when using the 150-W light source.

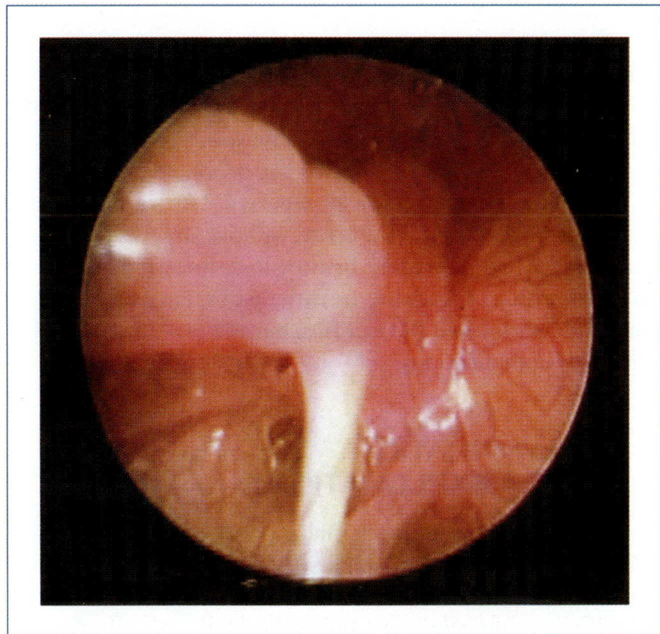

FIGURE 20–2 • Transtympanic endoscopic view of the superior mesotympanum: 1.9-mm, 30-degree angled Hopkins rod endoscope.

At the conclusion of the endoscopy, the myringotomy is inspected under the microscope to ascertain that the margins were minimally traumatized and lie nearly in apposition. Wide gaps or inadvertent tears may be repaired with adhesive

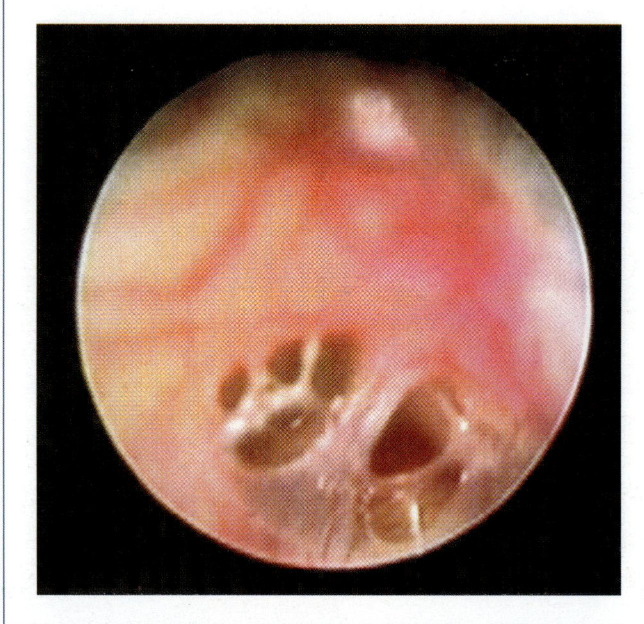

FIGURE 20–3 • Transtympanic endoscopic view of the round window niche: 1.9-mm, 30-degree angled Hopkins rod endoscope.

Steri-strip™, cigarette paper, or Gelfilm™. This problem is usually avoided by making a sufficiently long myringotomy initially. The patient is advised to follow water precautions and avoid nose blowing for 1 week after the procedure.[14]

The author has previously reported 112 transtympanic endoscopic procedures in the office, without any complications, including vertigo, persistent hearing loss, infection, or persistent perforation. Presently, transtympanic endoscopy is not commonly performed in the office but the procedure remains free of any complications.

PERILYMPHATIC FISTULA EXPLORATION

Surgical exploration for perilymphatic fistula was once considered the gold standard for establishing the diagnosis. It has been learned that mere observation of pooling of fluid in the round and/or oval window niches, the previously accepted criterion for determining the presence or absence of a fistula, is inaccurate. Tissue transudates or residual injected anesthetic can also accumulate in these niches and appear identical to a presumed fistula.[15] Endoscopic exploration may help reduce some of the artifacts by using a topical cauterizing anesthetic such as phenol. The middle ear can be inspected in an undisturbed state. Transtympanic exploration for fistula may be done entirely in the office, or, if done in the operating room, there is also the capability to elevate a tympanomeatal flap for fistula repair, if a fistula is discovered.

Studies have been done to determine if endoscopy, in comparison to microscopic examination, has sufficient resolution to detect the presence of a leaking fistula.[16] Endoscopic and microscopic findings have been compared in temporal bone specimens and in the operating room.[17] Seventeen patients with a clinical history and findings suspicious for fistula underwent combined transtympanic endoscopy and microsurgical exploration. The middle ear endoscopy was performed first, with no local anesthetic, and findings were determined. One mL of lidocaine (1% solution with 1:100,000 epinephrine) was then infiltrated into the external auditory canal, and a standard tympanomeatal flap was elevated. In 8 of the 17 patients, thorough endoscopic examinations showed no evidence of a fistula. However, with the immediately subsequent microsurgical exploration, active pooling of clear fluid in the round or oval window, which would ordinarily have been regarded as a fistula, was seen. The preceding endoscopic exploration was done carefully and actually yielded more complete exposure of each window niche with superior magnification and resolution when compared to microscopic views. It was concluded that the pooling of fluids seen only on microscopic view must be artifactual.

There were four cases of probable true perilymphatic fistula identified with both endoscopic and microsurgical examinations. The site of each fistula was imaged better with the endoscope than by a microscope. Each case involved true trauma: barotraumatic injury in three cases and perforating trauma in one case. There were five patients, all of whom had undergone previous surgery and had inadequate endoscopic examination as a result of bleeding that occurred during the lysis of middle-ear adhesions that resulted from the prior surgery (Figure 20–4).

The author has previously reported 75 transtympanic middle ear explorations for perilymphatic fistula in the office or in the operating room, identifying only five cases in which a fistula was seen. Other surgeons, using endoscopic techniques, have also reported a low incidence of fistulae, with Rosenberg and colleagues[18] seeing no cases in 13 endoscopic explorations and Pyykkö and colleagues[19] identifying only two fistulae in 350 endoscopies.

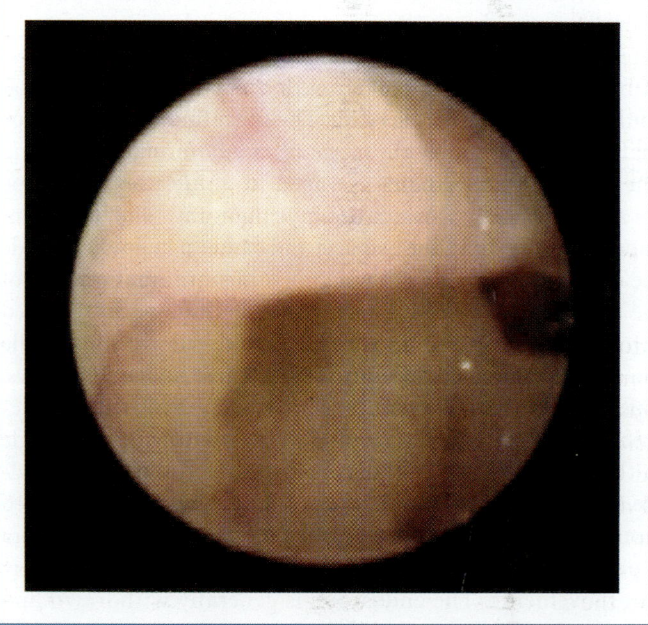

FIGURE 20–4 • Transtympanic endoscopic view of the round window perilymphatic fistula: 1.9-mm, 30-degree angled Hopkins rod endoscope.

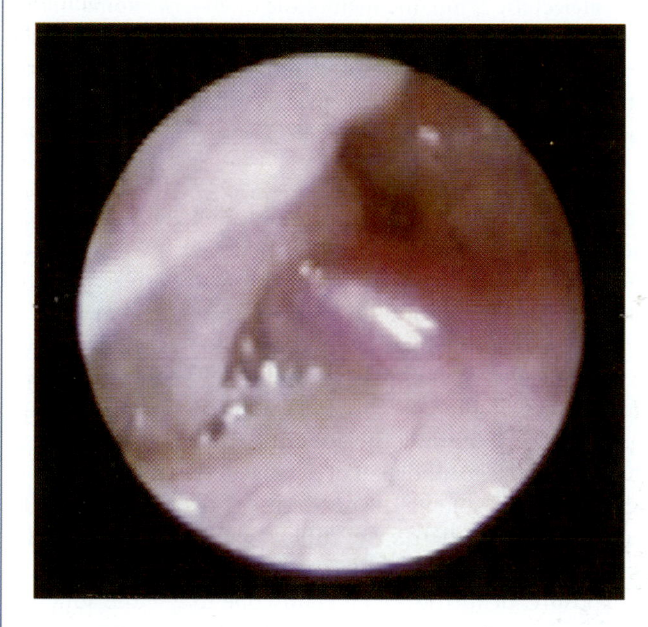

FIGURE 20–5 • Transtympanic endoscopic view of a persistent stapedial artery: 1.9-mm, 30-degree angled Hopkins rod endoscope.

Middle ear endoscopic techniques probably improve the ability to identify true perilymphatic fistulae and reduce the number of false-positive examinations. Open surgical exploration cannot eliminate the artifactual pooling of infiltrated anesthetics and surgically induced transudates. Endoscopy is an excellent adjunct to microsurgical exploration (Figure 20–5).

Fistulae in adults most likely occur with significant trauma, such as barotrauma, head injury, penetrating trauma, and otologic surgery. Exploration is indicated in patients with sensorineural hearing loss or persistent vertigo or dysequilibrium associated with the trauma. A positive subjective or objective fistula test was present in each of the true fistula cases seen by the author. The diagnosis of perilymphatic fistula should be made only after exclusion of other possible etiologies. Consideration of additional evaluation, such as laboratory tests and imaging studies, should be individualized.

ENDOSCOPY IN CHRONIC EAR SURGERY

Endoscopes are best employed in chronic ear surgery as an adjunct to the removal of cholesteatoma.[20–24] Residual disease tends to occur in the sites hardest to inspect with the operating microscope, including the epitympanum, the sinus tympani, and the facial recess. Endoscopes may help to detect residual disease in otherwise hidden recesses after microsurgical resection or may be used for a portion of the primary dissection of cholesteatoma. When cholesteatoma is limited to the attic, the aditus ad antrum, the facial recess, or the sinus tympani, endoscope-assisted surgery may eliminate the need for mastoidectomy in many cases. The enhanced ability to remove cholesteatoma reduces the incidence of residual disease and the frequency of planned second-stage procedures. In the event that a second-look operation is indicated, the procedure can most often be done as a transcanal approach with endoscopic assistance. The endoscopic view of the temporal bone recesses is far superior to the limited views obtained by microsurgical approaches.

The endoscope is not intended to replace microsurgical resection. It has several disadvantages. The endoscopes are held in the surgeon's nondominant hand, so that only one hand is free for surgery. The surgeon must often alternate between dissection and suction-aspiration of blood from the field, reducing operating efficiency compared to two-hand techniques. One should do as much dissection under the microscope as possible and reserve the endoscope for areas that are not easily seen microscopically. Most commonly, an entire case is performed without endoscopes, and the endoscopes may be introduced only at the end of the procedure to inspect the recesses for residual disease. In other cases, microsurgical resection of cholesteatoma matrix may be hindered by adhesions in a recess such as in the sinus tympani, and continued "blind" elevation may risk tearing the matrix and leaving residual disease (Figure 20–6). The adhesion may be seen endoscopically, allowing for expeditious

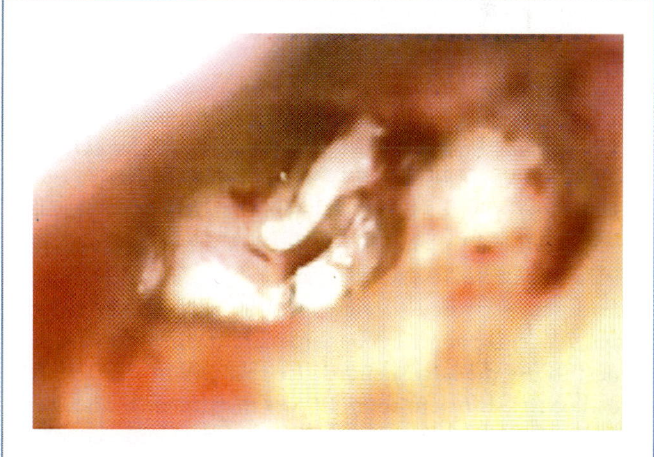

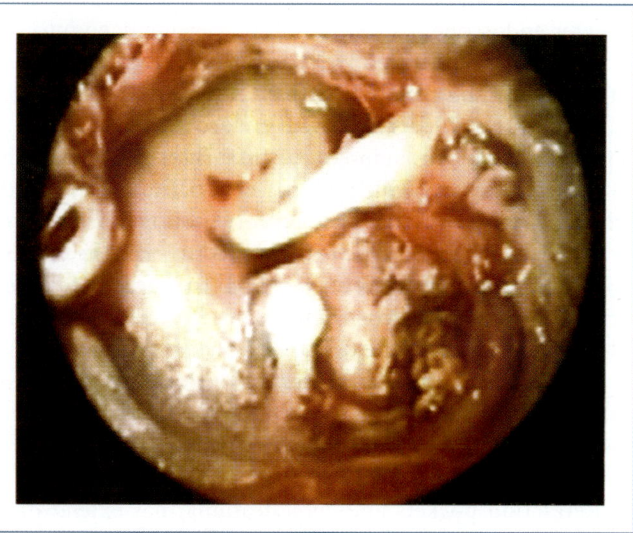

FIGURE 20–6 • *A*, Microscopic view of the left ear with cholesteatoma in posterior–superior pars tensa retraction pocket. *B*, A 4-mm, 0-degree Hopkins rod endoscopic view of the same ear.

lysis and resumption of microsurgical resection. It is often helpful to alternate between microscopic and endoscopic resections for this reason.

Cases of limited cholesteatoma or tympanic membrane atelectasis with deep retraction pockets are often approached by atticotomy or mastoidectomy. These are the standard microsurgical approaches to remove disease from the epitympanum, the mastoid antrum, the medial surface of the scutum and within the facial recess itself. Removal of the cholesteatoma matrix is frequently piecemeal, and second-stage procedures or serial imaging for residual disease are often recommended. These types of cholesteatoma cases are well suited to endoscopic resection, which may often be performed as a transcanal procedure or by postauricular exposure while working through the bony canal but without the need for an atticotomy or mastoidectomy. Cholesteatomas extending toward the tegmen but not deep into the antrum may be managed with the addition of an atticotomy to the extent necessary to see the superior aspect of the matrix sac or at least sufficiently to allow for intact dissection of the sac with angled instruments. The attic defect is reconstructed with cartilage graft. The matrix may be dissected under direct endoscopic imaging or by microscopic view and can often be removed completely intact, obviating the need for second-look surgery.

Technique

Use of the video monitor is preferred because the images are superior to those seen by viewing through the eyepiece. Prolonged endoscopic resection is optimized by using a monitor. If limited endoscopy is used only briefly, such as to inspect for residual disease, then viewing through the eyepiece is satisfactory and requires less setup time.

Endoscopy is used to view into the recesses so that the 30- and 70-degree angled endoscopes are the most often used. It is best to use the largest endoscope that will fit into the field while allowing sufficient room to pass instruments. The larger image and illumination afforded with the bigger endoscopes are preferred. Endoscopes of 30-degree angulation with a 2.7- or 4-mm outer diameter are often used. A 70-degree, 2.3-mm-diameter endoscope is most useful for viewing deep into the facial recess or aditus and yields excellent views far into the epitympanum and mastoid antrum. It requires considerable practice to use a 70-degree angled endoscope safely as there is no forward view. The endoscope is first inserted to nearly the full depth necessary while looking externally along the shaft of the endoscope with the naked eye and noting the location of the ossicles. The endoscope is then tilted to bring the ossicles into the monitor (or eyepiece) view, and the surgeon may then work through the endoscope or the monitor, carefully tilting the endoscope away from the ossicles into the appropriate recess, but always maintaining awareness of the location of the ossicles, which may now be out of view. The location of the ossicles should be periodically checked to confirm one's orientation and avoid inadvertent injury.

Retraction pockets and cholesteatoma that extend deep into the mastoid antrum or epitympanum are beyond the reach of endoscopic resection and are best managed by open microsurgical techniques. Removal of shallow pockets and cholesteatoma may be assisted with endoscopic resection. The elevation of the atelectatic tympanic membrane or cholesteatoma matrix is begun with conventional microsurgical techniques, generally starting by freeing up retractions into the attic or wherever the matrix may be loosely applied, such as the neck of the malleus or anterior or posterior to the incus.

Strategies in Removal of Cholesteatoma Matrix

Cholesteatoma matrix is not uniformly adherent to middle ear mucosa. Rather, it is adherent intermittently in areas and loosely applied in many other areas. When attempting to remove the matrix, it is best to look for the adhesions and systematically lyse them. The remaining matrix will then be loosely attached over the subsequent area and may be readily elevated until the next adhesion is encountered. Matrix elevation becomes an exercise in identifying and lysing the adhesive attachments. When an adhesion disappears under an overhang or in a recess out of line of sight, the adhesion may be lysed with angled instruments if it is believed that the matrix can still be maintained intact with a "blind sweep" technique. Otherwise, the options are to expand the exposure, or introduce an endoscope to lyse the adhesion and keep the matrix as intact as possible. It is not important to keep the lateral surface matrix intact. On the contrary, it may be opened to allow for debulking of the squamous debris interior, which facilitates the elevation of the deeper matrix by allowing it to be folded out of the way once it has been separated from the mucosa or underlying bone or soft tissues. When an adhesion cannot be readily separated from the adjacent mucosa, the mucosa itself may be removed to try to preserve continuity of the matrix.

Endoscopic Dissection Technique

Elevation with two-hand techniques is continued until adhesions within the epitympanum, aditus, facial recess, or sinus tympani restrict further elevation. If the matrix cannot be mobilized without risking a tear, the endoscope may be inserted to view the adhesions limiting the dissection. The adhesions may then be lysed with long-angled picks or suction that has been bent to 90-degree angle and used as a suction dissector. The endoscope is held in the nondominant hand, and one-handed dissection is performed using the dominant hand. It may be appropriate to obtain good hemostasis with Gelfoam™ soaked in 1 to 100,000 epinephrine solution placed in the middle ear for a few minutes prior to beginning endoscopic dissection. If bleeding occurs during the dissection, it will be necessary to alternate between suction and dissection. Frequent irrigation of the field aids with hemostasis. It may be beneficial to return to the microscope periodically to improve hemostasis, evacuate clots, and then continue with two-hand dissection until additional adhesions are encountered. The suction dissectors are useful in improving endoscopic dissection efficiency but are not commercially available at present. Careful elevation of retraction pockets usually results in the intact removal of even very thin matrix in most cases, and, when successfully accomplished, a second-stage procedure is unnecessary (Figure 20–7).

Small cholesteatomas may be excised using techniques similar to those used to manage retraction pockets. The squamous debris is first removed, and in many cases the cholesteatoma matrix may be delivered intact. Large, bulky cholesteatomas are

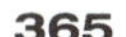

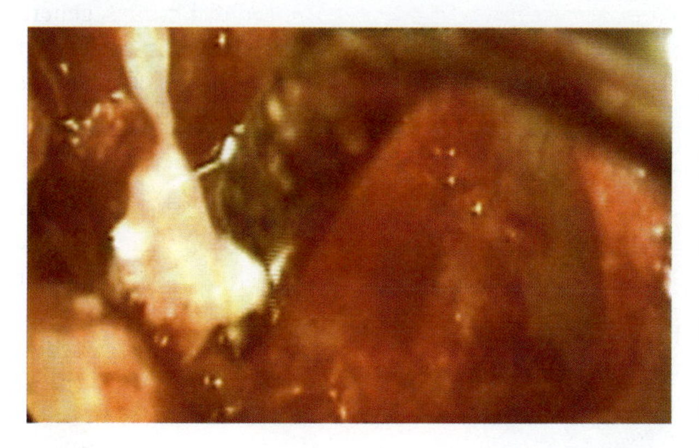

FIGURE 20–7 • Endoscopic dissection of cholesteatoma using a suction dissector.

best excised with conventional microsurgical techniques, but endoscopes may be useful in inspecting the epitympanum, the supratubal recess, the facial recess, the sinus tympani, and other recesses. If residual matrix is identified, removal may be accomplished either with endoscopic or microscopic dissection.

It is helpful to use a diamond bur to drill on the medial surface of the scutum, the epitympanic tegmen, and into the supratubal recess to ensure maximal exposure and complete eradication of the disease. In the unusual event that the posterior bony canal wall excessively obstructs the view into these areas, the drilling may be accomplished under endoscopic guidance (Figure 20–8).

Results in Endoscopic-Assisted Cholesteatoma Surgery

The author used endoscopic-guided surgery in 160 cases to assist in the eradication of cholesteatoma and each case had been planned for possible tympanomastoidectomy. These cases generally represent a subset of more difficult cholesteatomas as the endoscopes are not routinely required for eradication of disease in most cases. Three- to ten-year follow-up was available for all cases.

Patients were prepared for possible two-stage tympanomastoidectomy, but ultimately 9% had a transcanal tympanoplasty, 23% had postauricular tympanoplasty with atticotomy, and 68% had canal-wall-up tympanomastoidectomy. Fifty-three percent underwent planned, second-stage operations 6 or more months subsequently and another 3% underwent unplanned second-stage surgery for evidence of recurrent or residual disease. The second-stage operations were accomplished by a transcanal approach with endoscopic guidance in 75%. In 12.5% of the cases, residual cholesteatoma was found at the second stage, but 9.5% were expected due to the extent of disease at the primary surgery. There was a 1% incidence of long-term residual cholesteatoma. The overall rate of unexpected residual disease was 4%, a rate that is comparable with canal-wall-down mastoidectomy surgery. Endoscopic-assisted surgery for cholesteatoma was found to significantly reduce operative time, morbidity, need for second-stage operations, and likelihood of residual disease compared with historic controls.

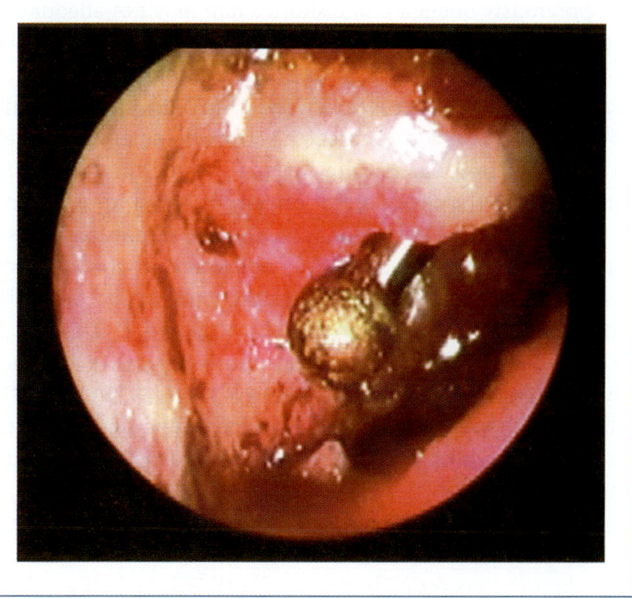

FIGURE 20–8 • Endoscopic view of the right mastoid cavity after intact canal mastoidectomy. A diamond drill is passed down the bony canal to smooth the tegmen bone and ensure cholesteatoma removal.

Canal-Wall-Up Versus Canal-Wall-Down Mastoidectomy

Canal-wall-down mastoidectomy has a fundamental advantage over the intact canal-wall technique in that the exposure of the sinus tympani, facial recess, and epitympanum is less restricted and the risk of residual disease is correspondingly reduced. Thomassin demonstrated that endoscopic visualization of recesses during canal-wall-up surgery may sufficiently improve residual disease removal as to become comparable with canal-wall-down surgery.[25] Initially, 44 of his patients underwent intact canal-wall mastoidectomy and 47.7% were found to have residual disease at the time of planned second-stage surgery. The subsequent 36 patients underwent endoscopic inspection for cholesteatoma during the primary operation, and the rate of residual disease dropped to 5.5% at the time of the second-stage procedure, an incidence on par with published results from canal-wall-down operations.

SECOND-LOOK MASTOIDECTOMY

Endoscopic techniques reduce the necessity for second-look procedures and also facilitate them when they are required. McKennan has advocated a small postauricular stab incision through which endoscopic inspection of the mastoid may be done,[10] and the view into the middle ear is usually obtained using angled endoscopes. Residual cholesteatoma, however, is most commonly found in the epitympanum, sinus tympani, or facial recess rather than in the mastoid antrum or cavity. For this reason, the author prefers a transcanal approach for second-look procedures.[26] A tympanomeatal flap is elevated through a transcanal approach, making the incision posteriorly in the bony external canal and midway between the tympanic ring and the cartilaginous junction. A longer flap will risk retraction of the canal skin into the mastoid cavity that has been previously opened and a shorter flap may not adequately cover the scutum defect and a supplemental graft may be required. Middle ear adhesions are lysed, and hemostasis is obtained, all under microscopic view. Once adequate exposure has been achieved, a 70-degree, 2.3-mm-diameter endoscope is introduced into the middle ear and rotated to give a panoramic view of the entire mesotympanum, the sinus tympani, the facial recess, the epitympanum, and the supratubal recess. Lysis of some adhesions is usually necessary to view through the attic and aditus far into the mastoid antrum and up to the tegmen. Satisfactory views are usually obtained. It is useful to alternate between endoscopic and microsurgical techniques to lyse adhesions and obtain hemostasis (Figures 20–9, 20–10, and 20-11). Figure 20-12 shows the healed tympanic membrane and external auditory canal after scutum reconstruction with a cartilage graft.

It is especially important to inspect the supratubal recess and sinus tympani carefully as they are the most hidden from view when the posterior bony canal wall is intact. If residual cholesteatoma is identified, small lesions may be removed with endoscopic dissection, but large deposits may require further drilling for exposure and microsurgical removal. Patients are counseled preoperatively about the possibility of reopening the postauricular incision if necessary for cholesteatoma removal.

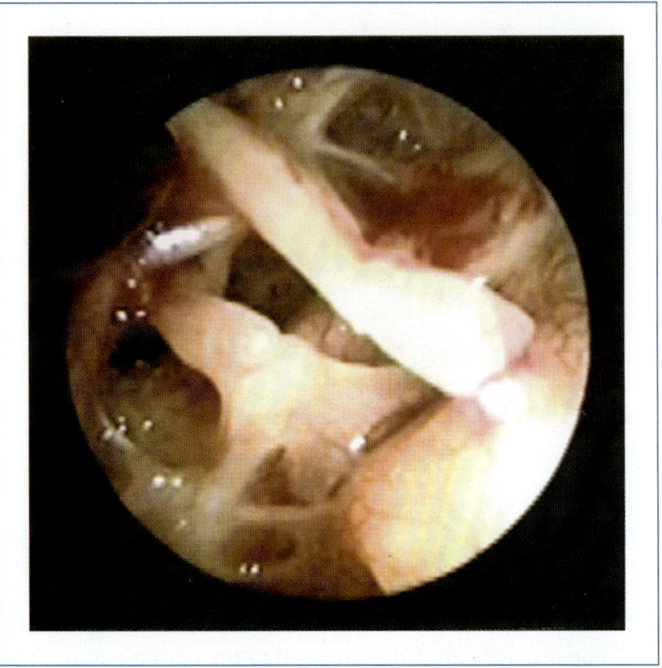

FIGURE 20–10 • A 2.3-mm, 70-degree Hopkins rod endoscopic view of the superior mesotympanum and epitympanum at primary surgery after removal of anterior epitympanic cholesteatoma from a right ear.

ENDOSCOPIC TYMPANOPLASTY

Anterior, marginal tympanic membrane perforations are frequently repaired using a postauricular approach to maximize exposure. The view of far anterior perforations may be especially difficult, and the anterior margin may be completely

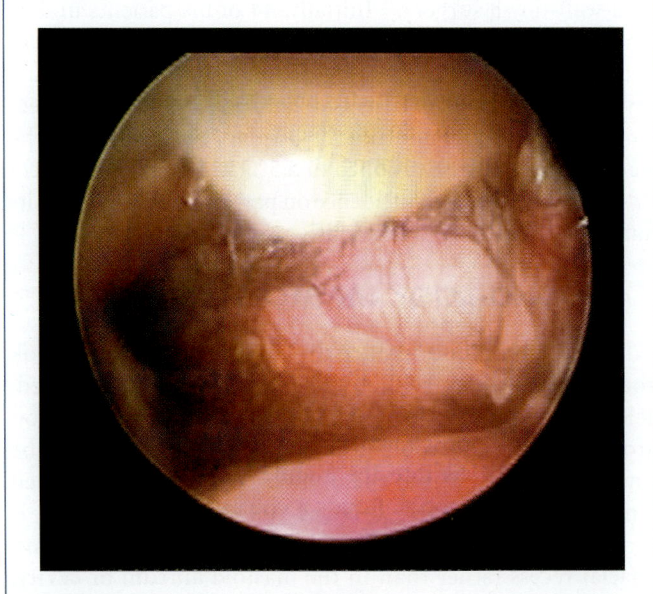

FIGURE 20–9 • A 2.3-mm, 70-degree Hopkins rod endoscopic view into the left ear of a "second-look" case after primary cholesteatoma removal from the cochleariform process and area medial to the malleus head.

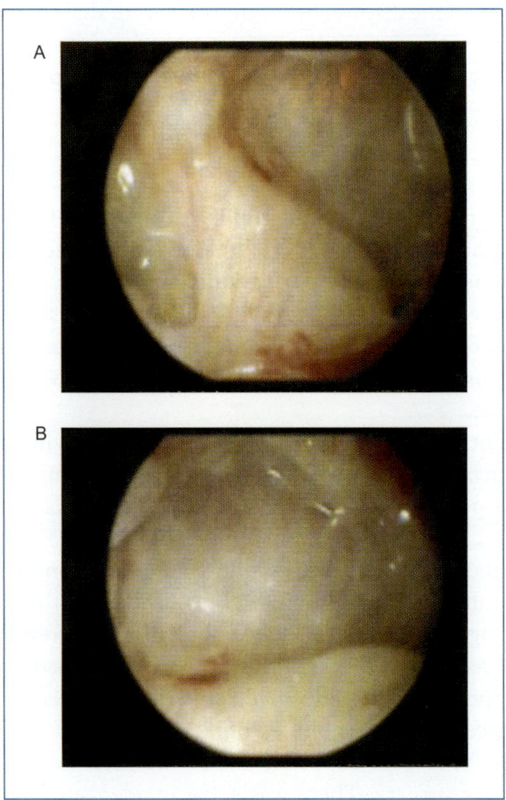

FIGURE 20–11 • Left ear second-stage procedure after cholesteatoma surgery 6 months prior. Middle ear silastic has been removed. Transcanal 2.3-mm, 70-degree Hopkins rod endoscopic views. *A*, Oval window and anterior epitympanum are free of residual cholesteatoma. *B*, Antrum and sinodural angle are free of residual cholesteatoma.

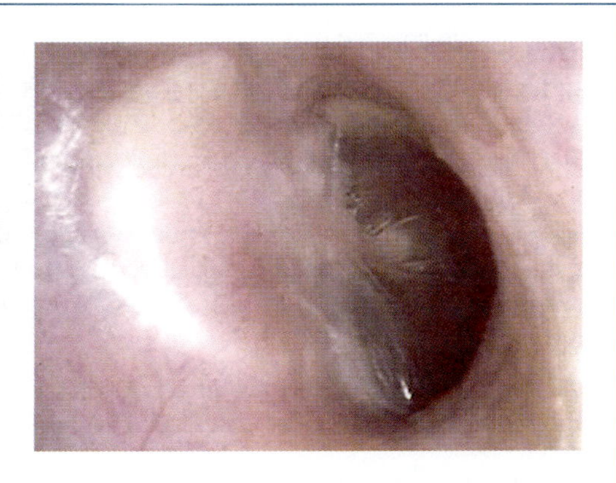

FIGURE 20–12 • Transcanal view of right ear with 4-mm, 0-degree Hopkins rod endoscopic view of reconstructed atticotomy with healed cartilage graft in place superior to the malleus.

hidden from direct view behind a prominent anterior canal bony overhang. Canalplasty of the anterior canal wall hump is usually recommended, either by a transcanal or postauricular approach. In some circumstances, a minimal technique may be desired and the anterior perforation edge may be readily seen with an endoscope.[27,28] If the anterior margin is minimal and blends with the anterior canal wall, there is increased risk that an underlay graft will have insufficient contact with the anterior drum remnant to hold it in place against the natural tendency for the graft to contract during healing. There are many techniques to deal with a far anterior, marginal perforation, including a fat graft, cartilage button graft *(see Chapter on Tympanoplasty)* or a lateral graft technique. A less commonly used method involves the use of a laser to "spot weld" the graft in place. A fiber-delivered laser (potassium titanyl phosphate [KTP], argon, and others) is convenient as the tip may be bent to accommodate any anterior bony overhang. KTP and argon lasers are in the visible spectrum and are not well absorbed without a chromophore, such as hemoglobin or applied dye (eg, methylene blue). Painting the area of intended laser exposure with a thin layer of methylene blue greatly aids the absorption of the laser energy. A line-of-sight, microscope-mounted, micromanipulator-steered laser, such as a conventional carbon dioxide (CO_2) laser, would not be practical in cases of limited exposure. However, recent advances in CO_2 laser handheld waveguides (hollow interiorly reflected tubes with diameters similar to fibers) could make its use possible in these cases.

ENDOSCOPIC ASSISTANCE IN STAPEDOTOMY

Laser stapedotomy minus prosthesis surgery is performed for conductive hearing loss due to otosclerosis without necessitating insertion of a prosthesis.[29] An otosclerotic focus, limited to the anterior one-third of the footplate, may be managed by laser vaporization of the anterior crus and a laser cut made linearly and transversely to divide the stapes footplate between the anterior one-third and the posterior two-thirds. These cuts free the posterior footplate and posterior crus, restoring sound transmission and retaining the native ossicular continuity without needing a prosthesis. The procedure differs from early mobilization techniques that fractured through the otosclerotic focus and the majority developed postoperative refixation. Division of the footplate posterior to the otosclerotic focus provides lasting air–bone gap closure.[29–31] Only rarely are the anterior crus and anterior footplate fully seen with the surgical microscope using a transcanal exposure, and the procedure may be facilitated with endoscopic assistance.

EUSTACHIAN TUBE ENDOSCOPIC SURGERY

Endoscopy of the eustachian tube may be performed from either the middle ear or nasopharynx and is giving new insights into tubal physiology and pathophysiology.[32,33]

The cartilaginous tube may be well studied by positioning an endoscope at the nasopharyngeal orifice, directing the angle of use superiorly into its lumen. Video capture of tubal function during swallows can be studied in slow motion to better understand the pathology cases of dysfunction. Endoluminal surgical procedures are now being performed on the basis of our growing understanding of many different mechanisms for failure of tubal ventilation.[33,34]

FUTURE PROGRESS

There is an ongoing need to develop specialized instruments to complement the minimally invasive endoscopic techniques that are rapidly being developed. Long, angled dissectors and suctions, laser probes, and forceps are being designed. Prototype-combined suction dissectors assist the one-hand techniques necessitated by handholding the endoscope.

An endoscope holder may prove useful in the future but should be used with caution to prevent catastrophic injury to the middle ear or ossicles in the event of unexpected patient movement. Fixation of any holder to the head of the patient will be necessary.

CCD cameras are becoming smaller and ultimately may be sufficiently tiny to place directly into the middle ear without the need for optical endoscopes, improving the flexibility and versatility of visualizing instrumentation and allowing more working space for surgical dissecting tools.

Surgery of the temporal bone and middle ear will become increasingly minimally invasive with anticipated improved patient outcomes, reduced morbidity, and enhanced maintenance or restoration of function.

References

1. Mer SB, Derbyshire AJ, Brushenko A, et al. Fiberoptic endoscopes for examining the middle ear. Arch Otolaryngol 1967;85:387–93.
2. Eichner H. Eline mother-and baby-scope-optic zur trommelfell-und mittelohr-endoskopie. Laryngol Rhinol Otol (Stuttg) 1978;57:872–6.
3. Nomura Y. Effective photography in otolaryngology—head and neck surgery: Endoscopic photography of the middle ear. Otolaryngol Head Neck Surg 1982;90:395–8.
4. Kimura H, Yamaguchi H, Cheng SS, et al. Direct observation of the tympanic cavity by the superfine fiberscope. Nippon Jibiinkoka Gakkai Kaiho 1989;92:233–8.

5. Chays A, Cohen JM, Magnan J. La microfibroendoscopie tubo-tympanique. Presse Med 1995;24:773–4.
6. Hopf J, Linnarz M, Gundlach P, et al. Die mikroendoskopie der eustachischen röhre und des mittelohres. Indikationen und klinischer einsatzpunkt. Laryngorhinootologie 1991;70:391–4.
7. Takahashi H, Honjo I, Fujita A, et al. Transtympanic endoscopic findings in patients with otitis media with effusion. Arch Otolaryngol Head Neck Surg 1990;116:1186–9.
8. Poe DS, Rebeiz EE, Pankratov MM, Shapshay SM. Transtympanic endoscopy of the middle ear. Laryngoscope 1992;102:993–6.
9. Thomassin JM, Korchia D, Duchon-Doris JM. Endoscopic guided otosurgery in the prevention of residual cholesteatomas. Laryngoscope 1993;103:939–43.
10. McKennan KX. Endoscopic "second look" mastoidoscopy to rule out residual epitympanic/mastoid cholesteatoma. Laryngoscope 1993;103:810–4.
11. Magnan J, Chays A, Lepetre C, et al. Surgical perspectives of endoscopy of the cerebellopontine angle. Am J Otol 1994;15:366–70.
12. O'Donoghue G, O'Flynn P. Endoscopic anatomy of the cerebellopontine angle. Am J Otol 1993;14:122–5.
13. Bottrill ID, Perrault DF Jr, Poe DS. In vitro and in vivo determination of the thermal effect of middle ear endoscopy. Laryngoscope 1996;106:213–6.
14. Poe DS. Transtympanic endoscopy of the middle ear. Oper Techn Otolaryngol Head Neck Surg 1992;3:993–6.
15. Friedland DR, Wackym PA. A critical appraisal of spontaneous perilymphatic fistulas of the inner ear. Am J Otol 1999;20:261–79.
16. Poe DS, Rebeiz EE, Pankratov MM. Evaluation of perilymphatic fistulas by middle ear endoscopy. Am J Otol 1992;13:529–33.
17. Poe DS, Bottrill ID. Comparison of endoscopic and surgical exploration for perilymphatic fistulas. Am J Otol 1994;15:735–8.
18. Rosenberg SI, Silverstein H, Wilcox TO, Gordon MA. Endoscopy in otology and neurotology. Am J Otol 1994;15:168–72.
19. Pyykkö I, Selmani Z, Ramsay H. Middle ear imaging in neurotological work-up. Acta Otolaryngol Suppl (Stockh) 1995;520:273–6.
20. Rosenberg SI. Endoscopic otologic surgery. Otolaryngol Clin North Am 1996;29:291–300.
21. Bottrill ID, Poe DS. Endoscope-assisted ear surgery. Am J Otol 1995;16:158–63.
22. Yung MM. The use of rigid endoscopes in cholesteatoma surgery. J Laryngol Otol 1994;108:307–9.
23. Bowdler DA, Walsh RM. Comparison of the otoendoscopic and microscopic anatomy of the middle ear cleft in canal wall-up and canal wall-down temporal bone dissections. Clin Otolarynol 1995;20:418–22.
24. Karhuketo TS, et al. Endoscopy and otomicroscopy in the estimation of middle ear structures. Acta Otolaryngol (Stockh) 1997;117:585–9.
25. Thomassin JM, Korchia D, Doris JM. Endoscopic-guided otosurgery in the prevention of residual cholesteatomas. Laryngoscope 1993;103:939–43.
26. Youssef TF, Poe DS. Endoscopic-assisted second-stage tympanomastoidectomy. Laryngoscope 1997;107:1341–4.
27. El-Guindy A. Endoscopic transcanal myringoplasty. J Laryngol Otol 1992;106:493–5.
28. Pyykkö I, Poe DS, Ishizaki H. Laser-assisted myringoplasty: Technical aspects. Acta Otolaryngol Suppl (Stockh) 2000;543:1–4.
29. Silverstein H. Laser stapedotomy minus prosthesis (laser STAMP): A minimally invasive procedure. Am J Otol 1998;19:277–82.
30. Poe DS. Endoscope-assisted laser stapedectomy: A prospective study. Laryngoscope Suppl 2000;110:1–36.
31. Silverstein H. Laser stapedotomy minus prosthesis (laser STAMP): absence of refixation. Presented at the American Otological Society, Palm Desert, CA, May 13, 2001.
32. Fabinyi B, Klug C. A minimally invasive technique for endoscopic middle ear surgery. Eur Arch Otorhinolaryngol Suppl 1997;1:S53–4.
33. Poe DS, Pyykkö I, Valtonen H, Silvolva J. Analysis of eustachian tube function by video endoscopy. Am J Otol 2000;21:602–7.
34. Poe DS, Abou-Halawa A, Abdel-Razek O. Analysis of the dysfunctional eustachian tube by video endoscopy. Otol Neurotol 2001;22:590–5.

Image-Guided Systems in Neurotology/Skull Base Surgery 21

M. Miles Goldsmith, MD, FACS

Traditional teaching of surgical technique emphasizes wide tissue exposure for progressive identification of surgical landmarks to safely navigate to the target. However, visualization beyond the exposed surface is often incomplete because the exposed surgical field lacks spatial clues orienting the surgeon to the underlying geometry of the target area.

In the past, integration of preoperative imaging information into the surgical field has been an intuitive process on the part of the operating surgeon. The surgeon relies on the ability to mentally reconstruct the image data in a three-dimensional fashion and transform this into the operative field. This ability may be adequate for simple routine cases with minimal distortion of normal anatomy. However, when routine anatomic landmarks are distorted by the pathologic lesion, the surgeon's ability to visualize damaged and functional anatomy is easily overcome.

The traditional open surgical approach has been dramatically impacted by the financial pressures of our managed care climate, as well as the rapid progression of technological advances within the health care system. So-called minimally invasive or minimal access surgical techniques have emerged that emphasize earlier functional recovery and cosmesis using a variety of technologies to minimize collateral tissue damage while achieving the surgical objective. Such minimally invasive surgical techniques often involve limited access and restricted visibility and thus mandate a precise knowledge of anatomy. Errors in localization of surgical position can result in damage to normally functioning tissue or failure to remove the pathologic lesion.

The emphasis on minimally invasive surgical techniques has increased the demand for sophisticated interactive radiographic guidance, which complements the eye that "sees the surface" with imaging to "see under the surface."[1] Real-time information from integrated multimodality image-based data can now be presented in an intuitive framework to facilitate precise preoperative visualization of pathologic anatomy as well as real-time interactive anatomic localization and targeting for surgical procedures.

The term *stereotactic surgery*, originally coined by Clarke in 1908,[2] refers to surgery incorporating devices that maintain spatial correspondence between the operating instrument and an image of the operative site. The term *virtual reality* has been described as the combination of human–computer interfaces, graphics, sensor technology, high-end computing, and networking to allow a user to become immersed in and interact with an artificial environment.[1] These terms are now very familiar to the modern-day surgeon as this technology is increasingly incorporated into preoperative planning, minimally invasive surgery, surgical education, and research.

In the field of otolaryngology, we have recently witnessed the rapid emergence of image-guided systems predominantly in surgeries of the anterior skull base (eg, functional endoscopic sinus surgery), and, to a lesser extent, these systems have found application in certain lateral skull base procedures. The purpose of this chapter is to present an overview of the history and technical aspects of current image-guided technology, its general and specific applications in the field of otology/neurotology, and its potential for the future.

HISTORY OF STEREOTAXY

Stereotaxy, before the age of computed tomography (CT), was based entirely on the use of equatorial head-frame systems.[2] Superimposition of frame-based Cartesian coordinate systems securely attached to the head, with calibration accomplished via orientation of the system to the anterior–posterior commissural line, provided an atlas for targeting cerebral lesions in animal models. Hoarsley and Clarke used these early stereotactic systems for placing electrodes in specific areas of animal brains and, although accurate for the purpose of their experiments, the system was not deemed sufficiently accurate or practical for human use.[2]

In 1947, Spiegel adapted the above stereotactic concepts to human use, employing pneumoencephalography and reference to internal tissues as opposed to external landmarks.[3] This technique was more precise than that of Hoarsley and Clarke,[2] but the methodology was tedious and laborious. With the increasing need to accurately localize deep intracranial structures, such as for the ablation of certain areas of the brain for the treatment of Parkinson's disease, there soon became a huge demand for more user-friendly stereotactic systems.

With the advent of CT, digital image databases, combined with more sophisticated surgical instrumentation, greatly enhanced the development of stereotactic surgery. Pioneered by Brown, Kelly, and other neurosurgeons, modern conventional stereotactic surgery employs a head frame to register image space to surgical space.[4–9] Preoperatively, digital image data via CT or magnetic resonance imaging (MRI) are obtained with a localization system (fiducials) attached to a head frame. The frame, which superimposes a Cartesian coordinate system on the head, provides attachment points for localization devices that are placed before imaging (Figure 21–1). Digital imaging allows the assignment of coordinates to any point in the image data. These image coordinates are then related to the coordinate system, which defines these points with respect to the head frame (stereotactic coordinates). Thus, stereotactic space is defined.

Although bulky and cumbersome, the head-frame systems have proven to be accurate in targeting intracranial lesions for stereotactic biopsy. The simplest form of preoperative planning with head-frame systems involves the selection of a point within the digital image of the head. This point will be transformed into a stereotactic coordinate for the purposes of surgically targeting a lesion, eg, to biopsy a brain tumor. More sophisticated preoperative planning may involve trajectory simulation to properly orient the surgeon and more safely guide the operative approach, minimizing collateral damage to normal tissues.

Since the accuracy of the head-frame systems is related to the rigid fixation of the frame to the skull, the frame must be securely bolted to the head, which causes considerable discomfort to the patient. This process often requires general anesthesia before the placement of the frame and the imaging; thus, the anesthesia time is lengthened and the potential for functional imaging is obviated. The frame is left on for the duration of surgery, committing both surgeon and anesthesiologist to a specific orientation with respect to the patient's accessible anatomy. The frame-based system presents a mechanical obstacle hindering a surgeon's ability to access particular areas, such as the posterior fossa and skull base. Because of these drawbacks, frame-based stereotaxy has not been widely used in the operating theater, particularly not for neurotologic applications.

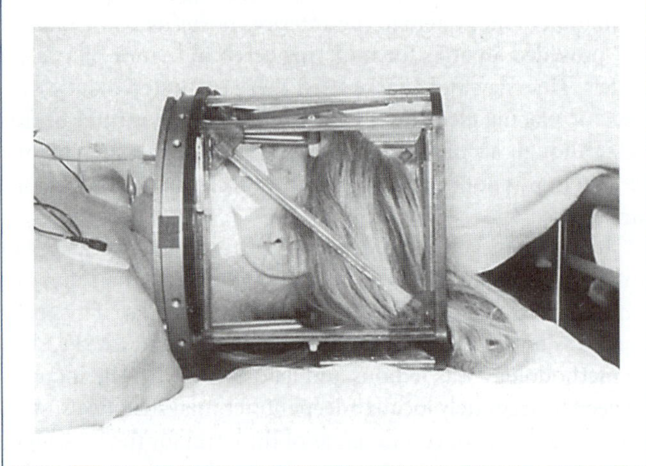

FIGURE 21–1 • Conventional head-frame stereotactic system.

FRAMELESS STEREOTAXY

More recently, frameless stereotactic systems have been devised as a more sophisticated and yet user-friendly means of providing comparable stereotactic accuracy without the use of the aforementioned bolted head frame. Current systems consist of two basic components: the sensor, which relays positional information, and a computer, which translates the sensor's positional information to a visual aid for the corroboration of real-time anatomic information. In frameless stereotaxy, the transformation from image coordinates to stereotactic coordinates is defined by three or more noncolinear points (fiducials) in common between the two coordinate systems. Depending on the sensor technology employed, these fiducials may involve anatomic landmarks or reference markers attached to the head at consistent and immovable sites.

A variety of three-dimensional digitizers, or sensor technologies, have been employed to transform the coordinates in surgical space to the corresponding image space. These three-dimensional sensor technologies can be classified into two broad groups: those that require a mechanical link between the pointer and the sensor technology (mechanically linked systems) and those that do not (nonmechanically linked systems).

Mechanically Linked Systems

Mechanically linked systems are based on arms that are mounted to the operating table.[10–13] These mechanical arms are equipped with sensitive potentiometers, or angle detectors, located within their joints. By sampling the output of rotary optical encoders at each point, a computer can determine the localization of the top of the arm and provide "arm coordinates" that are referenced to the base of the arm. Because the base of the arm is mechanically connected to the head, and the patient's head is registered to the image of the head by an appropriate method, a transformation can be calculated to map any common point in the two coordinate systems. For surgical purposes, real-time localization of the tip of the arm, or pointer, relative to preoperative images of the patient is possible. A variety of mechanically linked devices has been developed and is in the marketplace. These mechanically linked devices have proven to be accurate, although they are somewhat bulky and restrictive, depending on the size of the highly accurate joint detectors employed. Generally, these systems have more limited versatility of instrument use and are not as user-friendly as the more current nonmechanically linked systems. To date, they have found limited application in the field of otology and neurotology.

Nonmechanically Linked Systems

More recently, nonmechanically linked sensor systems have been developed for the registration of image data to the surgical patient. These systems rely on the active or passive detection of signals generated by various emitters that are attached to surgical instruments (Figure 21–2). Using similar traditional triangulation concepts employed in the satellite industry, these frameless stereotactic systems are able to localize and track surgical instruments in three-dimensional space. There are essentially three types of nonmechanically linked digitizing systems: ultrasonic, electromagnetic, and optoelectric.

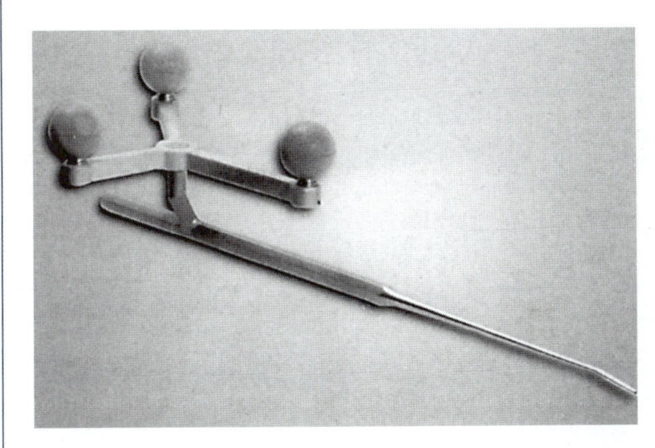

FIGURE 21–2 • Passive surgical instrument employed by optoelectric system (LandMarx, Medtronic/Xomed, Inc).

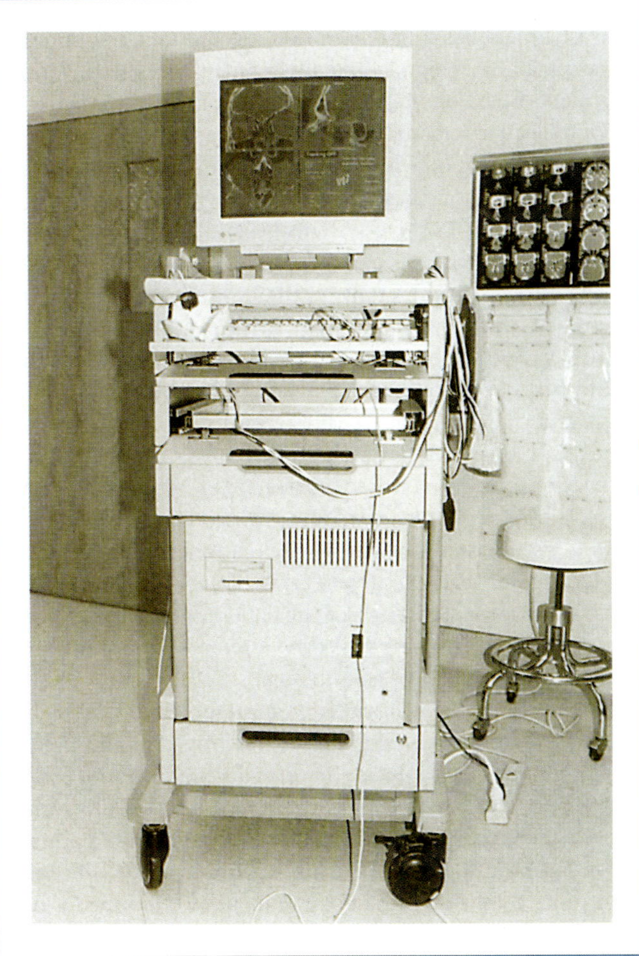

FIGURE 21–3 • Electromagnetic referenced system (InstaTrak, VTI, Inc).

Ultrasonic digitizers determine position by measuring the time flight of sound from an emitter to at least three microphones.[14] The main advantage of ultrasonic digitizing systems is that a free line of sight between the receptor and the emitter arrays need not be maintained. The distinct drawback to ultrasonic digitizers is that the speed of sound varies with temperature and humidity gradients, which may result in positional error. Furthermore, ultrasonic digitizers may be compromised by echoes within the operating room (OR) or by interference from extraneous radiofrequency emissions. For these reasons, sonic referenced systems are no longer used.

Electromagnetic reference systems (eg, InstaTrak System, GE Medical Systems, Lawrence, Massachusetts) share similar advantages to the ultrasonic digitizers in terms of not needing to maintain a free line of sight between receptor and emitter arrays (Figure 21–3). These systems are referenced by a headset, which is worn by the patient during the CT scan and again later during the surgical procedure. Registration of this device is more rapid and user-friendly than other commercially available frameless systems. However, electromagnetic referenced systems suffer the drawback of potential interference from other electromagnetic systems as well as certain ferromagnetic instrumentation in the operating arena. This interference, as well as minor inconsistencies in the repositioning of the headset for imaging and surgery, contributes to positional error and inaccuracy. These inaccuracies are relatively minor and inconsequential for most anterior skull base surgery (eg, endoscopic sinus surgery) where this system finds its primary application in otolaryngologic surgery. The automatic headset registration and referencing algorithm are currently not well suited for lateral skull base applications.

Optoelectric digitizers require an unobstructed path from the emitters to the overlying camera array.[15–17] Three cameras, containing a 1 x 4096 element linear charged-coupling device, are required to determine the three-dimensional position of infrared light-emitting diodes (LEDs) attached to the surgical instruments (Figure 21–4). The overlying camera array is positioned 1.5 to 2 m above the surgical field so that it can track the instrument-attached LEDs, and it thus detects and tracks the precise position of the surgical instrument in three-dimensional space.

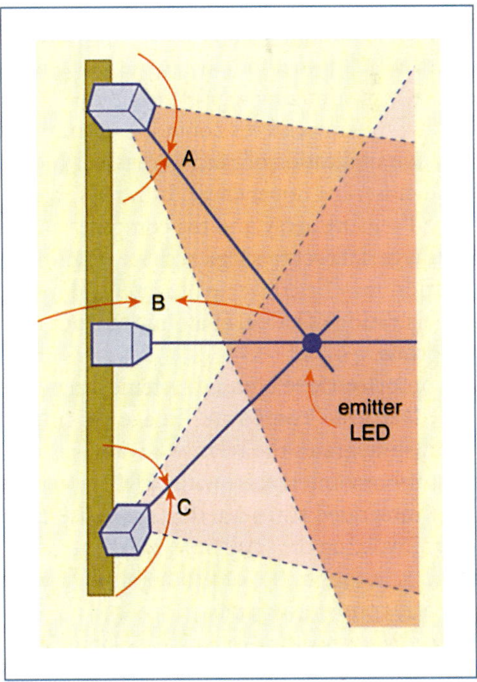

FIGURE 21–4 • In optoelectric systems, three cameras triangulate position of surgical instruments based on the angle of light received from infrared light-emitting diodes attached to the surgical instruments.

Multiple LEDs can be placed on different surgical instruments. Each instrument has a unique emitter spacing, and the computer software is able to recognize and differentiate between the various instruments based on the distance between the emitter pairs.

Optoelectric referenced systems are designated as active or passive, depending on whether the instrument reference points actively transmit or passively reflect the sensor medium (ie, infrared radiation). Active systems generally require wiring of the instruments, whereas passive systems do not.

The three commercially available optoelectric systems (LandmarX, Medtronic Xomed, Minneapolis, Minnesota; BrainLAB, Feldkirchen, Germany; Stryker Image Guidance System, Stryker Leibinger, Kalamazoo, Michigan) are quite transparent and adaptable to different surgical instruments of various geometric configurations, such as bipolar cautery, various suctions, powered microdebriders, and straight or curvilinear probes. A reference arc attached to the stabilized head allows adjustment in calibration with inadvertent movement of the OR table or overlying camera array. Three-dimensional and three-planar reconstructions of the data set are displayed on a video monitor, permitting real-time interactive and positional information for the operating surgeon.

The three above referenced commercially available systems are now contour referenced, meaning that the patient does not have to wear fiducial markers during the preoperative image scan. The registration of the image data set to surgical space is achieved by matching anatomic contour data points to corresponding image points using a contour probe. Recently, the BrainLAB and LandmarX systems have developed a new method of laser-contoured anatomic registration that does not use a contact probe. By attaching LEDs to a laser range finder and by moving the range finder over a part of the skull with anatomic diversity (such as the forehead), hundreds of points constituting a contour can be produced. This contour is then matched to a corresponding contour of the scalp extracted from the image data set.[15] This method of registration facilitates setup time while greatly minimizing registration error.

The Stryker system achieves contour registration through the intraoperative application of a facial "mask," which is applied to the forehead, nose, and upper cheek. Infrared LEDs are sensed by the overhead sensing array and the computer automatically registers the image data set to surgical space (Figure 21–5). The latter registration may be converted to lateral skull base anatomy by the registration of lateral anatomic contour coordinates by a contour probe.

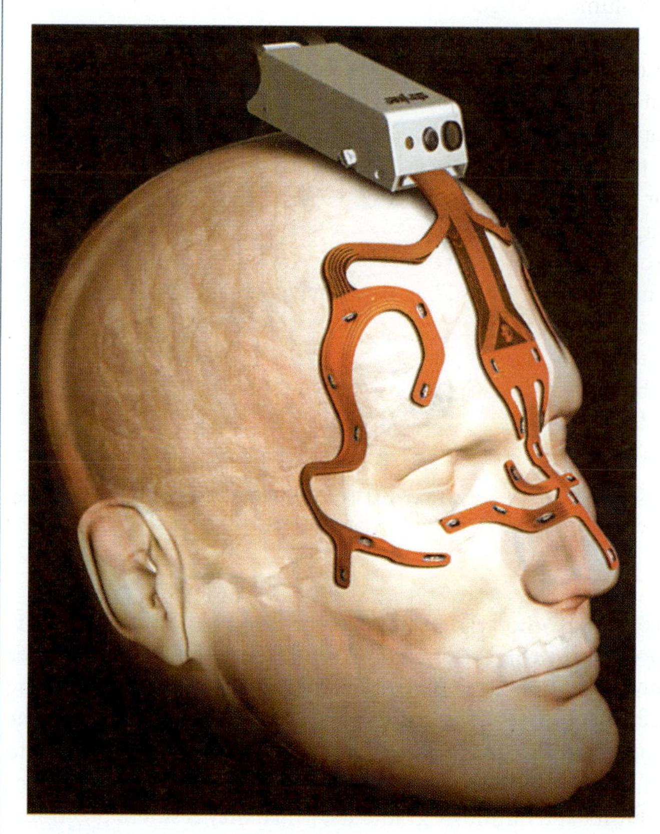

FIGURE 21–5 • The Stryker system achieves contour registration through intraoperative application of a facial "mask" applied to the forehead, nose, and upper cheek. Infrared LEDs are sensed by the overhead sensing array and the computer automatically registers the image data set to surgical space. The later registration may be converted to lateral skull base anatomy by the registration of lateral anatomic contour coordinates by a contour probe.

All three optoelectric referenced systems can now integrate CT and MRI data to a "composite" image for intraoperative navigation. This integrates the relative advantages of CT (better definition of bony interfaces) with MRI (better soft tissue contrast). The integrated scans are thus more useful for surgical procedures involving the skull base/brain interface, such as pituitary surgery, lesions of the cavernous sinus, and skull base tumors with intracranial extension.

Generally, the author has found these optoelectric referenced systems (BrainLAB, LandmarX, and Stryker) to be the most accurate of the frameless stereotactic systems. The registration algorithms are currently better suited for lateral skull base orientations than the electromagnetic system (InstaTrak). The electromagnetic referenced system is quite useful for anterior skull base applications such as endoscopic sinus surgery, but is less easily referenced for lateral skull base procedures. The electromagnetic systems have the advantage of fast and simple registration, but they have the disadvantage of requiring the patient to wear the rather uncomfortable headset for the preoperative image scan. Fiducial registration used to be problematic for the optoelectric systems, but this has been greatly facilitated by the aforementioned automated contour registration schemes. Maintaining line of sight with the overhead camera array of optoelectric systems can also be difficult in otologic/neurotologic procedures, depending on the size and orientation of the operating microscope to the surgical field. The latter concern is less apparent for the electromagnetic systems as they do not require a nonobstructed line of sight between sensor arrays and the detector.

VOLUMETRIC STEREOTAXY

Kelly and colleagues pioneered the next logical development in stereotactic surgery, interactive volumetric stereotaxy.[5–9] The name describes a process by which enhanced volumetric routines are reconstructed by the computer and stacked into a "volume" that can be displayed or manipulated in stereotactic space. Frameless stereotactic techniques have been adapted to operating microscopes by Kelly and Roberts so that image data can be displayed in the operating microscope in the correct scale, orientation, and position superimposed on the focal plane of the surgical field.[5–9,18] Kelly has recently adapted this system for interactive volumetric resection of intracranial tumors.[5,6] This system displays cross-sectional volumetric contours at progressive depths along the view line so that CT-defined margins of the tumor can be localized. The tissue volume can then be resected either passively or with laser ablation via the computer or actively by the surgeon. Although this system greatly enhances the integration of image data with the surgical field, it does not allow for soft tissue shifts caused by intraoperative manipulations because its information source is antecedent image data.

REAL-TIME INTRAOPERATIVE IMAGING

With all of the previously discussed frameless stereotactic systems, the computer algorithms and hence graphic image displays reflect antecedent imaging data. Intraoperative shifts and deformations of soft tissues can occur with surgical manipulations, swelling, or hemorrhage. These soft tissue shifts may thus distort accurate registration of image-based three-dimensional models with the patient's actual anatomy without full volumetric image update. This is particularly relevant for neurosurgical procedures such as the removal of intracranial tumors for which surgical manipulation may produce edema and soft tissue shift. This is less relevant for otolaryngologic and neurotologic surgical procedures within the stable confines of a "bony box," such as the sinus cavities or the temporal bone.

Only real-time intraoperative imaging can provide the necessary updated positional data to integrate with and modify the volumetric image data set. Such real-time imaging provides updates about the position of instrumentation relative to the surgical anatomy without the fiducial registration process of frameless stereotactic systems.

X-ray fluoroscopy, ultrasonography, and CT have permitted sufficient interactive visualization for percutaneous biopsies and some intravascular interventions, but are limited by the degree of spatial resolution of volumetric images as well as radiation exposure. Mobile CT scanners have recently been developed, which can be deployed in the operative suite (Xoran, Medtronic). Intraoperative CT is generally more useful in corroboration of bony interfaces than soft tissue shifts, and thus to date it is more applicable for anterior skull base applications, such as endoscopic sinus surgery.

Because of its improved soft tissue contrast, volumetric resolution, multiplanar and functional capabilities, and lack of ionizing radiation, MRI is ideally suited for real-time image-guided therapy. Mid-field open configurations with vertical magnets [1,19,20] are available that permit full surgical access to patients. When combined with computer algorithms similar to those employed by the frameless stereotactic systems, these MRI systems permit the tracking and video display of nonferromagnetic MR-compatible instrumentation in real time for open surgeries.

Various low- to high-field intraoperative MRI (iMRI) systems have been developed and investigated in the past 10 years. Two basic concepts have been explored: (1) iMRI in which the surgeon operates within the MRI field using MRI-compatible surgical instrumentation and (2) iMRI in which the surgical patient is intraoperatively transferred into the MRI field via table shift or physical transfer to a separate suite for imaging. In the latter instance, special MRI-compatible instrumentation is obviated.

An example of a high-field intraoperative system has been developed by a cooperative effort of the Siemens and BrainLAB companies, known as the BrainSUITE. It consists of a standard 1.5 Tesla MRI scanner, which is completely integrated with a state-of-the-art neuronavigation system into a dedicated high-tech surgical suite. The patient is placed on a rotatable operating table. During surgery, the head or operative area of the patient is placed outside the MRI field so that procedures can be performed with routine instrumentation. At any time during the operation the surgical procedure can be interrupted, and the patient can be placed into the magnet by simple rotation of the operating table. Due to its high-field capabilities, excellent intraoperative images can be acquired.

Another commercially available iMRI system is the PoleStar N20 system (Medtronic, Minneapolis). The PoleStar (Figure 21–6) is a more compact and flexible low field system, which does not require a dedicated OR suite, and it is compatible with standard OR equipment and surgical instruments. The PoleStar Suite's vertically oriented magnets fit under a standard operating table, and it will accommodate most patient positions (lateral, supine, and prone), as well as full access to the

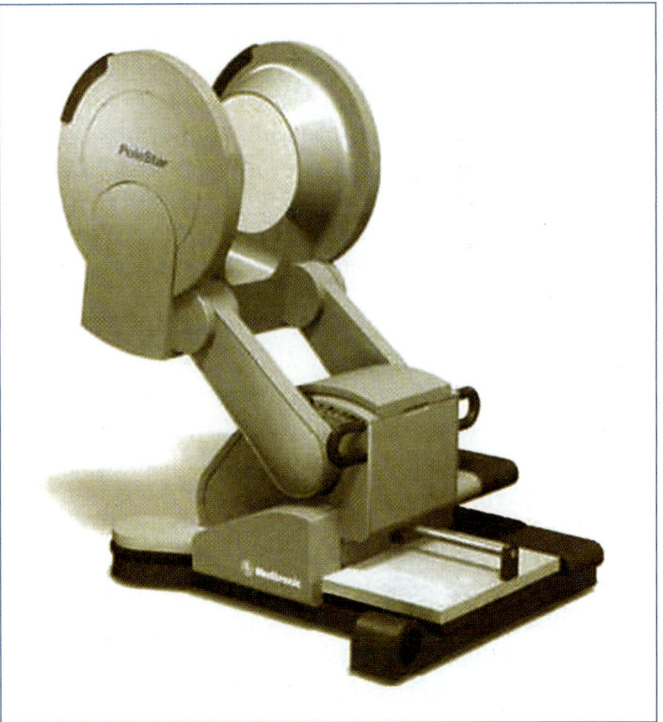

FIGURE 21–6 • An iMRI system—the PoleStar N20 system (Medtronic, Minneapolis) is a more compact and flexible low field system which does not require a dedicated OR suite and is compatible with standard OR equipment and surgical instruments.

patient when the magnet is stowed under the OR table. When its scanner is stowed in the magnet storage cabinet, the OR can be used as a conventional OR. This MRI system is fully integrated with the StealthStation frameless stereotaxic navigation system, which may be used as a stand-alone image-guidance system.

A most exciting application for these iMRI systems has been the removal of deep-seated brain tumors, particularly malignant intra-axial tumors.[21,22] Because surgical brain tumor margins are indistinct from normal tissues, real-time MRI may facilitate location of such tumor margins, thereby enhancing the likelihood of complete tumor resection while maximizing the integrity of surrounding normal brain.

Additionally, MRI can be used to control energy deposition of thermal ablative therapies because of the intrinsic sensitivity of MRI to both temperature and tissue integrity. Such thermal therapies have to date been applied to pathologies of the brain, spine, breast, and prostate.[21–23]

Multimodality preoperative image data sets from MRI, CT, positron emission tomography, and single-photon emission CT scanning can now be integrated with intraoperative imaging data into a single data source. From this resource, enhanced visibility and virtual reality representation can be accomplished using various three-dimensional interactive display systems.[1]

In summary, the intraoperative use of real-time MRI imaging in surgery is in its infancy and future developments in this technology will surely add to the rapidly evolving field of MRI-guided surgery. The aforementioned interventional MRI systems currently offer the most sophisticated and accurate image guidance for the OR of the future, providing updated real-time anatomic and functional data for diagnostic and therapeutic purposes. These systems are now commercially available though they are quite complex and expensive. Currently, the question is whether this extremely expensive high-tech tool represents a technical overkill restricted to only a very small number of elite surgical centers, or whether this will be a major breakthrough in minimally invasive surgical procedures. As an increasing number of iMRI units will be installed into operating theatres worldwide, the answer to the aforementioned question must await the burgeoning scientific evaluation of this technology.

ROBOTICS

Robots offer the advantages of reliability, repeatability, and control of tremor for the neurotologic surgeon. Autonomously acting robots in concert with image-guided systems have recently been investigated for mastoidectomy by Labadie et al. at Vanderbilt.[24] Preliminary studies have demonstrated that the robot can achieve low-level milling of the mastoid cavity in approximately 4 min, leaving the high-level tasks of drilling on vital structures to the neurotologic surgeon. Federspil and colleagues[25] have used robotics to accurately drill the receiving well for cochlear implants. More recently, robots have been explored for minimally invasive surgical approaches to the facial recess and cochleostomy for cochlear implantation.[26, 27] Conceivably, in the near future, robots could be used to facilitate minimally invasive access to other neurotologic anatomic structures, such as the internal auditory canal, the endolymphatic sac, and the semicircular canals. The efficacy of robotics is highly contingent upon the fiducial accuracy of the associated image-guided system, and widespread commercial use is limited by the high cost of these systems in their current form.

APPLICATIONS OF IMAGE-GUIDED SYSTEMS IN OTOLOGY/NEUROTOLOGY

Traditional temporal bone surgery has involved a "funnel concept" (Figure 21–7) of methodical and progressive identification of key anatomic landmarks en route to the surgical target. For example, with routine mastoidectomy, the surgeon proceeds stepwise with initial identification of the mastoid antrum, the middle fossa dural plate, and lateral semicircular canal to achieve an intuitive three-dimensional orientation within the surgical field. For the ordinary well-pneumatized mastoid, this funnel concept is routine and safely accomplished for the well-trained otologist without the need for real-time image guidance. However, for the nonroutine mastoid in which normal anatomic landmarks may be obscured by pathologic disease, previous surgery, or anatomic variation, real-time image guidance may prove very helpful in safely navigating to the surgical target while minimizing collateral damage to vital anatomic structures. Such examples would include the sclerotic mastoid and congenital malformations, such as cochlear dysplasia, enlarged vestibular aqueduct syndrome, and atretic ear malformations. In these situations, real-time image guidance may permit us to convert our traditional "funnel technique" to a "tunnel concept" of surgical navigation whereupon we may virtually "see" these vital anatomic landmarks via interactive imaging rather than by direct surgical exposure (Figure 21–8).

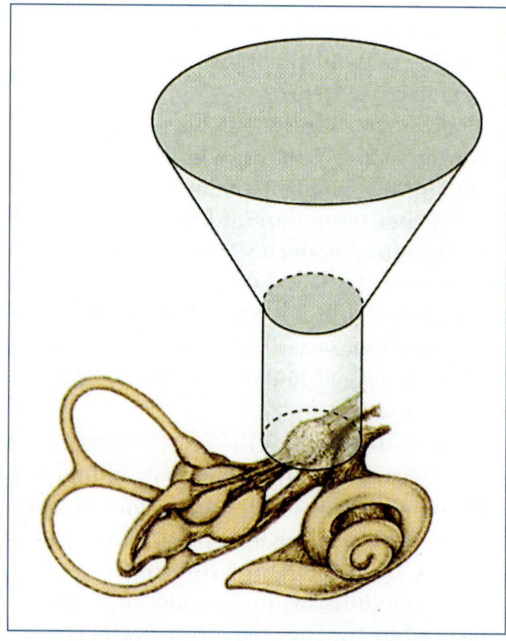

FIGURE 21–7 • Traditional temporal bone surgery involves a "funneling" to the surgical target via exposure and progressive identification of key anatomic landmarks.

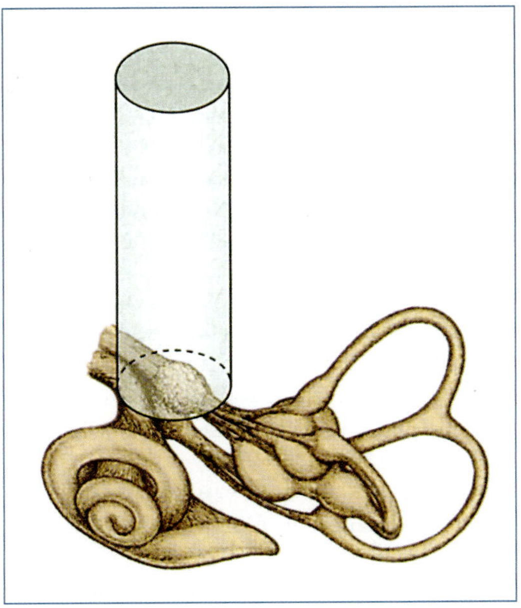

FIGURE 21–8 • With image guidance systems, a "tunneling" to the surgical target may be achieved, whereupon vital anatomic landmarks are identified via interactive imaging rather than by direct surgical exposure.

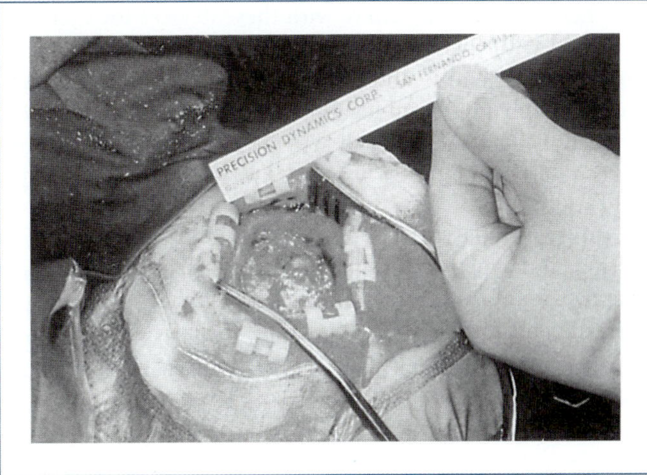

FIGURE 21–9 • Keyhole craniotomy for removal of a posterior fossa meningioma.

Identification of the internal auditory canal via the middle fossa approach is another such example of this concept. The traditional "funnel" techniques of Fisch and House involve the sequential identification of certain neural and/or labyrinthine structures en route to the internal auditory canal. Using highly accurate frameless stereotactic guidance, the "tunnel" approach would permit direct localization of the internal canal with a pointer via interactive three-planar and three-dimensional imaging, thus obviating the stepwise approach. Theoretically, this should shorten surgical time and enhance safety, provided that the critical issue of clinically verifiable accuracy is achieved. Absent accuracy, the opposite may be true.

Image-guided systems may greatly facilitate so-called keyhole surgical approaches to the posterior fossa and cerebellopontine angle. "Keyhole" is a term coined by neurosurgeons for the concept of operating through a minimal craniotomy using a variety of minimally invasive technologies to minimize collateral tissue damage—analogous to working through a keyhole. Interactive imaging is thus very useful in precisely orienting the minimal craniotomy necessary for achieving the desired surgical trajectory for accessing the surgical target (Figure 21–9). Postoperative healing is thus facilitated, and morbidity is decreased.

Another area of neurotologic application for these systems is the petrous apex. In this difficult to access, often poorly pneumatized anatomic area, we do not have a consistently defined series of anatomic landmarks for orientation as with conventional mastoidectomy or the middle fossa approach. Various pathologies of the petrous apex thus lie within very narrow confines bordered by vital structures, such as the carotid artery and cranial nerves. In these situations, image guidance systems provide valuable preoperative planning, trajectory simulation, and target and entry formulation in addition to real-time intraoperative localization of these anatomic structures.

In certain other areas of neurotologic/skull base surgery, frameless stereotactic systems may have less relevance. This largely relates to an accuracy issue related to soft tissue shifts during surgery. Because these devices are referenced to antecedent image data, without intraoperative updated information, inaccuracies develop as soft tissues are surgically manipulated. Thus, for procedures that are performed within an anatomic area confined to a "bony box," such as the mastoid, internal auditory canal, petrous apex, or sinus cavity, frameless stereotactic systems remain accurate without updated information. Outside of these bony confines, such as in the cerebellopontine angle and the soft tissue planes of the infratemporal fossa, these systems are subject to positional error because of operative soft tissue shifts. In the latter instance, real-time imaging (CT and/or MRI) is more applicable, but the complexity and expense of these systems has to date limited their widespread commercial use.

SUMMARY

Real-time image guidance employing computer interfaces and antecedent imaging can facilitate certain minimally invasive surgical approaches of the temporal bone. Current frameless stereotactic systems based on various referencing methodologies have individual advantages and disadvantages. In common among them all, the systems appear to be stable over time in the OR and are generally transparent in use, permitting free movement of the surgeon and of the patient's head during the course of surgery. Optoelectric referenced systems, both active and passive, generally appear to be the more consistently accurate of the systems and the more practical systems for lateral skull base procedures, whereas the electromagnetic referenced systems are generally more applicable for anterior skull base procedures. Optoelectric systems have the disadvantage of having to maintain unrestricted line of sight to the overhead sensing arrays. The electromagnetic system does not have the line-of-sight problem, but does have the problem of interference by ferromagnetic instrumentation and other electromagnetic systems in the operative suite.

There is a learning curve with these devices for everyone associated with their use, but software interactions are menu driven, user-friendly, and simple enough to allow the surgeon to simply point and localize during the operative procedure. Clinical accuracy for all systems is generally 1 to 3 mm, which is sufficient for most anterior skull base and neurotologic applications.

Interventional MRI represents the most sophisticated, exciting, and expensive of the image-guided systems available. Its chief advantage is the ability to provide real-time updated anatomic and functional information. Its chief disadvantages are its expense, complexity, and the need for special instrumentation depending upon the system used.

The OR of the future is witnessing a paradigm shift from open surgical visualization to virtual visualization through integrated image data. The inherent complexity of image-guided therapies will require an increasing dynamic cooperation and interplay between the disciplines of surgery and radiology. Through the advancement of these technologies, we have the possibility of improving the safety, efficacy, and cost-effectiveness of our diagnostic and therapeutic procedures.

Finally, it is important to remember that these adjunctive tools should never replace precise knowledge and visualization of anatomy when visualization is at all possible. That is, it is always preferable to visualize the runway before landing a plane rather than to rely solely on instrumentation.

References

1. Jolesz FA. Image-guided procedures and the operating room of the future. Radiology 1997;204:601–12.
2. Hoarsley V, Clarke RH. The structure and function of the cerebellum examined by a new method. Brain 1908;31:45–124.
3. Zinreich J. Imaging of inflammatory sinus disease. Otolaryngol Clin North Am 1993;26:535–47.
4. Brown RA. A computerized tomography-computer graphics approach to stereotaxic localization. J Neurosurg 1979; 50:715–20.
5. Kelly PJ. Volumetric stereotactic surgical resection of intraaxial brain mass lesions. Mayo Clin Proc 1988;63:1186–98.
6. Kelly PJ. Volumetric stereotaxis and computer-assisted stereotactic resection of subcortical lesions. In: Lunsford LD, editor. Modern stereotactic neurosurgery. Boston: Nijhoff; 1988. p. 169–84.
7. Kelly PJ, Alker GJ. A stereotactic approach to deep-seated central nervous system neoplasms using the carbon dioxide laser. Surg Neurol 1981;15:331–4.
8. Kelly PJ, Farnest I 4th, Kall BA, et al. Surgical options for patients with deep-seated brain tumors: Computer-assisted stereotactic biopsy. Mayo Clin Proc 1985;60:223–9.
9. Kelly PJ, Kall BA, Goerss SJ, et al. Computer-assisted stereotaxic laser resection of intra-axial brain neoplasms. J Neurosurg 1986;64:427–39.
10. Barnett GH, Barnett G II, Kormos DW, et al. Use of a frameless, armless stereotactic wand for brain tumor localization with two-dimensional and three-dimensional neuroimaging. Neurosurgery 1993;33:674–8.
11. Maciunas RJ, et al. Beyond stereotaxy: A computerized articulated localizing arm for all neurosurgical procedures [abstract]. Proc Am Assoc Neurol Surgeons 1990;254.
12. Watanabe E, Watanabe T, Manaka S, et al. Three-dimensional digitizer (Neuronavigator): New equipment for computed tomography-guided stereotaxic surgery. Surg Neurol 1987;27:543–7.
13. Watanabe E, Mayanagi Y, Kasugi Y, et al. Open surgery assisted by the Neuronavigator, a stereotactic, articulated, sensitive arm. Neurosurgery 1991;28:792.
14. Nitsche N, et al. Einsatz eines beruhrungsfreien computergestutzten Orientierungssystems bei Nasennebenhohlenoperationen. Otorhinolaryngol Nova 1993;3:57.
15. Bucholz RD, Ho HW, Rubin JP. Variables affecting the accuracy of stereotactic localization using computerized tomography. J Neurosurg 1993;79:667–73.
16. Bucholz RD, et al. Intraoperative localization using a three-dimensional optical digitizer. Proc Clin Appl Modern Imaging Technol 1894:1993.
17. Goldsmith MM, Bucholz RD, Smith KR, Nitsche N. Clinical applications of frameless stereotactic devices in neurotology: A preliminary report. Am J Otol 1995;16:475–9.
18. Roberts DW, Strohbehn JW, Hatch JF, et al. A frameless stereotaxic integration of computerized tomographic imaging and the operating microscope. J Neurosurg 1986;65:545–9.
19. Lufkin RB. Interventional MR imaging. Radiology 1995;197:16–8.
20. Gronemeyer DHW, Seibel RMM, Melzer A, et al. Future of advanced guidance techniques by interventional CT and MRI. Minimally Invasive Ther 1995;4:251–9.
21. Jolesz FA, Shtern F. The operating room of the future. Report of the National Cancer Institute Workshop, Imaging Guided Stereotactic Tumor Diagnosis and Treatment. Invest Radiol 1992;27:326–8.
22. Black PCL, Moriarity T, Alexander E, et al. Development and implementation of intraoperative magnetic resonance imaging and its neurosurgical applications. Neurosurgery 1997;41:831–43.
23. D'Amico AV, Cormack R, Tempany CM, et al. Real-time magnetic resonance image-guided interstitial brachytherapy in the treatment of select patients with clinically localized prostate cancer. Int J Radiat Oncol Biol Phys 1998;42:507–15.
24. Labadie RF, Majdani O, Fitzpatrick JM. Image-guided technique in neurotology. Otolaryngol Clin North Am 2007;40:611–624.
25. Federspil PA, Geisthoff UW, Henrich D et al. Development of the first force-controlled robot for otoneurosurgery. Laryngoscope 2003;113:557–62.
26. Labadie RF, Choudhury P, Cetinkaya E, et al. Minimally invasive, image guided, facial recess approach to the middle ear. Otol Neurotol 2005;26:557–62.
27. Baron S, Eilers H, Hornung O, et al. Conception of a robot assisted cochleostomy: First experimental result. In Proceedings of the 7th International Workshop on Research and Education in Mechatronics, REM2006. Stockholm (Sweden); June 15–16, 2006.

Surgery of the External Ear

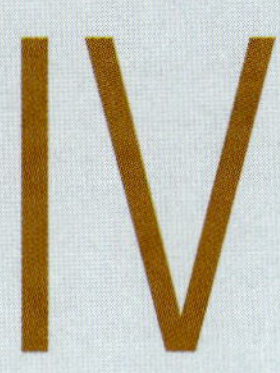

Diseases of the Auricle, External Auditory Canal, and Tympanic Membrane

22

Stephanie Moody Antonio, MD / Barry Strasnick, MD, FACS

The auricle and external auditory canal (EAC) serve to augment and transmit sound to the tympanic membrane. The shape of the EAC results in the optimization of sound conduction to the tympanic membrane in the frequencies of 2 to 4 kHz, those most important in human communication. Disorders of the pinna, EAC, and tympanic membrane are common entities in clinical otology. Successful diagnosis and management require a detailed knowledge of the embryology, anatomy, physiology, and bacteriology of these structures.

DEVELOPMENTAL CONSIDERATIONS

The auditory and vestibular systems develop as distinct anatomic units. During the 6th week of gestation, auricular development begins with the formation of the six "hillocks of His," mesenchymal proliferations originating from the first and second pharyngeal arches. The first arch contributes three hillocks, which eventually form the tragus, the root, and superior portion of the helix. The second arch also contributes three hillocks, destined to become the antihelix, antitragus, and lobule. The definitive auricle develops from the fusion of the hillocks and is usually complete by the 12th week of gestation. The auricle will not reach its adult shape, however, until the 20th gestational week, and it continues to grow for the first 5 years of life. Given the complexity of this process, it is not surprising that developmental abnormalities of the auricle are common.

The ectoderm of the first branchial groove invaginates to form the primitive EAC. As the cells continue to grow inward, they eventually meet endodermal tissue of the developing tubotympanum, a derivative of the first pharyngeal pouch. Mesodermal anlages encroach on this area of apposition from ventral and dorsal sites. The resulting solid core of tissue is named the meatal plug or plate. By the 28th week of fetal development, the plate resorbs and the EAC recanalizes. Ectodermal elements from the meatal plate form the epithelial lining of the EAC and the lateral tympanic membrane, whereas mesodermal elements contribute to the development of the cartilaginous EAC, ossification centers of the tympanic ring, and the ossicular chain. Failure of EAC recanalization results in congenital aural atresia.

ANATOMY

The Auricle

Fibroelastic cartilage, perichondrium, and skin comprise the auricular framework. The cartilage of the auricle is continuous with that of the lateral EAC. The skin of the topographically complex lateral surface of the auricle is firmly attached to the perichondrium; however, the skin of the posterior surface is less adherent due to a layer of loose areolar tissue between it and the perichondrium. The auricle is fixed to the temporal bone by its cartilaginous contribution to the external meatus, the three auricular ligaments (anterior, superior, and posterior), and by six poorly developed intrinsic muscles. Additionally, three distinctly better developed extrinsic muscles exist, also named anterior, superior, and posterior. Voluntary contraction of the extrinsic musculature is responsible for the ability possessed by some to "wiggle" the auricle. These muscles are innervated by the facial nerve.

Sensory innervation of the auricle is characterized by a great deal of overlap between multiple nerves.[1] The auriculotemporal branch of the mandibular division of the trigeminal nerve supplies sensation to the tragus and the helix and its crus; it also supplies sensation to the anterior and superior portions of the EAC and corresponding areas of the lateral surface of the tympanic membrane. Fibers from cervical sensory nerves (C2, C3), contained in the great auricular nerve, innervate the posterior surface of the auricle, the posterior region of the helix, the antihelix, and the lobule. Fibers from the 9th and 10th cranial nerves supply the majority of the conchal concavity, with additional contribution from the 7th cranial nerve.

The external carotid artery supplies blood to the auricle and external meatus via the postauricular and superficial temporal branches. Venous drainage parallels the arterial supply. The superficial temporal vein joins the retromandibular vein and ultimately the internal jugular system, whereas the postauricular vein joins the external jugular system. There also may be drainage to the sigmoid sinus via the mastoid emissary vein. The lymphatics of the anterior auricle and meatus drain into the preauricular and periparotid nodes. Lymphatics of the posterior auricle, however, empty into the retroauricular (mastoid) and infra-auricular nodes.

The External Auditory Canal

The EAC is an S-shaped tube measuring approximately 2.5 cm in length that extends from the concha to the tympanic membrane. The most lateral one-third of the canal is cartilaginous, whereas the medial two-thirds is osseous. The narrowest segment of the EAC, the isthmus, corresponds to the junction of the cartilaginous and bony portions. The canal's anteroinferior wall is slightly longer than the posterosuperior wall, creating an acute angle between the anterior canal wall and the tympanic membrane. The EAC is also slightly convex anteriorly, which can prevent complete examination of the tympanic membrane. Improved tympanic membrane visualization is achieved by retracting the auricle in a posterosuperior direction during otoscopy.

Skin and subcutaneous tissue cover the cartilage of the lateral EAC. Hair follicles and sebaceous and apocrine (ceruminous) glands exist within this subcutaneous tissue. These structures form an apopilosebaceous unit and produce a protective layer of cerumen. In contrast, the more medial, osseous EAC lacks glandular adenexae and consists only of the tympanic bone and a tightly adherent epidermis. The clinical significance of this difference lies in the fact that infected sebaceous cysts and furuncles occur only in the lateral EAC. The epidermis of the EAC is continuous with the squamous epithelial layer of the tympanic membrane. Infectious processes of the EAC may spread to the temporomandibular joint (TMJ) and periparotid soft tissue via inconstant dehiscences of the cartilaginous canal, the fissures of Santorini. An anteroinferior gap of the tympanic bone, named Huschke's foramen, may permit similar spread of infection to the preauricular tissue. This developmental dehiscence usually closes in late childhood but may persist into adulthood.[2]

Sensory innervation of the EAC is variable, with suspected contributions from cranial nerves V, VII, IX, and X. Generally, the auriculotemporal branch of the mandibular division of the trigeminal nerve innervates the anterior and superior walls of the EAC. Fibers from the facial, glossopharyngeal, and vagus nerves, traveling with the auricular branch (Arnold's nerve) of the vagus nerve, enter the EAC through the tympanomastoid suture to supply the posterior and inferior aspects of the canal.[1]

The blood supply of the EAC is the same as that of the auricle, with additional contributions from the deep auricular artery. This vessel, a branch of the internal maxillary artery, passes through the substance of the parotid gland and travels posterior to the TMJ capsule before penetrating the EAC in the region of the isthmus. Venous drainage is via the superficial temporal and posterior auricular veins that join the internal and external jugular systems, respectively. Lymphatics of the inferior EAC drain to the infra-auricular nodes, those of the posterior canal drain to the retroauricular nodes, and the periparotid, superficial, and deep cervical nodes receive drainage from the anterior region of the canal.

Cerumen is a mixture of desquamated epidermal cells and secretions from sebaceous and ceruminous glands of the EAC, including fatty acids, alcohols, triglycerides, cholesterol, cholesterol precursors, and amino acids. The composition of wax may be in part hereditary. Cerumen that tends to be wet as opposed to dry wax tends to contain more lipid and pigment. Cerumen lubricates the EAC and keeps the canal clean by trapping dirt and repelling water. Whether cerumen has further antimicrobial benefits is not entirely clear.

The Tympanic Membrane

The tympanic membrane is a thin fibrous sheet interposed between the EAC and middle ear. Its diameter measures approximately 9 mm and it is oriented obliquely at the lateral end of the external canal. Its appearance is one of a cone directed medially, the apex of which corresponds to its attachment to the umbo. Three cell layers form the tympanic membrane: a lateral epithelial lining that is continuous with the skin of the EAC, a middle fibrous layer composed of both radiating and circular fibers of connective tissue, and an internal mucosal layer. A coalescence of the fibrous layer at its rim, known as the fibrous annulus, helps anchor the tympanic membrane within the bony tympanic sulcus. The pars tensa refers to the majority of the membrane area, which is separated from the pars flaccida (Shrapnell's membrane) superiorly by the anterior and posterior alveolar folds. The lamina propria of the pars tensa is thin and strong, made up of abundant type II collagen. The medial layer of the pars flaccida contains thicker and more loosely arranged collagen fibrils, mainly type I collagen, and it is more elastic than the pars tensa.[3] The pars flaccida sits in a region of the tympanic ring deficient of bone, named the notch of Rivinus. Medial to the pars flaccida is Prussak's space, the most common site of primary cholesteatoma formation.

Sensory innervation to the lateral surface of the tympanic membrane mirrors that of the EAC. The auriculotemporal nerve supplies the posterior and inferior region of the tympanic membrane, and the auricular branch (Arnold's nerve) of the vagus nerve innervates its anterior and superior aspect, with additional fibers originating from the seventh cranial nerve. The tympanic branch (Jacobson's nerve) of the glossopharyngeal nerve provides sensation to the medial surface of the tympanic membrane.

The blood supply to the tympanic membrane is derived from vessels that supply the external canal and middle ear cavity. The deep auricular branch of the internal maxillary artery forms a peripheral ring from which arise branches destined for the tympanic membrane's lateral surface. The internal maxillary artery also supplies the internal surface of the tympanic membrane via its anterior tympanic branch.[4] Venous drainage tends to parallel corresponding arterial anatomy.

DISEASES OF THE AURICLE

Frostbite

The auricle, with its high ratio of surface area to mass is at increased risk for this type of injury. Blood vessels supplying this region lie superficially within the subcutaneous tissues, increasing their exposure to colder temperatures. Prolonged exposure blocks afferent sensory nerve transmission, reducing the patient's awareness of ongoing injury. The initial physiologic response is vasoconstriction. The frozen tissue appears yellow-white and waxy and is cold and hard. This appearance combined with the loss of sensation is diagnostic of frostbite. Extracellular ice formation during the freezing and thawing process results in cell dehydration and cell membrane rupture. The blood vessels are also damaged, resulting in extravasation of fluid and clotting. As tissues warm, extravasated fluid causes edema and bullae formation, and pain is the rule.

Management consists of rapid tissue warming via circulating warm water or warmed moistened dressings. Use of radiant heat is contraindicated as it may worsen the injury, especially if warming and refreezing takes place. The pinna should be dressed aseptically with 1% silver sulfadiazine cream, similar to management of a burn injury. Secondary infection is treated with antimicrobial agents directed against *Pseudomonas aeruginosa* and *Staphylococcus aureus*. In some cases, tissue initially appearing devitalized will recover after a period of observation and conservative management. Therefore, debridement of necrotic tissue should be delayed until a reliable line of demarcation develops.

Hematoma

Blunt trauma to the auricle may result in hematoma. The trauma causes a shearing injury, resulting in separation of auricular cartilage from its associated perichondrium and bleeding into this newly created space. The cartilage is subsequently deprived of its perichondrium-dependent blood supply and may become ischemic. Hematoma may present immediately following an injury or in delayed fashion as a painful swelling, which causes effacement of the normal topography of the auricle.

Management consists of evacuation. This may be accomplished by needle aspiration if the hematoma is acute and small in size. For larger collections, incision and drainage are required. The incision is placed along the helical fold, thereby minimizing the conspicuousness of the resultant scar, and the blood clot is expelled. Curettage may be used to completely remove all of the hematoma. Most important is the placement of a pressure dressing to prevent reaccumulation. Many prefer to use dental rolls secured with through-and-through sutures as bolsters on both the lateral and medial auricular surfaces. Close follow-up is necessary to address recurrences in a timely fashion. Failure to evacuate a hematoma leads to fibrosis and new cartilage formation. The resulting deformity is permanent and ranges from mild cartilaginous thickening to the severe "cauliflower" ear seen most frequently in wrestlers and boxers.

Perichondritis

Infection of the auricular perichondrium and underlying cartilage is a possible complication of surgery, trauma, or external otitis. Perichondritis presents with erythema, edema, and exquisite tenderness of the involved pinna. Progression of the infectious process can lead to abscess formation and loss of cartilage. The most common offending organism is *P. aeruginosa*. Diabetes and other causes of immunosuppression have been implicated as predisposing factors.[5]

If diagnosed early, perichondritis may be managed on an outpatient basis with oral antibiotics, aural toilet and debridement, and close observation. Because of its excellent cartilaginous penetration and high activity against *Pseudomonas* species, ciprofloxacin is the drug of choice. In children with early perichondritis, outpatient management with antibiotics can be initiated. Fluoroquinolones in children may be used with caution and with appropriate monitoring for toxicity.[6] If significant clinical improvement is not observed within the first 24 to 36 h of oral therapy, or if the patient presents initially with severe infection, parenteral antibiotic therapy is warranted. An auricular abscess requires prompt incision and drainage. Additionally, all necrotic cartilage and tissue should be debrided and cultures obtained. A drain under a conforming pressure dressing may help reduce permanent deformity.

Sebaceous Cyst

Sebaceous cysts form as a result of sebaceous gland obstruction. The lobule and retroauricular area are common locations for these soft, mobile masses. Normally, asymptomatic sebaceous cysts do not require treatment unless cosmetic deformity exists. Occasionally, however, the cyst will become acutely infected and require antibiotic therapy. Formal excision should be delayed until the infection has resolved. When excision is performed, the entire cyst capsule must be removed, or recurrence is likely.

Preauricular Sinus

The incidence of preauricular pits and sinuses is 5 to 6 per 1,000 births. Resulting from abnormalities in the fusion of the hillocks of His during auricular development, these lesions present as pit-like depressions anterior to the root of the helix and superior to the level of the tragus. Preauricular sinuses are bilateral in 25 to 50% of cases. Genetic inheritance is more likely involved in the case of bilateral sinuses. These lesions are prone to acute infection requiring antibiotic therapy. If infection does not respond to oral antibiotics, incision and drainage may be necessary. However, acute incision and drainage are ideally avoided since subsequent scarring and fibrosis will obliterate normal tissue planes and make future excision more difficult. When symptomatic or associated with recurrent infection, surgical resection of a preauricular sinus is indicated.

Other related lesions include preauricular skin tags and branchial cleft anomalies. Similar to preauricular sinuses, skin tags in this location represent duplication anomalies of the ectodermal hillocks of His. Although generally benign in their natural history, the skin tags may be excised for cosmetic purposes. First branchial cleft cysts, sinuses, and fistulas, on the other hand, result from duplication anomalies of the membranous EAC (Figure 22–1). A fistulous tract may exist between the skin of the neck and an intact EAC. The Work classification divides first branchial cleft sinuses into two types.[7] Type I anomalies contain only ectodermal derivatives, whereas type II anomalies possess tissues of both ectodermal and mesodermal origin. Management of first branchial cleft lesions consists of surgical resection. Caution is required when dealing with branchial cleft anomalies as their mesodermal origin results in an intimate association with the parotid gland, placing the facial nerve at risk during attempts at excision.

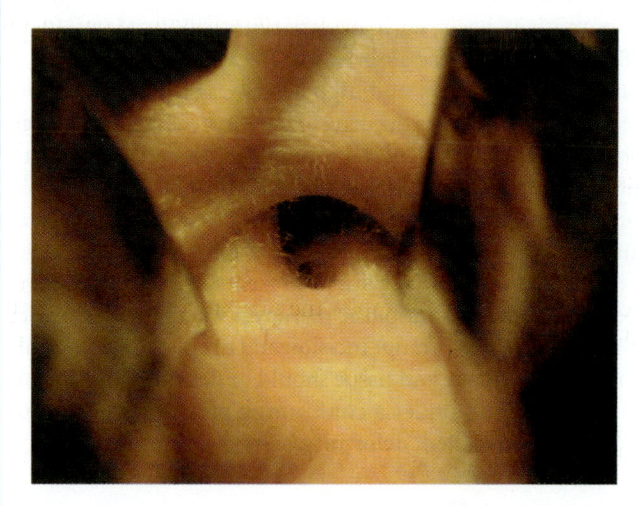

FIGURE 22–1 • Work Type I sinus of the inferior meatus of the external auditory canal.

Hearing loss may be associated with preauricular pits, branchial cleft anomalies, and other congenital external ear and EAC anomalies. For example, branchiootorenal syndrome, which is the second most common type of autosomal dominant syndromic hearing loss, manifests with conductive, sensorineural, or mixed hearing loss with branchial cleft cysts or fistulae, preauricular pits, and renal anomalies. CHARGE association, Townes-Brocks syndrome, branchiootorenal syndrome, Nager syndrome, Miller syndrome, and diabetic embryopathy also may include both auricular and renal anomalies. Patients who present with auricular anomalies should be examined for dysmorphic features such as facial asymmetry, colobomas, choanal atresia, branchial cysts, or sinuses or other abnormal features. Renal ultrasound may be indicated if syndromic features such as these are found. Isolated preauricular pits are infrequently associated with hearing loss and rarely associated with renal abnormalities.[8] Audiologic testing is warranted to rule out hearing loss, but follow-up audiologic testing is probably not indicated, unless there is a significant family history of hearing loss or other risk factors. Wang et al. suggest that a renal ultrasound should be performed in patients with preauricular pits, cup ears, or any other ear anomaly accompanied by other dysmorphic features, a family history of hearing loss, auricular and/or renal malformations, or maternal gestational diabetes; while in the absence of these findings, renal ultrasonography is not indicated.[9]

Surgical Technique for Resection of Preauricular Pit and Sinuses

Pits and sinuses that have been subject to infection or discharge are appropriately considered for resection. It is best to avoid operating on an actively infected pit or sinus.

Surgical Details: An elliptical incision is designed incorporating the pit. Some surgeons prefer a wide local excision with a supra-auricular approach, citing reduced recurrence. Placement of a lacrimal probe into the tract aids in determining its extent. After making the incision and beginning the dissection of the tissues, the probe may be stabilized by clamping it to the surrounding soft tissues. The tract is followed while avoiding violation to the medial extent, usually at the helical cartilage. Care should be taken to avoid violating the sinus and an adequate margin of tissue should be resected with the specimen. Preauricular sinuses tend to have multiple "fingers," which can cause recurrences if left behind. At the medial extent, a section of the cartilage is removed with the specimen to prevent recurrence.

Pitfalls and Complications: The most significant challenge with resection of preauricular sinuses is recurrence. Meticulous dissection is needed to completely remove the sinus and cyst. Some surgeons inject methylene blue to help delineate the extent of the lesion. Attempting to perform resection during acute infection will increase the risk of recurrence. Also, if the cyst has been infected on multiple occasions, tissue planes will have been disrupted, and it will be more difficult to achieve a complete excision. Thus, once a lesion has been infected, surgical treatment should be strongly considered. In cases of postoperative recurrent sinus or cyst, a wider resection incorporating tissue between the superficial temporal vessels, temporalis fascia, and conchal cartilage will improve the likelihood of removing all the epithelial remnants.

Keloid

Keloids are benign, hypertrophic, fibrous lesions that generally develop following trauma or surgery. They are more common in darkly pigmented people and are frequently found on the lobule as a result of ear piercing. An excess of extracellular matrix, particularly glycoproteins, characterizes the histologic appearance of keloids.[10] Treatment generally requires a combination of medical and surgical therapy. For small lesions or developing keloids, intralesional injections of triamcinolone acetonide may be used as first-line therapy. Because of their poor absorption through hypertrophic tissue, topical corticosteroids play a very limited role in the management of keloids. For larger and more mature lesions, excision is required. Intralesional corticosteroid injection is performed at the time of surgery and repeated every 4 to 6 weeks thereafter for a minimum of three postoperative injections. Patient compliance with this postoperative regimen is required to minimize the risk of recurrence. Some advocate additional preexcisional injections to ensure that patients understand and accept the need for multiple treatments and adhere to the prescribed postoperative regimen.[11] Despite combined excision and intralesional corticosteroid therapy, recurrence rates approach 50%.[12] Extremely gentle tissue management may reduce activation of the inflammatory response that can increase recurrence. Low-dose radiation therapy can be considered for cases resistant to conventional therapy, but the risk of radiation-induced malignancy in these predominantly young patients tempers our enthusiasm for this aggressive approach.

Tophi

Gout is a severe monoarticular inflammatory arthritis triggered by the presence of urate crystals in synovial joint fluid. Tophaceous deposition of urate crystals in and around joints is one of the hallmark physical findings associated with hyperuricemia. Frequently, patients will present with deposits in the helix, appearing as moderately painful, salmon-pink nodules. When compressed, tophi exude a whitish, chalky substance consisting of sodium biurate. Crystals appear negatively birefringent when examined under polarized light. Treatment of acute attacks of gouty arthritis focuses on pain relief and correction of the underlying abnormality in uric acid metabolism.[13] No specific surgical therapy directed at auricular tophi is necessary.

Chondrodermatitis Nodularis Chronica Helicis

Chondrodermatitis nodularis chronica helicis, or Winkler's nodule, is an intensely painful solitary nodule, usually found of the helix or antihelix of older men. They appear spontaneously and are thought to be caused by pressure or trauma-induced damage to underlying cartilage. The right side is more commonly involved, possibly due to favored sleeping position. The nodules are tender, round, well-defined-and firm, and usually pale, gray, or slightly erythematous. The edge may be raised and the center may be ulcerated or crusted. These lesions are best treated surgically with removal or shaving of the immediately involved cartilage.

Neoplasms

The external ear is a common site for benign and malignant processes of the skin, including actinic keratosis, papilloma, melanoma, basal cell carcinoma, and squamous cell carcinoma. The otologic surgeon should be aware of the differential diagnosis of skin lesions and apply appropriate management. Auricular cancers commonly originate in areas with maximal sun exposures, such as the helical rim or antihelix. Basal cell carcinoma is less likely to be associated with sun exposure and is a more common type of tumor found on the posterior surface of the auricle. The thin skin of the pinna provides very little resistance to spread to the underlying perichondrium, but embryonic lines of fusion may limit disease to an anatomical subunit, at least temporarily. Biopsy is required to make a diagnosis and should not be delayed. Management is varied and may include curettage, electrodissection, cryosurgery, topical 5-fluorouracil, local excision, or radiation therapy. The auricle is particularly amenable to surgical excision with Mohs' technique. After surgical excision, reconstruction is geared toward covering defects and restoring cosmesis and function. The technique is greatly influenced by the deficit tissue and can be as simple as allowing healing by secondary intention or skin grafting to rotating tissue flaps onto reconstructed structural elements.

Congenital Deformities of the Pinna

Congenital deformities of the pinna, including protruding ear and lop ear, are frequently encountered in otologic practice. The deformity may be unilateral or bilateral. Frequently, the auricular cartilage is of appropriate size but lacks a well-defined antihelical fold. An excessively high or spherical conchal cartilage contributes to the prominent ear. The entity has no significant otologic ramifications; rather, its importance is determined by the psychological disturbance endured by the patient. By the age of five, the auricle has essentially reached adult size, and children generally start school. Teasing from peers may become severe at this time, and surgical correction need not be delayed.

Although differences in opinion regarding "normative values" for auricular position and protrusion exist, Tolleth provided some general guidelines on which surgical correction can be based.[14] With the head oriented vertically, the desired position of the auricle is approximately one-ear length posterior to the lateral orbital rim. The level of the brow defines the preferred position of the top of the ear, whereas the base of the columella marks the appropriate inferior extent of the lobule. The axis of the auricle should not lie in the vertical plane; rather, it should be rotated 15 to 20 degrees in the posterior direction. A distance of 15 to 20 mm between the scalp and the outer edge of the helix provides an esthetically pleasing degree of auricular protrusion.

Surgical Technique for Correction of Protruding Ear

Preoperative Planning: The goals of otoplasty include correction of protrusion of the helix and lobe, create an antihelical fold, avoid overcorrection, and create auricles that are symmetric in appearance and position. A surgical plan will include a detailed analysis of the anatomy and a combination of techniques to address each component of the deformity. Preoperative photographs will assist in planning and counseling. A wide variety of techniques can be used to reshape the auricular cartilages, including abrasion and scoring or suture fixation. We prefer a modification of the technique described by Mustarde, employing a combination of posterior auricular skin excision and mattress sutures.[15] The technique is relatively simple and provides predictable results.

Surgical Details: The ear is again examined and the plan reviewed. Markings with ink are applied with a marker to define the crest of the antihelix and with a needle to define the suture sites. The location for the Mustarde sutures may also be made by placing marking sutures through the anterior skin while folding the ear into position (Figure 22–2A). An elliptical incision is made in the postauricular sulcus (Figure 22–2B). Most surgeons will plan to resect an ellipse of skin, but others do not, in which case a simple linear incision is made. The posterior auricular skin is elevated to the helical rim and triangular fossa, taking care to avoid nicking the cartilage (Figure 22–2C). The tissues are also elevated from the conchal cartilage toward the periosteum of the mastoid. The intrinsic and extrinsic muscles will need to be divided. Several Mustarde sutures (a row of horizontal mattress sutures) are placed through cartilage and anterior perichondrium to roll and create a smooth antihelical fold and approximate the scaphoid fossa closer to the concha (Figure 22–2D). A 5-0 or 6-0 nonabsorbable suture with a taper needle is used. Once a suture is set, it is temporarily tightened with just enough pull to fold the antihelix, but not necessarily to fully approximate the gap. The tie is clamped, while the next sutures are thrown. Once three or four sutures are in good position, they can be individually tied. Repetitive reevaluation of the created fold is done to ensure a good result. The helix should be

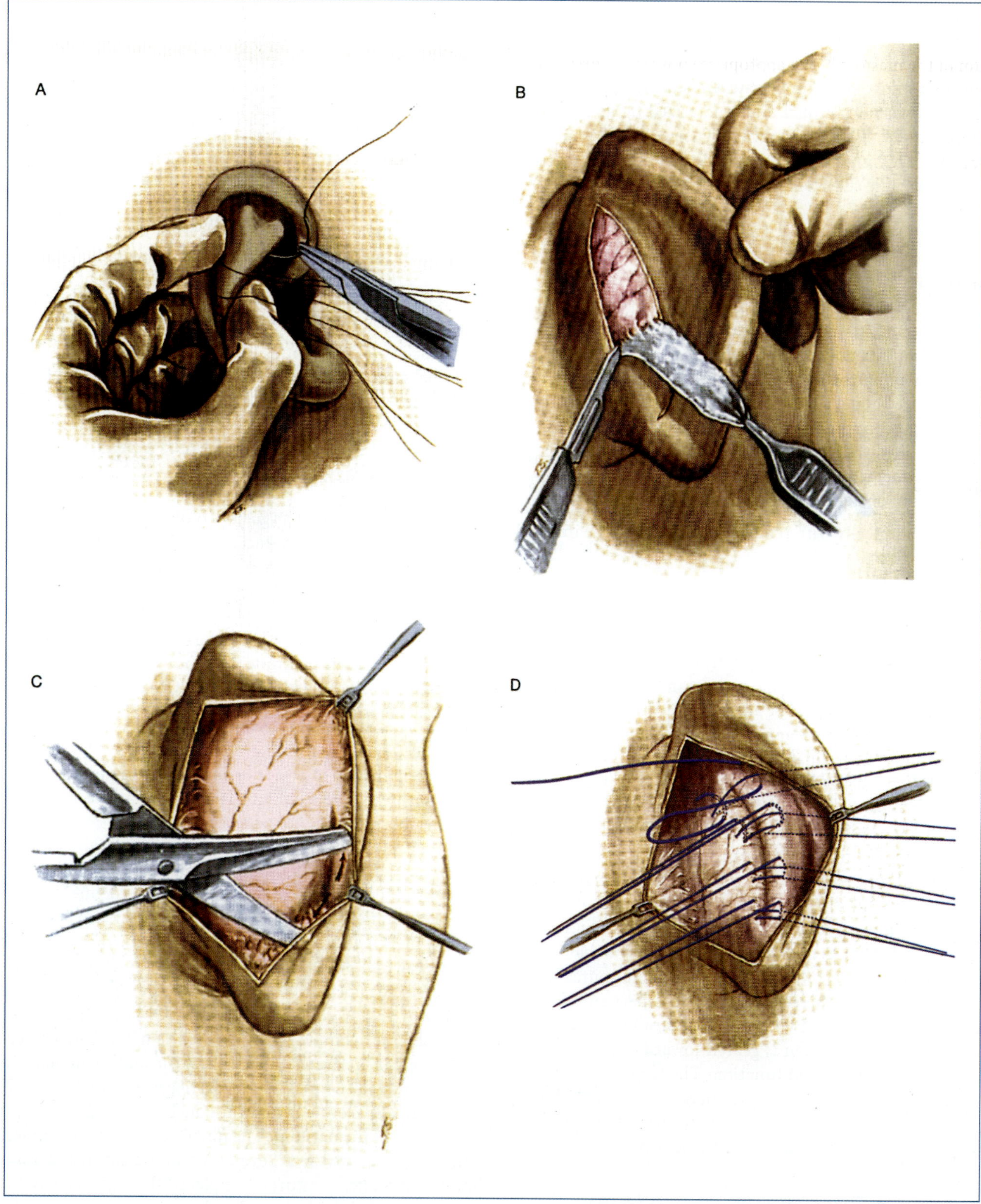

FIGURE 22–2 • Otoplasty. *A*, Marking the suture sites by a through-and-through silk suture (after raising the skin from the posterior aspect of the pinna). *B*, Postauricular elliptical skin incision. *C*, Elevating the postauricular skin to the helical rim. *D*, Placing multiple horizontal mattress sutures at the site of the marking sutures.

visable beyond the new antihelix. An excessively high concha is reduced by tacking the proximal conchal cartilage to the periosteum of the mastoid.[16] The appropriate position is first evaluated by holding the ear. A 4-0 or 5-0 suture should be used and more than one stitch used for support, as these sutures tend to bear more force. If needed, conchal cartilage can be thinned or excised. At this point, examine the upper pole of the ear and the lobule to ensure these areas do not appear excessively prominent. A prominent upper pole can be corrected with a stitch between the triangular fossa and the deep temporal fascia.[17] Redundant posterior auricular skin is excised in elliptical fashion and the incision is then closed. The ear is dressed by packing the auricular contours with cotton, padding the posterior surface, and placing a mastoid dressing.

Postoperative Care: The dressing should be removed at postoperative day 1 to examine for hematoma and signs of excessive pressure. It can then be replaced for a few days. The patient should be examined frequently in the postoperative period to check the ear position. Some surgeons ask the patient to wear a headband for 3 or 4 months.

Pitfalls and Complications: Otoplasty can be a very challenging procedure requiring multiple intraoperative adjustments and a full armamentarium of techniques to manage a multifaceted deformity and variable cartilage characteristics. Failure to understand the factors contributing to the deformity of each ear, which in some cases may be different between the two ears in one patient, can result in a less favorable outcome. If the cartilage overcomes the suture fixation, relapse can occur. This can be reduced by using several redundant sutures and by relaxing cartilage with thinning or scoring when needed. Prompt recognition of shifting or other postoperative deformity may be corrected with a molding dressing, headband, or steri-strips. Overcorrection results when the sutures are too tight, causing the helix to be invisible behind the new antihelix in the frontal view. Another undesirable outcome, telephone deformity, occurs if the upper and lower poles of the ear are not addressed or if too much conchal cartilage is removed. Resection or scoring can result in contour problems. Complications include hematoma, infection, chondritis, and suture bridging or extrusion.

DISEASES OF THE EXTERNAL AUDITORY CANAL

Exostoses and Osteoma

External auditory exostoses and osteomas are benign clinical entities characterized by hyperplastic growth of bone in the osseous EAC. Exostoses tend to be bilateral, broadly based protrusions originating from the anterior and posterior canal walls. In contrast, osteomas are more often unilateral, pedunculated growths located at suture lines and resulting in lesser degrees of EAC obstruction (Figure 22–3). Both types of lesions are most commonly noted incidentally in asymptomatic patients. However, as EAC obstruction worsens, symptoms of chronic debris trapping, recurrent otitis externa, and hearing loss develop.

External auditory exostoses occur with a high prevalence in patients with repetitive exposure to cold-water and cold-wind activities, such as swimming, surfing, or boating. A causal relationship between cold-water exposure and the development of exostoses was first proposed by van Gilse, who showed that irrigation of the EAC with water colder than 17°C results in prolonged meatal erythema.[18] Exposure to cold temperature is thought to produce a periosteitis, which seems to cause new bone growth.

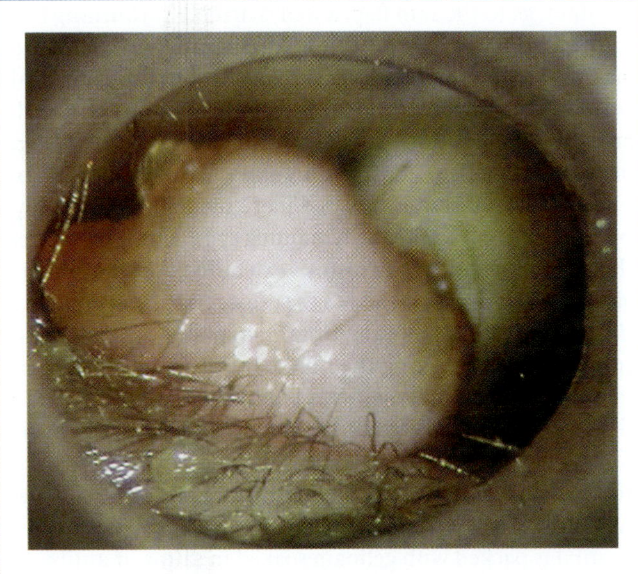

FIGURE 22–3 • Osteoma at bony-cartilaginous junction. In this case, the patient had recurrent cerumen impactions.

Surgical Technique for Removal of Exostosis and Osteoma

Indications and Preoperative Planning: Management of exostoses and osteomas consists of periodic cerumen disimpaction, debridement, and treatment of infection as necessary. Avoidance of further water exposure should be advised, but compliance with this recommendation is unlikely. Many surfers are, however, willing to wear earplugs or occlusive hoods to minimize water exposure. Surgical treatment is considered when the osteomas or exostoses occlude the canal and cause conductive hearing loss or recurrent otitis externa. Osteomas can often be resected with very limited procedures and a transcanal approach. Since they are often pedunculated, a curette may suffice to break the connection. Alternatively, they may be drilled.

Surgical Details for Removal of Exostosis: Exostosis removal is done through a postauricular approach. The ear canal is examined and injected with local anesthesia. If the level of the tympanic membrane can be appreciated, a mental note is made of its location. A posterior vascular strip is designed and made as long as possible. In some cases, the medial incision is made after some of the lateral canalplasty is done so that the flap can be made longer. A postauricular incision is made, and the periosteum is incised in a half-circle just behind the bony meatus in order to elevate the vascular strip and reflect the ear. The anterior skin is incised laterally and carefully elevated medially. The bony canal is drilled through 360 degrees, although the majority of bone removal will be on the anterior wall. To avoid damage to the skin flap, a well is drilled by thinning bone over the TMJ while leaving a thin "eggshelled" wall of residual bone between the well and the skin of the anterior canal wall. Work can continue by deepening this well, while continually monitoring the position of the tympanic membrane, the lateral process of the malleus and avoiding exposure of the TMJ. Next, the anterior canal skin is elevated more medially and finally, a curette is used to fracture the remaining eggshelled bone. Often, at this point, one finds the exostosis extending over the annulus. A piece of foil is placed medial to the exostosis to protect the skin and the tympanic membrane from injury, and the canalplasty if completed by removing the final bone at the medial extent. Curettage or very small diamond burs are used around the lateral process of the malleus to avoid touching the malleus with the drill. The anterior skin flap and vascular strip are replaced onto the canal wall. A split-thickness skin graft or fascial graft may be necessary if significant areas of exposed bone remain. The canal is packed with gelfoam soaked in saline or antibiotic. The incision is closed.

Postoperative Care: Antibiotic drops are applied to the packed ear canal twice daily. Water exposure is avoided. Packing material is removed during weekly or biweekly visits over 4 to 6 weeks.

Pitfalls and Complications: Risks of canalplasty for excision of exostoses include facial nerve injury, perforation of the tympanic membrane, infection, recurrence of exostoses, and sensorineural hearing loss. Facial nerve injury is avoided by using intraoperative facial nerve monitoring and by limiting posterior and inferior bone removal. Complete excision is safer with a postauricular approach and is therefore preferred over a transcanal approach, which will limit exposure and understanding of the presumed location of the facial nerve. The anterior canal wall skin and tympanic membrane should be protected from injury by good technique and by using a small disk made from foil suture packing material. Also, great care should be taken to identify and protect the lateral process of the malleus from drill trauma, which can induce sensorineural hearing loss.

Keratosis Obturans

Keratosis obturans is characterized by the accumulation of large keratin plugs in the osseous EAC, resulting in obstruction, acute pain, and hearing loss. The underlying epithelium is hyperplastic with an increased rate of desquamation and loss of normal migration. Additionally, it is often chronically inflamed. Interestingly, upwards of 90% of patients suffering from keratosis obturans also have a past history of bronchiectasis or sinusitis.[19,20] Clinically, keratosis obturans presents as occlusion of the external meatus by tightly compacted plugs of laminar desquamated keratin debris. Over time, the osseous external canal may become significantly widened, frequently to the point at which the tympanic membrane and annulus "stand out in relief." The tympanic membrane typically shows moderate degrees of thickening. Management consists of local debridement of the plug, occasionally requiring general anesthesia secondary to severe discomfort, and appropriate ototopical therapy to address residual tissue inflammation or secondary infection. Routine cleaning with acetic acid solution or irrigation with hydrogen peroxide and warm water may reduce accumulation of debris. Infrequently, patients will suffer from repeated canal occlusion and pain despite vigilant home maintenance, office surveillance, and debridement. In these difficult situations, canalplasty with skin grafting can be an effective treatment option by replacing chronically diseased epithelium with the healthy epidermis of a skin graft.

External Auditory Canal Cholesteatoma

Cholesteatoma of the EAC is similar to keratosis obturans in that each is characterized by the presence of keratin debris within the canal. They are, however, distinct clinical entities. Patients with EAC cholesteatoma are generally older and often present with unilateral disease with otorrhea, dull pain, and hearing loss. This rare variety of cholesteatoma can be acquired secondary to trauma, surgery, stenosis, or chronic inflammation or arise spontaneously.[21] The precise etiology of spontaneous EAC cholesteatoma is unclear, but pathologic studies consistently cite a localized periosteitis and bone sequestra formation.[22]

Clinically, EAC cholesteatomas cause focal erosion of the bony canal wall, usually in an inferior and posterior location. The accumulated debris is loose and random as opposed to the laminated plug of keratosis obturans. The severity can range from limited, superficial erosion and minimal debris accumulation to extensive involvement of surrounding structures, such as the TMJ, facial nerve, or mastoid. Complete microscopic examination of the cholesteatoma is critical in determining its extent. For localized lesions, frequent office debridement of necrotic bone and debris may suffice. For cholesteatomas eroding into the canal wall and when office management is difficult or painful, a canalplasty may successfully exteriorize the defect. External auditory canal healing can be aided by obliterating large defects with cartilage or cartilage-perichondrial grafts and/or covering exposed bone with skin or fascial grafts. Disease involving the mastoid may warrant tympanomastoidectomy to remove involved bone and repair associated defects.

Foreign Body

Children are frequently referred to otolaryngologists for the management of ear canal foreign bodies. Primary care physicians often discover the foreign body when evaluating a child for possible otitis, or it may be found incidentally during a well-child visit. Inorganic objects are commonly present. A greater challenge to manage in the office, however, are organic objects, such as popcorn and peanut fragments, which tend to absorb moisture and swell to completely obstruct the meatus. Foreign bodies are removed under microscopic visualization with a cerumen loop, right-angle pick, or suction. For the uncooperative child, removal under general anesthesia is required, given the risk of tympanic membrane and ossicular chain injury that can result from the sudden movement of a distressed patient. Occasionally, an endaural incision is necessary to remove a severely impacted object. Postoperative antibiotic drops should be used when an incision is required or extensive trauma to the skin of the external canal is observed.

Furuncle

Also known as acute localized otitis externa, acute furunculosis is the result of obstruction of pilosebaceous glands present in the subcutaneous tissue of the cartilaginous EAC. Elevation of the tightly adherent skin of the external canal causes exquisite pain and discomfort. The pinna and preauricular soft tissue may display associated cellulitic changes. Treatment of acute furunculosis consists of antibiotics directed against *S. aureus* and warm compresses. If significant fluctuance develops, incision and drainage are required and generally provide welcome pain relief. If possible, a small wick of packing material should be placed into the abscess cavity following drainage to prevent recurrence.

Aural Polyp

Aural polyps are well-circumscribed, soft, fleshy masses frequently found in the EACs of patients presenting with otorrhea and hearing loss. They are usually inflammatory and suggest active middle ear disease. An association between aural polyps and cholesteatoma, especially in children, is well established and may be as high as 45%.[23,24] Polyps are frequently seen in pediatric patients, the result of a foreign body reaction to pressure equalization tubes. Polyps may arise from middle ear mucosa and protrude into the external meatus through a tympanic membrane perforation or tube. Additionally, polyps may be a manifestation of myringitis, malignant otitis externa, temporal bone malignancy, or other neoplastic or inflammatory lesion, such as inflammatory pseudotumor or giant cell granuloma. Histopathologic analysis is therefore required when the etiology of a polyp is unknown.

Gentle aural cleansing and the application of antibiotic-corticosteroid–containing drops can effectively reduce a polyp's size and allow adequate examination of the medial EAC and tympanic membrane. Cauterization with silver nitrate can also be a helpful adjunctive measure in initial therapy. Aggressive debridement or avulsion of an aural polyp should be avoided as it may have attachments to a dehiscent facial nerve, the stapes footplate, or cholesteatoma overlying a labyrinthine fistula. Biopsy and histologic analysis should be performed on polyps of uncertain origin, both to rule out malignancy and possibly to help in diagnosing an underlying cholesteatoma. Patients who fail to respond to medical management require surgery. Removal and biopsy of aural polyps with middle ear involvement should be performed in conjunction with middle ear exploration, tympanoplasty, and possibly mastoidectomy to appropriately address the primary disease.

Dermatologic Processes

The EAC is basically a blind pouch lined with skin. Its epidermis is susceptible to the same dermatologic processes encountered elsewhere in the body. Because it encompasses a small space and its skin is so thin, dermatitic processes of the external meatus produce troubling symptoms. These conditions present with chronic itching, serous or mucoid drainage, fullness, and subjective hearing loss. During the acute phase, the skin of the EAC and concha may appear edematous, erythematous, and wet and may have vesicles, excoriations, and serous or mucoid otorrhea. Bacterial superinfections may occur, with associated purulent otorrhea and potentially, microabscesses and cellulitis. In the chronic disease state, the skin becomes lichenified and often has the appearance of dryness with flaking and excoriations. The EAC may display purely local disease, such as contact dermatitis, asteotosis, or neurodermatitis (lichen simplex chronicus). However, in some cases, EAC problems are a manifestation of a systemic condition, such as psoriasis, atopic dermatitis, seborrheic dermatitis, acne vulgaris, and sarcoidosis. Generally, all these conditions will respond to local care with topical steroid cream or ointment, antibiotic or antifungal preparations, and modification of exposure to moisture, dryness, or allergens as the case may be. Systemic steroids may be added for severe inflammatory disease. Surgical therapy for dermatologic conditions is limited. However, deep cysts of the EAC may manifest secondary to generalized acne vulgaris. Uncomplicated acne can be managed with salicylic acid cleansers, topical tretinoin or antibiotic, or intralesional steroid. Large cysts may easily become superinfected, then causing generalized pain, swelling, and inflammation of the EAC. Incision and drainage may be needed along with systemic antibiotics.

Bacterial and Fungal Otitis Externa

Cerumen plays an important protective role in EAC physiology. A relatively acidic pH and hydrophobic nature account for its bacteriostatic properties. A warm, moist environment favors bacterial growth, accounting for the increased incidence of acute otitis externa during summer months and in regions with tropical climates. Overzealous removal of cerumen not only compromises the natural defenses of the EAC, it may also cause sufficient trauma to allow for bacterial inoculation. Patients with pruritic dermatologic conditions often suffer from recurrent bouts of infection as a result of frequent scratching and excoriation of the canal skin.

Acute diffuse otitis externa (swimmer's ear) refers to bacterial infection and inflammation of the skin and subcutaneous tissue of the cartilaginous EAC. Characteristic symptoms include itching, pain, and tenderness of the pinna with associated hearing loss and aural fullness. Examination typically reveals erythema and edema of the external canal skin, which may spread to involve the concha and lobule. Seropurulent otorrhea often results in crusting of the EAC and concha. Manipulation of the pinna and mastication generally elicit pain. In advanced cases, worsening edema significantly narrows the external canal lumen, preventing visualization of the tympanic membrane, and associated inflammatory changes may spread to involve preauricular soft tissue.

Otomycosis refers to an acute fungal infection of the EAC. Candida and Aspergillus are the most common fungal species implicated in otomycosis. The initial symptoms of fungal otitis externa mirror those of bacterial otitis externa, with the exception that associated pain is less severe. Intense pruritus is the most common complaint in otomycosis. Examination typically reveals canal skin erythema and the presence of abundant fungal debris, often embedded in a cheesy material thicker than that seen in bacterial otitis externa. Recognizing the white, gray, or black filamentous elements characteristic of fungal growth is critical to make the diagnosis of otomycosis. When unsure, a potassium hydroxide preparation can be helpful in demonstrating branching filaments or budding yeasts.

Treatment of acute otitis externa requires the thorough removal of all purulent or fungal material and desquamated debris to allow penetration of antimicrobial therapy. The frequency of aural cleansing is dictated by the amount of debris present in the canal. When significant, debridement may be required several times per week. This is essentially the only role surgery plays in the management of otitis externa. Ototopical preparations containing acidifying agents and antibiotics active against *P. aeruginosa* and *S. aureus* address the infectious component of this process. When edema is severe, inserting a wick into the canal aids in the delivery of medication to its deeper portions. Wicks should be replaced every 2 to 3 days until canal patency is restored. Many otic preparations contain a corticosteroid, helpful in reducing inflammation and edema of the canal as well as associated pain. Oral antibiotics may be necessary when bacterial infection has extended to involve preauricular soft tissue. Pain control is another cornerstone in the treatment of otitis externa. Nonsteroidal anti-inflammatory medications or narcotic analgesics are required if over-the-counter analgesics fail to provide sufficient relief. Treatment of otomycosis requires appropriate topical antifungal medications. Many options are available, including M-cresyl-acetate (Cresylate™), 1% clotrimazole cream or solution, and vital dyes such as gentian violet. The majority of treatment failures, particularly in those cases managed by primary care providers, are believed to result from inadequate skin penetration of the prescribed ototopical medication, further emphasizing the importance of adequate EAC debridement.[25]

Efforts to prevent recurrent episodes of otitis externa focus on minimizing the moisture content within the EAC. Water precautions should be recommended. Occlusive earplugs are effective in preventing water entry into the canal. Directing a hair dryer at the EAC after water exposure followed by use of drying agents such as boric acid in ethyl alcohol can also be helpful.

The potential for ototoxicity must be considered when treating patients with tympanic membrane perforations or pressure equalization tubes. Instillation of ototopical drops into the middle ear of chinchillas was shown to result in cochlear toxicity.[26] Nevertheless, this appears to be an exceedingly rare complication in humans. In his review, Roland documented only four cases in the English literature of sensorineural hearing loss potentially related to topical antibiotic use.[27] A possible explanation is provided by the work of Schachern and colleagues, who demonstrated that the thickness of the round window membrane increases while in the presence of inflammation or infection.[28] Use of potentially ototoxic medications in nondiseased middle ears should therefore be employed with caution as they lack this potentially protective characteristic.

Malignant Otitis Externa (Skull Base Osteomyelitis)

Malignant otitis externa was first described by Meltzer and Keleman in 1959 and was later named by Chandler in 1958.[29,30] The term skull base osteomyelitis more accurately describes the pathophysiology of this life-threatening infection of the EAC and skull base. Usually seen in diabetic patients and those with other forms of immunocompromise, infection spreads from the skin and subcutaneous tissue of the cartilaginous canal to involve the tympanic bone. Skull base osteomyelitis spreads via the haversian system of compact bone, forming multiple abscesses and sequestra of necrotic bone. As infection progresses, periparotid and cervical soft tissues become involved. A facial nerve paralysis implies infection encasing the extratemporal portion of the nerve or involvement of the stylomastoid foramen. Palsies of cranial nerves IX, X, XI, and XII present as infection extends to involve the jugular foramen.

The cerumen of patients with diabetes has been shown to be of higher pH than that of nondiabetics, perhaps responsible for the increased incidence of external otitis in this population.[31] Impaired polymorphonuclear leukocyte function and microangiopathic disease typical of advanced diabetes contribute to the progression of otitis externa to skull base osteomyelitis in elderly diabetic patients.[32]

Patients with osteomyelitis of the skull base often report a previous history of otitis externa. Intense otalgia exceeding that expected for routine otitis is common and can be associated with otorrhea. Granulation tissue seen protruding into the EAC from the bony-cartilaginous junction is a cardinal sign of skull base osteomyelitis and should not be underestimated. Biopsy is required both to rule out malignancy and for culture purposes. Sedimentation rate will be elevated, but osteomyelitis may occur in the absence of fever and elevated white blood cell count. Computed tomographic scans help to evaluate the extent of bony involvement. Magnetic resonance imaging provides more detail regarding soft-tissue disease and, when combined with magnetic resonance angiography, can evaluate the patency of the dural sinuses. Technetium 99 and gallium 67 bone scans help in confirming the diagnosis of skull base osteomyelitis. Only the gallium scan, however, can be used to monitor response to therapy. Gallium scans image the activity of white blood cells and proteins at sites of active infection. This study will normalize as infection resolves, whereas the technetium scan may remain positive for many months.

Treatment of osteomyelitis of the skull base generally requires long-term administration of parental antibiotics in combination with daily aural debridement and vigilant management of diabetes and other compromising medical conditions. The vast majority of skull base osteomyelitis results from infection by *P. aeruginosa*. Double coverage directed against *Pseudomonas* is empirically begun after cultures have been obtained. Fluoroquinolones offer potent activity against *Pseudomonas* via oral administration and may be effective as monotherapy. However, recent resistance to fluoroquinolones has emerged, suggesting that monotherapy may not be adequate in some cases.[33] Surgical therapy is rarely required and is usually mandated by progression of infection despite aggressive medical management. The role of surgery should be limited to the debridement of necrotic bone and granulation tissue and the drainage of abscesses. Decompression of the facial nerve for cases complicated by facial paralysis appears to have no role in the management of skull base osteomyelitis as it fails to address the extratemporal location of nerve involvement.[34]

Atresia and Stenosis

Acquired stenosis and atresia of the EAC, also known as medial canal fibrosis, refers to a condition characterized by the cicatricial formation of fibroinflammatory tissue lateral to the tympanic membrane. A distinct clinical entity that must be differentiated from congenital aural atresia, acquired stenosis usually results from chronic infection and inflammation and may also represent a complication related to prior otologic surgery or EAC trauma.[35] As the developing stenosis progresses, affected patients suffer a worsening conductive hearing loss. Examination reveals edema and hypertrophy of the canal wall skin, and once fibrosis matures, the EAC becomes a blind, skin-lined pouch. The lateral aspect of the tympanic membrane frequently becomes incorporated into the scar tissue, obliterating any potential intervening space.

The best treatment of acquired stenosis of the EAC is prevention. Chronic otitis externa refers to a diffuse inflammatory process of the external canal of long duration. Its etiology remains unclear, but it appears to be the most frequent cause of medial canal fibrosis.[36] Bilateral in 50% of cases and twice as common in women than men, this entity is probably related to a combination of infection, allergy, and dermatoses.[37] A paucity of literature analyzing treatment options for chronic otitis externa exists, but management is primarily medical until complete medial canal fibrosis develops. A regimen consisting of topical corticosteroid and antibiotic preparations in combination with periodic, atraumatic cleansing may prevent the need for surgical intervention. Cauterization of granulation tissue may also aid in drying and halting the inflammatory process.

Surgical Technique for Repair of Acquired Stenosis of EAC

Preoperative Planning: Surgical therapy of acquired stenosis is indicated for correction of conductive hearing loss (hearing aids tend to exacerbate underlying inflammation) and to prevent or remove cholesteatoma in those stenosis related to trauma or prior surgery where an epithelialized tympanic membrane or canal may exist medial to the stenotic segment. Generally, canalplasty with a wide meatoplasty is the procedure of choice. This may be performed endaurally if adequate exposure can be obtained but usually requires a postauricular approach. Computed tomography may be helpful to determine the status of the middle ear, the presence of cholesteatoma medial to the stenosis, and define the pertinent anatomy.

Surgical Details: A vascular strip is designed and made with the medial incision at the level of the stenosis or blind sac (Figure 22–4 A to I). The flap should be made as long as possible. It may be helpful to make the medial incision from behind after making the postauricular incision. Similar to the incision for exostosis, the periosteal incision may be made as a semicircle, corresponding to the bony meatus. The flap is elevated and the ear is retracted anteriorly. Next, the anterior canal skin is either incised medially and "window-shaded" by elevating it as a laterally based flap or incised laterally and removed to be replaced as a free graft. The cicatrix can frequently be dissected free of the medial layer of the tympanic membrane, but, if not the drum remnant is resected. A drill is used to perform a wide canalplasty. For reconstruction, a fascial graft is taken from the temporalis muscle and used to reconstruct any perforation of the tympanic membrane, with either a medial or a lateral technique. The anterior canal skin is trimmed of disease and prepared for replacement. Usually, a skin graft will be needed. Ideally, skin is taken with a dermatome from the inner arm or thigh. Postauricular skin can be taken freely, but in the authors' experience the full thickness graft is too thick and shrinks to an undesirably small graft, leaving less than desirable bony coverage. Fascia can also be used to cover bone where inadequate skin is available. The tympanic membrane may be covered with a disk of Gelfilm™. The postauricular incision is closed and the canal is packed with gelfoam. A stent or rosebud packing fashioned from silk or silicone strips filled with gelfoam is helpful in many cases to encourage adherence of the grafts and vascular strip.

Postauricular Care: Antibiotic drops are used twice daily and the packing is removed over 4 to 6 weeks during biweekly visits. The packing can be removed and replaced and allowed to support the canal for 10 to 14 days or longer. Granulation tissue is carefully monitored and treated with chemical cautery. Close monitoring is needed as restenosis can occur very quickly. Postoperative infection should be managed aggressively as it will contribute to failure.

Pitfalls and Complications: Recurrence is a very distinct risk. All involved tissue must be removed and the bony canal enlarged to allow for some element of postoperative restenosis. Critical to the success of this procedure is resurfacing the osseous canal with epithelium. If bone is left exposed, and the formation of granulation tissue and healing by secondary intention are allowed, the rate of recurrent stenosis is unacceptably high. Usually, a split-thickness skin graft is employed, but a variety of pedicled flaps, as well as full thickness skin grafts, have been described.[38–40] Other risks include sensorineural hearing loss, conductive hearing loss, facial nerve injury, and tympanic membrane perforation. Intraoperative facial nerve monitoring may be used to reduce the risk of facial nerve injury.

Necrosis of the External Auditory Canal

Occasionally, one will encounter a benign-appearing, painless ulcer in the EAC, often near the bony-cartilaginous junction in the inferior or posterior canal (Figure 22–5). The edges of the ulcer may appear healthy without evidence of infection. The underlying bone is exposed, sometimes with sequestra, but does not appear infected. Over time, the lesion does not appear to progress. Culture and biopsy are negative. This type of presentation may be indicative of benign osteonecrosis of the EAC, after ruling out malignancy, infection, and primary cholesteatoma of the EAC. Radiation may also predispose to osteonecrosis of the EAC, but in this case, the process may be more progressive. This disorder may occur in the setting of breast cancer, prostate cancer, or multiple myeloma, often with a history of chemotherapy or bisphosphonate use. Bisphosphonates reduce osteoclast activity and are a frequently used therapy for bone metastases and tumor-induced hypercalcaemia,

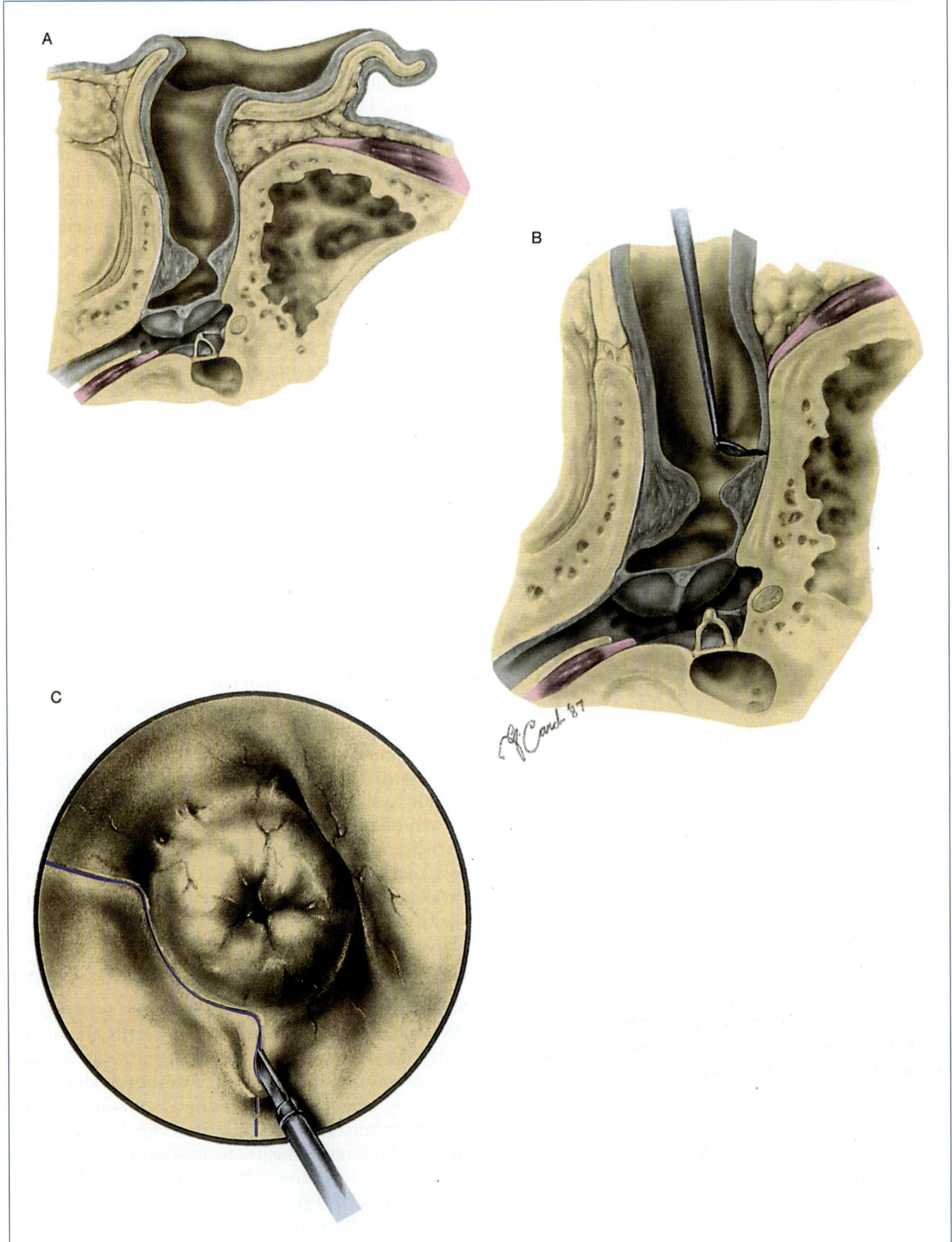

FIGURE 22–4 • Surgical treatment of acquired external canal stenosis. *A*, Cicatricial fibrous stenosis at the level of the bony external auditory canal. *B* and *C*, Vascular strip incisions are made as far medial as is safe and practicable.

Continued

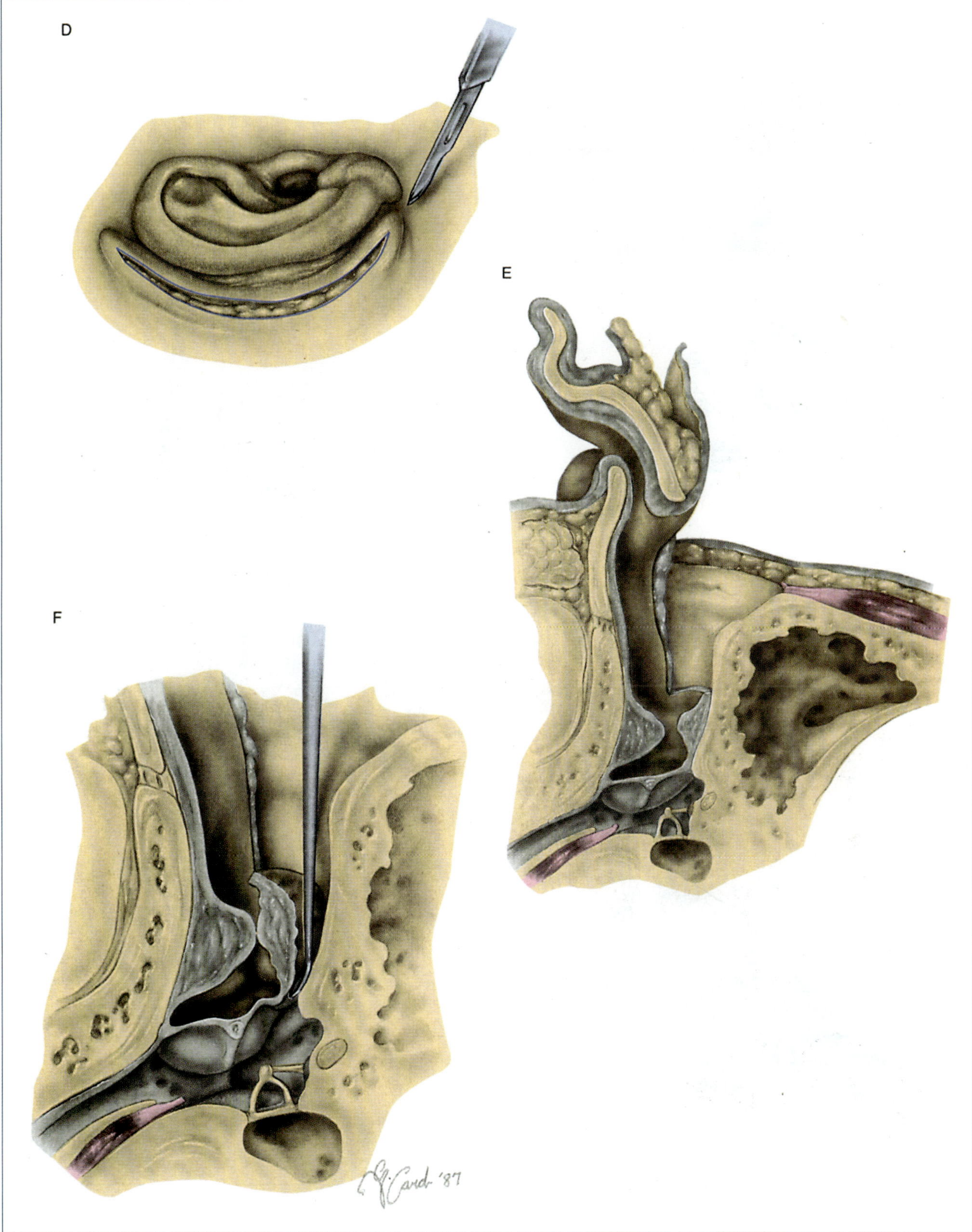

FIGURE 22–4 • *Continued. D*, A postauricular incision is made. *E*, The vascular strip is elevated out of the external canal. *F*, The mass of scar tissue is elevated from the posterior wall of the ear canal until the middle ear space is entered.

Continued

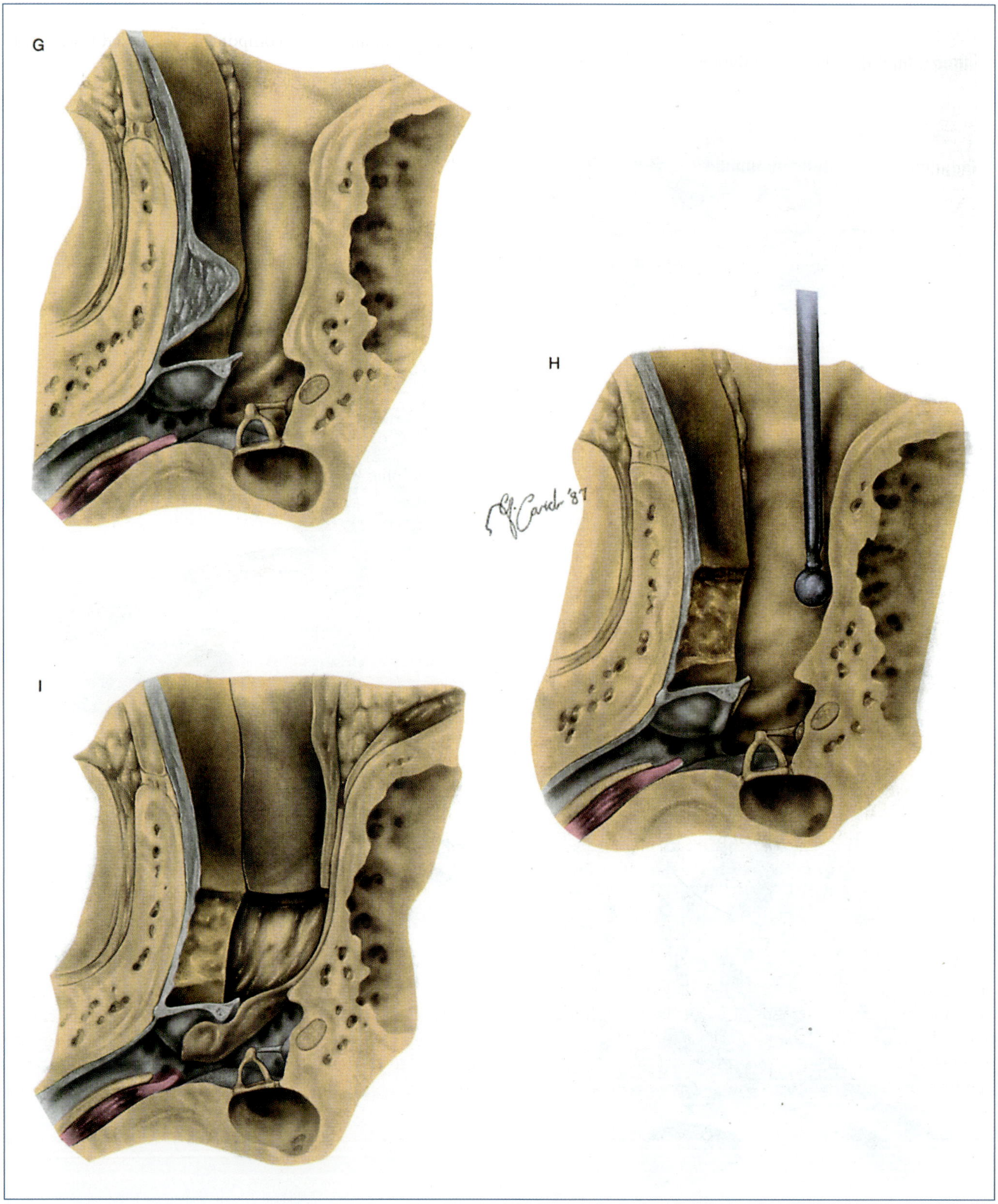

G

H

I

FIGURE 22–4 • *Continued*. *G*, Posterior fibrous stenosis excised. *H*, The stenotic scar tissue anteriorly is excised, leaving the anterior drum remnant if at all possible. The canal is enlarged with a drill until air cells can just be seen through bone. *I*, The drum and canal are grafted with fascia and the canal is filled with ointment.

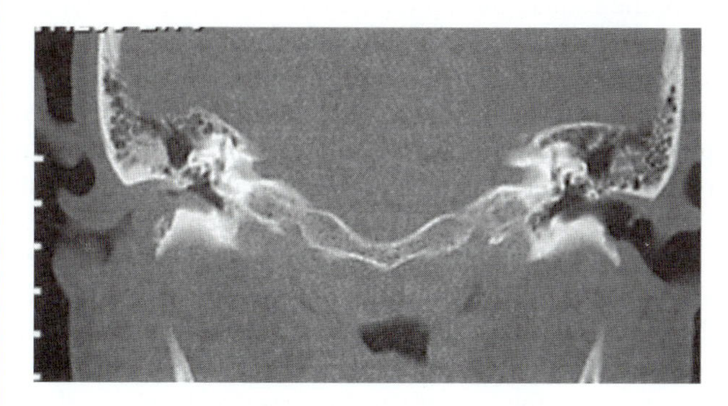

FIGURE 22–5 • Benign bilateral nonprogressive osteonecrosis of bony canal with overlying ulcers in a patient with a history of breast cancer.

osteoporosis, and Paget's disease. The reduced ability of bone to respond to physiological demands in the presence of radiation or bisphosphonate-induced reduced osseous remodeling and reduced blood flow may predispose to loss of bone and overlying skin. Traumatic and idiopathic cases have also been presented in the literature. Uncomplicated, nonprogressive, focal EAC necrosis can be managed with local, conservative cleaning and precautions. More extensive and progressive disease may respond to debridement. Local tissue grafts and skin grafts can be used to reconstruct defects if viable bone is uncovered.

Malignancies of External Auditory Canal

The EAC may be afflicted by cutaneous malignancies, most commonly, squamous cell carcinoma, followed by basal cell carcinoma and melanoma. Adenoid cystic carcinoma, ceruminal gland adenocarcinoma, as well as more rare tumors may also occur within the EAC. Malignancies of the EAC typically present as ulcerated or nodular skin lesions, which are associated with chronic bloody otorrhea. Temporal bone invasion is classically heralded by complaints of a deep-boring otalgia. Radiographic imaging helps define the extent of tumor invasion. Successful treatment usually requires wide excision by temporal bone resection, frequently combined with postoperative radiation therapy. Chemotherapy may also play a role. A thorough discussion of the management of this class of malignancy is beyond the scope of this chapter (see Chapter 23). However, it is important to keep benign and malignant processes in mind when forming a differential diagnosis for disorders of the EAC.

DISEASES OF THE TYMPANIC MEMBRANE

Bullous Myringitis

Bullous myringitis is a poorly understood condition characterized by inflammation of the tympanic membrane and the formation of serous or hemorrhagic bullae on its epithelial surface. Middle ear effusion may also be present. Most commonly, the disease is unilateral and results in severe otalgia, often disproportionate to findings seen on physical examination. Sensorineural hearing loss frequently accompanies bullous myringitis. In Hoffman and Shepsman's review of 15 patients with 21 affected ears, 67% showed evidence of sensorineural loss, either alone or as a component of a mixed loss.[41] Hearing loss associated with bullous myringitis is generally transient, and the majority of patients recover full auditory function.[42]

The etiology of bullous myringitis remains unknown. It often follows a nonspecific upper respiratory illness, and early studies indeed suggested a causal relationship with influenza infection.[43] Later, Rifkin and colleagues induced bullous myringitis in nearly half of the healthy subjects inoculated with *Mycoplasma pneumoniae*.[44] However, when examining the acute and postconvalescent sera of patients diagnosed with bullous myringitis, Merifield and Miller found no consistent changes in antibody titers to suggest an etiologic role for *M. pneumoniae* or a variety of common upper respiratory viruses.[45] It may be that the bullous lesions characteristic of this illness represent a nonspecific response to inflammation of the tympanic membrane and that bullous myringitis is not, in fact, a distinct entity.

Treatment of bullous myringitis has traditionally included decompression of the painful vesicles and oral analgesics. In cases complicated by sensorineural hearing loss, it is our practice to treat aggressively with antibiotics and systemic corticosteroids (prednisone 1 mg/kg/day for 7 days, then tapered) as if it represents a complication of otitis media. Myringotomy may be performed if a middle ear effusion accompanies bullae formation. Randomized trials comparing management options for bullous myringitis with associated sensorineural hearing loss do not exist.

Granular Myringitis

Another poorly understood condition, granular myringitis is characterized by chronic inflammation of the tympanic membrane leading to the replacement of its epithelial surface and, occasionally, adjacent deep meatal skin with proliferating granulation tissue. The predominant presentation of granular myringitis is a unilateral scant constant or recurrent, often malodorous otorrhea. Symptoms of pruritus and aural fullness are also common, but the ear is usually painless. Otoscopy reveals a mucoid, serous, mucopurulent, or frankly purulent discharge bathing the tympanic membrane. Careful aural cleansing is required to visualize characteristic granulation tissue, which may involve the tympanic membrane in focal patches, segmental distributions, or diffusely, where most of the pars tensa surface is replaced. Most agree that the tympanic membrane must be intact to diagnose granular myringitis and differentiate it from chronic suppurative otitis media, although occasionally perforations may occur in conjunction with myringitis. A mild conductive hearing loss is frequently noted on audiometric evaluation.

The etiology of granular myringitis is unknown. Acute infection or mechanical trauma leading to loss of the squamous epithelial layer of the tympanic membrane appears to be a critical event in the development of granular myringitis, which disrupts normal epithelial migration responsible for the healing properties of the tympanic membrane.[46] In their review, Blevins and Karmody found that 60% of patients with granular myringitis had previously undergone an otologic procedure.[47] Once the epithelial layer has been compromised, infection by those organisms commonly responsible for otitis externa, especially

Pseudomonas and *Staphylococcus*, further inhibits healing of the tympanic membrane. *P. aeruginosa*, *S. aureus*, Proteus, and *Staphylococcus* epidermis have been linked to the process.[48]

Management of granular myringitis often requires protracted therapy. Initially, external infection must be controlled. Antibiotic-steroid drops, diluted vinegar, antifungal agents, and oral quinolone antibiotics have also been used with some success. Once infection has been addressed, granulation tissue may be cauterized with silver nitrate, trichloroacetic acid, or phenol, if abundant, and is controlled with daily use of topical corticosteroid drops [0.05% fluocinonide (Lidex™)] until resolution is observed. Frequent office visits are often required until the process is under good control. Unfortunately, recurrence is typical. The role of surgery in the management of granular myringitis remains controversial. It is generally reserved for those refractory cases that fail prolonged topical therapy. The involved area of the tympanic membrane is excised and repaired with an underlay or overlay graft. Some authors have reported excellent success rates for surgical therapy of granular myringitis, but available data are sparse and limited by short follow-up periods.[48]

Traumatic Perforation

Acute perforations of the tympanic membrane generally result from episodes of acute otitis media or trauma. The majority of infectious perforations heal as the inciting condition resolves. Traumatic tympanic membrane perforation may result from blunt or penetrating injuries as well as rapid changes in barometric pressure (barotrauma). Slap injuries to the head, frequently encountered in cases related to assault or aquatic sports accidents, create a column of compressed air within the EAC of sufficient pressure to implode the tympanic membrane. Blast injuries inflict similar implosive forces on the tympanic membrane. Penetrating injuries are most frequently self-inflicted during overzealous cerumen removal. Barometric trauma commonly occurs following rapid airplane descent or deep-water diving or during hyperbaric oxygen therapy. Rather than causing a perforation, barotrauma generally results in hemorrhage of tympanic membrane vasculature. Thermal injuries to the tympanic membrane, commonly seen in welders and those struck by lightning, result in a small percentage of perforations. However, because of associated tissue necrosis, burn-related perforations have a high rate of nonhealing.

Most studies suggest that upward of 90% of traumatic perforations heal spontaneously within 3 months of injury.[49] Epithelial migration patterns on the tympanic membrane and within the EAC responsible for the removal of desquamated cells and keratin debris form the basis for the tympanic membrane's impressive healing properties. Studies by Litton and Alberti used India ink to mark epithelial elements on the tympanic membrane and documented cell migration that originates from the region of the umbo and proceeds in a centripetal fashion.[50,51] Following an acute injury, platelets gather to cause vasoconstriction and form a thrombus. An inflammatory response ensues, attracting neutrophils, macrophages, and bioactive cytokines to the wound. A matrix of proteoglycans and glycosaminoglycans is formed and allows for proliferation of the tympanic membrane's squamous epithelial layer across the perforation, forming a scaffold on which the mucosal and, later, the fibrous layers of the tympanic membrane can grow. The squamous elements responsible for bridging the perforation originate from "upstream" and must traverse the length of the defect. It is not surprising, therefore, that larger perforations are associated with delayed healing and higher rates of chronicity.

Patients who have suffered a traumatic tympanic membrane perforation often complain of mild hearing loss and aural fullness. Vertigo is uncommon and should prompt concern for a perilymphatic fistula. Audiometric assessment often shows conductive hearing loss of varying severity. Ritvik et al. suggest that the conductive hearing loss associated with a perforation is frequency dependent and varies directly with the size of the perforation, inversely with the volume of the middle ear space, and is not related to the location.[52] Management of traumatic perforations ranges from observation along with dry-ear precautions to early myringoplasty. Either approach will result in perforation closure in approximately 90% of cases. Those who practice expectant management of traumatic tympanic membrane perforations cite the high likelihood of spontaneous healing, whereas supporters of early intervention report quicker resolution of hyperacusis and prompt return of patients to their preferred lifestyles. Myringoplasty can be performed as an office-based procedure under local anesthesia. After injecting the external canal with 1% lidocaine, the margins of the tympanic membrane are everted and aligned with a pick. A patch of moistened cigarette paper or Gelfilm™ is then placed over the perforation. The patch helps prevent inversion of the tympanic membrane edges and promotes prompt healing. Use of ototopical medications in the setting of an uncomplicated traumatic tympanic membrane perforation is discouraged. There is a theoretical risk of ototoxicity. Additionally, the wet environment resulting from medication application impairs fibroblast proliferation and may therefore hinder perforation healing.

Tympanosclerosis

Tympanosclerosis is characterized by hyaline degeneration of the fibrous layer of the tympanic membrane and the middle-ear mucosa. Isolated involvement of the tympanic membrane is most common and is more appropriately named myringosclerosis, but tympanosclerotic plaques may also present within the middle ear cleft and mastoid. Tympanosclerosis is irreversible and results from infection or inflammation of the middle ear space. The incidence of tympanosclerosis in patients with a previous history of otitis media ranges from 14% to 43% in different clinical series.[53,54] In their review, Tos and Stangerup demonstrated an association between ventilation tube placement and tympanosclerosis.[55] Tympanosclerosis developed in 13% of ears with secretory otitis media treated with paracentesis compared with 59% treated with grommet tube insertion. Additionally, Kay and colleagues' recent meta-analysis of 134 studies regarding sequelae of tympanostomy tube insertion revealed a 32% incidence of postintubation tympanosclerosis compared with 10% of controls.[56]

Rarely does isolated tympanic membrane tympanosclerosis result in a clinically significant hearing loss requiring intervention. Middle ear tympanosclerosis, on the other hand, can cause ossicular fixation and result in more severe degrees of conductive hearing loss.

Retraction Pockets of the Tympanic Membrane

Retraction of the tympanic membrane is a common finding in both children and adults. Middle ear negative pressure (atelectasis) results in retraction or retraction pockets that range in severity from shallow nonprogressive and self-cleaning pockets to deep, adherent, and problematic retractions into the attic and mastoid. Even shallow retractions into the posteriosuperior region of the pars tensa can cause progressive hearing loss from erosion of the ossicular chain. Deeper attic retractions can remain asymptomatic for years while collecting keratin debris, expanding by erosion of bone, and eventually developing into extensive cholesteatoma. Sade's grading system is clinically useful for staging retraction of the tympanic membrane. Grade I retractions are simple, shallow, and nonadherent. Grade II retractions touch the incus and/or stapes with or without erosion. Grade III pockets retract to the promontory without adhesion and grade IV retractions are adherent to the promontory.[57]

The primary cause of atelectasis is eustachian tube dysfunction that results in the loss of normal middle ear ventilation and the development of negative pressure in the middle ear as the middle ear mucosa absorbs nitrogen from the air. The inherent structure of the posterosuperior portion of the pars tensa and the pars flaccida make these areas of the tympanic membrane more prone to retraction. The posterosuperior pars tensa has thinner, more sparsely distributed collagen and increased vascular supply. The pars flaccida is actually thicker than the pars tensa, but has thinner less-organized collagen fibers loosely arranged in a vascular lamina propria. Inflammation and infection damage the inherent collagenous support, making the tympanic membrane weaker and more susceptible to increased and persistent negative middle ear pressure and eventual retraction.[3,58,59] The atelectatic tympanic membrane is characterized by hyperkeratosis, edema and inflammation of the lamina propria, and loss of collagen organization.[60]

The dilemma at diagnosis is distinguishing stable from progressive disease. Problematic pockets will manifest with recurrent otorrhea, hearing loss, and cholesteatoma. Sometimes, a "trail sign" is evident as a line of keratin extending from the pocket onto and along the posterior wall of the EAC. This line of migrating keratin may represent cholesteatoma within the pocket. Other red flags include deep pockets where the medial extent cannot be appreciated, conductive hearing loss, recurrent otorrhea, polypoid tissue, or crusts or cerumen covering a pocket that is difficult to clean. Management options include observation, medical therapy, and surgery. Routine microscopic exams can over time identify stable disease. Shallow pockets should be cleaned of debris and cerumen. Acetic acid drops, mineral oil, or other cleansing and lubricating agents may reduce the accumulation of debris in the pockets. Eustachian tube function is supported by managing contributing factors, such as allergy, adenoid disease, and gastroesophageal reflux and by encouraging autoinflation. Progressive or risky pockets can often be managed by placement of a tympanostomy tube. Some advocate simple excision of the damaged tympanic membrane, which can then heal similar to a perforation with thicker collagen and scar, less prone to retraction, either with or without placement of a tube. Ostrowski and Bojrab describe a novel technique of laser-assisted contraction myringoplasty to address the redundant and weakened atelectatic tympanic membrane.[61] Other surgical options for progressive or complicated disease include tympanoplasty, cartilage tympanoplasty, and tympanoplasty combined with mastoidectomy. Postoperative recurrence is not uncommon with any of these techniques.

References

1. Hollinshead WH. Anatomy for surgeons: the head and neck. 3rd ed. Philadelphia: Lippincott-Raven; 1982. p. 159–67.
2. Donaldson JA, Duckert LG. Anson-Donaldson: surgical anatomy of the temporal bone. 4th ed. Lippincott Williams & Wilkins; 1992.
3. Stenfeldt K, Johansson C, Hellstrom S. The collagen structure of the tympanic membrane. Arch Otolaryngol Head Neck Surg 2006;132:293–8.
4. Schuknecht HF. Pathology of the ear. 2nd ed. Philadelphia: Lea & Febiger; 1993. p. 31–41.
5. Bassiouny A. Perichondritis of the auricle. Laryngoscope 1981;91:422–31.
6. Buck ML. Ciprofloxin use in children: A review of recent findings. Pediatric Pharmacotherapy, A monthly review for health care professionals of the children's medical center 1998;4(12):1–8. http://www.healthsystem.virginia.edu/internet/pediatrics/pharma-news/dec98.pdf (accessed February 17, 2008).
7. Work WP. Newer concepts of first branchial cleft defects. Laryngoscope 1972;82:1581–93.
8. Deshpande SA, Watson H. Renal ultrasonography not required in babies with isolated minor ear anomalies. Arch Dis Child Fetal Neonatal Ed 2006;91:29–30.
9. Wang RY, Earl DL, Ruder RO, Graham JM. Syndromic ear anomalies and renal ultrasounds. Pediatrics 2001;108(2):E32.
10. Kischer CW, Shetlar MR. Collagen and mucopolysaccharides in the hypertrophic scar. Connect Tissue Res 1974;2:205–13.
11. Sherris DA, Larrabee WF, Murakami CS. Management of scar contractures, hypertrophic scars, and keloids. Otolaryngol Clin North Am 1995;28:1057–67.
12. Farrior RT, Stambaugh KI. Keloids and hyperplastic scars. In: Facial scars, revisions, and camouflage. Thomas JF, Holt JR, editors. St. Louis: CV Mosby; 1989. p. 211–28.
13. Wortmann RL. Gout and other disorders of purine metabolism. In: Harrison's principles of internal medicine. Isselbacher, Kurt J, editors. 13th ed. New York: McGraw-Hill; 1994. p. 2079–88.
14. Tolleth H. A hierarchy of values in the design and construction of the ear. Clin Past Surg 1990;17:193.
15. Mustarde JC. The treatment of prominent ears by buried mattress suture—A ten years' survey. Plast Reconstr Surg 1967;39:382.
16. Furnas DW. Correction of prominent ears with multiple sutures. Clin Plast Surg 1978;5(3):491–5.

17. Lin SJ, Furnas DW. Ear, prominent ear. emedicine 2007. http://www.emedicine.com/plastic/TOPIC454.HTM (accessed February 18, 2008).
18. van Gilse PHG. Des observations ulterieures sur la genes des exostoses du conduit externe par l'irriations d'eau froide. Acta Otolaryngol (Stockh) 1938;26:343.
19. Corbridge RJ, Michaels L, Wright T. Epithelial migration in keratosis obturans. Am J Otolaryngol 1996;17:411–4.
20. Morrison AW. Keratosis obturans. J Laryngol Otolaryngol 1956;70:317–21.
21. Vrabec JT, Chaljub G. External canal cholesteatoma. Am J Otol 2000;21:608–14.
22. Piepergerdes JC, Kramer BM, Behnke EE. Keratosis obturans and external auditory canal cholesteatoma. Laryngoscope 1980;90:383–90.
23. Veitch D, Brockbank M, Whittet H. Aural polyp and cholesteatoma. Clin Otolaryngol 1988;13:395–7.
24. Gliklick RE, Cunningham MJ, Eavey RD. The cause of aural polyps in children. Arch Otolaryngol Head Neck Surg 1993;119:669–71.
25. Hannley MT, Dennery JC, Holzer SS. Consensus panel report: Use of ototopical antibiotics in treating 3 common ear diseases. Otolaryngol Head Neck Surg 2000;122:934–40.
26. Wright CG, Meyerhoff WL. Ototoxicity of otic drops applied to the middle ear in the chinchilla. Am J Otolaryngol 1984;5:166–76.
27. Roland PS. Clinical ototoxicity of topical antibiotic drops. Otolaryngol Head Neck Surg 1994;110:598–602.
28. Schachern PA, Paparella MM, Goycoolea MV. Thickness of the human round window membrane in different forms of otitis media. Arch Otolaryngol Head Neck Surg 1987;110:630–4.
29. Meltzer P, Keleman G. Pyocyaneus osteomyelitis of the temporal bone, mandible and zygoma. Laryngoscope 1958;69:1300–16.
30. Chandler JR. Malignant external otitis. Laryngoscope 1968;78:1257–94.
31. Driscoll PV, Ramachandrula A, Drezner DA, et al. Characteristics of cerumen in diabetic patients: A key to understanding malignant external otitis? Otolaryngol Head Neck Surg 1993;109:676.
32. Smitherman KO, Peacock JE. Infectious emergencies in patients with diabetes mellitus. Med Clin North Am 1995;79:53–77.
33. Djalilian HR, Shamloo B, Thakkar KH, Najme-Rahim M. Treatment of culture-negative skull base osteomyelitis. Otol Neurotol 2006;27(2):250–5.
34. Neal GD, Gates GA. Invasive Pseudomonas osteitis of the temporal bone. Am J Otol 1983;4:332–7.
35. El-Sayed Y. Acquired medial canal fibrosis. J Laryngol Otol 1998;112:145–9.
36. Selesnick S, Nguyen TP, Eisenman DJ. Surgical treatment of acquired external auditory canal atresia. Am J Otol 1998;19:123–30.
37. Roland PS. Chronic external otitis. Ear Nose Throat J 2001;80(Suppl 6):12–6.
38. Adkins WY, Ogusthorpe JD. Management of canal stenosis with a transposition flap. Laryngoscope 1981;91:1267–9.
39. Heeneman H. Surgical correction of the stenosed ear canal. J Otolaryngol 1979;8:461–2.
40. McCary WS, Kryzer TC, Lambert PR. Application of split-thickness skin grafts for acquired diseases of the external auditory canal. Am J Otol 1995;16:801–5.
41. Hoffman RA, Shepsman MA. Bullous myringitis and sensorineural hearing loss. Laryngoscope 1983;93:1544–5.
42. Lashin N, Zaher S, Ragab A, et al. Hearing loss in bullous myringitis. Ear Nose Throat J 1988;67:206–10.
43. Milligan W. Hemorrhagic types of ear disease occurring during epidemics of influenza. J Laryngol Otol 1926;41:493–8.
44. Rifkind D, Chanock R, Kravetz H, et al. Ear involvement (myringitis) and primary atypical pneumonia following inoculation of volunteers with Eaton agent. Am Rev Respir Dis 1962;85:479–89.
45. Merifield D, Miller G. The etiology and clinical course of bullous myringitis. Arch Otolaryngol 1966;84:41–3.
46. Makino K, Amatsu M, Kinishi M, et al. The clinical features and pathogenesis of granular myringitis. Arch Otorhinolaryngol 1988;245:224–9.
47. Blevins NJ, Karmody CS. Chronic myringitis: Prevalence, presentation, and natural history. Otol Neurotol 2001;22:3–10.
48. El-Seifi A, Fouad B. Granular myringitis: Is it a surgical problem? Am J Otol 2000;21:462–7.
49. Griffin WL. A retrospective study of traumatic tympanic membrane perforations in a clinical practice. Laryngoscope 1979:89;261–82.
50. Litton WB. Epithelial migration over the tympanic membrane and external auditory canal. Arch Otolaryngol Head Neck Surg 1963;77:254.
51. Alberti PWRM. Epithelial migration on the tympanic membrane. J Laryngol Otol 1964;78:808–30.
52. Mehta RP, Rosowski JJ, Voss SE, et al. Determinants of hearing loss in perforations of the tympanic membrane. Otology & Neurotology 2006:27(2):136–43.
53. Sheehy JL, House WF. Tympanosclerosis. Arch Otolaryngol 1962;76:151–7.
54. Bhaya MH, Paparella MM, Morizono T, et al. Pathogenesis of tympanosclerosis. Otolaryngol Head Neck Surg 1993;109:413–9.
55. Tos M, Stangerup SE. Hearing loss in tympanosclerosis caused by grommets. Arch Otolaryngol Head Neck Surg 1989;115:931–5.
56. Kay DJ, Nelson M, Rosenfeld RM. Meta-analysis of tympanostomy tube sequelae. Otolaryngol Head Neck Surg 2001;124:374–80.
57. Sade J, Berco E. Atelectasis and secretory otitis media. Ann Otol Rhinol Laryngol 1976;85(suppl 25):66–72.
58. Danner CJ. Middle ear atelectasis: What causes it and how is it corrected? Otolaryngol Clin N Am 2006;1211–9.
59. Ramakrishnan Y, Kotecha A, Bowdler DA. A review of retraction pockets: Past, present and future management. J Laryngol Otol 2007;121:521–5.
60. Sade J. Atelectatic tympanic membrane: Histologic study. Ann Otol Rhinol Laryngol 1993;102:712–6.
61. Ostrowski VB, Bojrab DI. Minimally invasive laser contraction myringoplasty for tympanic membrane atelectasis. Otolaryngol Head Neck Surg 2003;128:711–8.

Surgery for Cancer of the External Ear 23

Keith A. Casper, MD / Myles Pensak, MD, FACS

Malignancy of the auricle is most frequently of cutaneous origin. Cancer of the skin is the most common of all diagnosed malignancies. The exact incidence of nonmelanoma skin cancer is unknown due to the lack of reporting; however, published estimates identify nonmelanoma skin cancer as more common than all other cancers combined.[1] Current estimates for nonmelanoma skin cancer are greater than one million new diagnoses per year. The vast majority of these cases are basal cell carcinoma (800,000 to 900,000 per year) with squamous cell carcinoma occurring less frequently (200,000 to 300,000 cases per year).[1] Greater than 80% of cutaneous carcinomas occur in the head and neck region, and 5 to 10% are localized to the ear.[2]

Otolaryngologists are routinely involved in all aspects of care for auricular malignancies, including the diagnosis, resection, and reconstruction. The primary concern for all malignancy is eradication of disease in concordance with oncologic principles; however, the esthetic concerns of the auricle make the management of cancer of the external ear a challenging problem. This chapter reviews the diagnosis and management of malignancy originating from the auricle. Otologic tumors that originate or extend into the external auditory canal, middle ear, or temporal bone are discussed in subsequent chapters.

ANATOMY

Embryology

Development of the external ear commences during the 4th gestational week. The auricle initially begins as several tissue swellings arising from the first and second branchial arches. These swellings continue to develop into prominent ridges, "hillocks of His" that form the pinna. The first branchial arch hillocks eventually form the tragus, helix, and superior antihelix. The second branchial arch hillocks develop into the lateral aspect of the helix, the remainder of the antihelix, antitragus, and the lobule. The fusion planes between the first and second branchial arch derivatives theoretically create a barrier to tumor spread. Beginning the 8th week of gestation, the first branchial groove begins to expand medially creating the primary external auditory canal. The core of epithelial cells continues medially through the mesenchyme to terminate at the meatal plate. During the fifth month of gestation, the core of epithelial cells begins to canalize in a medial to lateral direction, eventually creating the external auditory canal. The lateral cartilaginous framework is derived from the mesenchymal tissue surrounding the developing canal, and the medial bony canal is formed from the tympanic portion as well as the squamous portion of the temporal bone (anterior, inferior, and lower part of the posterior canal walls) and the squamous portion (posterior and superior walls).

Auricle

The appearance of the auricle derives from its irregular framework of elastic fibrocartilage covered by perichondrium and skin. The skin is more loosely attached on the medial surface of the pinna than it is to the lateral surface. Numerous skin appendages are found on both surfaces of the auricle, including hair follicles as well as sebaceous and sudoriferous glands. There is a complex series of ridges and depressions that constitute the lateral surface of the auricle. The helix is the external rim of the auricle, whereas the antihelix parallels the helix but forms the transition to the conchal bowl. The scaphoid fossa is the concave region between the helix and antihelix. The triangular fossa is the depression located between the superior and inferior crura of the antihelix. The tragus is an extension of the cartilaginous anterior canal wall and is mirrored by the antitragus, which is located immediately superior to the lobule. The lobule is the inferior most extension of the pinna and is devoid of cartilage. The auricle is secured to the underlying cranium by three ligaments as well as the extrinsic muscles of the ear and the overlying skin. The auricle has six or more intrinsic muscles as well as several extrinsic muscles, all of which are innervated by the facial nerve. The auricle has a lavish blood supply with branches from the internal maxillary artery, the superficial temporal artery, as well as the posterior auricular artery. The lymphatic drainage of the external ear is to the preauricular nodes of the parotid gland and the mastoid and postauricular nodes, which then drain into the second echelon lymph nodes of the superior jugular chain.

Physiology

Basal cell carcinoma (BCC) and squamous cell carcinoma (SCC) are jointly referred to as nonmelanoma skin cancers. Although these cancers are often grouped together, a number of significant differences exist. Sun exposure (ultraviolet radiation [UV radiation]) is the most significant risk factor for the development of a cutaneous malignancy; however, the correlation with UV radiation is stronger for SCC than BCC.[3,4] Cutaneous SCC occurs in regions of the head and neck, receiving maximal irradiation.[4] Basal cell carcinoma most commonly occurs on the head and neck region as well; however, the distribution of BCC does not correspond to areas of maximum irradiation.[4] Basal cell carcinoma commonly occurs in areas of little sun exposure, such as the postauricular region.

The sun is the primary source of terrestrial UV radiation. Ultraviolet radiation is only a small segment of the electromagnetic spectrum. The entire electromagnetic spectrum ranges from 10^{-14} m (gamma radiation) to 10^4 m (radio waves).[5] Ultraviolet radiation occurs in the narrow spectrum with wavelengths in the 10^{-7} m range, specifically between 100 nm and 400 nm.[5] The ultraviolet waveband is further divided into three spectral regions, UVA, UVB, and UVC, based primarily on differing biological effects.[5] UVA radiation (320 to 400 nm) comprises the majority of the ultraviolet spectrum reaching the surface of the earth, and therefore, despite a lower overall energy, produces most of the damage to our skin. UVB radiation (290 to 320 nm) is the most efficient at inducing cutaneous changes but it makes up less than 10% of the solar UV radiation. UVC radiation (100 to 280 nm) is absorbed almost entirely by the stratospheric ozone, and therefore is minimally involved in solar damage to the skin.[5] Terrestrial UV radiation increases with decreasing latitude, reduced cloud cover, increasing altitude, as well as during the summer months and the midday period.[6] The importance of these factors can be explained by the primary phenomenon influencing the exposure of solar UV radiation, which is attenuation and scattering by the earth's atmosphere.[5]

Ultraviolet radiation affects the skin in numerous ways. UVB radiation causes direct genetic mutations by dimerizing pyrimidines in DNA at dipyrimidine sites.[7] This leads to characteristic mutations that can be identified and attributed to UVB radiation. UVA radiation causes cellular damage and nuclear injury via the formation of reactive oxygen species.[7] Mutations occur throughout the genome as a result of UV radiation; UV radiation-related tumor promotion occurs by way of damage to tumor suppressor genes including *p53* as well as aberrant expression of a host of chemokines, growth factors, proinflammatory mediators, and DNA repair enzymes.[8] The *p53* tumor suppressor gene is mutated in the majority of SCCA and BCCA.[9] Ultraviolet radiation also downregulates host immune function primarily by upregulating the action of suppressor T cells.[7,10] In the context of this decreased immunoregulation, ultraviolet-induced damage to keratinocyte DNA may continue undetected and may proliferate leading to significant irreversible damage.[7]

Ultraviolet radiation also induces other cutaneous changes. Actinic keratoses (AKs) are rough, scaly lesions that are typically 2 to 6 mm in diameter and occur on sun-exposed areas of the body. Actinic keratoses are thought to be precursors of cutaneous SCC in addition to markers of increased risk for nonmelanoma skin cancer, as they are sensitive indicators of cumulative UV radiation exposure.[7] The transformation rate of AKs to SCC has been estimated to be 0.01 to 0.24% per year.[11,12] However, it is estimated that 60% of cutaneous SCCs initially arise from an actinic keratosis. Other lesions that may be premalignant include keratoacanthomas and radiation keratoses.[13]

The Fitzpatrick classification system was initially developed to categorize skin types for the estimation of dosing parameters with UV radiation for psoriasis patients.[14] The Fitzpatrick classification system (Table 23–1) currently is utilized to identify people who are at a high risk for the development of cutaneous malignancy. Fair-skinned individuals (Fitzpatrick skin types I and II) are at highest risk, with a relative risk (RR) two to five times that of darker individuals.[15]

The public health concerns regarding skin cancer among organ transplant recipients (OTRs) continue to increase as the longevity of the grafts improve and the number of organ transplantation surgeries continues to increase.[8] Pharmacologic immunosuppression, required for long-term graft survival, increases the risk of skin cancer by interfering with immunosurveillance as well as by augmenting viral proliferation.[8] It is estimated that roughly 1% of all nonmelanoma skin cancers occur in OTRs.[16] In comparison to the general population, however, there is a significant increase in the relative risk of skin cancer among OTRs. This is especially apparent in younger OTRs (<50 years), where the relative risk is 200 times the age matched nonimmunosuppressed population.[16] In addition, skin cancer in OTRs also tends to be more aggressive and has a greater potential to metastasize and threaten life.[17] The mortality rate due to skin cancer among OTRs has been estimated at 5%, of which two-thirds has been attributed to SCC; in contrast, the mortality from nonmelanoma skin cancer in the general population has been estimated at less than 1 death per 100,000 individuals.[18] Greater than one quarter of deaths occurring at least 4 years after transplantation are attributable to skin cancer.[8]

TABLE 23–1 Fitzpatrick classification system

SKIN COLOR	SKIN TYPE	SUNBURN	TAN
White	I	Always	Never
	II	Easily	Minimally
	III	Rarely	Yes
	IV	No	Yes
Brown	V	No	Yes
Black	VI	No	Yes

Adapted from Fitzpatrick.[34]

Several genetic syndromes have been shown to increase an individual's risk of developing skin cancer. Nevoid basal cell syndrome (NBCCS or Gorlin's syndrome) is an autosomal dominant disorder causing a predisposition to BCC as well as several developmental anomalies. These patients often have characteristic facial features, including frontal bossing, hypertelorism, lengthened mandible, and drooping lips. They also can develop other anomalies including odontogenic keratocysts, bifid ribs, and calcification of the falx cerebri.[1,20] Approximately 0.4% of all cases of BCCA and 2% of patients with BCC under the age of 45 are affected with Gorlin's syndrome.[21] Nevoid basal cell syndrome has been linked with germ-line mutations in the human homologue of the *Drosophila* polarity gene patched (PTCH).[22] The frequency of PTCH mutations in NBCCS patients ranges from 40 to 80%.[23] Xeroderma pigmentosum (XP) is the most well-known disease of an expanding family of nucleotide-excision repair (NER) diseases.[24] The total number of genes directly involved in NER is estimated to be around 40 but only about a dozen of these genes have been identified in NER-related human diseases.[24] These diseases have numerous overlapping symptoms, which may include cancer, developmental delay, immunological defects, neurodegeneration, retinal degeneration, and premature aging.[24] Xeroderma pigmentosum is an autosomal recessive disorder; patients develop numerous skin malignancies at a very young age.[25] Xeroderma pigmentosum is also associated with photophobia, keratitis, and neurologic abnormalities, including deafness.[25] Unfortunately, the surgical treatment of these patients is often difficult due to the numerous malignancies that often result in significant deformity. Prevention with sun avoidance, sunscreen, and covering apparel is vital.

Differential Diagnosis

Malignancies involving the ear and temporal bone are typically classified according to the location as well whether they are primary malignancies or metastatic disease. The sites of origin for otologic malignancies include the auricle, external auditory canal, middle ear, and mastoid. Auricular neoplasms represent 50 to 70% of all otologic malignancies; in addition, approximately 20% of all temporal bone cancers are attributed to advanced auricular neoplasms.[26] The most common histologic subtypes of the auricle include basal cell carcinoma, squamous cell carcinoma, and malignant melanoma.

The reported incidence of BCC and SCC, as well as all cutaneous malignancies, has risen dramatically over the last half-century.[27] This phenomenon likely reflects both a greater awareness coupled with an increased vigilance on the part of physicians. Current fashion and beauty ideals with an emphasis on skin exposure and tanned skin have also increased our exposure to UV radiation. Although skin cancer can occur in any age group, the vast majority of patients presenting with a cutaneous malignancy are older. The mean age of patients with BCC or SCC is approximately 70.[28] The incidence of skin cancer is much lower in darker-skinned ethnic groups than in Caucasians, who represent 95% of patients.[28]

Basal cell carcinoma represents 65 to 85% of all head and neck cutaneous malignancies with a similar distribution in regards to auricular carcinomas.[29,30] Squamous cell malignancy is the second most common malignancy of the auricle followed by malignant melanoma. There is debate concerning the most common histologic subtype of the auricle. Several series have reported SCC to be the most common; regardless, the varying incidence is most likely due to differing referral practices and the retrospective nature of these studies.[31,32] There are differences in the distribution of these two malignancies on the auricle. Basal cell carcinoma is found primarily on the posterior surface of the auricle, followed by the preauricular and then the retroauricular areas. Squamous cell carcinoma occurs in order of decreasing frequency on the helical rim, antihelix and triangular fossa, and posterior pinna. When these lesions appear on the auricle, 72% of the BCCs and 61% of the SCCs are confined to a single subsite of the ear.[33]

Basal Cell Carcinoma

Basal cell carcinoma is the most common type of skin cancer. In addition, BCC is usually accepted as the most common subtype in auricular malignancies. Basal cell carcinoma arises from cells in the basal layer of the epidermis. The tumor is locally invasive, aggressive, and destructive, but has a limited capacity for metastasis.[34] The tumor cells often form lobules, cords, or nests extending from the basal layer of epidermis into more superficial as well as deeper layers. Histologically, BCC typically demonstrates proliferating atypical basal cells with little pleomorphism and large, oval hyperchromatic nuclei with minimal cytoplasm. There are several clinical variants of BCC: nodular, ulcerating, sclerosing (morpheaform), superficial, pigmented, and basaloid.[3,35] These variants differ in their gross clinical appearance, histologic appearance, and behavior.[35]

Nodular BCC is the most common variant, accounting for 54% of all BCC. Fortunately, this variant is the least aggressive subtype.[35] Tumors appear as a translucent or "pearly" lesion with a smooth surface and central telangiectasia. These lesions often present with bleeding due to the absence of a keratin layer on the surface of the tumor.

Ulcerating BCC represents 11% of all BCCs.[35] Histologically, there are strands or cords of tumor surrounded by a fibrous stroma, which makes the determination of tumor margins difficult. Clinically, ulcerating BCC appears as a lesion with central necrosis and a rolled border (rodent ulcer). The periphery is translucent and smooth, which leads many to believe that this variant represents a nodular BCC that has outgrown its blood supply.

Sclerosing BCC (also known as morpheaform BCC) appears as a superficial scar, which is often ill defined and skin colored; the margins are indistinct and frequently extend beyond what is suspected clinically. This variant is characterized by an infiltrating growth pattern.[34–36] It is almost universally found in the head and neck region. This variant accounts for approximately 1% of all BCCs but has the highest rate of recurrence.[36]

Superficial BCC (11%) appears as a thin plaque. It is often red or pink in color with a fine threadlike border.[34] Pigmented BCC (6%) may be blue, black, or tan. They may appear like a nodular or superficial spreading melanoma (SSM) except for the firmer quality.[34] Basaloid SCC shows malignant cells with some squamous differentiation and keratin formation. This malignancy is considered more aggressive but some series refute this.[3,36–39] In addition to the listed subtypes, there are numerous less frequent types of BCC, including adenoid, sebaceous, eccrine, and apocrine BCC.[3]

Squamous Cell Carcinoma

Squamous cell carcinoma is characterized by enlarged, atypical keratinocytes with a perversion of the normal maturation of cells from the spinous layer to the upper layer of the epidermis. The tumor cells can have a great deal of pleomorphism and numerous mitotic figures. The nuclei are hyperchromatic with large nucleoli. Squamous cell carcinoma is often subdivided according to the degree of differentiation. Well-differentiated lesions typically will have numerous deposits of keratin or "keratin pearls." Poorly differentiated tumors have less obvious histological findings, but they can be identified with cytokeratin markers to help with the diagnosis.[35]

As with BCC, there are numerous histological subtypes of SCC. These subtypes include, but are not limited to, the following: conventional, pigmented, acantholytic, spindle cell, verrucous, and basaloid. The pigmented variant is often mistaken histologically for melanoma. The spindle cell variant is rare, accounting for approximately 1.5% of SCC, and is seen more often in previously irradiated skin or chronic burns.[40] This malignancy demonstrates cells in a fusiform pattern with poorly defined borders and has a propensity to infiltrate into the surrounding fibrous stroma.[41] Verrucous SCC is a well-differentiated variant. Although not considered a risk for metastases, verrucous carcinoma can be locally destructive.[35]

Squamous cell carcinoma usually arises in epidermal precancerous lesions.[34] The surrounding skin often demonstrates actinic damage. Most commonly, the malignant lesion will have nondescript borders with central ulceration and crusting. Aggressiveness varies depending on the histologic subtype and degree of differentiation, but in general, most actinic-induced malignancies will have a more indolent course with a lower rate of distant metastasis.[34] The overall rate of metastasis is approximately 3 to 4%.[34] High-risk features of SCC (from any location) include a diameter greater than 2 cm; a depth greater than 4 mm; tumor involvement of bone, muscle, and nerve; location on ear, lip, or genitalia; tumors arising in a scar (Marjolin's ulcer); following ionizing radiation; and poorly differentiated tumors.[34] The rate of regional metastasis is higher in auricular SCC compared with other locations.

Malignant Melanoma

Malignant melanoma of the auricle is a curable disease when diagnosed early but can be one of the most lethal malignancies if addressed at an advanced stage. Similar to other cutaneous malignancies, cutaneous malignant melanoma (CMM) has dramatically increased in incidence over the last two decades. Otolaryngologists are often the first physicians to identify lesions involving the head and neck including melanoma; therefore, a thorough knowledge of the diagnosis and treatment of malignant melanoma is crucial.

Cutaneous malignant melanoma is the third most common malignancy of the auricle. Despite the lower incidence of CMM, the mortality rate is far greater than the nonmelanoma skin cancers. The incidence of auricular melanoma is 0.1 to 0.6 per 100,000.[42] Auricular melanoma accounts for 7 to 20% of all melanomas of the head and neck and approximately 1 to 4% of all cutaneous melanomas.[43] The estimated number of new cases of CMM in the United States for 2006 was 62,190; the estimated number of deaths in 2006 was 7,910.[2] The most common site of origin on the ear is the helix (60%) followed by the lobule (25%).[44] The average age of presentation for a patient with malignant melanoma is 65 to 79.[45] Like that of other cutaneous malignancies, the rate of melanoma is lower in dark-skinned individuals.[46] There is a lower incidence of auricular melanoma among women, which most likely is partially attributed to longer hair length providing coverage to the skin of the ear.[42,45]

Melanoma can be exceedingly difficult to diagnose histologically. The individual malignant cells may be undifferentiated or, in some cases, even amelanotic. Melanocytes are normally located in the basal layer of the epidermis. Malignant cells may display nuclear/cellular atypia, mitotic figures, and vesicular nuclei with prominent nucleoli.[47] In general, the four most common histologic subtypes are superficial spreading melanoma (SSM), lentigo maligna melanoma (LMM), nodular melanoma (NM), and acral-lentiginous elanoma (ALM). The most common types of melanoma involving the auricle are SSM (46%), LMM (26%), and NM (22%).[43] Other variants include desmoplastic and neurotrophic malignant melanoma but account for less than 5% of tumors.[48]

Superficial spreading melanoma is the most common variant. Its overall incidence is 4.4 per 100,000; it represents nearly one-third of all melanomas and 65 to 75% of all head and neck melanomas.[42,45] Grossly, the lesions may be thin but are raised, palpable, and pigmented, with fairly regular borders. Histologically, there are melanocytes in all layers of the epidermis. These tumors tend to grow in a radial direction for 1 to 6 years before beginning their vertical growth phase into deeper tissue layers.[47]

Lentigo maligna melanoma (LMM) accounts for 17 to 24% of all malignant melanomas and approximately 5 to 15% of head and neck melanomas.[42,45,47] Lentigo maligna melanoma is flat and barely palpable, with irregular shapes and borders. There are nests of atypical melanocytes that are confined to the lower epidermis. This neoplasm has a very long radial growth phase, lasting up to 20 years.[47]

Nodular melanoma represents 28% of all melanoma and 15 to 20% of head and neck melanomas.[42,45,47] Nodular melanoma is typically darkly pigmented and raised, with a polypoid or nodular appearance. The malignant cells show a very early vertical growth phase, with very little involvement of the epidermis.[47] These tumors are particularly aggressive because of their deep invasiveness.

Nonepithelial Skin Cancers

In addition to the previously discussed malignancies, other less common tumors can occur and should be considered in the differential diagnosis of auricular neoplasms. The remaining malignancies are a diverse compilation of tumors, which account for approximately 5% of auricular neoplasms.[41]

Merkel cell carcinoma is one of the most aggressive nonmelanoma skin malignancies. It is a believed to be a neuroendocrine tumor that arises from the pleuripotent Merkel cell found near the basal layer of the epithelium.[49] Merkel cell carcinoma often presents as a red, glossy nodule. This malignancy occurs in the head and neck region in approximately 50% of cases.[50] Histologically, the tumor appears similar to other neuroendocrine tumors—a small blue cell tumor with a hyperchromatic nuclei and a high nuclear-cytoplasmic ratio.[51] Electron microscopy, often helpful in establishing a diagnosis, shows perinuclear whorls of intermediate filaments.[52] The cells stain positively for neuron-specific enolase, neurofilament, and cytokeratin.[49] Merkel cell carcinoma is very aggressive, with a high propensity for recurrence and metastases. The recurrence rate after wide local excision ranges from 40 to 90%.[50,52,53] Regional metastases are present in 31 to 80% of cases.[53,54] Wide local excision with 2- to 3-cm margins is recommended.[53] Mohs surgery may be helpful for tumors located on the face and ear to preserve normal tissue. Prophylactic lymph node dissection or radiation therapy to the nodal regions at highest risk may decrease local recurrence but does not consistently affect overall survival.[53] In many high volume centers, sentinel lymph node biopsy is often used when there is no evidence of nodal disease instead of a staging/prophylactic neck dissection. Despite aggressive locoregional therapy, the five-year survival rate is only approximately 60%, primarily due to distant metastases.[55]

Adnexal carcinomas are exceedingly rare, accounting for less than 0.005% of all skin lesions.[56] Because of the rarity, there is little data regarding outcome and therapy. These lesions usually develop in older patients and often appear as slowly growing, nontender pink or yellow masses.[49] Despite their slow growth, these malignancies are locally aggressive and tend to invade the surrounding connective tissue. Recurrence rates are high despite wide local excision. Other malignancies that can occur on the auricle include malignant fibrous histiocytoma, atypical fibroxanthoma, dermatofibrosarcoma protuberans, angiosarcomas, and metastatic disease from other areas.

Diagnostic Techniques

The history and physical examination are the most important initial steps in the evaluation of lesions of the auricle. Patient questioning should include elucidation of prior skin cancers, cumulative sun exposure, occupation, prior transplantation or radiation, and pertinent family history. The physical examination should include a detailed head and neck examination. Evaluation of the lesion should include close inspection of surrounding tissue and inspection for possible involvement of underlying structures (eg, cartilage, temporal bone, and parotid gland). The size and location of the lesion should be assessed in the context of the potential cosmetic and functional sequela of resection. Determination of potential locoregional spread is important especially for bulky lesions.

The diagnosis of an auricular neoplasm requires a diligent clinical evaluation. These lesions can often be overlooked as benign, especially in elderly patients with extensively sun-damaged skin. Early detection results in a better outcome with less need for more radical surgery. For early detection, especially with regard to the diagnosis of malignant melanoma, remember *ABCD*: *A*symmetry in shape, *B*order irregularity, *C*olor variation, and *D*iameter greater than 6 mm. Lesions that meet these criteria or lesions that have increased in size or are ulcerated or bleeding are worrisome and should be biopsied.

Imaging studies are rarely needed for auricular neoplasms; however, they should be considered whenever there is bulky or extensive disease or palpable adenopathy. The modality of choice depends on the clinical scenario. A contrast-enhanced computed tomography (CT) can be utilized for evaluation of cervical metastasis or bony involvement. Magnetic resonance imaging (MRI) is the preferred imaging study for the evaluation of intracranial or skull base extension.

A biopsy is crucial for the definitive management of a malignant lesion. A full-thickness biopsy containing a portion of the epidermis, dermis, and subcutaneous tissue is required. The preferred method is an excisional biopsy; however, if the lesion is extensive, an excisional biopsy may not be feasible. In this scenario, a punch biopsy will allow preservation of the architecture of the lesion while providing important histologic information. It can provide reliable information regarding the depth of the lesion. This important information assists in determining the strategy and the extent of the definitive resection. Shave biopsies are discouraged because they often fail to demonstrate the full depth of the lesion.

Staging

There is no specific staging system for malignancies of the auricle. The American Joint Committee on Cancer (AJCC) includes auricular malignancies in their staging system for nonmelanoma lesions of the skin (Table 23–2). This system, however, has many limitations when applied to the ear. The thin skin of the ear allows tumors to reach the deeper subcutaneous levels much sooner than they would at other sites. These factors result in many tumors being assigned an advanced stage that do not have similar prognoses or require as radical a treatment as T4 tumors located elsewhere. In addition, the unique anatomy of the ear makes a staging system based on size less practical. Even small tumors located in certain areas such as the conchal bowl or preauricular region can require surgery that is more extensive. Finally, the AJCC system does not account for the varying histologic subtypes. SCC and BCC often behave very differently, and the histologic subtypes of each often greatly influence the relative aggressiveness of the tumor.

The staging of melanoma is based on tumor thickness and depth of invasion, as well as the presence of metastatic disease. The first prognostic staging system was devised by Clark in 1969 (Table 23–3).[57] This staging system analyzed the extent of tumor invasion based on the histologic layers of involvement.[57] Breslow devised another system based on the absolute depth of tumor invasion (see Table 23–3).[58] The 1997 AJCC staging system uses both systems.

The revised 2002 AJCC staging system (Table 23–4) differs from the prior system in five important ways: (1) the level of invasion (Clark's level) is replaced by tumor thickness as the prognostic variable of primary tumor invasion that best predicts survival,[59] (2) ulceration of the primary tumor is incorporated into the staging system and patients in each T stage subgroup are upstaged,[59] (3) the size of lymph nodes is replaced by the number of lymph nodes involved in the nodal staging,[59] (4) patients are categorized into clinical and pathologic staging

TABLE 23–2 AJCC staging system: Nonmelanoma Cancer of the skin

T stage			
Tx	Cannot assess primary tumor		
T0	No evidence of primary tumor		
Tis	Carcinoma in situ		
T1	Tumor ≤ 2 cm in greatest dimension		
T2	Tumor > 2 cm but not > 5 cm in greatest dimension		
T3	Tumor > 5 cm in greatest dimension		
T4	Tumor invades deep extradermal structures (bone, cartilage muscle)		
N stage			
Nx	Cannot assess regional nodes		
N0	No regional node metastasis		
N1	Regional lymph node metastasis		
M stage			
Mx	Distant metastasis cannot be assessed		
M0	No distant metastasis		
M1	Distant metastasis		
Stage 0	Tis	N0	M0
Stage 1	T1	N0	M0
Stage 2	T2, T3	N0	M0
Stage 3	T4	N0	M0
Stage 3	Any T	N1	M0
Stage 4	Any T	Any N	M1

AJCC, American Joint Committee on Cancer.

TABLE 23–3 Clark and Breslow staging systems

CLARK		BRESLOW	
Level I	Superficial epidermis	Stage I	<0.75 mm
Level II	Basal cell layer of epidermis	Stage II	0.75–1.5 mm
Level III	Papillary dermis	Stage III	1.5–1.99 mm
Level IV	Reticular dermis	Stage IV	2.0–3.99 mm
Level V	Subcutaneous tissue	Stage V	>4.0 mm

to incorporate lymphatic mapping data and micrometastatic disease within lymph nodes, and (5) subcategorization of stage IV metastatic disease is based on anatomic site and inclusion of an elevated serum LDH.[59] These changes reflect several variables that have more recently been shown to be significant in predicting survival.[59]

TABLE 23–4 Revised AJCC Melanoma staging system

Primary tumor	
Tx	Primary tumor cannot be assessed
T0	No evidence of primary tumor
Tis	Melanoma in situ
T1a	Melanoma ≤1 mm in thickness, no ulceration
T1b	Melanoma ≤1 mm in thickness, with ulceration
T2a	Melanoma 1.01–2.0 mm in thickness, no ulceration
T2b	Melanoma 1.01–2.0 mm in thickness, with ulceration
T3a	Melanoma 2.01–4 mm in thickness, no ulceration
T3b	Melanoma 2.01–4 mm in thickness, with ulceration
T4a	Melanoma >4 mm, no ulceration
T4b	Melanoma >4 mm, with ulceration
Regional lymph nodes	
Nx	Regional nodes cannot be assessed
N0	No regional lymph node metastases
N1	Metastases to one lymph node
N1a	Clinically occult (microscopic) metastasis
N1b	Clinically apparent (macroscopic) metastasis
N2	Metastases in 2–3 regional lymph nodes or intralymphatic regional metastasis without nodal metastases
N2a	Clinically occult (microscopic) metastasis
N2b	Clinically apparent (macroscopic) metastasis
N2c	Satellite or in-transit metastasis without nodal metastasis
N3	Metastasis in 4 or more regional nodes, or matted metastatic nodes, or in-transit metastasis or satellite(s) with metastasis in regional node(s)
Distant metastasis	
Mx	Distant metastasis cannot be assessed
M0	No distant metastasis
M1	Distant metastasis
M1a	Metastasis to skin, subcutaneous tissues or distant lymph nodes
M1b	Metastasis to lung
M1c	Metastasis to all other visceral sites or distant metastasis at any site associated with an elevated serum lactic dehydrogenase (LDH)

Medical Treatment

Treatment options for nonmelanoma skin lesions include ablative options (cryosurgery, electrodessication, surgical excision, Mohs micrographic surgery (MMS), laser surgery, or radiation therapy) and topical therapies (5% 5-fluorouracil [5-FU], imiquimod, or photodynamic therapy).[60] Topical 5-FU has been evaluated for the treatment of premalignant lesions as well as select cutaneous carcinomas. The 5-FU therapy for malignant lesions usually involves a 12-week treatment regimen, with reported cure rates of over 90% for superficial BCC and Bowen's disease (SCC in situ).[60] Given the prolonged treatment regimen and the variability success, this technique should only be used to treat patients in whom other methods of therapy are contraindicated. Intralesional interferon (IFN) has also been shown to be effective for treatment of nodular and superficial BCC.[61] Patients typically receive nine injections over a 3-week period. The side effects are typically minor such as flu-like symptoms, erythema, and pain; however, more significant adverse events such as leukopenia and thrombocytopenia have been reported. The rate of cure approaches 96% for superficial and nodular BCC.[61] This data suggest that the results of IFN treatment for BCC are comparable to most other methods of tumor ablation.[61] The use of photodynamic therapy for BCC and SCC has also been studied, but has not gained widespread use. It entails the administration of a photosensitizing drug that selectively localizes in the tumor and then, on exposure to light, causes tumor necrosis.

Rediation Therapy

Radiation therapy is a viable option for the treatment of cutaneous malignancies, and in the context of auricular neoplasms, radiotherapy offers several theoretical advantages over surgical excision. Radiation therapy avoids the creation of tissue defects in this anatomically complex area; it is an option for medically infirm patients who are unable to undergo ablative surgery or for patients who refuse surgery.

The size of the primary tumor is the major determinant of local control with primary radiotherapy.[62] Tumors of 2 cm or less in size have long-term control rates (10-year local control) of approximately 98%, lesions 2 to 5 cm in size have a 79% long-term local control rate.[62,63] Tumors greater than 5 cm in size have a 53% long-term local control rate (8 years).[62,63]

Radiation therapy is not recommended as primary therapy in patients younger than 50 years of age due to the late effects of radiation and the risk of a secondary malignancy in the radiation portal.[62] In addition, previous radiation can lead to more aggressive tumors, less clearly defined margins, and poorer surgical outcomes.[64] Postoperative radiation may be used in several clinical scenarios including positive surgical margins, perineural spread, invasion of bone or cartilage, extensive skeletal muscle infiltration, a positive lymph node measuring greater than 3 cm in size, extranodal extension, and multiple positive nodes.[62]

SURGICAL THEORY AND PRACTICE

There are many options available to the physician while deciding how to treat primary malignancies of the auricle. The choice of which modality to use depends on the location and size of the lesion, the overall health of the patient, the specific expertise of the physician, and the desires expressed by the patient after a detailed explanation of the various options and risks.

Indications and Contraindications for Surgery

Malignancy of the auricle is a surgical disease. Regardless of the histopathology or the excisional technique, the goal is complete surgical eradication of disease. Prior to surgery, detailed evaluation is crucial for appropriate surgical planning. Surgical planning entails elucidation of the extent of resection, both locally and regionally, as well as defining the reconstructive goals.

There are relatively few contraindications to surgical treatment of auricular neoplasms. The medical status of the patient is an important determinant for surgical candidacy; however, given the malignant nature of disease, unless the disease has metastasized or the lesion is locally advanced precluding a total resection, surgery should be the mainstay of treatment. Topical therapies can be offered for in situ disease or low-grade, limited nonmelanoma skin cancer in patients unwilling to undergo surgical resection. Radiation therapy is also an option for patients refusing surgical therapy or with locally advanced, unresectable disease.

Operative Techniques

Surgical Excision

Surgical extirpation of malignant lesions of the auricle is the most common form of treatment. The complex anatomy of the ear requires careful evaluation and planning to ensure an adequate oncologic resection and a cosmetically acceptable outcome. Many small lesions can be excised, with little or no repair required.

Auricular neoplasms tend to follow consistent patterns of growth along embryologic fusion planes. Tumors that arise along the helix typically spread superiorly or inferiorly along the helix before extending to the antihelix or the posterior surface of the auricle; in contrast, lesions that arise on the antihelix tend to expand in a concentric fashion.[29] The thin skin of the auricle allows tumors to invade the dermis and subdermis quickly and facilitates dissemination in those planes much sooner than expected. This rapid horizontal growth makes determining appropriate margins for resection difficult. Shockley et al. reported that 37% of auricular carcinomas excised using standard margins demonstrated tumor cells at the margin.[31] Bumsted et al. recommended 8-mm margins around BCC if the tumor is less than 3 cm and 1.5-cm margins for larger lesions.[65] Other surgeons have advocated smaller, 2- to 3-mm margins for solid, well-circumscribed BCCs less than 1 cm in size, 3- to 5-mm margins for those less than 2 cm in size, and even larger margins for high-risk morphologies.[3] The surgical margins for SCC should be even larger (1–2 cm).[65]

By excising the tumor based on gross surgical margins, a larger amount of normal tissue is resected as compared to MMS. Bumsted et al. analyzed defects created with traditional wide local excisions and concluded that 1.8 to 3.5 cm^2 of normal tissue was removed beyond what was required for a sound oncologic resection.[65] Despite this drawback, the advantages of traditional surgery are that it is easily performed, relatively quick, and does not require advanced training.

The outcomes for patients with auricular carcinoma treated with standard surgical excision are good. The overall cure rate is approximately 95% when surgical salvage is included.[31] However, the recurrence rate for auricular carcinoma treated with conventional surgical excision ranges from 10 to 16%,[44,66] a fact that must be taken into account when comparing conventional surgery to other methods of excision (Tables 23–5 and 23–6).

There are several factors that increase the chance of tumor recurrence. The location of the tumor on the ear is associated with differing rates of recurrence. The postauricular area and the preauricular area have high rates of recurrence.[29,30,65,66] The cure rates for SCC and BCC are higher for lesions located on the helix, antihelix, and posterior surface of the ear (Table 23–7). In addition, tumor size greatly affects the recurrence rate. Size greater than 3 cm increases the recurrence rate for BCC from 1 to 17% and for SCC from 2 to 31%.[66] In addition, as previously mentioned, the type of cancer and the histologic subtype can also increase the likelihood of recurrence.

Mohs Micrographic Technique

Mohs micrographic surgery was developed in 1941 by Dr. Frederick Mohs, a dermatologist at the University of Wisconsin.[67] His technique involves serial horizontal sectioning of the tumor and surrounding tissue with immediate microscopic analysis to confirm a histologically negative specimen margin. Once the initial tissue is removed, the edges are color coded to ensure precise orientation of the specimen; the specimens are then processed as frozen sections. The tissue specimen is cut horizontally, unlike the standard serial vertical sections, to ensure that all of the margins are evaluated. If any tumor cells are seen along the specimen margin, the physician can immediately excise more tissue from the localized region.

This technique has several advantages over traditional wide local excision. The horizontal sectioning allows analysis of the entire margin to evaluate for small, localized extensions of tumor cells that theoretically could be missed with normal pathologic examination. It provides a means of ensuring that the entire tumor is removed without relying on unnecessary excision of normal tissue, especially important in regions such as the ear, nose, and eyelid. These locations require the preservation of as much normal tissue as possible to maintain adequate cosmesis while concurrently minimizing tumor recurrence.

The oncologic outcomes of MMS compare favorably to other treatment modalities (see Tables 24–3 and 24–4). Overall, the cure rates for auricular carcinomas are approximately 98% for BCC and 92% for SCC.[65,68,69] The ability to precisely follow the tumor margin with MMS, affords this technique a lower recurrence rate for auricular malignancies compared with standard excision. The 5-year recurrence rate is approximately 1% for BCC and less than 3% for SCC; these rates are significantly lower than the recurrence rate of 10 to 16% for tumors treated with wide local excision.[44,66] Mohs micrographic surgery is the recommended method of treatment for cancers arising in cosmetically sensitive areas, recurrent or previously treated tumors, tumors with aggressive histologic subtypes, large lesions for which standard excision would require removal of significant amounts of normal tissue, and for tumors with poorly defined margins.[35]

TABLE 23–5 Five-year recurrence rates for primary basal cell carcinoma

TREATMENT	RECURRENCE RATE (%)
Wide local excision	10.1
Radiation	8.7
Curettage and electrodessication	7.7
Mohs' surgery	1.0

TABLE 23–6 Five-year recurrence rates for previously treated basal cell carcinoma

TREATMENT	RECURRENCE RATE (%)
Excision	17.4
Curettage and electrodessication	40.0
Radiation	9.8
Mohs' surgery	5.6

Adapted from Rowe, et al.[66]

TABLE 23–7 Five-year cure rates (%) for auricular carcinomas based on location

LOCATION OF TUMOR	BASAL CELL CARCINOMA	SQUAMOUS CELL CARCINOMA
Helix	99.2	99.1
Antihelix and crus	99.0	94.6
Posterior surface	97.7	90.5
Lobe	97.4	90.0
Preauricular and tragus	97.0	80.9
Concha	94.0	78.4
Postauricular sulcus	92.0	81.3

Adapted from Mohs, et al.[68]

Surgical Excision in Malignant Melanoma

Surgical extirpation with adequate margins is the primary treatment modality for malignant melanoma of the auricle. The excision should be full thickness, including the perichondrium and cartilage if necessary.[47] The required margin, however, is debated. A consensus panel sponsored by the National Institutes of Health (NIH) recommended a 1-cm margin of normal skin and subcutaneous tissue for melanomas less than 1-mm thick and a 1–2 cm margin for tumors of intermediate thickness and a 2 cm margin for tumors greater than 2 mm thick.[47,70–72] These recommendations, however, are based primarily on truncal and extremity lesions, where wide margins are more easily obtained without creating substantial cosmetic or functional deficits. Lesions involving the auricle often complicate the ability to obtain recommended margins. Frequently, an appropriate resection will entail a wedge excision or a partial amputation of the pinna.

The anatomic considerations of the head and neck region, and in particular the auricle, make MMS an appealing option. Mohs micrographic surgery has been advocated for resection of malignant melanoma due to the theoretical advantage of reducing the amount of normal tissue excised.[73] In contrast to SCC, malignant melanoma cells are typically more challenging to identify pathologically. Therefore, precise identification of the tumor margins is more complicated than with other skin cancers. The use of immunohistochemical stains often improves identification of melanoma cells involving the excised margins. Several studies from the dermatologic literature document equivalent overall survival and similar local recurrence rates for malignant melanoma excised via a micrographic technique as apposed to standard surgical margins.[73,74] Despite these more recent studies, the role of MMS in malignant melanoma remains a controversial topic and currently not the standard of care.

The overall cure rate for surgical excision of malignant melanoma of the ear approaches 68%; however, the success rate for early-stage disease is significantly higher.[70] Local recurrence occurs in approximately 6.5% of the cases and typically manifest 1 to 3 years after excision.[75] The early pattern of local recurrence mandates regular and frequent patient evaluation. Ideally, patients should be seen every 1 to 2 months during the initial postexcision period, followed by a biannual examinations for the subsequent 2 to 3 years.[47]

Management of Metastatic/Nodal Disease

The rate of metastasis for cutaneous carcinoma is low; however, auricular neoplasms, like those arising elsewhere on the face, have an increased risk of metastasizing compared with other locations.[66,69] Regional metastases occur in approximately 5 to 18% of auricular SCCs and in 2 to 6% of BCCs.[76,77] Distant metastases occur with even less frequency. The incidence of distant metastases is 0.3 to 3.7% for SCC and approximately 0.003 to 0.1% for BCC.[28,76,77] When nodal disease is present, it is most often located in the parotid and preauricular nodes.[28,77] Nodal disease involving the neck is less common, with the upper jugulodigastric region being the primary site of involvement. Byers et al. retrospectively analyzed 486 patients with auricular SCC and found that only 3 patients had nodal disease below the level of the omohyoid; none of these patients demonstrated skip metastases.[28] Several studies have noted that the suboccipital nodes are not involved in auricular cutaneous carcinomas.[28,77]

Multiple studies have looked at the factors predisposing patients to regional and distant metastases. There are conflicting data as to which factors are statistically important. Some authors have found the size and location on the ear (especially the preauricular region) to correlate with increased risk of nodal disease.[77–79] Other studies, however, negate these findings.[28,77] Several histologic subtypes are more likely to metastasize, including the basalosquamous variant and poorly differentiated carcinoma.[37,77] Other factors that have been implicated include perineural invasion, cartilage invasion, recurrent tumors, and immunosuppresion.[78,80,81]

Patients who present with clinically positive nodal disease should at a minimum receive a selective neck dissection. Sacrifice of the sternocleidomastoid muscle, cranial nerve XI, or jugular vein should be done only if the nodal disease cannot be safely removed otherwise. The majority of patients present with limited nodal disease, typically N1 disease.[28]

The treatment algorithm for the N0 neck is more variable. Elective lymph node dissection (ELND) has not been shown to increase survival over watchful waiting for patients with cutaneous carcinoma of the ear with no clinical evidence of nodal metastases. Elective lymph node dissection should be reserved for patients with multiple risk factors for nodal disease given the overall low rate of nodal metastases in auricular carcinoma. Byers et al. recommended proceeding with neck dissection in patients with poorly differentiated SCC measuring greater than 3 cm in largest diameter.[28] In addition, the data from this study supported the utilization of the supraomohyoid neck dissection due to the low rate of lower neck metastases (3 of 486 patients). Others have reported a greater percentage of level III and level IV neck disease; although, when lower nodal disease was present there were no skip lesions identified.[70] Therefore, it appears that a supraomohyoid neck dissection suffices for the N0 neck.

Regional Management of Metastatic Melanoma

Overall, the risk of occult, microscopic nodal metastases in cutaneous malignant melanoma is approximately 10 to 20%.[47,82] Earlier studies looking specifically at melanoma of the auricle describe a higher likelihood of regional metastases and a worse overall prognosis compared to other head and neck sites; these data, however, have been refuted in more recent studies.[47,89] The risk of nodal metastases correlates with tumor thickness/depth of invasion, presence of ulceration, and histologic subtype.[48,75,83] Tumor thickness and ulceration are the two most important predictors of outcome.[81–83] The risk of developing nodal metastases from a tumor less than 0.75 mm is nearly zero. However, the risk increases significantly in the setting of thicker tumors (Table 23–8). An older study by Byers et al., demonstrated that tumors of the auricle that are less than 3 mm in thickness have been shown to have a 21% chance of nodal disease; this risk increases to 61% for lesions thicker than 3 mm.[44]

The most common nodal areas involved in auricular melanoma are the parotid and upper jugulodigastric nodes. The retroauricular, preauricular, and submental nodes can also contain metastatic disease depending on the location of the primary lesion. The suboccipital nodes may also be at risk for involvement, particularly if the tumor is located on the

TABLE 23–8 Relationship of tumor thickness to outcomes in malignant melanoma

THICKNESS (mm)	RECURRENCE RATE (%)	METASTASES (%)	SURVIVAL (%)
< 0.75	2	0	85–99
0.75–1.49	5	20–25	65–88
1.50–3.99	15	51–57	58–71
> 4.0	20	62	25–57

Adapted from O'Brien, et al.,[48] Ringborg, et al.,[45] Medina,[85] Balch et al,[71] Fisher.[75]

posterior portion of the pinna or in the retroauricular area.[47,85] Although there are recognized patterns of nodal involvement, there is no uniform, sequential route of spread. One study demonstrated that 43% of patients with auricular melanomas and neck metastases will have no disease in the parotid nodes.[86]

Patients with clinically positive nodal disease should undergo a therapeutic neck dissection. Despite this recommendation, neck dissection in the presence of nodal disease does not improve survival due primarily to the high rate of eventual distant metastases (85%) in patients with clinically evident nodal disease at the time of presentation; however, neck dissection decreases the rate of regional recurrence.[87] Radical neck dissections have been advocated in the past, but in most cases a selective or modified radical neck dissection is usually sufficient for patients with nodal disease.[88,89] The type of neck dissection performed should depend on the location of the primary tumor and the extent of disease as well as the expertise of the surgeon. It is important that the neck dissection should include all the pertinent draining nodal basins.

Classically, the role of ELND in patients with clinically N0 disease was controversial. Overall, the percentage of patients with clinically N0 disease that harbor microscopic metastatic disease is quite low.[45] Primary tumors less than 1 mm in thickness have an exceedingly low rate of nodal metastases with a 5-year survival rate greater than 95%.[89] Therefore, neck dissection is not typically indicated. However, 70% of cases will have distant metastatic disease in lesions with 4 mm or greater invasion.[89] This is thought to negate the benefits of therapeutic neck dissection in the occasional patient presenting with a primary lesion greater than 4 mm without clinically evident regional metastases.[89] The controversy primarily involved tumors of intermediate thickness. A subset of these patients may benefit from elective neck dissection; however, numerous randomized trials have been unable to demonstrate a survival benefit for patients undergoing elective neck dissection. Therefore, routine ELND is not currently recommended in this population; sentinel lymph node biopsy (SLNB) is now the preferred diagnostic/screening modality.[89]

SLNB is a relatively minimally invasive screening technique for the at-risk nodal regions in patients that have no clinical evidence of cervical metastases. This technique involves identifying the primary nodal drainage basin for a specific tumor through the injection of isosulfan blue dye and/or a lymphoscintigraphy. The sentinel node is then identified and sent for pathologic analysis. The theory is that if the sentinel node is negative, the likelihood of further regional disease is low. If the node is positive, then a completion lymph node dissection can be undertaken. This technique provides the opportunity to avoid the potential morbidity of an ELND in a population with a relatively low rate of nodal disease.

SLNB is well accepted in the treatment of trunk and extremity melanoma, providing important staging and prognostic information.[89] A prospective multi-institutional trial demonstrated that the status of the sentinel nodes in stages I and II disease was the most important predictor of disease-free survival.[84,89,90] There are many studies of involving SLNB in the head and neck for malignant melanoma. In contrast to the lymphatic drainage patterns of the trunk and extremities, the lymphatic drainage patterns of the head and neck are variable and significantly more complex. In addition, the frequent involvement of the lymph nodes of the parotid gland complicates SLNB.[89] Currently, the data from studies of head and neck sites are conflicting; several studies demonstrate a high rate of SLN identification with a concordant low rate of false-negative results, whereas other studies demonstrate a high rate of regional recurrence after SLNB.[89–92] Despite the conflicting data, most high-volume melanoma centers are using SLNB in the setting of melanoma of the head and neck region.

Reconstruction of the Auricle

The complex anatomy of the auricle requires exquisite skill and planning for effective reconstruction of defects. Effort should be made during the oncologic resection to preserve as much normal tissue as possible. The approach to auricular repair can be divided into partial-thickness defects (removal of skin and perichondrium) and full-thickness defects (removal includes cartilage). For reconstructive purposes, the ear can be divided into several regions: the external scaffolding, including the helical rim and the antihelix; the central cartilaginous portion, which is composed primarily of the conchal bowl; the lobule; the preauricular region, which includes the tragus; and the retroauricular region.

Partial-Thickness Defects

Most partial-thickness defects can either be repaired with a split-thickness skin graft, a full-thickness skin graft, or can be allowed to heal by secondary intention. If there is greater than a 1-cm area of cartilaginous exposure, granulation tissue may not be able to completely fill the defect from the edges. Healing by secondary intention is useful in patients in whom close surveillance of the site is desired or in patients who have had or have multiple cutaneous malignancies and minimal skin is preserved for a local flap or grafting. Zitelli developed mnemonics for remembering areas appropriate for healing by secondary intention.[93] Locations favorable for good cosmetic results after healing by secondary intention include the concave surfaces of the nose, ear, eye, and temple (NEET).[93] In contrast, the convex surfaces of the nose, oral lips, cheeks, chin, and helix of the ear (NOCCH) develop unsightly, depressed scars.[93] Other areas of the forehead, the antihelix, the eyelids, and the remainder of the nose, lips, and cheeks (FAIR) give variable results.[93] If the defect is large, a skin graft helps prevent the contraction that occurs as the wound granulates. It is important to place skin grafts only in areas that have perichondrium or subcutaneous tissue remaining that can provide nourishment to the graft. If bare cartilage is exposed, some of the cartilage can be resected to allow access to the perichondrium on the other side, or a delayed approach can be pursued allowing granulation tissue to form prior to subsequent graft placement.

Defects of the Helical Rim and Antihelix

The majority of the full-thickness helical/antihelical defects can be closed primarily. Defects of the helix of up to 1 cm can be closed following a wedge excision (Figure 23–1).[94]

As the resection increases in size, closure results in pronounced bowing of the ear as the more medial cartilage is compressed. There are several options to eliminate this phenomenon and close larger defects. The most common technique involves the use of a chondrocutaneous advancement flap (see Figure 23–1).

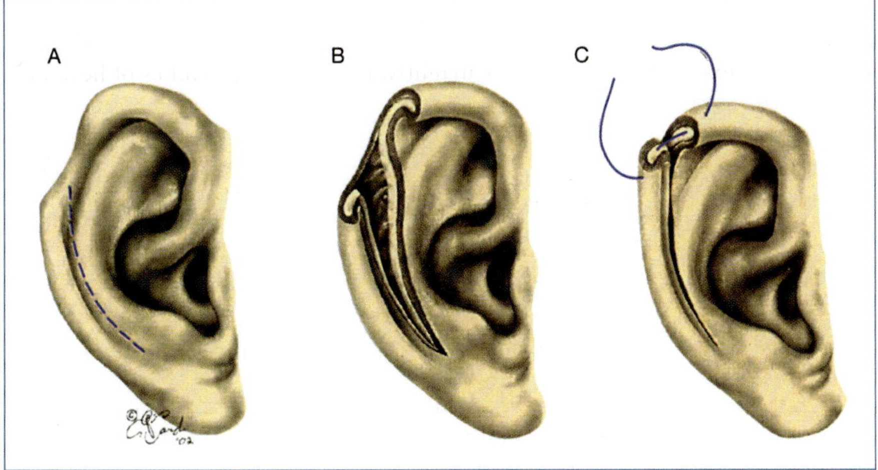

FIGURE 23–1 • Chondrocutaneous helical advancement. A vertical releasing incision is made in the antihelical area extending into the lobule if needed (*A* and *B*). The helical rim can then be rotated and closed with minimal deformity (*C*).

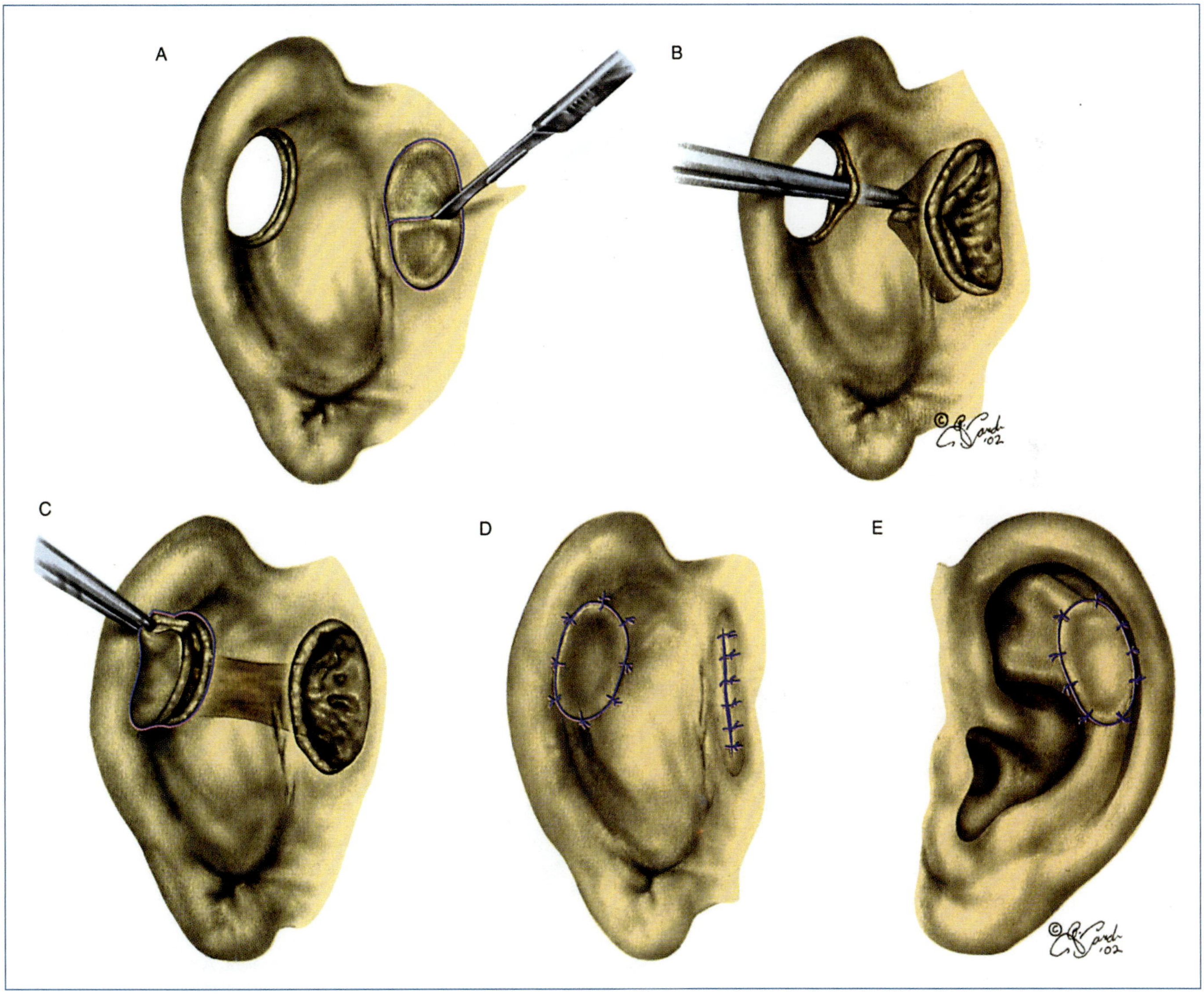

FIGURE 23–2 • Posterior island flap. Defects of the conchal bowl can be repaired by lifting a flap of skin and subcutaneous tissue (*A*), which can pedicled posteriorly and pulled through the defect (*B* and *C*). If skin is needed anteriorly and posteriorly, the flap can be folded on itself. The posterior defect is then closed primarily (*D* and *E*).

Many variations of this flap have been devised.[95,96] The basic idea entails the removal of a geometric portion of the more central cartilage to allow rotation of the outer rim. The space is then filled as cartilage is rotated up from below. Other alternatives include a composite cartilage graft with local skin flap coverage, preauricular flaps (if the defect is located along the anterior helix), or postauricular flaps for more posterior defects.[93–98]

Defects of the Concha

The central location of the conchal bowl makes it difficult to devise rotational flaps. In defects in which the posterior perichondrium and skin are intact, a skin graft may be the only reconstruction necessary. This approach is similar to that used to repair the defect created after a conchal cartilage graft is harvested. If there is a full-thickness defect, then tissue must be supplied from another location. One effective reconstructive option is the subcutaneous island pedicle flap.[95,99] In this flap, an island of skin is taken from the postauricular area and advanced forward connected to a deep connective tissue pedicle, which is secured to the conchal defect. The posterior wound is closed primarily (see Figure 23–2).

Preauricular and Postauricular Defects, Reconstruction of the Lobule

The vast majority of defects anterior to the external auditory canal can be closed primarily. If the tragus has been removed, reconstruction of the tragus may be performed with a cartilage graft, although the cosmetic results are often not as satisfactory as one would desire. Wide undermining in the postauricular area will provide considerable laxity in the tissue, and most wounds can be closed primarily. Otherwise, skin grafts work adequately in this well concealed location. The lobule contains no cartilage and therefore can be recreated by the advancement of soft tissue either from the ear itself or from the surrounding skin, which is then folded over on itself and divided at a secondary procedure (Figure 23–3).

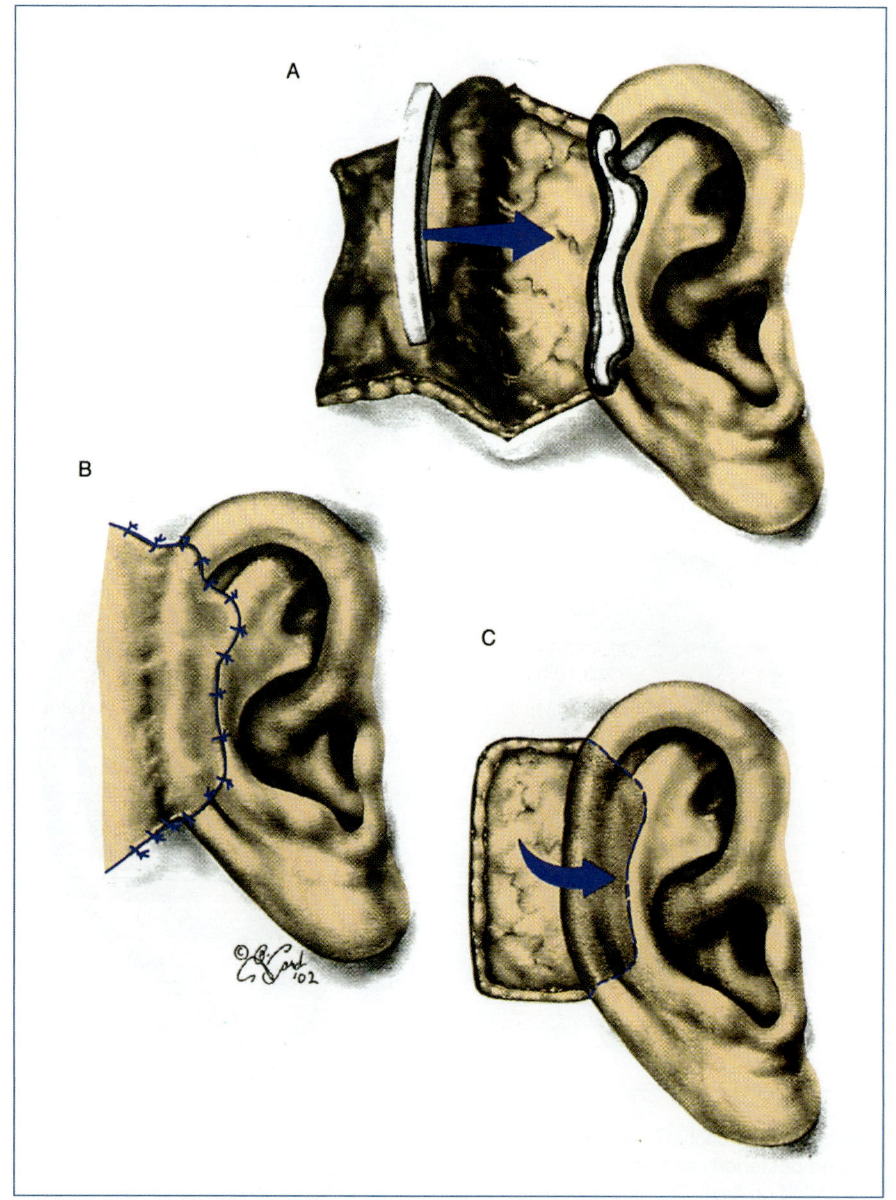

FIGURE 23–3 • Postauricular. For defects of the posterior helical rim, skin and soft-tissue coverage can be obtained by using tissue from the postauricularарea. A posterior based flap is raised and sutured over the defect (*A* and *B*). After 2 to 3 weeks, the pedicle is divided and closed primarily (*C*). If a cartilage grafting can be performed using the contralateral auricular cartilage prior to coverage with the flap.

CONCLUSIONS

Auricular malignancies are becoming increasingly common as exposure to solar radiation increases. Recently, there has been an increasing awareness by the public of the signs and symptoms of skin cancer in conjunction with a heightened sense of awareness by physicians. Early detection of skin cancer is the most effective form of treatment. When identified early, auricular malignancies are curable. More advanced disease, however, carries a poorer prognosis and requires a surgical resection that can potentially be cosmetically deforming. Mohs micrographic surgery is increasingly being used and it can provide a reliable means of preserving normal tissue during resection for SCC or BCC. Melanoma remains challenging to treat and is associated with a worse overall survival. If excision of a tumor of the auricle is required, careful surgical planning is critical for effective eradication of disease and successful reconstruction.

References

1. American Cancer Society. Cancer references–2007. New York: American Cancer Society; 2007. http://www.cancer.org/docroot/lrn/lrn_0.asp.
2. American Cancer Society. Cancer facts and figures–2007. New York: American Cancer Society; 2007. http://www.cancer.org/docroot/stt/stt_0.asp.
3. Nguyen AV, Whitaker DC, Frodel J. Differentiation of basal cell carcinoma. Otolaryngol Clin North Am. 1993;26:37–56.
4. Leman J, McHenry P. Basal cell carcinoma: Still an enigma. Arch Dermatol. 2001;137(9):1239.
5. Matts PJ. Solar ultraviolet radiation: Definitions and terminology. Dermatologic Clinics. 2006; 24:1–8.
6. Buzzell RA. Effects of solar radiation on the skin. Otolaryngol Clin North Am. 1993;26:1–11.
7. Hawrot A. Squamous cell carcinoma. Current Problems in Dermatology. 2003;15(3):91–133.
8. Lewis KG, Jellinek N, Robinson-Bostom L. Skin cancer after transplantation: A guide for the general surgeon. Surg Clin N Am. 2006;86:1257–76.
9. Ridky TW. Nonmelanoma skin cancer. J Am Acad Dermatol. 2007;57(3):484–501.
10. Streilein JW. Photoimmunology of non-melanoma skin cancer. Cancer Surv 1996;26:207–17.
11. Glogau RG. The risk of progression to invasive disease. J Am Acad Dermatol. 2000;42(1 Pt 2):23–4.
12. Marks R, Rennie G, Selwood TS. Malignant transformation of solar keratoses to squamous cell carcinoma. Lancet. 1988;1(8589):795–7.
13. Sanders GH, Miller TA. Are keratocanthomas really squamous cell carcinomas? Ann Plast Surg. 1982;9:306–9.
14. Fitzpatrick TB. The validity and practicality of sun reactive skin types I through VI. Arch Dermatol. 1988;124:869–71.
15. Johnson TM, Rowe DE, Nelson BR, Swanson NA. Squamous cell carcinoma of the skin (excluding lip and oral mucosa). J Am Acad Dermatol. 1992;26(3 Pt 2):467–84.
16. Moloney FJ, Comber H, O'Lorcain P, O'Kelly P, Conlon PJ, Murphy GM. A population-based study of skin cancer incidence and prevalence in renal transplant recipients. Br J Dermatol. 2006;154(3):498–504.
17. Martinez JC, Otley CC, Stasko T, Euvrard S, Brown C, Schanbacher CF, Weaver AL. Transplant-skin cancer collaborative. Defining the clinical course of metastatic skin cancer in organ transplant recipients: A multicenter collaborative study. Arch Dermatol. 2003;139(3):301–6.
18. Penn I. Tumors after renal and cardiac transplantation. Hematol Oncol Clin N Am. 1993;7(2):431–45.
19. Shumrick KA, Coldiron B. Genetic syndromes associated with skin cancer. Otolaryngol Clin North Am. 1993;26:117–37.
20. Gorlin RJ. Nevoid basal cell carcinoma (Gorlin) syndrome. Genet Med. 2004;6:530–9.
21. Farndon PA, Del Mastro RG, Evans DG, Kilpatrick MW. Location of gene for Gorlin syndrome. Lancet. 1992: 581–2.
22. Johnson RL, Rothman AL, Xie J, et al. Human homolog of patched, a candidate gene for the basal cell nevus syndrome. Science. 1996;272(5268):1668–71.
23. Kimonis VE, Mehta SG, Digiovanna JJ, Bale SJ, Pastakia B. Radiological features in 82 patients with nevoid basal cell carcinoma (NBCC or Gorlin) syndrome. Genet Med. 2004; 6(6): 495–502.
24. Cleaver JE. Cancer in xeroderma pigmentosum and related discords of DNA repair. Nat Rev Cancer. 2005 Jul; 5(7):564–73.
25. Gherardini G, Bhatia N, Stal S. Congenital syndromes associated with nonmelanoma skin cancer. Clin Plast Surg. 1997;24(4):649–61. Review.
26. Koriwchak M. Temporal bone cancer. Amer J Otolaryngology. 1993;14(6):623–26.
27. Estrem SA, Remmer G. Special problems associated with cutaneous carcinoma of the ear. Otol Clin North Am. 1993;26: 231–45.
28. Byers R, Kesler K, Redmon B, Medina J, Schwarz B. Squamous carcinoma of the external ear. Am J Surg. 1983;146(4):447–50.
29. Bailin PL, Levine HL, Wood BG, Tucker HM. Cutaneous carcinoma of the auricle and periauricular region. Arch Otolaryngol. 1980: 106:692–6.
30. Robins P, Nix M. Analysis of persistent disease on the ear following Mohs' surgery. Head Neck Surg. 1984;6:998–1006.
31. Shockley WW, Stucker FJ. Squamous cell carcinoma of the external ear: a review of 75 cases. Head Neck Surg. 1987;97(3): 308–12.
32. Thomas SS, Matthews RN. Squamous cell carcinoma of the pinna: A 6-year study. Br J Plast Surg. 1994;47(2):81–5.
33. Bailin PL, Levine HL, Wood BG, Tucker HM. Cutaneous carcinoma of the auricle and periauricular region. Arch Otolaryngol. 1980;106(11):692–6.
34. Fitzpatrick's Color Atlas and Synopsis of Clinical Dermatology–Section 11. In: Fitzpatrick TB, editor. New York: McGraw-Hill; 2005.
35. Kuijpers DI, Thissen MR, Neumann MH. Basal cell carcinoma: treatment options andprognosis, a scientific approach to a commonmalignancy. Am J Clin Dermatol. 2002;3(4):247–59.
36. Sloane JP. The value of typing basal cell carcinomas in predicting recurrence after surgical excision. Br J Dermatol. 1977;96(2): 127–32.
37. Borel DM. Cutaneous basosquamous carcinoma: Review of the literature and report of 35 cases. Arch Pathol. 1973;95: 293–7.
38. Jacobs GH, Rippey JJ, Altini M. Predictions of aggressive behavior in basal cell carcinoma. Cancer. 1982;49:533–7.
39. Von Domarus H, Steven PJ. Metastatic basal cell carcinoma: Report of five cases and review of 170 cases in the literature. J Am Acad Dermatol. 1984;10:1043–60.

40. Emmett AJ. Surgical analysis and biological behaviour of 2277 basal cell carcinomas. Aust N Z J Surg. 1990;60(11):855–63.

41. Sewell DA, Lai SY, Weber RS. Nonmelanoma skin cancer of the head and neck. In: Myers EN, Suen JY, editors. Cancer of the head and neck. Philadelphia: WB Saunders; 2003. p. 117–32.

42. Elder DE. Skin cancer: melanoma and other specific nonmelanoma skin cancers. Cancer. 1995;75 Suppl 1:245–56.

43. Jahn V, Breuninger H, Garbe C. Moehrle M. Melanoma of the ear: Prognostic factors and surgical strategies. Br J Dermatol. 2006;154(2):310–18.

44. Byers R, Smith J, Russell N, Rosenberg V. Malignant melanoma of the external ear. Am J Surg 1980;140:518–21.

45. Ringborg U. Cutaneous malignant melanoma of the head and neck. Analysis of treatment results and prognostic factors in 581 patients: A report from the Swedish Melanoma Study Group. Cancer. 1993;71:751–8.

46. Singh B, Bhaya M, Shaha A, Har-El G, Lucente FE. Presentation, course, and outcome of head and neck skin cancer in African Americans: A case-control study. Laryngoscope. 1998;108(8 Pt 1):1159–63.

47. Beaver M, Chang CJ. Melanoma. In: Jackler RK, Driscoll CLW, editors. Tumors of the ear and temporal bone. Philadelphia: Lippincott Williams & Wilkins; 2000. p. 56–66.

48. O'Brien CJ, Coates AS, Petersen-Schaefer K, et al. Experience with 998 cutaneous melanomas of the head and neck over 30 years. Am J Surg. 1991;162:310–4.

49. Marenda SA, Oto RA. Adnexal carcinomas of the skin. Otolaryngol Clin North Am. 1993;26:87–116.

50. Haag ML, Glass LF, Fenske NA. Merkel cell carcinoma. Diagnosis and treament. Dermatol Surg. 1995;21(8):669–83.

51. Brown MD. Recognition and management of unusual cutaneous tumors. Dermatol Clin. 2000;18(3):543–52.

52. Hitchcock CL, Bland KI, Laney RG Franzini D, Harris B, Copeland EM. Neuroendocrine (Merkel cell) carcinoma of the skin. Ann Surg. 1988;207:201–7.

53. Lawenda BD, Thiringer JK, Foss RD, Johnstone PA. Merkel cell carcinoma arising in the head and neck: optimizing therapy. Am J Clin Oncol. 2001 Feb;24(1):35–42.

54. Ott MJ, O'Brien CJ, Coates AS, et al. Multimodality management of merkel cell carcinoma. Arch Surg. 1999;134(4):388–92; discussion 392–3.

55. Pacella J, Ashby M, Ainsie J, Minty C. The role of radiotherapy in the management of primary cutaneous neuroendocrine tumors (Merkel cell or trabecular carcinoma): experience at the Peter MacCallum Cancer Institute (Melbourne, Australia). Int J Radiat Oncol Biol Phys. 1988;14:1077–84.

56. Smith CC. Metastasizing carcinomas of the sweat glands. Br J Surg. 1955;43:80–4.

57. Clark WH Jr, From L, Bernardino EA, Mihm MC. The histogenesis and biologic behavior of primary human malignant melanomas of the skin. Cancer Res. 1969;29:705–26.

58. Breslow A. Thickness, cross-sectional areas and depth of invasion in the prognosis of cutaneous melanoma. Ann Surg. 1970;172:902–8.

59. Kim CJ, Reintgen DS, Balch CM. AJCC Melanoma Staging Committee. The new melanoma staging system. Cancer Control. 2002;9(1):9–15.

60. Gross K, Kircik L. Kricorian G. 5% 5-Fluorouracil cream for the treatment of small superficial Basal cell carcinoma: efficacy, tolerability, cosmetic outcome, and patient satisfaction. Dermatol Surg. 2007;33(4):433–9.

61. Tucker SB, Polasek JW, Perri AJ, Goldsmith EA. Long-term follow-up of basal cell carcinomas treated with perilesional interferon alfa 2b as monotherapy. J Am Acad Dermatol. 2006;54(6):1033–8.

62. Ang KK, Wilder RB. Chapter 5. In: Cox JD, Ang K. editors. The skin. Radiation oncology: Rationale, technique, results. 8th ed. Philadelphia: Mosby; 2003. p. 127–143.

63. Petrovich Z, Parker RG, Luxton G, et al. Carcinoma of the lip and selected sites of head and neck skin. A cliical stuy of 896 patients. Radiother Oncol. 1987;8:11–117.

64. Smith SP, Grande DJ. Basal cell carcinoma recurring after radiotherapy: A unique difficult treatment subclass of recurrent basal cell carcinoma. J Dermatol Surg Oncol. 1991;17:26–30.

65. Bumstead RM, Ceilley RI, Panje WR, Crumley RL. Auricular malignant neoplasms: When is chemosurgery (Mohs' technique) necessary? Arch Otolaryngol. 1981;107:721–4.

66. Rowe DE, Carroll JR, Day CL Jr. Long term recurrence rates in previously untreated (primary) basal cell carcinoma: implications for patient follow-up. J Dermatol Surg Oncol. 1989;15:315–28.

67. Mohs FE. Chemosurgery: A microscopically controlled method of cancer excision. Arch Surg. 1941;42:279–95.

68. Mohs F, Larson P, Iriondo M. Micrographic surgery for the microscopically controlled excision of carcinoma of the external ear. J Am Acad Dermatol. 1988;9:729–37.

69. Niparko JK, Swanson NA, Baker SR, Telian SA, Sullivan MJ, Kemink JL. Local control of auricular, periauricular, and external canal cutaneous malignancies with Mohs' surgery. Laryngoscope. 1990; 100: 1047–51.

70. National Institutes of Health Consensus Development Conference statement on diagnosis and treatment of early melanoma. Am J Dermatopathol 1993;15:34–43.

71. Balch CM, Urist MM, Karakousis CP, et al. Efficacy of 2-cm surgical margins for intermediate thickness melanomas (1–4 mm). Ann Surg. 1993;218:262–9.

72. Schmalbach CE, Johnson TM, Bradford CR. The management of head and neck melanoma. Curr Probl Surg. 2006;43(11): 781–835.

73. Coldiron BM. Current management of skin cancer. Curr Opin Otolaryngol Head Neck Surg. 1997;5:214–22.

74. Arlette JP, Trotter MJ, Trotter T, Temple CL. Management of lentigo maligna and lentigo maligna melanoma: Seminars in surgical oncology. J Surg Oncol. 2004;86(4):179–86.

75. Fisher SR. Cutaneous malignant melanoma of the head and neck. Laryngoscope. 1989;99:822–36.

76. Glass AG, Hoover RN. The emerging epidemic of melanoma and squamous cell skin cancer. JAMA. 1989;262:2097–100.

77. Lee D, Nash M, Har-El G. Regional spread of auricular and periauricular cutaneous malignancies. Laryngoscope. 1996;106:998–1001.

78. Hayden RC III. Cutaneous squamous carcinoma and related lesions. Otolaryngol. Clin North Am 1993;26:57–71.

79. Balough BJ, O'Leary M, Martin P. Basal and squamous cell carcinoma of the auricle. In: Jackler RK, Driscoll CLW, editors. Tumors of the ear and temporal bone. Philadelphia: Lippincott Williams and Wilkins; 2000. p. 29–55.

80. Goepfert H, Dichtel WJ, Medina JE, et al. Perineural invasion of squamous cell skin carcinoma of the head and neck. Am J Surg. 1984;148:542–7.
81. Lewis J. Cancer of the ear. Laryngoscope. 1966;70:551–79.
82. Balch CM, Soong SJ, Gershenwald JE, et al. Prognostic factors analysis of 17,600 melanoma patients: Validation of the American Joint Committee on Cancer melanoma staging system. J Clin Oncol 2001;19:3622–34.
83. Day C, Mihm M, Sober A, et al. Prognostic factors of melanoma patients with lesions 0.76–1.69 mm in thickness: An appraisal of thin level IV lesions. Ann Surg. 1982;195:30–4.
84. Morton DL, Thompson JF, Cochran AJ, et al. MSLT Group. Sentinel-node biopsy or nodal observation in melanoma. N Engl J Med. 2006;355:1307–17.
85. Medina JE. Malignant melanoma of the head and neck. Otolaryngol Clin North Am. 1993;26:73–86.
86. Shah JP, Kraus DH, Dubner S, et al. Patterns of regional lymph node metastases from cutaneous melanomas of the head and neck. Am J Surg. 1991;162:320–3.
87. Ballantyne AJ. Malignant melanoma of the head and neck: An analysis of 405 cases. Am J Surg. 1970;120:425–31.
88. Byers RM. The role of modified neck dissection in the treatment of cutaneous melanomas of the head and neck. Arch Surg. 1986;121:1338–41.
89. Lentsch EJ, Mers JN. Melanoma of the Head and Neck. In: Myer EN, Suen JY, editors. Cancer of the head and neck. Philadelphia: WB Saunders; 2003. p. 133–53.
90. Gershenwald JE, Thompson W, Mansfield PF, et al. Multi-institutional melanoma lymphatic maping experience: The prognostic value of sentinel lymph node status in 612 stage I or II melanoma patients. J çlin Oncol. 1999:17:976–83.
91. Wells, KE, Rapapor DP, Cruse Cw, et al. Sentinel lymph node biopsy in melanoma of the head and nck. Plas recontr Surg. 1997: 100;591–94.
92. Alex JC, Krag DN, Harlow SP, et al. Localization of regiona lymph nodes in melanomas of the head and neck. Arch Otolaryngol Head Neck Surg. 1998;124:135–40.
93. Zitelli JA. Wound healing by secondary intention: A cosmetic appraisal. J Am Acad Dermatol. 1983;9:407–15.
94. Menick FJ. Reconstruction of the ear after tumor excision. Clin Plast Surg. 1990;17:405–15.
95. Chiu LD, Barber W, Chen A. J-shaped, conchal excision with rotation advancement for closure of large auricular wedge defects. Laryngoscope. 1996;106:116–8.
96. Millard DR Jr. Reconstruction of one third plus of the auricular circumference. Plast Reconstr Surg 1992;90:475–8.
97. O'Brien CJ, Uren RF, Thompson JF, et al. Prediction of potential metastatic sites in cutaneous head and neck melanoma using lymphoscintigraphy. Am Ju Surg. 1995:174:536–9.
98. Lawson VG. Reconstruction of the pinna using preauricular flaps. J Otolaryngol. 1984;13:191–3.
99. Fader DJ, Johnson TM. Ear reconstruction utilizing the subcutaneous island pedicle graft (flip-flop) flap. Dermatol Surg. 1999;25:94–6.

Surgery for Congenital Aural Atresia 24

Bradley W. Kesser, MD / Robert A. Jahrsdoerfer, MD

HISTORY

While atresia of the external auditory canal has been recognized for over 70 years,[1] reports of surgical repair of atresia do not surface until the late 1940s and 1950s.[2–8] Nager advocated tailoring the surgical technique to open the ear canal and restore hearing to the severity of the atresia.[9,10] For minor malformations (Group I; normal or stenotic canal with hypoplastic tympanic cleft and some malformation of the middle-ear structures), Nager described an endaural approach to widen the stenotic ear canal and address any middle-ear abnormalities. For Group II malformations (fistulous tract or complete atresia of the canal with a bony atretic plate and some degree of malformation of the middle-ear structures), Nager recommended opening the mastoid antrum, aditus, and attic to expose the lateral ossicular mass, freeing the ossicular chain, and using a split thickness skin graft to the mucoperiosteal membrane on the undersurface of the bony atretic plate. For more severe malformations (Group III; complete ear canal atresia with nonpneumatized mastoid and middle ear), he advised against surgery, or possibly a fenestration of the lateral semicircular canal.[10]

Schuknecht[11] also divided aural atresia patients into three groups based on severity and reviewed three methods for surgical reconstruction: (1) fenestration of the lateral semicircular canal,[3–5] (2) canalplasty,[6,7] and (3) type III tympanoplasty.[2,8] In all of these, the mastoid cavity is opened to access the ossicles and middle-ear space leaving the patient at risk for postoperative drainage and other problems associated with a cavity.

Jahrsdoerfer first described the anterior approach—avoiding opening the mastoid air cells—in 1978.[12] This approach, the standard in atresia surgery today, keeps the drilling anterior and superior by following the tegmen and the temporomandibular joint (TMJ) through the nonpneumatized bone of the atretic plate directly into the epitympanum and middle-ear space. The atretic bone is carefully picked away, the ossicles are freed, and temporalis fascia is used as an onlay graft with preservation of the native ossicular chain. Placement of a split thickness skin graft and meatoplasty complete the procedure. With a few minor modifications, this technique is used today and continues to deliver significantly improved hearing results without a mastoid cavity and with fewer complications.

The introduction of high-resolution computed tomography (HRCT) of the temporal bone has allowed the otologic surgeon to evaluate the aeration of the mastoid and middle ear, position of the tegmen, morphology of the ossicles, and course of the facial nerve with a high degree of accuracy. This technological development has singularly contributed to better patient selection for surgery and to more predictable surgical outcomes, and has broadened the scope of atresia surgery to include unilateral cases.[13–15]

Congenital aural atresia occurs once in every 10,000 births. Unilateral atresia is seven times more common than bilateral atresia. Aural atresia is associated with a recognizable syndrome (most commonly Treacher Collins, Goldenhar, and hemifacial microsomia) in about 10% of cases. In about 5% of nonsyndromic cases, the birth defect is inherited.

Bellucci separated major middle-ear malformations from minor malformations, defining minor malformations as those with a normal ear canal and tympanic membrane.[16] Minor malformations include congenital stapes fixation, congenital absence of the long process of the incus, malleus bar, congenital absence of the oval window, and single stapes crus. Major malformations, discussed in this chapter, refer to aural atresia—absence of an ear canal and tympanic membrane with some degree of underdevelopment of the middle-ear cleft and its structures.

Surgical correction of congenital atresia is a formidable operation and demands the best talent of the ear surgeon. Risks of facial nerve injury and sensorineural hearing loss are higher in the hands of the inexperienced operator. Even in the hands of the experienced otologist, stable long-term closure of the air–bone gap without canal stenosis can be difficult to achieve. However, in a patient with bilateral atresia, successful surgery that achieves normal hearing and allows the patient to discard his/her hearing device can be very gratifying for both the patient and otologist.

SURGERY FOR UNILATERAL VERSUS BILATERAL ATRESIA

The older literature reiterates the theme that only bilateral cases of congenital aural atresia should be operated on.[11] The reasoning behind this philosophy was that surgery would probably not produce serviceable hearing, and the risks of facial nerve injury and sensorineural hearing loss would outweigh any potential benefit. Moreover, postoperative meatal stenosis and the failure to maintain long-term hearing were cited as arguments against operating on patients with unilateral atresia. If unilateral cases were to be operated on, it was stated, they should be operated on only when the child had reached adolescence or young adulthood and could share in the decision.

Times have changed. With refinements in preoperative imaging and surgical technique, patients with unilateral atresia may be successfully operated on but only under strict criteria. This patient selection involves sorting out the high-risk (poor result) patients in whom the preoperative HRCT evaluation would indicate a low likelihood of success (defined as a postoperative speech reception threshold less than or equal to 30 dB HL). This threshold is attainable in 75 to 80% of patients carefully selected for surgery.

Criteria for surgical intervention may be more lenient in cases of bilateral atresia. In patients who are marginal candidates, it is appropriate to operate on at least one ear in an attempt to render serviceable hearing. However, impossible cases (cases in which there is no mastoid or middle-ear aeration, or cases in which the course of the facial nerve places it at great risk, or cases in which the tegmen rides too low) should be avoided.

A grading system, a 10-point scale in which individual anatomic structures are given points, was developed in an effort to select those individuals who have the best chance of successful atresia surgery.[13] The system is based on a preoperative HRCT scan of the temporal bones. In addition, the appearance of the external ear prior to microtia surgery is factored in, as external ear development correlates well with the degree of middle-ear development.[17]

To be a potential candidate, certain other criteria must be met. First, there must be audiometric evidence of normal cochlear function (normal bone conduction thresholds), and second, there must be imaging evidence of normal inner ear architecture. Since the inner ear develops embryologically from a completely separate anlage at a completely separate time from the middle and outer ear, cochlear function is typically normal in these patients. A contraindication of surgery would be a nonaerated middle ear and mastoid or a low-hanging tegmen (Figure 24–1). If the middle ear is not aerated, we do not recommend surgery. Lack of aeration may be temporary, such as middle-ear fluid, or it may be permanent, as the middle ear may be filled with primitive mesenchymal tissue of a fibrous gelatinous nature. This tissue is found in patients with absent or poor Eustachian tube function, in whom air has never reached the middle ear or mastoid. Repeat CT scanning (generally in one or two years) may help sort out temporary fluid versus more permanent primitive mesenchymal tissue; if this soft-tissue density persists for 2 years or more, surgery is not recommended. Otitis media with effusion will generally clear within 1 year revealing a well-ventilated middle ear and mastoid on subsequent HRCT scan.

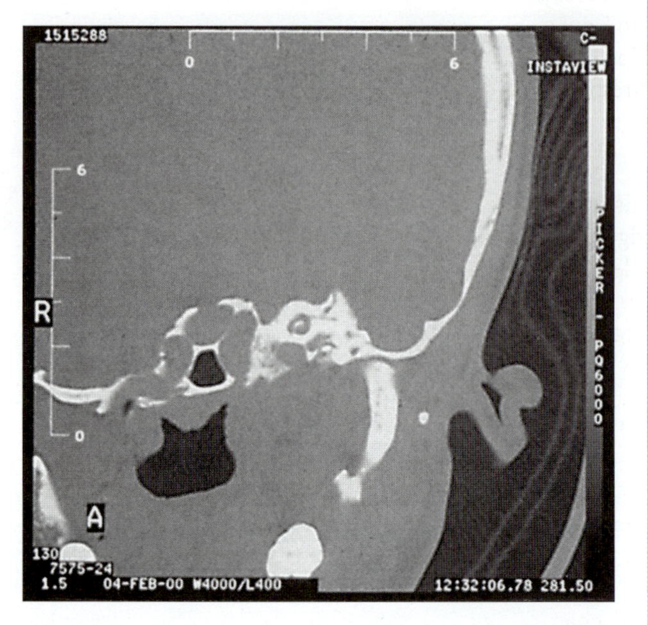

FIGURE 24–1 • Coronal computed tomography (CT) scan of a patient not a candidate for atresia surgery. There is no aeration of the middle ear or mastoid, and the tegmen hangs too low for creation of an ear canal.

TABLE 24–1 Grading system of candidacy for surgery of congenital aural atresia

PARAMETER	POINTS
Stapes present	2
Oval window open	1
Middle ear space	1
Facial nerve	1
Malleus/incus complex	1
Mastoid pneumatized	1
Incus-stapes connection	1
Round window	1
Appearance external ear	1
Total available points	10

From Jahrsdoerfer, et al.[13]

We still employ the Jahrsdoerfer grading scale shown in Table 24–1. The stapes is assigned two points as this is the most important ossicle on which the success of the operation hinges. In approximately 4% of patients, the stapes will be fixed; there is no way to diagnose this preoperatively. A fixed stapes requires that the operation be staged. The first stage includes the usual atresia repair with canalplasty, tympanoplasty, split thickness skin grafting, and meatoplasty; the second stage requires that the stapes be mobilized or a stapedectomy/stapedotomy be performed with ossicular chain reconstruction.

Most patients who are candidates for surgery will be graded 7 to 8 out of 10. This generally translates to an 80 to 90% chance of achieving normal or near-normal hearing (speech reception threshold ≤30 dB HL) through surgery.[18]

OTHER OPTIONS

It is important for the ear surgeon and the family to acknowledge that other options for hearing rehabilitation are available. For bilateral atresia patients, a long-term bone conducting hearing device (such as the BAHA Softband®, Cochlear Corp., Englewood, CO[19]) may be used, and most patients with this device develop excellent speech. An implantable bone conducting hearing device (BAHA System®, Cochlear Corp., Englewood, CO) is an excellent means of rehabilitating hearing in patients not candidates for atresia surgery or patients in whom atresia surgery has not significantly improved air conduction thresholds.[20–22] The BAHA System has been approved by the US Food and Drug Administration for patients over 6 years of age.

For patients who have undergone atresia surgery but did not achieve enough hearing gain to support language development or success in school, a conventional behind the ear or in the ear hearing aid in the newly epithelialized canal may also provide enough amplification to support normal receptive and expressive language and good progress in school. We do not require amplification for unilateral atresia patients as long as the contralateral ear shows normal hearing.

OPTIONS FOR REPAIR OF MICROTIA

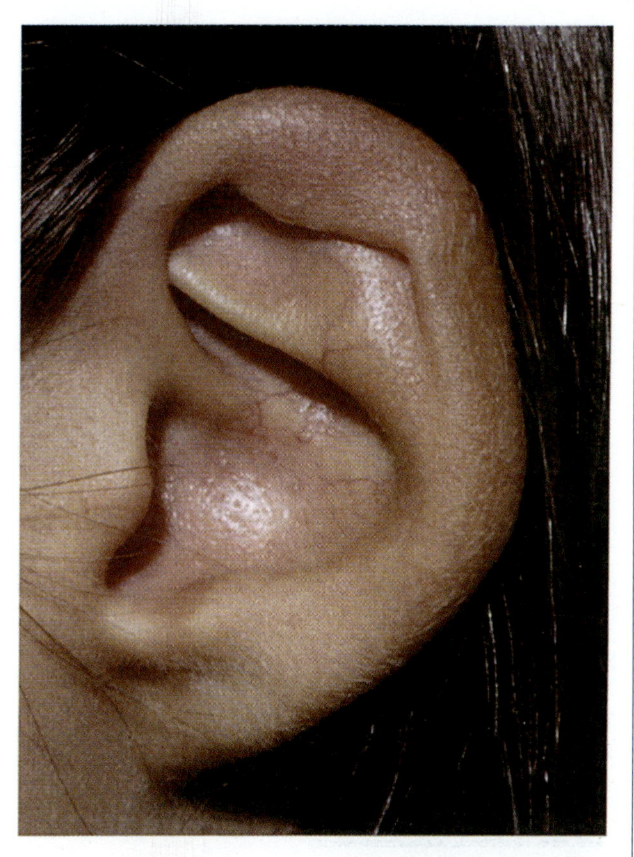

FIGURE 24–2 • Grade I microtia. The appearance of the ear is fairly well formed but smaller. *Courtesy of Burt Brent, MD.*

While most cases of Grade I microtia (Figure 24–2) do not require extensive reconstructive surgery, most patients and their families do elect to undergo reconstructive surgery for Grade III microtia. Fewer families choose to undergo reconstruction for Grade II microtia.

Repair of Grade II microtia (Figure 24–3) depends on the development of the auricle, the experience, judgment, and technical expertise of the reconstructive surgeon, and, of course, the desires and expectations of the patient and his/her family. In some cases of Grade II microtia, the auricular cartilage is not salvageable, and the reconstructive surgeon must "start from scratch" and harvest autologous rib cartilage (see below) to replace the cartilage remnant. It is the experience, skill, and judgment of the reconstructive surgeon as to whether the postoperative ear will be improved compared to the unoperated ear.

Options for repair of Grade III microtia (Figure 24–4) include prostheses, a porous polyethylene implant, and autologous rib cartilage. Silicone prosthetic ears may be affixed to the side of the skull either with medical adhesive glue (applied daily) or by titanium osseointegrated posts placed surgically.[23] Prostheses have the advantage of minimal morbidity with very lifelike cosmesis. Prosthetic ears have been a popular, if not preferred, method in failed surgical autogenous reconstructions, patients with severe soft-tissue/skeletal hypoplasia, patients with a low or unfavorable hairline, or patients with a total or subtotal auricular defect secondary to either trauma or malignancy.[24]

A porous polyethylene implant (Medpor®, Porex Surgical, Inc., Newnan, GA) has gained considerable popularity in the last several years in Grade III microtia repair. In the hands of the experienced reconstructive surgeon, this method of microtia repair also achieves excellent cosmetic results.[25] The procedure involves making a large Y-shaped incision with the anteroposterior limb 10 cm superior to the auricular remnant in the temporal scalp with one arm extending from the horizontal limb down to the remnant. Skin flaps are elevated, and a pocket is created in the appropriate position for the implant. The implant is measured, trimmed, and placed in the pocket, and a large temporoparietal fascia flap is elevated and brought down to cover the implant. The superior one-third of the implant will not have a skin covering, and this area is covered with a full thickness skin graft from the contralateral postauricular area. The Medpor microtia repair gains excellent projection and definition, but long-term durability studies are lacking.

Microtia repair using autologous rib cartilage is a challenging series of operations that few have mastered. The first stage involves harvesting autologous rib (usually the costal cartilage of the seventh and eighth ribs with a margin of the sixth rib cartilage) and sculpting the cartilage into the auricular framework.[26] The sculpted cartilage is placed in a subcutaneous pocket at the correct location and correct orientation on the lateral skull. Small suction drains are necessary to ensure that the thin skin sticks down to the cartilage. Lobule transposition follows approximately 3 months later, where the soft tissue remnant is translocated to the lobule position. The framework

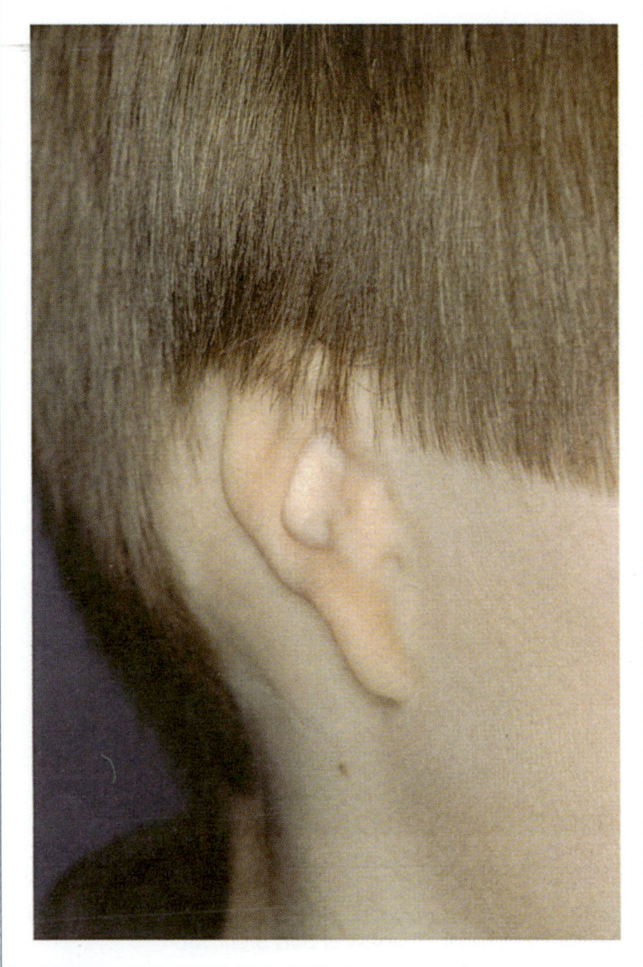

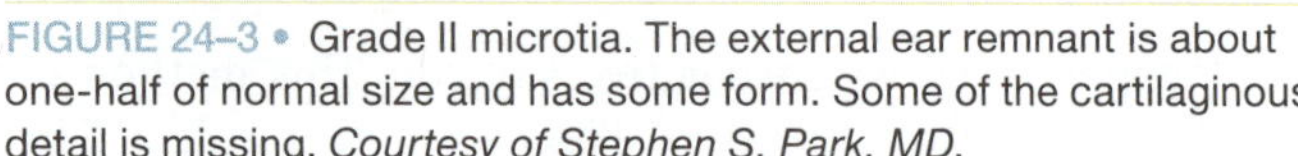

FIGURE 24–3 • Grade II microtia. The external ear remnant is about one-half of normal size and has some form. Some of the cartilaginous detail is missing. *Courtesy of Stephen S. Park, MD.*

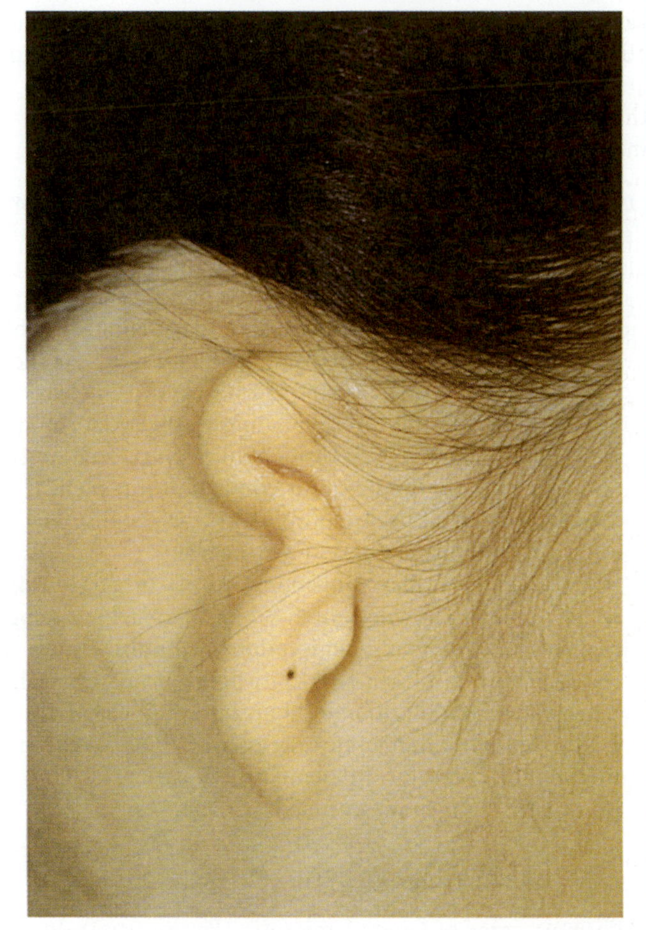

FIGURE 24–4 • Grade III microtia. Note the poorly formed ear remnant on the lateral face. Cartilage may or may not be present. *Courtesy of Stephen S. Park, MD.*

is next elevated off the lateral skull, and a relatively thick split thickness or full thickness skin graft is placed to create the postauricular sulcus in the third stage. Atresia repair can follow the third or fourth (and occasionally the second) stages. The tragus is created in the fourth stage.

A distinct advantage of rib graft microtia repair is that the cartilage is autologous tissue, and there is no concern for rejection. The cartilage and subcutaneous tissue also gain a robust blood supply, so there is little concern for exposure, infection, or extrusion for the atresia surgeon. In fact, the atresia surgeon must carve and remove a portion of the cartilage to ensure a widely patent meatus. The rib graft microtia repair has been criticized for lack of framework definition and poor projection, but in the hands of the experienced microtia surgeon, these risks are low.[26–29]

WHO SHOULD OPERATE FIRST—MEDPOR VERSUS RIB GRAFT?

Close communication between the reconstructive surgeon and otologist is critical to optimize results of both surgeries.[30] As mentioned, not all cases of microtia require a reconstructive surgeon. Grade I microtia, in which the ear is relatively well formed, usually does not require reconstructive surgery because this ear can rarely be improved on cosmetically; atresia surgery may proceed without any reconstructive work on the auricle (see Figure 24–2).

Grade II microtia, in which the external ear is about one-half of normal size but has reasonably good shape, may be operated on by the otologic surgeon first if the atresia is bilateral (see Figure 24–3). If the atresia is unilateral, it is a judgment call by the reconstructive surgeon, who must decide if his/her skills may improve the appearance of the external ear.

Grade III microtia, in which the external ear remnant is little more than a nub of skin or small piece of cartilage, must be operated on first by the reconstructive surgeon using autologous rib graft (see Figure 24–4). It is imperative that the reconstructive surgeon have a virgin field in which to place the sculpted rib cartilage; it is far easier for the reconstructive surgeon to build an ear in the absence of scar tissue and a compromised vascular bed than it is to build an ear around a hole in the side of the head. The otologic surgeon, however, drills the bony canal in the same location for every patient (see below); the reconstructed auricle may be safely moved and positioned to align with the bony canal. In fact, in approximately 50% of cases, the reconstructed auricle must be moved (usually in a posterosuperior direction) so that the meatus in the reconstructed auricle aligns with the newly created bony canal.

Anecdotally, atresia surgery following microtia repair with the Medpor implant has resulted in exposure of the implant, infection, and even extrusion. The implant does not acquire its own vascular supply and, therefore, if exposed during atresia surgery, will not heal or reepithelialize. One option recently undertaken is to perform the atresia repair before Medpor microtia repair. This sequence avoids the risk of exposure/extrusion of the polyethylene implant and allows the Medpor surgeon to reconstruct the new auricle around the newly created bony canal. At the time of atresia surgery, the ear canal skin graft is simply sutured to the patient's native skin on the side of the head where the bony canal exits. A recent report has demonstrated short-term results in patients undergoing atresia surgery *prior* to Medpor microtia repair comparable to results achieved in patients undergoing atresia surgery *after* rib graft microtia repair.[31] Despite this limited short-term success, the authors have serious concerns regarding the fate of the implant if the patient undergoing Medpor microtia repair following atresia repair needs a revision atresia operation (as many as 25–30% of patients will need revision atresia surgery[32]).

TIMING OF MICROTIA AND ATRESIA REPAIR

For the child with bilateral atresia, it is imperative that the hearing be tested [bone conduction auditory brainstem response (ABR) testing to ensure normal cochlear function] and followed at regular intervals, and that a bone conducting hearing device be placed as soon as possible after birth so that the child will develop receptive and expressive language skills. We generally do not recommend amplification for the child with unilateral atresia as long as the normal ear hears well. Normal hearing in one ear is sufficient for the development of normal speech and language skills, although it is becoming increasingly clear that children with unilateral hearing loss do have more subtle difficulties.[33,34]

External ear reconstruction is usually delayed until the child is about 6 to 7 years of age, with atresia repair following the series of operations required for rib graft microtia repair. This delay allows for growth of the rib cage, enabling sufficient costal cartilage to be harvested for sculpting the auricle. A child who is large for his/her age may be operated on earlier. For the child with Grade I or II microtia that does not require reconstructive surgery, atresia surgery can be performed at the age of 5 if the child is cooperative. Waiting until the child is 6 or 7 allows the child to achieve a level of maturity and cooperation absolutely critical for the postoperative dressing changes, packing removal, and ear canal cleaning to ensure a good result. A potentially poor result can be salvaged postoperatively in the office but requires the cooperation of the patient.

While reconstructive surgeons using the Medpor implant have implanted children as young as 3, we do not advocate atresia repair at that age because the child is simply too young to cooperate with the necessary postoperative packing removal and ear canal debridement. In addition, the authors feel that younger children may have a higher rate of meatal or canal stenosis necessitating revision surgery. The younger child certainly is not bothered psychologically by the ear deformity and is not yet in school where other children could tease him/her.

SURGICAL TECHNIQUE

Patient Preparation

The patient is placed in the supine position with the operated ear turned away. The arm on the ipsilateral side of the operated ear (split thickness skin graft donor arm) is tucked loosely so that in the middle of the case the arm can be removed from under the drapes and placed on an arm board for skin grafting. No blood pressure cuff is placed on the donor arm. A half-inch swath of hair is shaved around the ear. One percent lidocaine with 1:40,000 epinephrine is injected in the postauricular area. The ear is prepped and draped in standard fashion.

Although the surgery takes 3 to 6 h, urethral catheterization is not employed; the anesthesiologist adjusts fluid volume accordingly. A short-acting paralytic may be used for induction of anesthesia and intubation, but no paralytic may be administered during the operation as facial nerve monitoring is performed for all atresia operations. The anesthesiologist is requested not to use nitrous oxide as this gas diffuses into the middle ear and can cause increased positive pressure ballooning the fascia graft away from the ossicles.

Incision and Drilling

A postauricular incision is made and carried down to the temporalis fascia. A quarter-sized piece of fascia is harvested, scraped, and placed on the back table to dehydrate. Mastoid periosteal incisions are made along the linea temporalis and perpendicular anteriorly, along the glenoid fossa, down toward the mastoid tip. This anterior mastoid incision allows a cuff of periosteum to remain at the TMJ to which a tragal skin flap will be sutured at the end of the case to create the anterior canal wall. The mastoid periosteum is elevated and retracted posteriorly; the auricle is retracted anteriorly.

Elevation of the mastoid periosteum proceeds farther anteriorly to identify the glenoid fossa. It is critical to identify this fossa because it is an important landmark for drilling. Occasionally, there will be a dimple on the surface of the mastoid cortex to identify the site of drilling; alternatively, the cribriform area is often present as a reliable surface landmark.

Using the cribriform area, temporal line, and the glenoid fossa as surface landmarks, drilling is begun with #5 cutting burr with continuous suction irrigation, with care taken to stay anterior and superior (Figure 24–5). The tegmen is identified superiorly and followed medially. This superoanterior approach should hug the tegmen superiorly and the glenoid fossa anteriorly. Care is taken to stay out of the mastoid antrum and to open as few mastoid air cells as possible to prevent a large cavity and the risk of postoperative infection or mucosalization of the skin graft. As the drilling proceeds medially, dense, nonpneumatized atretic bone is encountered. This bone is carefully drilled away with progressively smaller diamond drill burrs. As the dissection stays superior, the goal is to enter the middle-ear cleft in the epitympanum, superior to the ossicles. This approach also avoids an aberrant facial nerve.

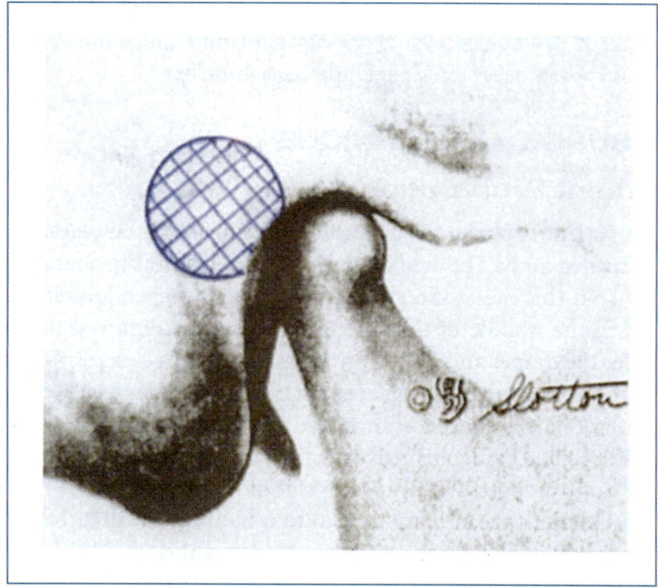

FIGURE 24–5 • Lateral view of temporal bone showing the area where drilling should begin. The glenoid fossa anteriorly and temporal line/tegmen superiorly are critical landmarks.

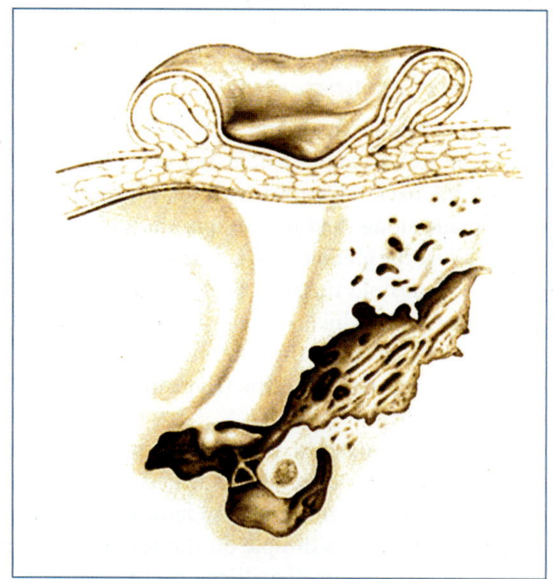

FIGURE 24–6 • Illustration of a sagittal view at the level of the epitympanum showing fused incus and malleus and bony attachment of the malleus neck to the atretic plate.

At a depth of about 1.5 cm, the air space of the middle ear is encountered, and the fused malleus–incus complex can be identified. The first landmark the surgeon encounters is usually the body of the incus; this can be confirmed by gentle palpation to assess mobility. The ossicular chain is typically fixed to the atretic plate medially and inferiorly at the level of the malleus neck (Figure 24–6). With a bit more bone removal, the "buttock sign" is identified—the fused head of the malleus and body of incus (Figure 24–7).

Drilling is continued over the atretic plate—with 3- and 2-mm diamond drill burrs with slow rotation—until the bone reaches eggshell thickness. The atretic bone overlying the middle

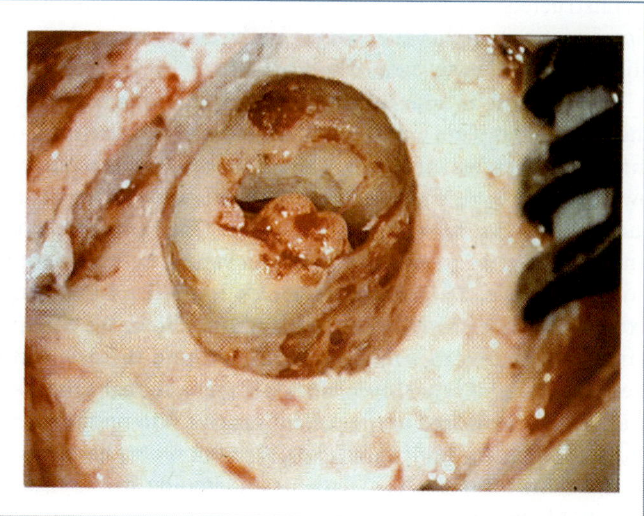

FIGURE 24–7 • "Buttock sign"—fused head of the malleus and body of incus as the atretic bone is removed and the epitympanum is opened (left ear).

ear and ossicles is carefully picked away with a Rosen needle or small dental excavator. Sharp dissection is often needed to lyse the periosteal attachments of the malleus to the underside of the atretic plate. There may also be a band of soft tissue, mostly periosteum, that courses through a bony defect in the wall separating the atretic plate from the TMJ; this band may be confused with the facial nerve. The facial nerve is most likely encountered while drilling posteriorly and inferiorly. In approximately 25% of cases, the facial nerve has a short vertical segment (sometimes nonexistent). Instead, the nerve makes a sharp curve anteriorly at the second genu. The facial nerve is most vulnerable to injury in this location.[35] Thin blood vessels coursing over the surface of the nerve seen through the thinned bone are a good clue to the location of the nerve. As mentioned, facial nerve monitoring is a necessity.

Once the atretic plate is removed, the ossicles are carefully assessed. Bone is removed 360 degrees around the ossicular chain to maximize mobility. The incus and malleus are almost always fused, although there may be some early demarcation of an incudomalleal joint. The handle of the malleus is often absent (Figure 24–8), and the neck of the malleus is usually in firm bony union with the undersurface of the atretic plate. Care must be exercised in removing the overlying fragments of bone so as not to sublux the ossicles or impart vibratory trauma to the inner ear. Bone around the fossa incudis is kept intact, and the anterior soft-tissue attachments between the malleus and anterior mesotympanic bone are also maintained to lend support to the ossicular chain. The last ligamentous attachment of the malleus to the atretic bone is incised with a #59 beaver blade or lysed with the laser.

The shape and direction of the incus long arm are highly variable. What is important is that the incus attaches to a stapes. The stapes superstructure may also be anomalous. In more extreme malformations, the superstructure may be monopedal with no connection to the incus. The mobility of the footplate must be determined. Congenital fixation of the stapes is found

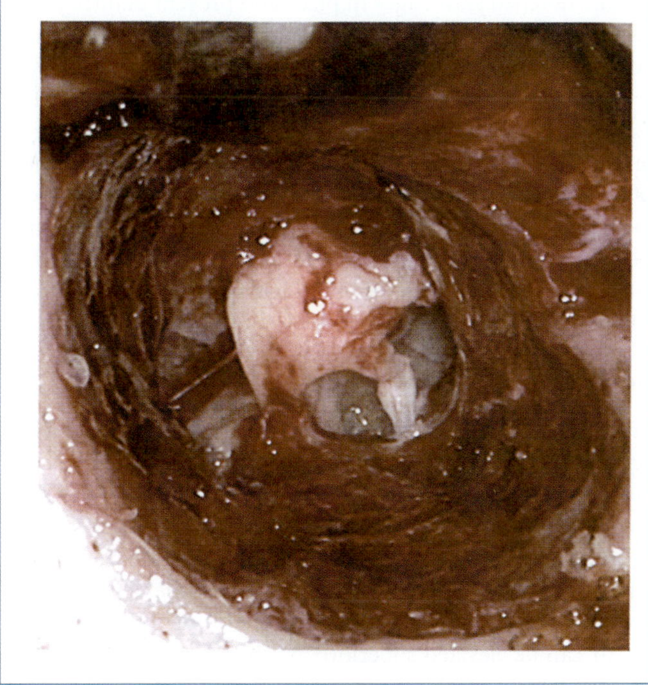

FIGURE 24–8 • Appearance of a typical ossicular chain after removal of all atretic bone. Note the absent malleus handle and fused malleus–incus complex (right ear).

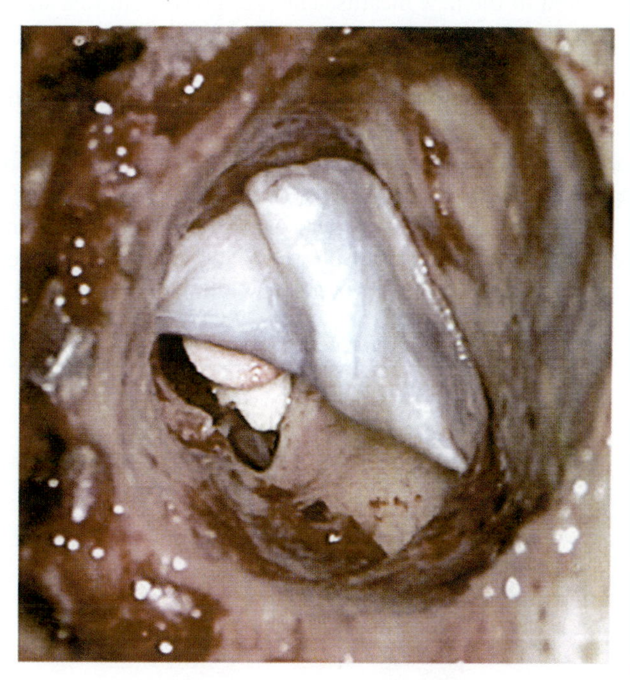

FIGURE 24–9 • Partial ossicular replacement prosthesis (PORP) under a temporalis fascia graft in patient with incudostapedial joint discontinuity. The lateral ossicular mass was removed (left ear).

in 4% of cases. It is common in congenital atresia to find a reasonably well-formed stapes with a mobile footplate. The oval window, in concert with the stapes footplate, may be smaller than normal, but this does not adversely affect either the reconstruction or the postoperative hearing result.

In cases of incudostapedial joint discontinuity, we prefer to remove the lateral ossicular mass and reconstruct with a notched partial ossicular replacement prosthesis (PORP). We have found this reconstruction to deliver superior hearing results compared to any other configuration (Figure 24–9).[36]

Fascia Grafting

The best possible circumstance in which to find the ossicles is for them to be intact (although malformed) and to move as a unit (see Figure 24–8). In this condition, the fascia graft may be placed directly on the ossicular mass. Bone must be drilled peripherally, away from the ossicular mass, to create as much room as possible for the fascia graft. The ossicular mass should be centered with regard to the new tympanic membrane. The new eardrum will be about 1 to 1.5 times the diameter of a normal tympanic membrane.

Prior to placing the fascia, the anesthesiologist is instructed to lower the expired oxygen to less than 25%. Room air fraction of inspired oxygen (FIO_2) is best. Lowering the expired oxygen (by lowering the inspired oxygen) reduces the ballooning of the graft. The fascia is trimmed to size (about 1.5 cm in diameter) and placed in an overlay fashion directly onto the ossicular mass. The edges of the fascia are reflected up onto the canal wall by about 1–2 mm in all directions (Figure 24–10). If large air cells have been opened, pieces of temporalis muscle are used to plug the defect.

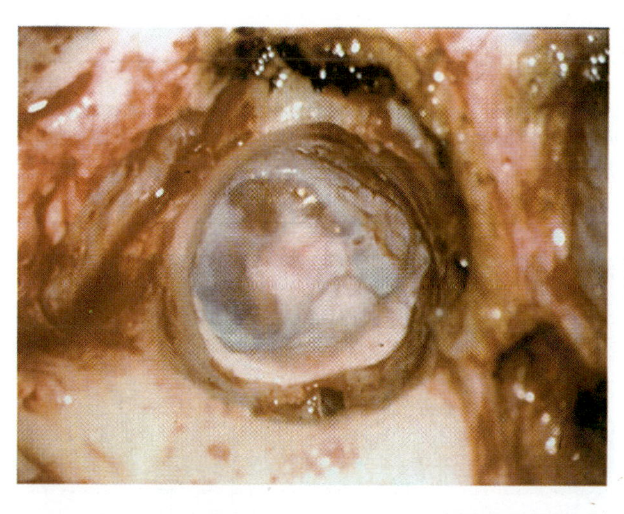

FIGURE 24–10 • Thin temporalis fascia placed in an overlay fashion with approximately 1–2 mm of fascia draped up onto the canal wall (left ear). Note the ossicular mass seen through the fascia.

Skin Grafting

A split thickness skin graft using the 2-inch dermatome blade and measuring 0.005 to 0.006 inches is harvested from the medial aspect of the ipsilateral upper arm. If the graft is any thicker, the skin graft tends to curl; buried squamous epithelium could produce a canal cholesteatoma. Too thin, and the graft does not withstand environmental pressures (eg, water) and can slough.

When the skin graft is harvested, an uneven thickness to its parallel borders is frequently noted. In this case, the thinner border is used at the level of the eardrum, and the thicker border is sutured to the new meatus. The skin graft is cut to a size of 4 × 5 cm and notched at the medial edge (Figure 24–11). The graft is carefully placed down into the canal, and the notched edges are aligned over the temporalis fascia so that the entire fascia graft is covered by squamous epithelium (Figure 24–12). The vertical slit faces anteriorly; this placement ensures that free edges will not grow into the mastoid air cells.

The key to a successful hearing result is a thin tympanic membrane and skin graft. Silastic of 0.04 inches is cut into a circular disk and placed over the new tympanic membrane to hold the notched skin edges in place and prevent blunting. The Silastic button also gives the surgeon something to pack against and helps prevent displacement of the skin graft.

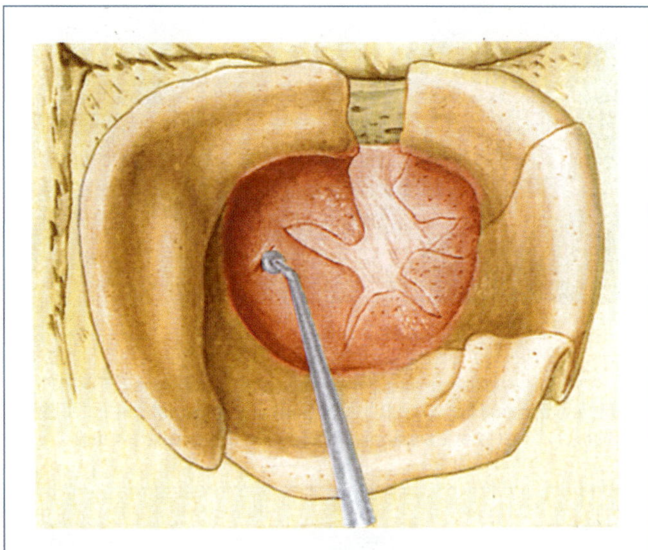

FIGURE 24–11 • The split thickness skin graft is notched at the medial end. The notches align to cover the temporalis fascia graft completely.

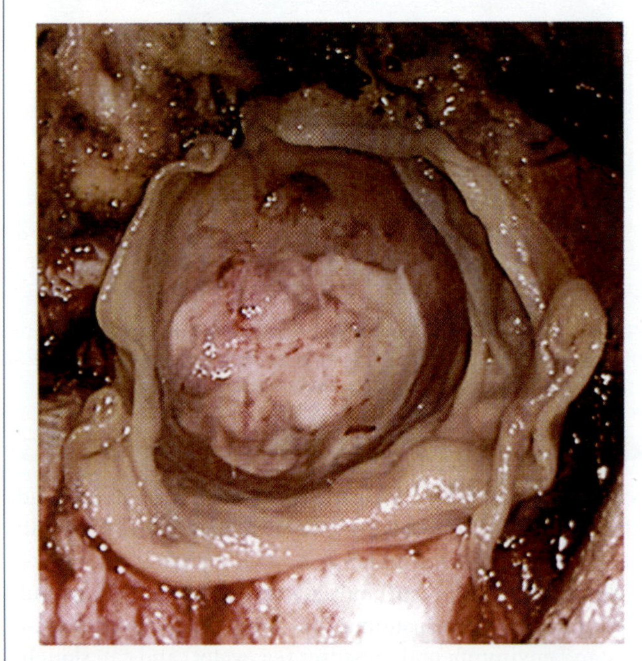

FIGURE 24–12 • Split thickness skin graft in position covering temporalis fascia (right ear). Note alignment of graft edges anteriorly.

Four to five Merocel® (Medtronic Corp., Jacksonville, FL) wicks are trimmed to three-fourth length and placed down into the ear canal onto the Silastic button (Figure 24–13). The new ear canal is packed to the level of the bony opening. The wicks are hydrated with an ototopical antibiotic solution (ofloxacin). The lateral skin graft is then folded over the hydrated wicks as the wicks hold the medial skin graft against the bony canal from which it will take its blood supply.

Meatoplasty

A hastily performed meatoplasty can ruin an otherwise flawless operation as it will result in meatal stenosis. Even a carefully constructed meatus can stenose, but if crafted with care, the risk is lower. The first priority is to ensure that the meatus and auricle align with the bony canal. The bony canal cannot move; the auricle needs repositioning to align the meatus to the bony canal in about half of the cases, usually in a posterosuperior orientation. The ear can be elevated superiorly by sharply releasing the skin and subcutaneous tissue over the parotid fascia anteriorly and over the sternocleidomastoid muscle inferiorly. Care must be taken to stay superficial and not enter the substance of the parotid gland, as a salivary fistula can be created.[37] The auricle can be moved posteriorly by excising a strip of skin from the postauricular incision and suturing the auricle to the new postauricular skin edge.

A U-shaped skin flap based anteriorly at the tragus is created by making a crescentic incision in the skin of the reconstructed auricle's conchal bowl. The skin is sharply elevated off the underlying cartilage and is hinged at the tragus. The skin flap is thinned and reflected anteriorly, and the underlying cartilage and soft tissue are cored out with a #11 blade. The skin flap is then brought through the new meatus medially and down to the cuff of TMJ periosteum that was created at the beginning of the operation with the mastoid periosteal incisions. The

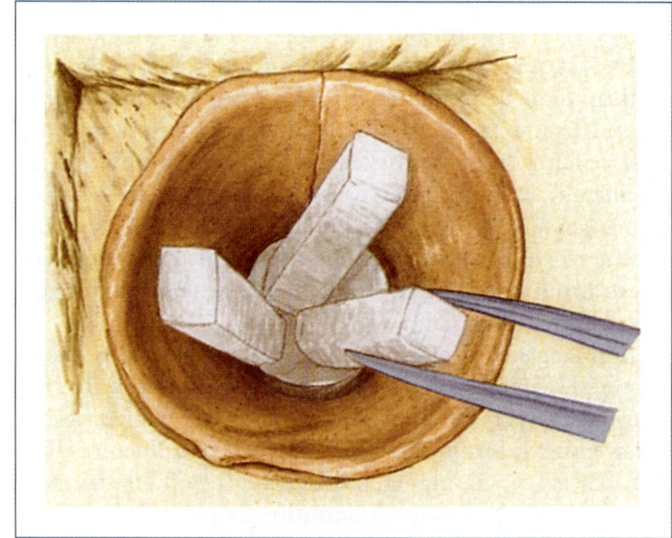

FIGURE 24–13 • Merocel wicks are placed down into the ear canal on the Silastic button and hydrated with an ototopical antibiotic preparation.

tragal skin flap is sutured to this cuff of tissue with 2-3 buried 4-0 undyed Vicryl sutures to create the lateral anterior canal wall. The postauricular incision is tacked down with interrupted 3-0 undyed Vicryl sutures, and the skin graft is delivered through the meatus and sutured to the patient's native skin at the edge of the conchal bowl with interrupted 5-0 fast absorbing gut sutures. The lateral canal is packed with full length Merocel wicks hydrated with ofloxacin solution. After closure of the postauricular incision, a mastoid dressing is applied.

Postoperative Care

The patient is admitted overnight and discharged on oral antibiotics (cephalexin) and pain medicine on the first postoperative day after the dressings are removed. Antibiotic ointment is placed over the postauricular incision and an antibiotic-soaked cottonball is changed at the meatus daily. The patient is seen in the office 1 week after surgery, and all sutures and packing are removed. A corticosteroid-antibiotic eardrop preparation is then used twice daily for 1 week with strict dry ear precautions. The canal is left open to the air.

A second postoperative visit is made 1 month later, and the canal is debrided of desquamated epithelium sloughed from the skin graft. Beneath the epithelial crust, the skin graft should be dry and healthy. The first postoperative audiogram is obtained at this visit.

It is important that the patient be followed every 6 to 12 months indefinitely for debridement of the desquamated epithelial crust. Although the skin graft is healthy, it is not self-cleaning. Failure to have the ear cleaned routinely may result in decreased hearing and chronic infection. There are no restrictions after the 1-month visit—patients may swim, but alcohol eardrops after swimming and once a week are advised.

Complications

Complications of atresia surgery can be minimized with proper selection of patients and with careful attention to surgical detail. Most common complications include meatal or canal stenosis in 15 to 20%, usually requiring revision surgery, and chronic drainage/infection in 10%, usually due to sloughing of the skin graft with "mucosalization" of the canal—requiring revision with a new skin graft or possible temporizing measures such as Gentian violet if the area is small. Less commonly, sensorineural hearing loss (5%) is most likely related to the high energy of the drill on the ossicular chain conducted to the cochlea; facial nerve injury occurs in 0.1%.[34] About 15 to 20% of patients will also lose the initial gains in hearing, due to either lateralization of the tympanic membrane or refixation of the ossicular chain. We counsel patients that approximately 15 to 20% will require a revision procedure at some point in the future, usually due to stenosis of the canal, loss of early hearing gains, or sloughing of the skin graft with chronic drainage.

RESULTS

The two most important factors in achieving consistently good hearing outcomes in atresia surgery are careful preoperative selection of patients and meticulous surgical technique at each step of the operation. Surgery is not recommended for patients with unilateral atresia and Jahrsdoerfer scores of 6 or below. Surgery is attempted on the patient with bilateral atresia and a score of 5 or 6, but excellent hearing outcomes are difficult. Even so, the patient may be able to wear a conventional hearing aid in the new canal to bring the hearing thresholds into the normal range. Surgery is not recommended for patients with scores of 4 or below. The most important anatomic feature for successful surgery is middle-ear aeration[18]; without an aerated middle-ear space, the patient is not considered a candidate for surgery.

A recent study has examined the predictive ability of the Jahrsdoerfer scale for hearing outcomes. In this series of 116 patients, patients with a score ≥7 had an 85 to 90% chance of achieving normal or near-normal hearing (as defined by an SRT ≤30 dB HL) in the short term; patients with lower Jahrsdoerfer scores had a 45 to 50% chance of achieving this result.[18]

One criticism of atresia surgery case series has been lack of long-term follow-up. Lambert examined the stability of hearing results after atresia surgery and found that almost two-thirds of patients maintained an SRT ≤30 dB HL for the longer follow-up (>1 year; mean, 2.8 years); about one-third required a revision procedure.[32] Similarly, De la Cruz reported a long-term (≥6 months) air–bone gap (ABG) of 30 dB or less in 51% of primary cases and 39% of revisions.[38] Digoy and Cueva also reported on the stability of hearing in their series of atresia patients, as hearing did not change between short and long term (>1 year): 50% of patients achieved an SRT of 30 dB HL or better.[39] These authors reported no difference in hearing outcomes between patients undergoing ossiculoplasty reconstruction (53%) versus those undergoing intact native chain reconstruction.[39] Conversely, Dobratz et al. did show a significant advantage to maintaining the patient's native ossicular chain when possible.[36] Revision surgery may not hold up as well long-term, as Chang et al. reported disappointing long-term hearing outcomes for patients undergoing revision atresia surgery.[40]

Surgeons 10 to 15 years ago counseled patients and families against repair of unilateral atresia, given the mediocre hearing gains and risk of major complications. Since the introduction of HRCT scanning with improved preoperative evaluation, the repair of unilateral atresia has become more widely accepted. Clearly, there is a learning curve for this challenging operation, and one report suggests a minimum of 32 ears to achieve proficiency in achieving good short-term hearing results, and 48 ears for good long-term hearing outcomes.[41] The anterior surgical approach as first proposed by Jahrsdoerfer[12] has withstood the test of time and scrutiny. As the seemingly subtle deficits of unilateral hearing loss in children are further elucidated, the repair of unilateral atresia will be more accepted and more often recommended.

SUMMARY

While technically challenging, surgery to construct an ear canal and restore the natural sound conducting mechanism of the middle and outer ear in patients with congenital aural atresia can be successful with careful attention to the preoperative selection of patients as candidates for the operation and with meticulous surgical technique at each step of the operation. Restoration of normal hearing in these patients is one of the most rewarding operations in our specialty.

References

1. Hrdlicka A. Seven prehistoric American skulls with complete absence of external auditory meatus. Amer J Phys Anthrop. 1933;17:355.
2. Pattee G. An operation to improve hearing in cases of congenital atresia of the external auditory meatus. Arch Otolaryngol. 1947;45:568–80.
3. Ombredanne. New proves of superiority of fenestration in surgery of aplasias of the ear. Ann Otolaryngol Chir Cervicofac. 1952;69(8–9):494–501.
4. Ombredanne M. 33 Operations for aplasia of the ear with atresia of the auditory canal: Technic, operative establishments and results. Acta Otolaryngol. 1952;41(1–2):69–109.
5. Woodman DG. Congenital atresia of the auditory canal; two stage operation with fenestration. AMA Arch Otolaryngol. 1952;55(2):172–81.
6. House HP. Management of congenital ear canal atresia. Laryngoscope. 1953;63(10):916–46.
7. Shambaugh GE, Jr. Developmental anomalies of the sound conducting apparatus and their surgical correction. Trans Am Otol Soc. 1952;40:217–31.
8. Ruedi L. The surgical treatment of the atresia auris congenita; a clinical and histological report. Laryngoscope. 1954;64(8): 666–84.
9. Nager GT. Aural atresia: Anatomy and surgery. Postgrad Med. 1961;29:529–41.
10. Nager GT. Congenital aural atresia: Anatomy and surgical management. Birth Defects. Origi. Artic. Ser. 1971;07(4):33–51.
11. Schuknecht HF. Reconstructive procedures for congenital aural atresia. Arch Otolaryngol 1975;101(3):170–2.
12. Jahrsdoerfer RA. Congenital atresia of the ear. Laryngoscope. 1978;88(9 Pt 3 Suppl 13):1–48.
13. Jahrsdoerfer RA, Yeakley JW, Aguilar EA, Cole RR, Gray LC. Grading system for the selection of patients with congenital aural atresia. Am J Otol. 1992;13(1):6–12.
14. Trigg DJ, Applebaum EL. Indications for the surgical repair of unilateral aural atresia in children. Am J Otol. 1998;19(5):679–84.
15. De la Cruz, A, Kesser B. Management of the unilateral atretic ear. In: Pensak M, editor. Controversies in otolaryngology-head and neck surgery. New York: Thieme Medical, 1999; 381–5.
16. Bellucci RJ. Congenital aural malformations: Diagnosis and treatment. Otolaryngol Clin North Am. 1981;14(1):95–124.
17. Kountakis SE, Helidonis E, Jahrsdoerfer RA. Microtia grade as an indicator of middle ear development in aural atresia. Arch Otolaryngol Head Neck Surg 1995;121(8):885–6.
18. Shonka DC, Livingston WJ III, Kesser BW. The Jahrsdoerfer grading scale in surgery for congenital aural atresia. Arch Otolaryngol Head Neck Surg 2008; 134(8)873–7.
19. Hol MK, Cremers CW, Coppens-Schellekens W, Snik AF. The BAHA Softband. A new treatment for young children with bilateral congenital aural atresia. Int J Pediatr Otorhinolaryngol 2005;69(7):973–80.
20. van der Pouw KT, Snik AF, Cremers CW. Audiometric results of bilateral bone-anchored hearing aid application in patients with bilateral congenital aural atresia. Laryngoscope 1998;108 (4 Pt 1):548–53.
21. Klaiber S, Weerda H. BAHA (bone-anchored hearing aid) in bilateral external ear dysplasia and congenital ear atresia. HNO. 2002;50(10):949–59.
22. Priwin C, Jonsson R, Hultcrantz M, Granstrom G. BAHA in children and adolescents with unilateral or bilateral conductive hearing loss: A study of outcome. Int J Pediatr Otorhinolaryngol 2007;71(1):135–45.
23. Wazen JJ, Wright R, Hatfield RB, Asher ES. Auricular rehabilitation with bone-anchored titanium implants. Laryngoscope 1999;109(4):523–7.
24. Thorne CH, Brecht LE, Bradley JP, Levine JP, Hammerschlag P, Longaker MT. Auricular reconstruction: Indications for autogenous and prosthetic techniques. Plast Reconstr Surg 2001;107(5):1241–52.
25. Romo T III, Presti PM, Yalamanchili HR. Medpor alternative for microtia repair. Facial Plast Surg Clin North Am 2006;14(2):129–36.
26. Brent B. Technical advances in ear reconstruction with autogenous rib cartilage grafts: Personal experience with 1200 cases. Plast Reconstr Surg 1999;104(2):319–34.
27. Brent B. Microtia repair with rib cartilage grafts: A review of personal experience with 1000 cases. Clin Plast Surg 2002;29(2):257–71.
28. Kawanabe Y, Nagata S. A new method of costal cartilage harvest for total auricular reconstruction: Part I. Avoidance and prevention of intraoperative and postoperative complications and problems. Plast Reconstr Surg 2006;117(6):2011–8.
29. Kawanabe Y, Nagata S. A new method of costal cartilage harvest for total auricular reconstruction: Part II. Evaluation and analysis of the regenerated costal cartilage. Plast Reconstr Surg 2007;119(1):308–15.
30. Jahrsdoerfer RA, Kesser BW. Issues on aural atresia for the facial plastic surgeon. Facial Plast Surg 1995;11(4):274–7.
31. Roberson JB Jr, Reinisch J, Colen TY, Lewin S. Atresia repair before microtia reconstruction: Comparison of early with standard surgical timing. Otol Neurotol 2009;30(6):771–6.
32. Lambert PR. Congenital aural atresia: Stability of surgical results. Laryngoscope 1998;108(12):1801–5.
33. Kiese-Himmel C, Kruse E. Unilateral hearing loss in childhood. An empirical analysis comparing bilateral hearing loss. Laryngorhinootologie 2001;80(1):18–22.
34. Wilmington D, Gray L, Jahrsdoerfer R. Binaural processing after corrected congenital unilateral conductive hearing loss. Hear Res 1994;74(1–2):99–114.
35. Jahrsdoerfer RA, Lambert PR. Facial nerve injury in congenital aural atresia surgery. Am J Otol 1998;19(3):283–7.
36. Dobratz E, Rastogi A, Jahrsdoerfer RA, and Kesser BW. To POP or not: Ossiculoplasty in congenital aural atresia surgery. Laryngoscope 2008;118(8):1452–7.
37. Miller RS, Jahrsdoerfer RA, Hashisaki GT, Kesser BW. Diagnosis and management of salivary fistula after surgery for congenital aural atresia. Otol Neurotol 2006;27(2):189–92.
38. De la Cruz A, Teufert KB. Congenital aural atresia surgery: Long-term results. Otolaryngol Head Neck Surg 2003;129(1):121–7.
39. Digoy GP, Cueva RA. Congenital aural atresia: Review of short- and long-term surgical results. Otol Neurotol 2007;28(1):54–60.
40. Chang SO, Choi BY, Hur DG. Analysis of the long-term hearing results after the surgical repair of aural atresia. Laryngoscope 2006;116(10):1835–41.
41. Patel N, Shelton C. The surgical learning curve in aural atresia surgery. Laryngoscope 2007;117(1):67–73.

Surgery of the Tympanomastoid Compartment

V

25. *Pathology and Clinical Course of the Inflammatory Diseases of the Middle Ear*
26. *Aural Complications of Otitis Media*
27. *Intracranial Complications of Otitis Media*
28. *Tympanoplasty: Tympanic Membrane Repair*
29. *Ossicular Chain Reconstruction*
30. *Canal-Wall-Up Mastoidectomy*
31. *Open Cavity Mastoid Operations*
32. *Surgery for Otosclerosis*
33. *Implantable Middle Ear and Bone Conduction Hearing Devices*

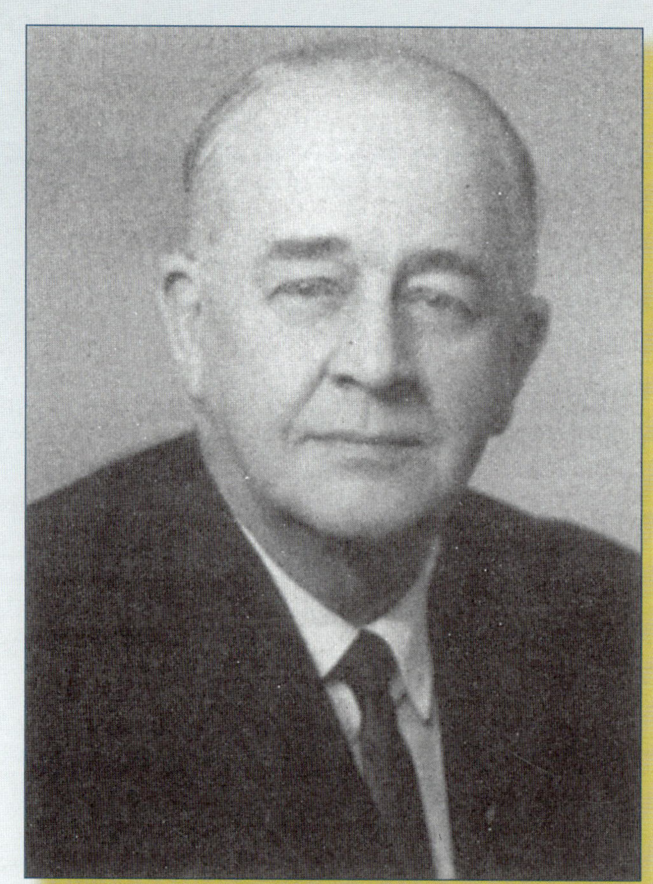

SIR TERENCE CAWTHORNE (1902-1970) • Eminent London aural surgeon who helped to bridge the transition from surgery for the evacuation of pus to surgery in a clean field under the operating microscope.

Pathology and Clinical Course of the Inflammatory Diseases of the Middle Ear

25

Quinton Gopen, MD

OVERVIEW

This chapter reviews the key features, pathology and clinical course of acute otitis media, otitis media with effusion, chronic otitis media including cholesteatoma, and selected granulomatous middle-ear diseases (tuberculosis, Wegener's granulomatosis, Langerhan's cell histiocytosis [LCH], and mycotic infections).

ACUTE OTITIS MEDIA

Acute otitis media is an acute inflammation of the middle-ear space. This inflammation typically occurs over several hours but must occur in less than 6 weeks to be classified as an acute process. Although the cause of inflammation is most typically infectious, the inflammation can also result from other etiologies such as autoimmune, neoplastic, traumatic, and metabolic. Infections can be due to viral, bacterial, or fungal pathogens. The most common viral pathogens include respiratory syncytial virus and rhinovirus but other viral pathogens such as coronavirus, influenza type A, adenovirus, and parainfluenzae have been implicated.[1] The most common bacterial pathogens include *Streptococcus pneumoniae*, *Haemophilus influenzae*, and *Moraxella catarrhalis* with Staphylococcal, Streptococcal, and Pseudomonal species less frequently identified. Fungal pathogens are usually *Aspergillus* and *Candida* species. It is not uncommon for a bacterial acute otitis media to result from superinfection of an initial viral process. Fungal infections are less usual but are an important consideration in immunocompromised individuals.

The clinical manifestations of acute otitis media include otalgia, hearing loss, and fever. If the tympanic membrane ruptures, purulent otorrhea may also be present. Technically, all cases of acute otitis media include mastoiditis as the middle-ear space is in continuity with the mastoid air cells. Clinically, however, these two terms refer to distinctly different processes. Acute mastoiditis clinically refers to acute coalescent mastoiditis and is differentiated from acute otitis media by abscess formation either within or superficial to the mastoid air cells. Computed tomography (CT) scans can be quite useful in making this distinction with identification of a subperiosteal abscess or coalescence of the mastoid air cells. A magnetic resonance imaging (MRI) scan, however, is not useful in this distinction as it does not image bone. Oftentimes an asymptomatic patient has either a CT scan or an MRI scan that demonstrates complete or subtotal opacification of the mastoid air cells without any bony erosion or abscess formation. Unfortunately, this finding is often erroneously termed "mastoiditis" by the radiologist, a designation that is clearly incorrect given the clinical setting.

Otoscopy reveals an erythematous tympanic membrane that is often bulging or ruptured with purulent drainage. Impedance tympanometry demonstrates a flat tympanogram and absent acoustic reflexes. Audiometric testing shows a conductive hearing loss.

The distinction between acute otitis media and acute mastoiditis can be made based on clinical features. Acute otitis media is not associated with auricular displacement, whereas acute mastoiditis is. Care must be taken to distinguish the auricular displacement of acute mastoiditis from the postauricular swelling due to otitis externa with cellulitis of the postauricular skin. Otitis externa with cellulitis has a faster clinical course (over several days) and has a reactive inflammatory opacification of the mastoid air cells without subperiosteal abscess or coalescence on CT scan. Acute mastoiditis has a slower time course (developing over 1 to 2 weeks) with septal breakdown of the mastoid air cells and/or subperiosteal abscess formation.

The pathologic manifestations of acute otitis media can be divided into four stages—hyperemic, exudative, suppurative, and resolution—depending on the timing and extent of the inflammatory response. The earliest response, the hyperemic response occurs upon the arrival of an antigen within the middle ear or mastoid. Antigens can enter via the Eustachian tube from infected nasopharyngeal secretions, through the systemic circulation, or through adjacent sites such as a perforated eardrum or a cutaneous infection. The invading antigen undergoes processing by immunocompetent cells residing in the middle-ear and mastoid spaces just as in other parts of the body. These immunocompetent cells include T-cells, macrophages, and B-cells bearing immunoglobulins IgM, IgG, and IgA. The initial hyperemic response to the antigen is characterized by hyperemia and edema of the tympanic membrane and middle-ear mucosa, and typically involves all three layers of the tympanic membrane.

If the early inflammatory response is insufficient to eradicate the offending antigen, the process often progresses to a second, exudative, stage (Figure 25–1). As the antigen is processed by the residing immunocompetent cells, immune factors are released to recruit other cells and cytokines from the systemic circulation. The release of interleukin-2, platelet endothelial cell adhesion molecule-1, and other mediators results in an increased expression of intercellular adhesion molecules within vein and venule walls. Inflammatory infiltrates such as B and T lymphocytes, macrophages, and polymorphonuclear cells rush in through these vessels rendered "leaky" via the expressed adhesion molecules and fill the middle-ear and mastoid spaces. IgG-bearing B-cells arrive first, quickly followed by IgM-bearing B-cells. T-helper cells arrive around 24 hrs later and increase in number over several days, peaking at between 2 to 3 weeks. IgA-bearing B-cells come later, usually around 3 weeks after the initial antigenic challenge. These newly recruited cells all participate in a complex cascade of cytokine release, including IL-1, IL-6, IL-8, TNF-α, and leukotriene B4, all of which have been implicated in acute otitis media.[2–5]

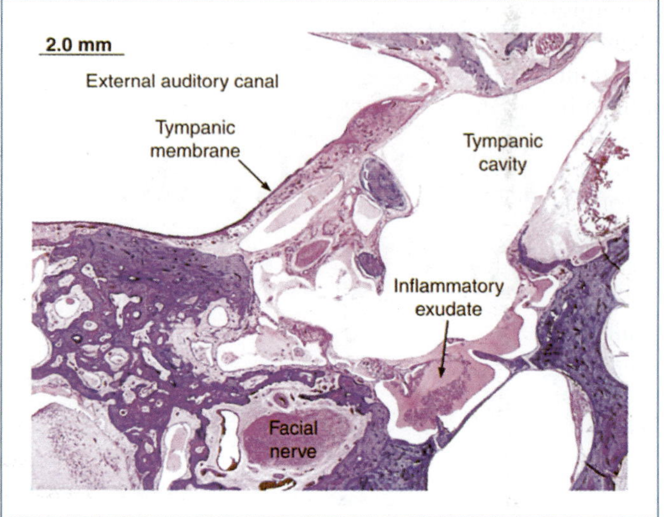

FIGURE 25–1 • Acute otitis media. Hematoxylin and eosin stained temporal bone slide through the mesotympanum at the level of the stapes footplate demonstrates an acute inflammatory exudate. The exudate contains polymorphonuclear cells as well as eosinophilic secretions as identified within the middle-ear space. The mucosal lining of the middle ear as well as the tympanic membrane are thickened. The process extends into the mastoid air cell system.

The next stage, suppuration, only occurs in bacterial infections. It reflects the immunologic response that destroys the offending bacterial organism, culminating in a purulent collection of fluid behind the eardrum. Bacterial destruction occurs via immunoglobulin coating of the bacteria with ensuing opsonization by macrophages as well as by involvement of the complement cascade. Tympanic membrane rupture can occur during this stage if the suppurative response is fulminant.

The final stage, resolution, varies in time of onset and rapidity of progress. Oftentimes, the accumulated fluid persists within the middle ear as the natural egress through the Eustachian tube orifice is blocked by mucosal edema. Once the acute process has resolved, if a sterile effusion persists, it is termed otitis media with effusion.

An excellent review of acute otitis media including the etiopathology, natural history, treatment, and complications is given by Bluestone.[6] Complications of acute otitis media are covered in Chapters 26 and 27.

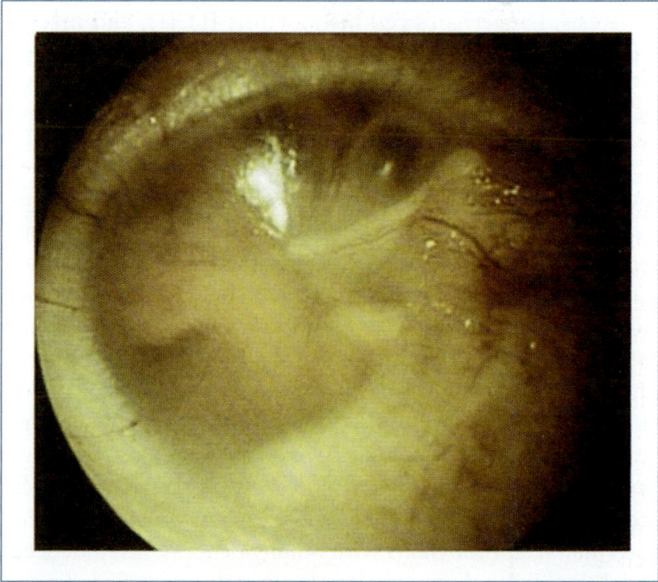

FIGURE 25–2 • Otitis media with effusion. This photograph demonstrates an amber-colored effusion behind an intact tympanic membrane. A small bubble can be seen near the light reflex.

Otitis Media With Effusion

Otitis media with effusion is defined as a serous or mucoid (nonpurulent) collection of fluid within the middle-ear space (Figure 25–2). In contradistinction to acute and chronic otitis media, otitis media with effusion is not classified according to length of duration. Otitis media with effusion can present over hours or last for decades. The mechanisms of formation and persistence of the fluid collection include chronic inflammation within the middle ear and Eustachian tube dysfunction. Historically, otitis media with effusion was considered a sterile effusion with only occasional bacterial species identified on culture. Because of the lack of evidence for pathogens in the fluid samples taken from the middle ear, Eustachian tube dysfunction was previously assumed the primary mechanism for formation of otitis media with effusion. As Eustachian tube dysfunction causes inadequate gas exchange into the middle-ear space, increasingly negative middle-ear pressures develop, resulting in the formation of a transudate that fails to clear.

Eustachian tube dysfunction arises from inflammatory disorders, muscular abnormalities, and anatomic factors. In children, the Eustachian tube is smaller, more flexible, and has a more horizontal orientation when compared to adults, which might help explain the relatively greater incidence of otitis media with effusion in children. Dysfunction can result from congenital anomalies, such as cleft palate or myopathies that affect the palatal musculature and consequently the dynamic excursion of the orifice of the eustachian tube. Inflammation is probably one of the more common causes of tubal problems resulting in mucosal edema with mucus production, and it can arise from any of a number of etiologies, such as allergic disease, laryngopharyngeal or gastroesophageal reflux, syndromic or smoking-related ciliary dysmotility, and middle-ear/nasopharyngeal biofilms. Anatomic obstruction of the Eustachian tube can result from prominent adenoid tissue, synechiae from surgery, or nasopharyngeal masses.

Importantly, however, evidence, particularly from biofilm research, has begun to mount indicating that otitis media with effusion may more reflect a chronic inflammatory state and that Eustachian tube dysfunction plays a secondary role. Biofilms are a matrix of polysaccharides formed by colonies of bacteria that protect these bacteria and form a more favorable environment for their existence. A common configuration of biofilms is a complex "tower and mushroom" conglomerate that coats the surface of a colony of bacteria.[7] These complex biofilms allow passage of nutrients and fluid as well as bacterial communication with one another via hormonal signals to optimize their function as a group. In a biofilm state, bacteria can persist in tissue and are shielded from eradication by the host defense system, even in the face of long-term antibiotic therapy. Furthermore, traditional swab cultures of the fluid within the middle-ear space are usually negative, as the biofilm-aggregated bacteria are not free-floating in the fluid but are sequestered onto the surface of the lining mucosa.

Several studies have supported the biofilm hypothesis of the etiology of otitis media with effusion. In 2001, Post demonstrated biofilms in a chinchilla model by injecting *H. influenzae* into the middle-ear space. Scanning electron microscopy (SEM) was used to examine the middle-ear mucosa and demonstrated biofilms. He also used SEM to document the presence of biofilms within tympanostomy tubes.[7] In 2006, Hall-Stoodley reported finding bacterial biofilms in the middle ears of pediatric patients with chronic otitis media. In this study, biopsies of middle-ear mucosa were taken from children undergoing tympanostomy tube placement for chronic otitis media. With visualization by confocal laser-scanning microscopy (which may be the most accurate way to detect biofilms), 92% of patients, but none of the 88 control patients, had biofilms present in the mucosal biopsies.[8] In 2008, with the use of transmission electron microscopy, Coates demonstrated intracellular bacterial infection of the middle-ear mucosal epithelial cells in pediatric patients diagnosed as having otitis media with effusion.[9]

The bacteria of a biofilm are sheltered and persist in a subclinical state, sequestered within the tissues and secreting endotoxins and exotoxins. These toxins can be found even months after the administration of culture-specific antibiotics. The bacteria, along with their toxins, initiate a complex cascade of inflammatory mediators including the proinflammatory cytokines TNF-α, TNF-β, IL-1b, IL-6, and IL-8 along with the immunoregulatory cytokines, IL-2, IL-4, IL-5, IL-10, and IFN-g. TNF-α and IL-1b are the two most important and are considered the primary cytokines responsible for the inflammatory response within the middle ear and mastoid. TNF-α, a cytokine produced by macrophages with a diverse spectrum of effects, has an important role in upregulating the production of other cytokines. IL-1b, also produced by macrophages, is considered a central mediator of inflammation by stimulating activation of a host of inflammatory cells, including fibroblasts, endothelial cells, osteoclasts, T-cells, B-cells, monocytes, and neutrophils.[10]

The inflammatory response starts in the submucosa of the middle-ear space. Initially, neutrophils, macrophages, and lymphocytes are recruited into action and are activated. Early mediators of inflammation include (1) arachidonic acid metabolites, (2) histamine, (3) platelet activating factor, (4) adhesion cell molecules of various types, and (5) the crucial cytokines TNF-α and IL-1b described earlier. In otitis media with effusion, this activity results in proliferation of the mucosal lining and secretion of mucus. In some cases, the basal cells of the mucosal layer undergo differentiation into goblet and ciliated cells, resulting in the production of an extremely thick and tenacious mucoid effusion consisting primarily of mucins. Mucins are glycoproteins that can bind proteins, including the outer membranes of bacteria, and help in the immune clearance of these and other pathogens.[10] It is primarily the mucin content that determines the viscosity of the effusion.

After the initial activation of the inflammatory process, mediators of ongoing inflammation such as complement 3a, INF-g, and IL-6 can be detected. The inflammatory response is ultimately downregulated by IL-2, IL-5, TGF-b, and IL-10. An excellent description of these events is given in Smirnova's 2002 review.[10]

Clinical manifestations of otitis media with effusion are hearing loss, aural fullness, and autophony. Patients may complain of crackling or popping noises as some air enters the middle ear. Otitis media with effusion typically lacks otalgia, but some patients may report the aural fullness as uncomfortable. Otoscopic findings vary, but often there is an amber-colored effusion that may have air bubbles. On pneumatoscopy, there is limited or no excursion of the tympanic membrane. Audiometric testing demonstrates a flat conductive hearing loss and tympanometry reveals a flat curve with normal ear canal volume and absent reflexes. On imaging (eg, CT scanning or MRI), opacification of the middle-ear and mastoid spaces without erosion of the mastoid septa is seen.

Pathologic manifestations include a serous or mucoid fluid collection of variable viscosity in the middle-ear and mastoid air cell spaces (Figure 25–3). Children tend to have more mucoid effusions, whereas adults have effusions that are more serous. The effusion lacks inflammatory cells, although bacterial colonization can occasionally be identified. There is no erosion of the mastoid air cell septa or of cortical bone. With otitis media with effusion of long duration, atrophy of the tympanic membrane as well as ossicular fixation and erosion can occur.[11]

Chronic Otitis Media

Chronic otitis media (COM) is an inflammatory process in the middle-ear space that results in long-term, or more often, permanent changes in the tympanic membrane including atelectasis, dimer (formerly "monomer") formation, perforation, tympanosclerosis, retraction pocket development, or

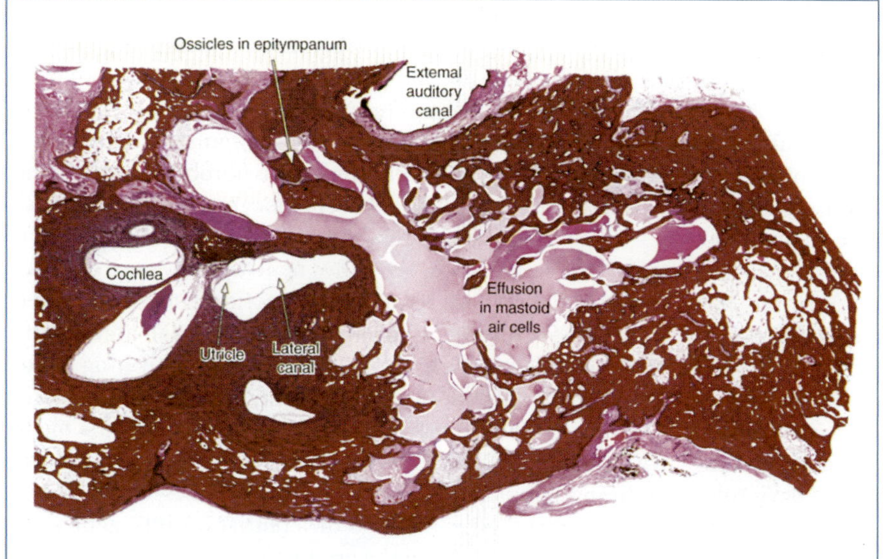

FIGURE 25–3 • Serous otitis media. Hematoxylin and eosin stained temporal bone slide through the epitympanum at the level of the head of the malleus and body of the incus demonstrates an eosinophilic effusion within the middle ear and mastoid air cell system.

cholesteatoma. There is variable involvement of the ossicular chain. Chronic otitis media results from long-term Eustachian tube dysfunction with a poorly aerated middle-ear space, multiple bouts of acute otitis media, persistent middle-ear infection, or other chronic inflammatory stimulus. Chronic otitis media can be classified as active, inactive, and inactive with frequent reactivation. The classification scheme followed here for COM was developed by Nadol[12] and is presented below (Table 25–1).

Inflammation of the middle ear and mastoid follows a spectrum of changes in a continuum. Consequently, the discussion of the sequence of inflammation and the cytokines involved provided above regarding acute otitis media and otitis media with effusion are relevant to COM and will not be repeated. Why some patients progress from the acute to the chronic state while others resolve in a timely fashion remains largely unknown.

The clinical presentation of COM varies with the underlying severity of the infection, the host response, and the time course over which it manifests. It is not uncommon for COM to be entirely asymptomatic, particularly in children who often do not complain of hearing loss. In general, the primary symptom of COM is conductive hearing loss, but patients may also present with otalgia, otorrhea, aural fullness, pulsatile tinnitus, and otorrhagia.

TABLE 25–1 Classification of chronic otitis media

Classification
Chronic active otitis media
With cholesteatoma
Without cholesteatoma
Chronic inactive otitis media
With perforation
With retraction pocket
Adhesive otitis media
With ossicular fixation or resorption
Chronic inactive otitis media with frequent reactivation

From Nadol JB.[12]

Chronic Active Otitis Media with Cholesteatoma

Cholesteatoma is an erosive process defined by trapped squamous epithelium that produces and accumulates desquamated keratin debris. Its annual incidence is estimated at 3 per 100,000 in children and 9.2 per 100,000 in adults, with a slight male predominance (1.4X female), based on a study of Finnish and Danish individuals.[13] Cholesteatoma can be divided into two general categories: congenital and acquired.

Bone erosion is present in the majority of mature cholesteatomas. Initially, bone erosion is confined to the ossicular chain and scutum. As the cholesteatoma expands, erosion of the otic capsule, fallopian canal, and tegmen can occur. The etiopathology of bone erosion is not well understood as it is complex and multifactorial. As the cholesteatoma contacts bone, the normal mucosal lining degenerates and inflammatory mediators of destruction such as macrophages, monocytes, and osteoclasts begin to appear in large numbers. Substantially increased populations of mast cells have been found in granulation tissue and in ossicles along their eroded surfaces.[14] Multinucleated osteoclasts have been identified as the cell responsible for bone resorption in cholesteatomas.[15–17]

Lipopolysaccharides, the primary component of bacterial cell walls, have been found in higher concentrations in patients with cholesteatoma and active bone destruction than in patients with cholesteatoma without bone destruction.[17] Lipopolysaccharides stimulate osteoclastic bone resorption by inducing maturation of preosteoclastic cells, but only if these cells are primed with a receptor activator NF-kB (RANKL).[18] Once activated, a variety of cytokines is secreted in elevated levels in cholesteatomas and perpetuates this process of osteoclastic activation and bone destruction. These cytokines include epidermal growth factor, TNF-α, IL-1a, IL-1b, IL-6, INF B, and PTHrP.[19–21] Nitric oxide, particularly nitric oxide type II, has been shown to enhance osteoclastic activation and is formed synergistically by the cytokines IL-1B, TNF-α, and

IFN-g.[22] The exact nature of their interaction and the other cytokines involved await elucidation, but an ongoing inflammatory response seems crucial.

Studies have also shown that cholesteatomas, unlike normal epithelium, no longer have the proper homeostasis of keratinocyte growth and programmed cell death (apoptosis). Measures of the proliferative marker Ki-67 show levels that are dramatically elevated in cholesteatoma when compared to normal postauricular skin from the same patient. Furthermore, measures of cell death, such as caspase-3, a marker for apoptosis, are not detected in cholesteatomas. These findings were confirmed using other markers of apoptosis such as the *t*erminal deoxynucleotide transferase mediated d*U*TP *n*ick *e*nd *l*abeling technique (TUNEL test).[23]

Biofilms have been implicated in cholesteatoma formation. Both gram-positive and gram-negative bacteria have been identified in a biofilm of extracellular matrix within keratin debris. Biofilms have been shown to have direct effects on epithelial cell signaling, such as induction of epidermal growth factors and upregulation of cytokines, specifically IL-6.[24] Theoretically, the altered epithelial cell signaling explains the imbalance in homeostatic growth of keratinocytes noted above, which then leads to a hyperkeratotic state, accelerating the formation of cholesteatoma matrix and keratin debris. Biofilm formation can also help explain the difficulty in eradicating the frequent infections that occur with cholesteatomas.

Congenital Cholesteatoma

Congenital cholesteatoma comprises squamous epithelium retained in the middle-ear space during embryologic migration of squamous cells. There is no connection to the tympanic membrane, which is normal in appearance and intact. The criteria for the diagnosis of congenital cholesteatoma are stringent and they include: (1) a normal tympanic membrane, (2) no history of prior ear infections, and (3) no history of prior ear surgery including tympanostomy tubes. Congenital cholesteatoma most commonly occurs in the anterosuperior quadrant of the middle-ear space reflecting the pathway of embryologic cell migration.

The typical clinical presentation consists of a painless, whitish mass behind the tympanic membrane along with a variably severe conductive hearing loss, depending on the size of the cholesteatoma (Figure 25–4). Imaging demonstrates a soft tissue mass in the middle-ear space that, as it enlarges, causes varying degrees of bony erosion of the tegmen, ossicular chain, mastoid, and otic capsule. A congenital cholesteatoma typically does not erode the scutum, in contradistinction to acquired cholesteatoma, which does erode the scutum.

The pathology of congenital cholesteatoma features a keratin cyst surrounded by epithelial cells that do not contact the tympanic membrane. The squamous epithelium surrounding the keratin debris can erode into the ossicular chain.

Acquired Cholesteatoma

Acquired cholesteatoma arises from squamous epithelium that has migrated into the middle-ear space via retraction of the tympanic membrane or through a perforation of the tympanic membrane. The trapped squamous epithelium produces keratin debris that are desquamated and accumulate, resulting in bone erosion with progressive enlargement.

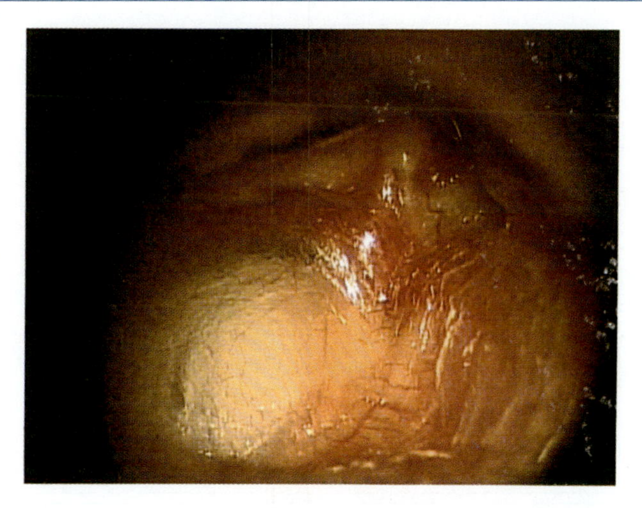

FIGURE 25–4 • Chronic otitis media with cholesteatoma (congenital). This photograph demonstrates a congenital cholesteatoma. The cholesteatoma can be seen posteriorly behind an intact eardrum.

An acquired cholesteatoma can be further subcategorized depending on its location. Attic cholesteatomas, resulting from retraction of the pars flaccida of the tympanic membrane, are the most common. Posterior-superior retractions extend into the posterior mesotympanum, facial recess, sinus tympani, and can pass through the aditus ad antrum into the mastoid air cells. Finally, pars tensa cholesteatomas, the least common type, result from retraction or perforation of the entire pars tensa of the tympanic membrane and invariably involve the eustachian tube orifice, the attic, and the mastoid.[25]

The clinical presentation of an acquired cholesteatoma is typified by retraction or perforation of the tympanic membrane with trapped squamous debris seen on otoscopy (Figure 25–5). The pars flaccida of the tympanic membrane is the most common site of cholesteatoma formation. Typically, a cholesteatoma causes conductive hearing loss as it affects the ossicular chain. A key diagnostic distinction detected by CT scanning is scutal erosion, present in acquired cholesteatoma, but absent in congenital cholesteatoma.

Pathologic examination demonstrates a keratin cyst with a tympanic membrane retraction or perforation in continuity with the cyst (Figure 25–6). In contradistinction, in a congenital cholesteatoma there is no connection between the tympanic membrane and the cholesteatoma. An epithelial lining surrounds the keratin cyst. A variety of inflammatory cells can be seen, along with evidence of infection and bacterial colonization.

Chronic Active Otitis Media Without Cholesteatoma

Chronic active otitis media without cholesteatoma is a chronic inflammatory process of the middle ear and mastoid. Clinically, it presents with chronic otorrhea that varies in amount, color, and consistency. Typically, otalgia is not severe and consists of a dull earache that waxes and wanes. Otorrhagia can occur, particularly with aural polyp formation. Hearing loss is virtually

FIGURE 25–5 • Chronic otitis media with cholesteatoma (acquired). This photograph demonstrates an acquired cholesteatoma. A retraction of the tympanic membrane within the attic contains keratin debris.

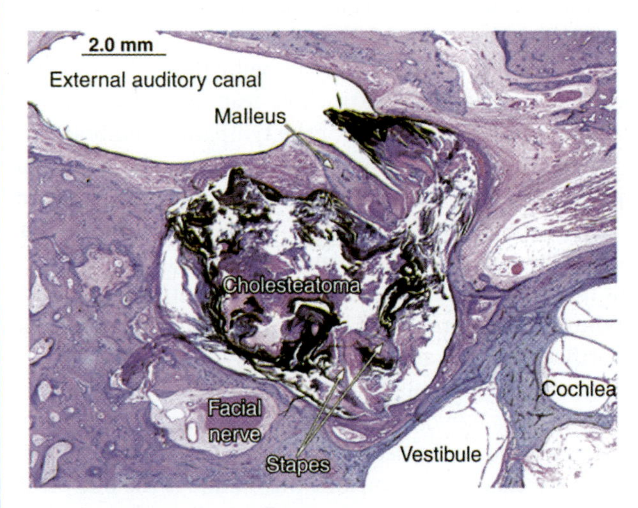

FIGURE 25–6 • Chronic otitis media with cholesteatoma. Hematoxylin and eosin stained temporal bone slide through the mesotympanum at the level of the stapes footplate demonstrates an acquired cholesteatoma. A keratin filled sac fills the entire middle-ear space eroding the stapes suprastructure. The entry point into the middle-ear cavity can be seen through the defect within the tympanic membrane.

always present and conductive. Chronic active otitis media without cholesteatoma is an indolent process that can persist for years, or indefinitely, in the absence of definitive management.

Pathologically, there is considerable inflammation in the middle ear and mastoid (Figure 25–7). Early in the course of inflammation, mucosal edema along with submucosal fibrosis and hyperemia are typical. An inflammatory infiltrate is present and usually comprises lymphocytes rather than polymorphonuclear cells. Plasma cells, histiocytes, and macrophages are also usually present. As the condition progresses, soft, friable granulation tissue begins to form, which consists of new capillaries

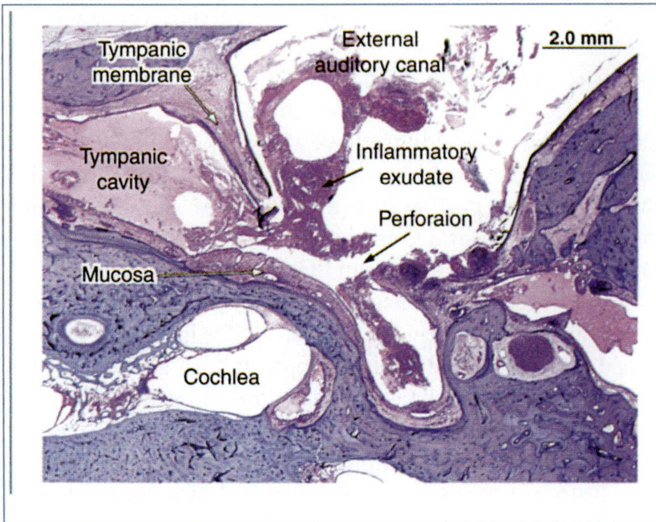

FIGURE 25–7 • Chronic otitis media without cholesteatoma—active. Hematoxylin and eosin stained temporal bone slide through the hypotympanum at the level of the basal turn of the cochlea shows an active inflammatory process. A perforation in the tympanic membrane is identified with an inflammatory exudate extending from the external auditory canal into the hypotympanic space. The mucosal lining as well as the remaining portion of the tympanic membrane are quite edematous.

and connective tissue as well as inflammatory cells. Variable amounts of mucoid and purulent otorrhea occur chronically. When inflammation persists, the hyperemic, inflamed mucosa forms aural polyps. These polyps can be impressive, filling the middle-ear space entirely or prolapsing through the tympanic membrane perforation and filling the entirety of the external auditory canal. With continued inflammation, the mastoid air cell tracts can become blocked, occasionally causing the formation of a cholesterol granuloma—a reaction of giant cells to cholesterol crystals from degraded blood products. Ossicular erosion can occur and is thought to follow similar mechanisms described earlier for cholesteatoma.

Chronic Inactive Otitis Media With Perforation

Chronic inactive otitis media with perforation is a permanent perforation of the tympanic membrane without any ongoing inflammatory process or infection in the middle ear or mastoid. The tympanic membrane has been ruptured in the past as part of previous acute or chronic inflammation. Perforations can be in the pars flaccida or pars tensa of the tympanic membrane, and can be marginal, central, subtotal, or total.

Pathologically, the tympanic membrane is perforated but there is no inflammation of the middle-ear space or mucosa (Figure 25–8). The perforation can be surrounded by healthy residual tympanic membrane or by tympanosclerosis, a dimeric membrane, or thick scar. The perforation can extend to the fibrous annulus and, rarely, involve it. The lamina propria of the tympanic membrane can thicken at the periphery of the perforation due to fibrous tissue proliferation.

Although the mucocutaneous junction (the junction of the squamous epithelial layer of the tympanic membrane and the mucosa of the medial tympanic membrane) is typically located at the edge of the perforation, in some cases, epithelial

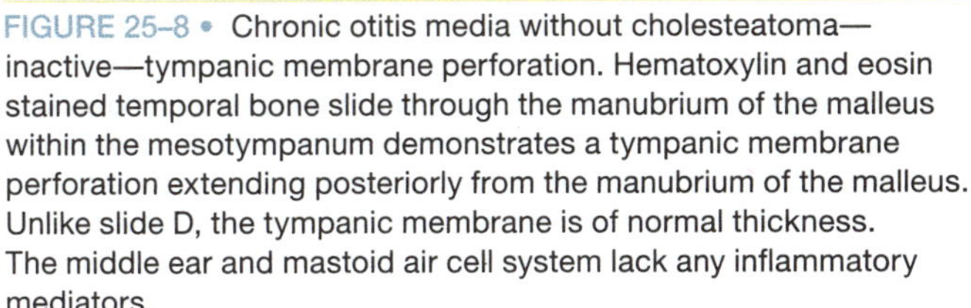

FIGURE 25–8 • Chronic otitis media without cholesteatoma—inactive—tympanic membrane perforation. Hematoxylin and eosin stained temporal bone slide through the manubrium of the malleus within the mesotympanum demonstrates a tympanic membrane perforation extending posteriorly from the manubrium of the malleus. Unlike slide D, the tympanic membrane is of normal thickness. The middle ear and mastoid air cell system lack any inflammatory mediators.

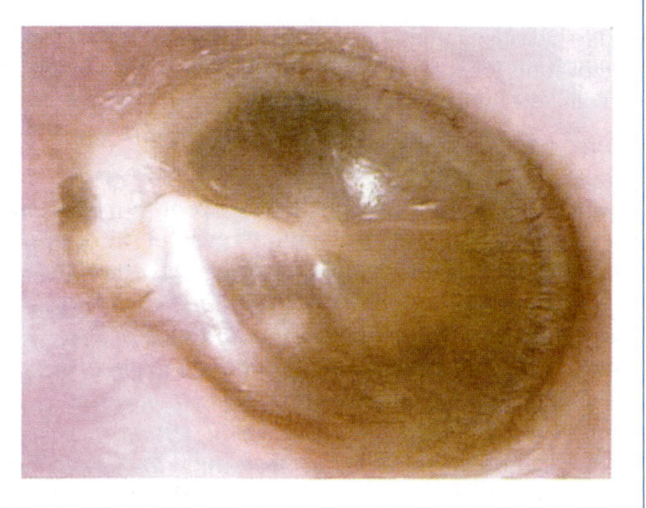

FIGURE 25–9 • Chronic otitis media without cholesteatoma—retraction pocket. This photograph demonstrates a retraction pocket in the pars flaccida region of the tympanic membrane down onto the neck of the malleus above the short process of the malleus. The tympanic membrane is also retracted down onto the incudostapedial joint. No keratin debris is collecting.

cells migrate medially through the perforation rather than stopping at the edge. The cause of this migration is not known, but it does have significant clinical implications. The appearance of an epithelial lining within the middle-ear space is different from the normal mucosal lining in that the squamous layer has a velvety or bumpy appearance under magnification. If the tympanic membrane is surgically repaired and the migrated epithelial cells not removed from the middle-ear space, an iatrogenic cholesteatoma forms.

Chronic Inactive Otitis Media With Retraction Pocket

Chronic inactive otitis media with retraction pocket implies that any ongoing inflammation has resolved but a portion of the tympanic membrane is retracted into the middle ear or attic (Figure 25–9). This situation can result from several conditions. One possibility is chronic Eustachian tube dysfunction, a condition that certainly can persist despite resolution of inflammation. The ensuing negative middle-ear pressure pulls the tympanic membrane medially, creating a retraction pocket. Negative pressure can also occur from a lack of ventilation through the aditus ad antrum, a so-called attic block. Once a retraction pocket has developed, a subclinical inflammatory state can evolve in the epithelial tissue, resulting in adhesions that tether the tympanic membrane to the ossicles, promontory mucosa, or medial aspect of the scutum. Ongoing inflammation can drive the retraction pocket further into the middle ear or mastoid, despite correction of the middle-ear pressure imbalance. Alternatively, irreversible adhesions can result from the acute inflammatory phase of infection. When a substantial portion of the tympanic membrane retracts and becomes adherent to the medial wall of the middle ear, it is termed adhesive otitis media (see below—chronic inactive otitis media with adhesive otitis media).

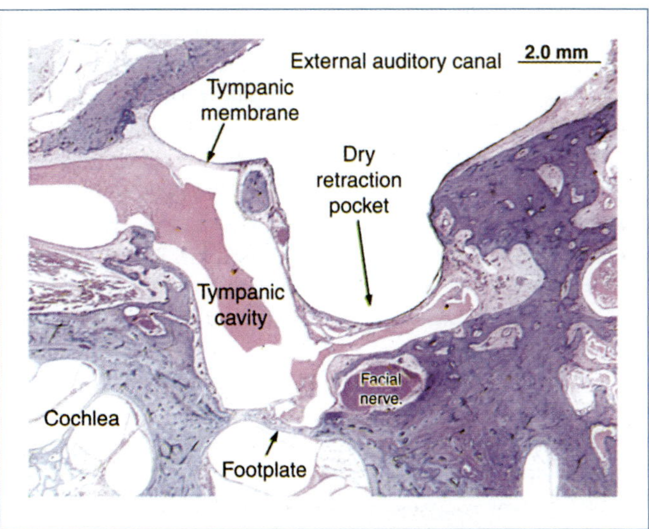

FIGURE 25–10 • Chronic otitis media without cholesteatoma—inactive—retraction pocket. Hematoxylin and eosin stained temporal bone slide at the level of the stapes footplate within the mesotympanum shows a retraction pocket of the tympanic membrane. The tympanic membrane is displaced inward in close approximation to the facial nerve. There are some subclinical eosinophilic exudates within the tympanic cavity.

Although retraction pockets are often precursors to cholesteatoma, some retraction pockets are quite stable and do not progress to cholesteatoma, even over a long period of time. A retraction pocket, by definition, does not have the retention keratin debris that is pathognomonic for cholesteatomas (Figure 25–10). Retraction pockets can involve any portion of the eardrum; but most often they involve the attic, the posterior quadrant, or a combination of both and is called a posterior-superior retraction pocket. Once a retraction pocket extends beyond clinical view, observation alone is deemed unwise as progression can go undetected. Such a retraction pocket can be an indication for surgical intervention even in the absence of overt cholesteatoma formation.

Chronic Inactive Otitis Media With Adhesive Otitis Media

Chronic inactive otitis media with adhesive otitis media comprises a stable, near total, or total retraction of the tympanic membrane onto the promontory, ossicles, and other middle-ear structures. Adhesions exist between the eardrum and these structures such that negative insufflation or even tympanostomy tube insertion cannot restore the drum to normal anatomic position (Figure 25–11). Negative pressure insufflation is accomplished by squeezing the air out of a Siegel pneumatic otoscope bulb before applying it to the ear, thus generating a negative pressure on the tympanic membrane. Adhesive otitis media can be stable, but it is difficult to predict which patients will worsen and go on to develop ossicular erosion from pressure necrosis, infection, or cholesteatoma formation.

Pathologically, the tympanic membrane is retracted into the middle-ear space and draped over the incus and stapes. The tympanic membrane thins and loses its lamina propria. An extreme form of adhesive otitis media is called epidermization of the middle ear (Figure 25–12), and it refers to a transformation of the normal mucosal lining of the middle ear into a squamous epithelial lining. No keratin debris are retained. Epidermization can follow either a profound retraction, which after adhesion development becomes incorporated into the middle-ear lining, or ingrowth of epithelial cells through an existing perforation, which then carpet the middle ear. Epidermization can involve either a portion of the middle ear or the entire middle ear. Epidermization can remain stable without necessarily evolving into a cholesteatoma. Progression, however, is variable and difficult to predict clinically.

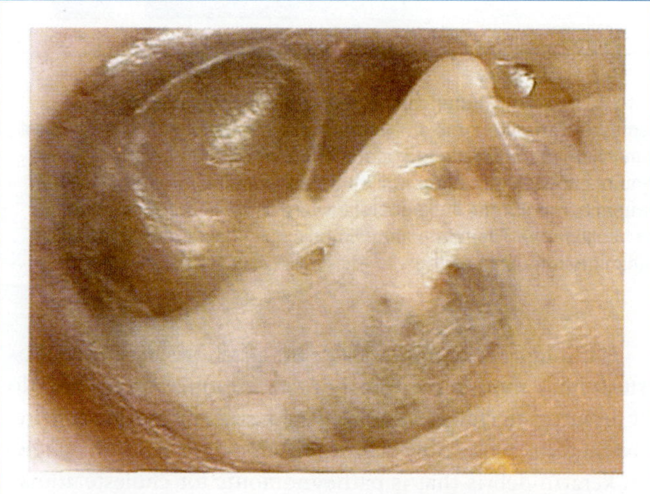

FIGURE 25–11 • Chronic otitis media without cholesteatoma—adhesive otitis media. This photograph demonstrates an atelectatic tympanic membrane which is retracted medially.

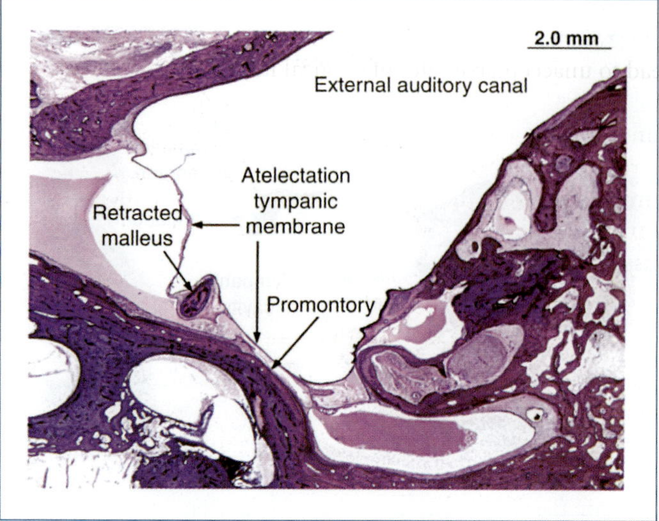

FIGURE 25–12 • Chronic otitis media without cholesteatoma—inactive—epidermization. Hematoxylin and eosin stained temporal bone slide at the level of the promontory within the mesotympanum demonstrates a thinned tympanic membrane draped onto the promontory of the cochlea. The malleus is substantially retracted medially and adhesed onto the promontory. The epidermal layer of the tympanic membrane is now covering the medial wall of the middle-ear space resulting in epidermization.

Chronic Inactive Otitis Media With Ossicular Fixation or Resorption

Chronic inactive otitis media with ossicular fixation or resorption is a complication of chronic otitis media. Some patients have substantial fixation of the ossicular chain, including the malleus, incus, and/or stapes in combinations. Ossicular fixation typically is the result of tympanosclerosis of the head of the malleus or the body of the incus in the attic, or of the stapes footplate around the annular ligament. Adhesions can also form medial to the tympanic membrane, impeding the normal mobility of the ossicular chain.

Ossicular resorption is common with chronic inactive otitis media. The incudostapedial joint is particularly vulnerable to resorption given the tenuous blood supply to the lenticular process of the incus, as well as its delicate structure. However, resorption can occur at any part of the ossicles, and often involves the long process of the incus and the capitulum and crura of the stapes. Involvement of the body of the incus and the manubrium of the malleus can occur but are less common. It remains unclear why some ears progress to ossicular fixation, whereas others develop ossicular erosions.

Chronic Inactive Otitis Media With Frequent Reactivation

Although the inflammation is not continuously active, frequent flare-ups are present. These episodes of reactivation or flare-ups usually are not caused by an inciting event, such as water exposure or an upper respiratory tract infection. Rather, although the patient is able to return to a clinically inactive state after each flare-up, a subclinical, inflammatory condition persists in the middle ear and mastoid air cell system. It is the subclinical inflammatory condition that waxes and wanes. Consequently, treatment must address this subclinical disease.

For example, simple tympanic membrane closure without addressing the subclinical mastoid inflammatory condition will lead to unacceptable rates of surgical failure.

Chronic inactive otitis media with frequent reactivation can persist indefinitely, progress to chronic active otitis media, or resolve into chronic inactive otitis media. Depending on the timing of histopathologic evaluation, the ear either appears actively infected or mimics inactive chronic otitis media (discussed earlier).

Granulomatous Diseases

The granulomatous diseases are, in general, uncommon but important. When a patient fails to respond to standard treatments for chronic otitis media, a high index of suspicion for a granulomatous disorder must be maintained. It is often helpful to obtain tissue in such cases for definitive diagnosis and appropriate treatment. A brief review of four granulomatous diseases is provided in the following sections.

Tuberculosis

Tuberculosis is an infection caused by *Mycobacterium tuberculosis* and is spread via respiratory droplets. In 2006, 13,767 cases of tuberculosis were reported in the United States or 4.6 cases per 100,000 individuals, according to the Center for Disease Control and Prevention, representing a decline of 3.2% from the preceding year. The prevalence of tuberculosis in foreign-born individuals was 9.5 times the rate in US-born individuals.[26] According to the World Health Organization, a new case of tuberculosis occurs each second. Furthermore, one-third of the world's population is currently infected with *M. tuberculosis*.[27]

Although virtually every organ system can be involved, pulmonary involvement and the resulting symptoms predominate, including chronic cough, hemoptysis, and dyspnea. Spread into the middle ear and mastoid occurs either through direct extension of the upper airway infection via the Eustachian tube, or by hematogenous seeding. The classic description of otic tuberculosis comprises a tympanic membrane with multiple perforations or one coalescent perforation. Intraoperative findings include thick, pale granulation tissue; but often the clinical and intraoperative findings are indistinguishable from ordinary chronic suppurative otitis media. The infection is usually painless and is often associated with serous or purulent drainage and a conductive hearing loss. Therefore, tuberculosis should be included in the differential diagnosis of a draining ear that is resistant to the usual topical therapy, especially if in a patient from an endemic area or the inner city. Although the diagnosis can be made through cell culture, *M. tuberculosis* is quite difficult to culture and is slow growing usually requiring at least 6 weeks for culture results to become positive. Real-time nucleic acid polymerase chain reaction (PCR) assays for tuberculosis are now available as a rapid tool for *M. tuberculosis* identification in samples. The purified protein derivative (PPD) test, a skin test for tuberculosis, along with a chest x-ray and sputum cultures can be used to screen patients for active pulmonary disease.

Treatment for active tuberculosis usually involves four drugs given concurrently—isonazid, rifampin, pyrizinamide, and ethambutol—for a minimum of 6 months, but more typically 1 year. Streptomycin also has activity against *M. tuberculosis*. Surgical treatment is limited to biopsies.

The hallmark histopathologic finding of tuberculosis is a caseating granuloma. Temporal bone histopathology varies widely. Tympanic membrane thickening, tympanic membrane perforation (multiple or coalescent), middle-ear hyperemia, inflammatory effusion, ossicular erosion, and temporal bone destruction have all been documented.[28]

Wegener's Granulomatosis

Wegener's granulomatosis was first described by Klinger in 1931, but Wegener is credited as the first to report it as a distinct clinical entity.[29,30] Wegener's granulomatosis is an idiopathic, granulomatous necrotizing vasculitis. Smaller vessels such as capillaries and small arterioles are typically involved. The incidence of Wegener's granulomatosis is 3.14 per million, with a slight female predominance and a predilection for Caucasians.[31,32] The peak age at onset ranges from 45 to 65 years.[32] Organ involvement includes the kidneys, lungs, and upper aerodigestive tract, with otic involvement occurring in 19 to 56% of patients.[33] Otic presentation includes conductive hearing loss, sensorineural hearing loss, tinnitus, vertigo, otalgia, facial nerve paresis, and otorrhea. There is usually a draining tympanic membrane perforation and the mucosa has prominent, often pale, edematous changes. The clinical picture of otic Wegener's disease is one of medically-refractory, purulent chronic otitis media. This initial presentation mimics tuberculosis except that there is usually a disproportionate degree of pain. Neurologic involvement is estimated at 15 to 30% with cranial nerve involvement at 7% in a 1993 review of 324 patients.[34,35] Current theories hypothesize that the antineutrophil cytoplasmic antibody c-ANCA forms against complementary peptide sequences to proteinase-3, termed PR3. These antibodies may be introduced or induced by exogenous infectious pathogens, with *Staphylococcus aureus* being implicated in many cases. *S. aureus* has a protein with a peptide sequence quite similar to that of PR3. The c-ANCA then causes damage by activating neutrophils, releasing free radicals and lytic enzymes.[36]

The original diagnostic criteria of Godman and Churg for Wegener's granulomatosis comprised a triad of upper respiratory tract granulomas, necrotizing vasculitis, and glomerulonephritis.[37] It is now recognized that there is a characteristic vasculitis that can be limited to just one organ. Biopsies can confirm the diagnosis, but in the ear, often show only nonspecific inflammation. Sinonasal biopsies have the highest specificity and sensitivity for the diagnosis. Diagnosis can be aided with a highly specific and sensitive serum marker, c-ANCA. However, up to 30% of cases can be c-ANCA negative, particularly in the more limited forms of the disease. Although in the past the prognosis was dismal, advances in treatment now result in a greater than 70% remission rate.

Treatment is initially directed toward the induction of remission with cyclophosphamide or methotrexate, combined with glucocorticoids. Maintenance of remission can be accomplished with methotrexate, azathioprine, and glucocorticoids. Antistaphylococcal antibiotics such as cotrimazole or trimethoprim have had mixed long-term results. Although the TNF-α blocker etanercept did not show efficacy in preliminary studies, the T-cell and B-cell inhibitor of differentiation, deoxyspergualin, showed promise in refractory cases leading to complete or partial remission in all cases.[38] Surgical management with either myringotomy or mastoidectomy has been associated with an exacerbation of the clinical course.[39]

The histopathology of Wegener's is characterized by non-caseating granulomas with necrotizing vasculitis of the small blood vessels. Temporal bone involvement includes granulation tissue in the middle-ear space, often at the Eustachian tube orifice, along with fibrous deposits in the submucosal layer of the middle ear and mastoid with necrotizing blood vessels surrounded by leucocytic infiltration. Also, proteinaceous material in the perilymphatic space, hair cell degeneration, edema of the spiral ligament, ossification of the cochlear turns, and thickening of the round-window membrane with invasion of the membranous labyrinth have been documented.[40,41]

Langerhan's Cell Histiocytosis

Langerhan's cell histiocytosis, also termed Histiocytosis X, is a granulomatous disease of unknown etiology. It can involve almost any organ system and has a wide scope of possible presentations (Table 25–2). One notable characteristic is the development of well-circumscribed, lytic lesions with scalloped edges seen on radiographic examination.

Otologic manifestations can be the initial presentation of the disease, including otorrhea, postauricular swelling, hearing loss, and vertigo.[33,42] Facial nerve involvement occurs in of 3% of all cases of LCH.[42]

Langerhan's cell histiocytosis is divided into three subtypes: Eosinophilic granuloma, Hand-Schuller-Christian disease, and Letterer-Siwe disease.

Eosinophilic granuloma is the localized form of LCH, lacking multiorgan, systemic involvement. It typically affects older children and young adults with a slight male-to-female predilection. It is characterized by osteolytic lesions, typically of the temporal and frontal bones. These bony lesions can be painful or asymptomatic. Treatment involves surgical excision, intralesional steroids, or low-dose (around 24 Gy) radiation therapy.[43] Adjuvant chemotherapy may be employed in individualized cases. The prognosis is excellent.

Hand-Schuller-Christian disease is a chronic, disseminated form of LCH that affects children and young adults. It is characterized by osteolytic lesions, typically of the mandible and skull. It also has systemic manifestations involving multiple organ systems (see Table 25–2). These systemic manifestations usually become evident within 6 months of the initial lesion.[44] Twenty-five percent of patients present with the triad of an osteolytic skull lesion, exopthalmos, and diabetes insipidus due to sphenoid roof erosion into the sella turcica.[45] Treatment is surgical excision, if possible, combined with chemotherapy and radiation therapy. The mortality rate approximates 30%.

Letterer-Siwe disease is the acute, disseminated form of LCH. It affects children less than 3 years of age. The presentation is acute with multiple bony lesions and extra skeletal systemic involvement such as fever, proptosis, hepatosplenomegaly, adenopathy, anemia, thrombocytopenia, and exfoliative dermatitis. Treatment is with chemotherapy using vinblastine, vincristine, methotrexate, cyclophosphamide, or other cytotoxic drugs along with intravenous high-dose corticosteroids. The prognosis is quite poor and the fatality rate is correspondingly high. Histopathologically, LCH is characterized by sheets of polygonal histiocytes (Langerhan's cells). These sheets of histiocytes rest in a background of inflammatory cells, such as eosinophils, lymphocytes, macrophages, and multinucleated giant cells. The Langerhan's cell is characterized by Birbeck granules (also called X bodies), which are trilaminar rod-shaped organelles in the nuclear cytoplasm as seen on electron microscopic evaluation. It is unclear whether the Langerhan's cell is neoplastic or reactive. These cells stain S-100 positive and/or CD1a positive, and have eosinophilic cytoplasm. Temporal bone involvement can manifest as erosion of the external auditory canal wall, mastoid cortex, bony labyrinth, squamous bone, zygomatic bone, or petrous bone.[46]

TABLE 25–2 Organ system involvement in Langerhan's cell histiocytosis

Bone	Flat/long bones, skull, ribs, vertebrae, pelvis, mandible, maxilla, scapulae
Otologic	Otorrhea, conductive hearing loss, sensorineural hearing loss, otalgia, facial paralysis, mastoiditis, otitis media, otitis externa
Ophthalmologic	Proptosis
Gastrointestinal	Hepatosplenomegaly, malabsorption
Oral	Gingival swelling, oral masses, loose or missing teeth
Lymphatic	Anterior cervical lymphadenopathy, other lymphadenopathy
Dermatologic	Scaly yellow-brown plaques, greasy popular rash with petechia, purpura, exfoliative dermatitis
Neuroendocrine	Diabetes insipidus, delayed growth, hypogonadism, truncal ataxia, tremors, seizures, cranial neuropathies
Hematologic	Anemia, leukocytosis, thrombocytopenia, elevated sedimentation rate
Pulmonary	Bilateral infiltrates with reticular or reticulonodular pattern, fibrosis
Constitutional	Fever, malaise

Mycotic Diseases

Fungal infection and inflammation can be divided into two broad categories: superficial and invasive. Superficial infections involve colonization of the external auditory canal and middle ear. These superficial infections result in minimal symptoms such as ear itching, otorrhea, and mild otalgia,[47] as often occurs in immunocompetent patients after topical or systemic antimicrobial therapy decreases the normal bacterial flora of the middle ear and ear canal skin. Although the most common site for superficial fungal colonization is the external auditory canal, the tympanic membrane, as well as the middle-ear space, can be involved.[48] *Candida* and *Aspergillus* are common superficial fungal pathogens. Otoscopy reveals spores that can be either white or black. Treatment is with debridement followed by topical antifungal agents such as clotrimezole 1% topical drops or lotrimin/triamcinolone ointment.

Invasive fungal infections usually occur in immunocompromised patients. *Cryptococcus* typically presents with neurologic symptoms, such as headache, confusion, depression, and agitation, with spread to the temporal bone in terminal cases. Aspergillosis most often begins as a pulmonary infection with direct seeding of the Eustachian tube and middle ear. Mucormycosis involves the sinonasal cavity and orbit and follows a fulminant course. All three pathogens have been found to involve the temporal bone but their development into an invasive fungal infection of the external ear canal, middle ear, or mastoid in an immunocompetent patient is an extremely rare event.[49–52] The presentation consists of acute, severe otalgia along with otorrhea, otorrhagia, and hearing loss, either sensorineural or conductive. Vertigo, facial paralysis, and other cranial neuropathies can also occur.[53] In invasive cases, Fungi of the order *Mucor* are most commonly implicated, followed by *Aspergillus* and *Cryptococcus*. Treatment consists of emergent surgical debridement and systemic antifungal therapy, such as amphotericin-B. Invasive fungal infections carry a high morbidity and mortality.

Histopathologically, the fungal infection can be identified by recognition of its characteristic appearance. *Candida* is dimorphic, meaning it exists in two forms; more common is the unicellular, nonfilamentous form, but *Candida* can also exist in a pseudohyphae form. *Cryptococcus* is a unicellular fungus that is nonfilamentous and spherical. *Aspergillus* has acutely branching septate hyphae. Mucor has branching hyphae but is nonseptate. Fungal infections can induce the development of caseating granulomas. Critical features of invasive fungal infections are vascular thrombosis and widespread tissue necrosis, which are never seen with superficial infections. Invasive fungal infections of the temporal bone include middle-ear involvement of the submucosa and tympanic membrane as well as infiltration of the nerves in the internal auditory canal, the membranous labyrinth, Rosenthal's canal with loss of cochlear neurons, and labyrinthine artery occlusion.[50,54]

ACKNOWLEDGMENTS

I would like to personally thank Dr. Saumil Merchant for his expertise and assistance in producing this chapter. I would also like to thank Robert Galla for processing the temporal bone slides and capturing the pathologic images.

References

1. Bulut Y, Guven M, Otlu B, et al. Acute otitis media and respiratory viruses. Eur J Pediatr 2007;166:223–8.
2. Chonmaitree T, Patel JA, Garofalo R, et al. Role of leukotriene B4 and interleukin-8 in acute bacterial and viral otitis media. Ann Otol Rhinol Laryngol 1996;105:968–74.
3. Leibovitz E, Dagan R, Laver J, et al. Interleukin 8 in middle ear fluid during acute otitis media: Correlation with aetiology and bacterial eradication. Arch Dis Childhood 2000;82:165–8.
4. Barzilai A, Dekel B, Dagan R, Passwell J, Leibovitz E. Cytokine analysis of middle ear effusions during acute otitis media: Significant reduction in tumor necrosis factor alpha concentrations correlates with bacterial eradication. Ped Inf Dis J 1999;18:303–10.
5. Barzilai A, Dekel B, Dagan R, Leibovitz. Middle ear effusion IL-6 concentration in bacterial and non-bacterial acute otitis media. Acta Paediatr 2000;89:1068–71.
6. Bluestone CD. Clinical course, complications and sequelae of acute otitis media. Ped Inf Dis J 2000;19:37–46.
7. Post JC. Direct evidence of bacterial biofilms in otitis media. Laryngoscope 2001;111:2083–94.
8. Hall-Stoodley L, Fen Ze H, Gieseke A, et al. Direct detection of bacterial biofilms on the middle ear mucosa of children with chronic otitis media. JAMA 2006;296:202–11.
9. Coates H, Thornton R, Langlands J, et al. The role of chronic infection in children with otitis media with effusion: evidence for intracellular persistence of bacteria. Otolaryngol Head Neck Surg 2008;138:778–81.
10. Smirnova M, Kiselev S, Gnuchev N, Birchall J, Pearson J. Role of the pro-inflammatory cytokines tumor necrosis factor-alpha, interleukin-1b, interleukin-6 and interleukin-8 in the pathogenesis of the otitis media with effusion. Eur Cytokine Network 2002;13:161–72.
11. Schuknecht HF. Infections. Otitis media with effusion. In: Pathology of the ear, 2nd edition. Philadelphia, PA: Lea and Febiger; 1993. p. 234.
12. Nadol JB. The chronic draining ear. Current therapy in Otolaryngol. Head Neck Surg 1987;18:18–22.
13. Kemppainen HO, Puhakka JH, Laippala PJ, Sipila MM, Manninen MP, Karma PH. Epidemiology and aetiology of middle ear cholesteatoma. Acta Otolarygol 1999;119:568–72.
14. Berger G, Hawke M, Ekem JK. Bone resorption in chronic otitis media. The role of mast cells. Acta Otolaryngol 1985;100:72–80.
15. Chole R. Osteoclasts in chronic otitis media, cholesteatoma and otosclerosis. Ann Otol Rhinol Laryngol 1988;97:661–6.
16. Jung J, Chole R. Bone resorption in chronic otitis media: The role of the osteoclast. ORL J Otorhinolaryngol Relat Spec 2002;64:95–107.
17. Peek F, Huisman M, Berckmans R, Sturk A, van Loon J, Grote J. Lipopolysaccharide concentration and bone resorption in cholesteatoma. Otol Neurotol 2003;24:709–13.
18. Nason R, Jung J, Chole R. Lipopolysacharide-induced osteoclastogenesis from mononuclear precursors: A mechanism for osteolysis in chronic otitis. JARO 2009;10:151–60.
19. Ahn JM, Huang CC, Abramson M. Localization of interleukin-1 in human cholesteatoma. Am J Otolaryngol 1990;11:71–7.
20. Schilling V, Negri B, Bujia J, Schulz P, Kastenbauer E. Possible role of interleukin 1-α and interleukin 1-β in the pathogenesis of cholesteatoma of the middle ear. Am J Otol 1992;13:350–5.
21. Yetiser S, Satar B, Aydin N. Expression of epidermal growth factor, tumor necrosis factor-alpha, and interleukin-1a in chronic

otitis media with or without cholesteatoma. Otol Neurotol 2002;23:647–52.

22. Jung J, Pashia M, Nishimoto S, Faddis, Chole R. A possible role for nitric oxide in osteoclastogenesis associated with cholesteatoma. Otol Neurotol 2004;25:661–8.
23. Huisman M, De Heer E, Grote J. Cholesteatoma epithelium is characterized by increased expression of Ki-67, p53 and p21, with minimal apoptosis. Acta Otolaryngol 2003;123:377–82.
24. Chole RA, Faddis BT. Evidence for microbial biofilms in cholesteatomas. Arch Otolaryngol Head Neck Sur 2002;128:1129–33.
25. Tos M. Incidence, etiology, and pathogenesis of cholesteatoma in children. Otol Rhinol Laryngol 1988;40:100–17.
26. Voelker R. Pattern of US tuberculosis cases shifting. JAMA 2007;297:685.
27. World Health Organization. Tuberculosis. http://www.who.int/topics/tuberculosis/en/. Accessed March 15, 2008.
28. Schuknecht HF. Tuberculous otitis media and mastoiditis. In: Pathology of the Ear, 2nd ed. Philadelphia, PA: Lea and Febiger; 1993. p. 200.
29. Klinger H. Grenzformen der Periareterits nodosa. Frankfurt Z Pathol 1931;42:455–80.
30. Wegener F. Uber eine eigenartige rhinogene granulomatose mit besonderer beteiligung des Arteriensystems und der Nieren. Beitr Pathol Anat Pathol 1939;102:36–68.
31. Mahr AD, Neogi T, Merkel PA. Epidemiology of Wegener's granulomatosis: Lessons from descriptive studies and analyses of genetic and environmental risk determinants. Clin Exp Rheumatol 2006;24:82–91.
32. Abdou NI, Kullman GJ, Hoffman GS, et al. Wegener's granulomatosis: Survey of 701 patients in North America. Changes in outcome in the 1990s. J Rheumatol 2002;29:309–16.
33. McCaffrey TV, McDonald TJ, Facer GW, DeRemee RA. Otologic manifestations of Wegener's granulomatosis. Otolaryngol Head Neck Surg 1980;88:586–93.
34. Dwyer J, Janzen VD. Wegener's granulomatosis with otological and nervous system involvement. J Otolaryngology 1969;10:6.
35. Nishino H, Rubino FA, DeRemee RA, Swanson JW, Parisi JE. Neurological involvement in Wegener's granulomatosis: an analysis of 324 consecutive patients at the Mayo Clinic. Ann Neurol 1933;33:4–9.
36. Jennette JC, Xiao H, Falk RJ. Pathogenesis of vascular inflammation by antineutrophil cytoplasmic antibodies. J Am Soc Nephrol 2006;17:1235–42.
37. Godman GC, Churg J. Wegener's granulomatosis: Pathology and review of the literature. AMA Arch Pathol 1954;58:533–53.
38. Erickson VR, Hwang P. Wegener's granulomatosis: Current trends in diagnosis and management. Curr Opin Otolaryngol Head Neck Surg 2007;15:170–6.
39. Takagi D, Nakiamaru Y, Maguchi S, Furuta Y, Fukuda S. Otologic manifestations of Wegener's granulamtosis. Larngoscope 2002;12:1684–90.
40. Friedmann I, Bauer F. Wegener's granulomatosis causing deafness. J Laryngol Otol 1973;87:449–64.
41. Yoon TH, Paparella MM, Schachern PA. Systemic vasculitis: A temporal bone histopathologic study. Laryngoscope 1989;99: 600–9.
42. Tos M. Facial palsy in Hand-Schüller-Christian's disease. Arch Otolaryngol 1969;90:563–7.
43. Olschewski T, Seegenschmiedt M. Radiotherapy of Langerhans' cell histiocytosis: Results and implications of a national patters-of-care study. Strahlenther Onkol 2006;182:629–34.
44. Merchant S, Nadol JB. Otologic manifestations of systemic disease In: Cummings Otolaryngology-Head and Neck Surgery, Cummings CW, editor, 5th edition. 2007.
45. Cunningham M, Curtin H, Jaffe R, Stool S. Otologic manifestations of Langerhans' cell histiocytosis. Arch Otolaryngol Head Neck Surg 1989;115:807–13.
46. Schuknecht HF. Histiocytosis X. In: Pathology of the ear, 2nd edition. Philadelphia, PA: Lea and Febiger; 1993. p. 411.
47. Kurnatowski P, Filipiak A. Otomycosis: Prevalence, clinical symptoms, therapeutic procedure 2001;44:472–9.
48. Vennewald I, Schonlebe J, Klemm E. Mycological and histological investigations in humans with middle ear infections. Mycoses 2003;46:12–8.
49. Chen D, Lalwani AK, House JW, Choo D. Aspergillus mastoiditis in acquired immunodeficiency syndrome. Am J Otol 1999;20:561–7.
50. McGill TJ. Mycotic infection of the temporal bone. Arch Otolaryngol 1978;104:140–4.
51. Ohki M, Ito K, Ishimoto S. Fungal mastoiditis in an immunocompetent adult. Eur Arch Otorhinolaryngol 2001;258: 106–8.
52. Bickley L, Betts R, Parkins C. Atypical invasive external otitis from Aspergillus. Arch Otolaryngol Head Neck Surg 1988;114:1024–8.
53. Gussen R, Canalis RF. Mucormycosis of the temporal bone. Ann Otol Rhinol Laryngol 1982;91:27–32.
54. Schuknecht HF. Mycotic infections. In: Pathology of the ear, 2nd edition. Philadelphia, PA: Lea and Febiger; 1993. p. 244–47.

Aural Complications of Otitis Media

26

Arvind Kumar, MD, FRCS / Richard Wiet, MD, FACS

As Shambaugh writes in his preface to *Surgery of the Ear*, "no branch of medical science has been altered more profoundly, advanced more rapidly, and benefited so greatly by sulfonamide and antibiotic therapy than surgery of the ear." The authors recall stories of the amazing transition Chicago witnessed as whole hospitals devoted to infectious disease began to close with the introduction of antibiotic therapy; this change echoed throughout otology.

Today a much more insidious problem exists. Young otologists are often surprised by the consequences of infection by virulent organisms, which can cause an alert patient with a disturbing otitis to become comatose and near death within 12 h. In this chapter, the authors aim to catalog and organize current thinking on the management of the intratemporal, extradural complications of otitis media with the hope that catastrophic complications can be avoided by prompt and appropriate intervention.

Otitis media is an inflammation of part or all of the mucoperiosteal lining of the tympanomastoid compartment comprising the Eustachian tube, the tympanic cavity, the mastoid antrum, and all the pneumatized spaces of the temporal bone. Complications of otitis media have been defined as spread of infection beyond the confines of the lining mucosa of the middle-ear cleft.[1] Both acute and chronic otitis media (COM) can cause complications (Table 26–1). In the preantibiotic era, 52% of complications were associated with virulent acute otitis media. Today, the majority of complications result from COM. Morbidity and mortality from complications can be minimized if there is a keen familiarity with the specific type of draining ear, the underlying pathology, and the early signs and symptoms of complications. These considerations are particularly significant now because the rarity of complications limits the individual experience of most otologists.

COMPLICATIONS OF ACUTE OTITIS MEDIA

Perforation of the Pars Tensa

Acute otitis media (AOM) of bacterial origin typically affects preschool children and the nasopharynx is usually the source of the infection. An initial inflammation of the middle-ear cleft is followed by suppuration, complication, and then resolution. In the inflammatory stage, hyperemia and edema of the mucoperiosteum is followed by exudation of serofibrinous fluid into the middle ear. As the fluid volume increases, pressure is exerted against the tympanic membrane (TM) and, if myringotomy is not performed, the bulging TM ruptures, usually in the anterior–inferior quadrant. Pain subsides, and toxicity and fever begin to abate. In most instances, subsequent to resolution of inflammation, the perforation heals spontaneously. In a Caucasian population, a perforation persists in about 2% of patients.

The hearing loss associated with such a permanent perforation is usually mild. The Weber lateralizes to the affected ear and the Rinne is positive bilaterally. The audiometric evaluation should bear out the tuning fork tests. The cause of conductive hearing loss from TM perforations is discussed in Chapter 3.

The TM perforation can be surgically repaired. What are the chances of success of myringoplasty in such cases? Eustachian tube dysfunction diminishes the chances for a successful myringoplasty. Unfortunately, an accurate preoperative evaluation of Eustachian tube dysfunction is not possible. The status of the opposite ear is no predictor of Eustachian tube

TABLE 26–1 Complications of suppurative ear disease

INTRATEMPORAL EPIDURAL COMPLICATIONS	INTRACRANIAL INTRADURAL COMPLICATIONS
• Leptomeningitis	• Leptomeningitis
• Acute mastoiditis	• Pachymeningitis
• Pachymeningitis	– Subdural abscess
– Epidural abscess	• Brain abscess
– Perisinus abscess and SST	• Otitic hydrocephalus
• Petrositis	
• Facial paralysis	
• Labyrinthitis	

function on the ipsilateral side. The best correlate of Eustachian tube dysfunction is mastoid pneumatization. The results of a technically well-done myringoplasty in a well-pneumatized mastoid exceed 95%.

Acute Mastoiditis/Subperiosteal Abscess

Acute mastoiditis is the extension of the middle-ear inflammation of AOM into the antrum and mastoid air cells. Such spread occurs because the mastoid antrum and the epitympanum communicate freely with each other through the *aditus ad antrum.* According to Nager[2] "a mild form of mastoiditis regularly accompanies an AOM in which the inflammatory process is limited to the mucoperiosteum." Therefore, this early stage of inflammation of the whole middle-ear cleft is better termed as *tympanomastoiditis.* Routine CT and MR scans of the temporal bone are often reported to show "mastoiditis" even though there is no clinical evidence of pain or tenderness over the mastoid or any radiologic evidence of bone destruction. To clarify the clinical significance of such apparent inconsistencies, it is worthwhile to trace the progression of tympanomastoiditis to a subperiosteal abscess: if during the course of tympanomastoiditis, the aditus is blocked by inflammatory tissue, mucopurulent material may become loculated within the antrum and the contiguous air cells of the temporal bone. If the infection is severe and the blockage of the aditus persists despite antibiotic therapy, retrograde thrombophlebitis may lead to edema and cellulitis of the soft tissues overlying the mastoid, underlying the ipsilateral retroauricular pain, swelling, and induration of acute mastoiditis. If the pus is not drained, either spontaneously or by surgical intervention, necrosis and demineralization of the bony trabeculae occur resulting in "coalescent mastoiditis" (Figure 26–1). From this stage on, disease progression follows a continuum depending on the direction in which the erosive process goes:

- Most commonly, the mastoid cortex is eroded and a subperiosteal abscess develops.
- With medial progression, the abscess involves the petrous pyramid; if the apex is involved, the classic symptoms and signs of Gradenigo's syndrome may develop.
- With anterior progression, the fallopian canal or the labyrinth can be compromised, resulting in facial paralysis and/or vertigo with or without sensorineural hearing loss.
- If the mastoid tip is eroded, a Bezold's abscess may develop.
- Progression toward the tegmen or Trautman's triangle may result in an epidural abscess.
- Invasion of the perilymph or cerebrospinal fluid space can evolve into meningitis.

In a multicenter study of 223 consecutive cases of mastoiditis/AOM, Luntz et al.[3] found that 88% occurred in children under the age of 8 years. Upon admission to hospital, 22% presented with one or more intratemporal or intracranial complications. The most commonly isolated organisms were *Streptococcus pneumoniae, Streptococcus pyogenes, Staphylococcus aureus, Staphylococcus* (coagulase negative), *Haemophilus influenzae, and Pseudomonas aeruginosa.* Cultures were positive for *Pseudomonas spp.* in 18 patients (8%), although it is important to note that in 50% of these cases, the specimen was taken from the external auditory canal. In nearly all these patients, recovery was uncomplicated, even though no antipseudomonal antibiotics were used in 12 of the 18 patients. These authors also found that antibiotic treatment of AOM is not a safeguard against acute mastoiditis. Early myringotomy was found to be associated with a less complicated course of mastoiditis.

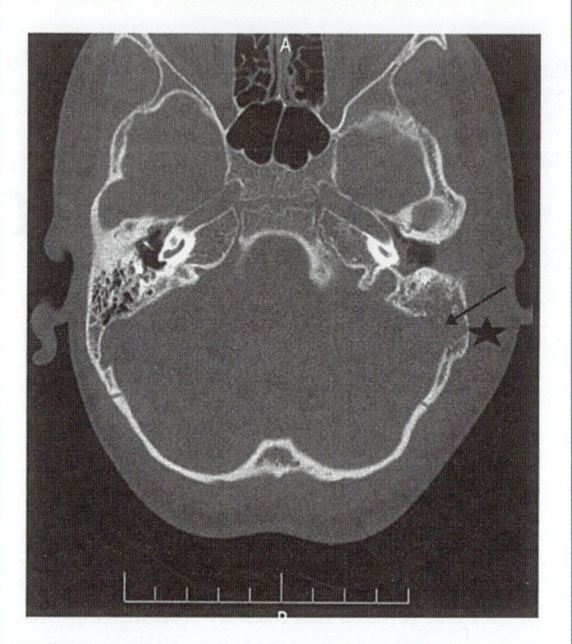

FIGURE 26–1 • Axial, bone-window temporal bone CT scan showing coalescent mastoiditis (*arrow*). Note the soft tissue swelling lateral to mastoid process (*star*).

Noncoalescent mastoiditis can be treated effectively using culture-specific intravenous antibiotics with myringotomy and placement of a tympanostomy tube. About 20% of patients so treated may nonetheless experience disease progression and ultimately need a cortical mastoidectomy. Close observation of such children is very important to anticipate and prevent serious complications.

Coalescent mastoiditis and subperiosteal mastoid abscess require careful evaluation and appropriate imaging studies. Management includes IV antibiotics, myringotomy, and cortical mastoidectomy. It is important to realize that in infants and young children, the stylomastoid foramen is located on the lateral surface of the mastoid as can be seen in Figure 26–2. The postauricular incision thus should be modified by not extending it inferiorly below the level of the floor of the external auditory canal, and facial nerve monitoring should be used.

Immunocompromised patients are particularly susceptible to coalescent mastoiditis.[4] The patient shown in Figure 26–3 was HIV-positive. Following an episode of AOM, he rapidly developed a zygomatic abscess.

Inadequately treated AOM can also lead to complications. Subacute otitis media, the consequence of inadequate therapy, comprises the resolution of the initial symptoms of

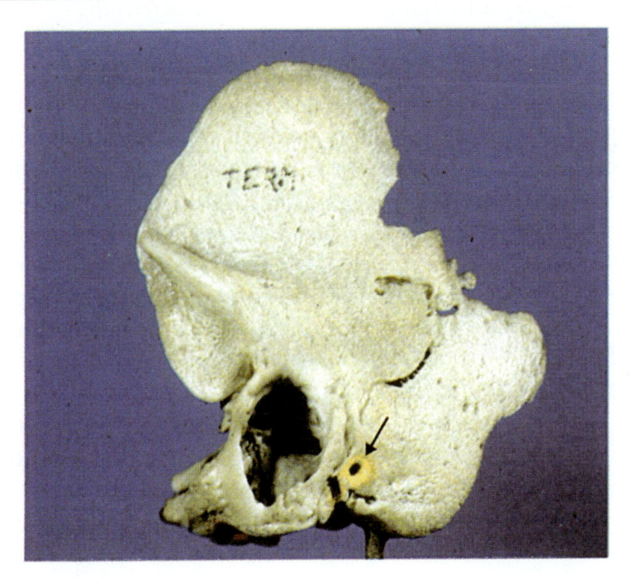

FIGURE 26–2 • Photograph of the lateral surface of the temporal bone of a full-term neonate. The mastoid process is not yet developed, and the stylomastoid foramen is located high on the lateral surface of the temporal bone (*arrow*).

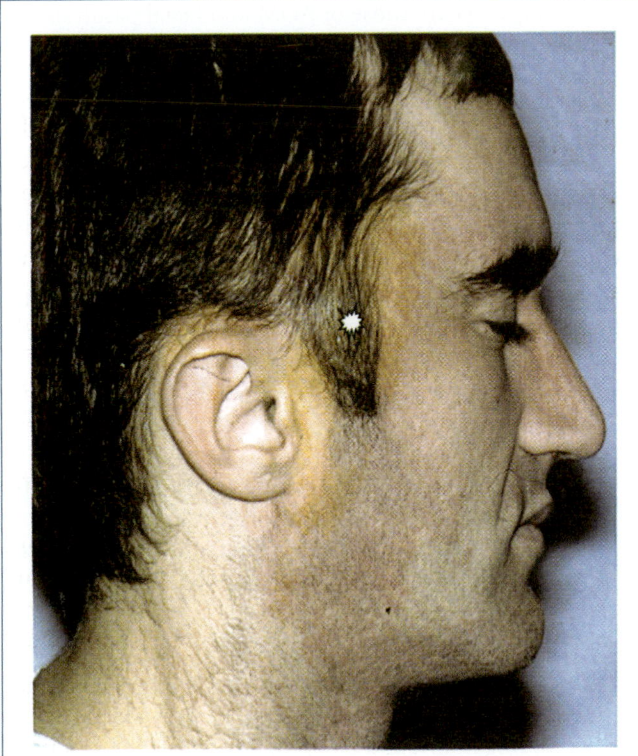

FIGURE 26–3 • Clinical photograph of an HIV-positive patient with an acute zygomatic abscess.

AOM, while disease progresses to the formation of an acute mastoid abscess without the usual accompanying toxicity. Holt and Gates[5] reported their experience with 9 patients with so-called masked mastoiditis, in which the patient presents with an intratemporal and/or intracranial complication. The history in such cases is one of persistent, mild irritability, diarrhea, and tugging at the ear after apparent resolution of an episode of AOM following antibiotic therapy. Dormant disease has been reported by Meyerhoff et al.[6] in temporal bones with otitis media. Based on clinical studies, it is postulated that anaerobic organisms such as *Peptococcus* spp. and *Bacteriodes* spp. thrive in the anaerobic environment of the mastoid in which the aditus is blocked by granulation tissue. These anaerobic organisms are of low virulence, and an indolent osteitis results that causes little or no pain. The patient depicted in Figure 26–4 presented with painless postauricular swelling. As is often the case, the TM was thickened[5] but intact. A CT scan (Figure 26–5) showed a subperiosteal abscess that required surgical drainage and cortical mastoidectomy. In their series of 9 cases of masked mastoiditis, Holt and Gates[5] found several associated complications, including epidural abscess (2), facial paralysis (1), meningitis and epidural abscess (1), meningitis (2), brain abscess (2), and cerebritis (1). It is important to maintain a high index of suspicion for this insidious disease and to have a low threshold for obtaining a CT scan of the temporal bones to rule out complications. When acute complications of otitis media are suspected, it is prudent to perform the CT scan with IV contrast to look for thrombophlebitis or intracranial involvement.

Petrositis

Petrositis (also known as petrous apicitis) is an inflammation of the pneumatized spaces of the petrous portion of the temporal bone and is a rare complication of AOM. In most individuals, the petrous apex is poorly pneumatized, but when pneumatization

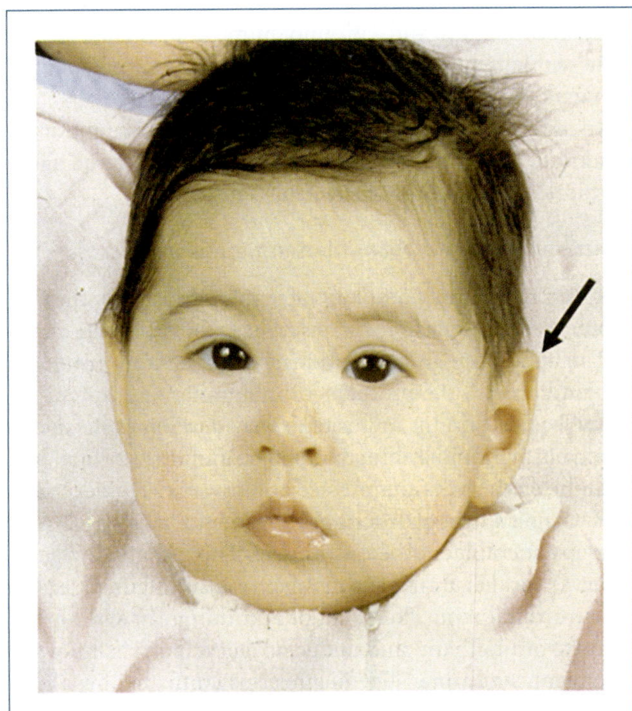

FIGURE 26–4 • Clinical photograph of baby with left "masked mastoiditis." Arrow points to the protruding left ear.

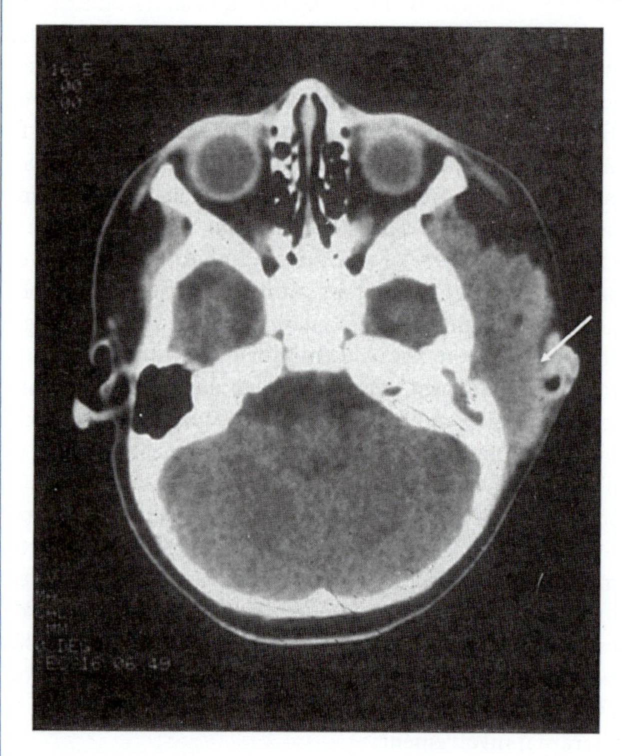

FIGURE 26–5 • Axial CT scan of the temporal bone of the same patient as in Figure 26–4.

does occur, air cells extend into the petrous pyramid in two main groups:

1. A posterior group of cells that are in continuity with the mastoid antrum and epitympanum, that cluster around the semicircular canals at the base of the pyramid, and that extend medially to the petrous apex.
2. An anterior group of cells that extends from the mesotympanum, hypotympanum, and protympanum and passes around the cochlea to the petrous apex.

Schuknecht[7] classified petrositis as *acute* and *chronic.*

Acute Petrositis: The pathology of acute petrositis is the same as acute tympanomastoiditis described above. In the majority of instances the inflammation resolves without producing any symptoms. If the products of inflammation are retained, the involved ear drains and osteitis may develop at the apex of the petrous pyramid leading to diplopia and retro-orbital pain. The abducens nerve is compressed as it traverses Dorello's canal under Gruber's (the petroclinoid) ligament, causing paralysis of the ipsilateral lateral rectus muscle. The ipsilateral trigeminal nerve, located at the petrous apex, is also inflamed, leading to retro-orbital pain. The triad of a draining ear with ipsilateral retro-orbital pain and abducens nerve palsy is known as Gradenigo's syndrome. The diagnosis is confirmed by a high-resolution temporal bone CT scan.

Chronic Petrositis: In addition to inflammatory changes, there is new bone formation and resorption. Osteitis adjacent to the otic capsule, dura, or veins may cause labyrinthitis, meningitis, epidural abscess, and brain abscess.

Management of petrous apicitis comprises the administration of systemic antibiotics and surgical drainage. The first step is a complete mastoidectomy with skeletonization of the semicircular canals. Then the petrous apex can be approached by several routes, depending on the location of the infection, the pneumatization of the temporal bone, and the status of the hearing. In a nonhearing ear, the translabyrinthine and transotic approaches are the easiest and offer excellent exposure of the petrous apex. Sacrifice of hearing may be justified if the clinical condition endangers the patient's life, and this approach is deemed to offer the best and safest means for management. If more anterior exposure is required, the transcochlear approach is the best option. In a hearing ear, a subtemporal or an infracochlear approach affords access to anteriorly located disease. The retrolabyrinthine or subarcuate routes allow drainage of posterior apicitis with preservation of hearing.

Facial Paralysis

Children are most susceptible to facial paralysis secondary to AOM. As with all other complications, antibiotics have reduced the incidence of facial paralysis. Most commonly, the first symptoms are those of AOM and facial paralysis follows several days later. Paralysis of the face is rarely the initial symptom.

Pathophysiology: The routes of spread of infection to the facial nerve are

1. via natural dehiscences in the fallopian canal, most often in its tympanic segment;
2. via natural pathways that connect the middle ear and the lumen of the Fallopian canal, such as the canal for the stapedius muscle, neurovascular connections, and mastoid air cells in close contact with the fallopian canal;
3. via direct infection of bone around the Fallopian canal (localized osteitis).

The organisms that cause facial paralysis are the same that cause AOM. Pus or osteitis around the dehiscent facial nerve most likely leads to inflammation and swelling of the nerve. Toxins and ischemia probably have an ancillary role.

Management:

1. The management aims to treat the underlying AOM with appropriate antibiotics for at least 10 days. At the same time, myringotomy, and if appropriate, insertion of a tympanostomy tube is helpful. The patient in Figure 26–6 was treated conservatively and the outcome, as can be seen, was satisfactory.
2. An intact canal wall mastoidectomy is indicated if coalescent mastoiditis develops and the response to conservative treatment is not satisfactory. Facial nerve decompression is not necessary in the vast majority of cases, particularly as complete facial recovery occurs in >95% of cases of paralysis secondary to AOM.

A

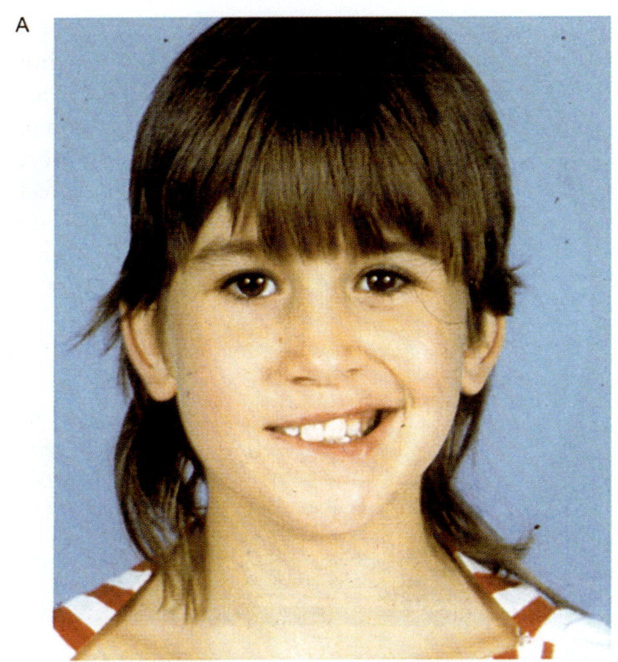

B

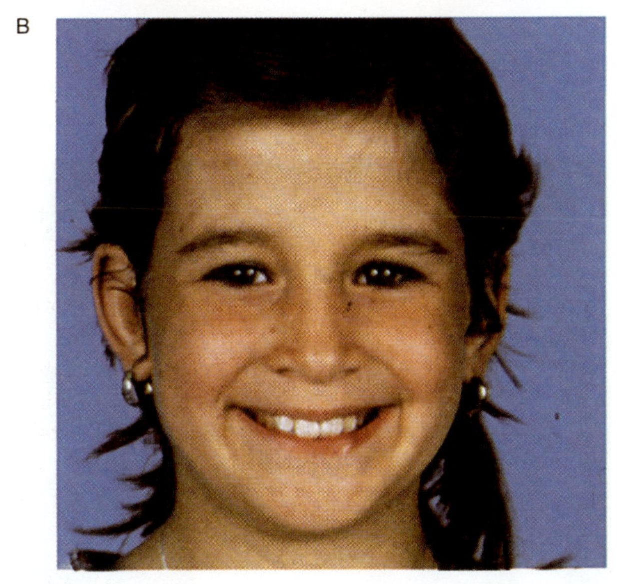

FIGURE 26–6 • *A*, Clinical photograph of a patient with right, infranuclear facial paralysis. *B*, Same patient after a 2-week course of treatment for AOM.

Labyrinthitis

Schuknecht[8] described three types of labyrinthitis:

1. Serous labyrinthitis
2. Otogenic suppurative labyrinthitis
3. Meningitic suppurative labyrinthitis

Serous labyrinthitis occurs during the course of acute or chronic otitis media. It is presumed that bacterial exotoxins enter the inner ear via the oval or round window or a labyrinthine fistula. As a complication of AOM the first two routes are more likely. According to Schuknecht,[8] in the acute phase there is no clinical method for differentiating serous from suppurative labyrinthitis. The diagnosis is retrospective. If vestibular and auditory functions are partially or completely retained, it can be assumed that the infection was serous. Margolis et al.[9] tested high-frequency hearing in children with history of AOM and in a matched control group. They found a higher incidence of high-frequency hearing loss in the AOM group.

In addition to antibiotic treatment of AOM, adjuvant corticosteroid therapy should be considered when labyrinthitis is suspected or diagnosed.

COMPLICATIONS OF CHRONIC OTITIS MEDIA

Today, complications are more commonly seen in the setting of chronic otitis media. A good understanding of the pathophysiology of COM enables an appreciation of which forms of COM lead to complications. Smyth[10] proposed that "middle-ear effusion (MEE) is the underlying cause of virtually all forms of chronic suppurative otitis media, ranging from benign uncomplicated perforations of the tympanic membrane, through atelectasia of the middle ear, to life threatening cholesteatomatous disease of the petrous bone." The long-term presence of MEE causes a portion of the TM to lose its fibrous and elastic layers; this loss is believed to be caused by enzymes present in the MEE. This portion of the TM appears thin and atrophic (Figure 26–7). Subsequently there are four possible outcomes:

1. The condition of the TM remains stable for many years and on examination a "healed scar" is seen.

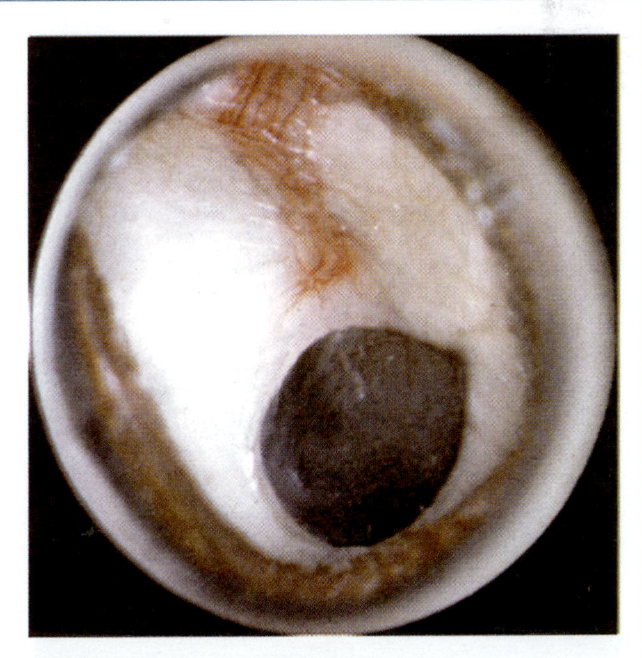

FIGURE 26–7 • Clinical photograph of a left TM showing myringosclerosis with a central dimeric area. *Courtesy of Dr. Richard Buckingham.*

2. The weak area breaks down during a subsequent episode of AOM, leading to a permanent perforation of the pars tensa of the TM. The status of the middle ear can often be assessed by viewing it through the perforation. When there is no mucosal disease, discharge, or evidence of ossicular erosion, the ear can remain stable (Figure 26–8). Alternatively, the mucosa may appear boggy and there may be discharge and granulation tissue. Granulation tissue may present as a polyp in the external auditory canal (EAC) (Figure 26–9).
3. If a large area of the TM becomes atrophic, the persistent negative middle-ear pressure can cause the atrophic TM to drape over the medial wall of the middle ear, the incus, and the stapes. The appearance of such an atelectatic TM is much like that of the thin plastic wrap used to protect food (Figure 26–10).
4. With atrophy of the posterior–superior quadrant of the TM, a retraction pocket develops. Enlargement of the pocket can result in erosion of the long process of the incus. With the development of adhesions that anchor the pocket to the middle-ear mucosa, the retraction pocket is no longer reversible. With loss of self-cleansing ability, the pocket accumulates squamous debris and becomes a cyst, which, with further enlargement, can extend medial to the body of the incus and the head of the malleus (Figure 26–11).

Therefore there are differences among draining ears, and successful management requires an understanding of the underlying pathology and its clinical presentation. Two main types of chronic suppuration, based on the embryology of the middle-ear cleft, have been described in the British literature:

1. Tubotympanic disease (safe or benign type)
2. Atticoantral disease (unsafe or malign type)

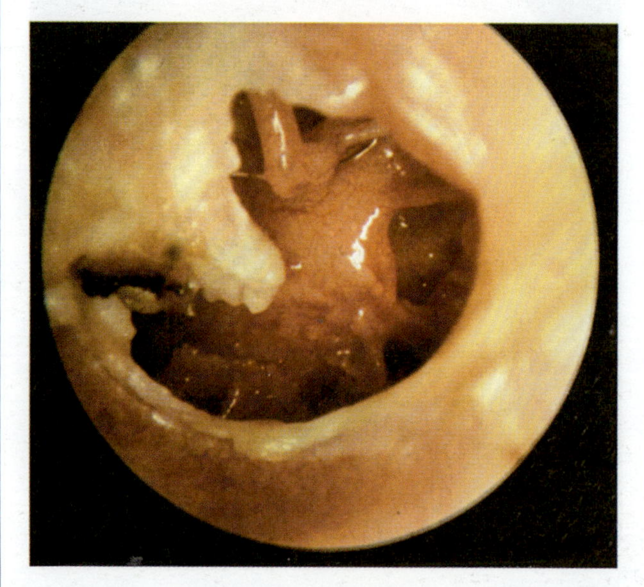

FIGURE 26–8 • Clinical photograph of a left TM showing a perforation of the pars tensa. *Courtesy of Dr. Richard Buckingham.*

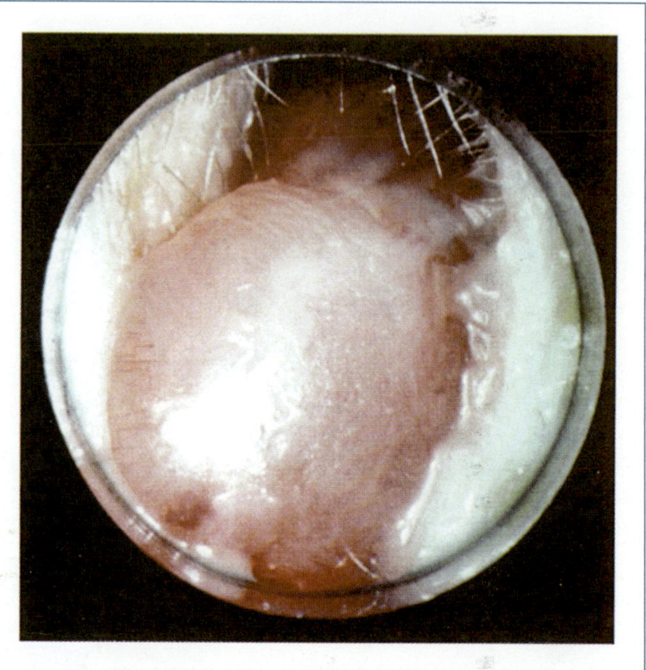

FIGURE 26–9 • Clinical photograph of right ear with an EAC polyp. *Courtesy of Dr. Richard Buckingham.*

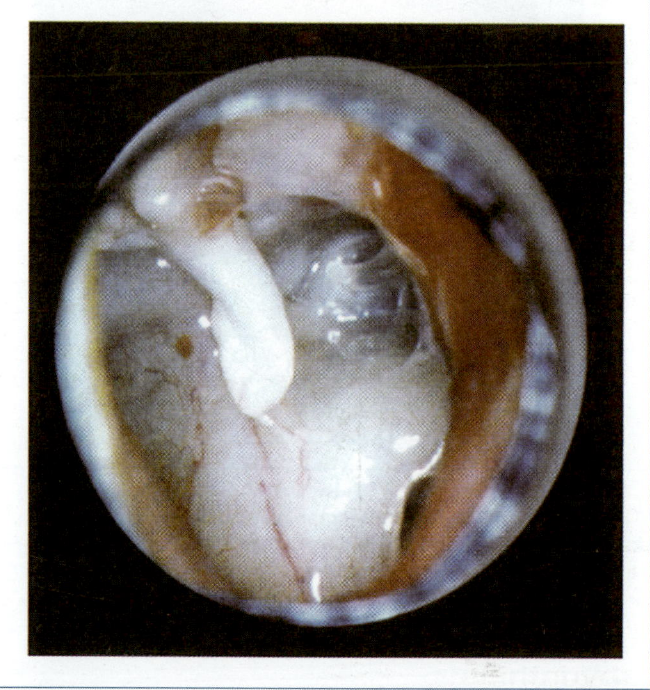

FIGURE 26–10 • Clinical photograph of a left ear showing an atrophic TM plastered on to the medial wall of the middle ear (atelectasis). *Courtesy of Dr. Richard Buckingham.*

Tubotympanic Disease

The tubotympanic recess is derived from the first branchial pouch, which is lined by respiratory epithelium. This form of disease is characterized by a perforation of the pars tensa in which the margins of the perforation are surrounded by a rim

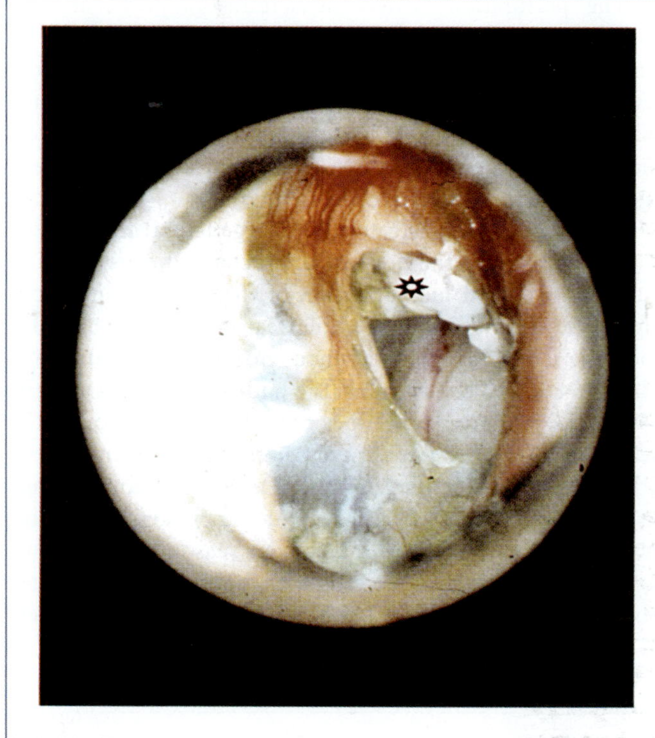

FIGURE 26–11 • Clinical photograph of a tympanic membrane with a posterior-superior quadrant retraction pocket that contains a cholesteatoma (*star*). *Courtesy of Dr. Richard Buckingham.*

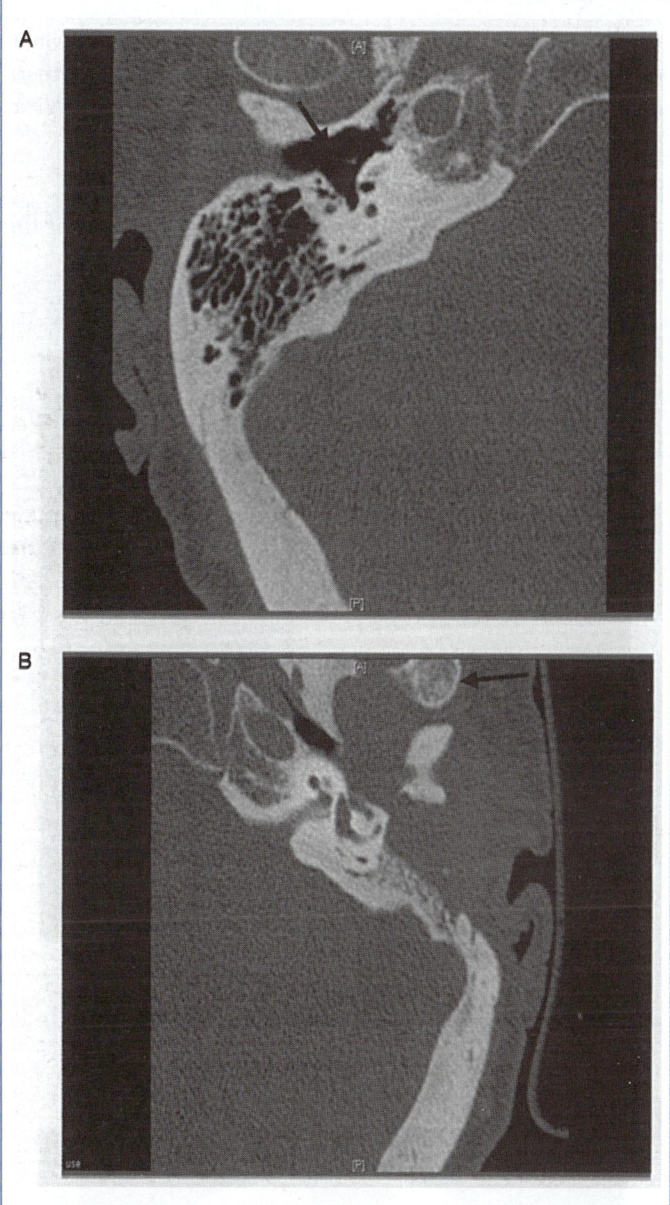

FIGURE 26–12 • *A,* Normal axial CT scan of a right temporal bone. *B,* Axial CT of a temporal bone with cholesterol granuloma in the middle ear, mastoid, and glenoid fossa. The condyle is displaced laterally (*arrow*).

of the pars tensa or the annulus. Disease in the middle-ear cleft is confined to the mucosa, and it is *rarely* the seat of complications. In our experience we have noted three types of tubotympanic disease:

1. A TM perforation is noted on a routine physical examination, and the patient is completely asymptomatic. Mawson and Ludman[11] have termed such a perforation as "inactive."
2. There is intermittent otorrhea that readily responds to conservative treatment with aural toilet and antibiotic drops.
3. There is intractable drainage that resists all conservative management. It is in such cases that florid granulation tissue occupies the entire middle-ear cleft, and if not treated surgically, a polyp may protrude into the EAC (Figure 26–9) or other complications may develop. Figure 26–12 shows the temporal bone CT scan of a patient who had undergone an intact canal wall mastoidectomy and tympanoplasty for tubotympanic disease 4 years earlier. Her presenting complaint was left-sided otalgia and painful mastication. The underlying problem was a cholesterol granuloma that had eroded the anterior wall of the middle ear and involved the glenoid fossa.

Can otogenic complications, such as brain abscess, occur in "safe" and noncholesteatomatous ears? Samuel et al.,[12] Rupa and Raman, [13] and Browning [14] reported series of cases in which complications occurred even though there was no cholesteatoma noted at surgery. A review of these articles shows that complications occurred in neglected cases of COM in which the underlying pathology seen at the time of surgery was florid granulation tissue in the middle-ear cleft.[14] Thus, it can be concluded that complications can occur in neglected cases of tubotympanic disease and that cholesteatoma is not typically associated with pars tensa perforations, even when complications occur.

Atticoantral Disease

The further embryologic development of the middle-ear cleft superior to the chorda tympani nerve occurs by penetration of the primordial mesoderm of the epitympanum and antrum by pavement epithelium. Chronic infection in this region is designated as atticoantral disease, is associated with cholesteatoma, and often leads to complications. In atticoantral disease, there are two types of presentation with their associated surgical implications:

1. A "perforation" in the pars flaccida (Figure 26–13).
2. A "perforation" of the posterior–superior quadrant of the pars tensa (Figure 26–14).

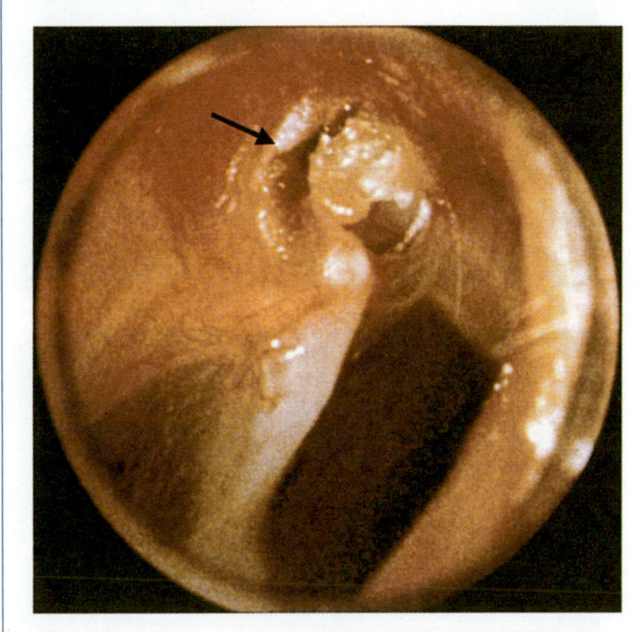

FIGURE 26–13 • "Perforation" of the pars flaccida (*arrow*).

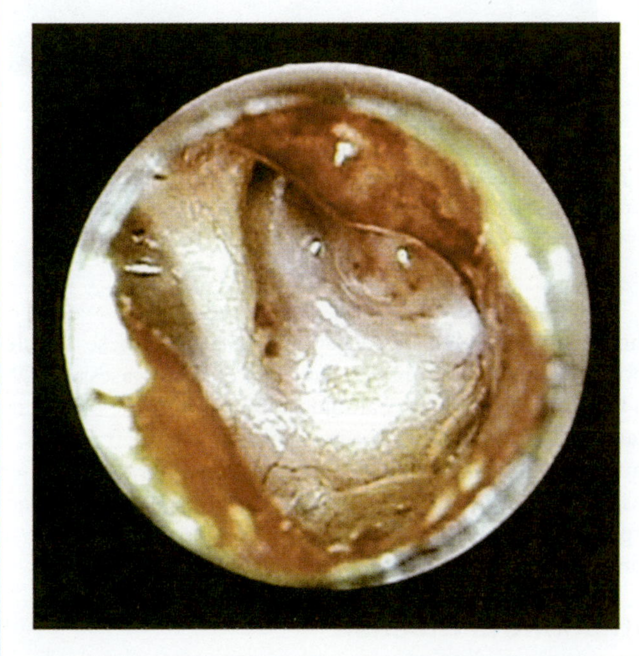

FIGURE 26–14 • "Perforation" of pars tensa, posterior–superior quadrant.

The "perforation" is, in reality, a retraction pocket and can be likened to the cut finger of a surgical glove (Figure 26–15). Its blind distal end lies deep in the middle-ear space, hidden from view by overlying bone. The erosive potential of cholesteatoma and its close proximity to important structures underlie the designation of "unsafe" to this disease. The clinical features of each type of COM are summarized in Table 26–2.

Pars flaccida cholesteatomas enlarge lateral to the head of the malleus and the body of the incus and cause erosion of the scutum and medialization of the malleus and incus (Figure 26–16). Pars tensa cholesteatomas (Figure 26–17) erode the long process of the incus or stapes early and then enlarge medial to the annulus, the body of the incus and the head of the malleus, sometimes causing lateralization of the malleus and incus. There is no erosion of the scutum as seen with pars flaccida cholesteatomas.[15] Our current understanding of the initial cause of these retraction pockets is negative pressure in the middle ear. It is for this reason that a shallow retraction pocket can be reversed with the placement of a tympanostomy tube. On the other hand, deep retraction pockets

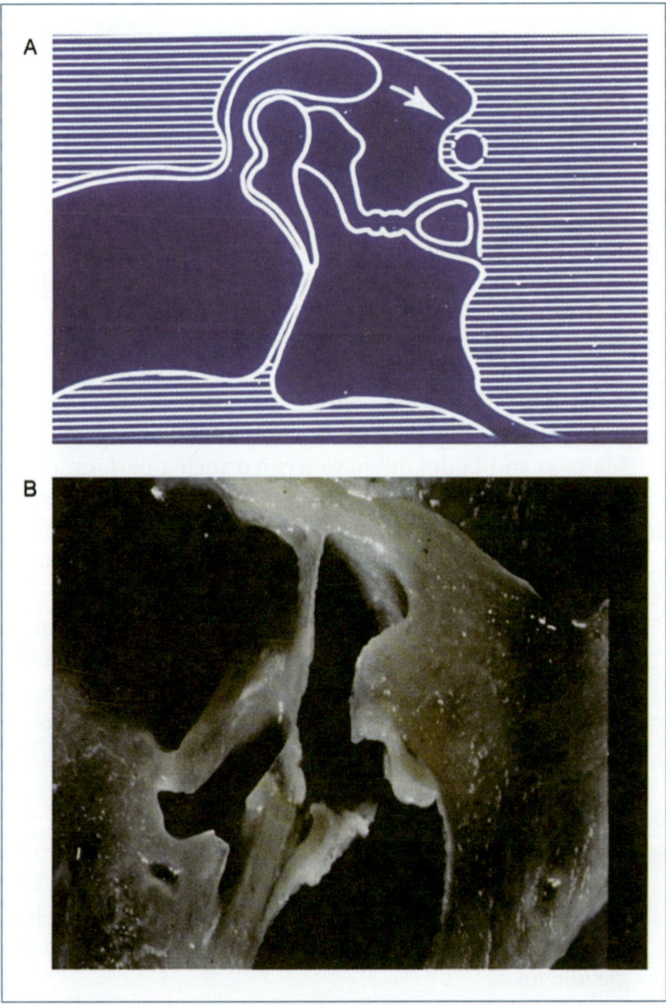

FIGURE 26–15 • *A,* Persistent negative middle-ear pressure leading to formation of retraction pocket. Note that the pocket cannot be seen during examination of the ear. *B,* A similar attic retraction seen in a postmortem specimen. *Courtesy of Dr. Richard Buckingham.*

TABLE 26–2 Clinical features of chronic otitis media

TUBOTYMPANIC DISEASE	ATTICOANTRAL DISEASE
Perforation: Confined to pars tensa	No perforation: Only retraction pocket, affecting pars flaccida or posterior-superior quadrant of pars tensa
Discharge: Profuse, mucoid, odorless and usually responds to conservative treatment	Discharge: Thick, scanty, foul smelling and usually does not respond to conservative treatment
Granulations: Uncommon. If present and unresponsive to treatment, may lead to complications	Granulations: Common around the mouth of retraction pocket
Polyp: Arises from exuberant granulations overlying the promontory. Polyp can enlarge into EAC and occupy its whole lumen	Polyp: Usually soft and fleshy and can easily be suctioned
Hearing loss: Conductive and usually mild	Hearing loss: Larger conductive hearing loss, with varying degrees of SNHL
Imaging: In active disease, haziness of the whole middle ear cleft and the pneumatization is usually truncated	Imaging: • Pars flaccida cholesteatoma shows erosion of scutum in bone window CT scan. Both axial and coronal views should be examined. • There is medialization of the ossicular chain. The mastoid pneumatization is truncated • Pars tensa cholesteatoma will show erosion of the posterior-superior wall, lateralization of the ossicular chain, haziness of the area medial to ossicular chain, possible erosion of the lateral semicircular canal. • The mastoid pneumatization is truncated. The scutum is not eroded
Complications: Very unusual except in neglected cases where there are florid granulations and drainage is unresponsive to treatment	Complications: Frequent and span one or more clinical conditions listed in Table 26–1
Cholesteatoma: Extremely rare	Cholesteatoma: Common finding
Bacteriology: *P. aeruginosa, S. aureus,* and *Proteus* species	Bacteriology: *S. aeruginosa, S. aureus, Bacteroides, Peptococcus, Peptostreptococcus*

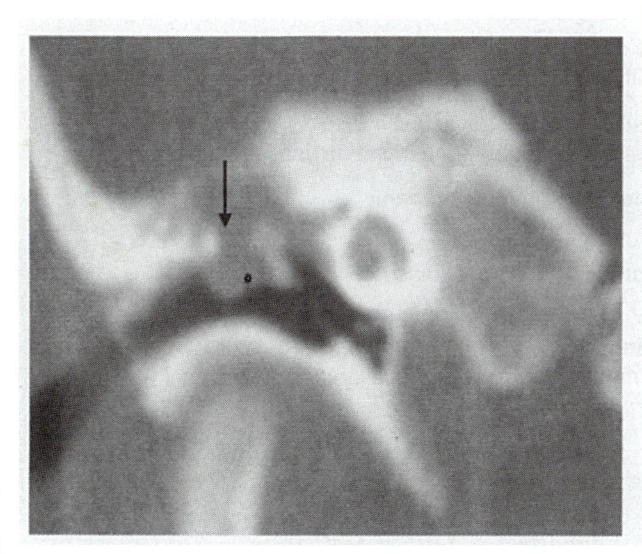

FIGURE 26–16 • CT scan of a temporal bone with the clinical diagnosis of pars flaccida cholesteatoma (*arrow*). Note the erosion of the scutum and medialization of the ossicular chain (*star*).

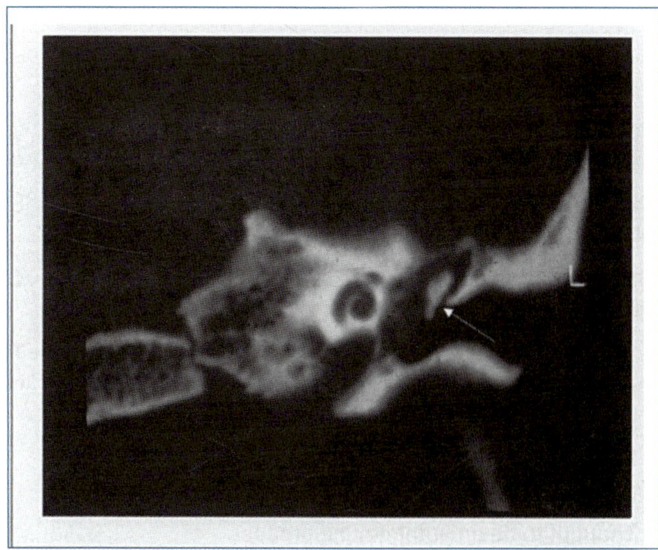

FIGURE 26–17 • CT scan of a temporal bone with the clinical diagnosis of a posterior–superior retraction pocket. Note that there is no erosion of the scutum (*arrow*) and there is lateralization of the ossicular chain (*arrow*).

do not respond to tympanostomy tube placement and may continue to deepen, despite normal middle-ear pressure. For this reason, it is suspected that an ongoing inflammatory process may play a role in the progression of retraction pockets. Deeper pockets tend to collect keratin. When infected, these cysts drain and granulation tissue develops around the sac. The stage is now set for bone erosion and possible complications. The predominant bacterial organisms associated with atticoantral COM are *Staphylococcus aureus*, gram-negative bacilli such as *β-proteus* and *Ps. aeruginosa, Kliebsella spp.* and *E.coli. Bacteroides fragilis* is cultured when the discharge is fetid. These two forms of COM have distinctive histopathological findings, as detailed by Nager[2] and summarized in Table 26–3.

Subperiosteal Abscess

With bony erosion, the mastoid cortex can be breached, most commonly at Macewen's triangle, and pus accumulates under the periosteum, resulting in pain and postauricular swelling and tenderness. Blunting of the postauricular crease and anterior–inferior displacement of the pinna are early signs. The postauricular area is tender and swollen, and the patient may have a fever. When the tip of the mastoid is eroded, swelling and tenderness occur in the upper neck. A Bezold's abscess develops when the abscess forms deep to the sternocleidomastoid muscle. In such cases, the patient complains of stiffness and tenderness of the neck. In some cases, the abscess bursts through the periosteum and skin manifesting in a draining, postauricular fistula.

Diagnosis: Diagnosis is easily confirmed with a noncontrast enhanced temporal bone CT scan using bone windows. Simultaneously, a contrast-enhanced CT scan of the brain should be obtained to rule out concurrent intracranial complications. More than one complication has been reported in as many as 44% of cases.

Management: Once the diagnosis is confirmed, IV antibiotic treatment directed against gram-negative and anaerobic bacilli is initiated. A tympanomastoidectomy is the definitive treatment, and this can be either a canal wall down procedure (CWD) or a canal wall up (CWU) mastoidectomy. Since the objective is to make the ear safe, we favor CWD mastoidectomy. It is critical to fashion a generous meatoplasty with the CWD

TABLE 26–3 Pathology of tubotympanic and atticoantral disease

TUBOTYMPANIC DISEASE	ATTICOANTRAL DISEASE
Perforation: Involves pars tensa, margins of which covered by stratified squamous epithelium	"Perforation": Is a retraction pocket of the pars flaccida or posterior-superior quadrant of the pars tensa
Mucoperiosteum: – Subepithelial layer thickened by inflammatory edema – Mucoperiosteum contains dense lymphocytic infiltration – Mucoperiosteum appears polypoid – Hyperplastic mucosa may form polyp, which may extrude into EAC and occupy its lumen	Mucoperiosteum: – Both mucoperiosteum and underlying bone are affected – There is regular osteitic erosion of the scutum, posterior-superior bony canal wall and ossicles – In addition osteitic defects can involve any of the walls of the middle ear cleft, including the whole labyrinth – Osteitic defects are frequently covered with inflammatory vascular granulations – New bone forms at the same time as it is destroyed by the osteitic process
Epithelial lining of middle ear cleft becomes cuboidal or high columnar ciliated, with proliferation of goblet cells	Cholesteatoma sac advances into middle ear cleft inducing osteitis and formation of granulation tissue
Exudate is mucopurulent with polymorphs, lymphocytes, plasma cells and macrophages	Exudate is purulent, and creamy
Cholesterol granulomas are frequently associated with this pathology	Cholesterol granulomas unusual
Tympanosclerosis: – Macroscopically, on the TM appear as chalky white plaques – In middle ear appear as drops of cooled candle wax – May cause ossicular fixation – Thought to be an autoimmune process – Hyaline degeneration of mucoperiosteum occurs with subsequent calcification and ossification – Complications unusual	Tympanosclerosis is unusual. However osteitis can give rise to intratemporal and/or intracranial complications

procedure. Depending on the circumstances, a postauricular drain can be placed.

Labyrinthine Fistula

Erosion of the labyrinth occurs in 7% of cases of COM[16] and is considered the most common intratemporal complication. Cholesteatoma, particularly of the posterior–superior pars tensa variety, is the most frequent cause of lateral canal fistulae. The lateral semicircular canal is particularly susceptible to erosion because of its prominence in the aditus and because it lies in the path of an enlarging cholesteatoma (Figure 26–18A). The most frequent symptom of a labyrinthine fistula is vertigo, often induced by straining against a closed glottis. Hearing loss or deafness, ipsilateral facial paresis/paralysis, and otalgia are frequent associated symptoms.

Diagnosis: The characteristic symptoms and the presence of spontaneous nystagmus should alert the surgeon to the presence of a fistula. The spontaneous nystagmus usually beats towards the nondiseased, contralateral ear. A fistula test, observing the eyes for nystagmus, should be performed. If the fistula is located on the nonampullated arc of the horizontal canal, positive pressure will cause cupular deviation toward the utricular sac; eg, with a fistula in the right ear the nystagmus will beat toward the right (Figure 26–18B). The definitive diagnosis of a fistula is made by a thin section bone window CT scan of the temporal bone in both the axial and coronal planes.

Management: With concurrent antibiotic therapy as described above, a tympanomastoidectomy, either CWD or CWU, comprises definitive treatment. However, the management of the labyrinthine fistula itself is controversial. Manolides et al.[16] and Sanna et al.[17] *advocate* CWU mastoidectomy and no manipulation of cholesteatoma matrix. At a second-stage procedure, the matrix, which turns into small cyst, is easily removed. In more than 96% of their patients a sensorineural hearing loss was thus avoided. Surgeons who advocate removal of cholesteatoma matrix at the initial surgery report on average sensorineural hearing loss in 10% of cases.[16] Several investigators have based the decision regarding whether or not to remove the cholesteatoma matrix on the intraoperative determination of the size or depth of the fistula. In our practice we do a CWD procedure and leave the matrix intact. This technique both preserves hearing and facilitates healing of the mastoid cavity, which in the final analysis is covered with stratified squamous, keratinizing epithelium without skin appendages. We could not find any studies to support the idea that preserved matrix exhibits ongoing erosive ability.

Labyrinthitis

The spread of infection into the labyrinth is most often associated with the bone-eroding atticoantral type of COM. The inflammatory process reaches the vestibule or cochlea via a fistula. The presenting symptoms are vertigo, pain, hearing loss, nausea, and vomiting. A 3rd degree, spontaneous nystagmus beating toward the nondiseased ear is usually present. The treatment of suppurative labyrinthitis in the initial stages is medical and prompt to avoid progression to meningitis. The prognosis for recovery of either vestibular or auditory function is poor. Under the cover of antibiotic treatment, the underlying COM is managed surgically. The long-term management of unilateral loss of vestibular function is achieved with physical therapy, and the unilateral deafness can be managed with the Baha® system (Chapter 33: Implantable Hearing Devices).

With increasing frequency, the causative organism in chronic suppuration of the ear is *M. tuberculosis*. Robertson and

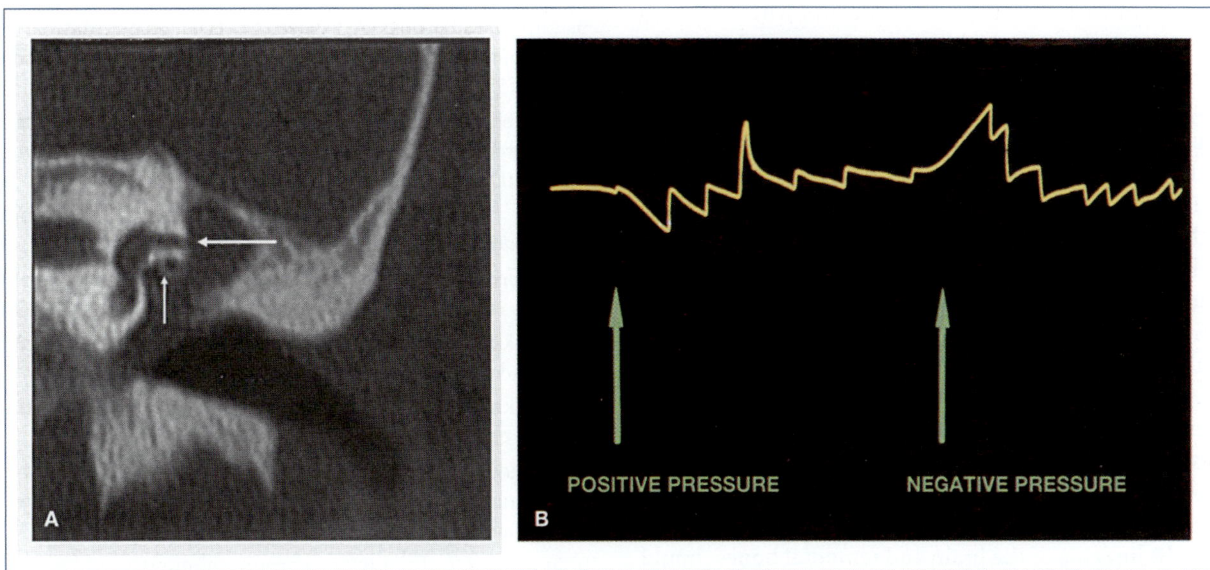

FIGURE 26–18 • *A,* The CT scan of a right temporal bone shows a bony defect over the nonampullated end of the lateral semicircular canal. *B,* ENG tracing shows that positive pressure produced a right-beating nystagmus and negative pressure produced a left-beating nystagmus.

Kumar[18] reported such an infection in a series of cases, and the following is an illustrative example:

An East Indian patient complained of ipsilateral facial asymmetry and otalgia, in addition to the classic symptoms of labyrinthitis. Examination of the right ear showed pus in the external canal, a thickened tympanic membrane, and a small perforation in the posterior–inferior quadrant. Examination of the facial nerve showed a complete right infranuclear facial paralysis. There was a spontaneous, 2nd degree left-beating nystagmus. A temporal bone CT scan showed opacification of the entire middle-ear cleft. The fallopian canal appeared intact throughout its course. A contrast-enhanced MRI scan of the brain showed enhancement of the cochlea, vestibule, and the tympanic and labyrinthine segments of the facial nerve. Audiometric evaluations documented a profound right-sided hearing loss. He had a positive purified protein derivative (PPD), common in immigrants from South Asia. At surgery, the tympanomastoid compartment was filled with granulation-tissue but there was no evidence of cholesteatoma. The fallopian canal, which was not dehiscent, was skeletonized from the geniculate ganglion to the stylomastoid foramen, but the cause of the facial paralysis was not obvious. Since the involved ear was nonhearing, the vestibule was opened by removal of the stapes and found to be filled with pale granulation tissue. Histopathology confirmed tuberculosis. Removal of the eggshell thin bone overlying the facial nerve showed inflammation in the same segments as indicated by MRI scanning. At the time of surgery, the cause of the paralysis was judged to be inflammation that had reached the nerve from at its medial aspect. After histological confirmation of tuberculosis, the patient was given a 1-year course of antitubercular treatment. At the end of 1 year his facial nerve function had returned to a III/VI on the House-Brackman scale, the otorrhea was controlled, and the dizziness resolved.

Facial Paralysis

When an infranuclear facial paralysis occurs with COM, in most cases, the underlying problem is atticoantral disease. In such cases, the exact cause or mechanism of the paralysis is unknown, largely because we have no histopathological data regarding the nerve. In the majority of cases the paralysis is associated with cholesteatoma, but as we have seen above, tubercular otitis media should also be kept in mind.[18] In nontubercular ears, the infectious process is believed to cause bony erosion of the fallopian canal, adjacent osteitis, direct infection of the nerve, and edema. The role of pressure by the cholesteatoma is less certain.

Facial nerve paralysis can either present abruptly or evolve over time. When present, the otologic surgeon should have a high index of suspicion for a labyrinthine fistula since the two structures are adjacent to each other. To assess the site and extent of involvement of the facial nerve and to identify other associated complications, both a temporal bone CT scan and contrast-enhanced MR imaging of the brain and temporal bones should be obtained. The MRI scan delineates the extent of involvement of the nerve and provides guidance for surgical decompression. The need for electrical tests is guided by the mode of onset of the paralysis and its duration.

Management: Prompt intervention is indicated when an individual with COM presents with facial nerve dysfunction. Initially, antibiotics and corticosteroids should be started to control the inflammatory process and to reduce facial nerve edema. In contrast to the nonsurgical management of facial paralysis due to AOM, the definitive treatment for paralysis due to COM is CWD mastoidectomy and decompression of the fallopian canal several millimeters distal and proximal to the affected portion. The nerve in the proximal and distal decompressed segments should appear normal. Should the epineurium be incised? Intuitively, such a move is expected to lead to the spread of infection into the substance of the nerve, and in the absence of any studies to demonstrate any advantage to epineurial lysis, it is no longer recommended. For the same reason, granulation tissue should not be followed into the nerve. Recovery of facial nerve function is not as dramatic as it is in a paralysis secondary to AOM. The grade of recovery will depend on the mode of onset of paralysis, the duration of paralysis, and the extent of disease.

The work of otologists of today is facilitated by a far more advanced diagnostic armamentarium that renders obsolete the older texts on management of ear infection. However, the lessons of the past cannot be forgotten. We must build on them. Progress has been especially rapid in neuroradiology, providing the physician with a more accurate picture of the problem. We certainly expect that in the years to come even more advanced systems will replace those of the present as we proceed in this twenty-first century.

References

1. Neely JG. Facial nerve & intracranial complications in otitis media. In: Jackler R, Brackmann BE, editors. Neurotology. 2nd edition. Philadelphia, PA: Mosby; 2005. p. 912–25.
2. Nager GT. Pathology of the ear and temporal bone. Baltimore, MD: Williams & Wilkins, 1993. p 220–97.
3. Luntz M, Brodsky A, Nusem S, et al. Acute mastoiditis—The antibiotic era: A multicenter study. Int J Ped Otorhinolaryngol 2001;57:1–9.
4. Soucek S, Michaels L. The ear in acquired immunodeficiency syndrome: II Clinical and audiological investigation. Am J Otol 1996;17:35–9.
5. Holt GR, Gates GA. Masked mastoiditis. Laryngoscope. 1983;93(8):1034–7.
6. Meyerhoff WL, Kim CS, Papparella MM. Pathology of chronic otitis media. Ann Otol Rhinol Laryngol. 1998;87:749–60.
7. Schuknecht HF. Infections. In: Pathology of the ear. Lea & Febiger, Philadelphia, 1993. p 218–20.
8. Schuknecht HF. Infections. In: Pathology of the ear. Philadelphia, PA: Lea & Febiger; 1993. p. 211–16.
9. Margolis RH, Saly GL, Hunter L, Lisa L. High frequency hearing loss and wideband middle ear impedance in children with otitis media histories. Ear Hear 2000;21(3):206–11.
10. Smyth GDL. Etiology of chronic suppurative otitis media. In: Smyth GDL, editor. Chronic ear disease. New York: Churchill Livingstone; 1980. p. 1–20.

11. Mawson S, Ludman H. Otitis media. In: Diseases of the ear: A textbook of otology. 4th edition. London: Arnold; 1979. p. 301–65.
12. Samuel J, Fernandes CM, Steinberg JL. Intracranial otogenic complications: A persisting problem. Laryngoscope 1986;96(3):272–8.
13. Rupa V, Raman R. Chronic suppurative otitis media: Complicated versus uncomplicated disease. Acta Otolaryngol. 1991;111(3):530–5.
14. Browning GG. The unsafeness of "safe" ears. J Laryngol Otol. 1984;98(1):23–6.
15. Valvassori GE. Imaging of the temporal bone. In: Mafee MF, Valvassori GE, Becker M, editors. Imaging of the head and neck. 2nd edition. New York; Stuttgart, Germany: Thieme; 2005. p. 74–89.
16. Manolides S. Complications associated with labyrinthine fistula in surgery of chronic otitis media. Otolaryngol Head & Neck Surg 2000; 123:733–7.
17. Sanna M, Zini C, Gamoletti R, Taibah AK, Russo A, Scandellari R. Closed versus open technique in the management of labyrinthine fistulae. Am J Otol. 1988;9(6):470–5.
18. Robertson K, Kumar A. Atypical presentations of aural tuberculosis. Am J Otolaryngol 1995;16:294–302.

Intracranial Complications of Otitis Media

27

Samuel C. Levine, MD, FACS / Chris De Souza, MD, FACS / Michael J. Shinners, MD

HISTORICAL PERSPECTIVE

Hippocrates noted in 460 BC that "acute pain in the ear with continued high fever is to be dreaded for the patient may become delirious and die."[1] In the preantibiotic era, complications from otitis media occurred abundantly, accompanied by a high morbidity. This was recognized by the Roman physician Celsius (25 AD) and the Arabian physician Avicenna (980–1037 AD).[2] It was Morgagni (1682–1771 AD) who recognized that the ear infection came first and the brain abscess was secondary.[2]

Brain abscess was the first complication of otitis media to be recognized and the first one successfully treated by operation. It was in 1768 that Morand reported a successful operation for brain abscess.[3] In 1856, Lebert accurately described the pathology of brain abscess, confirming the fact that it follows infection of the ear, not the reverse.[4] It was in 1881 that MacEwen reported a successful series of brain abscesses that were operated by him.[5] Körner, in 1908, was able to find 268 reported operations with 137 recoveries.[6]

The surgery of brain abscess had reached its peak of otologic interest by the time of Eagleton's text in 1922.[7] The management of this relatively common complication of otitis media remained chiefly in the hands of the otologic surgeon until sulfonamides began to be used for acute otitis media (AOM) in 1935 and penicillin was introduced in 1942. Thereafter, the incidence of brain abscess, which may already have begun to decline, decreased abruptly. The relative success of surgery for brain abscess remained in sharp contrast for many years to the almost invariably fatal outcome of purulent meningitis, the most dreaded complication of otitis media and the most frequent cause of death. Because therapy of generalized otitic meningitis was rarely successful, the efforts of the otologic surgeon were directed toward prevention. Whenever possible, bone-invading types of AOM and chronic otitis media (COM) were operated on before a complication had occurred. Careful clinical observation of patients with middle ear infections would not infrequently permit the detection of the earliest stages of beginning meningeal involvement. With prompt and thorough surgical drainage of the suppurative focus in the temporal bone, considerable success was achieved in arresting the meningeal invasion, in many cases while it was still localized, preventing the development of otherwise fatal generalized meningitis.[8] Despite these advances, meningitis remained the most frequent cause of death in otitis media, and otitis media was by far the most frequent cause of meningitis not due to *Neisseria meningitidis.*

The last of the three major intracranial complications of otitis media to be related to ear disease was infective thrombosis of the lateral sinus, first described in 1826. Thirty years later, Lebert accurately described the pathology of otitic sinus thrombosis.[9] In 1880, Zaufal proposed an operation for this complication and first attempted it in 1884, but the patient died.[10]

The surgical treatment of sinus thrombosis was finally established by the publications of Lane[11] in 1889 and Ballance in 1890.[12] However, a controversy over whether, as part of the surgical management, to ligate the jugular vein in all cases, in some cases, or in no case continued for many years, only to be resolved by the introduction of effective antibacterial and anticoagulant medication in favor of nonligation for most cases.

The two complications of otitis media caused by expansion within the temporal bone that often lead to a fatal intracranial extension, namely, purulent labyrinthitis and petrositis, were the last serious complications to be defined and effectively treated. A technique for draining the infected labyrinth was first described in 1895 by Jansen.[13] In 1904, Gradenigo described the syndrome of continuing aural discharge, severe fifth cranial nerve pain, and sixth nerve paralysis caused by infection of pneumatic cells in the petrous portion of the temporal bone with adjacent meningitis.[14] Kopetsky and Almour[15] in 1930 and Eagleton[16] in 1931 described the first systematic attempts to drain an abscess of the petrous apex. Other methods for reaching this relatively inaccessible area were soon described. For a few years, the literature contained numerous reports of successful operations for petrositis, many of them in patients with early meningitis. Just at the time that this frequent cause of otitic meningitis began to yield surgical therapy, it virtually disappeared from the scene of otologic experience as a result of effective antibacterial medication for AOM.

The frequency of complications of otitis changed dramatically with the introduction of effective antibiotics. In the 5-year period immediately preceding the introduction of these agents, from 1928 to 1933, approximately 1 in every 40 deaths in a large general hospital was caused by an intracranial complication of otitis media, with meningitis heading the list, sinus thrombosis second, and brain abscess last.[17] In a subsequent 5-year period (from 1949–1954), only 1 in every 400 deaths was the result of ear disease—an amazing 10-fold reduction in less than 20 years. The decrease in fatalities following AOM was greatest because this disease previously accounted for the majority of serious complications.

Of the three major intracranial complications of otitis media, the reduction in mortality has been greatest for thrombophlebitis of the lateral sinus, which has nearly disappeared as a cause of death.[17] This fact is easily understood because infection of the bloodstream was the usual mechanism of death from sinus thrombosis, and antibiotics act best in the bloodstream. The incidence of brain abscess has been greatly reduced by antibiotics. Purulent meningitis, though reduced, persists today as by far the most frequent intracranial complication of otitis media. However, it has changed from a nearly 100% fatal disease to one in which recovery can be expected in the majority of instances if diagnosed early and treated adequately.

The family physician has come to rely more on drugs to take care of ear disease than on careful clinical study and early otologic consultation. The diagnostic acumen of the otologist has been blunted by diminished experience and lessened familiarity with the symptoms of otitic complications. The situation has been made more difficult by the masking effect of antibiotics on the symptoms of continued infection.

Today the neurosurgeon is often the first to be called in consultation for intracranial complications. Most otologists work in combination as a team with a neurosurgeon. Treatment involves both specialties. Although the neurosurgeon should direct therapy of the complication, he/she must recognize the frequent otitic (sometimes nasal accessory sinus) origin and always request otologic consultation and help in the management, with surgical removal of the suppurative focus, which is usually in the ear.

The patient with chronic suppurative otitis media who is not doing well may indicate trouble. Earache with chronic otitis means that something has gone wrong, and if pus is under pressure in the middle ear cleft, an intracranial complication may be impending. Certainly, headache and drowsiness are signs of danger. One of the earliest signs of brain abscess is a visual field defect, which is almost invariably present if the patient is carefully examined. A fever suggests meningitis or sinus thrombosis. Awareness of the significance of the symptoms and signs results in earlier diagnosis, prompt treatment, and further reduction in mortality.

Although the incidence of the complications of otitis media has declined and a whole new range of antibiotics has been introduced, complications have not been eradicated completely. Complicating early identification and timely intervention when complications occur is the fact that most patients have been treated with one or more courses of antibiotic therapy.

FACTORS THAT INFLUENCE THE DEVELOPMENT OF COMPLICATIONS

Intracranial complications occur as the result of many factors, often acting simultaneously, causing the infection to spread from the ear and into the intracranial cavity. In general, intracranial complications occur when ear infections are either uncontrolled or inadequately controlled.

The tendency of middle ear infection to spread beyond the confines of the middle ear and its adjacent spaces is influenced by a number of factors, including the virulence of the infecting organism and its sensitivity to antibiotics, host resistance, the adequacy of antibiotic therapy, the anatomic pathways and barriers to spread, and the drainage of the pneumatic spaces, both natural and surgical.

The microbiology of middle ear infections remains relatively constant over time. *Streptococcus pneumoniae*, *Haemophilus influenzae*, and *Moraxella catarrhalis* cause most acute infections.[18] As new antibiotics are introduced, however, the patterns of antibiotic resistance seem to change and may vary from one location to another.

The microbiology of chronic infection is different from the acute process. Organisms such as *Pseudomonas aeruginosa* are much more common.[19] The treatment of a *Pseudomonas* infection requires a higher dosage of less routinely used antibiotics. The benign type of chronic otorrhea with mucoid discharge coming from a central perforation does not by itself invade bone and cause complications. There is, however, nothing to prevent a fresh virulent organism from entering such an ear and causing an acute exacerbation and a complication by the same mechanism as in any case of AOM. Unfortunately, the new organism is likely to display some greater resistance to antibiotics since the patient is likely to have received treatment for the otorrhea.

Immunocompromised individuals are at risk of developing not only otitis media but also complications of otitis media. The organisms causing the infection are more likely to be atypical pathogens. Individuals may be taking immunosuppressive medications, rendering them immunocompromised and susceptible to infection, or may have acquired immune deficiency syndrome (AIDS).

Intracranial extension of AOM occurs somewhat more often from poorly pneumatized than well-pneumatized temporal bones and even ears with a history of previous attacks of otitis media. The likelihood of a complication arising from chronic middle ear infections depends on the pathologic lesion causing the chronic otorrhea. The middle ear cleft has bony barriers that prevent the middle ear infection from extending intracranially. However, these barriers may be eroded by antecedent infections, granulation tissue, or cholesteatoma, thus allowing infection to spread into the cranial cavity from the middle ear. Trauma with fracture can create passages that allow infections to bypass these natural defenses.

The natural drainage of the mastoid cavity (approximately 5 cc in volume) is into a relatively smaller space, the middle ear cavity (capacity approximately 0.9 cc), which then drains through the Eustachian tube. Drainage may be inadequate, allowing infected secretions to accumulate and then erode through the middle ear cleft to extend intracranially.[20]

PATHWAY OF SPREAD IN THE PRODUCTION OF A COMPLICATION

As stated above, the infection spreads beyond the confines of the ear because it may be uncontrolled or poorly controlled. The infection from the middle ear cleft may enter the intracranial cavity through any of three routes.

Bone Erosion

Extension by bone erosion is the most frequent manner of spread, leading to a complication in cases of AOM in well-pneumatized temporal bones, and it is nearly always the manner of spread in cases of chronic suppurative otitis media (Figure 27–1A). In AOM, bone erosion is the result of coalescent mastoiditis. In COM, the bone erosion is usually caused by a cholesteatoma; less often, it is caused by chronic osteomyelitis.

The bone-eroding process first exposes the soft tissue of a neighboring structure. Protective granulations form on the structure as a last line of defense. Then, after a period of time that varies with the virulence of the organism, the pus under pressure finally penetrates the wall of protective granulations by pressure necrosis. Bone erosion as the pathway of spread may be recognized by the following characteristics:

- The complication occurs several weeks or more after the onset of AOM or in chronic otitis of long duration.
- A prodromal period of partial or intermittent involvement of the structure frequently precedes the diffuse involvement. Thus, a milder, intermittent facial weakness may precede complete facial paralysis; recurrent mild vertigo may precede diffuse purulent labyrinthitis, and localized meningismus may precede diffuse purulent meningitis.
- At operation, a dehiscence of the bone barrier is found between the suppurative focus and the neighboring structure. A layer of granulations covers the exposed soft tissue of the neighboring structure.
- The treatment of a complication by bone erosion is directed toward the complication and always includes surgical removal of the suppurative, bone-eroding focus in the temporal bone. If such removal is neglected, the complication is likely to recur or respond poorly to treatment.

A

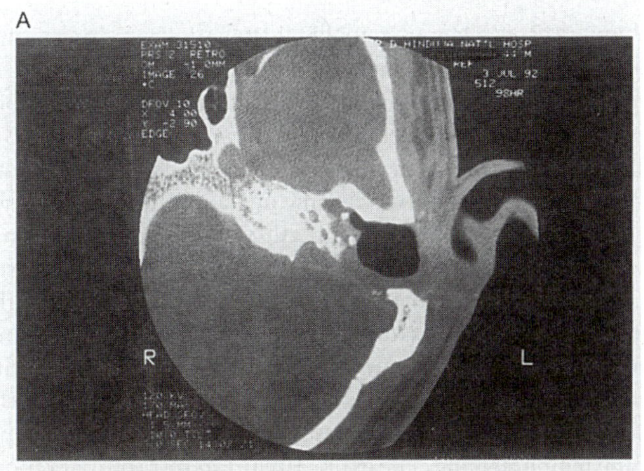

B

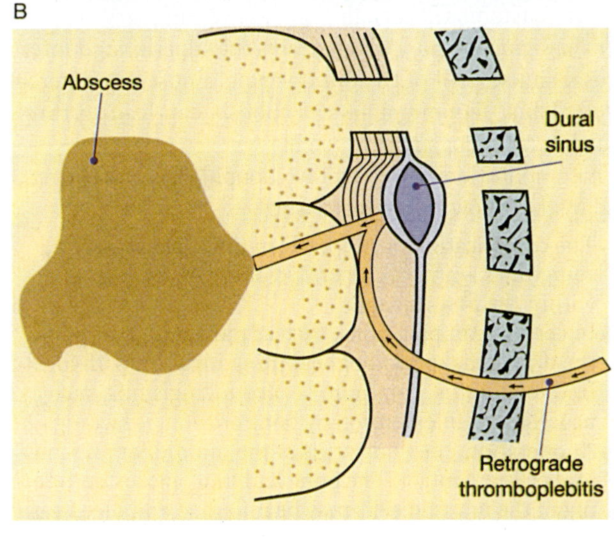

FIGURE 27–1 • *A*, Temporal bone CT scan, axial section. There is considerable erosion of the temporal bone and a high likelihood of an intracranial complication developing. *B*, Schematic representation of the development of a brain abscess from otitis media. Spread of infection can occur by direct extension or by retrograde thrombophlebitis.

Direct Extension Along Preformed Pathways

Extension by preformed pathways may occur in either acute exacerbations of COM or AOM. The preformed pathway may be a normal anatomic opening in the bony wall, such as the oval or round window, internal auditory canal, cochlear aqueduct, or endolymphatic duct and sac. The pathway may be a developmental dehiscence such as a patent suture or a dehiscent floor of the hypotympanum over the jugular bulb. The preformed pathway may be the result of a skull fracture or previous surgery. A perilymph fistula, either congenital or acquired, can also serve as a pathway. Occasionally, previous otitis media with coalescent mastoiditis heals but leaves a scar tissue tract to a neighboring structure. This tract acts as a preformed pathway for succeeding infections. Extension by a preformed pathway is not always easily diagnosed preoperatively. The diagnosis is suggested by the following characteristics:

- There is a history of repeated attacks of meningitis, skull fracture, operation on the temporal bone, or previously healed otitis media.
- The complication occurs early in the acute infection, thus resembling extension by thrombophlebitis.
- At operation, a dehiscence of the bone barrier not caused by bone erosion is found.
- The patient has an intracranial complication following suppurative labyrinthitis.

The treatment of a complication by a preformed pathway is directed toward the complication along with closure of the fistula and surgical evacuation of any collection of pus within the temporal bone. An example is beginning meningitis via the internal auditory canal from suppurative labyrinthitis; the labyrinth should be drained at the same time that the meningitis is treated by antibacterial medication.

Thrombophlebitis

In 1902, Körner demonstrated by histopathologic studies that it is possible for infection to pass from the lining mucosa of the middle ear and mastoid through intact bone by means of a progressive thrombophlebitis of small venules (Figure 27–1B).[6] This manner of spread may occur in acute middle ear infections or acute exacerbations of a chronic infection. Infection spreads through veins contiguous with either the infected pneumatized spaces of the temporal bone or the previously thrombosed dural venous sinus. There is a rich network of veins within the temporal bone that is in direct communication within the temporal bone and that, in turn, is in direct communication with the extracranial, intracranial, and cranial diploic veins. The extracranial veins are closely associated with the arterial supply of the temporal bone. The extracranial and intracranial venous systems anastomose through the mastoid emissary veins that enter the sigmoid sinus, which drains the superior and inferior petrosal sinuses. All of the dural venous sinuses are interconnected. Thus, sigmoid sinus thrombosis can lead to thrombophlebitis of other sinuses as well.

A complication caused by thrombophlebitis may be recognized by the following characteristics:

- The complication occurs early in the acute infection, sometimes within a day or two of the onset, usually within the first 10 days.
- In certain complications, such as purulent meningitis, the prodromal period of beginning invasion with localized meningitis, commonly called menigismus, such as is usually seen in extension by bone erosion, is lacking.
- At operation, the bony walls of the middle ear and mastoid cells are intact. The bone and mucoperiosteum lining of the mastoid cells may be inflamed and bleed easily, but there is no coalescent abscess, and the bone is not dehiscent.
- Hematogenous spread of infection usually results in meningitis. Whereas venous thrombophlebitis usually leads to cerebellar abscesses, arterial spread leads to temporal lobe abscesses and diffuse septicemia.

SPECIFIC COMPLICATIONS

It is uncommon for an intracranial complication to occur without a temporal bone complication occurring first. Common symptoms of an impending intracranial complication are as follows:

- Persistence of otorrhea. The otorrhea is particularly foul-smelling, and the pus becomes more viscous. The pus is thicker and creamier and may be blood stained. When intracranial complication is imminent, the discharge becomes scanty, indicative of poor drainage.
- Pain is an ominous sign that an intracranial complication is imminent. The pain is typically of a deep boring nature and is accompanied by a change in the quality of the pus emanating from the ear. Patients may also complain of a generalized headache that is "the worst headache" they have ever had.
- High-grade fever, altered sensorium, toxemia, photophobia, and irritability are other signs of impending intracranial complication.
- Neck stiffness and generalized malaise are signs that the organism has reached the cerebrospinal fluid (CSF) space.

The principles of ear surgery remain unchanged in these complications:

- Eradication of disease
- Establishment of adequate drainage for accumulated material.

Eradication of disease requires a thorough and complete mastoidectomy. All of the diseased air cells are exenterated. Pus, wherever it is encountered, is drained. All diseased or dead tissue is removed. There are some general remarks that can be made concerning all complications of mastoid disease. Specific recommendations are made in the following sections concerning each complication. Creating adequate drainage usually requires a canal-wall-down approach, with exceptions in certain situations. In the presence of AOM that has caused meningitis, usually antibiotics and a myringotomy with tube insertion suffice to provide adequate drainage. In the presence of overwhelming disease and cholesteatoma, most reports advocate canal-wall-down techniques in order to make the ear disease free. Equally important is creating a wide meatoplasty. A wide meatoplasty permits adequate drainage and allows easy inspection and cleansing of the mastoid cavity.

Each diagnosis of intracranial disease is defined and discussed individually. The diagnoses are presented in order of decreasing frequency. Meningitis is the most common complication in this group of diagnoses in most traditional articles. Brain abscess and lateral sinus thrombosis are the next most common. Finally, other diagnoses, including otitic hydrocephalus, and subdural and epidural processes are reviewed. Pathophysiology, including microbiology, unique symptoms, specific evaluation methods, and treatment, is outlined.

Meningitis

Generalized bacterial meningitis is defined as an inflammatory response to bacterial infection of the pia-arachnoid and the CSF of the subarachnoid space. Since the subarachnoid space is continuous around the brain, spinal cord, and optic nerves, infections of this space usually involve the entire cerebrospinal axis.

Localized meningitis may be defined as a localized inflammation of the dura and pia-arachnoid confined to the region adjacent to a suppurative focus or dural irritation, without viable organisms in the CSF.

Meningitis was the most frequent intracranial complication of otitis media in the preantibiotic era. With the introduction of antimicrobial drugs, recovery from meningitis improved from 10 to 86%[21] whereas recovery from otogenic meningitis was 59%.[22] Currently, community-acquired meningitis caused by *S. pneumonia* has fatality rates from 19 to 37%.[23] Other clinicians have confirmed that meningitis is the most common intracranial complication of AOM.[24] Some workers find that AOM is more likely to cause meningitis than COM.[25] *S. pneumoniae* infections of the meninges are often associated with AOM.[26]

Pathophysiology

Recovery of anaerobic organisms from the CSF suggests intraventricular rupture of a brain abscess. Polymicrobial infection of CSF resulting from otogenic complications is uncommon and accounts for less than 1% of cases.

Meningitis may result from infection spreading from the ear via retrograde thrombophlebitis, bone erosion, and preformed pathways. An important route through which infection can gain access to the CSF is via the labyrinth through the round and oval windows. Nager[27] and Kaplan[28] stressed that this mode of extension is via the perineural spaces to the internal auditory canal and less frequently via the endolymphatic ducts. Proctor[29] postulated that otitic meningitis occurs as the result of infection spreading via the labyrinth and petrous apex. Meningitis can develop following trauma to the ear with fracture, dural tear, and CSF leak. Meningitis can also occur following any middle ear and mastoid surgery.

Of all patients surviving bacterial meningitis, 5 to 35% experience bilateral sensorineural hearing loss.[30] Paparella described the pathophysiology of suppurative meningogenic labyrinthitis as having three phases. The acute phase is characterized by infiltration of leukocytes and is followed by the fibrous stage, which is characterized by fibrous proliferation within perilymph spaces. The ossification stage ensues, with the most significant disease in the basal turn of the cochlea near the round window. He stated that the pathologic features of meningogenic suppurative labyrinthitis are essentially the same as tympanogenic labyrinthitis.[31] In a human temporal bone study, Merchant verified the hypothesis that the cochlear modiolus and the cochlear aqueduct can serve as potential pathways for spread of infection from the meninges to the inner ear.[32]

Clinical Presentation

Otogenic meningitis often goes unrecognized. It is imperative for the physician who is treating a patient with meningitis to rule out a possible otologic cause. Most physicians will suspect an otologic cause in the presence of otorrhea or obvious long-standing ear disease. It is imperative to rule out otitis media in the patient who does not have otorrhea or long-standing otologic complaints.

Cawthorne[33] noted that the symptoms tend to be more rapid when associated with AOM. The earliest symptoms are headache, fever, vomiting, photophobia, irritability, and restlessness. Infants may have seizures. As the infection progresses, the headache increases, and vomiting becomes more pronounced. Neck stiffness, with resistance to flexing the neck so that the chin does not touch the chest, may start with minimal discomfort and progress. Brudzinski's sign, the inability to flex the leg without moving the opposite leg (or flexion of the neck resulting in flexion of the hip and knee), is a sign of meningitis. Similarly, Kernig's sign, an inability to extend the leg when lying supine with the thigh flexed toward the abdomen, is suggestive of meningitis.

Management

Computed tomographic (CT) scanning of the temporal bones demonstrates the status of the temporal bone and that of surrounding structures. High-resolution CT scanning is very useful and is the imaging modality of choice. Rapid CT scanning is now available that reduces the time to take a high-resolution scan of the temporal bones, which is particularly important in children in whom a congenital malformation of the ear needs to be ruled out. CT scanning helps rule out the presence of congenital ear malformations that permit leakage of CSF through an associated inner ear fistula. Bony details are best visualized with CT scanning.

Magnetic resonance imaging (MRI) provides better resolution of the brain substance and shows middle ear fluid and inflammatory changes in the brain and meninges. No bone detail is possible. The relationship of middle ear disease to the surrounding bone is not well visualized.

Either CT scanning or MRI can identify a mass effect that could lead to herniation. Thus, imaging usually precedes lumbar puncture. Although fundoscopic examination may show indistinct disk margins or even choking of vessels, it is sometimes difficult to perform in an uncooperative patient.

It is imperative to identify the causative organism and the source of infection. Accordingly, a lumbar puncture is performed to obtain CSF for bacteriologic analysis. In meningitis, the CSF is cloudy or yellow (xanthochromic); an elevated white blood cell count, low glucose, and high protein are expected. The pathogen is identified by microscopic examination of Gram-stained fluid with confirmation by culture; sensitivity testing aids in the selection of a suitable antimicrobial drug. A sample should be taken from the ear as well, especially if pus is present.

Treatment

Antimicrobial drugs are essential in the treatment of meningitis. Empiric antibiotic therapy should be initiated with a third-generation cephalosporin plus vancomycin.[23]

The advantages of third-generation cephalosporins are their bactericidal activity, ability to penetrate the blood-brain barrier and enter the CSF, their expanded activity against β-lactamase–producing organisms and gram-negative organisms, and low toxicity.[34] Vancomycin is now recommended secondary to the increase in prevalence of penicillin-resistant pneumococci.[23]

In a Cochrane review by van de Beek et al., corticosteroids significantly reduced rates of mortality, severe hearing loss, and neurologic sequelae associated with acute bacterial meningitis. In children with acute bacterial meningitis, corticosteroids reduced the rate of severe hearing loss from 11 to 6.6%. In adults with acute bacterial meningitis, corticosteroids reduced the mortality rate from 21.7 to 11.7%. A 4-day regimen of dexamethasone—0.6 mg/kg/day divided into four daily doses—is recommended. Dexamethasone should be started before or with the first dose of antibiotics.[35]

Role of Surgery

In AOM with an intact tympanic membrane, surgery consists of myringotomy with evacuation of the fluid from the middle ear, which is sent for examination and culture.

For the patient with coalescent mastoiditis or with a history of ear trauma and precipitous meningitis, a complete mastoidectomy with middle ear exploration should be performed. In the latter circumstance, the surgeon should look for and repair the route of CSF leakage. CT scanning usually reveals the fracture line, allowing the surgeon to identify the site of the leak.

If cholesteatoma is present, the default procedure should be a radical mastoidectomy because the goal of surgery is to make the ear disease-free and provide adequate drainage. A modified radical or a canal-wall-up mastoidectomy can be considered in select cases (Figure 27–2).

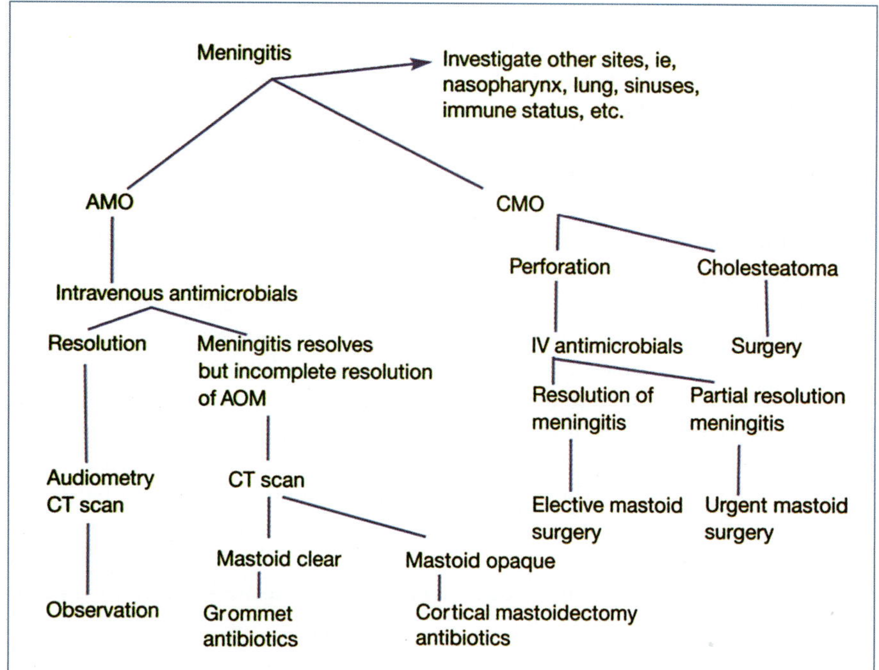

FIGURE 27–2 • Management of otogenic meningitis. CT, computed tomography; PE, pressure equalization; MRI, magnetic resonance imaging; MRV, magnetic resonance venography.

Brain Abscess

A brain abscess is a focal suppurative process within the brain parenchyma surrounded by a region of encephalitis.[26]

Brain abscess secondary to otitis media displays a bimodal age distribution, with peaks in the pediatric age group and in the fourth decade.[36] In most series, the male-to-female ratio has been approximately 3:1.[37] Otitis media was an important cause of brain abscess in the past but has been much less significant more recently. COM is much more likely to cause brain abscess than AOM,[38] and cholesteatoma now accounts for most cases.[39] Most authors report that otogenic brain abscesses are more likely to be located in the cerebrum (temporal lobe) than in the cerebellum;[40,41] however, the majority of cerebellar abscesses are associated with middle ear infections.[26] On the other hand, Murthy[42] and Dubey[43] found that otogenic abscesses occurred more frequently in the cerebellum. The mortality associated with brain abscess of otogenic origin in the antibiotic era continues to decline. Bento[44] and Migirov[24] recently reported a total of 14 patients with cerebral or cerebellar abscess without a mortality. Cerebellar abscesses have a greater likelihood of fatal outcome.[45] Permanent neurologic sequelae are commonly associated with brain abscesses. In Penido's review of intracranial complications of otogenic origin, the permanent neurologic sequelae that developed in all eight patients were secondary to brain abscess.[46]

Pathophysiology

Multiple organisms are usually present in brain abscesses.[47] Polymicrobial cultures with a high incidence of anaerobes are reported in various studies.[48] *Streptococcus* and *Staphylococcus* are common gram-positive organisms that are isolated from brain abscesses. *Escherichia coli* and *Proteus*, *Klebsiella*, and *Pseudomonas* species are typical gram-negative isolates. The microbiology of a brain abscess is influenced by the immune status of the host. It is interesting to note that *H. influenzae* is rarely found in otogenic brain abscesses.[33]

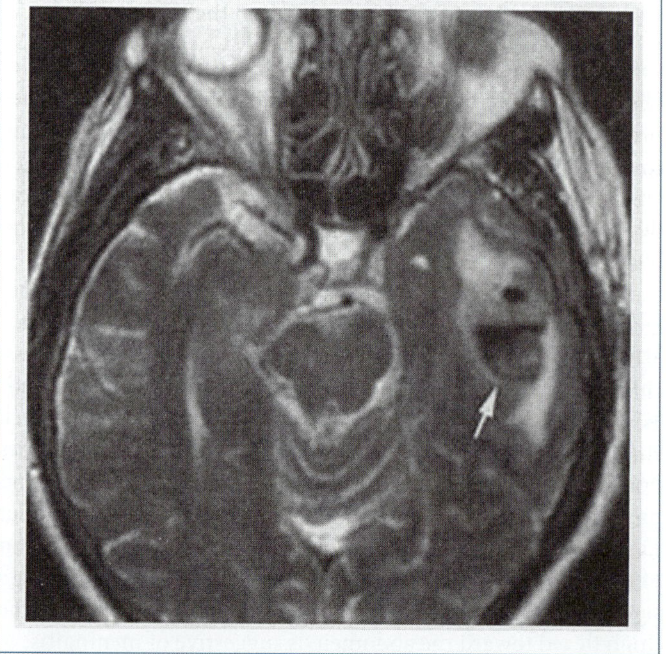

FIGURE 27–3 • A well-encapsulated brain abscess complicating otitis media.

Brain abscess can result from any of three processes: (1) a contiguous focus of infection, such as otitis media (Figure 27–3); (2) hematogenous spread from a distant focus of infection, such as chronic pyogenic lung disease; and (3) head injury or cranial surgery.

Otogenic brain abscesses are often the result of venous thrombophlebitis rather than direct dural extension.[49] Five

Stages	Number of days	Changes
Early cerebritis (invasion)	Days 1 to 3 following innoculation	Perivascular inflammatory response surrounding a developing necrotic center with edema
Late cerebritis ([localization] quiescent abscess)	4 to 10 days	Well-formed necrotic center, neovascularity in the periphery of the necrotic zone
Early capsule formation (enlargement: manifest abscess)	10 to 13 days	Well-developed layer of fibroblasts with persistent cerebritis and neovascularity
Late capsule formation (termation)	14 days	Thickening of capsule

FIGURE 27–4 • Stages of formation of brain abscess and changes that occur.

percent of brain abscesses occur soon after mastoidectomy,[37] eg, when an open mastoid cavity has been created but residual disease persists.[50]

Thrombophlebitis usually accompanies the formation of a brain abscess and must be managed appropriately. Osteitis or granulation tissue causes retrograde thrombophlebitis of dural vessels that terminate in the white matter of the brain,[51] producing encephalitis. This localized encephalitis progresses to necrosis and liquefaction of brain tissue (focal suppuration) with surrounding edema.[52] Within approximately 2 weeks, an abscess capsule surrounded by granulation tissue forms. Brain abscess formation is a continuum from cerebritis to a well-encapsulated necrotic focus; nonetheless, many authors[29,53] have described stages of the formation of a brain abscess (Figure 27–4). Encapsulation is more well defined on the cortical side as compared with the ventricular side, perhaps explaining the propensity of abscesses to rupture medially into the ventricular system rather than into the subarachnoid space (Figure 27–5).

The maturity of the brain abscess depends on the local oxygen concentration, the offending organism, and the host immune response.

Clinical Presentation

The patient appears very "toxic" and drowsy and often complains of deep bony pain. Occasionally, indolent mastoiditis can cause a brain abscess. Foul-smelling, creamy otorrhea indicates a fulminant, destructive process. Brain abscess formation is indicated by the presence of the triad of (1) headache, (2) high-grade fever, and (3) focal neurologic deficits. In more recent times, the complete triad is not frequently encountered. Symptoms may be present for 2 weeks before the brain abscess is fully formed.[26] Focal deficits depend on the location of the abscess. Cerebellar abscesses provoke dizziness, ataxia, nystagmus, and vomiting. Temporal lobe lesions may result in seizures. Associated signs of meningitis are usually present.[49] Papilledema is frequently seen in stage 3 of abscess formation.[54]

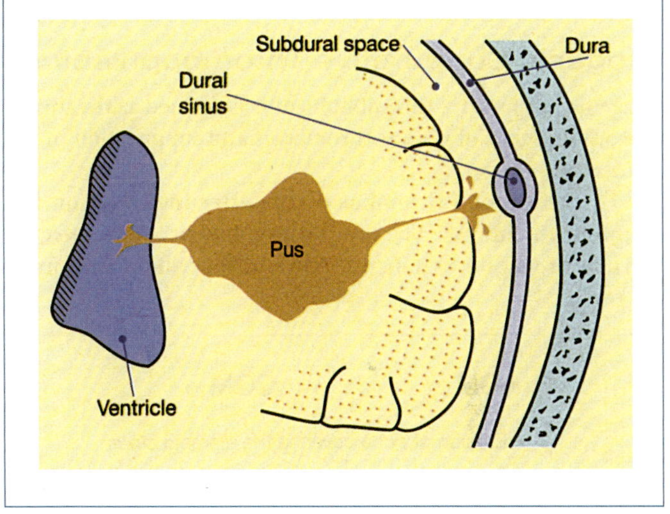

FIGURE 27–5 • Schematic illustration demonstrating brain abscess rupture into the ventricle and into the subdural space.

Imaging

CT scanning is very useful in the evaluation of the patient suspected of having an otogenic brain abscess. Scanning may allow for earlier detection of abscesses and improved outcomes.[55] The brain abscess appears as a hypodense area surrounded by an area of edema, a configuration known as the "ring" sign. Serial CT scanning can be used to follow the effects of treatment, determine if the abscess is resolving, and assist in the timing of surgical intervention.

MRI has also proven to be useful and is superior to CT scanning in detecting subtle changes in the brain parenchyma and in detecting the spread of the abscess into the subarachnoid space or into the ventricle.[56]

One limitation of MRI is that it cannot provide detailed information about the temporal bone; thus, a separate CT scan is required to assess the temporal bone.

Management

The patient must be hospitalized and treated with appropriate, high-dose antimicrobial medication immediately. The management of the brain abscess takes precedence over that of the primary infective source because the patient is seriously ill and the neurosurgical procedure may be the life-saving procedure. The patient should be first stabilized neurologically; only then should the ear causing the infection be operated on.

Currently, the management of brain abscesses is a controversial issue owing to improved imaging and more effective antibiotics. The decision to excise or drain a brain abscess is one such controversy. Williams recommends aspiration with high doses of appropriate antibiotics because he finds that this regimen is associated with fewer permanent neurologic sequelae.[57] Le Beau and colleagues recommend total excision because they find that this leads to lower mortality.[58] Another controversy exists as to whether neurosurgical intervention is required at all because the intravenous administration of newer and more effective antibiotics can result in the complete resolution of small brain abscesses, obviating neurosurgical intervention.[59]

Otogenic Suppurative Thrombophlebitis

Otogenic suppurative thrombophlebitis is defined as the simultaneous presence of venous thrombosis and suppuration in the intracranial cavity.

Formation of a thrombus occurs after the infection has spread to the intima. The mural thrombus becomes infected and may propagate; as it increases in size, it occludes the lumen. Embolization of septic thrombi or extension into tributary vessels may produce further disease.

Infectious thrombophlebitis of the sigmoid sinus is a well-known intracranial complication of otitis media. The advent of antibiotics has brought about a decline in the frequency of this condition[60] as well as the mortality rate to 0 to 10 % over the last 20 years.[61] Suppurative thrombophlebitis of the sigmoid sinus can be seen with AOM and COM.

Pathophysiology

The *β-hemolytic streptococcus* was the most common organism associated with this condition; however, more recently, cultures have revealed mixed flora, including *Bacteroides*, *Streptococcus* species, *methicillin-resistant Staphylococcus aureus (MRSA)*, *coagulase-negative staphylococcus*, mixed anaerobes, *Pseudomonas*, *Enterococcus*, and *Proteus*.[61,62]

Two pathophysiologic mechanisms for the formation of suppurative thrombophlebitis are given in Figure 27–6. Once thrombosis has occurred, propagation of the thrombus can extend intracranially or into the jugular vein and the right atrium of the heart. Intracranial extension results in brain abscess and thrombophlebitis of other vessels in the cranial cavity with their attendant sequelae. Intracardiac spread results in widespread dissemination of infection and fulminant septicemia.

Recent evidence suggests that patients developing lateral sinus thrombosis may have an elevated incidence of prothrombotic disorders when compared to the general population. Oestreicher-Kedem reviewed a series of seven children with lateral sinus thrombosis secondary to AOM and found five to have prothrombotic disorders with an elevated level of lipoprotein apolipoprotein being the most common finding.[62]

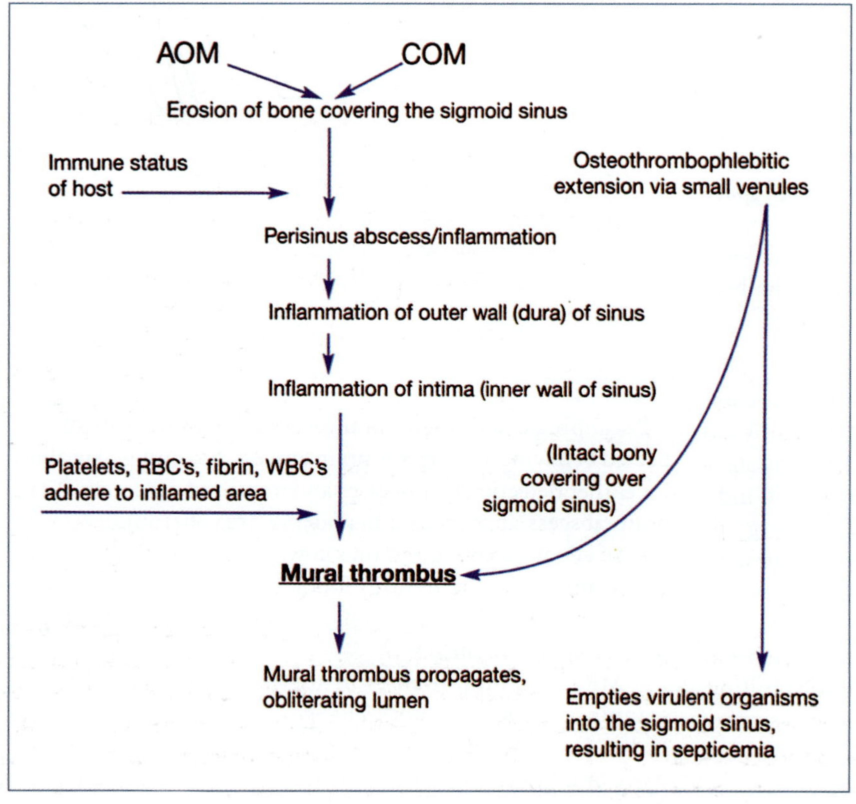

FIGURE 27–6 • Pathogenesis of thrombophlebitis in the sigmoid sinus. AOM, acute otitis media; COM, chronic otitis media; RBC, red blood cell; WBC, white blood cell.

Clinical Presentation

High-grade fever is a sign of suppurative thrombophlebitis. The fever may have a "picket fence" appearance or may be high grade without returning to baseline.[63] However, the presence of fever has become variable because many patients are partially treated with antibiotics. As reported in a recent study, as few as 33% of patients presented with fever and none with a "picket fence" appearance.[64] Typically, the patient will be toxic and restless, and will complain of otalgia. The otalgia, described as a deep, boring pain, usually heralds a worsening neurologic status. Otorrhea will be foul-smelling and usually blood stained.

If *β-hemolytic streptococci* are responsible for the infection, the patient may present with anemia, manifesting in pallor, and low hemoglobin levels. Proptosis, ptosis, chemosis, and ophthalmoplegia indicate that the thrombus has spread to the cavernous sinus. Tenderness and edema over the mastoid (Griesinger's sign) are pathognomonic for suppurative thrombophlebitis of the sigmoid sinus and reflect thrombosis of the mastoid emissary veins. Propagation of the thrombus into the internal jugular vein causes it to become hard, cord-like, and very tender to palpation, and results in a stiff neck. The lymph nodes along the internal jugular vein are enlarged and tender. Involvement of the torcular and sagittal sinuses can result in otitic hydrocephalus.

The frequency of central nervous system–specific findings at presentation has decreased. Manolidis reported that 8% of patients presented with papilledema, 33% with nuchal rigidity, and 42% with nausea.[64]

Imaging

CT scanning and MRI are the current imaging tools of choice in making the diagnosis. Before the advent of these imaging tools, cerebral angiography with observation of the venous phase was used to determine if thrombosis was present; however, cerebral angiography is no longer routinely performed because of its potential to dislodge the clot.[60]

CT scanning usually demonstrates the "delta sign"—an empty triangle at the level of the sigmoid sinus, consisting of the clot surrounded by a high-intensity rim of contrast-enhanced dura (Figure 27–7)—when thrombosis is present.[65] However, this sign is not always detectable, and not all thrombi can be documented by CT scanning.[66]

MRI is more sensitive than CT scanning in detecting thrombosis. When compared to MRI as the gold standard, CT scanning sensitivity ranges from 72 to 84%.[64,67] Magnetic resonance venography (MRV) shows blood flow, sinus obstruction, and subsequent reversal of flow(Figure 27–8).[65] MRI also provides higher resolution in detailing nerve tissue. Thus, MRI allows for earlier and more precise diagnosis of sinus thrombosis and better delineates both its extent and the involvement of surrounding structures. On gadolinium-enhanced MRI, the thrombus appears as a soft tissue signal associated with a vascular and bright appearance of the dural walls—the "delta" sign as seen with gadolinium-enhanced MRI.[68,69]

Early thrombus, as it is rich in deoxyhemoglobin, has an intermediate density on T1-weighted images and a low intensity on T2-weighted images. As the clot matures, methemoglobin forms and the MRI appearance changes so that the clot is hyperintense on both T1- and T2-weighted images.

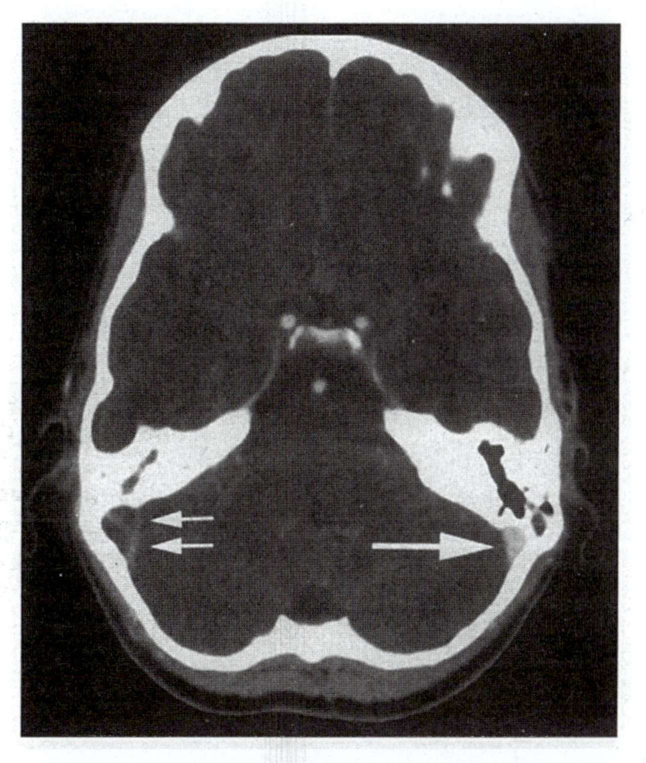

FIGURE 27–7 • A computed tomographic scan of sigmoid sinus thrombophlebitis. The pathognomonic "delta" sign is seen (2 small arrows). The contralateral sigmoid sinus is patent (single large arrow). *Reproduced with permission from Bradley DT, et al.*[65]

Management

Sigmoid sinus thrombophlebitis manifesting the classic signs and symptoms outlined above is unmistakable. However sigmoid sinus thrombophlebitis can present in an atypical manner and additional evaluation may be necessary. Queckenstedt's (or the Tobey-Ayer) test is used to detect lateral venous sinus thrombosis and is performed as follows: a spinal needle is inserted into the subarachnoid space, a manometer is attached, and the resting CSF pressure is recorded. The change in pressure produced by digital compression of first one internal jugular vein and then the other, and then both at the same time, is noted. When the pressure fails to rise after compression of the internal jugular vein on the side of the diseased ear and fails to fall when the vein is released, with a prompt contralateral response, the test is positive. A positive Queckenstedt's test is very strong evidence in favor of occlusion of the sigmoid sinus; however, it is not infallible. A false-positive test occurs when one sigmoid sinus is smaller than the other (usually the left one). A false-negative test occurs when there is unusually good collateral circulation around the obstructed sigmoid sinus via the mastoid emissary vein and the inferior petrosal sinus.

Any contraindication to performing a lumbar puncture (eg, elevated intracranial pressure) is also a contraindication to performing Queckenstedt's test. A positive blood culture provides good evidence of sigmoid sinus thrombosis, especially when accompanied by the clinical signs and symptoms of thrombosis.

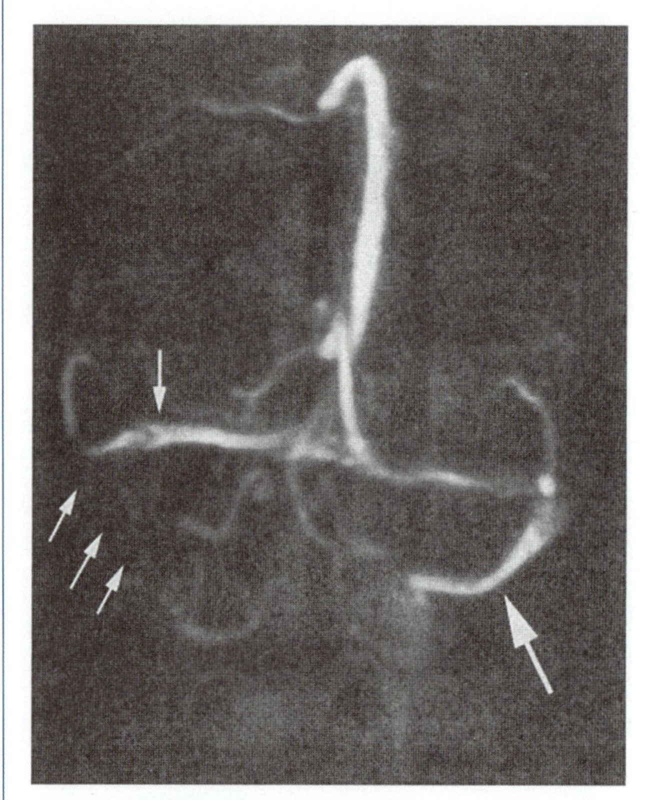

FIGURE 27–8 • Magnetic resonance venography image demonstrating loss of signal in the sigmoid sinus (multiple small arrows) indicative of sigmoid sinus thrombosis. Enhancement of the contralateral sigmoid sinus (large single arrow) and ipsilateral transverse sinus (single small arrow) representing sinus patency. *Reproduced with permission from Bradley DT, et al.*[65]

Treatment

Before the development of antibiotics, the treatment of lateral sinus thrombosis comprised surgery. A complete mastoidectomy was performed, and the entire sigmoid sinus was unroofed. Often a perisinus abscess was encountered and drained. Once the entire sinus was exposed, it was inspected and palpated; if it was soft and pliable, and the patient's symptoms were not serious, the sinus was left alone. However, if a rubbery clot was felt, then the sinus was carefully aspirated with a small-gauge needle and syringe. Lack of blood flow indicated a clot. The sinus was then opened in such a way that the medial dural wall was not traumatized. The clot was evacuated as completely as possible. Prior ligation of the internal jugular vein was carried out to prevent propagation of the thrombus into the heart.

Controversy remains regarding the extent of surgery required, and ranges from exposure of the sigmoid sinus to ligation of the internal jugular vein. Manolidis has attempted to clarify the surgical management of lateral sinus thrombosis by dividing patients into the categories of limited or extensive thrombosis. He further divided the lateral cranial venous system into five regions: transverse sinus, sigmoid sinus, jugular bulb, upper internal jugular vein to the confluence of the facial vein, and the lower jugular vein from the confluence of the facial vein to the subclavian vein. Limited thrombosis is confined to one or two regions whereas extensive thrombosis involves 3 or more contiguous regions. Three contraindications were applied when considering resection of the sinus: the affected side being the dominant flow system, limited thrombosis, and the presence of an intracranial complication that raises intracranial pressure. In limited thrombosis, the sinus is opened and the contents drained. In extensive thrombosis, the sinus is resected unless contraindicated.[64]

Historically, there has been debate about the use of anticoagulation. Two of the four patients treated in an Israeli study with 6 months of enoxaparin developed significant hematomas secondary to falls.[62] Shah discusses the management of two patients with lateral sinus thrombosis with postoperative low-molecular-weight heparin (LMWH) who developed hemorrhagic complications. Enoxaparin has the advantage of twice-daily subcutaneous administration. However, it is more difficult to monitor therapeutic ranges and its longer half-life compared to heparin make it difficult to fully and rapidly reverse the anticoagulation effect. Shah recommends proceeding with caution when using enoxaparin in the perioperative period for pediatric lateral sinus thrombosis.[70]

Otitic Hydrocephalus

Otitic hydrocephalus is the term suggested by Symonds[71,72] to describe the syndrome associated with otitis media characterized by increased intracranial pressure, normal CSF findings, spontaneous recovery, and no abscess. Although the term otitic hydrocephalus was coined by Symonds, the condition itself was first described by Quincke in 1897.[73] As there is no associated ventricular dilation, it is more appropriately termed "benign raised intracranial tension";[73] however, the term "otitic hydrocephalus" has persisted and is used in this chapter.

Otitic hydrocephalus is a rare complication of otitis media and stems from either AOM or COM. Otitic hydrocephalus has a favorable prognosis and is very commonly associated with sigmoid sinus thrombophlebitis; however, not all patients with sigmoid sinus thrombophlebitis develop otitic hydrocephalus.

Pathophysiology

The precise mechanism underlying the development of otitic hydrocephalus is unknown. Symonds[71,72] provided the explanation seen in Figure 27–9. An alternative theory postulates

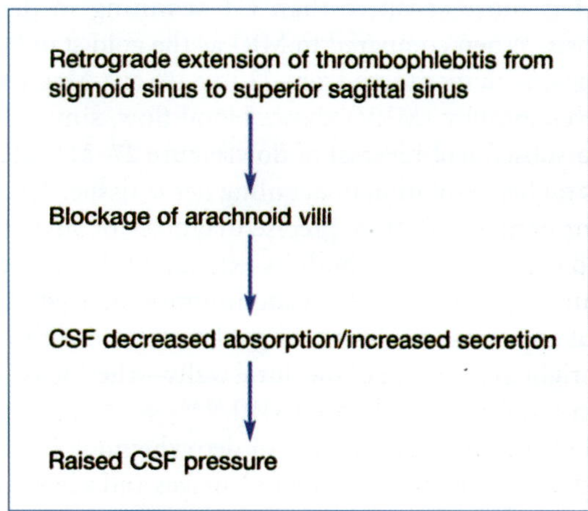

FIGURE 27–9 • Pathophysiology of otitic hydrocephalus. CSF, cerebrospinal fluid.

an increase in CSF volume.[74] Sahs and Joynt[75] theorized that the hydrocephalus is secondary to brain edema as brain biopsies reveal interstitial edema, yet electroencephalograms and neurologic function are normal. Weed and Flexner[76] postulated disruption in venous circulation as a cause since changes in CSF pressure are directly related to intracranial venous pressure.

Clinical Presentation

Headache, drowsiness, vomiting, blurring of vision, and diplopia are typical symptoms. Acute or chronic otitis media is also seen. Papilledema and sixth cranial nerve palsy are usually evident. Optic atrophy can eventually develop. Elevated CSF pressures with normal CSF biochemistry comprise the classic findings of otitic hydrocephalus. A lumbar puncture should be done with caution lest herniation of the cerebellar tonsils occur. MRI is the imaging modality of choice as it allows for superior evaluation of the venous sinuses.

Management

The goals of therapy are eradication of ear disease and lowering of the elevated intracranial pressure. O'Connor and Moffat[77] recommend decompression of the sigmoid sinus. CSF drainage procedures, such as shunts, have been recommended. Optic sheath decompression has been recommended to prevent optic atrophy.[78] Medical therapy includes corticosteroids, mannitol, diuretics, and acetazolamide.

Subdural Empyema

A subdural empyema is a collection of pus in the space between the dura mater and the arachnoid membrane. This condition was almost always fatal prior to the advent of antibiotic therapy. Today, subdural empyema is the rarest of the complications of otitis media.

Pathophysiology

The subdural space, normally a potential space rather than an actual one, is divided into several large compartments by the foramen magnum, tentorium cerebelli, base of the brain, and the falx cerebri (Figure 27–10). Since these spaces are anatomically confined, a developing empyema can quickly evolve into a fatal mass lesion (Figure 27–11).

Clinical Presentation

Headache of abrupt onset and unusually severe nature is typical of subdural empyema. Fever and vomiting are other symptoms that accompany this disease. The rapidity with which the patient deteriorates points to a subdural empyema.

MRI is the imaging modality of choice.[79] It has been found to be superior at detecting the presence and extensions of the infection and can also distinguish between epidural and subdural infection. Multiple, discrete, loculated subdural collections may occasionally be seen. MRI is particularly useful because of the absence of bone artifact, heightened contrast between bone, CSF, and brain parenchyma, as well as because of its multiplanar imaging capability.[80] MRI can also characterize subdural collections, allowing differentiation of sterile, bloody, and infected collections. CT is unable to perform these functions.

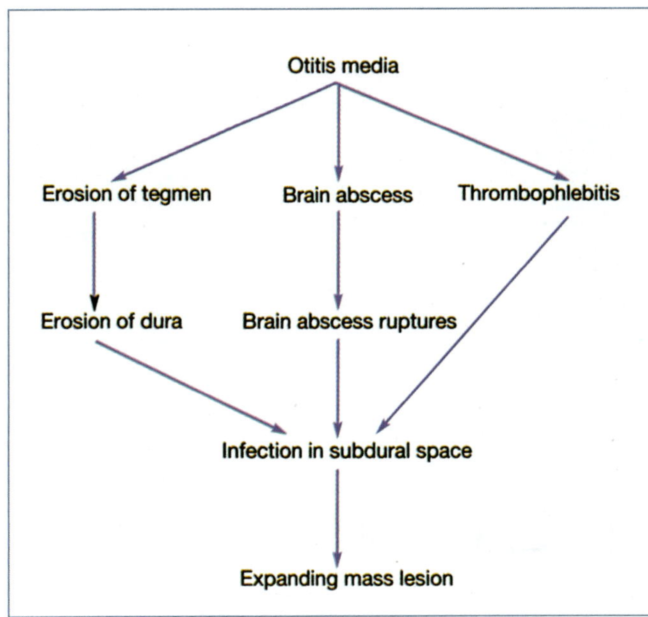

FIGURE 27–10 • Pathology of subdural empyema.

Treatment

Subdural empyema is a surgical emergency, and prognosis is related to the promptness of diagnosis and drainage. Lumbar puncture is contraindicated as it could precipitate herniation of the cerebellar tonsils. Emergency drainage with high-dose, intravenous antimicrobial medication is the treatment of choice. Once the patient has been stabilized neurologically, the underlying ear disease can be managed.

Epidural (Extradural) Abscess

The epidural (extradural) space is a potential space between the dura mater and the bone of the intracranial cavity. Infection here usually manifests with granulation tissue that is in direct continuity with the suppurative process. Large accumulations of pus are rare. Granulation along the dura mater is seen more commonly than an actual abscess (Figure 27–12A and B). An epidural abscess usually precedes other intracranial complications, especially sinus thrombophlebitis and brain abscess. Sinus thrombophlebitis is the complication that most frequently coexists with an epidural abscess.

Pathogenesis

Coalescent mastoiditis entails bone reabsorption, especially in the areas adjacent to the sigmoid sinus; these areas of bone give way, resulting in a pocket of granulation tissue/pus that expands along the sigmoid sinus. Ultimately, the granulation tissue also infects the sigmoid sinus. Chronic suppurative otitis media without cholesteatoma is usually associated with granulation tissue that invades the perisinus air cells. A single acute exacerbation of infection may cause silent extradural granulation tissue to progress into more serious complications.

Epidural abscesses are rarely symptomatic unless they are very large. Usually, they are noted as incidental findings during surgery performed for another complication; however, with the radiologic imaging modalities of today, epidural abscesses can be visualized prior to surgery.

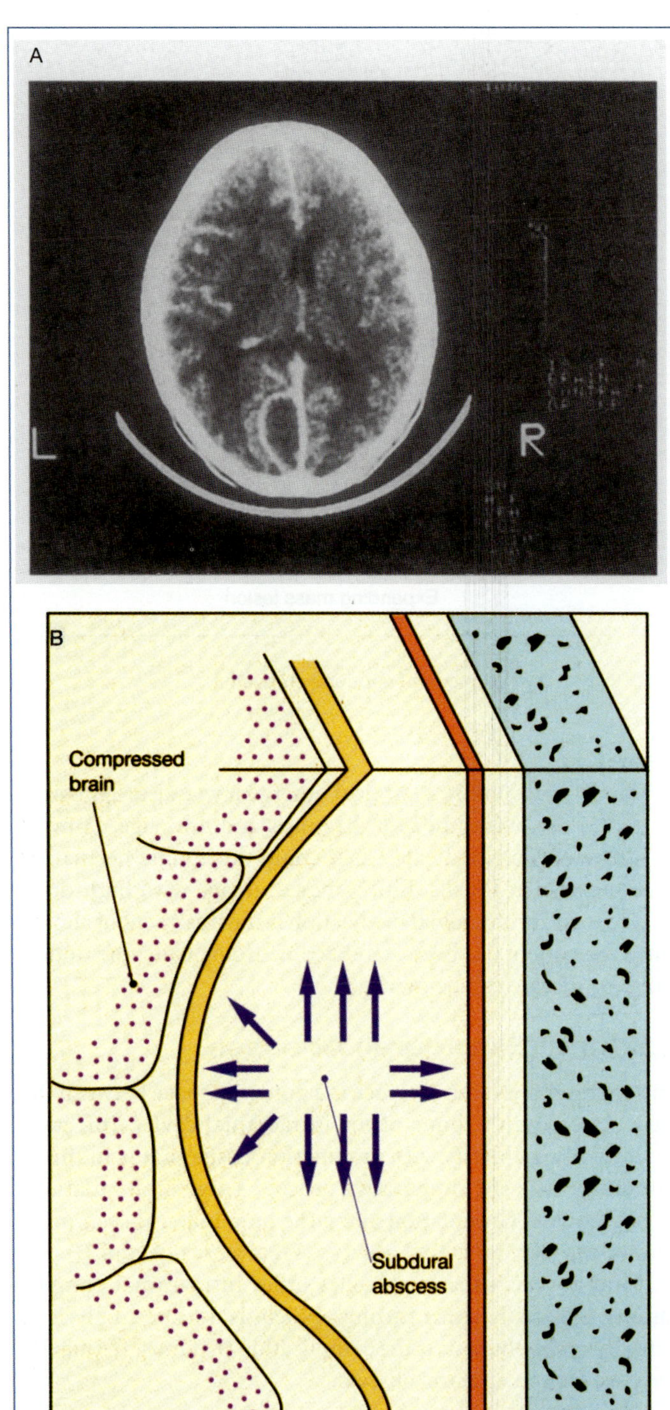

FIGURE 27–11 • *A*, A computed tomographic scan of a loculated subdural abscess in the falx. *B*, Schematic illustration of the mass effect related to an expanding abscess in the subdural space.

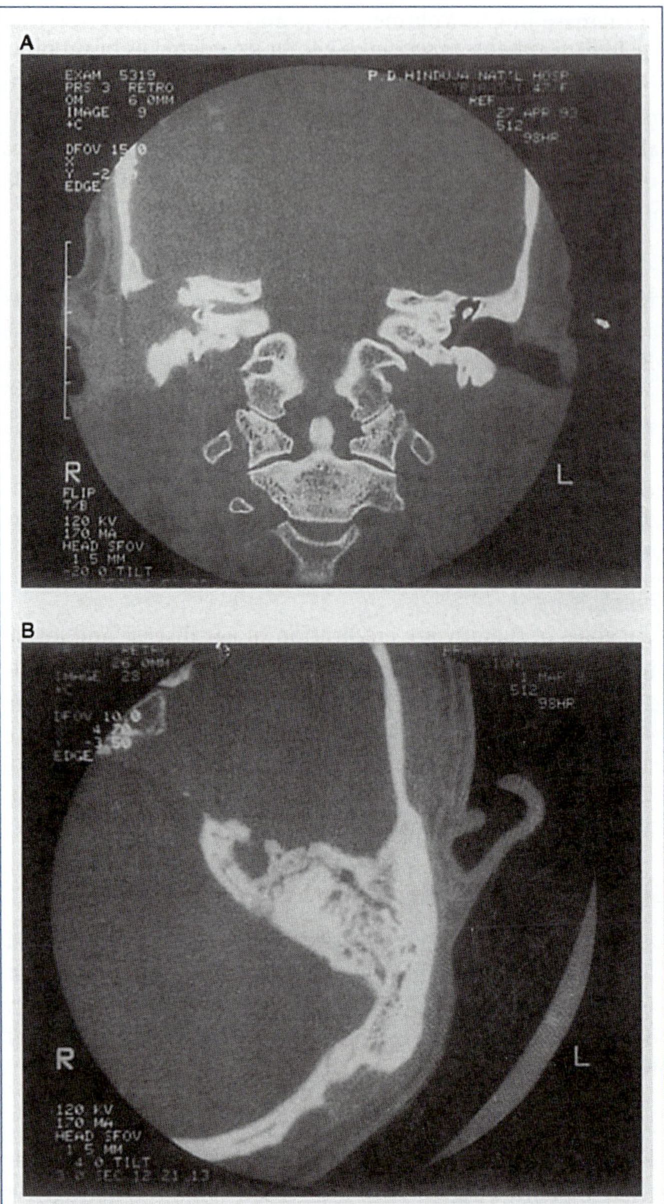

FIGURE 27–12 • *A*, Temporal bone computed tomographic (CT) scan, coronal section. There is mastoiditis and dural elevation, indicative of an epidural abscess. The contralateral temporal bone is normal. *B*, Temporal bone CT scan, axial section. Petrous apicitis is associated with a small epidural abscess.

Management

The discovery of granulation tissue penetrating bone or granulation tissue along the sigmoid sinus should prompt further exploration. The surrounding bone should be gently removed and the abscess drained. Care should be taken not to perforate the dura, which could result in a CSF leak and allow the infection to spread directly into the brain. Excessive granulation tissue should be gently trimmed.

References

1. Cawthorne T. The surgery of the temporal bone. J Laryngol Otol 1953;67:377–91.
2. Heine B, Beck J. Handbuch der Hals-Nassen-Ohr-enheilkunde. In: Denker A, Kahler O, editors. Berlin: 1927.
3. Morand S. Opuscules de chirugie. Paris, 1768.
4. Lebert. Ueber Entzundung der Hirn-Sinus. Virchows Arch 1856;9:381.
5. MacEwen W. Pyogenic infective diseases of the brain and spinal cord. Glascow: 1893.

6. Korner O. Otitischen Erkrankungen des Hirns, der Hirnhaute und der Blutleiter. Wiesbaden, 1908.
7. Eagleton WP. Brain abscess: Its surgical pathology and operative technique. New York: Macmillan, 1922.
8. Shambaugh GJ. The surgical treatment of meningitis of otitic and nasal origin. JAMA 1937;108:696.
9. Lebert. Ueber Gehirnabscesse. Virchows Arch 1856;10:78.
10. Zaufal E. Operation der Sinusthrombose und Versuche mit Cocain am Gehororgane. Prag Med Wochenschr 1884;9:474.
11. Lane W. Middle ear suppurations and their complications. BMJ 1889;1:998.
12. Ballance C. Pyemic thrombosis of the lateral sinus. Lancet 1890;1:1057.
13. Jansen A. Referat die Operations methoden bei den verschiedenen otitischen Gehirnkomplikationen. Verhandl Deutsch Otol Gesellsch 1895;4:96.
14. Gradenigo G. Sulla leptomeningite circoscritta e sula paralisi dell' adducente di origine otitica. Cior Accad Med Torino 1904;10:59.
15. Kopetsky SJ, Almour R. Suppuration of the petrous pyramid. Ann Otol Rhinol Laryngol 1931;39:996.
16. Eagleton WP. Unlocking the petrous pyramid for localized bulbar meningitis secondary to suppuration of the petrous apex. Arch Otolaryngol 1931;13:386.
17. Courville CB. Intracranial complications of otitis media and mastoiditis in the antibiotic era. I. Modification of the pathology of otitic intracranial lesions by antibiotic preparations. Laryngoscope 1955;65:31–46.
18. Bluestone CD, Stephenson JS, Martin LM. Ten-year review of otitis media pathogens. Pediatr Infect Dis J 1992;11:S7–S11.
19. Feinmesser R, Wiesel YM, Argaman M, Gay I. Otitis externa—Bacteriological survey. ORL J Otorhinolaryngol Relat Spec 1982;44:121–5.
20. Neely G. Complications of suppurative otitis media, Parts 1 and 2. Otolaryngol Head Neck Surg; Washington D.C.; 1978.
21. House H. Acute otitis media. A comparative study of the results obtained before and after the introduction of the sulfonamide compounds. Arch Otolaryngol Head Neck Surg 1946;43:371–5.
22. McLay K. Otogenic meningitis. J Laryngol Otol 1954;68:140–6.
23. van de Beek D, de Gans J, Tunkel AR, Wijdicks EF. Community-acquired bacterial meningitis in adults. N Engl J Med 2006; 354:44–53.
24. Migirov L, Duvdevani S, Kronenberg J. Otogenic intracranial complications: A review of 28 cases. Acta Otolaryngol 2005;125:819–22.
25. Gower D, McGuirt WF. Intracranial complications of acute and chronic infectious ear disease: A problem still with us. Laryngoscope 1983;93:1028–33.
26. Scheld W. Bacterial meningitis and brain abscess. In: Harrison's principles of internal medicine. Isselbacher K, editor. New York: McGraw-Hill; 1994. p. 2296–309.
27. Nager GT. Mastoid and paranasal sinus infections and their relation to the central nervous system. Clin Neurosurg 1966;14:288–313.
28. Kaplan RJ. Neurological complications of infections of head and neck. Otolaryngol Clin North Am 1976;9:729–49.
29. Proctor CA. Intracranial complications of otitic origin. Laryngoscope 1966;76:288–308.
30. Wellman MB, Sommer DD, McKenna J. Sensorineural hearing loss in postmeningitic children. Otol Neurotol 2003;24:907–12.
31. Paparella MM, Sugiura S. The pathology of suppurative labyrinthitis. Ann Otol Rhinol Laryngol 1967;76:554–86.
32. Merchant SN, Gopen Q. A human temporal bone study of acute bacterial meningogenic labyrinthitis. Am J Otol 1996;17:375–85.
33. Cawthorne T. Otogenic meningitis. J Laryngol Otol 1939;54: 444–70.
34. Jacobs RF, Wells TG, Steele RW, Yamauchi T. A prospective randomized comparison of cefotaxime vs ampicillin and chloramphenicol for bacterial meningitis in children. J Pediatr 1985; 107:129–33.
35. van de Beek D, de Gans J, McIntyre P, Prasad K. Corticosteroids for acute bacterial meningitis. Cochrane Database Syst Rev 2007:CD004405.
36. de Souza CE. Complications of otitis media in children. In: de Souza CE, editor. Pediatric otorhinolaryngology head and neck surgery. San Diego, London: Singular; 1999. p. 115–35.
37. Yen PT, Chan ST, Huang TS. Brain abscess: with special reference to otolaryngologic sources of infection. Otolaryngol Head Neck Surg 1995;113:15–22.
38. Myers EN, Ballantine HT Jr. The management of otogenic brain abscess. Laryngoscope 1965;75:273–88.
39. Sennaroglu L, Sozeri B. Otogenic brain abscess: Review of 41 cases. Otolaryngol Head Neck Surg 2000;123:751–5.
40. Samuel J, Fernandes CM, Steinberg JL. Intracranial otogenic complications: A persisting problem. Laryngoscope 1986;96:272–8.
41. Stuart E, O'Brien F, McNally W. Some observations on brain abscesses. Arch Otolaryngol Head Neck Surg 1955;104:542–3.
42. Murthy PS, Sukumar R, Hazarika P, et al. Otogenic brain abscess in childhood. Int J Pediatr Otorhinolaryngol 1991;22:9–17.
43. Dubey SP, Larawin V. Complications of chronic suppurative otitis media and their management. Laryngoscope 2007;117:264–7.
44. Bento R, de Brito R, Ribas GC. Surgical management of intracranial complications of otogenic infection. Ear Nose Throat J 2006;85:36–9.
45. Quijano M, Schuknecht HF, Otte J. Temporal bone pathology associated with intracranial abscess. ORL J Otorhinolaryngol Relat Spec 1988;50:2–31.
46. Penido Nde O, Borin A, Iha LC, et al. Intracranial complications of otitis media: 15 years of experience in 33 patients. Otolaryngol Head Neck Surg 2005;132:37–42.
47. Ingham HR, Slekon JB, Roxby CM. Bacteriological study of otogenic cerebral abscesses: chemotherapeutic role of metronidazole. BMJ 1977;2:991–3.
48. Brook I. Bacteriology of intracranial abscess in children. J Neurosurg 1981;54:484–8.
49. Nissen AJ. Intracranial complications of otogenic disease. Am J Otol 1980;2:164–7.
50. Keet PC. Cranial intradural abscess management of 641 patients during the 35 years from 1952 to 1986. Br J Neurosurg 1990; 4:273–8.
51. Maniglia AJ, VanBuren JM, Bruce WB, et al. Intracranial abscesses secondary to ear and paranasal sinuses infections. Otolaryngol Head Neck Surg 1980;88:670–80.
52. Kornblut AD. Cerebral abscess—A recurrent otologic problem. Laryngoscope 1972;82:1541–56.
53. Ward PH, Setliff RC, Long W. Otogenic brain abscess. Trans Am Acad Ophthalmol Otolaryngol 1969;73:107–14.

54. Buchheit WA, Ronis ML, Liebman E. Brain abscesses complicating head and neck infections. Trans Am Acad Ophthalmol Otolaryngol 1970;74:548–54.
55. Nalbone VP, Kuruvilla A, Gacek RR. Otogenic brain abscess: The Syracuse experience. Ear Nose Throat J 1992;71:238–42.
56. Maniglia AJ, Goodwin WJ, Arnold JE, Ganz E. Intracranial abscesses secondary to nasal, sinus, and orbital infections in adults and children. Arch Otolaryngol Head Neck Surg 1989;115:1424–9.
57. Williams MR. Open evacuation of pus: A satisfying surgical approach to the problem of brain abscess? J Neurol Neurosurg Psychiatry 1983;45:697–700.
58. LeBeau J, King S. Surgical treatment of brain abscess and subdural empyema. J Neurosurg 1973;38:198–203.
59. Brand B, Caparosa RJ, Lubic LG. Otorhinological brain abscess therapy—Past and present. Laryngoscope 1984;94:483–7.
60. Teichgraeber JF, Per-Lee JH, Turner JS Jr. Lateral sinus thrombosis: a modern perspective. Laryngoscope 1982;92:744–51.
61. Ooi EH, Hilton M, Hunter G. Management of lateral sinus thrombosis: Update and literature review. J Laryngol Otol 2003;117:932–9.
62. Oestreicher-Kedem Y, Raveh E, Kornreich L, et al. Prothrombotic factors in children with otitis media and sinus thrombosis. Laryngoscope 2004;114:90–5.
63. Wolfowitz BL. Otogenic intracranial complications. Arch Otolaryngol 1972;96:220–2.
64. Manolidis S, Kutz JW Jr. Diagnosis and management of lateral sinus thrombosis. Otol Neurotol 2005;26:1045–51.
65. Bradley DT, Hashisaki GT, Mason JC. Otogenic sigmoid sinus thrombosis: What is the role of anticoagulation? Laryngoscope 2002;112:1726–9.
66. Harris TM, Smith RR, Koch KJ. Gadolinium-DTPA enhanced MR imaging of septic dural sinus thrombosis. J Comput Assist Tomogr 1989;13:682–4.
67. deVeber G, Andrew M, Adams C, et al. Cerebral sinovenous thrombosis in children. N Engl J Med 2001;345:417–23.
68. Davison SP, Facer GW, McGough PF, et al. Use of magnetic resonance imaging and magnetic resonance angiography in diagnosis of sigmoid sinus thrombosis. Ear Nose Throat J 1997; 76:436–41.
69. Fritsch MH, Miyamoto RT, Wood TL. Sigmoid sinus thrombosis diagnosis by contrasted MRI scanning. Otolaryngol Head Neck Surg 1990;103:451–6.
70. Shah UK, Jubelirer TF, Fish JD, Elden LM. A caution regarding the use of low-molecular weight heparin in pediatric otogenic lateral sinus thrombosis. Int J Pediatr Otorhinolaryngol 2007;71:347–51.
71. Symonds C. Otitic hydrocephalus. Brain 1931;54:55–71.
72. Symonds C. Hydrocephalic and focal cerebral symptoms in relation to thrombophlebitis of the dural sinuses and cerebral veins. Brain 1937;60:531–50.
73. Foley J. Benign forms of intracranial hypertension: Toxic and otitic hydrocephalus. Brain 1955;78:1–41.
74. Calabrese VP, Selhorst JB, Harbison JW. CSF infusion test in pseudotumor cerebri. Trans Am Neurol Assoc 1978;103:146–50.
75. Sahs AL, Joynt RJ. Brain swelling of unknown cause. Neurology 1956;6:791–802.
76. *Weed* LH, Flexner LB. The relations of the inracranial pressure. Am J Physiol 1933;105:266–72.
77. O'Connor AF, Moffat DA. Otogenic intracranial hypertension. Otitic hydrocephalus. J Laryngol Otol 1978;92:767–75.
78. Horton JC, Seiff SR, Pitts LH, et al. Decompression of the optic nerve sheath for vision-threatening papilledema caused by dural sinus occlusion. Neurosurgery 1992;31:203–11; discussion 211–2.
79. Weingarten K, Zimmerman RD, Becker RD, et al. Subdural and epidural empyemas: MR imaging. AJR Am J Roentgenol 1989;152:615–21.
80. Baum PA, Dillon WP. Utility of magnetic resonance imaging in the detection of subdural empyema. Ann Otol Rhinol Laryngol 1992;101:876–8.

Tympanoplasty: Tympanic Membrane Repair 28

Aristides Athanasiadis-Sismanis, MD, FACS

INTRODUCTION

According to the American Academy of Ophthalmology and Otolaryngology Subcommittee on Conservation of Hearing 1965 definition, tympanoplasty is "a procedure to eradicate disease in the middle ear and to reconstruct the hearing mechanism, with or without tympanic membrane grafting."[1] This procedure can be combined with either an intact canal wall (ICW) or a canal-wall-down (CWD) mastoidectomy to eradicate disease from the mastoid area. The original tympanoplasty classification system of Wullstein (Figure 28–1) is used presently only in the vernacular of otology (eg, a "type III mechanism" or a "type I tympanoplasty").

HISTORY

The term tympanoplasty was introduced in 1953 by Wullstein to describe surgical techniques for reconstruction of the middle-ear hearing mechanism that had been impaired or destroyed by chronic ear disease.[2] The same year Zöllner reported on surgical techniques for improving the sound conduction mechanism of the middle ear following surgery for chronic ear disease.[3] One year earlier Wullstein had described an operation for repairing tympanic membrane perforations with split-thickness skin grafts.[4] Another major contribution of these two otologists was the introduction of the operating microscope in performing otologic surgery, which improved their results significantly.

Tympanoplasty can be considered the final step in the surgical conquest of conductive hearing loss and represents the culmination of over 100 years of evolution of surgical procedures on the middle ear to improve hearing. The first of these procedures was the stapes mobilization of Kessel in 1878, soon followed by Berthold's plastic repair of a perforated tympanic membrane in the same year and Kiesselbach's attempt in 1883 to correct a congenital meatal atresia. These very eventful years might well have been the beginning of a fruitful development of operations for conductive hearing loss, for the mechanics of the middle ear had been defined clearly by Helmholtz shortly before, in 1868. However, despite the early successes with stapes mobilization reported by Boucheron in 1888 and Miot in 1890, the new surgery for deafness declined and by the end of the 19th century died out, as determined opposition by the leaders in otology had arisen against all attempts to improve hearing by operations on the middle ear.

The strong opposition to surgery for deafness was reflected in the standard texts of otology and otologic surgery, which scarcely mentioned, or mentioned only to condemn, such operations. For example, Kerrison's 627-page *Diseases of the Ear*, published in 1930, devoted less than a single page to "Surgical Measures for Relief of Deafness," concluding that: "These operations, mentioned for their place in otological history, are quite obsolete today." It is even more surprising that Sir Charles Ballance, in his two-volume text fails to mention any sort of operation to improve hearing.

Reasons for the opposition to reconstructive surgery of the middle ear were no doubt the lack of surgical microscopes, imperfect sterilization techniques, and the absence of protective antibiotics, possibly resulting in infections and other iatrogenic injuries. There were few reports of serious infections following the early operations, but one can surmise that some very unfortunate unreported results contributed to the opposition. An additional reason for the skepticism for operations to improve hearing may have been the lack of audiometers for quantitative measurements of hearing before and after surgery.

Probably the greatest reason for the lack of interest in reconstructive operations on the ear was the intense preoccupation of the otologists of those days with infections of the ear and their complications. It is interesting that Schwartze[5] described the simple mastoid operation just 3 years before Kessel mobilized

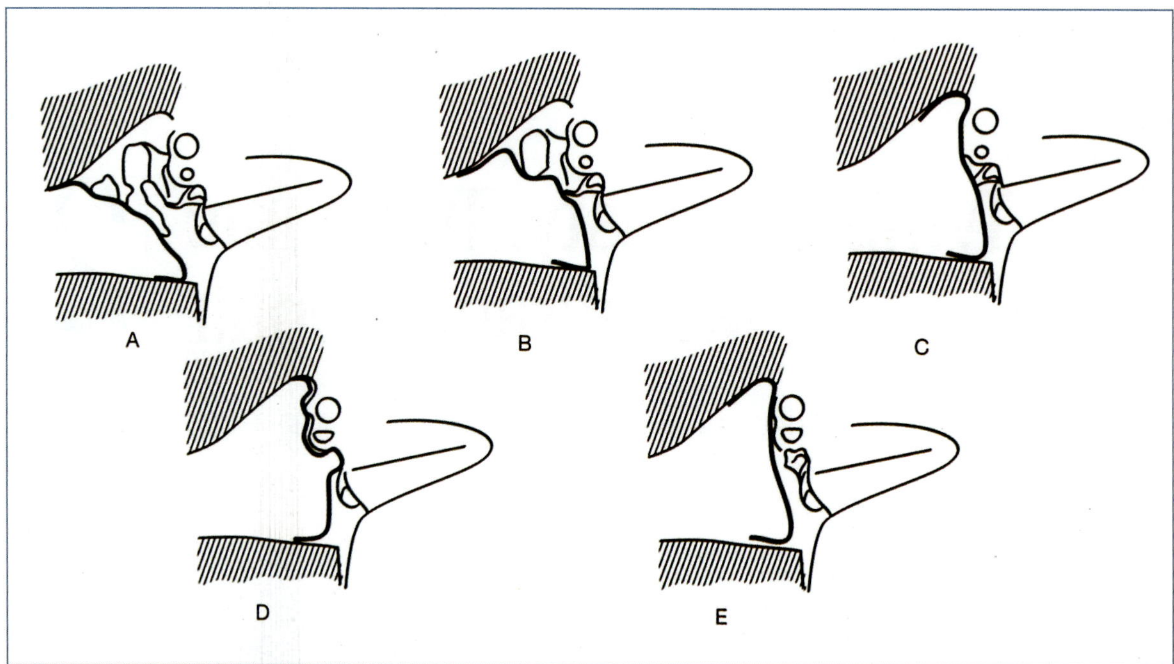

FIGURE 28–1 • Types of tympanoplasty according to Wullstein. *A*, Type I with restoration of the normal middle ear. *B*, Type II. Ossicular chain partially destroyed but preserved and continuity restored. Skin graft laid against the ossicles after removal of the bridge. *C*, Type III. Myringostapediopexy producing a shallow middle ear and a columella effect. *D*, Type IV. Round window protection with a small middle ear mobile footplate left exposed. *E*, Type V. Closed middle ear with round window protection; fenestra in the horizontal semicircular canal covered by a skin graft.

the stapes, and Kuster,[6] Zaufal,[7] and Stacke[8] described the radical mastoidectomy at exactly the time that Boucheron and Miot were reporting successes with stapes mobilization. It is evident that the climate of otologic thought was favorable toward procedures to control infection and quite unfavorable toward operations on the ear to improve hearing.

The revival of interest in the surgery of deafness began when Holmgren[9] with considerable courage in the face of the concerted opposition, began his long series of operations on the labyrinth for otosclerosis, demonstrating that, with modern methods of aseptic technique, the noninfected mastoid process and labyrinth could, after all, be opened safely. The surgical application of the operating microscope, first by Nylen[10] in 1921 as a monocular instrument, and then by Holmgren, who introduced the binocular operating microscope in 1922, was an important advance destined to play an increasing role in the perfection of fenestration, stapes operations, and tympanoplasty. Sourdille's[11] ingenious and successful tympanolabyrinthopexy for otosclerosis added to the reviving interest in surgery for deafness.

The real turning point in the reorientation of otologic surgery away from operations for infection toward reconstruction of the hearing mechanism occurred when Lempert[12] combined Sourdille's several-stage operation into a more practical one-stage fenestration operation. At this time, sulfonamide therapy of acute otitis media and otitic complications had begun to lessen the urgency and frequency of operations for acute mastoiditis. Lempert emphasized careful aseptic technique in the postoperative period as well as during the fenestration operation. With the later addition to sulfonamides of prophylactic penicillin, postoperative infections lost much of their threat. Most important of all, Lempert taught his operation to otologists from all parts of the world. It was inevitable, as the number of patients successfully treated by Lempert and his pupils increased to hundreds and then thousands, that the traditional and often bitter opposition started to decline. Thanks to Lempert, the climate of otologic thought finally became favorable toward surgery for deafness. This led first to the successful operations for congenital meatal atresia in 1947 by Patte[13] and Ombredanne[14] and finally to the revival of stapes mobilization by Rosen in 1953.[15]

It is a remarkable fact that during all these years, clinicians and surgeons failed to see clearly the applications to surgical techniques of the principles of the middle-ear sound-pressure transformer, as described by Helmholtz. Holmgren, Sourdille, and Lempert had no clear idea of how the fenestrated-ear functioned and why the fenestration operation could not restore hearing to normal. Likewise, Pattee and Ombredanne failed to appreciate the need to restore sound-pressure transformation by placing the substitute tympanic membrane in contact with the mobile stapes.

The mechanics of the fenestrated ear remained obscure until Bekesy and Juers began to study the problem. Juers[16] in 1948 noted that the tympanic membrane of the fenestrated ear must be intact "to protect the round window somewhat from sound pressure." Two years later, Davis and Walsh[17] defined the residual conductive hearing loss after successful fenestration as being "due to loss of the impedance-matching mechanism of the tympanic membrane, ossicular chain and oval window." The two basic principles of tympanoplasty had now been defined; namely, sound protection for the round window and sound-pressure transformation for the oval window.

It is interesting and surprising that tympanoplasty techniques for chronic otitis media began in Germany rather than in the United States, where fenestration surgery had reached a high degree of maturity and perfection.

In 1950 Moritz first described the use of pedicled flaps to construct a closed middle-ear cavity in cases of chronic suppuration, to provide sound shielding or protection for the round window in preparation for a later fenestration of the horizontal semicircular canal.[18]

The principles of Moritz's procedure were immediately apparent. Zöllner in 1951, and Wullstein in 1952, began to report of similar operations to provide sound protection for the round window and to reconstruct sound-pressure transformation for the oval window. Early on, Wullstein advocated free skin transplants rather than the pedicled grafts used by Moritz, and Zöllner soon after changed from pedicled to free grafts as well.[4,19]

The subsequent development of tympanoplastic techniques has gone through major changes. Soon after the introduction of split-thickness grafts it was realized that the accumulation of keratin debris and associated infections resulting in failures made their use impractical. Zöllner replaced free distant skin grafts with meatal skin, removed as free full-thickness grafts. Vein as grafting material was reported independently by Shea and Tabb in 1960.[20,21] Temporalis fascia was described by Heermann in 1961 and was introduced in the United States by Storrs in 1963.[22,23] Plastic prostheses for reconstruction of the ossicular chain were tried early on and abandoned by Zöllner and Wullstein; however, they continued to be used in the United States both for tympanoplasty and stapedectomy. Soon after, the tendency toward rejection and extrusion of the plastic prostheses used in tympanoplasties and stapedectomies became evident. Following these initial failures it was soon realized that wire prostheses made of stainless steel, platinum, or tantalum were better tolerated in the middle ear. Ossicular repositioning was described by Hall and Rytzner in 1957.[24] Homograft ossicles for reconstructing the ossicular chain in tympanoplasty became popular in the early 1960s.[25] Glasscock and House reported the first large series of homograft tympanic membrane procedures in 1968.[26] Biocompatible ossicular prostheses such as total ossicular replacement prostheses (TORPs), acting as a columella from the tympanic membrane to the oval window, and partial ossicular replacement prostheses (PORPs), connecting the stapes head to the tympanic membrane, have been in everyday use during the past 25 years.[27] During the past 25 years, otologists have used numerous types of ossicular prostheses made of various alloplastic materials such as Plastipore®, Proplast®, polyethylenes, polytetrafluoroethylene, ceramics, Teflon®, and hydroxylapatite. Ossicular chain reconstruction is presented in detail in Chapter 29.

PHYSIOLOGY OF MIDDLE EAR

When animals emerged from the sea onto dry land, a mechanical device was needed to overcome the air–water sound barrier. The middle-ear mechanism, developed from the discarded bronchial apparatus no longer needed for breathing, was the answer. By means of a rather large hydraulic ratio of a large tympanic membrane acting on a small stapes footplate, combined with a rather small lever ratio of longer handle of the malleus acting on the slightly shorter long-process of the incus, air-borne sound vibrations of large amplitude but small force are transformed into fluid-borne sound vibrations of small amplitude but large force. Békésy calculated the effective vibrating surface of tympanic membrane area compared with stapes footplate area to be 17 to 1 and the lever effect of ossicular chain 1.3 to 1. The 17 to 1 hydraulic ratio × the 1.3 lever ratio yields a total increase of pressure at the oval window of 22 times. This is termed the sound-pressure transformer ratio of the normal human ear and equates to approximately 27-dB gain.[28]

The round window in the normal ear acts as a relief opening at the opposite end of the cochlear duct from the stapes footplate to permit maximum to-and-fro vibratory movements of the noncompressible cochlear-fluid column in the rigid bony cochlea. In the normal ear, the round window membrane movements are largely passive in response to the stapes footplate movements. This is partly because the 22 times pressure increase at the oval window far exceeds any competitive pressure exerted on the round window from the tympanic cavity side. Furthermore, round window membrane movements are largely passive in response to the stapes footplate movements because the intact tympanic membrane "protects" the round window from competitive sounds, partly by damping and partly by a phase difference.

EFFECTS OF TYMPANIC MEMBRANE PERFORATIONS ON HEARING

In patients with tympanic membrane perforations the round window begins to play a more active and troubling role in the mechanics of hearing. A tympanic membrane perforation removes sound protection from the round window, with a tendency for sound to reach both windows at nearly the same moment, thus canceling the resultant movements of the perilymph. As long as the transformer ratio of the middle ear is larger, as in the case of small tympanic membrane perforation with an intact ossicular chain, the canceling effect of sound reaching the round window is small. As the perforation enlarges and the transformer ratio diminishes, the canceling effect of sound on the unprotected round window rises rapidly until a total perforation results in a loss of 40 to 45 dB. An interruption of the ossicular chain does not add much to the hearing loss of a large perforation, however, behind an intact tympanic membrane, it results in maximum conductive hearing loss of 60 dB because both windows are protected from sound, and there is no sound-pressure transformation for the oval window.

The ideal tympanoplasty restores sound protection for the round window by constructing a closed and air-containing middle ear, and rebuilds the sound-pressure transformation mechanism for the oval window by connecting a large tympanic membrane with the stapes footplate via either an intact or a reconstructed ossicular chain.

ETIOLOGY OF TYMPANIC MEMBRANE PERFORATIONS

Tympanic membrane perforations result mainly from infectious and traumatic etiologies.

Infectious Etiologies

Perforations resulting from acute otitis media heal spontaneously in the majority of cases. However, in rare instances a central perforation may remain, especially in cases with associated Eustachian tube dysfunction. Acute otitis media secondary to group A beta-hemolytic streptococcus is associated with a high incidence of tympanic membrane perforations and mastoiditis.[29]

Chronic otitis media with effusion treated with ventilating tubes can result in tympanic membrane perforation, atrophy, retraction, hearing loss, and tympanosclerosis.[30] Typical temporal bone pathologic findings in chronic otitis media with tympanic membrane perforation include: granulation tissue (97.4%), ossicular changes (90.5%), tympanosclerosis (19.8%), cholesterol granuloma (12.1%), and cholesteatoma (4.3%).[31]

Perforations secondary to tuberculous otitis media are rare and diagnosis is made with a positive middle-ear tissue biopsy for acid-fast bacilli and a positive *Mycobacterium* tissue culture.[32] Significant clinical features are pale granulations in the middle ear, a disproportionately severe hearing loss, facial paralysis, the presence of normal mastoid cellular development, and a past or family history of tuberculosis. Antituberculous treatment and surgery give good results.[33]

Traumatic Etiologies

Traumatic tympanic membrane perforations result from penetrating trauma, nonexplosive and explosive blast injuries, and iatrogenic causes. Decreased hearing, tinnitus, and aural fullness are common initial symptoms. Persistent dizziness or disequilibrium and tinnitus should alert the physician to the possibility of a concomitant inner-ear injury and may prompt middle-ear exploration. Thorough otologic, neurotologic, and audiologic evaluation is imperative for detection of any associated perilymphatic fistula, inverted perforation edges, displaced segments of the tympanic membrane in the middle-ear cavity and foreign bodies. For patients with inverted edges, under local anesthesia in the office, a piece of sterile Gelfoam® soaked in saline is placed into the middle ear through the perforation. The edges of the perforation are then everted and a properly trimmed piece of Gelfilm® or cigarette paper is placed on the tympanic membrane. Oral antibiotics are prescribed for one week if water or a foreign body has entered the middle ear. The patient is advised to avoid blowing the nose, take water precautions, instill Ofloxacin® otic drops twice a day, and return to the office in 3 to 4 weeks for re-evaluation.

Penetrating tympanic membrane injuries are usually self-induced and are secondary to cotton-tipped swab injuries, bobby pins and other objects used to relieve itching or clean the ear canal. These perforations usually heal spontaneously within 4 to 6 weeks, and during this period patients need to observe water precautions. Penetrating thermal injuries, such as a hot slag, carry a poor prognosis regardless of medical or surgical treatment.[34] Facial nerve injury and sensorineural hearing loss have been reported as a result of welding sparks.[35] Other causes include water activities such as skiing, and lightning strikes. Patients with perforations resulting from water activities are at risk for developing otitis media and should be treated with non-ototoxic antibiotic drops such as Ofloxacin® otic.

Nonexplosive blast injuries include such entities as a blow to the ear, usually a slap, which results in a sudden increase of air pressure that ruptures the tympanic membrane.[36–38] It has been reported that conservative management of nonexplosive blast-injury tympanic membrane perforations results in spontaneous closure in 94.8% of cases. High-frequency sensorineural hearing loss has been detected in 20% of these patients. Healing of the perforation is always associated with closure of the air–bone gap, while recovery of the sensorineural hearing loss is less frequent.[39] On the contrary, in a report of 124 tympanic membrane perforations resulting from explosive blast injuries, only 47 healed spontaneously.[40] Early intervention with eversion of the perforation edges and application of a paper patch has been recommended for these cases.[41] In a recent report regarding 541 blast-injury victims of the coalition forces in Iraq who underwent neuro-otologic examination, 35.2% were found to have tympanic membrane perforations. In 37.8% of cases, perforations were bilateral. Approximately 37% of the soldiers reported wearing ear protection, a precaution that was associated with a significantly reduced risk of tympanic membrane perforation.[42] In such cases, displaced tympanic membrane remnants in the middle-ear cavity should be detected early on and be removed in order to avoid cholesteatoma formation.

The most common iatrogenic perforations result from ventilating tubes for otitis media and have been reported to occur in 4.6% of patients following tympanostomy.[43] Perforation rates are higher for tubes of larger diameter and those with longer retention times. In a study comparing T-tubes to small grommets (the Donaldson tube), the perforation rates were 13.6% and 1.8% respectively.[44] Gelfoam®/Gelfilm® patching of the perforation at the time of ventilation tube removal has decreased the perforation incidence.[45,46]

Perforations following exploratory tympanotomy for stapedectomy and other middle-ear pathologies are rare.

GOALS AND EXPECTATIONS OF TYMPANOPLASTY

The two goals of tympanoplasty are to achieve a dry ear by eradicating middle-ear disease and hearing improvement by closure of any tympanic membrane perforation by grafting and/or ossicular reconstruction. The results of tympanoplasty are measured in terms of success or failure of graft-take and hearing improvement. In order to obtain a fair assessment of the long-term success of ear surgery, it is best to separate cases of benign central perforations from cases with cholesteatoma, previous tympanoplasty failure, severe mucosal disease, poor Eustachian tube function, and total loss of the ossicular chain. Individuals with benign perforations and simple ossicular chain deficits have a very good-to-excellent chance of obtaining a dry ear and hearing within the normal range. Such a patients may expect a 93 to 97% chance for a graft "take" and an 85 to 90% chance for a hearing gain to within 20 dB of bone level.[47,48] It must be remembered that a tympanoplasty may be considered partially successful if a dry, intact ear is obtained regardless of whether there is any hearing improvement. Patients with atelectatic ears and poor Eustachian tube function undergoing tympanoplasty may be benefited by insertion of long-term ventilating tubes.

INDICATIONS FOR TYMPANOPLASTY

Indications include tympanic membrane perforations and associated hearing loss, with or without middle-ear pathology such as tympanosclerosis, small retraction pockets, and cholesteatomas.

CONTRAINDICATIONS FOR TYMPANOPLASTY

Absolute contraindications for tympanoplasty include poor general health, malignant tumors of the outer/middle ear, uncontrolled cholesteatoma, unusual infections such as malignant otitis externa, and complications of chronic ear disease such as meningitis, brain abscess, or lateral sinus thrombosis.[49] Tympanoplasty is also contraindicated on the only or significantly better hearing ear in order to avoid the risk of irreversible sensorineural hearing loss. Operating on the better hearing ear in patients who can use a hearing aid in the opposite ear with satisfactory results may be considered in selected cases. Any acute exacerbation of chronic otitis media, chronic mucoid discharge associated with allergic rhinosinusitis, or chronic otitis externa should be controlled with appropriate treatment prior to tympanoplasty. A nonfunctioning Eustachian tube is a relative contraindication to tympanoplasty; although this is not always easily determined preoperatively. Smoking has been reported to be a significant negative prognostic factor and has been associated with a threefold increase in long-term graft failure.[50,51]

Indications for tympanoplasty in the elderly and children should be individualized. With modern anesthetic techniques, an older individual in relatively good general health can be operated on without any significant risk.[52] Unless there is a cholesteatoma or bilateral tympanic membrane perforations with significant conductive hearing loss, tympanoplasty in children can be delayed until the age of 8 or 10 when the incidence of otitis media decreases and a satisfactory outcome is more likely. When surgery becomes necessary in young children the author prefers using cartilage "shield" grafts, which are resistant even to continuous Eustachian tube dysfunction.[53] Hearing aid fitting is another option for such cases. History of recurrent otitis media or presence of otitis media with effusion in the contralateral ear are suggestive of a dysfunctional Eustachian tube and should alert the otolaryngologist to the possibility of a poor surgical outcome.[54]

Repeated surgical failures due to extensive middle-ear fibrosis, a nonfunctioning Eustachian tube, recurrent perforations, and prosthesis extrusion are better left alone. The patient should be given the option of a hearing aid, although recurrent ear drainage may be a major problem. The Baha® system has provided satisfactory results for patients who cannot tolerate conventional hearing aids due to recurrent otitis externa, draining mastoid cavities, and active chronic otitis.[55,56]

PREOPERATIVE EVALUATION

A complete history and head and neck examination should be performed on all patients prior to surgery. The otoscopic examination is best accomplished with the operating microscope. An audiogram within 3 months prior to surgery is essential and should consist of pure-tone air- and bone-conduction thresholds as well as speech-discrimination scores. All hearing test results should be confirmed with tuning fork testing.

For an actively draining ear, the external auditory canal and tympanic cavity should be cleaned of any purulent material with a small otologic suction under the surgical microscope and the patient should be instructed to take water precautions. For refractory cases, irrigating the ear with a solution of 1.5% acetic acid using a bulb syringe two to three times a day can be helpful. The solution should be brought to body temperature prior to irrigation in order to avoid a caloric effect. Following irrigation, the ear should be allowed to drain and antibiotic drops covering *Pseudomonas aeruginosa* should be instilled. Digital pressure over the ipsilateral tragus should then be applied several times to force the antibiotic solution deeper into the ear canal and middle ear. Oral antibiotics with activity against *Pseudomonas aeruginosa* may be considered for patients not responding to local treatment. Culture and sensitivity should be obtained for refractory cases, in immunosuppressed patients, and when an unusual infectious process, such as tuberculosis, is suspected. Cholesteatoma cases may fail to respond to local treatment prior to surgery and although most surgeons prefer to operate on a "dry" ear, there is no contraindication to performing a tympanoplasty in the face of active infection. Often cholesteatomas must be treated surgically in order to attain a dry ear.

In addition to the aforementioned measures, an effort should be made to control any conditions predisposing to failure such as obstructive adenoids and recurrent tonsillitis in children, allergic rhinitis, sinusitis, and nasal obstruction secondary to a deviated septum. These upper respiratory tract conditions can directly influence Eustachian tube function and therefore the outcome of any surgery in the tympanic cavity.

There is no preoperative test for Eustachian tube function. The Toynbee test and the Valsalva maneuver can detect patency of the Eustachian tube, a finding that does not correlate with normal function. Furthermore, poor Eustachian tube function prior to surgery may improve following tympanoplasty by removing middle-ear disease processes such as polyps, granulation tissue, infection, and the insertion of a sheet of absorbable Gelfilm® (gelatin film). For patients who develop middle-ear effusion following tympanoplasty, a myringotomy and ventilation-tube insertion can be done as an office procedure 2 months after surgery.[57]

IMAGING STUDIES

Dry, chronic central perforations require no preoperative imaging. In cases with cholesteatoma, atelectasis, and chronic drainage, high-resolution computed tomography (CT) of the temporal bones may be helpful in determining disease extension, possible intracranial involvement, degree of mastoid pneumatization, the type of surgical approach to be used, presence of labyrinthine fistulae, fallopian canal anatomy, as well as tegmental defects. If a tegmental defect is detected by CT, the diagnosis of brain herniation can best be established with a magnetic resonance imaging (MRI) study of the temporal bones.[30]

INFORMED CONSENT

Prior to surgery, patients should be properly informed regarding the nature of their disease process, treatment options, and the proposed surgical procedure, including expected outcomes, potential risks and complications, and the possibility of a second-stage procedure. Brochures describing the disease process and proposed surgical procedure and postoperative care are very useful.

OFFICE CHEMICAL MYRINGOPLASTY

This technique was introduced by Roosa in 1876[58] and was popularized by Derlacki in the 1950s who reported good results.[59] Cooperative patients with small (less than 4 mm) central tympanic membrane perforations may be considered for this procedure. Marginal perforations, a small ear canal, active infection, the presence of cholesteatoma, a conductive hearing loss due to an ossicular problem, and the presence of extensive tympanosclerosis in the tympanic remnant are contraindications for this procedure.

Under the microscope, the edges of the perforation are cauterized with trichloroacetic acid, applied by a metallic applicator with a very small amount of cotton wound tightly at its tip. Chemical cauterization destroys the squamous epithelium that has grown over the rim of the perforation and in so doing exposes fibroblasts and promotes healing of the lamina propria. Silver nitrate is alternative chemical agent that can be used for this purpose.[60] The perforation is then covered with a Gelfoam®, or Gelfilm® (Pharmacia & Upjohn company, Kalamazoo, Mi), or a cigarette-paper patch. Local antibiotic drops are prescribed and the procedure is repeated every 2 weeks until the perforation is healed. A 64% success rate has been reported with this technique.[60]

ALLOPLASTIC PATCHING

Toynbee in 1853[61] and Yearsley in 1863[62] first reported the use of alloplastic materials for hearing improvement in patients with tympanic perforations. Recently, a very soft silicone device in the shape of a sealed tympanostomy tube, placed in the office, has been found to be a safe and effective alternative for treating tympanic perforations with an intact ossicular chain when surgery is contraindicated or is refused by the patient.[63] Contraindications for this device are active middle-ear infection, cholesteatoma, and Eustachian tube dysfunction.

HISTOPATHOLOGY OF TYMPANIC MEMBRANE PERFORATIONS

In a histopathologic study of chronic tympanic membrane perforations, it was found that the squamous epithelium often extended medially from the perforation edge. Epidermal growth factor, hyaluronan, fibronectin, and other glycosaminoglycans, all of which are known to be present in wound healing, were only scantily present. These findings could explain the arrested healing and cessation of spontaneous closure associated with chronic perforations.[64] Accordingly, complete removal of the perforation rim prior to grafting is mandatory to avoid any entrapment of epithelium within the middle ear.

In experimental animal studies the epidermis is the first layer that closes a tympanic membrane perforation. Healing of the fibrous layer occurs secondarily, and the site of response in this layer is related to the vascular distribution in the tympanic membrane. This process begins within 48 hours and is complete within 9 days.[65] The epithelial layer of healed human tympanic membranes does not contain basal cells, confirming its origin from migration from the periphery and not by *in situ* proliferation.[66] Epidermal growth factor has been reported to promote healing of chronic tympanic membrane perforations.[67] In animal studies hyaluronic acid and heparin have been found to improve the healing rate as well as the quality of the scar.[68]

GRAFTING MATERIALS

Presently the most commonly used grafting material for repair of tympanic membrane perforations is temporalis fascia. Another grafting material, introduced by Moon in 1970 with excellent graft-take, is areolar tissue obtained from the area overlying the temporalis fascia.[69,70] This grafting material has been used extensively by Glasscock[47] and is highly recommended by the author because there is minimal or no bleeding during removal due to its location in an avascular plane, it is easier to handle during graft placement, and in case of failure the temporalis fascia is still available for use. Tragal and auricular cartilage as well as perichondrium are other very commonly used grafting materials.[53] Surgical results with these grafts are similar to those obtained with temporalis fascia.[71] Other reported autologous grafting materials associated with excellent results are fat and scar tissue.[72,73] Recently, treated acellular dermal homografts (AlloDerm®, LifeCell Corporation, Branchburg, NJ) and Tutopatch® (Tutogen Medical, Inc., Alachua, FL), a xenograft derived from bovine pericardium, have afforded results similar to those obtained with temporalis fascia, perichondrium, and cartilage.[74–76] These homografts may be considered for revision cases in which autogenous grafting material is no longer available. For cases with total perforation, cholesteatoma, or atelectasis, and especially for revision cases, the author prefers to use cartilage "shield" grafts obtained from the concha cymba. This technique is described in the cartilage tympanoplasty section of this chapter.

ANESTHESIA FOR TYMPANOPLASTY

General anesthesia is preferred for all chronic ear surgery procedures and is particularly helpful for children and excessively apprehensive patients. General anesthesia can be used in an outpatient setting as well. For such cases, long anesthesia machine circuits are used to allow the anesthesiologist to be positioned at the feet of the table. This allows adequate room for the surgeon's legs beneath the table. The blood pressure cuff should be placed on the arm opposite to the ear undergoing surgery so it does not interfere with the surgeon. If facial nerve monitoring is used, paralyzing agents should be avoided during anesthesia.

In cases of myringoplasty or when general anesthesia is contraindicated, local anesthesia with sedation can be used as well.

POSITIONING OF THE PATIENT

The patient is placed close to the edge of the table in order to prevent the surgeon from hyperextending his/her arms. The patient's body is properly strapped on the table and both arms are padded and tucked close to the body. The head is turned approximately 120 degrees away from the surgeon and is supported with a folded towel placed between the table and the contralateral cheek. No doughnut-shaped pillow is necessary. An operating table that can rotate along its long axis is essential in order to allow the whole body of the patient to move away from or towards the surgeon to achieve optimal visualization of the surgical field. Rotating the patient toward the surgeon allows better visualization of the posterior area of the surgical field, whereas rotating the patient away improves inspection of the anterior surgical field. A hydraulic chair is very helpful for the surgeon because it allows change of visualization angles with minimal effort.

POSITION OF THE NURSE AND SURGICAL MICROSCOPE

The nurse and the instrument table are placed across from the surgeon and the surgical microscope is positioned at the head of the table.

FACIAL NERVE MONITORING

Although facial nerve monitoring is not a substitute for thorough knowledge of facial nerve anatomy, the author uses it in the majority of otologic procedures. In cholesteatoma cases in particular, dissection and removal of the cholesteatoma matrix from the facial nerve can be done in a more controlled fashion, especially in cases with fallopian canal dehiscence.

PROPHYLACTIC ANTIBIOTICS

In an uncomplicated tympanoplasty case, prophylactic antibiotics are unwarranted. However, for a draining ear antimicrobial coverage is recommended prior to surgery.[77] Frequent irrigation of the surgical field during the surgery removes devitalized tissue and perhaps reduces bacterial colony counts and subsequent infection.

HEMOSTASIS

Complete hemostasis is imperative in otologic surgery and can be accomplished as follows.

- Discontinuation of aspirin and other anti-inflammatory medications 10 days prior to surgery. Discontinuation of anticoagulant treatment, such as Plavix®, requires prior clearance by the patient's primary care physician.
- Injection of the postauricular incision and ear canal with lidocaine 2% (Xylocaine®) with 1:100,000 epinephrine at least 10 minutes prior to making any incision.
- Availability of otologic electromicrobipolar and conventional cauteries.
- Gelfoam® soaked in undiluted epinephrine. A dry surgical field can be accomplished by leaving Gelfoam® soaked in epinephrine in the middle ear while obtaining the graft.
- Availability of diamond burrs of various sizes for control of bleeding from bone.
- Frequent irrigation of the surgical area with a saline solution.

PREPPING OF THE SURGICAL AREA

A 2–3 cm area of hair above and behind the auricle is shaved and then rubbed with an alcohol solution to degrease the skin. Tincture of benzoin is applied and 3M® (No. 1010) drapes are placed on the skin to keep the hair away from the surgical area. The postauricular area is injected with 3–4 cm^3 of lidocaine 2% (Xylocaine®) with 1:100,000 epinephrine for hemostasis. The surgical area is cleaned with iodine soap and solution, and blotted dry with a sterile towel. The patient is draped with sterile paper-drapes and a 3M® plastic drainage-bag with self-adhesive is applied at the most dependent segment of the surgical area. Irrigation-suction tubing and cautery lines are wrapped in a cloth towel and secured on the drapes with towel clips. A compartmentalized plastic-pouch is attached to the drapes of the Mayo stand to accommodate the suction tips and electrocauteries.

TYMPANOPLASTY APPROACHES

There are three tympanoplasty approaches: transcanal, postauricular, and endaural. Factors to be considered regarding the type of approach to be used include the size of the ear canal, the location and size of the perforation, and the surgeon's training and experience.

Transcanal Approach

Small posterior perforations can be repaired through the transcanal approach, especially when the size of the ear canal is large. By doing so the inconvenience of the mastoid dressing, and the slightly higher morbidity of the postauricular incision (pain, hematoma, and infection) are avoided.

In this approach, the edges of the tympanic membrane perforation are denuded of squamous epithelium and tympanosclerotic areas are completely removed from the remnant of the tympanic membrane (Figure 28–2). The middle ear is explored by elevating a tympanomeatal flap, similar to the one used in stapedectomy (Figure 28–3). Pathologic processes of the middle ear are removed, and the ossicular chain is inspected and repaired as necessary. Should polypoid mucosa or adhesions be removed, Gelfilm® (absorbable gelatin) is placed over the promontory to prevent adhesion formation. The middle ear is then packed with Gelfoam® (gelatin sponge), and the graft is placed medial to the tympanic membrane remnant, or tympanic annulus, and the manubrium of the malleus. Finally the tympanomeatal flap is returned to its original position and the medial aspect of the ear canal is packed with pledgets of Gelfoam® impregnated in antibiotic ointment. The patient is instructed to instill ofloxacin drops twice a day and to return to the office in 4 weeks for cleaning of the ear canal.

For persisting, small perforations, such as those following tympanostomy tube extrusion and myringoplasty failure, transcanal fat graft myringoplasty is the procedure of choice.[78,79] In the majority of patients, with the exception of children who require sedation, this procedure can be done under local anesthesia in the ambulatory surgery center.

The transcanal fat graft myringoplasty procedure proceeds as follows: local anesthetic is injected into the four quadrants of the ear canal and into the ear lobe. Through a small incision in the rim of the ear lobe, a small piece of adipose tissue is removed and kept in sterile saline solution. The incision is closed with several 5–0 Monocryl® sutures. Using microscopic visualization and a cup forceps, the edges of the perforation are denuded of epithelium. A piece of the previously removed adipose tissue larger than the perforation is inserted through the perforation in a dumbbell fashion. Antibiotic soaked Gelfoam® is placed over the graft. The patient is instructed to instill ofloxacin otic drops in the ear canal twice a day, avoid blowing of the nose and to observe water precautions. The ear canal is cleaned at the office at 4 weeks following surgery. This technique achieves excellent results if used in the appropriate case.[80]

Postauricular Approach

The postauricular approach is preferable for large perforations necessitating total replacement of the tympanic membrane, especially when the ear canal is small and for surgeons

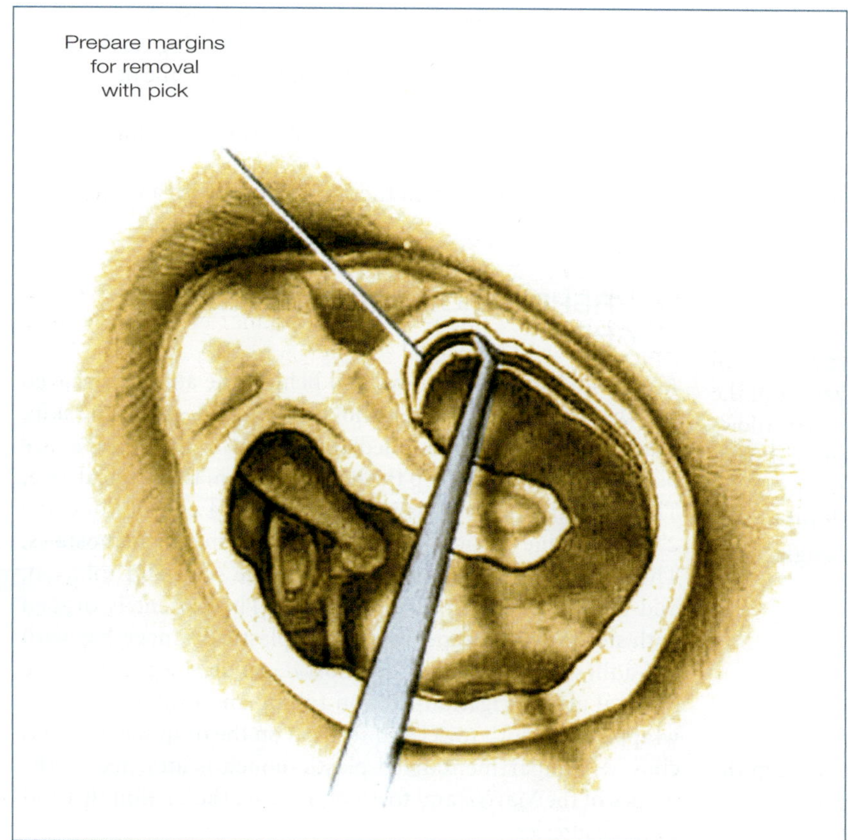

FIGURE 28–2 • Denuding perforation edges.

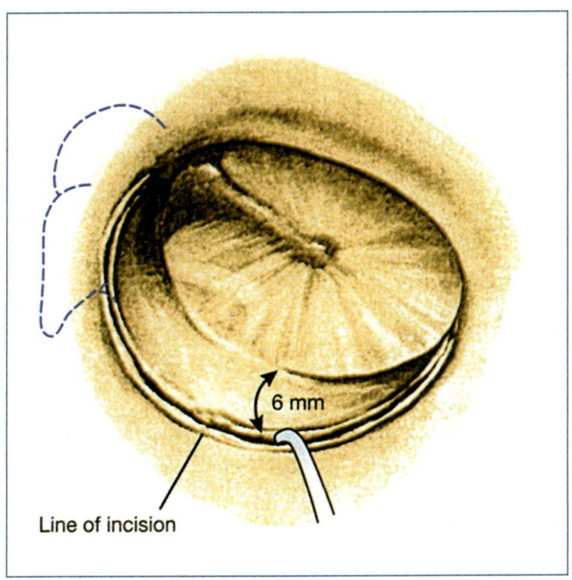

FIGURE 28–3 • Typical design for a tympanomeatal flap.

with limited experience working through the ear canal. For cases with a narrow ear-canal, usually due to a bulging of the anterior bony wall, canaloplasty should be performed at the time of tympanoplasty. Poor visualization of the anterior sulcus may result in improper graft placement and failure of the procedure.

Endaural Approach

This approach is popular in Europe for chronic ear surgery and stapedectomy. It was first described by Kessel in 1885 and was later popularized by Lempert.

The first incision in this approach is made along the entire posterior half of the ear canal at the bony–cartilaginous junction. A second vertical incision is made in the incisura and connects the previous incision and the area between the tragus and the root of the helix[81] (Figure 28–4).

TYMPANOPLASTY GRAFTING TECHINQUES

There are two tympanoplasty grafting techniques, underlay and overlay. Graft placement in the underlay technique is medial to the tympanic membrane remnant (or annulus) and manubrium of the malleus whereas in the overlay technique, graft placement is lateral to the tympanic membrane remnant and medial to the manubrium.

Both techniques give excellent results provided they are properly performed by experienced surgeons. The overlay technique has been associated with a higher incidence of blunting of the anterior sulcus and graft lateralization, which may result in significant conductive hearing loss. Other drawbacks of this technique are formation of epithelial pearls from a failure to completely remove the squamous epithelium of the ear canal or tympanic membrane remnant, and delayed healing, most likely resulting from completely removing and repositioning the skin of the ear canal. Upon repositioning the ear canal skin, areas devoid of epithelium may develop that can contribute to formation of granulation tissue and delayed healing. These potential complications are avoided in the majority of cases performed with the underlay technique. The overlay technique is overall a more technically demanding procedure and requires considerable experience.

Underlay Technique

The technique described in this chapter was initially reported by Glasscock in 1973[82] and is used by the author in the majority of tympanoplasty cases. Since facial nerve monitoring is performed during the procedure, short-acting paralytic agents can be used only at the induction of anesthesia. Administration of nitrous oxide gas should be avoided because it diffuses into the middle ear and can displace the graft.

After the ear has been prepped and draped, the external ear canal is injected with lidocaine 2% (Xylocaine®) with 1:100,000 epinephrine. A vascular strip incision is outlined by making an incision with a 72 Beaver® knife blade just lateral to the tympanic annulus, followed by one along the tympanomastoid suture line and one along the tympanomastoid suture line using a 67 Beaver® blade (Figure 28–5A). A postauricular incision, approximately 5 mm behind the postauricular sulcus, is performed and bleeding is controlled with electrocautery. By grasping the auricle firmly and pulling it forward and outward, identification of the loose areolar tissue in the avascular plane overlying the temporalis fascia is greatly facilitated (Figure 28–5B). A Weitlaner retractor is placed horizontally to hold the auricle forward and a Senn retractor is placed by the assistant under the superior part of the skin incision and pulled laterally to expose the temporalis fascia. Separation of the areolar tissue from the temporalis fascia is facilitated by injecting this area with local anesthetic solution. An incision is made at the level of the linea temporalis and is carried down to the level of the temporalis fascia; the areolar tissue is dissected using Metzenbaum scissors (Figure 28–5C). The harvested areolar tissue is squeezed out on a Polytef® (Teflon®) block and placed under a gooseneck lamp on the back table for dehydration (Video clip 28–1). A T-shaped incision is made in the musculoperiosteal tissues overlying the mastoid cortex with the horizontal component in the avascular plane of the linea temporalis and the vertical component between the mastoid tip and the midportion of the horizontal incision. Using a Lempert elevator, musculoperiosteal flaps are elevated posteriorly, superiorly, and anteriorly, the vascular strip is elevated out of the ear canal and is kept in place by repositioning the previously placed self-retaining retractor (Figure 28–5D). A second self-retaining retractor is placed vertically between the temporalis fascia and mastoid tip. This allows for excellent exposure of the ear canal, tympanic membrane, and middle ear from the postauricular region and eliminates the need of working through an ear speculum. In cases with a prominent tympanosquamous suture line it can be difficult to elevate the vascular strip out of the ear canal with this maneuver. In such instances, using the surgical microscope through the postauricular area, the attachment of the vascular strip to the tympanosquamous suture line is incised with a

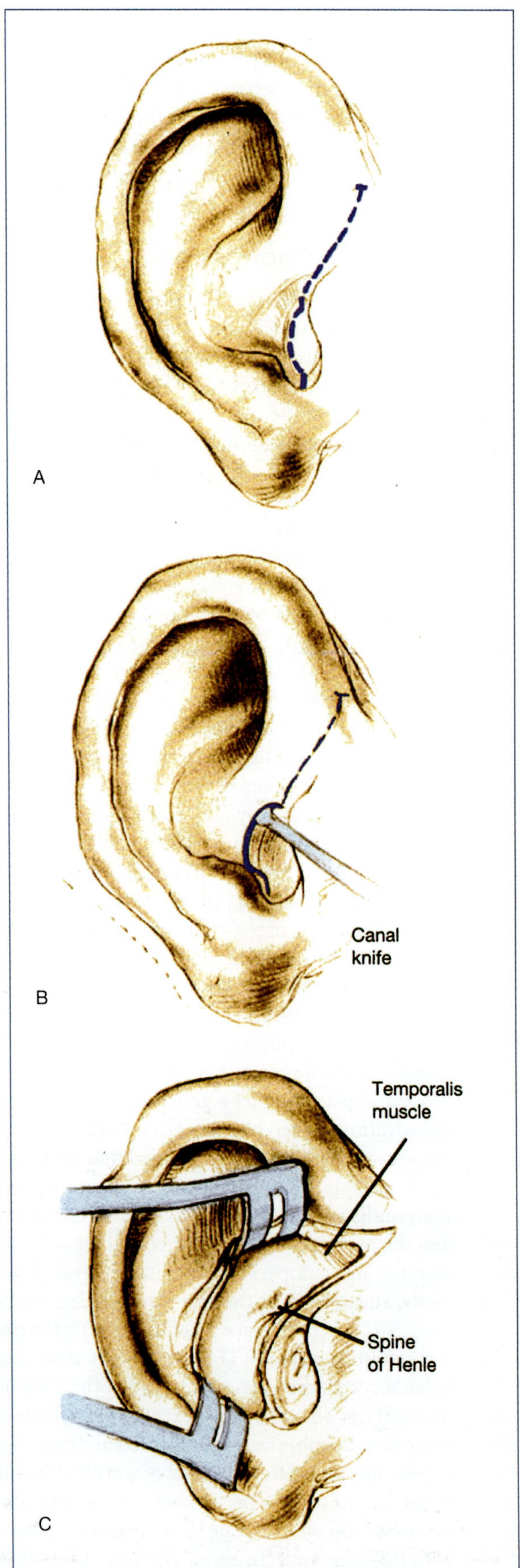

FIGURE 28–4 • *A*, Endaural incision. *B*, Separation of bony cartilaginous junction. *C*. Mastoid exposure via an endaural incision.

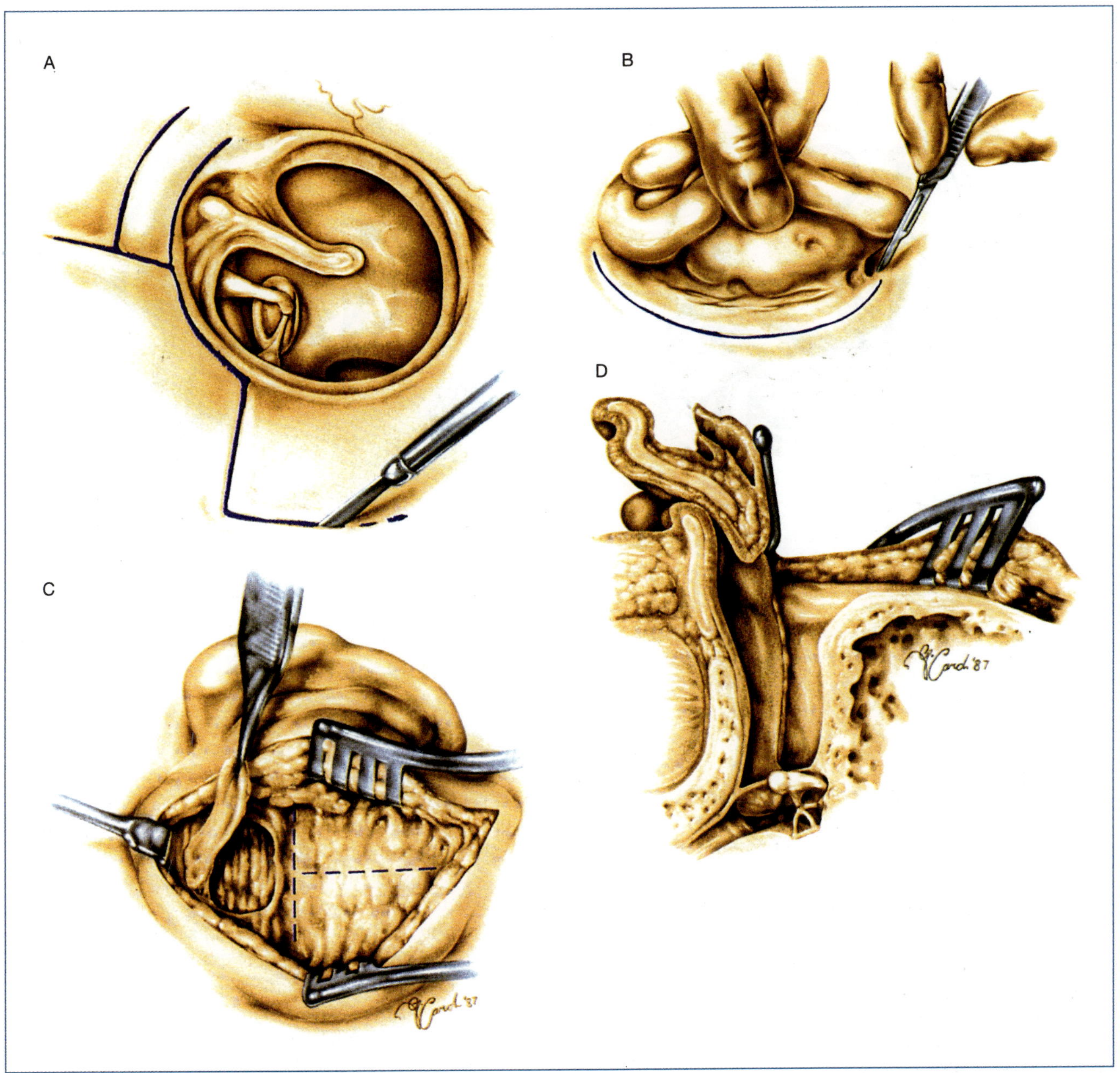

FIGURE 28–5 • *A*, The vascular strip is outlined with a No. 67 Beaver blade. *B*, A standard postauricular incision is used to expose the temporalis fascia. *C*, A larger piece of loose areolar temporalis fascia is removed, pressed, and dried under a heat lamp. Note the T incision used to expose the external auditory canal. *D*, The vascular strip is lifted out of the external auditory canal and placed under the anterior blade of a self-retaining retractor.

Continued

67 Beaver® blade and the strip is then gently elevated out of the ear canal (Video clip 28–2). Failure to recognize this situation may result in disruption of the vascular strip during elevation with the Lempert elevator.

At this point a canaloplasty is performed if visualization of the anterior sulcus is limited by an anterior wall bulge. The canaloplasty facilitates proper placement of the graft and adequate inspection of the tympanic membrane in the postoperative period. Next, the skin of the inferior ear canal is elevated to the fibrous annulus, developing the inferiorly based flap (Figure 28–5E), followed by elevation of the superior flap. The middle ear is entered, the status of the ossicular chain is determined, and any middle-ear pathology is removed (Figure 28–5F). In particular, markedly polypoid mucosa, granulation tissue, and cholesteatoma are removed from the middle ear. Mild mucosal polypoid changes generally revert to normal once the perforation is closed and other middle-ear pathology, such as cholesteatoma, has been removed. Cholesteatoma matrix around the stapes superstructure and over the promontory is removed at the very end

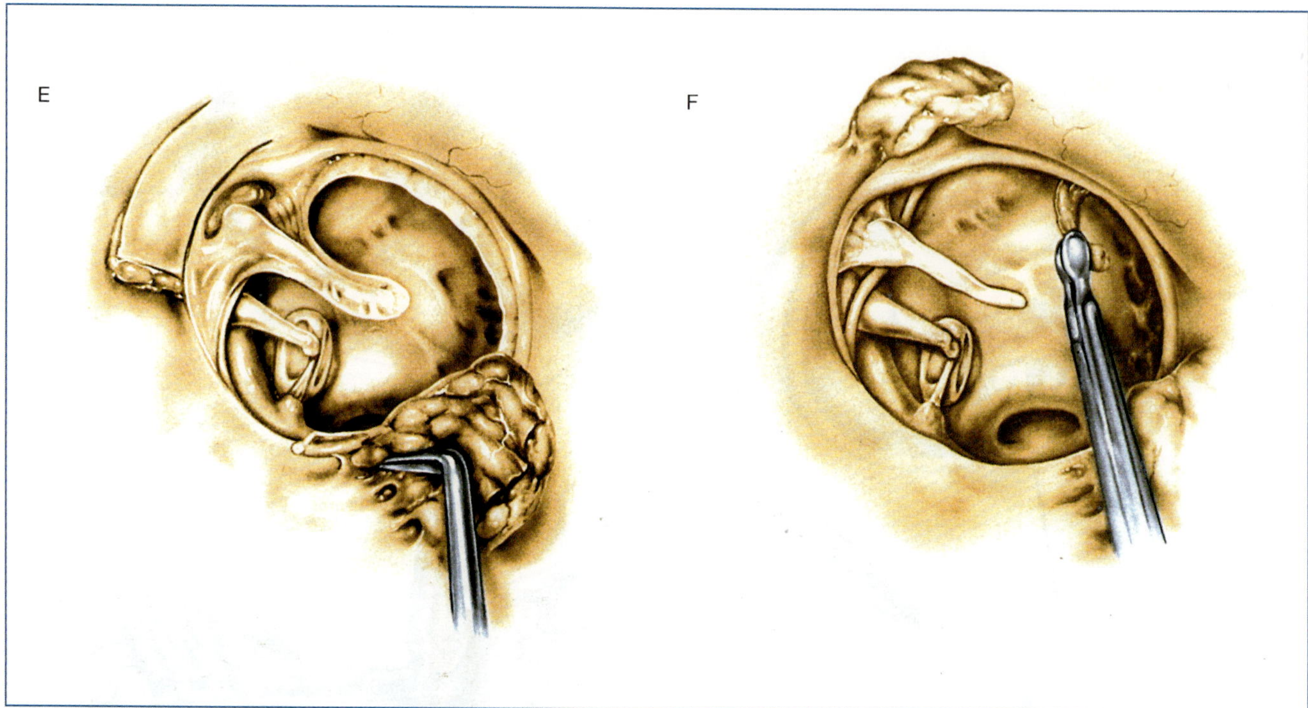

FIGURE 28–5 • *Continued. E*, The inferior flap is elevated to the fibrous annulus with a House No. 2 knife. *F*, Cup forceps remove mucosa from under the fibrous annulus.

of the procedure in order to avoid prolonged exposure of the inner in case of an accidental opening of the oval window or a fistula. Cholesteatoma matrix can be removed from the stapes superstructure using a micro cup forceps or a Crabtree dissector in a dissection motion proceeding from posterior to anterior and paralleling the stapedial tendon (Video clip 28–3). It is very important while this is being performed to avoid any injury to the stapes. In case minimal fracture of the stapes footplate occurs with leakage of perilymph, then the involved area should be gently packed with areolar tissue. If the matrix of the cholesteatoma is very adherent to the stapes superstructure or horizontal facial nerve, it can be left in place in order to avoid injury to these structures. Usually, during the second-stage procedure one year later, the cholesteatoma remnant has formed a "pearl" that can be removed much more easily. The surgeon should be vigilant for any dehiscent/high jugular bulb, exposed horizontal segment of the facial nerve, and dehiscent internal carotid artery in order to avoid major complications. Jacobson's nerve, the cochleariform process, the Eustachian tube orifice, the round window niche, and the stapedial tendon are very constant, reliable, and useful middle-ear landmarks, which, when encountered, can orient the surgeon. Should the surgeon become disoriented because of extensive middle-ear pathology, he/she should immediately stop working in the unknown area, identify a region of known anatomy, and then proceed to the area obscured by pathology. The sinus tympani cannot be visualized directly by any approach to the middle ear and can only be inspected indirectly, using a small mirror (Buckingham), or with an endoscope. Extension of disease into the facial recess may necessitate a mastoidectomy with opening of the facial recess. Upon completion of disease removal, Gelfilm® is placed over the medial wall of the middle ear to prevent adhesion formation and the middle ear is packed with absorbable Gelfoam®. The properly-sized dehydrated areolar tissue graft is placed medial to the tympanic membrane remnant draping posteriorly over the posterior canal wall. For cases with total tympanic membrane perforations, an incision is made in the superior aspect of the graft to facilitate insertion medial to the manubrium. Small pieces of Gelfoam® are placed over the graft for stabilization and the canal skin flaps are replaced to their original position. Antibiotic ointment is left over the Gelfoam® (Figure 28–6). In cases having cholesteatoma and/or a retraction pocket, tragal or conchal cartilage, with or without attached perichondrium, is used to reconstruct the tympanic membrane in the posterior–superior aspect and/or the attic to prevent recurrent retraction. Using a Lempert ear speculum the ear canal is inspected and the proper position of the canal skin flaps is ascertained. One or two Pope's® ear wicks (Merocel®) impregnated in antibiotic ointment are inserted into the lateral aspect of the ear canal to keep the flaps in proper position. The postauricular incision is closed in two layers with 3-0 Vicryl® and a rubber-band drain is left in the most dependent portion of the incision. A mastoid dressing is applied at the end of the procedure. The dressing and rubber-band drain are removed the next morning.

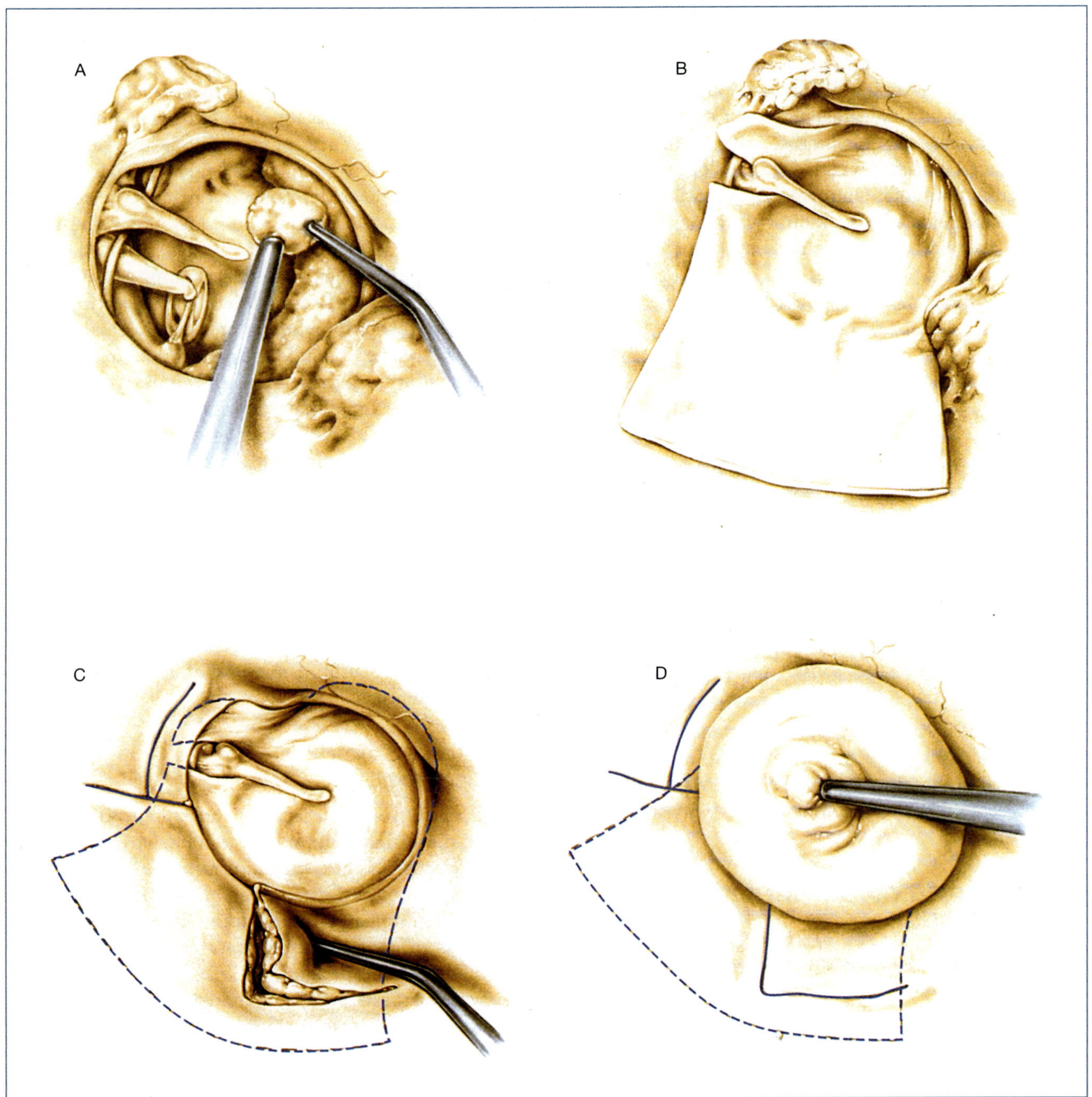

FIGURE 28–6 • *A*, Moist absorbable gelatin sponge (Gelfoam) is packed into the entire middle ear space, starting in the Eustachian tube orifice. *B*, The graft is placed into the middle ear so that it lies under the annulus anteriorly. *C*, When the inferior and superior flaps are replaced, the graft is held securely in position. *D*, The ear canal is filled with polymyxin B and bacitracin (Polysporin) ointment instead of packing at the end the procedure.

Overlay Technique

Exposure of the ear canal is accomplished through a postauricular approach as in the underlay technique. After the vascular strip is removed from the ear canal and is kept folded in the postauricular area with a self-retaining retractor, the skin of the ear canal medial to the bony–cartilaginous junction and the squamous epithelial layer of the lateral aspect of the tympanic membrane remnant are completely removed and kept in saline solution for use later in the procedure. The tympanic annulus is left in place and a canaloplasty is performed if necessary. Any middle-ear pathology is removed as in the underlay technique. The middle ear is packed with Gelfoam® and the graft is placed lateral to the tympanic annulus and medial to the manubrium to prevent lateralization. To accommodate proper placement medial to the manubrium, a slit is made in the superior aspect of the graft. The graft should be long enough to extend over the posterior canal wall. In order to avoid blunting of the anterior sulcus, caution is needed to avoid draping the flap over the anterior canal wall. The previously removed epithelium is placed in its original position and Gelfoam® packing is placed in the anterior sulcus to avoid a dead space and blunting by the formation of fibrous tissue. Gelfoam® is placed on the lateral aspect of the graft as well. Finally the vascular strip is returned to its original position and the ear canal is packed with one or two Pope's® ear wicks impregnated in antibiotic ointment. The postauricular incision is closed in the similar fashion with the underlay technique and a mastoid dressing is applied.

Canaloplasty

Canaloplasty is performed in cases with a bulge of the anterior bony wall that causes poor visualization of the anterior sulcus. Failure to secure good exposure of the anterior sulcus during tympanoplasty may result in failure due to improper graft placement.

The canaloplasty Figure 28–7A to D is performed as follows: with a Beaver® blade number 74, a horizontal incision is made medial to the anterior wall bulge and above the anterior sulcus. With a Beaver® blade number 67, two vertical incisions are placed on either side of the horizontal incision, and are extended laterally on the anterior canal wall encompassing the area of the obstruction. The created skin flap is elevated laterally up to the level of the bony–cartilaginous junction and the bony protuberance is exposed. Using continuous suction-irrigation and a high-speed drill the obstructing bone is removed until adequate exposure of the anterior sulcus is achieved. Meticulous dissection is needed in order to avoid injury to the glenoid fossa capsule. A prominent spine of Henle should also be removed when interfering with visualization (Video 28–4).

CARTILAGE TYMPANOPLASTY TECHNIQUES

Although temporalis fascia and perichondrium still remain the most commonly used grafts in tympanoplasty and the reported results are excellent, they both have the potential to atrophy resulting in failure, especially in such high-risk ears as those with atelectasis, cholesteatomas, and prior surgery.[83] Since Utech in 1959[84] and then Heermann[85] and Jansen[86] in the early 1960s reported their experience with cartilage grafts in tympanoplasty, many authors have described their use either as a palisade, perichondrium/cartilage island flap, or cartilage "shield" for cases at high risk for failure.[53,87–90] Conchal and tragal cartilage are the two most commonly used cartilaginous grafts, and they resist resorption and retraction even in the face of Eustachian tube dysfunction.[53] Another advantage of these grafts is the feasibility of ossicular reconstruction at the time of grafting.[53,87]

Perichondrium/Cartilage Island Flap and Palisade Techniques

The perichondrium/cartilage island flap and palisade technique have been popularized in the United States by Dornhoffer; the tragus or concha are the donor sites used in these techniques.[53]

In the perichondrium/cartilage island flap technique (Figure 28–8A to E), a piece of tragal cartilage measuring 15 mm in length and 10 mm in width is harvested. One side of the perichondrium is elevated leaving the reverse side attached. Using a knife, cartilage is removed to create an eccentrically located disk of cartilage measuring approximately 7 to 9 mm in diameter. Then a 2-mm strip of cartilage is removed vertically from the center of the cartilage to accommodate the manubrium. In cases with an intact ossicular chain, an additional triangular piece of cartilage is removed from the posterior–superior quadrant to accommodate the incus. The middle ear is packed with Gelfoam® anteriorly at the Eustachian tube but the promontory and ossicular chain are left devoid of any packing. The graft is placed in an underlay fashion with the cartilage facing the promontory and the free perichondrium extending posteriorly, draping over the bony canal wall (Figure 28–8D).

In the palisade technique the cartilage is sectioned into several slices, which are pieced together to reconstruct the tympanic membrane. The more curved cymba concha is considered a more suitable donor site,[53] although tragal cartilage is also an option. This technique has been found useful in the reconstruction posterior tympanic membrane perforations with associated ossicular disease necessitating synchronous reconstruction with PORPs or TORPs. In cases with cholesteatoma it can be used to reconstruct the scutum and posterior–superior quadrant to prevent recurrence.

Cartilage "Shield" Tympanoplasty

For the past 10 years, cartilage "shield" tympanoplasty(CST) has been the author's preferred technique for cases requiring total replacement of the tympanic membrane, cases with questionable or borderline Eustachian tube dysfunction, atelectatic ears, cholesteatomas, tympanoplasty failures, laterally displaced tympanic membranes and atresia cases.[87,90] The technique used is a modification of the one described by Duckert et al.[88] For primary and secondary acquired cholesteatomas, posterior perforations, especially when titanium ossiculoplasty is performed, the author prefers the palisade technique as described previously. The CST is considered by the author to be a less technically demanding and less time consuming procedure than the perichondrium/cartilage island flap technique.

The CST technique proceeds as follows: under general anesthesia vascular strip incisions are made in the ear canal followed by a postauricular incision. Areolar tissue overlying the temporalis fascia is harvested and the vascular strip is elevated out of the ear canal and kept in position using two self-retaining retractors. Access to the ear canal and tympanic membrane is accomplished via the postauricular area. A canaloplasty is performed in cases with bulging of the bony anterior canal wall to improve visualization of the anterior sulcus. The edges of the perforation are denuded and areas of tympanosclerosis are completely removed. The middle ear is explored, the status of the ossicular chain is determined and any pathology found is removed. At this point a mastoidectomy is performed if deemed necessary. A round piece

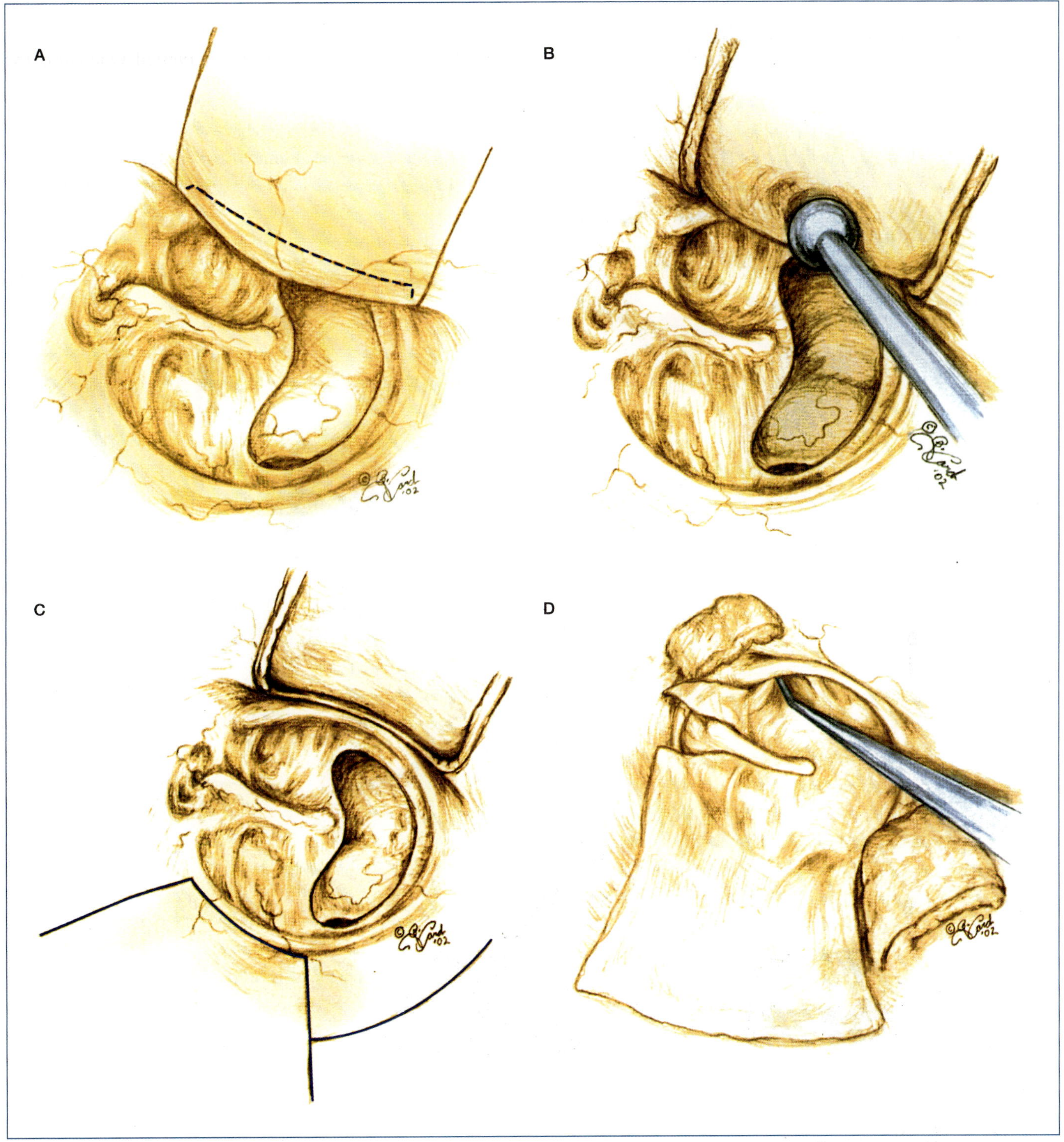

FIGURE 28–7 • The canaloplasty.

of cartilage, approximately the size of the tympanic membrane defect (10 mm), is harvested from the concha cymba area (Video clip 28–5). The initial size of the cartilage graft should be slightly larger than the tympanic membrane defect and it is gradually trimmed with scissors to the proper size. The perichondrium is stripped from both sides and a wedge of cartilage is excised to accommodate the manubrium. The middle ear is packed with Gelfoam® (Pharmacia and Upjohn Co., Kalamazoo, MI) and the cartilaginous graft, with its convex surface placed medially, is placed underneath the

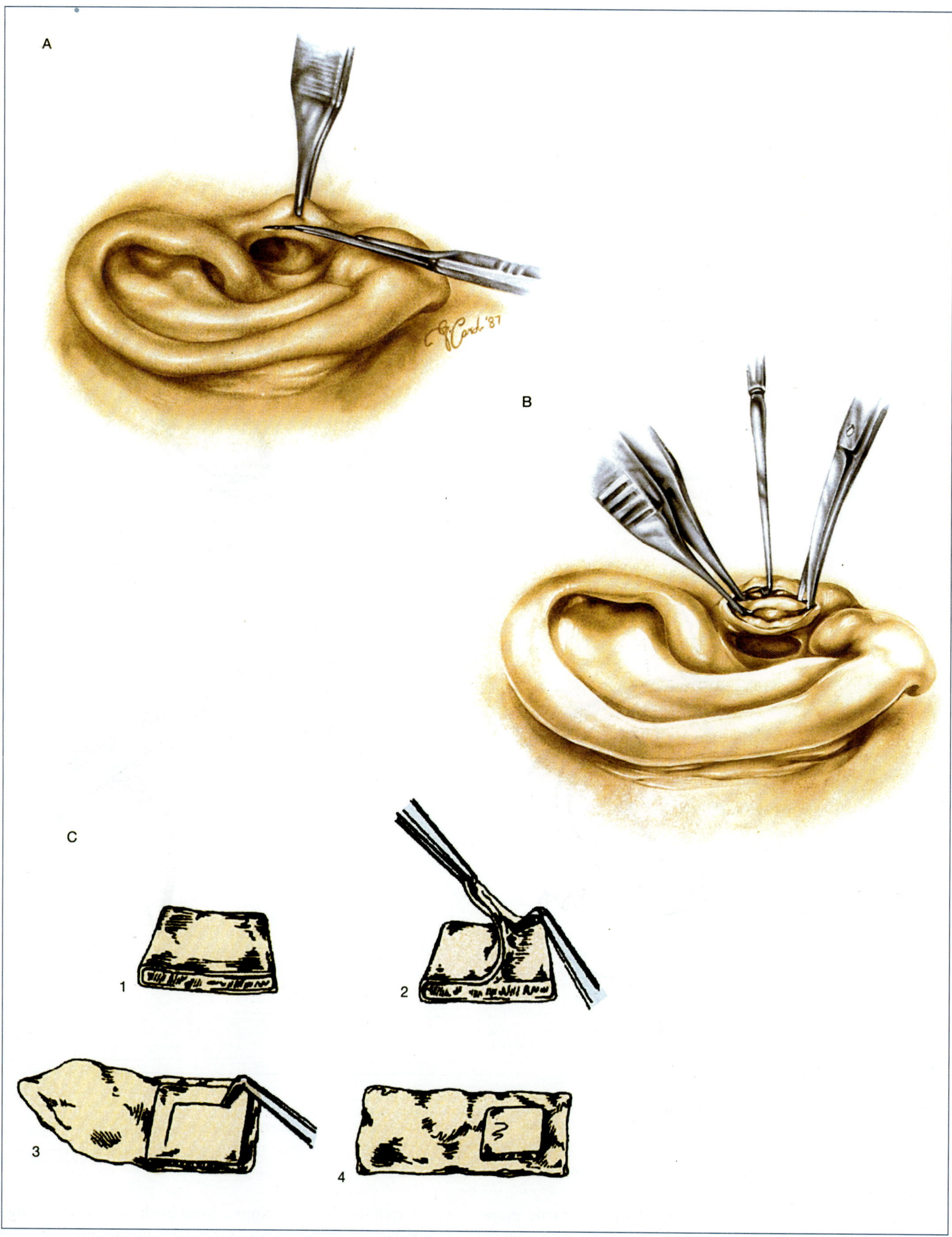

FIGURE 28–8 • *A*, An incision is made in the posterior aspect of the tragus and carried through perichondrium and tragal cartilage. This leaves cartilage remaining at the tip of the tragus to maintain its shape. *B*, A piece of tragal cartilage with perichondrium is removed with the use of small-pointed scissors. *C*, The perichondrium is reflected from the surface of the cartilage similar to a book cover and the cartilage is trimmed to size.

Continued

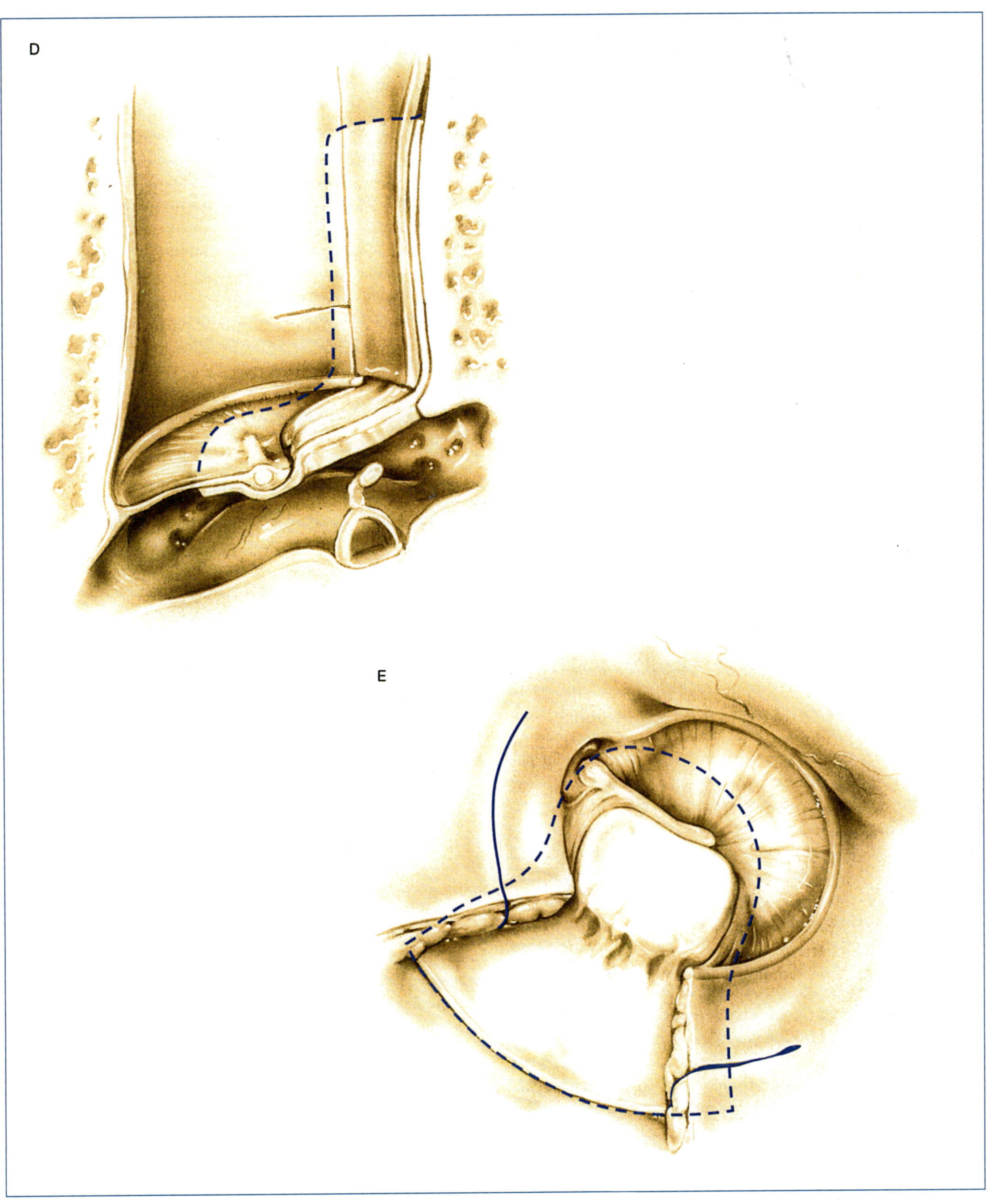

FIGURE 28–8 • *Continued. D*, The perichondrium is placed under the malleus anteriorly and on to the posterior canal wall posteriorly. *E*, This view demonstrates how the cartilage becomes incorporated into the substance of the tympanic membrane to prevent recurrence of the disease process.

manubrium by lifting it up with a small right angle hook while gently pushing the graft medially with a 22-gauge suction (Video clip 28–6). Subsequently, the periphery of the cartilage graft is placed medial to the tympanic membrane remnant or the fibrous annulus. If there is no fibrous annulus, the cartilage graft is placed at the level of the tympanic sulcus. There is no need to create a groove in the anterior bony wall to accommodate the graft. A very small gap (less than 1 mm) is allowed between the graft and the tympanic sulcus. It must be emphasized that a tight-fitting, oversized graft should be avoided because of reduction in eventual vibrational properties. For patients with medialization of the malleus, the tensor tympani tendon can be sectioned to lateralize the manubrium and allow medial placement of the graft. In case it is required ossicular reconstruction is performed with a TORP, a PORP or a type III tympanoplasty. The previously harvested areolar tissue is then placed over the cartilage graft and medial to the tympanic membrane remnant, or fibrous annulus, so any small gaps are bridged (Video clip 28–7). The vascular-strip flap is returned to its original position and two Pope's® ear wicks (Xomed Co., Memphis, TN) impregnated in antibiotic ointment are inserted in the ear canal to secure proper position of the vascular strip (Video clip 28–8). The postauricular incision is closed in two layers with 3.0 Vicryl® sutures, a rubber-band drain is left in the most dependent area of the incision, and a mastoid dressing is applied.

The concha cymba cartilage is within the operative field, has an average thickness of 0.8 mm and its concave contour resembles the conical shape of the normal tympanic membrane.[57] This cartilage has an average thickness similar to fossa triangularis cartilage (0.775 mm) and is thinner than tragal cartilage (1.016 mm).[57] In the technique described by Duckert et al.,[88] the perichondrium is left in place and the cartilage is thinned. The author, in order to achieve a thinner graft, strips the perichondrium from both sides of the cartilage graft. There has been neither graft lateralization nor collapse into the middle-ear space in the author's experience and therefore there is no need to create a groove in the bony sulcus for graft stabilization as recommended by Moore.[57] Despite the cartilage thickness, 78% of patients following CST have a type A or C tympanogram.[57] If a middle-ear effusion develops in the postoperative period, myringotomy with tubing can be performed.[53,57] Although the thickness of the cartilage graft may decrease the middle-ear space, this has not had any significant adverse effect on the hearing results. In postoperative temporal bone CT scans, space can been detected between the cartilaginous graft and the promontory.[87] In a considerable number of patients with no incus and a contracted middle-ear space, the cartilage thickness makes a type III tympanoplasty feasible, obviating the need for a PORP. Hearing results in such cases are similar to those obtained with PORPs.[90] A potential disadvantage of this technique is the cartilage opacity and possible concealment of recurrent/residual cholesteatoma and middle-ear effusion. These potential problems can be avoided by performing a second-look procedure in all cholesteatoma cases in 12 months following the initial surgery and a diagnostic myringotomy in case of suspected middle-ear effusion.[91]

Regardless of the tympanoplasty approach or technique used, involvement of the mastoid antrum with cholesteatoma necessitates either a CWD, or an ICW mastoidectomy. The ICW mastoidectomy can be used in the majority of cholesteatoma cases and is the preferred method over the CWD technique since it avoids the creation of an open mastoid cavity with the associated need for long term cleaning, restriction of water activities, and recurrent infections. This technique results in an ear that is anatomically and functionally closer to normal. However, this technique is associated with a higher incidence of residual and recurrent cholesteatoma; for this reason a second-stage procedure, usually one year later, is required. Residual cholesteatomas is defined as persistent cholesteatoma in the middle ear or mastoid cavity following incomplete removal. Recurrent cholesteatoma develops following complete removal due to retraction of the pars flaccida or the posterior–superior quadrant of the tympanic membrane. Both mastoidectomy techniques when properly performed give very satisfactory results.

TYMPANOPLASTY RESULTS

Graft-take and hearing results following tympanoplasty depend upon multiple factors. Eustachian tube dysfunction, presence of cholesteatoma or atelectasis, previous tympanoplasty failure, lateralized tympanic membrane, and smoking are negative prognostic factors. These factors make it difficult to compare tympanoplasty results reported in the literature. However, the success rate for graft-take is quite high and overall it is more than 90%. Tympanoplasty results are summarized in Table 28–1.

POSTOPERATIVE CARE

The patient is discharged on the day of the surgery or in case of uncontrolled nausea or vomiting, the patient is discharged the next morning. The mastoid dressing and drain are removed the day after surgery and the patient is instructed to instill antibiotic drops in the ear canal at bedtime. Showering is allowed provided the patient places a cotton ball impregnated with petroleum ointment in the outer-ear canal. Water should be kept away from the postauricular incision for 2 days. Nose blowing should be avoided until the tympanic membrane is healed. If sneezing is unavoidable, the mouth should be kept open. Oral antibiotics are prescribed for patients with ears that were infected at the time of surgery. The first postoperative visit is one week following surgery, during which the Merocel® ear wick (Pope's® ear wick) is removed. The Gelfoam® over the graft is gently suctioned away, if still present, at the second visit 3 to 4 weeks later. Persisting granulations of the ear canal are cauterized with a 25% solution of silver nitrate to promote healing. Hearing improvement may be noticed within 6 to 8 weeks following surgery. An audiogram is obtained 4 to 6 months after surgery. Postoperative instructions for patients are outlined in Appendix 1.

COMPLICATIONS

Most tympanoplasty complications are preventable by comprehensive preoperative planning, thorough knowledge of the

TABLE 28–1 Tympanoplasty results

AUTHOR (REF. NO.)	NO. OF PATIENTS	TECHNIQUE	TYPE OF GRAFT	GRAFT-TAKE (%)	POSTOPERATIVE PTA-ABG
Vartiainen E et al.[103]	404	Overlay and underlay	TF	88	<25 db in 87% of cases
Sheehy JL et al.[48]	472	Overlay	TF	97	<10 db in 88% of cases
Glasscock ME et al.[47]	1,556	Underlay	Autogenous and homograft TF	93	NA
Cueva RA[69]	406	Underlay	Areolar tissue	97.5	NA
Dornhoffer J[53]	533	Underlay	Perichondrium/ cartilage island flap Palisade	97.6	Pre-PTA-ABG 22.8 ± 12.3db Post-PTA-ABG 13.5 ± 9.4 db
Aidonis et al.[87]	62	Underlay	Concha cymba cartilage "shield"	98.4	Pre-PTA-ABGs 32.4 ± 14.1 db Post-PTA-ABG 24 ± 13.7 db ABG < 10 db in 86% of type I tympanoplasties

TF, temporalis fascia; NA, not available; PTA, pure-tone average; ABG, air–bone gap.

temporal bone anatomy, applying meticulous surgical techniques and close postoperative follow-up. Patients should be informed prior to surgery regarding potential complications and proper documentation should be made in the patient's chart. Alternate rehabilitation modalities such as a conventional or the Baha® system should be presented to the patient.

Intraoperative Bleeding

Bleeding from accidental injury of a high and uncovered jugular bulb may occur during exploration of the middle ear. Prompt application of a piece of Gelfoam® soaked in saline or Surgical® should be able to control bleeding since the jugular bulb is a low-pressure structure. In order to avoid pulmonary embolism, it is important for the packing not to be pushed into the lumen of the jugular bulb but rather to cover its surface while very gentle pressure is applied with a small moistened neurosurgical cottonoid.

Bleeding from the internal carotid artery can be catastrophic and should be avoided. A pulsating structure in the area of the Eustachian tube orifice is suggestive of an uncovered or aberrant internal carotid artery.

Facial Nerve Injury

It is the author's impression that during the last decade in this country, better otologic training of residents by fellowship-trained faculty has resulted in a significant decrease in iatrogenic facial paralysis. The fact that the more complicated cases are referred to otologists may have contributed to this decline as well.

Postotologic surgery facial paralysis is a devastating complication and is avoidable in the majority of cases. A facial nerve exposed in its tympanic segment is vulnerable to injury especially if involved with cholesteatoma or granulation tissue. Jacobson's nerve and the cochleariform process are very useful anatomic landmarks for locating the facial nerve in this situation. Facial nerve monitoring, although not a substitute for anatomic identification of the facial nerve, can help locate the facial nerve, guide the dissection, and confirm neural integrity.[92]

Postoperative facial paralysis is managed according to whether or not the nerve was positively identified during surgery. If the nerve was identified and not injured during the procedure, the patient may be followed with serial nerve excitability tests or electroneuronography. In the majority of such cases, the paralysis will resolve without any need for surgical intervention.[93] When the surgeon has failed to identify the facial nerve during surgery and its integrity is questionable, exploration should be performed as soon as possible. In cases of delayed facial paralysis the prognosis is very good and the patient can be followed with serial-nerve-excitability tests or electroneuronography. Reactivation of a previous *Varicella-Zoster* infection has been suspected as an etiologic factor in such cases.[94]

In a series of 22 patients who sustained an iatrogenic facial nerve injury, although the most common procedure performed that led to the injury was mastoidectomy (55%), in a significant number of cases injury occurred during the tympanoplasty part of the procedure (14%). The most common site of injury was the tympanic segment and in 79% of the patients, the injury was not detected at the time of surgery.[93]

When the facial nerve is transected more than half of its diameter, repair either with direct reanastomosis or with a cable nerve graft is recommended. For transections less than 50%, decompression is advised.[95] No patient with direct anastomosis or cable graft repair is expected to have better than a House-Brackmann grade III result.[95] In the majority of cases the greater auricular nerve can be used as a graft since it is located in close proximity to the surgical area and has the same diameter as the facial nerve.

Facial paralysis secondary to local anesthetic always subsides within several hours following completion of surgery.

Wound Infection/Perichondritis

These are very rare complications and present with pain, erythema, and swelling of the incision or auricle. Perichondritis can develop subsequent to the use of endaural incisions in the cartilaginous ear canal or after cartilage is harvested from the auricle for grafting. Intravenous antibiotics covering *Pseudomonas* and gram-positive organisms are indicated. Incision and drainage should be performed for cases with abscess formation. Meticulous surgical technique with special attention to minimal tissue damage and frequent irrigation with saline of the surgical field during surgery may prevent these complications.

Wound Hematoma

Hematomas form at the donor sites of grafts, usually the temporalis muscle area and auricle, and present with severe pain and swelling within the first postoperative day. Good hemostasis during surgery and the routine use of a rubber-band drain in all tympanoplasties performed through a postauricular approach may prevent this complication. Immediate opening of the incision and drainage is required.

Chorda Tympani Nerve Injury

Preservation of the chorda tympani nerve during tympanoplasty is necessary to avoid postoperative gustatory changes. Stretching of this structure is associated with more symptoms than transection. Complete recovery has been reported in 76% of cases.[96] Tympanoplasty candidates should be properly informed prior to surgery regarding this potential complication.

Tympanoplasty Failure

Persistent/recurrent perforation, blunting of the anterior sulcus, graft lateralization, epithelial pearls development, and conductive hearing loss may require revision tympanoplasty. Poor Eustachian tube function, inadequate visualization of the anterior sulcus, extensive tympanosclerosis of the tympanic membrane remnant, inadequate anterior support of the graft with Gelfoam®, previous overlay technique, and recurrent/residual cholesteatoma are common etiologies.

Blunting of the anterior angle and its associated conductive hearing loss is a complication usually associated with the overlay technique and may necessitate revision surgery. Meticulous technique is required during the primary procedure to avoid this complication.

Epithelial pearl formation on the graft or in the ear canal is also associated with the overlay technique. Meticulous removal of all squamous epithelium from the tympanic membrane remnant and the ear canal is necessary to avoid this complication. Opening of the pearl(s) and removal of the keratin debris can be done in the office in cooperative patients.

When the graft lateralizes by migrating away from the manubrium, conductive hearing occurs and revision surgery may be required. This complication may also arise when the graft is placed lateral to the manubrium at the primary surgery.

Results of revision tympanoplasty are satisfactory although slightly less successful than primary cases. In a recent study of revision tympanoplasty using the cartilage "shield' technique, there was statistically significant closure of the air–bone gap, with the majority of cases being less than 25 dB and the graft-take was 93.5%. Most of the Pure tone average (PTA) improvements were seen in cases with atelectatic middle ears and those with lateralized tympanic membranes. With the exception of cholesteatoma cases, significant improvement in PTA was made in all surgical groups, including those with and without mastoidectomy, and all types of ossicular reconstruction.[91] Table 28–2 summarizes the revision tympanoplasty results.

Recurrent/Residual Middle-Ear Cholesteatoma

Recurrent and residual cholesteatomas have been reported to occur in 14% and 12% respectively of cases undergoing tympanoplasty in conjunction with ICW mastoidectomy.[97] Cholesteatomas in children are more aggressive and the 3 and 5 year recurrence rates have been reported as high as 48% and 57% respectively.[98] In another study of 199 children with cholesteatoma in whom 215 procedures were performed, the residual cholesteatoma rate for the ICW technique was 20.5% and recurrent 8.9%. For the CWD technique, the residual and recurrent cholesteatoma rates were 23.8% and 19%, respectively. Eighty-eight percent of the procedures performed were ICW technique.[99] In 283 patients who underwent tympanoplasty with ICW mastoidectomy, the incidence of residual cholesteatoma was 13.43% and recurrent 7.77%. It was more common in children (25%) than in adults (11.72%), and was more frequently localized in the middle ear (47.54%) than in the epitympanum (40.98%) or in the mastoid (6.56%).[100]

It is evident that long-term follow up of cholesteatoma patients is imperative to detect recurrent and residual disease. When tympanoplasty is combined with ICW mastoidectomy, a "second look" procedure 12 months following the initial procedure is necessary to detect residual or recurrent cholesteatoma. In the second-stage procedure the vascular strip incision can be eliminated and the middle ear can be approached directly from the postauricular incision. Avoiding a vascular-strip incision provides a more stable tympanic membrane since its continuity with the posterior canal skin is not been disrupted. Ossicular reconstruction is performed at the second procedure.

TABLE 28–2 Revision tympanoplasty results

AUTHOR NAME (REF. NO.)	TYPE OF GRAFT	GRAFT-TAKE	HEARING RESULT
Boone et al.[104]	Tragal cartilage, perichondrium island, concha cymba palisade	94.7%	24.6 ± 13.8 db preop ABG 12.2 ± 7.3 db postop ABG
Sismanis et al.[91]	Cartilage shield, concha cymba	93.5%*	33.6 db ± 13 db preop ABG 25.7 db ± 11db postop ABG 56% of cases <25 db ABG
Moore[57]	Cartilage shield, fossa triangularis	100%	Mean postop PTA 32.5 db 98% of cases <30db ABG at 2 kHz
Kaylie et al.[105]	Temporalis fascia, tragal perichondrium	86%	50% of PORP cases <20 db ABG 60% of PORP cases <30 db ABG 68% of TORP cases <30 db ABG
Djalilian[106]	Pressed scar tissue	91%	21 db mean improvement in postop ABG
Veldman et al.[107]	Autogenous fascia, allografts**	90%	70.3 % of cases <30db ABG
Ghanem et al.[108]	Butterfly cartilage inlay graft***	92%	Mean pre- and postop ABG improvement from 23–21 db

PTA, pure-tone average; ABG, air–bone gap.
*97.8% with cholesteatoma cases excluded.
**Not specified.
***Mixed, primary, and revision cases.

Sensorineural Hearing Loss/Dizziness

This complication can be secondary to direct injury to the stapes resulting from manipulation of this structure during removal of disease. Should the stapes be partially avulsed, it should be repositioned in its original position and stabilized with a tissue graft. When cholesteatoma matrix is very adherent to the facial nerve, stapes or oval window, it can be left in place and removed at the second-stage procedure one year later. Usually at the second stage, a cholesteatoma pearl is found, which is easier to remove. Other causes of sensorineural hearing loss are labyrinthine fistula (usually on the promontory) and acoustic trauma resulting from the high-speed drill contacting the ossicular chain. Although it is not absolutely contraindicated to remove the fistula matrix during tympanoplasty, a more conservative approach is to leave it in place and remove it at a second-stage procedure one year later. This approach is more applicable to large fistulas that involve most of the promontory, especially if associated with infected cholesteatoma. Sensorineural hearing loss and dizziness present prior to surgery should alert the otolaryngologist to the potential of a labyrinthine fistula. In such cases a CT of the temporal bones may confirm this entity.[101] When a labyrinthine fistula is discovered accidentally during tympanoplasty, it should be immediately covered with temporalis fascia or areolar tissue. Removal of the fistula matrix has been reported to result in severe hearing loss in 11% of cases.[102] In such cases postoperative dizziness may be prolonged.

Appendix 1

Postoperative Instructions for Myringoplasty and Tympanoplasty (Modified After James Sheehy)[109]

Precautions

1. Do NOT drive home from the hospital, either arrange for someone else to drive you or some other means of transportation. Air travel is NOT permissible until four weeks after surgery.
2. Do NOT blow your nose until your doctor tells you that your ear is healed. To clear secretions in the nose, sniff secretion to the back of the throat and expectorate.
3. When sneezing, keep your mouth open.
4. Avoid water entering the ear canal until the doctor tells you that the ear is healed. To help avoid water entering the ear canal, place a piece of cotton saturated with Vaseline in the outer ear canal.
5. Two days after surgery, you may shower and allow water to flow over the incision site behind your ear.

Instructions for Inserting Ear Drops

You will be expected to use antibiotic drops as prescribed by your doctor, for 3 to 4 weeks after surgery. Five drops in the ear will help loosen the packing. Tip the head to the side, insert the five drops into the ear canal, and allow drops to remain in the ear canal for five minutes. Then place a piece of cotton in the outer ear canal.

When to expect hearing improvement

Hearing is not expected to improve immediately after surgery, and it may even decrease due to the packing in the middle ear and ear canal. Improvement can be noticed 6 to 8 weeks after surgery, but maximum improvement may take 4 to 6 months.

Normal Side Effects after Surgery

Hearing pulsating sounds, popping, clicking, sensation of liquid in the ear canal, ear fullness, and occasional sharp earaches are normal.

Dizziness. Minor dizziness may occur when moving the head for a few days after surgery. This minor dizziness should not concern you. If dizziness increases, contact your doctor.

Discharge from the ear. Bloody drainage from the ear canal should be expected for up to 4 weeks after surgery. Notify your physician immediately if drainage becomes yellow in color (pus).

Pain. Mild intermittent ear pain is common during the first 2 weeks after surgery. When chewing, pain above or in front of the ear is common. If you have persistent ear pain and increased swelling of the auricle, notify your doctor.

Numbness. Numbness of the auricle is very common when an incision is made behind the ear. This numbness disappears within 3 months in almost all cases.

References

1. Committee on Conservation of Hearing, American Academy of Ophthalmology and Otolaryngology. Standard classification for surgery of chronic ear disease. Arch Otol 1965;81:204.
2. Wullstein H. [Technic and early results of tympanoplasty.]. Monatsschr Ohrenheilkd Laryngorhinol 1953;87(4):308–11.
3. Zollner F. [Surgical technics for the improvement of sound conduction after radical operation.] Arch Ital Otol Rinol Laringol 1953;64(4):455–68.
4. Wullstein H. Funktionelle operationen im mittelohr mit hilfe des freien spaltlappen-transplantates. Arch Ohren- Nasen- u Kehlkopfh 1952;161:422.
5. Schwartze HH, Eysell CG. ueber die kunstliche eroffnung des warsenfortsatzes. Arch Ohrenh 1873;7:157.
6. Kuster E. Ueber die grundsatze der behandlung von eiterungen in starrwandigen hohlen, mit besonderer berucksichtigung des empyems der pleura. Deutsche med Wchnschr 1889;15:254.
7. Zaufal E. des trepanation des proc. mastoid nach kusterschen grundsatzen. Arch Ohrenh 1890;30:291.
8. Stacke L. Stacke's operationsmethode. Arch Ohrenh 1893;35:145.
9. Holmgren G. Some experiences in surgery for otosclerosis. Acta Otolaryng 1923;5:460.
10. Nylen CO. The microscope in aural surgery, its first use and later development. Acta Otolaryng, Suppl 1954;116:226–40.
11. Sourdille M. New technique in the surgical treatment of severe and progressive deafness from otosclerosis. Bull N Y Acad Med 1937;13:673.
12. Lempert J. Improvement of hearing in cases of otosclerosis: New one-stage surgical technic. Arch Otolaryng 1938;28:42.
13. Pattee GL. An operation to improve hearing in cases of congenital atresia of the external auditory meatus. Arch Otolaryng 1947;45:568.
14. Ombredanne M. Surgery of deafness: Fenestration in cases of congenital atresia of the external auditory canal. Oto-rhino Laryng Internat 1947;13:229.
15. Rosen S. Mobilization of the stapes to restore hearing in otosclerosis. N Y State J Med 1953;53(22):2650–3.
16. Juers AL. Observations on bone conduction in fenestrated cases. Ann Otol Rhin Laryng 1948;57:28.
17. Davis H, Walsh TE. The limits of improvement of hearing following the fenestration operation. Laryngoscope 1950; 60:273.
18. Moritz W. Horverbessernde operationen bei chronisch-entzundlichen prozessen beider mittelohren. Ztschr Laryng Rhin Otol 1950;29:578.
19. Zollner F. Radical operation with special reference to auditory function. Z Laryngol Rhinol Otol 1951;30(3):104–11.
20. Shea JJ Jr. Vein graft closure of eardrum perforations. J Laryngol Otol 1960;74:358–62.
21. Tabb HG. Closure of perforations of the tympanic membrane by vein grafts. A preliminary report of twenty cases. Laryngoscope 1960;70:271–86.
22. Storrs LA. Temporalis muscle fascia and denatured fat grafts in middle-ear surgery. Laryngoscope 1963;73:699–701.
23. Heermann H. Tympanoplasty with fascial tissue taken from the temporal muscle after straightening the anterior wall of the auditory meatus. HNO 1961;9:136–7.
24. Hall A, Rytzner C. Stapedectomy and autotransplantation of ossicles. Acta Otolaryngol 1957;47(4):318–24.
25. House WJ, Patterson ME, Linthicum FH Jr. Incus homografts in chronic ear surgery. Arch Otolaryngol 1966;84(2):148–53.
26. Glasscock ME III, House WF. Homograft reconstruction of the middle ear. A preliminary report. Laryngoscope 1968;78(7):1219–25.
27. Shea JJ, Homsy CA. The use of Proplast TM in otologic surgery. Laryngoscope 1974;84(10):1835–45.
28. Brown DV, Keith RW. Principles of audiology and auditory physiology. In: Hughes GB PM, editor. Clinical otology. New York: Thieme Publishers, Inc.; 2007. p. 35–43.
29. Segal N, Givon-Lavi N, Leibovitz E, Yagupsky P, Leiberman A, Dagan R. Acute otitis media caused by streptococcus pyogenes in children. Clin Infect Dis 2005;41(1):35–41.
30. Daly KA, Hunter LL, Lindgren BR, Margolis R, Giebink GS. Chronic otitis media with effusion sequelae in children treated with tubes. Arch Otolaryngol Head Neck Surg 2003;129(5):517–22.
31. Chole R, Sudhoff H. Chronic otitis media, mastoiditis, and petrosistis. In: Cummings CW, Flint PW, Harker LA, et al., editors. Cummings otolaryngology—head and neck surgery. Philadelphhia, PA: Elsevier Mosby; 2005. p. 2988–3012.
32. Cho YS, Lee HS, Kim SW, et al. Tuberculous otitis media: A clinical and radiologic analysis of 52 patients. Laryngoscope 2006;116(6):921–7.
33. Windle-Taylor PC, Bailey CM. Tuberculous otitis media: A series of 22 patients. Laryngoscope 1980;90(6 Pt 1):1039–44.
34. Frenkiel S, Alberti PW. Traumatic thermal injuries of the middle ear. J Otolaryngol 1977;6(1):17–22.
35. Panosian MS, Dutcher PO Jr. Transtympanic facial nerve injury in welder. Occup Med (Lond) 1994;44(2):99–101.
36. Lasak JM, Van Ess M, Kryzer TC, Cummings RJ. Middle ear injury through the external auditory canal: A review of 44 cases. Ear Nose Throat J 2006;85(11):722–4, 728.

37. Offiah C, Heran M, Graeb D. Lightning strike: A rare cause of bilateral ossicular disruption. AJNR Am J Neuroradiol 2007;28(5):974–5.
38. Zoltan TB, Taylor KS, Achar SA. Health issues for surfers. Am Fam Physician 2005;71(12):2313–17.
39. Berger G, Finkelstein Y, Harell M. Non-explosive blast injury of the ear. J Laryngol Otol 1994;108(5):395–8.
40. Miller IS, McGahey D, Law K. The otologic consequences of the Omagh bomb disaster. Otolaryngol Head Neck Surg 2002;126(2):127–8.
41. Helling ER. Otologic blast injuries due to the Kenya embassy bombing. Mil Med 2004;169(11):872–6.
42. Xydakis MS, Bebarta VS, Harrison CD, Conner JC, Grant GA, Robbins AS. Tympanic-membrane perforation as a marker of concussive brain injury in Iraq. N Engl J Med 2007;357(8):830–1.
43. Kalcioglu MT, Cokkeser Y, Kizilay A, Ozturan O. Follow-up of 366 ears after tympanostomy tube insertion: Why is it draining? Otolaryngol Head Neck Surg 2003;128(4):560–4.
44. Matt BH, Miller RP, Meyers RM, Campbell JM, Cotton RT. Incidence of perforation with Goode T-tube. Int J Pediatr Otorhinolaryngol 1991;21(1):1–6.
45. Hekkenberg RJ, Smitheringale AJ. Gelfoam/Gelfilm patching following the removal of ventilation tubes. J Otolaryngol 1995;24(6):362–3.
46. Puterman M, Leiberman A. Gelfoam plug tympanoplasty concomitant with removal of retained ventilation tubes. Int J Pediatr Otorhinolaryngol 2005;69(1):57–60.
47. Glasscock ME III, Jackson CG, Nissen AJ, Schwaber MK. Postauricular undersurface tympanic membrane grafting: A follow-up report. Laryngoscope 1982;92(7 Pt 1):718–27.
48. Sheehy JL, Anderson RG. Myringoplasty. A review of 472 cases. Ann Otol Rhinol Laryngol 1980;89(4 Pt 1):331–4.
49. Glasscock ME, III. Symposium: Contraindications to tympanoplasty. II. An exercise in clinical judgment. Laryngoscope 1976;86(1):70–6.
50. Uguz MZ, Onal K, Kazikdas KC, Onal A. The influence of smoking on success of tympanoplasty measured by serum cotinine analysis. Eur Arch Otorhinolaryngol 2008;265:513–6.
51. Becvarovski Z, Kartush JM. Smoking and tympanoplasty: Implications for prognosis and the middle ear risk index (MERI). Laryngoscope 2001;111(10):1806–11.
52. Saito T, Tanaka T, Tokuriki M, et al. Recent outcome of tympanoplasty in the elderly. Otol Neurotol 2001;22(2):153–7.
53. Dornhoffer J. Cartilage tympanoplasty: Indications, techniques, and outcomes in a 1,000-patient series. Laryngoscope 2003;113(11):1844–56.
54. Collins WO, Telischi FF, Balkany TJ, Buchman CA. Pediatric tympanoplasty: Effect of contralateral ear status on outcomes. Arch Otolaryngol Head Neck Surg 2003;129(6):646–51.
55. Badran K, Bunstone D, Arya AK, Suryanarayanan R, Mackinnon N. Patient satisfaction with the bone-anchored hearing aid: A 14-year experience. Otol Neurotol 2006;27(5):659–66.
56. Snik AF, Mylanus EA, Proops DW, et al. Consensus statements on the BAHA system: Where do we stand at present? Ann Otol Rhinol Laryngol Suppl 2005;195:2–12.
57. Moore GF. Candidate's thesis: Revision tympanoplasty utilizing fossa triangularis cartilage. Laryngoscope 2002;112(9):1543–54.
58. Roosa DB. Diseases of the ear. New York:William Wood & Co.; 1876.
59. Derlacki EL. Residual perforations after tympanoplasty: Office technique for closure. Otolaryngol Clin North Am 1982;15(4):861–7.
60. Goldman NC. Chemical closure of chronic tympanic membrane perforations. ANZ J Surg 2007;77(10):850–1.
61. Toynbee J. On the use of an artificial membrana tympani in cases of deafness dependent upon perforations or destruction of the natural organ. London: J. Churchill & Sons; 1853.
62. Yearsley J. Deafness, practically illustrated. London: J. Churchhill & Sons; 1863.
63. Kartush JM. Tympanic membrane Patcher: A new device to close tympanic membrane perforations in an office setting. Am J Otol 2000;21(5):615–20.
64. Spandow O, Hellstrom S, Dahlstrom M. Structural characterization of persistent tympanic membrane perforations in man. Laryngoscope 1996;106(3 Pt 1):346–52.
65. Johnson AP, Smallman LA, Kent SE. The mechanism of healing of tympanic membrane perforations. A two-dimensional histological study in guinea pigs. Acta Otolaryngol 1990;109(5–6):406–15.
66. Govaerts PJ, Jacob WA, Marquet J. Histological study of the thin replacement membrane of human tympanic membrane perforations. Acta Otolaryngol 1988;105(3–4):297–302.
67. Lee AJ, Jackler RK, Kato BM, Scott NM. Repair of chronic tympanic membrane perforations using epidermal growth factor: Progress toward clinical application. Am J Otol 1994;15(1):10–18.
68. Spandow O, Hellstrom S. [Healing of tympanic membrane perforation-a complex process influenced by a variety of factors.]. Acta Otolaryngol Suppl 1992;492:90–3.
69. Cueva RA. Areolar temporalis fascia: A reliable graft for tympanoplasty. Am J Otol 1999;20(6):709–11.
70. Moon CN Jr. Loose areolar connective tissue: A graft for otologic surgery. Laryngoscope 1973;83(5):771–7.
71. Gierek T, Slaska-Kaspera A, Majzel K, Klimczak-Golab L. [Results of myringoplasty and type I tympanoplasty with the use of fascia, cartilage and perichondrium grafts]. Otolaryngol Pol 2004;58(3):529–33.
72. Djalilian HR. Revision tympanoplasty using scar tissue graft. Otol Neurotol 2006;27(2):131–5.
73. Ozgursoy OB, Yorulmaz I. Fat graft myringoplasty: A cost-effective but underused procedure. J Laryngol Otol 2005;119(4):277–9.
74. Fayad JN, Baino T, Parisier SC. Preliminary results with the use of AlloDerm in chronic otitis media. Laryngoscope 2003;113(7):1228–30.
75. Fishman AJ, Marrinan MS, Huang TC, Kanowitz SJ. Total tympanic membrane reconstruction: AlloDerm versus temporalis fascia. Otolaryngol Head Neck Surg 2005;132(6):906–15.
76. Gerard JM, Gersdorff M. The Tutopatch graft for transcanal myringoplasty. B-ENT 2006;2(4):177–9.
77. Jackson CG. Antimicrobial prophylaxis in ear surgery. Laryngoscope 1988;98(10):1116–23.
78. Fiorino F, Barbieri F. Fat graft myringoplasty after unsuccessful tympanic membrane repair. Eur Arch Otorhinolaryngol 2007;264(10):1125–28.
79. Schraff SA, Markham J, Welch C, Darrow DH, Derkay CS. Outcomes in children with perforated tympanic membranes after tympanostomy tube placement: Results using a pilot treatment algorithm. Am J Otolaryngol 2006;27(4):238–43.

80. Landsberg R, Fishman G, DeRowe A, Berco E, Berger G. Fat graft myringoplasty: Results of a long-term follow-up. J Otolaryngol 2006;35(1):44–7.

81. Chole RA, Brodie HA. Surgery of the mastoid and petrosa. In: Bailey BJ, editor. Head and neck surgery-otolaryngology. Philadelphia, PA: Lippincott Williams & Wilkins; 2001:1799–1817.

82. Glasscock ME III. Tympanic membrane grafting with fascia: Overlay vs. undersurface technique. Laryngoscope 1973;83(5):754–70.

83. Buckingham RA. Fascia and perichondrium atrophy in tympanoplasty and recurrent middle ear atelectasis. Ann Otol Rhinol Laryngol 1992;101(9):755–8.

84. Utech H. Ueber diagnostische und therapeutische Moeglichkeitender Tympanotomie bei Schalleitungsstoerungen. Laryngol Rhinol 1959;38:212–21.

85. Heermann J. [Experiences with free transplantation of fascia-connective tissue of the temporalis muscle in tympanoplasty and reduction of the size of the radical cavity. Cartilage bridge from the stapes to the lower border of the tympanic membrane.]. Z Laryngol Rhinol Otol 1962;41:141–55.

86. Jansen C. Cartilage—Tympanoplasty. Laryngoscope 1963;73: 1288–301.

87. Aidonis I, Robertson TC, Sismanis A. Cartilage shield tympanoplasty: A reliable technique. Otol Neurotol 2005;26(5):838–41.

88. Duckert LG, Muller J, Makielski KH, Helms J. Composite autograft "shield" reconstruction of remnant tympanic membranes. Am J Otol 1995;16(1):21–6.

89. Anderson J, Caye-Thomasen P, Tos M. A comparison of cartilage palisades and fascia in tympanoplasty after surgery for sinus or tensa retraction cholesteatoma in children. Otol Neurotol 2004;25(6):856–63.

90. Kyrodimos E, Sismanis A, Santos D. Type III cartilage "shield" tympanoplasty: An effective procedure for hearing improvement. Otolaryngol Head Neck Surg 2007;136(6):982–5.

91. Sismanis A, Dodson K, Kyrodimos E. Cartilage "shield" grafts in revision tympanoplasty. Otology & Neurotology 2008;29(3): 330–3.

92. Noss RS, Lalwani AK, Yingling CD. Facial nerve monitoring in middle ear and mastoid surgery. Laryngoscope 2001;111(5):831–6.

93. Green JD Jr, Shelton C, Brackmann DE. Iatrogenic facial nerve injury during otologic surgery. Laryngoscope 1994;104(8 Pt 1): 922–6.

94. Safdar A, Gendy S, Hilal A, Walshe P, Burns H. Delayed facial nerve palsy following tympano-mastoid surgery: Incidence, aetiology and prognosis. J Laryngol Otol 2006;120(9):745–8.

95. Green JD Jr, Shelton C, Brackmann DE. Surgical management of iatrogenic facial nerve injuries. Otolaryngol Head Neck Surg 1994;111(5):606–10.

96. Michael P, Raut V. Chorda tympani injury: Operative findings and postoperative symptoms. Otolaryngol Head Neck Surg 2007;136(6):978–81.

97. Glasscock ME, Miller GW. Intact canal wall tympanoplasty in the management of cholesteatoma. Laryngoscope 1976;86(11):1639–57.

98. Stangerup SE, Drozdziewicz D, Tos M. Cholesteatoma in children, predictors and calculation of recurrence rates. Int J Pediatr Otorhinolaryngol 1999;49 (suppl 1):S69–S73.

99. Darrouzet V, Duclos JY, Portmann D, Bebear JP. Preference for the closed technique in the management of cholesteatoma of the middle ear in children: A retrospective study of 215 consecutive patients treated over 10 years. Am J Otol 2000;21(4):474–81.

100. Sanna M, Zini C, Scandellari R, Jemmi G. Residual and recurrent cholesteatoma in closed tympanoplasty. Am J Otol 1984;5(4):277–82.

101. Soda-Merhy A, Betancourt-Suarez MA. Surgical treatment of labyrinthine fistula caused by cholesteatoma. Otolaryngol Head Neck Surg 2000;122(5):739–42.

102. Romanet P, Duvillard C, Delouane M, et al. [Labyrinthine fistulae and cholesteatoma]. Ann Otolaryngol Chir Cervicofac 2001;118(3):181–6.

103. Vartiainen E, Nuutinen J. Success and pitfalls in myringoplasty: Follow-up study of 404 cases. Am J Otol 1993;14(3):301–5.

104. Boone RT, Gardner EK, Dornhoffer JL. Success of cartilage grafting in revision tympanoplasty without mastoidectomy. Otol Neurotol 2004;25(5):678–81.

105. Kaylie DM, Gardner EK, Jackson CG. Revision chronic ear surgery. Otolaryngol Head Neck Surg 2006;134(3):443–50.

106. Djalilian HR. Revision tympanoplasty using scar tissue graft. Otol Neurotol 2006;27(2):131–5.

107. Veldman JE, Braunius WW. Revision surgery for chronic otitis media: A learning experience. Report on 389 cases with a long-term follow-up. Ann Otol Rhinol Laryngol 1998;107(6): 486–91.

108. Ghanem MA, Monroy A, Alizade FS, Nicolau Y, Eavey RD. Butterfly cartilage graft inlay tympanoplasty for large perforations. Laryngoscope 2006;116(10):1813–16.

109. Sheehy JL. Tympanoplasty: The outer surface grafting technique. In: Brackmann DE, Shelton C, Arriaga MA, editors. Otologic Surgery. Philadelphia, PA: W.B. Saunders Company; 2001. p. 96–105.

Ossicular Chain Reconstruction 29

Aristides Athanasiadis-Sismanis, MD, FACS / Dennis S. Poe, MD, FACS

Reconstruction of the ossicular chain aims to surgically optimize the middle ear transformer mechanism so that sound energy is conducted from the environment to the inner ear fluid with only minimal loss. An understanding of middle ear mechanics is key to the proper design of the reconstruction of choice (the underlying principles are presented in detail in Chapter 3).

HISTORICAL ASPECTS

Attempts to rebuild the middle ear transformer mechanism began shortly after the introduction of tympanoplasty and great advances have been made in the physiological functioning and biocompatibility of autografts and implants. An ideal prosthesis should be made of a durable, biocompatible, and easy to manipulate material.

Ossicular repositioning was described in 1957[1] and continues to be used today. The early plastic prostheses suffered from high extrusion rates and stapes footplate fistulas. Homograft ossicles were convenient, especially for complete tympanic membrane and ossicular chain reconstructions, but ultimately were largely abandoned due to potential transmission of viral or prion diseases. Wire prostheses, made of stainless steel, platinum, or tantalum, were better tolerated in the middle ear but had problems with displacement and extrusion over time.

As the biomaterials science advanced, improved alloplastic ossicular prostheses were developed. The longest clinical experience exists with Plastipore®, an alloplast made from a high-density polyethylene sponge (HDPS) that has nonreactive properties and sufficient porosity to encourage tissue ingrowth. In 1976, a Plastipore stapes to tympanic membrane partial ossicular replacement prosthesis (PORP), for use in cases with an intact stapes superstructure, and a stapes footplate to eardrum total ossicular replacement prosthesis (TORP), for use when the stapes superstructure is absent, were developed.[2] A thermal-fused HDPS was also developed, known as Polycel®.[3] Histologic examination of HDPS alloplasts that have been implanted from 1 to 4 years has shown extensive invasion of the porous spaces with fibrocytes, small round cells, and foreign body giant cells. Often, an envelope was seen around the implant, composed of fibrous tissue with a lining membrane of mucosal epithelium.[4] Clinical experience showed the necessity to cover these alloplasts with cartilage to minimize extrusion.[3] Extrusion rates ranging from 3 to 5% have been reported in large series with 5 to 10 years of follow-up.[5,6] Most of the extrusions occurred within the first year postoperatively; however, some extrusions occurred up to 5 years postoperatively.[6] Brackmann attributed 70% of the extrusions in his series to middle ear pathology, such as atelectasis, middle ear fibrosis, and otitis media.[5] Satisfactory long-term results have been reported with the Plastipore prosthesis by various authors, and many surgeons continue to use them.[7,8]

Ceramic implants were introduced in 1979 with the anticipation that this new material would have a lower incidence of extrusion than the porous polyethylene implants.[9] Ceramic prostheses have been manufactured from both bioinert and bioactive materials. Bioactivity refers to the property of a material to react with surrounding soft and bony tissue, which affects how it will couple to an ossicle. Ideal bioactivity would permit or stimulate actual osseointegration, ie, direct growth of bone up to the implant and possibly even incorporating bone into the implant.[9] Unfortunately, the extrusion rate with the ceramic Bioglass™ was higher than expected at 8% over 5 years and many cases of fragmentation of the prostheses were found.[10]

Hydroxylapatite is a bioactive implant material with a calcium and phosphorous chemical composition similar to living bone and has been used successfully, since the early 1970s, in reconstructive procedures.[11] Satisfactory long-term results have been reported with this type of ossicular prosthesis.[12,13] The first hydroxylapatite prostheses were produced in a dense form, but subsequent lighter, porous hydroxylapatite became available, enhancing intraoperative stability and the likelihood of osseointegration. Histological evidence and surgical experience have shown that the biocompatibility of hydroxylapatite in the middle ear is excellent, with only moderate to minimal, and sometimes no, reactive fibrosis. Hydroxylapatite appears to be extremely well tolerated with osseointegration occurring in many cases and it can even come into direct contact with the tympanic membrane indefinitely without extrusion. Because of the tolerance of the tympanic membrane to hydroxylapatite, it was initially suggested that cartilage interposition between the implant and the tympanic membrane was unnecessary, but experience has shown that extrusion does occur with thin or retracted tympanic membranes. In one report, extrusion of hydroxylapatite prostheses occurred in 16% of patients when placed in direct contact with the tympanic membrane.[14] In cases with thin tympanic membranes, insertion of a tissue graft, such as fascia or perichondrium, between the prosthesis platform and the tympanic membrane may decrease the likelihood of extrusion. Full- or partial-thickness cartilage grafts are even more likely to prevent extrusion. Similarly, placing the head of the prosthesis medial to the manubrium, if present, can decrease extrusion.

Surgeons have noted that hydroxylapatite may develop undesirable fractures when drilled to customize fit. This brittleness results from the manufacturing process, which involves high-pressure compression of a powder form of the material into the solid final product. Despite the brittleness of hydroxylapatite prostheses, they can be trimmed to size with a diamond burr using copious irrigation and a very light touch.

In a recent study, hydroxylapatite and Plastipore PORPs and TORPs were the ossicular prostheses preferred by 48 and 16%, respectively, of otologists in the United States.[11] Both materials have withstood the test of time and are suitable for ossicular reconstruction. Hybrid prostheses combining these two materials have successfully taken advantage of the tolerance of the tympanic membrane with direct contact with hydroxylapatite and Plastipore's flexibility and ease of trimming to appropriate length. These hybrid prostheses, composed of hydroxylapatite heads, are also available with shafts made of Teflon, fluoroplastic, platinum, or stainless steel.[15–18]

Recently, prostheses made of glass ionomer cement, titanium, and gold have been reported to have promising results.[19–23] Titanium middle ear prostheses were introduced by Stupp in 1993,[24] after a long and successful experience with this material in dental, orthopedic, craniofacial, and neurosurgical procedures. Titanium is strong, lightweight, and has excellent biocompatibility, with a remarkable tendency to osseointegrate. The metal allows the use of laser-cutting tools to create prostheses with extremely precise design specifications. Titanium tends to extrude when placed in direct contact with the tympanic membrane and partial- or full-thickness cartilage graft interposition is recommended. At present, hydroxylapatite and titanium are the most commonly used prostheses and both have yielded good results.[11,23]

Most recently, bone cements, which are principally hydroxylapatite or other compounds of calcium and phosphate similar to bone matrix, have been used in the reconstruction of limited erosion of the distal incus and other small ossicular defects, as well as to help fixing of prostheses, such as a loose stapes prosthesis wire.[25–27]

PREOPERATIVE AND INTRAOPERATIVE CONSIDERATIONS

In many cases, the extent of ossicular problems can be estimated preoperatively by micro-otoscopy, computed tomography (CT) imaging, and audiometry, but the surgeon must be prepared to make intraoperative decisions upon appreciation of the full extent of reconstructive needs. Ossicular problems usually cause conductive hearing losses in the 25 to 40 dB SPL range, but maximal or minimal losses can be particularly revealing. A maximal conductive loss (60–65 dB) with an intact tympanic membrane implies complete separation of the ossicular chain. A tympanic membrane perforation with a 50 to 60dB conductive hearing loss, in the absence of chronic otitis media, suggests ossicular fixation. A minor subluxation or laxity in the ossicular chain can result in a downsloping, high-frequency conductive hearing loss that can be mistaken for a sensorineural loss if bone conduction testing is omitted.

Ossicular reconstruction is performed in otherwise healthy ears or in conjunction with a tympanoplasty and mastoidectomy for chronic ear disease. In the case of active chronic otitis media, it is important to treat the middle ear and mastoid disease as first priority and consider ossicular reconstruction secondarily, utilizing whatever remains after extirpation. The repair can be done primarily, at the time of initial surgery, or deferred to a later time in a second-stage operation.

Patient Selection and Staging

Long-term success with ossicular reconstruction depends on the control of chronic otitis media and the assurance of middle ear ventilation. In one report, five factors—surgery (open versus closed mastoidectomy), prosthesis type, presence of infection, tissue health, and Eustachian tube function—were found to be predictive of ossicular reconstruction success. These five factors allow for an accurate preoperative individual assessment when counseling patients regarding the likelihood of success or failure of a proposed ossicular reconstruction.[28] Of note, hearing results comparing Plastipore ($n=247$) versus hydroxylapatite ($n=265$) prostheses revealed no statistically significant differences between these popular implants.[28] Extrusion and displacement of ossicular prostheses have been consistently reported in association with Eustachian tube dysfunction, chronic infection, mucosal adhesions, and atelectasis.[5,29,30] For ears with known ventilation problems, long-term tympanostomy tube insertion or planned acceptance of atelectasis, with the reconstructed tympanic membrane placed directly onto the stapes superstructure or footplate, are reasonable options.

At the close of surgery for chronic otitis media the surgeon must make an individualized judgment, carefully weighing the risks and benefits, whether to proceed with ossicular reconstruction or defer it to a later stage. Ossicular reconstruction is typically deferred to improve the likelihood of success. At the author's institution, the incidence of prosthesis displacement has been found to be higher in cases undergoing synchronous total tympanic membrane replacement and ossicular reconstruction. For this reason, such cases are staged. Additionally, the presence of medical infirmities, advanced age, intraoperative complications, excessive intraoperative time, and other considerations may mitigate against adding the time and potential difficulties of ossicular reconstruction to the procedure. Hearing reconstruction can be deferred to a time when medical issues have been resolved, and hearing aids or assistive devices are always an option. In younger, healthy patients, the surgeon may be more inclined to add the ossicular repair to the primary operation than plan a staged reconstruction.

OSSICULAR STATUS AND RECONSTRUCTION OPTIONS

The Austin classification of ossicular problems is very practical and is based upon the presence or absence of the malleus handle (M+, M–) and stapes superstructure (S+, S–). According to this classification there are four types of ossicular defects: type A (M+, S+), type B (M+, S–), type C (M–, S+), and type D (M–, S–).[31] The most commonly encountered ossicular defect is erosion of the long process of the incus with intact malleus handle and stapes superstructure (type A), followed by types B, C, and D.

Due to the wide variability of techniques and implants available today, reconstructions are generally reported without reference to a particular classification and instead include a detailed description of the type of prosthesis used, how it is interposed between the ossicular defect, and the use of other interposed or stabilizing grafting materials. The original classification presented by Wullstein (see Figure 28–1 of chapter 28 in this book) remains in popular clinical use and serves to briefly communicate reconstruction type. Figure 28–1A depicts a type I reconstruction in which myringoplasty (surgery confined to the drumhead) or tympanoplasty (myringoplasty plus middle ear surgery) has been done and there is no need for ossicular chain repair. Figure 28–1B shows a type II reconstruction comprising erosion of the manubrium with a repair that consists of draping the tympanic membrane onto the remaining malleus and the long process of the incus; it is not commonly used today. Figure 28–1C depicts the direct placement of the tympanic membrane graft onto the stapes capitulum. Modern variations of this type III reconstruction include: (1) a *minor columella*, in which bone or a PORP is interposed between the capitulum and the undersurface of the tympanic membrane and (2) a *major columella*, in which bone or a TORP extends from the stapes footplate to the undersurface of the tympanic membrane. In the majority of cases today, a cartilage graft is placed between the prosthesis and the reconstructed tympanic membrane. A type IV reconstruction (Figure 28–1D) involves placing the tympanic membrane graft directly onto the stapes footplate, or around it, leaving the footplate exposed. The round window niche is covered to create a protective air-containing space. Type V reconstructions, as performed in the past, involve covering the middle ear to protect the round window and to allow sound transmission to pass to a fenestrated lateral semicircular canal that is either covered with cholesteatoma matrix left in place or that is covered with a tissue graft. The term as used in current parlance describes placement of a tympanic membrane graft over an open oval window (Figure 28–1E).

MIDDLE EAR MECHANICS APPLIED TO OSSICULAR RECONSTRUCTION

Ossicular reconstruction is considered an art in which the best results formerly occurred in the most experienced of hands. Although experience remains an important factor, our increased understanding of the science of reconstruction has greatly shortened the learning curve. A definitive discussion of the factors influencing ossicular reconstruction is presented in Chapter 3. Merchant and Rosowski's presentation of the basic science of the mechanics of ossicular reconstruction translate into five important principles that should guide surgeons intraoperatively. They can be summarized in a mnemonic: TRACS.

- Tension (T): The tension under which an implant is placed is an important determinant of hearing outcomes, and the surgeon has a significant ability to adjust this factor in most cases. Excessive laxity in the ossicular chain results in sound energy loss. The surgeon must learn to feel the appropriate tightness of fit for a prosthesis or autograft that optimizes hearing. The reconstruction should remain inherently stable once in position, without a tendency to topple. The surgeon can test stability by slightly displacing the prosthesis with gentle pressure—it should spontaneously return to position once the pressure is released. This degree of tension is usually achieved by adjusting the length of the prosthesis to be slightly greater than the visible gap, resulting in an ossicular chain with a stiffness the same as, or slightly greater than, the normal ossicular chain. Excessive tension dampens sound energy and worsens hearing results;[16] excessively loose-fitting prostheses are at risk for displacement and excessive mobility can cause scarring or adjacent ossicular erosion may further alter fit.
- Round (R): Round window protection is an important consideration when tympanic membrane grafting is close to the round window, eg, directly onto the stapes footplate, or if the oval window is left exposed. Sound waves reaching both the round and oval windows simultaneously with similar amplitudes result in hearing loss. Isolation of the round window maximizes sound transmission.
- Angle (A): A prosthesis (or autograft) should contact the tympanic membrane or malleus at an angle of 45 to 90 degrees. A more acute angle results in hearing loss. Incus interposition should not be performed if the stapes capitulum is at nearly the same height (from the promontory) as the malleus. Better results can be achieved with the use of a PORP. PORPs and TORPs should be positioned as vertically as possible while also contacting the tympanic membrane as close to its center as possible.
- Centered (C): A prosthesis should be positioned so that it contacts the tympanic membrane as close to the center as possible in order to take advantage of the maximal vibratory excursions at this location. Placement too close to the annular ring dampens sound transmission. Preservation of the manubrium takes advantage of its central tympanic membrane location and incorporating it into the ossicular reconstruction can significantly improve hearing results.[16,32,33] If the malleus is excessively medialized, hearing results can be optimized by placing the reconstruction into direct contact with the tympanic membrane. Alternatively, the malleus can be lateralized by dividing the tensor tympani tendon or by partially dividing and stretching it. Placing an ossicular graft or prosthesis against such a lateralized malleus has the advantage of adding to the stability and tension of the reconstruction. Flexible prostheses have an advantage that the head can be angled to optimize contact with the malleus, tympanic membrane, or both.

- Space (S): The airspace around the ossicular chain should be more than 0.3 mL. The normal middle ear space, excluding the mastoid, is approximately 1 mL. Efforts should be made to reconstruct this air-containing space when possible to optimize hearing and to prevent the development of adhesions. If Eustachian tube function is likely to remain inadequate, tympanostomy tube placement, even at the primary operation, is a consideration.

OSSICULAR RECONSTRUCTION TECHNIQUES AND RESULTS

For type A defects (M+, S+) three ossicular reconstruction techniques are available.

If the lenticular process of the incus is eroded, and if the manubrium is in close proximity to the stapes superstructure (a favorable relationship), a fitted (or sculpted) incus prosthesis is an excellent choice (Video 29–1). This technique has been described by Pennington[34] and Austin[31] and is performed as follows: After the incus is removed, it is held gently but firmly with the Sheehy ossicular holder and is shaped with an otologic drill using a light drilling technique. Any remaining long process is removed to minimize mass and to reduce the possibility of undesired fixation to the fallopian canal or promontory. A groove is made in its articulation with the malleus surface with a 1.5-mm diamond burr roughly following the natural groove of the joint and an acetabulum is created in its short process (Figure 29–1). The short process is trimmed to the desired length, which can be roughly measured by holding a 2-mm-diameter round knife adjacent to the gap between the capitulum and manubrium. In order to create appropriate tension, the sculpted incus must slightly exceed the size of the gap and push the malleus anterolaterally when in place (usually about 2.4 mm). The surface of the trimmed short process is flattened and drilled with a 0.5- or 0.7-mm diamond burr to create an acetabulum for the capitulum that is hollowed out as much as possible to create an oval-shaped defect without gouging the walls, which would allow the prosthesis to slip off of the capitulum. This oval shape allows the interposed incus to seek the optimal angle for its final position. To place the prosthesis, the sculpted incus is set to engage the manubrium in its groove and both ossicles are elevated laterally with a curved pick in the acetabulum. (Figure 29–2) The incus is rotated onto the capitulum and the pressure slowly released from the malleus, making sure that the incus does not exert excessive pressure on the stapes. Once in position, the incus is slipped superiorly along the malleus until it contacts tensor tympani tendon, where it will be maximally stable and hearing optimized. (Figures 29–3 and 29–4) When properly fitted, there should be just enough tension to hold the prosthesis firmly in place between the manubrium and the capitulum, with no need to pack the middle ear with Gelfoam®. The sculptured incus must be neither too long nor too short in order to prevent fixation or displacement, respectively. Results of this technique are excellent and air–bone gap closure has been reported to be within 20 dB in 68% of patients.[29] Once healed, the sculpted incus is usually visible on otomicroscopy as a shadow, or bulge, just posterior to the malleus Figure 29–5.

If the lenticular process of the incus is eroded, and if the manubrium is positioned far anterior to the stapes superstructure (an unfavorable relationship), sculpted incus placement is not recommended because of its inherent instability. The use

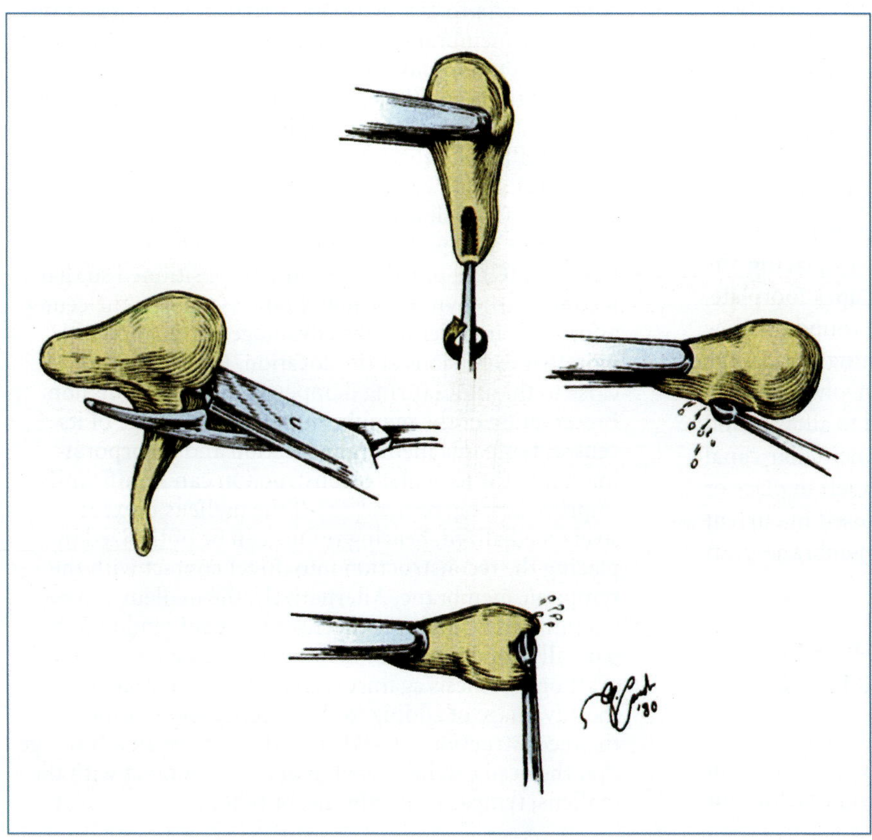

FIGURE 29–1 • Fashioning a sculpted incus interposition graft.

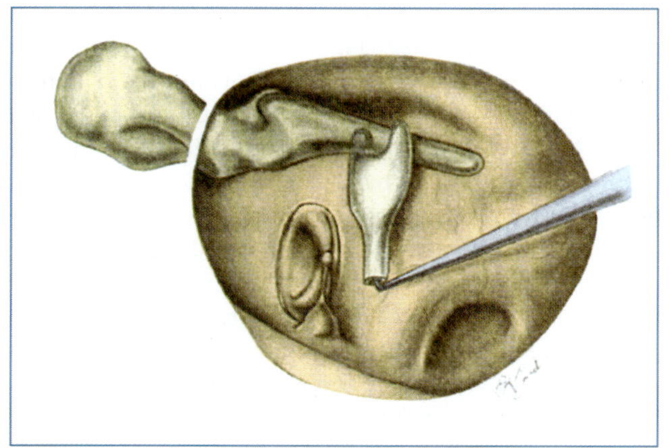

FIGURE 29–2 • Fitted incus prosthesis being positioned with a right angle hook.

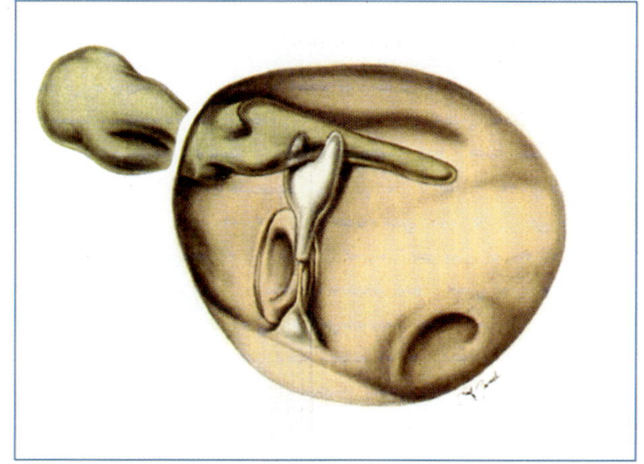

FIGURE 29–3 • Fitted incus prosthesis in position between the malleus and the capitulum of the stapes.

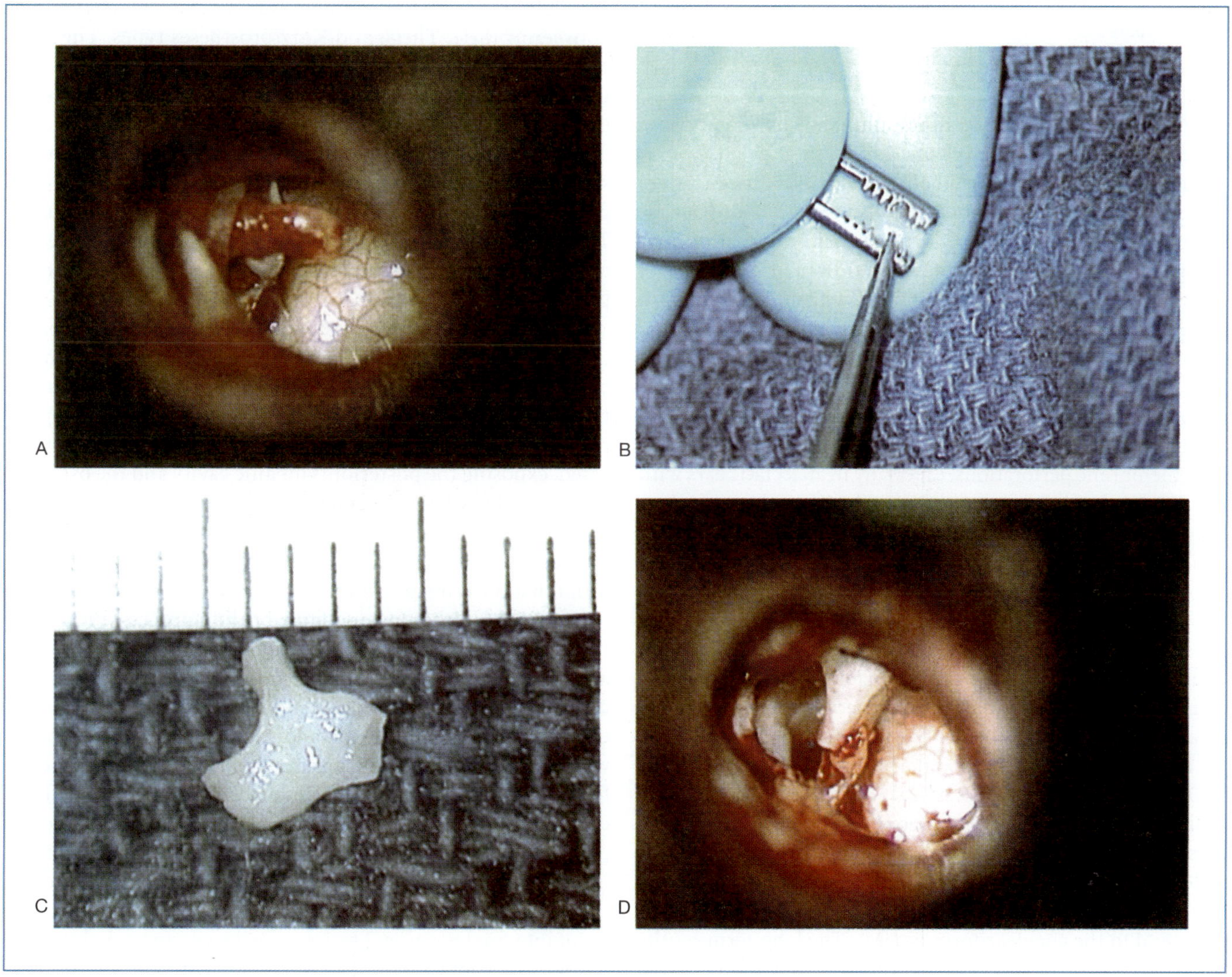

FIGURE 29–4 • *A*, Intraoperative microscopic view of a right ear with incudostapedial dislocation. *B*, The incus has been extracted and is being sculpted for use as an interposition graft. An oval acetabulum is fashioned in the short process. *C*, The completed sculpted incus. *D*, The incus interposition graft in position.

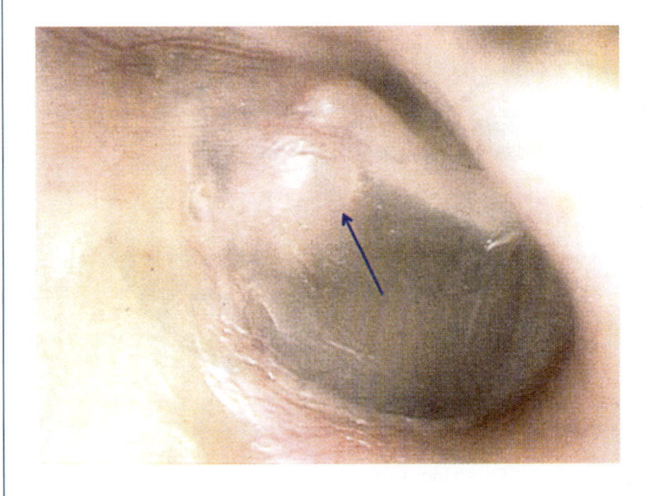

FIGURE 29–5 • Postoperative, microscopic view of same ear as Figure 29–4. The interposition graft is indicated by the arrow and is properly located superiorly along the manubrium. The air–bone gap postoperatively was 5 dB.

of a PORP has been reported to result in air–bone gap closure within 20 dB in 49% of such cases.[29]

In selected cases of erosion of the lenticular process of the incus, reconstruction can be accomplished with hydroxylapatite bone cement; early reports claimed achieving a 10-dB air–bone gap in about 50%, and under a 20-dB gap in 70 to 80%, of cases.[26,27] These cements are easy to work with and become firm within 5 mins, making them reasonable alternatives for small defect repair. It is important to strip away all the mucosa from the bony surfaces and allow them to dry before applying the cement or the material can become loose over time.[27]

It has been the senior author's experience in repairing tympanic membrane perforations, especially in atelectatic ears with type A ossicular defects, that the space between the capitulum of the stapes and the manubrium is limited and performing cartilage "shield" grafting results in a de facto type III tympanoplasty, often obviating the use of any prosthesis whatsoever. In a series of 52 such cases, a postoperative air–bone gap of less than 25 dB was achieved in 79%.[35] Hearing results of cartilage "shield" type III tympanoplasty compare favorably with other types of ossicular reconstruction and are depicted in Table 29–1.

For type B (M+, S–) as well as type D (M–, S–) defects, a TORP can be used (Video 29–2). For cases with a medially displaced manubrium, encountered often in chronic otitis cases due to unopposed medial traction of the tensor tympani tendon, lateralization of the manubrium can be accomplished by sectioning or partially sectioning and stretching the tendon just lateral to the cochleariform process. The long-term results with TORPs are generally not as satisfactory as with PORPs, as the medial strut can be displaced from the center of the stapes footplate, as there is nothing to secure it into position. A cartilage shoe can be helpful in this situation. To make the "shoe," a cartilage graft is cut to a 4 × 2 mm oval shape, the size of the oval window niche; a hole is made in its center to accommodate the base of the TORP, enhancing intraoperative and, hopefully postoperative, stability[39,40] (Figure 29–6). Long-term results with the "shoe" are not yet available.

For type C defects (M–, S+), a PORP can be used (Video 29–3). Analysis of long-term results in 233 patients undergoing ossicular reconstruction with the Goldenberg hydroxylapatite prosthesis revealed an air–bone gap of 21.1 dB in 56.8% of patients, with a 5.29% extrusion rate. Overall, 50.6% of patients met the criteria for successful hearing, which included no extrusion and a dry ear. Better hearing before surgery, presence of the manubrium, tympanoplasty alone, and canal-wall-up (CWU) tympanomastoidectomy were factors associated with successful hearing results.[11] A recent study comparing hydroxylapatite versus titanium ossiculoplasty determined that both prostheses gave good functional results and stability with low exclusion rates, with no statistically significant differences detected between the two,[41] as has been the senior author's experience. In a report of 140 ossiculoplasties with titanium prostheses, there was no statistical difference between Spiggle, Theis, and Kurz prostheses types. The presence or absence of the manubrium and the mucosal status of the middle ear had a statistically significant predictive value in the prognosis of ossiculoplasty.[42] Cartilage grafts placed medial to the tympanic membrane are effective in reducing the extrusion rates of titanium and hydroxylapatite TORP and PORP prostheses with one study reporting approximately a 4% rate.[43] The use of homograft ossicular grafts has been abandoned by many in this country due to the risk of transmission of viral, prion, and other diseases.[41]

When ossicular reconstruction is performed at the close of tympanoplasty, it should be coordinated with tympanic membrane reconstruction. Usually, the anterior mesotympanum is first packed with Gelfoam® and the tympanic membrane graft positioned. The posterior aspect of the graft can be gently elevated, exposing the posterior tympanic cavity and the ossicular remnants. Prostheses intended to engage the manubrium can be placed directly into contact with it or onto the graft covering its medial surface. As tension is estimated, it should be kept in mind that the tympanic membrane graft will thin and contract considerably in the postoperative healing process. Prostheses intended to contact the tympanic membrane will usually require a thinned, conchal or tragal cartilage graft interposition. The cartilage graft typically covers most of the posterior–superior quadrant of the middle ear and can extend onto the annulus without causing a significant hearing loss. Sizers are available for some of the titanium prostheses. These plastic or metal sizers are advantageous in that they can be inserted to judge the precise length necessary to produce the desired tension. Sizing is done with the cartilage graft in final position, medial to the tympanic membrane. The sizer is then removed and the implant is put into final position. Flexible prostheses can be slightly bent to optimize contact with the tympanic membrane and/or malleus. The prosthesis should remain in stable position as the cartilage graft is lowered onto its lateral surface and it should not at all be dependent on Gelfoam® packing for support. The tympanic membrane graft is draped into final position onto the posterior annulus and canal wall.

TABLE 29–1 Ossicular reconstruction results

AUTHOR	NUMBER OF PATIENTS	TECHNIQUE	POST-OPERATIVE PTA-ABG
Kyrodimos et al.[35]	52	Type III Cartilage "shield" Tympanoplasty	<20 dB in 54% <25 dB in 79%
Schember S, et al.[36]	111	PORP or TORP	PORP <20dB in 77% TORP <20dB in 52%
Gardner EK, et al.[37]	102	Titanium PORP or TORP	PORP <20 dB in 70% TORP <30 dB in 44%
Dalchow C, et al.[38]	1300	Titanium PORP or TORP	PORP and TORP <20 dB in 76%

PORP, partial ossicular reconstruction prosthesis; TORP, total ossicular reconstruction prosthesis.

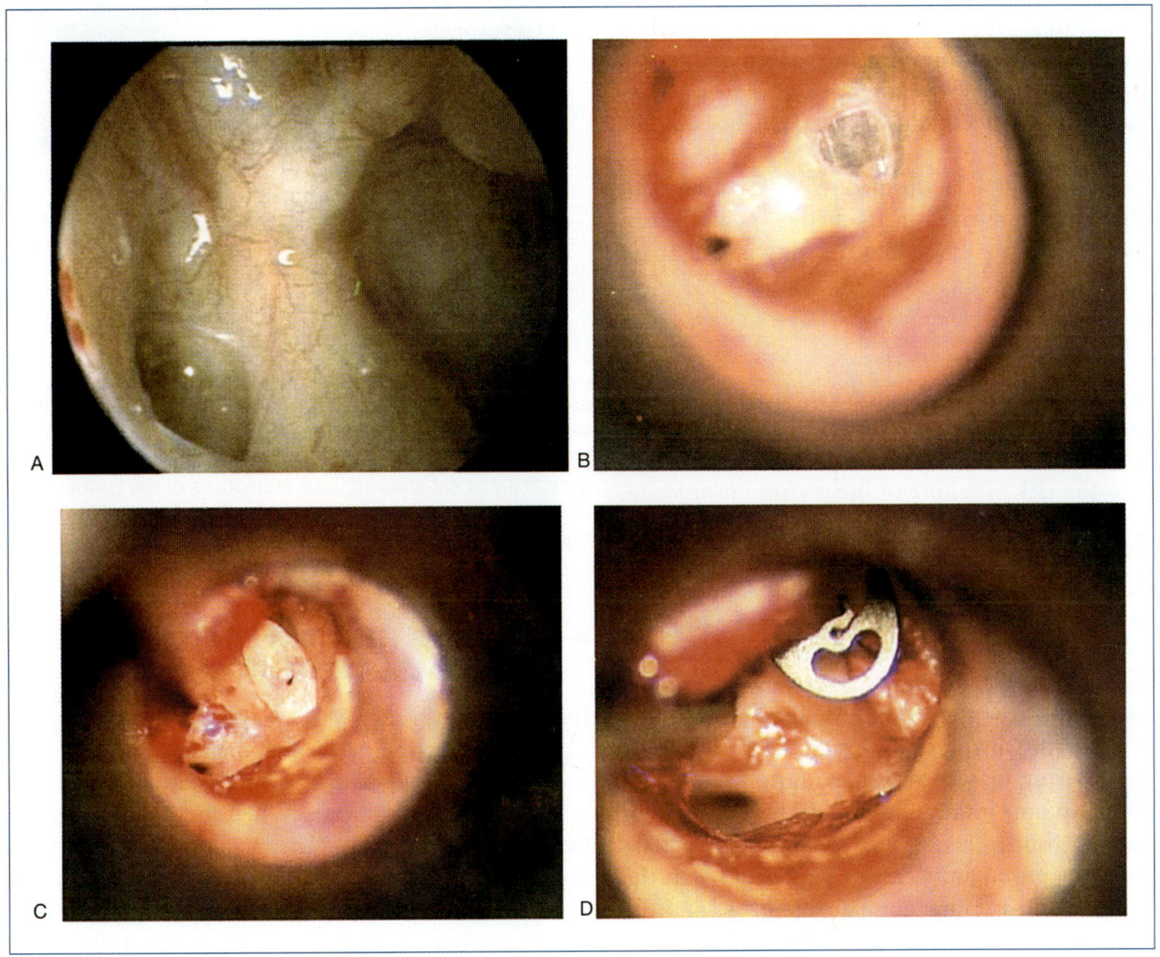

FIGURE 29–6 • *A*, A 70-degree, 2.3-mm-diameter endoscopic view of a left ear during a second-stage reconstruction following CWU tympanomastoidectomy for cholesteatoma. The oval window is seen inferiorly (on the left of the figure) and the epitympanum is seen superiorly (on the right). There is no residual disease. The stapes superstructure is absent. *B*, Microscopic view of the oval window. *C*, A cartilage shoe has been placed over the stapes footplate. Note the 0.6-mm-diameter central hole in the center of the cartilage graft that is intended to hold the TORP's medial foot. *D*, The TORP is in position, with its medial foot engaged in the cartilage shoe.

Malleus/Incus Fixation

Fixation of the incus/malleus complex is uncommon, difficult to diagnose preoperatively, and often mistaken for otosclerosis. Prior to surgery, pneumatic micro-otoscopy with a Siegel lens, observing for movement or fixation of the malleus umbo, is helpful in diagnosing this problem.[45] Tympanosclerosis, chronic infection, trauma, Paget's disease, ligament ossification, otosclerosis, and congenital and idiopathic disorders have been reported as etiologic.[45–47]

In tympanoplasty with or without mastoidectomy, an effective procedure to correct this problem is to remove the incus and use it as a sculptured prosthesis fitted between the manubrium and the stapes.[46] The manubrium is mobilized by amputating the malleus head at the level of the neck with a House malleus nipper. This approach is especially useful when there is a limited epitympanum due to low lying dura or meningoencephalocele repair.

Another approach to this ossicular problem is to free the head of malleus/incus complex through an atticotomy. A 2-mm free space around the malleus/incus complex is created with a microdrill and a thin sheet of silastic, or absorbable esterified hyaluronate (Epifilm®, Seprafilm®), is interposed and left in place to prevent refixation.[45,48] To prevent noise-induced hearing loss, contact of the drill with the ossicular chain should be avoided.

When mastoidectomy is performed in conjunction with tympanoplasty, repair of a fixed incus/malleus complex can be accomplished by gaining access into the epitympanic space through the transmastoid route.

Revision Surgery

Revision operations for ossicular reconstruction generally have a lower long-term success rate than primary repairs.[49–51] The initial failure is often due to problems with chronic ear disease that may add to the risk of failure of the revision procedure. Efforts to control the causes and sequelae of poor middle ear ventilation and chronic otitis media are important for success. In the absence of chronic ear disease, the failure is more likely to be due to a simple mechanical problem, such as a loose or displaced prosthesis and the prognosis may be more favorable. A preoperative CT scan is very helpful in ascertaining whether there is active middle ear disease and visualizing the status of the ossicular chain. During surgery, adhesions should be lysed gently and sharply, or with a laser, to minimize mucosal injury that could promote more adhesions. If there are a lot of adhesions, placing absorbable esterified hyaluronate or silastic sheeting over the promontory can be very helpful. In the event of a failed TORP, the stapes footplate should be carefully inspected for any fistula to the vestibule. If there is a fistula, it should be repaired with a tissue graft. There is a risk to placing a TORP onto a soft tissue graft overlying an oval window fistula during primary surgery as the prosthesis may be forced into the vestibule should the tympanic membrane retract over time as shown in Figure 29–7. Staging the reconstruction or placing the tympanic membrane graft directly onto the tissue graft and covering the oval window are some reasonable options.

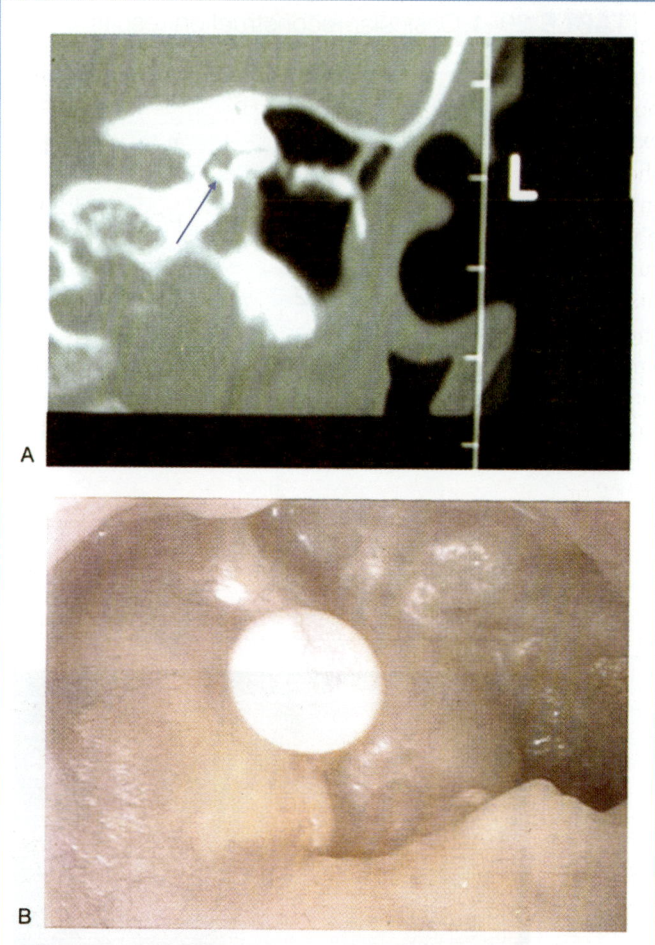

FIGURE 29–7 • *A*, High-resolution CT scan, coronal view, of a left ear showing a radiopaque, hydroxylapatite TORP protruding nearly to the medial wall of the vestibule. A CWU tympanomastoidectomy had been performed previously for cholesteatoma. *B*, Micro-otoscopic view of same ear showing total atelectasis of the tympanic membrane onto the floor of the middle ear and epitympanum. The TORP head rests flush with the promontory and fallopian canal.

RECONSTRUCTION IN CANAL-WALL-DOWN MASTOIDECTOMY

In canal-wall-down (CWD) mastoidectomy, the type of ossicular reconstruction performed depends upon the presence of the stapes superstructure and its relationship to the level of the horizontal facial nerve. When the stapes superstructure is located below the level of the facial nerve, a PORP or a sculptured ossicle, such as the malleus head, can be considered. In cases with an absent stapes superstructure, a TORP is a good option (Video 29–4). Postoperative atelectasis and adhesion formation are more common after CWD mastoidectomy, so ossicular reconstruction is best staged. When an adequate meatoplasty has been performed, a transmeatal approach can be used for ossicular reconstruction. A CWD meatoplasty ideally admits a 10- or 12-mm-diameter speculum that is stabilized with a holder. If the meatus is too small for adequate exposure, a postauricular approach can be used and consideration should be given for enlarging the meatus. The transmeatal approach begins with an incision parallel to the course of the facial nerve that creates an anteriorly based, tympanomastoid flap, beginning about 3 to 5 mm superior to the fallopian canal, passing posterior–superior to the horizontal semicircular canal, and extending inferiorly 3 to 5 mm posterior to the facial ridge. A shorter flap risks encroaching on the course of the facial nerve; in addition, the flap may contract to such an extent that it cannot cover the middle ear, requiring an additional graft for closure. The flap is raised by pushing tissue anteriorly and carefully inspecting for a dehiscent facial nerve, sharply lysing adhesions that hold it to bone. The usual technique of sliding a sharp knife along bone risks injury to the potentially dehiscent facial nerve. Once beyond the facial nerve, the flap is further elevated to expose the middle ear. Ossicular reconstruction proceeds depending on the type of defect present and usually requires a PORP or TORP (Figure 29–8).

OSSICULAR RECONSTRUCTION IN CANAL-WALL-UP VERSUS CANAL-WALL-DOWN MASTOIDECTOMIES

There are numerous advantages and disadvantages to these two types of mastoidectomy, but it remains inconclusive how they affect the ultimate results of ossicular chain reconstruction. The CWU operation preserves the normal anatomy of the external auditory canal and attempts to reconstruct the hearing mechanism within a nearly normal middle ear volume. In a CWD mastoidectomy, the facial ridge is lowered to a variable degree depending on the course of facial nerve, and the surgeon's intention and ability to lower the facial ridge. The volume of the middle ear around the ossicles, which has been shown by Merchant et al.[52] to be a critical factor in hearing reconstruction, can be quite variable near the critical minimal range for

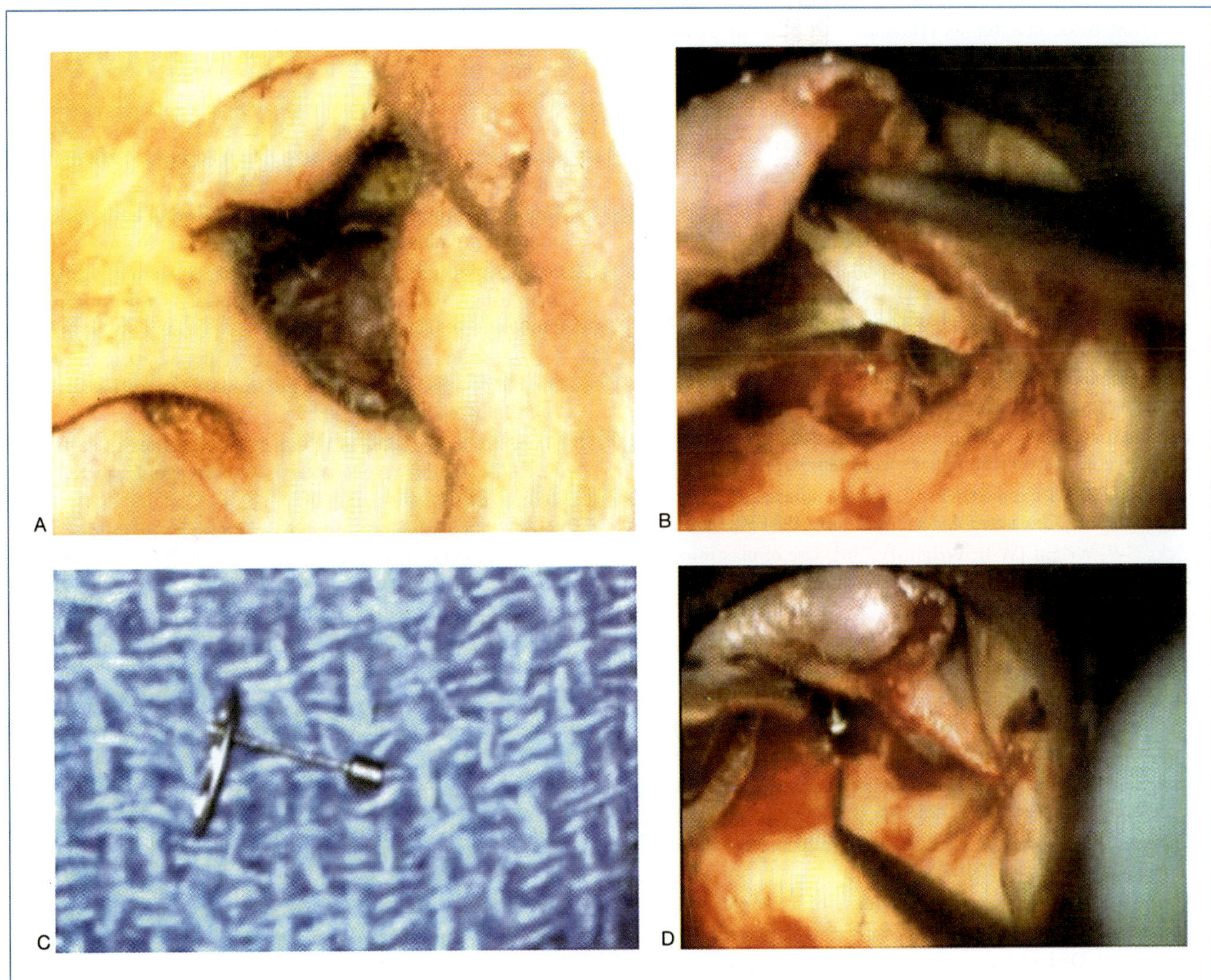

FIGURE 29–8 • *A*, Intraoperative view of a right ear in the surgical position undergoing second-stage ossicular reconstruction following CWD mastoidectomy. The meatoplasty is suitable for transmeatal approach. *B*, Microscopic view with elevated tympanic membrane flap. The round window is exposed and is being covered with a broad, partial-thickness tragal cartilage graft for sound protection. The stapes superstructure is absent. *C*, A Kurz® titanium TORP has been fashioned to appropriate length. *D*, The TORP is positioned over the footplate and the tympanic membrane flap, which includes a second, broad partial-thickness cartilage graft, is lowered onto the prosthesis.

optimal hearing transduction. Coverage of the round window is also important and variable with CWD procedures. The smaller middle ear volume and the selection of more severely diseased ears in CWD cases predisposes to the development of adhesions that further reduce middle ear volume. Therefore, there continue to be discrepancies among large series as to whether hearing results are similar between CWU and CWD[52] or whether CWD results are significantly worse. In CWU operations using a variety of prostheses that had long-term follow-up, the air–bone gap was found to be 20 db or better with a PORP in 64% of patients and with a TORP in 46% of patients.[53–57] Long-term results of CWD operations showed ≤20 dB air–bone gap in 43% of those with PORP and 23% of those with TORP reconstructions.[54,55,58]

It remains to be seen how the results of future long-term studies will be influenced by continuing advances in our understanding of middle ear mechanics. By paying careful attention to the principles of ossicular reconstruction and the lessons learned from basic science as translated to clinical practice, surgeons will be increasingly able to optimize hearing results for their patients.

References

1. Hall A, Rytzner C. Stapedectomy and autotransplantation of ossicles. Acta Otolaryngol (Stockh) 1957;47:318.
2. Shea JJ, Homsy CA. The use of proplast in otologic surgery. Laryngoscope 1974;84:1835.
3. Emmett JR, Shea JJ, Moretz WH. Long-term experience with biocompatible ossicular implants. Otolaryngol Head Neck Surg 1986;94:611.
4. Schuknecht HF, Shi SR. Surgical pathology of middle ear implants. Laryngoscope 1985;95:249–58.
5. Brackmann DE. Porous polyethylene prosthesis: Continuing experience. Ann Otol Rhinol Laryngol 1986;95:76.
6. Sheehy JL. TORPs and PORPs: Causes of failure—A report on 446 operations. Otolaryngol Head Neck Surg 1984;92:583.
7. Hicks GW, Wright JW Jr, Wright JW 3rd. Use of plastipore for ossicular chain reconstruction: An evaluation. Laryngoscope 1978;88:1024–33.
8. Brackmann DE, Sheehy JL. Tympanoplasty: TORPs and PORPs. Laryngoscope 1979;89:108–14.
9. Niparko JK, Kemink JL, Graham MD, Kartush JM. Bioactive glass ceramic in ossicular reconstruction: A preliminary report. Laryngoscope 1985;95:249–58.
10. Babighian G. Bioactive glass ceramic in ossicular reconstruction: A preliminary report. Am J Otol 1985;6:285–90.
11. Goldenberg R, Emmet JR. Current use of implants in middle ear surgery. Otol Neurotol 2001;22:145–52.
12. Wehrs RE. Hydroxylapatite implants for otologic surgery. Otolaryngol Clin North Am 1995;28:273–86.
13. Kartush JM. Ossicular chain reconstruction. Capitulum to malleus. Otolaryngol Clin North Am 1994;27:689–715.
14. Shinohara T, Gyo K, Saiki T, et al. Ossiculoplasty using hydroxyapatite prostheses: Long-term results. Clin Otolaryngol 2000; 25:287–92.
15. Goldenberg RA, Driver M. Long-term results with hydroxylapatite middle ear implants. Otolaryngol Head Neck Surg 2000; 122:635–42.
16. Goldenberg RA. Hydroxylapatite ossicular replacement prostheses: Results in 157 consecutive cases. Laryngoscope 1992; 102:1091–6.
17. Black B. A universal ossicular replacement prosthesis: Clinical trials of 152 cases. Otolaryngol Head Neck Surg 1991;104: 210–8.
18. Van Blitterswijk CA, Hesseling SC, Grote JJ, et al. The biocompatibility of hydroxyapatite ceramic: A study of retrieved human middle ear implants. J Biomed Mater Res 1990;24:433–53.
19. Maassen MM, Zenner HP. Tympanoplasty type II with ionomeric cement and titanium-gold-angle prostheses. Am J Otol 1998;19:693–9.
20. Milewski C, Giannakopoulos N, Muller J, et al. Tragus perichondrium-cartilage island transplant in middle ear surgery. Method and results after 5 years. HNO 1996;44:235–41.
21. Muller J, Geyer G, Helms J. Restoration of sound transmission in the middle ear by reconstruction of the ossicular chain in its physiologic position. Results of incus reconstruction with ionomer cement. Laryngorhinootologie 1994;73:160–3.
22. Schwager K. Titanium as an ossicular replacement material: Results after 336 days of implantation in the rabbit. Am J Otol 1998;19:569–73.
23. Wang X, Song J, Wang H. Results of tympanoplasty with titanium prostheses. Otolaryngol Head Neck Surg 1999;121: 606–9.
24. Stupp CH, Stupp HF, Grun D. Replacement of ear ossicles with titanium prostheses. Laryngorhinootologie 1996;75:335–7.
25. Ozer E, Bayazit YA, Kanlikama M, Mumbuc S, Ozen Z. Incudostapedial rebridging ossiculoplasty with bone cement. Otol Neurotol 2002;23:643–6.
26. Feghali JG, Barrs DM, Beatty CW, et al. Bone cement reconstruction of the ossicular chain: A preliminary report. Laryngoscope 1998;108:829–36.
27. Goebel JA, Jacob A. Use of Mimix hydroxyapatite bone cement for difficult ossicular reconstruction. Otolaryngol Head Neck Surg 2005;132(5):727–34.
28. Black B. Ossiculoplasty prognosis: The spite method of assessment. Am J Otol 1992;13:544–51.
29. Jackson CG, Glasscock ME 3rd, Schwaber MK, Nissen AJ, Christiansen SG, Smith PG. Ossicular chain reconstruction: The TORP and PORP in chronic ear disease. Laryngoscope 1983;93:981–8.
30. Brackmann DE, Sheehy JL, Luxford WM. TORPs and PORPs in tympanoplasty: A review of 1042 operations. Otolaryngol Head Neck Surg 1984;92:32–7.
31. Austin DF. Ossicular reconstruction. Arch Otolaryngol 1971;94(6):525–35.
32. Dornhoffer JL. Cartilage tympanoplasty. Otolaryngol Clin North Am 2006;39:1161–76.
33. Dornhoffer JL, Gardner E. Prognostic factors in ossiculoplasty: A statistical staging system. Otol Neurotol 2001;22:299–304.
34. Pennington CL. Incus interposition techniques. Ann Otol Rhinol Laryngol 1973;82(4):518–31.
35. Kyrodimos E, Sismanis A, Santos D. Type III cartilage "shield" tympanoplasty: An effective procedure for hearing improvement. Otolaryngol Head Neck Surg 2007;136(6):982–5.
36. Schmerber S, Troussier J, Dumas G, Lavieille JP, Nguyen DQ. Hearing results with the titanium ossicular replacement prostheses. Eur Arch Otorhinolaryngol 2006;263(4):347–54.

37. Gardner EK, Jackson CG, Kaylie DM. Results with titanium ossicular reconstruction prostheses. Laryngoscope 2004; 114(1):65–70.
38. Dalchow CV, Grun D, Stupp HF. Reconstruction of the ossicular chain with titanium implants. Otolaryngol Head Neck Surg 2001; 125(6):628–30.
39. Beutner D, Luers JC, Huttenbrink KB. Cartilage 'shoe': A new technique for stabilisation of titanium total ossicular replacement prosthesis at centre of stapes footplate. J Laryngol Otol 2008;122:682–6.
40. Babighian G. Cartilage shoe prosthesis for TORP stabilization. In: Manolidis S, editor. Vienna, 2006.
41. Truy E, Naiman AN, Pavillon C, Abedipour D, Lina-Granade G, Rabilloud M. Hydroxyapatite versus titanium ossiculoplasty. Otol Neurotol 2007.
42. De Vos C, Gersdorff M, Gerard JM. Prognostic factors in ossiculoplasty. Otol Neurotol 2007;28(1):61–7.
43. Doi T, Hosoda Y, Kaneko Tet al. Hearing results for ossicular reconstruction using a cartilage-connecting hydroxyapatite prosthesis with a spearhead. Otol Neurotol 2007;28:1041–4.
44. Glasscock ME, III, Jackson CG, Knox GW. Can acquired immunodeficiency syndrome and Creutzfeldt-Jakob disease be transmitted via otologic homografts? Arch Otolaryngol Head Neck Surg 1988;114(11):1252–5.
45. Seidman MD, Babu S. A new approach for malleus/incus fixation: No prosthesis necessary. Otol Neurotol 2004;25(5):669–73.
46. Moon CN, Jr., Hahn MJ. Primary malleus fixation: Diagnosis and treatment. Laryngoscope 1981;91(8):1298–1307.
47. Vincent R, Lopez A, Sperling NM. Malleus ankylosis: A clinical, audiometric, histologic, and surgical study of 123 cases. Am J Otol 1999;20(6):717–25.
48. Armstrong BW. Epitympanic malleus fixation: Correction without disrupting the ossicular chain. Laryngoscope 1976;86(8):1203–8.
49. Mangham CA, Lindeman RC. Ceravital versus plastipore in tympanoplasty: A randomized prospective trial. Ann Otol Rhinol Laryngol 1990;99:112–6.
50. Yung M. Long-term results of ossiculoplasty: Reasons for surgical failure. Otol Neurotol 2006;27:20–6.
51. Colletti V, Fiorino FG, Sittoni V. Minisculptured ossicle grafts versus implants: Long-term results. Am J Otol 1987;8: 553–9.
52. Merchant SN, McKenna MJ, Mehta RP, Ravicz ME, Rosowski JJ. Middle ear mechanics of Type III tympanoplasty (stapes columella): II. Clinical studies. Otol Neurotol 2003;24(2): 186–94.
53. Pfaltz CR, Pfaltz R, Schmid P. Reconstructive surgery in chronic otitis media. Statistical analysis of long-term results. ORL J Otorhinolaryngol Relat Spec 1975;37:257–70.
54. Deguine C. Longterm results in cholesteatoma surgery. Clin Otolaryngol Allied Sci 1978;3:301–10.
55. Charachon R. Temporal bone cholesteatoma. Am J Otol 1985;6:233–6.
56. Tos M. Modification of combined-approach tympanoplasty in attic cholesteatoma. Arch Otolaryngol 1982;108:772–8.
57. Sheehy JL, Crabtree JA. Tympanoplasty: Staging the operation. Laryngoscope 1973;83:1594–1621.
58. Ragheb SM, Gantz BJ, McCabe BF. Hearing results after cholesteatoma surgery: The Iowa experience. Laryngoscope 1987;97:1254–63.

Canal-Wall-Up Mastoidectomy 30

David S. Haynes, MD / Justin Wiffkopf, MD

INTRODUCTION

Descriptions of chronic and suppurative infections of the mastoid have been discovered dating back to ancient Greece. Prior to the advent of surgery and antibiotics, morbidity from acute mastoiditis was considerable. Mastoid surgery has evolved from simple trephination for acute infection, to the canal-wall-preserving mastoidectomy employed by most otologists today. Many variations on the basic mastoidectomy have been developed, and each has its proponents.

The complete (or simple) mastoid operation, as described by the authors, refers to a canal-wall-up (CWU) mastoidectomy, with complete removal of disease from the temporal bone lateral to the otic capsule. CWU mastoidectomy is usually accompanied by tympanoplasty, and when necessary, with ossicular chain reconstruction. These techniques, as well as canal-wall-down (CWD) mastoidectomy are not addressed in this chapter as each has its own dedicated chapter within this text.

HISTORY

Mastoid operations have been employed for over 300 years to control suppurative disease of the ear, but the first proposed mastoidectomy dates back more than four centuries. Ambrose Pare', a medieval barber-surgeon, was called upon to care for the young King Charles II of France. King Charles had become ill with a draining ear and subsequently developed high fevers and delirium. Pare' proposed to operate on the skull and drain the pus. King Charles' bride, Mary, Queen of Scots and France, agreed to the operation, but King Charles' mother, Catherine de' Medici, forbade it. King Charles succumbed to the infection and died, depriving Mary of her first husband and first throne.[1]

Jean Petit of Paris reported the first successful mastoid trephination operation in the late 1700s.[2] Trephination of the mastoid was abandoned soon after the King of Denmark died from complications of this surgery, used to treat his deafness and tinnitus.[3] The first postauricular incision was introduced in 1853 by Sir William Wilde of Dublin. Wilde described the postauricular incision for drainage of a postaural abscess, yet advised against operating on the mastoid unless facing a life-threatening infection.[4]

Interest in mastoid surgery revived in 1873, when Schwartze and Eysell reported the use of cortical mastoidectomy for management of acute mastoid infections.[5] Their success reintroduced to the world the idea of mastoid surgery as a safe option in the treatment of acute, often life-threatening, infections of the ear.

Zaufal expanded the concept of cortical mastoidectomy and, in 1890, described the radical mastoidectomy with the addition of removal of the tympanic membrane, ossicles, and posterior wall of the ear canal.[6] Bondy described opening the epitympanum and leaving the middle ear intact. In 1902, Sir Charles Ballance was the first to advocate the complete mastoid operation for control of advanced suppuration of the ear.[7] He described ligating the jugular vein and draining the lateral sinus, as well as grafting the mastoid cavity to facilitate better healing. The operation was accomplished using mallet and gouges. These tools remained the standard equipment and were used with remarkable finesse until Lempert popularized the use of a drill and loupe magnification in the 1920s.

The importance of the cortical mastoidectomy in the management of acute suppurative mastoid infections declined with the discovery and widespread use of sulfanilamide and penicillin. These antibiotics became increasingly employed in the early treatment of acute otitis media, often preventing the formation of localized collections of pus in the mastoid and the development of coalescent mastoiditis.

With the introduction of the Zeiss operating otologic microscope in 1953 and the description of the CWU mastoidectomy by Jansen shortly thereafter, the paradigm for mastoid surgery changed dramatically for acute and chronic mastoid infections.[8,9] With the advent of the CWU mastoidectomy, disease control as well as preservation of anatomy and function became a reality.

PATHOPHYSIOLOGY

Pathology

CWU mastoidectomy is used as a standard approach for cochlear implantation, excision of tumors, and surgery for vertigo. However, the primary role of CWU mastoidectomy is in the control of chronic otitis media, with and without cholesteatoma. Indeed, the initial mastoid procedures were for control of acute mastoiditis, which has dramatically decreased in incidence with the advent and wide usage of antibiotics. As the incidence of acute mastoiditis has markedly declined, relatively few mastoid procedures are required for this indication. In fact, in our practice, incision and drainage of subperiosteal abscess, and placement of tympanostomy tubes and antibiotics, without mastoidectomy, suffice in the treatment of most cases of acute mastoiditis. Thus in today's otology practice, CWU mastoidectomy is used to treat chronic ear disease.

Acute mastoiditis arises from untreated acute otitis media, or otitis media that fails to respond adequately to antibiotics. Coalescent mastoiditis is acute mastoiditis in which a localized collection of pus has accumulated in the mastoid, with evidence of erosion of the normal bony septae within the mastoid cavity. The natural history is that coalescent bony erosion typically evolves after several days or weeks of severe middle ear infection, although in young children, the course can be much more fulminant. Several signs and symptoms can suggest an underlying coalescent mastoiditis in the face a prolonged middle ear infection. Persistent purulent otorrhea for more than 3 weeks after an acute otitis media, pain behind the ear, or pain deep in the ear are indications that infection is failing to resolve and that coalescence may be developing. The tympanic membrane appears erythematous and thickened, often with loss of landmarks. An intermittent fever may be present and a leukocytosis may also be present. Many of these signs and symptoms may be seen in both acute otitis media and coalescent mastoiditis but their persistence 2 to 3 weeks after the onset of infection is more suggestive of coalescent mastoiditis. Definitive diagnosis of the bony septal erosion associated with coalescent mastoiditis is most often accomplished by computed tomographic (CT) scans. The developing mastoid abscess with pus under pressure may subsequently erode through the lateral mastoid cortex and present as a postauricular subperiosteal abscess. Coalescent mastoiditis requires urgent intervention. Should the infection continue to progress, it may further break through the confines of the mastoid cavity to produce complications of otitis media that are discussed in Chapters 26 and 27.

Subacute mastoiditis is a potentially dangerous consequence of partially treated acute otitis media. Following therapy with antibiotics, the clinical course may appear to improve or even completely resolve, yet there may be slow, silent progression of a coalescent abscess. Identifying subacute mastoiditis before the development of complications requires a high index of suspicion and a low threshold for obtaining a CT scan of the mastoid, should any worrisome signs or symptoms occur following initially successful treatment. In contrast to acute mastoiditis that develops over days to weeks, subacute mastoiditis evolves over several weeks.

Chronic suppurative otitis media (CSOM) is defined as chronic inflammation of the middle ear and mastoid. The disease manifests most commonly as hearing loss and intermittent otorrhea. CSOM can be seen with or without cholesteatoma. It is insidious in onset and usually painless, although an acute infection in CSOM with an intact tympanic membrane can present with pain. Vertigo is uncommon, and if present raises concern for a labyrinthine fistula or inflammation.

In the clinical setting, CSOM is most often associated with a tympanic membrane perforation, but can also be present behind an intact tympanic membrane. Meyerhoff et al. examined 123 temporal bone specimens with findings of CSOM and only 20% had tympanic membrane perforations.[10] Similarly, da Costa et al. reported that 19% of temporal bone specimens with CSOM had tympanic membrane perforation.[11]

Schuknecht initially described the pathology of CSOM and others have corroborated his findings.[12] The pathologic findings include osteitis, mucosal edema with submucosal gland formation, granulation tissue, tympanosclerosis, cholesterol granulomas, cholesteatoma, and tympanic membrane retraction and perforation.

Osteitis, or inflammation with osteoclastic resorption of bone, is often found involving the ossicles, otic capsule, and mastoid bone. Bone erosion from osteitis can result in ossicular discontinuity, dural exposure with or without brain herniation, meningitis, and labyrinthine fistula. In Meyerhoff's study, ossicular involvement was found in 81% of specimens, with the incus most commonly involved (81%), followed by the stapes (57%), and then the malleus (43%).[10] Ossicular changes were more prevalent in the study of 144 temporal bones with CSOM by da Costa et al.[11] Overall, 91% of temporal bone specimens had ossicular involvement. Interestingly, da Costa also classified the temporal bone specimens by intact or perforated tympanic membrane and 90% of the temporal bones with intact tympanic membranes had ossicular changes. Most of these specimens had gross abnormalities of the tympanic membrane, such as retractions, tympanosclerosis, and atelectasis.[11]

Ongoing osteitis, bone resorption, and deposition of new bone may lead to the development of a more narrowed and dense mastoid bone. Sclerotic mastoids make identification of underlying structures more difficult and therefore increase the risk of injury during surgery.

Granulation tissue within the middle ear cleft and mastoid is also a nearly omnipresent finding in CSOM, observed in 93 to 98% of temporal bone specimens.[10,11] The epitympanum and round window niche were the most frequent areas of involvement in temporal bone studies, but as is often the case, granulation tissue involvement of the entire middle ear cleft, to some degree, was conspicuous in all specimens. Granulation tissue blocking the aditus can prevent aeration of the mastoid and subsequent resolution of infection.

ETIOLOGY OF CHRONIC SUPPURATIVE OTITIS MEDIA

CSOM is believed to be caused by Eustachian tube dysfunction and the subsequent development of a persistent middle ear effusion. This effusion, serous or purulent, leads to mucosal edema and the formation of granulation tissue. Bacterial infection leads to purulent effusions that generate an inflammatory response in the middle ear and the chemical mediators produced lead to chronic changes of the mucosa and the tympanic membrane.[13] In the setting of chronic inflammation, the middle ear mucosa has also been found to develop submucosal glands that convert the mucosa to a secretory mucosa and thus contribute to the persistent effusion.[14]

Granulation tissue formation is initiated in the inflamed mucosa. Bacterial toxins and inflammatory mediators interact with the edematous mucosa and lead to ruptures of the basement membrane of the epithelia. Inflammatory cells in the underlying lamina propria now can enter the lumen of the middle ear and portions of the lamina propria also extrude through the basement membrane. This tissue is now capable of growth due to a variety of chemical factors, such as angiogenic growth factors and epithelial growth factors. The combined result leads to fibroblast recruitment, neovascularization, and polyp formation.[15]

The tympanic membrane is affected by the enzymes contained in the granulation tissue and the chronic effusion. The strength of the tympanic membrane is diminished as the enzymes break down its collagen skeleton. The weakening of the tympanic membrane and the negative pressure in the middle ear from Eustachian tube dysfunction leads to the development of retraction pockets in the tympanic membrane. Deepening of the retraction pockets ultimately leads to contact with the underlying mucosa or granulation tissue and fibrous bands often develop between the two, anchoring the membrane medially, or can result in perforation. Deep retraction pockets and perforations set the stage for the genesis of cholesteatoma, which appear to be a result of propagation of the inflammatory process that has been set into motion.[16]

DIAGNOSIS AND MEDICAL TREATMENT: ACUTE MASTOIDITIS

It is very important to obtain a thorough history of each patient's current otologic symptoms to properly evaluate the disease process. Acute mastoiditis begins as acute otitis media, often heralded by deep, often throbbing, ear pain, associated with pus in the middle ear. The tympanic membrane is erythematous and usually bulges laterally. There may be a perforation of the tympanic membrane, and if so, there is accompanying purulent otorrhea. Fever and leukocytosis are also common findings. These signs and symptoms are often present within the first several days of the infection. Acute mastoiditis results from progression of the acute middle ear infection in the mastoid and is associated with similar findings. Additionally, the mastoid may be tender to palpation and the postauricular skin may be erythematous. Coalescent mastoiditis is suspected when acute otitis media signs and symptoms persist, or recur, over days or weeks after the onset of infection, especially if there is associated disproportionate deep pain, mastoid tenderness, erythema, or swelling.

Treatment of acute mastoiditis begins with broad-spectrum antibiotics. Oral antibiotics may suffice if started early in the disease process. Ototopical antibiotics are added if there is a tympanic membrane perforation. If the infection progresses despite oral antibiotic treatment, or if there are signs of systemic sepsis, the patient should be admitted to the hospital for intravenous antibiotics; a tympanostomy tube should be inserted into the tympanic membrane if no perforation is present. A CT scan may be obtained to further delineate the extent of the disease. If the acute mastoiditis persists or progresses despite intravenous antibiotics and tympanostomy, a mastoidectomy is warranted in order to evacuate the localized collection of pus in the mastoid. Upon completion of the surgery, antibiotics are continued postoperatively for 1 to 2 weeks.

A subperiosteal abscess occurs when the pus within the mastoid erodes through the bony cortex, resulting in swelling and erythema in the postauricular region. Fluctuance may be present. The auricle often protrudes away from skull, in an inferior and anterior direction (Figure 30–1). A subperiosteal abscess is an indication for surgery to evacuate the accumulated pus and is accomplished by a cortical mastoidotomy or complete mastoidectomy, as necessary. Penrose drains are placed in the wound to allow drainage for several days postoperatively.

DIAGNOSIS AND MEDICAL TREATMENT: CHRONIC SUPPURATIVE OTITIS MEDIA

Most patients with CSOM present with a history of intermittent otorrhea, which is sometimes foul-smelling, and with some degree of hearing loss. Otalgia and headache are uncommon in CSOM and, if present, should raise the suspicion of intracranial involvement or other disease process, including malignancy. Likewise, the presence of vertigo should raise suspicion for labyrinthitis or fistula. It is also important to note in the patient's history any other significant past medical treatments or ear surgery.

A full head and neck examination should be completed on each patient, including an otomicroscopic evaluation when possible. Otorrhea often obscures the tympanic membrane. The condition of the external auditory canal (EAC) should be noted, including inspection for any edema or polyps. Additionally, careful evaluation should be made for any tympanic membrane perforations, retractions, atelectasis, or cholesteatoma. If a perforation is identified, the condition of the middle ear mucosa should be noted and further inspection should be made looking for evidence of scutal erosion, ossicular erosion, and granulation tissue as well.

A full audiometric evaluation is imperative when possible. Conductive hearing loss is common, but some patients may also exhibit sensorineural hearing loss (SNHL) that should be documented preoperatively. Several studies have found SNHLs ranging from 5 to 33 dB.[17] Conductive losses greater than 30 dB can suggest ossicular erosion. Occasionally, hearing can be preserved in the presence of ossicular erosion secondary to sound transmission directly to the oval window via the cholesteatoma.

Cholesteatoma combined with medically refractory CSOM is a nearly absolute indication for surgery, but often patients with CSOM do not have cholesteatoma and many cases may respond to appropriate medical therapy. When patients present with ongoing CSOM without cholesteatoma, medical treatment with ototopical antibiotics and aural toilet is employed in an effort to dry the ear and limit the inflammation. In patients who have failed multiple attempts at medical treatment or have symptoms suspicious of complications (vertigo, facial weakness, or headache), surgery should be entertained. Retraction pockets

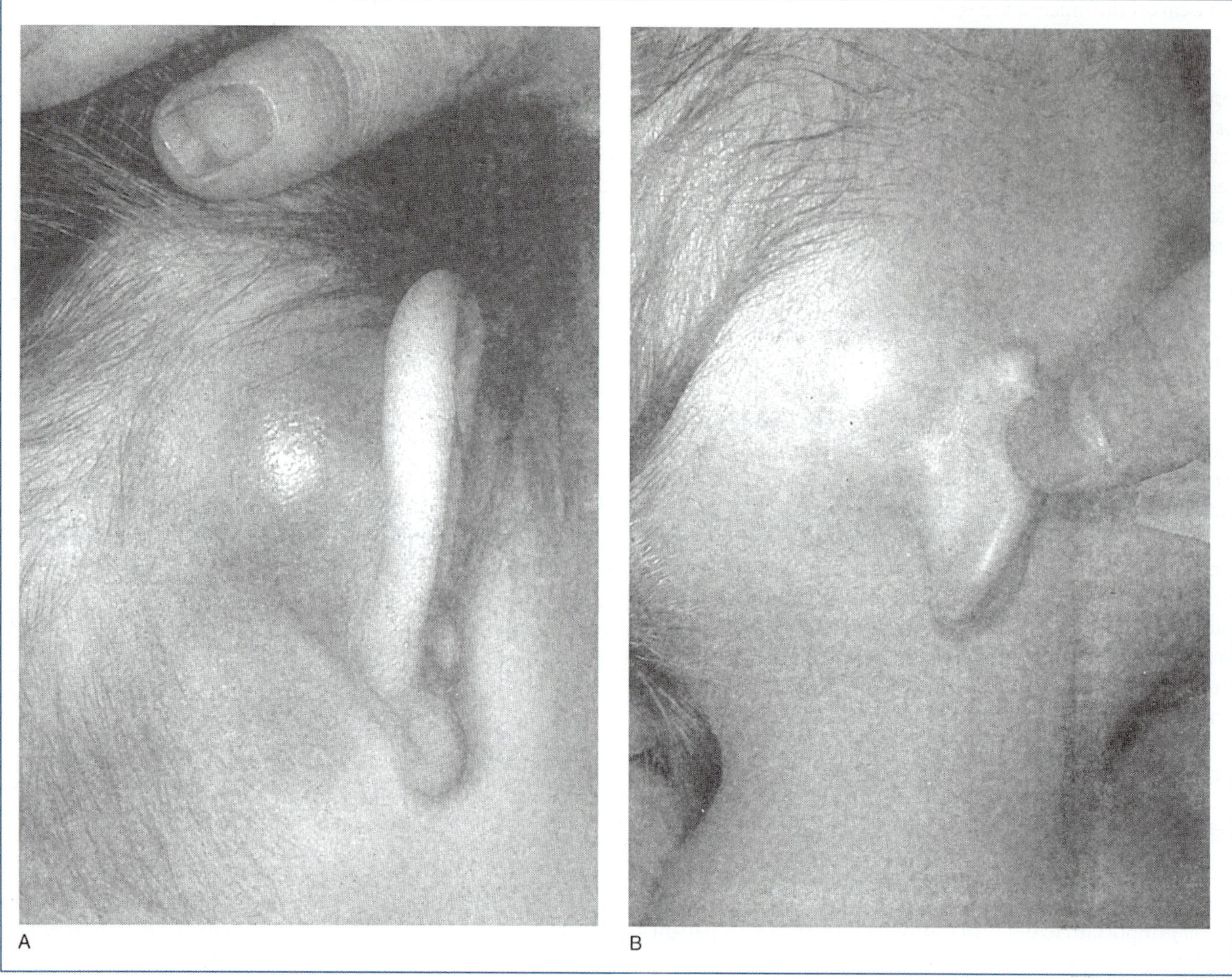

FIGURE 30–1 • *A* and *B*. Mastoid subperiosteal abscess. *Courtesy of Eiji Yanagisawa, MD, FACS.*

may be monitored if they do not collect debris, the patient has good hearing, and no progression is noted on serial examinations. Atelectatic ears without tympanic membrane perforation and otorrhea, but with significant conductive hearing loss, may be candidates for surgery.

The decision to operate should only be made after a thorough discussion with the patient about the nature of their disease, the risks of the surgery, the risk of further nonsurgical management, and expectations after the surgery. As CSOM is often an insidious, seemingly benign disease to the patient, many do not fully comprehend the potential consequences of leaving the disease untreated.

SURGICAL THEORY AND PRACTICE

Indications

The three priorities in surgery for CSOM are (1) eradication of disease, (2) prevention of disease recurrence, and (3) preservation or restoration of hearing. To this end, the choice of surgery is based on the extent of disease, the patient's health, the status of the contralateral ear, the surgeon's experience, and the patient's preference. Mastoidectomy in CSOM has three primary indications, eradication of disease and infection, approach for removal of cholesteatoma, and less important, establishing aeration. Some surgeons believe that previous tympanoplasty failures and perforated tympanic membranes with persistent suppurative drainage are indications for mastoidectomy, but in most cases, these conditions are remedied with a well-executed tympanoplasty alone. Small cholesteatomas isolated to the tympanic membrane or small congenital cholesteatomas also may not need a mastoidectomy for complete disease removal.

The choice for preserving or removing the posterior wall of the EAC, ie, CWU versus CWD mastoidectomy, has been extensively debated. In CWD surgery, the posterior EAC is removed to increase access to the middle ear and epitympanum and to exteriorize any unresectable cholesteatoma matrix, eg, cholesteatoma matrix overlying a lateral semicircular canal fistula. The open mastoid cavity that results from CWD surgery epithelializes over the next several months and requires frequent clinical visits, at least initially, to debride and maintain the cavity. Even when fully healed, the cavity often requires routine, lifetime follow-up. The increased surgical exposure afforded by removal of the canal wall has been reported to result in lower rate of disease recurrence versus a CWU mastoidectomy.[18] Others have reported that removal of the canal wall does not significantly impact the disease recurrence rate, but rather the anatomical position of the cholesteatoma more significantly impacts the recurrence rate.[19] Additionally, an open cavity is not as aesthetically appealing as the normal anatomy, and patients may become self-conscious of the enlarged meatus that accompanies the open cavity.

Preserving the canal in mastoidectomy results in a considerably reduced postoperative convalescence and rarely requires in-office debridement. The preservation of the canal wall avoids restrictions on water exposure and offers a greater selection of hearing aids versus the difficulties of wearing an aid in an open cavity. Traditionally, hearing outcomes have been considered better in CWU mastoidectomy versus CWD.[20] Indeed, this discrepancy may have more to do with the extensive nature of disease that results in a CWD procedure, rather than the presence, or lack thereof, of a posterior canal wall. Other authors have reported that hearing outcomes are not significantly different between the two procedures, and that the presence of ossicular erosion is more important in determining the hearing results.[20,21,22] Often, CWU surgeries are staged, requiring a second-look procedure typically in 6 to 12 months to assess for disease recurrence and to reconstruct the ossicles. Proponents of CWD procedures maintain that with this approach, second-look procedures are generally unnecessary.

Preservation of the canal wall is preferred in our practice. The decision to remove the wall is most often made during surgery, when the extent of the disease is fully appreciated. Intraoperative findings that may be indications for a CWD procedure include labyrinthine fistula, unresectable disease on the facial nerve or stapes footplate, a low-lying tegmen that limits access to the attic, unresectable sinus tympani disease, and an unreconstructable posterior canal wall defect. Removal of the canal wall does not improve access to the sinus tympani. Rarely, our preoperative evaluation may result in the decision to take down the canal wall. Obvious posterior wall erosion, larger labyrinthine fistula on CT scan, elderly or infirmed patients in which second look is unadvisable, and occasionally with disease in an only hearing ear, are preoperative conditions that may warrant a CWD procedure. CWD mastoidectomy is always discussed with the patient preoperatively during the informed consent process, should unexpected findings during surgery necessitate removal of the canal wall.

PEDIATRIC CHOLESTEATOMA

It is a general perception (but debated) that cholesteatoma is more aggressive in the pediatric population. While an immature Eustachian tube may facilitate tympanic membrane retraction and cholesteatoma, others have postulated that the increased amount of growth factors in children lead to faster growth rates in cholesteatomas. Additionally, children with CSOM often have better aerated mastoids than adults with CSOM and this increased aeration may facilitate the spread of cholesteatoma through the middle ear and mastoid, and complicate complete removal. Despite these generally accepted ideas, only one study has revealed any molecular difference between adult and pediatric cholesteatoma. Bujia et al. demonstrated a faster replication rate of keratinocytes in pediatric cholesteatoma versus adult.[23]

Recurrence rates after surgery for cholesteatoma in children vary widely in the literature, from 5 to 71%.[24] In one comparative study of 66 patients, Dodson et al. reviewed their experience and found that the overall recidivism (recurrent and residual disease) rate with pediatric CWU mastoidectomy was 42% versus 12% for CWD mastoidectomy.[21] Only 17% of patients treated with CWU mastoidectomy required conversion to CWD mastoidectomy for recidivistic disease (mean follow-up of 37.6 months). Despite the difference in recidivism, the authors continued to support the use of CWU surgery because of the lack of chronic mastoid cavity management issues. Hearing results in the two groups were similar. On the contrary, some authors maintain that the higher rates of recidivism with CWU mastoidectomy are an indication that CWD surgery is the prudent option for pediatric cholesteatoma. CWD mastoidectomy does not necessarily assure better recidivism rates as shown in a study by Shirazi et al., who recently reviewed their experience with 106 pediatric cholesteatoma cases (both acquired and congenital), with a mean follow-up of 6 years. Eight percent of CWU mastoidectomies required revision surgery for recurrent or residual disease, whereas 21% of CWD mastoidectomies required revision surgery. Interestingly, only 28% of the CWD revisions were for recurrent disease, the other 72% were for stenosis and granulation. Overall, the rates of recurrent disease in CWU versus CWD were 8% versus 6%, respectively, and were not statistically significant. Similar to other authors, they found that the status of the canal wall had little effect on the postoperative hearing results; rather the main determinant of postoperative hearing results in their study was stapes superstructure erosion.[25]

As with adults, we strive to preserve the canal wall in all pediatric cases when possible. The decision to remove the canal wall is primarily made during surgery. The intraoperative decision to remove the canal occurs most often after discovery of a semicircular canal fistula or significant erosion in the posterior canal wall. Scutal erosions are reconstructed with cartilage to prevent recurrent retraction. The tympanic membrane is reinforced with cartilage in all quadrants when severe disease is encountered. We have not observed this reinforcement to result in decreased postoperative hearing thresholds. Patients are brought back for a second-look procedure and ossicular chain reconstruction in 12 months.

The decision for a second-look procedure is made at the time of the initial surgery. Careful notation of extent and location of disease is conducted at the time of the initial procedure. Often the second-look procedure (and Ossicular Chain Reconstruction (OCR)) is via a transcanal middle ear exploration, as the primary areas of disease recurrence, namely the stapes, facial nerve, and sinus tympani, can be examined with this approach. A postauricular approach is indicated if extensive dural involvement or poor attic exposure is noted on the initial procedure.

We strongly believe that preservation of the posterior canal wall is important in children, whether it is maintained intact or reconstructed. In fact, we prefer to bring a child back for a third look for residual disease, if there is such a concern, rather than converting to an open cavity.

CONTRAINDICATIONS

Contraindications to performing a CWU mastoidectomy include an unreconstructable posterior canal wall defect, patients in whom proper follow-up is questionable, and unresectable matrix involving the labyrinth, facial nerve, carotid, dura, and sinus tympani. Active infection and otorrhea are not contraindications to surgery, but efforts should be made to treat the ear and make it as dry as possible preoperatively. The rate of postoperative infection is higher when an ear is operated while draining.

PREOPERATIVE MANAGEMENT AND PLANNING

As discussed previously, a thorough history and full head and neck exam with binocular otomicroscopy is imperative when feasible in the initial evaluation of each patient. In patients who have failed medical therapy or with cholesteatoma, the discussion of surgery is initiated.

CT scans are not obtained routinely in all patients. In patients with vertigo, facial palsy, pain, or other symptoms suggestive of complications, a CT scan is recommended to fully delineate the anatomy and disease. Revision surgery is also an indication for a CT scan, especially for patients whose previous procedure was not performed at our institution.

OPERATIVE TECHNIQUES

The techniques for the CWU mastoidectomy will be described below. A thorough description of the tympanoplasty, middle ear dissection, and ossicular chain reconstruction are addressed in other chapters within this text.

Preparation

All cases are performed under general anesthesia without paralytic agents and with continuous facial nerve monitoring. The tragus and postauricular skin are injected with 1% lidocaine with epinephrine (1:100,000) to provide hemostasis and local anesthesia. We use dental carpules with the dental syringe for all local anesthetic injections. This avoids any inadvertent injection of more concentrated epinephrine that is used topically during surgery. The authors then "prescrub" the ear and the entire side of the head, including hair, with betadine. The surgical site is then prepped and draped in sterile fashion. Preoperative antibiotics and steroids are used for every surgery. Additionally, 400 mg of ciprofloxacin (IV piggyback) is mixed with the saline irrigation (1 L) for use on all cases.

Incisions

The EAC and tympanic membrane are examined, irrigated with saline, and cleaned of debris. The canal skin is injected with 1% lidocaine with epinephrine (1:50,000) in the posterior, inferior, and superior quadrants. Vascular strip incisions are made in the ear canal (Figure 30–2). An incision is made along

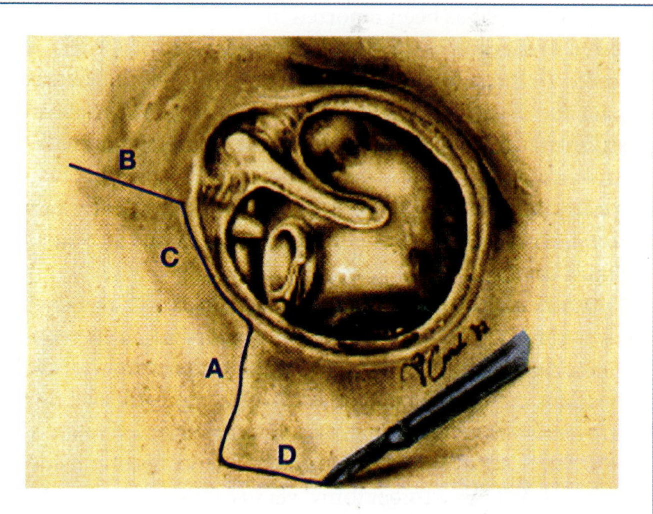

FIGURE 30–2 • Vascular strip incisions. *A*, Tympanomastoid suture line; *B*, tympanosquamous suture line; *C*, medial incision; *D*, radial incision.

the tympanosquamous suture line and then, in a similar fashion, just inferior to the tympanomastoid suture line. Another incision is then made between the medial extents of these 2 incisions, approximately 2 to 3 mm lateral to the bony annulus. A radial incision is made at the bony cartilaginous junction of the ear canal, perpendicular to the incision at the tympanomastoid suture line and extending inferiorly to the floor of the ear canal. The advantage of these incisions is that they create a laterally based skin flap that allows for retraction of much of the meatal tissue, thus improving exposure.

The postauricular incision is made from helical rim to mastoid tip, approximately 1 cm posterior to the sulcus (Figure 30–3). Care is taken to avoid making the incision in the sulcus as this can make closure more difficult and lead to unsightly deepening of the sulcus as the scar matures. In young children, the mastoid tip is not fully developed and the facial nerve is located in a more lateral position. It is important to bring the inferior aspect of the postauricular incision more posterior to avoid any potential for injury of the facial nerve as it exits the mastoid.

Beginning superiorly, the incision is carried down through the skin and subcutaneous fat to the layer of loose areolar tissue overlying the superficial layer of the true temporalis fascia. Within this avascular plane, lateral to the loose areolar tissue, the ear is reflected forward to the EAC.

The layer of loose areolar tissue is harvested for use in tympanoplasty (Figure 30–4). In revision cases when this layer of tissue may be absent, remaining scar tissue or true temporalis fascia can be harvested. Multiple revisions can result in a paucity of traditional grafting materials. In these situations, tragal perichondrium, conchal cartilage perichondrium, temporal bone periosteum, and vein graft, are all options for tympanoplasty materials. Alloderm is also a viable option, but rarely used.[26]

A T-shaped incision is made in the mastoid periosteum to expose the mastoid cortex (Figure 30–4). Using the electrocautery, an incision is made along the linea temporalis, to the

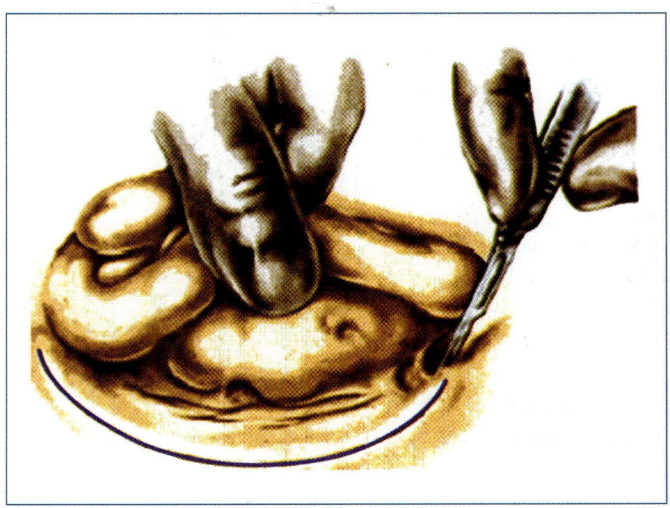

FIGURE 30–3 • Postauricular incision.

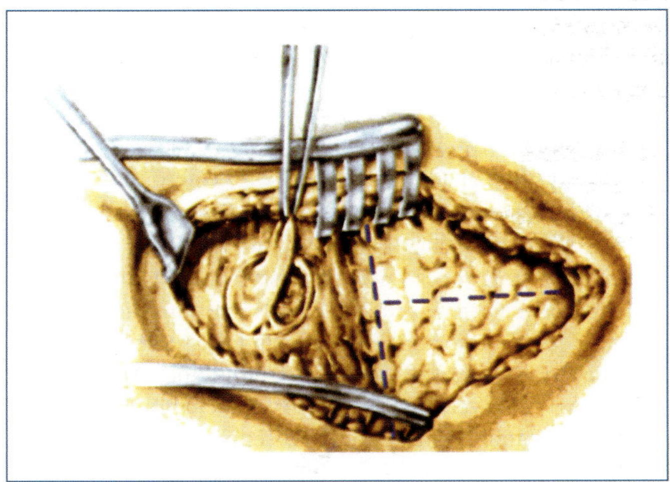

FIGURE 30–4 • Facial graft harvest and periosteal incisions.

level of the underlying bone. It is important to carry this incision superior to the level of the EAC for adequate exposure to facilitate middle ear and attic dissection. A second periosteal incision is made perpendicular to the linea temporalis and is carried down to the mastoid tip. In revision surgery where a prior mastoid defect exists, a C-shaped incision is preferred by the authors. After carefully palpating the mastoid defect, the incision is carried from anterior extent of the linea temporalis, to the mastoid tip, avoiding entry into the mastoid cavity by staying a few millimeters superior and posterior to the cavity. We feel that the C-shaped incision provides a better exposure of a previously drilled cavity and prevents inadvertent injury to important underlying structures that may be exposed from the prior surgery, such as the sigmoid sinus and middle fossa dura.

Using the Lempert elevator, the periosteum is elevated superiorly over the tegmen, posteriorly over the sigmoid sinus, and anteriorly to the level of the EAC meatus, where the vascular strip is identified and reflected posteriorly. Two self-retaining retractors are used perpendicular to each other to expose the entire mastoid and EAC for remainder of the surgery (Figure 30–5).

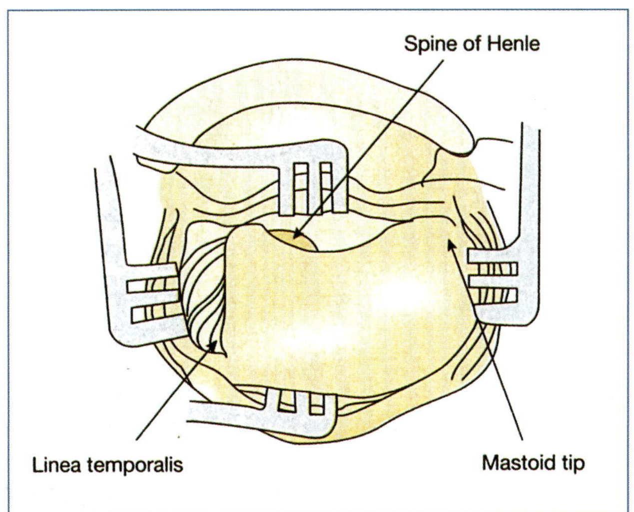

FIGURE 30–5 • Mastoid surface anatomy.

Middle Ear Dissection

The authors prefer to begin with middle ear dissection prior to mastoidectomy to control middle ear disease and ascertain the state of the ossicular chain. Ossicular discontinuity and/ or erosion may allow for removal of the incus and malleus to protect the stapes and footplate from injury prior to dissection of the attic.

The tympanomeatal flap is elevated anteriorly and is carefully dissected free from the ossicular chain. Any diseased portion of the tympanic membrane warrants removal to prevent graft failure. The exposed middle ear is then assessed to ascertain the extent of disease and the status of the ossicles and facial nerve. Cholesteatoma, if present, is gently dissected from the middle ear to expose the ossicles and facial nerve. The ossicular chain is considered intact until proven otherwise. When possible, cholesteatoma or severe retraction pocket is kept intact to prevent disease recurrence. Removal of part of the scutum and widening of the bony EAC with the diamond drill may improve exposure and facilitate disease removal. For extensive disease, the cholesteatoma is internally debulked and resected. Cholesteatoma or granulation tissue is dissected free from the ossicles, leaving the ossicular chain intact if possible. If preservation of the ossicular chain is not possible, separation of the incudostapedial joint is performed early to prevent injury to the stapes or inner ear.

Canalplasty

Often middle ear dissection and postoperative follow-up is facilitated by canalplasty, which is performed at the onset of the procedure. Using a 2-mm diamond burr, excess tympanic bone at the tympanomastoid and tympanosquamous suture lines is removed. If required, the entire EAC can be enlarged, from the 12 o'clock to 6 o'clock position posteriorly. Anterior canal wall bulges rarely require canalplasty, but removal may be done when needed to facilitate postoperative follow-up of the anterior tympanic membrane. Within the posterior–inferior quadrant of the EAC, Adad et al. found the facial nerve to be lateral to the plane of the annulus in 71% of temporal bone specimens, and of these, 73% were also anterior to the posterior edge of the annulus. The distance from the annulus to the facial nerve in the posterior–inferior quadrant of the EAC ranges from 1.9 mm to 5.7 mm, showing great variability in the course of the nerve.[27] Extreme care must be taken when drilling in this quadrant of the canal as this is the area of the canal where the facial nerve is at most risk to injury. Often removal of this small amount of bone greatly improves the exposure, ensuring better disease resection and graft placement.

Mastoidectomy

Basics

Mastoidectomy is conducted with the visualization afforded by the binocular-operating microscope, a high-speed drill, and suction-irrigation. We currently use a high-speed electric drill system. Fluted or cutting burrs are efficient at removing large amounts of bone in a small amount of time but are used with caution around important structures. Diamond burrs are very good at delicate dissection around important structures, thinning the bone off the sigmoid sinus, tegmen, facial nerve, and opening the facial recess. During the mastoidectomy, larger burrs are used first and the burr size is sequentially decreased as the areas of dissection get narrower. The largest burr possible should always be used as it is less likely to inadvertently penetrate an underlying structure and is yet more efficient for bone removal. The surgeon must always be aware of what the back of the burr may be touching. It is not recommended to drill under a ledge or in recesses in which there is not a view fully 360 degrees around the burr.

Effective use of the suction irrigator is important for safe and effective drilling. The irrigation clears the operative field of bone dust and blood and keeps the burr clean. Ample irrigation is imperative when using diamond burrs around the facial nerve to keep the bone cool and avoid thermal injury to the nerve. Diamond burrs are also effective at controlling bleeding in the bone by driving bone dust into the lumen of the small vessels.

Canal-Wall-Up Mastoidectomy

Initial dissection involves using a 5- or 6-mm cutting burr and removing bone along the linea temporalis to identify the underlying tegmen (Figure 30–6). The surgeon should look for the emergence of a pink hue under the bone as it is thinned over the tegmen, accompanied by a change (more "tinny") in the sound of the burr. The location of the tegmen varies with the anatomy of the individual. Once located, the surface of the tegmen is followed medially toward the antrum. The middle fossa dura is always delineated as it is the superior extent of the dissection. Inadvertent damage to the ossicles and lateral semicircular canal can result if the dura is not delineated properly.

After identification of the tegmen, cortical bone is removed behind the EAC, keeping the posterior wall of the EAC thin, but intact. Cortical bone is removed inferiorly to the mastoid tip and posteriorly to the sigmoid sinus and sinodural angle. Bone removal is continued in these three planes, progressing medially, and removing the cortical bone between them. As the bone over the sigmoid sinus is thinned, a bluish hue will

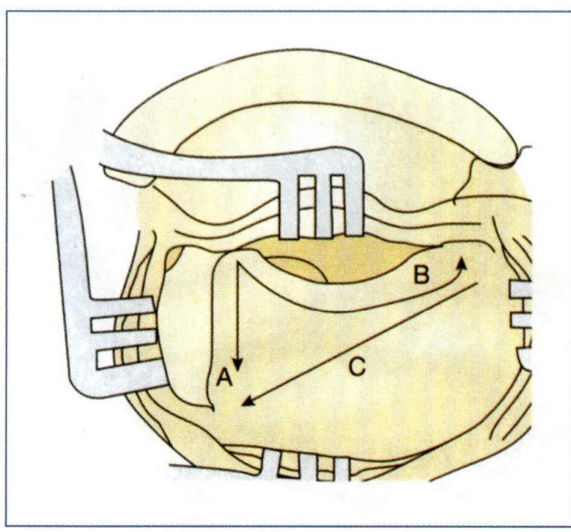

FIGURE 30–6 • Drill cuts used in start of mastoidectomy. *A*, Thin layer of tegmen bone is left over the middle fossa dura, remembering that tegmen height is variable depending on mastoid pneumatization. Cut *B*, perpendicular to the first and tangential to the external auditory canal is made from the zygomatic root to the mastoid tip. Cut *C*, is made from the mastoid tip to the sinodural angle.

become apparent beneath the bone, accompanied by a change in the sound of the burr. Decortication of the sinus or middle fossa dura is unnecessary unless involved with disease.

With the tegmen, sigmoid sinus, and posterior canal wall identified, the antrum can now be dissected, following the tegmen anteriorly. Koerner's septum, the embryologic remnant of the fusion plane between the petrous and the squamous bones is often encountered next. After penetrating Koerner's septum, the antrum is uncovered and the surgeon can identify the lateral semicircular canal (Figure 30–7). The enchondral bone of the otic capsule bone is more compact than the rest of the temporal bone and is easily identified by its smooth and often slightly amber appearance. In patients with CSOM, the antrum may be observed with cholesteatoma, granulation tissue, or edematous mucosa, obscuring the lateral semicircular canal and making its identification more difficult.

The next step is attic dissection, which is performed by following the tegmen anteriorly and by thinning the canal wall posteriorly and superiorly. Care is taken to avoid drilling a hole in the bony canal wall. The canal wall is thinned starting laterally and progressing medially. Rotating the operating bed toward the surgeon affords simultaneous viewing of the canal and the mastoid and aids in preventing injury to the wall during drilling.

Drilling out the zygomatic root and opening the attic is often better accomplished with a 3-mm cutting burr and a smaller suction irrigator. The tegmen is carefully followed and usually dips inferiorly as the epitympanum is approached from posterior to anterior. A smaller diamond burr is used for more medial dissection, especially if the ossicular chain is intact. The 3-mm diamond burr offers better control in this tight area and is less likely to skip, as the 3-mm cutting burr can often do in tight areas. The attic air cells are opened completely, fully exposing any epitympanic disease. Granulation and cholesteatoma can now be removed from the canal or attic vantage points. The cog is a flat, thin, bony projection from the tegmen, in the

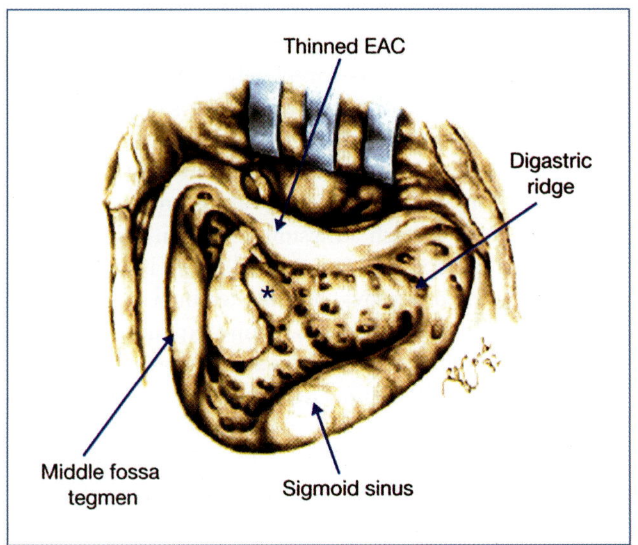

FIGURE 30–7 • Complete mastoidectomy in cholesteatoma dissection. Asterisk indicates lateral semicircular canal.

parasagittal plane, that appears to have a semicircle cut out of the inferior border. Located directly superior to the cochleariform process, with the tensor tympani tendon it creates a small, roughly round aperture that opens into the anterior epitympanum. If it is not specifically identified and removed, significant disease may be left in the anterior attic, which is one of the most common locations of residual disease. If disease extends into the mastoid tip, the tip can be easily drilled out with a large cutting burr. In most cases, cholesteatoma or chronic infection does not extensively involve the tip. It is our practice to not remove the mastoid tip air cell system unless disease dictates its necessity.

Preserving facial nerve function is paramount in ear surgery. The surgeon must be cognizant of its general location within the surgical field at all times. As the nerve travels distally from the geniculate ganglion, it passes superior to the cochleariform process and oval window. Posterior to the oval window, the nerve turns inferiorly to take on a more vertical course; this area is often referred to as the second genu of the facial nerve. The second genu is located a few millimeters anteromedial to the lateral semicircular canal, and is an anatomic landmark for localizing the facial nerve.

The authors do not localize the facial nerve in each mastoidectomy, but rather on a disease-specific basis. If after opening the antrum and ascertaining the extent of the disease, we encounter cholesteatoma filling the mastoid, then we determine the location of the facial nerve throughout its course to assure its integrity during the remainder of the surgery. If disease is limited to the antrum, we rarely elect to uncover the vertical segment of the facial nerve to determine its location. In these situations, the small benefit obtained in precisely localizing the nerve is offset by the potential harm that can be done to the nerve by drill trauma.

Acute Mastoiditis

The goal of mastoidectomy for acute, coalescent mastoiditis is the simple evacuation of pus from the mastoid, rather than a complete anatomical mastoid dissection, which would be difficult given the inflammation, granulation tissue, and bleeding that are encountered. The removal of the cortical mastoid bone begins using a large cutting burr and proceeds as described above until pus is encountered in the coalescent mastoid cavity. The coalescent cavity is often only several millimeters under the surface of the mastoid cortex. This cavity is widely opened and the pus is entirely evacuated from the mastoid. Copious irrigation with antibiotic-containing saline is done to maximally wash out the purulent material.

Facial Recess

The facial recess approach (posterior tympanotomy) is not required in all CWU mastoidectomy cases; rather it is employed only when dictated by the location of the disease. The facial recess is a triangular-shaped area bordered by the facial nerve posteriorly, the incus buttress superiorly, and chorda tympani nerve anterolaterally (Figure 30–8). Access to the mesotympanum can be gained by removing the bone in the facial recess. For additional exposure, the facial recess can be extended inferiorly by sacrificing the chorda tympani nerve. The entire

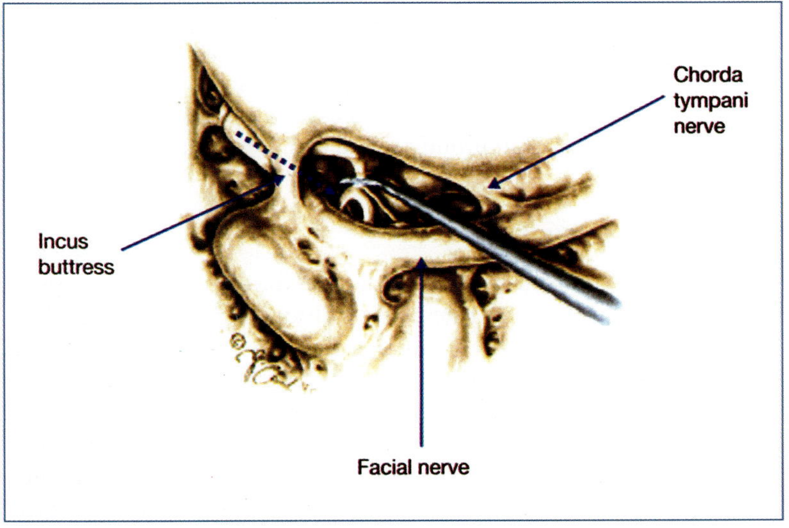

FIGURE 30–8 • Facial recess (*dashed line*) Short process of the incus helps identify the facial recess.

mesotympanum and hypotympanum can usually be accessed through the mastoid by the extended facial recess approach (Figure 30–9).

Prior to opening the facial recess, it is important to thin the posterior canal wall, if not previously accomplished. Identification of the facial nerve is imperative to minimize the risk of injury, should the nerve take an aberrant course. The lateral semicircular canal lies just superior to the facial nerve as it completes its transition to the vertical segment. The short process of the incus points to the facial recess. The digastric ridge is another anatomic landmark for the facial nerve.

Removing the bone over the facial nerve is best accomplished with a large diamond burr and copious irrigation. The burr strokes are always parallel to the course of the nerve. Using long, gentle strokes, the facial nerve is gently uncovered until it is observed through a thin layer of bone. Small vessels that accompany the nerve often bleed during this dissection, and are easily controlled with epinephrine-soaked Gelfoam™ (Pfizer Inc.) or bipolar cautery.

After identifying the facial nerve, the chorda tympani nerve is identified in similar fashion as it branches off the vertical segment of the facial nerve, and is traced superiorly toward the incus. With all borders of the facial recess delineated, the recess is opened with a 2-mm diamond burr, starting superiorly where the recess is widest. Care is taken to preserve a small piece of bone just inferior to the incus to protect it from the drill. With gentle removal of bone in an anteromedial direction, the recess will be opened exposing the middle ear.

The extended facial recess approach involves sharply sectioning the chorda tympani nerve as it branches off the facial nerve trunk and extending the recess ear inferiorly along the course of the facial nerve. The lateral boundary of the exposure becomes the annulus of the tympanic membrane.

Dissection of Cholesteatoma

Before dissecting the cholesteatoma sac from the mastoid bone, the sac should be opened and its contents should be evacuated, leaving the matrix in place. The consistency of cholesteatoma matrix is quite variable, ranging from a relatively thick and well defined capsule to loose squamous debris without any visible capsule. To minimize the risk of leaving residual disease, the matrix should be resected as completely as possible, elevating it as an intact sheet if at all possible. The sac is usually not uniformly adherent to the underlying mucosa or bone; rather, it is often in loose contact and fixed only intermittently by mucosal adhesions. The strategy for removal becomes a search for the adhesions, lysis of each adhesion, and then resumption of elevation of the matrix until the next adhesion is encountered. Lysis of an adhesion or removal of cholesteatoma extending into recesses or air cells may sometimes require expanding the surgical exposure or drilling out the focal air cells involved.

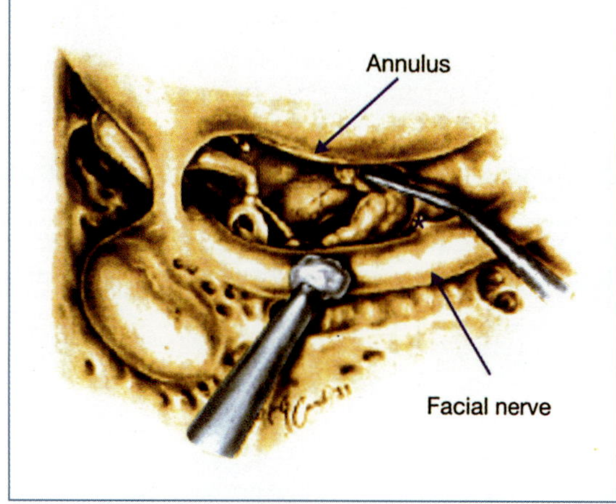

FIGURE 30–9 • Inferior extended facial recess. Asterisks indicate sacrificed chorda tympani nerves.

A small dimple or flattening in the matrix covering the bone over the lateral semicircular canal may belie a fistula. Suspicious areas can be palpated gently with a blunt instrument to ascertain if there is erosion of the bony labyrinth. Even if a small dimple is not seen in the matrix, meticulous dissection of the matrix from the otic capsule bone in this area is warranted to avoid inadvertently uncovering a previously undetected fistula. Fistulae of the lateral semicircular canal can be classified generally as small (smaller than 2 mm in diameter) and large (greater than 2 mm in diameter). Because erosion of the otic capsule bone occurs in a saucerized manner, fistulae smaller than 2 mm are unlikely to involve the endosteal membrane of the semicircular canal and likely have not compromised the endolymphatic compartment. If a large fistula is suspected during surgery, leaving the matrix intact and converting to a CWD procedure is recommended. Alternatively, if the suspected fistula is small, the offending matrix can be left intact and revisited in a second-look procedure 12 months later. At that time, with a more sterile environment, matrix removal may be attempted.

Smaller fistulae (or inadvertently uncovered fistulae) may be repaired at the initial procedure by covering the fistula with fascia or perichondrium. Antibiotics and corticosteroids are recommended for patients with suspected or confirmed fistulae. It should be noted that in patients with suspected fistula, the planned removal of matrix and repair of fistula should be deferred until the end of the procedure, whenever possible, after the removal of infection and cholesteatoma has been completed. Addressing a fistula with repair early in the procedure is usually not advisable, as subsequent drilling, irrigation, and disease removal necessary to complete the procedure risks further contamination of and damage to the membranous labyrinth. Significant morbidity may be reduced from inadvertently uncovering a fistula if it is recognized and addressed quickly. Often the patient will experience transient postoperative vertigo, but prompt initial action may limit any SNHL.

CLOSURE

Upon complete removal of disease, the ear canal and mastoid cavity are irrigated extensively with antibiotic-containing saline solution to remove any bone dust and remaining squamous debris. The middle ear and mastoid are temporarily packed with epinephrine-soaked Gelfoam for hemostasis.

Cartilage grafting is routinely used in patients with CSOM. Tragal cartilage is harvested and its perichondrium is removed. Under the microscope, the cartilage is thinned with a scalpel.

To repair a scutal defect, the perichondrium is dissected from the cartilage, but left attached at one edge. This perichondrium is used to anchor the cartilage graft to the remaining posterior canal wall. The perichondrium is laid against the canal wall lateral to the defect, securing the attached cartilage to the area to be reconstructed. In addition to the standard cartilage grafting of the posterior–superior quadrant of the tympanic membrane, other areas of the tympanic membrane may be supported by cartilage as well.

The epinephrine-soaked Gelfoam is removed and the middle ear is packed with saline-soaked Gelfoam. Multiple thinned cartilage grafts are placed in a patchwork array over the Gelfoam-packed middle ear to support the fascia graft. The scutum is reconstructed, if required. The fascia graft is placed medial to the tympanomeatal flap, lateral to the ossicular chain, and lateral to any cartilage grafts. Ossicular reconstruction is conducted if necessary, or left for the second-look procedure. The tympanomeatal flap is reflected posteriorly to cover the fascia graft. Any previously elevated canal skin is placed back to its natural position. Gelfoam is placed lateral to the tympanomeatal flap to secure its position.

The self-retaining retractors are removed and the vascular strip skin flap is unfurled and placed back into the ear canal. A nasal speculum is placed in the external auditory meatus to provide a view of the vascular strip and confirm proper placement. Long strips of Gelfoam are placed over the vascular strip incisions and the ear canal is filled with antibiotic ointment. The postauricular incision is closed in two layers. The periosteum is closed with 3-0 Vicryl sutures and the skin is closed with subcuticular 4-0 Vicryl sutures. The incision is covered in antibiotic ointment and a Glasscock ear dressing™ (Otomed) is applied.

POSTOPERATIVE CARE

Patients are sent home the day of surgery with antibiotics and pain medicine. The Glasscock ear dressing is removed the day after surgery. Patients are asked to keep a clean cotton ball in their ear, and replace it as necessary until their next follow-up appointment. Water precautions are maintained for 6 weeks. Patients return for their first postoperative visit in 3 weeks. The patient is examined for infection, granulation tissue, and polyps. Packing may be gently removed. Antibiotic/ steroid ear drops may be utilized. The second postoperative visit ranges from 2 weeks to 6–8 weeks, depending of the appearance of the ear at the first postoperative visit. At this appointment, the ear canal and tympanic membrane are examined, and an audiogram is obtained.

COMPLICATIONS

Most complications in mastoid surgery occur as a result of inadequate surgical exposure, granulations or bleeding obscuring the surgical field, or the failure to recognize anatomic variations. Most complications can be avoided by actively anticipating complications at all times and taking appropriate steps to avoid them as possible. Surgeons must familiarize themselves with anatomic variants and proceed with the expectation of encountering such variants at any time. Despite such efforts, complications may still occur in even the most experienced of surgical hands.

SURGICAL EXPOSURE

The surgical exposure should be sufficiently developed to adequately remove disease and to identify the important anatomic structures that should be preserved intact. Errors may occur when exposure is limited and the surgeon may become unknowingly disoriented. To prevent such problems, positive identification of important landmarks, such as the tegmen, lateral semicircular canal, facial nerve, cochleariform process, ossicles, etc., should be made and the surgeon should very frequently make a conscious visual sweep of the exposure to note the location of these landmarks in order to maintain orientation.

BLEEDING

Bleeding is not often a problem in mastoidectomy unless a significant injury to the dural sinuses or jugular bulb occurs. Rather, the small amount of bleeding that occurs during mastoidectomy tends to cause difficulty by obscuring the field of dissection, leading to a greater risk of injury to underlying structures. Bleeding should be controlled to the maximum extent possible. It is better to stop the procedure and pack the ear with Gelfoam™ soaked in epinephrine for a few minutes and then resume rather than to persist operating in a blood-obscured field.

Small injuries to the sigmoid sinus can result in copious bleeding. Often, bipolar cautery can control these small injuries. For more sizeable injuries, steps must be taken to prevent an air embolus from developing through the tear in the sinus. In such instances, gently place a finger over the tear in the sinus to prevent further bleeding and to prevent air from entering the sinus. With your finger in place, have the patient rotated toward you and placed in a head down position. Once in this position, the injury to the sinus is repaired. Gelfoam can be placed over the point of injury, covered with a small cotton pledget or cotton ball, and held in place with gentle pressure. Surgery can then continue, leaving the Gelfoam in place. Cotton must be removed prior to closure to avoid delayed granulation reaction and possible infection.

Small bleeding vessels emanating from the mastoid bone are easily controlled with a diamond burr. Larger vessels encountered can be addressed with the bipolar cautery or bone wax. Slow generalized oozing from the cavity is easily managed with epinephrine-soaked Gelfoam.

Postauricular hematomas may result from uncontrolled bleeding that is generated as the patient coughs or strains during the postoperative period. These are generally managed with direct pressure and a compressive mastoid dressing. The deep branch of the superficial temporal artery may be injured with the opening incision of the periosteum over the temporal line superior to the EAC and in rare cases can cause a delayed hematoma. Careful cautery of the anterior extent of the periosteal incision will usually avert such bleeding.

GRANULATION TISSUE

Granulation tissue presents a particularly difficult challenge as it may be extremely adherent to important underlying structures, such as the facial nerve, dura, or ossicles. Removal of granulation tissue from these structures should be done parallel and tangential to the structure to minimize the risk of avulsion. Facial monitoring has shown that traction along the direction of the facial nerve is much better tolerated than that in a perpendicular direction. Occasionally, granulation tissue is densely adherent to and indistinguishable from an inflamed, dehiscent facial nerve or dura and it is best to trim such granulations, leaving them in place rather than risk injury by complete removal. Residual granulation tissue usually resolves with the removal of cholesteatoma or other etiology of the inflammation.

FACIAL NERVE INJURY

Facial nerve injury is perhaps the most significant complication that can arise from otologic surgery. Facial nerve monitoring is used for all otologic cases at our institution (except myringotomy with tube insertion), but is not a substitute for knowledge of facial nerve anatomy. Initial assessment for facial nerve function postoperatively should be done in the operating room. During the reversal of anesthesia, flaring of the nasal ala is usually the first facial movement to recover and a more complete evaluation of function can be done once the patient has gained full consciousness in the post anesthesia care unit.

If injury to the nerve is recognized during surgery, the bone proximal and distal to the injured area is removed with a diamond burr to prevent nerve compression from the postinjury edema that is likely to occur. Proper management of a partially transected nerve is debated. Since only a minority of axons will ultimately heal across an anastamosis, it is generally recommended to preserve any remaining intact fascicles. Some surgeons have argued that when greater than 50% of the nerve is transected, superior results in facial function will be obtained by resecting the injured segment and grafting the nerve.[28] Most surgeons, however, have found better outcomes with preserving any remaining fascicles, unless there is truly a near complete transection.[29] In the unusual case of iatrogenic injury, we carefully assess the injury and try to preserve the intact portion of the nerve. Rarely is the nerve completely transected. In our opinion, leaving this portion intact and repairing the injured portion of the nerve is preferable. If a subtotal transection of the nerve is discovered, we prefer to decompress the nerve proximally and distally and assess the injury. If there is sufficient tissue, we attempt to bring the injured areas of the nerve together, without tension, using 9–0 nylon suture; we serially assess facial nerve function over the next 6 to 12 months. If a full transaction of the nerve is recognized during surgery, primary reanastamosis is attempted. When there is tissue missing, cable (interpositional) nerve grafting is employed, using the greater auricular nerve or sural nerve.

When no injury to the nerve is discerned during surgery but facial paralysis is encountered in the immediate postoperative period, it is prudent to wait and reassess facial function over the next 4 h. Temporary facial nerve paralysis can result from use of local anesthetic at the beginning of the case. If paralysis persists after 4 h, surgical exploration is warranted. In the operating room, the facial nerve is inspected from the

TABLE 30–1 Management of iatrogenic facial nerve injury

Intraoperative recognized facial nerve injury	
Minimal injury	Decompress fallopian canal proximal and distal to site
Partial transection	Preserve remaining fascicles, anastamosis of separated fascicles, decompress fallopian canal proximal and distal to site
Complete transection	Attempt primary anastamosis without tension, cable graft if necessary
Postoperative recognition of facial weakness, early	
Immediate postoperative	Reassess after 4 h to allow for injected anesthetic to wear off
Mild paresis	Observe. Steroids. Surgery if progresses rapidly to severe paresis or paralysis.
Severe paresis or paralysis	Return to operating room for exploration and repair
Postoperative recognition of facial weakness, delayed (more than 8 h postoperative)	
Mild paresis	Observe. Steroids (antivirals if 2–10 days postoperative)
Severe paresis or paralysis	Observe. Steroids (antivirals if 2–10 days postoperative). Surgery rarely indicated. Prognosis for complete spontaneous recovery may be reduced if there is absence of volitional activity on EMG and > 90% loss of ENoG amplitude compared to normal slide[31]

EMG, electromyography; ENoG, electroneuronography.

geniculate ganglion to the stylomastoid foramen. Areas that are suspicious for potential injury are decompressed as described above. Postoperatively, patients are treated with corticosteroids. Delayed (2 to 10 days postoperatively) facial paralysis is managed with steroids, antibiotics, and antiviral are considered. Antivirals such as famcyclovir, which has better blood-brain barrier penetration than acyclovir, may be effective if started within 72 hours of the onset of weakness (see Table 30–1). Latent viral activation is known to occur with neurosurgical procedures and may be one cause of delayed facial weakness in otologic surgery. Delayed paralysis rarely, if ever, requires surgery.[30]

SENSORINEURAL HEARING LOSS AND VERTIGO

SNHL after surgery can be attributed to trauma to an intact ossicular chain from middle ear dissection or from contacting the ossicular chain with the drill. Drill-related injuries often result in high-frequency losses. SNHL, with or without vertigo, may result from chemical labyrinthine injury. Serous labyrinthitis can occur if inflammatory cells or blood enter the perilymph following direct penetration of the oval window, round window, or labyrinthine fistula. Although not infectious, these components can disrupt the delicate homeostasis of the perilymph/endolymph relationship and can lead to SNHL and vertigo. SNHL may occur with a semicircular canal fistula, even if treated appropriately, especially if pus is encountered. Serous labyrinthitis often responds promptly to early corticosteroid treatment. For these reasons, in part, all patients in our practice are treated preoperatively with corticosteroids. If an oval window, round window, or labyrinthine defect is encountered intraoperatively, corticosteroids are continued postoperatively.

Suppurative labyrinthitis can occur when pus and/or bacteria gain access to the inner ear. Although more commonly associated with untreated, chronically infected ears, this may occur when operating in the setting of acute or chronic mastoiditis and, in addition to SNHL and vertigo, may result in postoperative fevers. Due to the infectious nature of this process, patients need to be placed on immediate antibiotics to prevent the spread of infection to the intracranial compartment.

INFECTION

Postoperative infection can be detrimental to the success of the operation and increase patient morbidity. Every attempt must be made to avoid infection. In our practice, preoperative antibiotics are always used, as well as antibiotic-containing saline irrigation (described earlier). The ear canal is also filled with Bactroban™ ointment to secure the flaps. We recommend antibiotics for 5 to 7 days postoperatively.

INTRACRANIAL INJURY

Exposure of the dura during mastoidectomy is common and is rarely a problem, even when large areas are uncovered. Adural tear with spinal fluid leak is repaired using a layered technique comprising fascia, cartilage, bone pate, Gelfoam, and often fibrinogen glue. This repair is generally more than adequate to stop any small spinal fluid leak. If cholesteatoma is present, meticulous care is needed to avoid cranialization of any cholesteatoma debris. If a small herniation of brain is encountered (less than 5 mm), gentle bipolar cautery of the tissue will result in its retraction back intracranially, and the defect is repaired as described above. Larger herniations of brain (greater than 5 mm) are often unable to be repaired effectively during the initial mastoidectomy. If a large brain hernia is encountered that cannot be effectively repaired as described above, a second procedure will be needed shortly after the initial mastoidectomy to repair the defect employing a middle fossa craniotomy approach, often with the assistance of a neurosurgeon. A planned second procedure allows time for proper informed consent to occur for the more invasive procedure. Delayed meningoencephaloceles, with or without spinal fluid leak, may occur if the dura is injured intraoperatively, even when unrecognized during the surgery. The most common causes of iatrogenic dural injury are laceration with a cutting burr and use of monopolar cautery on the dura, even with the lowest possible settings. These problems can be minimized by the use of careful drilling along the tegmen, use of a diamond drill when appropriate, and exclusive use of bipolar cautery on exposed dura or brain tissue.

CONCLUSIONS

CSOM is a destructive disease that typically requires surgical intervention to achieve its eradication. Cholesteatoma may accompany CSOM and is a definite indication for surgery. Astute otologists should be keenly aware of the characteristics of this disease process and its associated complications. As inflammation, bleeding, and disease complicate surgery, thorough knowledge of the mastoid anatomy is essential in safely performing any mastoid surgery. Both CSOM and cholesteatoma can be effectively controlled with tympanoplasty and mastoidectomy. Surgical intervention should be tailored to each individual patient. In our practice, CWU mastoidectomy offers many advantages over CWD mastoidectomy and is our procedure of choice.

References

1. Kemble J. Hero-Durst. London: Methuen; 1936.
2. Petit JL. Traite' des maladies chirurgicales. Paris:1774.
3. Balance CA. Essays on the survey of the temporal bone. London: Macmillan; 1919.
4. Wilde W. Practical observations on aural surgery and the nature of the ear. Dublin: Maclachlan; 1853.
5. Schwartze HH, Eysell CG. Ueber die kunstliche eroffnung des warzenfortsatzes. Arch Ohrenheilkd 1873;7:157.
6. Zaulfal E. Technik der trepanationdes proc. mastoid. nach kuster'schen grundsatzen. Arch Ohrenheilkd 1893;30:291.
7. Waldman EH, Lustig LR. Sir Charles Alfred Ballance: contributions to otology and neurotology. Otol Neurotol 2005;26:1073–82.
8. Krampe C. Zeiss operating microscopes for neurosurgery. Neurosurg Rev 1984;7(2–3):89–97.
9. Jansen C. Radikaloperation and typanplastik. Sitz Per Fortbild Anztekamn Oh 18, 1958.

10. Meyerhoff WL, Paprella MM, Kim CS. Pathology of chronic otitis media. Ann Otol Rhinol Laryngol 1978;87:749–60.
11. Da Costa SS, Paparella MM, Schachern PA, et al. Temporal bone histopathology in chronically infected ears with intact and perforated tympanic membranes. Laryngoscope 1992;102:1229–36.
12. Schuknecht H. Pathology of the ear. 1st ed. Cambridge, MA: Harvard University Press; 1974.
13. Palva T, Pekka K, Pala A, et al. Middle ear mucosa and chronic ear disease, IV. Enzyme studies of thick non-cholesteatomatous epithelium. Arch Otoloaryngol 1975;101:380–4.
14. Sade J. The biopathology of secretory otitis media. Ann Otol Rhinol Laryngol 1974;83 Suppl 11:59–70.
15. Roland PS. The formation and management of middle ear granulation tissue in chronic ear disease. Ear Nose Throat J 2004;83 Suppl 1:5–8.
16. Abramson M, Huang C. Localization of collagenase in human middle ear cholesteatoma. Laryngoscope 1977;87:777–85.
17. Paparella MM, Morizono T, Le CT, et al. Sensorineural hearing loss in otitis media. Ann Otol Rhinol Laryngol 1984;93:623–9.
18. Palva T. Surgical treatment of chronic middle ear disease. II. Canal wall up and canal wall down procedures. Acta Otol Laryngol 1987;104:487–94.
19. Tos M, Lau T. Late results for surgery in different cholesteatoma types. ORL J Otorhinolaryngol Relat Spec 1989;51:33–49.
20. Brown JS. A ten year statistical follow up of 1142 consecutive cases of cholesteatoma: The closed vs. the open technique. Laryngoscope 1982;92:390–6.
21. Dodson EE, Hashisaki GT, Hobgood TC, et al. Intact canal wall mastoidectomy with tympanoplasty for cholesteatoma in children. Laryngoscope 1998;108(7):977–83.
22. Toner JG, Smyth GD. Surgical treatment of cholesteatoma: A comparison of three techniques. Am J Otol 1990;11(4):247–9.
23. Buijia J, Holly A, Antol-candela F, et al. Immunobiological peculiarities of cholesteatoma in children: Quantification of epithelial proliferation by MIB 1. Laryngoscope 1996;106(7):865–8.
24. Stangerup Se, Drozdziewicz D, Tos M, et al. Recurrence of attic cholesteatoma: Different methods of estimating recurrence rates. Otolaryngol Head Neck Surg 2000;123(3):283–7.
25. Shirazi MA, Muzaffar K, Leonetti JP, et al. Surgical treatment of pediatric cholesteatomas. Laryngoscope 2006;116:1603–7.
26. Haynes DS, Vos JD, Labadie RF. Acellular allograft dermal matrix for tympanoplasty. Curr Opin Otol Head Neck Surg 2005;13(5):283–6.
27. Adad B, Rasgon B, Ackerson L. Relationship of the facial nerve to the tympanic annulus: A direct anatomic examination. Laryngoscope 1999;109(8):1189–92.
28. Lambert P. Mastoidectomy. In: Cumming's Otolaryngology head and neck surgery. 4th ed. Amsterdam: Elsevier; 2005. pp. 3075–86.
29. Weber, P. Iatrogenic complications from chronic ear surgery. Otolaryngol Clin North Am 2005;38(4):711–22.
30. Vrabec JT. Delayed facial palsy after tympanomastoid surgery. Am J Otol 1999;201(1):26–30.
31. Gantz BJ, Rubinstein JT, Gidley P, Woodworth GG. Surgical management of Bell's palsy. Laryngoscope 1999;109(8):1177–88.

Open Cavity Mastoid Operations

31

John F. Kveton, MD, FACS

Open cavity procedures can be broadly defined as those requiring the removal of the posterior wall of the external auditory canal. These procedures are identified by many names—canal-wall-down mastoidectomy, modified radical mastoidectomy, radical mastoidectomy, and the Bondy mastoidectomy—depending on how the middle ear and the disease are managed. The purpose of open cavity procedures is to exteriorize the mastoid cavity for future monitoring of recurrent cholesteatoma, provide drainage for unresectable temporal bone infection, and, occasionally, provide exposure for difficult-to-access areas of the temporal bone.

HISTORICAL NOTES

In 1873, Von Troltsch[1] was the first surgeon to suggest that Schwartze's[2] simple mastoidectomy technique needed to be modified to reduce persistent otorrhea after initial surgery. He had observed that remnants of cholesteatoma in the attic, antrum, or mastoid process would invariably result in chronic drainage. Von Bergmann[3] applied the term "radical" to any case in which the posterior and superior bony canal walls were removed to develop an open cavity. In 1890, Zaufal[4] described in detail the technique of the radical mastoidectomy to eradicate disease in the middle ear and mastoid. This operation converted the attic, antrum, mastoid process, tympanum, and external auditory canal into a common "radical cavity" that could be inspected and cleaned for the rest of the patient's life. Access to these areas involved in cholesteatoma would therefore prevent recurrence of bone-invading, life-threatening cholesteatoma. One year later, Stacke[5] described the addition of a plastic meatal skin flap, and the radical operation was referred to as the Zaufal or Stacke operation.

The effect of the radical operation on hearing was minimal in most cases in which it was employed. Initial severe necrotic otitis acquired in childhood had already destroyed much of the tympanic membrane, ossicles, and middle ear mucosa, allowing stratified squamous epithelium to extend from the external meatus into the tympanum, attic, antrum, and mastoid process as healing had occurred. Hearing was poor in these cases and so was not made worse by removal of the remnants of the tympanic membrane and ossicles or scraping of the middle ear mucosa in an attempt to close the Eustachian tube. Hearing, however, was at times quite good in patients who presented with cholesteatoma confined to the attic in which the pars tensa of the tympanic membrane was intact. Körner[6] recognized this situation in 1899 and suggested that the tympanic membrane and ossicles could be left in place during radical operations in certain cases of chronic otitis. In 1910, Bondy[7] described the indications and technique for a modification of the radical operation in cases involving a pars flaccida perforation with an intact pars tensa. In this technique, the superior osseous meatal wall and a portion of the posterior osseous meatal wall were removed without disturbing the intact tympanic membrane (except for the attic perforation), ossicles, or tympanic cavity. This technique thus exteriorized the attic and antral cholesteatoma into a permanently open "modified radical" cavity that could be cleaned through the external meatus without further destroying hearing.

Despite the clear indications that Bondy set forth, this modification of the radical mastoid operation was slow to become accepted into practice. In fact, as late as 1929, the Bondy modification was not even mentioned in a standard text of otologic surgery.[8] The overriding concern of otologic surgeons continued to focus on the prevention of intracranial complications of chronic otorrhea, regardless of the effect on hearing. The purpose of surgery was to produce a safe and hopefully dry ear, with little regard for a functioning ear.

Concern for preservation or improvement of hearing, in addition to the prevention of complications from chronic otorrhea, began to evolve after the introduction of Lempert's one-stage fenestration operation in 1938.[9] The early advocates of the Bondy modified operation soon were joined by otologic surgeons in the United States and abroad. The Bondy procedure rapidly evolved as the preferred method for the management of chronic otorrhea with cholesteatoma rather than the classic radical operation, as noted by Baron in 1944.[10] The introduction of tympanoplastic techniques by Zöllner[11] and Wullstein,[12] in the early 1950s, directed attention to reconstruction of the sound-conducting apparatus of the middle ear, further altering the philosophy regarding radical destructive procedures. Successful tympanoplasty required features such as an open, functioning Eustachian tube, normal middle ear mucosa, and portions of normal tympanic membrane and ossicles, present in many ears undergoing radical procedures. By contrast, the radical operation attempted to close the Eustachian tube and remove all remnants of the tympanic membrane, middle ear mucosa, and ossicles, eliminating any possibility of reconstruction. The introduction of tympanoplastic techniques, therefore, was responsible for the emergence of the modified radical mastoidectomy procedure.

Refinements in the modified radical mastoidectomy technique developed because of the drawbacks in the Bondy procedure. Recurrent or persistent aural discharge often occurred because of incomplete removal of infected mastoid air cells. Allowing the cholesteatoma matrix to remain in the attic frequently led to continued bone erosion and granulation tissue formation by the osteolytic enzymes produced by the matrix. Squamous debris accumulation, often resulting in recurrent infection, occurred because of incomplete tip cell removal and high facial ridge. These problems resulted in the Bondy procedure losing favor as the preferred open cavity technique.

The description of the intact canal wall tympanomastoidectomy for removal of cholesteatoma by Jansen[13] in 1958 placed further emphasis on the status of the middle ear in the surgical management of cholesteatoma. Using a postauricular incision, the mastoid air cells are exenterated and the facial recess is opened to access the middle ear. This approach provides improved exposure of the anterior epitympanum and the whole mesotympanum while allowing tympanic membrane reconstruction. Theoretically, maintenance of an aerated middle ear with a normal external auditory canal and tympanic membrane should result in improved postoperative hearing. Hearing restoration has not been consistent using this technique, underscoring the importance of a functional Eustachian tube and the dilemma associated with diagnosing a functional middle ear. The emphasis on Eustachian tube function prompted by the intact canal wall mastoidectomy aided in the evolution of the modified radical mastoidectomy from the Bondy procedure to the complete mastoidectomy with tympanoplasty. Through a postauricular approach, all mastoid air cells are exenterated, the facial nerve is identified, and the facial ridge is taken down to the level of the fallopian canal. Tympanoplasty is performed and a large meatoplasty is created. A dry, self-cleaning mastoid cavity can be maintained in 95% of cases if strict attention to these techniques is paid.[14,15] Epithelial pearls occur in 5 to 6% of cases and can usually be treated by in-office removal without anesthesia. Hearing results often are unchanged from preoperative levels.[16] The details of this technique will be described in greater detail in this chapter.

INDICATIONS FOR THE CLASSIC RADICAL MASTOID OPERATION

Antibiotic therapy, ventilating tube placement, and early identification of ear disease have reduced the incidence of secondary acquired cholesteatomas extensive enough to require treatment by a radical mastoidectomy. Even in the few remaining cases with a large tympanic membrane perforation associated with ossicular destruction and cholesteatoma, the Eustachian tube should not be obliterated, the middle ear mucosa should not be stripped, and the ossicular and tympanic membrane remnants should not be removed, as in the case of the classic radical mastoidectomy, because these structures can be used in future tympanoplasty. The middle ear space should therefore be sealed except when access to the mesotympanum is needed. Thus, indications for the classic radical mastoidectomy are limited to the following unusual situations:

1. Unresectable cholesteatoma extending down the Eustachian tube or into the petrous apex
2. Promontory cochlear fistula caused by cholesteatoma
3. Chronic perilabyrinthine osteitis or cholesteatoma that cannot be removed and must be cleaned or inspected periodically
4. Resection of temporal bone neoplasms with periodic monitoring

INDICATIONS FOR MODIFIED RADICAL MASTOIDECTOMY

Modified radical mastoidectomy is an effective method to manage cholesteatoma in a single-stage approach. Because there are potential disadvantages to the procedure, the author prefers to manage cholesteatoma with the staged intact canal wall technique whenever possible. If successful, this technique eliminates the need for periodic cleaning, avoids the caloric vertigo effect with water exposure, and provides the possibility of improved hearing. As described in Chapter 30, the intact canal wall technique is performed in two stages. The first operation is performed to remove all cholesteatoma and repair the tympanic membrane. Six months later, the second operation is performed to inspect the mastoid and middle ear for residual or recurrent cholesteatoma and to improve hearing by ossicular reconstruction. Since the canal-wall-up technique is technically more demanding, the modified radical mastoidectomy is recommended for the occasional otologic surgeon when confronted with a cholesteatoma extending into the attic, antrum, or mastoid process. The modified radical mastoidectomy should also be selected for patients who are unwilling to submit to the two-stage approach or are in circumstances for which the second procedure would be impractical.

The diagnosis of cholesteatoma in cases of chronic otorrhea deserves brief mention. Most cholesteatomas are associated with a pars flaccida or a marginal tympanic membrane perforation or retraction, in which stratified squamous epithelium extends into the attic. Rarely, a central perforation with mucoid discharge is associated with cholesteatoma in the middle ear and attic. An attic or pars flaccida perforation (actually an invagination) always means a cholesteatoma. Noninfected cholesteatoma debris may be present behind a dry attic perforation. Granulation tissue or a polyp protruding from an attic perforation indicates an infected cholesteatoma in the attic region.

The size of the attic defect bears little relation to the extent of the cholesteatoma in the attic, antrum, or mastoid. Preoperatively, the extent of the cholesteatoma can best be estimated by imaging studies. Noncontrast computed tomography (CT) of the temporal bone provides excellent definition of erosion of vital structures including the semicircular canals, cochlea, fallopian canal, dural plates, and sigmoid sinus. The diagnosis of attic cholesteatoma is made by noting erosion of the scutum with soft tissue accumulation in the attic on CT scan. Surgical planning is enhanced by identifying the degree of mastoid sclerosis and involvement of vital structures. Gadolinium-enhanced magnetic resonance imaging (MRI) may be used as an adjunct to CT to better define pathologic situations. In cases of extensive tegmen plate erosion on CT, MRI will demonstrate the presence of meningoencephalocele, dural inflammation, or intracranial infection. Sigmoid sinus thrombosis, suspected in cases of erosion of the posterior fossa dural plate and sigmoid sinus, may be confirmed by magnetic resonance angiography. Conservative management of cholesteatoma can be attempted when the attic defect is large and the cholesteatoma sac is shallow, allowing the accumulated desquamated debris to be removed by microdebridement and suction. Conservative management is contraindicated when

1. Radiographic evidence of an enlarged, smooth-walled antrum indicates a large cholesteatoma cavity.
2. Otorrhea persists after several cleanings.
3. A very small attic perforation makes cleaning painful, difficult, and unsatisfactory.
4. Cholesteatoma is observed behind the pars tensa.
5. There are symptoms or signs of erosion of vital structures, such as the fallopian canal, semicircular canals, cochlea, or dura.
6. There is hearing loss, either conductive or sensorineural, indicating progression of cholesteatoma.
7. The patient is uncooperative or is geographically unable to return for necessary management.

In actual clinical situations, the management of cholesteatoma is surgical. It is rare that an otologist will treat cholesteatoma medically. Modified radical mastoidectomy should be considered in cases of cholesteatoma in which there is a high risk of residual disease or risk of recurrence. The indications for modified radical mastoidectomy can be divided into absolute and relative indications. Absolute indications include unresectable disease, an unreconstructable posterior canal wall, failure of a first-stage canal-wall-up procedure because of poor Eustachian tube function, and inadequate patient follow-up. The relative indications for an open cavity procedure include disease in an only hearing ear or in a dead ear, medical illness, severe otologic or central nervous system complications, and neoplasms. An additional relative indication is poor Eustachian tube function.

CONTRAINDICATIONS FOR THE OPEN CAVITY MASTOID OPERATION

Removal of the posterior canal wall is contraindicated in cases of chronic otitis media without cholesteatoma. Unless the surgeon is certain of the diagnosis of cholesteatoma, the procedure should begin as a simple mastoidectomy, preserving the posterior canal wall until cholesteatoma is identified. Extensive debridement of mastoid or atticoantral infection can be accomplished with preservation of the posterior canal wall. Open cavity procedures are contraindicated in cases of acute otitis media with coalescent mastoiditis, persistent secretory otitis media, or chronic allergic otitis media. Tuberculous otitis media should be treated primarily with chemotherapy, with surgical intervention reserved for persistent drainage. Relative contraindications for open cavity procedures include wide exposure of the sigmoid sinus, dura, and the facial nerve caused by aggressive disease.

TECHNIQUE OF RADICAL MASTOIDECTOMY AND BONDY MODIFIED RADICAL MASTOIDECTOMY

The techniques of the radical mastoidectomy and the Bondy radical mastoidectomy are presented for historical interest and perspective. The objective of these procedures was to remove safely all bone-invading disease; create an accessible, exteriorized cavity for lifelong cleaning and care; and promote epithelialization of the cavity with healthy skin. Hearing improvement was of secondary importance.

The radical and Bondy operations began with exposure of the attic and antrum, followed by removal of the superior and posterior canal walls. By performing the "inside-out" mastoidectomy, the resultant cavity was smaller than if a complete mastoidectomy with tympanoplasty were performed. However, as a result of this approach, peripheral air cells were isolated from the eustachian tube. If the mucosa continued to produce mucus, it discharged into the mastoid cavity.

Atticotomy Bone Removal

The incision and atticotomy bone removal are the same for the classic radical mastoidectomy and for the Bondy modification. The endaural incision is made in two steps, with either a Lempert triangular knife or a Bard-Parker scalpel with a #15 blade, as follows:

1. Beginning at "12 o'clock" on the superior canal wall and about 1 cm from the outer edge of the canal, the first incision extends at about the same depth down the posterior canal wall in the incisura terminalis nearly to "6 o'clock," then at right angles outward about 2 or 3 mm to the edge of, but not into, the conchal cartilage.
2. Beginning again at "12 o'clock" on the superior canal wall where the first incision began, the second incision extends directly upward, still in the incisura terminalis, to a point about halfway between the meatus and the upper edge of the auricle. For greater exposure, this vertical incision can be extended as far upward as desired without encountering any important structure except for the temporalis muscle and branches of the superficial temporal artery and vein.

The two incisions, now continuous and at first through the skin only, are deepened to include periosteum, with the knife held at an angle so that it will not plunge into the bony canal. A broad periosteal elevator is inserted into the incision, directed posteriorly, and the periosteum over the entire mastoid process is elevated posteriorly and anteriorly only over the posterior root of the zygoma. Failure to elevate the periosteum sufficiently widely is a common cause of failure to obtain adequate exposure by this approach.

The self-retaining (Shambaugh) endaural retractor is inserted with retraction of periosteum, exposing the bone above and behind the osseous meatus, from the posterior root of the zygomatic process to 2 or 3 cm posterior to the suprameatal spine of Henle and from the temporal line above to the lower portion of the mastoid process below. Wide retraction of periosteum is essential to "mobilize the incision," as emphasized by Lempert.[9]

Atticotomy by means of a surgical cutting bur removes outer cortex just above and behind the meatus over a semilunar area. As the surgeon deepens the initial groove, he/she watches for the pink color shining through the bone and then for a little bleeding as the middle fossa dura is approached. An effort is made to avoid unnecessary dural exposure as the groove between the dura and the superior meatal wall is deepened. The notch of Rivinus is located by passing a narrow periosteal elevator inward along the superior osseous meatal wall. The epitympanum is encountered shortly before the groove reaches the depth of the notch of Rivinus, and if the preoperative diagnosis was correct, the white smooth wall of the cholesteatoma sac is identified. The middle fossa dura might resemble the wall of the cholesteatoma, requiring careful removal of bone anteriorly, inferiorly, and posteriorly before the surgeon is sure.

The sac is opened cautiously (in case dura is mistaken for the sac wall), the cholesteatoma contents are removed by suction and instrumentation, and the sac's furthest extensions anteriorly, superiorly, and posteriorly are explored with a blunt mastoid searcher. Bone cortex and overhang removal proceeds with a cutting bur, curet, or rongeur until the entire cholesteatoma sac lies exposed. In some cases, the cholesteatoma lining or matrix is smooth, with a thin layer of connective tissue between it and eburnated surrounding bone. More often, the cholesteatoma matrix is closely applied to bone with finger-like extensions into small cells and haversian canals. All cholesteatoma extensions must be followed to their end with the aid of the operating microscope. The entire matrix is removed, with the following exceptions:

1. Matrix firmly adherent to exposed dura or sigmoid sinus may be left rather than risk injury to these structures.
2. Matrix over a fistula of a semicircular canal may be left to avoid postoperative serous labyrinthitis. Some surgeons prefer to dissect matrix from the fistula and immediately apply a thin fascia graft.
3. Matrix firmly attached to exposed facial nerve may be left.
4. Matrix extending into the mesotympanum and covering the stapes footplate may be left at the initial operation rather than opening the vestibule, with the risk of serous or suppurative labyrinthitis. At a second operation, after the ear is dry and healed, cholesteatoma matrix can be dissected from the oval window, and tympanoplasty can proceed, as described in Chapter 28.

Bone Removal Beyond Cholesteatoma

Remembering that chronic otorrhea is the result of infected epidermal debris in the cholesteatoma sac, in most cases, evacuation of the sac, removal of matrix (epithelial lining), and curettage of softened osteitic bone adjacent to the matrix suffice to control the disease. The surgeon needs to exercise prudent judgment with regard to mastoid cells outside the cholesteatoma sac. These cells may be infected and osteitic (softened), with granulations requiring removal, but in many cases, mastoid cells are intact and need not be removed.

Taking Down the Bridge and the Facial Ridge

The remaining superior osseous meatal wall bridging the notch of Rivinus is removed in small bites with a narrow rongeur after first elevating the meatal skin from bone. With a small (000) curet, always working outward away from the fallopian canal and facial nerve, the anterior and posterior spines of the notch of Rivinus, composing the anterior and posterior buttresses of the bridge, are taken down. The tympanic segment of the facial canal is identified and kept in view while ossicles or remnants of ossicles are inspected. Wherever cholesteatoma envelops or extends onto the medial surface of the malleus head or incus, these ossicles must be removed. When cholesteatoma matrix lies against and lateral to these ossicles, the matrix may be left or carefully removed and the ossicles are left undisturbed. When the long process of the incus is absent and matrix lies against the mobile stapes head, with excellent hearing producing nature's myringostapediopexy, this portion of the matrix is left undisturbed.

The step in the radical or Bondy operations most often accomplished poorly is taking down the posterior osseous meatal wall, which, deeper in, houses the posterior bend and vertical facial nerve and thus is called the facial ridge. The approximate position of the facial nerve is located by three usually dependable landmarks: the bony horizontal semicircular canal above, the tympanomastoid suture in the posterior meatal wall, and the digastric ridge in the mastoid tip. Because the tip cells rarely require removal in radical and Bondy mastoidectomies, the surgeon needs to dispense with the digastric ridge in the mastoid tip as a dependable landmark.

The bony facial ridge is taken down slowly and carefully with a drill or curet, working under the operating microscope, always parallel to and never across the direction of the facial nerve, until the bowl of the surgical cavity after removal of disease is flush with intact (or perforated) tympanic membrane. A pinkish color and bleeding are encountered when the facial nerve is approached. It is better not to expose the nerve unnecessarily because a Bell's palsy–type paresis occurs more often when this nerve is exposed than when not. Whereas this paresis, beginning 1 to 6 or 7 days postoperatively, generally recovers completely in a matter of weeks, residual weakness with synkinesis and spasm can ensue, just as occurs after recovery of some cases of Bell's palsy.

Preparation of the Meatal Plastic Skin Flap

The plastic-pedicled skin flap that is turned back to cover the facial ridge and the floor of the completed operative cavity consists of the skin and periosteum of the entire superior osseous meatal wall and most of the posterior meatal wall. As the atticotomy proceeds and the bridge is being taken down, a narrow periosteal elevator separates the skin and periosteum from the superior and posterior meatal walls. With a curved meatal knife and iris scissors, an incision along the anterosuperior angle of the meatus frees the plastic flap anteriorly. The connective tissue band that enters the tympanosquamous suture needs to be cut, and posteriorly similar but less pronounced connective tissue in the tympanomastoid suture needs to be separated, beginning at the annulus and working outward. The outer edge of the meatal flap may need to be thinned to make it lie smoothly over the facial ridge.

Toilet of the Tympanum

In the classic radical mastoidectomy, the tympanic cavity is inspected minutely under the operating microscope. Healthy skin and remnants of tympanic membrane closing off the Eustachian tube are not disturbed, but any polyps, granulations, or remaining mucosa are removed. Instrumentation in the oval window and round window niches should be avoided because of the possibility of opening the labyrinth. If the Eustachian tube orifice is open and lined with mucosa, an attempt is made to close it in the classic radical operation after curetting its mucosa. In curetting the mouth of the Eustachian tube, remember that the internal carotid artery is separated from it only by a thin plate of bone. Should curettage produce brisk bleeding, the bleeding is usually from the venous plexus that surrounds the carotid artery in its journey through the temporal bone and not from the artery. In removing a mass of granulations from the stapes and the oval window, start at the pyramidal eminence and strip the granulations in a forward direction parallel to the stapedius tendon to keep from dislodging the stapes. Once the bone-invading infected cholesteatoma in the attic, antrum, and sometimes the mastoid process has been removed, any small granulations in the middle ear caused by the purulent drainage soon dry up with local conservative treatment.

Final Inspection of the Cavity

The completed open radical or Bondy cavity is irrigated with warm saline (Tis-U-Sol® or Ringer's) solution for hemostasis and for removal of any bone particles or other debris. Under the operating microscope, the cavity is inspected minutely for any remaining osteitis or cholesteatoma remnants. There must be no cortical overhang and no part of the cavity that is not perfectly accessible and exteriorized from the external meatus.

Atticotomy From Within the Meatus

For a small cholesteatoma sac, lateral to the incus and malleus head and with a large external meatus, it may be possible to perform an endomeatal atticotomy as follows:

1. A stapes type of meatal flap extended forward superiorly and outwardly is followed by removal of the meatal rim to exteriorize the small attic cholesteatoma sac.
2. The surgeon may then dissect the sac and remove it intact, or may leave the matrix and exteriorize the sac as a small Bondy radical cavity.
3. Should the surgeon find that the cholesteatoma pocket is larger than anticipated, he/she should proceed with an endaural incision and atticotomy, as described previously.

Placement of the Meatal Flap and Packing of the Cavity

The plastic flap of meatal skin is turned back to cover the facial ridge, taking care not to cover areas of remaining matrix or even areas that had been covered by matrix. A closed sleeve of surgical rayon or wide strips of surgical rayon are inserted to line the cavity, with cotton balls soaked in sulfisoxazole otic (or ophthalmic) solution placed firmly, but not tightly, to fill the cavity. At no point should cotton touch the raw surface. One or two sutures partially close the endaural incision, but the final meatal opening must be packed wide open to three or four times the original size so that when healing is complete, the final meatus is twice the former size, and the healed exteriorized cavity can easily be inspected and kept clean.

Skin Grafting the Radical or Bondy Cavity

Siebenmann[17] was the first to recommend skin grafting by the method of Thiersch to promote rapid healing of the radical cavity. Experience in nearly 100 fenestration operations treated in this manner convinced Shambaugh[18] that primary split-thickness skin grafting of the operative cavity is not desirable. When such a graft took by first intention, the epidermal lining of the healed cavity was closely applied to the bone without an intervening layer of connective tissue. Not only was the surface of the stratified squamous epithelium rough and uneven, but also it continued to desquamate excessively, and was very subject to localized areas of breakdown and granulations with discharge, and demonstrated a distinct tendency to invasion of crevices and cells requiring a later revision. With a thoroughly performed radical or Bondy operation with removal of matrix, the cavity nearly always heals without troublesome granulations or suppuration provided that careful sterile technique is observed in the operations and postoperative dressings. Should the surgeon wish to shorten the time of final healing, a skin graft may be applied to the cavity 2 or 3 weeks postoperatively after it has become lined by a thin layer of healthy granulations that then provide the desired subepithelial connective tissue layer.[19]

TECHNIQUE OF MODIFIED RADICAL MASTOIDECTOMY

Modified radical mastoidectomy, also known as complete mastoidectomy and tympanoplasty, is an evolutionary surgical development that attempts to incorporate the major goal of cholesteatoma surgery (i.e., exteriorization of disease) with sealing of the middle ear space to avoid chronic drainage from exposed mucous membrane. A primary feature of the modified radical procedure is complete removal of the posterior canal wall, the major reason for failure of the Bondy procedure. The Bondy procedure was predicated on the philosophy of limited dissection of the canal wall and mastoid region, and this technique, although often sparing hearing in the short term, resulted in recurrent cholesteatoma or at least persistent aural discharge because of subsequent infection of the remaining mastoid air cells. The radical mastoidectomy, although effectively dealing with the shortcoming of the Bondy procedure by more extensive bone dissection, results in chronic aural drainage because of the impossibility of removal of all remaining mucosa in the exposed middle ear. The modification of the radical procedure (i.e., adding the technique of tympanoplasty) potentially eliminates the expected intermittent discharge from the middle ear mucosa. Hearing, it should be noted, is a secondary consideration of the modified radical procedure.

Preoperative Assessment

The decision to perform a modified radical mastoidectomy rather than a staged intact canal wall approach depends on the extent and location of the disease, previous surgery, Eustachian tube function and patient age, medical condition, and aftercare preference. Careful microscopic inspection and cleaning of the ear aid in the decision. Pus, mucus, and cholesteatomatous debris should be removed under microscopic suction. Polyps can be removed with gentle traction with the suction or microcup forceps. Significant retraction should be avoided since the polyp may be attached to the facial nerve, matrix of a labyrinthine fistula, or stapes superstructure or footplate. Extensive destruction of the posterior canal wall with obvious cholesteatoma invading the mastoid indicates the need for modified radical mastoidectomy. Active suppuration should be controlled prior to surgery whenever possible. Acetic acid (1.5% solution) irrigations followed by antibiotic otic drops should be instituted for several weeks prior to surgery. Acetic acid solution is made by mixing one part of white vinegar to two parts of boiling water. After cooling, the solution is instilled into the ear several times using an infant nasal-bulb syringe to mechanically debride the area. Antibiotic eardrops are instilled after the irrigations, which should be performed two to four times daily. The author prefers to use neomycin or aminoglycoside-based corticosteroid otic preparations rather than the newer flouroquinolone preparations in these cases. In cases of extensive mucosal infection and cellulitis, a 10- to 14-day course of oral fluoroquinolones with gram-positive coverage is indicated prior to surgery.

Surgical Procedure

After induction of general anesthesia, the ear is prepared by pouring povidone-iodine solution into the ear canal and scrubbing the auricle and postauricular area with povidone-iodine. One percent lidocaine with 1:100,000 epinephrine is injected into the postauricular region and the ear canal for hemostasis. Incisions are made in the ear canal for the vascular strip (Figure 31–1A).[20] A postauricular incision is made about 1 cm behind the postauricular crease and a plane is developed between the subcutaneous tissue and the temporalis muscle and periosteum of the mastoid. Several large pieces of areolar tissue and temporalis fascia are harvested and set aside to dry. A horizontal incision is made superior to the temporal line through the temporalis muscle and a vertical incision is carried down to the mastoid tip, perpendicular to and bisecting the horizontal incision (Figure 31–1B). The mastoid bone is exposed using a Lempert elevator, and as the periosteum is raised into the ear canal, the vascular strip is elevated and reflected out of the ear canal anteriorly using a self-retaining retractor (Figure 31–1C). In revision cases, elevation of the scarred musculoperiosteum must be done carefully to avoid injury to exposed dura or sigmoid sinus. Canal wall flaps are elevated and rotated anteriorly (Figure 31–1D) prior to entering the middle ear. Disease in the mesotympanum is first removed, using the malleus handle and incus as landmarks. Cholesteatoma, polyps, and granulation tissue are removed from all areas except the posterosuperior quadrant; any atrophic tympanic membrane is removed and the middle ear is prepared for grafting. Once all available landmarks have been identified, the posterosuperior quadrant is inspected. If disease extends into the attic, dissection of disease ceases and Gelfoam with epinephrine is packed into the middle ear.

Bone Work

A simple mastoidectomy is now begun using a large cutting bur. The canal wall should be left up in all but the most contracted mastoid cavities. All mastoid air cells should be removed with exposure of the middle fossa and posterior fossa dural plates, the sigmoid sinus, digastric ridge, and bony canal wall (Figure 31–1E). Cholesteatoma and granulations filling the central mastoid tract can be removed at this time. As the labyrinth is approached, the lateral capsule of the cholesteatoma should be opened and the cholesteatoma should be removed, leaving the medial matrix of the cholesteatoma on the bony labyrinth. Under higher-power magnification, the matrix can be inspected for the telltale blue line or palpated for the presence of a labyrinthine fistula. The vertical segment of the facial nerve should now be identified, followed by opening of the facial recess (Figure 31–1F). This is best accomplished by using the digastric ridge and the lateral semicircular canal as landmarks. If the incus is involved with cholesteatoma, the incudostapedial joint is identified through the facial recess and cut and the incus is removed. The posterior canal wall can now be safely taken down with a rongeur and the facial ridge can be lowered until a thin layer of bone remains over the vertical segment of the facial nerve (Figure 31–1G). The chorda tympani nerve must be sacrificed. Disease can now be removed from the oval window region and horizontal segment of the facial nerve. The malleus, or any remnant of the malleus, is removed by cutting the tensor tympani tendon at the cochleariform process, which provides access to the anterior epitympanum. The anterior epitympanum should be drilled down to become continuous with the anterior canal wall. The inferior canal wall must be drilled away until the inferior canal wall and mastoid tip are confluent, with no bony overhang to obscure the mastoid tip. This dissection more widely exposes the middle ear, which can now be reinspected for residual disease. The sinus tympani is the most difficult region to investigate. If disease extends into this region, and if the stapes is absent, the pyramidal eminence can be removed with a small diamond bur. Right angle hooks, whirlybird dissectors, micromirrors, and surgical telescopes can aid in cholesteatoma removal from this region. Tympanoplasty should not be performed if there is a question of residual cholesteatoma in the sinus tympani or hypotympanum.

At this point, the cavity should be smooth-walled and free of active disease (Figure 31–1H). Copious irrigation is used to lower the bacterial count and aid in hemostasis. The cavity should approach an ovoid or rectangular shape, with

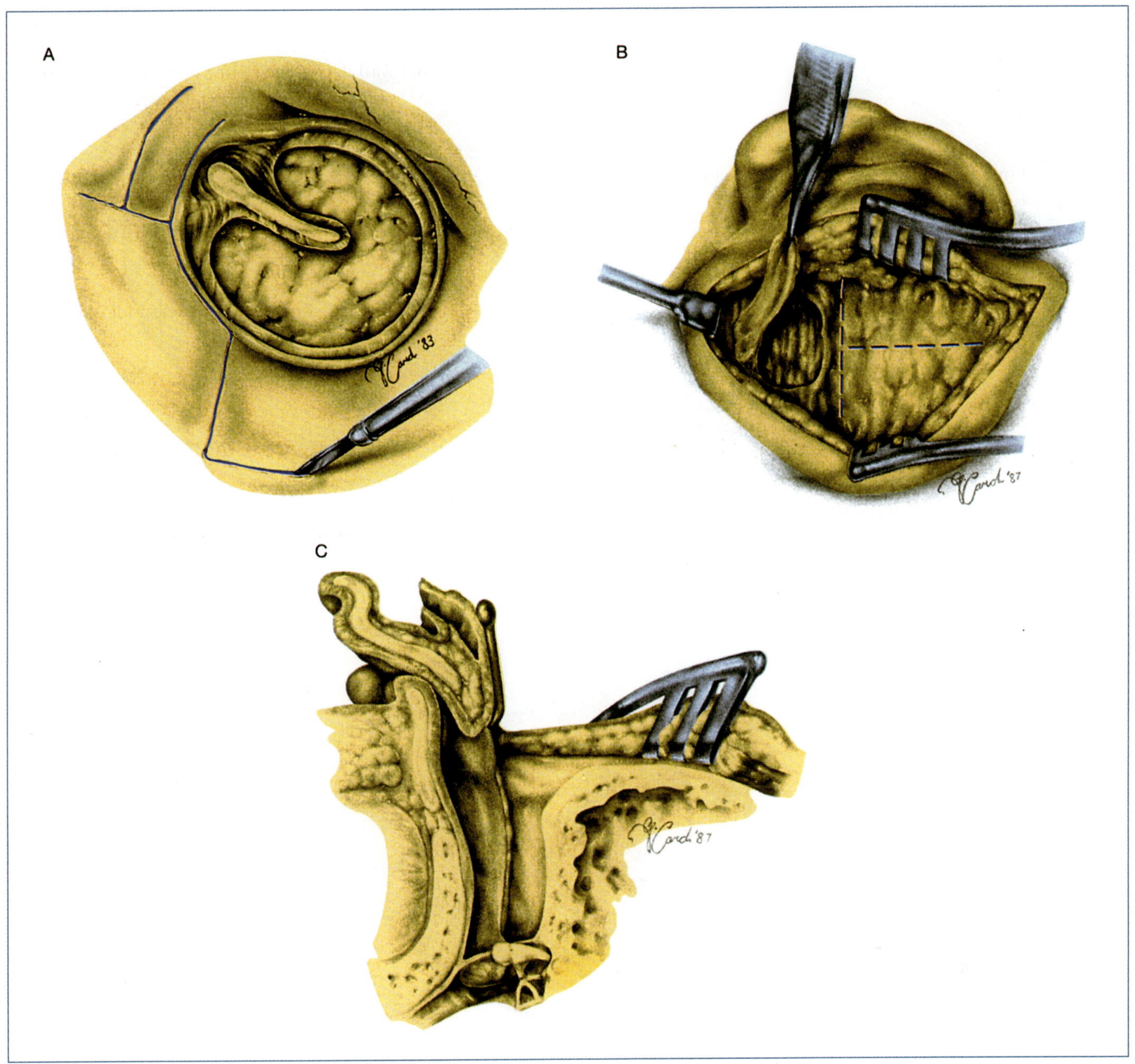

FIGURE 31–1 • *A*, Standard tympanoplastic canal incisions outline the vascular strip as well as the superior and inferior canal wall flaps. *B*, Loose areolar fascia is harvested from temporal muscle, and a T-shaped incision is made in soft tissue over mastoid. *C*, Exposure of mastoid in crosssection showing vascular strip held forward under anterior blade of retractor.

Continued

the facial ridge low. The stapes, if present, should be the only remaining ossicle. A portion of the anterior tympanic membrane may remain after removal of disease. The mastoid bowl has been saucerized and makes a gentle transition into the depths of the mastoid bone without ledges. This attention to detail helps ensure soft tissue obliteration of much of the cavity space.

Rarely, the mastoid is so contracted that the posterior canal wall is taken down as the antrum is exposed. This approach is potentially more dangerous to the facial nerve and ossicular chain and should be avoided whenever possible. Regardless of when the canal wall is removed, the remainder of the technique remains the same.

Meatoplasty

One percent lidocaine with 1:100,000 epinephrine is infiltrated into the conchal bowl. The entire posterior aspect of the conchal bowl is exposed using sharp dissection with an iris scissors through the fibrous periosteum and soft tissue. With a finger in the conchal bowl, a semilunar incision is made into the cartilage posteriorly until the knife tip is felt through the anterior skin. This crescent-shaped cartilage measures about 1.5 × 2 cm

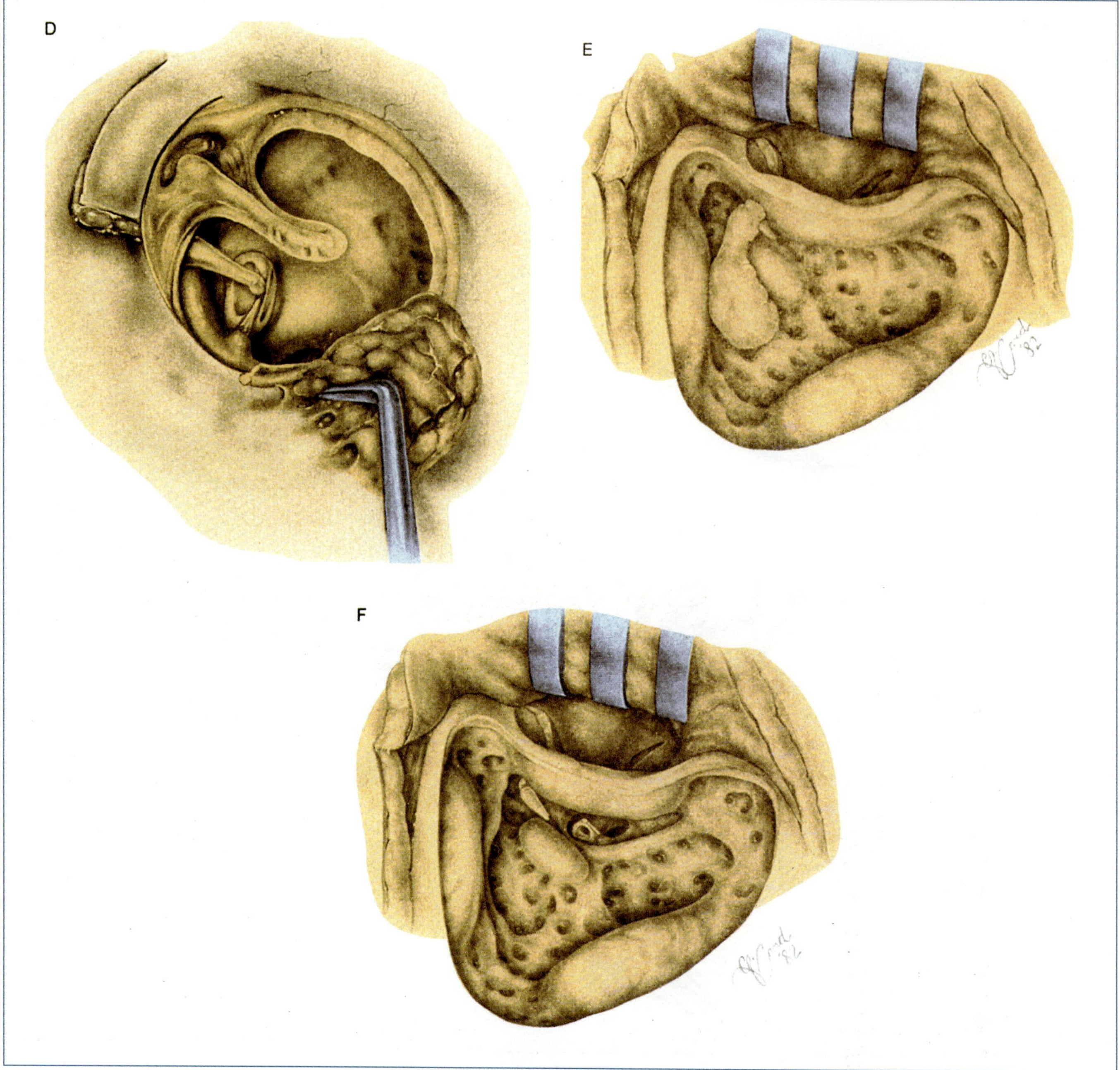

FIGURE 31–1 • *Continued. D*, The inferior flap is elevated to the fibrous annulus with a House #2 knife. *E*, With the posterior external auditory canal (EAC) wall preserved, a complete, simple mastoidectomy demonstrates the anatomy and the pathology. *F*, Through the facial recess, disease can be well managed in an intact canal wall (ICW) context. The malleus head and incus are shown for orientation only. They are customarily removed. Incudostapedial disarticulation is demonstrated.

Continued

(Figure 31–1I). A Körner flap is now developed by making incisions through the external auditory canal skin. An inferior incision is begun in the inferior canal at 6 o'clock, carried into the conchal bowl, and curved around the inferior margin of the bowl. A superior incision is made at 12 o'clock and carried between the tragus and the anterior helix. These incisions create a long (vascular strip) flap that is based in the posterosuperior aspect of the conchal bowl and will constitute the back wall of the mastoid cavity (Figure 31–1J).

Grafting

The auricle and flap are retracted anteriorly to expose the mastoid and middle ear. Epinephrine-soaked absorbable gelatin sponge is removed and the middle ear and Eustachian tube are packed with saline-moistened absorbable gelatin sponge to the level of the anterior annulus (Figure 31–1K). The fascia graft is placed medial to the anterior annulus and drum remnant, extending over the stapes to the facial ridge into the mastoid

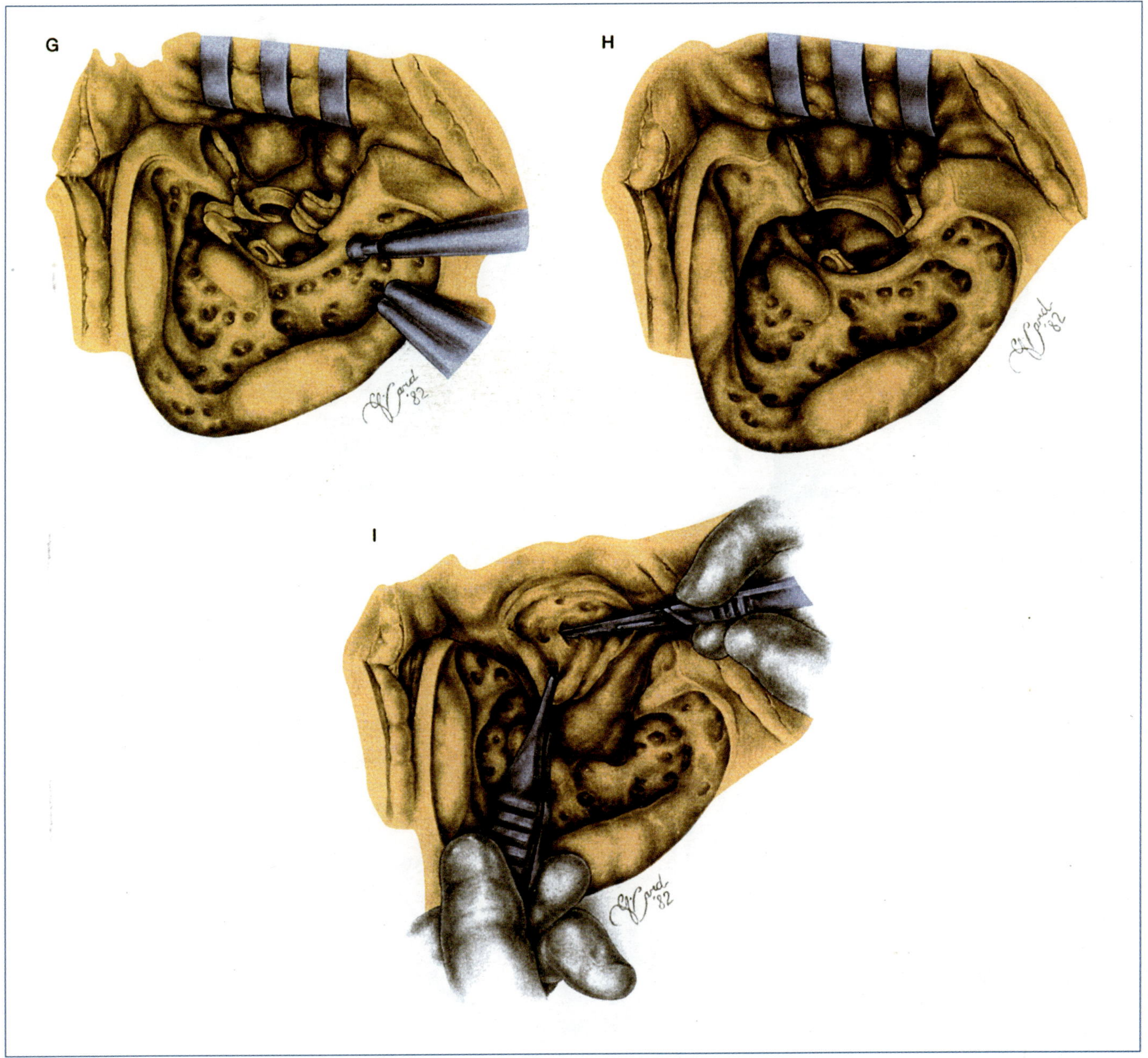

FIGURE 31–1 • *Continued. G*, The posterior EAC wall must be lowered to the visible facial nerve. The chorda tympani is sacrificed. Canal wall flaps are preserved. *H*, The facial ridge must be lowered to the visible facial nerve. The chorda tympani is sacrificed. Canal wall flaps are preserved. *H*, The facial ridge must be low. The inferior EAC wall must be drilled down so that the hypotympanum and mastoid tip are confluent. The same applies to the antero superior EAC wall and anterior epitympanum. The stapes is the only ossicular remnant. *I*, The meatoplasty begins by excising, from behind, conchal cartilage.

Continued

bowl (Figure 31–1L). As much of the mastoid bone as possible should be covered with fascia grafts to reduce granulations and speed epithelialization. In particular, perilabyrinthine, retrofacial, zygomatic, and peritubal cell tracts should be covered.

Ossicular reconstruction is limited in these cases. If the stapes is present, the fascia graft is placed directly onto the capitulum. If the stapes is lower than the facial ridge, the height can be augmented by using a malleus head goblet prosthesis atop the capitulum (Figure 31–1M and N). With an absent stapes, ossicular reconstruction with autologous tissue is preferred over alloplastic prostheses. Once the fascia graft is in place, the surface is covered with polymixin B and bacitracin ophthalmic ointment (Figure 31–1O and P).

The Körner flap must now be secured to the musculoperiosteum at the edge of the mastoid cavity. A 3.0 polyglactin 910 (Vicryl®) suture is placed subdermally at both edges of the base of the Körner flap and affixed posteriorly to the soft tissue. The tension of these sutures is adjusted until the meatus has the desired shape (Figure 31–1Q). Overtightening of the sutures, especially the superior suture will result in a protruding auricle.

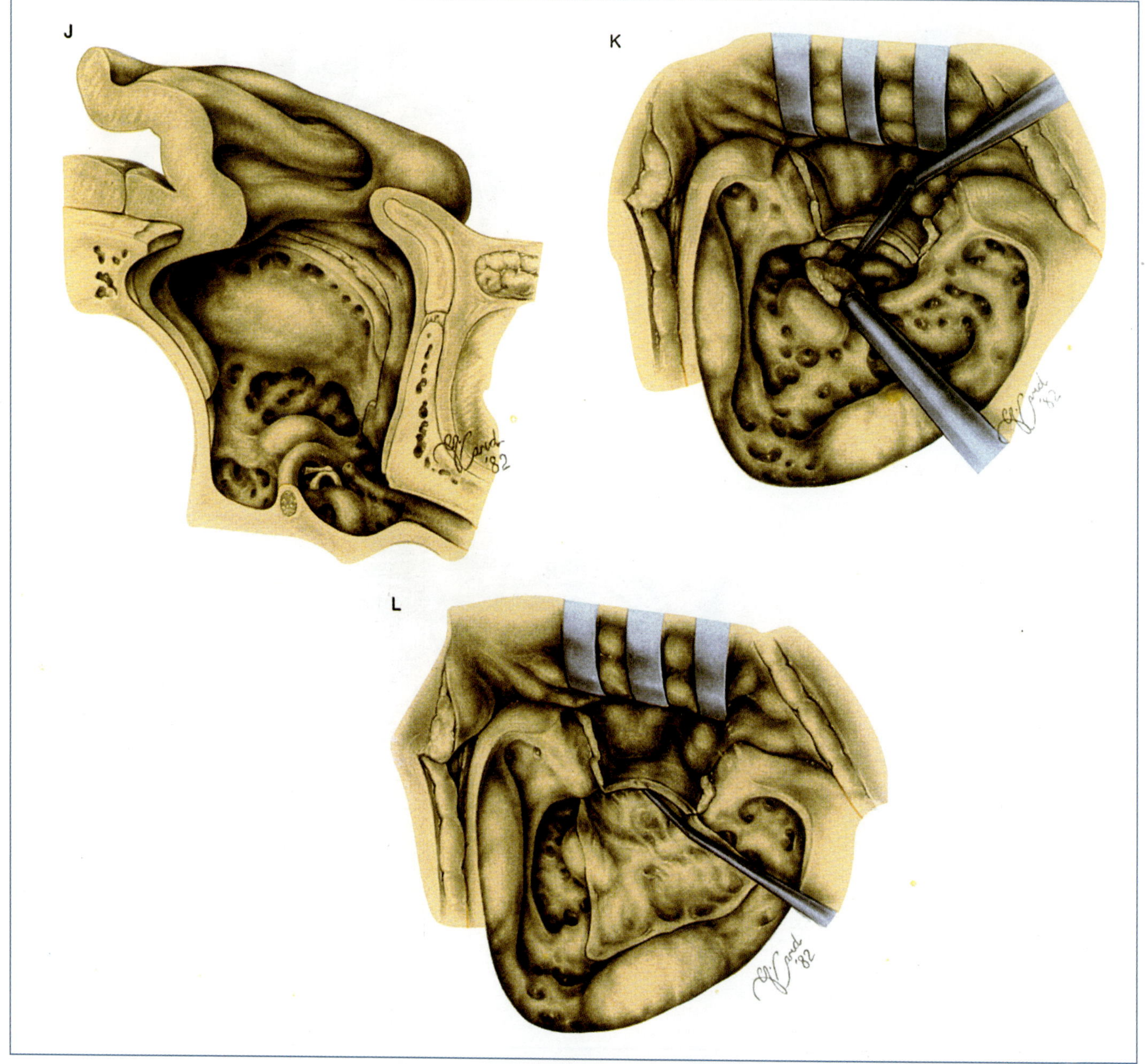

FIGURE 31–1 • *Continued. J*, Superior and inferior meatal incisions create a posterior Körner's flap, shown here as it will be sutured in place. *K*, An absorbable gelatin sponge (Gelfoam) bed is prepared for the tympanic membrane graft. Note the Körner's flap free in the meatus. *L*, The graft is placed medial to the tympanic membrane remnant, superiorly over the labyrinth and posteriorly over the facial ridge. The graft is applied directly atop the stapes superstructure.

Continued

The postauricular incision is closed with a subcuticular absorbable suture. The mastoid bowl is filled with ointment or packed with gauze, and a mastoid dressing is applied.

Postoperative Care

The mastoid dressing is removed on the first postoperative day. A large piece of cotton is kept in the meatus, and a postauricular dressing is placed. Copious drainage occurs through the meatus for about 1 week, requiring frequent cotton changes. The postauricular dressing is removed on the second postoperative day, and antibiotic ointment is applied to the incision for 1 week. The patient is instructed to keep the ear dry and avoid nose blowing. Pain medication is prescribed, but oral antibiotics are not used routinely. The patient returns in 2 to 3 weeks. At the first postoperative visit, any area that has not been grafted is covered by a layer of granulation tissue. Exuberant granulation tissue should be debrided and treated with silver nitrate. Silver nitrate should not be used near an exposed facial nerve to avoid facial palsy. The granulation tissue should then be painted

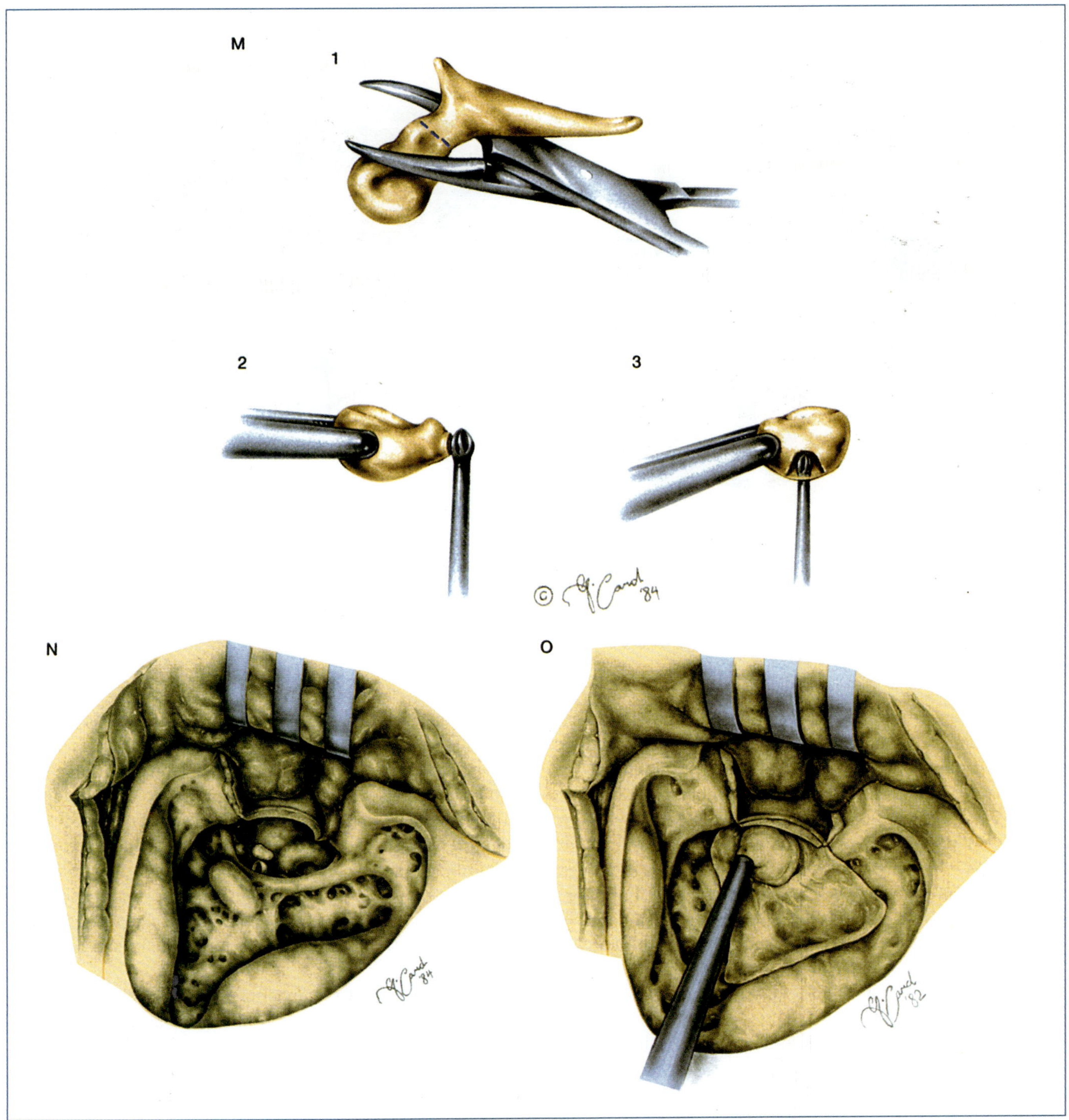

FIGURE 31–1 • *Continued*. *M*, When the facial ridge is high, a sculpted homograft malleus head can be constructed to augment the height of the stapes superstructure. *N*, The sculpted homograft fits atop the stapedial capitulum, ready for grafting. *O*, Ointment "packing" fills the cavity.

Continued

with 2% gentian violet and the patient is instructed to use antibiotic otic drops two or three times per day until the next (at 2 to 3 weeks) visit. Drainage decreases with ensuing visits as re-epithelialization occurs. As epithelialization progresses, acetic acid irrigations can replace the use of antibiotic otic drops. Once the cavity is healed, the patient should return for a yearly visit and is given full water sport privileges.

COMPLICATIONS OF OPEN CAVITY PROCEDURES

The complications associated with open cavity mastoid operations are identical to those possible in any procedure in which the mastoid bone is removed and structures in the middle ear are manipulated. These include deafness or further hearing loss,

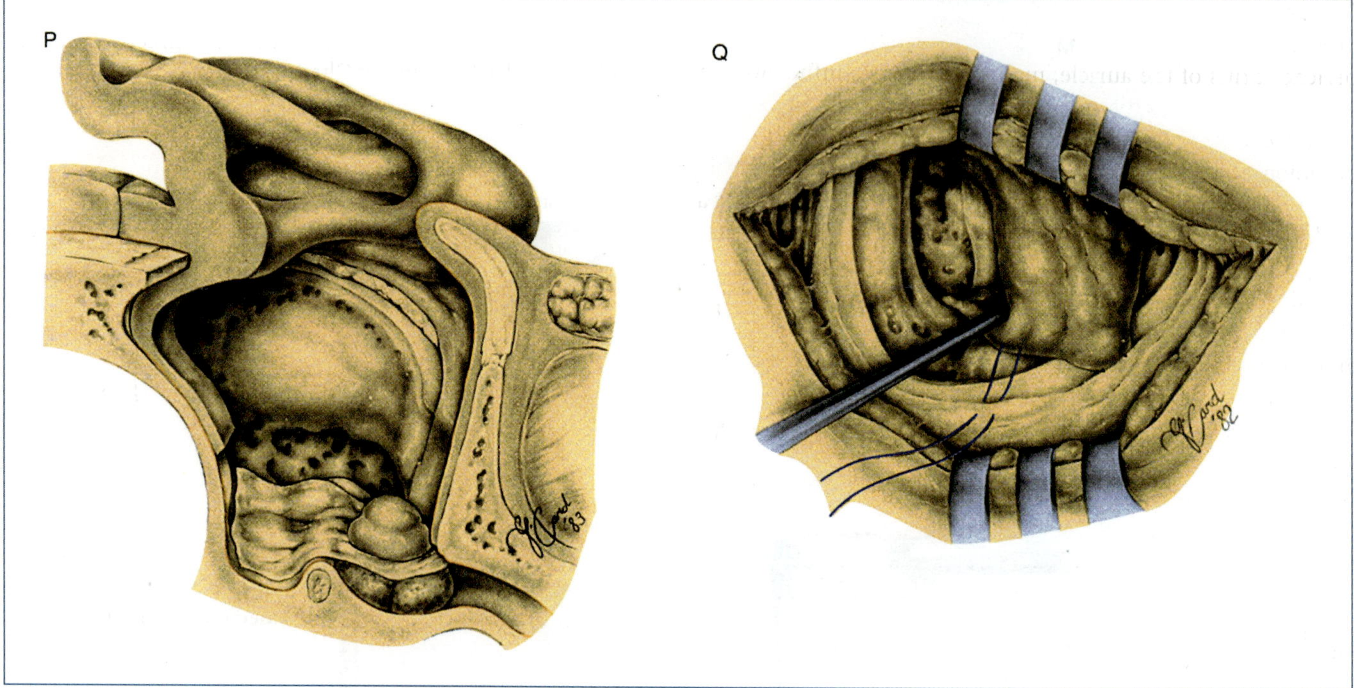

FIGURE 31–1 • *Continued. P,* In cross-section, the low facial ridge, graft bed, with graft and initial ointment, is demonstrated. The posterior meatal flap is illustrated in the desired position. *Q,* The posterior flap is sewn to the posterior soft tissue margins of the incision. Tension on the sutures can be adjusted to open the meatus but avoid tipping the auricle.

facial paralysis, vestibular symptoms, cerebrospinal fluid leak, infection, and recurrent cholesteatoma or drainage. The incidence of certain complications may be higher, though, because of the nature of disease within the mastoid bone that requires a more extensive procedure, such as an open cavity procedure. Facial nerve paralysis is the most common major complication associated with open cavity procedures. Although facial nerve injury is at times unavoidable because of the extent of disease, most cases of postoperative facial paralysis are a result of unrecognized facial nerve trauma at the hands of an unskilled otologic surgeon. Intraoperative facial nerve monitoring is performed during most otologic procedures, but should not be relied upon to identify the facial nerve. Normal surgical landmarks are often distorted in the diseased mastoid, and positive identification of vital structures is mandatory to perform a successful open cavity procedure. Surgical discipline must be maintained during the procedure to identify vital structures in a systematic fashion as the surgery progresses.

In particular, it is critical to identify the facial nerve throughout its course in the mastoid as soon as possible, which is best accomplished after the lateral semicircular canal and any ossicles within the posterior epitympanum have been identified. Especially in revision cases, the most effective way to locate the vertical segment of the facial nerve is to follow the digastric ridge to the stylomastoid foramen. The bony dissection may then proceed in a proximal direction to uncover the vertical segment as it approaches the second genu. This method also underscores the importance of preserving the posterior canal wall until late in the dissection since early identification of the nerve reduces the risk of injury as the canal wall is taken down. Early identification of the nerve also ensures that the facial ridge will be brought down appropriately (i.e., until the nerve sheath can be identified through a thin layer of bone remaining on the fallopian canal). In cases of disease obliterating the stylomastoid foramen, the fallopian canal can be identified by following the chorda tympani nerve distally to the facial nerve trunk. This junction is approximately 5 mm from the stylomastoid foramen. Less specifically, the distal portion of the second genu of the facial nerve is found just inferior to the level of the lateral semicircular canal.

The management of postoperative facial paralysis bears brief mention. Facial nerve injury must be considered when any noticeable loss of facial nerve function has been identified. Eye closure is often inappropriately relied on as an indicator of total facial nerve paralysis. The tonus of the orbicularis oculi muscle appears to persist longer than that of the remaining facial musculature, and it is not unusual for eye closure to persist for several days after facial nerve injury has occurred. (Witness the fact that eye closure persists in the immediate postoperative period for patients with known facial nerve transection after removal of an acoustic tumor.) Unless facial nerve injury was noted at the time of the surgery, the axiom "Never let the sun set on a facial paralysis" should be followed. The patient should be returned to the operating room as soon as possible for exploration and decompression of the facial nerve. Especially in difficult cases, it is the author's policy to maintain sterility in the operating suite until the patient displays normal facial movement on emergence from general anesthesia.

The second most common complication of open cavity procedures is wound infection. This infection usually results in perichondritis of the auricle, manifested by a painful, swollen auricle with copious discharge. Pseudomonas aeruginosa is the causative organism, and treatment comprises high-dose fluoroquinolones and antibiotic-corticosteroid drops.

A "chocolate" or mucous retention cyst can occur in a healed mastoid cavity as a result of a collection of serum within a mucous membrane–lined pocket. Simple aspiration of the mucoid, brownish serum will reduce the size of the cyst, but recurrence is usually the case. Definitive management requires exposure of the cyst and complete removal of the mucoperiosteal pocket.

Cholesteatoma recurrence in open cavity procedures occurs in 4 to 28% of cases[21] and is usually caused by inaccessible disease or a remnant of matrix that was amputated at the time of surgery. Through routine follow-up, these "pearls" of recurrent cholesteatoma can be readily identified and removed in the office. Extensive recurrent disease, with its attendant complications, is more commonly found behind an intact canal wall rather than in an open cavity.

Recurrent aural drainage from a previously healed and dry cavity is usually the result of poor aural toilet. Breakdown of the epithelial lining and formation of granulation tissue occurs when epidermal debris is allowed to accumulate and becomes infected. Careful microscopic debridement of granulation tissue and application of gentian violet followed by antibiotic-corticosteroid otic drops will lead to re-epithelialization and a dry ear. The development of scar bands within the mastoid defect can lead to keratin debris accumulation and subsequent infection. Transmeatal removal of the scar bands can often be accomplished under local anesthesia. In extensive cases, general anesthesia is necessary with transmeatal removal of the scar bands and re-epithelialization of the mastoid bowl. It is critical that the patient understand the need for periodic, usually annual, examination to prevent such occurrence.

SUMMARY

Open cavity mastoid procedures are indicated when canal-wall-up procedures are inadequate to control disease. The vast majority of these procedures will result in a modified radical mastoidectomy. The creation of a dry mastoid cavity primarily depends on surgical technique. Identification of the facial nerve is critical in this procedure. Lowering of the facial ridge to the level of the facial nerve and development of a large external auditory meatus are mandatory for successful outcome. Grafting of the middle ear eliminates mucous discharge and may improve hearing. Long-term postoperative care is minimal, with patients returning to normal activity, including water exposure.

References

1. Von Trroltsch AR. Lehrbuch der Ohrenheilkunde mit Einschlussder Anatomicdes Ohres. Leipzig: Fogel; 1873.
2. Schwartz HH, Eysell CO. Ueber die Kiinstliche eroffnung deswarzenfortsatzes. Arch Ohrenh 1873;7:157.
3. Von Bergmann E. Die chirurgische Behandlung von Himkrankheiten. Berlin; 1889.
4. Zaufal E. Technik der Trepanationdes Proc. Mastoid. NachKuster'schen Grundsatzen. Arch Ohrenh 1890;30:291.
5. Stacke L. Stacke's Operationsmethods. Arch Ohrenh 1893;35:145.
6. Korner O. Die eitrigen Erkrankungen des Schlafenbeins. Wiesbaden: Bergmann; 1899.
7. Bondy G. Totalaufineisselung mit Erhaltung von Trommelfell and Gehorknochelchen. Monatsschr Ohrenheilk 1910;44:15.
8. Kopetsky SJ. Otologic surgery. 2nd ed. New York: Paul B. Hoeber; 1929.
9. Lempert J. Improvement of hearing in cases of otosclerosis: new one stage surgical technic. Arch Otol 1938;28:42.
10. Baron S. Modified radical mastoidectomy. Arch Otol 1949; 49:280.
11. Zollner F. Die Radikal-Operatiion mit besonderem Bezug auf die Horfunktion. Ztschr Laryngol Rhinol Otol 1951;30:104.
12. Wullstein H. Funktionelle Operationen im Mitelohr mit Hilfedes freien Spaltlappen-Transplantates. Arch Ohren-Nasen-u Kehlkopfh 1952;161:422.
13. Jansen C. Ulur Radikaloperation Und Tympanoplastik. Sitz Ber Fontbild. Arztekamm. Ob. V. 18, February 1958.
14. Mukherjee P, Saunders N, Liu R, Fagan P. Long-term outcome of modified radical mastoidectomy. J Laryngol Otol 2004;118(8):612–6.
15. Kos MI, Castrillon R, Montandon P, Guyot JP. Anatomic and functional long-term results of canal walldown mastoidectomy. Ann Otol Rhinol Laryngol 2004;113(11):872–6.
16. Berenholz LP, Rizer FM, Burkey JM, Schuring AG, Lippy WH. Ossiculoplasty in canal wall down mastoidectomy. Otolaryngol Head Neck Surg 2000;123(1):30–3.
17. Siebenmann F. Die Radical-operation des Cholesteatoma mit-telst Anlegung breiter permanenter Oeffhungen gleihchzeitiggegen den Gehorgang and gegen dieretroauriculare Region. Berl Klin Wochenschr 1893;30:12.
18. Shambaugh GE Jr, Derlacki EL. Primary skin grafting of the fenestra and fenestration cavity. Arch Otol 1956;64:46.
19. Guilford FR, Wright WK. Secondary skin grafting in fenestration and mastoid cavities. Laryngoscope 1954;64:626.
20. Jackson CG, Glasscock ME, Schwaber MK, et al. Open mastoid procedures: Contemporary indications and surgical technique. Laryngoscope 1985;95:1037.
21. Hirsch BE, Kamerer DB, Doshi S. Single-stage management of cholesteatoma. Otolaryngol Head Neck Surg 1992;106:351.

Surgery for Otosclerosis 32

Ophir Handzel, MD, LLB / Michael J. McKenna, MD

INTRODUCTION

Otosclerosis is a disease of altered bone metabolism unique to the human temporal bone. The typical human otic capsule remodeling rate is extremely low. In otosclerosis, normal inhibition of bone remodeling is lost resulting in foci of bone remodeling. When remodeled bone bridges the stapediovestibular joint, it fixates the joint and impedes sound transmission manifested as conductive hearing loss. Sensorineural hearing loss (SNHL) can occur when bone remodeling extends to the cochlea.

The prevalence of otosclerosis varies among races, being common in Caucasians, less common in Southeast Asians and Native Americans, and rare in patients of African descent. The prevalence of clinically apparent otosclerosis is 0.3 to 0.5%.[1,2] Otosclerosis found on histology at autopsy is about ten times more prevalent than clinically manifested. Asymptomatic otosclerosis is present when bone remodeling does not hamper stapedial movement or does not affect the cochlea. Temporal bones studies have shown that the prevalence of histologic otosclerosis is 8.3 to 12% in Caucasians and 1% in blacks.[3,4,5] A more recent study found a lower prevalence of 3 to 4%.[6] The prevalence of clinical otosclerosis seems to be declining.[7] Although histologic otosclerosis has similar prevalence in both genders,[3,4,5] clinical otosclerosis has 1.4 to 2 times the incidence in women as compared to men. Otosclerosis will eventually involve both ears in 85 to 90% of patients.[8]

This chapter reviews the nature and development of otosclerosis, and historic and current methods of surgery for correction of the hearing loss associated with otosclerosis. Indications for surgery, description of the procedure, complications, and their management are elaborated. For some of the treatments, a number of viable options exist and this chapter reflects the management approach at the Massachusetts Eye and Ear Infirmary.

HISTORY OF SURGERY FOR OTOSCLEROSIS

Otosclerosis was first described in the early 18th century by Valsalva, who noticed a stapes ankylosed by ossification of its ligament in the course of dissecting a temporal bone of a deaf patient.[9] In 1869, von Tröltsch named the final inactive sclerotic stage of the disease, "otosclerosis." Siebenmann designated the active, hyperemic stage as "otospongiosis" in 1912. Toynbee surveyed 1659 temporal bones and characterized several types of stapes fixation and oval window involvement without fixation. Politzer recognized otosclerosis as a primary bone disease and not sclerosis secondary to a mucoperiosteal disease.[10]

Attempts to reverse hearing loss associated with stapes fixation dates to the late 19th century. In 1878, Kessel reported transtympanic mobilization and removal of the stapes. Subsequently, Boucheron (1888) and Miot (1890) reported their experience with patients who had undergone a similar procedure. Hearing improvement resulted in 74 of 126 patients. Blake (1892) and Jack (1893) at the Massachusetts Eye and Ear Infirmary in Boston removed the stapes and observed that in some patients hearing improved with healing of the tympanic membrane to the oval window niche. At this time, no attempts were made to seal the oval window niche or reconstruct the ossicular chain. However, at the 6th International Otologic Congress held in London in 1899, these types of surgeries were condemned as being useless (as hearing gain was often temporary) and dangerous. The exact reason for this statement is not known, but probably was based on complications that were not widely published; presumably infections that lead to the death of patients from meningitis.

Surgery to overcome fixation of the stapes was resumed in the 1930s by Holmgren's and then, Sourdille's multistage and Lempert's single-stage fenestration of the lateral semicircular canal. Fenestration surgery provided significant and lasting hearing improvement in large series of patients. Rosen, in 1952, reintroduced stapes mobilization, unaware of earlier work by Miot. In 1956, armed with the new technology of the binocular-operating microscope, Shea perfected stapedectomy and introduced the concept of ossicular chain reconstruction, first by means of a Teflon prosthesis and later by a polyethylene strut, while supporting both by a vein graft. Within a decade this procedure had become the standard operation for the treatment of otosclerosis. Those interested are encouraged to read *For the World to Hear* by Howard House,[11] who lived through the time of the introduction of many of these innovations and personally knew many of the individuals who made these important contributions to otology.

Various methods have been devised to overcome fixation of the footplate. The complete removal of the footplate (once commonly practiced) is now reserved for selected cases. It has been replaced by various methods of removal of more limited parts of the footplate and ultimately precise fenestration of the fixed footplate. Since its development in the early 1960s by Shea[12] in the United States and Marquet and Minon in Europe, small hole (fenestra) stapedotomy is probably the procedure of choice for most surgeons. The small fenestra were first created using a handheld microdrill and most recently by a laser.

Portman and Claverie in 1957 suggested utilizing part of the suprastructure of the stapes for bridging the gap from the incus to the oval window. Other variations on this theme include removal of the posterior footplate, as well as removal of the anterior fixed footplate maintaining ossicular continuity via the posterior crus.[13]

Dozens of various prosthesis types have been designed.[14] The Schuknecht type of stapedectomy fat-wire prosthesis was developed to address both the need to seal the open vestibule and to reconstruct the ossicular chain.[15] Later, with the popularization of small fenestra surgery, many other prostheses were made available, varying mostly in the materials of construction, in the mode of attachment to the incus and in the diameter of their vestibular contact.

PATHOLOGY

The normal otic capsule has an extremely low remodeling rate; compared to the 10% annual turnover rate of some of other bones, the rate for the normal otic capsule is no more than 2%.[16] Otosclerosis is a disease of abnormal bone remodeling occurring in the endochondral layer of the temporal bone. The normal temporal bone has embryonic cartilage rests called "globuli interossei." These rests are associated with sites of predilection in otosclerosis. The first histologic sign of otosclerosis is a change in the extracellular staining pattern that has been termed "blue mantle." This presumably unstable matrix begins to remodel giving rise to an otosclerotic focus. Immature bone is then laid and continued remodeling occurs, with prominent osteoblastic involvement ("otospongiosis"). The process is completed by maturation of the lesion into a sclerotic, dense, irregularly woven and poorly vascularized bone ("otosclerosis"). The disease process is not necessarily a continuous, linear process; active areas can become inactive and reactivated later and various stages of the disease can coexist in single focus.

Foci of otosclerosis can occur in any portion of the otic capsule; however, there are areas of predilection. Schuknecht and Barber studied the temporal bones of patients with clinically apparent otosclerosis.[17] Stapedial fixation by a focus anterior to the footplate was present in 96% of cases. Fixation is first caused by remodeling bone encroaching on the anterior footplate with subluxation of the posterior part of the footplate. As the process progresses and the lesion transgresses the stapediovestibular joint bony fixation of the footplate occurs. The former mechanism of fixation will result in hearing loss more pronounced in low frequencies, the latter apparent in all frequencies. In 49%, there was involvement of other areas as well: the round window niche in 30%, the cochlear apex in 12% and less frequent involvement of the walls of the internal auditory canal, around the cochlear aqueduct, semicircular canals, and the unusual disease limited to the footplate. Of special note is the involvement of the round window niche, found to be obliterated in 7% of histological specimens.[17] Obliteration of the round window niche can cause conductive loss, irrespective of the state of the stapes. Even with extensive disease, invasion of the membranous labyrinth is rare. The location and extent of the foci determines the clinical presentation: extent of the conductive loss and the presence or absence of SNHL. For a more detailed description and numerous photos of the histopathology of otosclerosis see Schuknecht's *Pathology of the Ear.*[18]

Gross appearance of otosclerotic foci is distinctly different from the normal otic capsule under the operative or examination microscope. Active, spongiotic lesions, having rich vascularization and hyperemic overlying mucosa may be seen through the tympanic membrane as a red discoloration of the promontory. This sign is named after Hermann Schwartze. Intraoperatively, a mature focus of otosclerosis is seen as a white, well-demarcated lesion compared to the ivory color of the otic capsule.

ETIOLOGY

The exact cause for the abnormal bone remodeling seen in the otosclerotic otic capsule has yet to be determined. Research regarding the genetics of otosclerosis and potential contribution of viral infection and the immune and endocrine systems has offered new insights in the etiology of this disease.[19]

Bone turnover is controlled by an intricate and complex mechanism. Cytokine factors that include osteoprotegerin (OPG), receptor activator for nuclear factor kappa B (RANK) and RANK ligand (RANK-L) play a major role in the system that directly controls bone turnover. Receptor activator for nuclear factor kappa B ligand is expressed by osteoblasts that are involved in bone turnover. Activation of its specific receptor RANK on osteoclasts promotes differentiation (in the presence of macrophage stimulating factor),[20] activation,[21] and survival[22] of osteoclasts. Bone remodeling is a process of bone resorption by osteoclasts and bone deposition by osteoblasts. Osteoprotegerin is a competitive inhibitor of RANK-L. High levels of OPG inhibit bone remodeling by inhibiting the differentiation, survival, and fusion of osteoclastic precursor cells, by suppressing activation and promoting apoptosis of osteoclasts.[23] Fibroblasts of the spiral ligament are a probable source of OPG, which is found in high levels in perilymph.[24] Osteoprotegerin may be dispersed throughout the otic capsule by the perilymphatic canalicular system traversing the bone.[25] The production of OPG in the cochlea may be the reason for the extremely slow turnover of bone in the otic capsule.[24,25] This cytokine regulatory mechanism may be influenced by genetic, endocrine, infectious, metabolic, biochemical, biomechanical, and other factors.

Otosclerosis has an underlying genetic cause, inherited in an autosomal dominant pattern with incomplete penetration of 20 to 40%. Monozygotic twins have a nearly 100% concordance rate of otosclerosis.[26] However, because information does not exist on the genetic transmission of histologic otosclerosis, it is not known whether the genetic basis of inheritance is related to the formation of an otosclerotic focus within the temporal bone or the tendency for a lesion to progress once it has begun, or both. There appears to be no significant difference in the degree of clinical severity between sporadic and familial cases.[27] To date, eight loci associated with otosclerosis have been identified and are designated *OTSC1-8*. The eighth locus has just recently been described.[28] Association analysis has revealed a significant association between both familial and sporadic cases of clinical otosclerosis and the COL1A1 gene using multiple polymorphic markers within the COL1A1 gene.[29] A preliminary study has demonstrated that osteoporosis may be more common in patients with otosclerosis, and these two common bone diseases may share some genetic and molecular pathologic mechanisms.[30] On the basis of the pattern of prevalence of otosclerosis and otitis media, it has been speculated that genetic susceptibility to otosclerosis may reduce susceptibility to otitis media.[31]

The evidence that has emerged thus far is suggestive of a possible persistent measles infection similar to what occurs in the central nervous system in subacute sclerosing panencephalitis.[32] Support of this hypothesis originates from ultrastructural and immunohistochemical evidence of measles-like structures and antigenicity in active otosclerotic lesions.[33,34,35] In addition, measles ribonucleic acid (RNA) has been found in archival and fresh footplate specimens with otosclerosis.[36,37,38] Elevated levels of antimeasles antibodies have also been reported in the perilymph of patients undergoing stapedectomy for otosclerosis as compared to controls.[39] Others have reported lower levels of circulating antimeasles antibodies in patients with otosclerosis as compared to healthy controls.[40] This hypothesis is further strengthened by recent evidence that the incidence of otosclerosis has declined since the introduction of measles vaccination.[7]

Hormones may influence otosclerosis. Otosclerosis is more prevalent in women compared to men by a factor of 1.4 to 2. It has been long held that pregnancy and lactation can accelerate otosclerosis, although reliable evidence for this is lacking.[41]

DIAGNOSIS

Otosclerosis is most often suspected to be the cause of a patient's hearing loss based on compatible history, physical examination, and audiometric testing. Definitive diagnosis is usually made at the time of surgery. The evaluation should exclude other causes of conductive or mixed hearing loss, including inactive chronic otitis media and tympanosclerosis. The diagnosis of a third mobile third window[42] such as superior semicircular dehiscence (SSCD) should be considered and excluded before surgery is undertaken.[43–45] Acoustic reflex testing at the time of audiometry is most recommended. Failure of stapes surgery to significantly reduce the air–bone gap should raise the suspicions of the existence of a third mobile window.

History

Typically, patients with otosclerosis will complain of a progressive hearing loss. In approximately three-quarters of cases both ears will be involved at presentation, although not necessary symmetrically. Most often, patients present in the third or fourth decade of life and 90% of patients present before the age of 50. The age at presentation may be slowly increasing.[46] Juvenile onset or presentation occurs, but rarely (<1% of cases in one series).[47] Other causes of juvenile-onset conductive hearing loss should be considered. Rarely, otosclerosis can manifest itself as a progressive SNHL, without a conductive loss. Approximately half of the patients will report a positive family history of hearing loss. A history of a relative who has had successful surgery for otosclerosis makes the diagnosis far more likely for a given individual.

Vestibular symptoms are reported by 10 to 30% of patients. Symptoms are highly variable, including *benign paroxysmal positional vertigo* (BPPV) and other paroxysmal vertigo attacks, dizziness, and unsteadiness. Severe episodic vertigo is usually not caused by otosclerosis. Patients with otosclerosis and history of vertigo have been found to have a reduction in Scarpa's ganglion cell counts compared to age-matched controls and to patients with otosclerosis free of vestibular symptoms.[48] Special attention should be paid to the potential coexistence of otosclerosis and Ménière's syndrome in a patient with clinical otosclerosis and vertigo. The hydropic saccule is at risk of injury during the operation with a high potential for SNHL. Hence, stapedectomy and stapedotomy are contraindicated in these patients. Patients may complain of tinnitus, which may sometimes improve with successful surgery.[49–51]

Physical Examination

A normal-appearing tympanic membrane in the setting of progressive conductive hearing loss is the hallmark of otosclerosis. In some cases, a vascular blush on the promontory can be appreciated (Schwartze's sign). Although reflective of an active disease process, Schwartze's sign is not considered a contraindication for surgery. Findings such as middle ear fluid, tympanosclerosis, retraction pockets, hypo- and hypermobility of the malleus, may point to other causes of conductive loss. The external auditory canal is surveyed for infections, exostoses, and other anatomic factors that may pose a problem during surgery. Exostoses limiting exposure should be repaired in a separate procedure prior to stapedectomy. Stapedectomy should follow healing of the canal.

Tuning forks of 512 and 1024 Hz should be used to assess hearing. The results of Rinne and Weber tests should correlate with the results of audiometry. Many surgeons consider a negative 512 Hz Rinne test a prerequisite to intervention. A limited otosclerotic focus at the anterior oval window niche may partially displace the footplate causing it to jam in the posterior oval window resulting in a mild low-frequency conductive hearing loss. At the time of surgery, fenestration attempts may result in a dislodged and floating footplate. Usually, by the time the Rinne test turn negative, fixation solidifies enough as to make this scenario less likely.

Audiometry

Complete audiometry including air and bone thresholds, speech discrimination, and acoustic reflexes is essential. Conductive, mixed, or rarely pure SNHL may be present. Early in the disease development of the typical air–bone gap loss is greatest in the low frequencies, which may be the result of an anterior otosclerotic focus that has resulted in posterior footplate displacement with partial subluxation and jamming of the footplate. With more advanced ankylosis of the footplate the loss equalizes across frequencies. The maximal conductive loss from stapes fixation is approximately 55 to 60 dB. The finding of a conductive hearing loss greater than 60 dB should raise suspicion of an ossicular discontinuity. A depression of bone conduction thresholds at 2000 Hz (Carhart's notch) is often seen in otosclerosis, but it is not considered pathognomonic. This elevated bone conduction is in fact a pseudo loss, an audiometric artifact and may be related to the resonance of the external auditory canal and middle ear in face of the fixed ossicle.[52] Following surgery, this notch usually disappears as part of overcorrection or closure of bone conduction by eliminating this artifact.

As mentioned, a third mobile window such as SSCD can present with low-frequency conductive loss similar to that seen in otosclerosis. These patients often have supranormal bone conduction in the low frequencies. Hence, measurement of bone conduction should not be stopped at 0 dB, but should include better than 0 dB thresholds. Acoustic reflexes will be absent in an otosclerotic ear, but present in an ear with air–bone gap due to a third mobile window. Hence, acoustic reflexes should be tested routinely as part of the evaluation of a conductive hearing loss.

Imaging

Imaging is not a routine part of the evaluation of a patient with suspected otosclerosis; however, it may be helpful in confirming or excluding the presence of other pathologies causing conductive loss. Sensitivity for detection of otosclerotic foci by high-resolution computed tomography (CT) scans is 85 to 87%.[53,54] Inactive and submillimeter foci are mostly responsible for false-negative scans.

SURGERY FOR OTOSCLEROSIS

Various procedures have been utilized to correct conductive loss associated with stapedial fixation. Currently, by far the most commonly performed procedure is stapedotomy: the creation of a small hole in the footplate with placement of a prosthesis from the incus to the vestibule. This is the procedure of choice at the Massachusetts Eye and Ear Infirmary (MEEI), and its detailed description follows. Awareness of other types of procedures is important, especially when performing revision stapedectomies.

Stapes surgery requires a specific set of acquired skills. It is estimated it takes an average of 50 or more[55,56] procedures to achieve reliable and consistent results. The declining numbers of stapedectomies may extend the time it takes for trainees to complete this learning curve.[56]

Indications

Surgery is considered in a patient with clinical otosclerosis when there are clinical indicators of stapes fixation and reasonable expectations that surgery will result in a perceptible benefit to the patient. An air–bone gap of 25 dB or more at frequencies of 250 Hz to 1 kHz and a negative Rinne at 512 Hz are considered to be good indicators. In cases of bilateral involvement, the worse hearing ear is usually operated first. The patient's preference can be used to guide side selection in symmetric loss. In those accustomed to aided hearing unilaterally, the nonaided ear may be chosen. Following a successful operation with stable results for at least a year, the contralateral ear can be operated upon. Concomitant sensorineural loss is not a contraindication for surgery. Even in patients requiring amplification after surgery, intervention may still be beneficial by allowing better performance with a hearing aid. In cases of advanced otosclerosis, measurement of true speech discrimination can be difficult, as the audiometer's output may not suffice for adequate presentation levels. Those patients may still significantly benefit from stapedectomy that should be considered in some patients with advanced otosclerosis prior to considering cochlear implantation (see below). In these circumstances, tuning forks can provide invaluable information.

Contraindications

Stapedectomy is contraindicated in patients with infected middle[57] or external ears. Perforation of the drum is a contraindication as well. Surgery is not to be done in an only hearing ear, with the exception of a patient with profound mixed hearing loss who is a candidate for cochlear implantation. In cases in which the contralateral ear has disease that may threaten hearing in the future, surgery is relatively contraindicated. In patients with vestibular symptoms, Ménière's syndrome must be ruled out before surgery, as previously mentioned. In those requiring an intact vestibular system for professional or other occupational activity, the potential impact of surgery needs to be considered. Advanced age is not a contraindication for surgery,[58] although the likelihood of success might be slightly reduced in patients older than 70 years.[59]

Informed Consent

Candidates for surgery should be informed about amplification as an alternative mode for improved hearing. Postponing surgery does not reduce the chances of success, nor increase the likelihood of complications. Hence, the patient need not act within a certain window of opportunity.

Informed consent must include description of the procedure and discussion of all potential risks: failure of the procedure to correct the conductive component of hearing loss, partial or complete SNHL (occurs in approximately 1% of surgeries), vestibular disturbances, perforation of the tympanic membrane, facial nerve injury, development of perilymphatic fistula (PLF), delayed failure after an initial good result, and disturbance of taste as a result of manipulation or sacrifice of the chorda tympani nerve. Patients with an occupational dependence on taste should consider this factor in the potential risk to the chorda tympani nerve, before submitting themselves to surgery. Patients wishing to engage in activities exposing them to significant pressure variations, such as pilots, divers, and parachuters, require proper counseling. Stapedotomy and stapedectomy are thought to increase the risk for barotrauma to the inner ear including PLF and its associated irreversible hearing and vestibular loss. Hence, it may be prudent to avoid these activities altogether after stapes surgery. That being said, some surgeons allow such activities with evidence of good eustachian tube function either clinically[60] or with a tympanometer pressure test of ±400 mm H_2O.[61]

Operative Note

The operative note of surgery for correction of otosclerosis must include several specific notations: the shape and mobility of the incus and malleus, the presence of otosclerosis, fixation of the stapes, patency of the round window, location of and the bone covering the facial nerve, and the status of the chorda tympani at the end of the procedure. Unusual perilymphatic flow should be noted as well. The type and size of the prosthesis used should be specified. These recordings may be of extreme importance when surgery for the contralateral ear is considered or in cases of consideration of revision stapedectomy.

Anesthesia

Choice of anesthesia depends on patient's and surgeon's preferences and the nature of surgery planned. Local anesthesia has the advantage of saving time compared to general anesthesia. Intraoperative patient reports of vestibular stimulation may be used as a safety measure to prevent excessive inner ear irritation; however, operations under general anesthesia do not carry increased risk for vestibular complication. General anesthesia provides assurance against pain and head movement.

Perioperative Antibiotics and Steroids

Most surgeons advocate antibiotic prophylaxis against common skin bacteria. Accordingly, one of the first-generation cephalosporins is appropriate for patients with no allergy to these agents and clindamycin for those with such allergy. Antibiotic treatment is continued for a week after the operation. Although there is no scientific evidence to support the use of antibiotics, they are commonly used in practice as otitis media in the immediate postoperative period can have devastating consequences.

Stapedectomy and stapedotomy are associated with an immediate and transient perioperative reduction in bone conduction attributable to serous labyrinthitis. To mitigate this reaction, steroids are commonly administered at time of operation and discontinued thereafter. There is evidence that steroids may reduced the severity of serous labyrinthitis after opening the perilymphatic space, but no clear proof that it has an effect on the results of stapes surgery.[62]

Surgical Technique

Positioning

Proper positioning of the patient is essential and allows for good visualization of the oval window niche and neighboring structures and ease of approach to the middle ear. Bringing the tympanic membrane to a near horizontal plane serves these goals. The head of the patients is turned toward the contralateral shoulder and tilted downward 10 to 15 degrees. This is best achieved by a surgical bed with a separate head rest. The surgeon position should be comfortable, preferably having his or her legs on the floor and back supported.

Exposure and Exploration

A speculum holder attached to the bed or the headrest allows free movement of both hands. Proper sizing of the speculum is important—if too small it will move against the external canal wall, restricting the view and the introduction of instruments. Too large a speculum will push the soft tissue of the cartilaginous canal medially, restricting the operative view. The speculum should wedge into the lateral aspect of the bony canal. Local anesthesia is achieved with a mixture of 1% lidocaine and 1:100,000 epinephrine. The four quadrants of the cartilaginous canal are injected with a 27-gauge needle. The bony external canal is injected with a beveled 30-gauge needle in the subperiosteal plane at 6 and 12 o'clock. Even under general anesthesia proper injection is crucial; it will reduce the chance of bleeding in an operation with low tolerance for visual obstruction of the surgical field.

The tympanomeatal flap can be fashioned in various shapes, triangular or trapezoid. It should allow good exposure of the posterior middle ear, and in its superior-posterior part provide coverage of the bone defect created by curetting during the operation. The flap is elevated to the annulus. Before entering the middle ear, the ear canal should be free of bleeding. The middle ear is entered inferior to the location of the chorda tympani nerve, carefully avoiding perforation of the drum. The annulus is elevated from its sulcus and together with the drum elevated from 6 o'clock inferiorly to the line of the manubrium superiorly. The flap is folded anteriorly where it should remain without creeping into the surgical field. Optimal exposure of the oval window niche requires visualization of the pyramidal eminence and the tympanic segment of the facial nerve prior to proceeding with removal of the suprastructure of the stapes. Most often, adequate exposure necessitates removal of the bony annulus in the posterior-superior quadrant. The bone is removed using a bone curette or a drill, with care not to injure the chorda tympani nerve and the incus.

Next, the middle ear pathology is delineated. Patency of the round window is examined and described in the operative note. The oval window niche is surveyed for evidence of otosclerosis. Mobility of the ossicular chain is checked. The malleus and incus are palpated and their mobility assessed. The movement of the stapes is examined by direct and gentle manipulation of the suprastructure. If the stapes is found to be fixed and the incus and malleus are mobile, the surgeon can proceed with stapedotomy. The incudostapedial joint is separated with a joint knife. The stapedial tendon is cut with scissors or with a laser as close as possible to the pyramidal eminence to minimize both visual and physical obstruction in the corridor through which the prosthesis will be introduced (Figure 32–1A). If the operating surgeon has a laser available, the posterior crus is divided as close to the footplate as possible to prevent obstruction of view of and approach to the footplate after removal of the suprastructure (Figure 32–1B). Section of the anterior crus (Figure 32–1C) is often not possible or necessary. The suprastructure is fractured downward toward the promontory and removed from the middle ear.

Fenestration

A hole in the fixed footplate is made to allow for the introduction of the prosthesis. The size of the fenestra is dependent in part by the prosthesis to be used and should be made just large

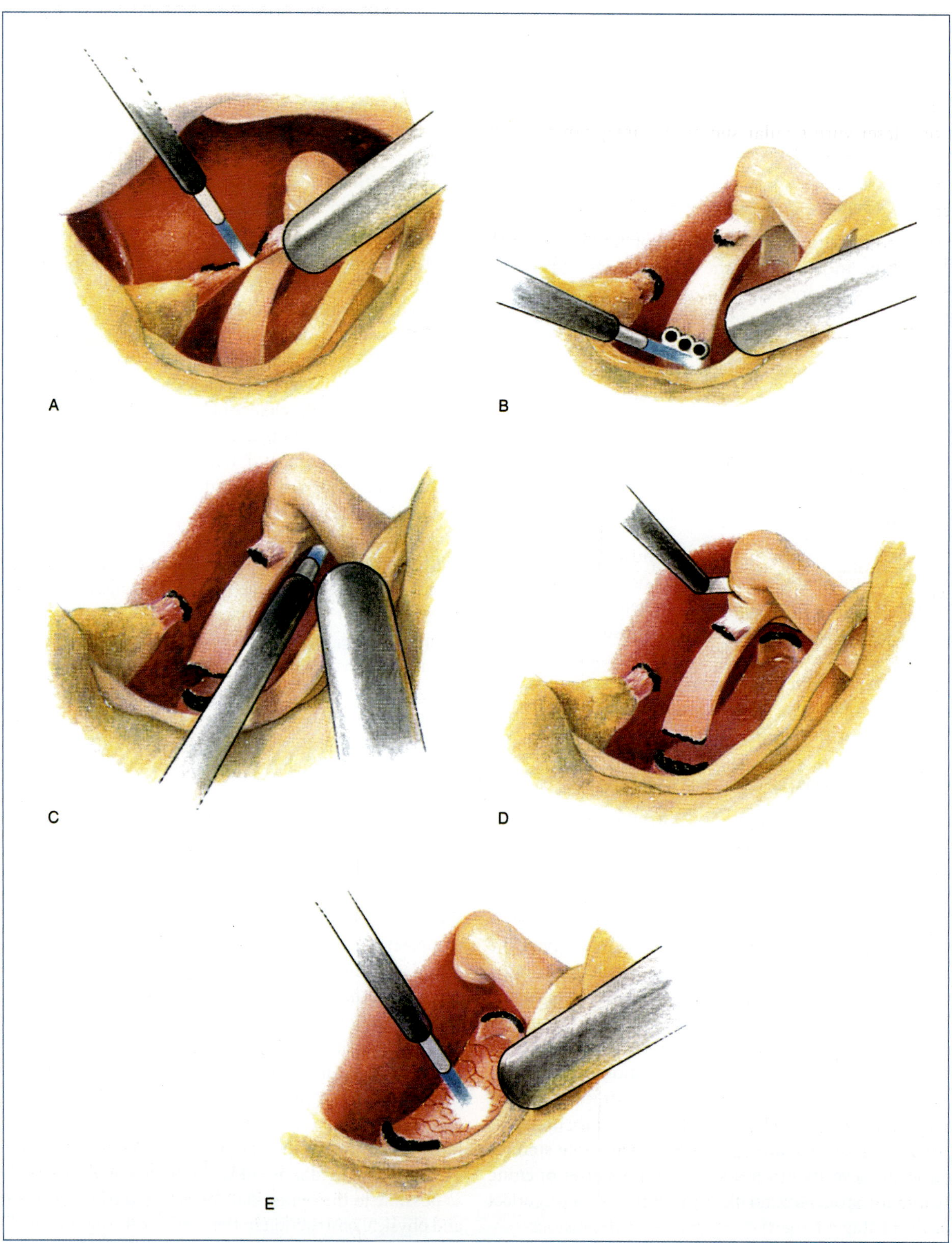

FIGURE 32–1 • Exposure of the stapes footplate using a handheld laser. For cutting, the tip of the laser is brought to immediate proximity to its target. A small-diameter suction is used to clear the field of fumes. *A*, Separation of the stapes tendon with a laser. Alternatively, the tendon can be cut with scissors. The tendon is separated as close as possible to the pyramidal eminence. *B*, Posterior crurotomy with a laser. The crus is separated as close as possible to the footplate to prevent impediment to the introduction and movement of the prosthesis. Sequential holes are created with the laser and separation is completed with a straight pick. Care is taken to prevent the laser from damaging the adjacent facial nerve. *C*, When possible, the anterior crus is separated as well. This can be achieved by pointing the laser between the crura toward the inner aspect of the anterior crus. Anterior crurotomy is often difficult to achieve and is not a mandatory step. *D*, Separation of the incudostapedial joint with a proprietary knife. Many surgeons prefer to separate the joint before incising the stapedial tendon in favor of more stability during disarticulation. The intact stapedial tendon counteracts separation movements that are directed from posterior to anterior. Excessive lateral movement of the incus is avoided. *E*, When needed thickened mucosa and blood vessels on the footplate can be coagulated using the defocused laser beam. The laser is held at a distance of 2 mm from its target. This will prevent bleeding during fenestration.

enough to accommodate the prosthesis freely. The fenestra in the footplate can be created with an electric microdrill (e.g., Skeeter) or a laser with similar success.[63] Lasers can cut and coagulate with great precision and without generating pressure or movement. These qualities are desirable for stapes surgery in a number of applications: fenestrating a thin footplate with the reduced risk of resultant floating footplate; having the ability to fenestrate a mobile footplate; and creating a fenestra with minimal movement of the footplate or perilymph thus reducing inner ear irritation and trauma. Although there are no studies that clearly demonstrate a difference in results between the use of drill and laser, for most otologic surgeons, the laser has proven to be a most useful tool.

The adventitious qualities of laser are shared by lasers both in the visible (argon or potassium titanyl phosphate [KTP-532]) and the invisible light range (carbon dioxide [CO_2]); both types have been used with similar success and complications rates.[64] Lasers in the visible light range are convenient in being deliverable through a flexible fiberoptic handheld piece and not requiring a separate aiming beam. Visible lasers are best absorbed by pigmented tissue and much less so by white tissue. Because they are delivered through a fiberoptic cable, the light energy disperses rapidly after leaving the tip thus allowing for both coagulation (Figure 32–1D) and cutting depending upon the distance between the tip and the target. Much experience has been gained with these lasers with good results and few complications, proving that with proper use visible light lasers are efficacious and safe for creation of a small fenestra stapedotomy. The current laser used at the MEEI is a KTP 532 with a beam width of 200 μm.

Carbon dioxide lasers have the advantage of not being absorbed in the perilymph, thus potentially reducing the risk to the structures within the vestibule. They have been used successfully for stapedotomy.[65,66] The disadvantages are the need for a separate aiming beam and the requirement of a microscope-attached delivery system with a direct sight line from the microscope to the footplate. Recently, a handheld, flexible CO_2 delivery system has been introduced.

With the KTP laser, fenestration is achieved by creating a rosette of five partially overlapping laser burn marks to achieve a fenestra that will accommodate a 0.6-mm piston (Figure 32–2A). The laser leaves a circular black char with central whitening representing a pinpoint hole allowing, at times, perilymph to egress the vestibule. After the first mark of the laser on the footplate is made, subsequent burns partially overlap the preceding spots to take advantage of the better absorption of the visible laser by the dark colored char. The surgeon should allow 2 or 3 sec to lapse between laser pulses to allow the perilymph to cool. It is better to create a slightly large fenestra than a slightly small one, as friction between the prosthesis and the bone edges of the fenestra can adversely impact the result. The fenestra is sized with a 0.6-mm rasp or measuring rod, which should easily pass through the fenestra without resistance (Figure 32–3).

Prosthesis Choice, Placement, and Attachment

Many prostheses designs are currently available.[67] They differ mostly in the mode of attachment to the incus, the diameter and length of the distal piston or rod, the material of construction,

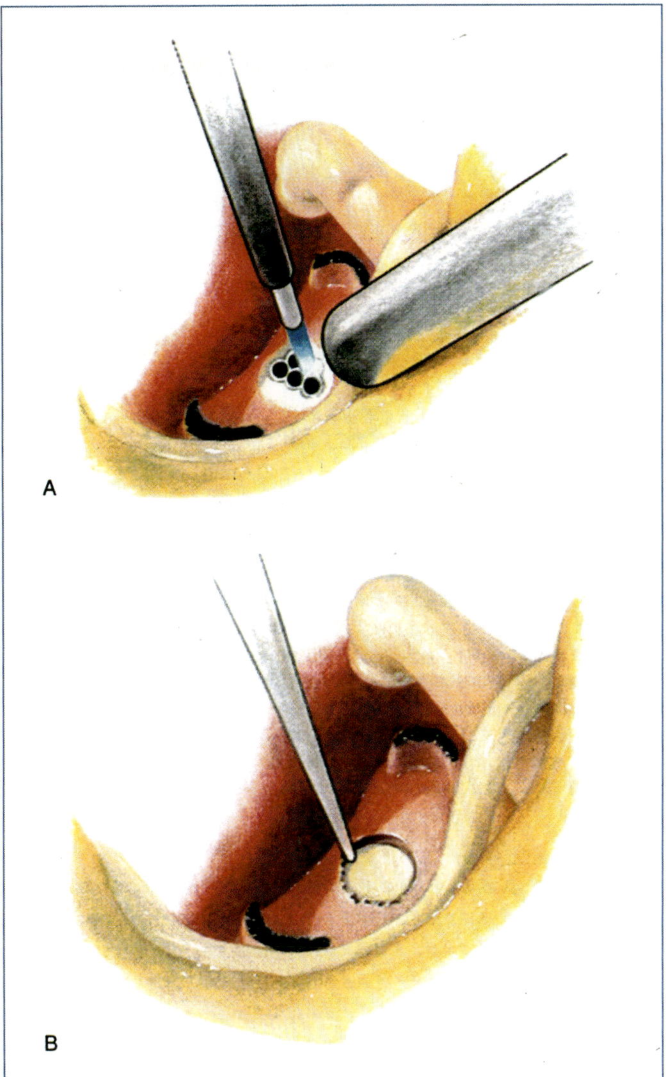

FIGURE 32–2 • Fenestration of the stapes footplate. *A*, A KTP-pulsed diode with a beam width of 200 μm is depicted. A rosette measuring five slightly overlapping holes is created to accommodate a 0.6-mm diameter prosthesis. *B*, The edges of the fenestra can be smoothed with a straight pick or a small rasp.

and weight (although the last variable has little influence on hearing results). A number of prostheses attach to the incus with a metallic loop that needs to be crimped for a stable fit around the incus; others attach without crimping. Robinson-type prostheses have a bucket that cradles the lenticular and long processes of the incus and a handle that stabilizes the prosthesis. The recently introduced shape memory alloy recoverable technology (SMART) piston prosthesis (Gyrus ENT, Bartlett, TE), makes use of the elastic memory of a nitinol metallic wire that coils around the incus in response to heating. Preliminary results reported with this prosthesis have shown equivalency in hearing results with other prostheses.[68,69] Some surgeons have expressed concern that the nickel component of the metal may not be as biocompatible within the ear as stainless steel and platinum.[68] Self-retaining prostheses that are clipped to the incus are available as well.[70] At the MEEI, the most commonly

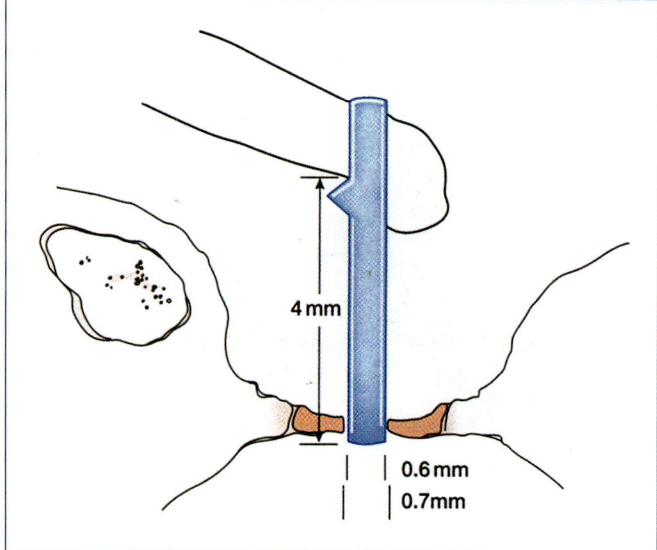

FIGURE 32–3 • The distance between the fenestra and the medial aspect of the incus is measured. A measuring gauge is placed level within the fenestra. An additional 0.25 mm is added to the measured distance as this is the appropriate protrusion of the prosthesis into the vestibule. The measuring rod can also be used to size the fenestra since its diameter is 0.6 mm. *From Nadol JB Jr, McKenna MJ, editors. Surgery of the ear and temporal bone. 2nd ed. Philadelphia: Lippincott Williams & Wilkins; 2005. p. 281. Reprinted by permission.*

used prosthesis is a platinum ribbon type. The ribbon makes a wider and more stable contact point with the incus compared to steel wire. Platinum is devoid of steel coiling memory and hence is easier to crimp. The platinum shaft connecting the ribbon to the piston base is a rounded wire and can be easily angulated after placement of the prosthesis for optimal incus to fenestra reach.

For sound transmission, larger prosthesis diameter should yield better closure of the air–bone gap, at least in low and middle frequencies,[71–73] although some studies have reported similar long-term results for 0.4 mm piston diameter prosthesis versus 0.6 mm.[74] Studies comparing the results with various types of commercially available prostheses are limited by confounding effects (such as the size of the fenestra and small sample size) and by ceiling effect as a reasonable air–bone gap closure is usually achieved regardless of the prosthesis size (see Chapter 3 for a more detailed discussion). Some surgeons prefer a 0.4-mm prosthesis to allow for fenestration of the stapes and crimping of the prosthesis to the incus before fracture and removal of the suprastructure.[75]

As magnetic resonance imaging (MRI) scans advance to create progressively stronger magnetic fields and have wider indications for use, concern for the safety of stapes and other middle ear prostheses has grown. A magnetic field can both heat and move a ferromagnetic prosthesis. All prostheses implanted over the past 17 years are safe for MRI scanning of 3 T.[76,77]

Prostheses are made in various lengths to accommodate variations in anatomy and pathology. The prosthesis should protrude into the vestibule up to a distance of 0.25 mm. The correct length of the prosthesis is the measured distance of the medial side of the incus to the opening in the footplate plus 0.25 mm (Figure 32–3). An additional 0.25 mm is added if the need for bending of the prosthesis is anticipated. A prosthesis of the appropriate length is selected based on the measurement of the fenestra diameter and the distance between the fenestra and incus. The surgeon ascertains sufficient opening of the loop of the prosthesis. The prosthesis is grasped by its loop with a smooth alligator forceps in an angle relative to the axis of the prosthesis, which allows its placement on the incus and fenestra in one movement. If the piston cannot be inserted to the fenestra in the initial effort, it is left in the oval window niche and manipulated to the fenestra in a separate maneuver. Tightening the ribbon or wire loop to the long process of the incus is done with a crimper. The crimping is done at the narrowest area of the long process, and then the prosthesis can be moved proximal along the incus to achieve a favorable angle. The crimper should be engaged with both its claws visible to the surgeon and having a deep purchase to the incus. Engagement that is too shallow or angulated backward may result in an elliptical loop around the incus that may allow differential movement of the incus against the prosthesis (Figure 32–4 and 32–5), which may result in a reduced hearing gain and long-term failure by erosion of the distal end of the incus. Common reasons for differential movement of the incus and the prosthesis are improper crimping or friction between the piston and the walls of the oval window niche or fenestra. The wire of the prosthesis can be manipulated with a right-angled hook to clear some obstacles and create a better and more perpendicular angle in relation to the entrance to the vestibule. The area around the prosthesis and the fenestra is packed with Gelfoam, blood or loose connective tissue, the latter obtained from the subdermal tissue of the lobule, postauricular area, or cartilaginous canal.

The tympanomeatal flap is restored to its anatomic position and surveyed for any perforations requiring grafting. The edges are inspected and unfurled. The flap is stabilized with Gelfoam or silk ribbons with sponge patch.

Total Stapedectomy

Although chronologically stapedotomy was introduced as an evolutunary improvement of stapedectomy, done properly both techniques can yield good results. In certain situations, stapedotomy is not possible and stapedectomy is performed, eg, a floating footplate, a comminuted fracture of the footplate, a footplate inadvertently removed during suprastructure dislocation through anterior crus attachment, and some revision surgeries. Stapedectomy is also a solution when the instruments required to create a small fenestra are lacking. Special care should be taken to minimize trauma to the inner ear when extracting the intact or fragmented footplate. The gap between the prosthesis and the oval window opening to the vestibule must be sealed with tissue graft, such as fat. Although the hearing results for stapedectomy and stapedotomy are similar, the occurrence, duration, and severity of vestibular symptoms are greater for stapedectomy.

Postoperative Care

Patients can usually be discharged from the hospital a few hours after surgery. They are instructed to keep their ears dry, to avoid strenuous physical activities (eg, heavy lifting,

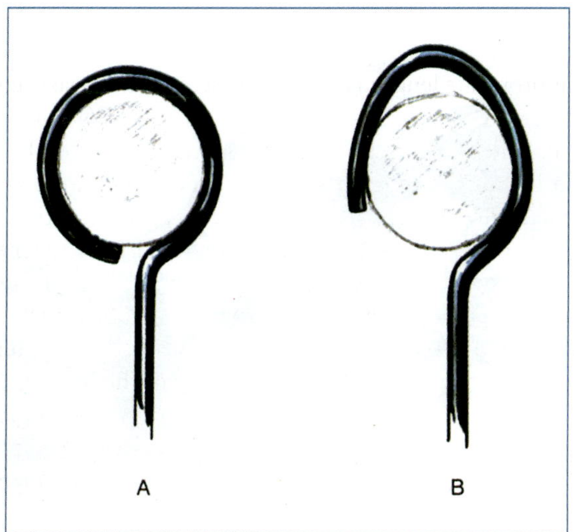

FIGURE 32–4 • Proper crimping is essential to long-term success of surgery. *A*, Proper crimping is depicted resulting in wire tightly conforming to the round shape of the incus. *B*, Improper crimping creates an oval shape that may allow differential motion between the incus and the prosthesis and delayed failure. *From Nadol JB Jr, McKenna MJ, editors. Surgery of the ear and temporal bone. 2nd ed. Philadelphia, PA: Lippincott Williams & Wilkins; 2005. p. 284. Reprinted by permission.*

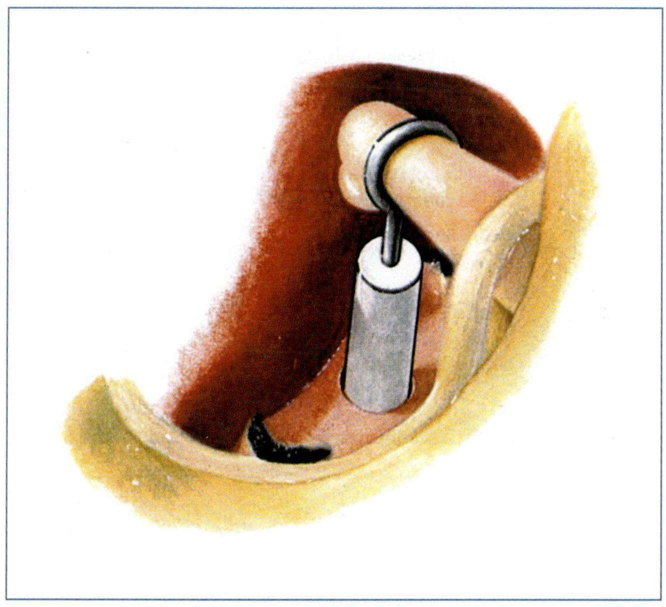

FIGURE 32–5 • A wire-piston positioned and crimped properly. The piston is perpendicular to the footplate fitting the fenestra snugly but moving freely. The wire is crimped tightly around the incus and perpendicular to its axis.

Valsalva maneuvers), to avoid nose blowing, and to sneeze with an open mouth. Air travel is permissible a couple of days after the operation. Oral antibiotics are continued for a week. If nonabsorbable packing is used, the patients are usually seen 1 week postoperatively for packing removal. Audiometric evaluation is performed 6 to 8 weeks following the procedure.

Results

As mentioned before, bone conduction is often improved after surgery with correction of the Carhart's notch. Hence, in evaluating the results of surgery, postoperative air–bone gap is calculated based on postoperative air and bone conduction measurements, as stipulated by the guidelines issued by committee on hearing and equilibrium of the American Academy of Otolaryngology—Head and Neck Surgery.[78] The results achieved by experienced surgeons comprise closure of the air–bone gap to 10 dB or less in 90% of patients with an incidence of profound SNHL of not more than 1%. In 90% of patients, closure of air–bone gap is stable for many years.[51,79]

COMPLICATIONS

Intraoperative Problems and Complications

Tears in the Tympanomeatal Flap

Common reasons for tears in the tympanomeatal flap are elevation of the flap in a limited segment, not in a broad front, and elevating the tympanic membrane without the annulus. These pitfalls are to be avoided.

Tears in the tympanic membrane are best repaired by placement of a medially placed tragal perichondrium or fascia graft. Small tears in the vicinity of the annulus can be closed with a piece of Gelfoam. Small linear tears in the canal skin flap typically need no repair but should be replaced in the correct orientation avoiding infolding of the edges of the tear.

Subluxation of the Incus

Subluxation and dislocation of the incus occurs most often during curettage of the bony annulus, separation of the incudostapedial joint, manipulation around the oval window, and crimping. Subluxation implies that part but not all of the attachments of the incus have been disrupted. In this case, chances are high for achieving a good functional result from completing the procedure with an incus attachment prosthesis, although crimping the prosthesis to a loose incus is more challenging. Some surgeons prefer to abort the procedure and attempt completion as a separate procedure after giving sufficient time for the incus to reattach to the malleus. However, if disarticulation or complete disruption of the joint occurs, as indicated by complete freedom of the incus to move in medial, lateral, anterior, and posterior directions, it is best to remove the incus and use a malleus attachment prosthesis.

Overhanging Facial Nerve

The location of the facial nerve should be visually verified as soon as the oval window area is exposed. The facial nerve can be dehiscent of its covering bone, but usually does not extend significantly out of the fallopian canal, i.e., prolapse or overhang the oval window (Figure 32–6). In a series of 1497 stapedectomies, prolapse of the facial nerve was found in 40 (2.6%); in 28 (1.9%) the prolapsed nerve covered more than 50% of the oval window niche. Only four operations had to be aborted for this reason.[80] If the prolapsed nerve abuts the promontory inferior to the oval window, surgery should not be completed. In the majority of cases, surgery can be completed by drilling a small fenestra that includes the inferior aspect of the annular

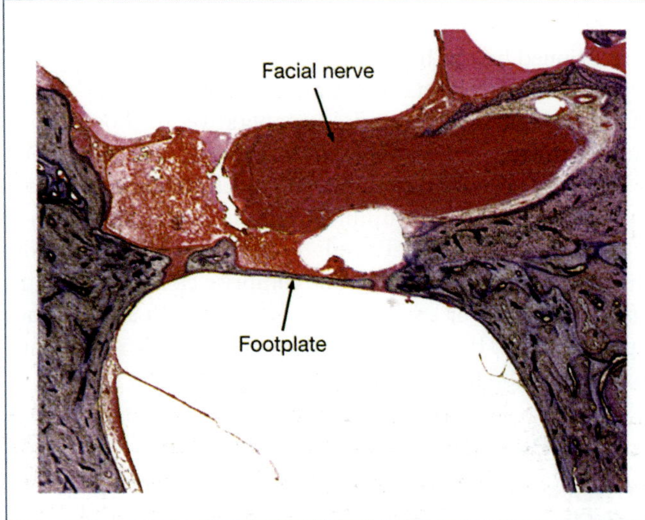

FIGURE 32–6 • Horizontal section of the oval window area. Facial nerve prolapsing from the fallopian canal may obstruct approach to the oval window. *From Nadol JB Jr, McKenna MJ, editors. Surgery of the ear and temporal bone. 2nd ed. Philadelphia, PA: Lippincott Williams & Wilkins; 2005. p. 291. Reprinted by permission.*

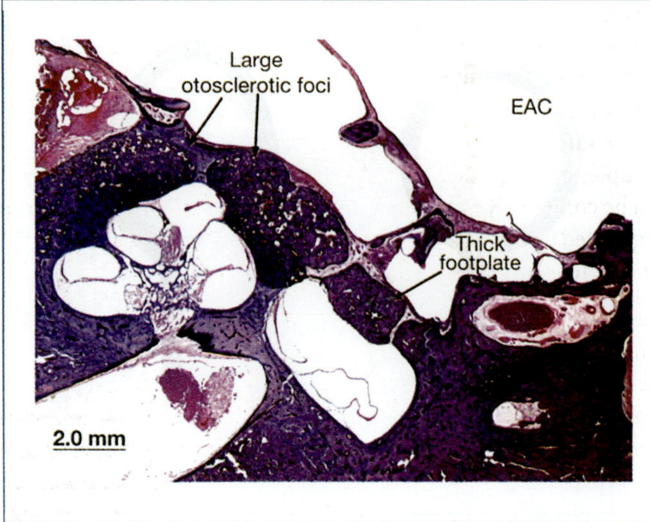

FIGURE 32–7 • Horizontal section of a temporal bone with extensive otosclerosis. The oval window niche is obliterated and the stapes footplate is severely thickened. This lesion cannot be perforated solely with a laser and will require thinning with a drill. EAC, external auditory canal. *From Nadol JB Jr, McKenna MJ, editors. Surgery of the ear and temporal bone. 2nd ed. Philadelphia, PA: Lippincott Williams & Wilkins; 2005. p. 292. Reprinted by permission.*

ligament. It is best to drill around the midpoint of the inferior margin, where the thickness of the promontory is greatest.[81] This technique is similar to the one used for extracting a floating footplate. Generally, with an overhanging facial nerve, the prosthesis must be longer than usual to accommodate bending inferiorly to avoid the nerve and being positioned perpendicular to the fenestra.

Obliterative Otosclerosis of the Oval Window

The oval window niche can be obliterated by severe thickening of the stapedial footplate and/or the margins of niche (Figure 32–7). In a series of 293 primary stapedectomies, obliterative otosclerosis was found in 14 (4.7%).[82] The laser is not efficient in removing such large amounts of bone. Fenestration can be achieved after first saucerizing the obliterated niche and thinning the obstructing bone. After blue lining the vestibule, the fenestration can be made with a 0.7-mm diamond burr. Measurements for prosthesis length are made just prior to fenestration. If obliterative otosclerosis is found in one ear, there is 50% chance of the same finding to be present in the other ear.[82]

Otosclerosis Involving the Round Window

The round window can be partially or completely obliterated by otosclerosis (Figure 32–8). Complete but not partial obliteration is associated with significant conductive hearing loss.[83] Attempts at removing this obstruction have resulted in SNHL and are contraindicated. During exploration of the ear, it is impossible to ascertain whether an otosclerotic obliteration is partial or complete. Even a minute opening to the round window membrane can be associated with good hearing. Hence, if the round window is found to be obliterated, the procedure should be completed and the finding noted in the operative note. If a residual conductive loss is present following surgery, revision surgery is not recommended as the likely cause is a completely obliterated round window.

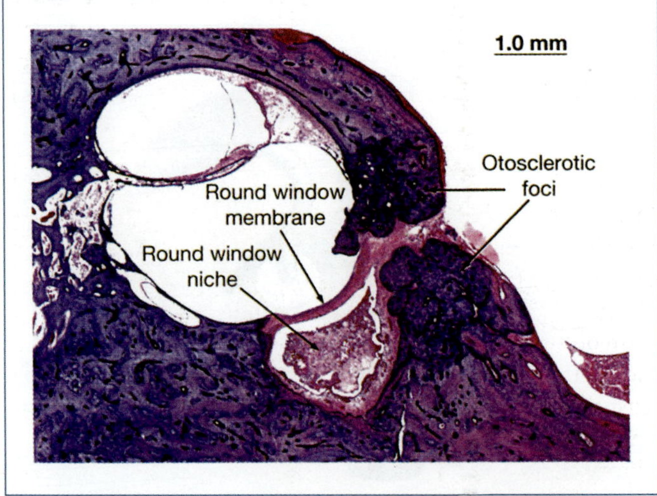

FIGURE 32–8 • Horizontal section of the round window area demonstrating otosclerotic obliteration of the round window. This may cause conductive hearing loss not amendable to surgical correction. *From Nadol JB Jr, McKenna MJ, eds. Surgery of the ear and temporal bone. 2nd ed. Philadelphia, PA: Lippincott Williams & Wilkins; 2005. p. 293. Reprinted by permission.*

Persistent Stapedial Artery

The stapedial artery develops and degenerates during the first trimester of pregnancy. The artery traverses the obturator foramen and after normal regression it is often seen as a small vessel running across the footplate. When the artery persists it arises from the internal carotid artery to either replace the middle meningeal artery or to branch into three arteries accompanying the branches of the trigeminal nerve. The incidence of persistent stapedial artery recorded in surgical observations is 1 of 5000 to 10,000 ears (Figure 32–9); based on temporal bone studies the incidence may be higher.[18] A persistent stapedial artery cannot be safely coagulated with bipolar cautery or laser. Often, it occupies only the anterior half of the footplate and fenestration can be completed in the posterior half. The procedure should be completed only if the space left by the artery is clearly sufficient for safe fenestration.

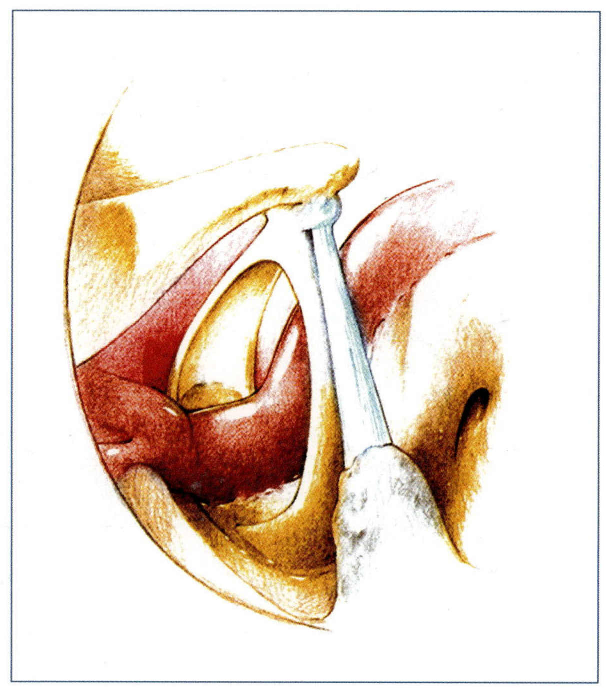

FIGURE 32–9 • A persistent stapedial artery may limit the approach to the footplate. Although the artery cannot be safely coagulated, usually the space left posterior to it will be adequate for safe completion of the procedure.

Malleus Ankylosis

The malleus head can be ankylosed to the wall or to the roof of the epitympanum by a spur or bar of bone. The etiology of this type of ankylosis has no association with that of otosclerosis, and may be the consequence of a developmental defect or new bone formation during inflammation of the middle ear cleft. The incidence of malleus fixation in the temporal bone collection at the MEEI is 0.5%.[84] Some surgical series report a slightly higher incidence of 1 to 2%. Physical examination and audiometry can raise the suspicion of malleus fixation. On pneumatic otoscopy, reduced mobility of the umbo, manubrium, or lateral process of the manubrium is noticed. If suspected, the diagnosis can often be confirmed by laser Doppler vibrometry. Myringosclerosis can be associated with malleus fixation. Most cases of fixation of the malleus are unilateral in contrast to otosclerosis. During exploration of the ear, the movement of each of the ossicles should be assessed independently by gentle palpation. Fixation of the malleus can be corrected during stapes surgery by removing the incus and head of malleus and reconstruction with a malleus attachment prosthesis.

Perilymph Gushers and Oozers

Fenestration of the footplate may be followed by fluid egress from the vestibule to the middle ear. Although named perilymph gushers and oozers, this is in fact flow of cerebrospinal fluid (CSF). Schuknecht suspected that oozers were a steady trickle of fluid, associated with a persistent cochlear aqueduct, which in the great majority of humans does not allow free flow.[85] A gusher is a strong and forceful flow (Figure 32–10) originating from a defect in the cribrose area of the fundus of the internal auditory canal. This defect is often associated with other inner ear anomalies and congenital fixation of the stapes and although high-resolution CT may be helpful, we have seen cases of perilymph gushers without abnormalities on CT. The rapid drainage of inner ears fluids can threaten sensorineural hearing, and needs to be addressed immediately. The fenestra is packed with tissue graft or a cotton pledget. Placing a lumbar drain and lowering spinal fluid pressure can be useful, especially when done preoperatively in suspected cases. Stapedectomy should be completed by using a perichondrium or vein tissue graft. X-linked recessive stapes gusher syndrome should be suspected in male patients with childhood onset of hearing impairment.[86]

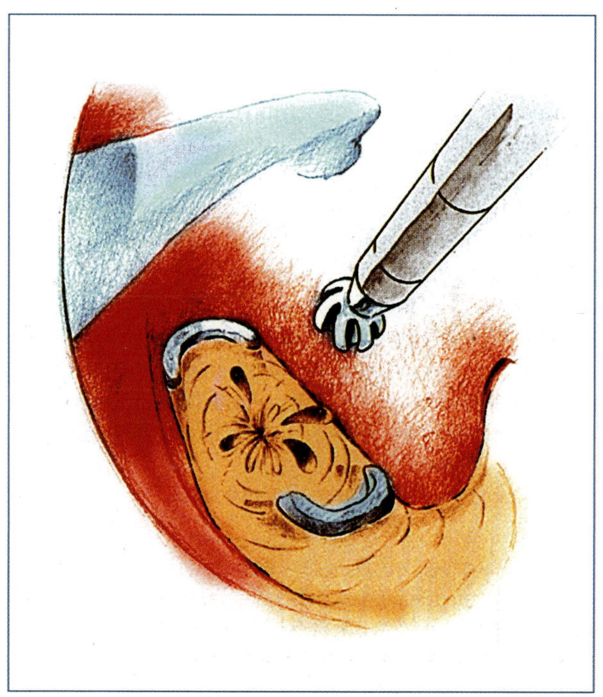

FIGURE 32–10 • Perilymphatic gusher. Fenestration results in a stream of CSF, which must be stopped promptly to prevent irreversible damage to the inner ear. CSF, cerebrospinal fluid.

Floating or Depressed Footplate

A footplate that is irretrievably depressed into the vestibule (Figure 32–11) will almost certainly cause immediate and in some cases, long-term vertigo. Once a footplate has settled in the vestibule there is no safe way to extract it without further jeopardizing the inner ear. If preoperative evaluation makes limited ankylosis likely the procedure may be deferred or extreme care should be exercised while manipulating the suprastructure. Fenestration by laser reduces the chances of a footplate disarticulation as the laser exerts no pressure. Another preventive measure is assessing the movement of the footplate before

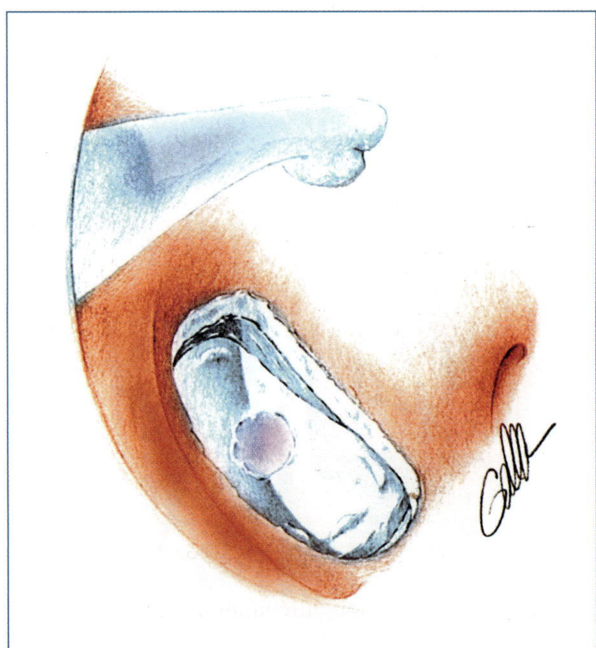

FIGURE 32–11 • A footplate floating in the vestibule, with the stapediovestibular joint completely separated, jeopardizing the integrity of the membranous labyrinth.

completing the fracturing and disengaging the suprastructure. If the footplate seems to be mobilized, every effort should be made to divide the crura prior to removal.

In the case of a floating footplate, fenestration can still sometimes be made with a laser. If that instrument is unavailable or the footplate too thick for the laser to penetrate, a small bur hole can be created inferior to the annular ligament and the footplate elevated with a small hook. The opening is then sealed with a tissue graft and an appropriately sized prosthesis is placed. If the footplate is depressed into the vestibule it should not be extracted, and the procedure is completed. However, results are highly variable. If the footplate is still attached at one end, it can sometimes be removed by a small hook engaged to a remnant of the crus on the nondepressed side. Small fragments of footplate or bone dust usually do not harm the inner ear.

Postoperative Complications

Facial Palsy

Immediate facial paralysis is related to local anesthesia or intraoperative trauma to the nerve. When facial paralysis is the result of local anesthesia, it is most often related to overzealous injection of the cartilaginous canal with injection of the stylomastoid foramen. Local anesthesia can also infiltrate to the middle ear from external auditory canal injection or by direct application to the middle ear. Temporary paralysis of the nerve results, but should recover completely within few hours. If weakness persists past a period of 3 h, a traumatic injury is the likely reason. The facial nerve can be damaged by a bone curette or drill during removal of the bony annulus, by fracturing the stapes toward the nerve rather than away toward the promontory, and by injuring an anomalous nerve. If the surgeon is certain of the integrity of the nerve, no further intervention is indicated rather than eye protection and potentially a course of systemic steroids. If the surgeon is uncertain of the state of the nerve and does not recall manipulating or traumatizing the nerve, exploration of the ear is required. On the very rare occasion that a transaction or other significant trauma to the nerve is found, repair with or without cable graft may be required.

Delayed facial nerve paralysis is uncommon, with a reported incidence of about 0.5%.[85] It appears 5 to 20 days following surgery and usually resolves in 1 or 2 months.[87,88] These patients are managed similarly to those with Bell's palsy.[87,88]

Chorda Tympani Dysfunction

The chorda tympani exits the posterior iter, usually to traverse the field of stapes surgery. Injury to the nerve may result in hypogeusia and dysgeusia, with evidence of atrophy of the fungiform papillae in the denervated area. Symptoms arise more often in stapes surgery and myringoplasty compared to surgery for chronic otitis media possibly as in the latter condition the nerve may be damaged by the disease prior to surgery.[89,90] Rarely the nerve does not need to be manipulated to obtain proper exposure and is not at risk. Infrequently, the nerve is situated as to prohibit surgery and needs to be cut. A severed nerve will cause temporary symptoms, which will improve in the course of 3 to 6 months with few or no long-term symptoms. In the course of typical stapes surgery, the nerve is manipulated to some extent, stretched or dried out. The dried nerve recuperates function quickly and completely. The stretched nerve may cause the most disturbing and potentially chronic symptoms of metallic taste, unpleasant taste, and altered taste of various foods. The stretched nerve seems to cause more disturbing symptoms compared to a severed nerve.[89,90] Hence, if the surgeon estimates during surgery that the nerve has been significantly stretched, it is better to sacrifice the nerve.

Otitis Media

Acute otitis media in the immediate postoperative period is worrisome as the risk of suppurative labyrinthitis and meningitis is high. In the rare occurrence of the latter complications, the patient experiences pain and fever; management includes removal of any ear canal packing and admission to the hospital. Treatment with broad-spectrum antibiotics is initiated and adjusted according to culture if available. Steroids may be helpful to minimize inner ear damage. Acute otitis media occurring after the immediate postoperative area (lasting approximately 6 weeks) is treated the same as for other patients.

Vertigo

Vertigo may appear during surgery, immediately following it, or in a delayed manner. The first type of vertigo may indicate an insult to the membranous labyrinth (Figure 32–12), or may be the result of air entering the vestibule. Air is most often introduced to the vestibule as a result of suctioning in the oval window or occasionally by the rapid expansion of perilymph from a laser pulse. Pneumolabyrinth generally resolves in 24 to 48 h. Blood causes chemical irritation and resolves in a matter of days. Vertigo extending beyond that time suggests a more serious insult to the inner ear and is often associated with SNHL. Even if hearing recovers, a vestibular deficit may remain, and should be tested for and taken into consideration before operating on the contralateral ear.

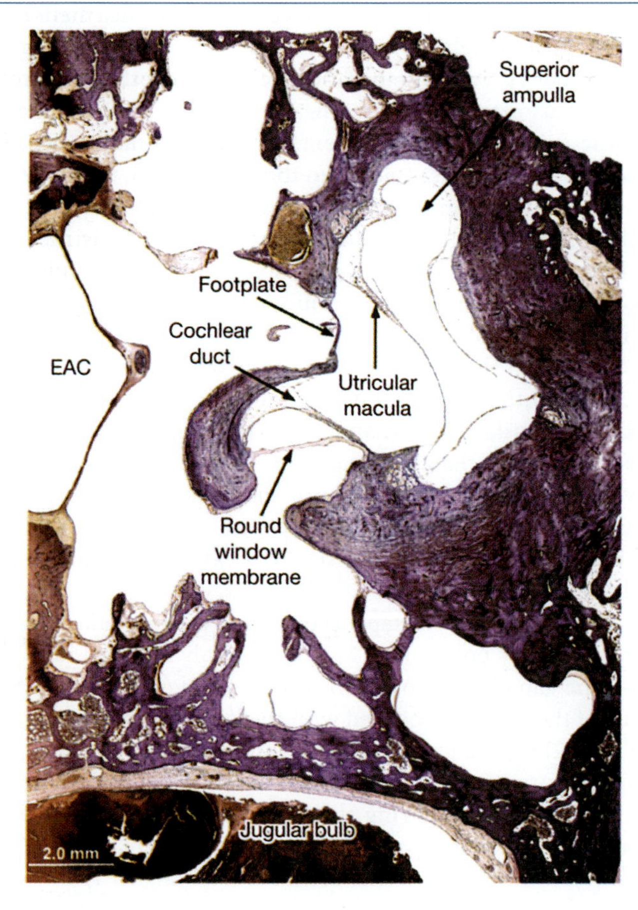

FIGURE 32–12 • A vertical section of a temporal bone. The proximity of the utricle to the undersurface of the footplate can be appreciated. This distance averages 2 mm. EAC, external auditory canal. *From Nadol JB Jr, McKenna MJ, editors. Surgery of the ear and temporal bone. 2nd ed. Philadelphia, PA: Lippincott Williams & Wilkins; 2005. p. 297. Reprinted by permission.*

Delayed vertigo after stapes surgery is rare and can be the result of benign positional paroxysmal vertigo[91] that can be treated by physical therapy or the result of a PLF.[92] A PLF can occur in the early or late post operative period.

Reparative Granuloma

A reparative granuloma is a mass of exuberant granulation tissue[18] developing in reaction to surgery, a foreign body (e.g., surgical glove powder, Gelfoam sterilized by formaldehyde, the prosthesis), or to perilymph.[93] It manifests in the 5th to 15th day after surgery. The associated symptoms and signs of labyrinthitis (dizziness, tinnitus, hearing loss, and nystagmus toward the nonoperated side) appear after an early period of hearing gain. Otoscopy reveals edema, thickening, and hyperemia of the skin flaps and tympanic membrane. Audiometry demonstrates a mixed hearing loss and decreased speech discrimination scores. Clinical suspicion of a reparative granuloma is an indication for immediate reexploration in order to attempt to reduce the likelihood and extent of permanent inner ear dysfunction. Steroids may be useful in this setting as well. The granulation tissue and prosthesis are removed, and the fenestra is sealed with a tissue graft. Early intervention may help patients recover some hearing. Vestibular symptoms usually resolve in weeks or months. Changes in surgical technique and materials used have made this once common complication rare.

Sensorineural Hearing Loss

Slight transient depression (<5 dB) in bone conduction immediately following the procedure is a common occurrence and attributable to mild serous labyrinthitis. Permanent SNHL can occur immediately following surgery or appear weeks or months after. Early loss, especially at high tones, is attributable to surgical trauma. Delayed SNHL should raise the suspicion of a PLF. A delayed fluctuating low-frequency loss may indicate post-traumatic hydrops. Up to 1% of patients undergoing stapes surgery suffer partial or even complete SNHL.

Conductive Hearing Loss

Conductive hearing loss after stapes surgery can appear unexpectedly immediately after the operation or more commonly delayed after initial good result. The etiology of immediate and delayed conductive loss and their respective treatment are different. Common reasons for immediate conductive loss after stapes surgery are (1) malfunctioning prosthesis, eg, one that is too short, (2) unrecognized malleus fixation, (3) unrecognized round window obliteration, (4) middle ear effusion, and (5) presence of unrecognized SSCD. Computed tomographic scanning can help in identifying SSCD and, at times, round window obliteration. Revision surgery may be considered after waiting for several months.

More commonly, conductive hearing loss appears at a variable time after a good initial closure or reduction of the air–bone gap. The most frequent findings for recurrent conductive hearing loss following stapes surgery are erosion of the incus at the site of prosthesis attachment (64%), malpositioned prosthesis (41%), bony (14%) or fibrous regrowth at the oval window area, and round window obliteration (23%).[93] Incus erosion initially manifests with a fluctuating loss intermittently improved by the Valsalva maneuver or changing head position. Eventually, complete discontinuity of the ossicular chain occurs resulting in a large air–bone gap. Incus erosion is due to resorptive osteitis from differential movement of the prosthesis and incus or foreign body reaction, as occurred with polyethylene struts. As the incus has good intraosseus blood supply, strangulation of the mucosa by crimping is not a likely cause.

REVISION STAPES SURGERY

Revision stapes surgery is technically more challenging, has a higher incidence of complications, and has lower success rates compared to primary stapes surgery.[94–96] There are a number of indications for revision stapes surgery.[65,96] Delayed or immediate postoperative conductive hearing loss of at least 20 dB in the speech frequencies can be an indication for revision surgery, depending on the hearing status of the contralateral ear. The best chance for improvement is in cases with initial hearing improvement after primary stapedectomy that later diminishes. Dizziness and unsteadiness can be caused by an excessively long prosthesis. Symptoms of PLF are an indication for intervention to alleviate symptoms and reduce the chances of further deterioration of inner ear function. In one series, 4 out of 10 patients suspected of having a PLF had the diagnosis confirmed at revision surgery.[96]

Local anesthesia in revision surgery allows the patients to report symptoms of inner ear trauma, however, the potentially extensive time of the procedure may warrant general anesthesia. As the chorda tympani nerve may be adherent to the tympanic membrane or the tympanomeatal flap, special attention must be paid to elevating the flap and to reflecting the drum anteriorly. Sharp dissection may be necessary to separate the nerve from the flap. Frequent findings at revision exploration are prosthesis malfunction at the incus, most often due to incus resorption or suboptimal prosthesis placement; prosthesis displacement from the oval window; an intact footplate; a short prosthesis; malleus fixation; and no abnormal findings in exploration.[65,96] More than one finding may be present, and each possibility should be assessed in a systematic manner. Assessing the exact cause of hearing loss requires good exposure of the oval window niche and the prosthesis. The laser is particular helpful in revision surgery when it can be used to divide adhesions, mucosal folds, and soft tissue surrounding the prosthesis in the oval window.

Details of revision surgery are dependent on the nature of pathology found on exploration of the middle ear and thus are not uniform. Often the lenticular process and the distal end of the long process of the incus are partially or completely eroded (Figure 32–13) or less frequently the incus is fixed or subluxed. If the anatomy is favorable, a replacement prosthesis can be positioned from the remainder of the incus to the vestibule with incus reattachment. Some surgeons have advocated reinforcement or augmentation by bone cement.[97] When the incus remnant is not suitable for prosthesis attachment, a malleus grip prosthesis can be used. Recommendations in order to maximize chances of successful malleus attachment include selecting patients with a normal tympanic membrane and plica mallearis (Figure 32–14), tight crimping, and using a prosthesis length that extends further into the vestibule (1 mm depth) compared to an incus attachment prosthesis.[98] A malleus attachment prosthesis is an option in patients with a fixed malleus head. After the prosthesis is attached to the manubrium, the malleus head is separated from the manubrium with a malleus nipper and removed. The periosteum of the manubrium is incised with a sickle knife, and the periosteum and plica mallearis are separated from the manubrium creating a space through which the hook of the prosthesis is introduced (Figure 32–14). Once crimped the wire at the tip of the hook is wrapped further around the manubrium with a fine hook— a technically challenging task—as the manubrium has a larger diameter and less round shape than the long process of the incus. A nitinol (SMART) malleus attachment prosthesis has been developed. The prosthesis must be bent or otherwise made to compensate for the anterior to posterior distance between the manubrium and the oval window.

Results of revision stapedectomy are, on an average, inferior to primary procedures. Most commonly reported rates of air–bone gap closure to 10 dB or better are 60 to 80%.[65,94,96] Some of the factors associated with the less favorable outcomes are more than one previous surgery in the revised ear; indications for surgery other than conductive hearing loss; findings of incus necrosis requiring the use of a malleus attachment prosthesis; and otosclerosis regrowth. At a reported rate of 0.8 to 7.7%,[65,94–96] SNHL is a small risk although higher than with primary procedures. The risk is higher in patients with SNHL following the previous procedure.

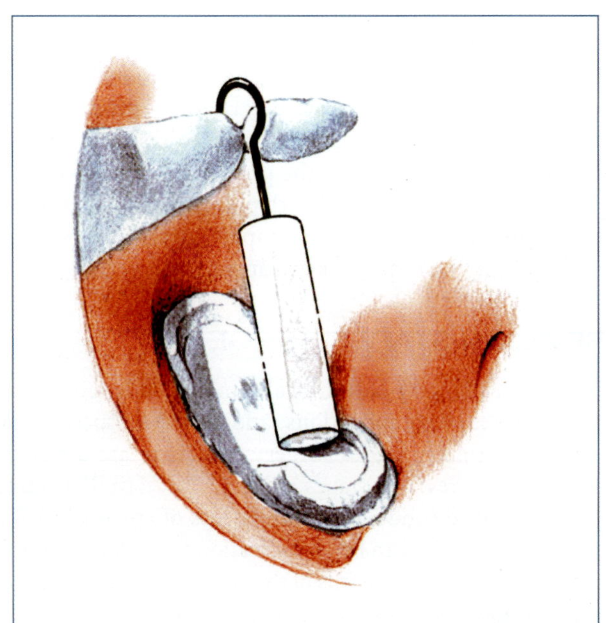

FIGURE 32–13 • Common finding in revision stapes surgery is resorptive osteitis of the incus, allowing the prosthesis to migrate laterally and out of the fenestra. With the prosthesis extruded, the fenestra may reseal with soft tissue. This is most often the result of inadequate crimping or interference with the free movement of the prosthesis.

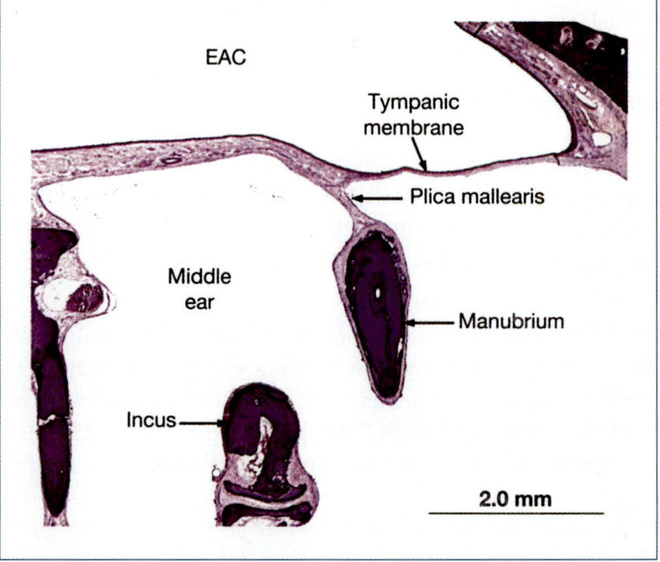

FIGURE 32–14 • A horizontal section through the drum and malleus. Along most of its length the manubrium is attached to the drum with a mucosal fold: the plica mallearis. Malleus attachment prosthesis can be placed by elevating the mucoperiosteum from the malleus in continuation of the plica mallearis to create a space of the prosthesis. Note the oval shape of the malleus, which contrasts the more rounded shape of the incus, hence requiring a different type of prosthesis. EAC, external auditory canal. *From Nadol JB Jr, McKenna MJ, editors. Surgery of the ear and temporal bone. 2nd ed. Philadelphia, PA: Lippincott Williams & Wilkins; 2005. p. 301. Reprinted by permission.*

TREATMENT OF OTOSCLEROSIS WITH COCHLEAR INVOLVEMENT

Sensorineural hearing loss is present in 20 to 30% of patients with otosclerosis. The loss is often progressive, gradual, irreversible, and worse in the high frequencies. It is speculated that cochlear otosclerosis reduces sensorineural hearing by interfering with the function of the spiral ligament.[99] At times, CT scans can demonstrate lucency around the cochlea representing demineralization around the cochlea, creating an appearance of a double ring or fourth turn of the cochlea.[100]

No agent has been proven to arrest or slow development of otosclerosis causing SNHL. Although the only controlled prospective study available for sodium fluoride demonstrated no better than a weak effect,[101] the drug is commonly used. Bisphosphonates may prove to be more efficacious in treating otosclerosis-induced SNHL.

Advanced otosclerosis can be an indication for cochlear implantation.[102,103] In some patients with evidence of profound loss, it may be prudent to first perform a stapedotomy prior to cochlear implantation.[102,104] In some patients, fitting a hearing aid after surgery will provide equal functional results as cochlear implantation.[104]

SUMMARY

Otosclerosis is a disorder of bone metabolism unique to the human temporal bone. Recent research has shed light on the etiology and pathogenesis of this disease. The disease is inherited in an autosomal dominant with incomplete penetrance pattern, and measles virus may play a role in the pathogenesis. Currently, treatment choices are limited to amplification and surgery for the correction of the conductive hearing loss associated with this condition. Medical treatment may be available in the future. Surgery for otosclerosis requires specific acquired skills. The most common procedure to correct stapedial fixation is the small fenestra stapedotomy with incus attachment prosthesis placed to re-establish sound transmission. Successful surgery reduces air–bone gaps to less than 10 dB and is achieved in 90% of patients. Noteworthy complications include SNHL (1%), chorda tympani nerve dysfunction, and vestibular injury. Patients with significant SNHL can be candidates for surgery even if they may require amplification after successful operation. Patients with far advanced otosclerosis may be candidates for cochlear implantation. Revision surgery is technically demanding, and is associated with lower success rates and slightly higher complication rates compared to primary surgery.

References

1. Pearson RD, Kurland LT, Cody DT. Incidence of diagnosed clinical otosclerosis. Arch Otolaryngol 1974;99:288–91.
2. Cawthorne T. Otosclerosis. J Laryngol Otol 1955;69:437–56.
3. Weber M. Otosklerose und umbau der labyrinthkapsel. Poeschel und Trepte, Leipzig, Germany.
4. Engstrom H. Uber das vorkmmen der otosklerose nebst exprimentellen studien uber chirurgische behandlung der krankheit. Acta Otolaryngol (Suppl.) 1940;43:1–153.
5. Guild SR. Histologic otosclerosis. Ann Otol Rhino Laryngol 1944;53:1045–71.
6. Decur F, et al. Prevalence of histologic otosclerosis: An unbiased temporal bone study in Caucasians. Adv Otorhinolaryngol 2007;65:6–16.
7. Vrabec JT, Coker NJ. Stapes surgery in the United States. Otol Neurotol 2004;25:465–469.
8. Nager GT. Pathology of the ear and the temporal bone. 1st ed. Williams and Wilkins; 1993.
9. Valsalva AM. Valsalvae opera et morgagni epistolae. Venetiis: Francescus Pitteri; 1741:2.
10. Politzer A. Die Otosclerose. In: Politzer A, editor. Lehrbuch der ohrenheilkunde für praktische ärtze und studierende. 2nd ed. Stuutgart: Ferdinand Enke Verlag; 1889. p. 233.
11. House HP, Hyman S. For the world to hear—a biography. 1st ed. Hope Publishing House; 1990.
12. Shea JJ Jr. Personal history of stapedectomy. Am J Otol 1998; 19(5 Suppl.):S2–S12.
13. Silverstein H. Laser Stapedotomy minus prosthesis (laser STAMP): A minimally invasive procedure. Am J Otol 1998;19:277–82.
14. Gjuric M, Rukavina L. Evolution of stapedectomy prostheses over time. Adv Otorhinolaryngol 2007;65:174–8.
15. Schuknecht HF, McGee TM, Colman BH. Stapedectomy. Ann Otol Rhinol Laryngol 1960;69:597–609.
16. Frisch T, Sorensen MS, Overgaard S, Bretlau P. Estimation of volume referent bone turnover in the otic capsule after sequential point labeling. Ann Otol Rhinol Laryngol 2000;109:33–9.
17. Schuknecht HF, Barber W. Histologic variants in otosclerosis. Laryngoscope 1985;95:1307–17.
18. Schuknecht HF. Pathology of the ear. Lea & Febiger; 1993.
19. Stankovic KM, McKenna MJ. Current research in otosclerosis. Curr Opin Otolaryngol Head Neck Surg 2006;14:347–51.
20. Quinn JM, Whitty GA, Byrne RJ, Gillespie MT, Hamilton JA. The generation of highly enriched osteoclast-lineage cell populations. Bone 2002;30:164–70.
21. Burgess TL, Qian Y, Kaufman S, Ring BD, Van G, et al. The ligand for osteoprotegerin (OPGL) directly activated mature osteoclasts. J Cell Biol 1999;145:527–38.
22. Lacey DL, Tan HL, Lu J, Kaufman S, et al. Osteoprotegerin ligand modules murine osteoclasts in vitro and in vivo. Am J Pathol 2000;157:435–48.
23. Ugasawa N, Takahashi N, Yasuda H, Mizuno A, et al. Osteoprotegerin produced by osteoblasts is an important regulator in osteoclasts development and function. Endocrinology 2000;141:3478–84.
24. Zehnder AF, Kristiansen AG, Adams AC, Merchant SN, McKenna MJ. Osteoprotegerin in the inner ear may inhibit bone remodeling in the otic capsule. Laryngoscope 2005;115:172–7.
25. Zehnder AF, Kristiansen AG, Adams AC, Merchant SN, Kujawa S, McKenna MJ. Osteopretegerin knockout mice demonstrate abnormal remodeling of the otic capsule and progressive hearing loss. Laryngoscope 2006;116:201–6.
26. Fowler EP. Otosclerosis in identical twins: A study of 40 pairs. Arch Otolaryngol 1966;83:324–8.
27. Morrison AW. Genetic factors in otosclerosis. Ann R Coll Surg Engl 1967;41:202–37.
28. Bel Hadj Ali I, Thys M, Beltaief N, Schrauwen I, et al. A new locus for otosclerosis, OTSC8, maps to the pericentromeric region of chromosome 9. Hum Genet 2008;123(3):267–72.
29. McKenna MJ, Kristiansen AG, Bartley ML, Rogus JJ, Haines JL. Association of COL1A1 and otosclerosis: Evidence for a shared

genetic etiology with mild osteogenesis imperfecta. Am J Otol 1998;19:604–10.

30. Clayton AE, Mikulec AA, Mikulec KH, Merchant SN, McKenna MJ. Association between osteoporosis and otosclerosis in women. J Laryngol Otol 2004;118:617–21.
31. Manolidis S, Alford LR, Smith RJ, Ball C, Manolidis L. Do the genes that cause otosclerosis reduce susceptibility to otitis media? Otol Neurotol 2003;24:868–71.
32. Ferlito A, Arnold W, Rinaldo A, et al. Viruses and otosclerosis: Chance association or true causal link. Acta Otolaryngol 2003;123:741–6.
33. McKenna MJ, Mills BG, Galey FR, Linthicum FH Jr. Filamentous structures morphologically similar to viral nucleocapsids in otosclerotic lesion in two patients. Am J Otol 1986;7:25–8.
34. McKenna MJ, Mills BG, Immunohistochemical evidence of measles virus antigens in active otosclerosis. Otolaryngol Head Neck Surg 1989;101:415–21.
35. McKenna MJ, Mills BG. Ultrastructural and immunohistochemical evidence of measles virus in active otosclerosis. Acta Otolaryngol Suppl 1990;470:130–40.
36. Karosi T, Konya J, Szabo LZ, Sziklai I. Measles virus prevalence in otosclerotic stapes footplate sample. Otol Neurotol 2004;25:451–6.
37. McKenna MJ, Kristiansen AG, Haines J. Polymerase chain reaction amplification of measles virus sequence from human temporal bone sections with active otosclerosis. Am J Otol 1996;7:827–30.
38. Niedermeyer H, Arnold W, Neubert WJ, Hofler H. Evidence of measles virus RNA in otosclerotic tissue. ORL J Otorhinolaryngol Relat Spec 1994;56:130–2.
39. Niedermeyer HP, Arnold W. Otosclerosis: A measles virus associated inflammatory disease. Acta Otolaryngol 1995;115:300–3.
40. Lolov SR, Encheva VI, Kyukchiev SD, Edrev GE, Kehayev IR. Antimeasles immunoglobulin G in sera of patients with otosclerosis is lower than that in healthy people. Otol Neurotol 2001;22:766–70.
41. Lippy WH, Berenholz LP, Schuring AG, Burkey JM. Does pregnancy affect otosclerosis. Laryngoscope 2005;155:1833–6.
42. Merchant SN, Rosowski JJ. Conductive hearing loss caused by third-window lesions of the inner-ear. Otol Neurotol 2008;29:282–9.
43. Mikulec AA, McKenna MJ, Ramsey MJ, et al. Superior semicircular canal dehiscence presenting as conductive hearing loss without vertigo. Otol Neurotol 2004;25:121–9.
44. Merchant SN, Rosowski JJ, McKenna MJ. Superior semicircular canal dehiscence mimicking otosclerosis hearing loss. Adv Otorhinolaryngol 2007;65:137–45.
45. Zhou G, Gopen Q, Poe DS. Clinical and Diagnostic characteristic of canal dehiscence syndrome: A great otologic mimicker. Otol Neurotol 2007;28:920–6.
46. Niedermeyer HP, Hausler R, Schwab D, Neuner NT, Busch R, Arnold W, Evidence of increased average age of patients with otosclerosis. Adv Otorhinolaryngol 2007;65:17–24.
47. Vincent R, Sperling NM, Oates J, Jindal M. Surgical findings and long-term hearing results in 3050 stapedotomies for primary otosclerosis: A prospective study with Otology-Neurotology Database. Otol Neurotol 2006;27:S25–S47.
48. Saim L, Nadol JB Jr. Vestibular symptoms in otosclerosis-correlation of otosclerotic involvement of vestibular apparatus and Scarpa's ganglion cell count. Am J Otol 1996;17:263–70.
49. Ayache D, Earally F, Elbaz P. Characteristic and postoperative course of tinnitus in otosclerosis. Otol Neurotol 2003;24(1):48–51.
50. Sobrinho PG, Oliveira CA, Venosa AR. Long-term follow-up of tinnitus in patients with otosclerosis after stapes surgery. Int Tinnitus J 2004;10(2):197–201.
51. Aarnisalo AA, Vasama JP, Hopsu E, Ramsay H. Long-term hearing results after stapes surgery. Otol Neurotol 2003;24:567–71.
52. Kaz J. Handbook on clinical audiology. 5th ed. Lippincott Williams and Wilkins; 2002. p. 22.
53. Vicente Ade O, Yamashita HK, Albernaz PL, Penido Nde. Computed tomography in the diagnosis of otosclerosis. Otolaryngol Head Neck Surg 2006;134:685–92.
54. Naumann IC, Porcellini B, Fisch U. Otosclerosis: Incidence of positive findings on high-resolution computed tomography and their correlation to audiological test data. Ann Otol Rhinol Laryngol 2005;114(9):709–16.
55. Hughes GB. The learning curve in stapes surgery. Laryngoscope 1991;101:1280–4.
56. Yung MW, Oates J, Vowler SL. The learning curve in stapes surgery and its implication to training. Laryngoscope 2006;116:67–71.
57. Falcone MT, Gajewski BJ, Antonelli PJ. Hearing loss with stapedotomy in otitis media. Otolaryngol Head Neck Surg 2003;129:666–73.
58. Ayache D, Corre A, Van Prooyen S, Elbaz P. Surgical treatment of otosclerosis in elderly patients. Otolaryngol Head Neck Surg 2003;129:674–7.
59. Iurato S, Bux G, Mevoli S, Onori M. Stapes surgery in the elderly. Adv Otorhinolaryngol 2007;65:231–6.
60. House JW, Toh EH, Perez A. Diving after stapedectomy: Clinical experience and recommendation. Otolaryngol Head Neck Surg 2001;125:356–60.
61. Huttenbrink KB. Clinical significance of stapedioplasty biomechanics: Swimming, diving, flying after stapes surgery. Adv Otorhinolaryngol 2007;65:146–9.
62. Riechelmann H, Tholen M, Keck T, Rettinger G. Perioperative glucocorticoid treatment does not influence early post-laser stapedotomy hearing thresholds. Am J Otol 2000;21:809–12.
63. Somers T, Vercruysse JP, Zarowski A, Verstreken M, Offeciers E. Stapedotomy with microdrill or carbon dioxide laser: influence on inner ear function. Ann Otol Rhinol Laryngol 2006;115(12):880–5.
64. Buchman CA, Fucci MJ, Roberson JB Jr. De La Cruz A. Comparison of argon and CO2 laser stapedotomy in primary otosclerosis surgery. Am J Otolaryngol 2000;21(4):227–300.
65. Lesinski SG. Revision Stapedectomy. Curr Opin Otolaryngol Head Neck Surg 2003;11:347–54.
66. Jovanovic S, Schonfeld U, Schere H. CO_2 laser stapedectomy with the "one-shot" technique-clinical results. Otolaryngol Head Neck Surg 2004;131(5):750–7.
67. Fritsch MH, Naumann IC. Phylogeny of stapes prosthesis. Otol Neurotol 2008;29:407–15.
68. Harris JP, Gong S. Comparison of hearing results of nitinol SMART prosthesis stapes piston prosthesis with conventional piston prosthesis: postoperative results of nitinol stapes prosthesis. Otol Neurotol 2007;28:692–5.
69. Brown KD, Gantz BJ. Hearing results after stapedotomy with nitinol piston prosthesis. Arch Otolaryngol Head Neck Surg 2007;133(8):758–62.

70. Wengen DF. A new self-retaining titanium clip stapes prosthesis. Adv Otorhinolaryngol 2007;65:184–9.
71. Rosowski JJ, Merchant SN. Mechanical and acoustic analysis of middle ear reconstruction. Am J Otol 1995;16(4): 486–97.
72. Teig E, Lindeman HH. Stapedotomy piston diameter is bigger better? Otorhinolaryngol Nova 1999;9:252–6.
73. Marches MR, Cianfrone F, Passali GC, Paludeti G. Hearing results after stapedotomy: Role of prosthesis diameter. Audio Neurotol 2007;12:221–5.
74. Shabana YK, Ghonim MR, Pedersen CB. Stapedotomy: Does prosthesis diameter affect outcome? Clin Otolaryngol 1999;24:91–4.
75. Herzog JA. 0.4 mm prosthesis stapedotomy: A consistent technique for otosclerosis. Am J Otol 1991;1:16–9.
76. Syms MJ. Safety of magnetic resonance imaging of stapes prosthesis. Laryngoscope 2005;115:381–90.
77. Fritch MH. MRI scanners and stapes prosthesis. Otol Neurotol 2007;28:733–8.
78. Committee on hearing and equilibrium guidelines for the evaluation of results of treatment of conductive hearing loss. Otolaryngol Head Neck Surg 1995;113:186–7.
79. Shea JJ. Stapedectomy—A long term report. Ann Otol Rhinol Laryngol 1982;91:516–20.
80. Neff BA, Lippy WH, Schuring AG, Rizer FM. Stapedectomy in patients with prolapsed facial nerve. Otolaryngol Head Neck Surg 2004;130:597–603.
81. Saunders NC, Fagan PA. Promontory drilling in stapedectomy: An anatomical study. Otol Neurotol 2006;27:776–80.
82. Ayache D, Sleiman J, Plouin-Gaudon I, Klap P, Elbaz P. Obliterative otosclerosis. J Laryngol Otol 1999;113(6):512–4.
83. Nadol JB Jr. Histopathology of residual and recurrent conductive hearing loss after stapedectomy. Otol Neurotol 2001;22:162–9.
84. Mehta RP, Harris JP, Nadol JB. Malleus fixation: Clinical and histopathologic findings. Ann Otol Rhinol Laryngol 2002;111:246–54.
85. Schuknecht HF, Reisser C. The morphologic basis of perilymphatic gushers and oozers. Adv Otorhinolaryngol 1988;39:1–12.
86. Cremeres CW. How to prevent a stapes gusher? Adv Otorhinolaryngol 2007;65:278–84.
87. Shea JJ Jr. Ge X. Delayed facial palsy after stapedectomy. Otol Neurotol 2001;22:465–70.
88. Salvinelli F, Casale M, Vitaliana L, Greco F, et al. Delayed peripheral facial palsy in stapes surgery: Can it be prevented? Am J Otolaryngol 2004;25(2):105–8.
89. Clark MP, O'Malley S. Chorda tympani nerve function after middle ear surgery. Otol Neurotol 2007;28:335–40.
90. Michael P, Raut V. Chorda tympani injury: Operative findings and postoperative symptoms. Otolarnygol Head Neck Surg 2007;136:978–81.
91. Atacan E, Sennaroglu L, Genc A, Kaya S. Benign paroxysmal positional vertigo after stapedectomy. Laryngoscope 2001;111(7):1257–9.
92. Albera R, Canale A, Lecilla M, Cavalot AL, Ferrero V. Delayed vertigo after stapes surgery. Laryngoscope 2004;114(5):860–2.
93. Kuhweide R, Van de Steene V, Vlaminck S, Casselman JW. Reparative granuloma related to perilymphatic fistula. Adv Otorhinolaryngol 2007;65:296–9.
94. Hammerschlag PE, Fishman A, Scheer AA. A review of 308 cases of revision stapedectomy. Laryngoscope 1998;108(12):1794–1800.
95. De La Cruz A, Fayad JN. Revision Stapedectomy. Otolaryngol Head Neck Surg 2000;123:728–32.
96. Lippy WH, Battista RA, Berenholz L, Schuring AG, Burky JM. Twenty-year review of revision stapedectomy. Otol Neurotol 2003;22:560–6.
97. Goebel JA, Jacob A. Use of Mimix hydroxyapatite bone cement for difficult ossicular reconstruction. Otolaryngol Head Neck Surg 2005;132:727–34.
98. Sarac S. McKenna MJ, Mikulec AA, Rauch SD, Nadol JB Jr, Merchant SN. Results after revision stapedectomy with malleus grip prosthesis. Ann Otol Rhinol Laryngol 2006;115(4):317–22.
99. Doherty JK, Linthicum FH Jr. Spiral ligament and stria vascularis changes in cochlear otosclerosis: Effect on hearing level. Otol Neurotol 2004;25:457–64.
100. Som PM, Curtin HD. Head and neck imaging. 4th ed. Mosby; 2003. p. 1249–53.
101. Bretlau P, Salomon G, Johnsen NJ. Otospongiosis and sodium fluoride. A clinical double-blind, placebo-controlled study on sodium fluoride treatment in otospongiosis. Am J Otol 1989;10: 20–2.
102. Rama-Lopez J, Cervera-Paz FJ, Manrique M. Cochlear implantation of patients with far-advanced otosclerosis. Otol Neurotol 2006;27:153–8.
103. Rotteveel LJ, Proops DW, Ramsden RT, Saeed SR, van Olphen AF, Mylanus EA. Cochlear implantation in 53 patients with otosclerosis: Demographics, computer tomographic scanning, surgery and complication. Otol Neurotol 25;2004:943–52.
104. Calmels MN, Viana C, Wanna G, Marx M, James C, Deguine O, Fraysse B. Very far-advanced otosclerosis: Stapedotomy or cochlear implantation. Acta Oto-Laryngologica 2007;127: 574–8.

Implantable Middle Ear and Bone Conduction Hearing Devices

33

Charles C. Della Santina, MD, PhD / Lawrence R. Lustig, MD

Although conventional hearing aids are the principal means of auditory rehabilitation for patients with sensorineural hearing loss (SNHL) or conductive hearing loss (CHL) that cannot be resolved via medical or operative treatment, more than 85% of hearing aid candidates reject them due to lack of sufficient perceived benefit, out-of-pocket expense, discomfort, and cosmetic concerns.[1] Even among the minority patients who do want to use hearing aids, medical complications of external auditory canal occlusion, such as chronic otorrhea and otitis externa, can complicate or prevent successful use of conventional hearing aids.

Implantable acoustic/mechanical hearing devices differ from conventional hearing aids in that they are partially or totally implanted and directly couple acoustic energy to the ossicular chain or cochlea. In exchange for the added surgical risks and costs associated with implantation, they offer several potential advantages over conventional hearing aids, including increased gain and dynamic range, reduced feedback, reduced maintenance, improved appearance, and freedom from ear canal occlusion. The balance between risks, costs, and advantages continues to evolve as implantable hearing device technology improves.

LIMITATIONS OF CONVENTIONAL HEARING AIDS

Conventional hearing aids are limited in their ability to amplify sound without generating feedback or imparting distortion, because these aspects of performance are physically interrelated (Table 33–1).

Insufficient Gain

For a patient with air conduction thresholds of 80 dB HL to perceive quiet sounds at a normal threshold of 0 dB HL, a hearing aid must amplify sound by a *gain* of 80 dB, generating a 10,000-fold increase in sound pressure wave amplitude and a 100,000,000-fold increase in sound power intensity.[2] This represents the limit of existing conventional hearing aids. For example, the maximum amplification at 1 kHz for a behind-the-ear (BTE) Phonak SuperFront PPCL4 power digital aid is about 75 to 82 dB.[3] As a rule, hearing aid gain and overall size scale up and down together, with the most powerful aids being large and the cosmetically less obtrusive aids offering less gain. The maximum gains for digital in-the-ear (ITE), in-the-canal (ITC), and completely-in-canal (CIC) aids currently are about 55 to 65 dB, 45 to 55 dB, and 35 to 50 dB, respectively.[3]

Acoustic Feedback

Feedback further limits the useful gain of conventional hearing aids to less than the maximum gains described above. Acoustic waves from the hearing aid speaker leak through the air space between the hearing aid body and the external auditory canal wall back to the microphone, where (for a subset of frequencies) they add to existing microphone input and are amplified further. The resulting positive feedback loop causes a low-frequency hum or high-frequency squeal. Feedback is typically worst for CIC aids, in which the microphone is closest to the speaker, and for ears with mastoid bowls, in which an airtight seal is difficult to obtain. At very high amplification, it is a problem even for BTE aids. Fitting aids tightly into the external auditory canal can decrease feedback, but this decrease comes at the cost of increased incidence of discomfort, otitis externa, autophony, and blockage of natural sound input.

Distortion of Spectral Shape and Phase Shifts

Typically optimized for performance in the band containing most speech signals (500–2,000 Hz), conventional hearing aids do not provide much amplification below ~250 Hz or above ~6,000 Hz. The resulting loss of "bass" and "treble" can give the sound percept an artificial character. Isolated severe hearing loss at low frequencies (as in Ménière's) or high frequencies (as in presbycusis) can be difficult to remediate with traditional aids without overamplifying the midrange frequencies at which

TABLE 33–1 Nonideal features of conventional aids

Insufficient amplification
Acoustic feedback
Spectral distortion
Nonlinear/Harmonic distortion
Occlusion of external auditory canal
Appearance/Visibility
Lack of directionality

a patient may have normal hearing. Even in the midfrequency range, steep changes in audiometric threshold at neighboring frequencies (eg, the notch often present in noise-induced hearing loss) cannot be perfectly fit due to inherent limitations in the rate of change of gain across frequencies. Too steep a change in amplifier gain across frequencies imparts phase shifts that distort the pitch and timbre of sounds. While the transition from analog circuitry to digital signal processing and programming has enhanced ability to fit each individual's audiometric profile, these fundamental limitations persist.

Nonlinear/Harmonic Distortion

For high-intensity hearing aid output, nonlinear distortion of the sound signal arises as the speaker is driven into the range of movements for which it begins to saturate or clip. The resulting distortion imparts aberrant spectral components into the sound percept, giving it an artificial or robotic character. While digital signal processing within an aid's amplification circuitry can mitigate distortion effects, distortion produced by a speaker generating loud sounds in air remain a fundamental limitation of all traditional hearing aids.

Occlusion Effects

To minimize feedback, most traditional hearing aids are fit to create an airtight seal with the external auditory canal wall, isolating the hearing aid's speaker in the occluded ear canal. Canal occlusion has several undesirable effects. First, it can be uncomfortable due to pressure on canal skin. Second, it increases the likelihood of otitis externa due to disturbance of wax egress and moisture retention, particularly in patients with tympanic membrane perforations or otorrhea due to chronic suppurative otitis media. Third, it causes autophony and a sense of aural fullness that can worsen with changes in ambient barometric pressure. Fourth, it blocks the normal pathway for sound entry to the ear. Finally, it disrupts the spectral shaping that normally occurs due to external auditory canal resonances. Open-fit hearing aids mitigate these canal occlusion side effects by dispensing with tightly fit occlusive canal molds and instead using thin, nonocclusive tubes for delivery of sound. To avoid feedback, these aids employ feedback cancellation circuitry and locate the microphone far from the speaker tube output (eg, on the BTE portion of the device). Open-fit hearing aids are an excellent option for individuals with isolated moderate high-frequency hearing loss. However, they perform less well when amplification at low and midrange frequencies is required.

Poor Appearance

Many patients reject hearing aids due to their appearance and social stigma. Even the 8% of hearing aid candidates wearing ITC aids listed poor cosmetic appearance as a major contributing factor in their decision not to use a hearing aid.[4] Hearing aids are difficult to conceal in patients who are balding or who wear their hair short. Miniaturization of electronics continues to improve hearing aids in this regard: CIC hearing aids are essentially invisible to the casual observer, and open-fit aids are unobtrusive. However, miniaturization typically comes at the cost of lower gain, more feedback, and higher cost. Ultimately, battery size becomes the limiting factor, with smaller batteries costing more and requiring more frequent replacement.

Poor Transduction Efficiency

Loss of energy due to impedance mismatching and transduction losses and is an inherent drawback of all conventional aids. The mechanical impedance (change in pressure for a given displacement) of the air-filled external auditory canal differs from that of the fluid-filled cochlea. When the tympanic membrane and ossicular chain are functioning normally, they act as an impedance-matching transformer by virtue of the relative areas of the tympanic membrane and stapes footplate, and by the lever action of the ossicular chain. The relatively large displacement, low-pressure movements of air against the tympanic membrane are transduced to the relatively small displacement, high-pressure movements of the footplate. Without a middle ear mechanism, most of the acoustic energy striking the stapes footplate reflects back into the air. Except for bone-conducting aids, all traditional hearing aids use a speaker to output an (amplified) acoustic wave into the air of the external auditory canal. When the middle ear apparatus is malfunctioning (as in otosclerosis, ossicular discontinuity, or tympanic membrane perforation), conventional hearing aids must overcome the impedance mismatch. The result is either reduced effective gain, increased distortion, or both.

Even when the ossicular chain is functioning normally (eg, in a patient with purely SNHL), transduction of acoustic energy from air at the input of a traditional hearing aid to stapes footplate motion is imperfect. Whenever a signal flows from one physical realm (eg, electrical current in a speaker) to another (eg, acoustic waves in air), some signal energy is lost and noise or distortion can add to the desired signal. There are several transduction steps for a traditional hearing aid—from acoustic waves in ambient air, to electrical current in a microphone, to a larger electrical current in a speaker wire or piezoelectric driver, to acoustic waves in air within the external auditory canal, to movement of the tympanic membrane and ossicular chain, to acoustic waves in perilymph, to hair cell stereociliary deflection and depolarization, and so forth. Most are unavoidable (although cochlear implants bypass these steps through direct cochlear nerve stimulation). However, directly coupling an actuator to the ossicular chain can bypass some of these transduction steps, boosting gain and reducing distortion. Nearly, all implantable acoustic/mechanical hearing devices make use of this approach.

IMPLANTABLE ACOUSTIC/MECHANICAL HEARING DEVICES

Implantable acoustic/mechanical hearing devices face most of the same challenges described above for conventional hearing aids, plus the added disadvantage of requiring surgery and thus being more costly. Considering the additional risk and costs, implantable hearing devices will only be an attractive option if they perform significantly better (in at least some respects) than the best available conventional aids a given patient could otherwise use.

Although the total number of hearing-impaired individuals is growing worldwide, the subset of hearing-impaired individuals who are currently considered good candidates for implantable rather than conventional aids by this criterion is limited to about 0.09% of the total.[4] Considering this comparatively small market against the expense of obtaining regulatory approval for implantable devices, the long-term viability of a small company offering a new implantable device is a factor both the patient and surgeon must critically evaluate when considering implantation. The sudden 2002 financial collapse of Symphonix Corp, the first company to clear the US Food and Drug Administration (FDA) hurdles and market their implantable middle ear hearing device in the United States, strongly underscored this point, as it transiently left a population of implanted patients (and their surgeons and audiologists) without a source for technical support. (Fortunately, subsequent purchase and successful rerelease of the Symphonix product line by the Med-El Corporation restored stable support for implantees in that instance.)

The following sections review common and distinctive features of the implantable acoustic/mechanical hearing devices in use in the US market as of 2008. Two recent reviews provide additional detail regarding these devices, technologies no longer in clinical use, and the history of middle ear implantable hearing devices.[5–7]

MIDDLE EAR IMPLANTS

Basic Design Features

Actuator Design

Conventional hearing aids function by receiving acoustic energy through a microphone, processing and amplifying the signal, and transmitting the signal through a speaker near the ear drum. This amplified sound then travels through the normal auditory pathway of the tympanic membrane and ossicles to the inner ear. Implantable middle ear hearing devices differ from conventional aids in how they impart sound vibration to the ossicular chain. In one of several mechanisms unique to each device, implantable middle ear hearing aids convert the electric signal movement of an actuator coupled to the ossicular chain. Two basic types of transducers that have been incorporated into the middle ear implantable hearing devices: *electromagnetic* and *piezoelectric*. Electromagnetic transducers generate a magnetic field using a wire coil carrying a current that encodes the microphone output. This magnetic field induces motion of a nearby magnet, which can either be separate from the coil and attached alone to the ossicles or integrated with the coil to become a vibrating compound mass affixed to the ossicles. Piezoelectric devices move ossicles using a piezoelectric crystal that bends or lengthens in time with changes in a signal voltage applied across it. Piezoelectric ossicular actuators generally yield greater power and less distortion than electromagnetic devices, but they are typically larger and require precise placement to ensure proper compressive force between the actuator (integrated into a housing rigidly connected to the temporal bone) and the ossicle it contacts.

Various implants employ a number of ways to couple vibration stimuli to the inner ear. Some employ a piezoelectric transducer to push on an ossicle, while others employ a magnet attached to an ossicle and vibrated via a signal current coursing through a wire coil. Either design can be adapted to contact the incus, stapes capitulum, stapes footplate, or round window membrane.

Total versus Partially Implantable Devices

Implantable middle ear hearing devices may be either partially or totally implanted. Partially implanted devices consist of an external processor comprising a microphone, speech processor, battery, and a transmitter coil that transcutaneously conveys signals and power to the internal device. This approach facilitates replacement of batteries, service and upgrade of processors, and minimization of internal device size, but requires patient acceptance of an external processor. By contrast, fully implantable systems house all of components within the implanted portion of the device, including the battery pack and a microphone. This frees the patient from wearing a visible external processor, but it increases the size and complexity of the implanted components, mandates surgical procedures for battery replacement each ~5 years, and complicates design and placement of the microphone.

Vibrant Soundbridge™ (Vibrant Med-El Corp.)

The Vibrant Soundbridge™ (Figure 33–1) was the first semi-implantable middle ear hearing device available in Europe (1998) and the United States (2000). Initially marketed by Symphonix, the product line was bought by the Med-El Corporation (Innsbruck, Austria) after Symphonix went bankrupt in 2002. Med-El resumed Vibrant Soundbridge™ sales in Europe by 2004 and in the United States in 2007.[8]

The device employs a "vibrating ossicular reconstruction prosthesis" (VORP) electromagnetic transducer, which is a magnet/coil combination typically attached to the long process of the incus and connected via a thin signal wire to an implanted receiver/amplifier. A signal current driven through the coil induces vibration of the magnet, which in turn shakes the long process of the incus to which it is attached. An external audio processor conveys power and signals to the implanted device via an inductive link. The external processor houses a microphone and standard zinc battery; it is held in place behind the ear by a permanent magnet.

The internal device typically is implanted using a standard transmastoid, facial recess approach to the middle ear. The internal receiver is placed in a bony trough in the retrosigmoid

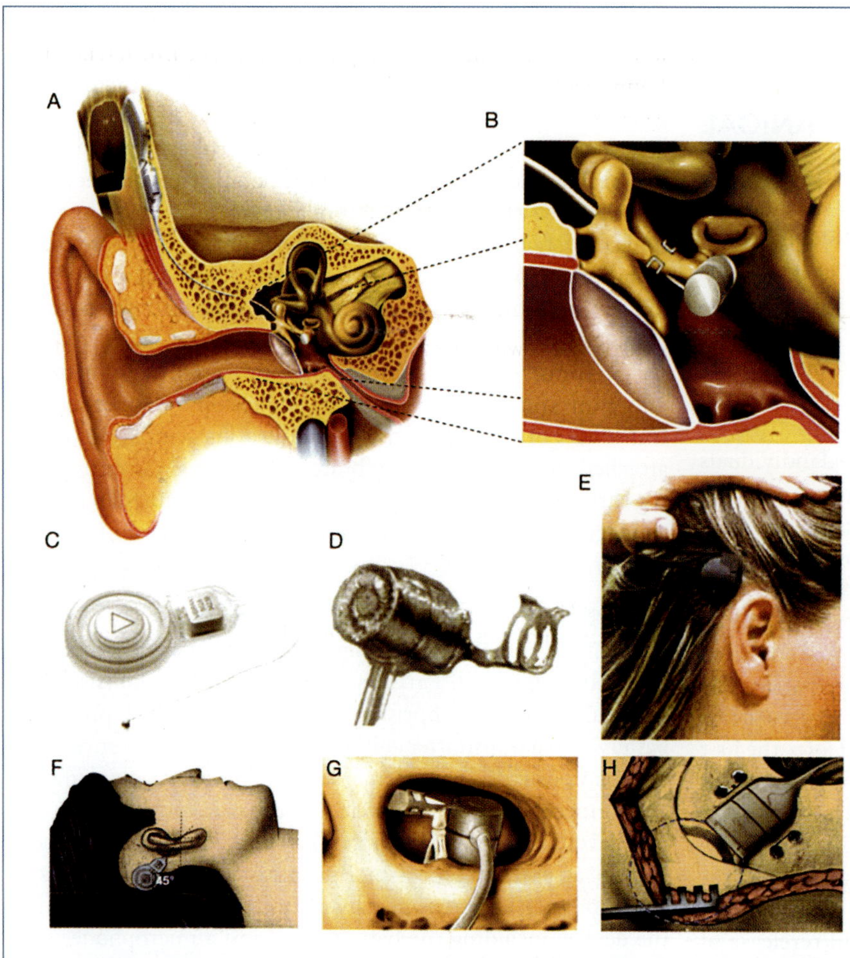

FIGURE 33–1 • The Vibrant Soundbridge™ semi-implantable hearing aid. *A*, An external microphone couples via an inductive transcutaneous link to the actuator, a "vibrating ossicular prosthesis" that couples to the incus long process (*B*). *C*, Implanted component of device. *D*, Vibrating ossicular prosthesis actuator. *E*, Programming unit and external circuitry. *F, H*, The inductive link is implanted against retromastoid cortical bone, similar to a cochlear implant. *G*, The VORP is clipped to the incus via a facial recess approach.

bone several centimeters behind the ear, similar to placement of a cochlear implant processor. The VORP™ is crimped into the long process of the incus. As in stapedectomy, crimping force during attachment of the prosthesis on the incus long process must reflect a balance between maximal vibration coupling and avoidance of incus ischemia and necrosis. Modifications of the typical surgical approach allow treatment of mixed hearing losses due to otosclerosis and/or ossicular erosion or agenesis through direct placement of the VORP™ on the stapes superstructure, round window, or oval window.

Short-term postoperative outcomes with the Vibrant Soundbridge™ compare favorably with optimally fit conventional hearing aids. A prospective, single-subject, repeated-measures multicenter study of 53 adult subjects with moderate to severe SNHL measured unaided hearing before and after implantation, functional gain, speech recognition, acoustic feedback, occlusion, patient self-assessment, and device preference in direct comparison between the Vibrant Soundbridge™ and appropriately fit acoustic hearing aids.[9] Implantation caused <10 dB change in residual hearing pure tone average (PTA) in 96% of subjects, while two subjects suffered a 12- to 18-dB worsening. Statistically significant improvement was observed in functional gain (threshold difference between aided and unaided condition) at all frequencies tested from 250 to 8,000 KHz, patient satisfaction, performance, occlusion, feedback, and device preference ($P<.001$). Greater than 10 dB improvement in functional gain was observed in 2, 4, and 6 kHz. Aided speech recognition in noise was statistically unchanged between the Vibrant Soundbridge™ and conventional aids cases, although 24% of subjects performed significantly better with the implanted device and 14% performed significantly worse. Multiple European studies have reported similar experience.[10,11]

As of 2008, over 2,500 patients have been implanted with the device worldwide over more than a decade, and long-term data for large cohorts reveal outcomes that are less ideal than early data but still favorable.[12] A multicenter study of the first 97 subjects implanted in France for whom 5- to 8-year follow-up was possible revealed that seven early recipients underwent reimplantation due to device failure (all before the 1999 redesign), seven underwent explantation without reimplantation, five others required revision surgery (four successfully), and eight others were nonusers (due to progression of loss, inadequate perceived benefit, or device failure).[12] Mean functional gain data remained unchanged from early postoperative values. The proportion of patients who said they would repeat the procedure (72%) remained the same as at 18 months postop, and ~40% said they would consider binaural implantation. The most common side effects were persistent aural fullness (27%) and persistent taste alteration (8%).

A 2005 summary from the device manufacturer on 1000 Vibrant Soundbridge™ implant cases described a 0.3% device failure rate since 1999 (excluding 27 of 200 devices of a prior design that failed before then) and a 5% incidence of revision

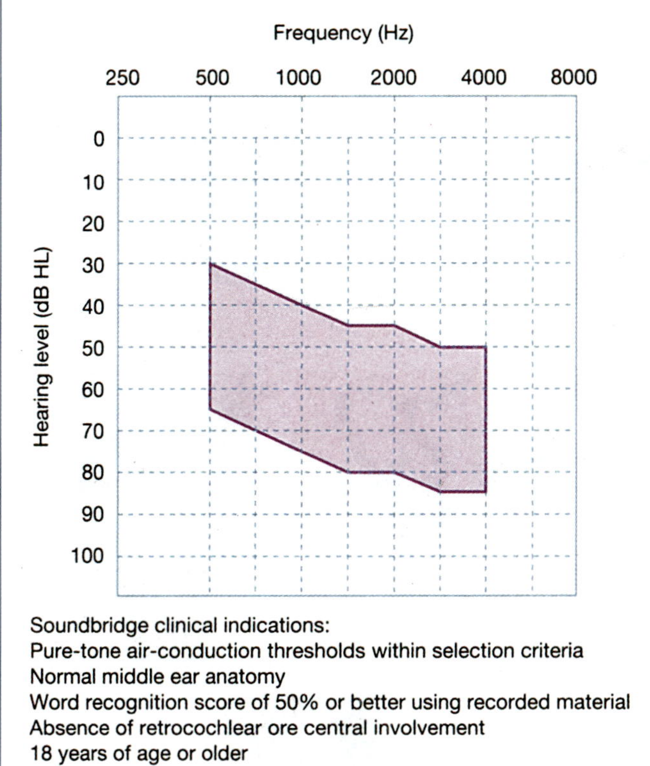

FIGURE 33–2 • Audiologic selection criteria for the Soundbridge™. The Soundbridge is indicated in patients with moderate to severe SNHL of up to 70 dB PTA hearing thresholds. The shaded area of the figure corresponds to the pure-tone audiometric implant criteria.

surgery due to inadequate performance (most of which were attributed to fibrosis, transducer malpositioning, or inadequate fixation).[13] Adequate performance was achieved after 12 of 16 revisions. Medical complications were uncommon, although a 1% rate of skin-flap necrosis was noted.

Because the VORP includes a magnetic component, the manufacturer recommends against magnetic resonance imaging (MRI) after VORP implantation. However, at least two implanted patients have undergone 1.5 T MRI without apparent injury or device damage.[14]

The Vibrant Soundbridge™ is suitable for patients with hearing loss of up to 70 dB PTA and is US FDA-approved for patients with moderate to severe SNHL, adequate aided speech discrimination, and medical contraindication or intolerance of a conventional hearing aid (Figure 33–2).[15] A clinical trial of the Soundbridge™ patients with mixed hearing loss (not yet a US FDA-approved indication) began in 2008.

Middle Ear Transducer (MET™) and Carina™ (Otologics LLC)

The Otologics Middle ear transducer (MET™) is an electromagnetic middle ear hearing aid using a mechanism initially developed by a group headed by John M Fredrickson, MD, PhD in collaboration with Storz Instrument Co. It is now manufactured by Otologics LLC.[16,17] The original, semi-implantable MET™ has been replaced by the fully implantable Carina™ currently in clinical trials (Figure 33–3).[18] Each uses the same actuator; the main difference between the two devices is that the Carina™ is a fully implantable device incorporating a subcutaneous microphone and battery sufficient to obviate the need for an external processor.

Whereas the Vibrant Soundbridge™ VORP relies upon vibration of a "floating mass" inertial load, the MET™/Carina™ mechanism moves the incus using a linear actuator rigidly connected to the edges of a limited mastoidectomy cavity. Within the actuator housing is an electromagnetic transducer converting signal current into axial movement of a rod extending out of the device to directly contact and move the incus body. This approach offers the potential to exert greater force on the incus than the floating mass approach; however, this comes at the expense of greater complexity in the implantation procedure, which must achieve precise positioning to ensure optimal compressive loading of the rod/incus junction.

Placement of Carina™ requires a general anesthetic and approximately a 2- to 3-hour operation (Figure 33–4).[18] Via a postauricular incision, a well is drilled to house the implant body and then a limited mastoidectomy is performed to expose the incus body and malleus head. A mounting stage similar to a titanium cranioplasty plate is attached over the opening using bone screws. A laser is used to make a small pit in the posterosuperior incus body, and then the linear actuator is maneuvered into the mounting system and its position is finely adjusted until its rod indents the incus pit with optimal compression force. The receiver capsule and transducer electronics are placed in the well, and the microphone is positioned subperiosteally at an intact region of mastoid cortex.

A multicenter, multinational trial of 282 adult patients with moderate to severe SNHL measured unaided hearing before and

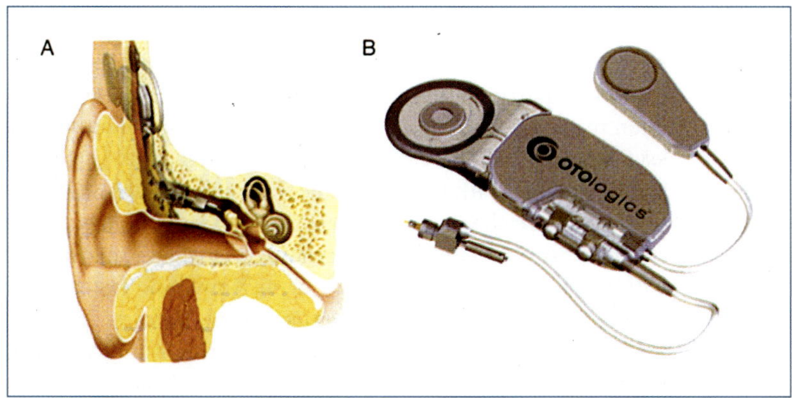

FIGURE 33–3 • Otologics Carina™. *A*, Anatomic placement. *B*, Internal and external components of the Otologics LLC Carina™ middle ear implant.

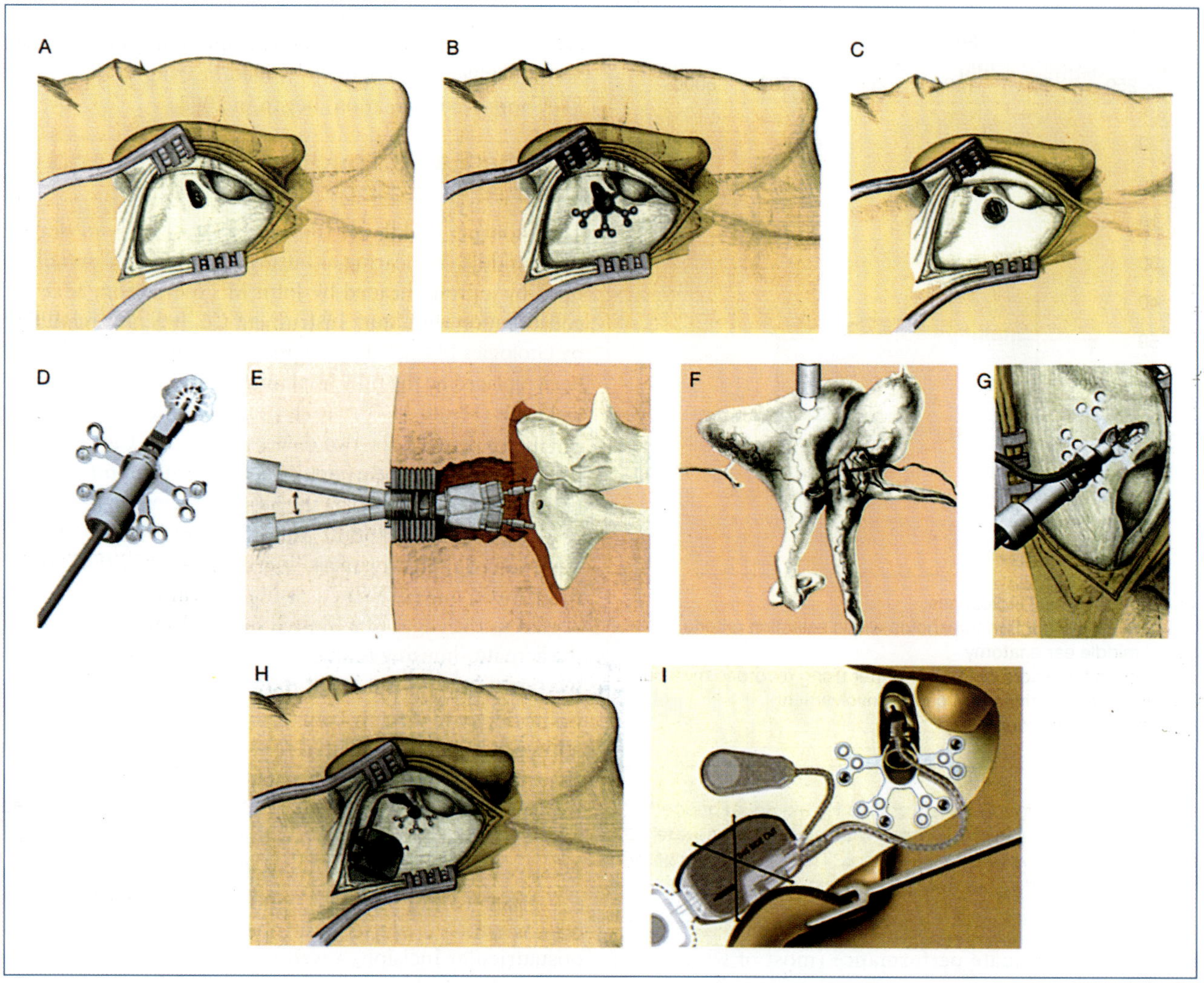

FIGURE 33–4 • Surgical implantation of the Otologics Carina™ begins with a limited antrotomy. (*A*) sparing cortical bone ledges for attachment of a metallic stage (*B*), which will steady a laser (*D*) for creation of a small hole in the posterosuperior incus. *E*, The laser is removed and replaced with the MET™ actuator, the tip of which inserts into the incudotomy (*F*). The actuator is secured to the stage (*G*), the remainder of the implanted device is secured to retromastoid cortical bone (*H*), and an external processor later connects to this area via a transcutaneous inductive link (*I*).

after implantation with the semi-implantable MET™, functional gain, speech recognition, and patient self-assessment.[17] A subset of 77 patients wore an optimally fit digital conventional hearing aid for at least 4 weeks preoperatively. Implantation caused no significant change in group mean air–bone gap; though an unspecified number of individuals suffered a "minor shift." Mean functional gain averaged across 0.5/1/2/4 kHz (for the subset of 160 subjects tested at 2 to 12 months postoperatively) was 28 dB. Speech recognition and subjective hearing assessment scores for the 77-subject cohort were not significantly different between the conventional digital aid and MET™. The rate of device failures, reoperation, and other complications were not described in that report.

A multicenter Phase I trial of 20 adults with up to 12 months use of the fully implantable Carina™ device revealed a <10 dB group mean threshold shift for all frequencies from 0.25 to 8 kHz at 3 months postop; this shift resolved by 12 months postop for all frequencies above 500 Hz.[18] Functional gain was lower than the preoperative "walk-in" hearing aid performance at all frequencies except 4 and 6 kHz at all test intervals. Word recognition scores remained close to preoperative aided levels, although significant decrements occurred due to microphone migration in some patients. These decrements improved with reprogramming. Patients' perceived benefit scores favored the implant particularly with regard to occlusion, appearance, and ease of use factors. Significant complications included device extrusion (partial in three devices and complete despite reoperation in two of those three) and device electronics failure in at least two subjects. The authors recommended against implantation in patients with thin or friable skin, and device fabrication processes were changed to address the electronics failure.

As a fully implanted device reliant on a rechargeable battery with a finite (~5-year) life, the Carina™ must be exposed via surgery for replacement of the battery every ~5 years.

The Carina ™ has received the CE mark for clinical use in Europe, and Phase II trials are underway in the United States. As

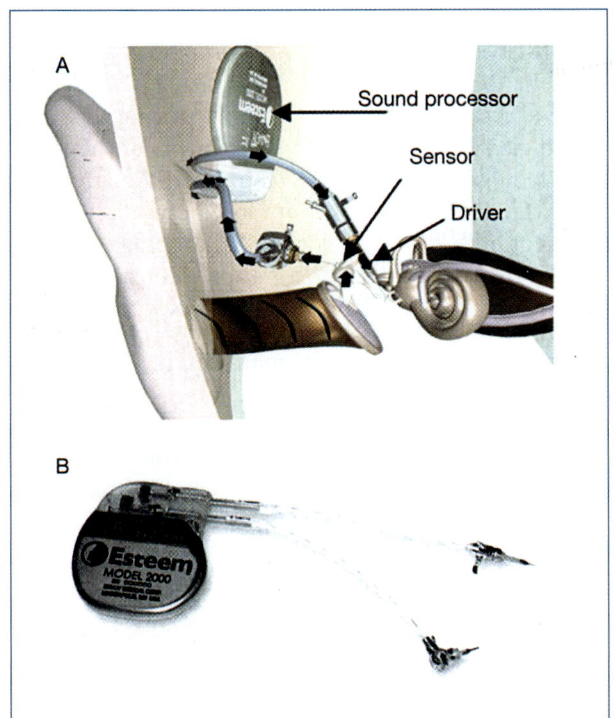

FIGURE 33–5 • The Esteem®/Envoy™ piezoelectric totally implantable hearing aid. *A*, Implantation technique. Instead of a microphone, sound enters the device via a piezoelectric transducer coupled to the malleus and tympanic membrane. A piezoelectric actuator produces amplified stapes motion. Note that the incus has been removed to prevent feedback. *B*, Complete device. *Images courtesy of Kem Jeanson, Envoy Medical Corp.*

of 2008, >50 patients had been implanted with the redesigned device and the failure modes identified during the Phase I trial had not recurred.[18] Variations on the size and length of the ossicular coupling have expanded the application of the Carina™ to patients with aural atresia and ossicular discontinuity, via direct attachment of the device on the stapes capitulum, stapes footplate, and round window.[19]

Esteem® Hearing Implant™ (Envoy Medical Corp.)

The Esteem®-Hearing Implant™ developed by Envoy Medical (formerly called the Envoy™ device and developed by St. Croix Medical, inc., Minneapolis, MN) is a fully implantable piezoelectric device that received the CE mark in Europe in 2006 and as of 2008 was in a Phase II clinical trial in the United States.[20,21] One especially notable design feature of the Esteem® is its use of the tympanic membrane and malleus as a microphone diaphragm; a piezoelectric sensor (essentially an actuator run in reverse) transduces malleus motion into a signal voltage, which is amplified and used to drive a second piezoelectric actuator in contact with the incus and/or stapes (Figure 33–5). Power is provided by a nonrechargeable lithium-ion battery designed to last 5 years between replacements, and control of the device is accomplished through a radio frequency transcutaneous link to a handheld device.

By using acoustic input measured at the malleus, the Esteem® should maintain the spectral shaping and sound-localizing characteristics of the pinna, external auditory canal, and tympanic membrane. However, implantation of the Esteem® requires partial removal of the incus to prevent feedback from actuator to sensor. This ensures a maximal CHL in the event of device failure or removal, unless a subsequent ossiculoplasty is performed. The internal battery must be replaced via a surgery every ~5 years.

The Esteem® is designed for patients with moderate to severe hearing loss. Indications include age ≥18 years, mild to severe (35 to 85 dB) SNHL between 0.5 and 4 kHz in the implanted ear that is equal to or worse than the hearing loss in the nonimplanted ear, a healthy ear with normal pneumatization and adequate space for device implantation on CT, normal tympanometry, and speech discrimination ≥60%.

A Phase I trial of the Envoy™ in the United States and Germany was completed in 2003.[20] By 1 year after implantation, three of the seven subjects continued to use the implant, three had been revised and then explanted, and one was awaiting revision surgery. For the three subjects with functioning implants, there was no significant change in bone thresholds, and the four-frequency PTA functional gain was 17 ± 6 dB, which was comparable to conventional hearing aids except at 3 kHz, where the Envoy™ performed less well than conventional aids. The drop in performance was attributed to a gradual ingress of moisture in the transducers.[20]

As of 2008, the device had received CE approval for European marketing, was available in several countries in and outside of Europe, and was undergoing a Phase II trial in the United States.[21]

IMPLANTED BONE CONDUCTION HEARING DEVICES

While many patients with conductive or mixed hearing loss can be effectively treated using standard surgical techniques, conventional hearing aids, or one of the middle ear implantable devices described above, others may not be well served by these options. This group includes patients with chronically draining ears despite multiple corrective attempts; inability to tolerate a hearing aid mold in a radical mastoid cavity; medical contraindications to surgical repair of a severe-to-profound predominantly CHL; canal atresia with unfavorable anatomy for atresia repair; and ear canal closure after radical mastoidectomy, lateral temporal bone resection, or extensive skull base surgery.

Conventional, nonimplanted bone-conducting hearing aids intended to serve these patients rely on a bone stimulator much like that used for audiometry. The stimulator is pressed firmly against postauricular skin over the mastoid cortex. Chronically applied, firm pressure on the skin and subcutaneous soft tissues typically results in pain, headache, and skin irritation. Sound fidelity is limited by soft tissue attenuation, variable placement of the vibrator, and flaccidity of the securing device (usually eyeglass frames). For these reasons, conventional bone conduction hearing aids have largely fallen out of favor with patients and clinicians, except in select circumstances. (Most notably, headband-mounted bone conduction stimulators serve a role in delivering auditory stimulation to infants with ear canal atresia whose temporal bones are not yet sufficiently calcified or thick enough to accommodate an osseointegrated device.[22]) For this group of patients, an osseointegrated bone-conducting stimulator can be an excellent option.

Implantable bone conduction stimulators work by vibrating the postauricular temporal bone. Because bone is an excellent short-range conductor of audio-band vibration, these vibrations reach the otic capsule with sufficient intensity to evoke basilar membrane and hair cell stereociliary deflections in time with the vibration. As illustrated by the Weber tuning fork test, CHL not only degrades air-conducted hearing relative to bone-conducted stimuli; it also effectively enhances bone-conducted hearing in the affected ear, probably because the acoustic impedance mismatch caused by loss of a middle ear transformer mechanism causes bone-conducted vibrations of the otic capsule to reflect off the stapes footplate.

Two such devices—the Audiant Bone Conductor (Medtronic Xomed, Inc.) temporal bone stimulator and the Baha® system (Cochlear Corp.)—have reached widespread clinical application. This section will review the former only briefly, because it is no longer available for sale, then focus on the latter.

Audiant™ Bone Conductor (Medtronic Xomed, Inc.)

The Audiant™ Bone Conductor™ manufactured by Xomed, Inc. (later Medtronic Xomed, Inc.) earned marketing approval by the US FDA in 1986 for patients with CHL and normal sensorineural hearing. It was implanted in over 2,000 patients before being removed from the market.[22,23]

The implanted portion of the Audiant™ comprised a titanium orthopedic bone screw attached to a titanium-aluminum-vanadium housing containing a permanent rare earth magnet. The external component included a microphone, amplifier, and power source connected to a transmitter coil held in position over the implant site by a second rare earth magnet.

Implantation was performed in the postauricular temporal bone near the sinodural angle. After elevation of a skin flap and identification of the sigmoid sinus, a 4-mm deep guide hole was drilled away from the sinus and tapped, and then the internal component was implanted flush with the skull surface via its integrated bone screw. After 8 to 12 weeks for healing, the external processor's transmitter coil was positioned over the implant and spacing between its permanent magnet and the underlying skin was adjusted, as needed, to excessive pressure and thus to reduce the risk of ischemic skin breakdown. Signal current in the external coil induced internal magnet vibration conveyed via the osseointegrated screw to cortical bone and thus to both otic capsules.

An initial report on the Audiant™ reported no complications and highly favorable outcomes, with a PTA functional gain of 25 dB for 19 recipients.[22] A subsequent report on 200 recipients revealed a mean 30 ± 9 dB improvement in 0.5 to 4 kHz PTA air–bone gap (to within 10 dB of closure) between the unaided and Audiant™-aided condition.

Complications of Audiant™ use mainly centered on soft tissue breakdown and failure to achieve desired results particularly in cases not meeting approved candidacy criteria.[23] In one series of 128 implants, 5 (4%) required removal for skin breakdown (2.3%), interference with MRI imaging, or patient dissatisfaction.[23] One other patient suffered experienced failure of osseointegration.

Growing experience and enthusiasm for the device quickly lead to off-label use and de facto liberalization of patient selection criteria to include patients with ipsilateral SNHL greater than the FDA-approved 25 dB PTA and patients with contralateral single-side SNHL. As of 1995, ~64% of the first 500 Audiant™ implantations performed in North America were in patients who did not meet FDA-approved candidacy criteria.[23] Inconsistent outcomes in such cases led to a 1995 recommendation against "overenthusiastic misapplication" in such scenarios.[23] Restriction of candidacy to patients with <25 dB PTA sensorineural hearing thresholds put the Audiant™ at a relative disadvantage compared with its main competitor, the percutaneous bone conduction Baha® system (see below). An unfavorable third-party payor environment in the United States for Audiant™ implantation reimbursement further restricted the number of patients implanted. As of 2008, Medtronic-Xomed was no longer marketing the Audiant™.

Baha® System (Cochlear Corp.)

The Baha® system (initially produced by Entific Corporation; now manufactured by Cochlear Corporation, Lane Cove, NSW, Australia) is currently the only US FDA-approved bone conduction hearing rehabilitation device available for clinical use (Table 33–2). It is a percutaneous osseointegrated bone conduction hearing rehabilitation instrument similar to the Audiant™ in the goal of delivering bone-conducted sound to an intact cochlea; however, its design differs in that it imparts bone vibration via a *percutaneous* metal post to which a microphone-amplifier-vibrator unit is directly attached.

Drawing upon Per-Ingvar Brånemark's discovery circa 1968 that titanium can bond directly to bone matrix without interposed soft tissue and result in an osseometallic interface of sufficient strength to support transgingival dental restorations, Brånemark, Tjellström, and colleagues at the Institute of Applied Biotechnology in Sweden developed percutaneous titanium implants intended for attachment of facial prostheses.[24,25] Extension of this approach to bone-stimulating vibrators led to the Baha®'s predecessor (the Noblepharma HC200) circa 1977.

Operative Technique

Insertion of osseointegrated implants for the Baha® generally takes place in a single stage (Figure 33–6) under local injection anesthesia typically delivered during a brief interval of sedation, although most children and some adults require general anesthesia and young children are often implanted via a two-stage procedure.[26] The implant site is typically chosen 50 to 55 mm posterior of the ear canal and preferably on or just below the linea temporalis. The ideal location is in a region of thin, relatively immobile skin, sufficiently posterior that subsequent attachment of the Baha® processor will not cause it to touch the pinna. Hair is shaved from the site and an adhesive drape is applied after skin preparation. A ~0.6-mm thick, ~2.5 × 2.5 cm skin flap is elevated using either a dermatome or scalpel. All soft tissue deep to this, including hair follicles, is excised down to (but not including) periosteum. An additional annulus of subcutaneous tissue is then excised for ~2.5 cm in all directions around the skin wound edges. The goal is to create a thin, immobile, dry, hairless ~1 cm rim of skin adjacent to the

TABLE 33–2 Baha®:Indications and Contraindications

INDICATIONS
1. Patient using a conventional BC hearing aid
2. Conventional AC hearing aid user with
a. chronic otorrhea
b. chronic otitis media/externa
c. uncontrollable feedback due to a radical mastoidectomy or large meatoplasty
3. Otosclerosis, tympanosclerosis, canal atresia with a contraindication to repair, eg,
a. only hearing ear
b. combination with 2a–c.
4. Single-side deafness with better ear BC PTA better than 45 dB HL and SDS >60%
CONTRAINDICATIONS
1. PTA BC thresholds (0.5 to 3.0 kHz) worse than 45 dB HL, SDS <60% in target ear
2. Emotional instability, development delay, or drug abuse
3. Age <5 years

AC, air conduction; BC, bone conduction; PTA, pure tone average; HL, hearing loss; SDS, speech discrimination score.

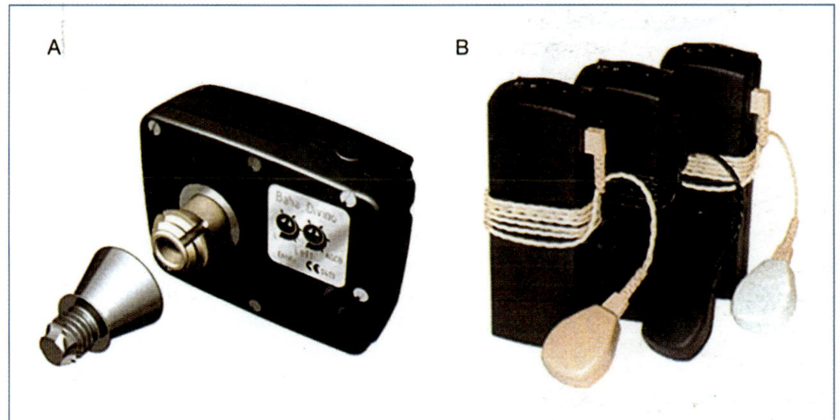

FIGURE 33–6 • Baha® by Cochlear Corporation. *A*, Divino (smallest of the three models), shown relative to the titanium osseointegrated screw and abutment (conical post) to which it attaches. Threaded portion of screw is 4 mm long. *B*, Cordelle body-worn processor (largest and most powerful of the Baha models).

planned implant site, analogous to the gingival around a tooth or cuticle adjacent to a finger nail, with a gradual increase in soft tissue thickness back to undisturbed tissues ~3 cm from the implant. This minimizes the area and relative mobility of the metal–skin interface (thus reducing the risk of infection) while creating a skin depression where the Baha® processor will reside (reducing the risk of acoustic feedback due to processor/skin contact). Periosteum is removed from a central ~1-cm region. A 3-mm deep guide hole is drilled at the planned implant site; if the hole's floor is solid, the hole is extended to 4 mm depth. The guide hole is used to align a countersink bur, which widens the guide hole and creates a shallow countersink in the adjacent bone surface. A self-tapping titanium bone screw with attached abutment (the percutaneous post to which a processor will be affixed 2 to 3 months postoperatively) is then advanced to full depth at a slow revolution rate and controlled insertion torque. Skin wound edges are sutured to underlying periosteum to coapt dead space; the skin flap is sutured back in its original position; a small hole is cut in the flap to allow it to slip around the abutment down to bone; and a gently compressive antibiotic-soaked dressing is applied and held in place with a plastic cap designed to snap on the abutment. After 5 to 7 days, the compressive dressing is removed. After waiting 8 to 12 weeks (for adults) or 12 to 16 weeks (for children >5 years old) for osseointegration, the Baha® processor can be snapped onto the abutment.

Although the procedure is straightforward, meticulous attention to technique is necessary to maximize the likelihood of osseointegration and minimize the chances of infection at the skin's interface with the abutment. In particular, bone must be kept clean and cool with copious irrigation during drilling and tapping to avoid osteocyte death and fibrosis; all drilling and implant insertion must occur along the same axis to avoid thread lock of the screw; and sufficient soft tissue must be excised to ensure a gradual descent of soft tissue thickness around the implant site. Without adequate irrigation, high-speed drilling typically used in otologic surgery can cause temperature elevations as high as 89°C, which can prevent subsequent osseointegration through death of osteocytes.[27] Variations in technique continue to evolve, mostly centered on ways to minimize soft tissue complications. Examples include stellate and linear incisions, use of full-thickness skin flaps, choice of dermatome or knife for flap elevation, various dressings, and early postoperative loading of the stimulating device.[28,29]

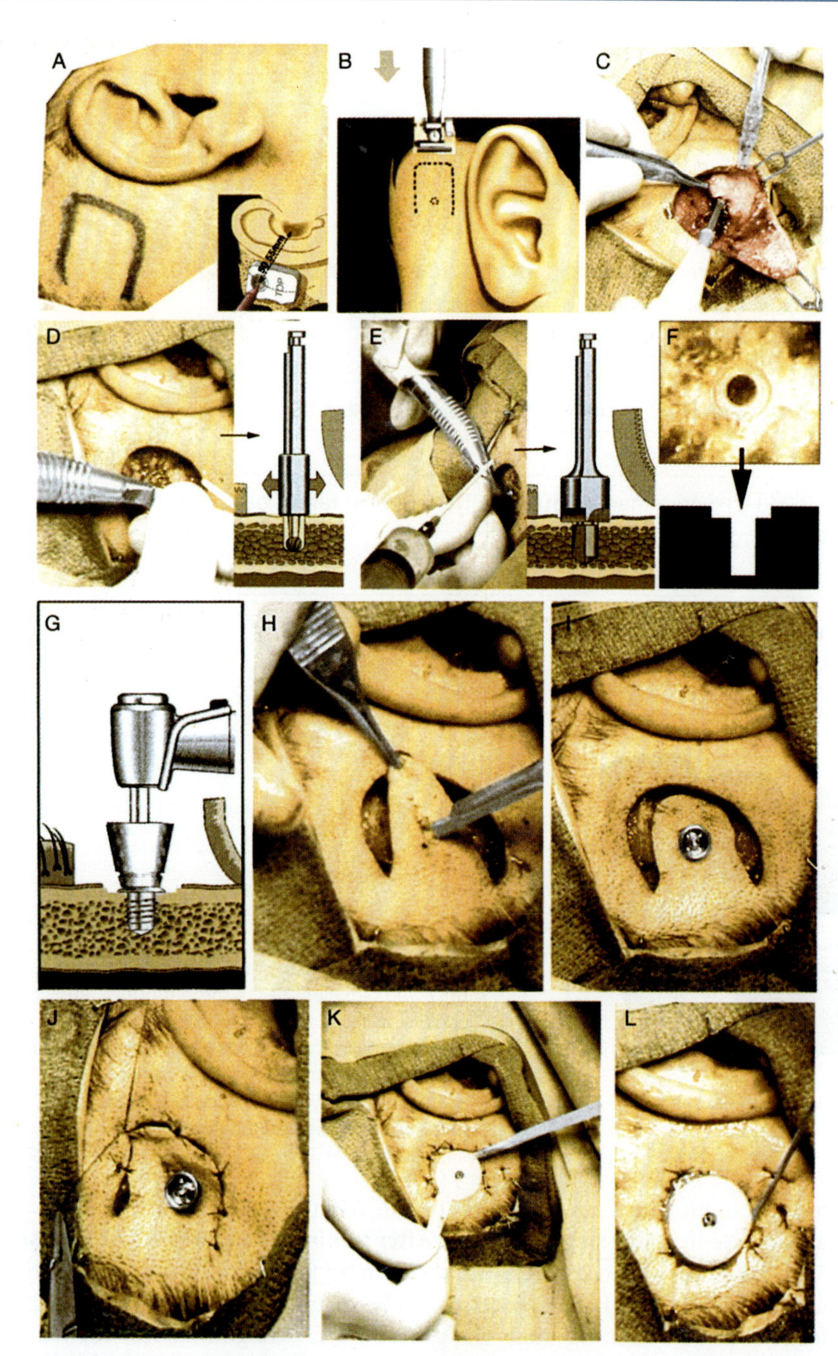

FIGURE 33–7 • Operative technique for placement of Entific Baha®™. *A,B*, A posterior-based skin flap is elevated and thinned until all hair follicles are removed from the flap center, typically using a dermatome. *C*, Soft tissues beneath and outward within ~2.5 cm of the flap are excised to create a smooth transition from surrounding tissue to the thin central skin flap. *D*, A 3- to 4-mm hole is drilled in mastoid or retromastoid cortex, typically at or just below the temporal line. *E, F*, A countersink creates a recessed surface for implant placement. *G*, A self-tapping titanium screw with integrated abutment (to which the Baha® processor will later attach) is implanted. *H–J*, The skin flap is replaced and sewn in place. *K, L*, A pressure dressing and healing cap are placed to apply gentle pressure to the skin flap, encouraging adhesion to the underlying periosteum and bone.

Outcomes

Håkansson et al.[30] reported on their 10-year experience in 147 patients who received the Baha®. Dividing patients into three groups based upon their PTA bone thresholds (0–45 dB, 46–60 dB, and >60 dB), the authors noted a strong relationship between PTA thresholds and successful outcome. In the group with the best cochlear reserve (PTA <45 db), 89% of patients reported subjective improvement with the implant, while 8% felt that their hearing was worse. By contrast, 61% and 22% of patients reported subjective hearing improvement, respectively in the groups with 46 to 60 dB and >60 dB bone conduction PTA. Average speech discrimination scores were 14% unaided, 67% with a conventional hearing aid, and 81% with the Baha®. Excluding subjects >60 dB bone conduction PTA, mean discrimination improved to 85%; excluding 46 to 60 dB PTA subjects raised mean discrimination to 89%. Based upon these results, the authors recommended a candidacy criterion of PTA <45 dB for the standard Baha® system. Subsequent development of more powerful Baha® processors (a slightly larger ear-level processor called the Intenso® and a belt-pack-powered device called the Cordelle®) has allowed liberalization of this criterion with successful outcomes in many cases up to ~60 dB bone-conducted PTA.

In a recent study of 115 children implanted over a 15-year period, parent-reported quality of life improved for every one of the 84 patients for whom a questionnaire was returned, and 97% of implanted children were daily users of the device.[31,32]

A review of the US experience with the Baha® has also been reported.[33] The most common indications for implantation included chronic otitis media and/or draining ears and external auditory canal stenosis or aural atresia. Patients who had undergone skull base surgery and had complete closure of the external auditory canal were also included. Overall, each patient had an average improvement of 32 dB +/− 19 dB with the use of the Baha®. Closure of the air–bone gap to within 10 dB of the preoperative bone conduction thresholds occurred in 80% of patients while closure to within 5 dB occurred in 60%. Nearly one-third of patients demonstrated "overclosure" of the preoperative bone conduction threshold of the better hearing ear.

Baha® implantation in patients with chronic suppurative otitis media who previously used hearing aids in mastoid bowls led to reduction of visit frequency for mastoid debridement and a consequent net cost savings.[34] A cost–benefit analysis of management options for external auditory canal atresia favored the Baha® over atresia repair.[35]

Baha® for Unilateral Sensorineural Hearing Loss

Though initially designed for patients with CHL, the Baha® system has proven valuable in rehabilitation of unilateral SNHL. Ipsilesional Baha® placement can capture sound and convey it to the intact cochlea via cranial vibration, accomplishing the same function of a conventional contralateral routing of signal (CROS) device without the need to wear a hearing aid in the intact ear. In one prospective trial of 23 adult subjects with unilateral deafness, patients were assessed after 1 month of using a CROS aid and then underwent Baha® implantation on the deaf side. The Baha® yielded improved patient satisfaction and speech recognition relative to CROS, while neither Baha® nor CROS significantly improved scores on a test of directional hearing.[36] Subsequent studies have demonstrated similar findings, suggesting that the Baha® outperforms conventional CROS aids in the setting of unilateral sensorineural deafness.[37]

Potential Complications

The most frequently encountered complication is a soft tissue inflammatory reaction around the percutaneous implant site. In a report on 456 patients, Tjellström and Håkansson noted a 3.4% incidence of adverse tissue reactions: 3 patients required implant removal for infection, 3 required revision surgery for infection, and 23 had tissue reactions requiring local treatment only.[26] A survey of the first 40 Baha® devices in the United States revealed that soft tissue complications were minimal and consisted of local inflammation at the percutaneous implant junction in 3 patients.[33]

As with any otologic procedure, Baha® complication rates vary with surgeon experience. Tjellstrom et al. reported a drop in soft tissue complication incidence from 6.8% in their first 60 patients to 3.5% in a separate cohort of 149 patients implanted a decade later.[38,39] Recent literature from a wide array of implant centers generally reflects higher rate of soft tissue complications, perhaps partly due to longer follow-up of previously trouble-free cases and partly due to the rapid expansion in the number of surgeons climbing the Baha® implantation learning curve. Falcone et al. reported a 22% incidence of skin growth over the abutment in a series of 90 adult cases.[39] In a retrospective review of 182 children over 15 years at one center, McDermott et al. found an implant failure rate of 14% despite use of a two-stage surgical approach, soft tissue complications in 17%, and revision surgery for skin growth over the abutment in 8%. Nonetheless, 97% of implanted children in that series remain daily Baha® users.[32]

Observations from these studies indicate that soft tissue reactions around percutaneous implants are best prevented by thinning periabutment skin, removing underlying soft tissue, and suturing dermis to subjacent bone to achieve immobility. Patient compliance with routine cleaning of the abutment site and close monitoring of adjacent skin is essential to success. Inadequate cleaning can lead to a vicious cycle in which increasingly severe periabutment inflammation increases the contact surface area between the abutment and adjacent skin or granulation tissue. This can ultimately lead to skin overgrowth sufficient to engulf the abutment beneath the skin surface, mandating surgical revision of the skin flap with more aggressive thinning of surrounding subcutaneous tissues. This problem is most common in patients with a thick (>1 cm) starting distance from skin surface to cranium. Wide resection of subcutaneous tissue is important in such patients. Topical steroid administration can help to thin down scar tissue threatening to engulf the abutment.

Due to cleavage of hair follicles during thinning of the underside of the skin flap, epithelial inclusion cysts and sebaceous cysts (due to collection of sebum from sebaceous glands cut open from below) sometimes require marsupialization in the office.

Complications other than adverse skin reactions are relatively rare. Osseointegration failure with subsequent device extrusion occurred in 4 (<3%) of 149 patients in one study of adults.[26] Additional complications cited for implant removal include poor cochlear function (5%), unexplained pain (2%), and uncooperative patients exhibiting poor compliance (2%).[33]

One disadvantage of any metallic implant is interference with subsequent imaging studies. Although the Baha® abutment causes some scatter artifact on CT, the implant is typically located out of the plane of axial and coronal slices through key temporal bone structures. Fortuitously, pure titanium produces relatively little degradation of images on MRI, and MRI is not contraindicated with the presence of a Baha® implant without its external processor.[40]

CONCLUSION

Totally and semi-implanted hearing aids can deliver improved sound quality, greater amplification, less distortion, better directional hearing, and better cosmetic appearance than conventional hearing aids. However, these highly desirable benefits come with tradeoffs including increased cost to both patient and insurer, risks of surgery, interference with imaging studies, the need to undergo subsequent procedures for battery replacement (in the case of totally implanted devices) and dependence on the sometimes uncertain long-term viability of manufacturers supporting implanted devices. Yet while conventional hearing aids continue to improve and while cochlear implantation criteria continue to expand, implantable acoustic/mechanical hearing devices will doubtlessly have a role to play in the care of patients whose hearing loss is not adequately addressed by those competing technologies.

References

1. 1977 Food and Drug Administration regulations: hearing aid devices—Professional and patient labeling and conditions for sale. Audiology Update 1993;12:3–5.
2. Blair B. Audio engineering handbook. New York: McGraw-Hill; 1988. p. 1–12.
3. http://www.phonak.com/professional/productsp/instrumentsp/classicp/superfront/superfrontppcl4.htm (accessed Sept 12, 2009).
4. Henrichsen J, Noring E, Christensen B, Pedersen F, Parving A. In-the-ear hearing aids. The use and benefit in the elderly hearing-impaired. Scand Audiol 1988;17:209–12.
5. Goode RL, Rosenbaum ML, Maniglia AJ. The history and development of the implantable hearing aid. Otolaryngol Clin North Am 1995;28:1–16.
6. Della Santina CC, Lustig LR. Surgically implantable hearing aids. In: Cummings CW, editor. Otolaryngology head & neck surgery. 4th edition. Philadelphia, PA: Elsevier Mosby; 2005. p. 2574–3602.
7. Goode RL. Current status and future of implantable electromagnetic hearing aids. Otolaryngol Clin North Am 1995;28: 141–6.
8. http://www.vibrantmedel.us/archive/layout/MEDEL_PR_Soundbridge.pdf (accessed March 12, 2008).
9. Luetje CM, Brackman D, Balkany TJ, et al. Phase III clinical trial results with the Vibrant Soundbridge implantable middle ear hearing device: A prospective controlled multicenter study. Otolaryngol Head Neck Surg 2002;126(2):97–107.
10. Fraysse B, Lavieille JP, Schmerber S, et al. A multicenter study of the Vibrant Soundbridge middle ear implant: Early clinical results and experience. Otol Neurotol 2001;22(6):952–61.
11. Fisch U, Cremers CW, Lenarz T, et al. Clinical experience with the Vibrant Soundbridge implant device. Otol Neurotol 2001;22(6):962–72.
12. Mosnier I, Sterkers O, Bouccara D, et al. Benefit of the Vibrant Soundbridge device in patients implanted for 5 to 8 years. Ear Hear 2008;29(2):281–4.
13. Labassi S, Beliaeff M. Retrospective of 1000 patients implanted with a Vibrant Soundbridge middle-ear implant. Cochlear Implants Int 2005;6(Suppl 1):74–7.
14. Todt I, Seidl RO, Mutze S, Ernst A. MRI scanning and incus fixation in Vibrant Soundbridge implantation. Otol Neurotol 2004;25(6):969–72.
15. Leysieffer H, Baumann JW, Mayer R, et al. A totally implantable hearing aid for inner ear deafness: TICA LZ 3001. HNO 1998;46:853–63.
16. Kasic JF, Fredrickson JM. The Otologics MET ossicular stimulator. Otolaryngol Clin North Am 2001;34:501–13.
17. Jenkins HA, Niparko JK, Slattery WH, Neely JG, Fredrickson JM. Otologics middle ear transducer ossicular stimulator: performance results with varying degrees of sensorineural hearing loss. Acta Otolaryngol 2004;124:391–4.
18. Jenkins HA, Atkins JS, Horlbeck D, et al. Otologics fully implantable hearing system: Phase I trial 1-year results. Otol Neurotol 2008;29(4):534–41.
19. Siegert R, Mattheis S, Kasic J. Fully implantable hearing aids in patients with congenital auricular atresia. Laryngoscope 2007;117:336–40.
20. Chen DA, Backous DD, Arriaga MA, et al. Phase 1 clinical trial results of the Envoy system: a totally implantable middle ear device for sensorineural hearing loss. Otolaryngol Head Neck Surg 2004;131:904–16.
21. http://www.envoymedical.com (accessed November 2, 2008).
22. Verhagen CV, Hol MK, Coppens-Schellekens W, Snik AF, Cremers CW. The Baha Softband. A new treatment for young children with bilateral congenital aural atresia. Int J Pediatr Otorhinolaryngol 2008;72(10):1455–9.
22. Hough J, McGee M, Himelick T, Vernon J. The surgical technique for implantation of the temporal bone stimulator (Audiant ABC). Am J Otol 1986;7(5):315–21.
23. Hough JV, Wilson N, Dormer KJ, Rohrer M. The Audiant Bone Conductor: update of patient results in North America. Am J Otol 1994;15(2):189–97.
24. Branemark PI, Adell R, Breine U, Hansson BO, Lindstrom J, Ohlsson A. Intra-osseous anchorage of dental prostheses. I. Experimental studies. Scand J Plast Reconstr Surg 1969; 3:81–100.
25. Albrektsson T, Branemark PI, Jacobsson M, Tjellstrom A. Present clinical applications of osseointegrated percutaneous implants. Plast Reconstr Surg 1987;79:721–31.
26. Tjellstrom A, Hakansson B. The bone-anchored hearing aid. Design principles, indications, and long-term clinical results. Otolaryngol Clin North Am 1995;28:53–72.
27. Eriksson RA, Albrektsson T, Magnusson B. Assessment of bone viability after heat trauma. A histological, histochemical and vital microscopic study in the rabbit. Scand J Plast Reconstr Surg 1984;18:261–8.
28. de Wolf MJ, Hol MK, Huygen PL, Mylanus EA, Cremers CW. Clinical outcome of the simplified surgical technique for BAHA implantation. Otol Neurotol 2008;29(8):1100–8.
29. Stalfors J, Tjellström A. Skin reactions after BAHA surgery: a comparison between the U-graft technique and the BAHA dermatome. Otol Neurotol 2008;29(8):1109–14.
30. Hakansson B, Liden G, Tjellstrom A, et al. Ten years of experience with the Swedish bone-anchored hearing system. Ann Otol Rhinol Laryngol Suppl 1990;151:1–16.
31. McDermott AL, Williams J, Kuo M, et al. Quality of life in children fitted with a bone-anchored hearing aid. Otol Neurotol 2009;30(3):344–9.
32. McDermott AL, Williams J, Kuo M, et al. The birmingham pediatric bone-anchored hearing aid program: A 15-year experience. Otol Neurotol 2009;30(2):178–83.
33. Lustig LR, Arts HA, Brackmann DE, et al. Hearing rehabilitation using the Baha® bone-anchored hearing aid: results in 40 patients. Otol Neurotol 2001;22:328–34.
34. Watson GJ, Silva S, Lawless T, Harling JL, Sheehan PZ. Bone anchored hearing aids: a preliminary assessment of the impact on outpatients and cost when rehabilitating hearing in chronic suppurative otitis media. Clin Otolaryngol 2008;33(4):338–42.
35. Evans AK, Kazahaya K. Canal atresia: "surgery or implantable hearing devices? The expert's question is revisited." Int J Pediatr Otorhinolaryngol 2007;71(3):367–74.
36. Lin LM, Bowditch S, Anderson MJ, et al. Amplification in the rehabilitation of unilateral deafness: speech in noise and directional hearing effects with bone-anchored hearing and

contralateral routing of signal amplification. Otol Neurotol 2006;27(2):172–82.

37. Holgers KM, Tjellstrom A, Bjursten LM, et al. Soft tissue reactions around percutaneous implants: a clinical study of soft tissue conditions around skin-penetrating titanium implants for bone-anchored hearing aids. Am J Otol 1988;9:56–9.

38. Baguley DM, Bird J, Humphriss RL, Prevost AT. The evidence base for the application of contralateral bone anchored hearing aids in acquired unilateral sensorineural hearing loss in adults. Clin Otolaryngol 2006;31(1):6–14.

39. Tjellstrom A, Granstrom G. One stage procedure to establish osseointegration. A zero to five years follow-up report. J Laryngol Otol 1995;108:593–8.

39. Falcone MT, Kaylie DM, Labadie RF, Haynes DS. Bone-anchored hearing aid abutment skin overgrowth reduction with clobetasol. Otolaryngol Head Neck Surg 2008;139(6):829–32.

40. Fritsch MH, Naumann IC, Mosier KM. BAHA devices and magnetic resonance imaging scanners. Otol Neurotol 2008;29(8):1095–9.

Surgery of the Inner Ear

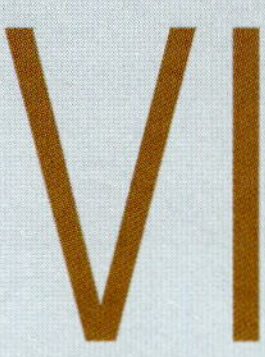

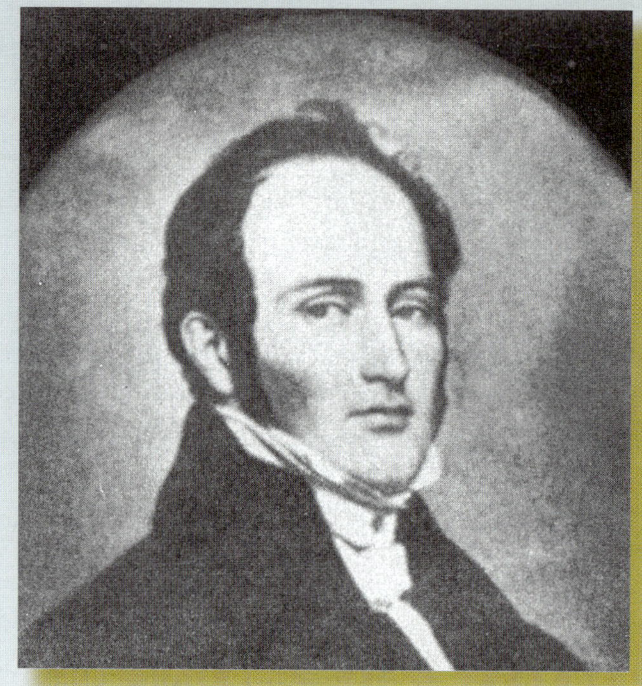

PROSPER MENIERE (1799-1862) • Described the symptomatology and proved the labyrinthine origin of episodic vertigo with deafness.

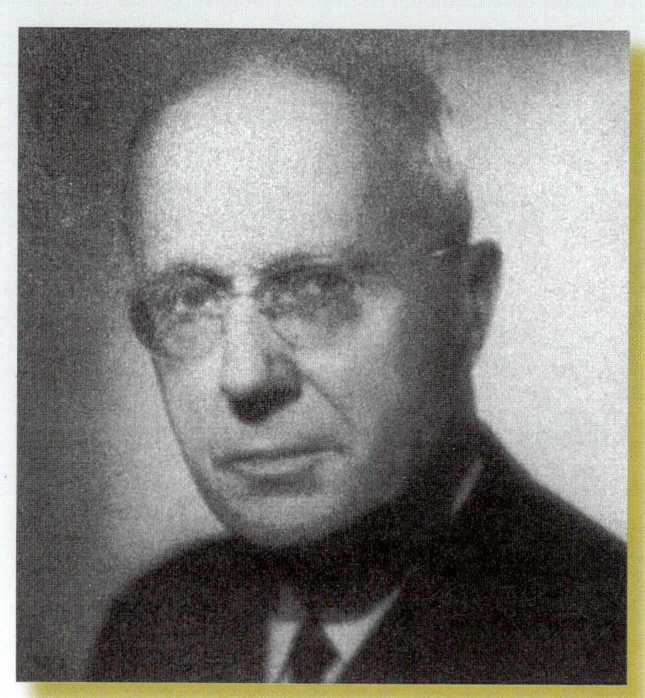

GEORGES PORTMANN (1890-1985) • Proposed surgical drainage of the endolymphatic sac for Ménière's disease.

Surgical Treatment of Peripheral Vestibular Disorders

34

Benjamin T. Crane, MD, PhD / Johan P. Carey, MD / Lloyd B. Minor, MD, FACS

INTRODUCTION

This chapter will review the surgical treatment of disorders that affect the vestibular end organs in the labyrinth. It begins with a brief review of historical understanding and treatment of peripheral vertigo, which is followed by a discussion of specific disorders and the procedures that have been used in the treatment of these disorders. It is important to note at the outset that most vestibular disorders are treated medically. Surgical treatment is only required in a minority of cases that fail medical treatment. The first step in evaluating a vestibular disorder that may require surgery is obtaining the history and performing a physical exam (see Chapters 6 and 9), followed by interpreting data from the relevant diagnostic tests (see Chapter 11) to derive an accurate diagnosis. It is rare, however, that the diagnosis itself leads immediately to a recommendation of surgery. The effects of symptoms on a patient's lifestyle and well-being have great influence in the selection and timing of different treatment options. In this regard, the factors influencing decisions about surgical interventions for disorders of the peripheral vestibular system are more diverse than those in many other areas of otology. The identification of a cholesteatoma, eg, readily leads to a recommendation for its surgical removal, unless there are extenuating circumstances precluding surgery. By contrast, two patients can have almost identical vertigo profiles due to Ménière's disease and similar findings on objective vestibular assessment but one patient may have little or no disruption of function from the vertigo, whereas the other patient may be debilitated.[1]

HISTORICAL BACKGROUND

Prior to the 1860s, dizziness and balance problems were thought to be exclusively central disorders, often referred to as "cerebral congestion" or classified as epilepsy. As early as the 1820s, the relationship of dizziness with eye movement was recognized; postrotatory nystagmus was observed in psychiatric patients after rotation in cages used to subdue them. Jan E. Purkinje hypothesized that this effect had a central origin. The field of clinical otology was very primitive at this time. John Harrison Curtis, who had a large, aristocratic practice in London (including the King) thought that deafness was caused by a cerumen deficiency, which he treated by painting creosote in the external auditory canal.[1] Vertigo was often treated with leaching, purging, and cupping. In the 1820s, there were the first hints that equilibrium may have a peripheral component. In 1824, Pierre Flourens published that after canal plugging, pigeons flew in circles in the same orientation as the ablated semicircular canal.[2]

The existence of peripheral vestibular disorders was proposed by Ménière in 1861.[3] Prosper Ménière, as director of a large deaf–mute institution in Paris, likely saw patients develop both vertigo and deafness immediately after trauma to the ear, allowing him to conclude that both symptoms have a common inner ear origin.[4] To support his conclusion, he presented the autopsy results of a young girl who developed sudden hearing loss and acute vertigo. On autopsy, Ménière found her brain was normal but the inner ear was filled with blood. Ironically, this patient likely had leukemia, not endolymphatic hydrops. Because of this finding it was commonly believed well into the 20th century that Ménière's disease was caused by hemorrhage. Prior to 1940, "Ménière's disease" was used as a generic term for any peripheral vertigo, especially if associated with hearing loss. The first insight into the true pathophysiology of Ménière's disease came in 1871, with Knapp's hypothesis that inner ear hydrops was similar to glaucoma.[5]

MÉNIÈRE'S DISEASE

Ménière's disease is the oldest of the peripheral vestibular diagnoses, and over time a large number of treatment options have been proposed. Early treatments focused on destruction of the end organ. In 1904, both the techniques of eighth cranial nerve section[6] and labyrinthectomy[7,8] were described. The concept of endolymphatic drainage was first reported by Portmann in 1926.[9] In the 1930s, Dandy proposed selective vestibular nerve section via a suboccipital approach and treated over 600 patients.[10] In this era, these procedures carried a high risk of deafness, facial nerve paralysis, and a considerable risk of mortality. Paradoxically, the surgical treatment of Ménière's disease indirectly led to better understanding of its pathophysiology. In 1938, upon histopathologic examination of the temporal bones of two vestibular nerve section patients who died in the perioperative period, Hallpike and Cairns noted endolymphatic system dilation with Ménière's disease, which they hypothesized to result from disruption of resorption.[11] This finding was independently and simultaneously reported by Yamakawa.[12] Subsequently, surgical treatment options focused on either attempting to correct the endolymphatic dilation or ablating the end organ.

Preoperative Considerations

Confirmation of the diagnosis is the first step in the evaluation of a patient in whom surgery is contemplated to treat the consequences of Ménière's disease. The presentation of classic Ménière's disease includes unilateral, low-frequency sensorineural hearing loss, aural fullness, tinnitus, and episodic vertigo that lasts for a few minutes to several hours.[13] The presence, characteristics, and severity of these symptoms can be variable and often overlap with other conditions, such as migraine[14] and vestibular schwannoma. Although tests can exclude diagnoses—for instance a magnetic resonance imaging (MRI) with gadolinium can exclude vestibular schwannoma—there currently is no "gold standard" test for Ménière's disease, and it remains a clinical diagnosis. The difficulty in establishing an accurate diagnosis of Ménière's disease has historically yielded a wide variation in the reported incidence of the disease, accuracy of diagnostic tests, and efficacy of treatment.[14]

The American Academy of Otolaryngology—Head and Neck Surgery (AAO-HNS) has published guidelines for the

TABLE 34–1 AAO-HNS Criteria for the diagnosis of Ménière's disease

MAJOR SYMPTOMS
Vertigo
• Recurrent, well-defined episodes of spinning or rotation • Duration from 20 min to 24 h • Nystagmus associated with attacks • Nausea and vomiting during vertigo spells common • No neurologic symptoms with vertigo
Deafness
• Hearing deficits fluctuate • Sensorineural hearing loss • Hearing loss progressive, usually unilateral
Tinnitus
• Variable, often low pitched and louder during attacks • Usually unilateral • Subjective
DIAGNOSIS OF MÉNIÈRE'S DISEASE
Possible Ménière's disease
• Episodic vertigo without hearing loss or • Sensorineural hearing loss, fluctuating or fixed, with dysequillibrium, but without definite episodes • Other causes excluded
Probable Ménière's disease
• One definitive episode of vertigo • Hearing loss documented by audiogram at least once • Tinnitus or aural fullness in the suspected ear • Other causes excluded
Definite Ménière's disease
• Two or more definitive spontaneous episodes of vertigo lasting at least 20 min • Audiometrically documented hearing loss on at least one occasion • Tinnitus or aural fullness in the suspected ear • Other causes excluded
Certain Ménière's disease
• Definite Ménière's disease, plus histopathologic confirmation

From Monsell et al.[15]

diagnosis of Ménière's disease. Guidelines are necessary because of the wide spectrum and severity of symptoms and the lack of standardization of the diagnosis in clinical studies. Initially proposed in 1972, these guidelines were revised in 1985, and again in 1995.[15] For the diagnosis of "definite" Ménière's disease, the following criteria must be fulfilled: the patient must have two or more episodes of spontaneous vertigo, each lasting at least 20 min; sensorineural hearing loss documented by audiogram; tinnitus or aural fullness in the affected ear; and other causes excluded (typically with a gadolinium-enhanced MRI of the internal auditory canals and cerebellopontine angles). The criteria for the diagnosis of Ménière's disease are summarized in Table 34–1.[15]

The criteria used to decide whether a patient is a good candidate for a procedure involve a determination that the symptoms are bothersome enough to justify the risks of that particular intervention. The results of quantitative vestibular testing, such as the caloric test, posturography, rotational testing, and others often do not correlate well with the severity of patient symptoms.[16] The severity of symptoms can be directly assessed through evaluation of responses on a questionnaire such as the Dizziness Handicap Inventory,[17] which quantifies the functional, emotional, and physical dimensions of dizziness. The Jacobson scale consists of 25 questions each of which can be answered with "no" (worth 0 points), "sometimes" (worth 2 points), or "yes" (worth 4 points); the range of scores is 0 to 100 with lower scores representing lesser impairment. The AAO-HNS has proposed criteria for determining the severity of Ménière's disease (Table 34–2).[15,18]

Patient's age should be considered when discussing surgical options. Although advanced age alone is not a contraindication, the risk of perioperative complications, such as pneumonia, myocardial infarction, stroke, and pulmonary embolus all increase with age. Furthermore, the time required to recover from ablative procedures will likely be longer in older patients.[19] Procedures that require access to the internal auditory canal may also have a higher incidence of postoperative complications, such as cerebrospinal fluid (CSF) leak, in older individuals.[20]

Finally, the status of the contralateral ear must always be considered. Estimates of the risk of developing Ménière's disease in the contralateral ear vary from 2 to 78%.[21] However, Perez et al. found that when strict criteria were applied to cases with long-standing, unilateral Ménière's disease, the risk of developing contralateral disease after 2 or more years of follow-up was less than 5%. Thus, ablative therapy is usually an appropriate consideration for long-standing, unilateral Ménière's disease when there is no clinical evidence of involvement of the contralateral ear at the time of therapy. However, the clinician and patient should discuss the fact that ablative treatment of one ear might limit options for treatment of the contralateral ear, should it become involved later.

Probably, the major reason for the difficulty in assessing the efficacy of treatment for Ménière's disease is the high spontaneous remission rate (60–80%) of the episodic vertigo that is a hallmark of the disease.[22] Thus, it can be difficult to determine if improvement following treatment is due to the treatment itself or the natural history of the disease. Often, the ability to meaningfully evaluate a treatment at a single institution is limited by small patient numbers and the results may not generalize to other sites if different patient selection criteria or techniques are used. The lack of uniform patient selection and treatment across institutions also limits the ability to conduct multi-institutional trials of surgical treatments.

Initial treatment of Ménière's disease should never be a procedure. The first line of treatment for Ménière's disease is a low-sodium diet, an established treatment for over 50 years.[23] Other lifestyle changes that may be beneficial include avoidance of alcohol, caffeine, and stress. Medical therapy with diuretics, such as triamterene with hydrochlorothiazide or acetazolamide is often used in combination with dietary changes. It should be remembered that without any therapy more than 50% of Ménière's patients improve within 2 years and more than 70% improve after 8 years.[24] However, this leaves 30% of patients who continue to have symptoms that may be relieved by surgery.[22] Additionally, the degree of hearing loss should be considered since many surgical procedures carry a risk of hearing loss, even if they are nonablative. Although Ménière's disease comprises the triad of tinnitus, hearing loss, and vertigo, it is usually the vertigo that is the most disabling and that prompts treatment.

Surgical treatment of Ménière's disease aims to achieve one or both of the two possible goals. One is to abolish or alter function of the labyrinth, which can be accomplished in a variety of ways, many of which result in reduction of function of the affected labyrinth, and may cause vertigo until vestibular compensation has re-established symmetric, resting neural activity in the central pathways.[25] Procedures that reduce or ablate vestibular function also carry the risk of hearing loss. The second goal involves modification of the underlying pathophysiology. This second aim is harder to achieve since the underlying physiology is still not well understood. Current surgical treatments tend to focus on altering the production or distribution of endolymph, or delivering steroids that may affect the course of the disease.[26]

Nonablative Procedures for Ménière's Disease

Intratympanic Injection of Corticosteroids

Corticosteroids have an anti-inflammatory effect on the labyrinth, as evidenced by their beneficial effect on the inner ear, in conditions of likely immune origin.[27] Steroids have been shown to influence ion transport in the labyrinth.[28] and can restore hearing in mice with progressive stria vascularis dysfunction.[29] It is possible that steroids have a therapeutic effect in Ménière's disease by either an anti-inflammatory or ion transport mechanism.

Intratympanic steroid injection is becoming an established therapy for Ménière's disease. Early reports found vertigo control rates of 80 to 96%,[30,31] but a subsequent prospective, randomized, blinded study failed to show benefit of intratympanic steroids in late-stage Ménière's.[32] However, it is plausible that more beneficial results may be obtained in the early stages of the disease. Other studies have reported a beneficial effect of intratympanic injection of dexamethasone in the control of the vertigo of Ménière's disease,[33,34] although the effect

TABLE 34–2 AAO-HNS Criteria for Ménière's disease severity

In 1996, the Committee on Hearing and Equilibrium reaffirmed and clarified the 1985 guidelines, adding initial staging and reporting guidelines.

VERTIGO

a. Any treatment should be evaluated no sooner than 24 months
b. Formula to obtain numeric value for vertigo: ratio of average number of definitive spells per month after therapy divided by definitive spells per month before therapy (averaged over a 24-month period) × 100 = numeric value
c. Numeric value scale

Numeric Value	Control Level	Class
0	Complete control of definitive spells	A
41–80	Limited control of definitive spells	B
81–120	Insignificant control of definitive spells	C
>120		D
Secondary treatment initiated		E

DISABILITY

a. No disability
b. Mild disability: intermittent or continuous dizziness/unsteadiness that precludes working in a hazardous environment
c. Moderate disability: intermittent or continuous dizziness that results in a sedentary occupation
d. Severe disability: symptoms so severe as to exclude gainful employment

HEARING

a. Hearing is measured by a four-frequency pure tone average (PTA) of 500 Hz, 1 kHz, 2 kHz, and 3 kHz
b. Pretreatment hearing level: worst hearing level during 6 months prior to surgery
c. Posttreatment hearing level: poorest hearing level measured 18–24 months after institution of therapy
d. Hearing classification:
   i. Unchanged = ≤10-dB PTA improvement or worsening or ≤15% speech discrimination improvement or worsening
   ii. Improved >10-dB PTA improvement or >15% discrimination improvement
   iii. Worse >10-dB PTA worsening or >15% discrimination worsening

IN1996, THE COMMITTEE ON HEARING AND EQUILIBRIUM REAFFIRMED AND CLARIFIED THE GUIDELINES, ADDING INITIAL STAGING AND REPORTING GUIDELINES.

Initial Hearing Level	
Stage	Four-tone average (dB)
1	≤25
2	26–40
3	41–70
4	>70

FUNCTIONAL LEVEL SCALE

Regarding my current state of overall function, not just during attacks.
1. My dizziness has no effect on my activities at all.
2. When I am dizzy, I have to stop for a while, but it soon passes and I can resume my activities. I continue to work, drive, and engage in any activity I choose without restriction. I have not changed any plans or activities to accommodate my dizziness.
3. When I am dizzy I have to stop what I am doing for a while, but it does pass and I can resume activities. I continue to work, drive, and engage in most activities I choose, but I have had to change some plans and make some allowance for my dizziness.
4. I am able to work, drive, travel, and take care of a family or engage in most activities, but I must exert a great deal of effort to do so. I must constantly make adjustments in my activities and budget my energies. I am barely making it.
5. I am unable to work, drive, or take care of a family. I am unable to do most of the active things that I used to do. Even essential activities must be limited. I am disabled.
6. I have been disabled for 1 year or longer and/or I receive compensation because of my dizziness or balance problem.

on hearing loss and tinnitus are minimal. Recently, a large retrospective study demonstrated satisfactory vertigo control in 91% of Ménière's patients followed for 2 years or more.[35] During this period, 63% had multiple injections. At the end of the 2-year period, 70% required no further injections, 26% continued to receive intratympanic steroids, and 3% went on to ablative therapy. A small, randomized trial found complete resolution of vertigo symptoms in 82% of patients receiving dexamethasone versus 57% with saline injection.[36] The risk of hearing loss or other complication from steroid injection is low. Dexamethasone is now a standard therapy for the control of the vertigo of Ménière's, although repeat injections are frequently required for recurrent symptoms. The optimal dosing frequency is unknown, but repeat dosing at 3 months is a reasonable starting point. Concentrations used have varied from 2 to 24 mg/mL; we use 12 mg/mL.

Partially Ablative Procedures for Ménière's Disease

Intratympanic Injection of Gentamicin

Intratympanic gentamicin injection has achieved vertigo control in patients with unilateral Ménière's disease who have been refractory to other treatments. In 1957, Schuknecht described streptomycin injection into the middle ear via a microcatheter placed through the tympanic membrane.[37] Control of vertigo was achieved, but severe hearing loss occurred in most treated ears.

Gentamicin has a high vestibulotoxicity relative to its cochleotoxicity; thus, it can be used to control vestibular symptoms while sparing hearing. Lange[38] administered gentamicin into the external auditory canal five times daily after placement of a tympanotomy tube. Vertigo was eliminated in 90% of his 92 patients, but hearing loss and level of vestibular function were not specified. Beck and Schmit sought to determine if complete ablation of vestibular function, as determined with ice-water caloric testing was necessary for vertigo control. They found that it was not, and that this end point led to severe to profound hearing loss in 58% of patients.[39] Nedzelski et al.[40,41] administered gentamicin three times daily through a catheter into the middle ear. Treatment was terminated when nystagmus was observed, unsteadiness developed, hearing worsened, or a maximum of 12 doses of gentamicin were given. Complete control of vertigo was achieved in 25 patients (83%) with substantial control in the remaining 5 patients. There was a 10% incidence of profound hearing loss in the treated ears.

Multiple daily doses of gentamicin were compared with weekly administration by Toth and Parnes,[42] in 1995. One group was treated with multiple doses of gentamicin daily for 4 days, and the other was treated with weekly doses up to a total of 4 weeks. Control of vertigo was about 80% in both groups, but hearing loss developed in 57% of the multiple-dose group and in only 19% of the weekly dose patients. The current trend is away from multiple doses of gentamicin and toward a single injection regimen, with additional doses only if needed to control symptoms ("titration therapy"). Harner et al. found that a single injection of gentamicin controlled vertigo in 41% of patients.[43]

Gentamicin likely gains access to the inner ear by diffusion through the round window membrane.[44] Access may be impaired by inflammation causing increased membrane thickness,[45] or obstruction with fat or fibrous tissue.[46] The concentration of gentamicin in the perilymph reaches 5 to 10% of that in the applied solution and has an elimination half-life of 75 min.[47] When gentamicin reaches the endolymph, it is selectively concentrated in hair cells and supporting cells.[48] Aminoglycosides destroy hair cell function by a variety of mechanisms. They block ion currents through the stereocilia,[49] cause adhesion of stereocilia,[50] and ultimately, cause the hair cells to degenerate or become extruded.[51] Gentamicin has a greater effect on type I than on type II hair cells,[52,53] which may reflect a more avid uptake of gentamicin.[54]

The term "chemical labyrinthectomy" is often applied to intratympanic gentamicin treatment, but it may not be an appropriate indication of the effect of gentamicin on the labyrinth. A single dose of gentamicin is sufficient to markedly reduce semicircular canal function as judged by the angular, vestibulo-ocular reflex in response to rapid, rotary head thrusts.[55] However, the reduction in function is not as severe as that seen after surgical labyrinthectomy or vestibular neurectomy. The reduction in the vestibulo-ocular reflex with head thrust correlates with initial relief of vertigo symptoms.[56] Hair cells may be able to self-repair after gentamicin.[57] Unlike surgical labyrinthectomy, almost one-third of patients will eventually require additional gentamicin.[58]

Intratympanic Delivery Techniques

Several techniques have been described to introduce medication into the middle ear. Delivery routes include direct injection though the tympanic membrane, injection through an inserted ventilation tube, injection through an indwelling catheter inserted into the middle ear, placing a sponge through the tympanic membrane, and injection directly into the round window niche. Minipumps have also been described. Efficacy does not seem to be affected by the delivery route.[59] Direct intratympanic injection can be done in the office and is probably the easiest method. Prior to injection, the tympanic membrane should be anesthetized. Preferred techniques include topical phenol applied with a Duperstein applicator to a pinpoint area of the tympanic membrane, injection of the external auditory canal with lidocaine, or topical Emla™ cream (Lidocaine 2.5%, Prilocaine 2.5%). A 25-gauge needle can be used to make a superior port to allow air to exit the middle ear and an inferior port for injection. The middle ear generally holds 0.5 to 0.8 mL of fluid. A brief episode of vertigo typically follows the injection, and can be mitigated by warming the solution to body temperature prior to injection. To maintain the fluid level over the round window membrane, the patient should lie in a slight Trendelenberg position with the treated ear up for 30 min, thus preventing the bulk of the injection from escaping through the Eustachian tube.

Local Overpressure Therapy

Endolymphatic hydrops has consistently been found upon histopathologic examination of the inner ears of patients with definite Ménière's disease.[60] However, the relationship of this postmortem finding to the symptoms of Ménière's disease is imperfect, as hydrops is also found in asymptomatic ears. Despite the uncertain link between disrupted endolymph and the symptoms of Ménière's disease, medical therapy and endolymphatic decompression surgery have attempted to address these symptoms by encouraging endolymphatic flow into the endolymphatic sac. The application of external pressure to the middle ear is a relatively recent approach to decreasing hydrops. As early as 30 years ago, overpressure in the middle ear was reported to decrease Ménière's symptoms in 4 of 5 patients during acute vertigo attacks.[61] The mechanism by which this therapy reduced vertigo was not clear, but one possible mechanism is that increased endolymph pressure facilitates its absorption.[62]

Since 2000, the Meniett™ device has been approved for use by the US Food and Drug Administration. The device is a handheld air pressure generator that the patient self-administers three times daily. The pressure is delivered in complex pulses of up to 20 cm of water over a 5-min period. The device requires ventilation tube placement in the tympanic membrane prior to starting therapy. A randomized controlled trial demonstrated that the Meniett™ device resulted in a significant decrease in vertigo for the first 3 months of therapy but afterward was similar to placebo.[63] The placebo device in these cases was an inactive device that did not administer pressure. Long-term treatment with the Meniett™ has yielded results similar to the natural course of Ménière's disease.[64]

It should also be noted that simple placement of a ventilation tube with no additional therapy has been reported in control of vertigo in many patients with Ménière's disease[65,66] to a degree similar to endolymphatic sac surgery.[67]

Endolymphic Decompression

Surgical decompression of endolymph for Ménière's was first described by Portmann in 1926,[9] more than a decade before the earliest histologic evidence of the existence of endolymphatic hydrops.[11,12] During the more than three-quarters of a century that this technique has been in use, there have been numerous variations on the concept. Despite extensive investigation into the pathophysiology of endolymphatic hydrops, its role in Ménière's disease is still an active area of controversy and debate. Several theories have been proposed to explain the potential benefit of endolymphatic sac decompression, which include release of external compression on the sac, neovascularization of the perisaccular region, allowing passive diffusion of endolymph, and creation of an osmotic gradient out of the sac.[68]

Some endolymphatic decompression techniques are no longer performed. Sacculotomy was proposed by Fick in 1964,[69] and consisted of using a needle to puncture the saccule through the stapes footplate. A later variation on this technique involved leaving a sharp prosthesis in the footplate that ruptured the saccule each time it expanded.[70] Long-term follow-up of patients so treated has shown an unacceptable degree of hearing loss. Endolymphatic decompression can be performed through the round window. The otic-periotic shunt is a tube placed through the round window membrane that perforates the basilar membrane.[71] Cochleosacculotomy aims to create a fracture dislocation of the osseous spiral lamina (and hence a permanent fistulization of the endolymph-containing cochlear duct) by inserting a hook through the round window membrane.[72] Both these procedures have a high rate of hearing loss.

Several variations in endolymphatic sac surgery have been described. Simple decompression, wide decompression including the sigmoid sinus,[73] cannulation of the endolymphatic duct, endolymphatic drainage to the subarchnoid space, drainage to the mastoid, and removal of the extraosseus portion of the sac[74] have all been advocated. A variety of prostheses have also been proposed, ranging from simple silastic sheets to tubes, and one-way valves designed to allow flow selectively into either the mastoid or the subarachnoid space.

Endolymphatic sac surgery begins with simple mastoidectomy and identification of the tegmen, sigmoid sinus, and facial ridge. Once these landmarks are established, the horizontal and posterior canals should be skeletonized and the bone over the posterior fossa thinned (Figure 34–1A). Only a thin covering of bone should be left over the facial nerve and the sigmoid sinus to allow adequate exposure of the posterior fossa dura. The bone over the posterior fossa should be completely removed using a diamond bur (Figure 34–1B). The endolymphatic sac lies on the dura medial to the vertical segment of the facial nerve and the retrofacial air cells. The superior aspect of the endolymphatic sac should be identified, and often lies just below a line (Donaldson's line) formed by extending the plane of the horizontal semicircular canal posteriorly to bisect the posterior semicircular canal. The procedure from this point varies according to which endolymphatic surgery is planned. Decompression of the sac requires only that the bone of the posterior fossa plate be removed (Figure 34–1C).

Endolymphatic shunting is most simply performed by incising the exposed sac and placing a stent to keep the incision open. The popular Paparella and Hanson technique[75] involves opening the edge of the sac, lysing any intraluminal adhesions, and probing the duct to insure that it is patent. A piece of Silastic® is placed through the incision in the sac allowing long-term drainage (Figure 34–2).

Shunting the sac into the subarachnoid space is more elaborate since it requires making a second incision in the posterior wall of the endolymphatic sac into the posterior fossa and a specially designed shunt tube.[76] After the initial, lateral incision is made in the sac, a small medial incision is made to allow a shunt to be placed into the basal cistern creating a passage into the subarachnoid space (Figure 34–3). The resulting CSF leak is controlled by placing a fascia graft over the lateral incision in the sac. Obliteration of the mastoid cavity with an abdominal fat graft is also an option. This technique has not been as popular in recent years due to its relative complexity, the higher risk of a postoperative CSF leak, and intracranial hematoma as a result of damage to arachnoid veins. A review comparing the efficacy of various sac procedures 2 years postoperatively revealed that they all had similar rates of vertigo relief, ranging from 49 to 66%.[77]

A double-blind, placebo-controlled study of 30 patients with 15 randomly selected for each operation[78] revealed that mastoidectomy alone has the same efficacy as endolymphatic shunting . In an attempt to prevent bias, Thomsen et al. operated at two different hospitals and had the patients follow-up at the other, thus blinding nursing staff and others to the type of surgery performed. The criterion Thomsen et al. used for

FIGURE 34–1 • Transmastoid endolymphatic sac surgery. *A*, Mastoidectomy is performed with identification of the tegmen, sigmoid sinus, antrum, facial nerve, horizontal semicircular canal, and posterior semicircular canal. The facial nerve, sigmoid sinus, and horizontal canal are skeletonized to allow wide exposure of the posterior fossa dura. *B*, The bony covering of the posterior fossa dura is removed between the sigmoid sinus and the posterior canal. *C*, The superior edge of the endolymphatic sac is identified; it usually lies at or below Donaldson's line, which extends posteriorly along the plane of the horizontal canal and bisects the posterior canal.

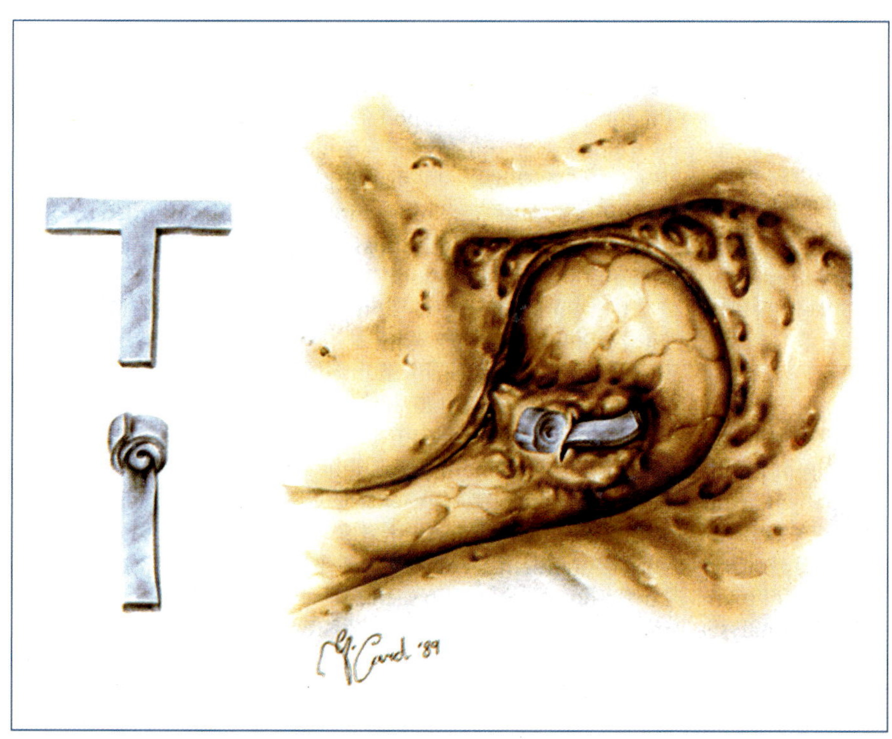

FIGURE 34–2 • Paparella technique for endolymphatic mastoid shunting. A T-shaped piece of silicone is coiled and placed into a lateral incision in the endolymphatic sac to create a drainage path to the mastoid cavity.

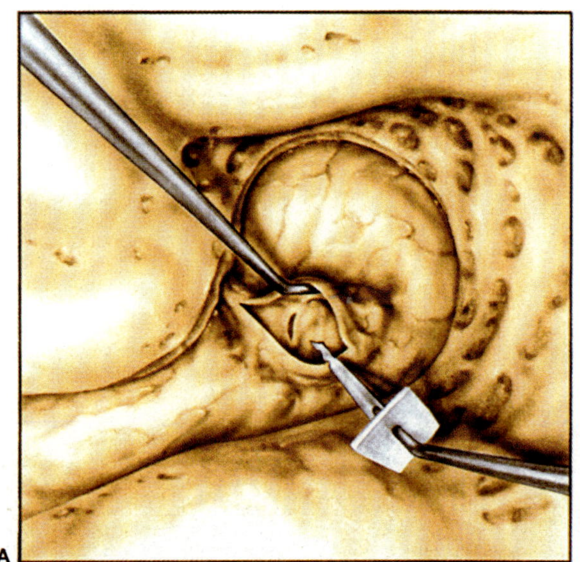

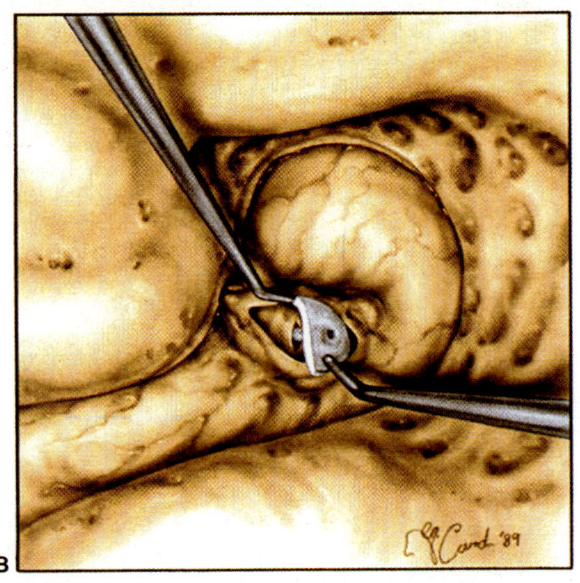

FIGURE 34–3 • Endolymphatic-subarachnoid shunt. *A*, After exposing and opening the lateral wall of the endolymphatic sac, the medial wall of the sac is incised to open the lateral prolongation of the basal cistern. Dissection in the cistern is carried out bluntly to avoid venous injury. *B*, A silicone (Silastic®) shunt is inserted to maintain drainage path between the endolymphatic sac and the basal cistern. The lateral endolymphatic sac should be carefully closed with a fascia graft to prevent cerebrospinal fluid leak.

success was absence of definitive vertigo spells, even if hearing worsens. Pillsbury et al. have argued that the shunt group would have had a significantly better outcome if patients who had success at relief of vertigo but worse hearing were considered failures.[79] It was also not clear which data—preoperative, postoperative, or the difference between—were used to compare the groups in the Thomsen et al. study.[80] A more recent analysis used the Wilcoxon signed rank test to compare the preoperative and postoperative groups.[81] From this new analysis, the shunt was found to achieve superior control of vertigo, tinnitus, and nausea ($P < 0.05$ for each). In the reanalysis, the only area in which the shunt did not offer a significant advantage over placebo was hearing improvement.

All of these procedures can be performed in an outpatient center, and patients can usually return to work within a week,—a recovery rate similar to mastoidectomy alone. Although the procedure is intended to be a hearing-sparing procedure with minimal morbidity, the risk of hearing loss may be as high as 5%;[82] in addition, there is a small risk of facial nerve damage associated with the procedure.

Some series have reported dramatic success with endolymphatic sac surgery, whereas other studies have shown it to be of no benefit. A survey of 19 patients after endolymphatic sac decompression revealed that 95% reported an improvement in vertigo.[83] Another study of 676 patients who had undergone endolymphatic sac surgery revealed that more than half of the patients continued to have vertigo.[84] Other studies have shown that 57% of patients who refused surgery, but only 40% of those who actually had endolymphatic shunt surgery obtained complete control of vertigo after 2 years follow-up.[24] The effect, if any, of sac surgery on vertigo control is likely less than intratympanic gentamicin, vestibular nerve section, or labyrinthectomy.[85] Despite the controversy over this procedure it continues to be commonly performed for vertigo.[86]

Vestibular Neurectomy

Several approaches to the vestibular nerve have been described. The earliest approach was the retrosigmoid, with the first large series by Walter Dandy in the 1930s.[10] The suboccipital approach is essentially identical but historical concerns regarding this approach developed due to poor results during the early years of surgery for vestibular schwannomas. The terms retrosigmoid and suboccipital are now used interchangeably. The middle fossa approach to the internal auditory canal and superior vestibular nerve was developed by William House in the early 1960s,[87] and was later modified to include inferior vestibular nerve section.[88] A retrolabyrinthine approach to sectioning of the vestibular nerve was introduced in 1980,[89] but concerns exist regarding this approach due to the poor exposure achieved relative to other techniques.[90] A transmeatal cochleovestibular neurectomy has also been described,[91] but has largely been abandoned due to the superior exposure and more consistent results afforded by other approaches. The middle fossa and retrosigmoid approaches remain the most commonly performed today.

Vestibular nerve section has a complete vertigo control rate of about 85 to 95% with 80 to 90% of patients maintaining their preoperative hearing immediately postoperatively.[92–94] The procedure offers much greater vertigo control rates than endolymphatic shunt procedures, but is also a more invasive and technically challenging procedure. Vestibular nerve section has been argued to have a lower risk of hearing loss when compared with gentamicin injection;[93] however, the risk of hearing loss with gentamicin seems to be greatest with high-dose protocols. Lower-dose gentamicin seems to carry a long-term risk of hearing loss similar to the natural history of Ménière's disease.[95]

The retrosigmoid approach to vestibular nerve section has the advantage of a generous exposure and a direct view of the seventh and eighth cranial nerves (Figure 34–4). The procedure

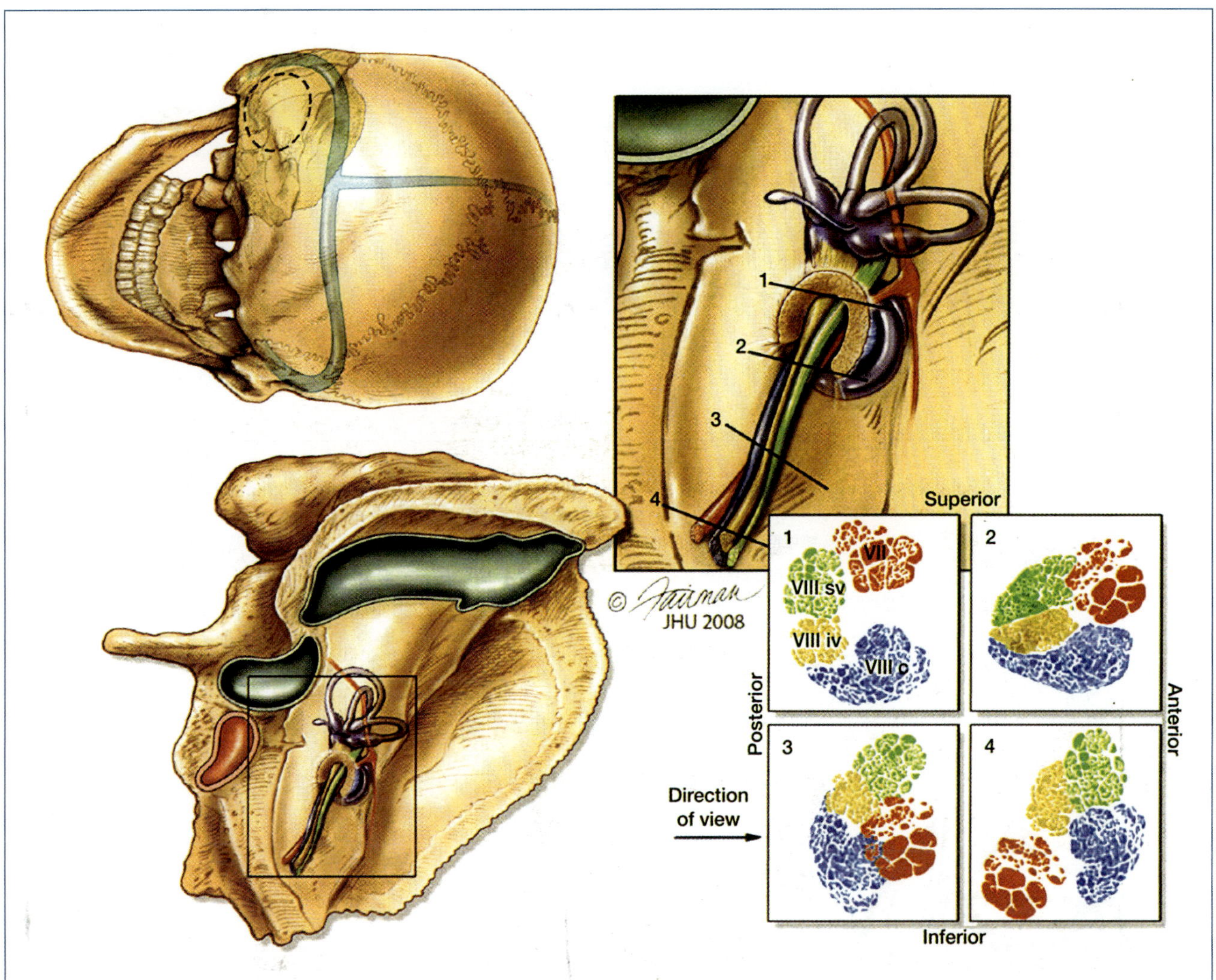

FIGURE 34–4 • Contents of the left internal auditory canal as viewed from the retrosigmoid approach. The upper left panel gives the orientation, with the right temporal bone shown in this same orientation on the lower left. The upper right panel details the seventh and eighth cranial nerves in their course from the brain stem. Cross-sections of the cranial nerves are shown on the lower right. The facial nerve (VII) is red, the cochlear nerve (VIII c) is blue, the superior vestibular nerve (VIII sv) is green, and the inferior vestibular nerve (VIII iv) is yellow.

begins with a standard suboccipital craniotomy having the sigmoid sinus as the anterior limit of exposure. The posterior fossa dura is opened, and the cerebellum is retracted to expose the cerebellopontine angle and petrous ridge. The cistern is decompressed with an incision that allows the cerebellum to fall medially obviating retraction. The vestibular, cochlear, and facial nerves are identified, and then the superior and inferior vestibular nerves can be sectioned (Figure 34–5). Afterward the dura is reapproximated, and the bone flap is replaced and covered as the wound is closed.

The middle fossa approach for vestibular nerve section is similar to that for vestibular schwannoma resection and has the advantage of requiring only minimal dural violation (Figure 34–6). A vertical incision is made above the auricle and the temporalis muscle is freed from squamous portion of the temporal bone. A small craniotomy is made in the squamous portion of the temporal bone. The middle fossa dura is elevated and a Fisch or House-Urban retractor is used to maintain temporal lobe elevation. The superior semicircular canal (arcuate eminence) and geniculate ganglion are identified on the floor of the middle fossa as landmarks for the internal auditory canal. The internal auditory canal is unroofed using a diamond bur, and the dissection is carried out to the lateral extent of the canal to identify "Bill's bar," which divides the facial nerve (anterior) from the superior vestibular nerve (posterior). The dura of the posterior aspect of the canal is incised and the superior vestibular nerve is identified. As the superior vestibular nerve is retracted, the inferior vestibular nerve can be identified, taking care to avoid the internal auditory artery and cochlear nerve. Often it is difficult to definitively separate the inferior vestibular nerve from the cochlear nerve, which can lead to remaining vestibular symptoms after surgery or hearing loss. Upon nerve sectioning, the internal auditory canal can be covered with fascia, the bone flap replaced, and the incision closed. The risk of

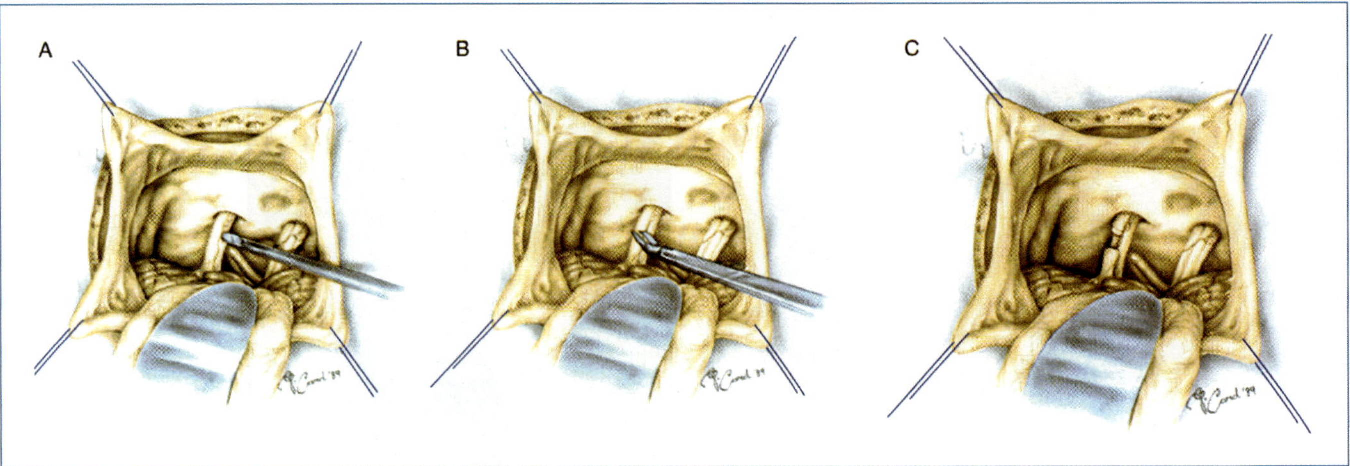

FIGURE 34–5 • Retrosigmoid approach to vestibular nerve section. The cerebellum is retracted medially giving a view of the superior and inferior vestibular nerves. *A*, The posterior fossa is exposed and nerves are identified. *B*, The superior vestibular nerve is separated from the more anterior facial nerve. *C*, The superior vestibular nerve has been sectioned.

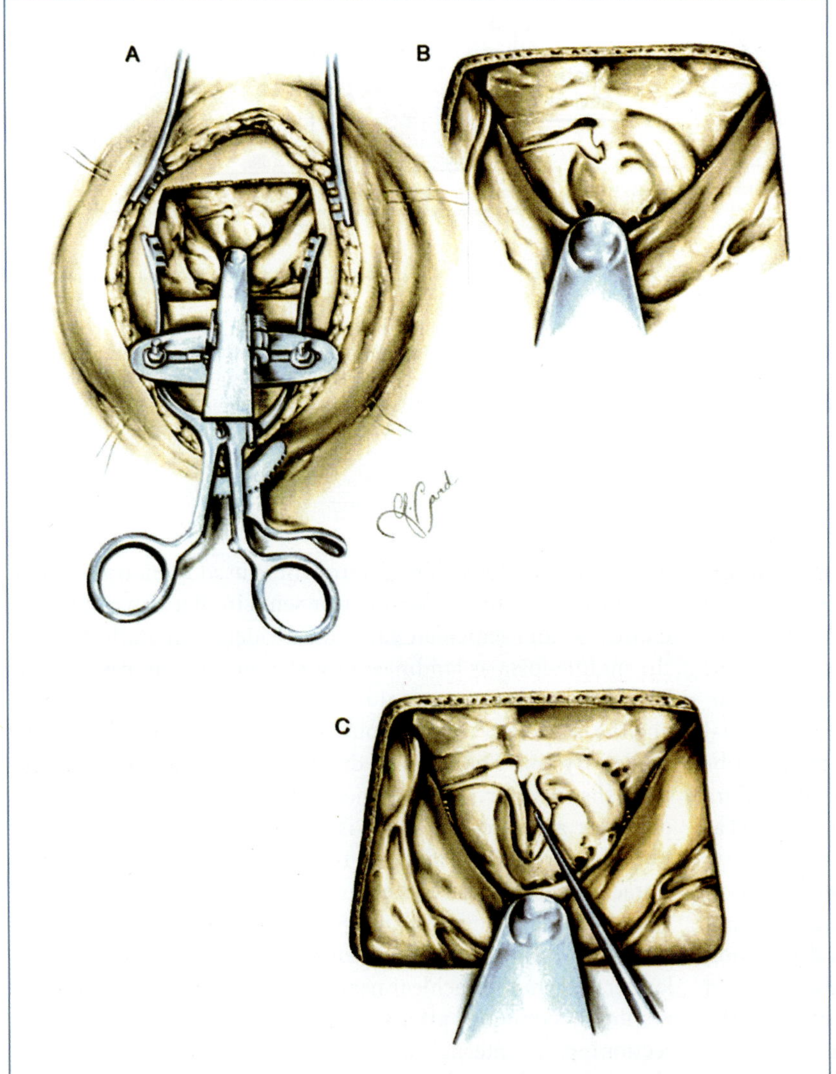

FIGURE 34–6 • Surgeon's view from the head of the table during the middle fossa approach to a vestibular nerve section. A right-sided procedure is shown with anterior toward the left. *A*, View of the middle fossa after the bone flap has been removed and the temporal lobe has been elevated. *B*, A diamond bur is used to thin the bone over the internal auditory canal between the arcuate eminence and geniculate ganglion. *C*, The internal auditory canal is opened revealing the facial nerve (anterior) and the superior vestibular nerve (posterior), which are separated by Bill's bar laterally. The superior vestibular nerve is carefully separated from the facial nerve in preparation for sectioning.

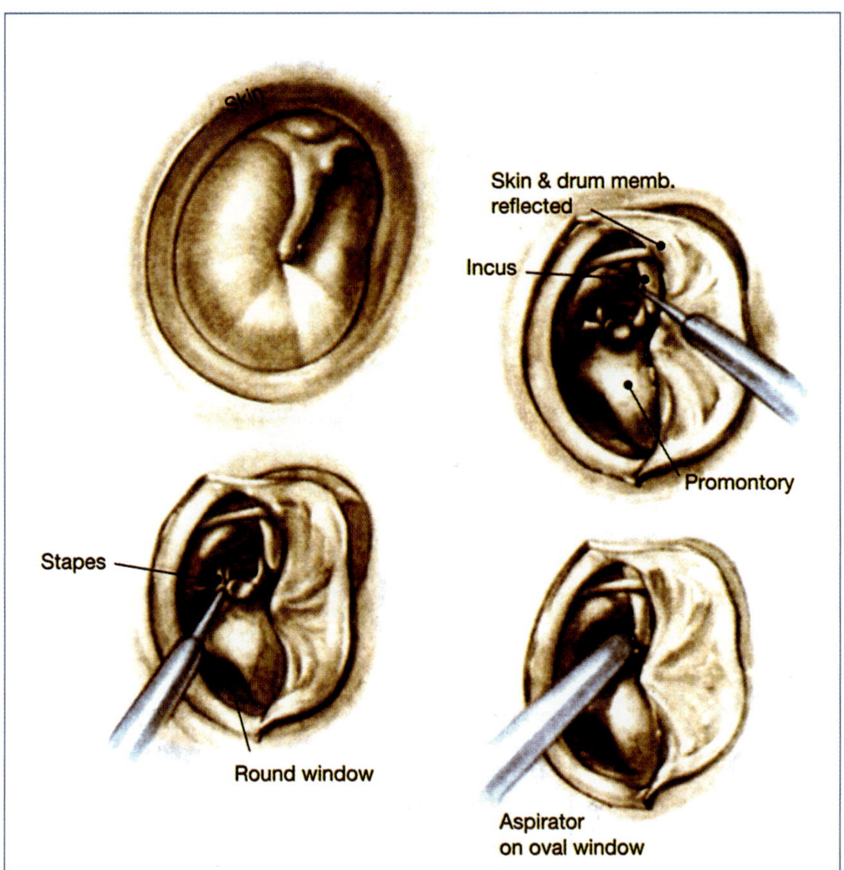

FIGURE 34–7 • Transcanal labyrinthectomy.

facial paresis is higher using a middle fossa approach than with the suboccipital approach,[96,97] causing many to abandon this technique in recent years.

Labyrinthectomy is the most destructive procedure in the treatment of Ménière's as it destroys both hearing and vestibular function. Ideal candidates for labyrinthectomy are those who have no hearing and have failed more conservative treatments, such as gentamicin injection. Despite its morbidity, the procedure has a higher rate of vertigo control than vestibular neurectomy [85] and has been reported to improve quality of life in 98% of patients.[98] There are two approaches: transcanal and transmastoid, although the transmastoid approach affords much better exposure and is more popular.

The transcanal approach (Figure 34–7) involves exposing the middle ear through a tympanomeatal flap.[72] The incus and stapes are removed to expose the oval window. A hook is then inserted into the vestibule to remove the neuroepithelium. A variation on this basic technique involves drilling out the promontory to connect the oval and round windows. The limitation of the transcanal approach is the poor access it yields to the posterior canal, located medial to the facial nerve; thus, complete ablation may not be achieved. The limited exposure also makes the procedure more technically difficult than the transmastoid approach.

The transmastoid approach to labyrinthectomy is more commonly performed and has the advantage of allowing direct visualization of the vestibular end organs as they are removed. The procedure starts with a standard mastoidectomy in which the horizontal canal and facial ridge are identified (Figure 34–8). Drilling superior to the horizontal canal between the labyrinth and the tegmen allows identification of the superior canal. The posterior canal is identified posterior to the horizontal canal. The canals can then be blue-lined and followed medially to the vestibule while removing the neuroepithelium under direct vision.

Complete loss of hearing is an expected outcome of labyrinthectomy. However, it may be possible to preserve hearing by packing the semicircular canals with bone wax[99,100] and using a diamond bur to remove the canal while preserving the vestibule. Although this approach has been demonstrated to have a high rate of hearing preservation in cases involving tumor removal,[101,102] less destructive procedures are indicated for patients with vertigo where hearing remains serviceable.

BENIGN PAROXYSMAL POSITIONAL VERTIGO

Benign paroxysmal positional vertigo (BPPV) is the most common cause of dizziness, accounting for about 40% of patient complaints of vertigo.[103] It is generally accepted that BPPV is caused by cupulolithiasis or canallithiasis. Typically, symptoms comprise brief (lasting less than 1 min) episodes of vertigo that occur after turning the head, especially when the head is facing upward, such as rolling over in bed. Canal repositioning

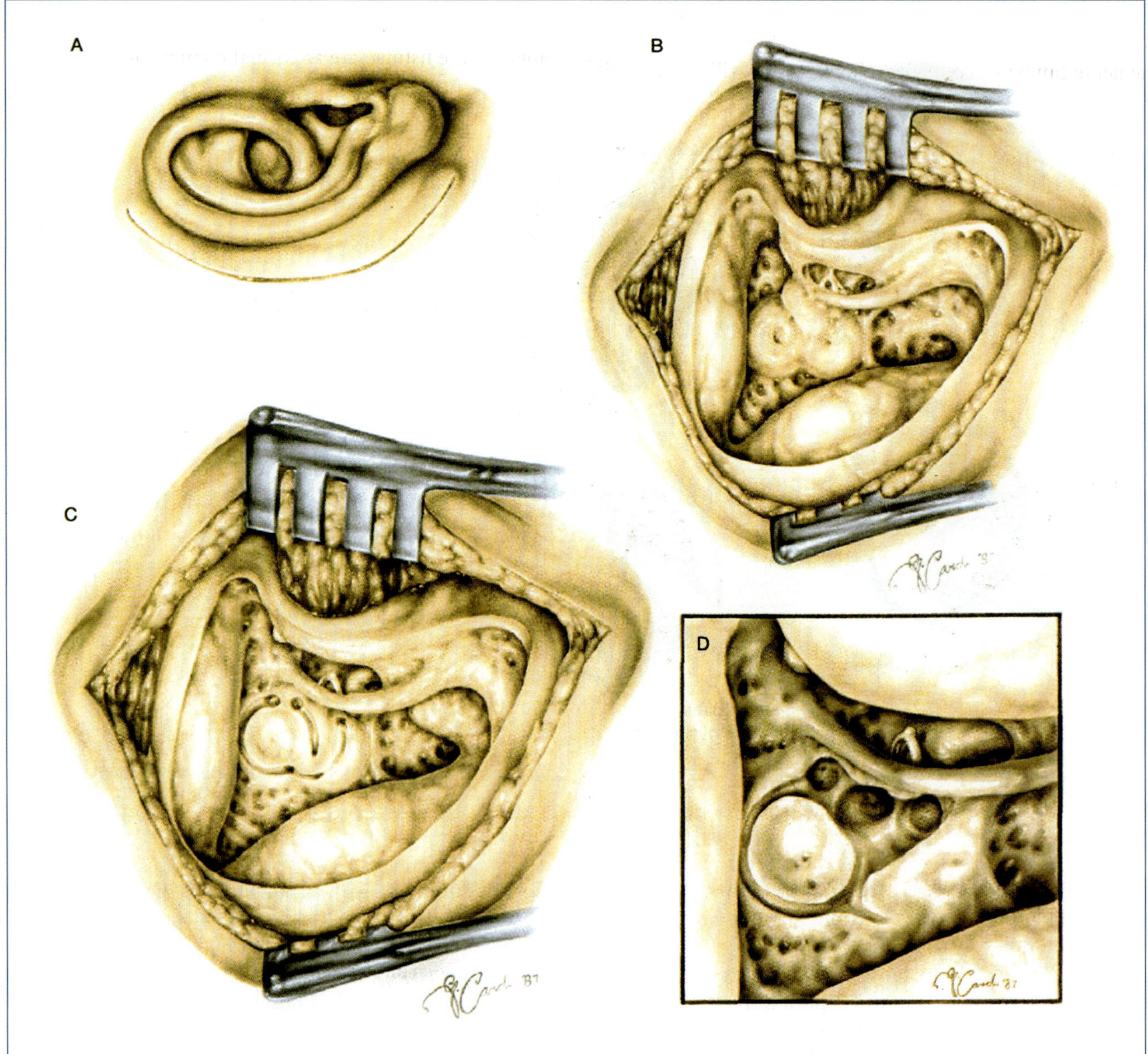

FIGURE 34–8 • Transmastoid labyrinthectomy. *A*, The approach begins with a standard postauricular incision. *B*, The mastoid cavity is opened with identification of the three semicircular canals and the facial nerve. The facial recess is shown opened, although this is an optional part of the procedure. *C*, The three semicircular canals are blue lined and traced to their ampullated ends. *D*, The ampullae and neuroepithelium of the three semicircular canals are exposed, along with the otolithic organs (the saccule and the utricle).

maneuvers such as those described by Epley,[104] control symptoms in 98% of the cases of BPPV. The vast majority of patients with BPPV can be treated successfully with canalith repositioning maneuvers (see Chapter 16). In rare cases, patients may continue to have refractory, disabling vertigo after multiple repositionings. Surgery is an option of last resort in these patients, since physical therapy with multiple canalith repositioning maneuvers is successful in almost all cases.

The posterior canal is most commonly involved in BPPV. Horizontal canal BPPV does occur and can be caused during a repositioning maneuver by free-floating otoconia that migrate from the vestibule into the horizontal canal. Superior canal BPPV occurs, but even more rarely. Thus, surgical treatment of BPPV has focused on cases involving the posterior canal that have been refractory to multiple canalith repositioning maneuvers.

Singular neurectomy was proposed by Gacek as a treatment for refractory BPPV.[105] During the three decades following its description, the procedure has been used at least 342 times, of which 252 were by Gacek himself.[106] The technique was initially performed under local anesthesia so that hearing and vertigo could be monitored, but it has also been done under general anesthesia. A transcanal approach exposes the entire round window niche, which may require removing some of the posterior portion of the external auditory canal. The bony overhang is removed until the scala tympani is visualized. Drilling is performed at the posterior margin of the membrane to a depth of 1 to 2 mm where the singular nerve should be identified. The nerve can be severed with a hook, which will cause a brief episode of vertigo and nystagmus. The procedure carries the risks of CSF leak and hearing loss. The incidence of hearing loss ranges from as low as 4%[106] to as high as 41%.[107] The procedure relieves symptoms in 75 to 96% of patients.[103]

Posterior semicircular canal occlusion was introduced as a treatment for BPPV in 1990.[108] This technique blocks the canal lumen so that it becomes unresponsive to angular acceleration. A total of 97 cases have been reported in the literature. Although the procedure was associated with brief, postoperative vertigo, 94 of the 97 patients were cured.[103] The operation begins with a mastoidectomy in which the bony posterior canal is identified. The occlusion is placed at the point furthest from the ampulla, just inferior to the region bisected by the horizontal canal. A diamond bur is used to drill to the membranous canal. A plug is created with bone chips or fascia and firmly inserted to completely fill the canal and compress the membranous duct.

Despite BPPV being a very common cause of dizziness, surgical therapy for this disease is decidedly uncommon, because most cases are successfully treated with repositioning maneuvers. In patients who present with severe, intractable BPPV, other causes of dizziness should be considered and ruled out prior to considering surgical therapy. Posterior fossa outlet obstruction, such as that associated with the Chiari malformation or with posterior fossa cysts, should always be considered in the differential diagnosis of refractory positional vertigo. These entities can be evaluated with appropriate imaging and interpretation of the associated nystagmus. The nystagmus of posterior fossa outlet obstruction does not parallel the plane of any specific semicircular canal, as does the nystagmus of BPPV.

ENLARGED VESTIBULAR AQUEDUCT

Enlarged vestibular aqueduct syndrome is the most common finding on computed tomography (CT) scan that is associated with a progressive hearing loss, often in association with minor head trauma. Although hearing loss is usually the symptom that brings these patients to the attention of otolaryngologists, they may also experience vertigo.[109] These periodic episodes of vertigo also can be triggered by minor head trauma or vigorous physical activity.[110] The vertigo can be associated with fluctuations in hearing, mimicking those seen in Ménière's disease. Despite these episodes of vertigo and progressive hearing loss, vestibular function tends to remain normal. Patients may develop vertigo many years after hearing loss.

Surgical treatment of the enlarged vestibular aqueduct has been attempted, in most cases with the primary goal of hearing preservation. The endolymphatic shunt is a procedure that has been attempted in this disorder, but has not been successful.[111] A second treatment option is extraluminal occlusion of the enlarged vestibular aqueduct, but this procedure has not altered the course of hearing loss.[112] Thus, at this time, vertigo related to enlarged vestibular aqueduct syndrome is not appropriately treated by surgery.

PERILYMPH FISTULAE

Labyrinthine fistulae are abnormal communications between the inner ear and surrounding structures. In the normal inner ear, the labyrinth is covered by dense bone. Labyrinthine fistulae can be organized into three main categories—leakage of perilymph from the inner ear to the middle ear, disruption of the bony labyrinth by disease such as cholesteatoma, and idiopathic bony dehiscence of the semicircular canals (e.g., superior semicircular canal dehiscence syndrome and posterior canal dehiscence). These disorders present with similar symptoms of hearing loss and episodic vertigo despite their different causes.[113] Since idiopathic bony dehiscence of the semicircular canals creates problems of pressure transfer but not of fluid (endolymph and perilymph) mixing they are discussed later.

Definitive leakage of perilymph from the inner ear to the middle ear can be caused by fractures of the temporal bone, congenital abnormalities of the inner ear such as the Mondini deformity, or after stapedectomy.[114] In definitive cases patching with a tissue graft can achieve the goals of hearing preservation and relief of vertigo. However, many cases of vertigo or hearing loss have been alleged to cause perilymph fistulae that are much more ambiguous ("spontaneous") and are associated with equivocal surgical findings.[115–117] Areas of possible fistulization are the fissula ante fenestram and a fissure from the round window niche to the ampulla of the posterior canal. Fissures in these areas tend to be common and their clinical significance is not clear.[118] It is difficult to know for sure if the small amounts of fluid seen during surgical exploration are truly perilymph. An assay for -2 transferrin (a protein unique to CSF) has been suggested, but it has a low sensitivity for small amounts of fluid.[119] The absence of observed leakage during surgery has been interpreted to mean either that no fistula exists, that the fistula may be intermittent, or that the fistula may be present but too small to be detected. In cases of a negative exploration, it is unclear if patching of the oval and round windows is of any value. Criteria for determining when a middle ear exploration for perilymph fistula may be beneficial have been difficult to establish since there is no definitive test to make the diagnosis. Applying pressure in the external auditory canal to see if eye movements are evoked (Hennebert sign) has been used. Measuring postural sway during pressure to the external auditory canal has also been proposed as a "fistula test."[120] Even if a spontaneous fistula exists spontaneous resolution may occur. Recently, many patients who were initially diagnosed with fistulae have been found to have superior canal dehiscence (SCD).[113]

Chronic ear disease can cause a bona fide fistula. Chronic otitis media can lead to cholesteatoma formation, which can cause erosion of the dense bone around the labyrinth. Patients who develop fistulae usually have a multiyear history of chronic ear disease, sometimes requiring several operations. In a recent review of 375 surgeries done for chronic otitis media,[121] labyrinthine fistulae were identified in 29 cases, 25 of which had had canal-wall-down mastoidectomy. The overall incidence of fistulae after canal-wall-down mastoidectomy was 13%. All of these patients experienced vertigo symptoms. However, of the 19 so tested, only 14 had a positive Hennebert sign with positive pressure. The horizontal semicircular canal was the most common site of fistula formation (76%), followed by the oval window and the promontory. In such cases, surgical closure of the fistula is recommended; cartilage, bone paste, and fascia can be used.

SUPERIOR CANAL DEHISCENCE SYNDROME

Superior canal dehiscence syndrome (SCDS)[122] is caused by the absence of bone over the superior canal. This bony dehiscence creates third "window" that allows the abnormal movement of endolymph during presentation of loud sounds (Tullio phenomenon[123]), tragal compression, nose blowing, or other sources of a pressure gradient between the ear and middle fossa. Loud sound or pressure often causes nystagmus in the same plane as the superior canal on the affected side. During straight-ahead gaze the nystagmus appears to be a combination of vertical and torsional rotation (Figure 34–9). When gaze shifts 45 degrees toward the side of the dehiscence, the pupil will move in a vertical direction. During gaze 45 degrees in the contralateral direction, the eye will rotate about an axis through the pupil. The Tullio phenomenon is not present in all cases of SCDS. In addition to dizziness and nystagmus, SCDS may be characterized by autophony (sensation of increased loudness of the patient's own voice), conductive hearing loss (which is not due to middle ear pathology), and/or pulsatile tinnitus. High-resolution CT scans with reconstructions in the plane of the superior canal and orthogonal to that plane should be done to confirm the diagnosis.

The pathophysiology of SCDS can be understood in terms of the creation of a "third mobile window" into the inner ear. Under normal circumstances, sound pressure enters the inner ear through the stapes footplate in the oval window and, after passing around the cochlea, exits through the round window. The presence of a dehiscence in the superior canal allows this canal to respond to sound and pressure stimuli. The direction of the evoked eye movements supports this mechanism. Loud sounds, positive pressure in the external auditory canal, and a Valsalva maneuver against pinched nostrils cause ampullofugal deflection of the superior canal that results in excitation of afferents innervating this canal. The evoked eye movements can involve a nystagmus that has slow components directed upward with torsional motion of the superior pole of the eye away from the affected ear (Figure 34–9). Conversely, negative pressure in the external canal, a Valsalva against a closed glottis, and jugular venous compression cause ampullopetal deflection of the superior canal that results in inhibition of afferents innervating this canal. The evoked eye movements are typically in the plane of the superior canal but in the opposite direction (downward with torsional motion of the superior pole of the eye toward the affected ear).

The severity of the patient's symptoms and the impact of these symptoms on lifestyle are major determinants in the consideration of surgery for SCD.[124] Some patients are discovered to have SCDS as an incidental finding on CT scan and do not have symptoms. Other patients have only autophony or conductive hearing loss. Such patients should be carefully counseled about the risks of a middle fossa surgery, prior to contemplating any surgical repair.

Surgical plugging of the affected superior canal can be beneficial in patients with debilitating symptoms due to this disorder. Two approaches to the plugging of SCD have been described. The middle cranial fossa approach was described first[122] and is the technique used by the authors of this chapter. An alternative approach that has more recently been described is SCD plugging via a transmastoid approach. Advocates of the transmastoid approach have noted that it avoids a craniotomy, involves no temporal lobe retraction, and may lead to better stability of the canal plug. Moreover, most otolaryngologists are more familiar with mastoidectomy.[125,126] The transmastoid approach was initially described in two patients in

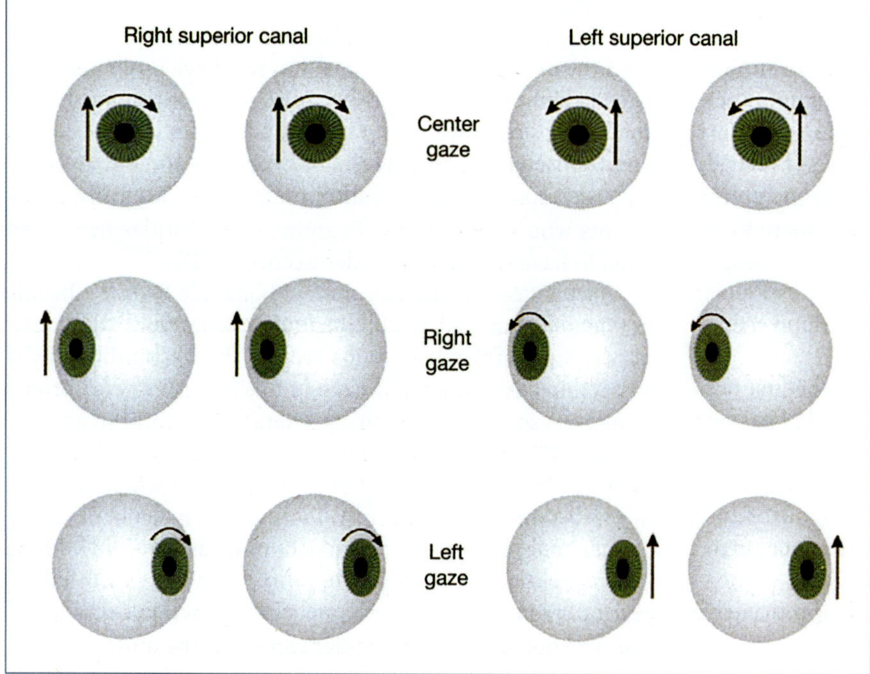

FIGURE 34–9 • Direction of slow phase of eye movement with superior canal excitation. Eye movement occurs in the plane of the superior canal regardless of gaze direction. There are both vertical and torsional components when the patient is looking directly ahead (center gaze). The torsional and vertical components can be separated by having the patient look to the right or left during stimulation.

2001, and although these patients were relieved of vertigo, one patient experienced significant sensorineural hearing loss after surgery.[127] More recently, additional reports of transmastoid superior canal plugging with minimal morbidity and improvement in symptoms have been published.[125,126,128]

We favor the middle fossa approach over the transmastoid approach for several reasons. The transmastoid approach does not permit direct confirmation of the dehiscence, and transmastoid plugging of a superior canal that was later found to be intact has been described.[125] The transmastoid approach may not be possible in patients with a low-hanging dura or extensive tegmen dehiscence.[125] In the transmastoid approach, the plug is placed closer to the sensory epithelia of the ampulla and the utricle, which may be more traumatic to these structures and risk disturbance of their baseline firing rates. Furthermore, opening the superior canal distal to the dehiscence may lead to plug placement in the common crus, causing loss of sensory function of the posterior canal as well.[129] Finally, the transmastoid approach

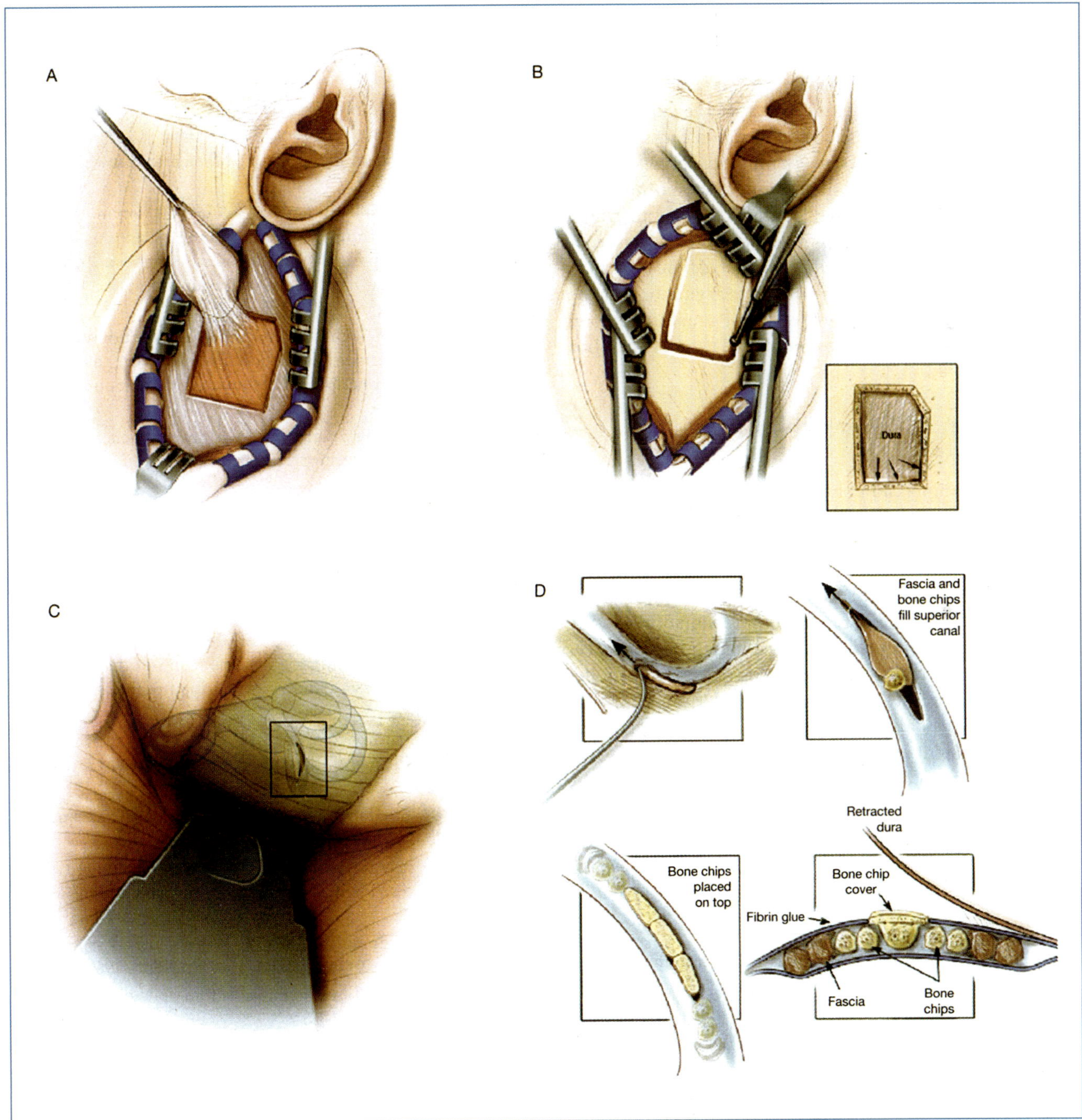

FIGURE 34–10 • Plugging of superior semicircular canal dehiscence. *A*, Temporalis fascia is harvested. *B*, Craniotomy is performed and the bone flap is gently freed from the dura. *C*, Dura is elevated revealing the superior canal dehiscence. *D*, Each end of the superior canal is packed with small pieces of the previously harvested fascia; these are held in place with bone chips.

requires drilling, irrigation, and suctioning on the bony canal. Once the canal is opened, these manipulations could contaminate or remove perilymph from the canal and cause collapse of the membranous labyrinth or serous labyrinthitis.

Therefore, our preferred technique for SCD repair is to plug the canal via a middle cranial fossa approach. The surgical approach begins with a middle fossa craniotomy similar to the approach previously described (Figure 34–6), although the craniotomy can generally be smaller than that used for approaches to tumors in the internal auditory canal (Figure 34–10). Fascia should be harvested from the temporalis muscle and bone chips should also be saved from the craniotomy for later use in plugging the superior canal. The dura should be carefully lifted from the tegmen while working medially to the location of the arcuate eminence. A Fisch or House-Urban retractor is used to maintain exposure while elevating the dura to expose the arcuate eminence, overlying the superior canal in the middle fossa. Patients with SCDS often have thin bone with multiple bony defects in the tegmen, which can make the precise location of the dehiscence difficult to find. We have found a three-dimensional image navigation system very helpful in locating the dehiscence without having to apply suction in the vicinity of the open canal, which would threaten to remove excess perilymph or tear the membranous canal duct. Once the superior canal is exposed, it is plugged by packing the canal with fascia patches and bone chips (Figure 34–10).

VASCULAR COMPRESSION SYNDROMES

Neurovascular compression by arterial loops has been implicated as the cause of many poorly understood symptoms, such as trigeminal neuralgia, hemifacial spasm, tinnitus, and vertigo. The House Ear Clinic[130] and the University of Pittsburgh[131] reported that 80% of patients had improvement in dizziness after microvascular decompression of the vestibulocochlear nerve. Despite this apparent high rate of success reported at a few centers, these procedures have not undergone controlled studies, and even the underlying diagnosis remains controversial. Cerebellopontine angle imaging has shown no consistent relationship between vascular loops and vertigo, and vessels in close proximity to the seventh or eighth cranial nerves in up to 30% of asymptomatic individuals.[132,133] Many approaches to microvascular decompression have been described, such as the retrosigmoid approach (see nerve section above).

References

1. Baloh RW. Charles Skinner Hallpike and the beginnings of neurotology. Neurology 2000;54:2138.
2. Flourens P. Recherches expérimentales sur les propriétés et les functions du systéme nerveux dans les animaux vertébrés. Paris, France: Crevot; 1824.
3. Ménière P. Sur une forme de sourdité grave dépendent d'une lésion de l'orelle interne. GazMed Paris 1861;16.
4. Baloh RW. Prosper Ménière and his disease. Arch Neurol 2001;58:1151.
5. Knapp H. A clinical analysis of the inflammatory affections of the inner ear. Arch Ophthalmol 1871;2:204.
6. Parry RH. A case of tinnitus and vertigo treated by division of the auditory nerve. J Laryngol Otol 1904;19:402.
7. Lake R. Removal of the semicircular canals in a case of unilateral aural vertigo. Lancet 1904;1:1567.
8. Milligan W. Ménière's disease: A clinical and experimental inquiry. J Laryngol Otol 1904;19:440.
9. Portmann M. The Portmann procedure after sixty years. Am J Otol 1987;8:271.
10. Green RE. Surgical treatment of vertigo, with follow-up on Walter Dandy's cases: Neurological aspects. Clin Neurosurg 1958;6:141.
11. Hallpike CS, Cairns H. Observations on the pathology of Ménière's syndrome. J Laryngol Otol 1938;53:625.
12. Yamakawa K. Über die pathologische veränderung bei eiem Ménière-Kranken. Z Otorhinolaryngol, Organ der Japan 1938;44:192.
13. Paparella MM, Mancini F. Vestibular Ménière's disease. Otolaryngol Head Neck Surg 1985;93:148.
14. Minor LB, Schessel DA, Carey JP. Ménière's disease. Curr Opin Neurol 2004;17:9.
15. Monsell EM, Balkany TA, Gates GA, et al. Committee on hearing and equilibrium guidelines for the diagnosis and evaluation of therapy in Ménière's disease. American Academy of Otolaryngology—Head and Neck Foundation, Inc. Otolaryngol Head Neck Surg 1995;113:181.
16. Gill-Body KM, Beninato M, Krebs DE. Relationship among balance impairments, functional performance, and disability in people with peripheral vestibular hypofunction. Phys Ther 2000;80:748.
17. Jacobson GP, Newman CW. The development of the dizziness handicap inventory. Arch Otolaryngol Head Neck Surg 1990;116:424.
18. Committee on hearing and equilibrium. Guidelines for the diagnosis and evaluation of therapy in Ménière's disease. Otolaryngol Head Neck Surg 1996;114:236.
19. Telian SA, Shepard NT. Update on vestibular rehabilitation therapy. Otolaryngol Clin North Am 1996;29:359.
20. Becker SS, Jackler RK, Pitts LH. Cerebrospinal fluid leak after acoustic neuroma surgery: A comparison of the translabyrinthine, middle fossa, and retrosigmoid approaches. Otol Neurotol 2003;24:107.
21. Perez R, Chen JM, Nedzelski JM. The status of the contralateral ear in established unilateral Ménière's disease. Laryngoscope 2004;114:1373.
22. Torok N. Old and new in Ménière disease. Laryngoscope 1977;87:1870.
23. Furstenberg AC, Lashmet FH, Talbot F. Ménière's symptom complex: Medical treatment. Ann Otol Rhinol Laryngol 1954;43:1035.
24. Silverstein H, Smouha E, Jones R. Natural history vs. surgery for Ménière's disease. Otolaryngol Head Neck Surg 1989;100:6.
25. Curthoys IS. Vestibular compensation and substitution. Curr Opin Neurol 2000;13:27.
26. Hughes GB, Barna BP, Kinney SE, et al. Autoimmune endolymphatic hydrops: Five-year review. Otolaryngol Head Neck Surg 1988;98:221.
27. Parnes LS, Sun AH, Freeman DJ. Corticosteroid pharmacokinetics in the inner ear fluids: An animal study followed by clinical application. Laryngoscope 1999;109:1.
28. Pondugula SR, Sanneman JD, Wangemann P, et al. Glucocorticoids stimulate cation absorption by semicircular canal duct epithelium

via epithelial sodium channel. Am J Physiol Renal Physiol 2004;286:F1127.

29. Trune DR, Kempton JB. Aldosterone and prednisolone control of cochlear function in MRL/MpJ-Fas(lpr) autoimmune mice. Hear Res 2001;155:9
30. Itoh A, Sakata E. Treatment of vestibular disorders. Acta Otolaryngol Suppl 1991;481:617.
31. Shea JJ Jr, Ge X. Dexamethasone perfusion of the labyrinth plus intravenous dexamethasone for Ménière's disease. Otolaryngol Clin North Am 1996;29:353.
32. Silverstein H, Isaacson JE, Olds MJ, et al. Dexamethasone inner ear perfusion for the treatment of Ménière's disease: A prospective, randomized, double-blind, crossover trial. Am J Otol 1998;19:196.
33. Sennaroglu L, Dini FM, Sennaroglu G, et al. Transtympanic dexamethasone application in Ménière's disease: An alternative treatment for intractable vertigo. J Laryngol Otol 1999;113:217.
34. Barrs DM, Keyser JS, Stallworth C, et al. Intratympanic steroid injections for intractable Ménière's disease. Laryngoscope 2001;111:2100.
35. Boleas-Aguirre MS, Lin FR, Della Santina CC, et al. Longitudinal results with intratympanic dexamethasone in the treatment of Ménière's disease. Otol Neurotol 2008;29:33.
36. Garduno-Anaya MA, Couthino De Toledo H, Hinojosa-Gonzalez R, et al. Dexamethasone inner ear perfusion by intratympanic injection in unilateral Ménière's disease: A two-year prospective, placebo-controlled, double-blind, randomized trial. Otolaryngol Head Neck Surg 2005;133:285.
37. Schuknecht HF. Ablation therapy in the management of Ménière's disease with topical gentamicin: A preliminary report. Acta Otolaryngol 1957;132:1.
38. Lange G. Gentamicin and other ototoxic antibiotics for the transtympanic treatment of Ménière's disease. Arch Otorhinolaryngol 1989;246:269.
39. Beck C, Schmidt CL. 10 years of experience with intratympanally applied streptomycin (gentamicin) in the therapy of Morbus Ménière. Arch Otorhinolaryngol 1978;221:149.
40. Nedzelski JM, Chiong CM, Fradet G, et al. Intratympanic gentamicin instillation as treatment of unilateral Ménière's disease: update of an ongoing study. Am J Otol 1993;14:278.
41. Nedzelski JM, Schessel DA, Bryce GE, et al. Chemical labyrinthectomy: Local application of gentamicin for the treatment of unilateral Ménière's disease. Am J Otol 1992;13:18.
42. Toth AA, Parnes LS. Intratympanic gentamicin therapy for Ménière's disease: Preliminary comparison of two regimens. J Otolaryngol 1995;24:340.
43. Harner SG, Driscoll CL, Facer GW, et al. Long-term follow-up of transtympanic gentamicin for Ménière's syndrome. Otol Neurotol 2001;22:210.
44. Smith BM, Myers MG. The penetration of gentamicin and neomycin into perilymph across the round window membrane. Otolaryngol Head Neck Surg 1979;87:888.
45. Hellstrom S, Johansson U, Anniko M. Structure of the round window membrane. Acta Otolaryngol Suppl 1989;457:33.
46. Alzamil KS, Linthicum FH Jr. Extraneous round window membranes and plugs: Possible effect on intratympanic therapy. Ann Otol Rhinol Laryngol 2000;109:30.
47. Hibi T, Suzuki T, Nakashima T. Perilymphatic concentration of gentamicin administered intratympanically in guinea pigs. Acta Otolaryngol 2001;121:336.
48. de Groot JC, Meeuwsen F, Ruizendaal WE, et al. Ultrastructural localization of gentamicin in the cochlea. Hear Res 1990;50:35.
49. Kroese AB, Das A, Hudspeth AJ. Blockage of the transduction channels of hair cells in the bullfrog's sacculus by aminoglycoside antibiotics. Hear Res 1989;37:203.
50. Takumida M, Bagger-Sjoback D, Harada Y, et al. Sensory hair fusion and glycocalyx changes following gentamicin exposure in the guinea pig vestibular organs. Acta Otolaryngol 1989;107:39.
51. Li L, Nevill G, Forge A. Two modes of hair cell loss from the vestibular sensory epithelia of the guinea pig inner ear. J Comp Neurol 1995;355:405.
52. Lopez I, Honrubia V, Lee SC, et al. Quantification of the process of hair cell loss and recovery in the chinchilla crista ampullaris after gentamicin treatment. Int J Dev Neurosci 1997;15:447.
53. Lindeman HH. Regional differences in sensitivity of the vestibular sensory epithelia to ototoxic antibiotics. Acta Otolaryngol 1969;67:177.
54. Lyford-Pike S, Vogelheim C, Chu E, et al. Gentamicin is primarily localized in vestibular type I hair cells after intratympanic administration. J Assoc Res Otolaryngol 2007;8:497.
55. Carey JP, Minor LB, Peng GC, et al. Changes in the three-dimensional angular vestibulo-ocular reflex following intratympanic gentamicin for Ménière's disease. J Assoc Res Otolaryngol 2002;3:430.
56. Lin FR, Migliaccio AA, Haslwanter T, et al. Angular vestibulo-ocular reflex gains correlate with vertigo control after intratympanic gentamicin treatment for Ménière's disease. Ann Otol Rhinol Laryngol 2005;114:777.
57. Zheng JL, Keller G, Gao WQ. Immunocytochemical and morphological evidence for intracellular self-repair as an important contributor to mammalian hair cell recovery. J Neurosci 1999;19:2161.
58. Carey J. Intratympanic gentamicin for the treatment of Ménière's disease and other forms of peripheral vertigo. Otolaryngol Clin North Am 2004;37:1075.
59. Chia SH, Gamst AC, Anderson JP, et al. Intratympanic gentamicin therapy for Ménière's disease: A meta-analysis. Otol Neurotol 2004;25:544.
60. Rauch SD, Merchant SN, Thedinger BA. Ménière's syndrome and endolymphatic hydrops. Double-blind temporal bone study. Ann Otol Rhinol Laryngol 1989;98:873.
61. Ingelstedt S, Ivarsson A, Tjernstrom O. Immediate relief of symptoms during acute attacks of Ménière's disease, using a pressure chamber. Acta Otolaryngol 1976;82:368.
62. Sakikawa Y, Kimura RS. Middle ear overpressure treatment of endolymphatic hydrops in guinea pigs. ORL J Otorhinolaryngol Relat Spec 1997;59:84.
63. Gates GA, Green JD Jr, Tucci DL, et al. The effects of transtympanic micropressure treatment in people with unilateral Ménière's disease. Arch Otolaryngol Head Neck Surg 2004;130:718.
64. Gates GA, Verrall A, Green JD Jr, et al. Meniett clinical trial: Long-term follow-up. Arch Otolaryngol Head Neck Surg 2006;132:1311.
65. Montandon P, Guillemin P, Hausler R. Prevention of vertigo in Ménière's syndrome by means of transtympanic ventilation tubes. ORL J Otorhinolaryngol Relat Spec 1988;50:377.
66. Sugawara K, Kitamura K, Ishida T, et al. Insertion of tympanic ventilation tubes as a treating modality for patients with Ménière's disease: A short- and long-term follow-up study in seven cases. Auris Nasus Larynx 2003;30:25.

67. Thomsen J, Bonding P, Becker B, et al. The non-specific effect of endolymphatic sac surgery in treatment of Ménière's disease: A prospective, randomized controlled study comparing "classic" endolymphatic sac surgery with the insertion of a ventilating tube in the tympanic membrane. Acta Otolaryngol 1998;118:769.
68. Shah DK, Kartush JM. Endolymphatic sac surgery in Ménière's disease. Otol Clin North Am 1997;30:1061.
69. Fick IA. Decompression of the labyrinth. Arch Otolaryngol 1964;79:447.
70. Cody DTR. The tack operation for endolymphatic hydrops. Laryngoscope 1969;79:1737.
71. House WF. Ménière's disease: management and theory. Otol Clin North Am 1975;8:515.
72. Schuknecht HF. Cochleosacculotomy for Ménière's disease: theory, technique and results. Laryngoscope 1982;92:853.
73. Otrowski VB, Kartush JM. Endolymphatic sac-vein decompression for intractable Ménière's disease: Long term treatment results. Otolaryngol Head Neck Surg 2003;128:550.
74. Gibson WP. The effect of surgical removal of the extraosseous portion of the endolymphatic sac in patients suffering from Ménière's disease. J Laryngol Otol 1996;110:1008.
75. Paparella MM. Endolymphatic sac drainage for intractable vertigo (method and experiences). Laryngoscope 1976;86:697.
76. House WF. Subarachnoid shunt for drainage of endolymphatic hydrops. Laryngoscope 1962;72:713.
77. Glasscock ME, Kveton JR, Christiansen SG. Current status of surgery for Ménière's disease. Otolaryngol Head Neck Surg 1984;92:67.
78. Thomsen J, Bretlau P, Tos M, et al. Placebo effect in surgery for Ménière's disease. A double-blind, placebo-controlled study on endolymphatic sac shunt surgery. Arch Otolaryngol 1981;107:271.
79. Pillsbury HC, 3rd, Arenberg IK, Ferraro J, et al. Endolymphatic sac surgery. The Danish sham surgery study: An alternative analysis. Otolaryngol Clin North Am 1983;16:123.
80. Vaisrub N. Placebo effect for Ménière's disease sac shunt surgery disputed [letter]. Arch Otolaryngol 1981;107:774.
81. Welling DB, Nagaraja HN. Endolymphatic mastoid shunt: A reevaluation of efficacy. Otolaryngol Head Neck Surg 2000;122:340.
82. Luetje CM. A critical comparison of results of endolymphatic subarachnoid shunt and endolymphatic sac incision operations. Am J Otol 1988;9:95.
83. Durland WF, Pyle M, Connor NP. Endolymphatic sac decompression as a treatment for Ménière's disease. Laryngoscope 2005;115:1454.
84. Glasscock ME, Jackson CG, Poe DS, et al. What I think of sac surgery in 1989. Am J Otol 1989;10:230.
85. Kaylie DM, Jackson CG, Gardner EK. Surgical management of Ménière's disease in the era of gentamicin. Otolaryngol Head Neck Surg 2004;132:443.
86. Silverstein H, Lewis WB, Jackson LE, et al. Changing trends in the surgical treatment of Ménière's disease: Results of a 10-year survey. Ear Nose Throat J 2003;82:185.
87. House WF. Surgical exposure of the internal auditory canal and its contents through the middle cranial fossa. Laryngoscope 1961;71:1363.
88. Glasscock ME. Vestibular nerve section. Arch Otolaryngol 1973;97:112.
89. Silverstein H, Norrel H. Retrolabyrinthine surgery: A direct approach to the cerebellopontine angle. Otolaryngol Head Neck Surg 1980;88:462.
90. Silverstein H, Norrel H, Haberkamp T. A comparison of retrosigmoid IAC, retrolabyrinthine, and middle fossa vestibular neuroectomy for treatment of vertigo. Laryngoscope 1987;88:165.
91. Silverstein H. Transmeatal labyrinthectomy with and without cochleovestibular neurectomy. Laryngoscope 1976;86:1777.
92. Silverstein H, Jackson LE. Vestibular nerve section. Otolaryngol Clin North Am 2002;35:655.
93. Colletti V, Carner M, Colletti L. Auditory results after vestibular nerve section and intratympanic gentamicin for Ménière's disease. Otol Neurotol 2007;28:145.
94. Thomsen J, Berner B, Tos M. Vestibular neurectomy. Auris Nasus Larynx 2000;27:297.
95. Wu IC, Minor LB. Long-term hearing outcome in patients receiving intratympanic gentamicin for Ménière's disease. Laryngoscope 2003;113:815.
96. Glasscock ME, 3rd, Kveton JF, Christiansen SG. Middle fossa vestibular neurectomy: An update. Otolaryngol Head Neck Surg 1984;92:216.
97. Zini C, Mazzoni A, Gandolfi A, et al. Retrolabyrinthine versus middle fossa vestibular neurectomy. Am J Otol 1988;9:448.
98. Diaz RC, LaRouere MJ, Bojrab DI, et al. Quality-of-life assessment of Ménière's disease patients after surgical labyrinthectomy. Otol Neurotol 2007;28:74.
99. Sekhar LN, Schessel DA, Bucur SD, et al. Partial labyrinthectomy petrous apicectomy approach to neoplastic and vascular lesions of the petroclival area. Neurosurgery 1999;44:537.
100. Horgan MA, Delashaw JB, Schwartz MS, et al. Transcrusal approach to the petroclival region with hearing preservation. Technical note and illustrative cases. J Neurosurg 2001;94:660.
101. Kaylie DM, Gilbert E, Horgan MA, et al. Acoustic neuroma surgery outcomes. Otol Neurotol 2001;22:686.
102. Smouha EE, Inouye M. Partial labyrinthectomy with hearing preservation: Frequency-specific data using tone-burst auditory brain stem response. Otolaryngol Head Neck Surg 1999;120:146.
103. Leveque M, Labrousse M, Seidermann L, et al. Surgical therapy in intractable benign paroxysmal positional vertigo. Otolaryngol Head Neck Surg 2007;136:693.
104. Epley JM. The canalith repositioning procedure: For treatment of benign paroxysmal positional vertigo. Otolaryngol Head Neck Surg 1992;107:399.
105. Gacek RR. Transection of the posterior ampullary nerve for the relief of benign paroxysmal positional vertigo. Ann Otol Rhinol Laryngol 1974;83:596.
106. Gacek RR, Gacek MR. Results of singular neurectomy in the posterior ampullary recess. ORL J Otorhinolaryngol Relat Spec 2002;64:397.
107. Epley JM. Singular neurectomy: Hypotympanotomy approach. Otolaryngol Head Neck Surg 1980;100:701.
108. Parnes LS, McClure JA. Posterior semicircular canal occlusion for intractable benign paroxysmal positional vertigo. Ann Otol Rhinol Laryngol 1990;99:330.
109. Schessel DA, Nedzelski JM. Presentation of large vestibular aqueduct syndrome to a dizziness unit. J Otolaryngol 1992;21:265.
110. Oh AK, Ishiyama A, Baloh RW. Vertigo and the enlarged vestibular aqueduct syndrome. J Neurol 2001;248:971.

111. Jackler RK, Luxford WM, Brackmann DE, et al. Endolymphatic sac surgery in congenital malformations of the inner ear. Laryngoscope 1988;98:698.

112. Welling DB, Martyn MD, Miles BA, et al. Endolymphatic sac occlusion for the enlarged vestibular aqueduct syndrome. Am J Otol 1998;19:145.

113. Minor LB. Labyrinthine fistulae: Pathobiology and management. Curr Opin Otolaryngol Head Neck Surg 2003;11:340.

114. Friedland DR, Wackym PA. A critical appraisal of spontaneous perilymphatic fistulas of the inner ear. Am J Otol 1999;20:261.

115. Shelton C, Simmons FB. Perilymph fistula: The Stanford experience. Ann Otol Rhinol Laryngol 1988;97:105.

116. Rizer FM, House JW. Perilymph fistulas: The House Ear Clinic experience. Otolaryngol Head Neck Surg 1991;104:239.

117. Meyerhoff WL. Spontaneous perilymphatic fistula: Myth or fact. Am J Otol 1993;14:478.

118. el Shazly MA, Linthicum FH Jr. Microfissures of the temporal bone: Do they have any clinical significance? Am J Otol 1991;12:169.

119. Buchman CA, Luxford WM, Hirsch BE, et al. Beta-2 transferrin assay in the identification of perilymph. Am J Otol 1999;20:174.

120. Shepard NT, Telian SA, Niparko JK, et al. Platform pressure test in identification of perilymphatic fistula. Am J Otol 1992;13:49.

121. Hakuba N, Hato N, Shinomori Y, et al. Labyrinthine fistula as a late complication of middle ear surgery using the canal wall down technique. Otol Neurotol 2002;23:832.

122. Minor LB, Solomon D, Zinreich JS, et al. Sound- and/or pressure-induced vertigo due to bone dehiscence of the superior semicircular canal. Arch Otolaryngol Head Neck Surg 1998;124:249.

123. Tullio P. Das ohr und die entstehung de sprache und schrift. Berlin: Urban Scharzenberg; 1929.

124. Minor LB. Clinical manifestations of superior semicircular canal dehiscence. Laryngoscope 2005;115:1717.

125. Agrawal SK, Parnes LS. Transmastoid superior semicircular canal occlusion. Otol Neurotol 2008;29:363.

126. Crovetto M, Areitio E, Elexpuru J, et al. Transmastoid approach for resurfacing of superior semicircular canal dehiscence. Auris Nasus Larynx 2008;35:247.

127. Brantberg K, Bergenius J, Mendel L, et al. Symptoms, findings and treatment in patients with dehiscence of the superior semicircular canal. Acta Otolaryngol 2001;121:68.

128. Kirtane MV, Sharma A, Satwalekar D. Transmastoid repair of superior semicircular canal dehiscence. J Laryngol Otol 2008;1.

129. Carey JP, Migliaccio AA, Minor LB. Semicircular canal function before and after surgery for superior canal dehiscence. Otol Neurotol 2007;28:356.

130. Brackmann DE, Kesser BW, Day JD. Microvascular decompression of the vestibulocochlear nerve for disabling positional vertigo: The House Ear Clinic experience. Otol Neurotol 2001;22:882.

131. Moller MB, Moller AR, Jannetta PJ, et al. Microvascular decompression of the eighth nerve in patients with disabling positional vertigo: Selection criteria and operative results in 207 patients. Acta Neurochir (Wien) 1993;125:75.

132. Sirikci A, Bayazit Y, Ozer E, et al. Magnetic resonance imaging based classification of anatomic relationship between the cochleovestibular nerve and anterior inferior cerebellar artery in patients with non-specific neuro-otologic symptoms. Surg Radiol Anat 2005;27:531.

133. De Carpentier J, Lynch N, Fisher A, et al. MR imaged neurovascular relationships at the cerebellopontine angle. Clin Otolaryngol Allied Sci 1996;21:312.

Cochlear Implants in Adults and Children

35

Peter S. Roland, MD

INTRODUCTION

Cochlear implants are the first true bionic sense organs. Cochlear implants, like the human hair cell, receive mechanical sound energy and convert it into a series of electrical impulses. The human cochlea is, in effect, an electromechanical transducer. This transformation is not trivial and some of the brightest engineering minds have spent hundreds of thousands of hours determining how this transformation should be accomplished so as to provide the human auditory cortex with the most meaningful information. Cochlear implants are not hearing aids. Hearing aids merely amplify mechanical sound waves and increase their energy content. Hearing aids do not fundamentally alter the nature of the signal.

Cochlear implants are playing an increasingly important role in the management of both adults and children with hearing impairment. Although the results remain variable and unpredictable for a given individual, a substantial proportion of implant recipients now recover high levels of open-set speech understanding. Cochlear implants permit implant recipients to reintegrate with the hearing world.

In the early days of implantation, there was considerable concern that the constant electrical stimulation produced by the implant would injure residual neural elements within the cochlea. This concern has been laid to rest. The preponderance of available scientific evidence has demonstrated that dendrite stimulation either enhances spiral ganglion cell survival or, at worst, has no effect on spiral ganglion cell counts at all.[1–3]

It has been estimated that only 10% of the normal spiral ganglion cell population of 35,000 is necessary for successful cochlear implant use.[4] Linthicum and Anderson demonstrated that of 46 temporal bones with total sensorineural hearing loss, 37 had more than 3,500 residual spiral ganglion cells and would be potential cochlear implant candidates based on that criterion.[5] Nadol has shown that the highest number of residual spiral ganglion cells are found following aminoglycoside toxicity and sudden sensorineural hearing loss. The lowest numbers of surviving spiral ganglion cells are seen in individuals with congenital/genetically mediated losses and following bacterial meningitis.[5] Nadol has shown a strong positive correlation between the diameter of the cochlear nerve and the total spiral ganglion cell count ($P \leq .001$). This finding offers the possibility of indirectly assessing the spiral ganglion cell population by measuring the size of the auditory nerve.[5]

Although the history of cochlear implantation in adults goes back well over 30 years, cochlear implantation in children is more recent. Implantation was initially limited to postlingually deafened children because it was widely believed that the device would have little utility for children with severe to profound congenital hearing loss.

Project Hope, combining the results of three different types of survey instruments, has estimated that there are at least 464,000 and possibly as many as 738,000 severe to profoundly hearing-impaired persons among the 22 million Americans with hearing loss. It estimated that about 5 of every 10,000 infants have severe to profound hearing loss and, using 1998 Bureau of Census data, 5,600 children under 2 years of age are profoundly hearing impaired.[6] Cheng has calculated that cochlear implants may be useful in as many as 200,000 children in the United States.[7]

IMPACT OF HEARING LOSS

The impact of severe/profound hearing loss on the US economy is substantial. Figures indicate that as much as $2.5 billion may be lost in workforce productivity. Approximately 42% of individuals with severe/profound hearing impairment between the ages of 18 and 44 years are unemployed, compared to 18% of the general population.[8,9]

In addition to lost productivity, there are direct costs associated with severe/profound hearing loss. For example, approximately $2 billion is spent to provide equal access for hearing impaired individuals as required by law.

More than $120 billion is spent in educational costs. Despite substantial resources invested in the education of severe/profoundly hearing-impaired individuals, 44% fail to graduate from high school as compared to 19% of normal-hearing students. Only 5% of severe to profoundly deaf individuals graduate from college, compared to 13% of normal-hearing children.[8] The cost of educating a severe to profoundly deaf child is vastly increased and approaches half a million dollars per child for kindergarten through grade 12, or 50 times the cost of educating a normal-hearing child.[10,11] The cost of cochlear implantation and associated rehabilitative services (ranging from $40,000 to $60,000) are modest in comparison. If cochlear implantation shifts only 1 child in 10 into a mainstream classroom, the savings in educational costs alone would pay all of the costs of implantation for all 10 implant recipients. Current evidence suggests that considerably more than 1 out of 10 children would be able to function within mainstream classrooms, and there is justifiable optimism that the high unemployment rates seen currently in individuals with severe to profound hearing loss can be lowered substantially as a result of widespread implantation.[9] There are already studies indicating that cochlear implantation can improve earnings for adults.[12]

Deaf Culture

The National Association for the Deaf (NAD) is an organization of deaf individuals who believe in "deaf culture." According to the NAD, "deaf people like being deaf, want to be deaf and are proud of their deafness." They do not regard deafness as a disability.[11] Deaf culturalists believe deaf individuals live and participate in a unique culture and that attempts to eliminate deafness is a form of cultural imperialism or even genocide.[13]

For the most part, deaf culturalists use American Sign Language (ASL). ASL is a distinctively different language from English with an entirely different grammatical structure. Facility in ASL does not translate into facility with even written English. Deaf culturalists believe that ASL is a "natural" communication system (the basis for this claim of "naturalness" is unclear) for deaf children and that spoken, written, or even signed English is "unnatural." Deaf culturalists believe that deaf children are natural members of deaf culture, and to restore their hearing is to deny them their natural birthright.[8,13]

Deaf culturalists, while claiming on the one hand that deafness is not a disability, derive support and benefit from billions of dollars in disability benefits. Insofar as cochlear implants are effective, deaf individuals who decline to use them have an "elective disability." Tucker has questioned the extent to which individuals with elective disabilities may call on society to provide supportive services and accommodations.[11]

The strongest advocates of deaf culture are quite explicit about the implications of their views: hearing parents have no "right" to make decisions about their deaf children if those decisions might result in hearing restoration. That right, they claim, belongs to the culture to which they "naturally belong" and should be made by deaf culturists on their behalf.[11,13] Some of these deaf culture activists regard cochlear implants in children as a form of "child abuse." These issues have been carefully examined by Balkany and colleagues with the following conclusion:

> However, the arguments of these leaders are internally contradictory: They hold that deafness is not a disability but support disability benefits for the deaf; they maintain both that cochlear implants do not work and that they work so well that they are "genocidal" (ie, they will eliminate deafness). Their position opposes the ethical principles of beneficence and autonomy as they relate to self-determination and privacy. Ethical standards hold that the best interest of the child precedes the interest of a special interest group and that parents have the responsibility to determine their child's best interest.[10]

Cost Effectiveness

Most cost-effectiveness studies use the "quality-adjusted life year" (QALY) as the basis for comparison. A QALY is an additional year of life with perfect quality of health. If health is only "50% of perfect," then only half a QALY is awarded for that extra year of life. It would take 5 extra years of life to equal one QALY if health quality during these years were only 20% of perfect. Since the life expectancy of cochlear implant recipients is not anticipated to change as a result of implantation, any increase in QALYs must result directly from improved health utility. Health utility can be measured using a variety of different instruments, including a visual analog scale and the Health Utility Index-2 (HUI-2). These scales have been used commonly in assessing the cost effectiveness of cochlear implants. The time trade-off instrument has been used only recently to assess the quality of life for children.

Krabbe and colleagues compared 45 postlingually deafened adult multichannel cochlear implant users with 46 deaf candidates on the waiting list for cochlear implants. Three health-related quality of life instruments were utilized: a specially developed cochlear implant questionnaire, the SF-36 health status questionnaire, and the HUI-2. All three questionnaires detected improvements in health-related quality of life attributable to cochlear implant use.[14]

In 1999 Palmer and colleagues prospectively evaluated cost effectiveness in 62 adult cochlear recipients.[15] Adults who received the implant had a health utility gain (using HUI) of 0.2. Ninety percent of the gain occurred within 6 months of implantation. Using standard models, a 0.2 improvement in health utility resulted in a cost of $14,670 per QALY. Cheng and colleagues published a series of articles assessing the cost effectiveness of cochlear implants. In their studies, half of the substantial loss of health utility (0.6) is recovered by a cochlear implant. Based on their estimates, the cost per QALY for a pediatric cochlear implant recipient varied between $5,197 and $9,029 depending on which survey instrument was used. Generally speaking a cost of $20,000 to $25,000 per QALY is considered a cost-effective intervention (ie, "a good deal"). For example, placement of a defibrillator has a cost of $34,836 per QALY. A total knee replacement is $59,292 per QALY. Cochlear implantation has been demonstrated to have one of the highest cost-effectiveness ratings of any current intervention. Overall, including indirect costs such as reduced educational expenses, the cochlear implant provides a savings to society of $53,198 per child.[7,15–17]

PREOPERATIVE EVALUATION

Initial screening for cochlear implant candidacy in postlingually deafened adults begins with pure-tone audiometry and speech discrimination testing. As a general rule, potential cochlear implant candidates will have a pure tone average greater than 50 dB and a standard speech discrimination score of less than 50 to 60%. The Ad Hoc Subcommittee of the Committee on Hearing and Equilibrium of the American Academy of Otolaryngology—Head and Neck Surgery has recommended that final candidacy determination be made using Hearing in Noise Test (HINT) sentence testing and consonant/nucleus/consonant (CNC) word testing. The HINT provides a reliable and efficient measure of speech recognition in quiet and noise. The HINT is not used in an adaptive mode for preevaluation/surgical candidacy purposes, but the adaptive mode is useful to assess results and compare outcomes. The CNC test is an open-set word recognition test that has the same phonemic distribution as English. High-quality disks can be obtained to standardize performance-measurements pre- and postoperatively and across institutions. Hearing in Noise Test sentence scores of less than 60% in quiet and CNC scores of less than 30% are used as general candidacy guidelines.

Postlingually deafened children are tested using the same measures as adults, but testing children with prelingual hearing loss is more difficult. Prelingually deafened children require special tests. Indeed, in the early years of cochlear implantation, adequate tests for assessing cochlear implant candidacy in prelingual children had to be developed. Existing tests were inadequate.

The Early Speech Perception (ESP) test assesses speech perception ability and is available in both a low verbal and a standard version. Speech perception ability is divided into three subtests to assess the child's capacity to (1) distinguish patterns in speech ("ball" versus "cookie" versus "airplane" versus "ice cream cone"), (2) identify spondee words ("hot dog," "cowboy," "airplane"), and (3) to discriminate monosyllabic words ("ball", "boot", "boat", "bat"). It is useful for children who have developed some language skills. A number of other tests are also used in the evaluation of young and prelingually deafened children, including the Craig Lip Inventory, the Meaningful Auditory Integration Scale (MAIS), and the Infant Toddler MAIS. This testing is specialized and requires a specially trained clinician.

Medical Evaluation

Once it has been determined that a person is a good audiologic candidate, a medical evaluation is necessary. The medical evaluation should determine that a candidate can undergo the operative procedure with acceptable risks. Radiographic imaging of the temporal bone should be obtained in order to identify any potential anatomic variations that might contraindicate the operation or require alterations to the usual surgical procedure.

Traditionally, radiographic evaluation of cochlear implant candidates has been performed using high-resolution computerized tomographic (CT) scanning. Recent refinements in magnetic resonance imaging (MRI) permit greatly enhanced resolution, and now MRI is also very useful in the preoperative assessment of cochlear implant candidates. There are pros and cons to both techniques. (Table 35–1) Each technique is capable of providing important information not provided by the other. Some thought should be given to the individual patient's circumstances and the potential difficulties that may be encountered in that individual before the decision is made as to which type of scan should be requested. Sometimes both types of imaging will be needed.

TABLE 35–1 CT or MRI?

	CT	MRI
Morphology of cochlea and semicircular canals	++	+++
Potency of cochlear duct	+	++
Status of cochlear nerve	-	+++
Anatomy of facial nerve and fallopian canal	++	+
Defect of the modiolar	+	+++
Defect of cribiform area	+++	++
Enlarged vestibular aqueduct	++	+++
Enlarged cochlear aqueduct	+++	+
Presence of round or oval window	+++	-
CNS abnormalities		+++

It has become clear that MRI is the most sensitive technique for identifying early labyrinthitis ossificans. Even high-resolution CT scanning may miss cochlear obstruction in up to 50% of candidates. Computed tomographic scanning cannot detect labyrinthine obstruction until frank ossification has developed. On the other hand, MRI relies on the presence or absence of a fluid signal within the labyrinthine bone. Consequently, anything that displaces or eliminates fluid from within the cochlea or semicircular canals, notably unossified fibrous tissue, will result in a detectable abnormality.[18–21] Consequently, MRI has become the diagnostic modality of choice for the detection of postmeningitic endocochlear obstruction.[22–24]

Magnetic resonance imaging can demonstrate an absent or hypoplastic cochlear nerve. Using currently available 1.5-T magnets, precise measurements of the size of the cochlear nerve are difficult, but higher-strength magnets may soon permit more exact quantification of cochlear nerve diameter.[22,23] Since cochlear nerve diameter appears to correlate with the number of surviving spiral ganglion cells, quantification of the size of the cochlear nerve may allow more exact prediction of postoperative outcome after cochlear implantation.[25] An absent cochlear nerve is one of the few absolute contraindications to cochlear implantation. Although a small internal auditory canal on CT scan suggests an absent cochlear nerve, absence of the cochlear nerve can definitely be verified on MRI using parasagittal reconstructions through the internal auditory canal (Figure 35–1).

Defects in the cribriform area of the cochlea, which present the likelihood of an intraoperative "gusher," can be identified on MRI scanning and warn the surgeon about this potential difficulty. Central nervous system (CNS) abnormalities that could adversely affect the outcome of implantation can also be well identified on MRI.

High-resolution CT scanning, however, permits more complete characterization of hypoplasia, aplasia, and incomplete partitioning defects (eg, the Modini deformity) (Figure 35–2 and 35–3), and enlarged vestibular aqueducts. High-resolution CT scanning permits fairly precise mapping of the fallopian

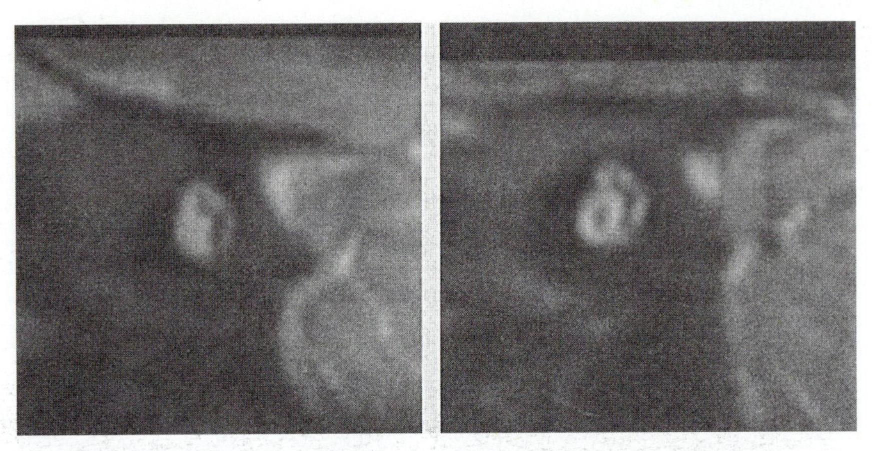

FIGURE 35–1 • Sagittal reconstruction of the internal auditory canal showing normal configuration and orientation of the nerves in the internal auditory canal above and the absence of the cochlear nerve on the sagittal reconstruction to the left. *Illustration courtesy of Dr. Timothy Booth.*

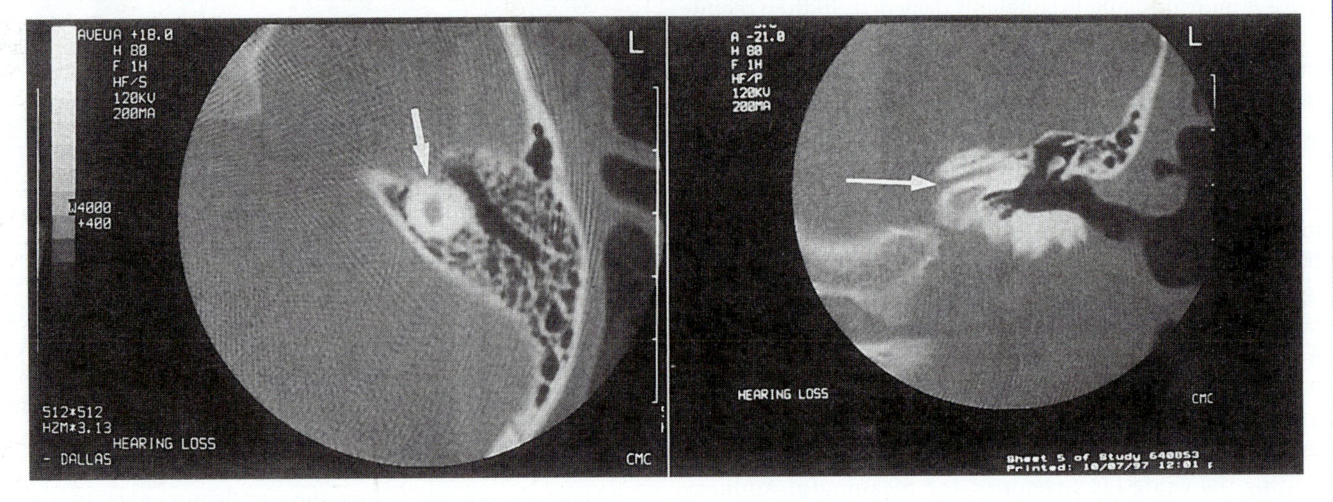

FIGURE 35–2 • Axial section on the right demonstrates a severe cochlear malformation in this case a common cavity deformity. (White arrow). There is no internal auditory canal visible through this section. The image on the left shows that there is a small canal present that is just large enough to accommodate the facial nerve. The cochlear and vestibular nerves are absent as is the vestibule and semicircular canals.

canal and facial nerve. A clear understanding of facial nerve anatomy is especially important in those persons with temporal bone developmental anomalies (eg, dysplastic semicircular canals) that increase the likelihood of anomalous facial nerve anatomy.

Psychological Evaluation

A psychosocial evaluation is no longer a routine part of the evaluation of the pediatric patient but should be considered in special circumstances. The purpose of a psychosocial evaluation is to determine the intellectual ability of the child, establish the child's expectations for postimplant performance, and identify family issues that may affect implantation or postimplant performance. If the child's intelligence is less than normal, the goals for the child, along with expectations, should be scaled back. Rehabilitative milestones for these recipients may be achieved more slowly. In severe to profoundly deaf children, nonverbal tests must be used. A revised form of the Wechsler Intelligence Scale is available for this purpose. Using these results, the psychologist, working with the speech pathologist and audiologist, will establish whether the child has developed the necessary cognitive and behavioral skills for successful device programming. Success is much more likely if the implant can be effectively programmed. If the child has not yet developed these skills, it is in some instances worthwhile postponing the implant long enough for the appropriate behavior to emerge. Intensive therapy can be directed toward the child's particular deficits to help him/her develop the necessary skill set.

Family issues that may affect the success of the implant such as marital stress, depression, or abuse must be identified and resolved. If the cochlear implant candidate is an adolescent, then special attention must be given to make sure that the parent's wishes and those of the adolescent are not substantially different. For example, an adolescent well integrated into a signing community may agree to an implant as a result of parental

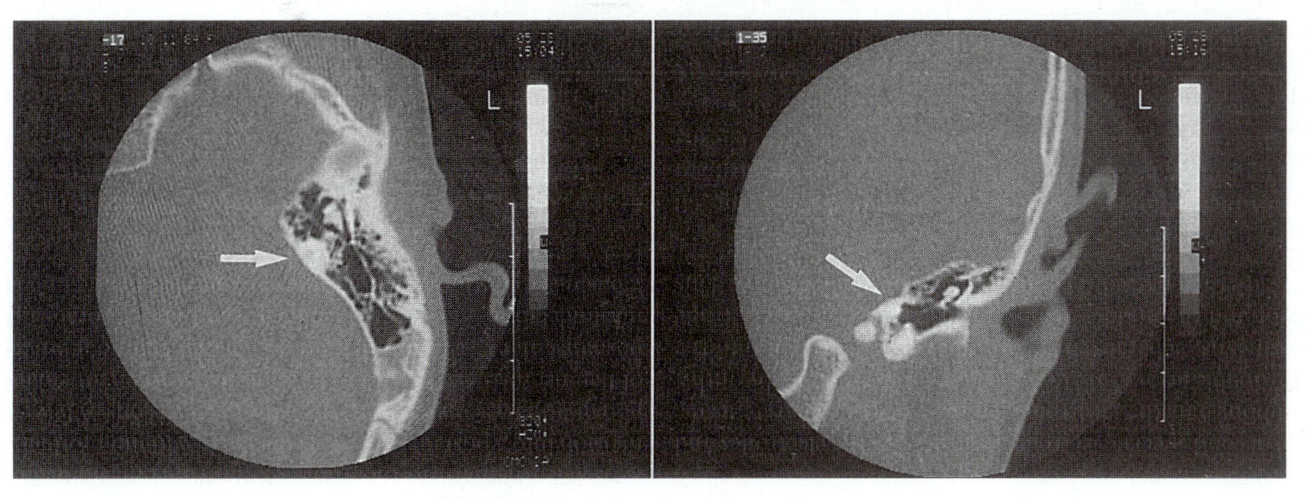

FIGURE 35–3 • The axial section on the right shows the complete absence of the cochlea. There is only some sclerotic bone where the cochlea should be. There is a complete absence of the internal auditory canal on both the axial and the coronal section (image on the right). Although no evidence of the internal auditory canal is apparent on these films, the patient had normal facial nerve function indicating that the facial nerve was in fact intact.

pressure when he/she really does not want one. If implanted, he/she is likely to become a nonuser.

Family dynamics are assessed during the psychosocial evaluation. Sometimes significant problems of family's interaction are recognized that can be improved with appropriate therapy. Such therapy often continues long after the implant has been placed and successfully programmed. Improved family dynamics can significantly enhance a child's ability to become a successful implant user.

Perhaps the most important part of the psychosocial evaluation is to assess both the recipient's and his/her family's expectations for the device. Almost nothing creates more trouble in the postoperative period as do unrealistic expectations on the part of cochlear implant recipients or their family members. The evaluating clinician must assess both the open and the "hidden" expectations of potential recipients and/or their families for the device. If expectations are unrealistic, they should be modified prior to implantation. When expectations are realistic, the chance of disappointment, anger, and rejection of the device is greatly diminished.

Multihandicapped Candidates

The assessment of multihandicapped individuals can be especially challenging. Handicaps most commonly associated with congenital hearing loss include mental retardation, visual and motor delays, epilepsy, autism, cerebral palsy, attention-deficit disorder, and a variety of syndromic abnormalities including CHARGE association (coloboma of the eye, heart anomaly, choanal atresia, retardation, and genital and ear anomalies), Usher's syndrome, and Pendred's syndrome.

Lesinski and colleagues have evaluated 47 children who were implanted and had one or more associated handicaps. Eighty-two percent of these children were successfully programmed.[26] Isaacson and colleagues evaluated five children with significant disabilities. Benefits were realized in the children with disabilities, but they did less well overall.[27] Waltzman and colleagues have evaluated 29 children between the ages of 2 and 12 years with significant handicaps. These children received significant benefit, but development was slower and less stable.[28]

Although associated handicaps are not in and of themselves a contraindication to cochlear implantation, children with multiple handicaps should be carefully evaluated by a team that understands not only the nature of their handicaps but the requirements for programming and successful use of a cochlear implant.

Which Ear to Implant

The selection of which ear to implant can be difficult. In the earliest days of cochlear implantation, the worse hearing ear was generally selected. It was argued that the implantation itself would destroy residual hearing (and it does in at least 50 % of cases) and that the better hearing ear should be conserved in case the implant did not work.[29] Over the years that philosophy has changed. As experience with cochlear implants has grown, confidence in them has increased. Experience to date indicates that the ability to eliminate patients who will not benefit from the implant has become quite good. Consequently, many programs currently select the better hearing ear. It is reasoned that the better hearing ear is likely to have a higher population of residual neural elements and hence offer the possibility of better performance. Most implant surgeons have had the experience of implanting the worse hearing ear, with the result that the patient has achieved no benefit. In such cases, one is inclined to wonder if the results would have been better if the better hearing ear had been implanted. Moreover, it is now often believed that if the residual hearing in the better hearing ear could provide significant benefit, then the patient would not be an appropriate implant candidate. Despite such reasoning, it has not been possible to verify, on the basis of quantitative outcome data, that implanting the better hearing ear produces superior results. Indeed, there is some evidence that results are just as good when the poorer ear is implanted, especially if the difference between it and the better ear is small.[30] Although this may well be true when differences between ears are small, the question remains unanswered when the difference between the ears is large.

Outcome data on cochlear implantation have shown repeatedly, and with a fairly high degree of reliability, that the longer the duration of deafness, the worse the postoperative performance. Consequently, differences in length of deafness between ears are often used to select the ear to receive the implant. The most recently deafened ear is chosen.

Anatomic considerations may guide side selection. If one ear is significantly dysplastic or hypoplastic, the contralateral ear may be selected.

Differences in cochlear patency, when present, are often determinative. While long-standing labyrinthitis ossificans is generally symmetric, initially it may progress more rapidly in one ear than in the other. The least obstructed labyrinth should be chosen.

Sometimes a previous procedure in one ear makes the other ear more desirable. Canal wall down mastoidectomy in one ear would make the contralateral side more appealing because the standard operative procedure would not require modification.

Occasionally there is a marked difference in vestibular function between ears. Previous trauma (surgical or otherwise) may have significantly reduced labyrinthine function on one side. If so, that side should be chosen so as to preserve the ear with the better vestibular function. If, however, the ear with reduced labyrinthine function is also the worse hearing ear or the ear with the longer duration of deafness, the decision becomes more difficult. In such circumstances, it may be justified to implant the ear with better vestibular function if, in the opinion of the implanting surgeon, a significantly better hearing outcome is likely to be obtained.

Ultimately, auditory information must reach the cerebral cortex to be useful. Even when peripheral auditory function is identical, there may be significant differences in the amount of CNS activation obtained by stimulating one side as opposed to the other. New techniques in brain imaging such as single-photon emission CT (SPECT), functional MRI, PET, and refined cortical auditory electrophysiology may allow differences in CNS activation to be identified preoperatively.[31-34]

Age of Implantation

Cochlear implantation in children began in the second half of the 1980s under the close supervision of the US Food and Drug Administration (FDA). It was initially limited to postlingually deafened children because it was widely believed that the device would have little utility for children with congenital hearing loss. Over the decades, the indications have expanded based on documented outcomes submitted to and reviewed by the FDA.

The age of implantation has slowly been lowered from 2 years through 18 months to 1 year of age. Initial objections to implanting very young children were partially based on the perceived potential for electrode migration/extrusion secondary to skull growth. This concern was addressed by Roland and colleagues, who used computer graphic analysis to assess electrode position on serial postoperative radiographs. Children were followed from 1 to 75 months, and no change in electrode position was noted.[35]

Almost all experts in the area of speech and language development have believed, on an intuitive basis, that younger age of implantation will be associated with improved outcomes. Slowly, evidence to support their intuitions is accumulating.[36–38] Connor et al. have evaluated 100 children who received implants between 1 and 10 years of age. Growth curve analysis indicated that there was an additional value for earlier implantation over and above advantages attributed to length of use. They concluded that there were clearly advantages to implanting children before the age of 2½ years.

Their conclusion is consistent with the information developed by Sharma and her colleagues using long latency cortical-evoked responses. Maturation of long-latency cortical responses (as measured by decreased latency) occurs reliably when children are implanted before the age of 3-1/2 years and occurs rarely in children implanted after the age of 7 years.[39–41]

Researchers at the University of Michigan have demonstrated that the postimplantation speech recognition scores of 48 seven-year-olds varied according to the length of time the child had been implanted. The longer the child had had the implant, the better the speech recognition scores. They evaluated an additional 53 children 36 months after their implant had been placed. Holding the length of use fixed, they demonstrated that the children's performance improved as age at time of implant decreased. Moreover, at a fixed post implant age, children implanted at younger ages demonstrated better performance.[42] Svirsky and colleagues have shown that postimplantation, the rate of expressive and receptive language learning approaches that of normal-hearing children. He was, however, unable to demonstrate "catch-up effects." Consequently, younger age at implantation would leave a narrower gap between normal-hearing and implanted children.[43] Moog and Geers have shown that normal levels of language and reading are associated with earlier age of implantation.[44] Cheng and colleagues' meta-analysis showed that more rapid gains in speech perception are associated with earlier age in implantation.[17] Connor et al. have shown that there is a substantial benefit for both speech and vocabulary outcomes when children receive their implant before the age of 2 ½ years.[38]

Reservations have also been voiced about implanting older patients. Concerns about effectiveness and cost utility have been raised. Although ganglion cell loss is a feature of many forms of presbycusis, it rarely reduces ganglion cell populations below the 3,500 (about 10% of normal) cells necessary for speech recognition. Data on speech recognition scores in elderly patients who have received cochlear implants verify that the elderly are as likely to achieve as successful hearing outcomes as younger patients.

A number of other concerns have been raised about the geriatric population. It has been suggested that they are at greater risk for soft tissue complications because of decreased blood flow in scalp tissues, related not only to microvascular disease but also to an increasing incidence of diabetes.

However, no such increase of soft tissue complications has been verified.[46] Because elderly individuals recover less promptly from vestibular injuries, it has been hypothesized that the impact of cochlear implant on ambulation and falling could be disproportionately severe in an elderly population. No data have been produced to support this concern, and Labadie and colleagues have shown no differences in hospital stays between geriatric and younger patients.[46] If enough vestibular function was destroyed to affect ambulation, one would expect a delay in hospital discharge. It has been noted that depression, social isolation, and anxiety are more prevalent in both the deaf and the elderly, and it has been speculated that the combination of both could mitigate against successful rehabilitation.

Several studies have evaluated the effectiveness of cochlear implants in the elderly. Labadie and colleagues have demonstrated that both geriatric and younger patients have statistically significant increases in Central Institute for the Deaf (CID) and CNC scores (there was no difference between groups). Satisfaction with the device has also been demonstrated as increased self-confidence and improved quality of life.[47]

Candidacy Guidelines

As cochlear implants have achieved documented improvements in open-set speech recognition scores, FDA guidelines for implantation have been expanded. At first, FDA guidelines suggested that potential recipients should have pure-tone averages (PTAs) of 90 dB or greater. The guideline has been lowered to 70 dB in recent clinical trials. It was initially suggested by the FDA that appropriate implant candidates should have HINT sentence scores of less than 20% in quiet. This criterion has now been substantially relaxed, and individuals with less than 50% correct responses to HINT sentences in quiet are considered appropriate candidates. It is worth emphasizing that FDA-approved criteria are guidelines and do not constrain an experienced implant team from making thoughtful exceptions. There is a move toward using CNC words as a criterion, primarily to avoid ceiling effects during postoperative evaluation.

Auditory Neuropathy

Auditory neuropathy (auditory dys-synchrony) is a recently identified type of sensorineural hearing loss. It is defined as a condition in which otoacoustic emissions are present but auditory brain stem response (ABR) waveforms are absent in the context of normal middle ear functions. It is hypothesized that the condition occurs because cochlear hair cells are discharging dys-synchronously, such that no identifiable action potential develops in the cochlear nerve. Hearing loss in this condition is variable, perhaps because of variable degrees of dys-synchrony. The degree of functional hearing impairment accompanying auditory neuropathy is difficult to assess. In the early years following the identification and description of the disorder, it was believed the amplification would be futile and provide no benefit. It is now recognized that some children will benefit significantly from hearing aids.[48–50] Cochlear implants, in theory, could restore synchrony by bypassing the cochlear hair cells and stimulating the auditory nerve directly and synchronously.[51,52] Labadie and colleagues have reported that the sound field threshold improved from an average of >70 dB preoperatively to better than 37 dB postcochlear implantation in four patients with auditory neuropathy. Electrical ABR showed detectable waveforms on apical, middle, and basal turn stimulation.[46] Shallop and colleagues have shown good results for cochlear implantation in five children with auditory neuropathy at 1-year follow-up. All had significant improvements in sound detection, speech perception, and communication skills. Shallop and colleagues interpreted the presence of a robust N1 on neural response telemetry (NRT) as an indication that synchrony was at least partially restored. Otoacoustic emissions remained in the contralateral ear but were eliminated in the operated ear after implantation.[53]

Bilateral Implantation

There are several potential benefits from using two implants:[54–57]

1. Bilateral listeners benefit from the "head shadow effect." At any given time, in a normal listening environment, each ear receives signals with different signal-to-noise ratios (SNRs).
2. Bilateral listeners can pick the ear with the best SNR and enhance their ability for speech understanding. This benefit becomes apparent in noisy environments, in which individuals with unilateral hearing experience greater difficulty in speech understanding.
3. Unilateral hearing makes sound localization almost impossible. Normal-hearing listeners use both interaural time delays and interaural intensity differences to localize sound. Normal-hearing listeners can detect as little as 1 to 2 degrees of difference in the origin of a sound signal. It has been documented that bilateral implant users can gain significant sound localization using both time discrimination and interaural intensity cues. It has been demonstrated that an average temporal resolution of 50 μs was achievable in four of eight bilaterally implanted patients, which should be adequate for 10 degrees of angle resolution in a free-field environment. One patient had a 25 μs resolution. Normal-hearing patients have, at best, 9 μs of resolution. On average, it is about 15 μs. The extent to which improved sound localization might enhance speech perception in noise remains to be determined.[58–62]
4. Improved speech understanding, especially in noise: D'Haese and colleagues have documented benefit in a group of 22 patients with bilateral implants.[63] Speech recognition in noise was improved when both implants were used simultaneously, and the difference was statistically significant. Comprehension of monosyllables delivered in quiet was also significantly better when using both implants rather than using either implant alone. D'Haese and colleagues were able to conclude that some of this benefit was attributable to factors other than merely the head shadow effect, including binaural unmasking, "squelch" effect, and diotic summation.[63,54,57]

Although bilateral cochlear implantation is no longer controversial, a number of questions remain to be answered, including the following:

1. Should one "use up" both ears, especially in a child? Although the recipient may adapt and obtain more benefit from bilateral cochlear implantation, it is reasonable to assume that over the period of a typical child's life (70+ years), significant improvements in technology will be made. Will hair cell regeneration be possible? And if so, will the opportunity be lost in an implanted ear? Should the second ear be held in reserve to take advantage of such technological improvements? Will the nonstimulated ear suffer neural degeneration and/or neural pathway degeneration if left unstimulated for many years?
2. Can bilateral implantation produce significant bilateral vestibular injury?
3. Is bilateral implantation cost-effective?

The move toward bilateral implantation evolved slowly and with great caution in the United States. But a consensus has now emerged that the benefits of bilateral implantation outweigh the potential harm and is the treatment of choice for many, if not all, cochlear implant candidates.[61]

Electroacoustic/Hybrid Implants

Hybrid implants combine a cochlear implant and a hearing aid in the same ear. Such a combined or "hybrid device" is being developed for individuals who retain useful hearing in the lower frequencies (ie, less than 1,000 cycles per second) but have a severe to profound loss in the higher frequencies. Such individuals often have poor speech discrimination scores, especially in noise. Both conventional hearing aids or cochlear implants alone provide only marginal improvements in speech discrimination for such individuals. A combined electroacoustic device is designed to electrically stimulate those regions of the apical cochlea that subserve higher frequencies (and where residual hair cell populations are very low) while permitting the individual to continue to hear (with or without a hearing aid) lower frequency sound acoustically. Successful implementation of such a strategy requires that residual hearing in the ear receiving the implant is retained. Several devices with electrode arrays of varying lengths have been developed and are in clinical trials. The ideal length of electrode for such individuals has not been established. Shorter electrodes may reduce the risk of hearing loss, but longer electrodes potentially can stimulate larger areas of the cochlea and may be needed if the individual loses additional hearing at the time. Surgeons placing hybrid cochlear implants use special "soft surgery" techniques in order to minimize hearing loss. Overall, the rate of conservation appears to be quite good—85–90%.[64–66]

Most individuals implanted with a hybrid device have experienced improvements in speech understanding. A significant number of patients have noted very dramatic gains in speech understanding in noise. Improvements in speech discrimination of 20–30% are not uncommon.

Additional gains from hybrid device implementation are very significant improvements in music appreciation compared to cochlear implant users; melody recognition approaches normal in hybrid implant recipients. Melody recognition in conventional cochlear implant recipients is generally poor.[65–68]

DEVICE SELECTION

Three devices are currently implanted in the United States (Table 35–2). Many programs offer all three devices. Each device has advantages and disadvantages and choosing among them can be difficult. To date, no systematic differences in performance between devices have been demonstrated. Consequently, the final decision is often made on the basis of patient preference.

Coding Strategy

A speech coding strategy defines the method by which pitch, loudness, and timing of sound are translated into a series of electrical impulses. There are a variety of coding strategies currently in use. All of the three devices available in the United States are capable of using more than one type of strategy. Strategies can be categorized into two types: simultaneous or nonsimultaneous.

Simultaneous Strategies

Simultaneous strategies permit the activation of more than one electrode at the same time.

Only the Advanced Bionics device is capable of simultaneous stimulation. The utility of simultaneous activation is contested, and the currently available outcome data is equivocal. Nonetheless, many implant professionals and potential recipients believe that simultaneous stimulation can improve speech outcomes and provide a more natural quality of sound.

When two electrodes are activated simultaneously, there is a potential that their signals will interfere with each other, a phenomenon known as "channel interaction." The lower the intensity of an emitted signal, the lower the likelihood that it will interact with a signal from a neighboring channel. When an electrode is close to the ganglion cells within the modiolus, it takes less energy to stimulate the cell. Consequently, simultaneous strategies appear to benefit from modiolus-hugging electrode arrays (see later).

Nonsimultaneous Strategies

Continuous interleaved sampling (CIS) strategies stimulate each active electrode serially. Every electrode is stimulated in turn, one after the other. No electrode is bypassed or stimulated out of order. Assuming that each electrode stimulates a different frequency within the cochlea, the cochlea receives complete information about the frequency composition of the incoming signal, even for frequencies that are not represented in the incoming signal. It is clear that, up to a certain point, the rapidity with which this sequential stimulation occurs affects speech recognition. Although there has been an inclination to believe that "the faster the better," it has not been possible to unequivocally demonstrate that "very fast" CIS strategies produce improved speech recognition.

All three currently available devices can be programmed using a CIS strategy. However, the rates at which stimulation occur are different.

TABLE 35–2 Comparison devices

	NUCLEUS 24 FREEDOM DENVER, CO	ADVANCED BIONICS HI-RES SYLMAR, CA	MED-EL PULSAR INNSBRUCK, AUSTRIA
Manufacturer	Cochlear Sydney, Australia • Nearly 100,000 implanted world-wide • Nucleus 22 approved in 1982 • First multichannel behind-the-ear device (BTE)	Advanced Bionics • 26,000+ implanted worldwide • Makes other neurostimulators • Advanced Bionics device approved in the United States in 1991	MED-EL Innsbruck, Austria • Over 15,000 worldwide • Developing implants since 1975
FDA-approved age for each implant	All approved for 12 months, except Nucleus 24 ABI at age 12 years	12 months	12 months
Length of electrode array	Contour advance = 15 mm Contour straight = 17 mm Double array—2 × 8.25 mm active length ABI = electrode pad 8.5 × 3.0 .0.7 mm	HiFocus jl = 25 mm HiFocus Helix precoiled = 24 mm	31 mm
Type of electrode	CA—perimodiolar electrode array with soft tip CS—straight array Double array—for individuals with significantly ossified cochlea, 2 electrodes of 11 channels each ABI—3 rows on the carrier pad	Straight array that can be placed into a perimodiolar position by use of an attached or separate electrode. Focused stimulation	Soft, flexible straight array designed for lateral wall stimulation
Special electrode arrays	Yes	Yes; precoiled	A split array is available for fully ossified cochleae, medium array (20 mm) available for midlength insertion, compressed array (14 mm) for cochlear malformations
Number of electrodes	24 (2 are ground electrodes)	16	26: 24 active contacts plus 1 additional ground electrode and 1 additional EAP electrode
Number of channels	Freedom 22	16 (addition of "virtual" channels could bring count up to 31)	12 (each electrode pair = 1 channel)
Processing speed. Maximum potential stimulation rate in pulses per second (PPS)	Freedom has up to 32,000 Recommendation is 900 pps per channel	250,000 pps	TEMPO + = 18,180 OPUS = 50,700
MRI compatibility	MRI compatible to 1.5 T with replaceable magnet removed	1.5 T with magnet removed	FDA-approved in United States for 0.2T without magnet removal MRI safe at 1.0 and 1.5 T internationally without magnet removal Approval must be obtained prior to scan

Continued

TABLE 35–2 Comparison devices—Continued

	NUCLEUS 24 FREEDOM DENVER, CO	ADVANCED BIONICS HI-RES SYLMAR, CA	MED-EL PULSAR INNSBRUCK, AUSTRIA
Speech processor and headpiece	4 wearing options Mini behind the ear (BTE) Standard BTE Babyworn (battery not at ear level to reduce weight and size) Bodyworn All wearing options can use rechargeable or disposable batteries Directional and Omni directional microphone	Platinum series bodyworn processor HiResolution Harmony BTE Water resistant Built in telecoil 16-bit CD quality processor Adaptive front end adapts to sound environment automatically	Both body worn and ear level processor Omni-directional microphone
Accessory equipment	Telephone adapter FM cable Personal audio cable TV/hi-fi cable Lapel microphone Monitor earphones Battery charger Pouch or harness for children Spare cable in a variety of lengths and colors	Telephone adapter T-mic in the ear microphone Telecoil Belt clip for adults Battery charger Battery charger car adapter Off ear power options, rechargeable and disposable Variety of pouches or harnesses for children Spare cable MP3 adapters Color covers	Body worn processor: 2 belt clip options 2 battery chargers Pouch or harness for children Spare cable in a variety of lengths and colors BTE processor: 4 battery packs for BTE that can be worn in 5 different ways; Fixation bar and belt clip options FM cables Personal audio cable Telephone adapter Lapel microphone MP3 adapter Dry-aid kit Battery charger Variety of earhook sizes
Program storage capacity	Bodyworn Processor can store 4	3 programs	Up to 9 programs (mostly 3 programs with 3 volume settings for each program are chosen)
Speech Processing	Freedom can use ACE™, CIS, & SPEAK. There are multiple Smart Sound™ pre-processing strategies for optimized listening.	CIS, MPS, HiResolution-S 16, HiResolution-P 16, HiRes Fidelity-S 120, HiRes Fidelity-P 120	CIS (TEMPO=), high-definition CIS and fine structure processing (OPUS)
Warranty	Implanted components: 10 years External component: 3 years Sound processor, battery pack and headpiece each covered for 1-time loss in the initial 3-year warranty. Service contracts available for additional coverage beyond the 3-year initial warranty on external equipment.	10 year ICS warranty 3-year warranty on speech processors 3-year warranty on headpieces 1 time loss/damage free replacement (warranted against water damage-excluding immersion) Extended warranty and loss/damage coverage available	Implanted components: 10 yr External components: 3 yr Limited accidental damage and loss coverage is available or all devices at additional cost Extended service contract available upon expiration of external equipment warranty

Feature extraction strategies do not attempt to encode complete frequency information about the incoming signal; rather, they attempt to "extract" the frequency information that will be most useful to the CNS for the purposes of speech understanding. Once those features of the incoming signal believed to be most important for speech understanding have been selected by the processor, they are presented to the electrodes. The electrodes are not activated sequentially because only those electrodes that represent frequencies "extracted" from the incoming signal are activated. These strategies are often called "roving strategies" because they "rove" around the electrode array, activating only those electrodes needed to supply the relevant information. Only late-generation feature extraction strategies are currently used. The MED EL COMBI 40® (MED EL Co., Innsbruck, Austria) can be programmed using an "N of M" feature extraction strategy, whereas the Nucleus 24® (Cochlear Corporation, Melbourne, Australia) device can be programmed using spectral peak (SPEAK) or advanced combination encoder (ACE). The ACE is, in effect, a fast form of SPEAK. The programming audiologist can adjust the number of frequencies selected from a given incoming signal (called "maxima") and the rate at which those features are presented to the electrode array.

Although there are theoretical reasons to believe that one strategy may be superior to another, no systematic differences between the most advanced strategies for any device have yet been demonstrated.

Styling

Other features that may be important for patients in device selection are appearance and styling. Each device looks different, and one may be more attractive to a given individual than another. Since compelling differences in performance cannot be demonstrated, the use of aesthetic criteria in deciding between devices is not entirely irrational.

Modiolus Hugging Electrode

It is widely believed that if the stimulating electrodes are closer to the auditory nerve cells, then stimulation will be more efficient and more efficacious. The ganglion cells reside in the core of the cochlear spiral, an area termed the modiolus. Consequently, there has been an ongoing effort to move the stimulating electrodes as close to the modiolus as possible. Electrodes that are in close approximation to the modiolus are referred to as modiolus-hugging electrodes. Both Cochlear Corporation and Advanced Bionics have modiolus-hugging electrode arrays that feature a self-coiling electrode array with "memory." The electrode array comes with a stylette, which keeps the electrode array relatively straight and relatively stiff so that it can be easily inserted. Once the electrode is inserted, the stylette is withdrawn and the electrode array "springs back" into its original, coiled configuration. Coiling wraps the electrode array tightly around the modiolus. Both techniques appear to be effective.

Modiolus hugging electrodes produce lower threshold comfort levels.[69] Since channel interaction is a potentially significant problem with simultaneous strategies, it is not surprising that the number of cochlear implant recipients who prefer to use the simultaneous strategy has significantly increased since Advanced Bionics has started using a modiolus-hugging array. Since the amount of current required to stimulate cochlear neurons is significantly reduced in modiolus-hugging array, battery life may be extended when such arrays are used. Battery life is an important issue in the emerging competition for a totally implantable device. It has not been demonstrated, however, that modiolus-hugging electrodes produce improved speech recognition compared to laterally placed arrays (nonmodiolus-hugging).

Megnetic Resonance Imaging

1. Although concerns about postoperative MRI scanning are not a major issue for most patients, they are a very important issue for a select minority. Individuals with CNS disorders that have traditionally been followed using MRI techniques are the most likely to be concerned. Magnetic resonance imagining has traditionally been considered contraindicated in cochlear implant recipients because of the potential for interaction between the two magnets. There are four possible interactions that could occur between the implanted magnet and a strong external magnetic field: (1) movement of the stimulator/receiver or electrode array, (2) generation of noxious or even injurious auditory stimuli, (3) generation of heat, and (4) demagnetization. These interactions have been investigated and are partially understood.[70]
2. It seems clear that the energies produced by commonly utilized magnetic fields ($\leq$1.5 T) will not produce sufficient heat to be troublesome.
3. Patients that have had MRI scans with cochlear implants in place have not reported injurious or disturbing auditory sensations.
4. Although there is some concern about movement in stronger magnetic fields, it does not appear to be a problem in magnetic fields of lower strengths ($<$1.5 T), and it may be that external stabilization of the device can limit the potential for movement of the stimulator/receiver even in stronger fields.
5. Demagnetization does occur, in vitro, with as much as 10% of the magnetic strength lost with each scan. The degree of demagnetization depends on the length of time the device is scanned and the strength of the magnetic field.

Investigators at the University of Vienna have evaluated 11 patients in a 1-T magnet. Each patient was evaluated 1 day before planned explantation. Auditory perception was evaluated before and after examination, and all explanted devices were assessed for function. There was no detectable movement of the electrode or the receiver coil in any of the patients, and there was no measured temperature change. There were no adverse stimuli reported by any subject. They concluded that the presence of a MED-EL cochlear implant was not a firm contraindication to MRI.[71]

Baumgartner et al. reported the results of scanning 30 patients at 1-T without magnet removal. There were no adverse consequences in implants.[72]

Several solutions have been offered by different manufacturers.

Advanced Bionics® (Sylmar, CA) manufactures a special version of the Advanced Bionics implant that has no magnet. It needs to be specially ordered in advance. The external headpiece is held to the magnetless stimulator/receiver with a special earpiece. To function correctly, the stimulator/receiver must be implanted closer to the auricle, so special care needs to be taken during the operative procedure. Weber and colleagues have reported results in 11 individuals with magnetless devices—the headpieces were stable and worked well.[73,74] One patient, implanted in England, has also been reported to be a successful user.[75]

The Cochlear Corporation (Melbourne, Australia) manufactures the Nucleus device with a removable magnet. The magnet can be extracted through an incision made directly over the stimulator/receiver and then replaced later. The required incision is small and it appears that the magnet can be easily removed as an outpatient procedure using only local anesthesia.

The recently introduced MED-EL Pulsar® implant is available in a titanium silastic housing which permits magnet removal if MRI is necessary.

The electromagnetic interference between the MED-EL Combi 40+ device and a 1.5-T scanner was within acceptable limits except for torque, which was questionable. Scanning at 0.2-T was clearly safe, and the MED-EL device has received FDA permission approval for use in a low-strength magnetic resonance scanner. However, there is a "blackout zone" extending 2 to 4 cm around the device in every direction. Consequently, magnetic resonance scanning, even though it can be performed safely, will not provide meaningful information about those areas of the skull base and brain close to the implant.[70]

Special Electrode Arrays

For a number of years, MED- EL has manufactured special electrode arrays for special clinical situations. A "compressed array" is available that includes the same number of electrodes as the standard array but compressed into about 60% of the distance. The compressed array is useful for patients with labyrinthitis ossificans when only a portion of the cochlear duct is available for implantation. If a "drill out" procedure is performed, it is usually possible to get the entire compressed array into the accessible portion of the cochlea. The compressed array is also useful for common cavity deformities of the cochlea. Electrode arrays placed in a single, common cavity tend to "curl up" so that the distal portion of the electrode curls over on itself and the electrodes overlap. There is less overlap of electrodes using the compressed electrode array. MED-EL offers a special (custom order) array for common cavities that carries the electrodes in the middle of the array. A double cochleostomy is necessary. The distal end of the array is brought out of the second cochleostomy so that the electrode comes to lie against the medial wall of the common cavity where the neural elements are believed to reside.

A second special electrode array divides the electrodes and puts about half the electrodes on each of two separate leads. Such "double arrays" are designed for subjects with labyrinthitis ossificans. Separate cochleostomies are performed into the inferior and the middle turn of the cochlea, and the electrode arrays are then passed separately into each cochleostomy. This design allows a greater number of electrodes to be inserted than could be inserted using a technique limited to drilling out only as much of the basal turn as can be reached through a single, round window cochleostomy. Both the MED-EL and Cochlear Corporation offer such arrays.

The Cochlear Corporation straight array has electrode placement that is closer together than even the MED-EL compressed array, but because there are more electrodes, the length of the entire array is longer than the MED-EL compressed array. The straight array is available as an alternative to the standard modiolus hugging Contour® array.

THE SURGICAL PROCEDURE

Preoperative Consideration

Roughly half of the pediatric cochlear implantations performed in the United States are performed on an outpatient basis and half as an inpatient. Liu and colleagues have shown that outpatient cochlear implantation is safe.[76] However, its acceptance by parents is less than universal. It is tolerated but not necessarily desired. Follow-up surveys have shown that the later in the day the operation finishes and the further away the patients live, the less likely parents and recipients are to be satisfied with the outpatient setting.

Prophylactic Antibiotics

While no double-blind studies have been conducted to justify the efficacy of perioperative antibiotics, they are administered by nearly all surgeons. Intravenous antibiotics should be given at least 20 minutes before the incision is made. Antibiotics should be continued for the first 24 hours postoperatively and then discontinued.

Incision and Skin Flap

A variety of incisions have been used. Initially, cochlear implants were almost always performed using the same type of C-shaped incision used for routine mastoidectomy but significantly enlarged so that the incision line did not overlap the implanted stimulator/receiver (Figures 35–4 and 35–5). It is widely believed that the incision should not cross the edges of the device. If the incision must cross over the stimulator/receiver, it should cross it at right angles and not parallel one of its edges. Although this admonition is widely promulgated in descriptions of surgical technique, it is frequently violated in practice.

In the mid-1990s, the inverted U-shaped incision became increasingly popular. The inverted U had several advantages. Theoretical considerations suggest that most of the blood flow to the skin of the postauricular area comes from inferiorly upward and that the blood supply to an inverted U-shaped flap is better. It is hard to incorporate a previous mastoidectomy incision into a postauricular C-shaped flap without producing a potentially avascular area between the two incisions. A few cases of flap necrosis are known to have occurred when an enlarged postauricular C-shaped incision was placed behind a previous mastoidectomy incision. It is much easier to incorporate a previous mastoidectomy incision into an inverted U; the previous

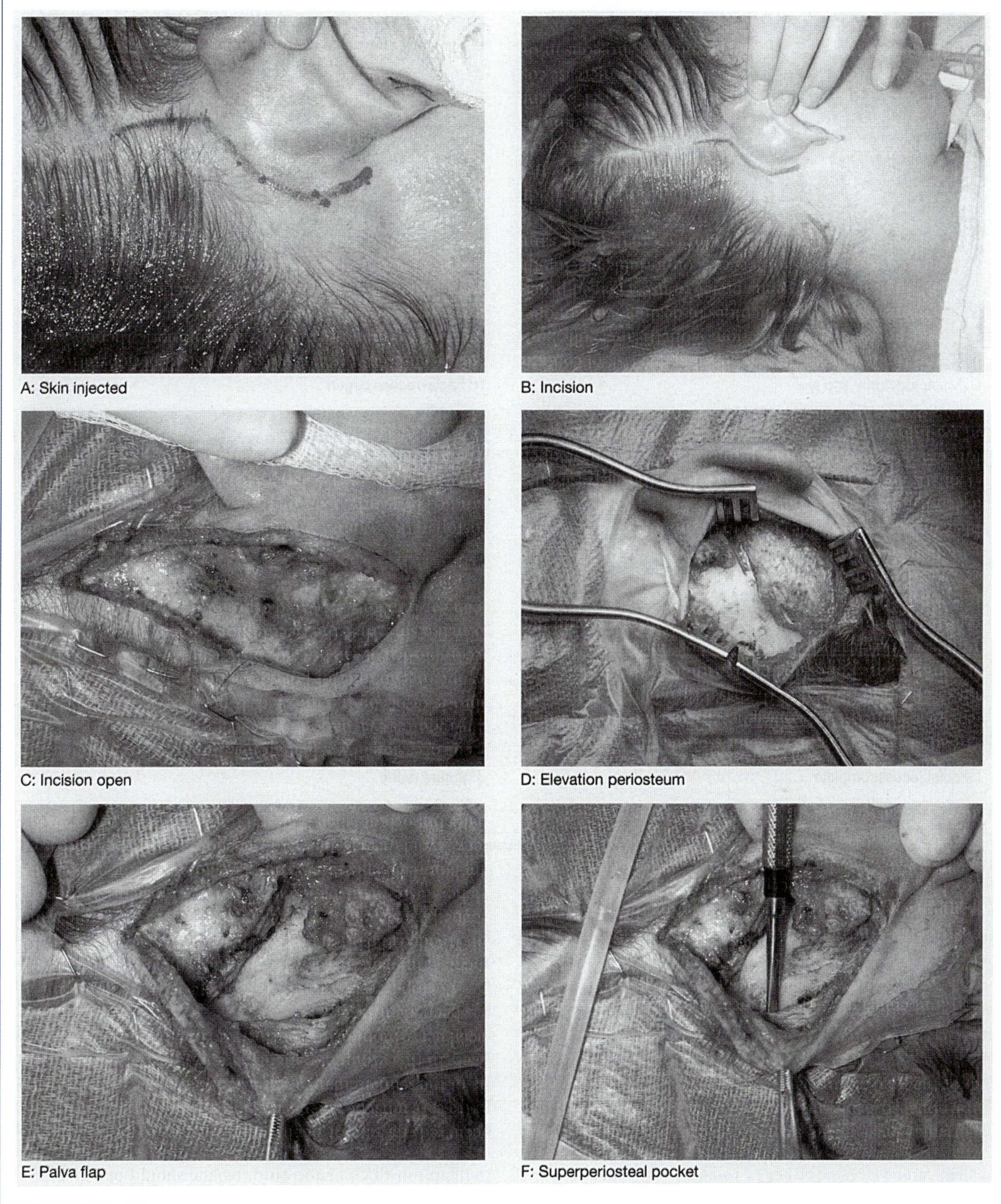

FIGURE 35–4 • A series of photographs indicating the steps in cochlear implantation.

Continued

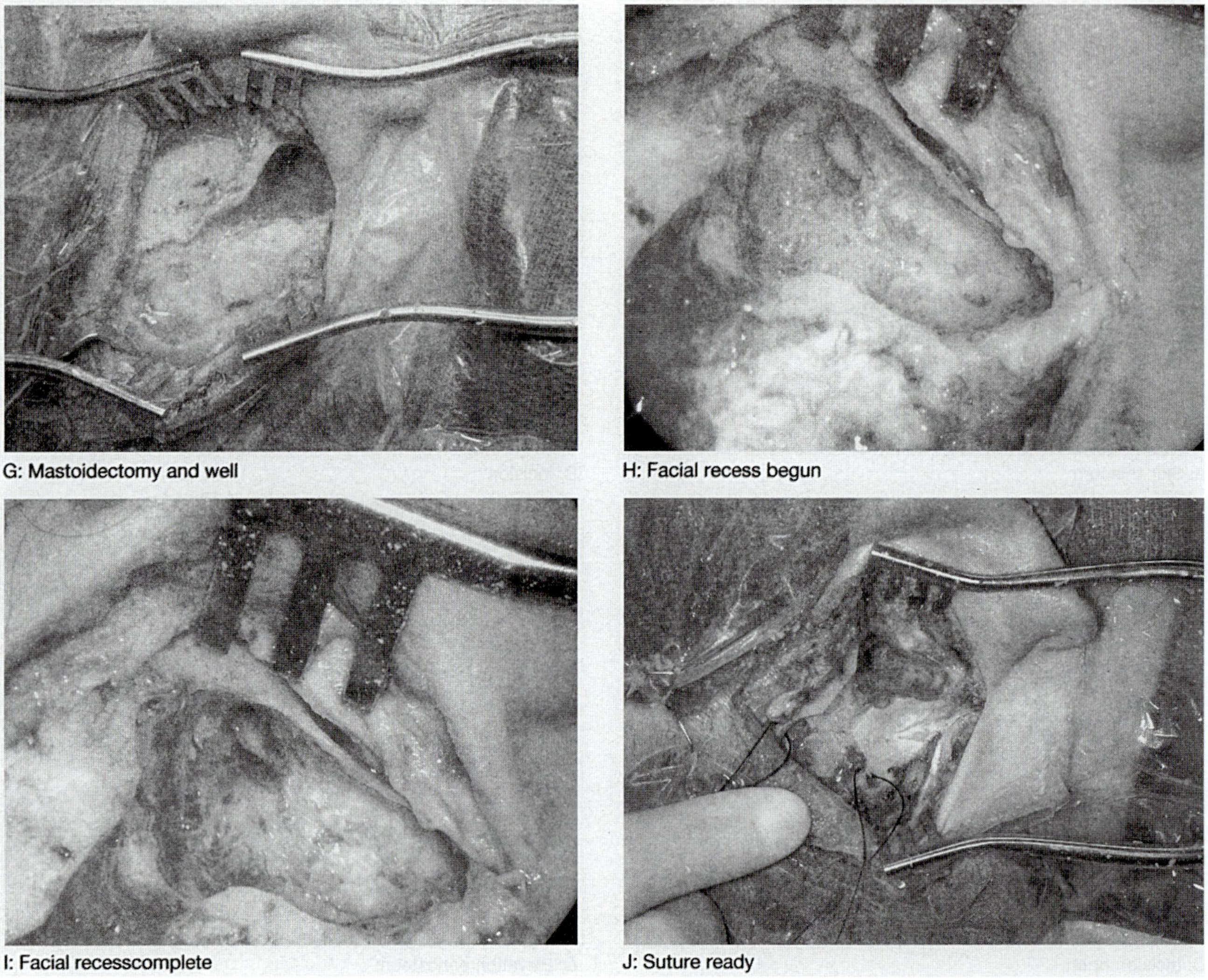

G: Mastoidectomy and well

H: Facial recess begun

I: Facial recesscomplete

J: Suture ready

FIGURE 35 –4 • *Continued.* A series of photographs indicating the steps in cochlear implantation.

Continued

mastoidectomy incision simply becomes the anterior limb of the inverted U.

As ever more experience in implantation was obtained, the posterior limb of the inverted U was abandoned and an incision that looked a bit more like an inverted L or an inverted J became more common. Over the last decade or so, incisions have become progressively shorter and more cosmetically acceptable. Many implant surgeons have reduced the incision to a 3–4 cm postauricular incision placed behind the postauricular fold.

Once the incision has been completed, the flap is elevated. The flap can be elevated either as a single layer or in two layers. If two layers are separately elevated, the superficial layer should be elevated first and the deep tissues, which include the periosteum of the mastoid, temporalis fascia, and temporalis muscle, should be left intact. The periosteum of the mastoid should then be elevated as an anteriorly based Palva flap, which can then be sutured back into position at the end of the case to protect the electrode array in the mastoid cavity. The Palva flap is developed by elevating the deep tissue overlying the mastoid cortex while leaving it attached to the posterior canal skin. The Palva flap should be as large as possible and, hopefully, will cover the take off point of the electrodes for the Nucleus and Advanced Bionics devices (Figure 35–6).

Thought should be given to flap thickness. It is difficult for the external device to be held to the implanted stimulator/receiver if the skin thickness overlying the stimulator/receiver is greater than 6.0 mm. Thinning should be done cautiously, however. Excessive thinning can lead to flap necrosis and exposure of the device. If the surgeon is faced with the choice of having the flap too thick or too thin, he/she should opt to leave the flap a little bit thicker. The flap can be thinned separately as a secondary procedure if necessary, and this is much easier than trying to deal with an exposed device.

The Well

A portion of the skull as flat as possible should be selected for placement of the stimulator/receiver, especially for those devices sealed in ceramic containers (Med-El and Advanced Bionics)

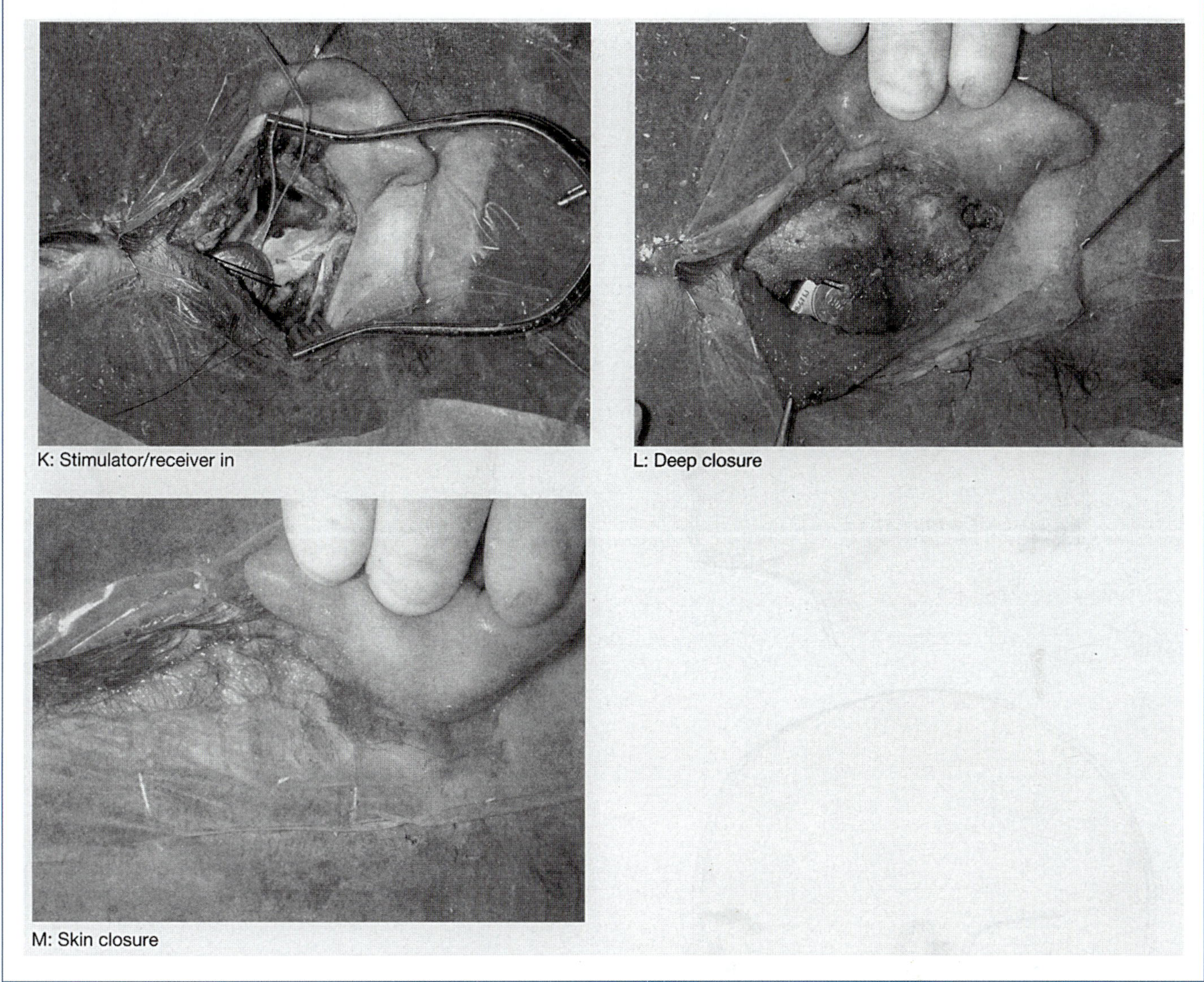
K: Stimulator/receiver in

L: Deep closure

M: Skin closure

FIGURE 35–4 • *Continued.* A series of photographs indicating the steps in cochlear implantation.

(Figure 35–7). In small children, this may necessitate placement a bit more superiorly, in the area of the temporal squama, than in adults, where reasonably flat spots can often be found over the occipital portion of the skull base. If an ear-level processor is to be used, the stimulator/receiver should be placed 2.5 cm posterior to the posterior border of the external auditory canal to avoid interfering with placement of the ear-level processor. Once the site has been selected, the surgical drill is used to create a defect in the skull contoured to exactly fit the implanted device exactly.

The skull of small children, especially children between 1 and 2 years of age, may be only 2 and 3 mm in thickness. For these children, the implant often rests on exposed dura. Some surgeons seek to leave an "island" of bone in the center of the area of exposed dura, whereas other surgeons are comfortable removing all the bone from the dura.

A channel in the bone must be formed so that the electrode leads can pass freely from the stimulator/receiver into the mastoid cavity. There should be no sharp edges or constraints at the point of takeoff of the electrode leads from the stimulator/receiver.

A recent trend is to omit the well entirely. Some surgeons regard drilling the well and tie down holes as the most dangerous part of the procedure: CSF leaks and epidermal hematoma can occur. Moreover, the benefit is principally cosmetic. If the well is omitted, a tight subperiostal pocket is essential to prevent movement and a bony ridge or tie down needs to be placed in front of the device to prevent anterior displacement.

Mastoidotomy

Once a site has been created to accommodate the stimulator/receiver, a mastoidectomy is performed (see Figure 35–7). The mastoidectomy cavity should not be saucerized. The edges should be left as acute as possible. These edges will help retain the electrode leads within the confines of the mastoid cavity. Once the mastoidectomy is complete, the facial recess is identified and widely opened. The most inferior portion of the facial

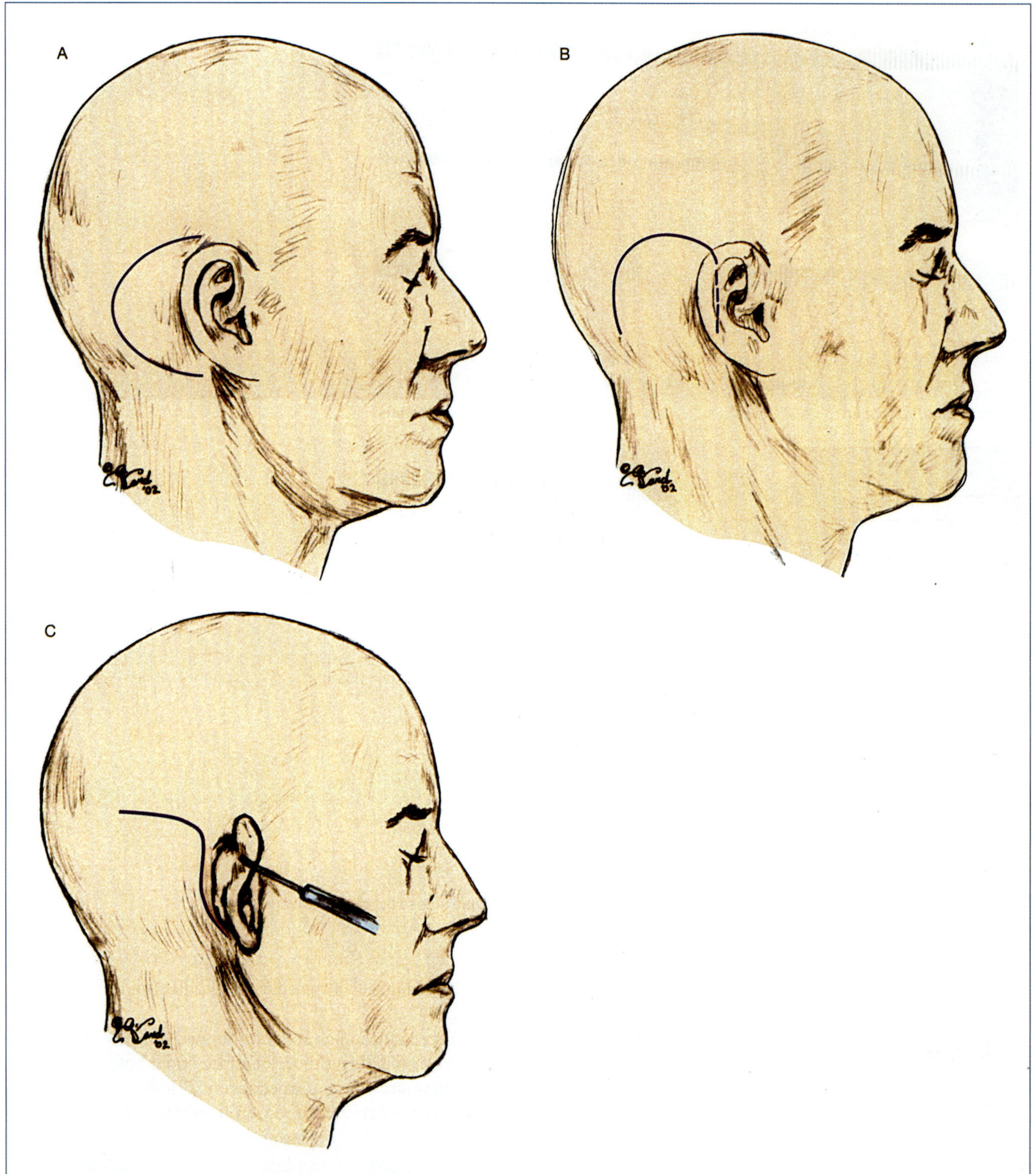

FIGURE 35 –5 • The three types of cochlear implant incisions utilize or illustrated including the "C" incision, the inverted "U," and the "hockey stick" incision.

recess is of greatest importance for visualization of the round window niche.[77] Some bone medial to the facial nerve must generally be removed. If this bone is left in place, exposure of the round window niche will be suboptimal, and it may not be possible to see even the anterior boundary of the round window niche.

Almost all anomalous facial nerves are displaced anteriorly and medially. Just distal to the oval window, they turn directly into the hypotympanum and run just inferior to or directly over the round window area. Consequently, when the facial nerve is absent from its usual position, it does not form the posterior boundary of the facial recess. If, as the facial recess is opened, it

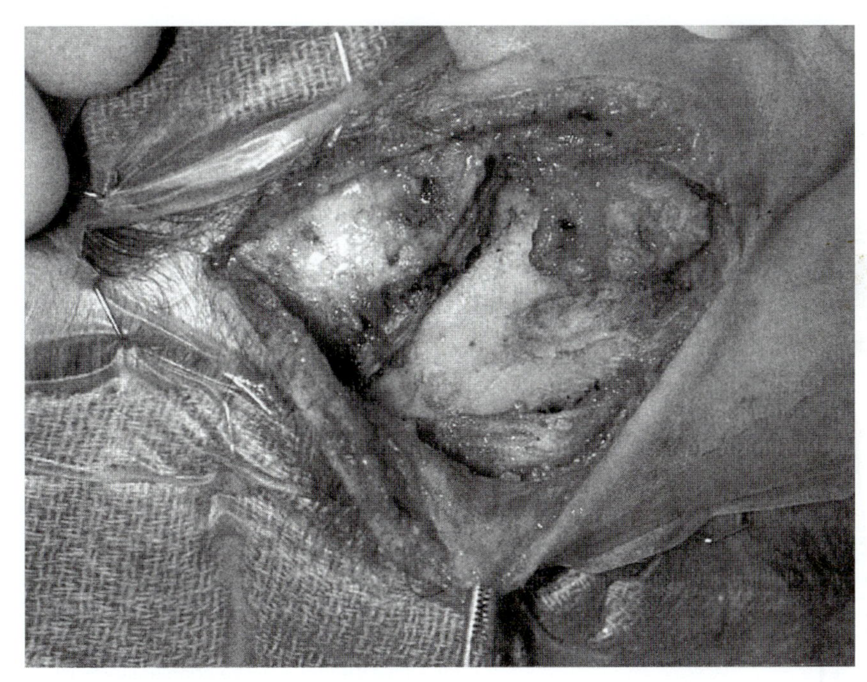

FIGURE 35–6 • Skin flaps have been elevated and the mastoid exposed.

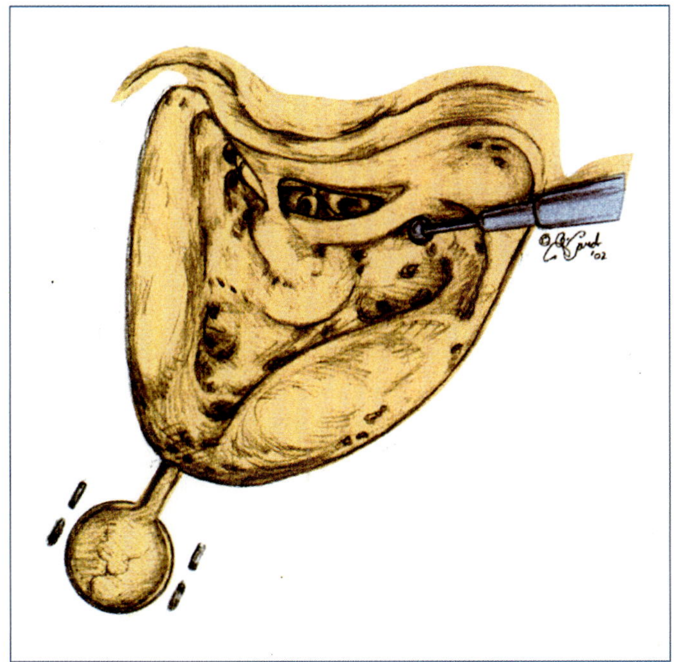

FIGURE 35–7 • A well has been drilled to accommodate the electronics package of the cochlear implant and a mastoidectomy with facial recess has been performed.

seems that the recess is unusually large, a facial nerve anomaly should be suspected. The recess will be large because its usual posterior medial boundary, the facial nerve, is missing from its normal position, and has been displaced medially and a bit anteriorly.

Cochleostomy

Once the facial recess has been widely opened, the round window niche can be clearly seen. It is often useful to remove the anterior lip of the round window niche so that the anterior attachment of the round window membrane itself can be visualized. Most experienced surgeons now make the cochleostomy inferior to the inferior attachment of the round window membrane to avoid the "hook" of the cochlea. This allows a straighter, more direct insertion of the electrode array into scala tympani (Figure 35–8). Although insertion through the round window (RW) was abandoned in the early years of cochlear implantation, it has regained popularity in recent years. A "pure" RW insertion avoids the trauma and bone dust associated with a classic promontory cochleostomy and is especially attractive if hearing conservation is the goal. Insertion through the RW ensures entrance into scala tympani.[78,79]

The size of the cochleostomy will vary among devices. Earlier generations of Advanced Bionics devices required a cochleostomy of 2 mm or more. Most currently available devices can be easily inserted through a cochleostomy of between 0.8 and 1.2 mm in diameter.

Insertion of the Electrode Array

As soon as the actual device is brought into the operative field, monopolar cautery should be removed. Use of monopolar cautery near the device risks damaging it and rendering it nonfunctional. Bipolar cautery can be used safely.

Opinions vary as to whether the electrode array should be inserted before or after fixation of the stimulator/receiver. Some very experienced surgeons believe that they can manipulate the electrode array more easily and have a greater chance of an atraumatic and complete insertion if the stimulator/receiver is not yet attached to the skull and can be moved freely as the electrode is passed into the scala tympani. Other surgeons find it easier to insert the electrode array once the stimulator/received has been fixed into its bony recess (Figure 35–9).

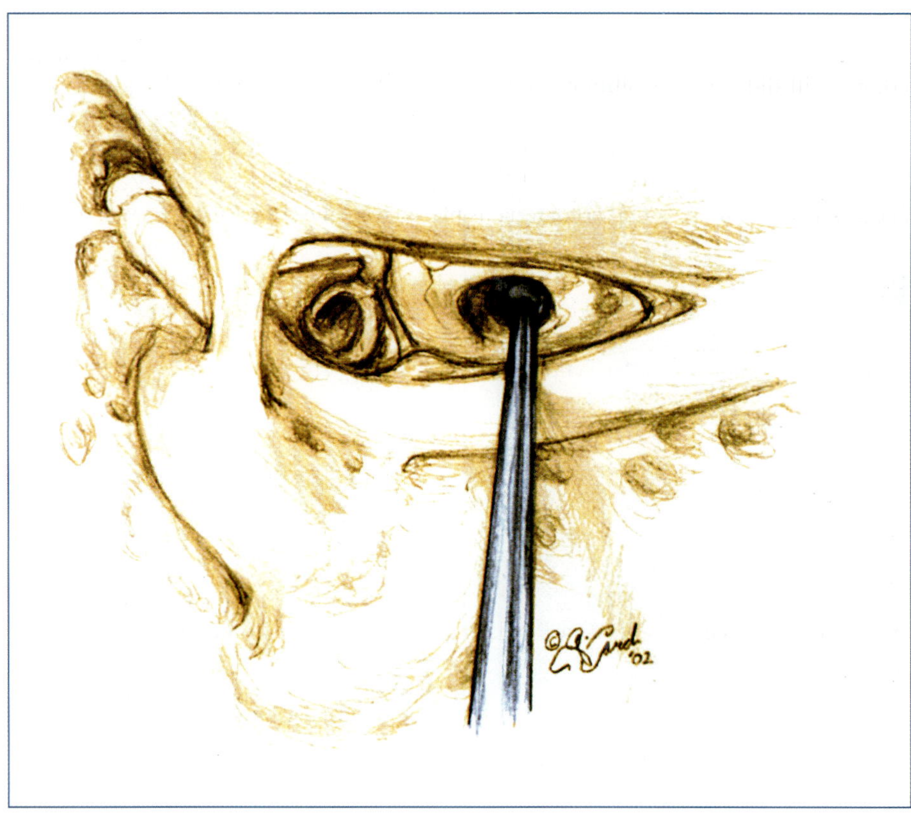

FIGURE 35–8 • The cochleostomy is performed through the facial recess just anterior and a little bit superior to the inferior attachment of the round window membrane.

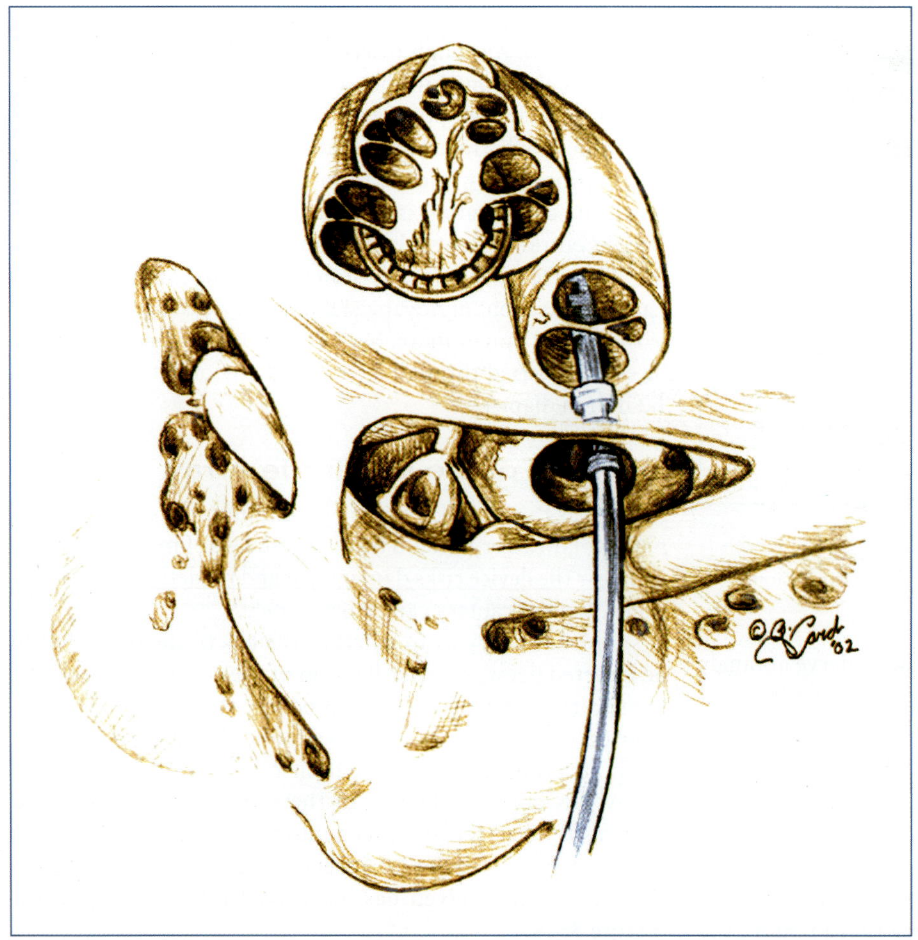

FIGURE 35–9 • This cross-sectional drawing shows that the electrodes are next to the modiolus, which contains the ends of the vestibular nerve.

The electrode array should be inserted as atraumatically as possible, and force should never be used. The tip of the electrode array should be directed inferiorly so that it will slide easily along the lateral (antimodiolar) wall of the scala tympani. Each manufacturer provides a special set of tools for insertion of their electrode, and directions for appropriate insertion technique differ according to device.[80,57] In addition, directions change from time to time, and the recommended technique for electrode insertion for each device should be briefly reviewed prior to beginning the operative procedure.

Some surgeons prefer to place a lubricant into the scala tympani prior to inserting the electrode array. The two most commonly used lubricants are a mixture of half glycerin and half water and a viscoelastic material such as Healon® or Provisc®. Lubricants may allow easier passage of the electrode array into the cochlea. Lubricants also encourage bone dust and other debris to "float out" of the scala tympani prior to electrode insertion and perhaps minimize the development of postoperative osteoneogenesis.[81–84]

Incomplete insertions are now uncommon except when there is an anomaly of cochlear morphology or labyrinthine ossification.

Once the electrode array has been satisfactorily inserted, the cochleostomy should be sealed with a small piece of soft tissue.

Fixation

If the stimulator/receiver has not yet been fixed to the skull base, its fixation should now be accomplished. The traditional way of securing the stimulator/receiver is by sutures. Drill holes are made above and below the receptacle site, and sutures are passed through these holes and over the implant. Drill holes must be made very cautiously. It is easy, especially in a young child, to penetrate the dura with the sharp end of a perforating burr and create a cerebrospinal fluid leak. More worrisome is the possibility of injury to a subdural vein resulting in postoperative intracranial hemorrhage. The number, type, and position of the sutures have varied substantially. Most commonly, a single suture is placed across the device (Figure 35–10). Alternatively, a strip of material is placed over the stimulator/receiver to hold it firmly in its well. The strip is secured with miniplates or screws. Nonabsorbable materials such as Gortex® and absorbable materials like AlloDerm® have been used. Some implant surgeons prefer this technique because it provides secure fixation and is quick. However, the materials involved are expensive and add considerably to the amount of foreign body placed into the wound. European surgeons have long used glues and cements to fix both the stimulator/receiver and the electrode array. Some surgeons no longer use any type of fixation. They rely on a tight subperiosteal pocket to immobilize the stimulator/receiver and prevent displacement. Some surgeons in the United States do not fix the electrode leads in any way.

Some implant systems have a second, separate lead leaving the stimulator/receiver, which serves as a separate ground electrode. This ground electrode needs to be placed beneath the temporalis muscle, directly on the squamous portion of the temporal bone. If placed directly into the muscle, repeated muscle contraction will result in breakage of the ground electrode.

Closure

Closure should be accomplished in layers. A three-layer closure begins with separate, interrupted sutures to close the deep layer and to return the Palva flap to its anatomic position over the mastoid cavity. If possible, the Palva flap should cover the take off of the electrode leads from the stimulator/receiver. Inverted, interrupted sutures are then used to approximate the

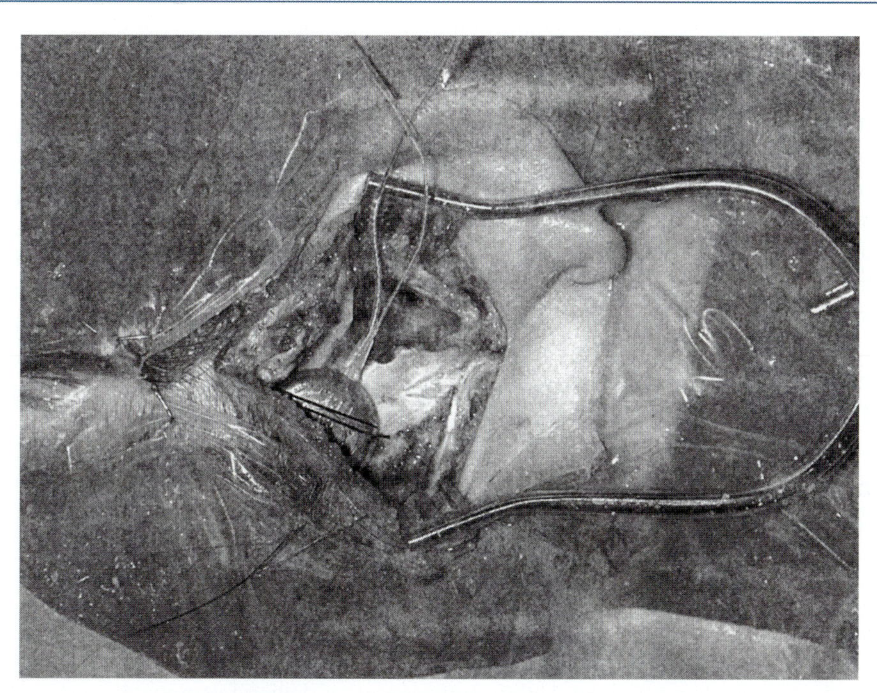

FIGURE 35–10 • The implant is in position with the electrode array inserted into the cochlea and the flying ground electrode beneath the temporalis muscle.

subcuticular layer of the skin closure. Staples, fast-absorbing suture, nonabsorbable sutures, and tissue adhesive have all been used for the final closure layer.

Middle Cranial Fossa Approach

Coletti and colleagues have advocated a middle cranial fossa approach to cochlear implantation as an alternative to the traditional transmastoid approach.[85] They have implanted 11 postlingually deafened adults through the middle cranial fossa approach. They believe that by opening the basal turn of the cochlea at its most superior point and by using a double electrode array, they have been able to place electrodes both antegrade toward the apex and posteriorly toward the round window. They assert that they have achieved deeper penetration with more extended coverage of the length of the cochlear duct in this fashion.

In addition to the potential for stimulating larger areas of the cochlea, Colletti and colleagues noted that this technique avoids ossification limited to the basal turn of the cochlea, the most common area of ossification. Although the middle fossa technique would clearly bypass isolated ossification of the basal turn near the round window, its unclear how one would deal with extensive ossification through a middle fossa approach. Moreover, deep insertion is not necessarily better. The spiral ganglion cells, which subserve the most apical turn of the cochlea, may actually reside closer to the middle turn, with only their dendrites extending out apically.

Colletti and colleagues are especially enthusiastic about a middle cranial fossa technique in individuals who have open, canal wall down mastoidectomy cavities.[85] They discussed at some length the difficulties in placing an implant in such cavities. They believe that staged procedures, months apart, should be used and that, even so, there is considerable risk of contamination and postoperative infection. Colletti and colleagues appear to overestimate the difficulties in dealing with an open cavity. Although many surgeons prefer to use a staged procedure in such circumstances, others are comfortable placing the implant and closing the external auditory canal at the same operation.[86]

The number of surgeons capable of performing a middle cranial fossa operation and placing a cochlear implant by that route is certainly limited, and the operation has at least theoretical risks not associated with the typical transmastoid technique. It is worth noting that hospitalization for Colletti's 11 patients ranged from 5 to 13 days. This would substantially increase cost and would be unattractive to most patients and surgeons in the United States.[85]

The technique is intriguing and may offer some advantages in special situations. It should be studied further.

POSTOPERATIVE COMPLICATIONS: EARLY COMPLICATIONS

Intraoperative facial nerve injury is feared by both patients and surgeons alike. Fortunately, this complication is rare. The incidence of temporary postoperative weakness is unknown, but probably even a transient paresis is uncommon. Although isolated case reports verify that permanent facial paralysis has occurred, its rate of occurrence appears to be less than 1%. Extra care must be taken when implanting patients with dysplasia of the semicircular canals as a facial nerve anomaly is more likely in this group of patients. Some surgeons who do not use facial nerve monitoring routinely do use it if a cochlear anomaly has been identified.

Postoperative alteration of taste is quite common after cochlear implant surgery. The chorda tympani nerve is occasionally divided and often irritated because the facial recess must be opened widely enough to get a good look at the round window niche. Taste disturbance is generally transient, and cochlear implant recipients rarely complain about it 6 months after surgery. Avoidance of injury to the chorda tympani nerve is especially important when bilateral implantation is performed.

The incidence of postoperative bleeding or hematoma formation after cochlear implant surgery is quite low but does occur occasionally. A hematoma of more than 5 or 10 cc probably requires evacuation to prevent its becoming organized and fibrotic or becoming infected. If possible, it should be drained by opening an inferior portion of the incision. If that cannot be accomplished, it can be cautiously aspirated. Care must be taken to make sure that the needle does not in any way injure the cochlear implant. Repeated aspiration is sometimes necessary.

Infection

Postoperative wound infection is generally trivial and can be handled by gently opening the wound in the area of the infection and treating the patient with appropriate antibiotics. A broad-spectrum antibiotic should be used initially. In adults, a quinolone is perhaps the best choice. In children, the use of a second- or third-generation cephalosporin is a good initial selection. The antibiotic can then be changed if necessary based on culture and sensitivity results. Almost all perioperative wound infections respond to appropriate antibiotic therapy, and it is rarely necessary to remove the device because of postoperative wound infection.[87,88] When wound infection is persistent, presence of a biofilm may be to blame.[89]

Wound Dehiscence

Wound dehiscence can occur and is more likely in an active child than in an adult. If the area of dehiscence is small, the wound can be left to heal by secondary intention or the child can be returned to the operating room for secondary closure. Again, simple postoperative wound dehiscence is unlikely to result in a device exposure and is unlikely to require device removal.

Flap necrosis, on the other hand, is a most serious complication and frequently will require device removal.[90,91] Flap necrosis can occur as the result of overly aggressive thinning of the flap, a flap design that has not given adequate consideration to previous incisions, or as a consequence of infection. At minimum, flap necrosis requires re-covering the device. Temporoparietal fascial flaps, along with various scalp rotation flaps, can be used for this purpose, depending on the circumstances.

Early Device Failure

Device failure can occur immediately: an "out of the box" failure. Unless intraoperative device telemetry is performed, out-of-the box failures will not be recognized until programming is attempted.

Out-of-the-box failures may be the result of factory defects or a consequence of damage during surgical manipulation. Buckled, broken, or exposed electrodes can result in failure of the entire electrode array or may leave only one or several electrodes nonfunctional. To prevent such failures, cochlear implants should always be handled gently. One must remember to discard the monopolar cautery once the implant is brought into the field. If the operating surgeon, for any reason, believes that the device is not going to function perfectly, the implant should be returned to the factory and a backup device should be used.

If the electrode array is not within the cochlea, the device may appear to function properly (although impedances may be suspiciously high) when it is checked by device telemetry but, of course, will not program because the electrodes are not in the vicinity of the auditory nerve (Figures 35–11 and 35–12). One advantage of NRT (see later) is that it can be used to assess physiologic efficacy and thereby verify placement. Extracochlear implantation can occur when hypotympanic air cells are mistaken for the scala tympani. This mistake is easier to make than one might think. It can be prevented by taking great care to be sure that one has the expected view of the round window niche and membrane before opening into scala tympani. Unless the surgeon is sure that he/she has inserted the device into the cochlea, interoperative radiographs should be obtained.

The electrodes can come to rest in a position outside the cochlea because the electrode array has moved or migrated after an initially correct placement. As every cochlear implant surgeon has noted, the electrode leads have some "spring" to them. Depending on the position of the proximal portions of the electrode leads in the mastoid, the array may tend to "spring back" out of the cochlea after each attempt to advance it. If the proximal portion of the electrode leads is not properly positioned in the mastoid cavity, these recoil forces can result in partial or complete withdrawal of the electrode array from the scala tympani. The most common cause of displaced electrodes, however, is movement of the electrode array after a "drill out" procedure (see later). Unless the electrode array is securely fixed, it will tend to become displaced; see below for a method of preventing this type of movement.[37,92]

If the implanting surgeon has any reason to believe that the electrode is not in a good position, a lateral skull film to ascertain its placement should obtained before the procedure is terminated.

Cerebrospinal Fluid Leak

A CSF leak can occur as the result of penetration of the dura when placing the stimulator/receiver. This is most likely in young children in whom the skull is very thin. It is perhaps more likely to occur with placement of the drill holes for the tie down sutures than with any other portion of the operation.

Cerebrospinal fluid gushers can occur when the scala tympani is opened to place the electrode array. Gushers are most likely to occur in the presence of modiolar defects. Modiolar defects are one of the most common forms of congenital anomaly seen within the cochlear implant population. Cerebrospinal fluid gushers are more the rule than the exception in severe cochlear dysplasia, such as common cavity deformity. Generally, the CSF leak can be controlled by packing the common cavity or vestibule with muscle. Drill out procedures for severe labyrinthitis will also occasionally result in CSF leak. The hard bone of the fully ossified otic capsule leaves few landmarks, and a surgeon may inadvertently wander into the middle fossa, posterior fossa, or internal auditory canal in attempting to create a trough in the presumed position of the scala tympani.

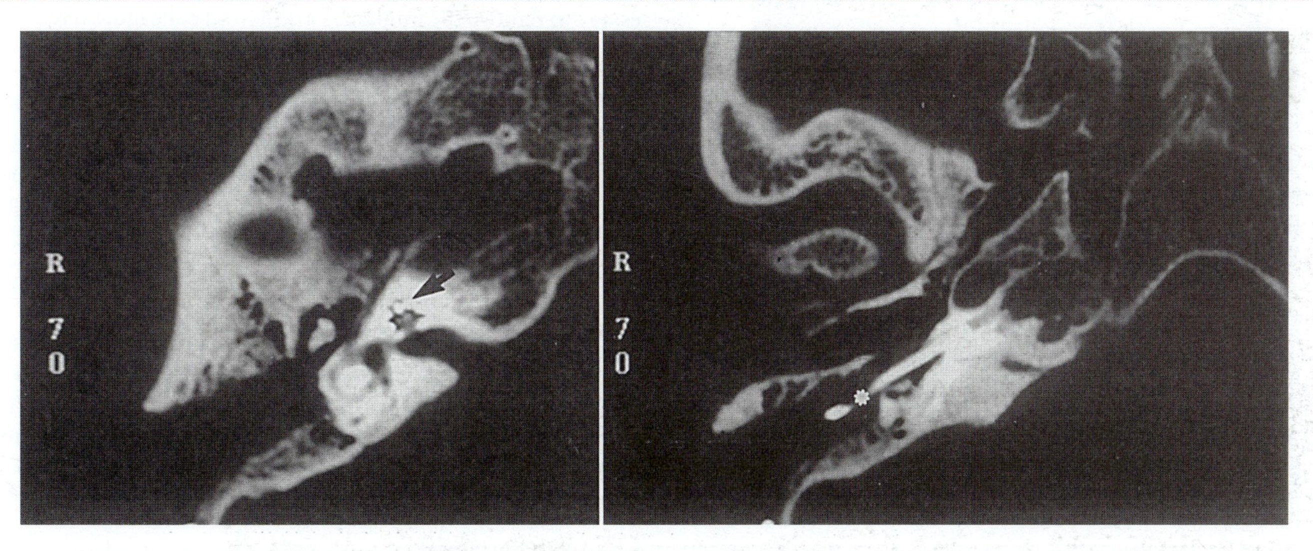

FIGURE 35–11 • A computed tomographic (CT) scan showing the well-positioned electrode array. The axial scan on the left shows the individual electrodes within the lumen of the cochlea (*black arrow*). The image on the right is also an axial CT scan. The asterisk indicates the electrode lead, which can be followed into the vestibule.

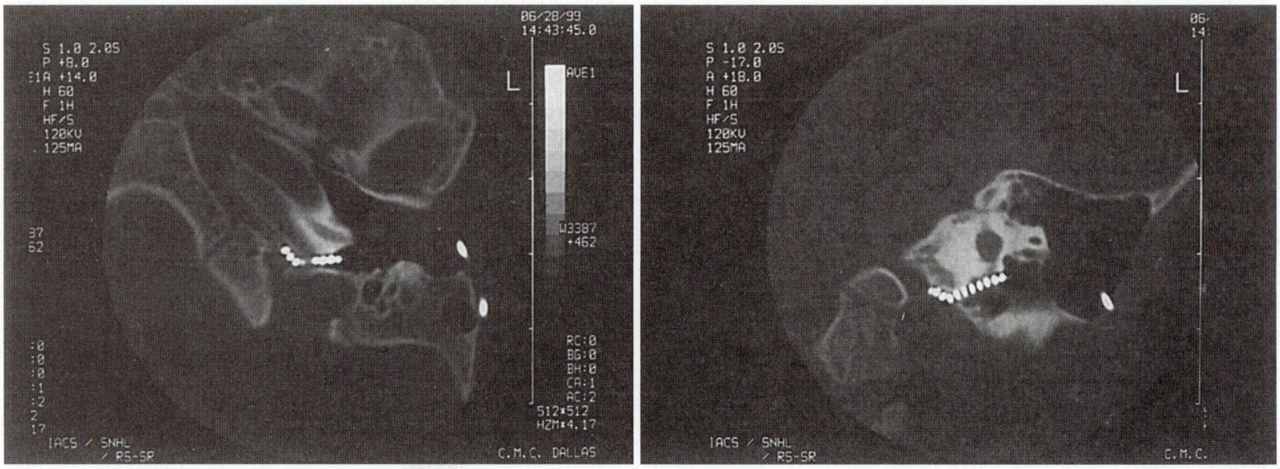

FIGURE 35 -12 • A malpositioned electrode array. The patient has a common cavity deformity. The axial CT scan on the right shows that the electrode array is posterior and medial to the common cavity and not within it. The coronal image on the left indicates that it also passes inferiorly to the common cavity deformity.

If occluding the vestibule or common cavity does not control the leak, the ear must be closed by plugging the eustachian tube, filling the middle ear and mastoid with fat and oversewing the external auditory canal.

From time to time, the operating surgeon will think that he/she has adequately controlled the egress of CSF only to find that there is CSF otorrhea or rhinorrhea postoperatively. Spinal drainage will often reduce CSF pressure and allow these areas to heal without a second operation, but reoperation is occasionally necessary.

Balance Disturbance

The incidence of vertigo and dizziness postoperatively is surprisingly low. Overall, fewer than 10% of patients experience significant dizziness. There is some reason to believe that the incidence of postoperative vertigo may vary a bit according to the extent to which the implant fills the scala tympani. When recipients do experience significant postoperative vertigo, it usually resolves within a few weeks. A few geriatric patients have had postoperative ataxia that resolves only over a period of several months. Papsin and colleagues, using the balance subtests of a test of standardized motor proficiency (Bruininks-Oseretsky), determined that children with cochlear implants performed slightly more poorly than normal children.[114] Surprisingly, however, they performed slightly better when the implants were on than when the implants were off.

Buchman et al. showed that unilateral implant recipients showed improvements in objective measures of postural stability using computerized dynamic platform posturography despite the fact that VOR testing demonstrates some decreases in response.[93–95]

Meningitis

Postoperative meningitis can occur but appears to be a little more likely after cochlear implantation than after other otologic procedures. Individuals who have perioperative CSF leak or a congenital inner ear malformation are at higher risk. If meningitis is suspected, a lumbar puncture should be performed after a CT scan has eliminated the risk of herniation. Antibiotics should be withheld until cultures have been obtained. As soon as the diagnosis has been verified by lumbar puncture, broad-spectrum antibiotic therapy can be initiated.

POSTOPERATIVE COMPLICATIONS: LATE COMPLICATIONS

One of the most feared late complications of cochlear implantation is extrusion or exposure of the device. As mentioned above, it is widely believed that keeping sutures lines as far as possible from the edge of the implant significantly reduces the incidence of excursion or exposure, although data to support this claim are not available. Once exposure has occurred, it is not always necessary to remove the implant. Parkins and colleagues have listed two criteria for successful salvage of an exposed prosthesis:[96]

1. Repair must remove enough skin and cicatrix to avoid suture lines that parallel the implant edge closer than 1–1/2 cm.
2. A pericranial flap should be rotated to fully cover the device with or without a temporoparietal flap as the initial layer of closure.[96]

Pain

Occasionally, patients will complain of postoperative pain at the site of the implant for months after the operation. This pain appears to be related to a form of periosteitis. It generally responds well to long-term use of nonsteroidal antiinflammatory agents (3 to 6 weeks).

Displacement

Late device migration or displacement is uncommon. Displacement can occur as a result of physical injury. Electrodes can be displaced as the result of scar tissue formation. Device displacement and migration can be best assessed on fine-cut CT scans of the temporal bone, which will often allow visualization of the electrode array as well as the stimulator receiver.

Late Device Failure

Late failure of stimulation is usually the result of internal device failure. Some of these failures are the result of trauma, but others appear to occur spontaneously. The external components of the device should first be replaced with loaner components. If that solves the problem, then the problem lies in the external component. If, however, replacement of external components results in no improvement, then a fine-cut CT scan should be obtained to make sure that the stimulator/receiver is still appropriately positioned, that the electrodes have not migrated, and no wires are broken. If the CT scan offers no explanation, then a company representative should be contacted for an "integrity check." Integrity checks seek to determine the electrical integrity of the device. Unfortunately, they are often inconclusive. One is then left unsure as to whether there has been some dramatic change in the patient's auditory system or if there has been an internal device failure ("soft" failure). Often the only way to resolve this dilemma is to replace the device and see if performance is improved.[97] Most commonly, it is.

Otitis Media

Prior to experience in implanting children, there was a great deal of concern that otitis media would present serious problems to children with cochlear implants. It was feared that every episode of otitis media would lead to infection of the implant and that chronic infection would require frequent device removal. This has not turned out to be the case. Luntz and colleagues evaluated 60 children, 74% of whom had had at least one episode of otitis media prior to implantation. All postoperative infections resolved with routine systemic antibiotic therapy without any additional complications. All children who experienced an episode of acute otitis media after implantation (16%) had an episode before the implant was placed.[98] Luntz and colleagues' experience is representative of the experience of others.

Meningitis

Cochlear implant recipients are at higher risk for the development of meningitis than children with normal hearing.[99–104] It is unclear, however, whether they are at higher risk for meningitis than other children with severe to profound hearing loss. It should be remembered that as many as 10% of children received cochlear implants because they have already had meningitis. Children with morphologic abnormalities of the labyrinth area are already at increased risk. Overall, the chances of a cochlear implant recipient developing meningitis appear to be roughly 1 in 1,000 if one excludes patients in whom an intracochlear "positioner" was used. (The positioner was a small, carefully shaped Silastic® obturator that slid into the scala tympani lateral to the electrode array and pushed it inward toward the modiolus. This device was withdrawn from the market several years ago and is no longer available.)

Almost all deaths associated with meningitis in cochlear implant recipients have been from pneumococcal infections.[105] Consequently, the Center for Disease Control and Prevention (CDC) has made very specific recommendations for pneumococcal vaccination in cochlear implant recipients. Specifically, these recommendations are: (1) all children should receive three doses of Prevnar® vaccine before the age of one. This recommendation is for all children, not just cochlear implant recipients. (2) Children with cochlear implants aged 2 years or older who have completed the pneumococcal conjugate vaccine (Prevnar®) should receive one dose of the pneumococcal polysacchride vaccine (Pneumovax® 23). If they have just received the pneumococcal conjugate vaccine, they should wait at least two months before receiving the pneumococcal polysaccharide vaccine. (3) Children's with cochlear implants between 24 and 59 months of age who have never received either the pneumococcal conjugate vaccine or the pneumococcal polysaccharide vaccine should receive the pneumococcal conjugate vaccine 2 or more months apart and then receive at least one dose of the pneumococcal polysaccharide vaccine at least two months later. (4) Persons aged 5 years and older with cochlear implants should receive one dose of the pneumococcal polysaccharide vaccine.

The issue of whether individuals need a "booster" dose of the pneumococcal polysaccharide vaccine remains unanswered. Some experts in the field strongly believe that a booster dose at 5 years or so is necessary. On the other hand, if the pneumococcal vaccine is given too frequently, the effect can be paradoxical; resistance can actually be reduced. Up-to-date information can be obtained from the CDC website.

Because their risk of meningitis is increased, children who have cochlear implants and develop otitis media should be treated aggressively and monitored very carefully.

SPECIAL PROBLEMS

Cochlear Dysplasia

A considerable proportion of children with severe to profound hearing loss have cochlea malformations. Malformations range from very mild incomplete partitioning defects through common cavity deformities to complete aplasias (Figures 35–2 and 35–3). The most commonly seen defects are enlarged vestibular aqueducts and defects of the modiolus. These defects do not necessarily adversely affect the outcome of cochlear implantation, nor do they necessarily require an alternation of surgical technique or the use of special electrode arrays.

More severe defects require some alteration of implantation technique.[106]

Common cavity deformities present special challenges because the extent and position of residual neuroepithelium is unknown. Common cavity deformities are more than likely to be associated with a defective modiolus, allowing abnormal communication between the common cavity and the internal auditory canal. The defect not only makes a CSF gusher more common, it also potentially allows the electrode array to slide directly into the internal auditory canal.

Some types of common cavity deformities make insertion through the round window area difficult or impossible. If the usual points of access to the cochlea are not available, the electrode array can be inserted directly through the lateral semicircular canal into the common cavity defect, as has been described by McElveen and colleagues.[107]

Facial nerve anomalies are more common in children who have significant cochlea dysplasia than in children who do not. The facial nerve is much more likely to be abnormal if the cochlea and semicircular canals are both involved in the malformation (Figure 35–13).[73] Most facial nerve anomalies involve anterior displacement of the nerve. The facial nerve may pass directly over the oval window niche (or where the oval niche should have been). Occasionally the nerve will pass anterior to the oval window niche over the promontory.

Although there have been a number of case reports and two questionnaire-based surveys on the results of cochlear implantation in children with cochlear dysplasia, no large series of patients with dysplasia has been reported. Graham, after reviewing the available information, believes that the range of potential outcomes is similar for children with cochlear dysplasia.[43] Nonetheless, most experienced implant centers warn the parents of children with significant cochlear deformities that the chances of success are somewhat reduced and that their expectations should be scaled back.[108–114]

Labyrinthitis Ossificans

About 5% of children who have had bacterial meningitis suffer profound hearing loss (Figure 35–14). Up to 80% of those children develop some degree of ossification. It appears that the infection spreads from the subarachnoid space to the labyrinth via the cochlear aqueduct. Consequently, labyrinthine ossification occurs first and is worst where the cochlear aqueduct enters the labyrinth: at the basal end of the scala tympani close to the round window.[115] Three stages of labyrinthitis ossificans can be identified: acute, fibrous, and ossification. The ossification process begins as early as 3 weeks after the onset of meningitis and it may progress over as long as 9 months.[116,117] Fortunately, the auditory nerve is preserved despite even advanced levels of ossification. Nadol has shown that the number of spiral ganglion cells decreases with increasing ossification and duration of deafness.[4]

Children who have lost hearing as the result of meningitis need to be closely monitored for the development of ossification. Since the earliest form is fibrous, CT scanning may not demonstrate it. An MRI scan is more sensitive because it can detect the absence of fluid within the obstructed cochlear duct and does not depend on the formation of new bone (Table 35–2).

There are several ways of managing a cochlea obstructed with fibrous tissue or new bone formation. If ossification is limited to the basal turn of the cochlea in the area of the round window, persistent drilling through the usual cochleostomy will penetrate the area of ossification until an open scala tympani can be identified. In such cases, the electrode array can be inserted as usual.

The earliest method of handling more extensive cochlear ossification was simply to continue drilling straight into the basal turn of the cochlea as far as possible—generally a distance of 6 to 8 mm. The surgeon then had to settle for as much of the electrode array as could be placed into this short segment of drilled-out, inferior basal turn. Four to eight electrodes were usually the most that could be inserted.

If there appears to be relatively extensive ossification of the basal turn of scala tympani, an attempt should be made to insert the electrode array into the scala vestibuli. Although the scala vestibuli is somewhat smaller than the scala tympani,

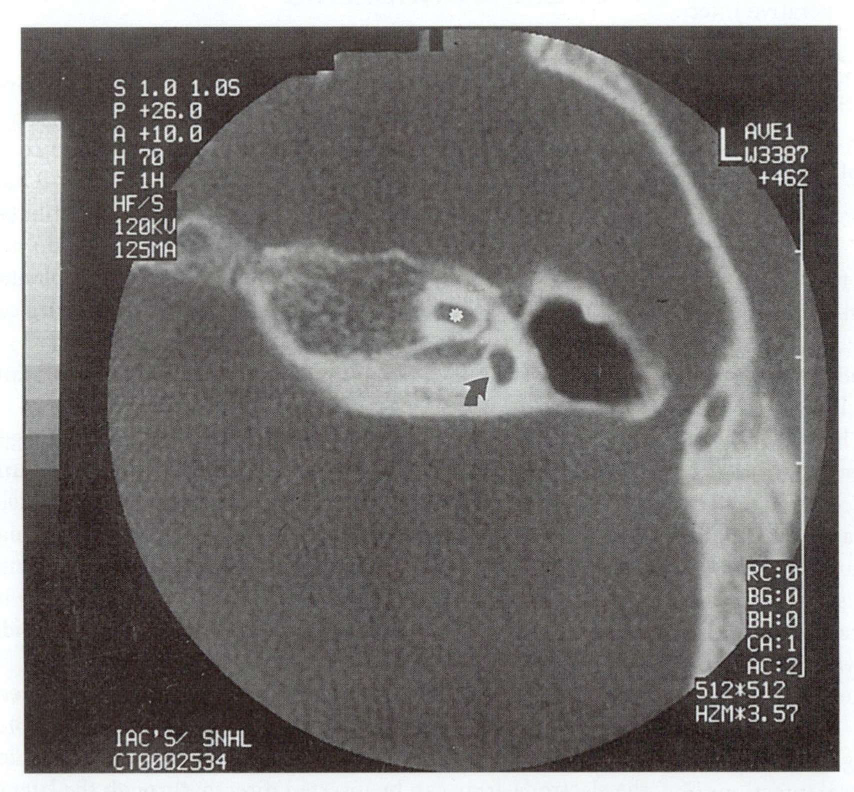

FIGURE 35–13 • The asterisk lies in the common cavity of a markedly dysplastic cochlea. The black arrow points to the only vestigial remnant of the semicircular canal: a single sac.

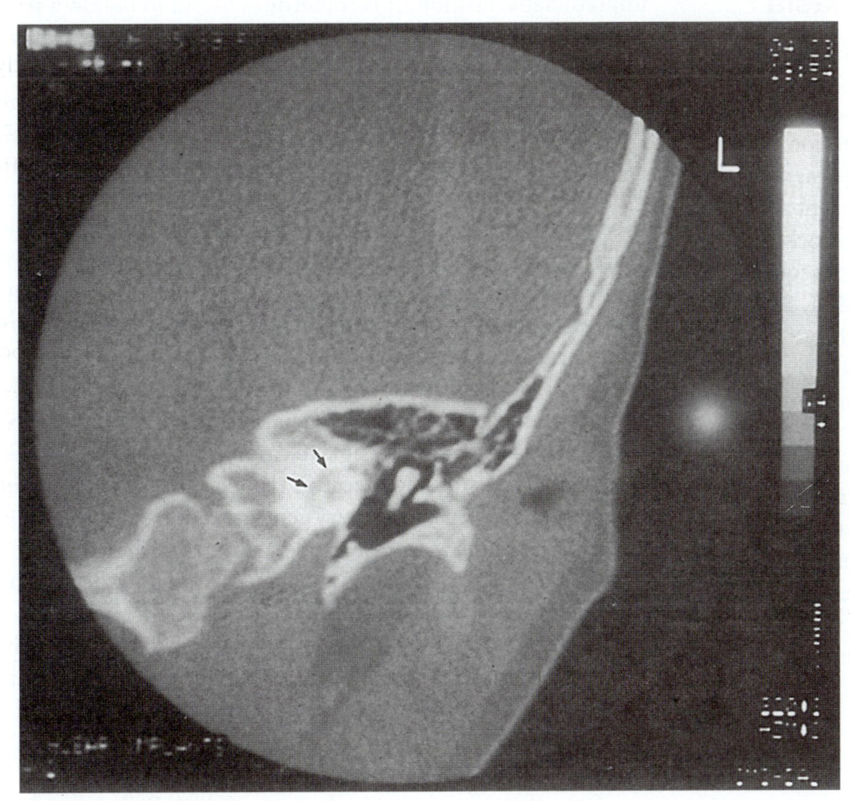

FIGURE 35 –14 • Coronal section through the cochlea. The arrows indicate haziness in the lumen of the membranous cochlear labyrinth, indicating early ossification.

the combined cross-sectional area of the scala tympani and scala media are about the same as that of the scala tympani.[118] Consequently, there is enough room to accommodate the electrode array, if Reissner's membrane is sacrificed. To access the scala vestibuli, the original cochleostomy should be extended posteriorly and superiorly toward the inferior limit of the oval window. If the scala vestibuli is also obliterated, a classic "drill out" procedure should be considered.

The classic drill out procedure was first described by Balkany and colleagues and allowed placement of many more electrodes into the ossified cochlea.[119] The posterior wall of the external auditory canal is removed, the soft tissue of the external auditory canal is excised, and the ear is closed. The entire lateral wall of the basal turn of the cochlea is then systematically removed, creating a trough in what had been the basal cochlear turn. Care must be taken to avoid the carotid artery anteriorly and to avoid penetrating the floor of the middle cranial fossa superiorly. As much as 300 to 360 degrees of the basal turn of the cochlea can be opened in this way. These early drill out procedures had a 50% failure rate because the electrode "pulled away" from the cochlea in the immediate postoperative period. Balkany and colleagues have recently described three modifications to this drill out procedure, two of which are designed to eliminate displacement of the electrode array.[120] The operation begins by identifying the round window and drilling anteriorly into the basal turn as usual. Drilling is continued approximately 6 to 8 mm anteriorly directly into the basal turn. A tympanomeatal flap is then designed, incised, and elevated, and the middle ear space is entered through the external auditory canal. The tympanomeatal flap should be superiorly based. The incus is removed and the drum is separated from the malleus. After identifying the middle ear landmarks, the previously drilled tunnel in the cochlea is entered approximately 4 mm anterior to the round window niche. This leaves a "bridge" of that bone intact that will secure the electrode array. The trough is then continued anteriorly and superiorly up the ascending bend of the basal turn, to the level of the semicanal of the tensor tympani muscle. It is then followed posteriorly to the anterior edge of the oval window and then inferiorly to complete the opening of the basal turn. Great care must be taken to avoid the carotid artery anteriorly and the facial nerve posteriorly. The electrode array is then passed into the original cochleostomy and the tip is retrieved in the open basal turn. The residual intact "bridge" of bone helps prevent electrode migration. Pieces of the incus are then used to wedge the tip of the electrode array into the trough. The cochlea around the electrode array is packed with fat.

A final option for management of the ossified cochlea is to use a split- or double-electrode array. To place the double array, a cochleostomy is made anterior to the round window membrane as usual. It is extended anteriorly superiorly directly into the ossified basal turn for about 8.0 mm. Care must be taken to avoid the internal carotid artery. The incus is removed along with the incus buttress. The stapedial crura are carefully cut and removed so as not to avulse the stapes footplate. A second cochleostomy is then performed immediately above the oval window just below the cochleariform process. It is drilled to a depth of 7.0 mm paralleling the tympanic portion of the facial nerve. The two electrode arrays are then placed into the two cochleostomies separately. The cochleostomies are sealed with soft tissue.[121]

Cochlear Nerve Aplasia/Hypoplasia

MRI scanning can be used to detect the presence and size of the cochlear nerve within the IAC or cerebellopontine angle. Radiographic absence of a cochlear nerve has been regarded as an absolute contraindication of cochlear implantation. However, recent experience indicates that stimulable cochlear fibers may be present in these individuals despite their apparent absence on imaging studies. It may be that these stimulable cochlear fibers do not separate from the vestibular nerve and, consequently, are not visualized as a separate neural bundle on MRI. Experience has shown that some patients with absent cochlear nerves on MRI do receive benefit from cochlear implants. In those few patients who have absent cochlear nerves on radiographic imaging but do have detectable behavioral or ABI responses, cochlear implants should be provided using the usual behavioral criteria. In those individuals who have "no response audiograms," the decision is more difficult. If a positive response is identified on electrical ABR (promontory stimulation), then it is reasonable to implant. Some surgeons have reported positive results of cochlear implantation even when electrical ABR testing was negative. Consequently, negative ABR testing cannot be regarded as a reliable absolute contraindication to cochlear implantation.[111,122–124]

REVISION SURGERY

There are several reasons for reoperating in the area of an existing cochlear implant:

1. There has been device failure.
2. A technologically outdated device needs to be removed and an updated device inserted.
3. The device becomes extruded or exposed. Revision operation may or may not require explantation and/or reimplantation.
4. The skin flap must be revised, usually because it is too thick.
5. An additional procedure is being performed in the area of the implant, eg, auricular reconstruction.

If the surgery in the area of the implant does not involve explanting the device, then great care must be taken to maintain its integrity and functionality. First, monopolar cautery must not be used. In its stead, the Shaw® knife (a heated scalpel blade) has been found useful.[125] Caution should be exercised to avoid injury to the electrodes. It is important to know the type of device that has been implanted if one is to have some idea of where the electrodes will be located. For example, the Advanced Bionics device has the electrode takeoff at its anterior-most portion. The electrode takes off as a single lead. On the other hand, the MED-EL device has two electrodes that leave from the side of the device. The takeoff of the electrodes will be inferiorly positioned when the implant is placed on one side of the head and superiorly when the implant is placed on the contralateral side.

The electrode leads generally take a fairly straight path from the device into the mastoid and through the facial recess. The flying ground electrode, however, may lie in an unpredictable position, often looping back on the stimulator/receiver in an unpredictable fashion. It is sometimes useful to obtain a plain, lateral, skull radiograph to be sure of exactly where the stimulator/receiver is located and where the various electrode leads lie.

The stimulator/receiver is usually found in a mesothelially lined pouch that is relatively easy to identify. There is usually little scar tissue formation between the stimulator/receiver and the surrounding soft tissues. Consequently, soft tissues are easy to separate from the stimulator/receiver. In the case of children, there will be often be substantial amounts of bony regrowth. Bony regrowth may cover the lateral portions of the implant. Not infrequently some drilling must be performed to release the stimulator/receiver from its bony niche.

The amount of scarring and the density of mucosal adhesions found in the area of the facial recess and middle ear are variable. It is generally possible to carefully follow the electrode leads from the stimulator/receiver through the facial recess into the cochlea. However, even very gentle traction on the electrode leads will withdraw the electrode array from the cochlea. Its utility as a guide through the facial recess and into the previous cochleostomy is then lost.

If the revision operation is designed to save an existing device after exposure or infection, then long-term postoperative antibiotics are necessary. If skin organisms are involved in the infection, as much as 6 weeks of therapy may be required (Niparko J. Personal Communication. 2001).

Reimplantation is generally successful.[59,60] Balkany and colleagues have reported on 16 patients who underwent reimplantation. The most common reason was device failure. After the results with the new device had been compared to the results with the old device, the reimplantation procedure was compared with the initial operation in terms of length of insertion, number of electrodes programmed, and postoperative audiometric results. Among their 16 subjects, there were no significant differences between the initial implant and the reimplanted device.[29,126,127]

Henson and colleagues reviewed 28 patients who had been reimplanted. Both the initial devices and the reimplanted devices were Nucleus 22 implants. Thirty-seven percent had improved performance, 26% showed no significant change in performance, and 37% showed poorer performance. Subjectively, 57% felt that their hearing was better and 43% thought it was poorer. There was no correlation between performance and cause of device failure, length of use of the old device, surgical complications, change of electrode insertion depth, or preoperative variables such as age, etiology, or duration of deafness.[128]

Parisier and colleagues retrospectively analyzed 27 consecutive multichannel cochlear implant reinsertions. Open-set speech recognition scores and speech perception ability remained stable or improved compared with the results before implantation.[129]

POSTOPERATIVE CONSIDERATIONS FOR SURGEONS

Device Activation

Two to four weeks postoperatively, when the wound is well healed, the cochlear implant is activated. This is a process frequently referred to as "hook up." The first decision that must be made during the hook-up process is to determine the stimulation mode. Every "channel" requires an active electrode paired with a ground electrode. It was initially believed that greater frequency specificity and therefore improved speech recognition would result from narrow band, highly specific stimulation of the cochlea. It was believed that widespread dispersion of current would result in activation of a large number of neurons and obscure frequency specificity. Consequently, each active electrode was paired with another electrode on the intracochlear electrode array, which served as its ground electrode. The active electrode can be coupled to any other electrode on the array: the electrode next to it or the electrode furthest away. When the active electrode is grounded to another intracochlear electrode, stimulation mode is referred to as "bipolar." The distance of the ground electrode to the active electrode is expressed as "bipolar +1", and "bipolar +2" etc.

Although intuition suggested that narrow bands of stimulation (ie, bipolar mode) would be most effective, experience has challenged that assumption. Most patients are programmed in a monopolar mode. Each electrode within the cochlea is grounded to an extracochlear electrode, resulting in wide current spread throughout the cochlea with every stimulation. Monopolar stimulation requires the availability of an electrode outside the cochlea. All currently available receivers have such electrodes. The ground electrode may be a separate electrode attached to a separate lead, may be built into the back of the stimulator/receiver, or both.

Initial programming of the device also requires that the threshold level and most comfortable loudness level be determined for each active electrode. This is a laborious process, taking up to several hours in adults. Together, measures of threshold and comfortable loudness levels set the electrical dynamic range within which all auditory signals will fall. Frequency bands are then assigned to each electrode pair by the software program. In the young, prelingually deaf child, this can be a very complicated matter requiring many days. A recent improvement in the area of cochlear implantation is the development of objective methods to assess threshold. These include NRT, estimation of stapedial reflex, and electrical ABR.

Neural response telemetry (NRT) uses radio frequency telemetry to measure the action potential in the auditory nerve. It differs from the older device telemetry (which evaluated only the internal electronics of the implant itself) because it can objectively evaluate the physiological response to the device. Neural response telemetry can be obtained both intraoperatively and postoperatively. The stimulus intensities necessary to generate an action potential in the auditory nerve can be determined and then used to provide target settings for the speech processor. Shallop and colleagues have confirmed a particular relationship between comfort settings and NRT thresholds in children.[130] Behavioral thresholds and comfort levels correlate well with NRT thresholds when the appropriate correction factor is applied.[131] The correction factor needed to program all electrodes is consistent across the electrode array and consequently, can be determined from behavorial programming of a single electrode. Once the correction factor has been accurately determined, it can be applied to all electrodes in the NRT-generated map. Programming of young children can be done more accurately and more quickly using NRT.[132–136]

An electrical ABR can be used in a similar fashion. The mean ABR threshold was predictive of the average comfort level in a study by Brown, but there was a fair amount of intersubject variability.[137]

A third method by which an objective estimate of comfort levels can be obtained is using the stapedius reflex. Intraoperatively, the stapedius muscle can be seen contracting in response to high stimulus intensities. When the stimulus used to elicit the reflex is electrical, the response is referred to as an electrical stapedius reflex. When the electrical stapedius reflex is performed intraoperatively to test the implant and contraction of the stapedius muscle is noted visually, the test is referred to as a visual electrical stapedius reflex test. Although the usual understanding of the protective nature of the stapedius reflex would lead one to believe that the presence of a stapedius reflex would correlate best with uncomfortable loudness levels, it has now been shown that it actually correlates better with the most comfortable loudness level.[53,130,138–140]

Facial Nerve Stimulation

The most common form of nonauditory stimulation associated with cochlear implantation is stimulation of the facial nerve. Facial nerve twitching as a consequence of activated cochlear implant electrodes is not uncommon. Bigelow and colleagues noted this in 8% of 58 patients implanted at the University of Pennsylvania. Kelsall and colleagues evaluated 14 patients (7% of implant recipients) at their institution. Both investigators found that the electrodes in the midbasal turn were the most common electrodes involved, presumably because of their anatomic proximity to the labyrinthine portion of the facial nerve. The overall incidence among implant recipients varies from 1 to 14.9%, with most recent studies suggesting an incidence of about 7%.[141–143] Facial nerve stimulation is most commonly seen in individuals with bony abnormalities of the cochlea, especially cochlear otosclerosis. Congenital abnormalities of the cochlea, cochlear labyrinthitis ossificans, and extensive new bone formation in the cochlea as a result of electrode placement can all increase the risk of facial nerve stimulation.

Demineralization of the otic capsule as a consequence of otosclerosis leads to an especially high incidence of facial nerve stimulation, 38% as reported by Rotterveel in 53 patients.[143,144] Decreased mineralization of the otic capsule significantly decreases the impedance of the otic capsule to the spread of electric current. Ramsden has reported that most cases of facial nerve stimulation can be managed by reprogramming the electrode array to "drop out" the rogue electrodes with little or no decrease in performance. Smullen et al., however, have indicated that if one electrode produces stimulation, on average 9.6 electrodes cause stimulation of the facial nerve. Consequently, 10 or more electrodes may need to be dropped out of the program to avoid facial nerve stimulation. Facial nerve stimulation is not necessarily immediate in onset. In Smullen's series, 11% of patients with facial nerve stimulation had the onset more than 12 months after implantation. Additionally, some patients experience a progressive increase in the number of electrodes causing facial nerve stimulation.

The electrodes most commonly at fault are electrodes closest to the geniculate ganglion, typically electrodes 16–17 in the Nucleus Corporation's Freedom 22® electrode array. These electrodes are in the superior segment of the basal turn close to the spiral ganglion.

Smullen et al. have demonstrated that patients with perimodiolar electrodes can tolerate higher loudness levels before facial nerve stimulation occurs than patients who have straight (laterally aligned) electrode arrays. This suggests that a modiolus-hugging electrode may be more suitable for patients at risk for facial nerve stimulation.[142]

Bigelow and colleagues reported that preoperative CT scanning can often identify those potential cochlear implant recipients at greatest risk. Gold and colleagues have suggested that sodium fluoride may reduce the risk and incidence of facial nerve stimulation in otosclerotic patients.[145,146]

Postoperative Rehabilitation

Postoperative rehabilitation is an important part of cochlear implantation. In children, especially prelingually deafened children, it is absolutely critical and makes the difference between a successful transition to implant use and a failure. The topic is significantly slighted in this chapter written principally for surgeons. However, it is imperative that every implant surgeon recognize that for many implant recipients, aggressive and intensive rehabilitation is absolutely essential. Rehabilitation focuses on making sure that the recipient can adequately use the information provided by the implant. The rate at which rehabilitation is accomplished varies substantially between one recipient and another. Clearly, the postlingually deafened individual with deafness of brief duration will progress much more quickly than the prelingually deafened adult. Most rehabilitative services are provided by specially trained speech-language pathologists. It should be recognized that this is a relatively specialized area and the general speech-language pathologist may not be able to adequately meet the needs of the cochlear implant recipient. Parents play a critical role in rehabilitating children and their active involvement in the rehabilitation process greatly accelerates the development of both expressive and receptive language skills.

RESULTS

Postlingually Deafened Adults

It is now recognized that postlingually deafened adults will achieve open-set word recognition in most cases. Because the efficacy of cochlear implants in postlingually deafened adults is no longer disputed, few results have been published recently.

In the recently completed Nucleus Freedom® trial, substantial improvement was seen after only 6 months of use. The average HINT sentence score rose from <5% to almost 80%.[147]

Gstoettner and colleagues have evaluated the benefit reached by 21 consecutive postlingually deafened adults who received the MED-EL COMBI 40+® device. At 12 months post-implant, sentence understanding averaged >85%.[148] Data on MED-EL's new Pulsar® implant is just now becoming available and is very promising.[149]

Whereas overall hearing results have improved dramatically in the last decade, individual hearing results remain variable and unpredictable.

Children

Waltzmann and colleagues evaluated 36 prelingually deafened children who received Nucleus® devices and were less than 5 years old. All children developed significant open-set speech recognition, and 37 of the 38 children use oral language as their sole means of communication.[150] Blamey and colleagues evaluated 47 prelingually deafened children with a mean unaided PTA of 106 dB using a cochlear implant and compared those children with 40 children with a mean PTA of 78 dB who used hearing aids. Both groups were treated in an oral/aural rehabilitation setting. They were closely followed and repeatedly evaluated over a 3-year period. Their results suggest that all children will reach 90% open-set speech recognition but that they will all enter secondary school about 4 to 5 years delayed unless they receive intensive language therapy.[151] Tomblin and colleagues have shown that grammatical development is significantly enhanced in prelingually deafened children who receive cochlear implants compared to those that do not.[152]

An important, practical way to assess the effectiveness of cochlear implantation is to establish use versus nonuse rates. Presumably, children who find cochlear implants useful will use them. Those children who do not find cochlear implants useful will not use them. Archbold and colleagues followed 161 children for 3 years. All were users. Parents rated 89% of the children as full-time users and 11% "most of the time users." Teachers rated the children slightly higher: 95% were rated full-time users and only 4% were rated "most of the time users." Neither parents nor teachers rated any child an occasional user or a nonuser.[153]

A number of variables have been considered in trying to account for the variability in outcome. Cheng and colleagues have shown that hearing outcomes are independent of the cause of deafness in children.[45] The length of the electrode array and the number of active electrodes does not appear to be important beyond a certain threshold number. Once 8 to 10 electrodes have been successfully inserted into the cochlea, the number of electrodes no longer correlates with postoperative performance. It has been hypothesized, and seems logical, that greater depth of insertion will increase performance but no validation of this hypothesis has been forthcoming. Hodges and colleagues have shown that insertion of the Nucleus 22® device beyond 22 rings did not improve performance in 31 patients.[29]

Length of deafness appears to be an important variable and has had predictive value in a number of studies. Together with preoperative CID sentence scores, Rubinstein and colleagues have shown that duration of deafness accounts for 70% of the variance seen in cochlear implant recipients.[6,87,88,154]

The mode of communication appears to have a significant impact on outcome. Hodges and colleagues have shown that children using oral-only modes of communication experience better outcomes than children using total communication. Indeed, in their study it was the most important predictor of success.[9,29] Geers and Nicholas, in an evaluation of 180 cochlear implant recipients, found that children in an environment that required them to depend on spoken language (rather than sign language) received more benefit from their cochlear implants.[155]

On the other hand, Robbins and colleagues evaluated 23 profound prelingually deafened children and found no difference between those using oral communication and those using total communication.[156]

Speech and Language Aquisition

Not only has improved speech perception (hearing) as the result of cochlear implantation been clearly demonstrated, but an improved ability to develop expressive speech and language skills has also been documented. However, evidence to support dramatically improved expressive language skills in cochlear implant recipients is accumulating a bit more slowly.[37] Moog and Geers evaluated 22 prelingually deafened children who received cochlear implants. They all had speech intelligibility scores that were statistically better than children managed with hearing aids, and half had language scores that fell within the average range for normal-hearing children.[44] Tobey and colleagues have shown that speech intelligibility correlates with the level of speech recognition and is better if children have received auditory verbal therapy than if they have been managed in a total communication environment.[157] Robbins and colleagues compared 23 prelingually deafened cochlear implant children to 89 deaf children treated without a cochlear implant (not with ossification) using the Reynell Developmental Language scale. Cochlear implant recipients exceeded by 7 months the gains predicted on the basis of previous maturation studies. Language development rate was about the same as in normal-hearing children.[156,87] Svirsky and colleagues compared 43 cochlear implant children to 52 children who used hearing aids. Cochlear implant users had better speech intelligibility than did the hearing aid users, and auditory verbal children had better speech intelligibility than children managed with total communication.[43] Miyamoto and colleagues reported that children with cochlear implants had much higher reported gains in expressive language skills after implantation than would have been predicted on the basis of an observed cohort of 89 unimplanted deaf children.[158]

Geers et al, in a cohort of over 181 children implanted before the age of 5, determined that over half these children produced and understood English on a level comparable with that of their hearing age mates. They further noted that such outcomes were not reliably achieved by children with profound hearing loss who used hearing aids and that sign language did not provide the linguistic advantage that had been anticipated. Notably, children who were not taught sign language and who did not use it regularly had superior language skills.

Cochlear implants, in summary, allow a child to recover a normal ability to acquire speech and language once the implant has been placed but do not fully overcome the detrimental effects of early auditory deprivation.[67] Thus, the gap between chronological age and language age, which progressively increases in unimplanted children, remains constant after cochlear implantation (see Figure 35–14).

ACKNOWLEDGMENTS

Special thanks is extended to Pam Henderson, my administrative assistant, whose tireless efforts saw this manuscript through multiple revisions. Without her cheerful collaboration, the task could not have been completed.

References

1. Miller AL. Effects of chronic stimulation on auditory nerve survival in ototoxically deafened animals. Hear Res 2001;151(1–2):1–14.
2. Leake PA, Hradek GT, Snyder RL. Chronic electrical stimulation by a cochlear implant promotes survival of spiral ganglion neurons after neonatal deafness. J Comp Neurol 1999;412(4):543–62.
3. Shepherd RK, Matsushima J, Martin RL, Clark GM. Cochlear pathology following chronic electrical stimulation of the auditory nerve: II. Deafened kittens. Hear Res 1994;81(1–2):150–66.
4. Nadol JB, Jr. Patterns of neural degeneration in the human cochlea and auditory nerve: Implications for cochlear implantation. Otolaryngol Head Neck Surg 1997;117(3 Pt 1):220–8.
5. Linthicum FH, Jr., Fayad J, Otto SR, Galey FR, House WF. Cochlear implant histopathology. Am J Otol 1991;12(4):245–311.
6. Blanchfield BB, Feldman JJ, Dunbar JL, Gardner EN. The severely to profoundly hearing-impaired population in the United States: prevalence estimates and demographics. J Am Acad Audiol 2001;12(4):183–9.
7. Cheng AK, Rubin HR, Powe NR, Mellon NK, Francis HW, Niparko JK. Cost–utility analysis of the cochlear implant in children. JAMA 2000;284(7):850–6.
8. Blanchfield BB, Feldman JJ, Dunbar J. The severely to profoundly hearing impaired population in the United States: Prevalence and demographics. Policy Anal Brief H Ser 1999;1(1):1–4.
9. Mohr PE, Feldman JJ, Dunbar JL, Conkey-Robbins A, Niparko JK, Rittenhouse RK, Skinner MW. The societal costs of severe to profound hearing loss in the United States. Int J Technol Assess Health Care 2000;16(4):1120–35.
10. Balkany T, Hodges AV, Goodman KW. Ethics of cochlear implantation in young children. Otolaryngol Head Neck Surg 1996;114(6):748–55.
11. Tucker BP. Deaf culture, cochlear implants, and elective disability. Hastings Cent Rep 1998;28:6–14.
12. Francis HW, Koch ME, Wyatt JR, Niparko JK. Trends in educational placement and cost–benefit considerations in children with cochlear implants. Arch Otolaryngol Head Neck Surg 1999;125(5):499–505.
13. Haimowitz S. Deaf culture. Hastings Cent Rep 1999;29(2):5.
14. Krabbe PF, Hinderink JB, van den BP. The effect of cochlear implant use in postlingually deaf adults. Int J Technol Assess Health Care 2000;16(3):864–73.
15. Palmer CS, Niparko JK, Wyatt JR, Rothman M, de LG. A prospective study of the cost–utility of the multichannel cochlear implant. Arch Otolaryngol Head Neck Surg 1999;125(11):1221–8.
16. Wyatt JR, Niparko JK, Rothman M, deLissovoy G. Cost utility of the multichannel cochlear implants in 258 profoundly deaf individuals. Laryngoscope 1996;106(7):816–21.
17. Cheng AK, Grant GD, Niparko JK. Meta-analysis of pediatric cochlear implant literature. Ann Otol Rhinol Laryngol Suppl 1999;177:124–8.
18. Arriaga MA, Carrier D. MRI and clinical decisions in cochlear implantation. Am J Otol 1996;17(4):547–53.

19. Ellul S, Shelton C, Davidson HC, Harnsberger HR. Preoperative cochlear implant imaging: Is magnetic resonance imaging enough? Am J Otol 2000;21(4):528–33.
20. Phelps PD, Proops DW. Imaging for cochlear implants. Journal of Laryngology & Otology 1999;24(Supplement):21–3.
21. Maxwell AP, Mason SM, O'Donoghue GM. Cochlear nerve aplasia: Its importance in cochlear implantation. Am J Otol 1999;20(3):335–7.
22. Adunka OF, Jewells V, Buchman CA. Value of computed tomography in the evaluation of children with cochlear nerve deficiency. Otol Neurotol 2007; 28(5):597–604.
23. Parry DA, Booth T, Roland PS. Advantages of magnetic resonance imaging over computed tomography in preoperative evaluation of pediatric cochlear implant candidates. Otol Neurotol 2005;26(4):976–82.
24. Buchman CA, Joy J, Hodges A, Telischi FF, Balkany TJ. Vestibular effects of cochlear implantation. Laryngoscope 2004;114(10 Pt 2 Suppl 103):1–22.
25. Nadol JB, Jr., Hsu WC. Histopathologic correlation of spiral ganglion cell count and new bone formation in the cochlea following meningogenic labyrinthitis and deafness. Ann Otol Rhinol Laryngol 1991;100(9 Pt 1):712–6.
26. Lesinski A, Hartrampf R, Dahm MC, Bertram B, Lenarz T. Cochlear implantation in a population of multihandicapped children. Ann Otol Rhinol Laryngol Suppl 1995;166:332–4.
27. Isaacson JE, Hasenstab MS, Wohl DL, Williams GH. Learning disability in children with postmeningitic cochlear implants. Arch Otolaryngol Head Neck Surg 1996;122(9):929–36.
28. Waltzman SB, Scalchunes V, Cohen NL. Performance of multiply handicapped children using cochlear implants. Am J Otol 2000;21(3):329–35.
29. Hodges AV, Dolan AM, Balkany TJ, Schloffman JJ, Butts SL. Speech perception results in children with cochlear implants: Contributing factors. Otolaryngol Head Neck Surg 1999;121(1):31–4.
30. Chen JM, Shipp D, Al-Abidi A, Ng A, Nedzelski JM. Does choosing the "worse" ear for cochlear implantation affect outcome? Otol Neurotol 2001;22(3):335–9.
31. Roland PS, Tobey EA, Devous MD, Sr. Preoperative functional assessment of auditory cortex in adult cochlear implant users. Laryngoscope 2001;111(1):77–83.
32. Coez A, Zilbovicius M, Ferrary E, et al. Cochlear implant benefits in deafness rehabilitation: PET study of temporal voice activations. J Nucl Med 2008;49(1):60–7.
33. Lee JS, Lee DS, Oh SH, et al. PET evidence of neuroplasticity in adult auditory cortex of postlingual deafness. J Nucl Med *2003;44(9):1435–9.*
34. Tobey EA, Devous MD, Sr., Buckley K, et al. Functional brain imaging as an objective measure of speech perception performance in adult cochlear implant users. Int J Audiol 2004;43 Suppl 1:S52–S56.
35. Roland JT, Jr., Fishman AJ, Waltzman SB, Alexiades G, Hoffman RA, Cohen NL. Stability of the cochlear implant array in children. Laryngoscope 1998;108(8 Pt 1):1119–23.
36. Holt RF, Svirsky MA. An Exploratory Look at Pediatric Cochlear Implantation: Is Earliest Always Best? Ear Hear 2008; 29(4):492–511.
37. Miyamoto RT, Hay-McCutcheon MJ, Kirk KI, Houston DM, Bergeson-Dana T. Language skills of profoundly deaf children who received cochlear implants under 12 months of age: A preliminary study. Acta Otolaryngol 2008;128(4):373–7.
38. Connor CM, Craig HK, Raudenbush SW, Heavner K, Zwolan TA. The age at which young deaf children receive cochlear implants and their vocabulary and speech-production growth: Is there an added value for early implantation? Ear Hear 2006;27(6):628–44.
39. Dorman MF, Sharma A, Gilley P, Martin K, Roland P. Central auditory development: Evidence from CAEP measurements in children fit with cochlear implants. J Commun Disord. 2007;40(4):284–94. Epub 2007 Mar 14.
40. Sharma A, Martin K, Roland P, Bauer P, Sweeney MH, Gilley P, et al. P1 latency as a biomarker for central auditory development in children with hearing impairment. J Am Acad Audiol 2005;16(8):564–73.
41. Sharma A, Dorman MF, Kral A. The influence of a sensitive period on central auditory development in children with unilateral and bilateral cochlear implants. Hear Res 2005;203(1–2):134–43.
42. Kileny PR, Zwolan TA, Ashbaugh C. The influence of age at implantation on performance with a cochlear implant in children. Otol Neurotol 2001;22(1):42–6.
43. Svirsky MA, Robbins AM, Kirk KI, Pisoni DB, Miyamoto RT. Language development in profoundly deaf children with cochlear implants. Psychol Sci 2000;11(2):153–8.
44. Moog JS, Geers AE. Speech and language acquisition in young children after cochlear implantation. Otolaryngol Clin North Am 1999;32(6):1127–41.
45. Cheng AK, Niparko JK. Cost–utility of the cochlear implant in adults: a meta-analysis. Arch Otolaryngol Head Neck Surg 1999;125(11):1214–8.
46. Labadie RF, Carrasco VN, Gilmer CH, Pillsbury HC, III. Cochlear implant performance in senior citizens. Otolaryngol Head Neck Surg 2000;123(4):419–24.
47. Buchman CA, Fucci MJ, Luxford WM. Cochlear implants in the geriatric population: benefits outweigh risks. Ear Nose Throat J 1999;78(7):489–94.
48. Rance G, Barker EJ. Speech perception in children with auditory neuropathy/dyssynchrony managed with either hearing AIDS or cochlear implants. Otol Neurotol 2008;29(2):179–82.
49. Rance G, Barker E, Mok M, Dowell R, Rincon A, Garratt R. Speech perception in noise for children with auditory neuropathy/dys–synchrony type hearing loss. Ear Hear 2007;28(3):351–60.
50. Rance G, Barker EJ, Sarant JZ, Ching TY. Receptive language and speech production in children with auditory neuropathy/dyssynchrony type hearing loss. Ear Hear 2007;28(5):694–702.
51. Mason JC, De MA, Stevens C, Ruth RA, Hashisaki GT. Cochlear implantation in patients with auditory neuropathy of varied etiologies. Laryngoscope 2003;113(1):45–9.
52. Peterson A, Shallop J, Driscoll C, Breneman A, Babb J, Stoeckel R, Fabry L. Outcomes of cochlear implantation in children with auditory neuropathy. J Am Acad Audiol 2003;14(4):188–201.
53. Shallop JK, Peterson A, Facer GW, Fabry LB, Driscoll CL. Cochlear implants in five cases of auditory neuropathy: Postoperative findings and progress. Laryngoscope 2001;111(4 Pt 1): 555–62.
54. Brown KD, Balkany TJ. Benefits of bilateral cochlear implantation: A review. Curr Opin Otolaryngol Head Neck Surg 2007;15(5):315–8.
55. Galvin KL, Mok M, Dowell RC, Briggs RJ. 12-month post-operative results for older children using sequential bilateral implants. Ear Hear 2007;28(2 Suppl):19S–21S.

56. Galvin KL, Mok M, Dowell RC. Perceptual benefit and functional outcomes for children using sequential bilateral cochlear implants. Ear Hear 2007;28(4):470–82.
57. Buss E, Pillsbury HC, Buchman CA, et al. Multicenter U.S. bilateral MED-EL cochlear implantation study: speech perception over the first year of use. Ear Hear 2008;29(1):20–32.
58. van HR, Bohm M, Pesch J, Vandali A, Battmer RD, Lenarz T. Binaural speech unmasking and localization in noise with bilateral cochlear implants using envelope and fine-timing based strategies. J Acoust Soc Am 2008;123(4):2249–63.
59. Cullen RD, Fayad JN, Luxford WM, Buchman CA. Revision cochlear implant surgery in children. Otol Neurotol 2008;29(2):214–20.
60. Seeber BU, Fastl H. Localization cues with bilateral cochlear implants. J Acoust Soc Am 2008;123(2):1030–42.
61. Balkany T, Hodges A, Telischi F, et al. William House Cochlear Implant Study Group: Position statement on bilateral cochlear implantation. Otol Neurotol 2008;29(2):107–8.
62. Litovsky R, Parkinson A, Arcaroli J, Sammeth C. Simultaneous bilateral cochlear implantation in adults: A multicenter clinical study. Ear Hear 2006;27(6):714–31.
63. Schleich P, Nopp P, D'Haese P. Head shadow, squelch, and summation effects in bilateral users of the MED-EL COMBI 40/40+ cochlear implant. Ear Hear 2004;25(3):197–204.
64. Luetje CM, Thedinger BS, Buckler LR, Dawson KL, Lisbona KL. Hybrid cochlear implantation: Cinical results and critical review in 13 cases. Otol Neurotol 2007;28(4):473–8.
65. Gantz BJ, Turner C, Gfeller KE. Acoustic plus electric speech processing: Preliminary results of a multicenter clinical trial of the Iowa/Nucleus Hybrid implant. Audiol Neurootol 2006;11 Suppl 1:63–8.
66. Roland PS, Gstottner W, Adunka O. Method for hearing preservation in cochlear implant surgery. Operative Techniques in Otolaryngology-Head and Neck Surgery 2005;16(2):93–100.
67. Gfeller K, Turner C, Oleson J, et al. Accuracy of cochlear implant recipients on pitch perception, melody recognition, and speech reception in noise. Ear Hear 2007;28(3):412–23.
68. Gstoettner W, Kiefer J, Baumgartner WD, Pok S, Peters S, Adunka O. Hearing preservation in cochlear implantation for electric acoustic stimulation. Acta Otolaryngol 2004;124(4):348–52.
69. Frijns JH, Briaire JJ, Grote JJ. The importance of human cochlear anatomy for the results of modiolus-hugging multichannel cochlear implants. Otol Neurotol 2001;22(3):340–9.
70. Teissl C, Kremser C, Hochmair ES, Hochmair-Desoyer IJ. Magnetic resonance imaging and cochlear implants: Compatibility and safety aspects. J Magn Reson Imaging 1999;9(1):26–38.
71. Youssefzadeh S, et al. MR compatibility of Med El cochlear implants: clinical testing at 1.0 T. J Comput Assist Tomogr 1998;22(3):346–50.
72. Baumgartner WD, Youssefzadeh S, Hamzavi J, Czerny C, Gstoettner W. Clinical application of magnetic resonance imaging in 30 cochlear implant patients. Otol Neurotol 2001;22(6):818–22.
73. Weber BP, Lenarz T, Dillo W, Maneke I, Bertram B. Malformations in cochlear implant patients. Am J Otol 1997;18 (6 Suppl):S64–S65.
74. Graham J, Lynch C, Weber B, Stollwerck L, Wei J, Brookes G. The magnetless Clarion cochlear implant in a patient with neurofibromatosis 2. J Laryngol Otol 1999;113(5):458–63.
75. Graham J. A Scheibe cochlea deformity with macrocephaly: a case for single channel implantation. J Laryngol Otol 1999;113(6):609–10.
76. Liu JH, Roland PS, Waller MA. Outpatient cochlear implantation in the pediatric population. Otolaryngol Head Neck Surg 2000;122(1):19–22.
77. Hamamoto M, Murakami G, Kataura A. Topographical relationships among the facial nerve, chorda tympani nerve and round window with special reference to the approach route for cochlear implant surgery. Clin Anat 2000;13(4):251–6.
78. Briggs RJ, Tykocinski M, Xu J, Risi F, Svehla M, Cowan R, Stover T, Erfurt P, Lenarz T. Comparison of round window and cochleostomy approaches with a prototype hearing preservation electrode. Audiol Neurootol 2006;11 Suppl 1:42–8.
79. Roland PS, Wright CG, Isaacson B. Cochlear implant electrode insertion: The round window revisited. Laryngoscope 2007;117(8):1397–402.
80. Roland PS, Wright CG. Surgical aspects of cochlear implantation: mechanisms of insertional trauma. Adv Otorhinolaryngol 2006;64:11–30.
81. Mens LH, Oostendorp TF, Hombergen GC, den BP. Electrical impedance of the cochlear implant lubricants hyaluronic acid, oxycellulose, and glycerin. Ann Otol Rhinol Laryngol 1997;106(8):653–6.
82. Roland JT, Jr., Magardino TM, Go JT, Hillman DE. Effects of glycerin, hyaluronic acid, and hydroxypropyl methylcellulose on the spiral ganglion of the guinea pig cochlea. Ann Otol Rhinol Laryngol Suppl 1995;166:64–8.
83. Donnelly MJ, Cohen LT, Clark GM. Initial investigation of the efficacy and biosafety of sodium hyaluronate (Healon) as an aid to electrode array insertion. Ann Otol Rhinol Laryngol Suppl 1995;166:45–8.
84. Lehnhardt E. Intracochlear electrode placement facilitated by Healon. Adv Otorhinolaryngol 1993;48:62–4.
85. Colletti V, Fiorino FG, Carner M, Sacchetto L, Giarbini N. New approach for cochlear implantation: Cochleostomy through the middle fossa. Otolaryngol Head Neck Surg 2000;123(4):467–74.
86. Gray RF, Ray J, McFerran DJ. Further experience with fat graft obliteration of mastoid cavities for cochlear implants. J Laryngol Otol 1999;113(10):881–4.
87. Rubinstein JT, Gantz BJ, Parkinson WS. Management of cochlear implant infections. Am J Otol 1999;20(1):46–9.
88. Rubinstein JT, Parkinson WS, Tyler RS, Gantz BJ. Residual speech recognition and cochlear implant performance: Effects of implantation criteria. Am J Otol 1999;20(4):445–52.
89. Pawlowski KS, Wawro D, Roland PS. Bacterial biofilm formation on a human cochlear implant. Otol Neurotol 2005;26(5): 972–5.
90. Kumar A, Mugge R, Lipner M. Surgical complications of cochlear implantation: A report of three cases and their clinical features. Ear Nose Throat J 1999;78(12):913–9.
91. Leach J, Kruger P, Roland P. Rescuing the imperiled cochlear implant: a report of four cases. Otol Neurotol 2005;26(1):27–33.
92. Connell SS, Balkany TJ, Hodges AV, Telischi FF, Angeli SI, Eshraghi AA. Electrode migration after cochlear implantation. Otol Neurotol 2008;29(2):156–9.
93. Cushing SL, Chia R, James AL, Papsin BC, Gordon KA. A test of static and dynamic balance function in children with cochlear implants: the vestibular olympics. Arch Otolaryngol Head Neck Surg 2008;134(1):34–8.
94. Jin Y, Nakamura M, Shinjo Y, Kaga K. Vestibular-evoked myogenic potentials in cochlear implant children. Acta Otolaryngol 2006;126(2):164–9.

95. Enticott JC, Tari S, Koh SM, Dowell RC, O'Leary SJ. Cochlear implant and vestibular function. Otol Neurotol 2006;27(6):824–30.
96. Parkins CW, Metzinger SE, Marks HW, Lyons GD. Management of late extrusions of cochlear implants. Am J Otol 1998;19(6):768–73.
97. Balkany TJ, Hodges AV, Buchman CA, et al. Cochlear implant soft failures consensus development conference statement. Otol Neurotol 2005;26(4):815–8.
98. Luntz M, Hodges AV, Balkany T, Dolan-Ash S, Schloffman J. Otitis media in children with cochlear implants. Laryngoscope 1996;106(11):1403–5.
99. Pettersen G, Ovetchkine P, Tapiero B. Group A streptococcal meningitis in a pediatric patient following cochlear implantation: report of the first case and review of the literature. J Clin Microbiol 2005;43(11):5816–8.
100. Cohen N, Ramos A, Ramsden R, et al. International consensus on meningitis and cochlear implants. Acta Otolaryngol 2005;125(9):916–7.
101. Cohen NL, Roland JT, Jr., Marrinan M. Meningitis in cochlear implant recipients: the North American experience. Otol Neurotol 2004;25(3):275–81.
102. Arnold W, Bredberg G, Gstottner W, et al. Meningitis following cochlear implantation: Pathomechanisms, clinical symptoms, conservative and surgical treatments. ORL J Otorhinolaryngol Relat Spec 2002;64(6):382–9.
103. Reefhuis J, Honein MA, Whitney CG, et al. Risk of bacterial meningitis in children with cochlear implants. N Engl J Med 200331;349(5):435–45.
104. Summerfield AQ, Cirstea SE, Roberts KL, Barton GR, Graham JM, O'Donoghue GM. Incidence of meningitis and of death from all causes among users of cochlear implants in the United Kingdom. J Public Health (Oxf) 2005;271):55–61.
105. Wei BP, Robins-Browne RM, Shepherd RK, Azzopardi K, Clark GM, O'Leary SJ. Assessment of the protective effect of pneumococcal vaccination in preventing meningitis after cochlear implantation. Arch Otolaryngol Head Neck Surg 2007;133(10):987–94.
106. Luntz M, Balkany T, Telischi FF, Hodges AV. Surgical techniques for cochlear implantation of the malformed inner ear. Am J Otol 1997;18(6 Suppl):S66.
107. McElveen JT, Jr, Carrasco VN, Miyamoto RT, Linthicum FH, Jr. Cochlear implantation in common cavity malformations using a transmastoid labyrinthotomy approach. Laryngoscope 1997;107(8):1032–6.
108. Zanetti D, Guida M, Barezzani MG, et al. Favorable outcome of cochlear implant in VIIIth nerve deficiency. Otol Neurotol 2006;27(6):815–23.
109. Mylanus EA, Rotteveel LJ, Leeuw RL. Congenital malformation of the inner ear and pediatric cochlear implantation. Otol Neurotol 2004;25(3):308–17.
110. Arnoldner C, Baumgartner WD, Gstoettner W, et al. Audiological performance after cochlear implantation in children with inner ear malformations. Int J Pediatr Otorhinolaryngol 2004;68(4):457–67.
111. Govaerts PJ, Casselman J, Daemers K, De BC, Yperman M, De CG. Cochlear implants in aplasia and hypoplasia of the cochleovestibular nerve. Otol Neurotol 2003;24(6):887–91.
112. Zhao XT, Han DM, Li YX, et al. [Cochlear implantation in patients with inner ear malformations, clinical analysis of 25 cases]. Zhonghua Yi Xue Za Zhi 2003;83(2):103–5.
113. Luntz M, Balkany T, Hodges AV, Telischi FF. Cochlear implants in children with congenital inner ear malformations. Arch Otolaryngol Head Neck Surg 1997;123(9):974–7.
114. Papsin BC. Cochlear implantation in children with anomalous cochleovestibular anatomy. Laryngoscope 2005;115(1 Pt 2 Suppl 106):1–26.
115. Bhatt S, Halpin C, Hsu W, Thedinger BA, Levine RA, Tuomanen E, Nadol JB, Jr. Hearing loss and pneumococcal meningitis: An animal model. Laryngoscope 1991;101(12 Pt 1):1285–92.
116. Brodie HA, Thompson TC, Vassilian L, Lee BN. Induction of labyrinthitis ossificans after pneumococcal meningitis: An animal model. Otolaryngol Head Neck Surg 1998;118(1):15–21.
117. Nabili V, Brodie HA, Neverov NI, Tinling SP. Chronology of labyrinthitis ossificans induced by Streptococcus pneumoniae meningitis. Laryngoscope 1999;109(6):931–5.
118. Gulya AJ, Steenerson RL. The scala vestibuli for cochlear implantation. An anatomic study. Arch Otolaryngol Head Neck Surg 1996;122(2):130–2.
119. Balkany T, Gantz BJ, Steenerson RL, Cohen NL. Systematic approach to electrode insertion in the ossified cochlea. Otolaryngol Head Neck Surg 1996;114(1):4–11.
120. Balkany T, Bird PA, Hodges AV, Luntz M, Telischi FF, Buchman C. Surgical technique for implantation of the totally ossified cochlea. Laryngoscope 1998;108(7):988–92.
121. Bauer PW, Roland PS. Clinical results with the Med-El compressed and split arrays in the United States. Laryngoscope 2004 March;114(3):428–33.
122. Bamiou DE, Mahoney CO, Sirimanna T. Useful residual hearing despite radiological findings suggestive of anacusis. J Laryngol Otol 1999;113(8):714–6.
123. Acker T, Mathur NN, Savy L, Graham JM. Is there a functioning vestibulocochlear nerve? Cochlear implantation in a child with symmetrical auditory findings but asymmetric imaging. Int J Pediatr Otorhinolaryngol 2001;57(2):171–6.
124. Ito J, Sakota T, Kato H, Hazama M, Enomoto M. Surgical considerations regarding cochlear implantation in the congenitally malformed cochlea. Otolaryngol Head Neck Surg 1999;121(4):495–8.
125. Roland JT, et al. Shaw scalpel in revision cochlear implant surgery. Ann Otol Rhinol Laryngol Suppl 2000;185:23–5.
126. Balkany TJ, Hodges AV, Gomez-Marin O, Bird PA, Dolan-Ash S, Butts S, Telischi FF, Lee D. Cochlear reimplantation. Laryngoscope 1999;109(3):351–5.
127. Balkany T, Hodges AV, Goodman K. Ethics of cochlear implantation in young children. Otolaryngol Head Neck Surg 1999;121(5):673–5.
128. Henson AM, Slattery WH, III, Luxford WM, Mills DM. Cochlear implant performance after reimplantation: A multicenter study. Am J Otol 1999;20(1):56–64.
129. Parisier SC, Chute PM, Popp AL, Suh GD. Outcome analysis of cochlear implant reimplantation in children. Laryngoscope 2001;111(1):26–32.
130. Shallop JK, Facer GW, Peterson A. Neural response telemetry with the nucleus CI24M cochlear implant. Laryngoscope 1999;109(11):1755–9.
131. Abbas PJ, Brown CJ, Shallop JK, et al. Summary of results using the nucleus CI24M implant to record the electrically evoked compound action potential. Ear Hear 1999;20(1):45–59.
132. Arnold L, Lindsey P, Hacking C, Boyle P. Neural response imaging (NRI. cochlear mapping: Prospects for clinical application. Cochlear Implants Int 2007;8(4):173–88.

133. van DB, Botros AM, Battmer RD, et al. Clinical results of AutoNRT, a completely automatic ECAP recording system for cochlear implants. Ear Hear 2007;28(4):558–70.
134. Potts LG, Skinner MW, Gotter BD, Strube MJ, Brenner CA. Relation between neural response telemetry thresholds, T- and C-levels, and loudness judgments in 12 adult nucleus 24 cochlear implant recipients. Ear Hear 2007;28(4):495–511.
135. Pedley K, Psarros C, Gardner-Berry K, et al. Evaluation of NRT and behavioral measures for MAPping elderly cochlear implant users. Int J Audiol 2007;46(5):254–62.
136. King JE, Polak M, Hodges AV, Payne S, Telischi FF. Use of neural response telemetry measures to objectively set the comfort levels in the Nucleus 24 cochlear implant. J Am Acad Audiol 2006;17(6):413–31.
137. Brown CJ, Hughes ML, Lopez SM, Abbas PJ. Relationship between EABR thresholds and levels used to program the CLARION speech processor. Ann Otol Rhinol Laryngol Suppl 1999;177:50–7.
138. Shallop JK, Ash KR. Relationships among comfort levels determined by cochlear implant patient's self-programming, audiologist's programming, and electrical stapedius reflex thresholds. Ann Otol Rhinol Laryngol Suppl 1995;166:175–6.
139. Clark GM. Cochlear implants in the Third Millennium. Am J Otol 1999;20(1):4–8.
140. Cohen NL. Surgical techniques to avoid complications of cochlear implants in children. Adv Otorhinolaryngol 1997;52: 161–3.
141. Kelsall DC, Shallop JK, Brammeier TG, Prenger EC. Facial nerve stimulation after Nucleus 22-channel cochlear implantation. Am J Otol 1997;18(3):336–41.
142. Smullen JL, Polak M, Hodges AV, et al. Facial nerve stimulation after cochlear implantation. Laryngoscope 2005;115(6): 977–82.
143. Ramsden R, Rotteveel L, Proops D, Saeed S, van OA, Mylanus E. Cochlear implantation in otosclerotic deafness. Adv Otorhinolaryngol 2007;65:328–34.
144. Rotterveel LJ, Proops DW, Ramsden RT, Saeed SR, van Olphen AF, Mylanus EA. Cochlear implantation in 53 patients with otosclerosis: demographics, computed tomographic scanning, surgery, and complications. Otol Neurotol 2004; 25(6):943–52.
145. Bigelow DC, Kay DJ, Rafter KO, Montes M, Knox GW, Yousem DM. Facial nerve stimulation from cochlear implants. Am J Otol 1998 March;19(2):163–9.
146. Gold SR, Miller V, Kamerer DB, Koconis CA. Fluoride treatment for facial nerve stimulation caused by cochlear implants in otosclerosis. Otolaryngol Head Neck Surg 1998;119(5):521–3.
147. Balkany T, Hodges A, Menapace C, et al. Nucleus Freedom North American clinical trial. Otolaryngol Head Neck Surg 2007;136(5):757–62.
148. Gstoettner WK, Hamzavi J, Baumgartner WD. Speech discrimination scores of postlingually deaf adults implanted with the Combi 40 cochlear implant. Acta Otolaryngol 1998;118(5):640–5.
149. Arnoldner C, Riss D, Brunner M, Durisin M, Baumgartner WD, Hamzavi JS. Speech and music perception with the new fine structure speech coding strategy: preliminary results. Acta Otolaryngol 2007;127(12):1298–303.
150. Waltzman SB, Cohen NL, Gomolin RH, et al. Open-set speech perception in congenitally deaf children using cochlear implants. Am J Otol 1997;18(3):342–9.
151. Blamey PJ, Sarant JZ, Paatsch LE, et al. Relationships among speech perception, production, language, hearing loss, and age in children with impaired hearing. J Speech Lang Hear Res 2001;44(2):264–85.
152. Tomblin JB, Spencer LJ, Tye-murray N. A preliminary study of grammatical development in prelingually deaf children with and without cochlear implant experience. Cochlear Implants Article 14D. 2001.
153. Archbold S, O'Donoghue G, Nikolopoulos T. Cochlear implants in children: An analysis of use over a three-year period. Am J Otol 1998;19(3):328–31.
154. Peters BR, Litovsky R, Parkinson A, Lake J. Importance of age and postimplantation experience on speech perception measures in children with sequential bilateral cochlear implants. Otol Neurotol 2007;28(5):649–57.
155. Geers AE, Nicholas J, Tye-murray N, et al. Effects of communication mode on skills of long-term cochlear implant users. Ann Otol Rhinol Laryngol Suppl 2000;185:89–92.
156. Robbins AM, Svirsky M, Kirk KI. Children with implants can speak, but can they communicate? Otolaryngol Head Neck Surg 1997;117(3 Pt 1):155–60.
157. Tobey EA, Geers AE, Douek BM, et al. Factors associated with speech intelligibility in children with cochlear implants. Ann Otol Rhinol Laryngol Suppl 2000;185:28–30.
158. Miyamoto RT, Svirsky MA, Robbins AM. Enhancement of expressive language in prelingually deaf children with cochlear implants. Acta Otolaryngol 1997;117(2):154–7.

Surgery of the Internal Auditory Canal/Cerebellopontine Angle/ Petrous Apex

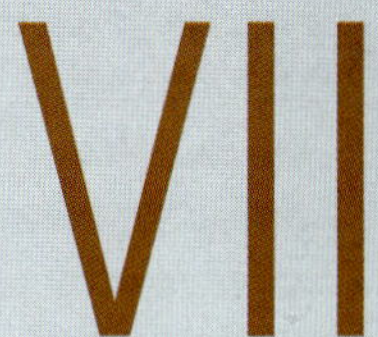

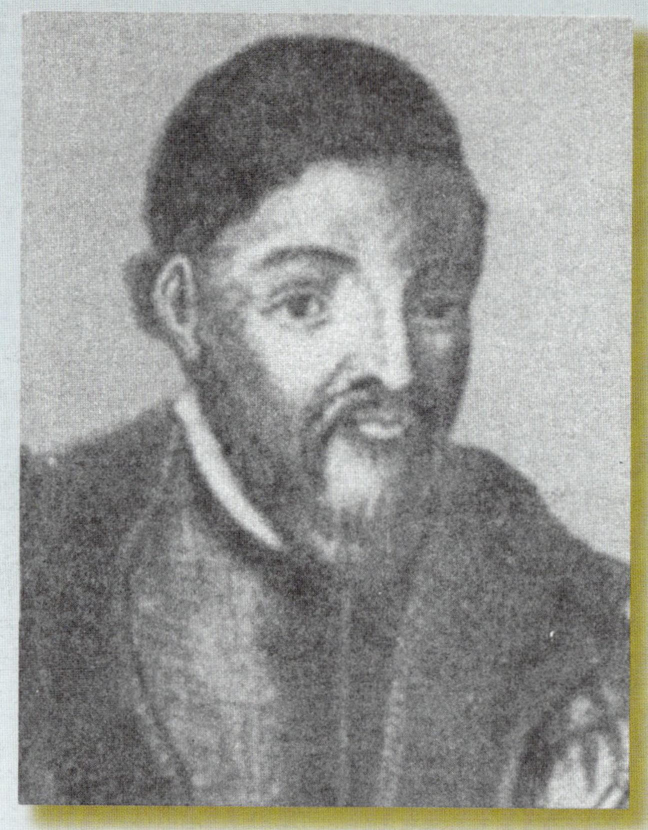

GABRIEL FALLOPIUS (1523–1562) •
Described the fallopian canal for the intratemporal portion of the facial nerve.

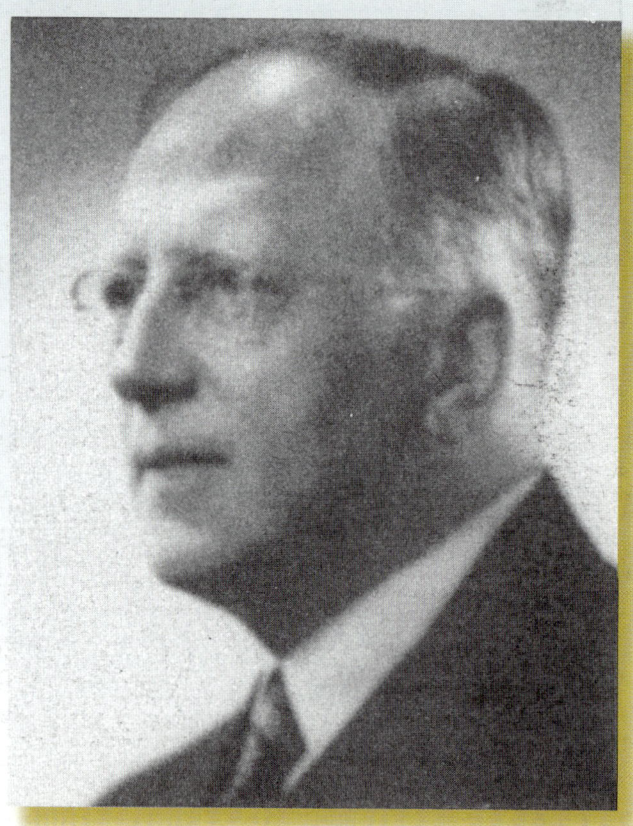

STERLING BUNNELL (1882–1957) •
In 1927, performed the first successful intratemporal suture of the facial nerve and in 1930, the first successful facial nerve graft within the temporal bone.

Surgery of the Facial Nerve 36

Bruce J. Gantz, MD / Samuel P. Gubbels, MD /
Ravi N. Samy, MD

Facial nerve dysfunction causes noticeable disfigurement and emotional distress to those suffering from it. Facial paresis and paralysis affect both voluntary and involuntary motion and can be a detriment to social interaction. More than any other cranial nerve, the facial nerve affects nonverbal humanistic expression, which is a significant component of communication. Facial palsy may also interrupt normal daily functions, such as eating and drinking; more importantly, it may disrupt the protective function of the eye. Before discussing the diagnosis and treatment of facial nerve disorders, one must understand the nerve's complex anatomy, physiology, and function. Management of facial nerve dysfunction is individualized and may include observation, administration of pharmacologic agents, surgical intervention, physical therapy, and psychological counseling.[1] These will be discussed in detail later in the chapter.

ANATOMY

An understanding of the anatomy of the facial (seventh cranial) nerve is essential to diagnose and treat facial nerve dysfunction. The nerve contains approximately 7,000 to 10,000 fibers.[2,3] The facial nerve originates from the facial motor nucleus, which lies in the lateral portion of the anterior pons and is composed of four cell groups. Facial nerve function is highly organized at the central nervous system level. Some level of topographic organization probably continues as the nerve courses peripherally. The facial nerve hooks around the nucleus of the sixth cranial (abducens) nerve. As a result, brainstem lesions involving the seventh nerve also usually involve the sixth nerve.

The facial nerve exits the brainstem at the pontomedullary junction caudal to the fifth cranial (trigeminal) nerve and approximately 1.5 mm anterior, medial, and superior to the eighth cranial (vestibulocochlear) nerve (Figure 36–1).[4,5] The facial nerve is smaller in diameter than the vestibulocochlear nerve (1.8 mm versus 3 mm). The facial nerve then crosses the cerebellopontine angle (CPA) (a distance of 15 to 17 mm) with the eighth cranial nerve and the nerve of Wrisberg (nervus intermedius).[6] The nervus intermedius not only carries secretory fibers to the lachrymal, sublingual, and submaxillary glands, but it also carries afferent fibers conveying taste from the anterior two-thirds of the tongue and sensation from the posterior wall of the external auditory canal (EAC) (see Figure 36–1).[7]

The facial nerve passes through the porus of the internal auditory canal (IAC). The superior and inferior vestibular nerves lie immediately posterior and inferoposterior to the facial nerve, respectively. The cochlear nerve lies caudal to the facial nerve in the IAC. By the lateral end (fundus) of the IAC, the facial nerve has merged with the nervus intermedius. The length of the IAC portion of the nerve is approximately 8 to 10 mm.[6] The facial nerve enters the labyrinthine segment of its fallopian canal through the meatal foramen, which is the narrowest portion of the entire canal and measures approximately 0.68 mm in diameter.[8] The labyrinthine segment (4 mm in length) makes up the first segment of the bony fallopian canal and is the narrowest and shortest portion of the canal.[9] In addition to the small diameter of the meatal foramen, a dense arachnoid band encircles the nerve at the lateral end of the IAC. This band contributes to the anatomic "bottleneck" that can constrict the nerve in disorders that induce edema of the nerve, such as Bell's palsy. Thus, the meatal foramen and labyrinthine segment of the nerve play a pivotal role in the pathophysiology of facial paralysis, as will be discussed later in this chapter. The labyrinthine segment is posterocephalad to the cochlea, anteromedial to the ampulla of the superior semicircular canal, and cephalad to the vestibule.[2] Subsequently, the fallopian canal takes a long (approximately 30 mm), tortuous course through the temporal bone.[10] The fallopian canal provides a bony covering for the facial nerve that is longer than that of any other nerve. This bony encasement protects the nerve but also renders it vulnerable to certain diseases and disorders (Figure 36–2).[7]

At the geniculate ganglion (GG), the facial nerve takes a sharp (75 degree) posterior turn at the first (internal) genu. The GG contains bipolar ganglion cells for the sensory functions of the nervus intermedius. The greater superficial petrosal nerve (GSPN) arises from the GG and emerges through the hiatus of the fallopian canal (facial hiatus) onto the floor of the middle fossa. The GSPN contains secretory fibers to the lacrimal gland

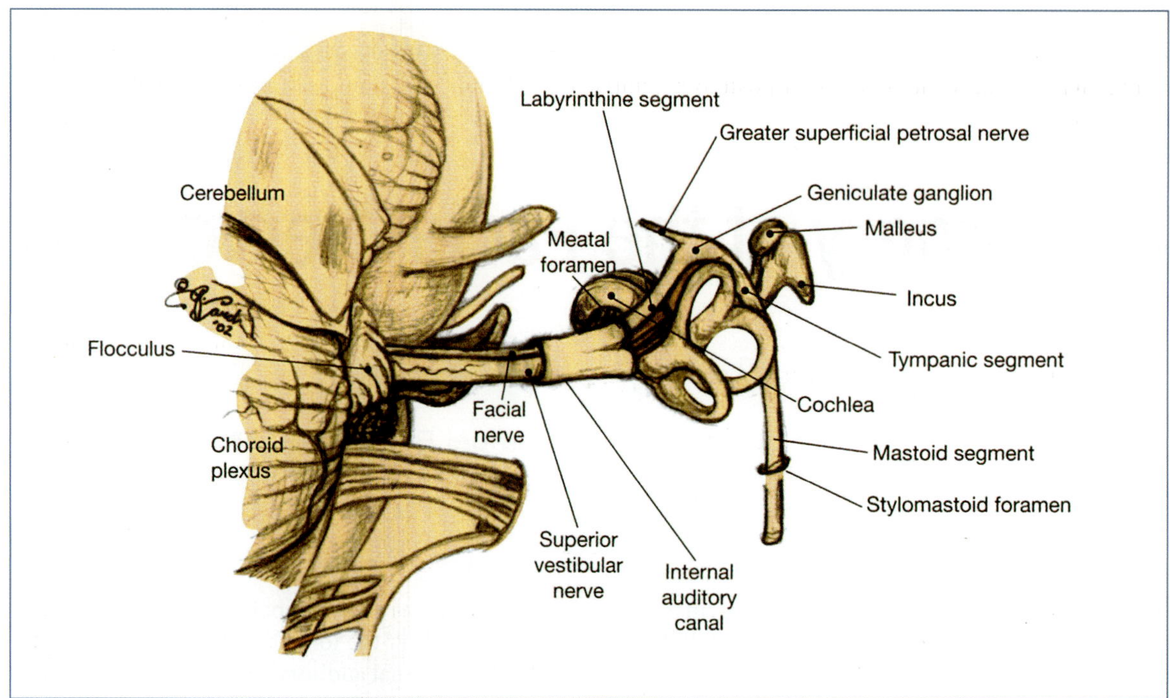

FIGURE 36 –1 • The course and relationships of the left facial nerve from the pontomedullary junction to the intratemporal course.

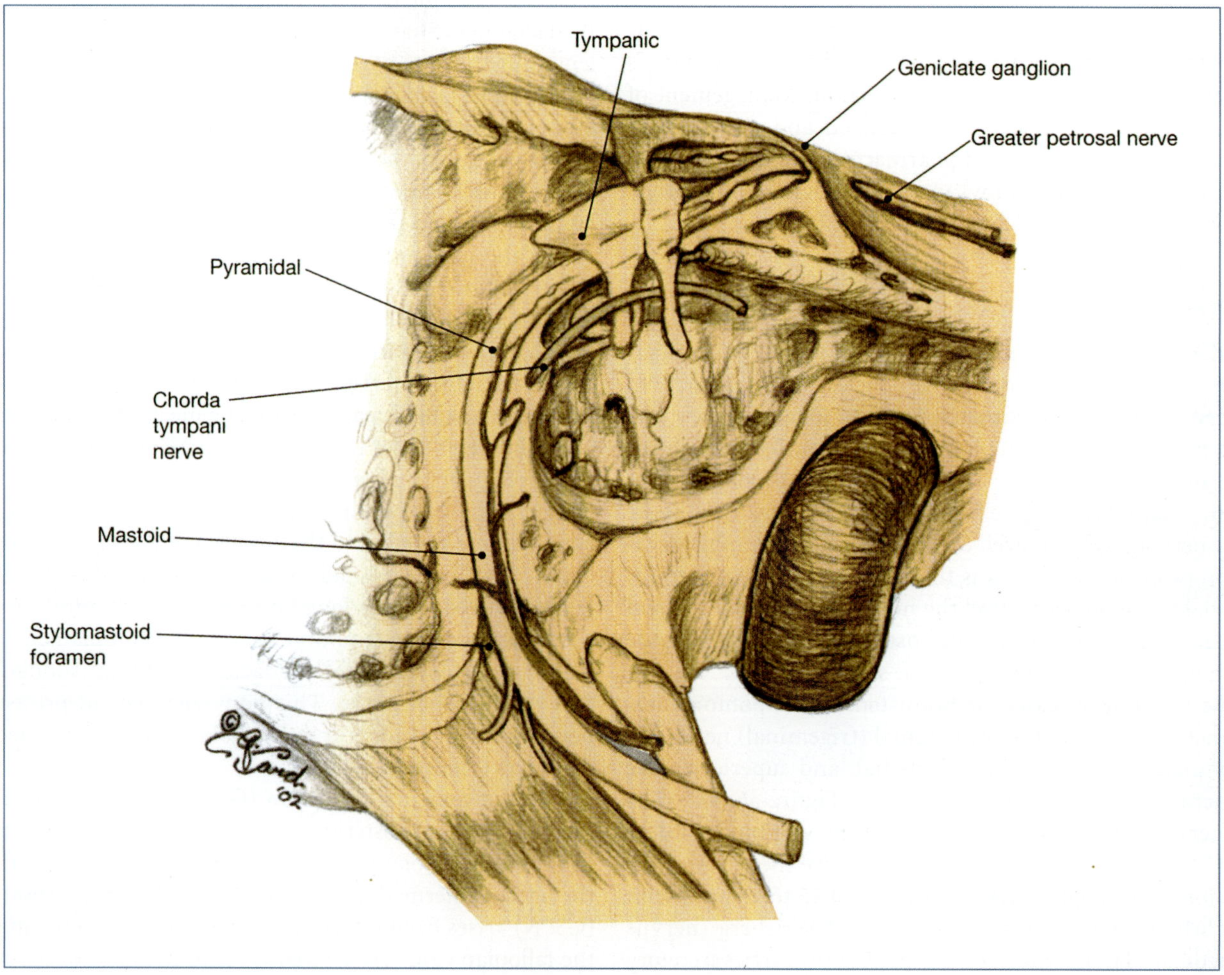

FIGURE 36 –2 • Overview of the facial nerve in its intratemporal course.

that synapse in the pterygopalatine ganglion; postganglionic fibers then innervate the lacrimal gland.[2]

From the GG, the facial nerve courses posteroinferiorly in its tympanic (horizontal) segment, which measures 11 mm in length and is the second segment of the fallopian canal. As the nerve runs posteriorly, a portion of the tympanic segment becomes the cephalad margin of the oval window niche. The nerve then makes a second turn (the second or external genu). At this point, the facial nerve gives off a branch to the stapedius muscle. The facial nerve then proceeds vertically in the mastoid cavity (vertical/mastoid segment), which measures 13 mm in length. Approximately midway in its mastoid segment, the facial nerve gives off the chorda tympani nerve (Figure 36–3). However, the points of origin of the nerve to the stapedius muscle and the chorda tympani nerve can be quite variable—anywhere between the second genu and the stylomastoid foramen.[11] The preganglionic, parasympathetic fibers present in the chorda tympani nerve synapse in the submandibular ganglion; postganglionic fibers innervate the submandibular and sublingual glands.[2] The facial nerve leaves the temporal bone and the fallopian canal via the stylomastoid foramen, lying between the mastoid tip and the styloid process. As the nerve approaches the stylomastoid foramen, it becomes encircled by the fibrous tendon of the digastric muscle, which becomes part of the nerve sheath and firmly attaches the nerve to surrounding structures. Surgical release of the nerve requires sharp dissection of the surrounding muscle to avoid neural injury. At the pes anserinus in the parotid gland, the extratemporal portion of the nerve divides into the temporofacial and cervicofacial trunks. The major peripheral branches arising from the trunks are the temporal, zygomatic, buccal, marginal mandibular, and cervical.

Minor variations and major anomalies often occur in the course of the facial nerve, predisposing the nerve to inadvertent surgical injury. The most common variation is a dehiscence of the fallopian canal, found in over 50% of temporal bones.[7] The most frequent site of dehiscence is the horizontal segment (91%). An uncovered nerve may herniate inferiorly and obscure the stapes.[12] During embryologic development, the fallopian canal originates from the primordial otic capsule and Reichert's cartilage (second branchial arch). Although ossification of these structures normally begins during gestation and is completed by the end of the first year of life, incomplete ossification often occurs, resulting in exposure (dehiscence) of the nerve.[13] More serious anomalies of the different segments of the intratemporal facial nerve are seen in congenital malformations of the middle and outer ear.[14] In addition, duplications of the facial nerve (bifurcations, trifurcations) have been reported in the mastoid and other segments of the nerve without other associated congenital malformations.[15,16] The discussion of specific malformations and the relative risk to the facial nerve is beyond the scope of this chapter.

HISTOLOGY

Each nerve fiber, consisting of a nerve cell body and an axon, is surrounded by an insulating layer of myelin secreted by Schwann cells. A single nerve fiber is surrounded by numerous Schwann cells, which also provide metabolic support. The

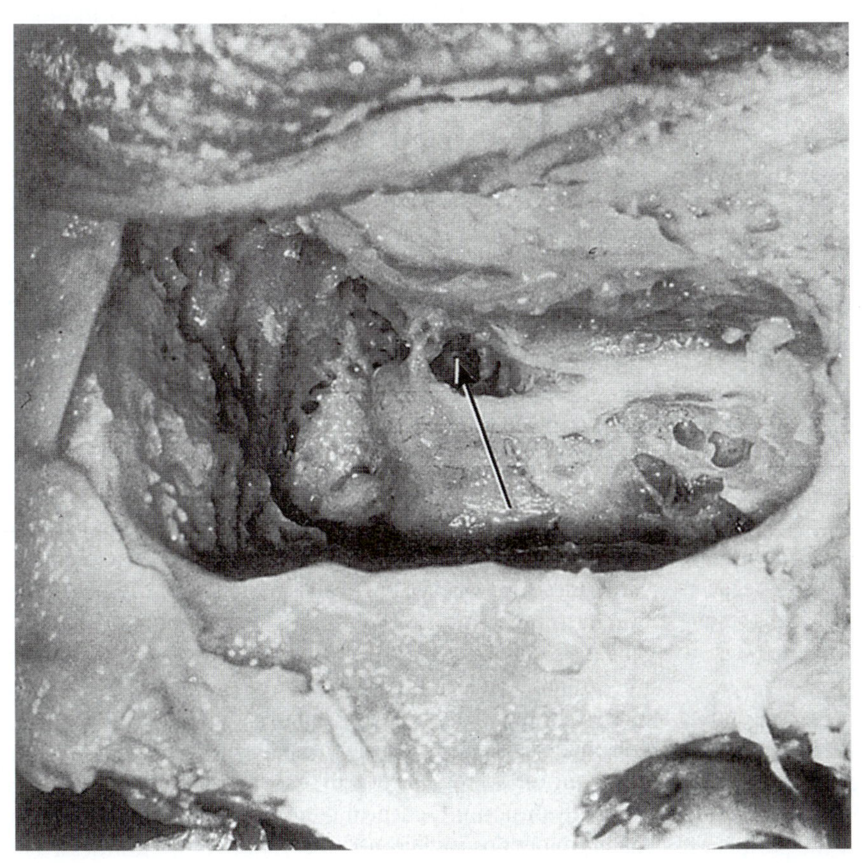

FIGURE 36–3 • The facial recess (arrow) lies between the facial and chorda tympani nerves. The incudostapedial joint is visible just to the right of the arrowhead. *Reproduced with permission from Gulya AJ, Schuknecht HF. Anatomy of the temporal bone with surgical implications. 2nd ed. Pearl River, NY: Parthenon Press; 1995.*

axon relies upon its parent neuron for nutrient replenishment through axoplasmic flow, which proceeds at the rate of 1 mm/day. Each nerve fiber is surrounded by multiple connective tissue layers, endoneurium, forming a tubule. Multiple tubules are bound together in bundles by additional connective tissue (perineurium). Additional connective tissue (epineurium) forms the nerve sheath.[7] The three connective tissue layers are complex in function and anatomy. They play important functions, including resisting stretching, maintaining tensile strength and intraneural pressures, providing insulation and circulation, and minimizing functional deterioration even in the presence of gradually applied deforming forces (eg, vestibular schwannomas or cholesteatomas).[2,7] It is important to note that the cisternal and intracanalicular segments of the nerve are devoid of epineurium, leaving the nerve especially vulnerable to injury with manipulations in these areas.

VASCULAR SUPPLY

The principal arterial supply of the facial nerve is provided by three main sources: (1) the labyrinthine artery, a branch of the anterior inferior cerebellar artery (AICA) (the AICA may lie anterior to cranial nerves VII and VIII or between them in the IAC or CPA); (2) the superior petrosal artery, a branch of the middle meningeal artery; and (3) the stylomastoid artery, a branch of the postauricular artery.[5] These three branches have numerous anastomoses and constitute the extrinsic vascular system, which runs in the epineurium. Veins accompany the arteries in the fallopian canal. An intraneural vascular plexus (intrinsic system) originates from the extrinsic system. This plexus can support segments of the nerve when it is mobilized from the fallopian canal, even when the extrinsic system is disrupted.[7] Lymphatic vessels are located in the epineurial layer.[2,7,17]

PATHOPHYSIOLOGY

In 1943, Seddon described three types of progressive nerve injury: neuropraxia, axonotmesis, and neurotmesis.[18] When pressure is placed on a nerve, the transmission of nerve impulses may be blocked. If the pressure is not sustained for long, release of the pressure usually results in a rapid and complete recovery of function with no residual dysfunction and no distal wallerian degeneration.[19] This type of injury is known as neuropraxia. Axonotmesis is a more severe injury and involves sectioning of an axon or sufficient pressure to block axoplasmic flow.[7] Although endoneurial tubules are preserved, distal wallerian degeneration occurs. Neurotmesis describes total nerve transection (all three protective sheaths are involved). In actuality, there is usually a mixture of the different types of injury unless there has been complete nerve transection. Wallerian degeneration usually occurs over a 72- to 96-h period following injury. Distal nerve excitability is therefore usually maintained for 3 to 4 days following severe injury.[72,19]

A more detailed classification of neural injury was proposed by Sunderland in 1951.[20] He proposed five progressively severe degrees of nerve injury, as opposed to the three types of nerve injuries described by Seddon. However, the Sunderland classification pertains only to traumatic injuries of the peripheral nerve and not to viral, inflammatory, or infiltrative lesions.[21] A first-degree injury is reversible and allows complete recovery. In second-degree injury, wallerian degeneration occurs, but endoneurial architecture is preserved; recovery is usually complete. In third-degree injury, wallerian degeneration and disruption of endoneurial architecture occur. There is incomplete recovery, usually complicated by functional sequelae. Second- and third-degree injuries are approximately equivalent to axonotmesis. Fourth-degree injury reflects significant nerve injury. Only the epineurium is intact, and recovery tends to be poor.[7] Fifth-degree injury involves complete and total disruption of nerve continuity; recovery cannot occur without surgical intervention. In general, the quality of the return of facial movement is inversely proportional to the amount of neural degeneration caused by injury.[22] As facial nerve function returns, most patients and physicians first notice a return of tone to the facial musculature that precedes a return of gross movement.[7]

If the injury is third degree or worse, there is disruption of the endoneurium, perineurium, and/or the epineurium. If recovery does occur, the axon develops a growth cone that begins to bring nutrients to the cell body. Branching of a regenerating axon with protoplasmic threads entering several empty neural tubules usually occurs. In other words, regenerating axon sprouts can enter the endoneurial tube of another axon, resulting in innervation of an inappropriate muscle.[7] Thus, a single axon can innervate widely separated facial muscles, resulting in synkinesis—simultaneous movement of different facial muscles.[2,7] Synkinesis may be cosmetically disfiguring and has been treated temporarily by chemodenervation with botulinum toxin. Animal studies using vincristine have shown a delay in reinnervation of selected muscles. Vincristine may someday be used in patients to prevent the development of synkinesis.[23,24]

Although the rate of axon regeneration is generally thought to be 1 mm/day, the rate of regeneration and overall recovery depend on several variables, including the etiology and severity of the paralysis, the degenerative process, and individual neuronal factors (eg, the longer the duration of degeneration, the poorer the quality of facial nerve recovery). Numerous cellular and systemic factors also affect the recovery process. Patient's age, level of nutrition, blood supply, comorbidities (eg, diabetes mellitus), and concurrent wound infection also influence the quality of regeneration.[72]

CARE OF THE EYE

Before turning to a discussion of facial nerve disorders and their treatment, the most important function of the facial nerve, protection of the eye, must be reviewed. Although facial paralysis is cosmetically displeasing, causes functional discomfort, and impairs communication, the most significant associated complication involves the eye. If the eyelids do not function well, the conjunctiva is not lubricated properly,[7] and the eye becomes dry. If eye dryness occurs in conjunction with other abnormalities, such as decreased lacrimation (eg, owing to GSPN disruption) and/or decreased corneal sensation (because of trigeminal nerve dysfunction), corneal complications are likely to occur, including exposure keratitis, ulceration, and blindness. Thus, one must instruct the patient in proper eye care.

The ultimate objectives in management of the eye are, in order, (1) corneal protection with preservation of vision and eye function, (2) comfort, and (3) cosmetic restoration.[25] If the facial nerve has been severed and an interposition graft inserted, it may take 6 months or longer for orbicularis oculi function to return. During this long period of time, lid loading with gold weight placement, an easily reversible procedure may be performed. Some surgeons prefer a lateral tarsorrhaphy, which can be either temporary or permanent. When significant lower lid laxity develops in a patient with facial paralysis, especially in elderly patients with poor skin tone, lateral canthoplasty should be considered as an adjunctive measure.

For patients whose facial function is likely to return in a short period of time, care of the eye can be accomplished using conservative measures. The patient is instructed to instill artificial tears frequently, even every hour if needed. Many commercially available preparations include various additives to increase the viscosity and slow the rate of clearance and evaporation from the conjunctiva, providing a longer period of moisturization without the blurring of vision that occurs with petroleum-based lubricants. The patient and his/her family member should monitor for conjunctival injection, a sign of irritation and dryness. The complaint of a foreign body sensation also indicates dryness. The patient should use a long-lasting ophthalmic lubricant at night or during the day if asleep. (Some patients prefer routine use of ointment during the day as well.) The patient may consider using a moisture chamber or taping of the eye whenever asleep. Wind protection, through the use of glasses, is recommended. If concerns of impending ocular damage arise, an urgent ophthalmologic consultation is required. Thus, treatment is highly individualized and is affected by the expected duration of paralysis.[2] Patients with an impaired blink reflex on the side of the facial paralysis are at increased risk of complications due to drying of the eye due to the lack of corneal sensation. Aggressive eye care and monitoring is advisable and there should be a lowered threshold for ophthalmological consultation when impaired corneal sensation accompanies a facial paralysis.

EVALUATION OF FACIAL NERVE FUNCTION

Numerous methods of grading facial nerve palsy have been developed since the 1940s.[1] Although no gold standard or universally accepted system exists, the most commonly used scale is the House-Brackmann (HB) facial nerve grading system, which differentiates six grades of facial function (I–VI).[26] The American Academy of Otolaryngology-Head and Neck Surgery has adopted this system to standardize the reporting of disorders of the facial nerve and treatment results. Prior to the adoption of this scale, scientific analysis of data lacked a uniform and objective measure.[2,27] The use of this scale represents a major stride in the objective analysis of facial nerve data (Table 36–1). However, the HB scale is not a perfect grading system because of the problems of interobserver and intraobserver variability.[28–30] Also, the grading system is applicable only to disorders of the nerve proximal to the pes anserinus.[5] The scale is not appropriate for single-branch injuries, such as a penetrating injury to the face affecting only the buccal branch. Future improvement in grading the status of facial nerve function may involve the use of digitalized images or computerized dynamic functional analysis.[31] Additionally, others have suggested the inclusion of

TABLE 36–1 House-Brackman nerve grading system

GRADE	DESCRIPTION	CHARACTERISTICS
I	Normal	Normal facial function in all areas
II	Mild dysfunction	Gross: slight weakness noticeable on close inspection; may have very slight synkinesis At rest: normal symmetry and tone Motion: forehead—moderate to good function; eye—complete closure with minimum effort; mouth—slight asymmetry
III	Moderate dysfunction	Gross: obvious but not disfiguring difference between two sides; noticeable but not severe synkinesis; contracture and/or hemifacial spasm At rest: normal symmetry and tone Motion: forehead—slight to moderate movement; eye—complete closure with effort; mouth—slightly weak with maximum effort
IV	Moderately severe dysfunction	Gross: obvious weakness and/or disfiguring asymmetry At rest: normal symmetry and tone Motion: forehead—none; eye—incomplete closure; mouth—asymmetric with maximum effort
V	Severe dysfunction	Gross: only barely perceptible motion At rest: asymmetry Motion: forehead—none; eye—incomplete closure; mouth—slight movement
VI	Total paralysis	No movement

Adapted from House JW, Brackmann DE. Facial nerve grading system. Otolaryngol Head Neck Surg. 1985;93(2):146–7.

TABLE 36–2 Repaired facial nerve recovery scale

SCORE	FUNCTION
A	Normal facial function
B	Independent movement of eyelids and mouth, slight mass motion, slight movement of forehead
C	Strong closure of eyelids and oral sphincter, some mass motion, no forehead movement
D	Incomplete closure of eyelids, significant mass motion, good tone
E	Minimal movement in any branch, poor tone
F	No movement

Adapted from Gidley et al.[32]

a patient-based system to measure overall impairment and disability, which would assist in evaluating quality-of-life issues affected by facial disfigurement.[1]

At the University of Iowa, we use a different grading system, known as the repaired facial nerve recovery scale (RFNRS), for nerve resections repaired by neurorrhaphy or interposition grafting (Table 36–2).[32] Like the HB scale, the RFNRS has six grades but uses letters instead of numbers (grades A to F). There is some correlation between the two grading systems, with grade A approximately equivalent to grade I, grade B to grade II, and so on.[26] The HB scale is not useful in assessing transected or repaired nerves for three reasons: (1) all repairs cause mass movement; (2) most patients can eventually close their eyes and have good oral sphincter function; and (3) almost no patients are able to raise their eyebrow or forehead. The HB system works well as long as there is an intact nerve sheath or incomplete nerve injury (ie, Sunderland grades I–IV).[32]

EVALUATION OF PATIENTS WITH FACIAL NERVE DISORDERS

There is no substitute for a thorough history and physical examination in the evaluation of a patient with a facial nerve disorder. Factors that are assessed include date of onset, rapidity of progression, comorbidities, risk factors, duration of symptoms, and associated symptoms.

For example, a description of otalgia associated with auricular vesicles is a sign of Ramsay Hunt syndrome and not of Bell's palsy. The physical examination includes a thorough head and neck examination, with an assessment for cervical lymphadenopathy and parotid gland pathology, which is suggestive of a malignant process. The auricle and external ear are examined closely for lesions consistent with Ramsay Hunt syndrome. The tympanic membrane and mesotympanum are examined with an otomicroscope (with pneumatic evaluation). All branches of the facial nerve are examined. If the forehead branches are intact but all other branches are paralyzed, a central etiology is likely. Involvement of a single branch tends to indicate a lesion distal to the pes anserinus in the parotid. Evaluation of the cerebellum and other cranial nerves is also performed. Other components of the general physical examination are performed as warranted by symptomatology.

Laboratory studies are performed as warranted. For bilateral facial palsy, additional testing includes the following: a complete blood count (looking for infection, leukemia), erythrocyte sedimentation rate (vasculitis), blood chemistry (diabetes mellitus), human immunodeficiency tests, fluorescent treponemal antibody tests (syphilis), or a lumbar puncture with cerebrospinal fluid (CSF) examination (Lyme disease, multiple sclerosis, Guillain-Barré syndrome).[22,33]

Audiometry plays an important role in the evaluation of facial paralysis. Every patient undergoes a pure-tone air and bone conduction audiogram, testing of speech reception threshold and speech discrimination, and tympanometry. Findings on the audiogram should be symmetric; if they are not, a retrocochlear workup is performed. For example, a unilateral sensorineural hearing loss on the same side of the facial paralysis may indicate a tumor in the IAC or CPA (or possibly Ramsay Hunt syndrome).[18] Additional audiometric studies, such as acoustic reflex decay or auditory brainstem response testing, can also be used to detect retrocochlear lesions. If vestibular complaints or abnormalities are detected, an electronystagmogram (ENG) and rotary chair testing are performed.

If the patient presents with the classic findings and history of Bell's palsy, radiographic imaging is not performed. However, if symptoms, signs, audiometry, or any additional testing is abnormal, imaging studies are obtained. Radiographic studies are also performed if no return of facial function is noted within 6 months of the onset of Bell's palsy, which is suggestive of a tumor. Plain films and polytomography no longer play a role in diagnosis. Fine-cut computed tomographic (CT) scans of the temporal bone (in the axial and coronal planes) and magnetic resonance imaging with gadolinium (Gd-MRI) play complementary roles. Gadolinium MRI of the brain and brainstem is useful in establishing the presence of lesions in the CPA or IAC, such as a facial nerve neuroma or vestibular schwannoma. The soft tissue detail of the MRI complements the CT scan's high-resolution views of the osseous structures of the temporal bone, including the fallopian canal and its anatomic relations. Computed tomographic evaluation of the temporal bone is helpful in determining the presence of intratemporal tumors, cholesteatomas, and fractures. In some instances, MR angiograms and/or conventional arteriography are indicated if there is a concern about the presence of a vascular lesion, such as a glomus tumor.

Topodiagnostic testing (eg, taste and saliva testing, Schirmer's tear test, stapedial reflex) is of historical significance only and, because of questionable accuracy and clinically imprecise administration, has been replaced by more objective and accurate investigations. Topodiagnostic tests evaluate different functions of the nerve to determine the site of the abnormality or lesion. However, since the loss of nerve impulse propagation is an electrophysiologic event, an electrodiagnostic test is employed to determine the site of injury and prognosis, helping separate which patients will fully recover from those likely to exhibit incomplete return of function.[34,35]

ELECTROPHYSIOLOGIC TESTING

Electrical testing evaluates the condition of the nerve and establishes the degree of dysfunction. Electroneurography (ENOG) and electromyography (EMG) are the two most precise and objective electrical diagnostic tests used to assess facial paralysis. They have replaced maximal stimulus and nerve excitability testing and other subjective electrical tests. Electrical testing is not employed if a patient exhibits paresis since the presence of even minimal voluntary motion indicates minor injury with a high probability of full recovery.

Electroneurography can estimate the amount of severe nerve fiber degeneration. It is most useful between 4 and 21 days after the onset of complete paralysis.[22] Since it takes 3 days for wallerian degeneration to occur after a severe injury, ENOG is not performed until the fourth day. The interpretation of much of the initial diagnostic information gathered with ENOG was based on the observation of patients with Bell's palsy. Subsequently, ENOG has been used in a variety of other conditions, including trauma and acute otitis media; however, it does not appear to be as useful in Ramsay Hunt syndrome owing to the multiple sites of injury in this disorder.[19,36,37]

Electroneurography uses an evoked, supramaximal electrical stimulus to activate the facial nerve as it exits the temporal bone at the stylomastoid foramen. The technique of performing ENOG can influence the results.[22,38] The technical aspects of test performance must be standardized if ENOG is to provide relevant clinical information regarding prognosis of facial nerve function and recovery.[39] Electroneurography provides an objective recording of the evoked biphasic compound muscle action potential (CMAP), which occurs with facial movement. The CMAP is measured with surface electrodes and its presence relies on the synchronous discharge of multiple viable nerve fibers. Supramaximal stimulation is used to obtain the maximum amplitude of the CMAP, which correlates with the number of remaining fibers that can be stimulated. The CMAP from the paralyzed side is compared with the CMAP of the normal side, which serves as control (mean CMAP of healthy nerves is approximately 5,320 μV).[39] A percentage of degenerated nerve fibers is calculated. Degeneration of greater than 90% occurring within the first 14 days of complete paralysis indicates poor recovery in >50% of patients.[35] In addition to the percentage of degeneration, the rate of degeneration is important. Patients who reach a severe level of degeneration in 5 days have a poorer prognosis than those who reach it in several weeks. In other words, if 90% degeneration does not occur by 3 weeks after the onset of Bell's palsy, a good prognosis is indicated.[22]

Electroneurography is not useful after 3 weeks of paralysis as it can lead to a false-negative result due to a phenomenon called deblocking. Deblocking occurs as recovering or regenerating fibers discharge asynchronously in response to a stimulus. Due to the lack of synchronization of neuronal discharge, no CMAP (as measured by the surface electrodes during electroneurography) is generated despite the ongoing recovery that is occurring.[40] EMG testing is performed in cases of long-standing (>3 week duration) facial paralysis or when 90% or greater neural degeneration has been recorded on ENOG.[41] Voluntary EMG measures motor activity using needle electrodes placed in the orbicularis oris and orbicularis oculi muscles when the patient is asked to make forceful facial contractions. In the setting of acute paralysis (<3 week duration), the finding of active motor unit potentials in the presence of complete paralysis and >90% degeneration on ENOG means that deblocking is occurring and that the prognosis for return of normal facial motion is good. In cases of long-standing facial paralysis, one looks for defibrillation potentials that suggest motor end-plate denervation or for polyphasic potentials that suggest reinnervation on routine EMG.

COMMON DISEASES AND DISORDERS OF THE FACIAL NERVE

Facial nerve dysfunction can stem from a variety of causes and may involve the supranuclear tract to the brainstem (intracranial course), the intratemporal segments, or the extratemporal portions. The disorder may even involve multiple segments of the nerve. The paralysis can be idiopathic or caused by trauma, systemic infection, acute or chronic otitis media, metabolic disorders, toxins, vasculidites, neurologic disorders, neoplasms (both benign and malignant), radiation therapy, and numerous other causes.[21] Owing to the limited space in this chapter, only the most commonly associated causes will be presented. The diagnosis and management of Bell's palsy, as discussed below, will serve as a paradigm in the treatment of other facial nerve disorders.

IDIOPATHIC FACIAL PARALYSIS (BELL'S PALSY)

Bell's palsy is named after the British physician Sir Charles Bell, who described the onset, physical findings, and course of the disease in 1821.[42] However, some historical records have shown that Nicolaus A Friedrich of Wurzburg published an account of three patients with idiopathic peripheral facial nerve paralysis 23 years before Bell's report (1798).[43] Although Bell's palsy is the most common cause of facial palsy (nearly three-fourth of cases),[44] with an incidence of 20 to 30 cases per 100,000 individuals per year,[45] it is still a diagnosis of exclusion.[35]

Bell's palsy is an acute, unilateral, peripheral facial paralysis. Although frequently called idiopathic facial paralysis, a viral etiology is the most likely cause; numerous studies have identified herpes simplex virus 1 (HSV-1) as the causative agent,[46–48] and it has been found in patients who have undergone decompression for Bell's palsy.[49] In an animal model of Bell's palsy, it has been demonstrated that HSV inoculation can cause a transient facial paralysis.[50] Polymerase chain reaction (PCR) assays have been performed on fresh and stored geniculate ganglions obtained from temporal bone specimens and have detected HSV-1.[34,46,51] (In a similar fashion, the presence of varicella-zoster virus [VZV] DNA has been shown in patients affected by herpes-zoster oticus, also called Ramsay Hunt syndrome.)[52]

There is no sex predilection for Bell's palsy. A person of any age may be affected, with those in the fifth and sixth decades of life most at risk.[53] The age of the patient is also important because older patients tend to have a poorer recovery. Right- and left-sided disease occurs equally and bilateral involvement (simultaneous or consecutive) has been described.[54] Recurrence is seen in 7 to 12% of patients;[55,56] however, recurrence should heighten suspicion for another etiology, such as a tumor involving the facial nerve. Pregnancy, and particularly the development of pre-eclampsia during pregnancy increases the risk of developing acute facial palsy.[57–59] Approximately 10% of patients have a family history of Bell's palsy. A substantial proportion of patients have an upper respiratory tract infection preceding (by 7–10 days) the onset of paralysis and a seasonal variance in the incidence of Bell's palsy has been noted in some epidemiological areas.[45,60,61]

The facial paralysis in Bell's palsy may be abrupt in onset and can progress to complete paralysis over 1 to 7 days. However, the paralysis is not slowly progressive (over weeks to months), a finding more consistent with a primary facial nerve tumor or malignant process. Other symptoms that tend to rule out Bell's palsy include facial twitching, hearing loss, vestibular dysfunction, otorrhea, and severe, unrelenting otalgia.[35]

The pathophysiology of Bell's palsy involves nerve swelling within the inelastic fallopian canal. The edema and inability to expand beyond the bony confines creates a conduction block, preventing axoplasmic flow. The site of inhibition of nerve impulse propagation is at the narrowest portion of the fallopian canal, the meatal foramen (0.68 mm)[8] (Figure 36–4).

The natural history of Bell's palsy dictates recovery, usually beginning within 3 weeks. Full recovery typically occurs within 6 months. Unfortunately, approximately 15% of patients experience severe deformity, with minimal return of facial movement. Another 15% of patients experience asymmetric movement and/or synkinesis.[62] Thus, despite a good prognosis for 70% of patients, there are approximately 8,000 people in the United States each year with permanent and disfiguring facial weakness.[63] Identification of patients at risk of poor recovery must be accomplished within 2 weeks of onset of complete paralysis if surgical intervention is to be an option.

The medical management of Bell's palsy has been the subject of a great deal of debate. Central to this debate has been the use of steroids in Bell's palsy with many studies finding improved facial nerve outcomes when steroid treatment was initiated early in the course of the disease.[53,63–69] Some studies have called the efficacy of steroid treatment into question,[70,71] especially in children.[69,72–74] It is important that medical treatment be initiated within the first two weeks if they are to be of any benefit. The authors treat patients with Bell's palsy with high-dose oral corticosteroids (prednisone 1 mg/kg or 60 to 80 mg orally, each day) for 10 days, followed by a brief taper. Patients with a history of diabetes mellitus or hypertension or those at risk for these corticosteroid-induced complications are advised to monitor their blood sugar and blood pressure. An oral medication is also given to decrease the chance of gastrointestinal ulceration from the corticosteroids (eg, histamine-2 blocker or proton pump inhibitor).

A number of studies have suggested that the combination of antiviral medications with steroids may be superior to the use of steroids alone in Bell's palsy.[63,75–79] Other investigators have been unable to detect a significant improvement in outcomes with the use of antivirals.[80–82] Given the paucity of side effects seen with antiviral medications and the benefit that has been demonstrated in some studies, the authors treat all patients with valacyclovir (500 mg orally, three times a day). Valacyclovir is the prodrug of acyclovir and is more rapidly and extensively absorbed than acyclovir. Care of the eye, as previously discussed, is instituted as needed. Treatment (other than eye care) is probably unnecessary if facial function is improving on its own at the time of presentation and these

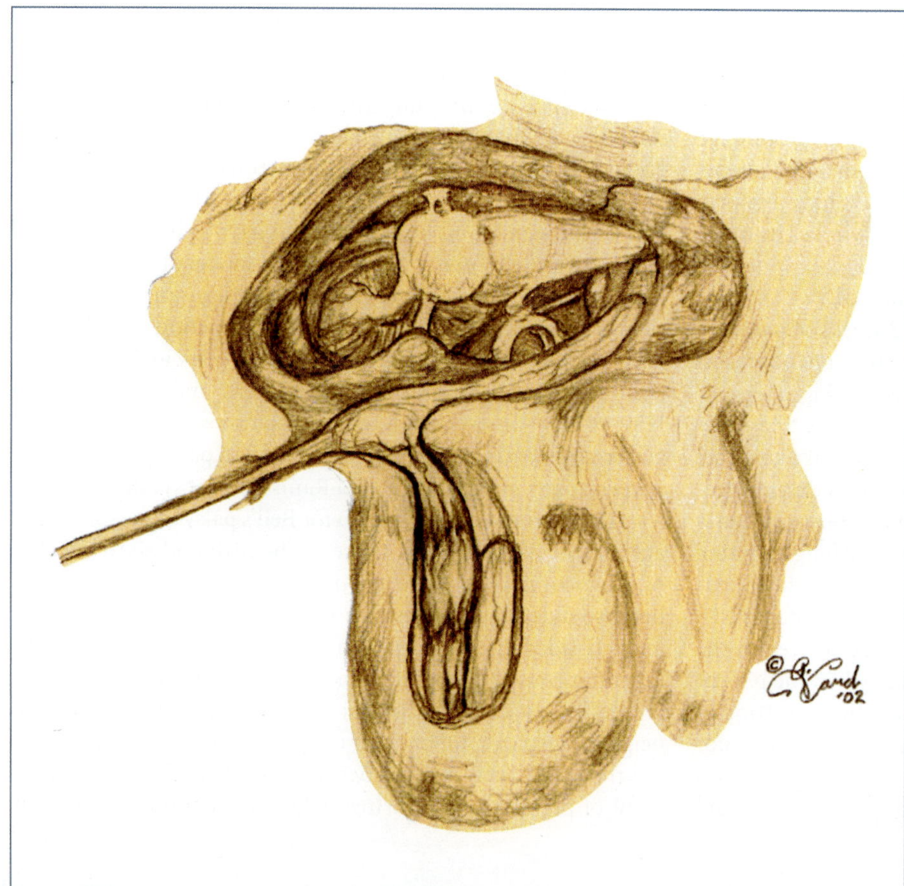

FIGURE 36–4 • Diagram of the labyrinthine segment and meatal foramen. This unique anatomy predisposes the nerve to injury by the pathophysiologic process (edema) of Bell's palsy.

patients are simply counseled and seen again for follow-up in 1 month.

When patients are seen in the acute phase of the disease, medical therapy is initiated and intermittent (every 2 to 3 days) examinations are performed to assess for progression of the disease process to complete facial paralysis. If the patient either progresses to complete paralysis or presents with complete paralysis, an ENOG is obtained 3 days after occurrence of complete paralysis. If degeneration is <90%, the corticosteroids and the antiviral agent are continued for the full treatment course. Electroneurographic testing is repeated every 1 to 3 days until >90% degeneration is detected and no voluntary motor unit potentials are noted on EMG; at that time, surgical decompression is an option. However, if >90% degeneration occurs after the 2-week window, surgery is not an option.[83] After 14 days of paralysis, surgical decompression does not alter the outcome, and its potential risks outweigh any potential benefit. Electromyographic testing, but not ENOG testing, is performed if patients present more than 3 weeks after the onset of paralysis and have no facial movement.

Surgical management of Bell's palsy has evolved along with the understanding of the pathophysiology of the disease.[5] Facial nerve decompression was first suggested in 1923 but not performed until 1931.[84] Since that time, surgical decompression has been very controversial.[85] A landmark multicenter, prospective study was published by the senior author.[83] In this study, middle cranial fossa (MCF) decompression more than doubled the chances of good facial nerve recovery (HB grade I or II) compared to medical treatment alone. The findings were highly statistically significant ($P = .0002$). Thus, at the University of Iowa, all patients with more than 90% neuronal degeneration within 2 weeks of onset, who are under 65 years of age and without any medical contraindications, are counseled to undergo MCF surgical decompression of the meatal foramen, labyrinthine segment, GG, and proximal tympanic portion. However, facial nerve decompression is a very technically challenging procedure and should be performed only in centers experienced in the MCF approach.[5] Transmastoid decompression does not provide access to enable adequate decompression of the meatal foramen or labyrinthine segments of the facial nerve and therefore does not have any role in the treatment of Bell's palsy. Our algorithm for management of Bell's palsy is outlined in Figure 36–5.

TRAUMATIC FACIAL PARALYSIS

Temporal bone fractures, blunt or penetrating head and neck trauma, and iatrogenic surgical injury are all common causes of facial nerve injury. Motor vehicle accidents account for a

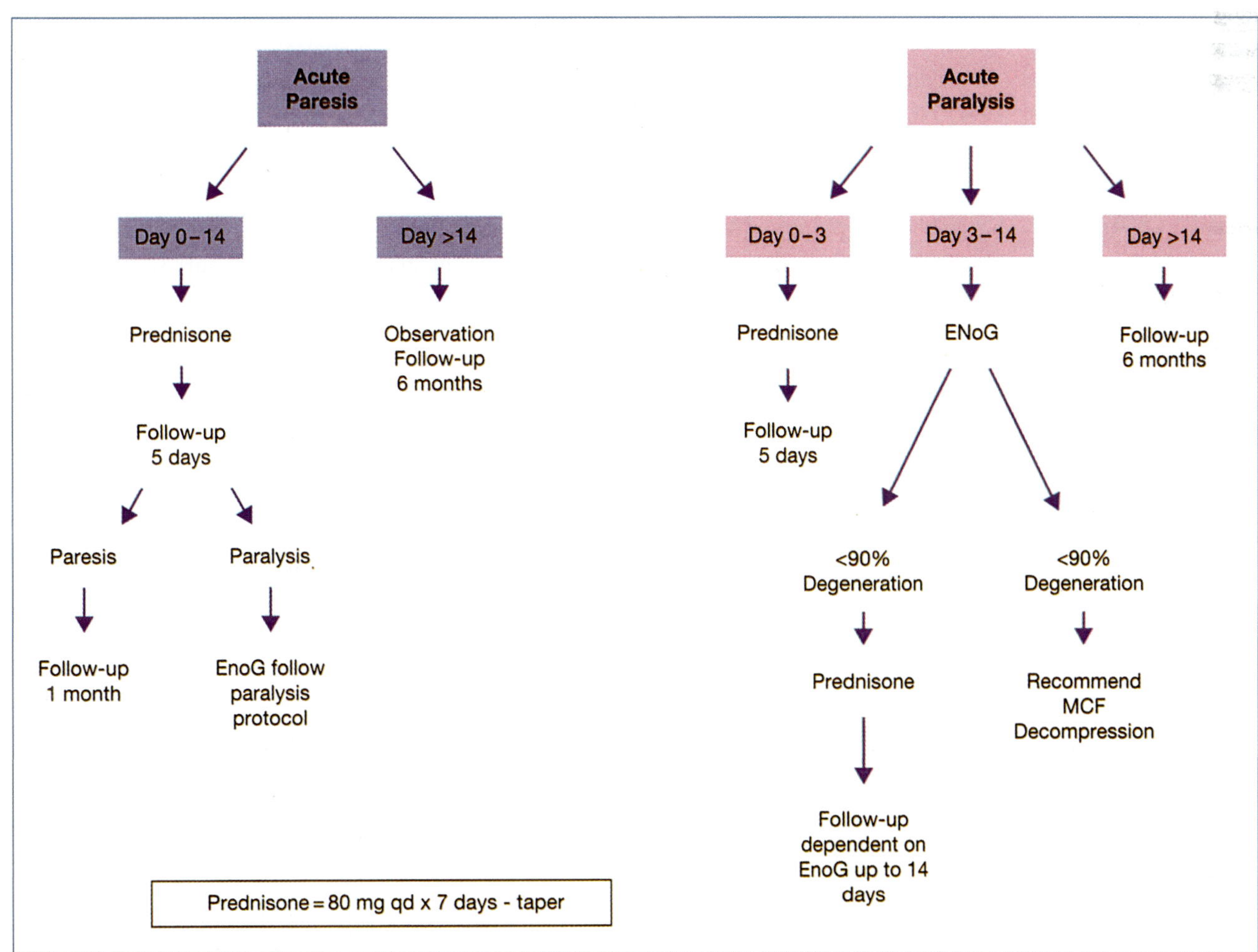

FIGURE 36–5 • Bell's palsy management algorithm. ENOG, electroneurography; MCF, middle cranial fossa. *Adapted from Gantz BJ and colleagues.*[41]

substantial proportion of the injuries, although the incidence of posttraumatic facial palsy is decreasing due to the use of seat belts and airbags.[86] The treatment of trauma-related dysfunction depends on many of the same factors listed above for Bell's palsy. After a thorough history and physical examination, an audiogram and electrodiagnostic tests are performed. Additionally, radiologic studies (temporal bone CT scans—fine-cut, axial, and coronal planes, bone window) assist in the determination of the site of the injury, which may involve multiple segments; unfortunately, imaging may not always be able to pinpoint the area of injury.

Animal experiments have shown that traumatic injuries requiring surgical repair exhibit 90% or greater neural degeneration within 1 week after the onset of the injury. In addition, the timing of the onset of the paralysis gives a clue as to the mechanism of injury; delayed paralysis most likely reflects nerve edema from the trauma (or viral reactivation), whereas immediate paralysis suggests nerve disruption or a severe compression injury, such as a bone fragment.[22] In some cases, it may be difficult to establish whether the onset of paralysis was immediate since the patient may be unconscious on arrival to the hospital. Electrodiagnostic testing, however, can be performed on an unconscious patient when suspicion of a traumatic facial paralysis exists after waiting for a period of 72 h to allow for Wallerian degeneration to occur, prior to electroneurography. Occasionally, bilateral paralysis is not noted because of an absence of asymmetry.[7]

Temporal bone fractures are classified as either longitudinal (along the long axis of the petrous pyramid), transverse (at right angles to the petrous pyramid), or mixed/complex/oblique. Trauma to the temporal and parietal regions of the skull tends to produce longitudinal fractures, which make up the majority (90%) of temporal bone fractures. These fractures cause conductive hearing loss by traversing the tympanic membrane and the tympanic cavity and by causing a hemotympanum. Facial paralysis occurs in 20 to 25% of longitudinal fractures, usually in the perigeniculate region, where a shearing force can disrupt the nerve, penetrate the nerve sheath, or stretch the nerve.[22]

Occipital trauma causes transverse fractures, which make up less than 10% of temporal bone fractures. Transverse fractures manifest with sensorineural hearing loss and vestibular dysfunction owing to involvement of the otic capsule or the IAC. Although less common than longitudinal fractures, they are more likely to cause facial nerve damage, occurring in up to 50% of fractures.[22] In transverse fractures, the facial nerve is usually injured at its labyrinthine segment.

In general, traumatic injury to the facial nerve often requires exploration and nerve repair. As will be discussed later in this chapter, grafts are used frequently in nerve repair, although grafting in a traumatized temporal bone may be difficult. The surgical approach is determined by the portion of the facial nerve affected and the amount of residual hearing. Potential surgical routes include the translabyrinthine, transcanal, transmastoid, or middle fossa approaches (which may be used singly or in combination).[86] In cases of immediate facial paralysis associated with extratemporal facial nerve trauma (laceration), repair should be performed within 72 h of an injury, allowing identification of distal segments electrically before Wallerian degeneration occurs.[22] When complete facial paralysis occurs associated with temporal bone fracture or trauma, electrophysiological testing is performed starting after 72 h and the decision to intervene surgically is made based on the criteria listed above (See Electrophysiological Testing).[22,87] If possible, exploration and repair are performed within the first week of injury before granulation tissue formation and scarring have occurred as these can complicate repair of the nerve.[22] Only in cases of complete facial paralysis associated with an obvious fallopian canal fracture and nerve transection clearly evident on CT might one proceed with surgical intervention without first performing electrophysiological testing.

In many cases of facial nerve injury associated with blunt temporal bone trauma, the paralysis may not be discovered or confirmed for a number of days given the high incidence of brain or other injuries that may have required the patient to be intubated and sedated after the trauma. In these cases or in cases of delayed facial paralysis after blunt temporal bone trauma, electrodiagnostic testing can help guide decision-making regarding the need for surgical intervention. Many surgeons employ similar testing criteria used for surgical candidacy in cases of Bell's palsy as a guideline for operative intervention in these cases.[22,88–90] Surgical decompression of all nerve segments affected by the temporal bone fracture should be performed using the middle fossa, transmastoid, or translabyrinthine (in cases where no serviceable hearing remains) routes as appropriate. In cases where no radiologically identifiable affected nerve segment can be found, surgery should aim to decompress the labyrinthine segment of the nerve at a minimum with consideration given to total facial nerve decompression.[22]

Iatrogenic injury to the facial nerve may occur even in the hands of the most qualified otologic surgeon and can occur in the absence of direct trauma. For example, thermal facial nerve damage may occur due to a diamond burr when inadequate irrigation has been used during drilling. Similarly, removal of disease (cholesteatoma, tumor, granulation tissue) adjacent to the facial nerve can alter the vascular supply of the nerve and result in ischemia with temporary paralysis.[7] In middle ear surgery, the most common site of injury is the tympanic segment due to the high incidence of fallopian canal dehiscence in that region. During mastoid surgery, the facial nerve is most commonly injured at the second genu. There are several factors that contribute to iatrogenic facial nerve injury. The injury may result from a lack of technical skill or inadequate anatomic knowledge.[6] In some cases, the injury may occur as a result of congenital malformation, such as dehiscence or duplication. In addition, scarring from previous surgery or erosion of the fallopian canal with exposure of the nerve due to the disease process (eg, cholesteatoma) may render the nerve more vulnerable to inadvertent injury.[6]

Management of iatrogenic facial nerve paralysis relies on an honest evaluation on the part of the surgeon, as to the status of the facial nerve during the procedure. If the patient awakens with an unanticipated facial paralysis after middle ear or mastoid surgery, urgent attention is mandatory. Often the paralysis is caused by the persistent effects of the local anesthetic, and the patient should recover completely within a few hours. The mastoid dressing and canal packing, if present, should be removed or loosened during this period of observation in case excessive pressure is present and impinging on an exposed nerve. If the paralysis persists beyond a few hours, one must decide whether the nerve may have been injured. If the surgeon has any suspicion of an intraoperative injury and the paralysis persists beyond a few hours, exploration should be performed. If the surgeon identified the nerve during surgery and is sure that the nerve is intact, the paralysis probably represents dysfunction caused by edema. Management includes corticosteroid treatment, electrodiagnostic testing, and serial clinical examinations. Some surgeons recommend observation and serial ENOG testing starting at postoperative day 3. If >90% degeneration is found on ENOG on day 3, then exploration is performed. If on exploration it is found that injury disrupted more than 50% of the nerve diameter, the injured portion is resected and either end-to-end anastomosis or interposition grafting is performed. Similarly, if facial nerve disruption is noted during surgery, it should be repaired immediately through end-to-end anastomosis or an interposition graft (ie, intraoperatively) if more than 50% of the nerve was transected.[5] In cases where less than 50% of the nerve was transected during surgery, no direct repair should be undertaken; however, the fallopian canal should be decompressed for one centimeter proximal and distal to the site of injury to accommodate the neural edema that will occur as the area heals. In all cases of iatrogenic facial nerve injury, it is prudent to consult with a colleague experienced in ear surgery to assist with evaluation, decision-making and management.

All surgery involving, or near to, the facial nerve has the potential to injure the nerve. Thus, intraoperative neurophysiologic monitoring (EMG) plays an important role in the prevention of facial nerve injury in otologic and neurotologic surgery. Available monitors have both visual and auditory real-time feedback for use by the operating team.[91] Because electrical monitoring is transiently disabled when electrocautery is being used, surgical draping with a clear plastic drape such that half of the face is visible will allow the surgical nurse to monitor facial movement as an adjunct to neurophysiological monitoring. During neurotologic/skull base surgical procedures (eg, removal of CPA tumors such as vestibular schwannomas), the facial nerve can be injured easily, especially if the tumor is large or adheres to the nerve. Although neurophysiologic monitoring is the "standard of care" in skull base surgery, studies have shown that facial nerve monitoring can aid in the surgical decision-making process and help avert potential injury to the nerve in tympanomastoid surgery as well.[92,93] Although monitoring is no substitute for experience gained in the temporal bone laboratory or operating room, it is a valuable tool that can be useful to surgeons at all levels. Monitoring may help in identification and localization of the facial nerve, guide in safer dissection and drilling, and minimize nerve irritation from direct trauma and traction.[91,94] Monitoring is also useful in locating the site of nerve conduction block in acute facial paralysis as the block is located between the area that responds and the area that does not respond to electrical stimulation.[92] Electrical stimulation at the end of the procedure can be used to confirm the integrity of the nerve.[91] Research has shown that intraoperative electrophysiologic measures of the CMAP correlate with postoperative facial function after vestibular schwannoma resection.[95,96]

Facial paresis or paralysis occurring in a delayed fashion after otologic and neurotologic procedures (delayed facial paralysis) is a well-described phenomenon likely due to viral reactivation within the geniculate ganglion as a result of surgical manipulation. A number of studies have described delayed facial paralysis after tympanomastoid, stapes, cochlear implant, vestibular nerve section, and acoustic neuroma procedures (refs). Delayed facial paralysis occurs most commonly after surgery for acoustic neuroma (2.2–29% of cases)[97–102] but has been described after vestibular neurectomy(0–18%),[103–105] stapedectomy/stapedotomy (0.5–1%),[106–108] endolymphatic sac procedures (1%),[108] cochlear implantation (0.4–0.7%),[108,109] and tympanomastoid surgery (0.38–1.4%).[110–112] Delayed facial paralysis typically occurs between the third and twelfth postoperative day but can present after an interval of several weeks.[102,109,113] A number of studies based on serologic investigations[102,105–107,114] as well as animal experimental data[50,115] suggest that delayed facial paralysis occurs due to reactivation of latent herpes virus particles within the facial nerve as a result of thermal or mechanical manipulations near the nerve during surgery. The majority of patients who experience delayed facial paralysis can be expected to return to normal or near-normal function (HB I–II)[97,99,101,105,109,112] after a period of one to two months, though slow recovery of function may occur in some patients. Some authors have advocated the use of antivirals in the prevention and treatment of delayed facial paralysis after neurotologic procedures,[102,105] though prospective controlled trials will be needed to determine the efficacy of medical therapy given the high rate of spontaneous recovery.[99,101] Prophylactic surgical decompression of the fallopian canal at the labyrinthine segment during translabyrinthine and middle fossa acoustic neuroma surgery has been demonstrated in one study to result in a better recovery profile versus tumor removal without bony decompression, though no difference in the incidence of delayed facial paralysis was noted.[100]

TUMORS INVOLVING THE FACIAL NERVE

Both benign and malignant tumors can affect the facial nerve—in the intracranial cavity, within the temporal bone, and in the parotid gland. Approximately 5% of facial nerve dysfunction is caused by the presence of a tumor.[7] One must differentiate intrinsic from extrinsic facial nerve tumors (eg, a primary facial nerve tumor versus tumor contiguous to the facial nerve or metastatic disease). Extrinsic tumor involvement is much more common than intrinsic as numerous benign and malignant neoplasms occur in and around the temporal bone. Within the temporal bone itself, skull base neoplasms and metastasis from breast and lung cancer are common neoplasms causing facial paralysis in adults, whereas hematologic malignancies (leukemia, lymphoma) are the most common etiologies in children.[21] Management of all of these lesions is beyond the scope of this chapter, as is a complete listing; however, some of the more common tumors are facial schwannomas, congenital cholesteatomas, hemangiomas, glomus tumors, vestibular schwannomas, squamous cell carcinoma, and parotid gland neoplasms. This chapter focuses on lesions of the facial nerve proximal to the stylomastoid foramen.

The most common sign of tumor involvement is a slowly progressive facial paralysis. A facial palsy progressive beyond 3 weeks since onset and with no return of function by 6 months is considered to be caused by tumor until proven otherwise.[7] Benign tumors compress the facial nerve, whereas malignant lesions invade the nerve. Thus, it is sometimes possible to dissect a benign tumor from the nerve without damaging the nerve. However, with malignant neoplasms, the nerve is resected with the tumor.

Early diagnosis of facial palsy caused by tumor relies on a high index of suspicion. In addition to a slowly progressive paralysis, several other clinical features should heighten suspicion of a tumor involving the facial nerve. Twitching of the facial nerve in association with palsy is not seen in Bell's palsy. In addition, recurrent palsy may reflect the presence of a tumor. Pain, although seen in Bell's palsy or Ramsay Hunt syndrome, can also be seen with tumors involving the facial nerve. Involvement of other cranial nerves in addition to the facial nerve is also suggestive of a neoplasm.[7] Evaluation for a neoplastic etiology causing facial palsy includes both CT and MRI scanning.

Vestibular schwannomas are benign tumors and are the most common lesions of the IAC and CPA. Facial paralysis is an unusual manifestation of these tumors and generally signifies an advanced stage of tumor growth. Vestibular schwannomas rarely invade the facial nerve, which generally appears to tolerate the gradual compression seen with these tumors without clinically evident dysfunction. The presence of facial nerve symptoms in a patient with a CPA or IAC mass should raise suspicion for a facial nerve tumor and the patient should be appropriately counseled regarding the intraoperative decision-making that might be encountered if this proves to indeed be the case. In addition, it is possible for a patient with a vestibular schwannoma to have a concomitant Bell's palsy as the true etiology of facial nerve dysfunction. Facial nerve dysfunction may also occur due to local vascular compromise[116] due to tumor enlargement in the IAC.

Nerve sheath and vascular neoplasms make up the greatest percentage of intrinsic facial nerve tumors (although they are relatively rare as a group). These tumors, including facial schwannomas (neuromas), meningiomas, hemangiomas, and glomus tumors,[21] may present with facial weakness relatively early in their course.[116] In general, facial nerve schwannomas are uncommon, slow-growing neoplasms that arise from the nerve sheath anywhere from the CPA to the peripheral branches of the facial nerve.[117] Most facial nerve schwannomas are intratemporal and most often involve the labyrinthine or geniculate segments.[117,118] A recent retrospective review demonstrated that facial nerve schwannomas were more likely to involve multiple segments than a single segment.[118] Management decisions are based on the patient's desires, age, degree of facial function, tumor location, and hearing status.[5] The goal in the management of these tumors is to maximize long-term facial nerve function while minimizing morbidity. At most centers, management typically entails tumor resection with grafting. However, at our institution, a review of 21 patients with primary/intrinsic facial nerve tumors showed that observation is possible, especially for patients with HB grade I or II facial function. Surgical decompression is an option for patients with HB grade II to III facial function. Resection and grafting are recommended for grade IV or worse, in agreement with other authors recommendations.[119,120] Conservative management with either observation or decompression is often an appropriate option since the best facial nerve function result after resection and grafting is an RFNRS grade C, owing to the presence of mass motion. Nonetheless, treatment is individualized; a patient with brainstem compression from a facial neuroma but with HB grade I function would still undergo resection with grafting.

The most common malignant tumor involving the facial nerve is squamous cell carcinoma of the head and neck. The tumor may be a primary tumor of the temporal bone (squamous cell carcinoma of the auricle), an extension from a regional tumor (squamous cell carcinoma of the skin), or a metastatic lesion (eg, from the oral cavity, nasopharynx, etc). Basal cell carcinoma is a locally invasive lesion that usually occurs on the auricle and, if left untreated, can involve the facial nerve. Other malignant neoplasms include sarcomas, melanomas, and adenoid cystic carcinomas of the parotid gland, which have a significant propensity for neural invasion.

INFECTION

Many infections can cause facial paralysis, such as mumps, mononucleosis, and poliomyelitis.[6] Besides Bell's palsy, the most common infectious causes of facial nerve paralysis are acute otitis media (sometimes complicated by mastoiditis), chronic otitis media (with or without cholesteatoma), Lyme disease, necrotizing otitis externa, and herpes-zoster oticus.

Facial paralysis as a complication of otitis media has become rare owing to ready access to medical care and antibiotics.[6] Hospital admission with close observation and institution of systemic antibiotics (initially intravenous followed by oral) are necessary to bring the infection under control. A myringotomy with tympanostomy tube placement is required to allow for drainage and to prevent the development of further complications, such as a mastoiditis or intracranial spread. Fluid is obtained for Gram stain, culture, and pathology (if so desired). Antibiotic selection is then tailored to culture results. Systemic corticosteroids are probably helpful, and their use is based on the premise that at least some of the dysfunction is caused by edema. In some cases, the paralysis is due to a congenital dehiscence of the fallopian canal, a finding present in 55% of normal temporal bones.[12] A CT scan is performed to determine whether there is an associated coalescent mastoiditis, in which case, a mastoidectomy is required. Fortunately, in most instances, recovery of facial nerve function is complete when paresis or paralysis occurs in the setting of acute otitis media. Electrodiagnostic testing should be performed to document the degree of neural injury in cases of complete facial paralysis. If greater than 90% neural degeneration occurs within 2 weeks, the mastoid and tympanic segments are decompressed. Decompression in the face of acute infection is extremely difficult and should be performed only by very experienced surgeons.

Facial paralysis complicating chronic otitis media with or without cholesteatoma is rare, even if the disease destroys the fallopian canal and compresses the facial nerve. Occasionally, granulation tissue can cause irritation of the nerve, edema, and dysfunction. Treatment is surgical; topical or systemic antibiotics are used as adjunctive modalities to control otorrhea and bacterial superinfection. As with acute otitis media, other complications of chronic otitis media include hearing loss, vestibular dysfunction, and intracranial sequelae. A recent study found that 80% of patients who had developed facial nerve dysfunction in the setting of a cholesteatoma had incomplete recovery after treatment of the underlying disease.[121]

Lyme disease is caused by a spirochete Borrelia burgdorferi and has been reported in many parts of the world. Infection by this spirochete can cause a myriad of systemic complications and disorders. However, the most common neurologic manifestation of this disease is facial nerve paralysis. A recent population-based study in Scandinavia found that 65% of cases of pediatric facial nerve paralysis were due to Lyme disease and lymphocytic meningitis was found on CSF analysis in the vase majority of the cases.[122] One study showed that patients suffering from Lyme disease who presented with facial palsy had longer-lived neurologic symptoms than other patients with Lyme disease, especially if antibiotic treatment was delayed.[123] Most, if not all, patients who develop facial nerve palsy due to Lyme disease will have constitutional or other neurological symptoms on presentation.[124] Serologic diagnosis, possibly supplemented by a lumbar puncture and CSF analysis should be considered in cases of peripheral facial palsy when other findings suggestive of Lyme borreliosis (meningeal irritation, bilateral facial paralysis, recent tick bite, erythema migrans) are present.[125] Antibiotic therapy (doxycycline, amoxicillin, cefuroxime) is typically recommended as treatment.[126] though some groups have not found antibiotic treatment to significantly improve facial nerve outcomes in the setting of Lyme disease.[125] An infectious disease consultation is recommended in view of the potential of this spirochete to cause widespread systemic damage.[6]

Necrotizing otitis externa (NOE) classically occurs in elderly patients with poorly controlled diabetes mellitus or in patients who are immunosuppressed (eg, human immunodeficiency virus). Necrotizing otitis externa begins in the EAC and, if left untreated, progresses to involve the temporal bone (causing facial paralysis) and skull base, eventually involving the lower cranial nerves and intracranial cavity. If not dealt with quickly and effectively, NOE can be fatal. It is most commonly caused by *Pseudomonas aeruginosa* but may be caused by other bacteria and fungi as well. Diagnosis includes radiologic imaging (CT and MRI as the situation dictates) and nuclear imaging studies (gallium and technetium bone scans). Dry ear precautions, EAC débridement, topical antibiotics, and long-term intravenous antibiotics are used in treatment. Antibiotics are continued until the gallium scans show no evidence of infection. For those cases that fail to improve with medical therapy, hyperbaric oxygen therapy has shown promise. Surgery (radical débridement of the temporal bone and skull base) is used only in recalcitrant cases and is performed in an attempt to save the patient's life.

Herpes-zoster oticus (Ramsay Hunt syndrome) underlies approximately 3 to 12% of facial paralyses in adults and 5% in children.[6] Ramsay Hunt syndrome, the second most common cause of facial paralysis, has a much poorer prognosis than Bell's palsy and represents reactivation of the virus in the geniculate ganglion. Varicella-zoster virus–infected patients may have a viral prodrome followed by severe otalgia. Vesicles appear in the ear canal and on the auricle within 3 to 5 days of the onset of the paralysis. Patients may also develop sensorineural hearing loss and vestibular dysfunction. The facial paralysis is usually rapidly progressive and other cranial nerves, including V and IX through XII, can be involved. Polymerase chain reaction assays have been used for the early diagnosis of VZV infection and to differentiate it from Bell's palsy.[127] Varicella-zoster virus infections without skin lesions (zoster sine herpete) can occur and can be mistaken for Bell's palsy.

Unfortunately, in nearly half of the cases, Ramsay Hunt syndrome leaves the patient with significant residual facial nerve dysfunction. However, early treatment with steroid and antiviral medication has reduced the long-term sequelae. The combination of antiviral with corticosteroid treatment, has been shown to be more effective than corticosteroids alone.[77,127–130] Since the active phase of Ramsay Hunt syndrome persists for a longer period of time than that of Bell's palsy, the duration of corticosteroid and antiviral is longer than for Bell's palsy (3 weeks versus 2 weeks). Bacterial superinfection of the vesicles may occur and should be treated with oral antibiotics.[21] Due to "skip" regions and diffuse neuritis of the facial nerve, surgical decompression is not recommended in Ramsay Hunt syndrome.

FACIAL PARALYSIS IN CHILDREN

Although facial nerve abnormalities in children include congenital and acquired pathologies, the principles of management are essentially the same as those for adults;[6] however, an identifiable clinical or radiologic cause can be identified in a much higher proportion of children than adults (72% versus 20% respectively).[131,132] The incidence of neonatal facial palsy is approximately 1 to 2 per 1,000 deliveries, most of which (80%) are related to birth trauma. Forceps delivery or cephalopelvic disproportion can injure the nerve in its vertical segment or as it exits the stylomastoid foramen; the lack of development of the mastoid tip predisposes the facial nerve to injury during delivery and during mastoid surgery in neonates and infants.[6] The facial paralysis is usually unilateral and partial. Other factors associated with acquired facial paralysis in children include birth weight exceeding 3.5 kg, intracranial hemorrhage, intrauterine trauma, primiparity, prolonged second stage of labor, and maternal exposure to teratogens (eg, thalidomide).[133] Signs of traumatic paralysis include periauricular ecchymosis and hemotympanum. Bell's palsy is a common cause of facial palsy in children, as in adults; however, the spontaneous recovery rate for children is higher than for adults. Most of the acquired facial palsies (90%) recover without treatment.[6,134]

In the newborn, the differentiation of acquired versus congenital facial paralysis must be made. Congenital facial paralysis has a poor prognosis and does not require urgent treatment. The evaluation and management of the palsy include physical examination for other anomalies or neurologic dysfunction, ENOG, EMG, and radiologic imaging. Electroneurography should be performed within the first 48 h of life. If the distal nerve can be stimulated, the paralysis is most likely caused by trauma; recovery of function is highly likely. One etiology of congenital paralysis is Möbius' syndrome, which can be unilateral or bilateral and involves cranial nerves VI and VII. Möbius' syndrome probably stems from nuclear agenesis.[6] Other congenital disorders associated with facial nerve palsy are hemifacial microsomia and its variant, Goldenhar's syndrome (oculoauriculovertebral dysplasia). Additional congenital syndromes, especially those involving first and second branchial arch abnormalities, can be associated with facial palsy. Miscellaneous causes of facial palsy include bony dysplasia (osteopetrosis: Albers-Schönberg disease) and Melkersson-Rosenthal syndrome (idiopathic recurrent facial palsy associated with fissured tongue and recurrent facial/labial edema).[133]

Facial nerve function that fails to recover after birth, a family history of craniofacial abnormality, other abnormalities (especially neurologic), bilateral palsy, absence of electrical response, and a silent EMG are all consistent with congenital paralysis. A muscle biopsy may be indicated to determine prognosis and management.

SURGERY OF THE FACIAL NERVE

The entire length of the facial nerve, from the brainstem to the parotid segments, is amenable to surgical intervention. When discussing anticipated results with the patient prior to surgery, it is extremely important that the patient have realistic expectations. Unfortunately, the restoration of normal facial motion (in particular, involuntary movement) is beyond the capabilities of modern techniques. The restoration of a dynamic smile with symmetry at rest is an achievable goal;[22] however, such a successful outcome demands that the surgeon have detailed knowledge of the three-dimensional anatomy of the temporal bone,[6] which requires many hours of practice in the temporal bone dissection laboratory.

There are two general surgical methods for rehabilitating a paralyzed face, dynamic and static.[7] Facial reanimation has the best outcome when facial nerve integrity can be re-established and directed by the facial nucleus. Even when this can be accomplished, the wide range of possible results must be clearly explained to the patient. The choice of procedure depends on the circumstances of each individual case. Dynamic rehabilitation may involve multiple procedures, performed singly or in combination: surgical exposure of the nerve with decompression, grafting, end-to-end anastomosis, and nerve or neuromuscular transfers.

Facial nerve electrophysiologic monitoring and visual monitoring (through a clear drape by the scrub nurse) are used intraoperatively. The importance of visual observation—with visualization of the entire profile, including the forehead, eye, mouth, and chin—cannot be overemphasized and serves as a back-up to intraoperative EMG. Due to the electrical feedback or the muting function that occurs with use of electrocautery on intraoperative EMG devices, it is possible that potentially damaging facial nerve stimulation can be undetected by the monitor and may only be reliably detected by the scrub nurse's visual facial monitoring. To facilitate visual observation, the endotracheal tube is taped to the side of the mouth opposite the surgical procedure.[43]

Proper instrumentation is critical to the conduct of a successful procedure. An operating microscope offers unparalleled visualization. When working in the immediate vicinity of delicate structures such as the facial nerve, the largest diamond bur that the operative site can safely accommodate is used. Copious irrigation clears the operative area of debris and dissipates friction-induced heat, which can induce temporary and permanent facial palsy. Although diamond burs are generally safer than cutting burs near the facial nerve (especially for surgeons in training), diamond burs generate more heat.[135] The final eggshell layer of bone overlying the nerve is removed with a blunt elevator to prevent direct, bur-induced damage to the nerve.[6] If neurolysis (incision of the sheath) is planned, disposable microblades are used. Cauterization near the nerve is done sparingly (if at all) with bipolar electrocautery at a low current level.

Regardless of what must be done to the facial nerve, the basic exposure in the temporal bone involves opening the fallopian canal without disruption of nearby neurovascular, intracranial, or inner ear structures. Depending on the site of the lesion and preoperative hearing, the nerve may be exposed via the MCF, translabyrinthine, and/or transmastoid approaches.

For the MCF approach, the patient lies supine with the involved ear facing the ceiling. The surgeon sits at the head of the operating table while the anesthesiologist is at the foot. Prior to induction, antithromboembolic stockings and pneumatic compression devices are placed on the legs to minimize the occurrence of deep venous thrombosis or pulmonary embolism. Facial nerve and auditory brainstem monitoring leads are applied. The anesthesiologist is not allowed to use long-acting paralytic agents. An arterial line, temperature probe, and urinary catheter are placed. The patient is given a dose of prophylactic antibiotics and corticosteroids. The end-tidal carbon dioxide level is dropped to approximately 25 mm Hg by hyperventilation. The side of the head is shaved and the proposed incision site is infiltrated with local anesthetic with epinephrine. The operative site is prepared and draped.

A posteriorly based skin flap measuring approximately 6 × 8 cm is created within the hairline above the ear (Figure 36–6). This flap can be extended into the postauricular area if a transmastoid approach is also needed. The incision is carried down to the level of the temporalis fascia, a large piece of which is harvested for later use to cover the MCF floor. An anteriorly based temporalis muscle flap is elevated from the outer cortex of the skull. Care is taken to prevent injury to the frontal branch of the facial nerve, which lies on the undersurface of the superficial temporalis (temporoparietal) fascia. At this time, the patient is given 250 cc of 20% mannitol over 30 min to induce a diuresis, reducing intracranial pressure and facilitating retraction of the temporal lobe. A 4 × 5-cm craniotomy, located above the zygomatic root and positioned with two-thirds of its width anterior to the external auditory meatus, is created with a cutting and diamond burrs, which allows visualization of dura at all times and minimizes the risk of a dural tear, as can more easily happen with a craniotome. The bone flap is dissected from the temporal lobe dura; care is taken to protect the middle meningeal artery that is sometimes encased within the bone. Dura is elevated from the MCF floor in a posterior to anterior and a lateral to medial direction. Posteromedially, the petrous

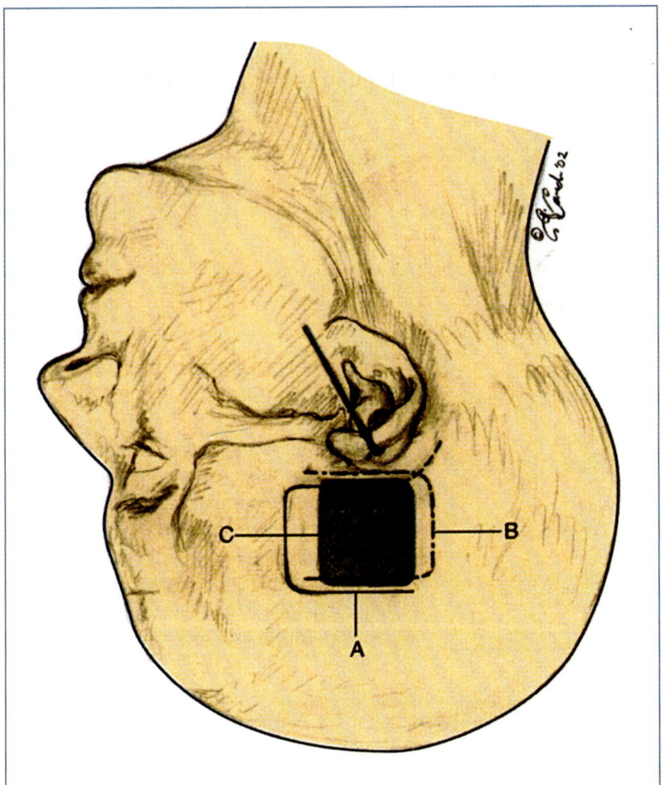

FIGURE 36–6 • The incisions used in the skin and muscle for the middle cranial fossa approach. *A*, Posteriorly based skin flap. *B*, Anteriorly based temporalis muscle flap. *C*, Bone flap.

ridge is identified. The ridge is the medial limit of dissection as the dura is elevated anteriorly to the foramen spinosum, which is traversed by the middle meningeal artery. The microscope is then brought in to view the surgical field. The greater superficial petrosal nerve is identified. Any open air cells are occluded with bone wax to prevent a postoperative CSF leak.

The House-Urban retractor is placed to maintain extradural retraction of the temporal lobe (Figure 36–7). The retractor blade tip is carefully placed at the medial margin of the petrous ridge. The superior semicircular canal (SSC) is identified by slowly removing bone over the arcuate eminence; identifying the yellow-white dense bone of the otic capsule is helpful. If the arcuate eminence is not evident, mastoid air cells are opened posteriorly. Drilling progressively anteriorly reveals the dense otic capsule bone. The otic capsule is slowly removed to "blue line" the SSC. Otic capsule drilling should be done in the direction of the SSC, which is perpendicular to the petrous ridge. Locating the SSC allows identification of the rest of the vital structures of the temporal bone: the IAC, cochlea, GG, and tympanic cavity. A preoperative Stenver's view helps to determine the depth of the SSC from the MCF floor.[6]

The IAC is located by removing bone at a 45- to 60-degree angle anteromedial to the SSC (Figure 36–8) and is followed laterally to the meatal foramen and labyrinthine segment of the facial nerve. The labyrinthine segment and GSPN are used to locate the GG. The thin bone of the tegmen tympani is removed to expose the ossicles lying in the attic. The facial nerve is followed laterally from the GG into the middle ear as far as its tympanic segment at the cochleariform process. The MCF approach is the only route that can gain the necessary exposure of the labyrinthine segment, IAC, and CPA while preserving hearing. At the same time, the MCF approach affords access to the tympanic segment. The MCF approach can be used in combination with the transmastoid approach for access to the entire intratemporal course of the facial nerve; it can be used for facial nerve decompression in longitudinal fractures of the temporal bone and in Bell's palsy, the removal of vestibular schwannomas that do not impinge on the brainstem, and the removal of facial nerve tumors limited to the areas listed above.

Once the surgical procedure is completed, the IAC defect is covered with a temporalis muscle plug; a bone chip can be used to cover any large MCF floor defects to prevent postoperative dural herniation or encephalocele. Care is taken to apply bone wax to air cells in the petrous apex prior to closure to help prevent postoperative CSF leakage. The retractor is removed and

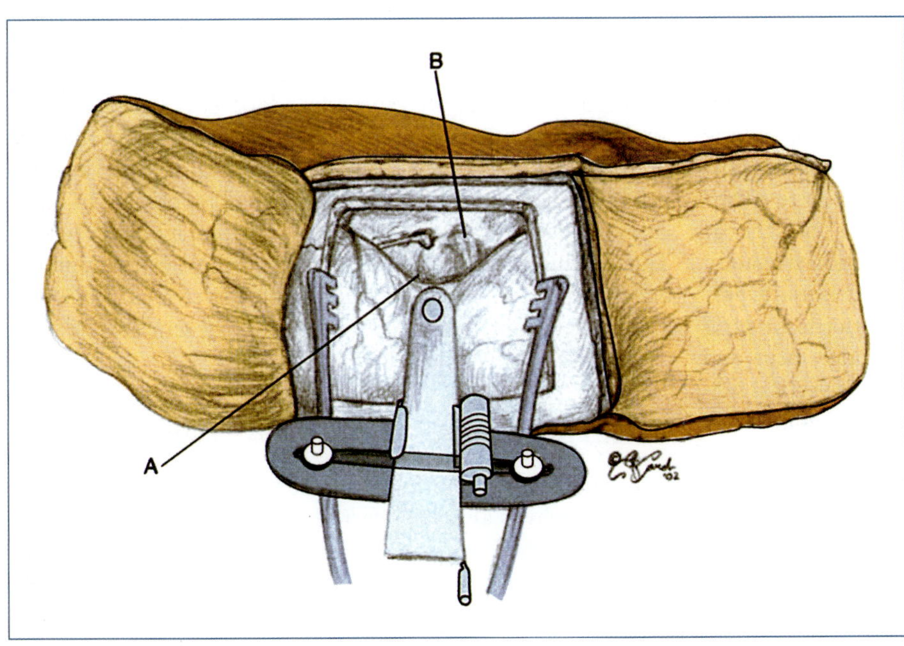

FIGURE 36–7 • Placement of the House-Urban retractor to view the middle cranial fossa floor. *A*, Petrous ridge. *B*, Arculate eminence.

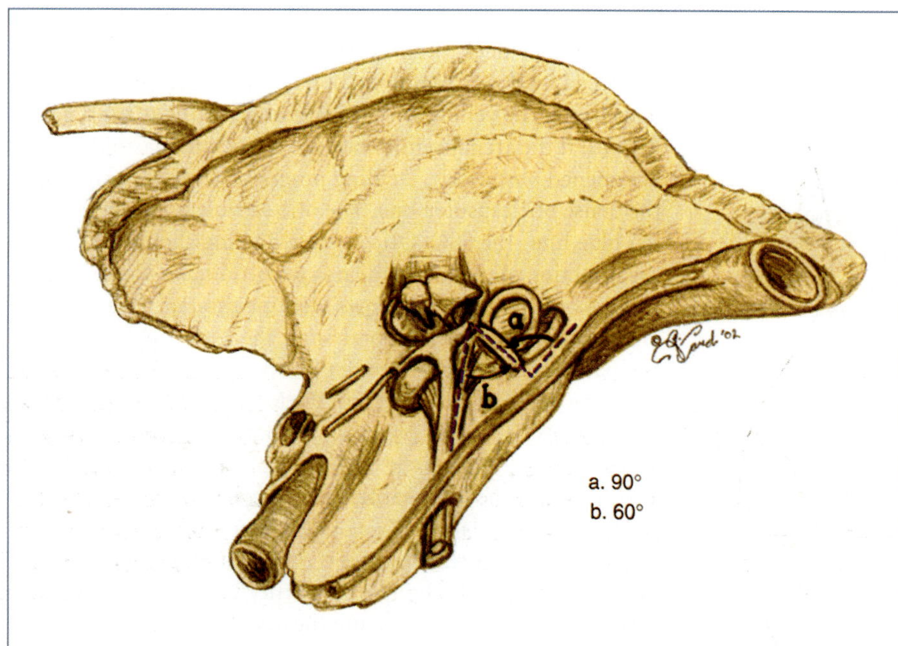

FIGURE 36–8 • View of the middle cranial fossa floor and the relationships between the superior semicircular canal, internal auditory canal, cochlea, and middle ear. *A*, Relationship between superior semicircular canal and petrous ridge. *B*, Relationship between superior semicircle canal and internal auditory canal.

temporalis fascia is placed on the MCF floor. Hyperventilation is stopped. The bone flap is replaced and the wound is closed in layers. A bulky mastoid dressing is applied. The patient is monitored in the intensive care unit overnight with hourly neurologic checks and is transferred to a routine surgical ward the following day. Antibiotics and corticosteroids are administered for 48 h postoperatively. In addition, the patient is kept on fluid restrictions for 24 h postoperatively to minimize the risk of postoperative temporal lobe edema. The patient is checked for CSF leakage on postoperative day two. If CSF leakage occurs, a lumbar drain is placed and the patient is kept in bed with their head elevated for 5 days. If the CSF leak still continues, the wound is re-explored to locate the site of the leak.

Patients are encouraged to ambulate early in the postoperative period to minimize the risk of a pneumonia or deep vein thrombosis/pulmonary embolism. Patients are discharged home when they are stable, ambulating well, tolerating oral intake, and without evidence of CSF leak. The length of stay in the hospital averages 3 days postoperatively.

To approach the facial nerve via the translabyrinthine or transmastoid approach, the initial setup of the patient and the operating room is basically the same. However, a routine postauricular incision is made in the hairline and a 2- to 3-cm-wide Palva flap is created. A self-retaining retractor holds the ear forward. A large cutting bur and continuous suction-irrigation are initially used. A complete mastoidectomy is initially performed, with exposure of the middle and posterior fossa dural plates, sinodural angle, sigmoid sinus, digastric ridge, incus, and lateral semicircular canal. The landmarks for the vertical segment of the facial nerve are the horizontal semicircular canal, fossa incudis, chorda tympani nerve, and the digastric ridge. The facial recess (the region bounded by the facial and chorda tympani nerves and the fossa incudis) is opened. This exposure gives access to the tympanic segment of the nerve. A diamond bur is used to delineate the course of the nerve by leaving only an eggshell layer of bone (Figure 36–9). Occasionally, the incus and head of the malleus must be removed to obtain adequate exposure, and ossicular reconstruction with a partial ossicular reconstruction prosthesis decreases the resulting conductive hearing loss. Once the exposure has been completed, the eggshell bone over the facial nerve is gently removed and the sheath can be opened.

The translabyrinthine approach begins with the transmastoid exposure described above but additionally incorporates a labyrinthectomy to access the IAC, labyrinthine segment, and GG. This approach can also allow complete mobilization of the facial nerve from the brainstem to the stylomastoid foramen.

HEMIFACIAL SPASM

Hemifacial spasm can be debilitating and makes it difficult for the patient to eat, talk, and interact socially. Usually, the entire face is affected by spasms and contractures. Hemifacial spasm is distinct from simple blepharospasm or neurologic disorders such as the myokymia of multiple sclerosis.[7] Some cases of hemifacial spasm are caused by a loop of AICA or another artery or vein pressing on the facial nerve; treatment involves placing a Teflon® sponge between the offending vessel and the nerve via the posterior fossa (retrosigmoid) approach. In other cases, the facial nerve spasm reflects irritation by a CPA tumor. Thus, evaluation includes a thorough neurotologic examination and imaging. At our institution, patients undergo Gd-MRI with a constructive interference steady state (CISS) series to assess for a CPA lesion or a vascular loop.

NERVE REPAIR AND GRAFTING

Restoration of the continuity of the facial nerve by a primary neurorrhaphy is always preferred over nerve grafting if it can be accomplished without tension. Primary neurorrhaphy and nerve grafting alone can restore facial tone and voluntary movement but not involuntary emotional expression. Primary repair

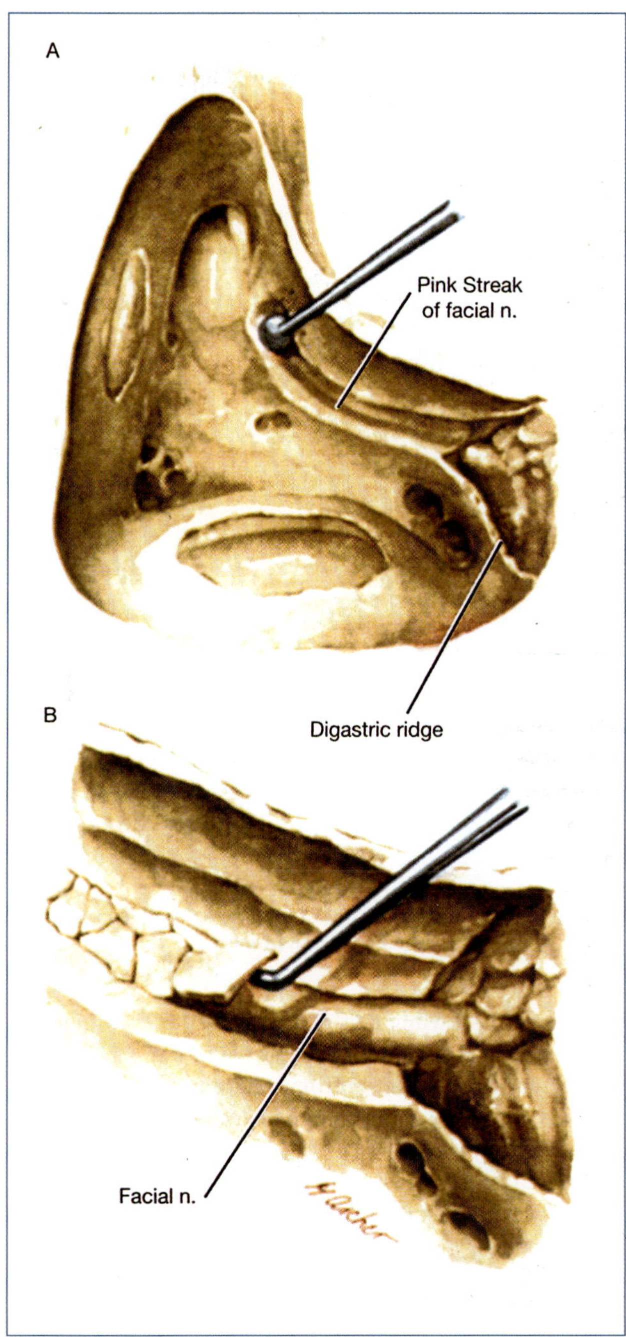

FIGURE 36-9 • *A*, Diamond bur used to delineate course to facial nerve. *B*, Eggshell pieces of bone taken off the facial nerve to allow access to the nerve for grafting, rerouting, or decompression.

or grafting can be performed on the intracranial, intratemporal, and extratemporal portions of the facial nerve; however, there are limitations, and perfect restitution of facial movement cannot be achieved. There are two main limitations: proliferation of connective tissue at the anastomotic sites and nondirected growth of regenerating fibers.[136]

When a segment of the facial nerve is disrupted (eg, by tumor or trauma), the best functional results are obtained with cable grafting. Grafting is also recommended if there is tension at the anastomotic site of a primary nerve repair. Immediate neurorrhaphy optimizes results compared with delayed repair, a finding confirmed experimentally in pigs.[137] The time beyond which nerve repair or grafting is abandoned in favor of other reconstructive methods is approximately 18 to 24 months.[7] Electromyography helps determine whether any muscle function remains and thus provides information about the advisability of dynamic versus static rehabilitation. Electroneurography is of no use for assessing the degree of neural degeneration when performed after three weeks from the injury to the facial nerve (See above).

The surgical approach chosen is based on the site needing repair and whether hearing is present. The interposed graft is aligned with the severed ends of the facial nerve (Figure 36–10). The anastomosis is performed under the operating microscope for the best results; atraumatic technique is required. When available, a surgically exposed and enlarged fallopian canal can help secure the anastomosis. When anastomosis is performed between the labyrinthine and the tympanic segments, the GG is bypassed to shorten the gap (possibly permitting an end-to-end anastomosis) and to prevent misdirected growth of the regenerating nerve fibers along the GSPN.[136] It is best to "freshen" the ends of both the nerve and graft by making an oblique (45 degrees) cut with a sharp knife, increasing the surface area for the anastomosis.[32] Epineurium is removed in the region of the anastomosis to minimize the formation of fibrous tissue. The nerve ends are secured with three sutures (in a tripod arrangement) of 8-0 to 10-0 monofilament suture (eg, nylon or polypropylene) in the epineurium.[22] Additional sutures cause additional trauma and connective tissue proliferation.[136] In grafting the intracranial portion of the nerve (owing to the absence of epineurium, as well as brain and CSF pulsation and overall technical difficulty), only one to three sutures are placed. Sutureless anastomosis, using tissue adhesive or even blood, has been advocated.[4,136] Some surgeons have proposed using collagen tubules or splints, whereas others believe that they cause additional fibrosis and negatively affect the final result. When grafting is performed, the graft should be approximately 25% longer than needed to allow for a tension-free anastomosis (in a lazy-S configuration). A silk suture can be used to measure the gap between the nerve ends.[4]

A retrospective review has been performed of 27 patients who underwent facial nerve grafting associated with a neurotologic procedure at our institution.[32] Fourteen patients had grafts at the brainstem. Over 90% of patients had some facial function by 8 months follow-up. Patients who had grafts performed distal to the meatal foramen seemed to have better function overall, although the difference was not statistically significant.

The effect that radiation has on the function of nerve grafts is unknown. Some believe that radiotherapy is so detrimental to the outcome of facial nerve graft function that dynamic or static sling procedures should be performed, instead of grafting, in all patients who are to undergo postoperative radiation therapy. However, the outcome achieved with such sling procedures is usually inferior to nerve grafting. In a recent retrospective study of patients who underwent nerve grafting followed by radiation therapy to approximately 6,000 cGy, no difference was noted in facial nerve function that could be attributed to the radiation therapy.[138] In addition, the use of a nerve graft followed by radiation therapy does not preclude the use of other reconstructive techniques if the graft fails.

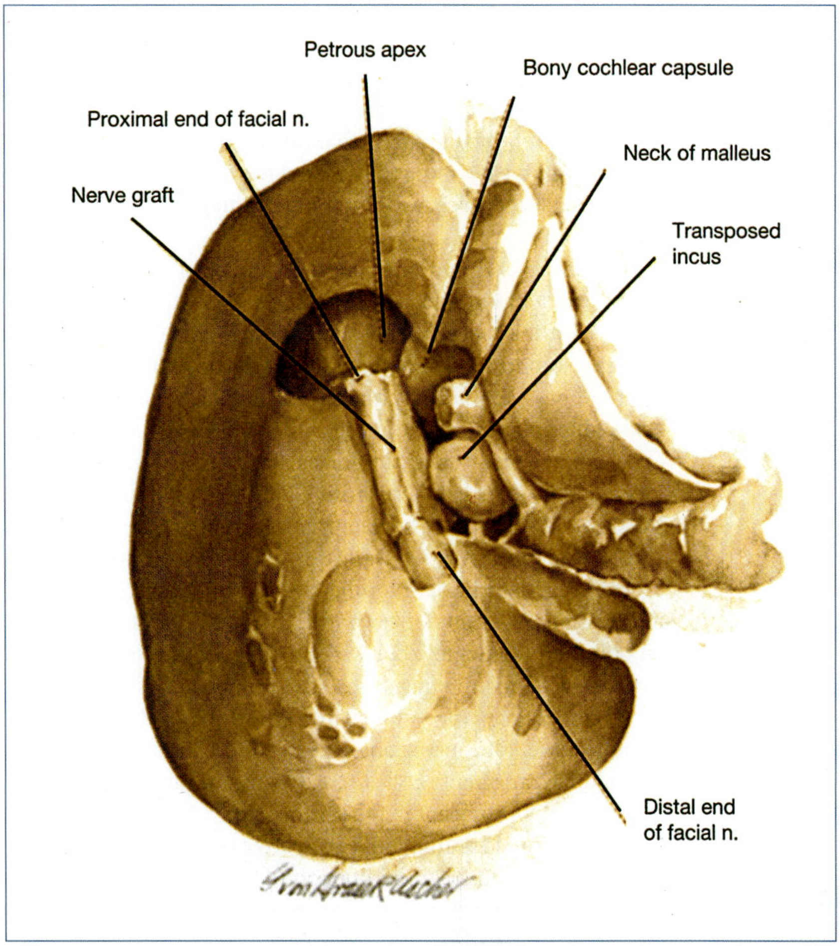

FIGURE 36 –10 • View of nerve graft as performed via a transmastoid approach.

Two sensory nerves are used primarily in facial nerve grafting: the greater auricular and the sural (Figure 36–11). The greater auricular nerve is used most frequently. It approximates the size of the facial nerve, is in the field of surgery, and provides a graft of up to 12 cm in length. The greater auricular nerve is located by drawing a line perpendicular to a line drawn between the mastoid tip and the angle of the mandible;[6] it lies immediately beneath the platysma muscle, on the sternocleidomastoid muscle. Extreme care is used in handling the graft. Once the graft has been harvested, it is placed in a physiologic solution. The graft should be removed only after the preparatory work on the facial nerve stumps is complete, improving the survival of the Schwann cells of the donor nerve.[136]

The sural nerve, which supplies sensation to the lateral lower leg and foot, is also used for grafting. This nerve can provide a graft of up to 35 cm in length and has branches that can be used to reconstruct the branching pattern of the facial nerve.[22] Due to its length, the sural nerve is particularly useful in cross-facial anastomosis.[136] The sural nerve is found posterior to the lateral malleolus, adjacent to the saphenous vein.

FACIAL REANIMATION

There are many factors important in reanimation: cause and degree of paralysis, timing/duration of paralysis, and patient factors (age, general health, patient expectations, life expectancy, nerve condition, and healing capacity). The ultimate goals of reanimation include eye closure, oral competence, muscle tone/facial symmetry at rest, voluntary movement/ symmetry with animation, minimal synkinesis, and involuntary (mimetic) movement. Although no technique is considered ideal, neurorrhaphy or nerve grafting is thought to be the best currently available. Occasionally, however, neither is feasible nor preferable (eg, lack of proximal nerve for anastomosis). For primary repair or grafting to be successful, an intact peripheral facial nerve trunk and functioning facial musculature are needed. However, additional options for dynamic repair exist, such as nerve transfer/crossover, muscle transposition, and free muscle transfer.

An alternate method of dynamic repair uses a substitution nerve graft, the most common of which is the hypoglossal to facial (XII–VII) nerve graft. Originally, the procedure comprised an end-to-end anastomosis of the proximal hypoglossal nerve to the distal facial nerve. The procedure has been modified by only partially sectioning the hypoglossal nerve and interposing, by end-to-side anastomoses, a greater auricular nerve graft between the hypoglossal and facial nerves. Since the hypoglossal nerve is transected only halfway, tongue function can be preserved. Even though the risk of injuring the grafted hypoglossal nerve has been minimized with the use of the greater auricular "jump" graft, a functional, contralateral hypoglossal nerve still must be present, and the presence of any lower cranial neuropathies is a relative contraindication for this procedure. This procedure is performed through a preauricular

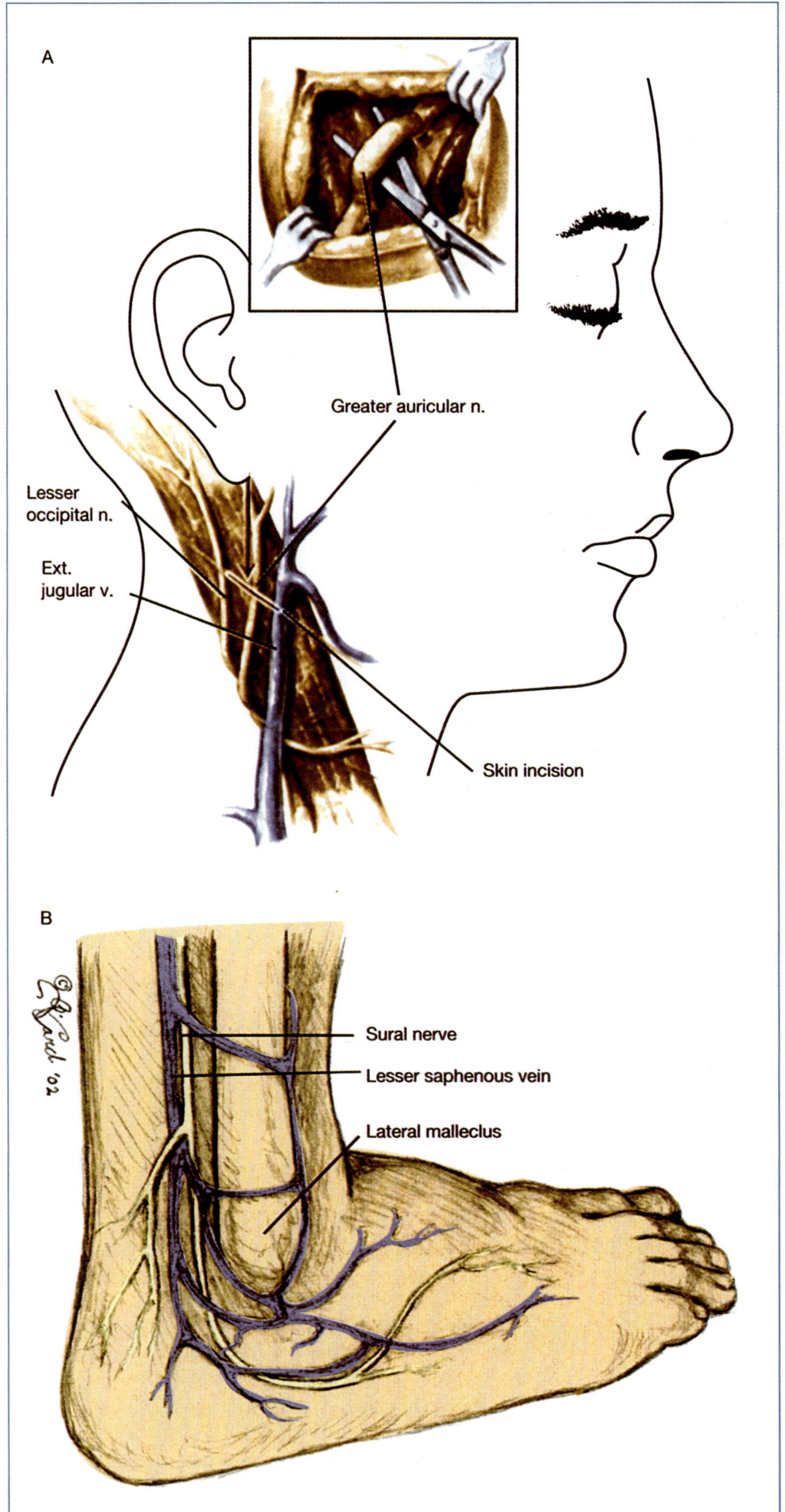

FIGURE 36–11 • The two most commonly used nerves for nerve grafting: the greater auricular nerve (*A*) and the sural nerve (*B*).

incision with a cervical extension. The facial nerve is located and transected at the stylomastoid foramen after raising a soft tissue flap over the parotid; the hypoglossal nerve is identified as it crosses the external carotid artery and is dissected proximally and distally. The hypoglossal nerve is partially transected in preparation for grafting and a greater auricular nerve graft longer than the gap is harvested.[7] After preparing the graft it is suture to the proximal portion of the transected hypoglossal nerve in end-to-side fashion followed by end-to-end anastomosis of the graft with the distal facial nerve as described above. Recovery of facial movement begins at approximately 6 months. Seventh to twelfth nerve grafting is a relatively simple procedure that provides strong neural input and results in acceptable dynamic function. The disadvantages of this technique include mass movement and potential tongue hemiatrophy, which rarely results in chewing, swallowing, or speech difficulties. The VII–XII anastomosis is preferable to the facial to spinal accessory nerve anastomosis.

If there is no functional neuromuscular system, surgical reconstruction involves muscular transposition rather than primary nerve repair, grafting, or XII–VII grafting. A variety of transposition procedures have been described, including transposition of both pedicled (temporalis, masseter) and free muscle (gracilis, rectus abdominus, abductor hallucis, pectoralis minor, latissimus dorsi) grafts.[21] In adults, the pedicled grafts are most commonly used. Free muscle transfer with a neurovascular anastomosis (using the contralateral facial nerve for innervation) is the mainstay of treatment of children with congenital disorders (such as Möbius' syndrome or Goldenhar's syndrome).[21] The cross-face graft usually interposes the sural nerve between the distal buccal branch on the functioning side to the nonfunctioning side; however, variations exist. Unfortunately, free muscle transfer procedures are of limited effectiveness.

Muscle transposition most commonly employs the temporalis muscle because of its good location, length, contractility, and vector of pull. The masseter and digastric muscles are used less often. The temporalis muscle is good for reanimation of the mouth in patients with long-standing (at least 1 year in length) paralysis.[139] It is a proven and useful technique for facial reanimation in patients in who nerve grafting or cranial nerve substitution procedures are not possible. It has also been used in conjunction with other procedures, such as placement of a gold weight in the upper eyelid. Temporalis transposition is a dynamic technique that allows patients to have a voluntary smile. Static (adynamic) versions of this technique use Gortex® or fascia lata, which is attached to the zygoma and then run subcutaneously to the corner of the mouth to support the sagging facial musculature. Overcorrection is required at first owing to relaxation of the tissues with time. Although static slings afford relative symmetry at rest, they provide no movement.

ADJUNCTIVE MEASURES

The patient and the surgeon must realize that, unfortunately, even the best postoperative result does not achieve perfection in cosmesis and facial symmetry. This lack of perfection provides a stimulus for continued basic and clinical research. In the meantime, there are additional steps that may be taken to further enhance the patient's appearance, including facial reconstructive procedures (eg, facelift, browlift, blepharoplasty), makeup prostheses, hairstyles, and the use of glasses to mask incisions Facial nerve rehabilitation, with the use of biofeedback, has also shown some promise, giving the patient a sense of hope, control and participation in the ultimate outcome of facial nerve function and appearance.

COMPLICATIONS OF FACIAL NERVE SURGERY

Before embarking on surgery of the facial nerve, the patient must be educated in detail regarding the disease process, the surgeon, and the expected results to obtain a truly informed consent. The surgeon must discuss potential risks, complications, hazards, and alternatives. However, the patient must be made aware that these potential problems are rare if the surgery is performed by a well-trained and skilled otologic, neurotologic, and skull base surgeon. The complications of surgery in general are first discussed (ie, anesthetic complications, bleeding, pain, myocardial infarction, etc). The major complications unique to facial nerve surgery are injury to the nerve itself and injury to the surrounding structures (semicircular canals, ossicles, cochlea, sigmoid sinus, etc). Depending on the approach, conductive and/or sensorineural hearing loss and vestibular dysfunction can occur. Additional risks posed by neurotologic/skull base approaches include intracranial hematoma, neurologic deficit (stroke or cranial nerve injury), CSF leak, seizures, meningitis, death, deep venous thrombosis, and pulmonary embolism.

References

1. Kahn JB, et al. Validation of a patient-graded instrument for facial nerve paralysis: the FaCE scale. Laryngoscope 2001;111(3):387–98.
2. Jackson CG. Facial nerve paralysis: Diagnosis and treatment of lower motor neuron facial nerve lesions and facial paralysis. AAOHNSF. Rochester, 1986.
3. Van Buskirk C. The seventh nerve complex. J Comp Neurol 1945;82:303–33.
4. Fisch U, et al. Intracranial facial nerve anastomosis. Am J Otol 1987;8(1):23–9.
5. Rubenstein J, Gantz B. Facial nerve disorders. In: Clinical otology. Hughes G, Pensak M, editors. New York: Thieme; 1997. p. 367–380.
6. Gantz BJ, Wackym PA. Facial nerve abnormalities. In: Pediatric facial plastic and reconstructive surgery. Smith J, Bumstead R, editors. New York: Raven Press; 1993. p. 337–347.
7. Glasscock M, Shambaugh G. Facial nerve surgery. In: Surgery of the ear. Glasscock M, Shambaugh G, editors. Philadelphia: W.B. Saunders; 1990. p. 434–465.
8. Ge XX, Spector GJ. Labyrinthine segment and geniculate ganglion of facial nerve in fetal and adult human temporal bones. Ann Otol Rhinol Laryngol Suppl 1981;90(4 Pt 2):1–12.
9. Lindeman H. The fallopian canal. An anatomical study of its distal part. Acta Otolaryngol Suppl 1960;158:204–11.
10. Sunderland S, Cossar DF. The structure of the facial nerve. Anat Rec 1953;116(2):147–65.
11. Haynes DR. The relations of the facial nerve in the temporal bone. Ann R Coll Surg Engl 1955;16(3):175–85.

12. Baxter A. Dehiscence of the fallopian canal. An anatomical study. J Laryngol Otol 1971;85(6):587–94.
13. Anson BJ, Harper DG, Warpeha RL. Surgical Anatomy of the Facial Canal and Facial Nerve. Ann Otol Rhinol Laryngol 1963;72:713–34.
14. Nager GT, Proctor B. The facial canal: normal anatomy, variations and anomalies. II. Anatomical variations and anomalies involving the facial canal. Ann Otol Rhinol Laryngol Suppl 1982;97:45–61.
15. Savic D, Djeric D. Anomalies of the mastoid portion of the facial canal and their surgical importance. Ann Otolaryngol Chir Cervicofac 1986;103(1):27–30.
16. Theissing J. Facial nerve anomalies found at surgery (author's transl). HNO 1975;23(10):310–2.
17. Lundborg G. Ischemic nerve injury. Experimental studies on intraneural microvascular pathophysiology and nerve function in a limb subjected to temporary circulatory arrest. Scand J Plast Reconstr Surg Suppl 1970;6:3–113.
18. Seddon H. Three types of nerve injury. Brain 1943;66:237.
19. Gantz BJ. Evaluating acute facial paralysis using electroneurography and intraoperative evoked electromyography. In: AAO-HNS. Annual Meeting, 1983.
20. Sunderland S. A classification of peripheral nerve injuries producing loss of function. Brain 1951;74(4):491–516.
21. Perry B, Gantz BJ. Diagnosis and management of acute facial palsies. Adv Otolaryngol Head Neck Surg 1999;13:127–162.
22. Gantz BJ. Traumatic facial paralysis. In: Gates GA, editor. Current therapy in otolaryngology head and neck surgery. Toronto: BC Decker; 1987. p. 112–115.
23. Paydarfar JA, Paniello RC. Functional study of four neurotoxins as inhibitors of post-traumatic nerve regeneration. Laryngoscope 2001;111(5):844–50.
24. Yian CH, Paniello RC, Gershon Spector J. Inhibition of motor nerve regeneration in a rabbit facial nerve model. Laryngoscope 2001;111(5):786–91.
25. Jelks GW, Smith B, Bosniak S. The evaluation and management of the eye in facial palsy. Clin Plast Surg 1979;6(3):397–419.
26. House JW, Brackmann DE. Facial nerve grading system. Otolaryngol Head Neck Surg 1985;93(2):146–7.
27. House JW. Facial nerve grading systems. Laryngoscope 1983;93(8):1056–69.
28. Ahrens A, et al. Rapid simultaneous comparison system for subjective grading scales grading scales for facial paralysis. Am J Otol 1999;20(5):667–71.
29. Kanerva M, Poussa T, Pitkaranta A. Sunnybrook and House-Brackmann Facial Grading Systems: intrarater repeatability and interrater agreement. Otolaryngol Head Neck Surg 2006;135(6):865–71.
30. Rickenmann J, et al. Comparative value of facial nerve grading systems. Otolaryngol Head Neck Surg 1997;117(4):322–5.
31. Neely JG, et al. Computerized quantitative dynamic analysis of facial motion in the paralyzed and synkinetic face. Am J Otol 1992;13(2):97–107.
32. Gidley PW, Gantz BJ, Rubinstein JT. Facial nerve grafts: from cerebellopontine angle and beyond. Am J Otol 1999;20(6):781–8.
33. Birkmann C, et al. Bell's palsy: electrodiagnostics are not indicative of cerebrospinal fluid abnormalities. Ann Otol Rhinol Laryngol 2001;110(6):581–4.
34. Carreno M, et al. Amplification of herpes simplex virus type 1 DNA in human geniculate ganglia from formalin-fixed, nonembedded temporal bones. Otolaryngol Head Neck Surg 2000;123(4):508–11.
35. Gantz BJ. Idiopathic facial paralysis. In: Gates GA, editor. Current therapy in otolaryngology head and neck surgery. Toronto: BC Decker; 1987. p. 62–66.
36. Denny-Brown D. Pathologic features of herpes zoster: a note on geniculate herpes. Arch Neurol Psychiatry 1944;20:149–159.
37. Honda N, et al. Swelling of the intratemporal facial nerve in Ramsay Hunt syndrome. Acta Otolaryngol 2002;122(3):348–52.
38. Sittel C, et al. Variability of repeated facial nerve electroneurography in healthy subjects. Laryngoscope 1998;108(8 Pt 1):1177–80.
39. Gantz BJ, et al. Electroneurographic evaluation of the facial nerve. Method and technical problems. Ann Otol Rhinol Laryngol 1984;93(4 Pt 1):394–8.
40. Fisch U. Maximal nerve excitability testing vs electroneuronography. Arch Otolaryngol 1980;106(6):352–7.
41. Sillman JS, et al. Prognostic value of evoked and standard electromyography in acute facial paralysis. Otolaryngol Head Neck Surg 1992;107(3):377–81.
42. Bell C. On the nerves, giving an account of some experiments on their structure and function, which led to a new arrangement of the system. Philos Trans 1821;111:398–424.
43. Bird TD, Nicolaus A. Friedreich's description of peripheral facial nerve paralysis in 1798. J Neurol Neurosurg Psychiatry 1979;42(1):56–8.
44. Peitersen E. Bell's palsy: the spontaneous course of 2,500 peripheral facial nerve palsies of different etiologies. Acta Otolaryngol Suppl 2002;(549):4–30.
45. Hauser WA, et al. Incidence and prognosis of Bell's palsy in the population of Rochester, Minnesota. Mayo Clin Proc 1971;46(4):258–64.
46. Burgess RC, et al. Polymerase chain reaction amplification of herpes simplex viral DNA from the geniculate ganglion of a patient with Bell's palsy. Ann Otol Rhinol Laryngol 1994;103(10):775–9.
47. Furuta Y, et al. Reactivation of herpes simplex virus type 1 in patients with Bell's palsy. J Med Virol 1998;54(3):162–6.
48. Lazarini PR, et al. Herpes simplex virus in the saliva of peripheral Bell's palsy patients. Rev Bras Otorrinolaringol (Engl Ed) 2006;72(1):7–11.
49. Murakami S, et al. Bell palsy and herpes simplex virus: Identification of viral DNA in endoneurial fluid and muscle. Ann Intern Med 1996;124(1 Pt 1):27–30.
50. Sugita T, et al. Facial nerve paralysis induced by herpes simplex virus in mice: An animal model of acute and transient facial paralysis. Ann Otol Rhinol Laryngol 1995;104(7):574–81.
51. Takasu T, et al. Detection of latent herpes simplex virus DNA and RNA in human geniculate ganglia by the polymerase chain reaction. Acta Otolaryngol 1992;112(6):1004–11.
52. Wackym PA. Molecular temporal bone pathology: II. Ramsay Hunt syndrome (herpes zoster oticus). Laryngoscope 1997;107(9):1165–75.
53. Katusic SK, et al. Incidence, clinical features, and prognosis in Bell's palsy, Rochester, Minnesota, 1968–1982. Ann Neurol 1986;20(5):622–7.
54. Cwach H, Landis J, Freeman JW. Bilateral seventh nerve palsy: A report of two cases and a review. S D J Med 1997;50(3):99–101.
55. Pitts DB, Adour KK, Hilsinger RL Jr. Recurrent Bell's palsy: Analysis of 140 patients. Laryngoscope 1988;98(5):535–40.
56. May, M. Differential diagnosis by history, physical examination and laboratory results. In: The facial nerve. May M, editor. New York: Thieme; 1986. p. 181–216.

57. Falco NA, E Eriksson. Idiopathic facial palsy in pregnancy and the puerperium. Surg Gynecol Obstet 1989;169(4):337–40.
58. Cohen Y, et al. Bell palsy complicating pregnancy: a review. Obstet Gynecol Surv 2000;55(3):184–8.
59. Hilsinger RL Jr, Adour KK, Doty HE. Idiopathic facial paralysis, pregnancy, and the menstrual cycle. Ann Otol Rhinol Laryngol 1975;84(4 Pt 1):433–42.
60. Leibowitz U. Epidemic incidence of Bell's palsy. Brain 1969;92(1):109–14.
61. Adour KK, Wingerd J. Nonepidemic incidence of idiopathic facial paralysis. Seasonal distribution of 419 cases in three years. JAMA 1974;227(6):653–4.
62. Peitersen E. The natural history of Bell's palsy. Am J Otol 1982;4(2):107–11.
63. Grogan PM, Gronseth GS. Practice parameter: Steroids, acyclovir, and surgery for Bell's palsy (an evidence-based review): Report of the Quality Standards Subcommittee of the American Academy of Neurology. Neurology 2001;56(7):830–6.
64. Ramsey MJ, et al. Corticosteroid treatment for idiopathic facial nerve paralysis: A meta-analysis. Laryngoscope 2000;110 (3 Pt 1):335–41.
65. Adour KK, et al. Prednisone treatment for idiopathic facial paralysis (Bell's palsy). N Engl J Med 1972;287(25):1268–72.
66. Shafshak TS, Essa AY, Bakey FA. The possible contributing factors for the success of steroid therapy in Bell's palsy: A clinical and electrophysiological study. J Laryngol Otol 1994;108(11):940–3.
67. Williamson IG, Whelan TR. The clinical problem of Bell's palsy: is treatment with steroids effective? Br J Gen Pract 1996;46(413):743–7.
68. Wolf SM, et al. Treatment of Bell palsy with prednisone: A prospective, randomized study. Neurology 1978;28(2):158–61.
69. Brown JS. Bell's palsy: a 5 year review of 174 consecutive cases: An attempted double blind study. Laryngoscope 1982;92(12):1369–73.
70. May M, et al. The use of steroids in Bell's palsy: A prospective controlled study. Laryngoscope 1976;86(8):1111–22.
71. Salinas RA, et al. Corticosteroids for Bell's palsy (idiopathic facial paralysis). Cochrane Database Syst Rev 2002(1):CD001942.
72. Prescott CA. Idiopathic facial nerve palsy in children and the effect of treatment with steroids. Int J Pediatr Otorhinolaryngol 1987;13(3):257–64.
73. Salman MS, MacGregor DL. Should children with Bell's palsy be treated with corticosteroids? A systematic review. J Child Neurol 2001;16(8):565–8.
74. Unuvar E, et al. Corticosteroid treatment of childhood Bell's palsy. Pediatr Neurol 1999;21(5):814–6.
75. Adour KK, et al. Bell's palsy treatment with acyclovir and prednisone compared with prednisone alone: A double-blind, randomized, controlled trial. Ann Otol Rhinol Laryngol 1996;105(5):371–8.
76. Axelsson S, Lindberg S, Stjernquist-Desatnik A. Outcome of treatment with valacyclovir and prednisone in patients with Bell's palsy. Ann Otol Rhinol Laryngol 2003;112(3):197–201.
77. Dickins JR, Smith JT, Graham SS. Herpes zoster oticus: Treatment with intravenous acyclovir. Laryngoscope 1988;98(7):776–9.
78. Hato N, et al. Valacyclovir and prednisolone treatment for bell's palsy: A multicenter, randomized, placebo-controlled study. Otol Neurotol 2007.
79. Morrow MJ. Bell's Palsy and Herpes Zoster Oticus. Curr Treat Options Neurol 2000;2(5):407–416.
80. De Diego JI, et al. Idiopathic facial paralysis: A randomized, prospective, and controlled study using single-dose prednisone versus acyclovir three times daily. Laryngoscope 1998;108 (4 Pt 1):573–5.
81. Ramos Macias A, de Miguel Martínez I, Martin Sanchez AM. Incorporacion del aciclovir en el tratamiento de la paralisis periferica: Un estudio en 45 casos. Acta Otolaryngol Espanola 1992;43:117–120.
82. Sullivan FM, et al. Early treatment with prednisolone or acyclovir in Bell's palsy. N Engl J Med 2007;357(16):1598–607.
83. Gantz BJ, et al. Surgical management of Bell's palsy. Laryngoscope 1999;109(8):1177–88.
84. Adour KK, Diamond C. Decompression of the facial nerve in Bell's palsy: A historical review. Otolaryngol Head Neck Surg 1982;90(4):453–60.
85. Friedman RA. The surgical management of Bell's palsy: A review. Am J Otol 2000;21(1):139–44.
86. Darrouzet V, et al. Management of facial paralysis resulting from temporal bone fractures: Our experience in 115 cases. Otolaryngol Head Neck Surg 2001;125(1):77–84.
87. Esslen E. Electromyography and electroneurography. In: Facial nerve surgery. Fisch U, editor. Birmingham, AL: Aesculapius; 1977. p. 93–100.
88. Chang CY, Cass SP. Management of facial nerve injury due to temporal bone trauma. Am J Otol 1999;20(1):96–114.
89. Jenkins H, Ator G. Traumatic facial paralysis. In: Otologic surgery. Brackmann DE ,Shelton C, editors. Philadelphia: W.B. Saunders; 2001. p. 318–331.
90. Sanus GZ, et al. Hearing preserved traumatic delayed facial nerve paralysis without temporal bone fracture: neurosurgical perspective and experience in the management of 25 cases. Surg Neurol 2008.
91. Kwartler JA, et al. Facial nerve monitoring in acoustic tumor surgery. Otolaryngol Head Neck Surg, 1991;104(6):814–7.
92. Gantz BJ. Intraoperative facial nerve monitoring. Am J Otol 1985;Suppl:58–61.
93. Wilson L, Lin E, Lalwani A. Cost-effectiveness of intraoperative facial nerve monitoring in middle ear or mastoid surgery. Laryngoscope 2003;113(10):1736–45.
94. Noss RS, Lalwani AK, Yingling CD. Facial nerve monitoring in middle ear and mastoid surgery. Laryngoscope 2001;111(5):831–6.
95. Neff BA, et al. Facial nerve monitoring parameters as a predictor of postoperative facial nerve outcomes after vestibular schwannoma resection. Otol Neurotol 2005;26(4):728–32.
96. Axon PR, Ramsden RT. Assessment of real-time clinical facial function during vestibular schwannoma resection. Laryngoscope 2000;110(11):1911–5.
97. Megerian CA, McKenna MJ, Ojemann RG. Delayed facial paralysis after acoustic neuroma surgery: Factors influencing recovery. Am J Otol 1996;17(4):630–3.
98. Magliulo G, D'Amico R, Di Cello P. Delayed facial palsy after vestibular schwannoma resection: Clinical data and prognosis. J Otolaryngol 2003;32(6):400–4.
99. Grant GA, et al. Delayed facial palsy after resection of vestibular schwannoma. J Neurosurg 2002;97(1):93–6.
100. Sargent EW, Kartush JM, Graham MD. Meatal facial nerve decompression in acoustic neuroma resection. Am J Otol 1995;16(4):457–64.

101. Lalwani AK, et al. Delayed onset facial nerve dysfunction following acoustic neuroma surgery. Am J Otol 1995;16(6):758–64.

102. Franco-Vidal V, et al. Delayed facial paralysis after vestibular schwannoma surgery: role of herpes viruses reactivation—Our experience in eight cases. Otol Neurotol 2004;25(5):805–10.

103. Garcia-Ibanez E, Garcia-Ibanez JL. Middle fossa vestibular neurectomy: a report of 373 cases. Otolaryngol Head Neck Surg 1980;88(4):486–90.

104. de la Cruz A, McElveen JT Jr. Hearing preservation in vestibular neurectomy. Laryngoscope 1984;94(7):874–7.

105. Vrabec JT, Coker NJ, Jenkins HA. Delayed-onset facial paralysis after vestibular neurectomy. Laryngoscope 2003;113(7):1128–31.

106. Shea JJ Jr, Ge X. Delayed facial palsy after stapedectomy. Otol Neurotol, 2001. 22(4):465–70.

107. Salvinelli F, et al. Delayed peripheral facial palsy in the stapes surgery: can it be prevented? Am J Otolaryngol 2004;25(2):105–8.

108. Kitahara T, et al. Delayed facial nerve palsy after otologic surgery. Nippon Jibiinkoka Gakkai Kaiho, 2006;109(7):600–5.

109. Fayad JN, et al. Facial nerve paralysis following cochlear implant surgery. Laryngoscope 2003;113(8):1344–6.

110. Bonkowsky V, et al. Delayed facial palsy following uneventful middle ear surgery: a herpes simplex virus type 1 reactivation? Ann Otol Rhinol Laryngol 1998;107(11 Pt 1):901–5.

111. Vrabec JT. Delayed facial palsy after tympanomastoid surgery. Am J Otol 1999;20(1):26–30.

112. Safdar A, et al. Delayed facial nerve palsy following tympanomastoid surgery: incidence, aetiology and prognosis. J Laryngol Otol 2006;120(9):745–8.

113. Gianoli GJ, Kartush JM. Delayed facial palsy after acoustic neuroma resection: the role of viral reactivation. Am J Otol 1996;17(4):625–9.

114. Gianoli GJ. Viral titers and delayed facial palsy after acoustic neuroma surgery. Otolaryngol Head Neck Surg 2002;127(5):427–31.

115. Sawtell NM, Thompson RL. Rapid in vivo reactivation of herpes simplex virus in latently infected murine ganglionic neurons after transient hyperthermia. J Virol 1992;66(4):2150–6.

116. Wexler DB, Fetter TW, Gantz BJ. Vestibular schwannoma presenting with sudden facial paralysis. Arch Otolaryngol Head Neck Surg 1990;116(4):483–5.

117. Chiang CW, Chang YL, Lou PJ. Multicentricity of intraparotid facial nerve schwannomas. Ann Otol Rhinol Laryngol 2001;110(9):871–4.

118. Kertesz TR, et al. Intratemporal facial nerve neuroma: Anatomical location and radiological features. Laryngoscope 2001;111(7):1250–6.

119. McMonagle B, et al. Facial schwannoma: results of a large case series and review. J Laryngol Otol 2008:1–12.

120. Shirazi MA, et al. Surgical management of facial neuromas: Lessons learned. Otol Neurotol 2007;28(7):958–63.

121. Makeham TP, Croxson GR, Coulson S. Infective causes of facial nerve paralysis. Otol Neurotol 2007;28(1):100–3.

122. Tveitnes D, Oymar K, Natas O. Acute facial nerve palsy in children: how often is it lyme borreliosis? Scand J Infect Dis 2007;39(5):425–31.

123. Kalish RA, et al. Evaluation of study patients with Lyme disease. 10–20-year follow-up. J Infect Dis 2001;183(3):453–60.

124. Ljostad U, et al. Acute peripheral facial palsy in adults. J Neurol 2005;252(6):672–6.

125. Vorstman JA, Kuiper H. Peripheral facial palsy in children: test for lyme borreliosis only in the presence of other clinical signs. Ned Tijdschr Geneeskd 2004;148(14):655–8.

126. Eppes SC, Childs JA. Comparative study of cefuroxime axetil versus amoxicillin in children with early Lyme disease. Pediatrics 2002;109(6):1173–7.

127. Furuta Y, et al. Early diagnosis of zoster sine herpete and antiviral therapy for the treatment of facial palsy. Neurology 2000;55(5):708–10.

128. Murakami S, et al. Treatment of Ramsay Hunt syndrome with acyclovir-prednisone: Significance of early diagnosis and treatment. Ann Neurol 1997;41(3):353–7.

129. Stafford FW, Welch AR. The use of acyclovir in Ramsay Hunt syndrome. J Laryngol Otol 1986;100(3):337–40.

130. Uri N, et al. Herpes zoster oticus: Treatment with acyclovir. Ann Otol Rhinol Laryngol 1992;101(2 Pt 1):161–2.

131. May M, Hardin WB. Facial palsy: Interpretation of neurologic findings. Laryngoscope 1978;88(8 Pt 1):1352–62.

132. Alberti PW, Biagioni E. Facial paralysis in children. A review of 150 cases. Laryngoscope 1972;82(6):1013–20.

133. Rubinstein J B Gantz. Facial nerve disorders. In: Clinical otology. Hughes G, Pensak M, editors. New York: Thieme Medical Publishers; 1997. p. 367–380.

134. Falco NA, Eriksson E. Facial nerve palsy in the newborn: incidence and outcome. Plast Reconstr Surg 1990;85(1):1–4.

135. Abbas GM, Jones RO. Measurements of drill-induced temperature change in the facial nerve during mastoid surgery: A cadaveric model using diamond burs. Ann Otol Rhinol Laryngol 2001;110(9):867–70.

136. Fisch U. Facial nerve grafting. Otolaryngol Clin North Am 1974;7(2):517–29.

137. Barrs DM. Facial nerve trauma: optimal timing for repair. Laryngoscope 1991;101(8):835–48.

138. Brown PD, et al. An analysis of facial nerve function in irradiated and unirradiated facial nerve grafts. Int J Radiat Oncol Biol Phys 2000;48(3):737–43.

139. May M, Sobol SM, Brackmann DE. Facial reanimation: The temporalis muscle and middle fossa surgery. Laryngoscope 1991;101(4 Pt 1):430–2.

Vestibular Schwannoma 37

Mark D. Packer, MD / D. Bradley Welling, MD, PhD, FACS

HISTORICAL ASPECTS

The entity now referred to as a vestibular schwannoma (previously acoustic neuroma, neurinoma, or neurilemmoma) was first observed at autopsy in 1777. Sir Charles Bell published the first clinical case report of a vestibular schwannoma in 1833.[1] His patient had a large tumor in the left cerebellopontine angle that had caused unilateral deafness, facial paralysis, temporal and masseter muscle paralysis (fifth cranial nerve), difficulty in speech and swallowing (tenth cranial nerve), and respiratory difficulty (brain stem) that led to the patient's demise.

Although deemed inoperable because of surgical inaccessibility, a vestibular schwannoma was successfully removed for the first time in 1894 by the pioneer otologic and neurologic surgeon Sir Charles A. Ballance.[2] The occasional operations that followed in the next two decades carried a mortality rate of around 80%. By the early 1900s, the diagnostic accuracy for brain tumors had progressed to the point that patients with particular symptoms were definitely found to have brain lesions.[3] At that time, supratentorial lesions could be differentiated from infratentorial masses, but it was still not possible to differentiate cerebellar from extracerebellar lesions.[3] Gradually, however, the various distinguishing characteristics of posterior fossa tumors were appreciated, and in 1902, Henneberg and Koch introduced the term cerebellopontine angle tumor.[4]

Cushing, in his classic monograph, *Tumors of the Nervus Acusticus and the Syndrome of the Cerebellopontine Angle*, carefully described and defined the clinical features of cerebellopontine angle tumors.[5] He categorized the progressive symptoms seen with gradually enlarging lesions into six stages:

> [It] can be gathered that the symptomatic progress of the average acoustic tumor occurs more or less in the following stages: First, the auditory and labyrinthine manifestations; second, the occipitofrontal pains with sub-occipital discomforts; third, the incoordination and instability of cerebellar origin; fourth, the evidence of involvement of adjacent cerebral nerves; fifth, the indications of increase in intracranial tension with a choked disc (papilledema) and its consequences; sixth, dysarthria, dysphagia, and finally cerebellar crises and respiratory difficulties.[5]

Cushing emphasized that unilateral hearing loss is the initial manifestation of a vestibular schwannoma and that the examiner must ascertain the status of the patient's hearing. The majority of Cushing's early patients had large (stage 4 or 5) tumors. He foresaw the need for early diagnosis to avoid the sequelae of tumor enlargement. In his 1917 publication describing the outcomes of his first 30 operations,[5] Cushing reported a surgical mortality rate of 30%—a dramatic reduction. In his 1932 publication, Cushing reported a further decrease in mortality rate to 4%[6]; however, most patients underwent subtotal, intracapsular tumor removal, and many subsequently required additional surgery to manage recurrences.

Dandy modified Cushing's techniques and in 1925 reported complete tumor removal with a further reduction in the mortality rate in his series of patients.[7] Dandy developed the unilateral cerebellar approach to the cerebellopontine angle, sacrificing the lateral third of the cerebellum to improve exposure of the angle. Although he applied the Halstedian principles of meticulous hemostasis and gentle tissue handling, Dandy made no effort to preserve the facial nerve, nor, apparently, did he appreciate the consequences of ligating the anterior inferior cerebellar artery.

The next significant advance in vestibular schwannoma surgery occurred in 1949, the year in which Atkinson published his autopsy studies documenting that occlusion of the anterior inferior cerebellar artery was the principal cause of operative mortality in vestibular schwannoma surgery.[8] By World War II, most otolaryngologists were aware of the appropriate evaluation of a unilateral hearing loss. Using radiographs and vestibular studies, tumors typically were identified in Cushing stage 2 or 3.

In the 1950s, as noted by House, the nationwide operative mortality rate for acoustic neuroma surgery in the United States remained high; approaching 40% in many locales.[3] This high mortality rate prompted House to investigate the translabyrinthine approach to vestibular schwannomas.

Early in the history of surgery for vestibular schwannoma, Panse proposed an approach through the labyrinth.[9] However,

Quix, who chiseled away the entire labyrinth with a mallet and gouge after a radical mastoidectomy approach, was the first to actually use this approach.[10] Although the bleeding from the superior petrosal sinus necessitated termination of the operation, it was completed 4 days later. After the walls of the internal auditory canal (IAC) were chiseled away, the carotid artery was exposed, and the tumor was removed. Quix predicted that this translabyrinthine approach would bring the small vestibular schwannoma within the realm of the otologist. Cushing warned that "while the otologist doubtless will be the first to recognize and diagnose these cases, there is no possible route more dangerous or difficult than this one...proposed by Panse."[6] His warning effectively dampened enthusiasm for the translabyrinthine approach to vestibular schwannoma removal for several decades.

In 1961, House,[11] using the middle fossa approach to the IAC described by Clerc and Battise 7 years earlier,[12] successfully removed a small, intracanalicular vestibular schwannoma. Soon House realized that the translabyrinthine approach was preferable for all but the smallest tumors in patients with serviceable hearing. In 1964, House reported 47 consecutive translabyrinthine complete or subtotal microsurgical removals without a fatality—a record never before achieved for these common and eventually lethal tumors.[13] The preservation of facial nerve function in the majority, the virtual absence of cerebellar trauma, and the amazingly brief convalescence compared with posterior fossa operations led to a remarkable series of more than 1,000 operations for vestibular schwannomas of all sizes by House and his associates. Glasscock and others have duplicated these extremely low morbidity and mortality rates.[14]

House's great interest in vestibular schwannomas, coupled with his early diagnosis and improved surgical techniques, prompted other otologists and neurosurgeons to attempt new procedures. In 1973, Smith and colleagues[15] advocated a microscopic suboccipital approach similar to that proposed by Rand and colleagues[16] for preservation of hearing in vestibular schwannoma excision. Several neurosurgeons, MacCarty, eg, have reported their considerable experience with the suboccipital approach and the microscope.[17]

Rhoton advocated the suboccipital approach for hearing preservation.[18] Later, Wade and House reported their hearing preservation results using the middle fossa approach for 20 vestibular schwannoma patients[19]; hearing was preserved in 35% of patients.

The morbidity and mortality rates of vestibular schwannoma surgery continue to improve. The operating microscope, first used by Nylén and introduced to the United States by Shambaugh, revolutionized neurotologic and neurosurgical technique, enabling better visualization and preservation of neural structures. More recently, intraoperative monitoring and stimulation of the facial nerve have enabled better identification, dissection, and preservation of this structure during vestibular schwannoma removal .[20,21] Furthermore, the advent of sophisticated diagnostic techniques, such as magnetic resonance imaging (MRI), has enabled the diagnosis of Cushing stage 1 tumors, that is, while still confined to the IAC. Such early diagnosis has improved the likelihood of hearing preservation with tumor removal. As predicted by Cushing,[5,6] early diagnosis has resulted in decreased morbidity and mortality rates.

The clinical characteristics of, and diagnostic strategies for, vestibular schwannomas are discussed in this chapter. Additionally the molecular biology of these tumors, as currently understood, is reviewed. Lastly, the therapeutic options, surgical approaches for removing vestibular schwannomas, and operative complications are described.

PATHOLOGY

Vestibular schwannomas are benign, well circumscribed, but unencapsulated tumors that arise from the Schwann cells of the vestibular nerve, hence the term vestibular schwannoma or vestibular neurilemmoma. Historically, the superior vestibular nerve sheath was thought to be the site of origin, giving rise to nearly two-thirds of tumors.[22] More recent reviews of our, and other's series shows the inferior vestibular nerve to be the predominant site of origin for these tumors.[23,24] The nerve of origin is identifiable in 33 to 74% of cases, and, when clearly seen, shows the tumor originating from the inferior vestibular nerve over twice as often, and in up to 94% in some reports. Rarely, the cochlear portion of the eighth cranial nerve or the facial nerve is the site of schwannoma origin.

It has been taught that vestibular schwannomas arise at the Obersteiner–Redlich junctional zone of the vestibular nerve, the region at which the Schwann cells and neuroglial supporting cells meet. Schwann cells tend to accumulate at the junctional zone, their progression to the brain stem slowed by neuroglial supporting cells. "Whorl-like" Schwann cell nests, as well as eosinophilic bodies, and ganglion cells are found at the junctional zone, as described by Prisig and colleagues in their study of serially sectioned temporal bones. They hypothesized that Schwann cell nests could be the forerunners of vestibular schwannomas.[25] This theory is not universally accepted.[26] Imaging and surgical observations of early tumors show that they more frequently originate near the fundus of the IAC, lateral to the junctional zone. The events that lead to the development of schwannomas are further discussed below. Interestingly, vestibular schwannomas have been reported to occur in 2.4 to 3.5% of temporal bones examined .[22,27] This high incidence likely reflects a selection bias as incidental schwannomas are found on MRI in asymptomatic patients in 0.2% of the population.[28] Screening of patients with asymmetric sensorineural hearing loss and/or unilateral tinnitus showed pathology on 14% of scans, pathology that could account for the auditory symptoms in 4.5 to 5.5%, and diagnosed IAC tumors in 3.1% of 1,080 symptomatic patients.[29] In other series, screening identified IAC masses in 2.5 to 3.5% (2.5% of 152) patients, rates similar to the temporal bone findings.[30]

Most vestibular schwannomas originate in the region of the IAC, enlarging the porus and extending into the cerebellopontine angle.[31] The color and the consistency of the schwannomas depend on the size of the tumor and the degree of tumor degeneration. Typically, tumors are either yellow or pinkish gray and have a rubbery consistency. Large tumors more often are mottled, owing to hemorrhage and fibrosis, and may have cystic regions, owing to necrosis and degeneration within the tumor.

However, some tumors appear to have an intrinsic cystic nature, not reflective of necrosis. Truly cystic tumors account for 4% of vestibular schwannomas. The literature differs on whether or not the facial nerve outcome is worse in cystic schwannomas.[32,33] Our experience agrees that cystic tumors are more refractory to both surgical and radiation management than solid tumors.

Microscopic examination of a vestibular schwannoma reveals a well circumscribed, but unencapsulated tumor, with the nerve of origin compressed at its periphery.[31] Structurally, vestibular schwannomas are composed of two histological patterns: Antoni A and Antoni B. Antoni A regions are compact and cellular, with elongated spindle cells and whorling or palisading nuclei aligned in rows (Verocay bodies). Antoni type B histology is loose and much less cellular, with a spongy appearance (Figure 37–1). Most vestibular schwannomas consist of predominantly type A histology, intermingled with areas of type B, but the proportion of these components varies. Vascularity is prominent, and thickened or hyalinized vessel walls are typical. As the tumor grows, myxoid areas, histiocytic infiltration, necrosis, and fibrosis are also seen.

Initially, a tumor confined to the IAC produces no symptoms as it slowly fills the canal. With continued growth, however, it begins to press on the cochlear, vestibular, and facial nerves, as well as the labyrinthine vessels. Tinnitus and neural hearing loss both manifest with progressive compression of the cochlear nerve. Sudden sensorineural loss may occur from acute labyrinthine vessel compression or spasm. Loss of vestibular nerve function occurs slowly with tumor growth, and vestibular symptomatology usually is subtle because of the compensatory ability of the contralateral vestibular system. With continued tumor enlargement, the IAC gradually expands. The (motor) facial nerve is more resistant to tumor compression; accordingly, facial weakness is generally seen only with large tumors, or smaller tumors of facial nerve origin. The facial nerve may even be stretched to a gossamer band on the tumor surface without impairment of function.

As the tumor encroaches into the cerebellopontine angle, it may assume a pear shape. Continued enlargement leads to compression of the superiorly located fifth cranial nerve, which results in ipsilateral anesthesia (e.g., absent corneal reflex). Large tumors may also compress the lower cranial nerves, resulting in neuropathy of the ninth, tenth, eleventh, and even twelfth nerves. If the tumor is not detected and removed, hydrocephalus, visual disturbance, and death from tonsillar herniation may ensue.

MOLECULAR BIOLOGY

The molecular events underlying the formation of vestibular schwannomas were elucidated by the study of families with neurofibromatosis 2 (NF2). Neurofibromatosis type 2 is a highly penetrant, autosomal-dominant disorder with

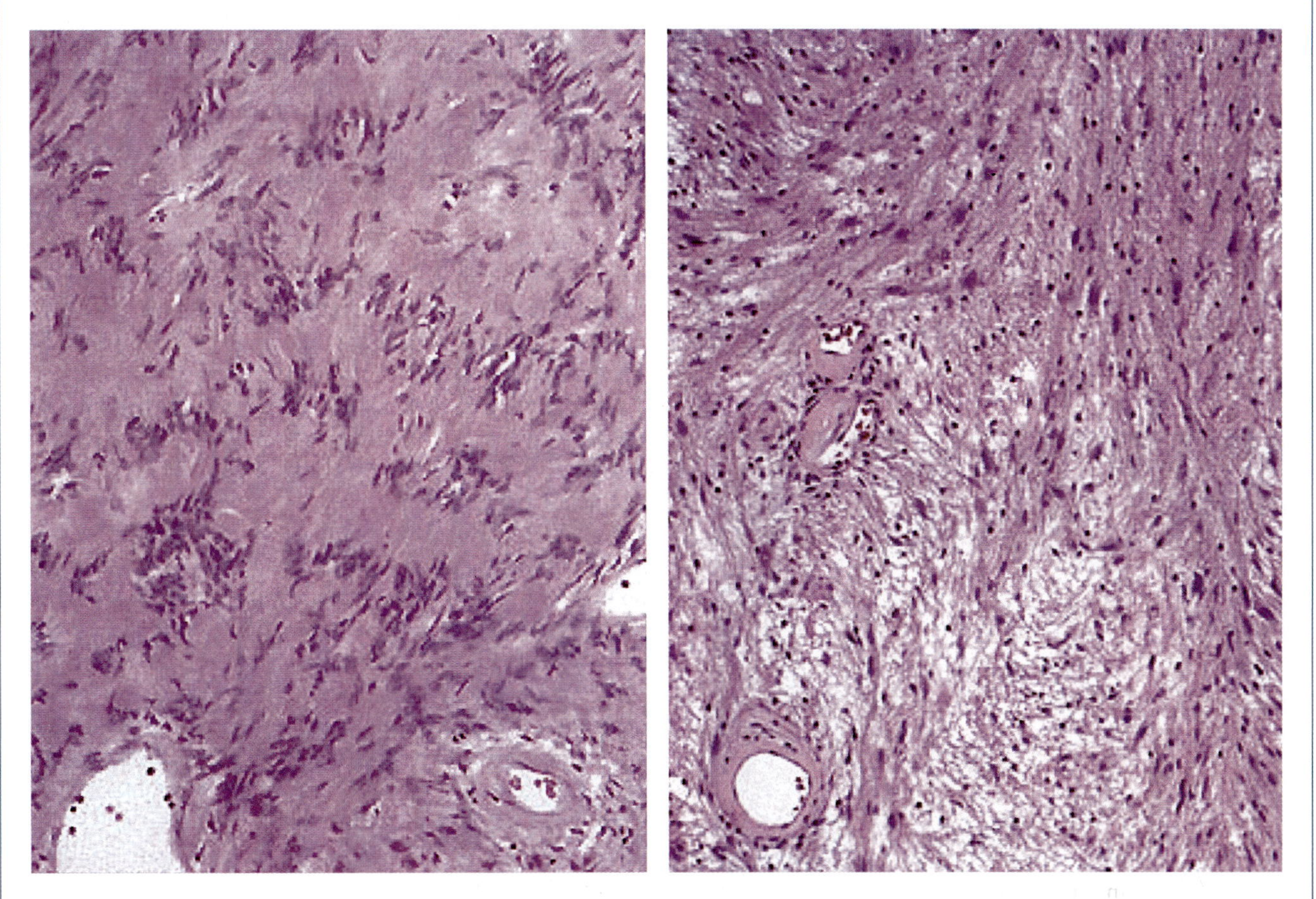

FIGURE 37–1 • Note the more cellular "Antoni A" pattern on the left with palisading nuclei surrounding pink areas (Verocay bodies). On the right is the "Antoni B" pattern with a looser stroma, fewer cells, and myxoid change. *Photo used by permission and courtesy of Dr. Keith Kaplan (http://rad.usuhs.edu/medpix/.*

variable expressivity. Patients with NF2 have approximately a 95% chance of developing bilateral vestibular schwannomas (Figure 37–2). In addition, meningiomas, ependymomas, spinal cord and peripheral schwannomas are observed with increased frequency. The gene responsible for NF2 was mapped to chromosome 22q12 by Seizinger and colleagues.[34] The gene was independently identified by Rouleau and colleagues,[35] and Trofatter and colleagues,[36] and was found to encode a cytoskeletal protein named schwannomin (or merlin) that appears to have a role in modulating cellular motility, proliferation, and adhesion.[37] Overexpression of the normal NF2 gene product inhibits actin-cytoskeleton-mediated processes including cell motility, spreading, and attachment.[38] Furthermore, control of Schwann cell proliferation is lost with inactivation of the NF2 gene. This suggests that a schwannomin/ merlin deficiency disrupts some aspect of intracellular signaling, which then leads to cell cycle progression.[39,40] These data suggest a tumor suppressor role for the NF2 gene product.

Vestibular schwannomas are usually sporadic, resulting from Schwann cell transformation within the vestibular division of the eighth cranial nerve. It is believed that mutations inactivating both alleles of the NF2 gene are responsible for the development of sporadic tumors. Patients with NF2 inherit one defunct copy of the NF2 gene through a germline mutation. Inactivation of the second allele in the Schwann cell results in the loss of NF2 tumor suppressor function and schwannoma formation.

Interestingly, mutations within the NF2 gene have been identified in up to 90% of vestibular schwannomas.[41] In our series, NF2 gene mutations were identified in 66% of unilateral tumors and 33% of bilateral tumors.[42] Analysis of the NF2 gene promoter has revealed that there are regulatory elements in the NF2 5' flanking regions.[43]

The protein product of the NF2 gene, merlin, acts as an important regulator of contact-dependent cellular proliferation. When phosphorylated by Racl with PAK2 (p21-activated kinase), merlin is inactivated, which is growth permissive. PKA (phosphkinase A) also phosphorylates merlin at an N-terminal site, which affects its interaction with the actin cytoskeleton. When dephosphorylated at Ser518 by myosin phosphatase, merlin becomes active and growth suppressive. Dephosphorylation changes merlin's configuration and allows an N-terminal to C-terminal self association. Merlin migrates to the cell membrane and interacts with cadherin or CD44 resulting in contact inhibition.

As shown by Hansen[44] and Doherty,[45] merlin inhibits activation of cell proliferation by suppressing the ErbB2 receptors. A potential mechanism to treat schwannomas when merlin has been inactivated would be with ErbB2 receptor inhibitors, several of which are available for the treatment of other malignancies. Likewise Jacob et al. have demonstrated activation of the AKT pathway by AKT phosphorylation in vestibular schwannomas and have proposed AKT inhibitors as another means of slowing or stopping schwannoma growth. In vivo studies are currently underway to further elucidate the AKT pathways.[46]

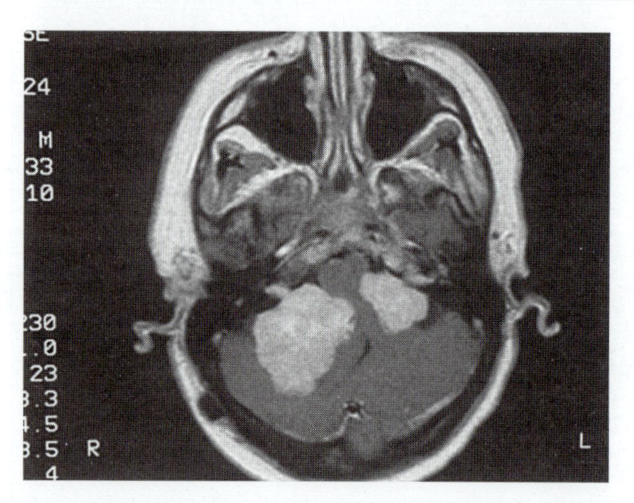

FIGURE 37–2 • Axial T1-weighed magnetic resonance imaging with gadolinium of bilateral vestibular schwannomas associated with NF2 compressing the brainstem and shifting it from the midline.

DIAGNOSIS

Early symptoms leading to the diagnosis of vestibular schwannomas may depend on the exact location of the tumor along the vestibular nerve. If the tumor arises in the IAC, it produces tinnitus and hearing loss early in its course. Should the lesion have its origin in the cerebellopontine angle, tinnitus and hearing loss might not become evident until the tumor has attained a larger size. Occasionally, patients ignore symptoms if other concomitant pathology exists. Thus, relatively large tumors continue to be found, even in an era in which the diagnosis of small tumors is possible.

The differential diagnosis of a vestibular schwannoma includes any entity that produces a unilateral sensorineural hearing loss and/or tinnitus. Vestibular schwannomas are the most common lesions of the cerebellopontine angle. The three next most common lesions are meningiomas, primary cholesteatomas, and arachnoid cysts. Schwannomas originating from the cochlear division of the eighth nerve, or from the seventh nerve, as well as, IAC lipomas, hemangiomas, and vascular loop compressions are less frequently encountered. Any of these lesions may mimic a vestibular schwannoma and can be differentiated by MRI and/or computed tomography (CT).

Early diagnosis depends on a high index of suspicion by the physician. Any patient with unilateral sensorineural hearing loss and/or unilateral tinnitus, with or without balance disturbance, should be suspected of having a vestibular schwannoma. These patients should have a basic neurotologic evaluation consisting of a thorough history, physical examination, and routine audiometric studies. If the basic neurotologic evaluation reveals any suspicious findings, special audiometric and vestibular studies may be obtained, remembering that gadolinium-enhanced MRI is the most sensitive modality to diagnose vestibular schwannomas; therefore, imaging is required for these patients.

HISTORY

The typical patient with a vestibular schwannoma experiences unilateral tinnitus followed by slowly progressive sensorineural hearing loss. A history of sudden sensorineural loss, however, is seen in 10 to 15% of patients with such lesions, and fluctuating hearing is rarely elicited. Seldom does the patient complain of true vertigo. Mild imbalance is not uncommon because, as the tumor grows, it slowly destroys vestibular function. While the contralateral vestibular system generally compensates for the slow ipsilateral loss, patients may notice mild unsteadiness. Aural fullness may be sensed due to hearing loss or tumor bulk. Decreased facial, corneal, or aural sensation, headache, tremor, ataxia, gait disturbance, visual loss, dysphagia, aspiration, hoarseness, shoulder and tongue weakness may be elicited with larger tumors. The family history should be assessed for NF2.

NEUROTOLOGIC EXAMINATION

In addition to the routine head and neck examination, all patients suspected of having a vestibular schwannoma require a complete neurotologic examination. Neurotologic screening includes an evaluation of audiovestibular, cerebellar, and cranial nerve function. The examiner first notes the presence or absence of any spontaneous nystagmus, gaze nystagmus, and vertical nystagmus. Frenzel lenses are helpful in preventing the patient from visually fixating, and suppressing a nystagmus of peripheral origin. Horizontal gaze nystagmus is occasionally observed, and the quick component is usually directed away from the affected ear. Rotary nystagmus and positional nystagmus can also be seen with the affected ear in the dependent position. Vertical nystagmus is always pathologic and suggests a central vestibular disorder such as brain stem compression or cerebellar involvement by a tumor. Romberg testing may elicit drift, and Fukuda stepping rotation, to the side of the lesion. Finger-to-nose testing may draw out dysmetria (fine movements) or past pointing; similarly an ataxic gait or abnormal heel-to-shin test all establish cerebellar involvement.

Multiple cranial nerves may be affected by a cerebellopontine angle tumor, and the number of nerves involved is usually directly proportional to the size of the tumor. Eighth nerve dysfunction is suggested by tinnitus, vestibular symptoms, and hearing loss. The tuning fork examination helps detect a sensorineural hearing loss on the suspect side. Involvement of the fifth cranial nerve by larger tumors may diminish the corneal reflex and cause ipsilateral facial hypesthesia. Although large tumors frequently affect fifth cranial nerve sensory function, they seldom cause wasting of the muscles of mastication. Similarly, the sensory function of the seventh cranial nerve is affected earlier, and more frequently, than its motor function. Involvement of the more vulnerable sensory fibers of the seventh nerve can educe Hitzelberger's sign, hypesthesia or pain of the posterior wall of the external auditory canal. Hemifacial spasm is rarely seen. It is unusual for vestibular schwannomas to affect cranial nerves other than the eighth, fifth, and seventh; however, large cerebellopontine angle tumors may also directly affect neighboring lower cranial nerves, or indirectly affect cranial nerve function through compression of the fourth ventricle causing elevation of intracranial pressure (ICP) and papilledema compressing the optic nerve. Thus, a complete cranial nerve examination is advised.

AUDIOMETRIC STUDIES

Early diagnosis of vestibular schwannomas relies on accurate assessment of auditory function including pure-tone air and bone conduction thresholds and speech discrimination. A reliable audiogram showing an asymmetric sensorineural hearing loss with disproportionately poor speech discrimination is suggestive of a potential vestibular schwannoma. A patient with a vestibular schwannoma may have very little or no hearing loss if the tumor is small, or if it originates in the cerebellopontine angle unrestricted by the bony canal. Occasionally, a large cerebellopontine angle tumor can be found in a patient who has normal hearing and a 100% discrimination score.

A number of special audiometric tests have been used historically to evaluate patients with abnormal audiograms that raise suspicion of retrocochlear lesions. Using a standard impedance bridge, the stapedial reflex decay test elicits the stapedial reflex with a suprathreshold tone burst. Decay of the reflexive stiffening of the tympanic membrane to half-amplitude in 5 sec or less is suggestive of retrocochlear pathology. Of historical interest is the Performance Intensity Function for Phonetically Balanced Words (PIPB) test, which evaluates speech discrimination at progressively higher sensation levels. As the presentation level increases, the speech discrimination score should also increase until a maximum score is obtained. If discrimination decreases as the presentation level increases the phenomenon of "rollover" occurs, which is consistent with a retrocochlear lesion. Burkey and colleagues suggested that patients with abnormal special auditory tests undergo an imaging study looking for retrocochlear pathology.[47] The stapedial reflex decay and PIPB tests are not routinely used in screening currently because more sensitive and specific tests are available.

One of the most sensitive audiometric tests available is the auditory brain stem response (ABR) (for detailed information, see Chapter 10). Early studies with ABR reported better than 90% sensitivity for the diagnosis of vestibular schwannomas.[48,49]

An interaural wave V latency difference of greater than 0.2 milliseconds, or prolonged interpeak latencies greater than 4.4 milliseconds for I–V, 2.3 milliseconds for I–III, or 2.1 milliseconds for III–V, suggests a retrocochlear disorder such as a vestibular schwannoma (Figure 37–3). The complete absence of wave V also suggests retrocochlear pathology.

A major limitation in the utility of ABR in the evaluation of vestibular schwannomas is that the patient must have no greater than a 70-dB hearing threshold. The sensitivity of the ABR to intracanalicular acoustic tumors less than 1 cm, ranges from 58 to 89%. In an attempt to improve the cost effectiveness of retrocochlear screening, we and other authors recommend using MRI for patients with suspicious histories and abnormal audiometric findings.[50–52] Others have recommended ABR as the initial screening study in low- to intermediate-risk patients, or those with contraindications to MRI.[53,54]

Attempts to overcome the diagnostic limitations of ABR have improved its reliability. Adjusting the wave V latency to account for hearing loss at 4 kHz have lowered false positive and false negative rates, improving sensitivity of this testing.

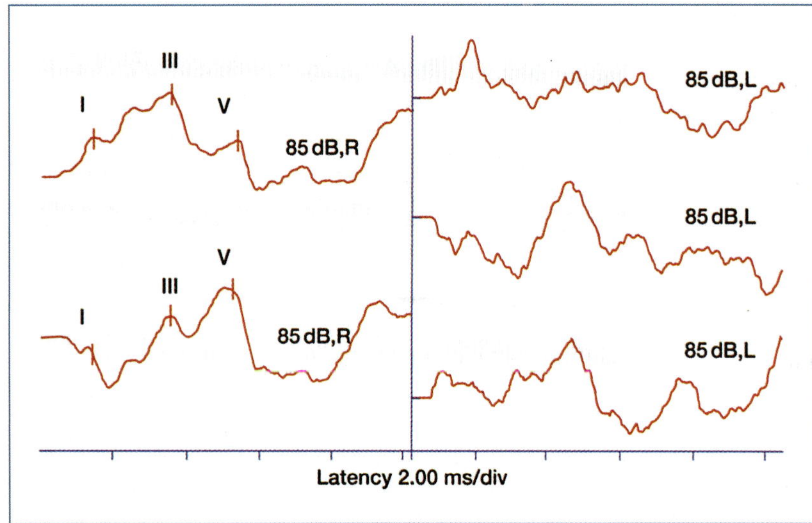

FIGURE 37–3 • Auditory brainstem response tracing of a left ear with a vestibular schwannoma compared with the contralateral (right) normal hearing ear. Note the delayed latency of wave V compared with the normal ear (right) and the poor waveform morphology.

Adjusting wave V limits by 0.1 millisecond/10 dB for hearing thresholds above 30 dB at 4 kHz has been recommended.[55] The use of 1 kHz tonal ABR in those with high-frequency hearing loss has been validated as a reliable method to screen patients with hearing loss above that level for retrocochlear pathology.[56]

Don and colleagues reported a modification of the standard ABR, called the stacked ABR.[57] This measure calculates the wave V amplitude by temporally aligning the wave V of each derived-band ABR and then summating the time-shifted responses. The stacked ABR is reported to be sensitive to the presence of small intracanalicular tumors and to have excellent specificity for the absence of tumors in patients with normal hearing. These authors recommend stacked ABR for vestibular schwannoma screening when MRI is unavailable or not tolerated by the patient.

VESTIBULAR STUDIES

As a vestibular schwannoma slowly destroys vestibular function in the affected ear, gradual compensation takes place.[58] Therefore, patients with vestibular schwannomas rarely complain of vertigo but often note slight unsteadiness or clumsiness. Although historically the finding of decreased vestibular function on caloric testing ipsilateral to a sensorineural hearing loss has been useful in suggesting the diagnosis of a vestibular schwannoma, at present, it is not sensitive enough to be helpful diagnostically.[50] Caloric testing measures the response of the lateral semicircular canal, which is innervated by the superior vestibular nerve; accordingly, a small inferior vestibular nerve schwannoma might not cause an abnormal caloric response.

Linthicum and Churchill described a simple method for examining the caloric response without sophisticated equipment.[59] The patient's head is placed at a 30-degree angle, and a small amount of ice water is placed in the external auditory canal for 20 sec. They used Frenzel lenses to examine the eyes for nystagmus. Absent or diminished nystagmus suggests a reduced vestibular response.

A more sophisticated method of determining vestibular function uses the Hallpike and Cairns[60] technique with electronystagmography (ENG) and bithermal caloric testing (see Chapter 11 for additional information). Eye tracking tests can reveal central vestibular dysfunction in the presence of a large tumor. Spontaneous nystagmus not apparent to the naked eye may be seen with Frenzel lenses or detected by ENG.

As more sensitive diagnostic modalities have developed (e.g., MRI and ABR testing), ENG is no longer used in the initial evaluation of most patients. However, when a small tumor has been identified in a patient with useful hearing, ENG may add prognostic information by identifying the nerve of origin when a hearing preservation operation is considered, although its prognostic value is not universally accepted in the literature.

The significance of identifying the nerve of origin is that hearing preservation may be more difficult in the removal of a tumor that arises from the inferior vestibular nerve due to its proximity to the cochlear nerve. During tumor dissection, an interruption of the cochlear nerve blood supply can result in postoperative hearing loss. Magnetic resonance imaging can occasionally differentiate the nerve of origin of smaller intracanalicular tumors. When MRI cannot determine the nerve of origin, ENG may provide useful information. A reduced vestibular response in the involved ear suggests a superior vestibular nerve tumor. Therefore, ENG results may influence selection of the surgical approach and provide prognostic information regarding hearing preservation.

A functional test for the inferior vestibular nerve could theoretically compliment an ENG, and enhance the ability to determine a vestibular schwannoma's nerve of origin. The vestibular evoked myogenic potential (VEMP) is receiving much attention for such capability. A VEMP is elicited by high-intensity sound stimulation of the saccule. The resultant vestibulospinal, or more accurately the sacculo-collic, reflex is recorded electrically as a biphasic p-13 n-23 potential from the ipsilateral sternocleidomastoid muscle. The hypothesis that an absent or reduced VEMP with a normal ENG is an indication of a lesion of the inferior vestibular nerve, or vice versa, is helpful in some cases, but idealistic.[61–63] Vestibular evoked myogenic potential responses have some cochlear nerve origin and are influenced by the level of ipsilateral hearing. The VEMP responses may be normal even when a tumor has its origin on the inferior vestibular nerve, and can be reduced or abolished by a compressive superior vestibular nerve tumor. The VEMP responses may be more influenced by the size or position of a vestibular schwannoma in the IAC than by the nerve of origin.[64] Further study of the ability of VEMP testing to accurately predict the nerve of origin is necessary.[65]

IMAGING

Although audiometric and vestibular testing raise suspicions for a vestibular schwannoma, imaging studies provide the definitive diagnosis. Contrast-enhanced T1-weighted MRI is the gold standard but high-resolution T2 images are also excellent at detecting IAC lesions. Fortunately, painful techniques carrying significant morbidity, such as posterior fossa myelography, and gaseous or opaque contrast CT, are rarely necessary today. These imaging studies have been replaced by MRI and are used only when MRI is contraindicated.

Computed Tomography

One-millimeter CT scanning in both the axial and coronal planes provides excellent detail of the temporal bone and IACs. Erosion of the IAC from expansion of a vestibular schwannoma is well visualized by the exquisite bony detail provided by CT.[66] Subtle bone erosion in the cochlea or vestibule may also be detected with an intralabyrinthine schwannoma. However, CT provides less soft tissue detail than MRI. In addition, to visualize most tumors, CT must be performed with the administration of an intravenous contrast agent. Tumors less than 1 cm are often missed by CT, even when contrast is used. Larger tumors causing brain stem compression, displacement of the fourth ventricle, and hydrocephalus, are readily appreciated by CT. For these reasons, and since CT is fast, and is more sensitive to differentiate acute intracerebral bleeds than MRI (that may present with similar symptomatology as acute hydrocephalus or brain stem compression), it may be considered for use in patients to whom intervention will only be offered if the tumor is exerting significant pressure on the brain stem. For patients intolerant of MRI, or when it is contraindicated, air-contrast CT is capable of showing intracanalicular tumor.[67] For this, air is inserted into the subdural space by way of a lumbar puncture. Following removal of cerebrospinal fluid (CSF), 7 to 10 cm^3 of air (or oxygen) is injected into the subarachnoid space, and the patient is positioned so that the air rises to the posterior fossa where it can outline a small intracanalicular tumor. Both sides are examined to rule out bilateral lesions. Following the procedure most patients will complain of a temporary headache.

Magnetic Resonance Imaging

When a patient's history or audiometric evaluation provides a moderate-to-high level of suspicion for a retrocochlear lesion, MRI is the diagnostic modality of choice to detect vestibular schwannomas, regardless of size. Magnetic resonance imaging reveals exceptional resolution of the full course of the seventh and eighth cranial nerves, from brain stem to end organ. Magnetic resonance images are obtained before and after administration of the paramagnetic contrast agent gadolinium. T1-weighted images show vestibular schwannomas hyperintense relative

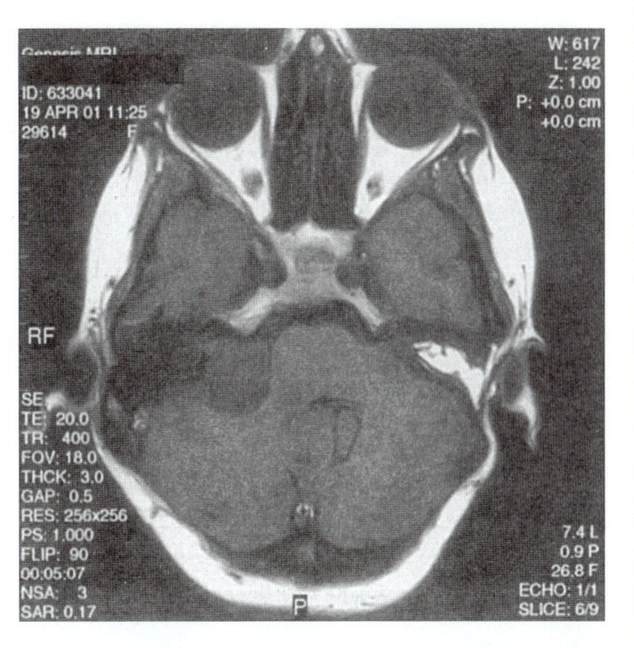

FIGURE 37–4 • Vestibular schwannoma as seen with T1-weighted magnetic resonance imaging. The tumor is so intense with gray matter.

to CSF and iso- to hypointense to gray matter (Figure 37–4). T2-weighted images show these tumors hypointense to CSF and hyperintense to gray matter. Additionally, the fluid-filled inner ear and CSF of the IAC are bright and clearly visualized on T2-weighted sequences. Cystic tumors often have high-signal intensity on T2-weighted sequences because fluid fills the cystic components of the tumor (Figure 37–5A and B). Gadolinium-enhanced, T1-weighted images of a vestibular schwannoma reveal marked tumor enhancement, and are considered to be the gold standard for imaging vestibular schwannomas (Figure 37–6). The sensitivity of gadolinium-enhanced MRI permits detection of schwannomas as small as 1–2 mm.[68]

Magnetic resonance imaging using a heavily T2-weighted fast spin echo (FSE) technique shows excellent contrast between bone, neural structures, and CSF. Images of the IAC contents are clearly visualized without the added cost or time of repeating the sequences following contrast administration. Fast spin echo T2-weighted studies can be completed much quicker than a contrast-enhanced scan. Vestibular schwannomas are hypointense compared to CSF on T2-weighted FSE sequences, and an intracanalicular tumor appears as a filling defect in the IAC (Figure 37–7). Investigators comparing gadolinium-enhanced, T1-weighted MRI with T2-weighted FSE sequences have reported that the latter modality can reliably detect mass lesions within the IAC and cerebellopontine angle and efficiently screen patients with sensorineural hearing loss.[69,70] It has been suggested that FSE MRI could be used as a highly sensitive and specific, yet cost-effective screening method, reserving the use of gadolinium to confirm suspected tumors.

More recently, the goal of imaging has shifted from early diagnosis of a tumor to determining prognostic information pertinent to surgical planning. If a mass is deemed favorable for

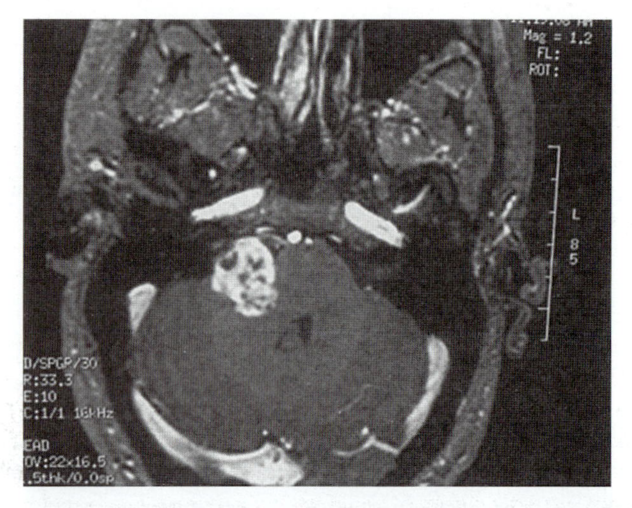

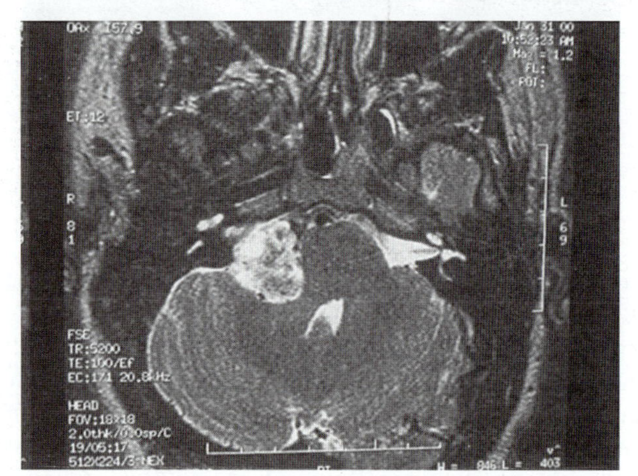

FIGURE 37–5 • Magnetic resonance imaging images of cystic vestibular schwannomas. *A*, Axial T1-weighted magnetic resonance imaging with gadolinium contrast. There is an enhancing right-sided cerebellopontine angle tumor with areas of central low intensity that correspond with cysts within this pathologically confirmed vestibular schwannoma. *B*, Axial T2-weighted magnetic resonance imaging. The tumor is more hyperintense than the typical T2 signal characteristics of a vestibular schwannoma. Additionally, there are focal areas of increased signal intensity that correspond with the intratumoral cysts.

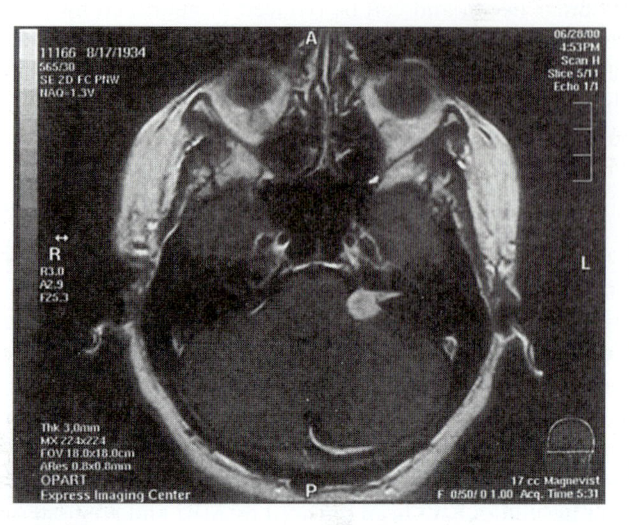

FIGURE 37–6 • Vestibular schwannoma, as seen with gadolinium-enhanced, T1-weighted magnetic resonance imaging. The vestibular schwannoma enhances brightly.

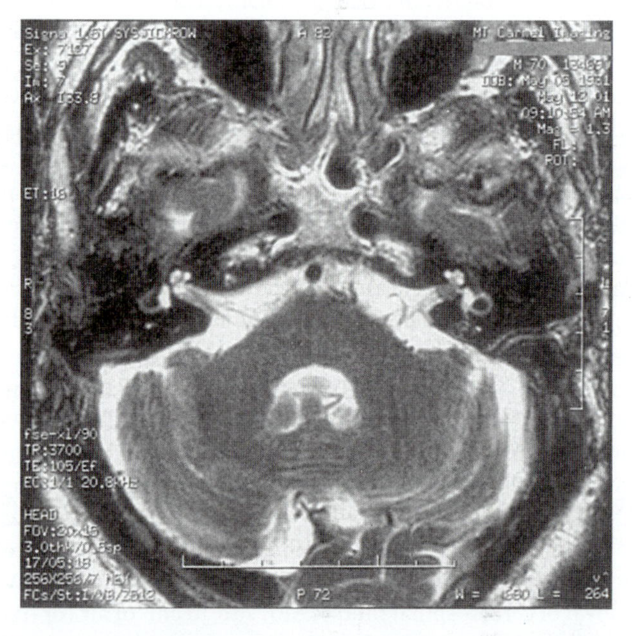

FIGURE 37–7 • Fast spin echo magnetic resonance image of an intracanalicular vestibular schwannoma. The tumor is hypointense to cerebrospinal fluid and appears as a filling defect within the internal auditory canal.

a hearing preservation operation due to its nerve of origin, position in the IAC, or relation to the other neural structures, then it would seem that patients could make a more calculated decision between observing the tumor, and choosing a more active course of treatment. Manipulation of the MR protocols and post imaging software packages are achieving some of these goals. Three-dimensional Fourier transform FSE manipulation was able to accurately determine the nerve of origin in 15–20 tumors as confirmed by surgery.[71] Tumors impacting the fundus of the IAC limited the ability of this technique. Presence of CSF lateral to a tumor in the IAC shows bright against the tumor void on T2-weighted images and is referred to as a "fundal cap." Absence of a fundal cap and impaction of the fundus of the IAC by tumor are harbingers of hearing loss. Assessment of fundal involvement was significantly enhanced by 3D-constructive interference in steady-state (CISS) sequencing when compared to standard post contrast T1-weighted imaging due to superior high-contrast resolution.[72] When evaluating the posterior fossa, 3D-fast imaging using steady-state acquisition (FIESTA) has been shown to improve cisternal imaging of cranial nerves V–XII as compared to FSE T2-weighting.[73] Finally, tumor volume was the only parameter significantly predictive of hearing preservation when compared to linear measures, audiometric parameters including

ABR latencies, caloric measures, as well as qualitative parameters such as fundal involvement, nerve of origin, and morphological features on ABR.[74] Despite the progress in imaging resolution and capabilities, most data continues to be collected using small numbers and retrospective constructs. Prospective imaging of adequate power is necessary to draw conclusions regarding the prognostic capabilities of these techniques.

Patients with claustrophobia may not tolerate the confinement required for MRI; however, mild sedatives or open MRI units make the study tolerable for most patients. Owing to the strong magnetic field, patients with metallic prostheses, such as cardiac pacemakers and cochlear implants, cannot undergo MRI. Manufacturing variability in some series of stapes prosthesis has shown ferromagnetic properties in lines that were labeled as MRI-compatible by the manufacturer.[75] Most stapes prostheses can tolerate the 1.5-Tesla magnet of MRI; however, these prostheses are likely to contraindicate imaging in more powerful magnets.[76]

In summary, MRI is the diagnostic test of choice for patients in whom a vestibular schwannoma is suspected. Fast spin echo MRI is a cost-efficient screening tool. Stacked ABR may also be useful for screening when the degree of suspicion is not as high, or in circumstances that prohibit MR imaging.

TREATMENT OPTIONS

The three options for the management of vestibular schwannomas are surgical excision, stereotactic radiation, and observation. Each treatment has its advantages and disadvantages. To a great extent, the decision is based on patient preference and the findings of observational studies. There is no randomized, controlled clinical trial that has objectively assessed outcomes of these treatment options. Consequently, clinical decision making can be difficult. Fortunately, in comparison with the morbidity and mortality of past decades, the outcomes of all three treatment options are quite good.

Observation

The indolent nature of many vestibular schwannomas has long been recognized, leading some physicians to recommend observation without immediate intervention as a reasonable treatment option.[77–82] The reported number of tumors that will grow over time ranges from 30 to 82%.[77,83,84] In a recent study, growth occurred in 66% of patients followed over a 5-year period.[84] The advantages of nonintervention for patients whose vestibular schwannomas do not exhibit growth are evident, no intervention may be required if critical growth does not occur over their life span.

Even with this conservative treatment option, there are inherent dangers. For example, although tumor growth rates average 2 mm per year, some tumors may grow up to 25 mm per year. As discussed below, the literature contains conflicting reports regarding the ability to predict future growth based on past growth patterns. A tumor may grow more quickly than the norm, compromising the ability to preserve hearing and facial nerve function with intervention, and may even endanger the patient's life.[83] Charabi and colleagues reported a 6% death rate owing to tumor-induced brain stem herniation in patients with vestibular schwannomas managed by observation.[85] Such a mortality rate has not been reported in other large series.[86,87] Patients who enter the observation period with salvageable hearing may lose hearing if the tumor grows. In one study, 28 patients were classified as candidates for a hearing preservation operation; 21 (75%) of the patients fell out of this classification during the observation period owing to tumor growth and/or deterioration of hearing.[85]

Surveillance protocols vary but typically, an MRI is obtained 6 months after the diagnostic scan, and yearly thereafter if there is no imminent danger of brain stem compression. Observation is considered reasonable treatment of an only-hearing ear when serviceable hearing remains and brain stem function is not immediately at risk.[87] Observation is also reasonable for reliable patients when the tumor is small, the patient is elderly (> 65 years) or medically infirm, or as a matter of patient's preference. Some patients prefer the idea of using the hearing they have as long as they can, as opposed to the risk of a radiation-induced or surgical loss.

Growth Rate Prediction

The ability to accurately predict schwannoma growth rates by evaluating factors such as tumor size at discovery, association with NF2, patient age, or interval growth over the initial observation period, would be helpful in making treatment decisions. Unfortunately, it is disputed which factors are predictive of growth rate. Tumor growth during the first year has been reported to be predictive of subsequent growth by Bederson and colleagues,[88] but Charabi and colleagues reported that growth patterns change during extended observation periods.[83] Ogawa and colleagues found the growth rate of unilateral vestibular schwannomas to be slower than that of the bilateral vestibular schwannomas of NF2.[89] The growth rate of recurrent tumors was also faster than that of primary tumors. In counterpoint, Levo and colleagues found that unilateral schwannomas grow more rapidly than schwannomas associated with NF2.[82] During their observation, the average growth rate of unilateral vestibular schwannomas was 3.5 mm per year compared to 1.5 mm per year for NF2 tumors. A prospective study by the NF2 Natural History Consortium showed a similar growth rate of 1.3 mm per year.[90]

The relationships between tumor growth rates and patient age or tumor size have also been analyzed. The younger the patient or larger the tumor, the greater the growth rate.[89] Diensthuber and colleagues proposed using a clinical growth index to estimate vestibular schwannoma growth rate.[91] An index calculated by dividing the tumor length by the length of the clinical history also showed statistically significant negative correlations between the clinical growth index and tumor size or patient age. This indicates that older patients with smaller intrameatal tumors may be good candidates for observation.

Study of the indicators of cellular proliferation showed a slightly higher nuclear proliferation labeling index (0.4 to 17.6%; mean = 2.7%) in NF2-associated schwannomas than in unilateral vestibular schwannomas (0 to 9%; mean = 2.2%).[92] Cystic tumors have been described as having faster than usual growth rates due to the rapidly enlarging cystic portion.[93] Recent studies conservatively following large numbers of patients for at least one year show no growth in 42 to 66%. Approximately 24–39% grew slowly, 4% grew rapidly, and 3–19% regressed.[94,95]

A better understanding of the fate of hearing with conservative management would also be prognostically useful when determining treatment strategies. Quaranta and colleagues studied the effect of watchful waiting on hearing loss and tinnitus in a group of 70 patients.[95] Over an average 33-month observation period, useful hearing was maintained in 71% of patients with class A hearing, and 60% with class A or B hearing. Raut and colleagues showed that prospective observation of a cohort of 72 patients followed for a mean duration of 80 months had hearing loss irrespective of tumor growth.[96] Over this time period 32% of patients failed observation and were actively treated for rapid growth of their tumor, or for increased signs or symptoms. They did not identify any factors predictive of failure of observation or tumor growth. They showed that tumors confined to the IAC grew significantly slower than tumors of the cerebellopontine angle, but statistical hearing deterioration occurred in both groups. Hearing preservation surgery could also benefit from preoperative parameters with prognostic value. In a retrospective evaluation of attempted hearing preservation in 29 patients following middle cranial fossa tumor resection, Gjuric et al found that only preoperative tumor volume analysis significantly predicted hearing outcomes.[74] Linear volume measurements, fundal involvement, and audiovestibular testing parameters were unable to predict postoperative hearing.

Stereotactic Radiation Therapy

In 1951, the Swedish neurosurgeon Leksell developed the first open stereotactic instrument by focusing multiple radiation beams on a single target. He reported his experience with closed cranial treatment of a variety of lesions over the next several years.[97] Currently, stereotactic radiation is the principal alternative active treatment for vestibular schwannomas (as opposed to microsurgical resection). The terms "Gamma Knife®, Cyber Knife®, and XKnife™" are often applied misnomers that may be confusing to patients. "Stereotactic radiation" is the preferred term as it is more descriptive of the treatment.

The goals of stereotactic radiation therapy are the long-term prevention of tumor growth, maintenance of neurologic function, and prevention of new neurologic deficits. Noren reported growth control, usually with shrinkage, in 95% of unilateral tumors.[98] The development of cranial neuropathies shows a direct relation to radiation dose. Miller and colleagues reported a facial neuropathy rate of 38% when delivering 20 Gy to the tumor periphery, but only 8% when the margin dose was reduced to 16 Gy ($p = .006$).[99] Multivariate analysis revealed that the only factor associated with increased risk of posttreatment facial neuropathy was a tumor margin dose greater than or equal to 18 Gy. Facial nerve preservation rates up to 98% have been reported as radiation dosage to the tumor periphery have been reduced to less than 16 Gy.[98–102] Similarly, the incidence of trigeminal neuropathy was reduced from 29 to 15% by decreasing the marginal dose from 20 to 16 Gy. By further limiting the dose to 12 Gy or less hearing preservation has been reportedly achieved in 65 to 70%, and tinnitus is rarely made worse.[98] Although delayed-onset cranial neuropathies can occur, no new neurologic deficits appear more than 28 months after stereotactic radiation.[100]

Linear accelerators have also been used to deliver stereotactic radiation to vestibular schwannomas, and are reported to achieve results similar to the Gamma Knife.[101,103] There are no noted advantages in hearing protection or facial nerve function to date demonstrated by fractionated stereotactic regimens.

Stereotactic Rediation Advantages

Potential advantages of stereotactic radiation over microsurgical resection include decreased hospitalization time, a quicker return to work, and, in some countries, a reduced cost of treatment.[104] Additionally, stereotactic radiation may be considered for elderly or medically infirm patients in whom tumor growth has been documented. The risks associated with microsurgical dissection, including infection and CSF leak, are avoided because of the minimally invasive nature of the treatment. Patients who demonstrate tumor recurrence after surgical removal may undergo salvage radiation therapy.[105] However, such tumor recurrence occurs only in 0.3 to 0.8% of patients treated in centers with considerable microsurgical experience.[106,107]

Stereotactic Radiation Disadvantages

A relative disadvantage of stereotactic radiation lies in the need for prolonged surveillance with repeated MRIs and the associated cost over a long follow-up course. Treated tumors may harbor viable tumor following a course of treatment and some have shown growth requiring salvage microsurgery.

Potential disadvantages of stereotactic radiation include radiation-induced hydrocephalus, even after treatment of tumors as small as 18 mm.[108] This complication, which is associated directly with tumor size,[101] was much more common in early reports; its occurrence has been reduced recently between 1.4 and 9.2%.

Some surgeons have reported great difficulty preserving the facial nerve in the surgical salvage of schwannomas that have failed radiation.[109] This difficulty has been disputed by others.[110,111]

Another consideration in stereotactic radiation therapy is the potential for sudden hearing loss, likely owing to swelling that occurs soon after radiation.[112] When observed, additional decline in auditory nerve function may occur over several years following radiation. In one study, useful hearing was preserved in 10 of 10 patients immediately after radiation treatment but declined to 8 of 10 patients at 6 months, 6 of 10 patients at 1 year, and 5 of 10 patients at 2 years.[113]

Stereotactic radiation for vestibular schwannomas associated with NF2 represent a special challenge because of the risk of complete deafness. Subach and colleagues reported an overall tumor control rate of 98% in 45 NF2-associated vestibular schwannomas treated with stereotactic radiation using a mean tumor margin dose of 15 Gy (range 12 to 20 Gy). During the median follow-up period of 36 months, 16 tumors (36%) regressed, 28 (62%) remained unchanged, and 1 (2%) grew. Useful hearing was preserved in 6 (43%) of 14 patients, and this rate improved to 67% after the radiation dose was reduced. Normal facial nerve function (House-Brackmann grade I) was preserved in 25 (81%) of 31 patients. Normal trigeminal nerve function was preserved in 34 (94%) of 36 patients.[114] A study by Ito and colleagues suggested that tumor diameter and the diagnosis of NF2 were risk factors associated with increased hearing loss following stereotactic radiation. Larger populations and longer follow-up are necessary to draw rigorous conclusions.[111]

Radiation-Induced Malignancy

Radiation treatment in low doses, and for benign processes, has been associated with malignant transformation of affected tissues. The risk of a previously benign schwannoma undergoing malignant degeneration is a concern, especially for younger patients that will require decades of observation. In 1998 Noren reported an estimated 0.1% worldwide rate of malignant change of 8,000 vestibular schwannomas treated with stereotactic radiation since 1969.[98] Patients whose tumors underwent malignant transformation died despite microsurgical excision. Histopathologic analysis revealed a malignant, spindle cell neoplasm with numerous mitotic figures. Rhabdoid elements detected by immunohistochemical analysis confirmed the diagnosis of a malignant triton tumor or sarcoma.[115,116] Schwannomas surgically removed after stereotactic radiation failure have also shown atypical and viable schwannoma cells as well as other foci showing delayed radiation changes such as nucleolar and cytoplasmic enlargement and proliferation of endothelial cells.[117,118] Although the incidence of malignant transformation is low, observation periods documented in the majority of studies are short relative to the time course range of radiation induced malignant degeneration. Further assurance or concerns rests on the unfolding longevity of experience with these techniques at current dosing parameters. It must also be recognized that malignant schwannomas or triton tumors may occur spontaneously in the absence of a prior history of irradiation.[119,120]

In a study of 2,311 patients with a history of childhood irradiation for enlarged tonsils and adenoids, Shore-Freedman and colleagues found 29 schwannomas, 2 neurofibromas, and 1 ganglioneuroma, representing a 1.4% incidence of tumors. Because of the frequency of tumor development and the strict localization of the tumors to the area of treatment, it was concluded that they were radiation induced. Analysis of the latency of these tumors indicates that they continue to occur for at least 30 years after the radiation exposure. In the same group of individuals, there have been 54 confirmed salivary gland tumors (40 benign and 14 malignant).[121]

Stereotactic radiation may be less likely to induce neoplastic change than fractionated radiation, and glandular tissue, which is prone to radiation-induced neoplasia, is not in the radiation field used for vestibular schwannomas. Thus, the overall risk of malignancy is less than for fractionated radiation. The overall risk of neoplastic change would appear to be less in patients over the age of 60 years; therefore, some clinicians, in keeping with the National Institutes of Health Consensus Development Conference report,[122] do not recommend radiation unless patients are elderly or otherwise medically infirm. The ultimate answer to the question of the long-term safety of stereotactic radiation will require at least a 30-year follow-up period. The risk of malignant degeneration must be weighed against the risk of complications of surgery, such as stroke or death, and the outcomes stratified by similar tumor size, location, and patient's health profile.

Finally, stereotactic irradiation treats lesions of the CPA based on the probability of their diagnosis as predicted by their radiographic appearance and their anatomic location. No confirmatory histopathologic analysis is available with this strategy, therefore the possibility of delaying the diagnosis and or treatment of a malignant lesion elsewhere may rarely occur.

Radiation Versus Observation

Shirato and colleagues reported a comparative study of observation versus stereotactic radiotherapy in the management of vestibular schwannomas.[123] Twenty-seven patients underwent observation as initial treatment, and 50 received stereotactic radiation. Small-field, fractionated radiotherapy (36 to 44 Gy in 20 to 22 fractions over 6 weeks) was delivered with or without a subsequent 4-Gy boost. The tumor control rate in the radiation group, when delivered at these high levels, was significantly better than that of the observation group. Mean tumor growth was 3.87 mm per year in the observation group and −0.75 mm per year in the stereotactic radiation group. Forty-one percent of the observation group and 2% of the stereotactic radiation group required salvage therapy. They concluded that stereotactic radiotherapy provided better tumor control and a similar rate of hearing deterioration than did observation.[123] Intervention assignment was not randomized, however, representing an important bias in the study. Also, the number of tumors that were growing at the time of patient entry into the study was not defined.

In summary, although acceptable outcomes have been reported with stereotactic radiation therapy for the treatment of vestibular schwannomas, long-term outcomes at current levels of radiation have not been well documented.[98–102] The average dose of radiation to the tumor margin has been progressively reduced since the technique was initially described, resulting in improved cranial nerve function and fewer brain stem complications. Unfortunately, these studies do not account for tumors that would not have grown without any treatment. We believe that longitudinal follow-up is required before definitive conclusions can be drawn regarding the ultimate rate of tumor control using reduced stereotactic radiation doses.[99]

Microsurgery

Historically, microsurgical excision has been the treatment of choice for vestibular schwannomas. There are four microsurgical approaches for vestibular schwannoma removal: the middle cranial fossa, the translabyrinthine, the suboccipital (retrosigmoid), and a combined approach. A multidisciplinary approach to the microsurgical removal of vestibular schwannomas has developed in tertiary referral centers. This amiable working relationship between the neurotologist and the neurosurgeon has led to improved hearing preservation rates and facial nerve outcomes.

Approach Selection

Access to the IAC via a middle fossa craniotomy is used when the possibility for hearing preservation exists. In our practice, hearing preservation is attempted when the pure-tone average is 30 dB or less and the speech discrimination is greater than 70%. However, in patients with NF2 or poor hearing in the contralateral ear, the criteria need not be so stringent. Small tumors restricted to the IAC are best accessed with the middle fossa approach. Generally, tumors of 1–1.5 cm can be successfully exposed and removed through the middle fossa route. The middle fossa approach affords excellent access to the fundus of the IAC while preserving the otic capsule, and is ideal for laterally situated tumors. However, tumors with substantial extension into the cerebellopontine angle can be removed through the middle fossa approach if the superior petrosal sinus is ligated and the temporal lobe is further retracted.

The translabyrinthine approach directly traverses the temporal bone and otic capsule and is therefore preferred for patients without useful hearing preoperatively. This approach can be used for tumors of all sizes, provides excellent exposure of the cerebellopontine angle, and affords the widest exposure of the facial nerve, extending from the vertical segment within the temporal bone to the root entry zone at the brain stem. Furthermore, visualization of adjacent cranial nerves is facilitated by the wide exposure of the translabyrinthine approach. A relative advantage of the translabyrinthine approach over the middle fossa and suboccipital approaches is the avoidance of cerebellar or temporal lobe retraction. Cerebellar retraction is occasionally necessary for very large tumors. The fragility of blood vessels increases with age, thus increasing the likelihood of intraparenchymal bleeding with brain retraction.

The suboccipital (retrosigmoid) approach accesses the posterior fossa through a craniotomy inferior to the transverse sinus and posterior to the sigmoid sinus. Generally, the neurotologist views the suboccipital approach as a hearing preservation approach for medially located tumors. This approach affords superior exposure of the cerebellopontine angle when compared with the middle fossa approach. The posterior wall of the IAC is drilled away to expose the medial IAC. The fundus of the canal cannot be fully visualized without drilling into the otic capsule. This can jeopardize complete tumor removal and hearing preservation if laterally based tumors require blind dissection. Tumors of all sizes can be removed through the suboccipital approach, and this is the traditional technique used by neurosurgeons. Cerebellar retraction is required.

The combined approach is used for tumors of the cerebellopontine angle that are greater than four centimeters, or that traverse intracranial compartments. Hearing preservation is not an objective with tumors of this size, but rather brain stem decompression and the prevention of increased ICP. Glasscock and Hays described a one-stage approach combining the translabyrinthine and suboccipital access for the treatment of giant tumors. This enabled additional cerebellar retraction and enhanced exposure of very large tumors.[58] The combined approach can be staged, performing tumor debulking, medial facial nerve identification, and brain stem decompression through the suboccipital approach, and then, at a later date, completing tumor removal with the addition of a translabyrinthine dissection. Identification of the lateral aspect of the facial nerve with the translabyrinthine dissection may facilitate facial nerve preservation with the removal of these large tumors.

Special considerations for the surgical planning of patients with NF2 arise due to the rapid growth rates and aggressive behavior of these tumors. The importance of preserving hearing in at least one ear is paramount. Likewise, bilateral brain stem compression seen in NF2 poses a greater threat to vital brainstem function and cerebrospinal fluid flow. There is controversy in the literature regarding the difficulty of surgical removal of unilateral vestibular schwannomas as compared to NF2-related schwannomas. Samii and Matthies reported microsurgical results in 120 tumors removed from 82 NF2 patients through a suboccipital approach. Overall, hearing was preserved in 36% of ears, and anatomic facial nerve preservation was achieved in 85%. Two deaths occurred.[124] They concluded that the chances of anatomic and functional nerve preservation are lower for patients with NF2 than for patients with unilateral tumors.

Slattery and colleagues reported the outcomes of 18 NF2 patients (23 tumors) who underwent surgical excision of vestibular schwannomas. Measurable hearing was preserved in 65% of patients. House-Brackmann grade I or II facial function was maintained in 100% of patients with normal preoperative facial nerve function. Unlike Samii and Matthies, they concluded that in patients with NF2, hearing and facial nerve function outcomes are similar to those for patients with sporadic, unilateral vestibular schwannomas. They agreed that early intervention was crucial in obtaining favorable outcomes.[125] Early detection with aggressive screening is strongly associated with favorable outcomes.[126,127]

MICROSURGICAL RESECTION

Middle Cranial Fossa Approach

The surgeon is seated at the head of the bed during middle fossa surgery (Figure 37–8). The head is turned opposite the side of the lesion, and the operative site is shaved. Facial nerve electrodes are placed in the obicularis oris and oculi muscles, and the facial nerve monitor is tested to ensure that it is functioning appropriately. Mannitol (1 g/kg) is given intravenously at the start of the case to decrease CSF pressure. If there is no contraindication, the patient is also given 10 mg of dexamethasone intravenously. Antibiotic prophylaxis covering skin pathogens is given prior to the skin incision. The surgical site is prepared and draped for neurotologic surgery in the usual fashion.

The skin incision is made with a #15 scalpel and extends 1 cm anterior to and approximately 12 cm superior to the tragus. The superior limb of the incision is angled (approximately 15 degrees) anteriorly. The temporalis fascia is divided sharply, and the temporalis muscle is incised with electrocautery to the skull. A periosteal (Lempert) elevator is used to elevate the musculoperiosteum anteriorly and posteriorly. Dura hooks are placed to retract the temporalis muscle. The root of the zygoma is identified at this point as it serves as the center of the inferior limit of the craniotomy. The anesthesia team should be instructed to hyperventilate the patient to a carbon dioxide (CO_2) level of 25–28 mm Hg to further facilitate brain relaxation.

A 4 × 4 cm craniotomy is drilled using a 5-mm cutting bur or craniotome. The craniotomy window should extend 2 cm anterior and 2 cm posterior to the zygomatic root and 4 cm in the vertical dimension. The surgeon should switch to a diamond bur when the dura is approached to prevent dural tears. The bone flap is gently elevated off the dura and placed in an antibiotic solution. Bleeding dural vessels are controlled with bipolar cautery. Exposed air cells within the zygomatic root should be sealed with either muscle or bone wax prior to the completion of the case to prevent a potential passage for CSF egress.

Using the operating microscope and a dural elevator, the temporal lobe and dura are gently elevated from the skull base.

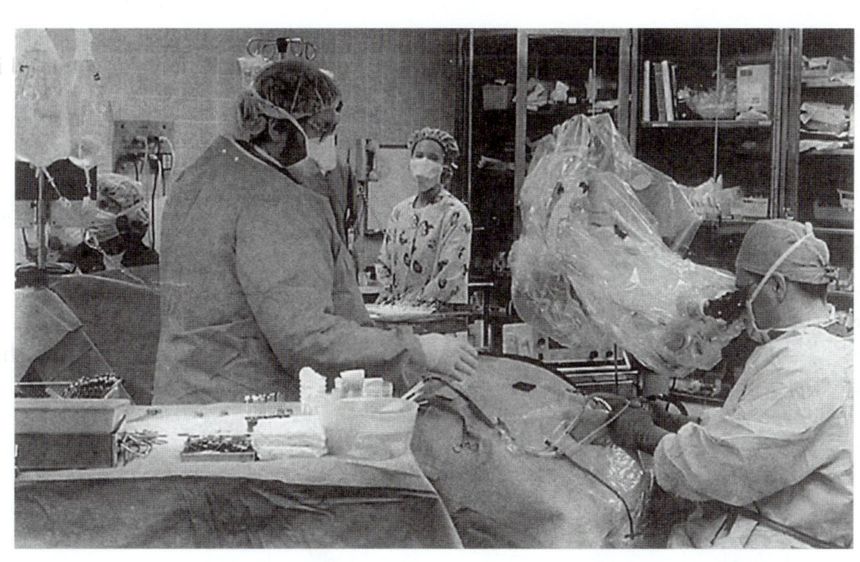

FIGURE 37–8 • The operating room setup for middle fossa surgery. Note that the surgeon is seated at the head of the bed and the anesthesiologist at the foot.

Elevation should proceed carefully in a posterior to anterior direction to avoid injuring a dehiscent geniculate ganglion, which is seen as high as in 18% of cases. Elevation proceeds to the anterior extent of the craniotomy, taking care not to lacerate the middle meningeal artery. Should the artery be lacerated, it is controlled with bipolar cautery. The temporal lobe and dura are elevated medially until the superior petrosal sinus and petrous pyramid are identified. As full exposure is accomplished, the arcuate eminence and greater petrosal nerve are identified. The greater petrosal nerve can be stimulated (at approximately 0.1 to 0.3mA) to "back-stimulate" the facial nerve. This maneuver helps to avoid confusion with the lesser petrosal nerve, which is located laterally and parallels the course of the greater petrosal nerve along the floor of the middle cranial fossa.

The House-Urban middle fossa retractor is placed to facilitate retraction of the temporal lobe. Cottonoid sponges should be placed between the blade of the retractor and the dura for protection. Using a #4 diamond bur and suction irrigation, drilling begins in the region of the arcuate eminence, and the superior semicircular canal is "blue-lined." Bisecting the angle between the greater superficial petrosal nerve and the superior semicircular canal gives the approximate location of the meatal plane and underlying IAC. Using successively smaller diamond burs, the IAC is identified medially near the porus. The depth of the IAC can be gauged by the coronal MR image. Bone is then removed laterally along the IAC, taking care to avoid fenestrating the cochlea or superior semicircular canal. The vertical crest (Bill's bar), which separates the anteriorly located facial nerve from the posteriorly located superior vestibular nerve, is identified at the fundus. The labyrinthine section of the facial nerve is identified as it exits the lateral end of the internal canal and heads toward the geniculate ganglion.

When the superior plane of the IAC is exposed 180 degrees, the bone work is complete and the surgical site is irrigated to remove any bone dust that might obscure visualization. The dura of the IAC is incised along its posterior border, avoiding the facial nerve. The dural margins are reflected anteriorly and posteriorly, and the facial nerve is identified on the superior surface of the tumor (Figure 37–9A). The nerve should be positively identified using the facial nerve stimulator set at 0.05 mA. As a result of the mass effect of the tumor, the facial nerve may occasionally be displaced anterior, inferior, or, rarely, even posterior to the tumor. Should this be the case, it is recommended that the nerve be positively identified at its lateral and medial limits prior to tumor dissection.

Using a sickle or Fisch knife, the facial nerve and tumor are gently separated. Often, the tumor can be gently retracted away from the facial nerve with the suction tip, facilitating exposure of the plane between the nerve and the tumor (Figure 37–9B). Once the facial nerve has been completely separated from the tumor, a 0.5-mm hook can be used to avulse the superior vestibular nerve lateral in the canal where it enters the temporal bone. The tumor is then carefully dissected free from the facial and cochlear nerves in a lateral to medial direction. The inferior vestibular nerve is usually intimately associated with the tumor and should be included with the specimen. Once the tumor is free from the IAC, the medial stalk of the vestibular nerve is sectioned with sharp microscissors (Figure 37–9C), leaving the facial and cochlear nerves exposed and intact in the IAC (Figure 37–9D). A plug of temporalis muscle is placed over the IAC, and the temporal lobe is allowed to expand. The bone flap is replaced, and the wound is closed in layers in a watertight fashion. A compression dressing is applied.

During hearing preservation surgery, the surgeon must remember that several important structures must be preserved. In addition to preserving the cochlea, labyrinth, and cochlear nerve, the labyrinthine artery within the IAC should be preserved. The surgeon should be aware of the fact that the anterior inferior cerebellar artery may loop into the IAC. Should this be the case, it is vital to gently dissect the vessel free from surrounding structures maintaining its integrity to prevent the sequelae of ischemic stroke.

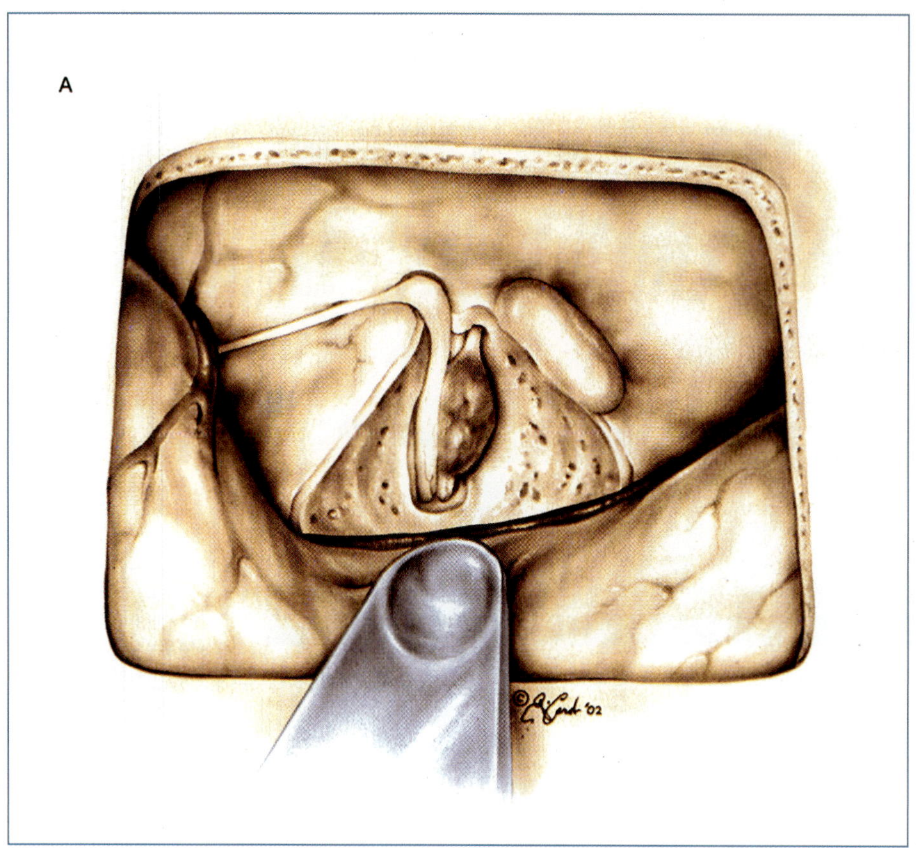

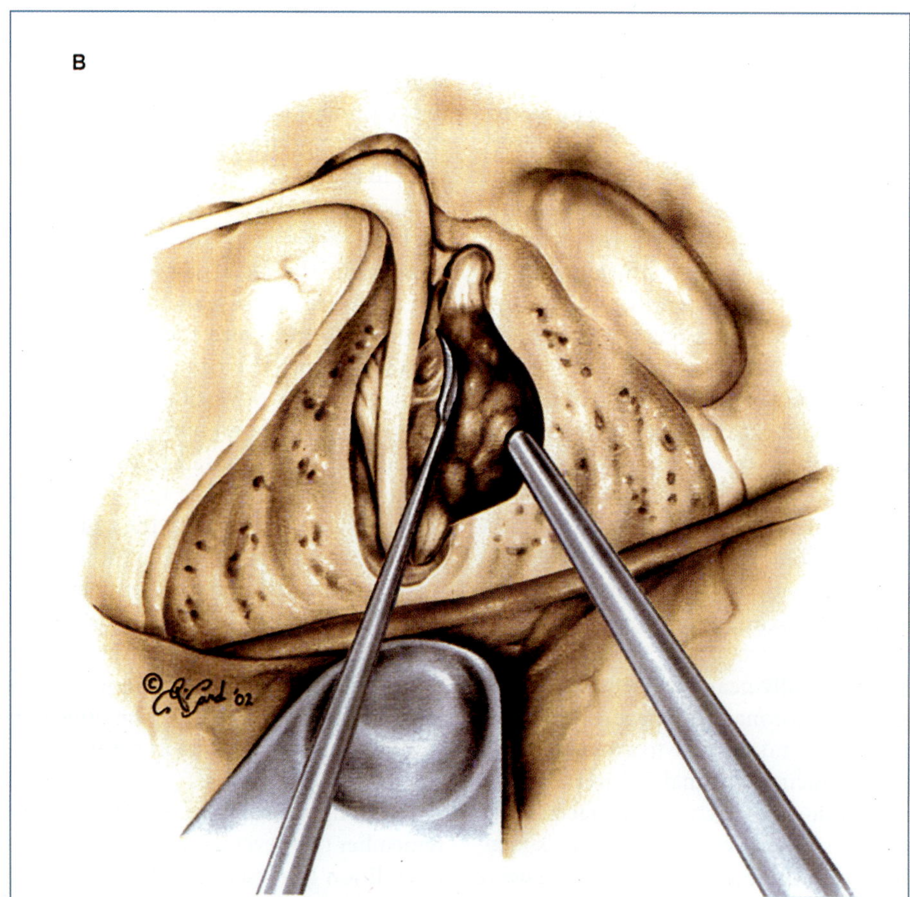

FIGURE 37–9 • *A*, Middle fossa exposure of a right vestibular schwannoma. The internal auditory canal and its dura have been opened. The facial nerve is identified on the superior surface of the tumor. *B*, A suction tip is used to retract the tumor, and the plane between the facial nerve and tumor is developed. The facial nerve must be completely separated from the tumor prior to avulsing the superior vestibular nerve and dissecting the tumor from the cochlear nerve.

Continued

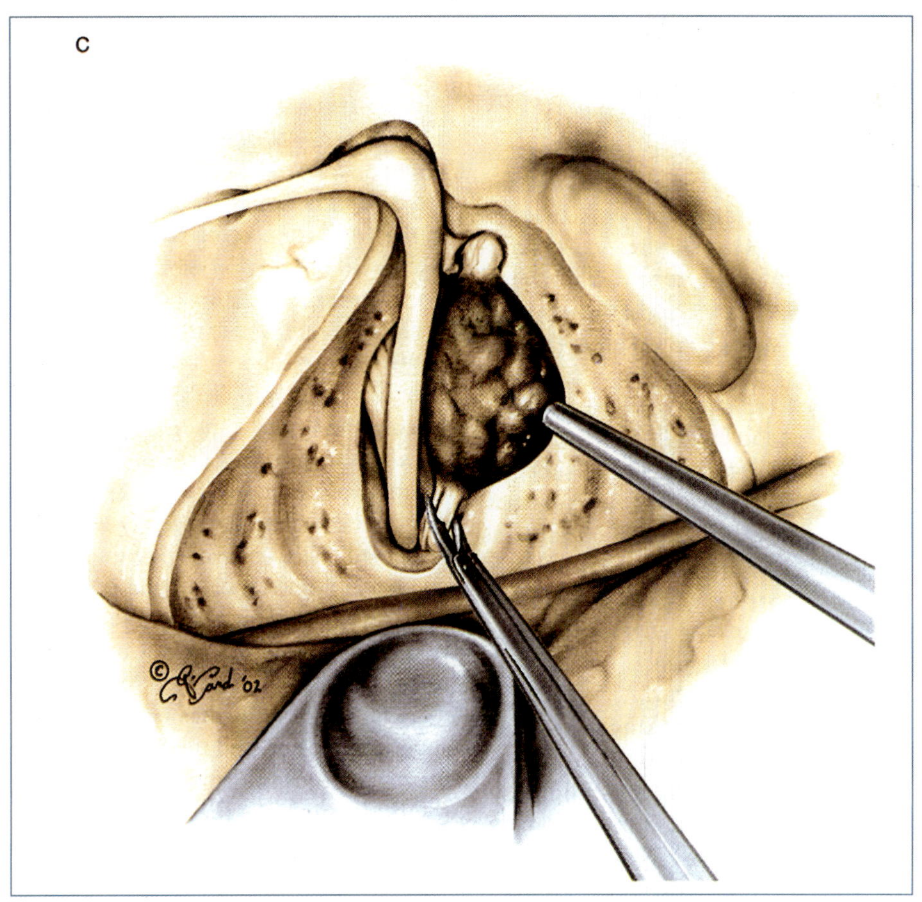

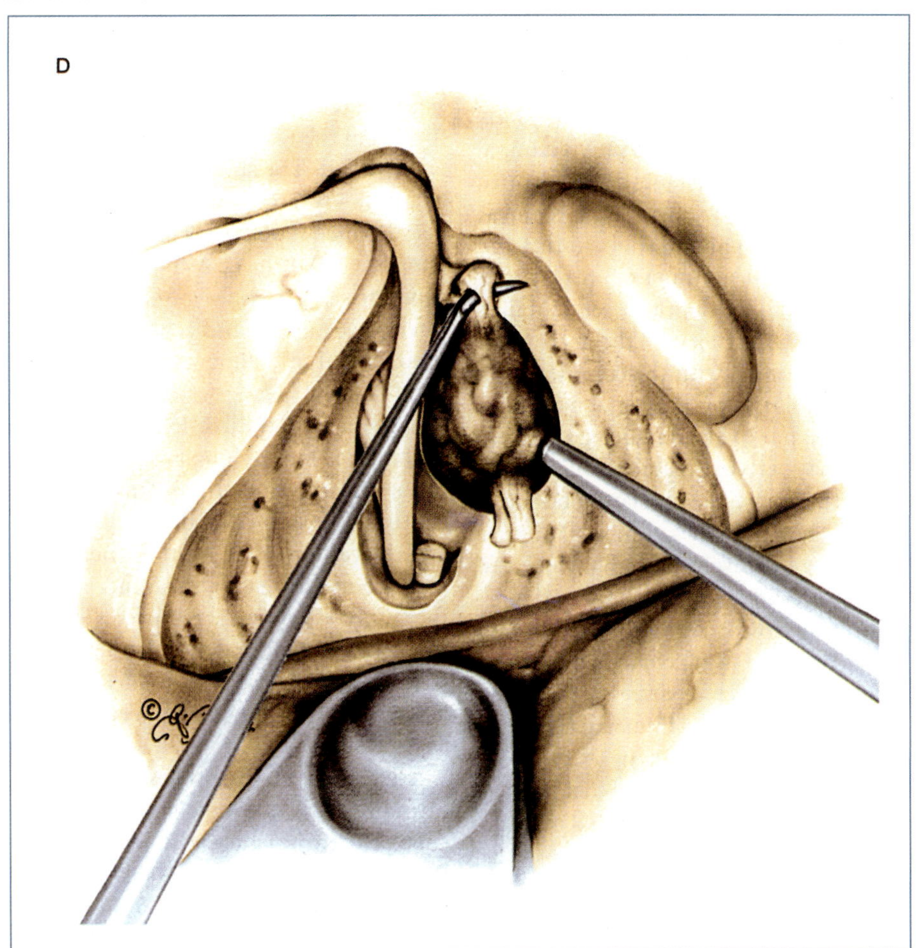

FIGURE 37–9 • *Continued. C*, Once the tumor is dissected free from facial and cochlear nerves, the medial stalk of the vestibular nerve is sectioned with microscissors. *D*, The facial and cochlear nerves remain in the internal auditory canal after tumor dissection.

Translabyrinthine Approach

The patient is placed in the supine position with the head turned away from the operative site. The hair is shaved above and behind the ear and the facial nerve monitor is attached along with other appropriate anesthetic monitors. Additionally, the left lower quadrant of the abdomen is prepared and draped for harvest of an abdominal adipose graft. The left lower quadrant is used to avoid creating the appearance of an appendectomy scar.

A postauricular, C-shaped incision is made approximately 4 cm behind the postauricular crease (Figure 37–10A). The postauricular flap is elevated anteriorly in the subcutaneous plane. A generous temporalis fascia graft is harvested, prepared on a cartilage cutting block, and placed on the back table along with a small temporalis muscle plug that is placed in an antibiotic solution for later use to pack and close off the middle-ear space. Dura hooks retract the edges of the skin flap anteriorly, and the musculoperiosteum is incised with electrocautery in a T- or C-shaped fashion. An elevator is used to elevate the musculoperiosteum, making sure not to tear the skin of the external auditory canal. Initially, a complete mastoidectomy is performed, exposing the middle and posterior fossa dural plates, sigmoid sinus, sinodural angle, antrum, and digastric ridge (Figure 37–10B). Next the vertical portion of the facial nerve is identified with a fine diamond bur, the facial recess is opened, and the incus is removed to facilitate later packing of the eustachian tube and middle ear (Figure 37–10C).

All bone is removed from the middle fossa dural plate, sinodural angle, and the sigmoid sinus at this point to provide ample working room to complete the labyrinthectomy and identify the IAC. Additionally, it is important to carry bone removal approximately 1 cm posterior to the sigmoid sinus so that the sinus can be retracted during subsequent tumor removal. Using a diamond bur and suction irrigation, the three semicircular canals are systematically removed, starting with the horizontal, moving to the posterior, and finishing with the common crus and superior canal (Figure 37–10D). After the horizontal canal is removed with a fine diamond bur to avoid injuring the horizontal segment of the facial nerve, a coarse diamond bur may be used to complete the labyrinthectomy. The jugular bulb should be well-defined; however, it is best to leave a thin shell of protective bone over this structure to prevent bleeding. Once the canals have been drilled away, the bone from the superior, inferior, and posterior aspects of the IAC is removed with successively smaller fine diamond burs and using copious irrigation. At the fundus, the transverse crest, which separates the superior and inferior vestibular nerves, is identified. The macula cribrosa superior (Mike's dot) facilitates identification of the lateral-most extent of the IAC and the superior vestibular nerve that lies just posterior to the vertical crest (Bill's bar) and the facial nerve at this point. Figure 37–10E, depicts the operative exposure at the completion of bone removal.

The posterior fossa dura is incised with a sharp knife blade or microscissors anteromedial to the sigmoid sinus and the incision is carried medially to the superior edge of the porus acousticus in a line just inferior to the superior petrosal sinus. A lower incision is created to the inferior edge of the porus in a line superior to the jugular bulb. A collagen sponge is placed under a cottonoid strip to protect the cerebellum. Microscissors are used to cut away the dura from the upper and lower edges of the IAC, connecting the incisions with the posterior fossa dura incisions, further exposing the cerebellum, tumor, and the neurovascular structures of the cerebellopontine angle. Small tumors are removed at this point without reducing them in size (Figure 37–10F). Large lesions require internal reduction before they can be extracted (Figure 37–10G). This begins with coagulating the tumor capsule vessels with a bipolar cautery and incising the capsule. Care should be exercised to cauterize only tumor capsule vessels. Larger vessels, such as the anterior inferior cerebellar artery, are gently swept off the tumor surface and preserved. The center of the tumor can be gutted using a variety of techniques, including laser vaporization, aspiration with a CUSA® (Cavitron Ultrasonic Surgical Aspirator, Valleylab, Boulder, CO) or microdebrider, or simply using microcup forceps.

Once the tumor has been reduced in size, the posterior, superior, inferior, and medial aspects of the tumor capsule are dissected from the surrounding arachnoid, cerebellum, and the brain stem. As the tumor is mobilized, cottonoid strips are gently placed between the tumor capsule and surrounding structures. Reducing the tumor capsule may facilitate identifying its medial relationship to the brain stem. The medial end of the facial nerve is identified at the brain stem with the aid of the facial nerve stimulator.

The remainder of the tumor is removed beginning at the fundus of the IAC and progressing medially. The vertical crest is identified. The superior vestibular nerve is gently displaced to allow visualization of the more anteriorly located facial nerve, which is positively identified with the facial nerve stimulator (set at 0.05 mA). A right-angled hook is used to avulse the superior vestibular nerve and fully expose the facial nerve. The inferior vestibular and cochlear nerves are also released from their lateral attachments, and the plane between the tumor and the facial nerve is established. Tumor is removed from the canal in a medial direction, dissecting it away from the facial nerve. The House-Hough facial nerve dissector facilitates separating the anterior tumor capsule from the nerve. Dissection continues until the facial nerve is seen entering the brain stem and the tumor is free from the nerve. At this point, microscissors are used to sever the V nerve from the brain stem, and the tumor specimen is removed. The facial nerve is stimulated at the brain stem to determine its integrity, and the cerebellopontine angle is irrigated to identify any bleeding. Hemostasis is obtained with bipolar cautery and topical hemostatic agents as necessary.

The tensor tympani tendon is severed from the cochleariform process to allow palpation and packing of the eustachian tube. Nu Knit® guaze (Johnson & Johnson Gateway, LLC, Piscataway, NJ) and bone wax are compressed and pushed into the eustachian tube orifice to prevent postoperative CSF rhinorrhea, using care not to perforate the tympanic membrane. The middle ear is packed with pieces of temporalis muscle. The temporalis fascia is then draped over the posterior external

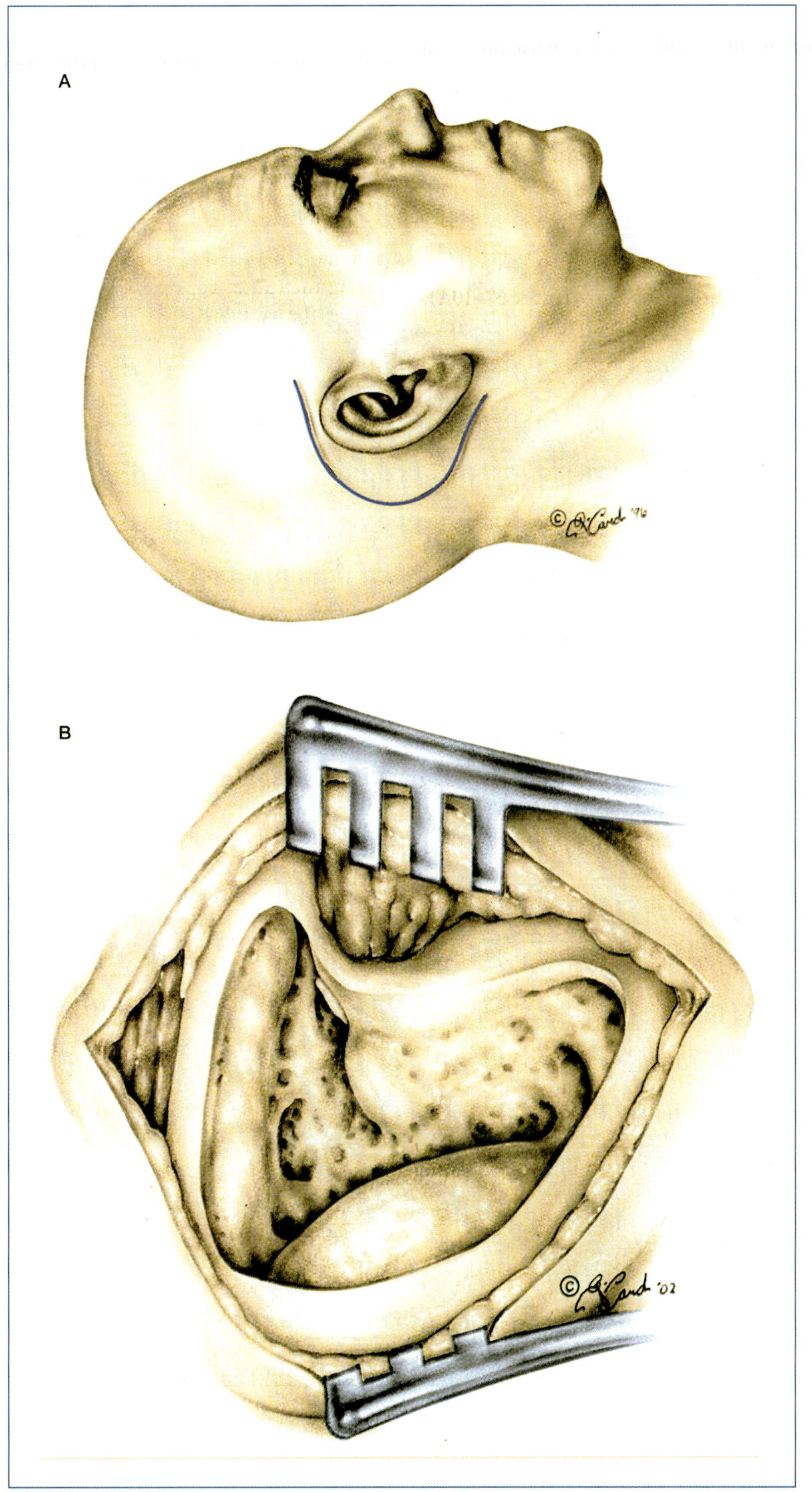

FIGURE 37–10 • *A*, Translabyrinthine removal of a vestibular schwannoma. The postauricular incision is made approximately 4 cm posterior to the postauricular crease. *B*, A complete mastoidectomy is performed.

Continued

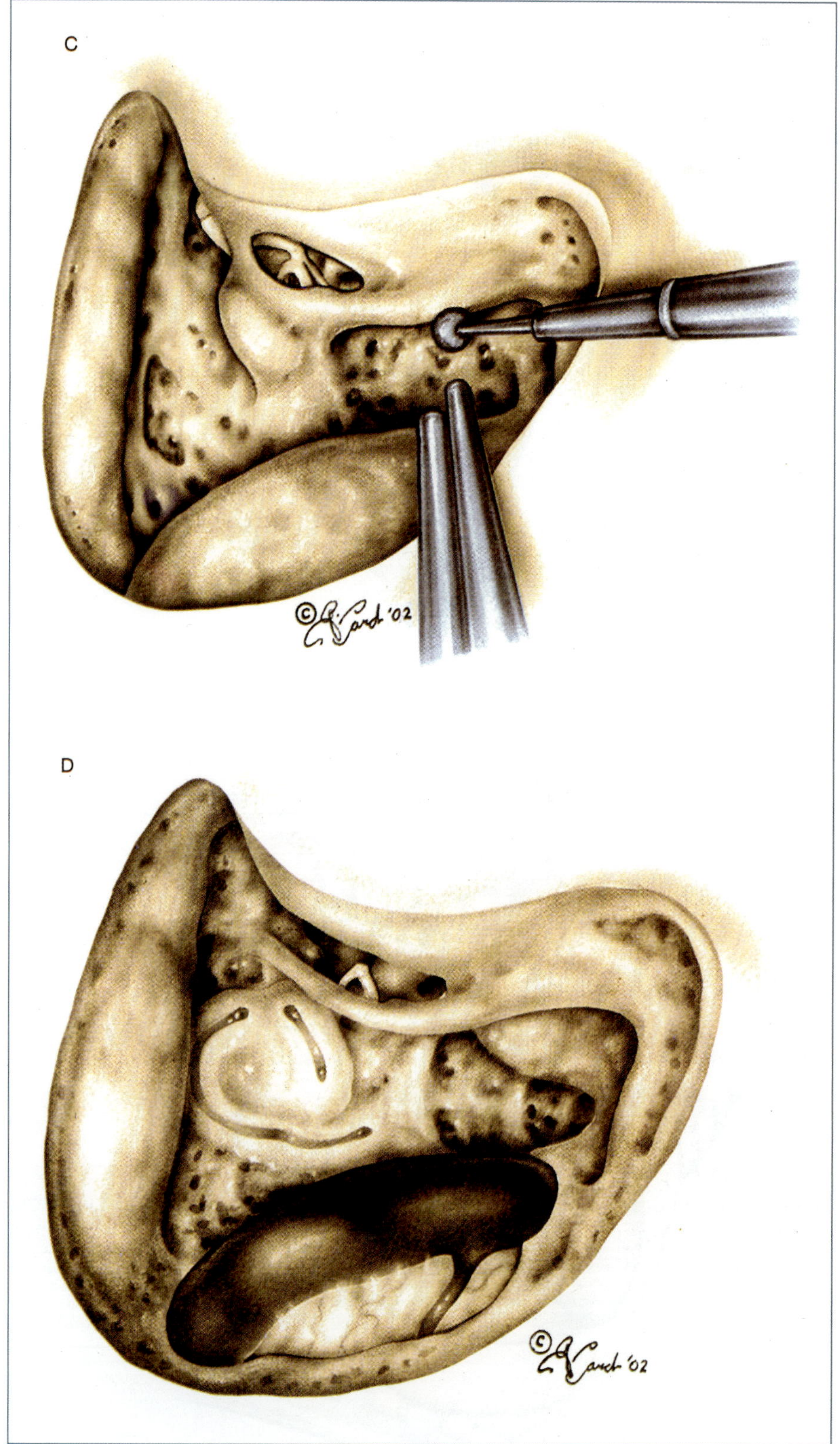

FIGURE 37–10 • *Continued. C*, The vertical portion of the facial nerve is identified and the facial recess is opened to gain access to the eustachian tube. *D*, The incudostapedial joint is separated and the incus removed. The malleus head is nipped, and the eustachian tube is occluded. The bone remaining over the sigmoid sinus and middle fossa dura is removed. A labyrinthectomy is performed.

Continued

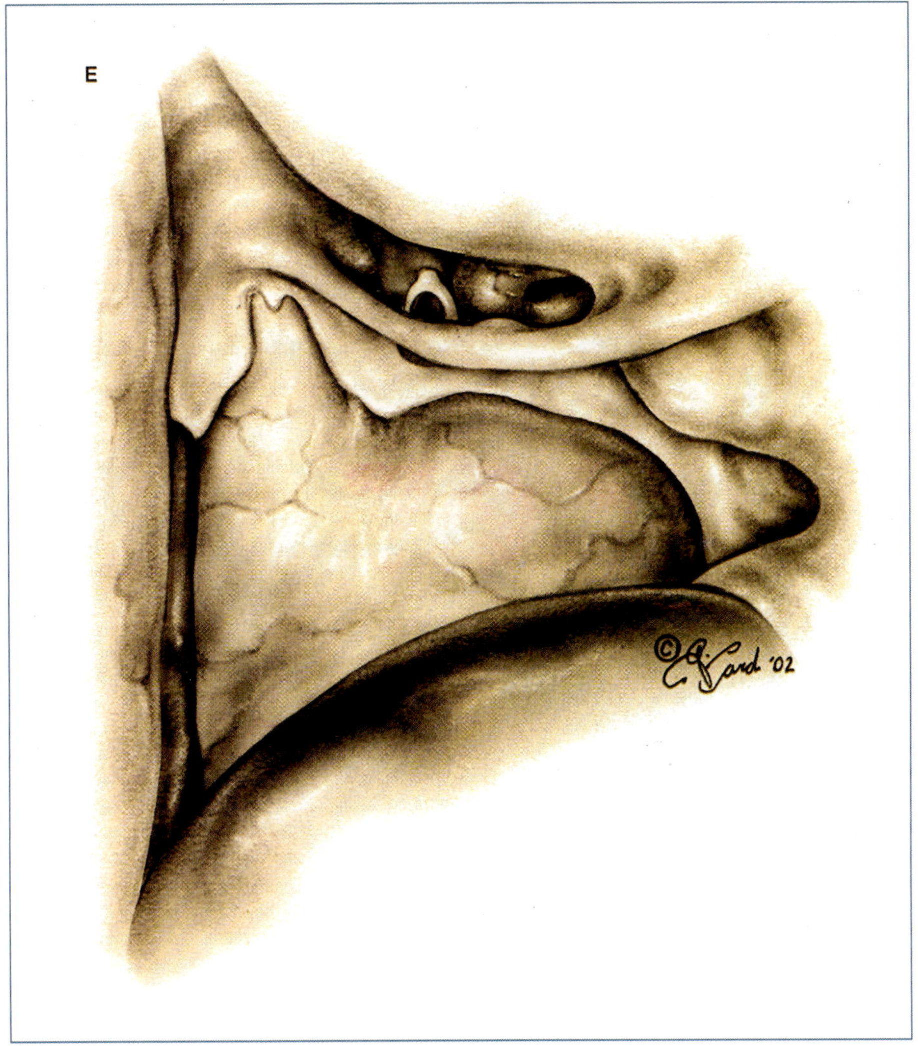

FIGURE 37–10 • *Continued. E*, The translabyrinthine approach after bone removal has been completed. The posterior fossa dura is incised with microscissors to expose the tumor.

Continued

auditory canal to cover potential routes of CSF egress such as the aditus ad antrum, the oval or round windows at the vestibules, or the sinus tympani. Any other open air-cell tract along the root of the zygoma, petrous apex, or hypotympanum should be occluded with bone wax. Abdominal fat is harvested, cut into approximately 2-in. strips in bacitracin irrigant, and then layered in to fill the surgical defect. Care must be exercised when filling the dural opening adjacent to the facial nerve to prevent its avulsion. Tissue glues such as Tisseel® (Baxter Healthcare Corporation, Glendale, CA) can be used. Titanium mesh, lactosorb, and medpor plating systems have been used to recontour the cranial defect and keep the fat graft immobile against CSF pulsations. Whether or not this will add to decreased CSF otorhinorrhea or increased cosmetic healing is yet to be seen. The musculoperiosteum is closed over the fat with interrupted absorbable suture. Another layer of interrupted absorbable suture is used to close the subcuticular layer, and the skin is closed with a continuous running-locking nylon suture. Every effort is made to ensure a watertight closure to prevent a postoperative CSF leak. A mastoid-type compression dressing is placed. The patient is extubated and taken to the neurologic intensive care unit where immediate, and sequential exams are observed overnight.

Suboccipital Approach

The suboccipital (retrosigmoid) approach to the cerebellopontine angle was first advocated by Dandy.[7] The microscope has been incorporated routinely and the approach improved on by removal of the posterior lip of the IAC to identify the facial and cochlear nerves and for complete tumor removal under direct visualization.

The procedure is performed on a supine patient placed in Mayfield pinions with the chin slightly tucked, and the head turned laterally. Two potentially catastrophic disadvantages to the seated position are air embolism and lumbar disk rupture; therefore, the supine or lateral position is preferred. Hyperventilating the patient to a CO_2 level of 25–28 mmHg, the use of intravenous mannitol (1 g/kg) at the start of the case, and hypotensive anesthesia with judicious use of intravenous fluids all help reduce ICP and intraoperative bleeding.

A curvilinear incision is made approximately four fingerbreadths behind the postauricular crease (Figure 37–11A

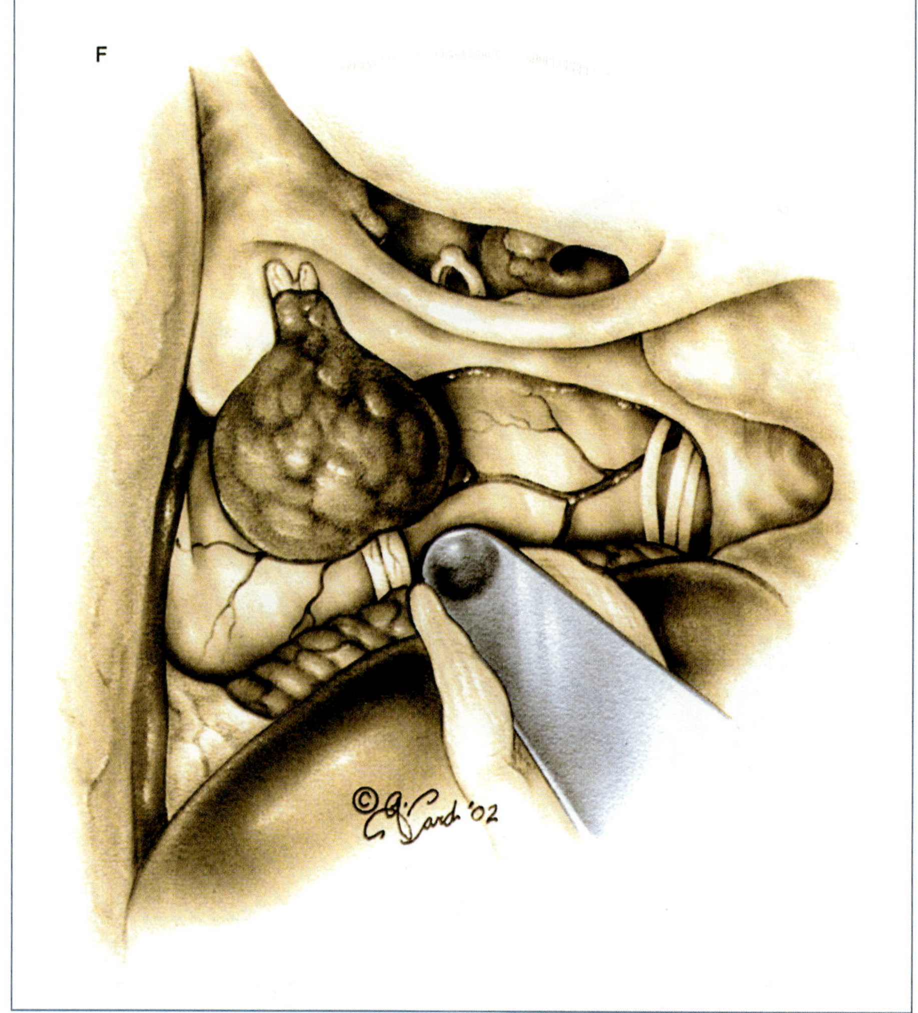

FIGURE 37–10 • *Continued. F*, The dura of the posterior fossa and internal auditory canal is opened, exposing the tumor. Smaller tumors may be removed at this point without a reduction in size.

Continued

and B). The musculoperiosteum and cervical musculature are incised vertically down to the skull. The Lempert periosteal elevator is used to sweep this tissue anteriorly and posteriorly to provide exposure for the craniotomy. An approximately 4 × 4 cm craniotomy is then created posterior to the occipitomastoid grove, and the bone flap is preserved for later replacement. The superior limit of the craniotomy is the transverse sinus, and the anterior extent is the sigmoid sinus. Inferiorly the atlas is palpated and care is taken to avoid injury to the vertebral artery as it emerges laterally from foramen transversarium and bends to course intracranially. The dura is initially incised with a #15 blade, and a cottonoid sponge is placed through the dural opening to protect the cerebellum. The remainder of the incision is made with microscissors, and the dura is retracted with stay sutures (Figure 37–11C). Moistened microgelatin foam is placed on the outer surface of the retracted dura to prevent desiccation during the procedure. The anterior and inferior portions of the cerebellum are gently retracted to expose the cerebellopontine cistern. An arachnoid knife is used to pierce the arachnoid, allowing egress of CSF and promoting cerebellar relaxation. The cerebellum is gently retracted to expose the cerebellopontine angle and tumor (Figure 37–11C). Cottonoid sponges are placed over a biologic collagen sponge (bicol®), or oxidized cellulose (Surgicel) placed between the cerebellum and the retractor to decrease trauma to the surface of the cerebellum.

Larger tumor capsules are incised, and the tumor is gutted and reduced, as previously described. The posterior, superior, inferior, and medial aspects of the tumor are gently dissected free from the cerebellum and brain stem, and the seventh and eighth nerves are identified at their root entry zones. If the tumor is small, it is completely dissected from the facial and cochlear nerves prior to removing the posterior lip of the IAC.

Cottonoid sponges are placed around the porus to keep bone dust out of the cerebellopontine angle. The dura overlying the posterior petrous apex can be removed prior to drilling the IAC, or it can be incised with the diamond bur (Figure 37–11D). Starting with a 3-mm diamond bur, the posterior lip of the IAC is drilled as far laterally as possible without damaging the otic capsule structures. Staying 2 mm medial to the operculum and not advancing beyond the blue-lined common crus helps avoid postoperative hearing loss. Review of the preoperative MRI can

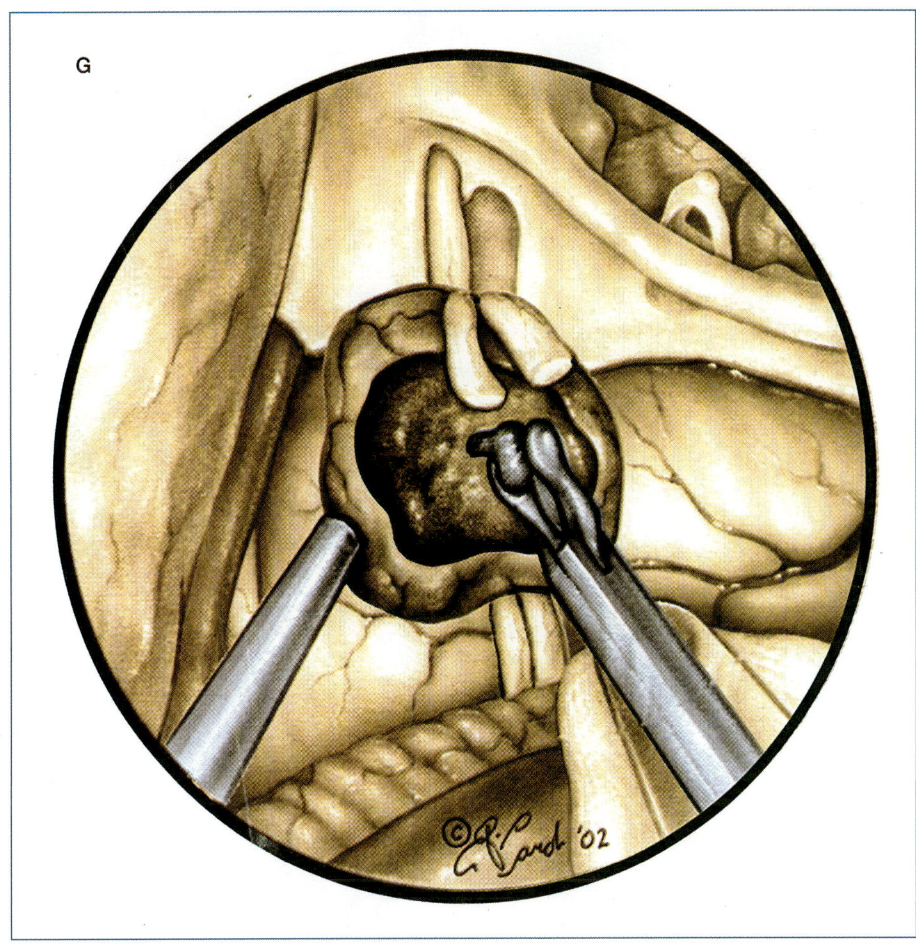

FIGURE 37–10 • *Continued. G*, Larger tumors must be reduced in size prior to removal. After debulking, the tumor capsule is separated from the surrounding structures. The vertical crest is identified, and the superior vestibular nerve is retracted inferiorly to identify the facial nerve. The vestibular nerves are avulsed, and the facial nerve is dissected free from the tumor in a lateral to medial direction.

help determine the amount of bone that can safely be removed without risking the inner ear.

Once exposed, the dura of the IAC is incised and opened. The superior and inferior vestibular nerves and tumor are identified within the canal. Gentle inferior retraction of the superior vestibular nerve reveals the facial nerve, which is positively identified with the facial nerve stimulator (set at 0.05 mA). The vestibular nerves are avulsed, and the plane between the tumor and facial and cochlear nerves is developed (Figure 37–11E). The tumor is gently dissected from the facial and cochlear nerves in a lateral to medial direction. The nerves are followed into the cerebellopontine angle, as in the translabyrinthine approach (Figure 37–11F). The surgeon must take care to preserve the labyrinthine artery in hearing preservation cases.

Once the tumor has been completely removed, all cottonoid sponges are removed. The surgical field is copiously irrigated and hemostasis is obtained. The bone around the IAC is carefully inspected for air cells, and if visualized, they are occluded with bone wax. The dural leaves of the IAC are replaced and covered with a piece of muscle to help prevent postoperative CSF leakage. The dura is closed in a running fashion with 4–0 silk, the bone flap is replaced and plated to the posterior calvarium, and the muscular layer is closed in layers with an absorbable suture. The skin is closed with a running 3–0 nylon suture (or stainless steel surgical clips), and a sterile pressure dressing is applied. The patient is extubated and monitored overnight in the neurologic intensive care unit.

The intraoperative use of a 30-degree endoscope can improve visualization of the lateral IAC, reducing the risk of leaving residual tumor in the fundus. The use of endoscopes eliminates reliance on blind tumor dissection of the fundus, or the sacrifice of hearing for direct visualization.[128]

Management of Large Vestibular Schwannomas

Giant (4.0 cm or larger) vestibular schwannomas require special perioperative, intraoperative, and anesthetic precautions to prevent serious complications. As with any surgery, existing medical conditions are optimally managed prior to surgery. Furthermore, the consulting internist is informed that the operative, and hence anesthetic time, may be prolonged. Patients and their families are informed that the primary goal of surgery is to preserve their life and that saving facial nerve function is a secondary goal.

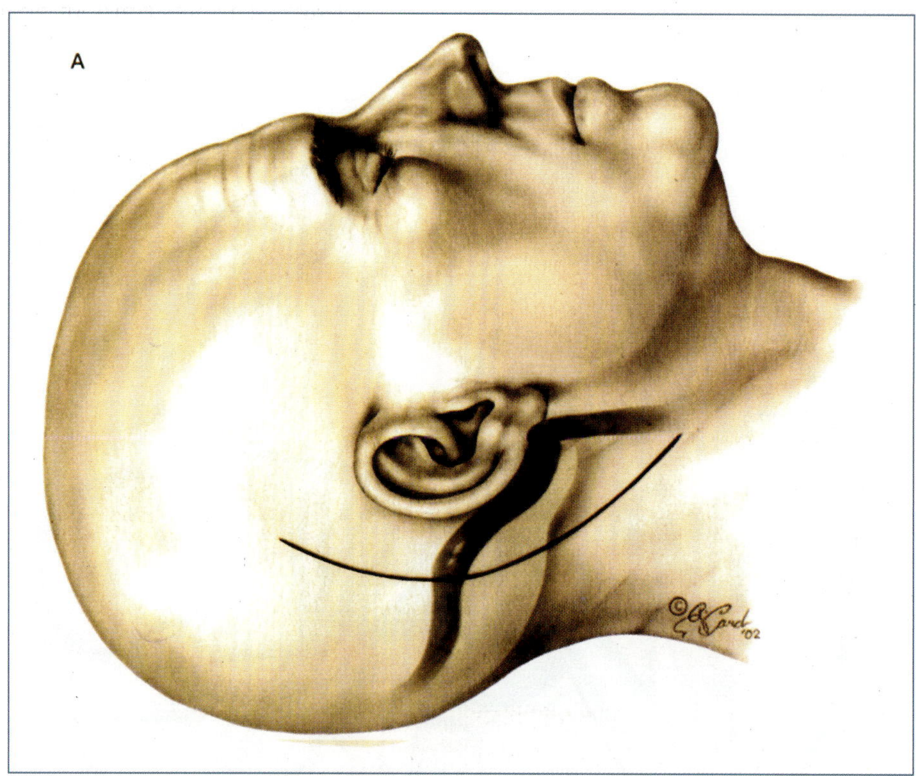

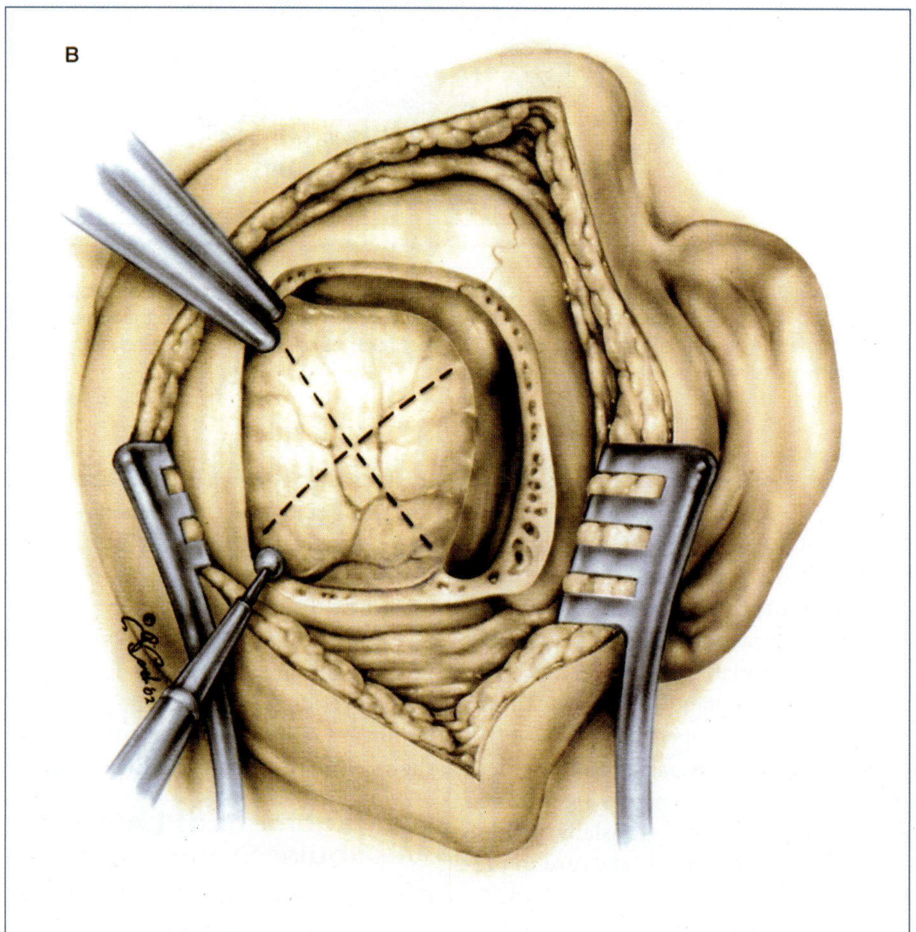

FIGURE 37–11 • Suboccipital removal of a vestibular schwannoma. A curvilinear incision is made approximately four fingerbreadths behind the postauricular crease. Note the relationship of the incision to the sigmoid sinus, transverse sinus, and cerebellum. *A*, The incision margins are retracted, and a 4 × 4-cm craniotomy is created. The superior limit of the craniotomy is the transverse sinus, and the anterior limit is the sigmoid sinus. *B*, Mannitol and hyperventilation provide brain relaxation, and the posterior fossa dura is opened. The cerebellopontine cistern is decompressed and the cerebellum is retracted to expose the cerebellopontine angle and tumor.

Continued

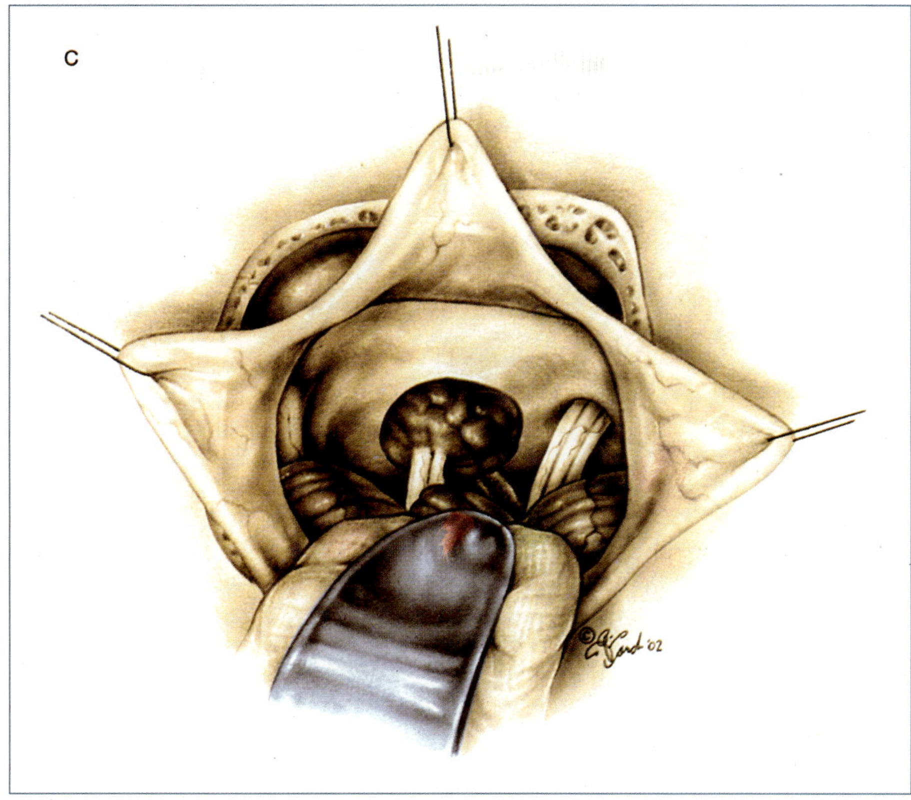

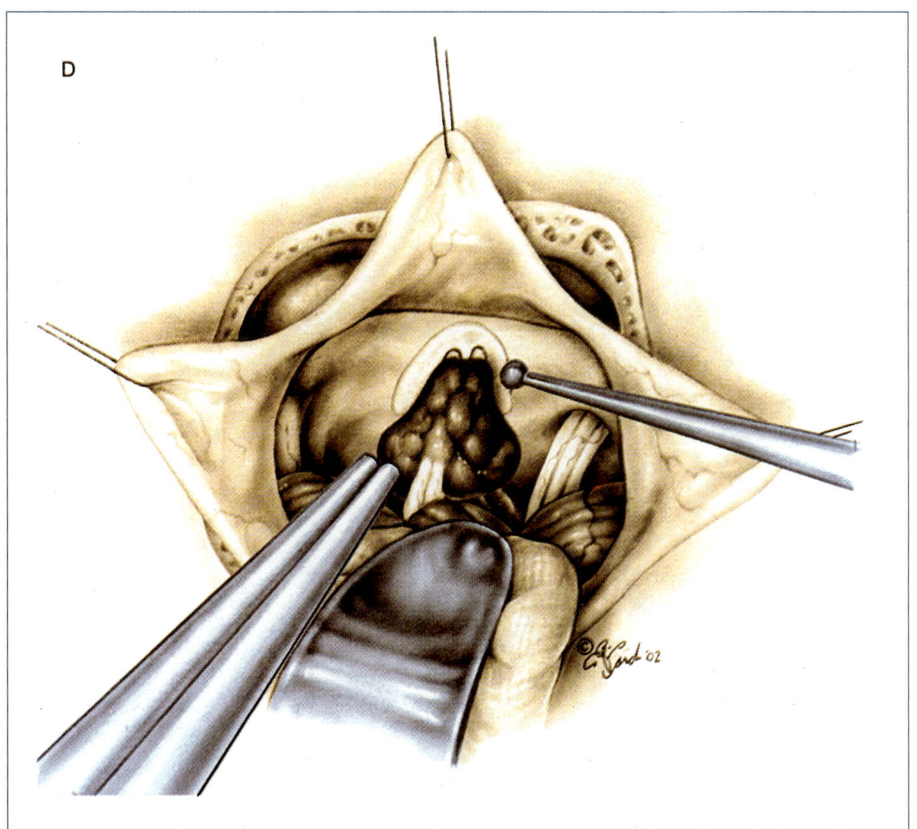

FIGURE 37–11 • *Continued. C*, Using a 3-mm diamond bur, the posterior lip of the internal auditory canal is drilled away. Staying 2 mm medial to the operculum and not advancing beyond the blue-lined common crus helps avoid violating otic capsule. *D*, The facial nerve is identified. The vestibular nerves are sectioned, and the tumor and vestibular nerves are dissected from the facial and cochlear nerves.

Continued

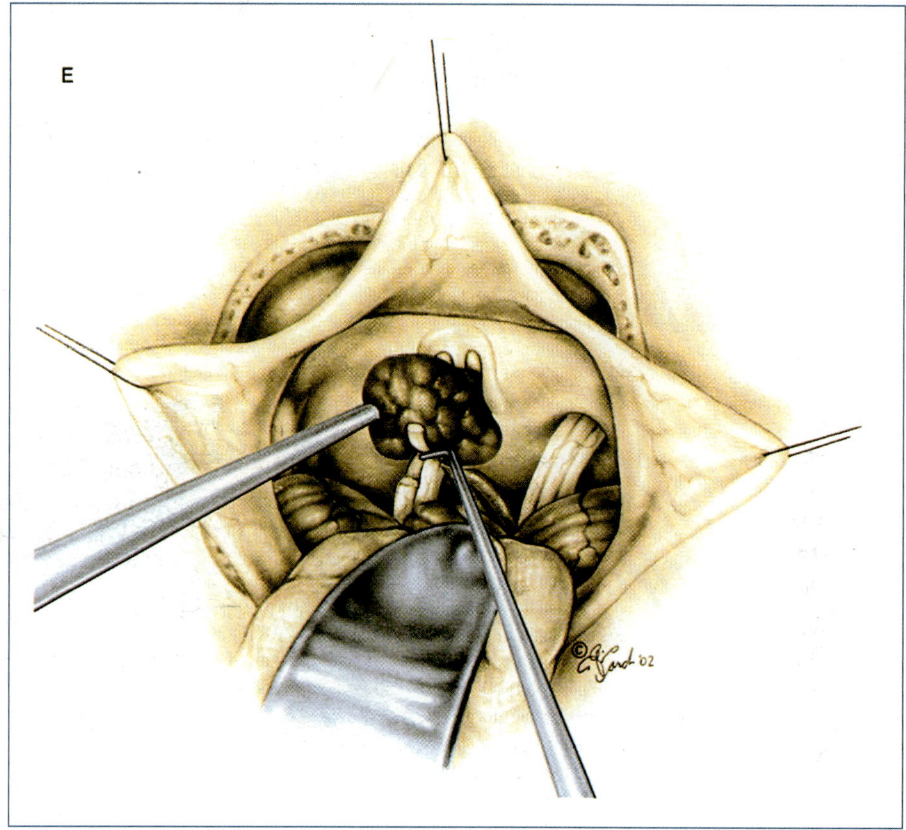

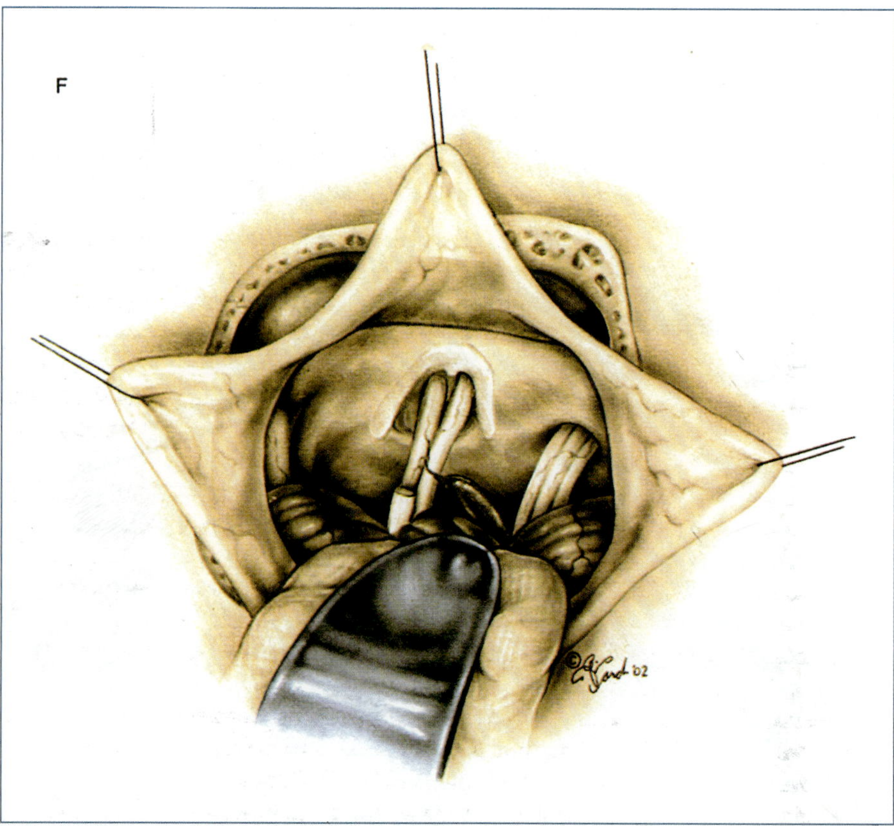

FIGURE 37–11 • *Continued. E*, The tumor removal is completed, with preservation of the facial and cochlear nerves. *F*, With the tumor resected the truncated proximal vestibular portion of the vestibulocochlear nerve is observed posterior to the intact facial and cochlear nerves which are separated by the falciform crest at the fundus of the internal auditory canal.

Large tumors generally cause significant brain stem compression. In addition, compression of the fourth ventricle may lead to increased ICP and hydrocephalus. Patients with symptomatic hydrocephalus or radiographic edema should be admitted and treated for several days with high-dose dexamethasone prior to surgery in an attempt to reduce brain edema. When hydrocephalus is present or suspected, a neurosurgical consultation should be obtained for additional treatment of elevated ICPs by placement of a ventriculoperitoneal shunt prior to definitive surgery, and to coordinate operative care. Failure to decompress hydrocephalus prior to placement of a lumbar drain or opening the posterior fossa can lead to brain herniation and death.

After the induction of general anesthesia and placement of appropriate monitoring devices, a central venous catheter is inserted due to the heightened risk of air embolism by the presence of a ventriculoperitoneal shunt. The central line can be used therapeutically to evacuate air from the right heart should an air embolism occur. Additionally, intravenous mannitol (1 g/kg) is given early in the case, and hyperventilation to a CO_2 level of 25 mm Hg is used to decrease ICP. Additional diuresis can be accomplished with intravenous furosemide as necessary. Blood chemistries must be evaluated intraoperatively to detect and correct any induced electrolyte or acid–base disturbances.

The patient is placed supine and secured in Mayfield pinions to maintain stability throughout the case. Utilization of image guidance systems can be helpful in the treatment of large cerebellopontine angle tumors. During the procedure, the anesthesiologist and surgeon must communicate and be cognizant of the signs of brain stem dysfunction, such as an alteration in heart rate or a rise in blood pressure. If brain stem signs appear, all surgical manipulation near the brain stem is stopped, and surgery resumes only after vital signs have returned to baseline. Additionally, care is taken to avoid occlusion of the sigmoid sinus; loss of this venous channel can provoke cerebral edema. Likewise, positioning of the table with a slight Fowler tilt can decrease venous engorgement, dependent edema, and enhance visibility by reducing oozing.

Combined Approach

The one-stage, combined translabyrinthine–suboccipital approach described by Glasscock and Hays[58] was developed for the removal of giant vestibular schwannomas. The postauricular flap is larger than the one used for the translabyrinthine approach to expose more of the occipital bone and is retracted forward by dura hooks (Figure 37–12A). A translabyrinthine approach is carried out as previously described (Figure 37–12B). Next bone is removed for approximately 4 cm posterior to the sigmoid sinus (Figure 37–12B). The dura over the cerebellum is incised and retracted with stay sutures. Cottonoid sponges are placed over the cerebellum, the cerebellopontine cistern is decompressed, and a posterior fossa retractor is inserted to gently retract the cerebellum (Figure 37–12C). The tumor margins are freed from the surrounding tissues with cottonoid sponges, and the tumor center is removed to decompress the tumor (Figure 37–12D). The capsule is cut away as the tumor size decreases. All vessels entering the tumor are coagulated with bipolar cautery. The capsule is carefully dissected free from

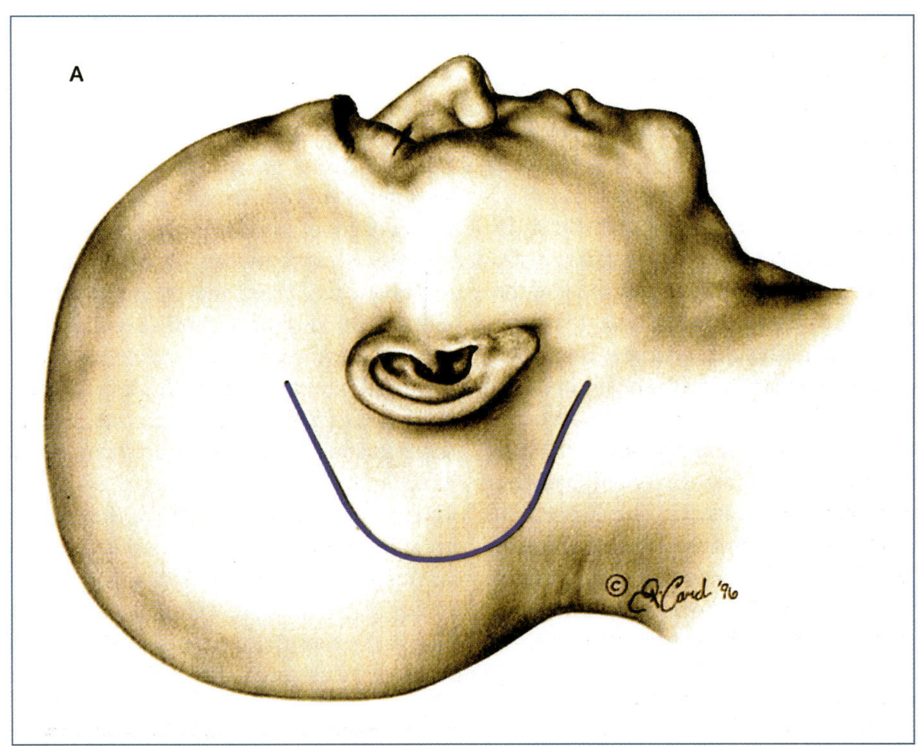

FIGURE 37–12 • *A*, The combined approach for removal of giant vestibular schwannomas. A large postauricular flap is created.

Continued

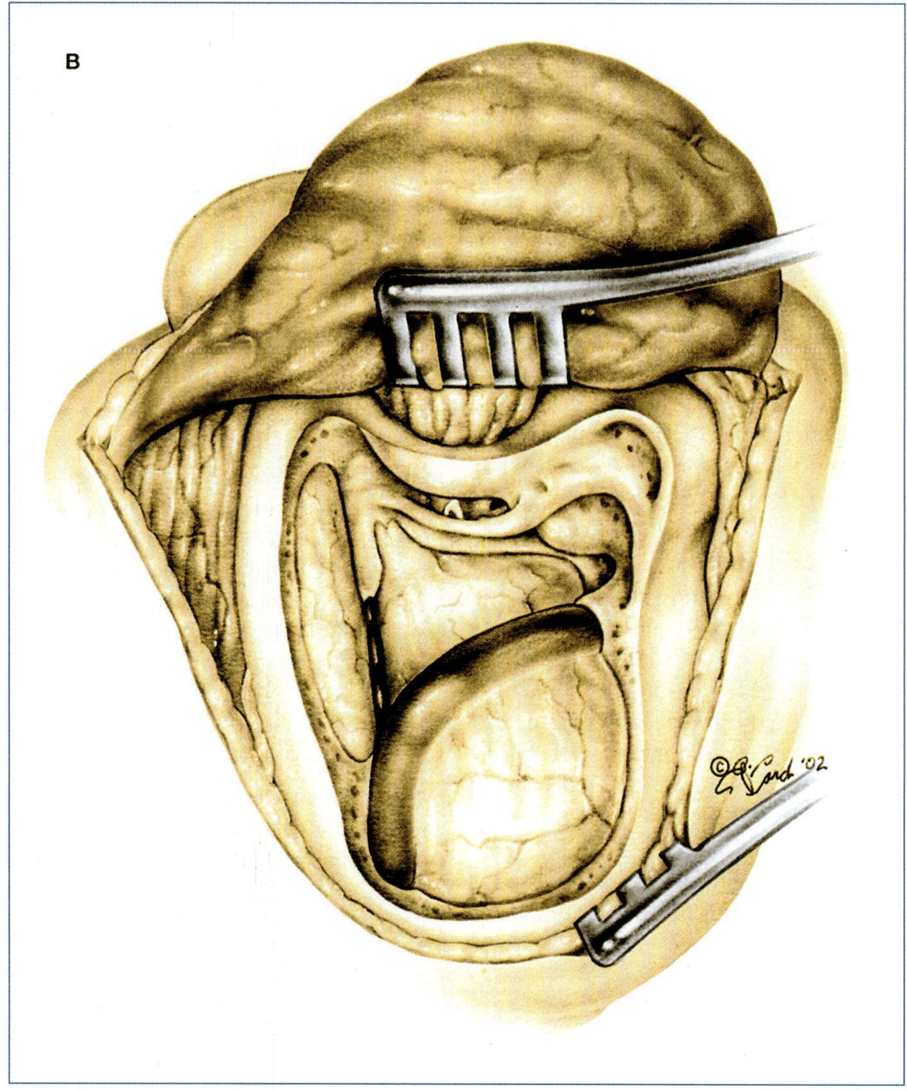

FIGURE 37–12 • *Continued. B*, The translabyrinthine approach is accomplished first.

Continued

the brain stem, and cottonoids are placed to protect the brain stem. The tumor is reduced to 2 cm or less, and the facial nerve is identified at the brain stem. At this point, the remainder of the surgery is performed through the translabyrinthine approach as described (Figure 37–12E to I). The facial nerve is identified laterally in the IAC and traced medially toward the brain stem. The tumor is separated from the facial nerve and removed as the dissection continues. On complete tumor removal, the cerebellopontine angle is irrigated and hemostasis is obtained with bipolar cautery and topical hemostatic agents. The eustachian tube and middle ear are packed, abdominal adipose tissue is placed within the surgical defect, and the dura is closed with a running 3–0 silk. The wound is closed in the usual manner, and the patient is observed in the neurologic intensive care unit.

Management of Neurofibromatosis Type 2

Early identification and treatment of family members found to have NF2 is crucial in optimizing the quality of life for these individuals. When tumors are identified while small and in the setting of good hearing, hearing preservation with surgical excision may be successful and provide long-term hearing and facial nerve benefits. When bilateral small tumors are present the side selected for initial treatment should be the side with the best opportunity for hearing preservation success. The outcome of the initial intervention dictates the treatment course of the contralateral ear. If hearing is preserved and shown to be audiometrically stable for 6 months and the contralateral tumor is small with good hearing, a hearing preservation operation may be attempted on the second side. If the hearing is lost on the initial attempt, a more conservative strategy must be employed for the contralateral tumor. This side may be observed, and or decompressed in an attempt to prolong useable hearing. During tumor removal for these patients it is wise to preserve the cochlear nerve whenever possible as cochlear implantation has been shown to be beneficial for long-term auditory rehabilitation.[129]

When tumors are identified later, and hearing or cochlear nerve preservation is not a likely option auditory brain stem implant of the cochlear nucleus at the time of tumor removal has been shown to be effective in providing environmental

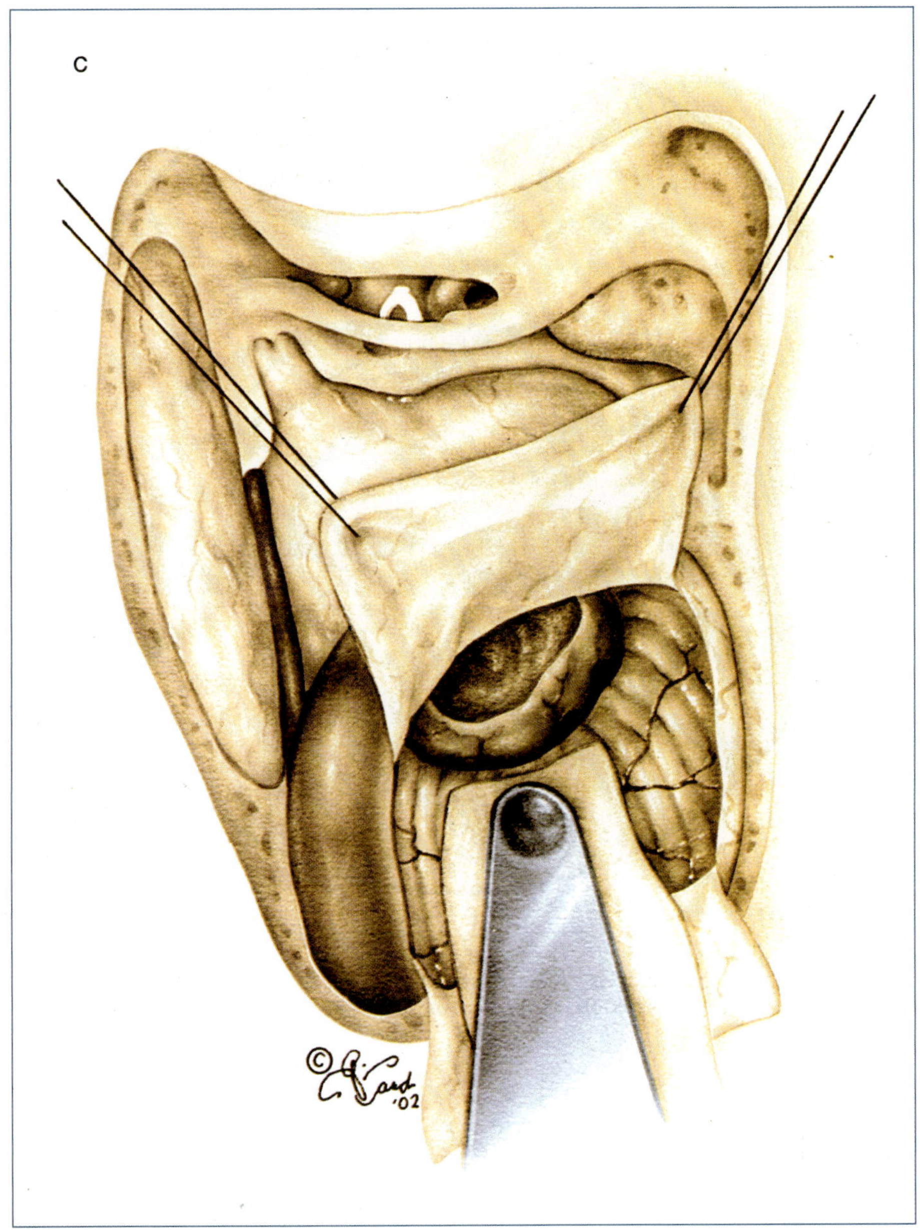

FIGURE 37–12 • *Continued. C,* A 4 × 4-cm area of bone is removed posterior to the sigmoid sinus and inferior to the transverse sinus to enable exposure of the posterior portion of the tumor.

Continued

sound cues that greatly enhance lip reading voice modulation capabilities. As these patients will need ongoing MRI surveillance of concurrent, residual or future tumors, removal of the implant magnet will prevent inconvenient procedures prior to future scanning.

Surgical Results

Mortality and morbidity rates have progressively declined, as noted above. Glasscock and colleagues reported a mortality rate of less than 1% for the surgical excision of vestibular schwannomas.[130] Our series is in agreement.[107] The most significant factor influencing mortality rate is early tumor diagnosis through heightened physician and patient awareness. Routine use of the operating microscope, facial nerve monitoring, development of the translabyrinthine approach, improved neuro-otologic/-anesthetic techniques, intensive care monitoring, and development of reliable imaging have all enhanced survivability and preservation of function in vestibular schwannoma patients. Early detection by high resolution, gadolinium-enhanced MRI has led to decreased morbidity by enabling treatment of tumors at early stages facilitating preservation of hearing and facial nerve function. Intraoperative facial nerve monitoring is associated with improved postoperative function and is considered "standard of care" treatment.[131,132] Preservation of facial nerve function is, to a great extent, size dependent,[133–135] although the tumor type also plays a role. Significantly poorer facial

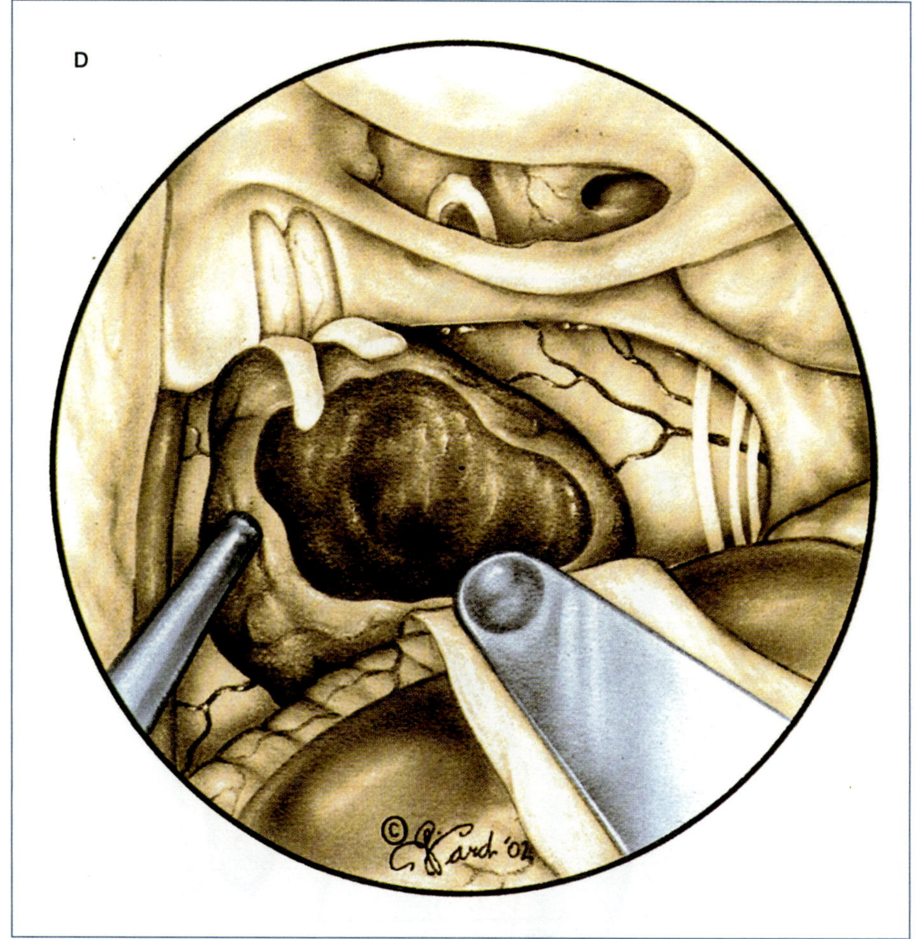

FIGURE 37–12 • *Continued. D,* Once brain relaxation has been obtained, the posterior fossa dura is opened, the cerebellopontine cistern is decompressed, and the cerebellum is retracted. The tumor is gutted to reduce its size.

Continued

nerve function has been shown when tumors present with headache, ataxia, or when facial function is compromised preoperatively.[136] Our series, similar to others, shows preservation of House-Brackmann grade I or II results in 88% of all tumors.[107,131,132] Near total excision, leaving an area of small residual tumor along the facial nerve in larger or inflammatory tumors may offer adequate tumor control and improved facial nerve outcomes in patients where aggressive resection may not be warranted.

Hearing preservation is also directly related to early detection and tumor size. Preservation rates range from 26 to 80% dependent on preoperative hearing class, size and location of tumor, patient's age, and approach used.[107,133,134,137,138] Optimal results are obtained when small tumors not impacting the fundus can be approached without violating the inner ear, sparing traction on the cochlear nerve and leaving canal vasculature intact. In well-selected patients with tumors smaller than 1.5 cm or tumor volumes smaller than 2.0 cm^3 that demonstrate a fundal cap on T2-weighted or 3D-CISS MRI, hearing preservation has been more consistently obtained ranging from 58 to 80%. Further attempts to prognosticate hearing preservation probabilities based on demographic, nerve of origin, audiometric or radiographic information has not revealed absolute clarity. Superior vestibular nerve tumors are seen to have improved hearing outcomes, however, tumors more often originate from the inferior vestibular nerve. When VEMP signals are preserved, hearing preservation is more often seen, and complete disappearance of the VEMP response is generally only been seen when the nerve of origin is the inferior vestibular nerve. The position of the tumor in the IAC regardless of the site of origin, and the hearing status of the patient, definitely influences VEMP findings and predictability.

Cerebrospinal fluid leak rates have declined to less than 10% with improved wound closure techniques.[139] The use of autologous fibrin glue has not been shown to significantly reduce CSF leak rates[140,141]; however, pooled fibrin glue may have some advantages.[142] Despite various closure techniques the CSF leak rate has plateaued at below 10%. This finding is consistent despite changes in techniques, and materials, and so may be more of an issue of battling recalcitrant rises in ICP.[143] It will be interesting to see if cranioplasty closure of the translabyrinthine defect with titanium mesh, or other plating systems will prevent CSF from pulsating through the fat graft and lower the incidence of CSF otorhinorrhea.

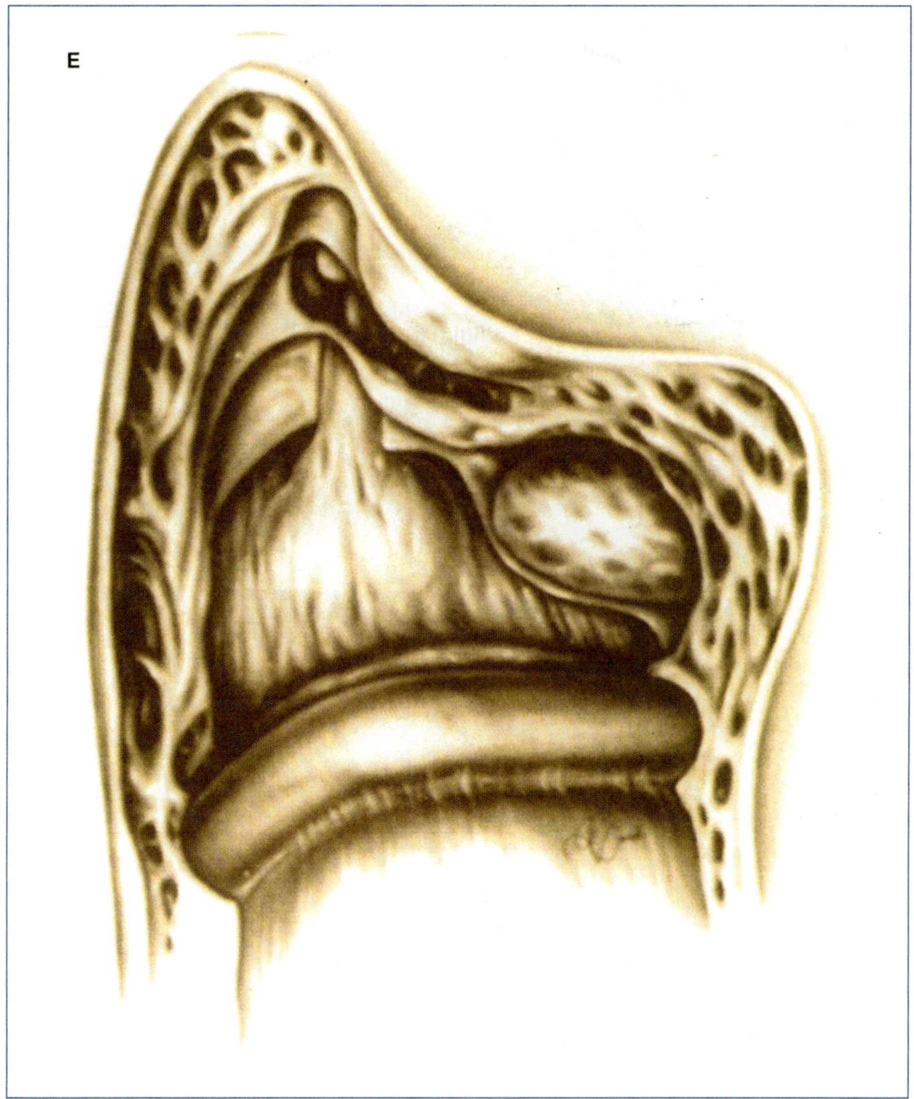

FIGURE 37–12 • *Continued. E*, Once the tumor has been reduced in size, the table is rotated back toward the surgeon, and the dura of the posterior fossa and internal auditory canal is opened.

Continued

MENINGIOMA OF THE TEMPORAL BONE

Meningiomas are the second most common neoplasm in the cerebellopontine angle and therefore deserve brief discussion. Meningiomas are nonmetastasizing but often locally invasive benign neoplasms. They arise from the endothelial lining cells of the arachnoid villi found in the walls of the cranial venous sinuses and their tributary veins. Although meningiomas constitute approximately 18% of primary brain tumors, only about 3% of meningiomas arise from the petrous pyramid, about equally from its middle and posterior fossa surfaces.[144] Occasionally, it may be difficult at presentation to differentiate a meningioma from a vestibular schwannoma. Symptoms produced by meningiomas are most often secondary to adjacent cranial nerve and brain compression. Tumors arising from the middle fossa surface of the petrous pyramid cause facial or eye pain and sensory and motor changes in the distribution of the fifth cranial nerve. Involvement of the fourth cranial nerve manifests with diplopia. As the lesion enlarges, seizures and sensory and motor aphasia may occur. The otolaryngologist is rarely the initial physician consulted by these patients. Meningiomas arising from the posterior surface of the petrous pyramid may present with the cerebellopontine angle syndrome, clinically mimicking a vestibular schwannoma. A meningioma arising within the IAC produces symptoms indistinguishable from those of a vestibular schwannoma; however, a meningioma usually originates outside the canal and involves adjacent cranial nerves and the cerebellum before affecting the eighth cranial nerve.

It is difficult to distinguish between vestibular schwannomas and meningiomas by audiovestibular testing. Imaging can often differentiate the two tumors. Meningiomas have more marked homogeneous enhancement on contrast CT than vestibular schwannomas and characteristically contain areas of calcification. Meningiomas are usually isointense or slightly

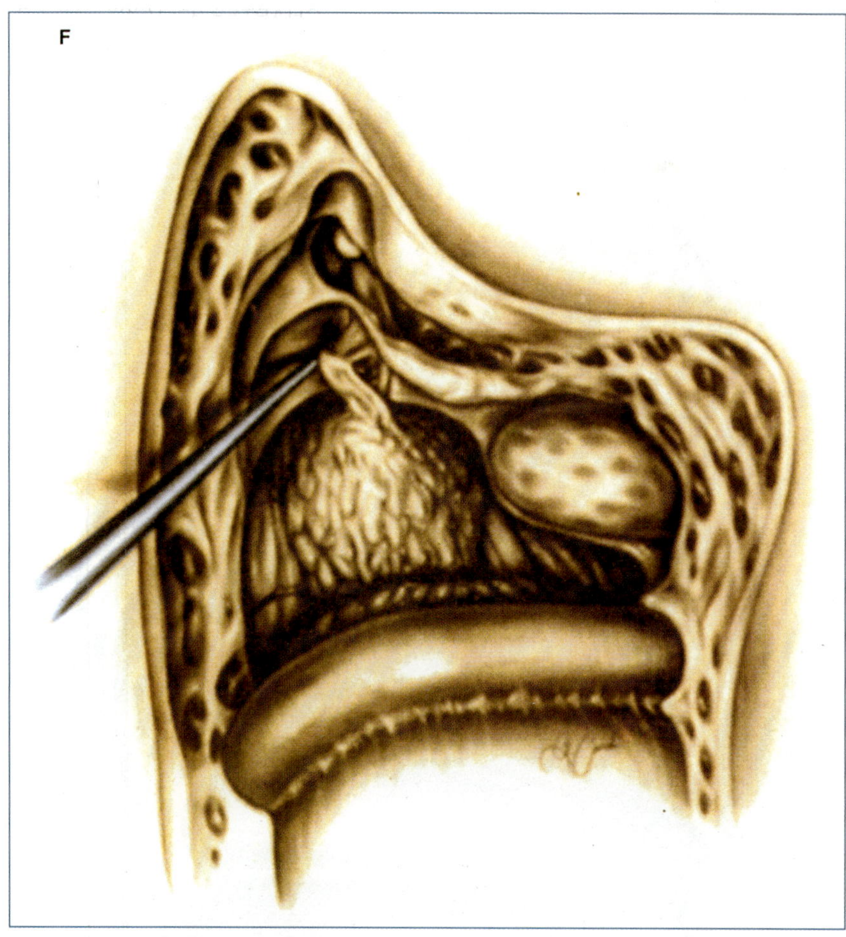

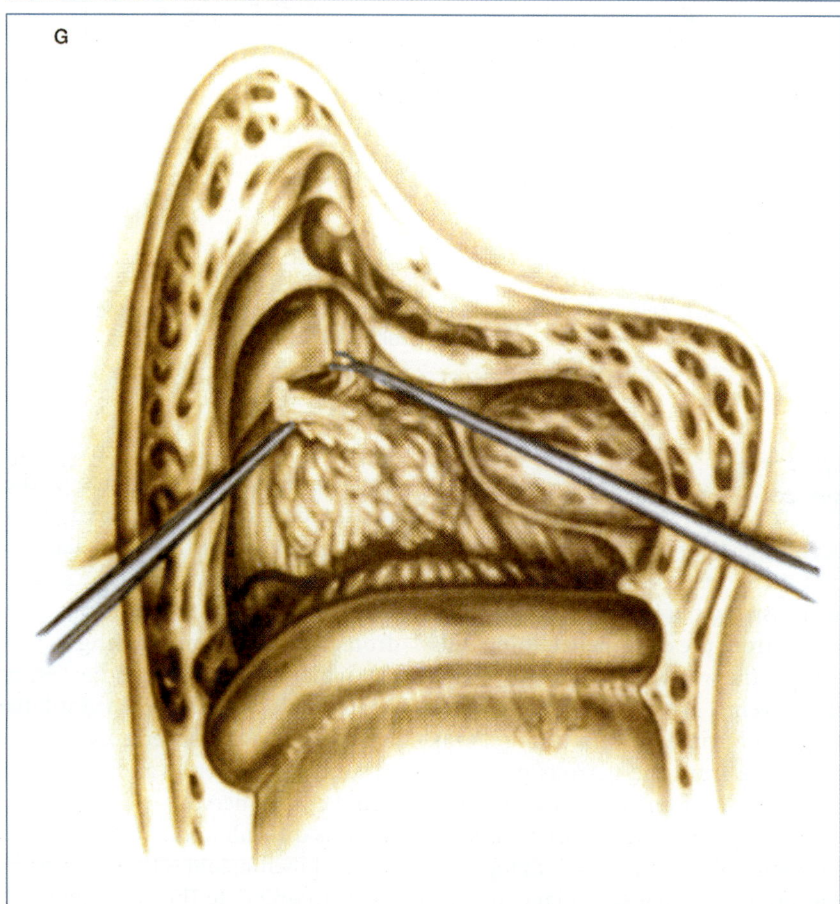

FIGURE 37–12 • *Continued. F*, The vertical crest is identified, and the superior vestibular nerve is avulsed from its canal, revealing the facial nerve anterior to Bill's bar. *G*, The plane between the tumor and facial nerve is established, and the tumor is dissected free.

Continued

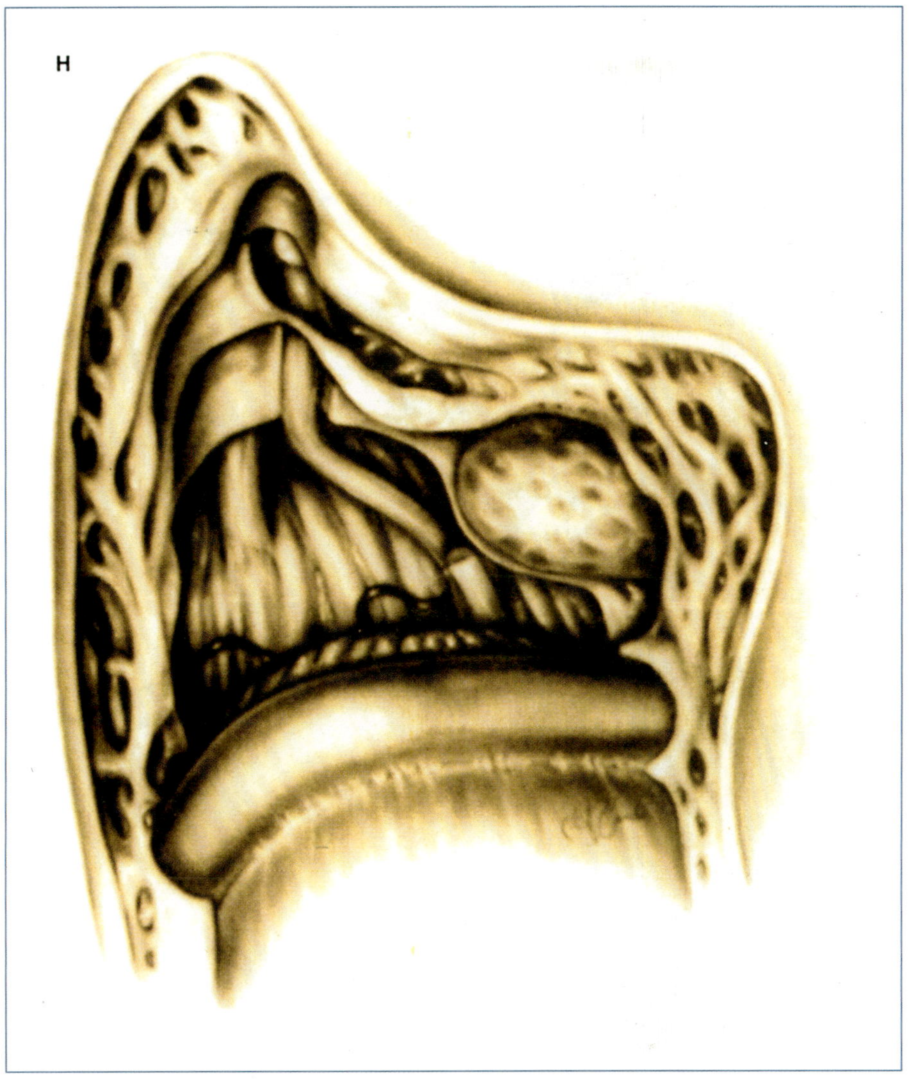

FIGURE 37–12 • *Continued. H,* The dissection is complete. The facial and superiorly located trigeminal nerves are seen in the cerebellopontine angle.

Continued

hypointense to gray matter on T1-weighted MRI sequences, with variable intensity on T2-weighted images.

Both vestibular schwannomas and meningiomas enhance with gadolinium on T1-weighted images, but the vestibular schwannoma usually enhances more markedly. The shape of the lesion is also very useful in differentiating these tumors. Radiographically, meningiomas have a broad base of attachment to the posterior petrous pyramid and demonstrate a dural "tail," a finding vestibular schwannomas rarely show (Figure 37–13). The angle between the meningioma and the dura tends to be obtuse whereas the same angle in a vestibular schwannoma is acute. Bone underlying meningiomas undergoes hyperostotic changes. Calcifications of meningiomas are seen as radiolucent foci on MRI. Vestibular schwannomas are generally centered over the IAC expanding the porus and extending into the CPA. Meningiomas may overlie the canal, but do not often expand it.

Meningiomas confined to the cerebellopontine angle are managed identically as described for the suboccipital approach to vestibular schwannomas. In cases in which hearing is severely impaired, or for large tumors, the translabyrinthine approach may be used. Interestingly, the facial nerve is often splayed over the posterior aspect of the tumor, in contrast to vestibular schwannomas, in which the nerve is most often found anteriorly. This finding is likely related to the differing origin of these tumors. Meningiomas are typically slow-growing tumors, and surgical resection usually relieves symptoms. Long-term follow-up is necessary to validate complete removal.

Meningiomas that are located in the far anterior reaches of the cerebellopontine angle can be approached in a number of ways. The transcochlear approach has been used to gain access to this portion of the angle (Figure 37–14A to E).[145] Traditionally, on completion of a translabyrinthine approach,

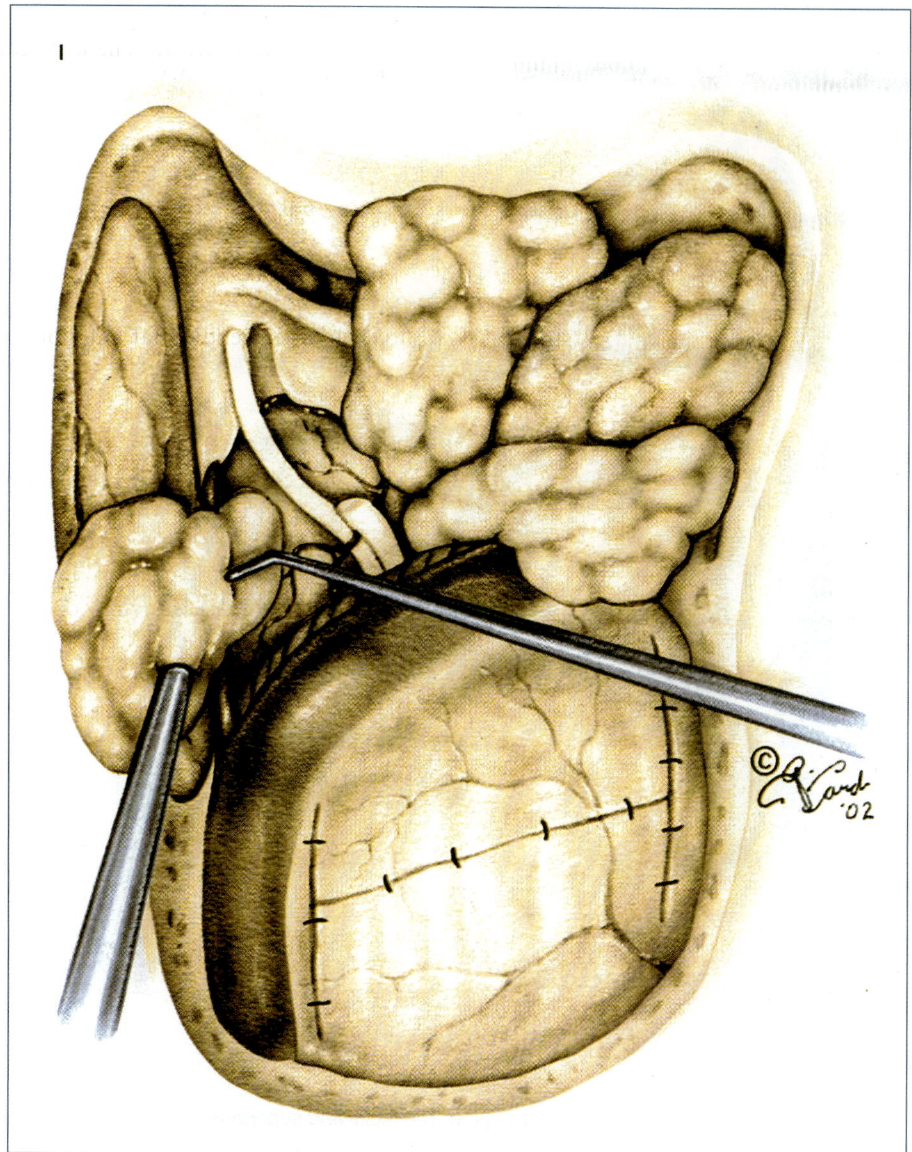

FIGURE 37–12 • *Continued. I*, Temporalis fascia is placed over the fossa incudis and facial recess. The posterior fossa durotomy is reapproximated and abdominal fat cut into strips is layered into the translabyrinthine defect to prevent CSF otorrhea.

the facial nerve is dissected from its fallopian canal and translocated posteriorly. The bone of the cochlea is drilled away, as is the bone medial to the carotid artery in the petrous apex. This bone removal expands access for tumor dissection anteriorly along the clivus.

Another approach to far anterior tumors is accomplished without facial nerve transposition. A transcochlear approach is still used; however. The cochlea is accessed after radical mastoidectomy with the tympanic membrane removed and the external auditory canal closed. Care is taken to remove all sqaumous epithelium with this exposure.

House and colleagues have described an adapted middle fossa approach to lesions of the far anterior cerebellopontine angle.[146] In this approach, the internal carotid artery and the cochlea are delineated. The bony space between these two structures is opened, providing access to the anterior portion of the cerebellopontine angle as well as control of the carotid artery.

COMPLICATIONS

Knowledge, avoidance, and identification of the possible complications of vestibular schwannoma surgery, and appropriate management should they occur, enable the best possible surgical outcome. Not surprisingly, the larger the tumor and the older or more medically complicated the patient, the greater the morbidity and mortality.

Intraoperative Complications

Cranial Nerve Injury

As pointed out by Glasscock and colleagues, there is a positive correlation between tumor size and facial nerve injury.[130] Facial nerve outcome is poorest with large tumors. Understanding facial nerve anatomy and identifying the nerve as one proceeds through the dissection helps in facial nerve preservation. As in any temporal bone procedure, the nerve is identified and

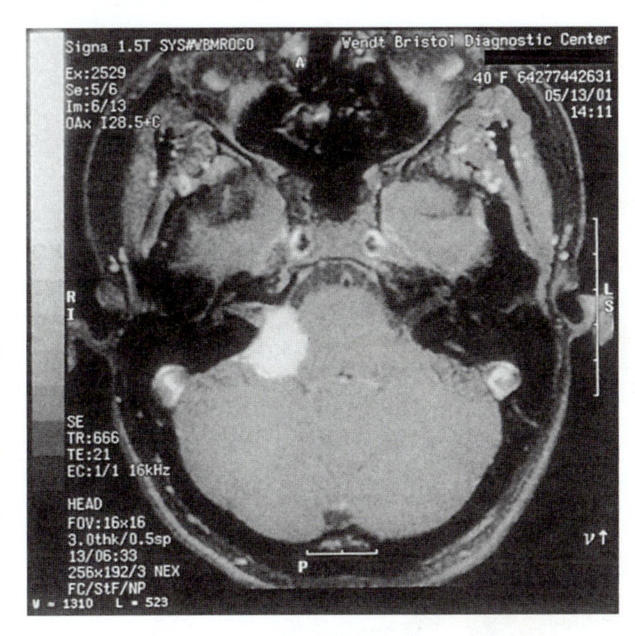

FIGURE 37–13 • A cerebellopontine angle meningioma as seen on a gadolinium-enhanced, T1-weighted magnetic resonance image. Note the broad-based attachment to the posterior fossa dura and the small posterior dural "tail."

skeletonized with a diamond drill during the translabyrinthine approach. Nerve trauma during labyrinthectomy is avoided by appreciating the relationship between the nerve and the lateral and posterior semicircular canals. During the middle fossa approach, the surgeon must be cognizant that the facial nerve is most often located superficial to the tumor, and care must be exercised when incising the IAC dura. Furthermore, the plane between the tumor and the nerve should be established early during middle fossa surgery to avoid traction on the nerve as the tumor is removed. During all approaches, reducing the size of large tumors decreases traction on the nerve. Furthermore, use of the facial nerve integrity monitor positively facilitates nerve identification and preservation.

In the event of facial nerve transection, immediate repair, if possible, should be accomplished. Primary neurorrhaphy is likely to yield the best postoperative functional results. Rerouting the facial nerve or placing a greater auricular nerve interposition graft may be necessary to provide a tension-free anastomosis. Nerve transection in the cerebellopontine angle can be very difficult to repair, but is possible and can deliver satisfactory results. When impossible, a facial-hypoglossal anastomosis is performed at a later date. Postoperative eye care including artificial tears, ocular lubricants, and eye humidity chambers is instituted, and early upper lid gold weight placement is encouraged. More elderly patients may also need a lower lid shortening or tarsal strip procedure to reduce pronounced ectropion. A concurrent fifth cranial nerve injury with corneal anesthesia can be devastating and needs the care and attention of an ophthalmologist.

During hearing preservation cases, intraoperative ABR may be used to monitor wave V. Alterations in the ABR should result in immediate cessation of any surgical manipulation until the tracing returns to baseline. The cochlear nerve must be dissected carefully, and the labyrinthine artery must be preserved. During the removal of larger tumors, the lower cranial nerves must be identified and preserved. Excessive surgical manipulation of these nerves may lead to difficulties with speech and swallowing postoperatively, requiring aspiration precautions, which may include temporary or permanent true vocal fold medialization. The fifth nerve is also at risk during the removal of larger tumors and must be atraumatically freed from the tumor. Tumors extending far anteriorly may involve the sixth nerve. If abducens palsy occurs, appropriate ophthalmologic consultation should be obtained.

Bleeding

A thorough history and physical examination should bring out medicines, medical conditions, and bleeding tendencies that should be fully worked up and planned for prior to the operation. Factor deficiencies, factor V leiden, genetic bleeding disorders, liver diseases, drug or alcohol abuse, and many medications including over the counter medications should be reviewed and stopped or worked up prior to the surgery.

Intraoperative bleeding is minimized through coordinated care with the neuroanesthesiologist, as well as by meticulous identification and preservation or hemostasis of vessels. Care must be exercised when removing bone from the sigmoid sinus. Diamond burs are much less likely to cause laceration, and the use of a Freer elevator to remove the thin layer of bone from the sigmoid and superior petrosal sinus after drilling causes less trauma. When the sigmoid sinus is lacerated, bipolar cautery is usually ineffective unless the laceration is very small; however, when the sinus is lacerated, immediate compression and measures to stop the bleeding decrease the risk of air embolus. Placement of a piece of Gelfoam (Pfizer, New York, NY) or Surgicel (Johnson & Johnson Gateway, LLC, Piscataway, NJ) directly over the bleeding site, followed by pressure with a cottonoid, usually stops the bleeding. If this approach fails, extraluminal sinus occlusion is preferable to intraluminal occlusion. A thin shell of bone should always be left covering the delicate jugular bulb to avoid bleeding. Should bleeding occur, the same techniques are used as for the sigmoid sinus. Caution should be exercised if intraluminal occlusion is used near the jugular bulb because compression of the pars nervosa can cause neuropathy of the lower cranial nerves. Significant bleeding from the superior petrosal sinus is controlled by intraluminal packing with oxidized cellulose Surgicel (Johnson & Johnson Gateway, LLC, Piscataway, NJ).

Arterial bleeders from the tumor surface are controlled with bipolar cautery, and bleeding from the center of the tumor during reduction is managed with oxidized cellulose packing. Small veins within the cerebellopontine angle are preserved to prevent venous congestion; however, they can be bipolar cauterized if necessary. All arteries within the cerebellopontine angle are treated with respect and carefully dissected from the tumor surface. Cautious, deliberate dissection is carried out in this region, and arteries to the brain stem are never intentionally sacrificed.

A full grasp of the intratemporal carotid artery anatomy is mandatory when using the transcochlear approach. The carotid artery is identified to enable dissection within the anterior

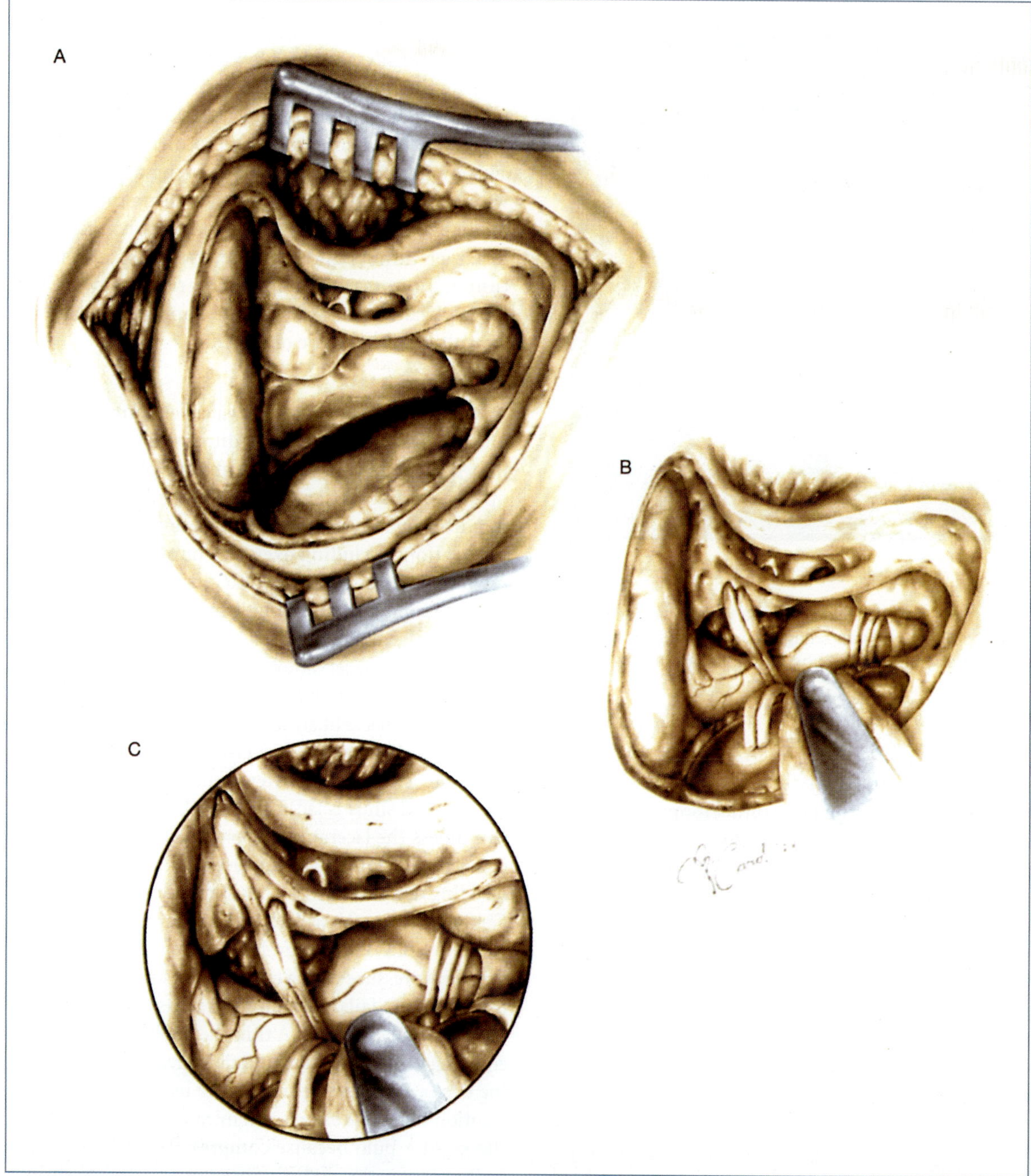

FIGURE 37–14 • *A*, Transcochlear approach to the anterior cerebellopontine angle. The internal auditory canal has been exposed using the standard translabyrinthine approach. *B*, The posterior fossa and internal auditory canal dura have been opened. The superior and inferior vestibular nerves have been released from their lateral attachments, enabling visualization of the superiorly located facial nerve and the inferiorly located cochlear nerve. The meningioma can be seen within the confines of the anterior cerebellopontine angle, anterior to the facial and cochlear nerves. *C*, The labyrinthine segment of the facial nerve is identified, and the entire intratemporal course of the facial nerve is exposed. The nerve is skeletonized prior to mobilization.

Continued

portion of the cerebellopontine angle. Diamond burs are used when removing the cochlea and delineating the carotid artery. In case of laceration a vascular surgeon's assistance should be obtained intraoperatively. An assessment of vessel backflow in the distal stump is used to estimate collateral flow through the circle of Willis. Shunting and primary repair should be accomplished if possible.

Brain Edema

Brain edema occurs most commonly with the suboccipital approach secondary to cerebellar retraction. Prior to opening the dura, ICP should be reduced with intravenous mannitol and hyperventilation. Intravenous dexamethasone is used to prevent the development of edema. The cerebellopontine cistern must be accessed to allow the egress of CSF and provide

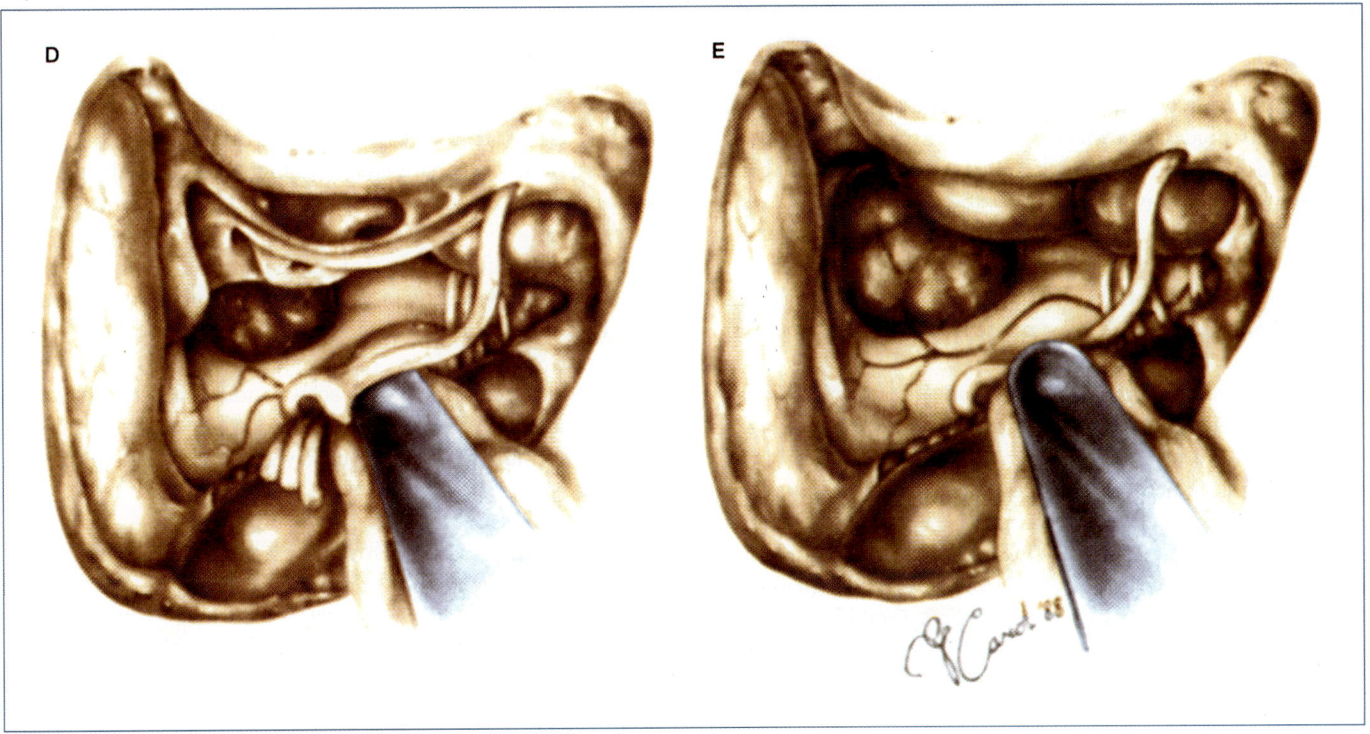

FIGURE 37–14 • *Continued. D, E,* The greater petrosal nerve is transected anterior to the geniculate ganglion, and the facial nerve is mobilized posteriorly. The otic capsule is drilled away with a diamond bur, and the internal carotid artery is delineated. Bone removal proceeds anteriorly to the internal carotid artery, giving access to the petrous tip and clivus.

further cerebellar relaxation prior to any surgical manipulation. Protecting the surface of the cerebellum from the retractor with a layer of nonadherent material such as bicol covered with cottonoid sponges also decreases trauma. Should significant edema occur, exposure will be limited, and the procedure may need to be terminated. In extreme cases, a portion of the cerebellum may need to be resected to decrease the rise in ICP. It is important to remember that the retracted temporal lobe is also at risk of becoming edematous in the course of middle fossa surgery.

Venous Air Embolism

Venous air embolism occurs when air is sucked into a venous sinus, emissary vein, or diploic vein. A large air embolus may travel to the right heart and ultimately the pulmonary circulation, causing cor pulmonale, insufficient gas exchange, and death. When a patient's head is above the heart, the intraluminal pressure of the head and neck venous system is subatmospheric, and an air embolus is more likely to occur. Therefore, the sitting position, once favored for the suboccipital approach, is discouraged in favor of the supine position.

When a venous sinus is lacerated, immediate compression and measures to stop the bleeding, decrease the risk of air embolism. Likewise, bleeding diploic spaces and mastoid emissary veins should be sealed immediately with bone wax. Air embolism is diagnosed by fluctuating blood pressure and a characteristic churning heart murmur. Once identified, the patient is placed in the left lateral decubitus position, and the air embolus is aspirated from the right heart through a Swan-Ganz catheter. Slightly lowering the patient's head encourages return of venous flow and decreased air entry through the wound. Additionally, nitrous oxide administration is discontinued, replaced by 100% oxygen.

Cardiac Arrhythmias

Tumor dissection from the brain stem can cause cardiac rhythm disturbances and altered hemodynamics. Typically, tachycardia and hypertension are observed with brain stem stimulation, and if either develops, the surgeon must cease tumor dissection immediately and not proceed again until vital signs have stabilized. The vagus nerve may be manipulated during the removal of large tumors, resulting in bradycardia and hypotension. Again, all surgical manipulation must stop until vital signs have returned to baseline.

Brain Herniation

Giant vestibular schwannomas may cause obstructive hydrocephalus (owing to compression of the fourth ventricle), leading to intraoperative herniation. It is essential that hydrocephalus be identified preoperatively. Increased ICP secondary to hydrocephalus presents with nausea, vomiting, headache, and visual disturbance. Funduscopic examination reveals papilledema. Prior to surgery, the neurotologist and neurosurgeon should determine the potential risk of herniation. When the risk is high, a ventricular drain should be placed prior to tumor removal. Ventriculoperitoneal shunts have inherent complications as well, such as infection and bleeding. Accordingly, the shunt is placed only in the high-risk patient.

Postoperative Complications Hemorrhage

Regardless of approach, copious irrigation must be employed prior to wound closure to ensure that all clots are removed, and all bleeding sources must be identified and controlled. Bipolar cautery and topical hemostatic agents are used as necessary, and wound closure is begun only when there is no evidence of bleeding. Hemorrhage may be epidural, subdural, or intraparenchymal, the last of which is usually owing to overzealous retraction. Preferably, the patient is awakened and extubated at the completion of the procedure so that a neurologic examination can be accomplished. Neurologic status is frequently checked in the intensive care unit.

Postoperative hemorrhage is usually accompanied by altered mental status and vital signs within the first 24 h after surgery. Deterioration may occur quickly, and prompt attention is critical. Patients in stable condition may be imaged, but time should not be wasted obtaining a CT scan if the patient's status is rapidly deteriorating. Opening the incision at the bedside under sterile conditions can decompress the brain and can be life saving. The source of hemorrhage is then identified and controlled in the operating room.

Brain edema may present early in the postoperative period with increased ICP, confusion, and altered mental status similar to hemorrhage. Often the edema is a consequence of cerebellar retraction in the suboccipital approach or of temporal lobe retraction in the middle fossa approach. Computed tomographic scanning can make the diagnosis if the patient's condition is stable and intravenous mannitol and steroids are administered to decrease ICP. Early operative intervention may be required to control postoperative brain edema. Severely edematous cerebellar tissue may require resection. In addition, a ventricular drain may be necessary to manage hydrocephalus.

Infarction

Infarction may be secondary to arterial or venous occlusion. Mechanisms of occlusion include vessel division, coagulation, compression and thrombosis, and vasospasm.[147] Overzealous bipolar cautery can disrupt the blood supply to the brain stem; therefore, only vessel branches directly feeding the tumor may be coagulated. The anterior inferior cerebellar artery is a major contributor to pontine and cerebellar circulation and is often intimately associated with vestibular schwannomas and the eighth nerve. Interruption of this vessel causes extensive infarction of the pons and the "lateral pontomedullary syndrome," consisting of unilateral labyrinthine infarction, cerebellar infarction, ipsilateral Horner's syndrome, ipsilateral facial and contralateral body sensory loss, contralateral hemiparesis, and, often, death. Therefore, when encountered, this vessel must always be gently swept off the tumor and preserved. If vasospasm occurs during manipulation, topical papaverine should be applied to promote vasodilatation.

Intraparenchymal infarction of the cerebellum or temporal lobe is usually related to brain retraction. Cerebellar infarction presents with brain edema, confusion, mental status changes, and cerebellar signs. Temporal lobe infarction may present with an expressive aphasia. To avoid infarction, it is essential to ensure brain relaxation. Intravenous mannitol should be given early in the procedure and an adequate diuresis confirmed. In addition, intravenous furosemide may be given if necessary. Hyperventilation to a P_{CO2} of 25 mm Hg can further decrease ICP. Dural opening and brain retraction should only be accomplished once proper brain relaxation has been established. A temporal lobe seizure may manifest secondary to the retraction or any resultant edema or hemorrhage. This requires a neurological consultation with possible period of anticonvulsant therapy.

Occlusion of the vein (or veins) of Labbé can precipitate temporal lobe venous infarction, cerebral edema, seizure, altered mentation, expressive aphasia, and even death. These veins drain into the distal transverse sinus and are therefore rarely encountered in vestibular schwannoma surgery. However, intraluminal packing of a lacerated transverse or proximal sigmoid sinus should be avoided to prevent injury to these veins.

Cerebrospinal Fluid Leak

The incidence of CSF leakage after vestibular schwannoma resection has been reported to be between 6 and 15%.[148] A CSF leak presents as clear, watery rhinorrhea, otorrhea, or leakage through the incision. Postoperative meningitis occurs more often in the presence of CSF leak, emphasizing the importance of its prevention. Patients with well-pneumatized temporal bones are at an increased risk; therefore, any open air cells must be sealed with muscle, fascia, or bone wax at the end of the case. A compression dressing is left in place for the first 72 h after surgery.

In the course of the translabyrinthine approach, the middle ear is entered, creating a potential route for CSF rhinorrhea. Therefore, the eustachian tube should be identified by partially opening the facial recess and removing the incus and head of the malleus. The eustachian tube is packed with Nu Knit (Johnson & Johnson Gateway, LLC, Piscataway, NJ), bone wax, muscle, or fascia, and the middle-ear space is obliterated with muscle. Care should be exercised when opening the facial recess and packing the middle ear to prevent damage to the tympanic annulus or membrane because such injury can lead to CSF otorrhea. Strips of abdominal fat are used to fill the posterior fossa dural defect. These strips are gently placed into the cerebellopontine angle, with the lateral two-thirds protruding into the mastoid cavity. The remainder of the cavity is filled with fat, and the incision is closed in a layered, watertight fashion.

At the close of a middle fossa procedure, a muscle or fascia graft is placed over the IAC and is covered in turn with a layer of Gelfoam. The weight of the temporal lobe holds the packing in place. During the suboccipital approach, the dural flaps must be kept moist throughout the procedure to facilitate later closure. If a watertight closure cannot be achieved, a pericranial graft is used to bridge the remaining gap. The incision is closed in multiple, watertight layers. Again, any open air cells must be sealed with tissue or bone wax.

Should CSF leakage occur through the incision, the site of leakage is oversewn sterilely at the bedside with a running-locking suture, and the compression dressing is replaced. Head of bed elevation, bed rest, and stool softeners are instituted. Insertion of a lumbar drain is necessary if these measures fail.

The management of CSF rhinorrhea depends on the surgical approach used. Re-exploring the surgical site and ensuring that the eustachian tube is occluded may most quickly address CSF rhinorrhea after translabyrinthine surgery. Lumbar drainage for 3 to 5 days may also be successful. Cerebrospinal fluid rhinorrhea after the middle fossa approach usually responds to lumbar drainage, with surgical intervention less frequently necessary. A CT scan is obtained prior to the insertion of a lumbar drain to rule out hydrocephalus, and no more than 10 to 15 cc of CSF is drained each hour. Additionally, sterile technique is paramount in placing and caring for a lumbar drain to prevent meningitis. A CSF sample for cell count, glucose, and protein should be examined if infection is suspected.

With persistent CSF rhinorrhea, a CT scan should be obtained to evaluate the presence of an air cell tract that extends from the petrous apex to the medial aspect of the eustachian tube; this tract may have to be obliterated via a transcochlear approach or middle fossa approach.[149]

Meningitis

The third most common complication of vestibular schwannoma surgery (after facial nerve paralysis and CSF leakage) is meningitis. Meningitis presents with fever, headache, neck and back stiffness, photophobia, and mental status changes. A concomitant CSF leak is not uncommon. After a CT scan has been obtained to rule out hydrocephalus, a lumbar puncture should be performed and broad-spectrum, intravenous antibiotics (with good CSF penetration) started. The CSF is sent for Gram stain, cell count, protein and glucose content, and culture and sensitivity. A marked white cell count elevation, decreased glucose, and increased protein content are typical of bacterial meningitis. The Gram stain results can be obtained quickly and enable antibiotic adjustment. Consultation with an infectious diseases specialist is recommended, and ototoxic antibiotics are avoided if possible. In addition, wound infections should be cultured and the appropriate antibiotics started to prevent progression to meningitis.

Aseptic (or chemical) meningitis may occur and is more common than its bacterial counterpart.[150] The meningeal inflammation may be secondary to bone dust, blood, or other irritants. Regardless of the cause, headache and fever are present, and chemical meningitis may closely mimic bacterial meningitis. Therefore, bacterial meningitis is ruled out as previously described, and antibiotics are started. In aseptic meningitis, CSF analysis reveals an elevated white cell count and protein; however, the glucose level usually is normal. No organisms are identified by Gram stain and culture. Bacterial meningitis must be absolutely ruled out prior to cessation of antibiotic therapy. The addition of a corticosteroid or a nonsteroidal anti-inflammatory agent may help alleviate the symptoms.

Tension Pneumocephalus

Postoperative pneumocephalus is often seen on scans obtained early in the postoperative period and resolves without treatment. In contrast, the rare complication of tension pneumocephalus results from air trapping within the cranial cavity and may present with symptoms of increased ICP and mental status changes.[151,152] A CT scan can make the diagnosis and rule out other causes of increased ICP. This complication is much more likely when a ventriculoperitoneal shunt has been placed to manage the hydrocephalus of a large tumor blocking the fourth ventricle. If there is a communication with the mastoid air-cell system, air can be drawn into, and trapped within, the cranium, causing tension pneumocephalus. If discovered, appropriate treatment consists of occlusion of the eustachian tube and mastoid, which may also require transcochlear obliteration of air cells in the petrous apex. Rarely, it may be necessary to evacuate the excessive accumulation of air.

Miscellaneous Complications

Appropriate measures should be taken to prevent the complications inherent to all surgical procedures. Pneumatic compression boots are routinely placed prior to starting the surgical procedure and are left in place until the patient is ambulatory to prevent deep venous thrombosis formation and pulmonary embolism. Histamine2 blockers should be instituted when corticosteroids are used to prevent gastrointestinal bleeding. Incentive spirometry and chest physiotherapy help avert postoperative pneumonia. Furthermore, indwelling intravenous catheters are replaced every 72 h, and urinary catheters are removed as soon as possible to avoid iatrogenic infection.

References

1. Bell C. The nervous system of the human body. Washington, DC: Green; 1833.
2. Ballance C. Some points in the surgery of the brain and its membranes. London: Macmillan & Co.; 1907.
3. House WF. A history of acoustic tumor surgery, 1900–1917: The Cushing era. In: House WF, Luetje CM, editors. Acoustic tumors. Vol 1. Diagnosis. Baltimore: University Park Press; 1979.
4. Henneberg, Koch. Uber "Centrale" Neurofromatese und die Geschwultse des kleinhirnbruckenwinkels (Acusticus neurome). Arch f Psychiat 1902;36:251.
5. Cushing H. Tumors of the nervus acusticus and the syndrome of the cerebellopontine angle. Philadelphia: WB Saunders; 1917.
6. Cushing H. Intracranial tumors. Springfield, IL: Charles C. Thomas; 1932.
7. Dandy WE. An operation for the total removal of cerebellopontine (acoustic) tumors. Surg Gynecol Obstet 1925;41:29.
8. Atkinson WJ. Anterior inferior cerebellar artery. J Neurol Neurosurg Psychiatry 1949;12:137.
9. Panse R. Clinical and pathological observations. IV. A glioma of the akusticus. Arch Ohrenh 1904;61:251.
10. Quix F. Ein Fall von operierter Acusticus-Geschwulst mit Durstellung mikrophotographischer Lichtbilder und Besprechung der Operationstechnik. Monatsschr Ohrenh 1915;717.
11. House WF. Surgical exposure of the IAC and its contents through the middle cranial fossa. Laryngoscope 1961;71:1363.
12. Clerc P, Battise R. Access to the intrapetrous structure from the intracranial aspect. Ann Otolaryngol 1954;21:20.
13. House WF. Report of cases, monograph. Transtemporal bone microsurgical removal of acoustic neuromas. Arch Otolaryngol 1964;80:617.
14. Glasscock ME, Hays JW. The translabyrinthine removal of acoustic and other cerebellopontine angle tumors. Ann Otol Rhinol Laryngol 1973;82:415.

15. Smith MF, Miller RN, Cox DJ. Suboccipital microsurgical removal of acoustic neuromas of all sizes. Ann Otol Rhinol Laryngol 1973;82:407. 42

16. Rand RW, Dirks DD, Morgan DE, et al. Acoustic neuromas. In: Youmans JR, editor. Neurological surgery. Vol 3. Philadelphia: WB Saunders; 1973.

17. MacCarty CS. Acoustic neuroma and the suboccipital approach (1967–1972). Mayo Clin Proc 1975;50:15.

18. Rhoton AL. The suboccipital approach to removal of acoustic neuromas. Head Neck Surg 1979;1:313.

19. Wade PJ, House WF. Hearing preservation in patients with acoustic neuromas via the middle fossa approach. Otolaryngol Head Neck Surg 1984;92:184–93.

20. Delgado TE, Bucheit WA, Rosenholtz HR, Chrissian S. Intraoperative monitoring of facial muscle evoked responses obtained by intracranial stimulation of the facial nerve: A more accurate technique for facial nerve dissection. Neurosurgery 1979;4: 418–21.

21. Silverstein H, Smouha E, Jones R. Routine identification of the facial nerve using electrical stimulation during otological and neurotological surgery. Laryngoscope 1988;98:726–30.

22. Henschen F. Concerning the history and pathogenesis of cerebellopontine angle tumors. Arch Psychiatry 1915;56:21.

23. Jacob A, Robinson LL Jr, Bortman JS, Yu L, Dodson EE, Welling DB. Nerve of origin, tumor size, hearing preservation, and facial nerve outcomes in 359 vestibular schwannoma resections at a tertiary care academic center. Laryngoscope 2007;117:2087–92.

24. Khrais T, Romano G, Sanna M. Nerve origin of vestibular schwannoma: a prospective study. J Laryngol Otol 2008;122: 128–31.

25. Prisig W, Eckermeier L, Mueller D. As to the origin of vestibular schwannomas. Seminar on the diagnosis and management of acoustic tumors and skull base tumors. Ear Research Institute, Los Angeles, CA (February 28–March 3, 1978). Cited in Bebin J. Pathophysiology of acoustic tumors. In: House WF, Luetje CM, editors. Acoustic tumors. Vol 1. Diagnosis. Baltimore: University Park Press; 1979. p. 52.

26. Xenellis JE, Linthicum FH Jr. On the myth of the glial/schwann junction (Obersteiner-Redlich zone): Origin of vestibular nerve schwannomas. Otol Neurotol 2003;24:1.

27. Hardy M. Crowe SJ. Early asymptomatic acoustic tumor: report of 6 cases. Arch Surg 1936;32:292.

28. Vernooij MW, Ikram MA, Tanghe HL, Vincent AJ, et al. Incidental findings on brain MRI in the general population. NEJM 2007;357:1821–8.

29. Dawes PJ, Mehta D, Arullendran P. Screening for vestibular schwannoma: Magnetic resonance imaging findings and management. J Laryngol Otol 2000;114:584–8.

30. Baker R, Stevens-King A, Bhat N, Leong P. Should patients with asymmetrical noise-induced hearing loss be screened for vestibular schwannoma? Clin Otolaryngol 2003;28:346–51.

31. Gruskin P, Craberry J. Pathology of acoustic tumors. In: House WF, Luetje CM, editors. Acoustic tumors. Vol 1. Diagnosis. Baltimore: University Park Press; 1979.

32. Sinha S, Sharma BS. Cystic acoustic neuromas: surgical outcome in a series of 58 patients. J Clin Neurosci 2008;15:511–5.

33. Jones SE, Baguley DM, Moffat DA. Are facial nerve outcomes worse following surgery for cystic vestibular schwannomas? Skull Base 2007;17:281–4.

34. Seizinger BR, Martuza RL, Gusella JF. Loss of genes on chromosome 22 in tumorigenesis of human acoustic neuroma. Nature 1986;322:644–7.

35. Rouleau GA, Merel P, Lutchman M, et al. Alteration in a new gene encoding a putative membrane-organising protein causes neurofibromatosis 2. Nature 1993;363:515–21.

36. Trofatter JA, MacCollin MM, Rutter JL, et al. A novel moesin-, ezrin-, radixin-like gene is a candidate for the neurofibromatosis 2 tumor suppressor. Cell 1993;72:791–800.

37. Welling DB, Packer MD, Chang LS. Molecular studies of vestibular schwannomas: a review. Curr Opin Otolaryngol Head Neck Surg 2007;15:341–6.

38. Gutmann DH, Sherman L, Seftor L, et al. Increased expression of the NF2 tumor suppressor gene product, merlin, impairs cell motility, adhesion, and spreading. Hum Mol Genet 1999;8: 267–75.

39. Gussela JF, Ramesh V, MacCollin M, et al. Merlin: the neurofibromatosis 2 tumor suppressor. Biochim Biophys Acta 1999;1423:29–36.

40. Gutmann DH, Haipek CA, Burke SP, et al. The NF2 interacter, hepatocyte growth factor-regulated tyrosine kinase substrate (HRS), associates with merlin in the "open" conformation and suppresses cell growth and motility. Hum Mol Genet 2001;10:825–34.

41. Zucmann-Rossi J, Legoix P, Dersarkissian H, Cheret G, et al. NF2 gene in neurofibromatosis type 2 patients. Hum Mol Genet 1998;7:2095–101.

42. Welling DB. Clinical manifestations of mutations in the neurofibromatosis type 2 gene in vestibular schwannomas (acoustic neuromas). Laryngoscope 1998;108:178–89.

43. Welling DB, Akhmametyeva EM, Daniels RL, et al. Analysis of the human neurofibromatosis type 2 gene promoter and its expression. Otolaryngol Head Neck Surg 2000;123:413–8.

44. Clark JJ, Provenzano M, Diggelmann HR, Xu N, Hansen SS, Hansen MR. The ErbB inhibitors trastuzumab and erlotinib inhibit growth of vestibular schwannoma xenografts in nude mice: a preliminary study. Otol Neurotol 2008;29:846–53.

45. Doherty JK, Ongkeko W, Crawley B, Andalibi A, Ryan AF. ErbB and Nrg: potential molecular targets for vestibular schwannoma pharmacotherapy. Otol Neurotol 2008;29:50–7.

46. Jacob A, Lee TX, Neff BA, Miller S, Welling B, Chang LS. Phosphatidylinositol 3-kinase/AKT pathway activation in human vestibular schwannoma. Otol Neurotol 2008;29:58–68.

47. Burkey JM, Rizer FM, Schuring AG, et al. Acoustic reflexes, auditory brain stem response, and MRI in the evaluation of acoustic neuromas. Laryngoscope 1996;106:839–41.

48. Selters WA, Brackmann DE. Acoustic tumor detection with brainstem electric response audiometry. Arch Otolaryngol 1977;103:181.

49. Glasscock ME, Jacksom GJ, Josey AF, et al. Brainstem evoked response audiometry in a clinical practice. Laryngoscope 1979;89:1021.

50. Welling DB, Glasscock ME, Woods CI, et al. Acoustic neuroma: a cost-effective approach. Otolaryngol Head Neck Surg 1990;103:364–70.

51. Ruckenstein MJ, Cueva RA, Morrison DH, et al. A prospective study of ABR and MRI in the screening for vestibular schwannomas. Am J Otol 1996;17:317–20.

52. Schmidt RJ, Sataloff RT, Newman J, et al. The sensitivity of auditory brainstem response testing for the diagnosis of acoustic neuromas. Arch Otolaryngol Head Neck Surg 2001;127:19–22.

53. El-Kashlan HK, Eisenmann D, Kileny PR. Auditory brainstem response in small acoustic neuromas. Ear Hear 2000;21:257–62.

54. Robinette MS, Bauch CD, Olsen WO, et al. Auditory brainstem response and magnetic resonance imaging for acoustic neuromas: cost by prevalence. Arch Otolaryngol Head Neck Surg 2000;126:963–6.

55. Rosenhamer HJ, Lindström B, Lundborg T. On the use of click-evoked electric brainstem responses in audiological diagnosis. III. Latencies in cochlear hearing loss. Scand Audiol 1981;10:3–11.

56. Telian SA, Kileny PR. Usefulness of 1000 Hz tone-burst-evoked responses in the diagnosis of acoustic neuroma. Otolaryngol Head Neck Surg 1989;101:466–71.

57. Don M, Masuda A, Nelson R, Brackmann D. Successful detection of small acoustic tumors using the stacked derived-band auditory brain stem response amplitude. Am J Otol 1997;18:608–21.

58. Glasscock ME, Hays JW. A one-stage combined approach for the management of large cerebellopontine angle tumors. Laryngoscope 1978;88:1563.

59. Linthicum FH, Churchill D. Vestibular test results in acoustic tumor cases. Arch Otolaryngol 1968;88:56.

60. Hallpike CS, Cairns H. Observations on pathology of Meniere's syndrome. J Laryngol Otol 1938;53:56.

61. Tsutsumi T, Tsunoda A, Noguchi Y, Komatsuzaki A. Prediction of the nerves of origin of vestibular schwannomas with vestibular evoked myogenic potentials. Am J Otol 2000;21:712–5.

62. Oghalai JS, Chen L, Brennan ML, Tonini R, Manolidis S. Neonatal hearing loss in the indigent. Laryngoscope 2002;112:281–6.

63. Diallo BK, Franco-Vidal V, Vasili D, Négrevergne M Darrouzet P, et al. The neurotologic evaluation of vestibular schwannomas. Results of audiological and vestibular testing in 100 consecutive cases. Rev Laryngol Otol Rhinol 2006;127:203–9.

64. Hamann C, Rudolf J, von Specht H, Freigang B. Vestibular evoked muscle potentials dependency on neural origin and the location of an acoustic neuroma. HNO 2005;53:690–4.

65. Suzuki M, Yamada C, Inoue R, Kashio A, Saito Y, Nakanishi W. Analysis of vestibular testing in patients with vestibular schwannoma based on the nerve of origin, the localization, and the size of the tumor. Otol Neurotol 2008;29:1029–33.

66. Valvassori GE. Cerebellopontine angle tumors. Otolaryngol Clin North Am 1988;21:337–48.

67. Lipkin AF, Jenkins HA. Role of contrast computed tomography in the diagnosis of small acoustic neuromas. Laryngoscope 1984;94:890.

68. Valvassori GE, Palacios E. Magnetic resonance imaging of the IAC. Top Magn Reson Imaging 2000;11:52–65.

69. Daniels RL, Swallow C, Shelton C, et al. Causes of unilateral sensorineural hearing loss screened by high-resolution fast spin echo magnetic resonance imaging: review of 1,070 consecutive cases. Am J Otol 2000;21:173–80.

70. Annesley DJ, Laitt RD, Jenkins JP, et al. Magnetic resonance imaging in the investigation of sensorineural hearing loss: Is contrast enhancement still necessary? J Laryngol Otol 2001;115:14–21.

71. Inoue Y, Ogawa K, Momoshima S, Kanzaki J. The diagnostic significance of the 3D-reconstructed MRI in vestibular schwannoma surgery: prediction of tumor origin. Eur Arch Otorhinolaryngol 2002;259:73–6.

72. Kocaoglu M, Bulakbasi N, Ucoz T, Ustunsoz B, Pabuscu Y, et al. Comparison of contrast-enhanced T1-weighted and 3D constructive interference in steady state images for predicting outcome after hearing-preservation surgery for vestibular schwannoma. Neuroradiology 2003;45:476–81.

73. Hatipoglu HG, Durakoglugil T, Ciliz D, Yüksel E. Comparison of FSE T2W and 3D FIESTA sequences in the evaluation of posterior fossa cranial nerves with MR cisternography. Diagn Interv Radiol 2007;13:56–60.

74. Gjuric M, Mitrecic MZ, Greess H, Berg M. Vestibular schwannoma volume as a predictor of hearing outcome after surgery. Otol Neurotol 2007;28:822–7.

75. Syms MJ, Petermann GW. Magnetic resonance imaging of stapes prostheses. Am J Otol 2000;21:494–8.

76. William MD, Antonelli PJ, Williams LS. Middle ear prosthesis displacement in high-strength magnetic fields. Otol Neurotol 2001;22:158–61.

77. Fucci MJ, Buchman CA, Brackmann DE, et al. Acoustic tumor growth: implications for treatment choices. Am J Otol 1999;20:495–9.

78. Glasscock ME 3rd, Papps DG Jr, Manolidis S, et al. Management of acoustic neuroma in the elderly population. Am J Otol 1997;18:236–41; discussion 241–2.

79. Nedzelski JM, Schessel DA, Pfleiderer A, et al. Conservative management of acoustic neuromas. Otolaryngol Clin North Am 1992;25:691–705.

80. Yamamoto M, Hagiwara S, Ide M, et al. Conservative management of acoustic neurinomas: Prospective study of long-term changes in tumor volume and auditory function. Minim Invasive Neurosurg 1998;41:86–92.

81. Silverstein H, McDaniel A, Norrell H, et al. Conservative management of acoustic neuroma in the elderly patient. Laryngoscope 1985;95(7 Pt 1):766–70.

82. Levo H, Pyykko I, Blomstedt G. Non-surgical treatment of vestibular schwannoma patients. Acta Otolaryngol Suppl (Stockh) 1997;529:56–8.

83. Charabi S, Thomsen J, Tos M, et al. Acoustic neuroma/vestibular schwannoma growth: past, present and future. Acta Otolaryngol (Stockh) 1998;118:327–32.

84. Massick DD, Welling DB, Dodson EE, et al. Tumor growth and audiometric change in vestibular schwannomas managed conservatively. Laryngoscope 2000;110:1843–9.

85. Charabi S, Thomsen J, Mantoni M, et al. Acoustic neuroma (vestibular schwannoma): Growth and surgical and nonsurgical consequences of the wait-and-see policy. Otolaryngol Head Neck Surg 1995;113:5–14.

86. Hoistad DL, Melnik G, Mamikoglu B, et al. Update on conservative management of acoustic neuroma. Otol Neurotol 2001;22:682–5.

87. Bhatia S, Karmarkar S, Taibah A, et al. Vestibular schwannoma and the only hearing ear. J Laryngol Otol 1996;110:366–9.

88. Bederson JB, von Ammon K, Wichmann WW, et al. Conservative treatment of patients with acoustic tumors. Neurosurgery 1991;28:646–50; discussion 650–1.

89. Ogawa K, Kanzaki J, Ogawa S, et al. The growth rate of acoustic neuromas. Acta Otolaryngol Suppl (Stockh) 1991;487:157–63.

90. Masuda A, Fisher LM, Oppenheimer ML, Iqbal Z, Slattery WH. Natural History Consortium. Hearing changes after diagnosis in neurofibromatosis type 2. Otol Neurotol 2004;25:150–4.

91. Diensthuber M, Lenarz T, Stöver T. Determination of the clinical growth index in unilateral vestibular schwannoma. Skull Base 2006;16:31–8.

92. Aguiar PH, Tatagiba M, Samii M, et al. The comparison between the growth fraction of bilateral vestibular schwannomas in neurofibromatosis 2 (NF2) and unilateral vestibular schwannomas using the monoclonal antibody MIB 1. Acta Neurochir 1995;134:40–5.
93. Falcioni A, Piccirillo E, Mancini F. Cystic vestibular schwannoma. Am J Otol 2000;21:595–6.
94. Al Sanosi A, Fagan PA, Biggs ND. Conservative management of acoustic neuroma. Skull Base 2006;16:95–100.
95. Quaranta N, Baguley DM, Moffat DA. Change in hearing and tinnitus in conservatively managed vestibular schwannomas. Skull Base 2007;17:223–8.
96. Raut VV, Walsh RM, Bath AP, et al. Conservative management of vestibular schwannomas: Second review of a prospective longitudinal study. Clin Otolaryngol Allied Sci 2004;29:505–14.
97. Leksell L. A note on the treatment of acoustic tumours. Acta Chir Scand 1971;137:763–5.
98. Noren G. Long-term complications following Gamma Knife radiosurgery of vestibular schwannomas. Stereotact Funct Neurosurg 1998;70 Suppl 1:65–73.
99. Miller RC, Foote RL, Coffey RJ, et al. Decrease in cranial nerve complications after radiosurgery for acoustic neuromas: a prospective study of dose and volume. Int J Radiat Oncol Biol Phys 1999;43:305–11.
100. Kondziolka DS, Lunsford LD, McLaughlin MR, et al. Long-term outcomes after radiosurgery for acoustic neuromas. NEJM 1998;339:1426–33.
101. Martens F, Verbeke L, Piessens M, et al. Stereotactic radio-surgery of vestibular schwannomas with a linear accelerator. Acta Neurochir Suppl 1994;62:88–92.
102. Ogunrinde OK, Lunsford LD, Kondziolka DS, et al. Cranial nerve preservation after stereotactic radiosurgery of intracanalicular acoustic tumors. Stereotact Funct Neurosurg 1995;64 Suppl 1:87–97.
103. Kwon Y, Kim JH, Lee DJ, et al. Gamma Knife treatment of acoustic neurinoma. Stereotact Funct Neurosurg 1998;70 Suppl 1:57–64.
104. van Roijen L, Nijs HG, Avezaat CJ, et al. Costs and effects of microsurgery versus radiosurgery in treating acoustic neuroma. Acta Neurochir 1997;139:942–8.
105. van Roijen L, Nijs HG, Avezaat CJ, et al. Costs and effects of microsurgical versus radiosurgical treatment of vestibular schwannoma. In: Third International Conference on Acoustic Neurinoma and Other CPA Tumors. Rome, Italy, 1999.
106. Shelton C. Unilateral acoustic tumors: how often do they recur after translabyrinthine removal? Laryngoscope 1995;105(9 Pt 1):958–66.
107. Welling DB, Slater PW, Thomas RD, et al. The learning curve in vestibular schwannoma surgery. Am J Otol 1999;20:644–8.
108. Thomsen J, Tos M, Borgesen SE. Gamma Knife: Hydrocephalus as a complication of stereotactic radiosurgical treatment of an acoustic neuroma. Am J Otol 1990;11:330–3.
109. Slattery WH 3rd, Brackmann DE. Results of surgery following stereotactic irradiation for acoustic neuromas. Am J Otol 1995;16:315–9; discussion 319–21.
110. Pollock BE, Lunsford LD, Kondziolka DS, et al. Vestibular schwannoma management. Part II. Failed radiosurgery and the role of delayed microsurgery. J Neurosurg 1998; 89:949–55.
111. Ito K, Kurita H, Sugasawa K, et al. Analyses of neuro-otological complications after radiosurgery for acoustic neurinomas. Int J Radiat Oncol Biol Phys 1997;39:983–8.
112. Chang SD, Poen J, Hancock SL, et al. Acute hearing loss following fractionated stereotactic radiosurgery for acoustic neuroma. Report of two cases. J Neurosurg 1998; 89:321–5.
113. Ogunrinde OK, Lunsford LD, Flickinger JC, et al. Cranial nerve preservation after stereotactic radiosurgery for small acoustic tumors. Arch Neurol 1995;52:73–9.
114. Subach BR, Kondziolka DS, Lunsford LD, et al. Stereotactic radiosurgery in the management of acoustic neuromas associated with neurofibromatosis type 2. J Neurosurg 1999;90:815–22.
115. Comey CH, McLaughlin MR, Jho HD, et al. Death from a malignant cerebellopontine angle triton tumor despite stereo-tactic radiosurgery. Case report. J Neurosurg 1998;89:653–8.
116. Thomsen J, Mirz F, Wetke R, et al. Intracranial sarcoma in a patient with neurofibromatosis type 2 treated with Gamma Knife radiosurgery for vestibular schwannoma. Am J Otol 2000;21:364–70.
117. Sangueza OP, Requena L. Neoplasms with neural differentiation: a review. Part II: malignant neoplasms. Am J Dermatopathol 1998;20:89–102.
118. Bonetti B, Panzeri L, Carner M, et al. Human neoplastic Schwanncells: changes in the expression of neurotrophins and their low-affinity receptor p75. Neuropathol Appl Neurobiol 1997;23:380–6.
119. Crandon IW, et al. Malignant triton tumour of the spine: a case report. West Indian Med J 1995;44:143–5.
120. Han DH, Kim DG, Chi JG, et al. Malignant triton tumor of the acoustic nerve. Case report. J Neurosurg 1992;76:874–7.
121. Shore-Freedman E, Abrahams C, Recant W, et al. Neurilemomas and salivary gland tumors of the head and neck following childhood irradiation. Cancer 1983;51:2159–63.
122. Acoustic neuroma. NIH Cons Statement 1991;9(4):11–13.
123. Shirato H, Sakamoto T, Sawamura Y, et al. Comparison between observation policy and fractionated stereotactic radiotherapy (SRT) as an initial management for vestibular schwannoma. Int J Radiat Oncol Biol Phys 1999;44:545–50.
124. Samii M, Matthies C. Management of 1000 vestibular schwannomas (acoustic neuromas): the facial nerve—Preservation and restitution of function. Neurosurgery 1997;40:684–94; discussion 694–5.
125. Slattery WH 3rd, Brackmann DE, Hitselberger W. Hearing preservation in neurofibromatosis type 2. Am J Otol 1998;19:638–43.
126. Welling DB. Clinical manifestations of mutations in the neurofibromatosis type 2 gene in vestibular schwannomas (acoustic neuromas). Laryngoscope 1998;108:178–89.
127. Glasscock ME, Hart MJ, Vrabec JT. Management of bilateral acoustic neuroma. Otolaryngol Clin North Am 1992;25: 449–69.
128. Wackym PA, King WA, Poe DS, et al. Adjunctive use of endoscopy during acoustic neuroma surgery. Laryngoscope 1999;109:1193–201.
129. Neff BA, Wiet RM, Lasak JM, et al. Cochlear implantation in the neurofibromatosis type 2 patient: Long-term follow-up. Laryngoscope 2007;117:1069–72.
130. Glasscock ME, Kveton JF, Christianson S, et al. A systematic approach to the surgical management of acoustic neuroma. Laryngoscope 1986;96:1088.
131. Lalwani AK, Butt FY, Jackler RK, et al. Facial nerve outcome after acoustic neuroma surgery: A study from the era of cranial nerve monitoring. Otolaryngol Head Neck Surg 1994;111:561–70.
132. Lenarz T, Ernst A. Intraoperative facial nerve monitoring in the surgery of cerebellopontine angle tumors: Improved

preservation of nerve function. ORL J Otorhinolaryngol Relat Spec 1994;56:31–5.

133. Kaylie DM, Gilbert E, Horgan MA, et al. Acoustic neuroma surgery outcomes. Otol Neurotol 2001;22:686–9.

134. Wiet RJ, Mamikoglu B, Odom L, et al. Long-term results of the first 500 cases of acoustic neuroma surgery. Otolaryngol Head Neck Surg 2001;124:645–51.

135. Lanman TH, Brackmann DE, Hitselberger WE, et al. Report of 190 consecutive cases of large acoustic tumors (vestibular schwannoma) removed via the translabyrinthine approach. J Neurosurg 1999;90:617–23.

136. Fundova P, Charabi S, Tos M, et al. Cystic vestibular schwannoma: surgical outcome. J Laryngol Otol 2000;114:935–9.

137. Arts HA, Telian SA, El-Kashlan H, Thompson BG. Hearing preservation and facial nerve outcomes in vestibular schwannoma surgery: Results using the middle cranial fossa approach. Otol Neurotol 2006;27:234–41.

138. Slattery WH 3rd, Brackmann DE, Hitselberger W. Middle fossa approach for hearing preservation with acoustic neuromas. Am J Otol 1997;18:596–601.

139. Leonetti J, Anderson D, Marzo S, et al. Cerebrospinal fluid fistula after transtemporal skull base surgery. Otolaryngol Head Neck Surg 2001;124:511–4.

140. Lebowitz RA, Hoffman RA, Roland JT Jr, et al. Autologous fibrin glue in the prevention of cerebrospinal fluid leak following acoustic neuroma surgery. Am J Otol 1995;16:172–4.

141. Hoffman RA. Cerebrospinal fluid leak following acoustic neuroma removal. Laryngoscope 1994;104(1 Pt 1):40–58.

142. Gillman GS, Parnes LS. Acoustic neuroma management: A six-year review. J Otolaryngol 1995;24:191–7.

143. Becker SS, Jackler RK, Pitts LH. Cerebrospinal fluid leak after acoustic neuroma surgery: A comparison of the translabyrinthine, middle fossa, and retrosigmoid approaches. Otol Neurotol 2003;24:107–12.

144. Rubenstein LJ. Tumors of the central nervous system. In: Firminger HI, editor. Atlas of tumor pathology. Washington (DC): Air Force Institute of Pathology; 1972.

145. House WF, Hitselberger WE. The transcochlear approach to the skull base. Arch Otolaryngol 1976;102:334–42.

146. House WF, Hitselberger WE, Horn KL. The middle fossa transpetrous approach to the anterior superior cerebellopontine angle. Ann J Otol 1986;7:1.

147. Almeida GM, Bianco E, Sousa AS. Vasospasm after acoustic neuroma removal. Surg Neurol 1985;23:38–40.

148. Brennen JW, Rowed DW, Nedzelski JM, et al. Cerebral spinal fluid leak after acoustic neuroma surgery: influence of tumor size and surgical approach on incidence and response to treatment. J Neurosurg 2001;94:217–23.

149. Grant IL, Welling DB, Oehler MC, et al. Transcochlear repair of persistent cerebrospinal fluid leaks. Laryngoscope 1999; 109:1392–6.

150. House WF, Hitzelberger WE. The neuro-otologist's view of the surgical management of acoustic neuroma. Clin Neurosurg 1985;32:214–22.

151. Kithata LM, Katz JD. Tension pneumocephalus after posterior fossa craniotomy: report of four additional cases and review of postoperative pneumocephalus. Neurosurgery 1983;12: 164–8.

152. Miller CF, Furman WR. Symptomatic pneumocephalus after translabyrinthine acoustic neuroma excision and nitrous oxide anesthesia. Anesthesiology 1985;58:281–3.

Auditory Brainstem Implant 38

Steven R. Otto, MA / Derald E. Brackmann, MD / William E. Hitselberger, MD / Elizabeth H. Toh, MD / Robert V, Shannon, PhD / Lendra M. Friesen, MS

Frequently, loss of integrity of the auditory nerve after removal of vestibular schwannomas in neurofibromatosis type 2 (NF2) leaves patients completely deafened. Other communication methods such as signing and lipreading have provided some assistance but obviously cannot restore useful hearing sensations. The auditory brainstem implant (ABI) was developed to bypass the auditory nerve and directly stimulate the cochlear nucleus complex. Useful auditory sensations have resulted[1,2] and the multichannel version of the ABI (Nucleus®, Cochlear Corporation, Englewood, Colorado) successfully completed US Food and Drug Administration (FDA) clinical trials in July, 2000 and received approval for commercial release. This chapter summarizes the history, surgical, and clinical aspects of ABI implantation and perceptual performance. The techniques have been refined in nearly 250 patients implanted with various implementations of the ABI since 1979 at House Ear Institute (HEI, Los Angeles, California). Twenty-five patients received the initial single-channel ABI, the next 71 patients received the 8-electrode ABI, and subsequent patients have received a 21-electrode ABI system (the Nucleus ABI24).

We also developed and conducted FDA clinical trials of a multichannel penetrating electrode system designed to increase the precision of auditory neural stimulation within the cochlear nucleus matrix. General technical and theoretical considerations regarding ABI implantation and management of patients with NF2 have been summarized elsewhere.[3–5]

HISTORY OF DEVELOPMENT

In 1979, William House and William Hitselberger (Figure 38–1) first implanted an electrode to stimulate the cochlear nucleus of a patient with NF2 facing deafness after removal of a vestibular schwannoma. The patient was persistent in her requests that this be tried in the hope that it would allow her to continue to have some hearing sensations. The electrode was a simple ball type, and electrical stimulation was supplied by a modified body-worn hearing aid. Useful auditory sensations resulted, but the electrode proved somewhat unstable and was shortly removed. A two-electrode (later three) mesh-type array was subsequently developed by Huntington Medical Research Institute (HMRI, Pasadena, California) and was used successfully in 25 recipients until 1992. The speech processors were modified 3M/House-type cochlear implant processors that provided patients with sound awareness, ability to discriminate some environmental sounds, and significantly improved understanding of speech in conjunction with lipreading. Experiments also suggested that multichannel stimulation was feasible and would be potentially beneficial with a multiple-electrode array. This led to the development and successful use of the present multichannel ABI.

PATIENT SELECTION

At least 90% of individuals with NF2 exhibit bilateral vestibular schwannomas.[6] Treatment of these and other tumors associated with NF2 has significantly prolonged the life span of such patients. Although performance with the ABI has not reached cochlear implant levels, the auditory information provided can significantly enhance quality of life and the ability to function in occupational and social environments.

The ideal goal in management of NF2 remains hearing preservation through early diagnosis and treatment. However, the ABI provides an alternative to a desperate attempt to preserve nonserviceable hearing when large tumors are present and hearing conservation is unlikely.

The multichannel ABI is approved for use in individuals with NF2 who are at least 12 years of age. There are no preoperative audiologic criteria because the surgical procedure for tumor excision and electrode array placement eliminates any remaining hearing. Implantation may occur during first- or second-side vestibular schwannoma removal or in patients with previously removed tumors bilaterally. A small but significant number of patients (9% at HEI) has failed to experience auditory responses from the implant, primarily because of anatomic difficulties. First-side implantation can provide a second opportunity (if necessary) to achieve a functioning system when the second acoustic tumor is removed.

Since completion of the clinical trials phase, the ABI is now available to a wider range of potential recipients. Realistically,

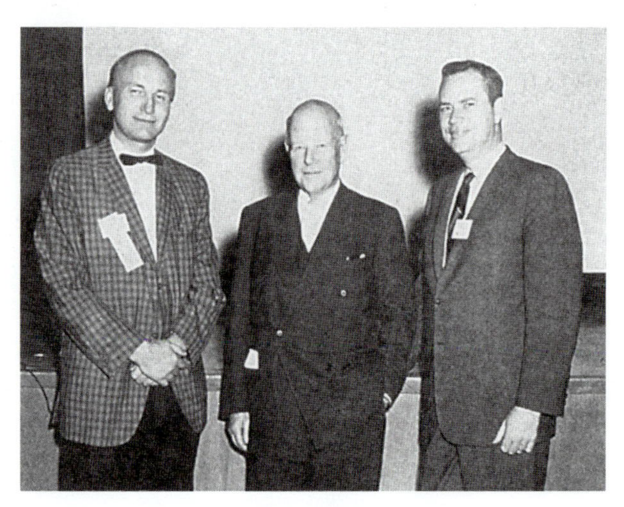

FIGURE 38–1 • Pioneers in auditory brainstem implantation. William E. Hitselberger (left) and William F. House (right) with early supporter and colleague Herbert Olivecrona (middle) of Sweden.

however, the ABI may not be for everyone. A number of non-implant-related factors including general health, vision, social activity, and anatomic status (as seen on magnetic resonance imaging [MRI]) can influence ABI benefit. Patient's age can also be a factor. For example, teenage implantees in general have been less successful regular and enthusiastic users than older recipients. Patients with limited vision also have shown relatively less benefit since the ABI works best in conjunction with lipreading; however, a few blind ABI recipients have benefited from their ABIs. Candidates for ABIs should be apprised of the potential effects of these factors on their ability to benefit from the device.

PREOPERATIVE EVALUATION AND COUNSELING

Preoperative determination of informed consent regarding the ABI is extremely important to the success of an ABI program. The goal of preoperative evaluation and counseling is to help prepare patients for the loss of hearing after tumor removal and lay the groundwork that will help them acclimate to a new way of hearing with the ABI. Prospective recipients and their families should have appropriate expectations regarding the potential benefits and limitations of the device. A frank and thorough explanation of what is involved in using and improving with an ABI is necessary. Inadequate preparation can significantly delay and complicate acceptance and use of the implant.

A major criterion for successful integration and use of the device is a high level of motivation and determination to make maximal use of whatever auditory sensations the ABI provides. Willingness to participate in the postoperative follow-ups is also very important in optimizing device function. Preoperative counseling provides an opportunity to explore motivation issues and to explain the need for judicious compliance with the follow-up protocol. Special counseling may also be helpful in patients having difficulties coping with deafness and other disabilities related to NF2. Such difficulties can distract patients from learning to use an ABI.

Patients should also be counseled preoperatively about the likelihood that they will experience mild nonauditory sensations such as tingling or dizziness on some electrodes, as well as the slight but significant possibility that the ABI may not provide any auditory sensations. Our focus has been to maintain a tone of hopeful and cautious optimism in preoperative counseling of our patients. This has worked well in eliminating unpleasant surprises and properly setting the stage for postoperative rehabilitation.

The participation of an experienced, skilled, and coordinated multidisciplinary team is necessary for the successful treatment and management of patients with NF2. Each team member is essential to the success of an ABI program. Chief among these is the surgeon's skill and experience in removing acoustic tumors, preserving necessary structures, and accurately placing the electrode array. Electrophysiologic monitoring expertise contributes to proper identification of the implant site. Postoperatively, implant audiology expertise is required to program the speech processor and optimize perceptual performance. Even under ideal circumstances, adapting to and learning to use an ABI is an ongoing process that typically extends over a longer period than in cochlear implantation. New recipients should be encouraged that performance almost always improves greatly with experience.

DEVICE

Hitselberger and colleagues originally used a cochlear implant ball-type electrode in their first ABI recipient.[7] Subsequently, patients received a 2 × 8-mm fabric mesh array with two or three platinum ribbon electrodes. In 1992, HEI collaborated with Cochlear Corporation and Huntington Medical Research Institute (Pasadena, California) in the development of an eight-electrode multichannel ABI system. This was further upgraded to the present 21-electrode (Nucleus ABI24) system and receiver/stimulator shown in Figure 38–2A. The electrode array comprises a flexible perforated silicone and mesh substrate with 0.7-mm platinum disk electrodes. This facilitates conformation of the array to the surface of the cochlear nucleus and promotes long-term stability. The ABI24 receiver/stimulator allows up to 2,400 pulse/second/electrode (ppse) of pulsatile stimulation and advanced sound-processing encoders.

The ABI24 system includes the Nucleus Freedom™ sound processor and a transmitter coil (Figure 38–2B). The processing strategy is the Nucleus SPEAK™ (spectral peak) strategy. This processor, also used in cochlear implantation, uses circuitry that analyzes input sound frequencies and codes the salient acoustic information to sequentially activate electrodes on the array. There is flexibility in the number of spectral maxima that can be transmitted, in the sequence and number of electrodes that can be activated, in the stimulus rate, and in available speech-processing strategies (including the Nucleus Advanced Combination Encoder™ [ACE]).

Basic function of the Freedom processor is as follows. The processor incorporates a series of 21 contiguous-input analysis

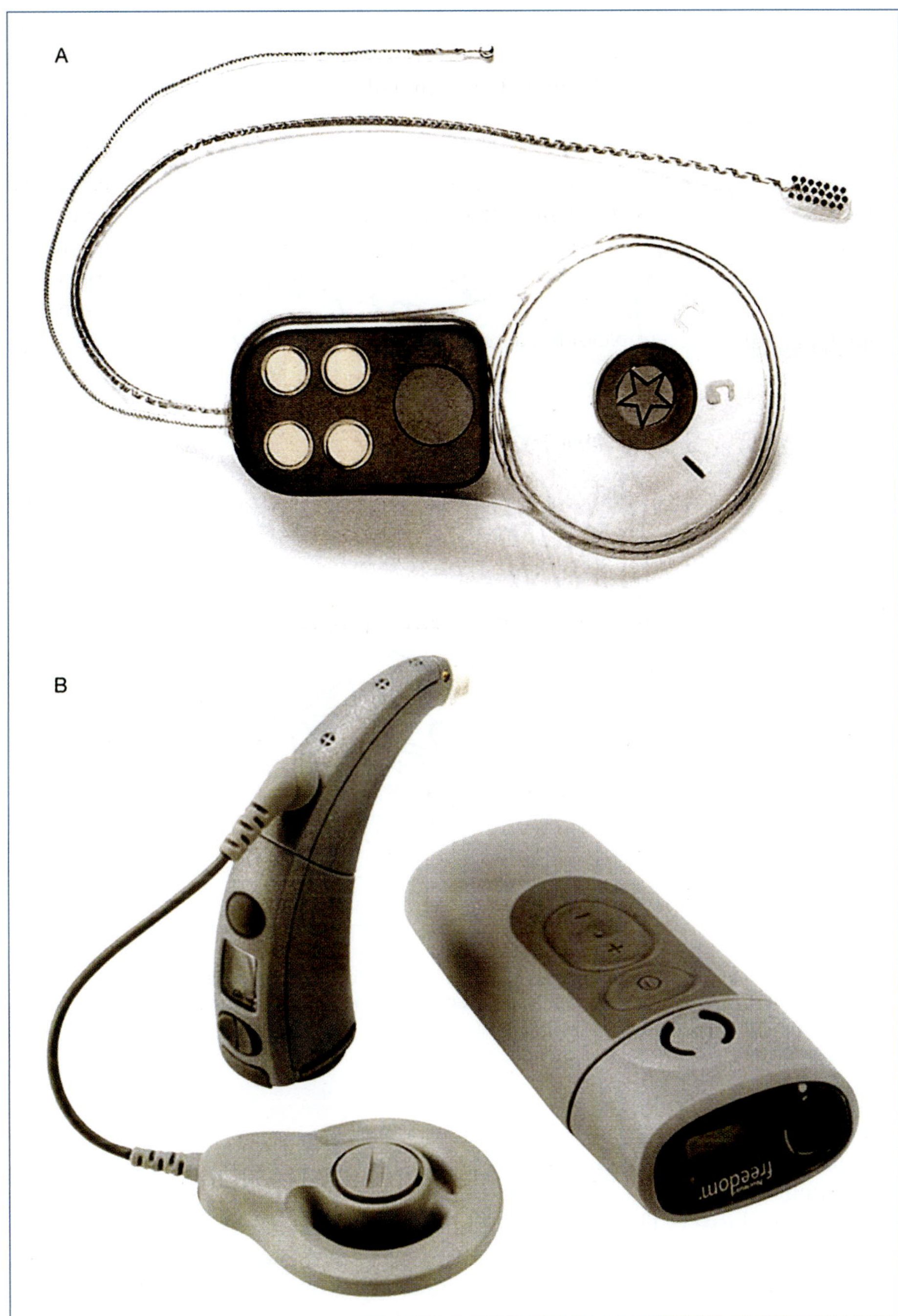

FIGURE 38–2 • *A*, The Nucleus ABI24 auditory brainstem implant receiver/stimulator with 21-electrode surface array (and remote ball ground electrode) for the cochlear nucleus complex. *B*, Auditory brainstem implant Freedom (Nucleus) speech processor with transmitter coil and the body-worn controller for increased battery life.

filters. These filters split the input sound spectra, and the resulting output is linked to selectable electrodes on the array. A major part of processor setup involves determining (via scaling and ranking of electrode-specific pitch) what an appropriate linking arrangement should be for individual patients. This varies greatly, but the general goal is to link low-frequency sounds with electrodes that sound lower in pitch and likewise with higher-frequency sounds. This strategy also optimizes speech and environmental sound perception in cochlear implants, but the process is relatively straightforward with this device because of the highly consistent tonotopic arrangement of neural processes in the cochlea. With an ABI, individual variations in cochlear nucleus anatomy, neuronal survival, and electrode placement result in a much more complex relationship. Therefore, programming ABI speech processors can take more time than programming cochlear implant recipients.

The research penetrating electrode ABI (PABI) system has two electrode arrays with a 10- (or 12-) electrode surface-type array, plus an array with 8 (or 10) penetrating needle-type microelectrodes. It uses the same external sound processor equipment and strategies as the regular surface ABI.

ANATOMIC CONSIDERATIONS

The dorsal and ventral cochlear nuclei are the targets for placement of the ABI electrode array. Although the nuclei are hidden by the cerebellar peduncle, surface landmarks are useful in identifying this region. Frequently, however, these structures may be distorted by tumor. Figure 38–3 shows the major structures of the pontomedullary junction and the translabyrinthine approach surgical field of view. Important landmarks include

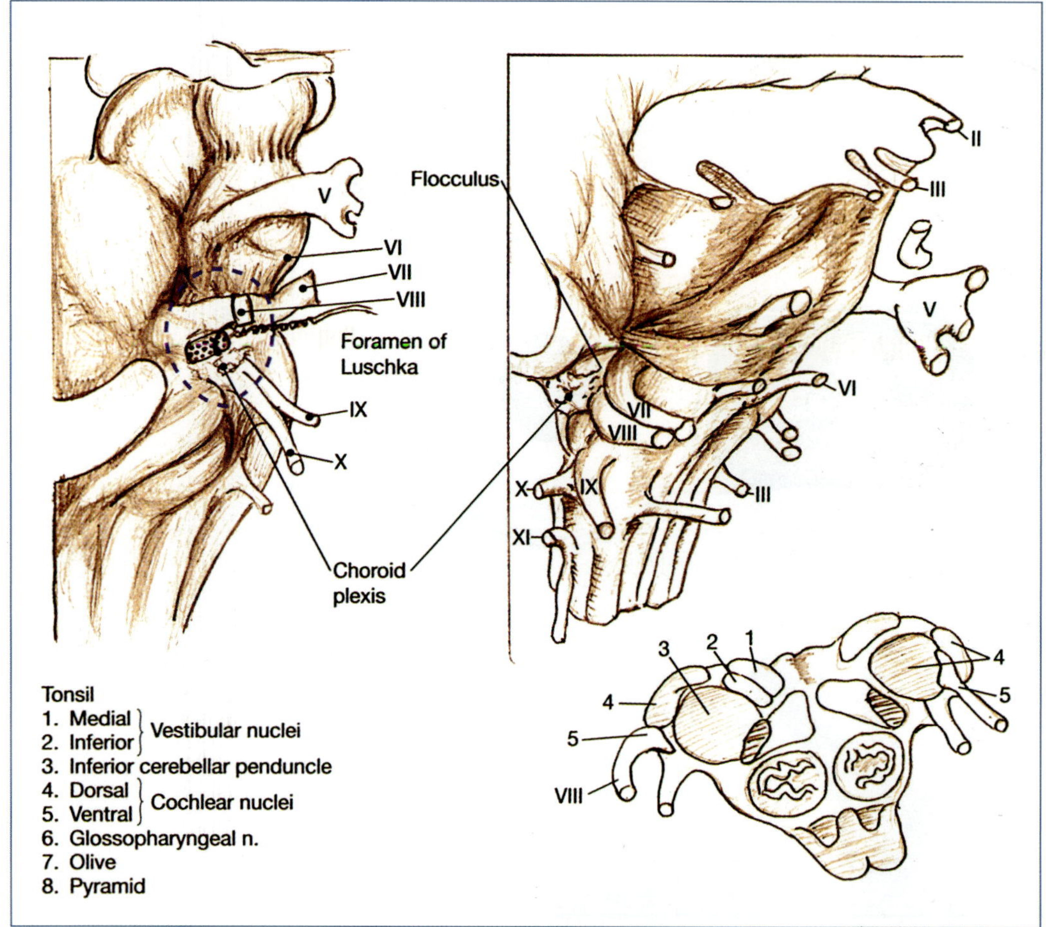

FIGURE 38–3 • Schematic view of the cochlear nuclei region demonstrating relative location of various landmarks. Dashed area represents approximate surgical view. Electrode array is fully inserted into proper position. *Adapted from Otto SR, Hitselberger WE, Telischi FF, et al. Auditory brainstem implant. In: Brackmann DE, Shelton C, Arriaga MA, editors. Otologic surgery. 2nd ed. Philadelphia, PA: WB Saunders; 2001. p. 594–603.*

the terminus of the sleeve-like lateral recess forming the foramen of Luschka, inferiorly the root of the glossopharyngeal (ninth) nerve, and superior to the foramen the vestibulocochlear and facial nerve roots.

Normally, the intact choroid plexus marks the entrance to the lateral recess (foramen of Luschka), and the taenia obliquely traverses the roof of the lateral recess, marking the surface of the ventral cochlear nucleus. These structures may not be clearly identifiable when a large tumor distorts the lateral surface of the pons and medulla. In such cases, the stump of the eighth nerve may be traced to the opening of the lateral recess. The ninth cranial nerve can also be used as a reference point for the lateral recess. A concavity sometimes visualized between the eighth and ninth nerves should not be confused with the introitus of the recess.

Within the lateral recess and on its superior aspect are found the dorsal and ventral cochlear nuclei. The electrode array is positioned well within the recess to provide positional stability. Electrical stimulation of the ventral cochlear nucleus, the main relay for eighth nerve input, and the major portion of the ascending auditory pathway is probably the primary source of auditory sensations even though some part of the array also lies adjacent to the dorsal cochlear nucleus.

SURGICAL CONSIDERATIONS

The translabyrinthine craniotomy provides the best access for tumor removal and exposure of the lateral recess of the fourth ventricle. A typical translabyrinthine acoustic tumor removal process is followed except that recording electrodes are placed for monitoring electrically evoked auditory brainstem responses (EABRs) and any activity from cranial nerves VII and IX. Also, a standard postauricular incision is used and the device is placed into a pocket in the temporal area (Figure 38–4). Intravenous antibiotics, eg, cefuroxime (Zinacef®, GlaxoSmithKline) 3 g, are administered prophylactically on induction of anesthesia. Monitoring of the EABR assists with confirmation that the electrode array is properly positioned. Slight adjustments of the array may be necessary to minimize responses that suggest activation of nonauditory neural structures. For EABR monitoring, subdermal needle electrodes are inserted at the vertex of the head, over the seventh cervical vertebrae, and at the hairline of the occiput. For electromyographic recording of nonauditory activation, the facial nerve is monitored in the standard fashion,[8] and bipolar electrodes are inserted in the ipsilateral pharyngeal (soft palate) muscles to monitor activity from cranial nerve IX.

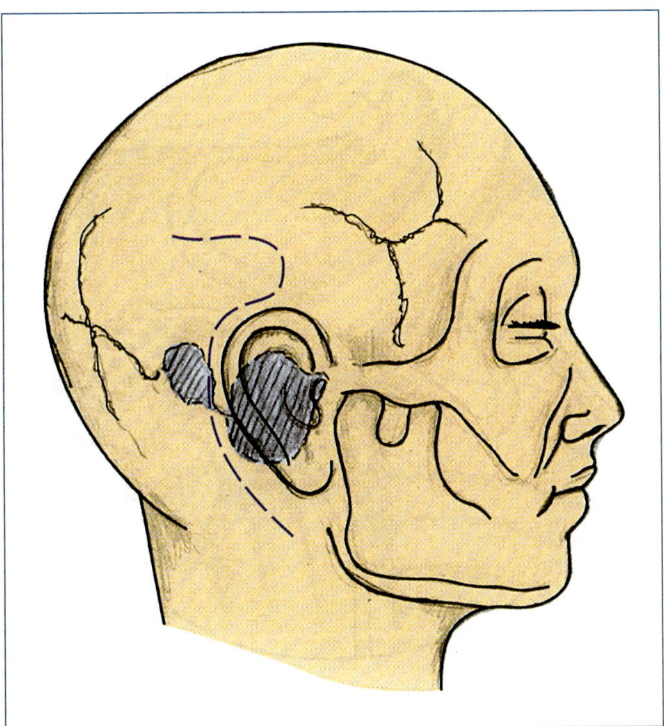

FIGURE 38–4 • Location of the incision with respect to the planned site of receiver/stimulator. The superior extension may be deleted and the implant placed into a subcutaneous pocket.

After the receiver/stimulator has been secured and the array placed, a transmitter coil is placed over the receiver antenna. The EABR obtained with biphasic pulsatile stimulation of the cochlear nucleus differs from responses obtained using acoustic stimulation and from electrical stimulation using cochlear implants.[9] An experienced electrophysiologist interprets these waveforms intraoperatively and provides feedback to the neurosurgeon regarding placement.

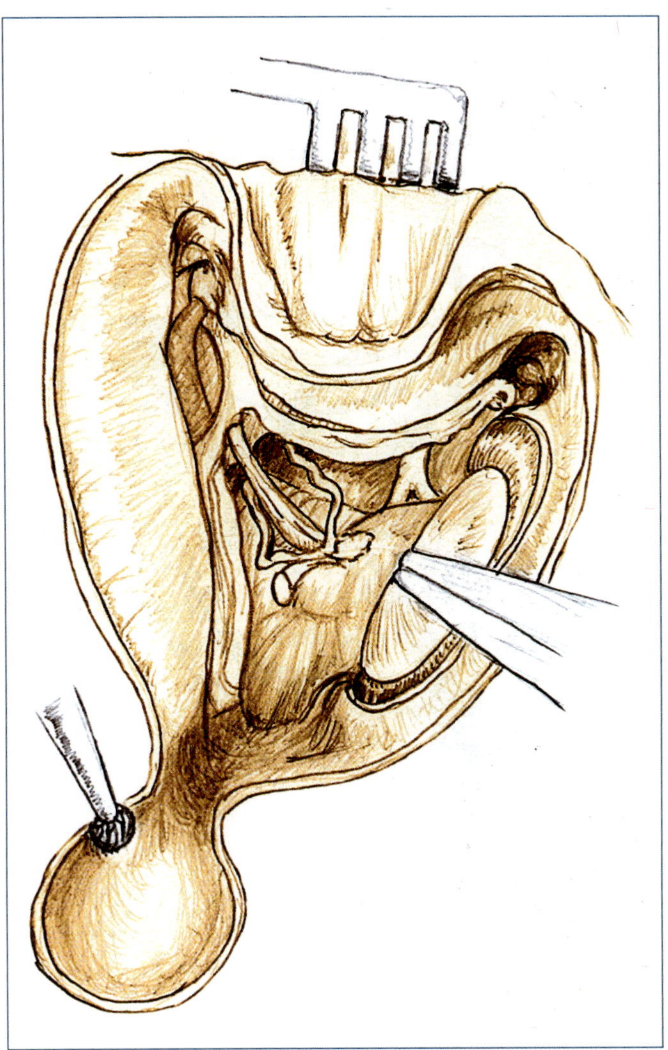

FIGURE 38–5 • Schematic surgical view of the completed translabyrinthine craniotomy, trough for receiver/stimulator wires, and receiver/stimulator seat being drilled.

IMPLANTATION PROCEDURE

Tumor dissection proceeds in the normal fashion via a translabyrinthine craniotomy. After complete tumor removal and adequate hemostasis, the site for the internal receiver posterosuperior to the mastoid cavity is determined, and temporalis muscle in this area is elevated off the parietal skull and excised. Using a replica of the receiver/stimulator as a guide, a circular area of bony cortex in this area is flattened using cutting burs, and a trough is created between the implant seat and the mastoid cavity for placement of the electrode wires (Figure 38–5). Suture tunnel holes are then created on either side of the receiver/stimulator, which is then fixed with nylon suture prior to electrode array positioning so that manipulation of the leads does not alter electrode placement (Figure 38–6). Once the internal receiver has been implanted, only bipolar electrocautery should be used for hemostasis since current transmission through the implant to the brainstem is a potential hazard with monopolar electrocautery.

The location of the lateral recess may be confirmed by noting the egress of cerebrospinal fluid (CSF) as the anesthesiologist induces the Valsalva maneuver in the patient. This technique should be reserved as a final check after the opening to the recess has been located using standard landmarks since CSF will be drained quickly, and the advantage of this technique is lost with multiple Valsalva maneuvers.

After identifying the foramen of Luschka, the electrode array is mounted on a Rosen needle and inserted into the lateral recess with the electrodes oriented superiorly (Figure 38–7). With experience, we have found that the implant functions better, with fewer nonauditory side effects, when the electrodes are placed fully within the lateral recess.[4] After placement, selected electrodes in the array are activated to confirm their position over the cochlear nucleus. They are tested for the presence of EABRs, stimulation of adjacent cranial nerves (VII and IX), and changes in vital signs. The position of the electrode array usually needs very slight adjustment to maximize auditory stimulation and minimize electromyographic responses from the other nerves. In case of activation of nerve IX, a small insulating pad of Teflon felt is interposed between the electrodes and the nerve.

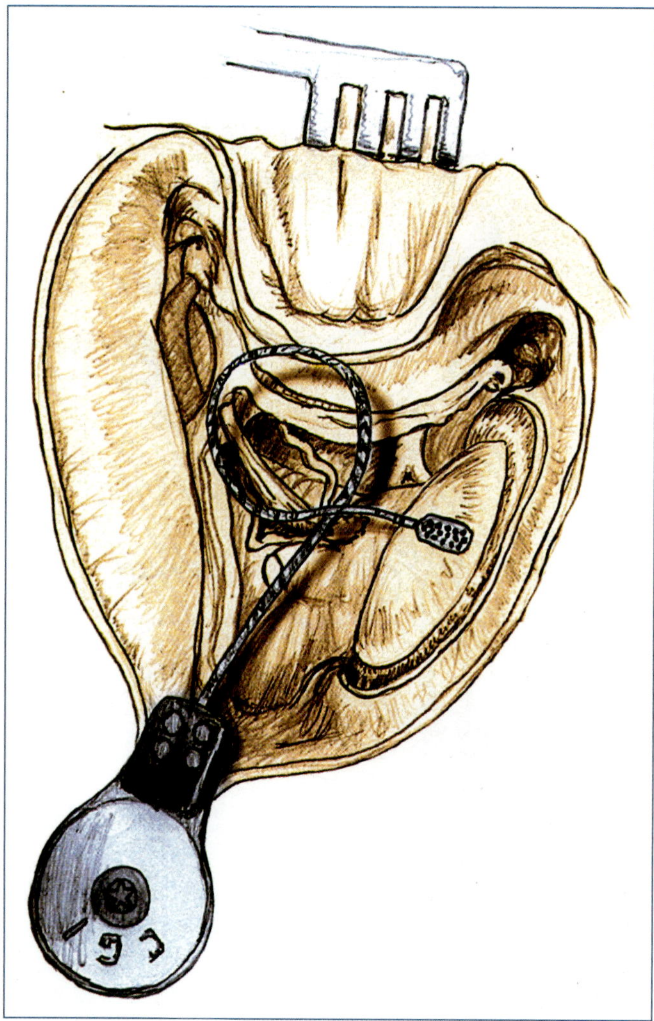

FIGURE 38–6 • Schematic view of the receiver/stimulator in place.

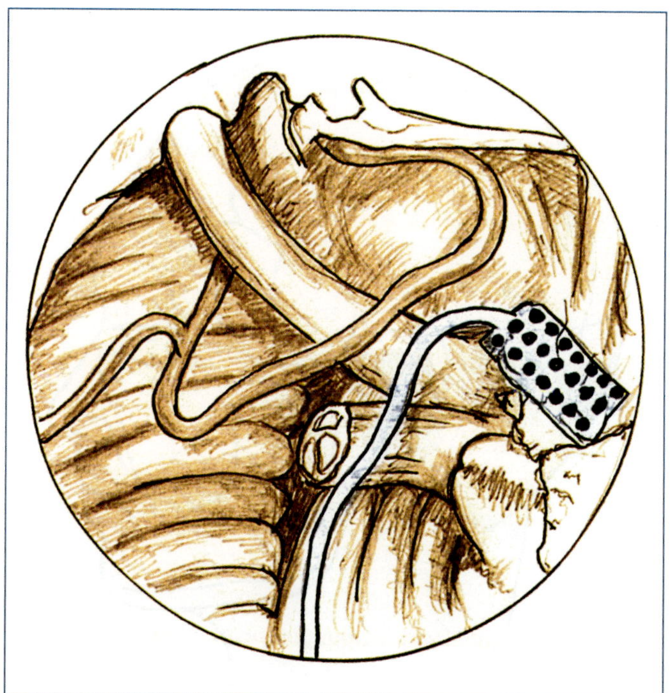

FIGURE 38–7 • Schematic surgical view of the auditory brainstem implant electrode array being passed into the lateral recess (magnified view from Figure 38–5).

The electrode array is secured using a small piece of Teflon felt packed into the meatus of the lateral recess. Subsequent ingrowth of fibrous tissue eventually stabilizes the array in position. The electrode wiring is positioned within the mastoid cavity and bony trough (Figure 38–8). The eustachian tube and middle ear are then packed with oxidized cellulose (Surgicel®) and muscle. Abdominal fat is used to obliterate the mastoid defect.

At this time, the magnet in the receiver/stimulator is removed to allow for future surveillance MRI. Since the magnet is typically removed from the receiver/stimulator at the time of implantation, there may be difficulty in identifying the location of the receiver/stimulator at the time of initial stimulation. Improper positioning of the external transmitter coil in such cases may lead to the false impression of device failure or stimulation failure on the part of the patient. We now routinely tattoo the center location of the circular receiver/stimulator antenna at the time of surgery to facilitate its location postoperatively. The incision is then closed in layers without drainage.

POSTOPERATIVE CARE

Postoperative care after auditory brainstem implantation is similar to that following routine craniotomies for acoustic tumor removal. A large mastoid-type dressing is left in place for 3 days. Careful attention to any moisture on the bandages allows prompt identification of CSF leak through the postauricular wound. The device is typically activated for the first time 4 to 8 weeks after implantation. This allows resolution of edema in the skin flap overlying the receiver/stimulator, which would otherwise prevent an adequate signal from reaching the implant. In actual use, implant patients must shave this area and apply a thin tape and metal disk ("retainer" disk) to which the magnetic transmitter coil adheres. The patient, or a companion, must be trained to ensure proper and consistent positioning of the transmitter coil over the implant receiver/stimulator. Many complaints about poor signal or deterioration in sound quality can be traced to improper positioning of the retainer disk.

POSTOPERATIVE COMPLICATIONS

The most significant complication in the immediate postoperative period is CSF leak. Unlike routine translabyrinthine surgery, in which the fluid usually takes the nasal route via the eustachian tube, the ABI electrode and wires provide a pathway along which CSF can travel under the skin flap. We have noted a marked reduction in the leak rate after transitioning to the fully implantable receiver from the percutaneous connector used with the single-channel ABI. Prevention of a leak begins with meticulous dural approximation. Although the dural opening cannot be closed in a watertight manner, it should be approximated as closely as possible and strips of abdominal fat are used to plug the residual dural defect.

Surgicel® and muscle are commonly employed for eustachian tube and middle ear closure and autologous fat packs the mastoid cavity. Titanium mesh is placed over the fat to hold it

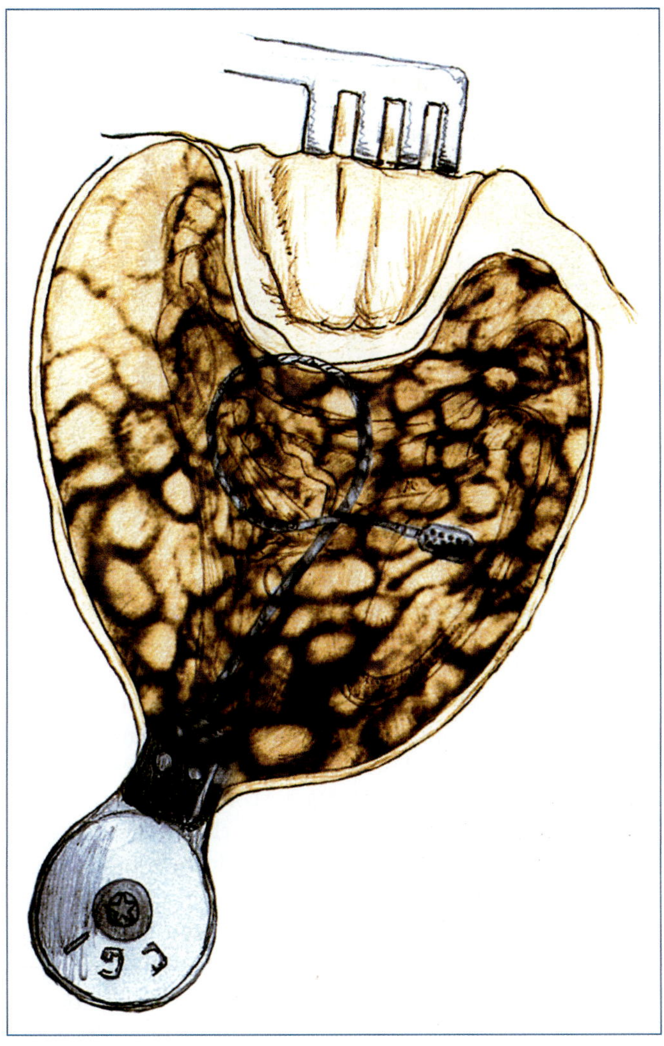

FIGURE 38–8 • Schematic view of the implant, electrode wires, and fat in place, prior to skin closure.

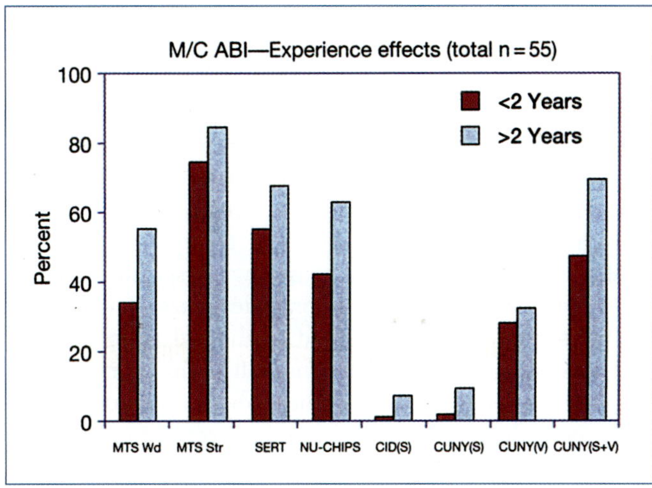

FIGURE 38–9 • Mean speech perception scores from patients with less than 2 years experience versus those with 2 years or more experience. MTS Wd, monosyllable, trochee, spondee word recognition; MTS Stress, monosyllable, trochee, spondee stress recognition; SERT, sound effects recognition test; NU-CHIPS, Northwestern University Children's Recognition of Speech Test; CID, Central Institute for the Deaf sentences; CUNY, City University of New York sentences; S, sound only; V, vision only; S+V, sound plus vision.

in position. Finally, a multilayered closure of the wound reduces the risk of CSF leak through the incision.

Despite these precautions, patients with ABIs appear more prone to CSF leak than those undergoing translabyrinthine procedures without implantation. Leaks from the nose and wound usually respond to reapplication of a mastoid pressure dressing and bed rest. A lumbar-subarachnoid drain is inserted for persistent leaks. When these maneuvers fail to control a leak, we perform a blind sac closure of the ear canal with removal of the external auditory canal skin, tympanic membrane, malleus, and incus. The eustachian tube is then closed with Surgicel packing and bone wax, and the middle ear is filled with muscle. This is a safer way to control spinal fluid leaks than surgical exploration and repacking of the wound. Meningitis can occur either spontaneously or as a result of postoperative CSF leak. This unusual complication, when identified promptly, responds to antibiotics and control of the leak.

RESULTS

Comprehensive performance results from the initial group of multichannel ABI recipients have been reported elsewhere.[2] With some notable exceptions, speech perception with the ABI typically does not reach the very high levels generally attained with modern cochlear implants. However, the auditory sensations in combination with lipreading can be highly beneficial in facilitating oral communication. With regular and continued use of the ABI, recipients typically show substantial improvements in performance over time that may continue for many years. Regular use of the device greatly enhances performance, and patients should be counseled about this necessity preoperatively.

Sixteen percent of our multichannel ABI recipients scored at least 20% correct on sound-only sentence recognition tests. Several of these individuals were also able to communicate on the telephone to a limited extent. Three of 88 multichannel ABI recipients achieved sentence recognition scores of more than 50% using sound only in the first year;[2] however, it took several years for some other patients to show significant "open-set" ability.

Figure 38–9 shows mean speech perception scores on a number of tests for two groups of ABI recipients: those with less than 2 years experience versus those with 2 years experience or more. These results from the FDA clinical trials were obtained from patients using the previous eight-electrode array. The group with longer duration of use shows substantial improvement in scores. This indicates that performance continues to improve beyond 2 years after ABI connection. Several patients continued to improve even after 7 years. Patients with unrealistic expectations or those with useful hearing remaining on their second tumor sides often did not use their ABIs regularly and typically did not show improvements. When remaining hearing was lost, such as after second-side tumor removal, regular use of the ABI increased, and improvements usually occurred. First-tumor side implantation was beneficial in that it allowed patients to adjust to ABI sound gradually before becoming completely reliant on it.

Speech perception with the ABI, as with cochlear implants, may be related to the presence of electrode-specific pitch sensations.[10] The majority of ABI recipients experienced these percepts; however, the range, magnitude, and relative ranking varied greatly.[2] This may be attributable to variations in anatomy, neuronal survival, and proximity of the surface electrodes to auditory neurons. The number of electrodes available for use is also patient-dependent. It is influenced in part by the presence of mild nonauditory sensations caused by the spread of activation to other nearby nonauditory brainstem sites. Nonauditory sensations typically have included tingling, dizziness, and a slight sensation of jittering of the visual field. By altering stimulus pulse duration or selecting other ground electrodes, it was usually possible to eliminate these side effects. In most cases, nonauditory sensations also decreased in magnitude over time. Primarily because of anatomic difficulties (eg, a large lateral recess, distortion or damage caused by large tumors, or inadequate adherence of the array to the brainstem surface), about 9% of our patients did not receive useful hearing after implantation. In a few such cases, we implanted another multichannel ABI when second-side tumors were removed, and this was successful.

Programming ABI speech processors requires experience. Pitch percepts, number of useable electrodes, and other factors can influence performance. The goal was to optimize the reception of important spectral cues. As part of the process, pitch sensations on available electrodes were scaled and ranked using classic psychophysical methods. An attempt was made to align the electrodes in proper pitch rank order relative to the frequency analysis bands in the sound processor. Such processor "maps" were considered to be properly "pitch ranked." Pitch percepts and nonauditory sensations fluctuated to some degree over time, and periodic reprogramming contributed to maintaining and improving performance. Patients who for some reason missed an appointment for this purpose often soon complained of a decrease in performance.

We reviewed the relationship between the number of useable electrodes, electrode pitch, and performance. With the present surface electrode array, a strong relationship was not found,[11,12] suggesting that other cues such as temporal information may also be important. With the relatively large (0.7- to 1-mm diameter) surface electrodes, it was probably difficult to activate tuned neurons within the body of the cochlear nucleus with high specificity. Nevertheless, patients generally did better if they had at least three or four available electrode "channels" and if these electrodes were correctly assigned to speech processor analysis bandwidths. All of the best performers also experienced a wider range of pitch sensations (>30 pitch scale units, 100-point scale) across electrodes.

Data relevant to this issue are presented in Figure 38–10. We tested vowel and consonant recognition in sound only with four different processor configurations in one of our best and most experienced (7 years) patients. She had an overall pitch scale range of approximately 35 units. In one processor configuration, all nine of her electrodes were used, but they were incorrectly (randomly) pitch ranked. Additionally, two-, four-, and nine-electrode configurations were programmed in which the electrodes were correctly pitch ranked. Vowel and consonant

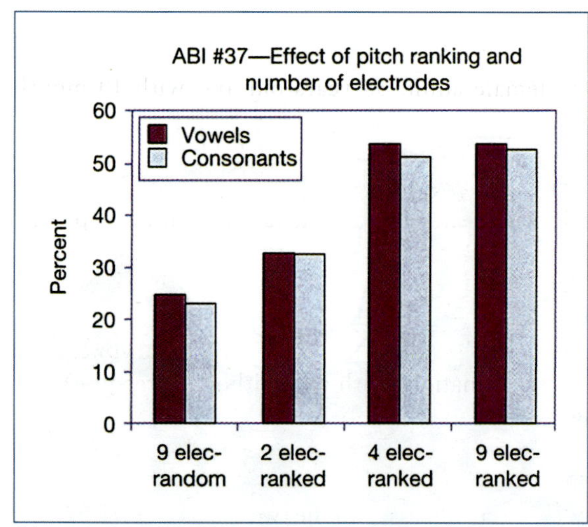

FIGURE 38–10 • Effect of electrode pitch ranking and number of electrodes (elec) on vowel and consonant recognition (sound only) in a top-performing auditory brainstem implant recipient.

recognition was poorest with the randomly pitch ranked nine-electrode configuration. Even the configuration using only two properly ranked electrodes resulted in better scores than the nine-electrode random configuration. Scores were nearly equivalent (52 to 55%) with the four- and nine-electrode processors. We subsequently tested two other good performers and found a similar pattern of scores.

Programming ABI sound processors can be more time consuming than cochlear implants,[10] but streamlining the process by de-emphasizing pitch ranking may be deleterious. The best configuration that could be relatively quickly obtained for the above patient was the four-electrode version. Qualitatively, she commented that this version sounded simpler in a musical sense—"like individual notes rather than chords." She further remarked that learning to use an ABI is an ongoing process, and that the four-electrode configuration might be easier for beginning users.

Cochlear implants can provide high levels of performance relative to the ABI, in part because of closer proximity to the tonotopic distribution of axonal processes in the modiolus. Microstimulation of brainstem auditory neurons in animals, such as with prototype needle electrodes, has been shown to be effective in accessing the tonotopic gradient.[13] This led to the development of the penetrating microelectrode ABI, about which more will be discussed in the final section, "RECENT DEVELOPMENTS."

OTHER RESEARCH EFFECTS OF STIMULATION RATE

The 21-electrode ABI allows higher stimulation pulse rates than the earlier eight-electrode version. In cochlear implants, stimulation rate has received considerable attention, with some investigators finding significant improvements in performance as the stimulation rate was increased.[14,15] Speech recognition results were measured in one ABI patient with the 21-electrode ABI as a function of the stimulation rate. One objective was to determine if immediate performance gains were possible with higher-rate speech-processing strategies.

One female adult, 58 years old and with 10 months of implant experience, was tested in this study using the Nucleus ACE processor. She had nine electrodes programmed in her processor for everyday use. These electrodes were 2, 3, 4, 5, 6, 7, 8, 9, and 10. Since she had very little range in pitch perception among these electrodes, they were simply arranged in ascending numerical order with progressively higher-frequency analysis bandwidths.

Speech perception tests consisted of medial vowel and consonant discrimination (with and without lipreading) and the Northwestern University Children's Perception of Speech test (NU-CHIPS).

Three conditions were selected using two, four, and eight electrodes (electrodes used in the two-electrode processor: 2, 6; four-electrode processor: 2, 4, 6, 8; and eight-electrode processor: 2, 3, 4, 5, 6, 7, 8, 9). Processors were programmed with the fastest and slowest rates available, plus at least one intermediate rate. In the two-electrode conditions, only the fastest and slowest rates were tested because of time constraints. Stimulation rates ranged from 250 to 2,400 ppse, depending on the number of electrodes used.

Figure 38–11 shows consonant, vowel, and word recognition results from the ABI recipient as a function of the stimulation rate for two-, four-, and eight-channel continuous interleaved sampling processors. The lower open symbols present results using the ABI alone, and the filled symbols present results using the ABI plus lipreading. The dotted line in each panel presents the performance achieved by this patient with her own everyday SPEAK™ (Nucleus) processor (ie, a nine-electrode processor with which she had more than 6 months experience). Little difference in performance was observed between the two-, four-, and eight-electrode processors, and no clear pattern was evident as a function of stimulation rate.

Consonant recognition was relatively constant as a function of stimulation rate and was similar to the low-performance level obtained with the patient's own everyday processor. There appears to be a slight decrease in vowel recognition as stimulation rate was increased. Word recognition on the NU-CHIPS test also appears to be relatively unchanged as a function of stimulation rate. Subjectively, the subject did not report any clear preferences for fast or slow rates. Thus, the results from short-term experiments in this single patient do not provide any incentive to pursue high-rate stimulation strategies.

RECENT DEVELOPMENTS

Penetrating Electrode Auditory Brainstem Implant

Many patients with regular surface ABIs have demonstrated good speech recognition performance, and some relationship with electrode-specific pitch percepts has been observed. Therefore, a PABI system using needle microelectrodes was developed in an effort to increase this type of perceptual information and hopefully improve speech recognition performance. One of the findings of this work has been that several patients performed best using a combination of surface and penetrating microelectrodes.

Each electrode type offers advantages, and the two seem to work synergistically. The larger current field of surface electrodes increases the likelihood of obtaining auditory sensations, and the more focused current field from the tip of the needle microelectrodes has provided auditory sensations 1 to 2 nC lower than surface electrodes. A wide range of pitch percepts also have resulted from penetrating electrodes, however the more focused stimulation also means that auditory neurons may not come in contact with the stimulating surface. Therefore, penetrating electrodes have had a higher incidence of failing to produce auditory sensations, or of not producing a comfortably

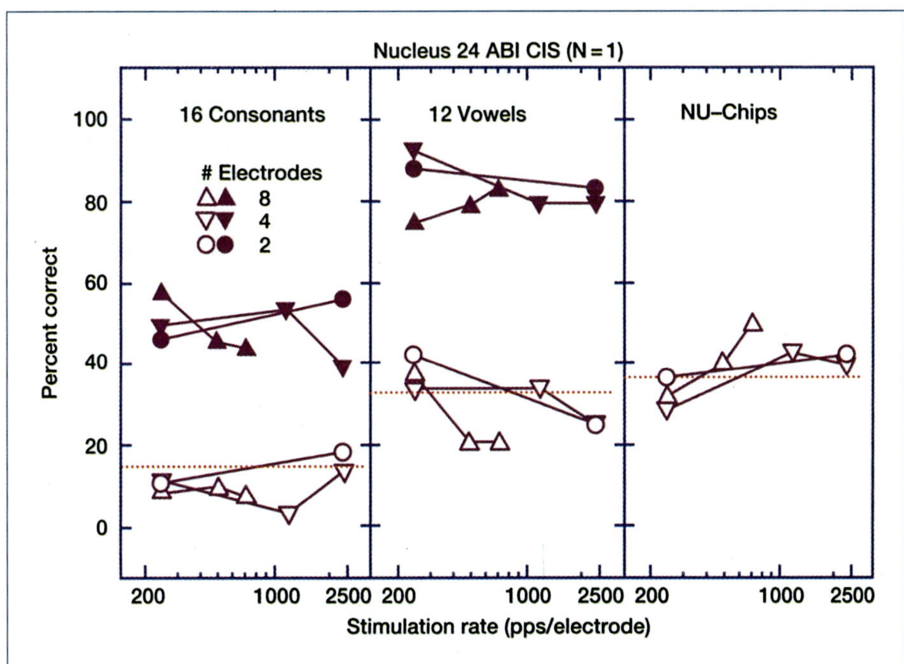

FIGURE 38–11 • Consonant, vowel, and word recognition scores for one auditory brainstem implant (ABI) recipient as a function of stimulation rate for two-, four-, and eight-electrode continuous interleaved sampling (CIS) sound processors. Open symbols, ABI alone; filled symbols, ABI plus lipreading; dotted line, patient's own nine-electrode processor.

loud level of sound at the maximum charge limit. Nevertheless, one patient did not experience any auditory sensations on his surface electrodes, but he did experience auditory sensations on 6 of 10 of his penetrating electrodes. In this instance, presence of the penetrating electrodes spared him from facing a future completely devoid of sound. A significant issue with the penetrating electrode array is that a slight deviation (only a millimeter or so) from the optimum location for placement may lead to no auditory responses at all. The surface array is much more forgiving in this respect, because of the overall size of the array (2.5 × 8.5 mm) and the size of the electrodes themselves (0.7 mm diameter). Also, while normally it is helpful to use intraoperative EABR to help verify placement of surface electrodes, this technique has been of little use with penetrating electrodes because of insufficient neural activity to be detected by distant scalp monitoring electrodes. While neural response telemetry (NRT) has been useful in detecting near-field activity in cochlear implants, it was not found to be useful in ABIs (and presumably PABIs).[16] When neural responses were correlated with perceptual responses in awake ABI recipients, NRT waveform morphology often appeared "cochlear implant-like" regardless of whether patients felt side effects, heard sounds, or experienced no sensations at all. It was impossible to differentiate auditory from nonauditory action potentials, which makes sense because any type of neuron (and there are many types in the brainstem) can generate action potentials.

Auditory Midbrain Implant and Inferior Colliculus Implant

Auditory brainstem implant recipients have generally not shown the excellent levels of performance obtainable with modern cochlear implants, possibly due to the fact that they do not have auditory nerves, or because of some undetected damage to the brainstem region from the vestibular schwannoma or the surgical removal. At least two studies have examined the effect of bypassing the lower brainstem by stimulating the inferior colliculus (IC) with either a surface electrode array (the auditory midbrain implant [AMI])[17] or a penetrating array (the inferior colliculus implant [ICI]).[18] Patients have been implanted with both types of devices (Spring, 2007) and auditory sensations were obtained (R.Shannon, personal communication). A variety of electrode-specific pitch could be obtained, and the sound sensations were found to be useful in combination with lipreading for communication. No sound-only word recognition has been achieved, however, but it is still relatively early to assess long-term capabilities with these midbrain implants.

SUMMARY

The multichannel ABI has received FDA approval for commercial release as a viable means of providing useful hearing sensations to individuals deafened by bilateral vestibular schwannomas (NF2). The sound information provided by the device facilitates sound awareness, recognition, and spoken communication when used in conjunction with lipreading. A small percentage of ABI recipients also experience significant degrees of speech understanding even without lipreading. Methods of programming ABIs and processing speech sounds can influence performance and benefit, and further work in this area is ongoing. In the future, the ABI may be useful in treating deafness from other causes affecting the peripheral auditory neural pathway. Evaluation in humans of new microstimulation techniques with an ABI array designed to probe the matrix of the auditory brainstem has shown some degree of benefit, as has the capability of stimulating the auditory midbrain to provide prophylactic hearing.

ACKNOWLEDGMENTS

The authors are grateful to Michael Waring for editorial assistance on electrophysiology and to the patients and staff of House Ear Clinic for their time and effort on behalf of ABI research.

References

1. Eisenberg LS, Maltan AA, Portillo F, et al. Electrical stimulation of the auditory brainstem structure in deafened adults. J Rehabil Res Dev 1987;24:9–22.
2. Otto SR, Brackmann DE, Hitselberger W E, et al. Multichannel auditory brainstem implant: Update on performance in 61 patients. J. Neurosurg 2002;96:1063–71.
3. Brackmann DE, Hitselberger WE, Nelson RA, et al. Auditory brainstem implant: I. Issues in surgical implantation. Otolaryngol Head Neck Surg 1993;108:624–33.
4. Shannon RV, Fayad J, Moore JK, et al. Auditory brainstem implant: II. Postsurgical issues and performance. Otolaryngol Head Neck Surg 1993;108:634–42.
5. Briggs RJ, Popovic EA, Brackmann DE. Recent advances in the treatment of neurofibromatosis type II. Adv Otolaryngol Head Neck Surg 1995;9:227–45.
6. Riccardi VM. Neurofibromatosis. Neurol Clin 1987;5:337–49.
7. Hitselberger N, House WF, Edgerton BS, Whitaker S. Cochlear nucleus implant. Otolaryngol Head Neck Surg 1984;92:52–4.
8. Niparko JK, Kileny PR, Kemink JL, et al. Neurophysiologic intraoperative monitoring: II. Facial nerve function. Am J Otol 1989;10:55–61.
9. Waring MD. Refractory properties of auditory brain-stem responses evoked by electrical stimulation of human cochlear nucleus: evidence of neural generators. Electroencephalogr Clin Neurophysiol 1998;108:331–4.
10. Otto SR, Ebinger K, Staller SJ. Clinical trials with the auditory brain stem implant. In: Waltzman S, Cohen N, editors. Cochlear implants. New York: Thieme Medical Publishers; 2000. p. 357–65.
11. Kuchta J, Otto SR, Shannon RV. The number of electrodes and perceptual performance in auditory brainstem implants. Abstract of presentation at 2001 Conference on Implantable Auditory Prostheses, Pacific Grove, CA, August 2001.
12. Kuchta J, Otto SR, Shannon RV. Pitch perception and perceptual performance in auditory brainstem implants. Abstract of presentation at 2001 Conference on Implantable Auditory Prostheses, Pacific Grove, CA, August 2001.
13. McCreery DG, Shannon RV, Moore JK, et al. Accessing the tonotopic organization of the ventral cochlear nucleus by intranuclear microstimulation. IEEE Trans Rehabil Eng 1998;4:1–9.

14. Brill SM, Hochmair I, Hochmair ES. The importance of stimulation rate in pulsatile stimulations strategies in cochlear implants. Presented at the XXIV International Congress of Audiology, Buenos Aires, August 1998.

15. Brill SM, Schatzer R, Nopp P, et al. JCIS:CIS with temporally jittering stimulations pulses: effect of jittering amplitude and stimulation rate on speech understanding. Presented at the 4th European Symposium on Paediatric Cochlear Implantation, s-Hertogenbosch, The Netherlands, June 1998.

16. Otto SR, Waring MD, Kuchta, J. Neural response telemetry and auditory/non-auditory sensations in 15 recipients of auditory brainstem implants. J Am Acad Audiol 2005;16:219–27.

17. Colletti V, Shannon RV, Carner M, et al. The first successful case of hearing produced by electrical stimulation of the human midbrain. Otol Neurotol 2007;28:39–43.

18. Lenarz T, Lim HH, Reuter G, et al. The auditory midbrain implant: a new auditory prosthesis for neural deafness—Concept and device description. Otol Neurotol 2006;27:838–43.

Stereotactic Radiosurgery and Radiotherapy for Temporal Bone Tumors

39

P. Ashley Wackym, MD, FACS, FAAP / Christina L. Runge-Samuelson, MD, PhD / David R. Friedland, MD, PhD

None of the authors have a financial interest in any of the companies discussed in this chapter.

Management of many skull base tumors has evolved in recent years away from microsurgical resection and toward control of growth using radiosurgery or radiotherapy. This is particularly true for vestibular schwannomas, i.e., acoustic neuromas, and is increasingly applicable to glomus jugulare tumors. The most commonly used modality for such treatment is gamma knife radiosurgery although other conformal radiation treatment systems are available. Gamma knife surgery is advantageous in requiring a single session for treatment of most skull base lesions, which increases its appeal to both surgeon and patient. This chapter will focus primarily on the methods used in treating skull base tumors with gamma knife surgery.

Gamma knife surgery, similar to microsurgery, has advantages and disadvantages, which must be thoroughly discussed with the patient.[1,2] For the patient, it is beneficial to undergo an outpatient procedure rather than microsurgical management that requires a much longer postoperative recovery. Further, gamma knife surgery outcomes show excellent tumor control and, with current methods, low cranial nerve morbidity. Gamma knife surgery is a viable treatment modality for the appropriate patient as defined by age, medical history, tumor characteristics, and physical findings. As such, many neurotologists now offer gamma knife surgery as part of their armamentarium for managing vestibular schwannomas and glomus tumors.[3]

NONVESTIBULAR SCHWANNOMA APPLICATIONS

Although the majority of stereotactic radiosurgery performed by the neurotologist will be for vestibular schwannoma, other neoplasms and pathologies may be amenable to radiotherapy.[4] This section will focus on a few of the more common non-schwannoma pathologies for which the neurotologist may be the primary surgeon.

Paragangliomas, more specifically glomus jugulare tumors, are becoming more commonly addressed with primary radiotherapy than with surgical resection. The other chemodectomas such as glomus vagale and carotid body tumors are located too low in the neck for most gamma knife units in use today. Further, these tumors do not typically carry the same morbidity as glomus jugulare tumors and are still commonly addressed surgically. In an effort to reduce the cranial nerve palsies that often accompany glomus jugulare resection, gamma knife surgery has been employed.

An evaluation of 42 patients with primary or recurrent/persistent glomus jugulare tumor undergoing gamma knife surgery showed excellent tumor response.[5] Approximately one-third of tumors shrank and two-thirds showed no size change. A single 3.9 cm tumor was found to have increased 99 months after treatment with 12 Gy at the margin and was re-treated. Progression-free survival was 100% at 7 years and 75% at 10 years. Six patients had complications related to treatment. Five of 26 patients with intact hearing at the time of treatment had subjective decline within the first year. Objective measures of hearing were not performed. One patient had facial paresthesias, one had vocal fold paralysis (the re-treated subject), one had vertigo and imbalance, and one had posttreatment migraine requiring admission.

A meta-analysis of glomus jugulare treatment and outcomes compared stereotactic radiosurgery to surgical resection.[6] Neurological deficits in those treated with gamma knife, CyberKnife or linear accelerator (LINAC), showed no change in 58.2%, improved in 39%, and permanently worsened in 2.8%. Such deficits included complaints of hearing loss, dizziness, dysphagia, voice change, shoulder dysfunction, and headache. Overall, there was an 8.5% incidence of cranial nerve complication with 75% of these being transient. Permanent deficits occurred in three of the 141 patients, all of which involved facial motor dysfunction; none of which reached House-Brackmann grade VI. Tumor control was achieved in approximately 98% of individuals at 39 months.

Conventional surgery for glomus jugulare had a complete resection rate of approximately 92%, some of which represented more than one operation for resection. The recurrence rate at a mean of 82 months was 3.3%. The mortality rate was 1.3% for conventional surgery compared with 0% for radiotherapy. Cranial nerve deficits varied widely among surgical reports but on average the facial nerve was affected in 4.4 to 11% of the patients; the glossopharyngeal nerve in 26 to 42%; the vagus nerve in 13 to 28%; the spinal accessory nerve in 25 to 26%, and the hypoglossal nerve in 5 to 21%. Other morbidities included a cerebrospinal fluid (CSF) leakage rate of 8.3%, aspiration in 5.5%, and wound infection in 5.5%. Although cranial nerve deficits occur more frequently with conventional surgery, most reports note that the long-term impact of such dysfunction is relatively small. It is important for the surgeon to take into account patient function, age, and general health, and tumor size when discussing and weighing treatment options for glomus jugulare tumors.

Meningiomas are the second most common benign neoplasm of the cerebellopontine angle and can often present with deficits similar to vestibular schwannomas. Total resection results in excellent tumor control rates and, for all cranial locations, shows a 15-year progression-free survival rate of approximately 68 to 75%.[7,8] Experience with partially resected or inoperable meningiomas, however, has shown that radiation therapy can produce excellent tumor control in the majority of cases. The use of stereotactic radiosurgery as a primary treatment to avoid or reduce the incidence of surgical and neurological deficits is increasingly common.

Elia and colleagues reviewed stereotactic radiosurgery outcomes for meningioma published since 2001.[8] In over 1,500 patients the 5-year progression-free control rate was 93.4%. The complication rate ranged from 2.5 to 13% and included neurological and vascular injuries. Many of these were for tumors around the optic chiasm and carotid arteries and included dosages up to 20 Gy. Kreil and colleagues recently published their series on the treatment of 200 skull base meningiomas with gamma knife surgery.[9] There were 21 patients with cerebellopontine angle lesions. Of 20 patients with preoperative hearing loss (not quantified), one improved and 19 remained stable; none showed deterioration. Tinnitus remained unchanged in seven patients. Vertigo was present in 25 skull base meningiomas and improved in eight patients and worsened in none. Given the low incidence of complication and the high rate of tumor control, stereotactic radiosurgery should be strongly considered in tumors around sensitive neural structures and in patients medically unsuitable for conventional surgery.

In addition to tumors, the neurotologist is often consulted for facial pain syndromes, most notably trigeminal neuralgia. Functional stereotactic radiosurgery using gamma knife has been employed in the treatment of trigeminal neuralgia. In the series of meningiomas reported by Kriel, there were 25 patients with preoperative trigeminal neuralgia due to tumor, of which 16 improved.[9] There were two induced cases of trigeminal neuralgia but these were transient. Such findings indicate that radiation to the trigeminal nerve can induce functional changes.

Gorgulho and De Salles reviewed surgical and stereotactic treatments for trigeminal neuralgia.[10] Among current treatments, long-term improvement was noted in 70 to 75% of microvascular decompressions, 58 to 77% of radiofrequency rhizotomies, 32% of balloon compressions, 17 to 50% of glycerol rhizotomies, and 45 to 57% of stereotactic radiosurgeries. Immediate improvement was noted in over 90% of patients with stereotactic radiosurgery. Recurrence rates were highest with glycerol rhizotomy and much lower and very similar among the other modalities. Stereotactic radiosurgery was noted to be particularly attractive because it is the least invasive of these methods.

Many different treatment protocols for trigeminal neuralgia have been attempted.[10] In their review, Gorgulho and De Salles identified several patterns with regard to gamma knife treatment for trigeminal neuralgia that affect outcomes. The root entry zone of the trigeminal nerve, not the nerve proper, should be the preferred target as dosage delivery to this area seems to correlate with pain relief. A minimal dosage of 70 Gy and maximal dosage of 90 Gy should be prescribed. The incidence of posttreatment numbness with this prescription dose ranges from 3 to 55% but bothersome numbness persists in only about 4 to 12%. Treating a longer section of the trigeminal nerve proper does not improve pain control and increases the incidence of posttreatment numbness. Likewise, higher dosage to the nerve does not improve pain control and increases numbness. The overall incidence of complications with stereotactic radiosurgery for trigeminal neuralgia is significantly lower than all other techniques. As with other benign diseases, potential long-term effects of radiation treatment need to be considered in younger individuals.

VESTIBULAR SCHWANNOMA APPLICATIONS

Patient Selection

Selection of treatment requires a complex decision-making process, which should consider the advantages and disadvantages of gamma knife surgery compared with observation or microsurgical resection. There are the preferences of the informed patient, the comfort and experience of the surgeon, the patient's medical history and condition, and the characteristics of the tumor. While there are no definitive measures defining or restricting the use of gamma knife surgery, particular guidelines can inform the decision-making process.

Although a tissue diagnosis is not typically acquired prior to gamma knife treatment, radiographic and clinical diagnoses of vestibular schwannoma and glomus jugulare are sufficient to initiate a discussion of gamma knife therapy. Other potential neoplasms amenable to gamma knife treatment by the neurotologist are cerebellopontine angle meningiomas, posterior fossa and jugular foramen nonvestibular schwannomas, temporal bone metastatic lesions, and primary vascular neoplasms. An absolute contraindication to gamma knife treatment is a tumor that extends too far inferiorly to enable placement into the centrum of the collimator helmet. Gamma knife surgery is also contraindicated in large tumors causing life-threatening brain stem and central aqueduct compression. Such large tumors, in the absence of clinically significant problems, provide a relative contraindication to gamma knife surgery as posttreatment swelling can cause obstructive hydrocephalus requiring emergent intervention. Typically, vestibular schwannomas greater than 2.5 cm in the cerebellopontine angle should be cautiously approached if gamma knife proves the best option given other medical concerns. Most surgeons will not treat vestibular schwannomas greater than 3.0 cm in maximum axial dimension within the cerebellopontine angle because of the risk of posttreatment obstructive hydrocephalus.

Other guidelines for gamma knife treatment require clinical judgment as to the medical condition of the patient, the expected growth and potential morbidity of the tumor, the functional status of the patient, audiometric and vestibular performance, age, and expected life span of the patient. Individualized treatment plans depend on a frank and thorough dialogue between physician and patient as to the options available, risks and benefits of each approach, and expected outcomes based upon evidence-based reviews or an analysis of each institution's outcomes.

Preoperative Counseling

Informed consent for gamma knife surgery requires the surgeon to discuss alternative options such as observation and microsurgical resection.[2] The risks and benefits of these alternatives should be frankly described and compared to gamma knife treatment. Many patients have received information from the Internet or from physicians with limited experience with gamma knife and may have erroneous information. Common misconceptions include the expectation that gamma knife surgery completely removes the tumor and that hearing will improve, or conversely that cranial nerve morbidities are insignificant. These need to be addressed with evidence-based reports and information.

One statistic, which is particularly alarming to patients considering gamma knife surgery, is that there have been eight cases of malignancy within vestibular schwannomas (as of 2002).[11] Four of these patients had been previously treated with radiosurgery. While it remains possible that these four malignancies developed after the radiation treatment, it is more likely that these malignant tumors were misdiagnosed as benign at the outset of evaluation and treatment.

Delayed development of radiation-induced neoplasms was addressed by Pollock and colleagues in 1998.[12] They reviewed more than 20,000 patients treated with radiosurgery worldwide and found no increased incidence of new neoplasm development (i.e., benign or malignant). A retrospective cohort study comparing the Sheffield, England radiosurgery patient database with the national mortality and cancer registries identified a single new astrocytoma among those treated.[13] Based on their national incidence figures, 2.47 cases would have been predicted. The risk of radiosurgery induced malignancy in patients with neurofibromatosis type 2 (NF2) and von Hippel-Lindau disease was similarly studied.[14] Of 118 NF2 and 19 von Hippel-Lindau disease patients, totaling, respectively, 906 and 62 patient-years of follow-up data, only two cases of intracranial malignancy were found. Both of these were in NF2 patients. One was thought to have arisen before the radiosurgery; the other was a glioblastoma diagnosed three years after radiosurgery. Gliomas may occur in as many as 4% of NF2 patients and the single case may not represent an increased risk. It was suggested that the late risk of malignancy arising after irradiation must be put in the context of the condition being treated, the treatment options available to these individuals, and their life expectancy.

Despite the findings of the studies just reviewed, it is important to counsel patients about the possibility of malignant transformation or induction. A handful of tumors suggestive of radiation induced malignancy have been reported among the tens of thousands who have undergone gamma knife treatment. Lustig and colleagues reported the development of a squamous cell carcinoma following radiation treatment of vestibular schwannoma.[15] Hanabusa and colleagues reported the malignant transformation of a vestibular schwannoma following gamma knife surgery.[16] There was histologic evidence of vestibular schwannoma following a retrosigmoid resection. Four years after this resection, recidivistic tumor was identified, and the patient was subsequently treated with gamma knife surgery. Six months posttreatment, the tumor had grown, and the patient underwent surgical resection via a combined retrosigmoid-translabyrinthine approach. Abnormal mitotic figures were observed on histologic sections, and the diagnosis of malignancy was assigned.

SURGICAL TECHNIQUES

Gamma Knife Surgery

The first gamma knife unit (Elekta Instrument AB, Stockholm, Sweden) was installed in Stockholm, Sweden in 1968, and it was not until 1987 that the first gamma knife (model U) was installed in the United States at the University of Pittsburgh. The gamma knife model B (1996) is the unit most currently used throughout the United States. The gamma knife model C was introduced three years later and the major upgrade consisted of an automatic positioning system (APS). The unit is otherwise quite similar to the model B and both contain 201 radioactive isotope cobalt 60 (^{60}Co) sources and beam channels. Because of physical restraints, these units can only treat lesions intracranially or along the skull base. During 2008, a completely redesigned gamma knife unit, named Perfexion, was introduced. It uses 192 ^{60}Co sources, has a single collimator helmet with variable diameters, and can treat lesions within the entire head and neck, down to the level of the clavicles.

The basic principle of gamma knife surgery is to provide focused radiation to the tumor while minimizing radiation delivery to surrounding tissues. As such, a semicircular shield called the collimator helmet is used to generate 201 individual gamma radiation "beams." In the center of the helmet, where the beams intersect, radiation delivery is maximal, but along each individual radiation tract tissue exposure is relatively low. When the collimator helmet is locked into position, the 201 openings of the collimator helmet coincide with the cobalt sources. There is a shielded chamber within which the ^{60}Co sources are contained, and stainless steel shielding doors protect the treatment room from the ^{60}Co sources. There is a treatment couch with an adjustable mattress that slides into the gamma knife unit together with the collimator helmet and the patient. Figure 39–1 schematically shows the orientation of the components of the gamma knife model 4C and the overall appearance of the gamma knife model 4C.

When treatment is initiated, the treatment couch is automatically moved from its idle position into the treatment unit together with patient and helmet. Once the couch is docked in its treatment position, the helmet collimator and corresponding collimators in the unit form a beam channel, allowing the radiation that is continuously emitted by the sources to reach the patient. At the end of each irradiation "shot," the couch is automatically withdrawn, either to its idle position or to a position outside the radiation focus to reposition the patient for the next irradiation "shot." There are four interchangeable helmets by means of which the size of the collimator (that part of the treatment unit that shapes the beam) can be changed among 4, 8, 14, and 18 mm. The combination of four different-sized collimators and repositioning the patient in the three-dimensional space defined by the stereotactic headframe are effective to deliver the radiation dose selectively and conformally to radiosurgical targets of any shape.

Frame Attachment

The stereotactic head frame is used to coordinate the location of the tumor within the collimator helmet. As such, proper placement is of utmost importance to providing adequate treatment. There are two general principles guiding head frame placement for gamma knife surgery. First, the target should be as close to the center of the frame as possible. This prevents possible collisions of the frame with the sides of the collimator helmet especially when trying to align laterally extended tumors in the center of the unit. Second, the frame attachment should be stable. This prevents movement and ensures accuracy and correlation among the pretreatment imaging study, workstation treatment plan, and delivery of focused radiation. These principles should be addressed at the time of frame attachment. In lateral targets, such as vestibular schwannomas or glomus tumors, the frame should be shifted toward the tumor side. In skull base tumors, the frame should also be positioned lower than for treatment of more superior intracranial lesions. Anterior-posterior alignment should also be accounted for and can be adjusted by varying the lengths of the pins used to secure the frame. To ensure stability, avoid screw fixation in bone flaps, cranioplasty materials, burr holes, or skull defects.

The method of anesthesia used during frame placement is surgeon- and patient-dependent. In our program, either sedation with Versed (midazolam) and Sublimaze (fentanyl), or monitored anesthesia with propofol, followed by injection of local anesthetic at the pin sites is used. Figure 39–2A shows the typical array of tools used for the frame attachment. A variety of screw lengths allows the surgeon to choose those ideally suited for the individual location of the posts and tumor. The placement of the frame should begin with an accurate orientation of the location of the target within the patient's head. Ideally, the target should be located within the fiducial range and placed centrally within the frame, thereby avoiding later collisions with the collimator helmet and granting sufficient accuracy for the stereotactic target definition.

The stereotactic frame is assembled and preliminarily supported by using external auditory canal support pins, a Velcro band, or a stereotactic fiducial box. When using a fiducial box to facilitate frame placement, it is important to use the magnetic resonance imaging (MRI) fiducial box, rather than the computed tomography (CT) or angiography fiducial box, since this is the smallest of the three plexiglass fiducial boxes (Figure 39–2B and C). Asymmetric frame placements are possible and do not impair the accuracy of imaging. The frame can be shifted from

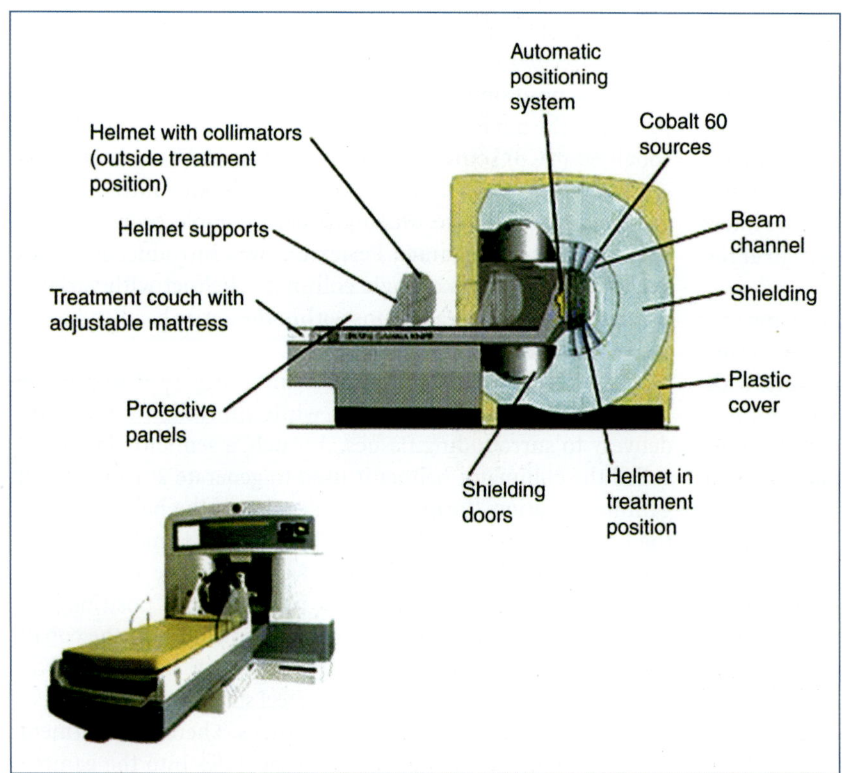

FIGURE 39–1 • Gamma knife radiosurgery. Schematic illustration of the Gamma Knife Model 4C which utilizes the automatic positioning system. Inset: Gamma Knife Model 4C. *Published with permission, copyright © 2009, Elekta Instrument AB (Stockholm, Sweden).*

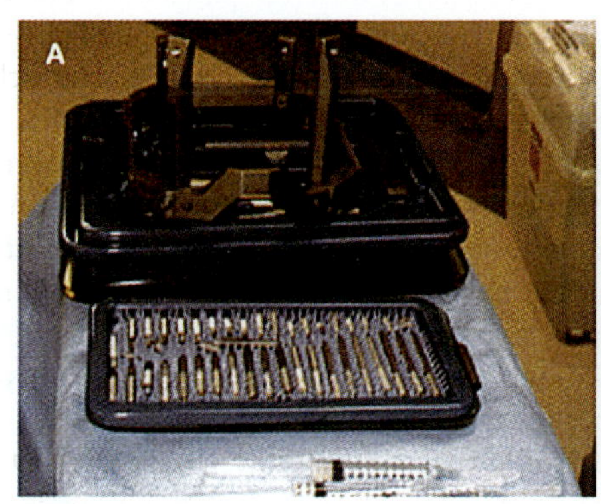

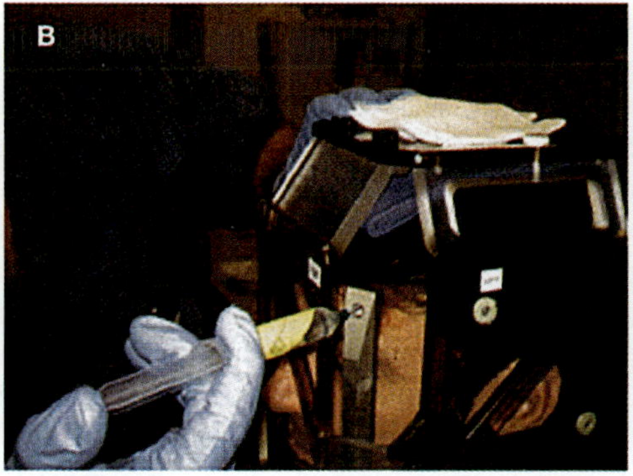

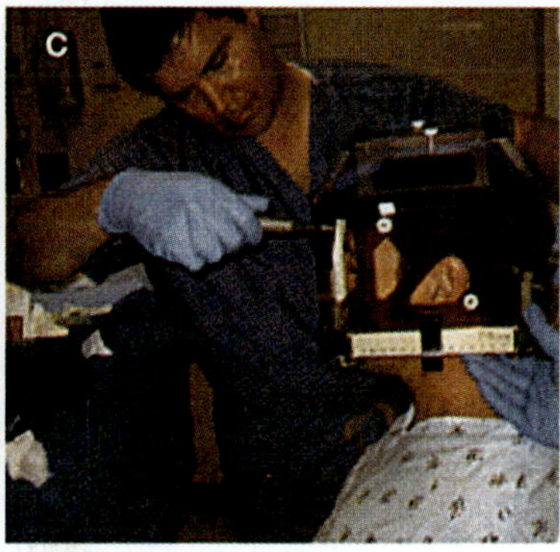

FIGURE 39–2 • *A*, Stereotactic headframe at the time of assembly. Pins used for fixation prior to imaging, treatment planning, and gamma knife radiosurgery are seen in the foreground. *B*, With a towel placed on the vertex of the head, the magnetic resonance imaging (MRI) fiducial box is balanced on the head while topical anesthetic is infiltrated at the pin sites. *C*, While the headframe and attached plastic MRI fiducial box is secured to the skull using the pins, an assistant stabilizes the assembly in place. Note the tightening of pins in opposing vectors. *Published with permission, copyright © 2009, P.A. Wackym, MD.*

side to side or can be moved as far as possible to the front or back to facilitate centering of the tumor. The frame is stabilized against the patient by an assistant and the surgeon should adjust the lengths of the posts to maintain relative tumor position. A low position of the anterior posts can help avoid anterior collisions with the collimator helmet for skull base posterior fossa tumors. In critical positions, collisions can sometimes be avoided by using the curved posts in the anterior position.

Once the post positions are determined, the screws can be inserted. The surgeon and assistant should work on diagonally opposing screws to provide the best stability without changing the desired frame position. For asymmetric frame placement, apply the longest screws first, thereby defining the desired distance of the target to the frame. Protrusion of the screws from the posts should be kept to a minimum to avoid collisions. Approximately 8 to 10 mm is considered to be sufficient but at our institution, we prefer to limit this projection to 4 to 6 mm. If a screw extends further, it should be exchanged for a shorter screw to avoid potential collisions with the collimator helmet during treatment.

Measurements of the frame and placement are then performed to allow the computer to identify any potential collisions after the plan is formulated. These measurements are required for the frame and skull section in Leksell GammaPlan treatment planning software. Measurements include the length of the four posts and the length of the screws that protrude from the posts. Additionally, the volume of the head is measured using the plastic collimator bubble, simulating the relationship of the frame to the treatment collimator helmet. This concludes frame placement and the patient may proceed to imaging.

Imaging

Treatment planning requires imaging of the tumor with respect to the frame as determined by specific fiducial boxes. The MRI fiducial box clips to the frame and care should be taken to ensure that it is flush and square during imaging. The MRI fiducial box has a z-shaped channel on each side filled with copper sulfate to generate position markers for each axial slice. The box should be checked prior to each use to ensure the channels are filled with solution and no air bubbles are present. The patient, with head frame and fiducial box, is secured into the head holder on the MRI sliding table. For imaging vestibular schwannomas and glomus tumors, we typically order axial 3D SPGR (spoiled gradient recalled) acquisition with T1 weighting and double dose IV contrast. Before the patient leaves, the scanner images are reviewed and the distance between fiducial registration markers is validated for accuracy.

Many centers acquire only MRI scans for treatment planning. We prefer to also acquire a noncontrast CT scan through the temporal bone to aid in planning. There is evidence of distortion of MRI images and correlation with CT scans at the time of planning can aid in reducing radiation delivery to critical structures such as the cochlea and facial nerve.[17] A CT fiducial box is affixed to the frame, the patient is secured in the holder attached to the table, and an axial scan through the temporal bone and skull base is acquired. Both CT and MR images are imported into the Gamma Knife workstation. Axial scans are defined, and coronal and sagittal reconstructions are generated for each type of imaging study.

Treatment Planning

Leksell GammaPlan is the dedicated software treatment planning system for Leksell Gamma Knife. Dose planning for gamma knife surgery means precisely conforming the isodose distribution to the target. The isodose distribution is built-up by a number of individual shots or isocenters. The Leksell GammaPlan software is designed to help the operator as much as possible to perform this procedure and is quite straightforward to use.

Currently, for vestibular schwannomas, the routine prescription is 12 to 14 Gy delivered to the 50% isodose line. The 50% isodose line shows where 50% of the prescribed dose lies. In the case of gamma knife treatments, the dose is frequently prescribed to the 50% isodose line. This ensures that the periphery of the tumor will receive at least the prescribed dose, that the dose will be higher than the prescribed dose inside the tumor, and that the dose will fall off rapidly outside the tumor, thus sparing critical structures. We also build three-dimensional (3D) volumes of the entire cochlea, basal turn of the cochlea, modiolus, and the internal auditory canal to assess radiation doses delivered to each of these structures.

Dose planning using Leksell GammaPlan involves composing shots to develop a conformal isodose. By definition, this includes the whole target but spares the surrounding healthy tissue. Figure 39–3 shows an example of a vestibular schwannoma. The target is well positioned on the screen and magnified for good visibility. When the shot menu is opened, one can select the size of the collimators. The size of the collimator is selected based on the tumor shape and the gaps in coverage of the 50% isodose line displayed over the tumor. Shots are placed sequentially to cover the target as effectively as possible. Changing the position of the shots, adding additional shots, and adjusting the relative weight of shots quickly lead to a conformal dose plan.

The dose plan can be checked using Leksell GammaPlan with the 3D image or the measurement tools, such as dose volume histograms. While the subject of conformity index is beyond the scope of this chapter, an excellent review of available methods has been published.[18] Leksell GammaPlan indicates the point in the stereotactic space where a global maximal dose can be found. Leksell GammaPlan also calculates the individual shot times. Once the treatment plan has been determined to be appropriate by the gamma knife team (surgeon, radiation oncologist, and radiation physicist), the stereotactic coordinates and irradiation times are printed and used during the gamma knife treatment.

Fine-tuning is made with small adjustments in shot position and weight, allowing optimization of the dose plan. Leksell GammaPlan allows the creation of different plans for the same target. This allows the surgeon and oncologist to follow different strategies and later compare plans and select the best plan for the actual treatment. Treatment plans can utilize as few as one or two shots, such as when treating trigeminal neuralgia, or over 10 shots when treating a large vestibular schwannoma within the cerebellopontine angle and filling the internal auditory canal. With the automated Leksell Gamma Knife C, plans with 20 shots or more can easily be implemented in a timely manner, since the model C does not require manual adjustments of coordinates in between each shot by the gamma knife treatment team. This allows improved conformity and selectivity of gamma knife surgery, potentially reducing the risk of complications.

To shape the dose distribution to avoid critical structures, one or more of the 201 collimators can be replaced with a closed shield called a plug. One can select spherical areas called shields with different diameters and place them over risk centers in the brain, cranial nerves, or cochlea. Once the shields are put in place, the Leksell GammaPlan software closes off all beams that would irradiate through the shielded area. The result is a modified dose plan in the low isodose lines with only little effect on the target peripheral isodose. The beam channels that need to be plugged can be seen in the plug pattern. The plug patterns can be merged for all shots of the same size so that the operator only has to plug the helmets for the treatment once.

In the final plan, the peripheral dose is set to a value, which is assessed as optimal for a particular patient. Indication, size, and location of the target are taken into account, as well as clinical experience. The peripheral isodose is usually set to the 50% isodose line. This is exactly half the maximum dose in the target, referred to as the hot spot (Figure 39–4). Along the 50%

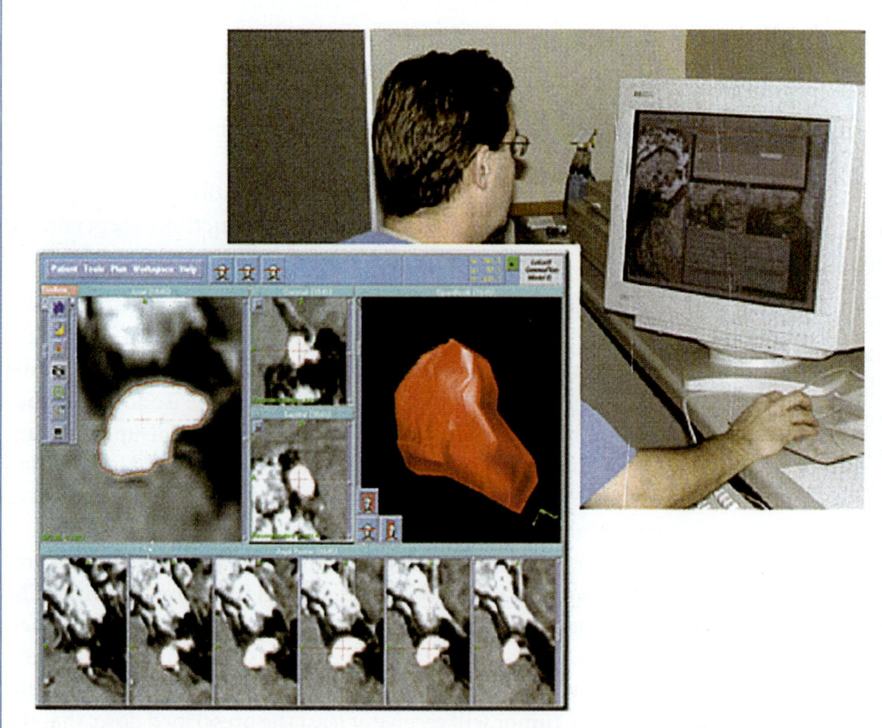

FIGURE 39–3 • Initial treatment planning at the gamma knife workstation involves building a three-dimensional model of the tumor. Determination of the conformation of the treatment plan follows placement of the shots and assignment of the radiation dose delivered to the specified isodose line. *Published with permission, copyright © 2009, P.A. Wackym, MD.*

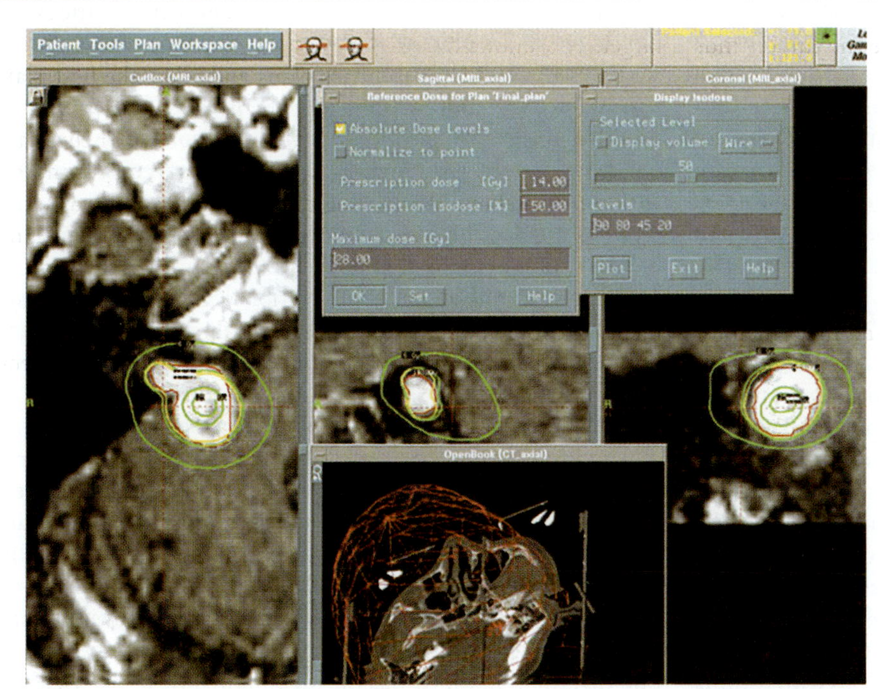

FIGURE 39–4 • Gamma knife radiosurgery. Selecting the Absolute Dose Level and Display Isodose options allows verification that the maximal radiation dose is not delivered near critical structures, such as the facial nerve. In this example, 14 Gy delivered to the 50% isodose line was prescribed. As shown, the maximum dose (28 Gy) is delivered to the center of the tumor (smallest circle). The largest circle represents the 20% isodose line where 6 Gy of radiation is delivered. *Published with permission, copyright © 2009, P.A. Wackym, MD.*

isodose line the dose gradient is usually the steepest ensuring sufficient dose within the target, while the dose level outside falls steeply, sparing the surrounding healthy tissue. Leksell Gamma Plan can also display the absolute dose values if desired. It will show the point in the stereotactic space where the global maximum dose can be found. With vestibular schwannoma, it is valuable to complete this exercise, as the maximal dose at the "hot spot" should be positioned well away from the facial nerve and cochlea. In addition, plotting the absolute dose lines will help in determining the actual level of radiation delivered to surrounding structures.

When the dose planning is completed, Leksell GammaPlan checks the shots for collisions with the collimator helmet and sorts the plan according to collimator size. The team performs quality assurance steps to check the accuracy of the *X*, *Y*, and *Z* coordinates and to ensure the plan treats the correct side. All relevant data are documented including details of the treatment plan, targets, dose volume histograms, snap shots, and images. When the treatment setup has been finalized, the treatment protocol is exported to Leksell Gamma Knife. This is via a special secured direct serial connection. Leksell GammaPlan only accepts valid and verified treatment plans for export. In addition, a protective design limits the transfer of a treatment plan to the Leksell Gamma Knife to one patient at a time. Once the data have been transferred to the operator's console, it is verified, and the patient can be treated.

For the model C unit, the operator does not have to enter the treatment room during a run. However, with the model B, the treatment team enters the treatment room after each shot is delivered and manually adjusts the *X*, *Y*, and *Z* coordinates, as well as the gamma angle, ie, the pitch of the head, if necessary. With both the model B and model C, the team has to change the collimator helmet manually when necessary, as dictated by the treatment plan. Detailed treatment and physics protocols are viewed and printed out.

Treatment

Treatment can be performed automatically using the automatic positioning system or manually using trunnions. For the model B, manual setting of the *X*, *Y*, and *Z* coordinates as well as the gamma angle if necessary is accomplished by the treatment team. The *Y* and *Z* coordinates are set with the *Y*, *Z* slides on the *y*-bar attached to the coordinate frame, whereas the *X* coordinate and the gamma angle are set with the trunnions. It is imperative to have a check and balance in place that consists of visual verification of each coordinate by a different team member. *Y*-coordinates need to be verified prior to setting the *Z*-coordinate, as the latter will obscure the scale on the *y*-axis. It is preferable to set the *X*-coordinate of the trunnion on the shorter side first, as this will provide more room to manipulate the patient and head frame within the collimator helmet. These coordinates need to be manually changed between each shot on the model B unit.

With the automatic positioning system (APS), the treatment is controlled from the operator console. Once the treatment starts, the selected run is carried out automatically. Before repositioning, the couch will move out a short distance to bring the patient out of treatment focus. At this point, the APS will move the patient's head to the next target position. A run consists of all shots for a specific collimator helmet size. Additional runs are performed after manually changing the collimator helmet.

After all runs have been completed, the head frame is removed. The anterior fixation sites are dressed with antibiotic ointment and adhesive bandages. The posterior sites are dressed with antibiotic ointment. Often pressure needs to be held to control bleeding and occasionally a staple may need to be used on the posterior sites. Typically patients will experience a transient headache after removal of the frame and some develop nausea and emesis. We typically premedicate with decadron and ondansetron prior to frame removal. Patients are observed for several hours posttreatment and discharged home with pain medication and follow-up appointments.

Gamma Knife Surgery Outcomes in Vestibular Schwannoma

Just as is the case with other forms of medical and surgical therapy, the techniques and outcomes of gamma knife surgery for vestibular schwannomas have evolved and improved over time. Tumor control and facial nerve motor preservation occurs with virtually all vestibular schwannoma patients treated with current gamma knife protocols. Areas of continued focused investigation include the effects of radiosurgery on hearing and balance, and methods of improving outcomes.

The University of Pittsburgh group has the largest clinical experience in treating vestibular schwannomas with gamma knife surgery. Lunsford and colleagues summarized their experience with 829 vestibular schwannomas treated between 1987 and 2002.[19] This extensive clinical experience included an average tumor volume of 2.5 cm^3 and a median margin dose to tumor of 13 Gy. They reported tumor control in 97% of patients at 10 years, and facial nerve (motor) dysfunction in <1% of patients. Trigeminal nerve symptoms occurred in <3% of patients and typically occurred with large tumors reaching the level of the trigeminal nerve. No reporting of balance function was included in their analyses.

The reporting of hearing preservation has limited representation in the entire 829 patients. Hearing outcomes data were presented in only 267 patients and "5-year actuarial rates of hearing level preservation and speech preservation" were reported in 103 patients. They reported "unchanged hearing preservation" in 50 to 77% of these patients, and this method of reporting auditory performance points to the difficulty in interpreting the outcome of most of the studies reporting hearing outcome in patients with vestibular schwannoma who have been treated with gamma knife surgery. They also stated that "for patients with intracanalicular tumors, hearing preservation rates in those treated with 12.5 to 14 Gy at the margin showed 90% preservation of serviceable hearing."[20] Unfortunately, pretreatment and longitudinal data are not available in these reports.

Prasad and colleagues from the University of Virginia reported their series of 200 vestibular schwannomas treated with gamma knife surgery over a 10-year interval in 2000.[21] Of these patients, 153 patients had follow-up data including 96 with primary treatment and 57 with secondary treatment. They reported no hearing pregamma knife in 105 patients, including 53 of 96 primary treatment and 52 of 57 secondary treatment patients. The Gardner-Robertson grading system and subjective assessment of hearing was used; however, no pure-tone average or speech discrimination data were reported. Unfortunately, their data set included audiometric data from only 48 patients, and the intervals of audiometric testing were not reported. Despite these limitations, they found that, except for one patient, no change in hearing was observed in the first two years after gamma knife surgery. Their data also showed that the greatest change in Gardner-Robertson grade occurred between 2 and 4 years post–gamma knife surgery; however, without understanding the assessment intervals, the precise onset of the hearing loss is unknown. No outcomes regarding balance function were reported.

Kim's group at the Seoul National University reported the hearing outcomes in 25 patients with vestibular schwannomas with serviceable hearing.[22] The median tumor volume was 3.0 cm^3 (0.16 to 9.1 cm^3), and the dose used was 12 ± 0.7 Gy at the 49.8 ± 1.1% isodose line. They reported the hearing outcomes using the Gardner-Robertson grading system, pure-tone averages, and speech discrimination scores. Pregamma knife, interim postgamma knife, and last postgamma knife data were reported. Similar to our experience, they found that in 16 patients the hearing deteriorated > 20 dB 3 to 6 months post–gamma knife surgery and that this hearing loss continued for 24 months. The only prognostic factor for hearing deterioration that they identified was the maximum dose to the cochlear nucleus.

In our Acoustic Neuroma and Skull Base Surgery Program, we have established a clinical pathway for all of our patients undergoing gamma knife surgery for primary or secondary treatment of their vestibular schwannomas. As pretreatment, they undergo a complete videonystagmography test battery, a complete audiologic assessment, and facial nerve electromyography. At 6-month intervals posttreatment, each patient undergoes a gadolinium-enhanced MRI as well as an audiologic test battery and caloric testing to assess peripheral vestibular function. In addition to other standard reporting methods, we have also presented the data in a longitudinal manner for their objective auditory thresholds (Figure 39–5), speech discrimination ability (Figure 39–6), and degree of vestibular paresis (Figure 39–7). We have recently published an expanded cohort of 54 patients with a median follow-up interval of 54.7 months.[23] This report focused on the longitudinal outcomes in vestibular function and changes in the Dizziness Handicap Inventory before and after gamma knife surgery.

It is clear that most of the change in hearing and balance function occurs during the first 12 months after gamma knife surgery; however, continued but less rapid worsening of function can occur for longer intervals. These objective measurements correspond well to the transient facial nerve dysfunction, trigeminal nerve dysfunction, tinnitus, and disequilibrium occurring in our patients with vestibular schwannomas undergoing gamma knife surgery.[3,17,23] A possible mechanism underlying these changes is that there is an initial increased size of the tumor after radiosurgery. Typically this posttreatment edema persists for 6 months; however, this may remain for up to 1 year.[3,17,23] The labyrinthine artery, a branch of the anterior inferior cerebellar artery, provides essentially all of the blood supply to the cochlea and vestibule and it is possible that the postradiation edema compromises this blood supply to the inner ear, although our linear regression analyses have not borne this out. Alternatively, devascularization of the stria vascularis is a likely

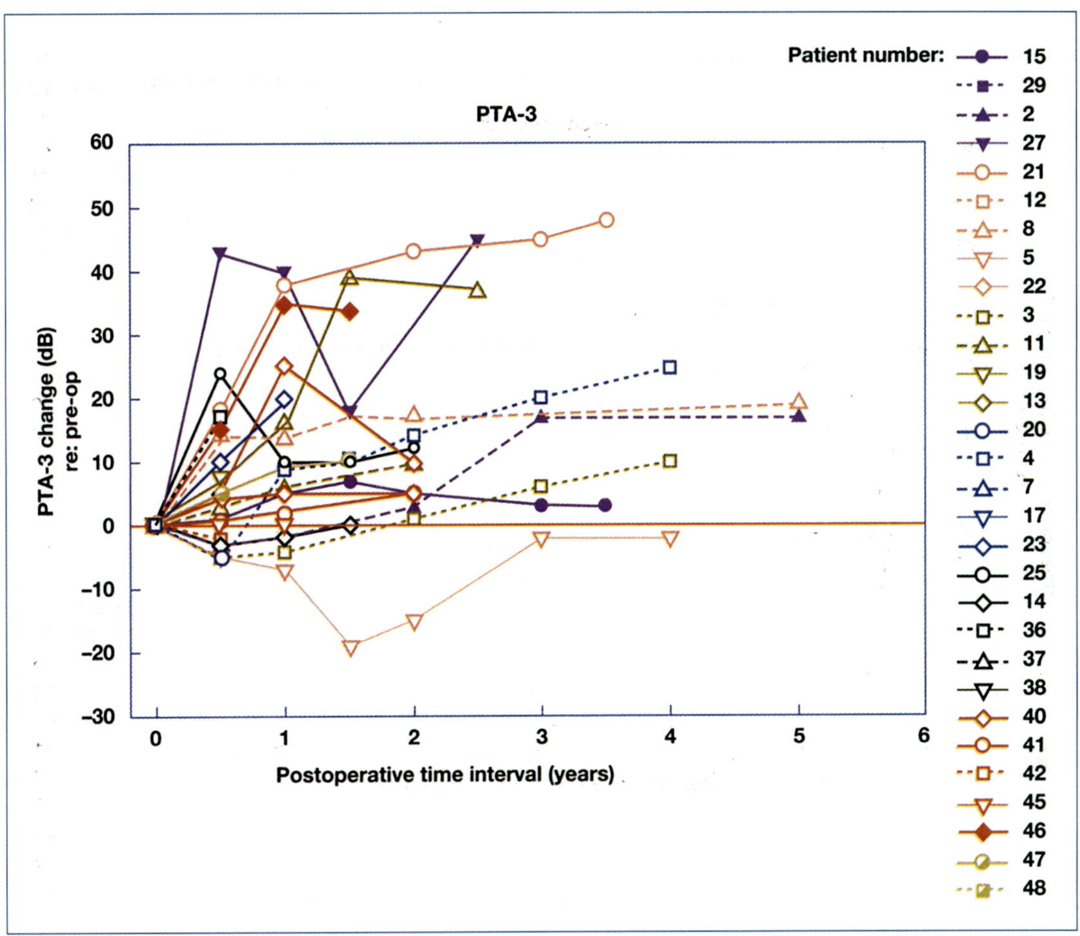

FIGURE 39–5 • Auditory function over time after gamma knife radiosurgery treatment of unilateral vestibular schwannomas. Three-frequency averages of pure-tone thresholds (PTA-3) in dB HL at 0.5, 1, and 2 kHz were determined for all patients with measures at the preoperative time and at least one postoperative interval. The PTA-3 difference was calculated for each time interval relative to the preoperative PTA-3. The differences are plotted as a function of postoperative time interval, with zero representing the preoperative time (red line). A positive difference value indicates a higher or poorer, postoperative PTA-3. In general, over time, the vast majority of patients were found to have PTA-3s that were poorer or similar to preoperative PTA-3s, although a few individuals showed some initial improvement (eg, subject 5). The greatest changes in PTA-3 were measured at 6 to 12 months posttreatment although continued changes were observed up to 5 years posttreatment. *Published with permission, copyright © 2009, P.A. Wackym, MD.*

mechanism responsible for this posttreatment hearing loss, particularly since we have seen a much greater impact on auditory thresholds than with speech discrimination, as is the case with strial presbyacusis (Figures 39–5 and 39–6).

Several of our patients treated with gamma knife have had tumor control or regression and improvement of hearing and vestibular function. This is clearly divergent from the natural history of vestibular schwannomas. In contrast, worsening of auditory and vestibular function and the development of disequilibrium has occurred in a number of our patients. Continued systematic studies of these patients and expansion of the cohort of patients studied are important to determine the efficacy of gamma knife surgery and to compare to other forms of radiotherapy, as well as microsurgery and expectant management. Recognition of symptoms such as disequilibrium and knowledge regarding the expected time course of vestibular paresis progression are important not only for patient counseling, but to provide the opportunity to intervene with vestibular rehabilitation or nonspecific vestibular suppression until compensation has been completed, should this be needed clinically.[23]

One final issue to consider is tumor growth after radiosurgery (Figure 39–8). It is important to appreciate that there is an increased size of the tumor after radiosurgery. In fact, we observed a statistically significant increase in tumor size for patients whose tumors extended outside of the internal auditory canal 6 months after gamma knife surgery and a statistically significant decrease at one year posttreatment.[3,17] Typically, posttreatment edema persists for 6 months; however, this may remain for up to 1 year. Consequently pretreatment counseling should include this information. There have been anecdotal cases discussed and occasionally reported that describe increased tumor size early after radiosurgery. The challenge is in making a decision about whether to resect these tumors and when.[2,12,24–28] Pollock and colleagues emphasized the need to demonstrate sustained tumor growth by serial MRI before making the decision to operate and also to review the case with

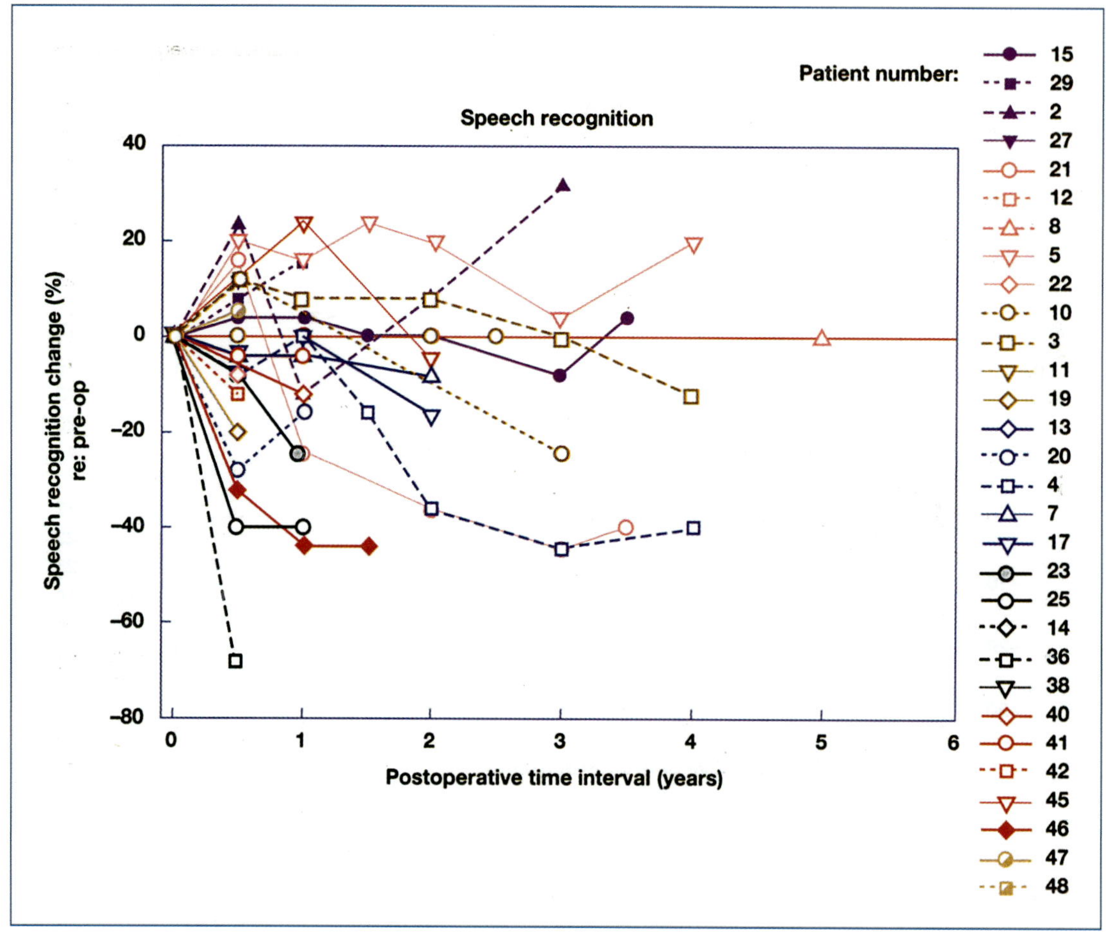

FIGURE 39–6 • Speech recognition testing was performed using the Northwestern University Auditory Test No. 6 (NU-6) monosyllabic words. The stimuli were presented at 40 dB sensation level, i.e., above speech recognition threshold, or if this was too loud, at the patient's most comfortable listening level. Speech recognition was scored in percent correct. As with PTA, the differences between pre- and postoperative speech recognition were calculated and plotted as a function of postoperative time interval, with zero representing the preoperative time (red line). Positive values are consistent with an improvement in speech recognition. Approximately half of the patients showed improvement in speech recognition at 6 months posttreatment, while the other half showed a decrease in performance. Of those patients who experienced a reduction in speech discrimination ability, there was a greater range of change than that observed in the patients who enjoyed an improvement in speech discrimination ability. It should be noted that the greatest changes in speech discrimination ability occurred at 6 to 12 months post–gamma knife surgery. However, over time, the patients generally demonstrate speech recognition performance similar to or poorer than pretreatment performance. *Published with permission, copyright © 2009, P.A. Wackym, MD.*

the surgeon who performed the radiosurgery before a surgical decision is made.[12]

Another related controversy is whether facial nerve dissection and preservation are more difficult during microsurgical resection after radiosurgery. On one end of the spectrum, descriptions of no increased difficulty have been reported;[12] and, on the other end of the spectrum,[25–28] markedly increased difficulty in separating the tumor from the facial nerve and poorer facial nerve function outcome have also been reported. The report of Watanabe and colleagues included a histopathologic analysis of the resected facial nerve.[26] They found microvasculitis of the facial nerve, axonal degeneration, loss of axons, and proliferation of Schwann cells. In light of the mechanism of delayed effects following radiosurgery, these findings are not surprising. Moreover, these findings emphasize the need for the neurotologist to be certain that the treatment plan avoids high radiation doses to the facial nerve. Recall as described earlier that a dose of 12 Gy delivered to the 50% isodose line means that the maximum tumor dose is 24 Gy. If the treatment plan delivers this maximal dose to the area of the facial nerve, it should be expected that greater radiation effects will be observed. For this reason, if the neurotologist and the patient have made a decision to resect a tumor previously treated with radiosurgery, it is important to review the treatment plan to determine the amount of radiation delivered to the facial nerve to counsel the patient appropriately preoperatively.

ALTERNATIVE RADIOSURGICAL TECHNIQUES

As noted earlier, tumor size and location may dictate that a method other than Gamma knife surgery be considered. Indeed, alternative methods of radiosurgery are available for treating a

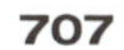

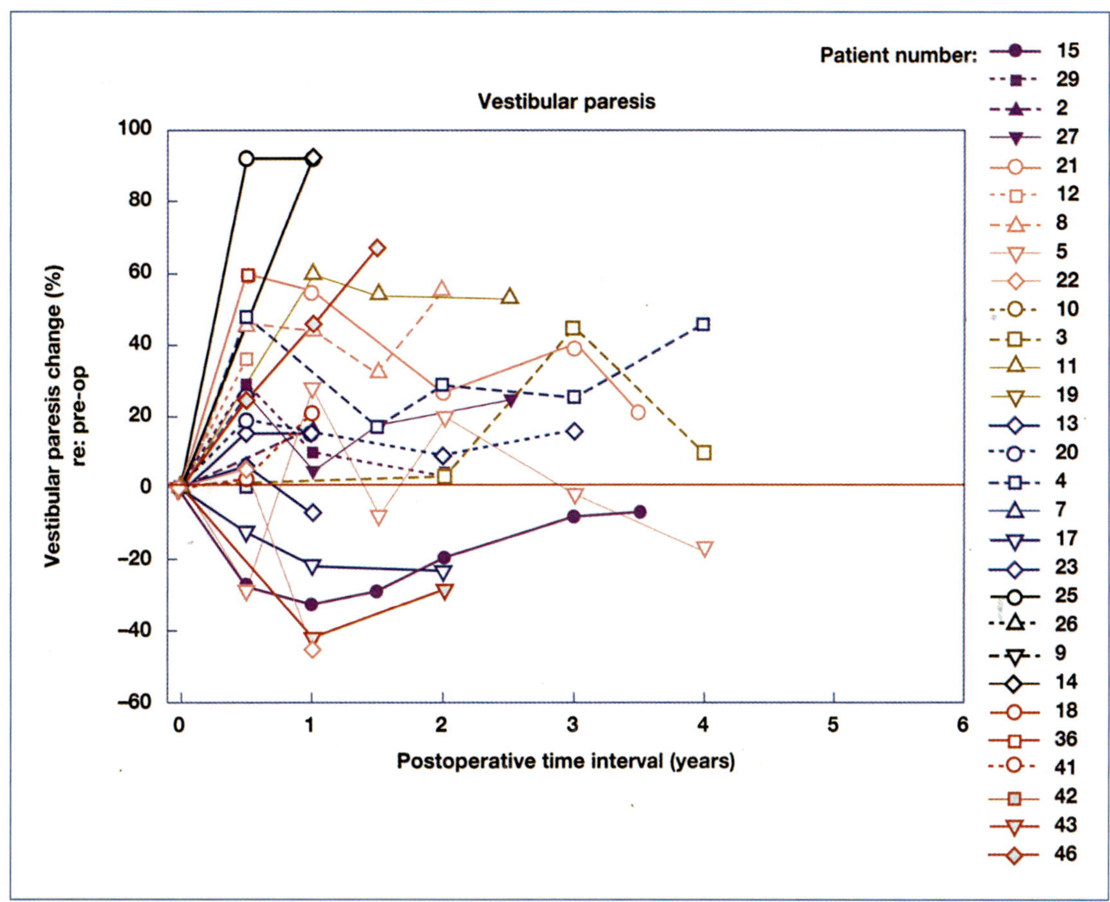

FIGURE 39–7 • Vestibular paresis was determined with bithermal caloric testing. A positive difference value indicates greater vestibular paresis post–gamma knife radiosurgery. Zero represents the preoperative value (red line). Both degradation and improvement in vestibular paresis are observed across patients. Within a patient, the postoperative degree of vestibular paresis generally tends to remain stable over time after the relatively large initial change observed at the 6- to 12-month posttreatment assessment. In those patients who had continued reduction in their vestibular function, there was continued difficulty with disequilibrium until vestibular compensation was complete and the vestibular paresis stabilized. *Published with permission, copyright © 2009, P.A. Wackym, MD.*

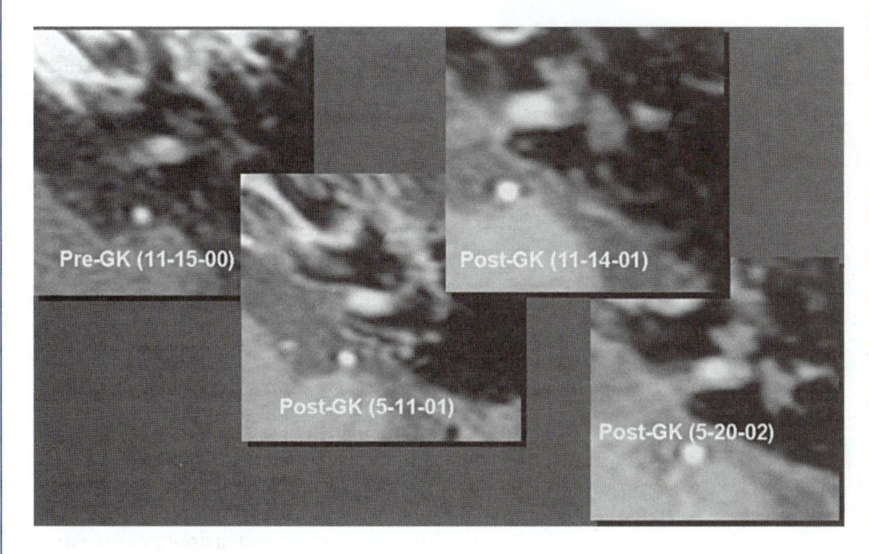

FIGURE 39–8 • Gamma knife radiosurgery. Example of serial magnetic resonance imaging studies of a small left vestibular schwannoma. Note at 6 and 12 months post–gamma knife radiosurgery, the tumor is larger than pretreatment. By 18 months, the tumor is smaller. *Reproduced with permission, copyright © 2009, P.A. Wackym, MD.*

wide variety of skull base neoplasms. These include the Peacock (NOMOS Inc., Cranberry Township, PA), the SmartBeam IMRT (Varian Medical Systems Inc., Palo Alto, CA), the Precise (Elekta, Inc., Stockholm, Sweden), and the CyberKnife (Accuray, Sunnyvale, CA). Among the more common of these modalities is CyberKnife, which will be briefly reviewed here.

CyberKnife Stereotactic Radiosurgery

Overview if Treatment Planning

The CyberKnife stereotactic radiosurgery system utilizes a compact 6-MeV LINAC, a computer-controlled robotic arm with six degrees of freedom, and an image-guidance technology that does not depend on a rigid stereotactic frame and thereby enables treatment of extracranial sites (Figure 39–9). Potential benefits of this approach include: (1) increased access to and coverage of any target volume including the ability to treat lesions in and around the cranium that are unreachable with other systems, for example, in the lower posterior fossa and foramen magnum; (2) enhanced ability to avoid critical structures; (3) capability to treat lesions in the neck and spine; (4) ability to treat lesions throughout the body; (5) delivery of highly conformal dose distributions; (6) option of fractionating treatment; and (7) potential to target multiple tumors at different locations during a single treatment, eg, skull base and neck.

The CyberKnife® treatment planning system is designed to support the radiosurgery team in determining the optimal plan, including beam weight, targeting positions, dose distributions, and other factors for each patient's treatment. The CyberKnife stereotactic radiosurgery system permits the following planning and delivery options: (1) inverse planning; (2) nonisocentric delivery; and (3) hypofractionation. In contrast to most gamma knife procedures, CyberKnife is CT-based. MR images can be fused with the CT to provide optimal information on soft tissue as well as skeletal anatomy. CT angiography can be used when vascular skull base lesions such as arteriovenous malformations or extensive glomus jugulare tumors are to be treated with this technique.

The flexibility of the robotic arm supporting the linear accelerator allows the CyberKnife to implement a wider range of treatment plans than other systems. Furthermore, because the system does not require the use of a stereotactic head frame temporarily attached to the patient's head, it allows scanning, treatment planning, and quality assurance to take place at any time prior to treatment itself. The CyberKnife system provides a range of treatment options, including the ability to use either forward or inverse treatment planning. With forward treatment planning, the radiation oncologist determines what dose to deliver from a particular targeting position. The total dose within the lesion is then calculated by the system software. With inverse treatment planning, the radiation oncologist specifies total dose to be delivered to the tumor. The surgeon and radiation oncologist are then able to set boundaries to protect adjacent critical structures. The software subsequently determines targeting positions and the dose to be delivered from each targeting position. While other stereotactic radiosurgery systems offer the inverse planning option, the number of possible plans is limited by the constraints of the delivery system.

Dose Distribution

The CyberKnife system offers a choice of a nonisocentric or an isocentric treatment approach. With other stereotactic radiosurgery systems, a fixed calculated isocenter is used. Isocentric treatment, or multiisocentric treatment, involves filling the lesion with a single or multiple, overlapping spherically shaped dose distributions. Isocentric treatment is effective for spherical lesions. However, with irregularly shaped lesions, isocentric delivery can produce significant dose heterogeneity. In this case the surgeon and radiation oncologist must account for the relationship of the maximum dose to critical structures such as the facial nerve or cochlea. Similarly, they must identify regions which may be undertreated by delivery of inadequate doses.

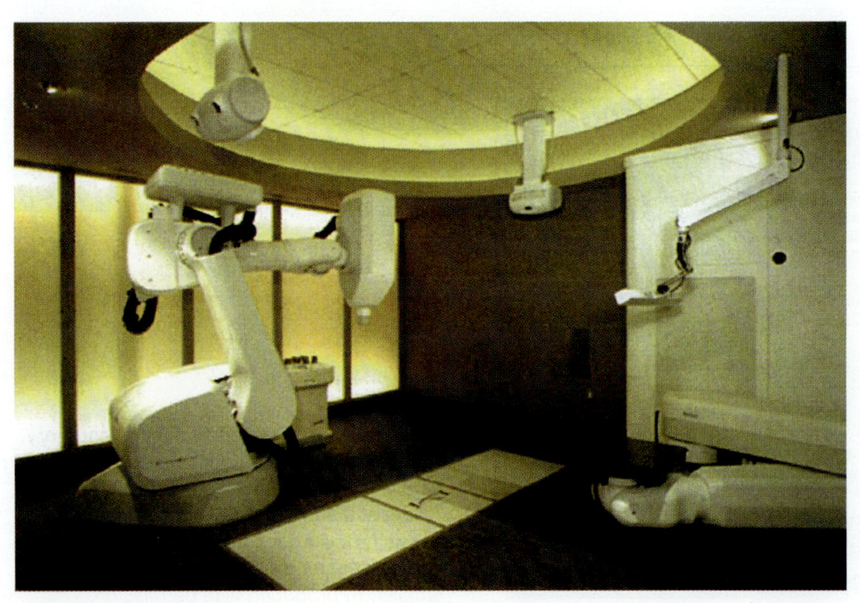

FIGURE 39–9 • Ceiling-mounted diagnostic-energy x-ray sources emit low-dose x-rays through the patient's tumor treatment area. Amorphous silicon image detectors capture x-ray images from ceiling-mounted diagnostic-energy x-ray sources to produce live radiographs. The operating system (typically located adjacent to the treatment room) correlates patient location detected by image guidance system with reconstructed CT scan and directs the robot to adjust position accordingly. The compact linear accelerator mounted on a computer-controlled robotic arm, which adjusts position to maintain alignment with the target, compensating for any patient movement and uses X-band technology for mobility. *Published with permission, copyright © 2009, Accuray (Accuray Incorporated, Sunnyvale, CA).*

Nonisocentric treatment plans are also possible with the CyberKnife system. The delivery of these treatment plans is possible because of the robotic arm which, because of the six degrees of freedom (discussed below) enables the delivery of radiation to complex treatment volumes. The beams originate from arbitrary points in the workspace and are delivered into the lesion. The result is a nonisocentric concentration of beams within the lesion and asymmetric irradiation. Nonisocentric treatment allows the avoidance of critical structures while providing complete coverage of the lesion at the prescribed isodose.

With the CyberKnife system, the treatment plan can utilize fractionated or hypofractionated approaches. Fractionated treatment is possible because localization of the lesion is achieved using image guidance technology. Dose delivery over two to five treatment sessions, termed hypofractionation, is another option with the CyberKnife system. Although not directly applicable in managing tumors within the posterior fossa, it has been suggested to be particularly useful in the treatment of large tumors. The argument for fractionation is that lowering the dose for each of a number of treatments, as opposed to a single, larger dose, allows healthy tissue to rejuvenate between treatments. The advantage of fractionated or a single radiation dose remains an active area of investigation and debate. Because of the rigid fixation that occurs with securing the stereotacic headframe in gamma knife surgery, fractionated or hypofractionated delivery of radiation is not possible. Furthermore, it remains to be determined if equal accuracy can be achieved by these two systems or if there is an advantage of fractionation or hypofractionation in the treatment of skull base tumors.

Localization

The CyberKnife system's use of stereotactic principles for tumor localization differs from other stereotactic radiosurgery systems by using an image guidance technology that depends on the skeletal structure of the body as a reference frame. In addition, it continually monitors and tracks patient position during treatment. The CyberKnife's operating system correlates live radiographic images with preoperative CT scans to determine patient and tumor position repeatedly over the course of treatment. The imaging information is transferred from the computer's operating system to the robot so that it may compensate for any changes in patient position by repositioning the LINAC.

Treatment Delivery

The CyberKnife system's computer-controlled robotic arm has six degrees of freedom. The robot can position the LINAC to more than 100 specific locations or nodes. Each node has 12 possible approach angles, translating to over 1200 possible beam positions. The treatment planning system determines a set sequence of approach angles, beam weights, and dose distributions. The calculated plan can be incrementally improved by the physicist and physicians. The actual delivery follows a step-and-shoot sequence. The patient is placed in a position approximating that of the CT scan. Image detectors acquire radiographs of the tumor region. The image guidance system software then compares the real time radiographs with the CT information to determine location of the tumor. This information is transmitted to the robot to initialize the pointing of the LINAC beam. The robotic arm then moves the LINAC through the sequence of preset nodes surrounding the patient. At each node, the LINAC stops, and a new pair of images are acquired from which the position is determined again. Corrected position is transmitted to the robot which adapts beam pointing to compensate for any movement. LINAC delivers the preplanned dose of radiation for that position. The entire process is repeated at each node. The total time from imaging to robot compensation is about 7 to 10 sec. The total treatment time depends on the complexity of the plan and delivery paths but is comparable to standard LINAC treatments. Each treatment session ranges from 30 to 90 min. Physicians may elect to treat with a single dose, a hypofractionated dose, typically of two to five sessions, or a more traditional fractionated regimen. Outcomes following CyberKnife treatment of vestibular schwannomas are emerging at this time.[29]

SUMMARY

Stereotactic radiosurgery and radiotherapy are increasingly utilized in the management of skull base tumors and other disorders. Whether driven by the consumer, or the surgeon, the field continues to evolve rapidly. Advances are being made in improving accuracy, effective radiation dose, and parameters necessary to maximize patient outcome. These methods have advantages and disadvantages that must be openly discussed with patients having vestibular schwannomas or other skull base tumors. It remains the responsibility of the surgeon to provide a balanced view as to the relative risks and benefits of observation, microsurgery, stereotactic radiosurgery or radiotherapy, or a combination of these methods.

References

1. Kondziolka D, Lunsford LD, McLaughlin MR, Flickinger JC. Long-term outcomes after radiosurgery for acoustic neuroma. N Engl J Med 1998;339:1426–33.
2. Wackym PA. Stereotactic radiosurgery, microsurgery, and expectant management of acoustic neuroma: Basis of informed consent. Otolaryngol Clin North Am 2005;38:653–70.
3. Wackym PA, Runge-Samuelson CL, Poetker DM, et al. Gamma knife radiosurgery for acoustic neuromas performed by a neurotologist: Early experiences and outcomes. Otol Neurol 2004;25:752–61.
4. Knisely JPS, Linskey ME. Less common indications for stereotactic radiosurgery or fractionated radiotherapy for patients with benign brain tumors. Neurosurg Clin N Am 2006;17:149–167.
5. Pollock BE. Stereotactic radiosurgery in patients with glomus jugulare tumors. Neurosurg Focus 2004;17:63–67.
6. Gottfried ON, Liu JK, Couldwell WT. Comparison of radiosurgery and conventional surgery for the treatment of glomus jugulare tumors. Neurosurg Focus 2004; 17:22–30.
7. Goldsmith B, McDermott MW. Meningioma. Neurosurg Clin N Am 2006;17:111–120.
8. Elia AE, Shih HA, Loeffler JS. Stereotactic radiation treatment for benign meningiomas. Neurosurg Focus 2007;23:1–9.
9. Kreil W, Luggin J, Fuchs I, et al. Long term experience of gamma knife radiosurgery for benign skull base meningiomas. J Neurol Neurosurg Psychiatry 2005;76:1425–1430.
10. Gorgulho AA, De Salles AAF. Impact of radiosurgery on the surgical treatment of trigeminal neuralgia. Surg Neurol 2006;66:350–356.

11. Bari ME, Forster DM, Kemeny AA, et al. Malignancy in a vestibular schwannoma. Report of a case with central neurofibromatosis, treated by both stereotactic radiosurgery and surgical excision, with a review of the literature. Br J Neurosurg 2002;16:284–9.
12. Pollock BE, Lunsford LD, Kondziolka D, et al. Vestibular schwannoma management. Part II. Failed radiosurgery and the role of delayed microsurgery. J Neurosurg 1998;89: 949–55.
13. Rowe J, Grainger A, Walton L, et al. Risk of malignancy after gamma knife stereotactic radiosurgery. Neurosurgery 2007;60:60–5.
14. Rowe J, Grainger A, Walton L, et al. Safety of radiosurgery applied to conditions with abnormal tumor suppressor genes. Neurosurgery 2007;60:860–4.
15. Lustig LR, Jackler RK, Lanser MJ. Radiation-induced tumors of the temporal bone. Am J Otol 1997;18:230–5.
16. Hanabusa K, Morikawa A, Murata T, Taki W. Acoustic neuroma with malignant transformation. Case report. J Neurosurg 2001;95:518–21.
17. Poetker DM, Jursinic PA, Runge-Samuelson CL, Wackym PA. Distortion of magnetic resonance images used in gamma knife radiosurgery treatment planning: Implications for acoustic neuroma outcomes. Otol Neurotol 2005;26:1220–8.
18. Paddick I. A simple scoring ration to index the conformity of radiosurgical treatment plans. Technical note. J Neurosurg 2000;93(Suppl 3):219–22.
19. Lunsford LD, Niranjan A, Flickinger JC, et al. Radiosurgery of vestibular schwannomas: Summary of experience in 829 cases. J Neurosurg 2005;Suppl 102:195–9.
20. Niranjan A, Lunsford LD, Flickinger JC, et al. Dose reduction improves hearing preservation rates after intracanalicular acoustic tumor radiosurgery. Neurosurgery 1999;45:753–62.
21. Prasad D, Steiner M, Steiner L. Gamma surgery for vestibular schwannoma. J Neurosurg 2000;92:745–59.
22. Paek SH, Chung H-T, Jeong SS, et al. Hearing preservation after gamma knife radiosurgery of vestibular schwannoma. Cancer 2005;104:580–90.
23. Wackym PA, Hannley MT, Runge-Samuelson CL, et al. Gamma knife surgery of vestibular schwannomas: Longitudinal changes in vestibular function and measurement of the Dizziness Handicap Inventory. J Neurosurg 2008; 109 (Suppl):137–43.
24. Pitts LA, Jackler RK. Treatment of acoustic neuromas. N Engl J Med 1998;339:1471–73.
25. Ho SY, Kveton JF. Rapid growth of acoustic neuromas after stereotactic radiotherapy in type 2 neurofibromatosis. Ear Nose Throat J 2002;81:831–3.
26. Watanabe T, Saito N, Hirato J, et al. Facial neuropathy due to axonal degeneration and microvasculitis following gamma knife surgery for vestibular schwannoma: A histological analysis. J Neurosurg 2003;99:916–20.
27. Lee DJ, Westra WH, Staecker H, et al. Clinical and histopathologic features of recurrent vestibular schwannoma (acoustic neuroma) after stereotactic radiosurgery. Otol Neurol 2003;24:650–60.
28. Friedman RA, Brackmann DE, Hitselberger WE, et al. Surgical salvage after failed irradiation for vestibular schwannoma. Laryngoscope 2005;115:1827–32.
29. Chang SD, Gibbs IC, Sakamoto GT, et al. Staged stereotactic irradiation for acoustic neuroma. Neurosurgery 2005;56: 1254–61.

Surgery for Cystic Lesions of the Petrous Apex

40

Gordon B. Hughes, MD / Joung Lee , MD /
Paul M. Ruggieri, MD / Martin J. Citardi, MD

The petrous apex lies anterior to the internal auditory canal; its pneumatization is indirectly proportional to the amount of bone marrow within the apex. The more the bone marrow, the less the air, and vice versa. Approximately one-third of adults have apical pneumatization, which usually is symmetric bilaterally. The petrous apex has three surfaces: anterior (superior), which forms the floor of the middle cranial fossa; posterior, which faces the posterior cranial fossa; and inferior, which lies along the horizontal plane. The most vital structure of the apex is the internal carotid artery, which enters through the inferior meatus and passes anteriorly and medially to reach the cavernous sinus. The Eustachian tube and tensor tympani muscle are located just lateral to the artery. On the anterior surface, the greater superficial petrosal nerve (GSPN) passes through the facial hiatus, carrying preganglionic parasympathetic fibers to the sphenopalatine ganglion. Near the anterior apex, the Gasserian ganglion of the trigeminal nerve rests in Meckel's cave, and the abducens nerve courses along with the superior petrosal sinus through a tight fold of dura known as the petroclinoid ligament to form Dorello's canal.

Cholesterol granuloma, cholesteatoma (epidermoid cyst), and mucocele account for 99% of primary cystic lesions of the petrous apex, with cholesterol granuloma being the most common (Table 40–1).[1,2] These lesions can be confused with normal bone marrow in a poorly pneumatized petrous apex,[3] trapped fluid (effusion) within an apical cell,[4] and an arachnoid cyst.[5] Magnetic resonance imaging (MRI) and computed tomography (CT) can usually distinguish among these lesions. Rare primary lesions of the petrous apex include unifocal Langerhans' cell histiocytosis (eosinophilic granuloma),[6] chordoma, chondrosarcoma, and osteoclastoma. Secondary lesions include osteomyelitis, direct tumor spread, metastatic tumor, sphenoid mucocele, and aneurysm of the internal carotid artery.[7] Because primary and secondary neoplasms, encephaloceles, middle ear cholesteatoma, and osteomyelitis extending to the apex have been covered in previous chapters, this chapter will concentrate on the diagnosis and management of primary "cystic" lesions of the petrous apex: cholesterol granuloma, cholesteatoma (epidermoid cyst), and mucocele.

PATHOLOGY

Cholesterol granuloma is a foreign body giant cell reaction to cholesterol deposits, with chronic inflammation, fibrosis, and vascular proliferation all contained within a fibrous capsule.[8,9] Cholesterol granulomas are 10 times more common than cholesteatomas and 40 times more common than mucoceles. Two theories have been proposed for the development of cholesterol granuloma. In the obstruction–vacuum theory, obstruction of a previously aerated space leads to gas trapping and resorption, vacuum formation, hemorrhage into the mucosal surface, inflammation, breakdown of red blood cells, and formation of cholesterol crystals.[10–13] With formation of cholesterol crystals, the inflammatory cascade is initiated with bony resorption and foreign body reaction (Figure 40–1). In the exposed marrow theory, during development aggressive pneumatization of the apex forms pathologic communications between the mucosa-lined air cells and the marrow they gradually replace, creating hemorrhage into the apical air cells. Red blood cells break down, cholesterol crystals form, and the inflammatory cascade begins.[14,15]

Cholesteatoma (epidermoid cyst) consists of an epithelial wall, fibrous subepithelium, and keratin debris (Figure 40–2). The presence of epithelium distinguishes cholesteatoma from cholesterol granuloma. Epidermoid rests are thought to arise near the foramen lacerum either directly during fetal development[16] or indirectly from inward migration of external meatus ectoderm.[17,18] Epidermoid cysts can be distinguished from dermoid cysts that have skin adnexae (eg, sweat glands). As the cholesteatoma expands, bone erosion may result from osteolytic enzymes at the junction of the epithelium and fibrous subepithelium.

A mucocele results from obstruction of drainage from a highly pneumatized petrous apex and also can produce an expansile cystic lesion. The mucocele can be distinguished from cholesteatoma by the absence of keratinizing epithelium and from the cholesterol granuloma by the absence of cholesterol crystals and dense fibrous capsule (Figure 40–3). Some clinicians consider chronic trapped effusion (see retained fluid, later

TABLE 40–1 Lesions of the petrous apex

Primary Cholesterol granuloma Cholesteatoma (epidermoid cyst) Mucocele Trapped fluid (effusion) Eosinophilic granuloma Mesenchymal tumor (chondroma, chondrosarcoma, osteoclastoma, fibrous dysplasia)
Secondary Direct spread of neoplasm (nasopharyngeal carcinoma, vestibular or jugular foramen schwannoma, trigeminal neuroma, glomus tumor, clival chordoma, meningioma) Metastasis or hematogenous spread (metastatic tumor, lymphoma) Infection (osteomyelitis, necrotizing external otitis) Other (arachnoid cyst, aneurysm of internal carotid artery, sphenoid mucocele)

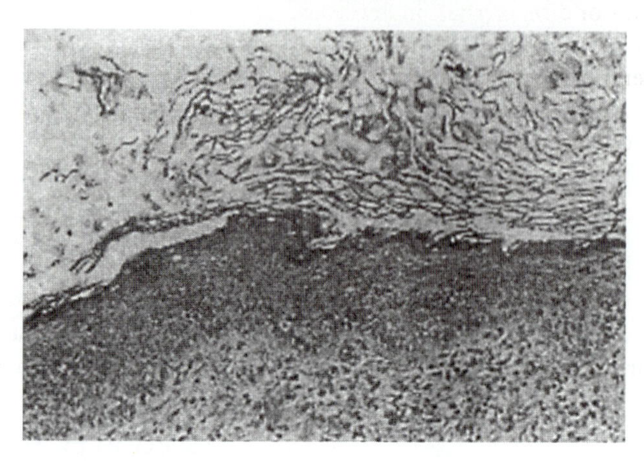

FIGURE 40–2 • Cholesteatoma. This cross-section of cholesteatoma shows keratin debris, keratinizing epithelium, and fibrous subepithelium. (Hematoxylin and eosin stain; ×200 original magnification.)

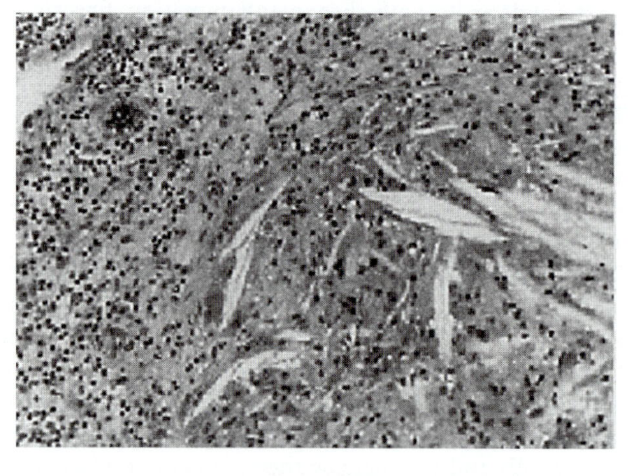

FIGURE 40–1 • Cholesterol granuloma. The oblong, needle-shaped clefts contain crystals of cholesterol esters that have been dissolved during histologic processing of the specimen. Foreign body–type giant cells have formed about some of the crystals, and many lymphocytes and histiocytes also are present. (Hematoxylin and eosin stain; ×200 original magnification.)

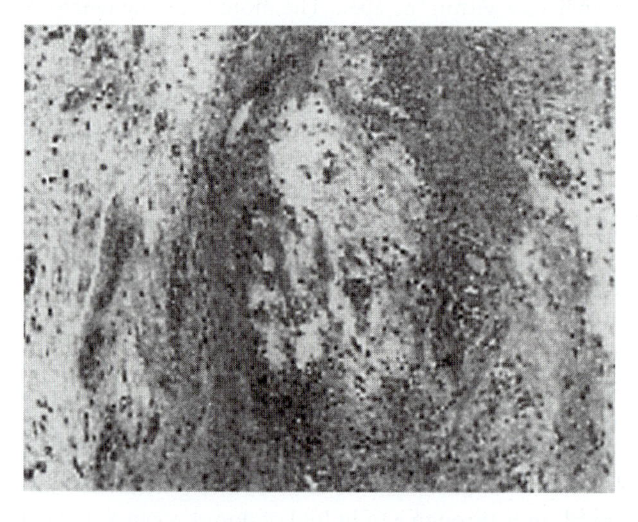

FIGURE 40–3 • Mucocele. The mucocele consists of extravasated mucous (mucous release reaction) with a surrounding inflammatory infiltrate. The mucocele can be distinguished from cholesteatoma by the absence of keratinizing epithelium and from cholesterol granuloma by the absence of cholesterol crystals. (Hematoxylin and eosin stain; ×200 original magnification.)

in the text), mucocele, and cholesterol granuloma to represent varying stages of severity of the same pathologic entity. The same reasoning implies that chronic, symptomatic, trapped fluid may not represent a benign "leave me alone"[4] lesion but instead may require surgery.

Other lesions of the petrous apex that can be confused with cystic lesions are retained fluid and asymmetric fatty marrow. Symptoms of petrous apicitis also can overlap those of cystic lesions. *Retained fluid* is a serous effusion trapped in apical air cells.[4] By definition, retained fluid does not destroy bone; however, headache and pressure symptoms may prompt surgery if serial CT scanning does not show resolution. The clinical entity of retained fluid is poorly understood but may be analogous to chronic serous mastoiditis or may be an initial step toward cholesterol granuloma formation. *Asymmetric fatty marrow* in the petrous apex is usually noted as an incidental finding on radiographic imaging.[3] It is the residual fatty marrow in the nonpneumatized or less-pneumatized apex that causes concern. Correct identification of this normal variant is essential to prevent misdiagnosis or unnecessary workup and treatment.[1,19] In a review of 500 CT scans, Roland et al.[3] found 34 patients with some asymmetry of pneumatization of the petrous apex. *Petrous apicitis* can result from acute or chronic otitis media; chronic otitis media is a more common cause with *Pseudomonas aeruginosa* being the predominant bacterium.[20–22] Petrous apicitis should be suspected whenever a chronic suppurative ear is associated with deep pain. The pain usually is a result of either dural involvement over the apex or direct irritation of the Gasserian ganglion in Meckel's cave. Petrous apicitis also should be suspected when cranial nerve palsies occur. The classical syndrome of Gradenigo's triad consists of discharging ear, deep retroocular pain, and abducens paralysis.[23]

CLINICAL PRESENTATION

Symptoms

Petrous apex findings (lesions) can be asymptomatic and discovered coincidentally on MRI. Leonetti and colleagues performed a retrospective chart review to categorize a group of petrous apex findings that were noted incidentally on MRI in 88 patients.[24] These incidental findings, which were unrelated to the presenting clinical manifestations, included asymmetric fatty bone marrow (n = 41), inflammation (n = 19), cholesterol granulomas (n = 14), cholesteatomas (n = 9), and neoplasms (n = 5). Follow-up imaging and clinical surveillance of these patients did not demonstrate any significant change in the incidentally detected lesions. In all cases, the incidental MRI findings represented benign pathology. Therefore, the clinician should bear in mind that a petrous apex "lesion" noted on MRI may or may not directly relate to the patient's presenting signs and symptoms; the physician should not overreact to an MRI finding that may, in fact, be coincidental.

Most published reports of symptomatic petrous apex lesions include primary and secondary neoplasms and list hearing loss as the most common presenting symptom.[1,7,11] Non-neoplastic, primary cystic lesions of the apex, however, more often present with headache, head pain, or aural pressure. Headache is usually ipsilateral and retro-orbital or temporoparietal but also can be referred to the occiput or vertex. Hearing loss occurs when the eustachian tube is compressed (conductive loss) or the internal auditory canal or inner ear is invaded (sensorineural hearing loss) and can be accompanied by tinnitus. Less often, inner ear involvement or vestibular nerve irritation can produce light-headedness or true vertigo. Trigeminal nerve compression can produce hypesthesia or paresthesia, especially along the distribution of the mandibular branch (V_3). Facial palsy and spasm from seventh cranial nerve compression and diplopia from sixth cranial nerve compression are uncommon. Ophthalmoplegia from anterior extension into the cavernous sinus is rare. Syncope also is rare and suggests carotid artery compression. Otorrhea can result from secondary infection and drainage of the cystic lesion.

Sings

Otoscopy is usually normal but can reveal drum retraction, middle ear effusion, or drainage. Hypesthesia of cranial nerve V and palsy of cranial nerves VI or VII are uncommon. The patient may have imbalance in performing the Romberg test or tandem gait. Often the head and neck examination is completely normal.

AUDIOMETRIC AND VESTIBULAR EVALUATION

The audiogram can be normal or reveal conductive, sensorineural, or mixed hearing loss. Vestibular testing can detect canal paresis from inner ear involvement. We usually obtain an audiogram but rarely an electronystagmogram.

RADIOLOGIC EVALUATION

Cholesterol granuloma is not only the most common cystic lesion of the petrous apex, it is also the only one that is invariably hyperintense on both T_1- and T_2-weighted images on MRI (Table 40–2 and Figure 40–4). Both cholesteatoma and mucocele are hypointense on T_1 views.[10,25,26] Fast-spin T_2 images of cholesteatoma will reveal a hyperintense, homogeneous mass (Figure 40–5). Magnetic resonance imaging, however, lacks bone detail. A CT scan can show whether the cyst is expansile. An expansile cyst usually requires surgery; a nonexpansile cyst usually does not. A CT scan also differentiates potentially surgical cysts of the apex from nonsurgical, asymmetric fatty marrow and trapped fluid (effusion). Trapped fluid (effusion) will have low signal intensity on T_1-weighted image and high signal intensity on T_2-weighted image on MRI and nonexpansile fluid attenuation (opacification) within a pneumatized petrous apex on CT (Figure 40–6).[4] Asymmetric fatty marrow will have high signal intensity on T_1-weighted images and intermediate intensity on T_2-weighted images on MRI and a nonexpansile, nonpneumatized petrous apex on CT (Figure 40–7).[4] Petrous apicitis on CT appears as a nonexpansile lesion that may have irregular margins and bony destruction and does not enhance on contrast administration. On MRI, petrous apicitis demonstrates low signal intensity on T_1-weighted images and high signal intensity on T_2-weighted images. Both CT contrast and MRI contrast may show rim enhancement if a true abscess has formed. Diffusion-weighted echoplanar MRI in the future may better distinguish between cholesterol granuloma and cholesteatoma.[27]

TABLE 40–2 Radiographic features of petrous apex cyst, tumor, fluid and marrow

LESION	MRI (T_1)	MRI (T_2)	ENHANCING	EXPANSILE
Cholesterol granuloma	High	High	No	Yes
Cholesteatoma	Low-medium	High	No	Yes
Trapped fluid	Low/variable	High	No	No
Tumor	Low-medium	High	Yes	Yes

MRI, magnetic resonance imaging.

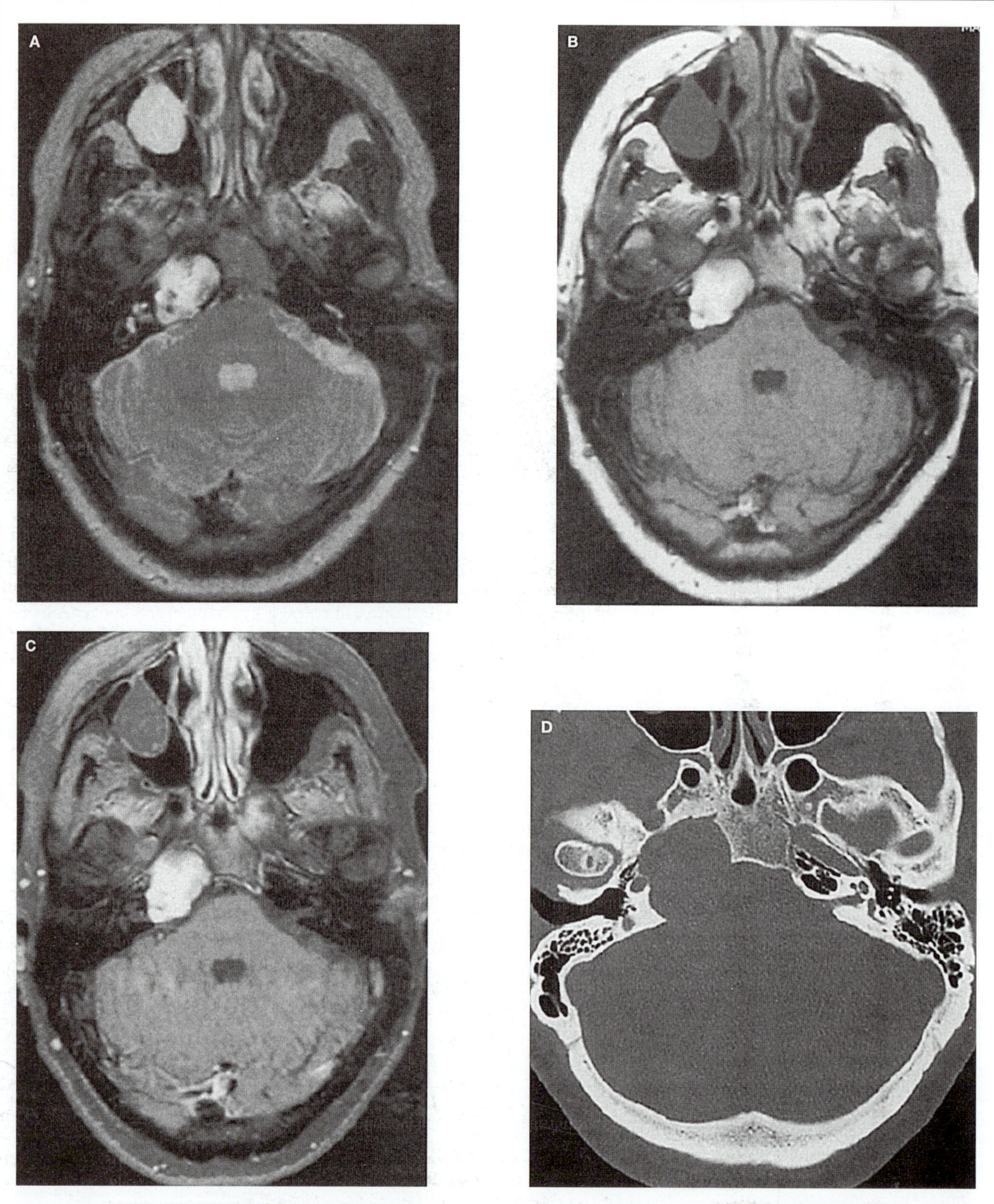

FIGURE 40–4 • Cholesterol granuloma. *A*, Axial T_2-weighted fast spin-echo magnetic resonance image (MRI) demonstrates a large, well-defined heterogeneously hyperintense mass in the right petrous apex that appears to be mildly expansile and impinges on the right carotid canal. A right maxillary sinus mucocele or polyp is noted coincidentally. *B*, The mass is also prominently hyperintense on the corresponding axial T_1-weighted spin-echo image. The signal intensity characteristics on T_1 and T_2 are quite typical for a cholesterol granuloma, presumably caused by prior hemorrhage. *C*, Fat suppression eliminates the high signal intensity of the fat in the normal petrous apex to make the lesion more obvious but has no impact on the signal of the cholesterol granuloma itself. No enhancement can be appreciated along the periphery of the mass because of the degree of hyperintensity of the contents on the unenhanced T_1-weighted images. *D*, On the axial computed tomographic image, the mass is more obviously expansile and protrudes into the cerebellopontine angle cistern. There is a thin rim of surrounding, reactive sclerosis as would be expected with a slowly growing process.

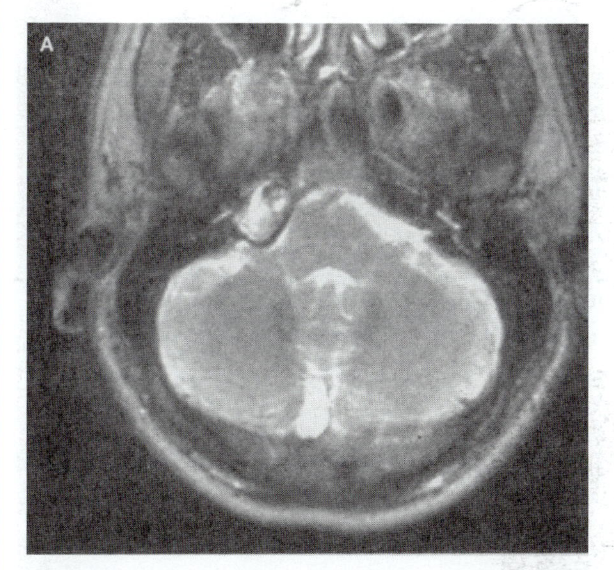

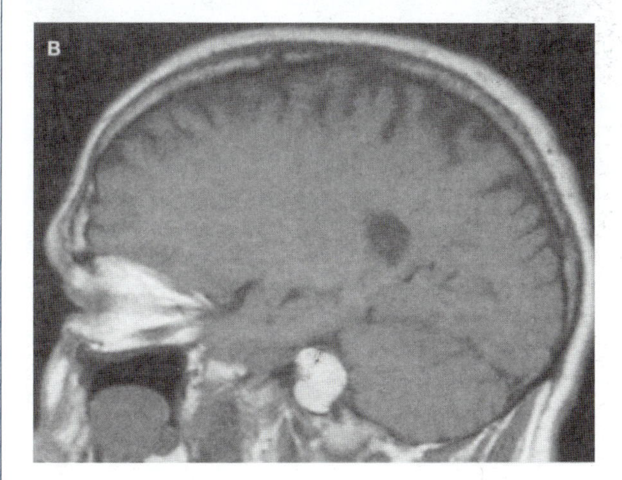

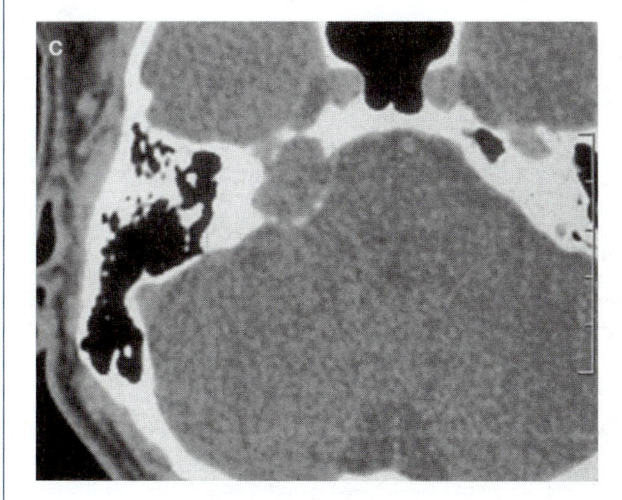

FIGURE 40–5 • Cholesteatoma. *A,* Magnetic resonance image (MRI), axial view, fast-spin T_2 image without contrast demonstrates a hyperintense, homogeneous, expansile lesion of the right petrous apex. *B, C,* Sagittal MRI, axial CT views of same lesion.

CLINICAL EVALUATION

Ipsilateral retro-orbital pain is relatively specific for petrous apex disease, but some patients present with ear pain or pressure and temporoparietal headache. Because headache and head pain from petrous apex cystic lesions are the most common presenting symptoms and otoscopy is often normal, the differential diagnosis of referred "ear" pain should be considered, especially when a small, nonexpansile petrous apex cyst is present on MRI but may not be the primary cause of the symptoms.

The facial nerve refers pain to the external ear canal and postauricular region. The second and third cervical nerves refer pain to the postauricular and mastoid regions. Trigeminal referred otalgia arises from lesions involving the oral cavity and floor of the mouth, teeth, mandible, temporomandibular joint (TMJ), palate, and preauricular skin. Glossopharyngeal referred otalgia arises from the tonsil, base of the tongue, soft palate, nasopharynx, eustachian tube, and pharynx. Vagal referred otalgia arises from the hypopharynx, larynx, and trachea. Differential causes of referred otalgia include migraine, TMJ syndrome, cervical myalgia, fibromyalgia, dental abscess, head and neck malignancy (particularly occult neoplasm of the nasopharynx, sinus, tonsil, base of the tongue, and hypopharynx), temporal arteritis, inflammatory sinusitis, carotidynia, trigeminal neuralgia, glossopharyngeal neuralgia, and gastroesophageal reflux disease.

Patients with ear pain and/or temporoparietal headache should have careful examination of the auricle and otoscopic examination of the external and middle ear. If the ear is normal, the anterior nares, oral cavity, oropharynx, laryngohypopharynx, neck, and scalp should be examined. The TMJ, temporal artery, tonsillar fossa, base of the tongue, carotid artery, and neck muscles should be carefully palpated for tenderness, mass, or spasm. The teeth can be percussed for tenderness. In selected cases, radiographic examination of the teeth, jaw, and sinuses can be obtained. If no cause is identified at this point, we recommend MRI of the brain and base of the skull (including infratemporal fossa) in both axial and coronal views, with and without gadolinium contrast enhancement.

MRI can reveal a petrous apex cystic lesion, encephalocele, or arachnoid cyst. CT scanning can be obtained to identify bone destruction or bone marrow fat in asymmetric pneumatization. CT can also be useful in delineating hypotympanic air cells in situations for which an infracochlear drainage procedure is considered (see in a later section). A cystic lesion of the petrous apex may be the only abnormality on clinical and radiographic evaluation. If other causes of ear pain and headache have been excluded (sometimes a treatment trial for migraine is warranted), then surgery can be considered. Surgery is indicated when the patient is symptomatic, when other causes are ruled out, and particularly when CT scan shows the lesion to be expansile and eroding bone. Patients with expansile lesions usually present with headache or head pain, and less often with neurologic symptoms. If the clinician is uncertain whether an apical cyst is the cause of symptoms, CT or MRI can be repeated in 6 months to check for cyst growth and bone destruction. If surgery is recommended, risks and benefits depend on the type

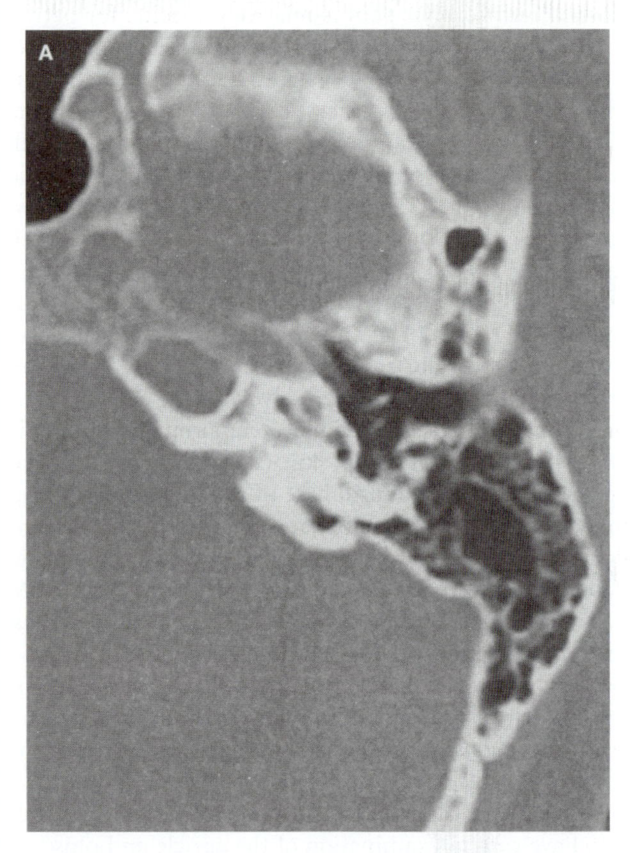

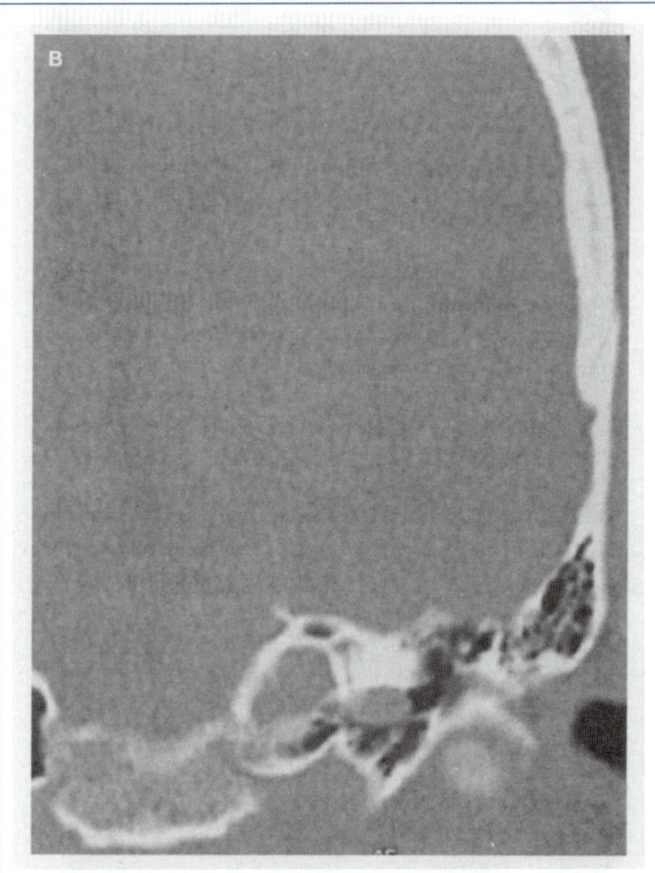

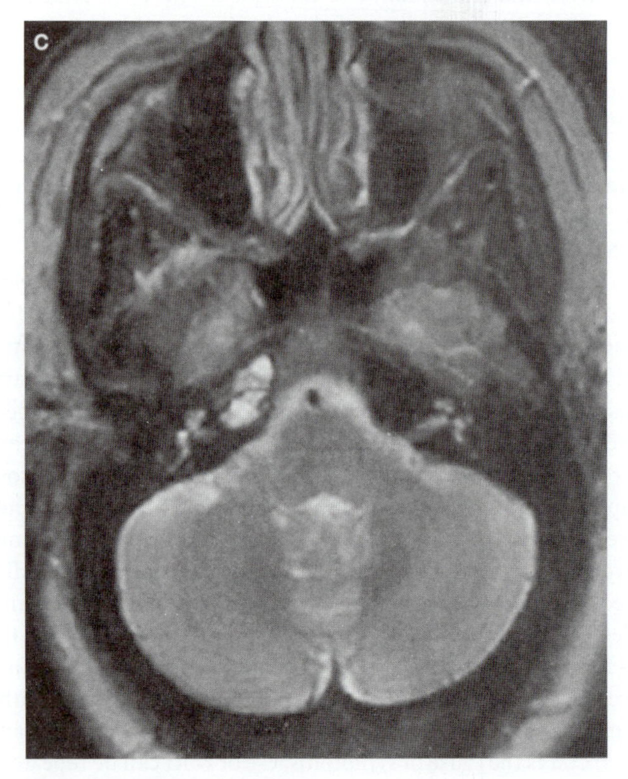

FIGURE 40–6 • Retained fluid (effusion). *A*, Axial high-resolution computed tomographic (CT) scan demonstrates a sharply marginated mass in the left petrous apex. There is a thin rim of sclerosis that is best appreciated along the anterior margins, suggesting a slow-growing lesion. Although confluent in nature, there is no apparent bony expansion into the epidural space. Magnetic resonance imaging (MRI) could be done to confirm the cystic nature of the lesion. *B*, Corresponding coronal CT scan confirms the confluent nature without apparent expansion. *C*, Axial T_2-weighted MRI from a different patient with retained fluid in the air cells of the right petrous apex. This lesion does not have the same cystic appearance as the lesion in the patient in Figure 40–6, A and B. The linear hypointense foci in the large bright lesion represent visible septae and/or inflammatory reactive changes in the air cells that contrast against the long T_2 of the fluid.

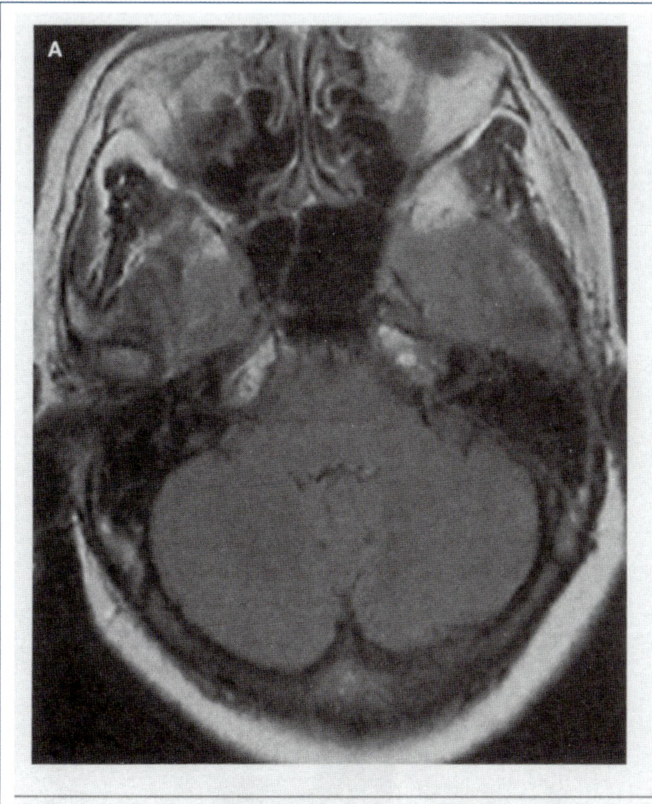

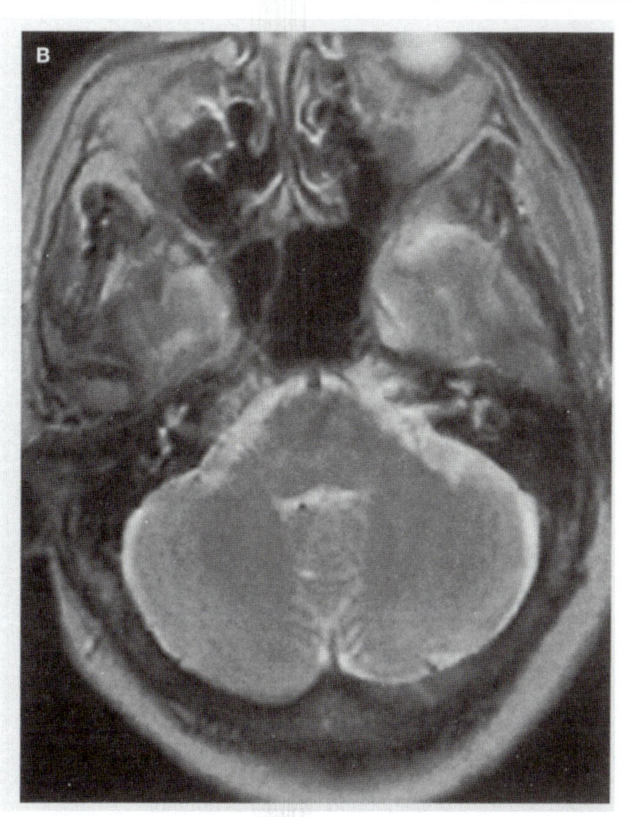

FIGURE 40–7 • Fatty bone marrow. *A*, Axial fast fluid-attenuated inversion recovery image with mildly hyperintense signal in each petrous apex that is symmetric and identical in signal to the subcutaneous fat and the fat in the marrow of the occipital bone. *B*, On the axial fast T_2-weighted image, the petrous apices are mildly hyperintense but relatively symmetric and comparable to the signal of the marrow in the occipital bone.

and size of the cyst, surgical excision or drainage, level of hearing, and approach selected.

SURGICAL APPROACH

For hearing preservation, the middle cranial fossa, infracochlear (hypotympanic), and transsphenoidal approaches can be used for management of benign, non-neoplastic, and cystic lesions of the petrous apex.[28] For very large lesions, when additional exposure and control of the carotid artery are required, the transcochlear approach can be used with extension into the infratemporal fossa if necessary.[29] Because MRI provides very sensitive, early detection of smaller apical lesions, the transcochlear-infratemporal fossa approach is rarely needed. Surgical management of cholesteatoma differs from that of cholesterol granuloma and is covered more fully in the section on Discussion.

The middle cranial fossa (transpetrosal) approach (Figure 40–8) to the petrous apex[30] is used to excise rather than simply drain the cyst and is the procedure of choice when the cyst location and lack of hypotympanic pneumatization make the infracochlear approach difficult. The middle cranial fossa approach provides good access to the cyst for total excision in many cases except those cysts that extend inferiorly or those that encircle the carotid artery. After general anesthesia is administered, a subarachnoid drain is placed, and 80 cc of cerebrospinal fluid (CSF) are removed slowly to relax the temporal lobe during elevation to expose the middle fossa floor. The drain is then clamped and removed at the end of surgery. The patient is placed supine with the head in points, and facial and auditory monitoring electrodes are placed. A subtemporal, 6-cm vertical incision extends superiorly from the zygomatic process, 1 cm anterior to the external auditory canal (see Figure 40–8). A 3-cm × 2.5-cm bone flap is removed, and the temporal lobe is elevated extradurally to reveal the foramen spinosum anteriorly, arcuate eminence posteriorly, and superior petrosal sinus medially. Temporal lobe traction is gently maintained with a Greenberg retractor. The GSPN is identified and followed posteriorly to the geniculate ganglion, which is confirmed with the facial nerve stimulator. The basal turn of the cochlea lies just anterior and medial to the ganglion and must be avoided to minimize the risk of postoperative hearing loss.

Between the foramen spinosum and arcuate eminence, the GSPN divides the petrous apex into the lateral Glasscock's triangle and the medial Kawase's triangle.[30,31] Glasscock's triangle is formed laterally by a line from the foramen spinosum toward the arcuate eminence, ending at the facial hiatus, medially by the GSPN, and at the base, the mandibular division of the trigeminal nerve. Kawase's triangle is formed laterally by the GSPN, medially by the petrous ridge (superior petrosal sinus), and has its base anteriorly near the cavernous sinus. The middle fossa approach uses Kawase's triangle to identify petrous apical cysts. The GSPN is preserved to avoid postoperative dry eye; however, in large lesions, the GSPN can be sacrificed to

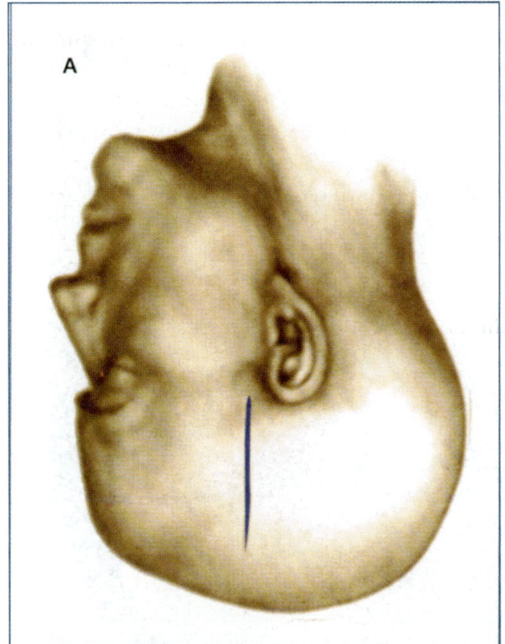

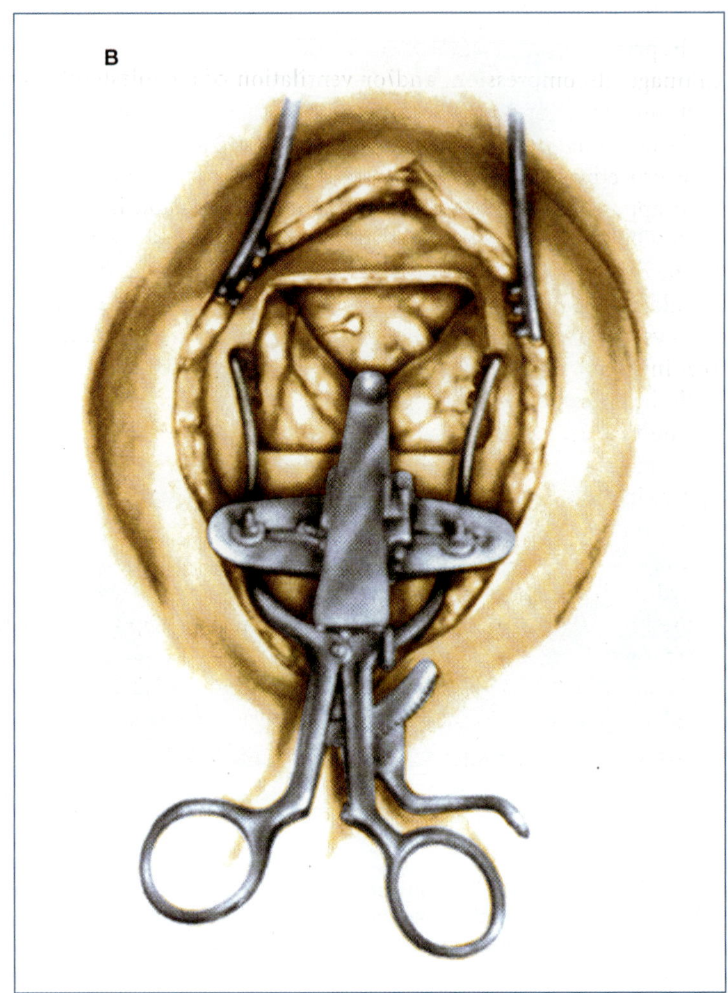

FIGURE 40–8 • Middle cranial fossa approach, right ear, surgical position. A 6-cm vertical incision is made 1 cm anterior to the external auditory canal and superior to the zygoma. A temporal craniotomy is performed one-third posterior and two-thirds anterior to this line. Dura is elevated to the middle meningeal artery anteriorly, arcuate eminence posteriorly, and superior petrosal sinus medially to expose Kawase's and Glasscock's triangles. Bone of the floor of the middle cranial fossa is removed anterior to the basal turn of the cochlea and internal auditory canal (see text for cyst removal and wound closure).

provide greater exposure. Manipulation of the GSPN should be minimized to avoid potential postoperative facial weakness. Just deep to the GSPN is the petrous carotid artery, which can be distinguished from cyst wall by its location, pulsation, and more reddish color. Just lateral to the artery is the Eustachian tube, which also should be preserved if possible. Any entry (intentional or accidental) into the eustachian tube must be recognized and appropriately repaired or packed to prevent postoperative CSF otorhinorrhea in the event that the dura is violated during craniotomy or during extradural middle fossa floor dissection.

Removal of bone proceeds anterior to the basal turn of the cochlea, down to the cyst wall with identification and preservation of the GSPN, carotid artery, and eustachian tube. The wall of the most common cystic lesion, cholesterol granuloma, is usually bluish and nonpulsatile but can be fibrotic and surprisingly thick. The cyst wall is exposed as much as possible and then opened. Thick, brown-black fluid fills the cholesterol granuloma and is suctioned out. The walls of the cyst are gently probed with a blunt dissector to identify the anatomic extent of the cyst. Mattox[32] recommends fiber-optic endoscopic visualization and cleaning of the cyst interior at this point. Traversing the center of larger cysts is the carotid artery, which must be carefully preserved. The cyst wall is removed by blunt dissection as much as the artery will permit. The posterior extension of the cyst may encroach on the cochlea and internal auditory canal. When bony drilling for cyst exposure passes deep to the basal turn of the cochlea, 2- to 3-mm additional bone then can be removed posteriorly toward the internal canal without violating the cochlea. Here also the cyst wall can be preserved to minimize postoperative sensorineural hearing loss.

The retractor is removed, and the temporal lobe is allowed to re-expand onto the middle fossa floor. The bone flap is refixed with miniplates and screws. The temporalis muscle fascia layer is closed with #2–0 Neuralon suture, the subcutaneous tissues with #3–0 Vicryl suture, and the skin with running (not locked) #3–0 Dermalon suture. A local drain is not needed. A large, sterile compression dressing is applied over the ear and side of the head. If the lesion is a cholesterol cyst or mucocele caused by inadequate ventilation through the air cells (or if the eustachian tube is packed), a pressure-equalizing (PE) tube can be placed across the drum. If it is an epidermoid cyst, a PE tube is not placed. The subarachnoid drain is removed in the operating room. Systemic antibiotics are not needed. The patient usually is ready for discharge after 2 or 3 days, at which time the dressing is removed. Postoperatively at 10 days, the skin sutures are removed, and an audiogram can be obtained.

The infracochlear-hypotympanic approach (Figure 40–9) to the petrous apex[33] is a more conservative procedure to provide drainage, decompression, and/or ventilation of a cholesterol cyst, mucocele, or trapped fluid (effusion), but not excision, and would not be used for an epidermoid cyst (cholesteatoma). This procedure is relatively safer and simpler than the middle fossa approach because it avoids dissection and possible injury to the GSPN, facial nerve, and Eustachian tube and has less risk to the carotid artery and inner ear. Preoperatively, a CT scan should be obtained to reveal adequate pneumatization between the cyst wall and the hypotympanum. General anesthesia is administered, and the patient is placed in the supine position with the operated ear upward, as in chronic ear surgery. Points, monitoring leads, and subarachnoid drainage are not needed. A superiorly based, radial incision is made in the ear canal approximately 8 mm lateral to the annulus. A postauricular incision is then carried down to temporalis areolar tissue and fascia, and a 2- × 2.5-cm piece of either tissue is obtained and dehydrated on a block for later use. The mastoid periosteum is incised in a standard "T" fashion, and the anterior flap is elevated toward and down the posterior canal wall until the radial incision is reached. The auricle and lateral external auditory canal skin are retracted anteriorly. The inferior three-quarters of the medial canal skin are then elevated to enter the middle ear but are left attached to the umbo of the malleus. A drill is used to remove additional inferior tympanic ring to enlarge the hypotympanic exposure. Drilling then proceeds inferior and medial to the cochlea, between the anterior carotid artery and the posterior jugular bulb. As the cholesterol granuloma is entered, dark fluid is removed. The air cells connecting the middle ear with the apex can be gently curetted or drilled to enhance postoperative drainage. A short, Silastic® catheter is placed into the connecting air cells. Temporalis fascia or areolar tissue is used to line and reinforce the enlarged inferior annular ring, and the tympanic membrane is replaced in its normal position. A PE tube can be placed and the canal filled with antibiotic ointment. The postauricular tissues are closed in two layers using absorbable suture. A sterile mastoid dressing is left on for one night, and the patient can be discharged home later that day or in the morning the next day. Systemic antibiotics are not needed.

The transsphenoidal approach is useful in selected cases.[34,35] The anatomic relationship between the cyst and sphenoid sinus must be favorable to consider this surgical strategy; ie, the cyst must lie just deep to the posterolateral sphenoid wall. From a practical perspective, this anatomic configuration reflects the impact of cyst size and sphenoid pneumatization. A relatively large cyst is more likely to have a close relationship to the sphenoid sinus, and similarly, a well-pneumatized sphenoid sinus is more likely to be immediately adjacent to even a small cyst. If there is any suggestion of cavernous sinus (or carotid artery) between the cyst and sphenoid sinus walls, a transsphenoidal procedure should not be considered.

The traditional transsphenoidal technique involves a transseptal route to the sphenoid sinus with microscopic visualization; however, more recently, pure endoscopic techniques have supplanted microscopic, transseptal-transsphenoidal procedures at many institutions. Intraoperative surgical navigation,[36,37] especially with fusion of CT and MRI images greatly facilitates the transsphenoidal procedure. The steps to achieve surgical drainage of the cyst are straightforward. After extended sphenoidotomy, the lateral and superior walls of the sphenoid sinus are examined for indentations of the pituitary gland, optic nerve, maxillary nerve, and carotid artery. Surgical navigation will simplify recognition of often subtle characteristics of the contour of the sphenoid sinus wall. Cyst drainage is achieved by merely opening the sphenoid sinus wall overlying the cyst. The mucosa ideally is sharply divided and reflected. Gentle palpation with a curette will often open the cyst, but more aggressive bone removal with a diamond drill may be required. After creation of the initial opening, through-cutting instruments may be used to enlarge it. Care must be taken to avoid injury to the nearby cavernous sinus and carotid artery, since inadvertent trauma can lead to catastrophic consequences. Placement of soft stent, which can be left in place for a few weeks or even months, may reduce the risk of closure.

The transcochlear approach (Figure 40–10) to the petrous apex[29,38] provides greater exposure and control of the carotid artery for large lesions but is rarely required for benign primary apical cysts when they are detected early by MRI. The translabyrinthine–transcochlear approach (subtotal petrosectomy, Figure 40–11) is a variation that combines transmastoid and cervical approaches. In both the transcochlear and translabyrinthine approaches, the patient is positioned supine with the head turned to the side. Facial nerve monitor leads are placed. Points, auditory monitoring, and subarachnoid drainage are not needed. The lower left quadrant of the abdomen is prepared for a fat graft. First, the skin of the lateral ear canal is incised radially. Then an anteriorly based, gently curved "C"-shaped incision is carried from the temporoparietal area down two finger-breadths behind the auricle and then continued into a natural skin crease of the neck. As the flap is elevated to the ear canal at the level of the temporalis fascia superiorly and periosteum inferiorly, a small flap of mastoid periosteum anteriorly based on the ear canal also is elevated with the flap. The skin flap, periosteal flap, auricle, and lateral ear canal are elevated to the anterior border of the parotid gland. The cartilaginous canal is everted and closed, and the periosteal flap is sutured medially across the canal remnant to provide a second layer closure. Through the neck incision, the carotid artery, jugular vein, and related cranial nerves are identified and followed superiorly to the base of the skull. A complete mastoidectomy is performed, and the bony canal wall, tympanic membrane, and ossicles are removed. Middle ear mucosa is removed, and the eustachian tube is obliterated. The facial nerve is removed from its canal from the geniculate ganglion proximally to the stylomastoid foramen distally and is rerouted anteriorly to enhance transcochlear exposure to the apex. As the cochlea is removed, the carotid artery is carefully exposed and followed through its petrous portion to the clivus.[39,40] If additional anterior exposure and mobilization of the artery are required, the transcochlear approach can be extended into the infratemporal fossa by dislocating or sectioning the mandibular condyle forward

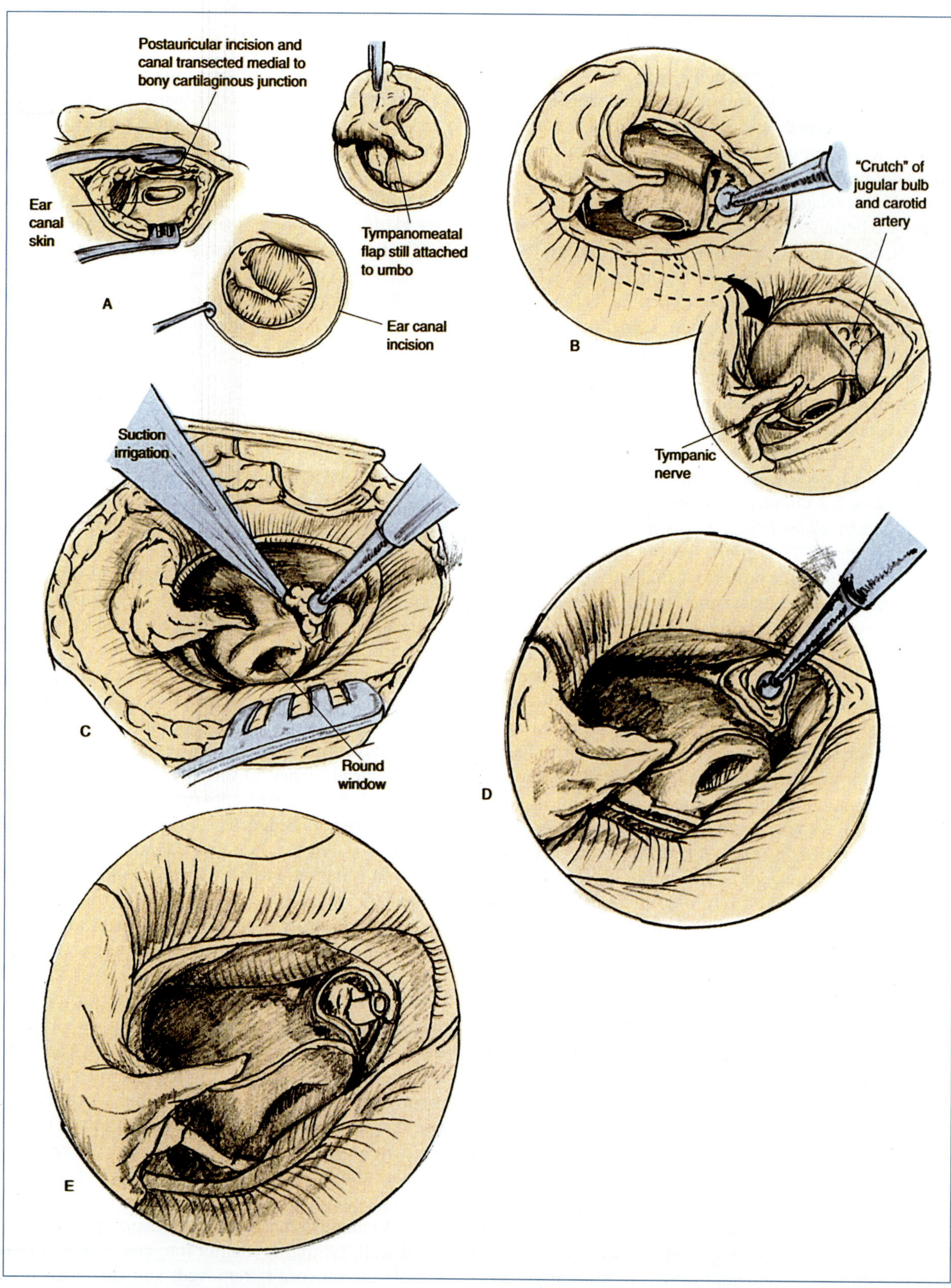

FIGURE 40–9 • Schematic view of the infracochlear-hypotympanic approach, right ear, surgical position. *A*, Superiorly based, radial incision is made transcanal. A postauricular incision is made and temporalis fascia harvested. The pinna and lateral canal skin are retracted forward. The remaining medial canal skin and tympanic membrane are elevated superiorly with the eardrum attached to the malleus. *B*, The bony external auditory canal is enlarged inferiorly to expose the hypotympanum. Bone is removed medially inferior to the cochlear promontory to identify the carotid artery anteriorly and the jugular bulb posteriorly. *C*, Hypotympanic bone removal proceeds medially between the carotid artery and jugular bulb into the anterior petrous apex air cells (D and E). The cholesterol granuloma cyst is reached and drained. A silastic catheter is placed into the cyst to maintain drainage. Temporalis fascia is used to reinforce the inferior canal defect in an underlay grafting technique, the tympanic membrane is returned to its normal position, and the ear canal is filled with antibiotic ointment (if Eustachian tube function has returned to normal, a PE tube may not be required). The postauricular incision is closed.

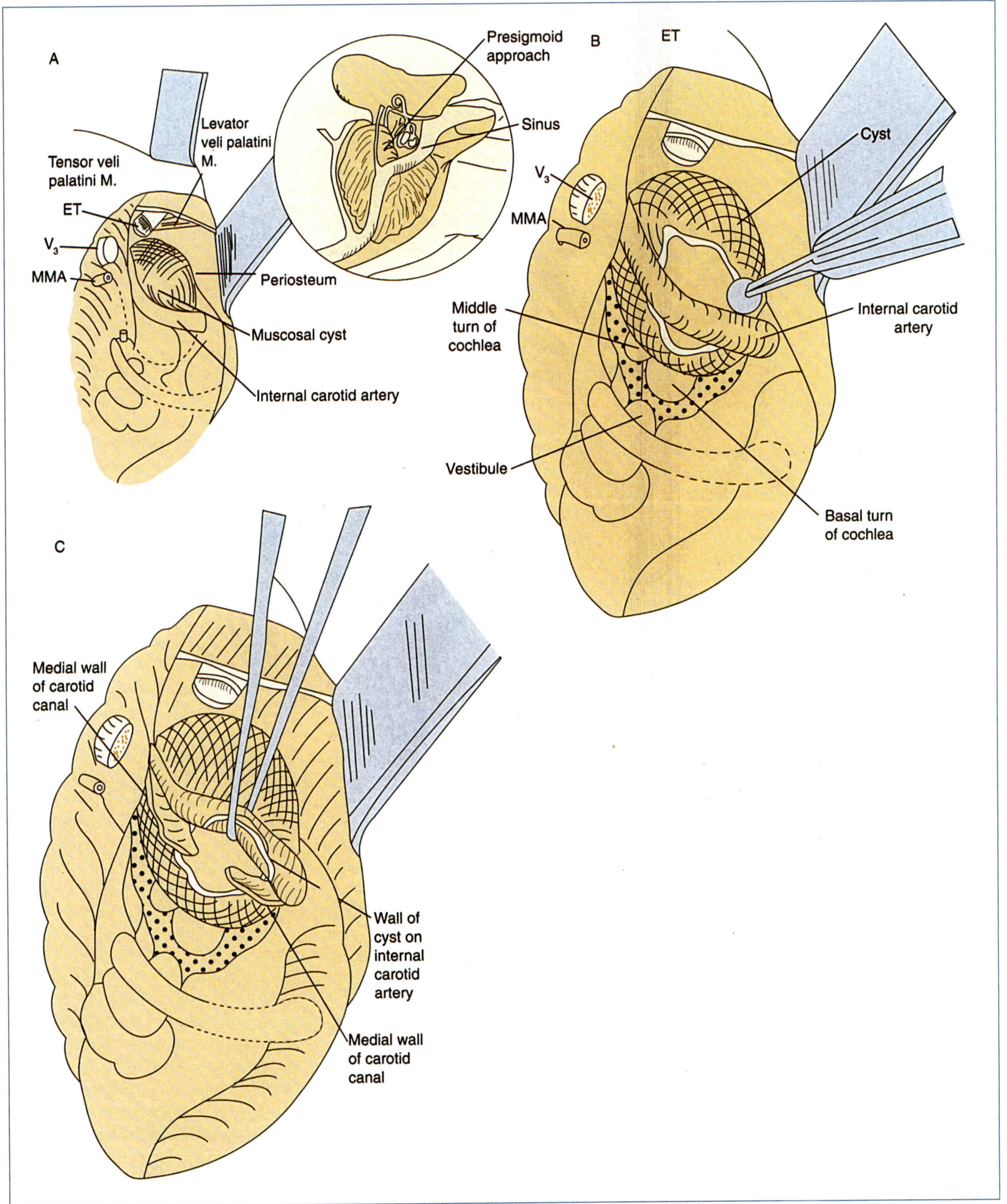

FIGURE 40–10 • Schematic view of the transcochlear approach, right ear, surgical position. *A*, The ear canal is transected and an anteriorly based, "C"-shaped flap is elevated forward to the parotid gland. The canal is then everted and closed. A radical mastoidectomy is performed with rerouting of the facial nerve anteriorly (optional), removal of the cochlea, and identification of the carotid artery. The cholesterol granuloma cyst (or cholesteatoma) is seen anterior and medial to the artery. *B*, The cyst is opened and drained. Additional bone is removed around the cyst. The Eustachian tube (ET) is transected and packed. The mandibular division of the trigeminal nerve can be divided if necessary for additional exposure. *C*, The cyst wall is resected by working anterior and posterior to the carotid artery. The artery can be retracted gently if necessary. The surgical defect is obliterated with abdominal fat and the wound closed.

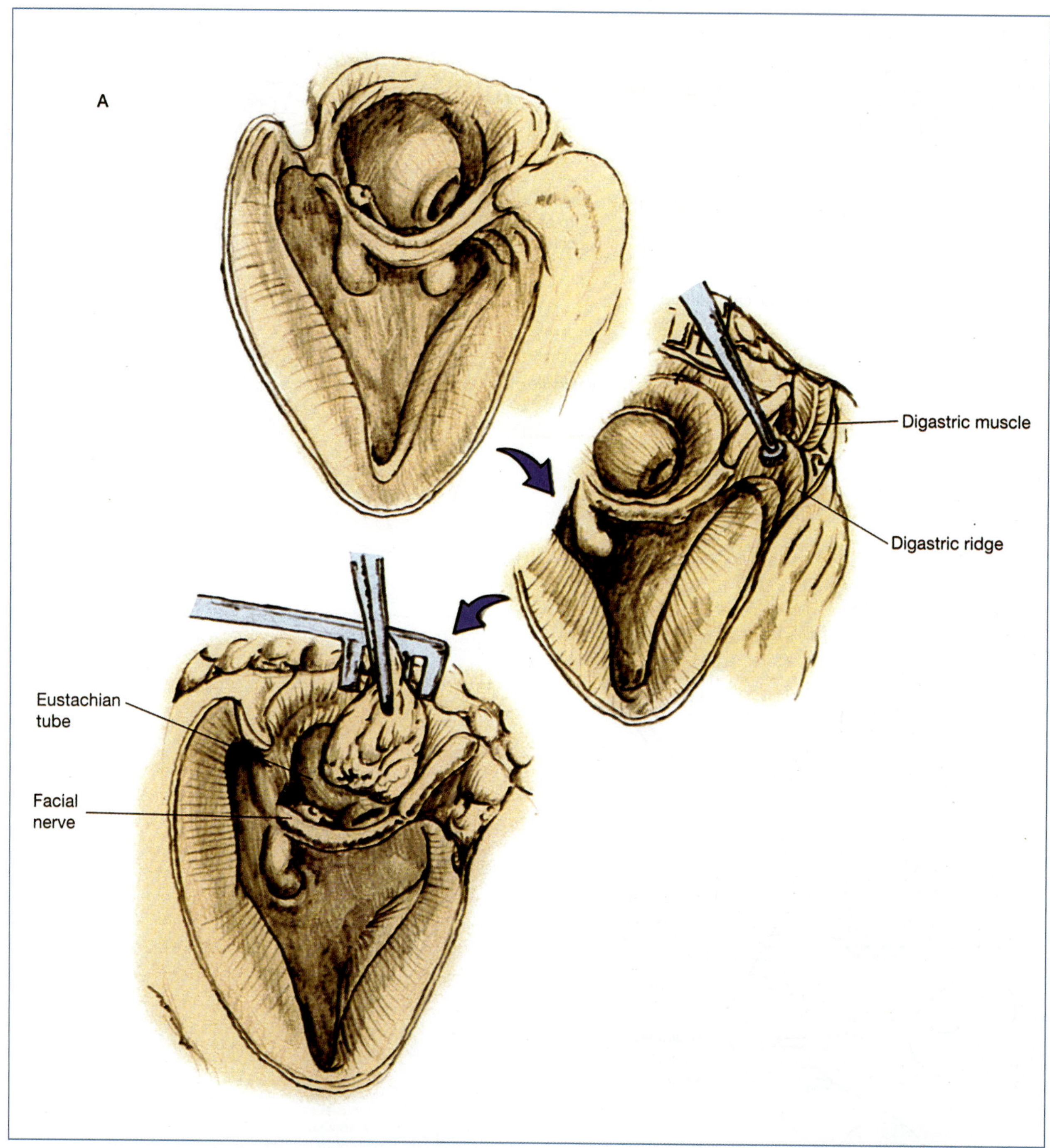

FIGURE 40–11 • Schematic view of the translabyrinthine/transcochlear approach (subtotal petrosectomy), right ear, surgical position. *A*, The ear canal is transected and a standard postauricular incision is made. The canal skin is everted and closed.

Continued

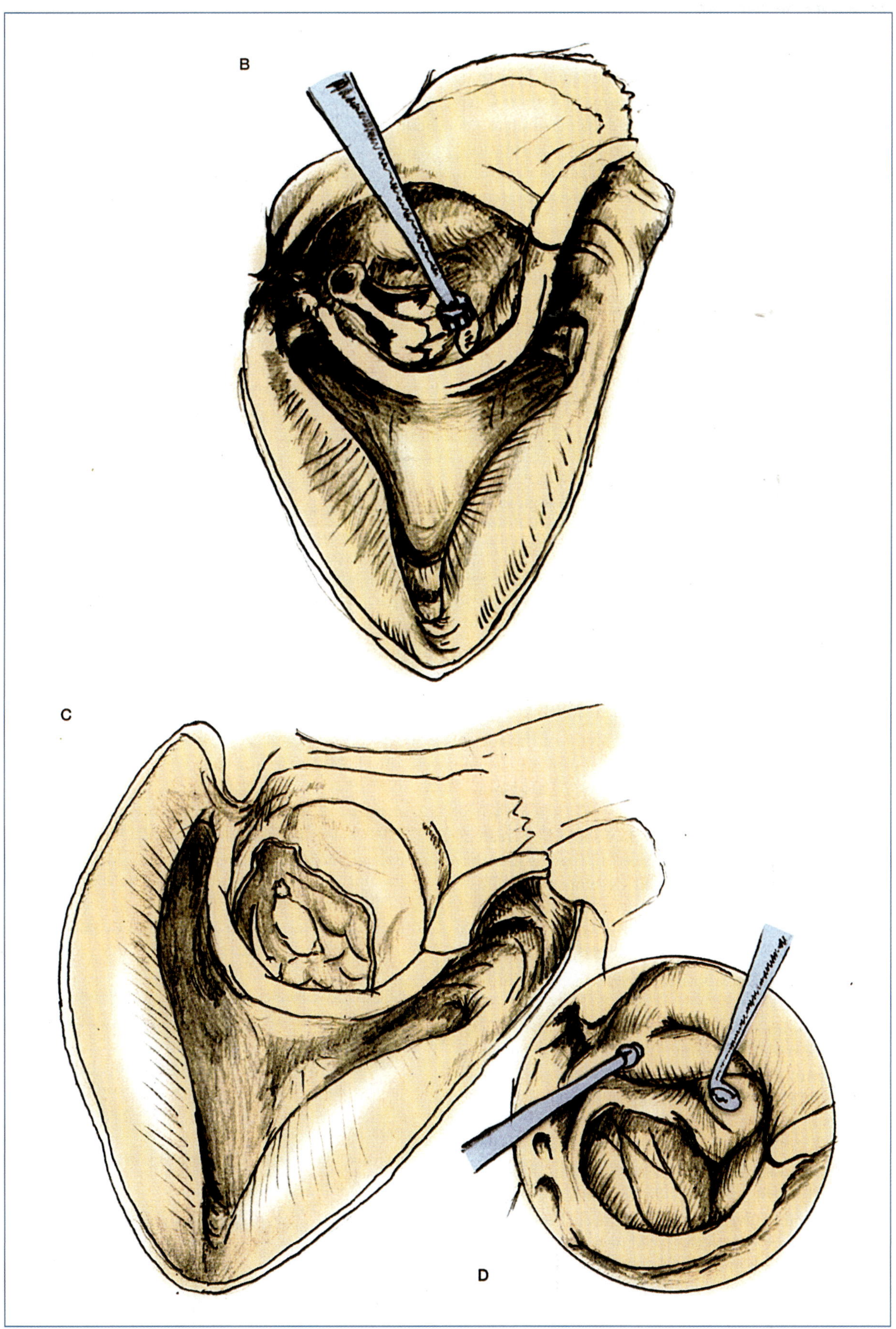

FIGURE 40–11 • *Continued. B*, A radical mastoidectomy is performed with removal of the remaining canal skin and tympanic membrane. The bony labyrinth and cochlea are removed. The facial nerve can be rerouted anteriorly (optional). *C*, The cholesterol granuloma cyst (or cholesteatoma) is resected posterior to the carotid artery. The eustachian tube is obliterated and the remaining middle ear mucosa is removed. *D*, The defect is obliterated with abdominal fat and a flap of temporalis muscle is rotated inferiorly and secured laterally to the fat. The postauricular incision is closed.

and by sectioning the mandibular branch of the trigeminal nerve, eustachian tube, and middle meningeal artery. Cyst removal is extradural. The temporal bone defect is obliterated with abdominal fat covered by a temporalis muscle rotation flap. Suction drainage catheters are left in place (away from the facial nerve), and the flap is closed in two layers. Systemic antibiotics are optional.

DISCUSSION

Management of a cystic lesion of the petrous apex can be difficult and controversial.[41] Is the cyst causing the symptoms or is it coincidental? When is surgery indicated? If it is cholesterol granuloma, should it be drained or resected? If it is cholesteatoma, is subtotal removal helpful? Does total resection for either lesion justify the morbidity of a transcochlear/infratemporal fossa approach with carotid artery dissection?

Is the petrous apex abnormality causing the symptoms, or is it coincidental? When the head, neck, and neurotologic examinations in the office are normal, we recommend a gadolinium-contrasted MRI of the brain, base of the skull, and infratemporal fossa in both axial and coronal views. The clinician should bear in mind that an "abnormal" petrous apex finding on MRI may or may not be the cause of symptoms.[24] A comparison of T_1- and T_2-weighted images often provides the diagnosis, and the size of the lesion suggests whether it is expansile. When in doubt, however, the clinician also should order a CT scan to further characterize the lesion.

When is surgery indicated for a cystic lesion of the apex? Surgery is indicated when the patient is symptomatic, when other causes are excluded, and particularly when CT also shows that the lesion is expansile and eroding bone. Patients with small lesions often have no symptoms; they should be treated conservatively. MRI or CT can be repeated in 6 or 12 months for comparison or sooner if the patient develops symptoms. Patients with expansile lesions present most often with headache or head pain and less often with middle ear effusion, sensorineural hearing loss, and/or dizziness. If the history and examination do not indicate another cause, surgery should be recommended.

General principles of surgical management are to (1) adequately drain or resect the lesion, (2) preserve hearing when possible, and (3) minimize the risk of cranial nerve and carotid artery injury and CSF leak. Should cholesterol granuloma be drained or resected? Drainage through the hypotympanic/infracochlear approach is fast, safe, and simple but, in our experience, may not provide long-term control of symptoms. Resection (total or near total) through the middle fossa has more risk to hearing if the surgeon inadvertently enters the cochlea or internal auditory canal, more risk to the facial nerve, and more risk to the carotid artery, which may be surrounded by cyst. We carefully identify and protect the carotid artery, leaving small remnants of cyst wall on the artery when necessary to minimize risk. Conservative, near-total removal offers good long-term control with minimal morbidity from surgery. Therefore, we recommend that the surgeon present both middle fossa and infracochlear/hypotympanic options to the patient and then help guide the final decision depending on the preference of the patient and the specifics of each case. If symptoms recur after a hypotympanic drainage procedure, the hypotympanic catheter can again be examined and replaced surgically (sometimes it slips or plugs), or resection can be recommended through the middle cranial fossa.

Is total removal of cholesteatoma necessary to provide long-term relief? Simple drainage is not helpful since the pathogenesis of (solid) cholesteatoma is different from that of (fluid) cholesterol granuloma. Total resection is frequently possible when the lesion is small and separate from the carotid artery; however, small lesions usually are not symptomatic. Large, expansile lesions warrant surgery but surround the carotid artery and tend to recur if not totally removed. The risk to the carotid artery can be minimized by increasing exposure through the transcochlear/infratemporal fossa approach, which allows gentle manipulation and circumferential dissection of the petrous carotid artery but sacrifices hearing. However, the morbidity of this combined approach is not justified unless the ear is already deaf and the cholesteatoma is massive. We generally recommend subtotal resection of cholesteatoma through a middle fossa approach when the expansile lesion is still confined to the temporal bone and when hearing is good. Residual cholesteatoma may not grow because of interruption of its blood supply, can be followed by serial MRI, and can later be reoperated. Presenting symptoms can be controlled and morbidity minimized by this more conservative approach.

References

1. Muckle RP, De La Cruz A, Lo W. Petrous apex lesions. Am J Otol 1998;19:219–25.
2. Arriaga MA, Brackmann DE. Differential diagnosis of primary petrous apex lesions. Am J Otol 1992;13(3):470–4.
3. Roland PS, Meyerhoff WL, Judge LO, Mickey BE. Asymmetric pneumatization of the petrous apex. Otolaryngol Head Neck Surg 1990;103(1):80–8.
4. Moore KR, Harnsberger HR, Shelton C, Davidson HC. 'Leave me alone' lesions of the petrous apex. Am J Neuroradiol 1998;19:733–8.
5. Cheung SW, Broberg TG, Jackler RK. Petrous apex arachnoid cyst: radiographic confusion with primary cholesteatoma. Am J Otol 1995;16:690–4.
6. Goldsmith AJ, Myssiorek D, Valderrama E, Patel M. Unifocal Langerhans' cell histiocytosis (eosinophilic granuloma) of the petrous apex. Arch Otolaryngol Head Neck Surg 1993;119:113–6.
7. Amedee RG, Gianoli GJ, Mann WJ. Petrous apex lesions. Skull Base Surg 1994;4(1):10–14.
8. Byrd MC, Hughes GB, Ruggieri PM, Lee J. Cystic lesions of the petrous apex. In: Hughes GB, Pensak ML, editors. Clinical Otology, 3rd ed. New York: Thieme Medical Publishers; 2007. p. 339–46.
9. Mosnier I, Cyna-Gorse F, Grayeli AB, et al. Management of cholesterol granulomas of the petrous apex based on clinical and radiologic evaluation. Otol Neurotol 2002;23(4):522–8.
10. Curtin HD, Som PM. The petrous apex. Otolaryngol Clin North Am 1995;28:473–96.
11. Flood LM, Kemink JL. Surgery in lesions of the petrous apex. Otolaryngol Clin North Am 1984;17:565–74.

12. Martin TP, Tzifa KT, Chavda S, Irving RM. A large and uncharacteristically aggressive cholesterol granuloma of the middle ear. J Laryngol Otol 2005;119(12):1001–3.
13. Rosca T, Bontas E, Vladescu TG, St Tihoan C, Gherghescu G. Clinical controversy in orbitary cholesteatoma. Ann Diag Path 2006;10(2):89–94.
14. Jackler RK, Cho M. A new theory to explain the genesis of petrous apex cholesterol granuloma. Otol Neurotol 2003;24: 96–106.
15. Pfister MHF, Jackler RF, Kunda L. Aggressiveness in cholesterol granuloma of the temporal bone may be determined by the vigor of its blood source. Otol Neuotol 2007;28(2):232–5.
16. Gacek RR. Diagnosis and management of primary tumors of the petrous apex. Ann Otol Rhinol Laryngol Suppl 1975;84(18):1–20.
17. Profant M, Steno J. Petrous apex cholesteatoma. Acta Otolaryngol 2000;120:164–7.
18. Atlas MD, Moffat DA, Hardy DG. Petrous apex cholesteatoma: Diagnostic and treatment dilemmas. Laryngoscope 1992;102:1363–8.
19. Chang P, Fagan PA, Atlas MD, Roche J. Imaging destructive lesions of the petrous apex. Laryngoscope 1998;108:599–604.
20. Visosky AMB, Isaacson B, Oghalai JS. Circumferential petrosectomy for petrous apicitis and cranial base osteomyelitis. Otol Neurotol 2006;27(7):1003–13.
21. Koral K, Dowling M. Petrous apicitis in a child: Computed tomography and magnetic resonance imaging findings. Clin Imaging 2006;30(2):137–9.
22. Cundiff JG, Djalilian HR, Mafee MF. Bilateral sequential petrous apicitis secondary to an anaerobic bacterium. Otolaryngol Head Neck Surg 2006;135(6):969–71.
23. Chole RA, Donald PJ. Petrous apicitis clinical indications. Ann Otol Rhinol Laryngol 1983;92:544–51.
24. Leonetti JP, Shownkeen H, Marzo SJ. Incidental petrous apex findings on magnetic resonance imaging. Ear Nose Throat J 2001;80:200–6.
25. Alexander AE Jr, Caldemeyer KS, Rigby P. Clinical and surgical application of reformatted high-resolution CT of the temporal bone. Neuroimag Clin N Amer 1998;8(3):631–50.
26. Pisaneschi MJ, Langer B. Congenital cholesteatoma and cholesterol granuloma of the temporal bone: Role of magnetic resonance imaging. Top Mag Res Imag 2000;11(2):87–97.
27. Fitzek C, Mewes T, Fitzek S, Mentzel HJ, Hunsche S, Stoeter P. Diffusion-weighted MRI of cholesteatomas of the temporal bone. J Mag Res Imag 2002;15(6):636–41.
28. Gianoli GJ, Amedee RG. Hearing results in surgery for primary petrous apex lesions. Otolaryngol Head Neck Surg 1994;111(3):250–7.
29. Fisch U, Mattox D. Pyramid apex: Mucosal cyst and epidermoid cyst. In: Microsurgery of the Skull Base. Fisch U, Mattox D, editors. New York: Thieme Medical Publishers; 1988. p. 304–13.
30. Miller CG. Transtemporal approach to the petrous apex. Neurosurg 1993;33:461–9.
31. Steward DL. Choo DI, Pensak ML. Selective indications for the management of extensive anterior epitympanic cholesteatoma via combined transmastoid/middle fossa approach. Laryngoscope 2000;110(10):1660–6.
32. Mattox DE. Endoscopic-assisted surgery of the petrous apex. Otolaryngol Head Neck Surg 2004;130(2):229–41.
33. Brackmann DE, Giddings NA. Drainage procedures for petrous apex lesions. In: Brackmann DE, Shelton C, Arriaga MA, editors. Otologic Surgery. Philadelphia, PA: WB Saunders; 1994. p. 572–7.
34. Chandra RK, Palmer JN. Epidermoids of the paranasal sinuses and beyond: Endoscopic management. Amer J Rhinol 2006;20(4):441–4.
35. Oyama K, Ikezono T, Tahara S, Shindo S, Kitamura T, Teramoto A. Petrous apex cholesterol granuloma treated via the endoscopic transsphenoidal approach. Acta Neurochirurgica 2007;149(3):299–302.
36. Van Havenbergh T, Koekelkoren E, De Ridder D, van de Heyning P, Verlooy J. Image guided surgery for petrous apex lesions. Acta Neurochirurgica 2003;145(9):737–42.
37. Gunkel AR, Vogele M, Martin A, Bale RJ, Thumfart WF, Freysinger W. Computer-aided surgery in the petrous bone. Laryngoscope 1999;109(11):1793–9.
38. Sanna M, DeDonato G, Taibah A, Russo A, Falconi M, Mancini F. Infratemporal fossa approaches to the lateral skull base. Keio J Med 1999;48(4):189–200.
39. Bockmuhl U, Khalil HS, Draf W. Clinicoradiological and surgical considerations in the treatment of cholesterol granuloma of the petrous pyramid. Skull Base J 2005;15(4):263–7.
40. Naguib MB, Sanna M. Subtemporal exposure of the intrapetrous internal carotid artery. An anatomical study with surgical application. J Laryngol Otol 1999;113(8):717–20.
41. Franklin DJ, Jenkins HA, Horowitz BL, Coker NJ. Management of petrous apex lesions. Arch Otolaryngol Head Neck Surg 1989;115:1121–5.

Surgery of the Skull Base

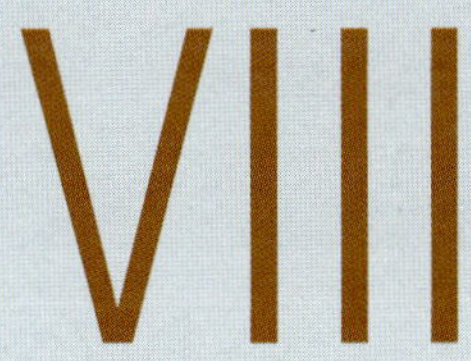

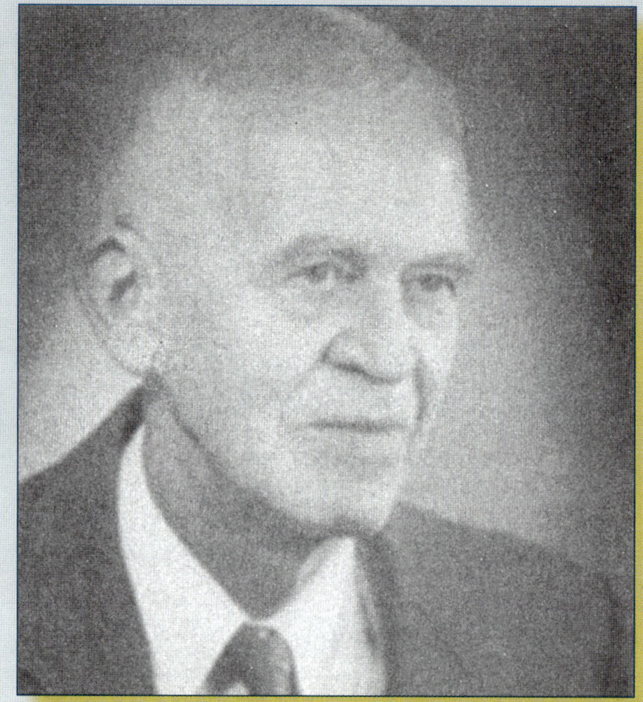

STACY RUFUS GUILD (1890-1966) •
Discovered the glomus jugularie, the site of origin of the most common neoplasm of the middle ear.

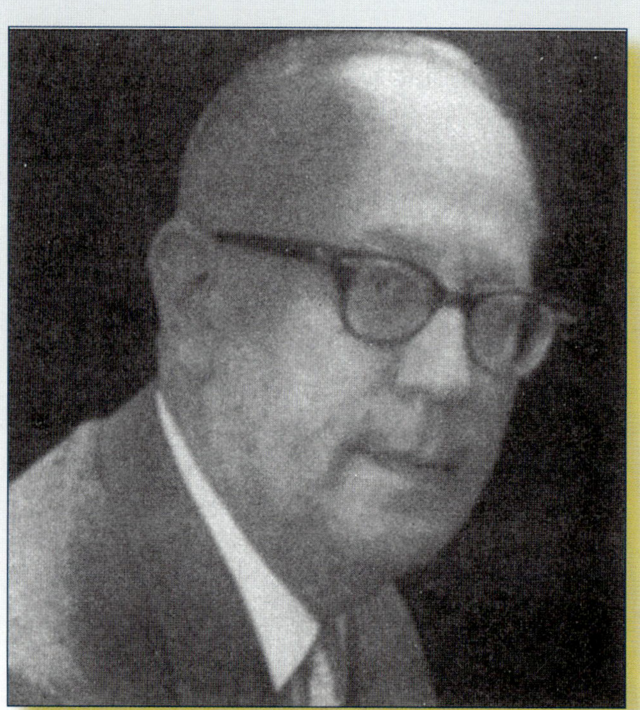

HARRY ROSENWASSER (BORN 1902) •
First described a vascular tumor of the middle ear as arising from the glomus jugularie.

Surgery for Benign Tumors of the Temporal Bone

41

C. Gary Jackson, MD, FACS / John P. Leonetti, MD / Sam J. Marz, MD

The evolution of surgery of the temporal bone (TB) has been based on and derived from technological advances concerned with the eradication of inflammatory disease of the middle ear (ME) and mastoid. Antibiotics, microsurgery, and amazing developments in neuroangiography and imaging have advanced neurotologic capabilities at an astonishing pace.

Even so, tumors of the TB continue to confound advanced management strategies and capacities. As part of the skull base, the TB is relatively inaccessible. Furthermore, regional consequences of TB pathology usually occur late. The deepest recesses of the TB appear to be anatomically privileged sites with pathology clinically betrayed only when it reaches the ME or the complex anatomy, which directly relates to its position at the lateral cranial base.

The embryology of TB is complex, reflecting the contribution of all germ layers. Consequently, a great variety of tumor cell types is possible, including both benign and malignant variants. Each is often unique and quite rare, disallowing any clinical familiarity with their diagnosis and/or management. Contemporary surgical protocols for benign lesions, notably glomus tumors (GTs), have led the way to a capacity that consistently emphasizes total tumor removal as well as maximization of postsurgical quality of life through minimization of cosmetic and neurologic loss. With neurosurgeons, head and neck surgeons, reconstruction specialists, and neuroradiologists, a collaborative approach to benign lesions has evolved; nonetheless, TB malignancy continues to be a formidable problem. Patients still die with progressive local disease, intolerable pain, neurologic loss, and all of the attributes of inanition so characteristic of the patient with terminal head and neck cancer.

This chapter examines tumors of the TB, cataloging rarer lesions and focusing on the most common benign lesion, the GT. The management concepts for GTs can be applied to rarer lesions.

ANATOMIC OVERVIEW

The four elements of the TB are petrosa (the petrous portion), squama (the squamous portion), mastoid bone, and tympanic bone. It constitutes the inferolateral skull base and is nearly completely formed at birth, completing development by age 3 years. In addition to its osseous structure, the TB contains almost every type of human tissue—epithelial, neural, epidermal, vascular, cartilaginous, and glandular.[1] Almost any tumor conceivable can arise within the TB. On its lateral-inferior surface lies the bony and cartilaginous external auditory canal (EAC). Lymphatics from the auricle and EAC drain into the parotid and pre- and retroauricular lymph nodes. Venous drainage is into the internal jugular vein.

The middle fossa dura overlies the superior surface. Anteromedially, the TB relates to the eustachian tube (ET), internal carotid artery (ICA), and the petrous ridge, with its superior petrosal sinus. The petrous apex houses the geniculate ganglion (GG), an embryologically diverse structure, which is a common site of origin of a variety of neoplasms. The nasopharynx has an important anatomic relationship with the TB. Posterior-medially is the petrous portion housing the internal auditory canal (IAC) and its contents. Anteriorly lie the glenoid fossa, the semi-canal of the tensor tympani muscle, and canal for the ICA. The infratemporal fossa (IFTF) is further anterior. The jugular bulb joins the internal jugular vein and the sigmoid sinus and is situated in the pars venosa of the petro-occipital fissure. Just anterior to the bulb is the pars nervosa containing cranial nerves IX, X, and XI. Adjacent to the bulb is the caroticojugular plate separating the jugular bulb from the ICA.[2]

The pneumatized spaces of the TB serve as a veritable superhighway for the spread of tumor, which varies as much in degree and extent as does the pneumatic pattern itself. The tympanic membrane (TM) offers some resistance to the medial spread of EAC pathology. The bone of the labyrinth is moderately resistant to tumor and serves as a temporary barrier. Along with the neurovascular structures, the foramen of Huschke, an incomplete closure of the tympanic ring, may also serve to permit tumor extent beyond the confines of the TB intracranially, into the parotid, into the IFTF, and vice versa. In addition to the major periauricular lymphatic drainage mentioned earlier, which is highly relevant in disease of the EAC, the ear is further served by upper cervical, deep jugular, postauricular, and posterior deep lymphatics. Although the inner ear has no known lymphatic drainage, the ME, mastoid, and ET drain into the deep jugular and retropharyngeal lymph nodes.[1] The significance of the lymphatics to TB tumors and their management is poorly understood.

TUMORS OF THE TEMPORAL BONE

A wide diversity of tumor types is encountered within the TB, each rarely; in fact, the occurrence of some tumors of the TB is so isolated as to constitute case report material. An outline based on anatomic site serves to superficially classify these lesions:

I. Tumors of the EAC
A. Benign
1. Osteoma
2. Exostosis
3. Fibrous dysplasia
4. Langerhans' cell histiocytosis (formerly called histiocytosis X)
5. Papilloma
6. Nerve sheath neoplasm
7. Paraganglioma
8. Hemangioma

II. Tumors of the ME
A. Benign
1. Adenoma
2. Meningioma
3. Chordoma
4. Paraganglioma
5. Hemangiopericytoma
6. Schwannoma

III. Tumors of the inner ear/petrous apex
A. Benign
1. Paraganglioma (GT)
2. Lipoma
3. Schwannoma
4. Hemangioma
5. Hemangiopericytoma
6. Cholesterol cyst of the petrous apex (formerly called granuloma)
7. Endolymphatic sac tumor

Next to the acoustic neuroma, the GT is the most common tumor encountered by today's neuro-otologists. Thankfully, TB carcinoma remains rare.

In general, benign TB lesions are slow-growing and insidious, producing minimal complaints until well advanced. The progression of these lesions can be so slow that neurologic symptoms undergo simultaneous compensation and therefore may be unnoticed by the patient. Inexorably and ultimately, these lesions produce cranial neuropathy and cause hearing loss, vestibular dysfunction, swallowing problems, dysphagia with glottic incompetence, facial nerve (FN) paresis, and ophthalmic disorders. Benign jugular foramen tumors can also cause referred otalgia, odynophagia, facial pain, or headaches.

The benign TB tumor is conceptually well represented by the GT, the diagnosis and management of which are applicable to rarer lesions.

Alternatively, patients presenting with otalgia, bloody or mucopurulent otorrhea, unresponsive external otitis, an EAC lesion/granulation tissue, or progressive cranial neuropathy, especially in the elderly with a long-term history of chronic otitis media, must be evaluated for malignancy and promptly biopsied. We deal with malignancy here generically only to differentiate it from its more benign counterpart.

Management of both benign and malignant disease is directed by disease type and extent. Complicated solutions are reserved only for complicated situations. Total tumor removal is paramount and, if possible, should be executed by protocols sufficiently flexible in scope to allow reasonable conservation of vital structures. When conservation is deemed impossible, strategies for defect reconstruction and cranial nerve rehabilitation must be planned preoperatively. A discussion of specific tumors follows the exposition of management concepts for benign lesions, as exemplified by the GT.

Glomus Tumors

Although GTs are generally benign and follow an indolent course, morbidity and mortality can occur by virtue of their location at the skull base adjacent to the posterior cranial fossa and the lower cranial nerves subserving coordination of deglutition and phonation.

Heretofore, the ability to diagnose these tumors far exceeded the ability to treat them. The evolution of treatment modalities has finally achieved parity with diagnostic technology. By consensus, the management of cranial-cervical GTs is surgical. The oncologically sound, primary objective is complete tumor resection for cure. Owing to the technical capacity of the day, issues of resectability have given way to issues of functional outcome, that is, the quality of postsurgical survival. The reconstruction of sizable defects, along with the rehabilitation of cranial nerve deficits, serves to minimize the most common ground on which surgery is most frequently criticized, the perceived risk of functional incapacity. Morbid consequences can be reliably predicted and outcomes controlled. Issues of intracranial extension (ICE) are well understood.

Nevertheless, the surgery versus radiation therapy (RT) and stereotactic radiosurgery (STS) debate continues to rage. The data to resolve this dilemma do not exist. Radiation therapy and STS offer low-morbidity conservation management strategies that ask the patient to coexist with a biologically altered tumor. This chapter reviews the surgical standardization that conceptually dominates GT surgery. Intracranial extension, management, defect reconstruction, and cranial nerve rehabilitation are addressed. Radiation therapy and STS are placed into perspective and covered in detail in Chapter 39.

Glomus Tumor Classification

To direct surgical planning and provide standards for reporting surgical results, a GT classification is necessary.

Oldring and Fisch,[3] in 1979, recognized this need and proposed an A, B, C, and D tumor classification system. This system was upgraded in 1982[4] to include ICE as subclasses of Types C and D lesions.

The Glasscock-Jackson[5] system of GT classification retained the familiar and clinically utilitarian tympanic and jugulare subclasses, expanding subclasses by tumor extent. Intracranial extension is expressed as a superscript; for example, GJ-Type IV$^{2.0}$ refers to a Type IV lesion with 2.0-cm ICE (Table 41–1).

Glomus Tumor Biology

The nomenclature of GT is in some disarray. The term "glomus" is a misnomer.[6] The initial thought that the tumor originated from true glomus complexes[6] has been discredited. It is now recognized that GTs arise from paraganglions, which are normally occurring structures usually found in close association with sympathetic ganglions along the aorta and its main branches. The chief cells of the paraganglions are of neural crest origin and are components of the diffuse neuroendocrine system (DNES). Glenner and Grimley[6] distinguished the adrenal paraganglion (the adrenal medulla) from extra-adrenal paraganglions. Paraganglion tumors (paragangliomas) also follow this classification. Recognizing the above, nonetheless the terms paraganglioma, GT, glomus tympanicum (GTy), and glomus jugulare (GJ) will be used interchangeably in this chapter.

The cranial-cervical (branchiomeric) paraganglions are distributed along the arterial vasculature and cranial nerves of the ontogenetic gill arches.[6] The branchiomeric paraganglions of prime interest to neuro-otologists are the jugulotympanic and intercarotid paraganglia. The intravagal paraganglion, as it is not intimately associated with arterial vasculature,[7] is not classified as a branchiomeric paraganglion.

The jugulotympanic paraganglions are ovoid, lobulated structures measuring 0.1 to 1.5 mm in diameter.[8] Vascularized by the inferior tympanic branch of the ascending pharyngeal artery, they number on average three per side and are found in association with Jacobson's and Arnold's nerves. The number of paraganglions does not correlate with race or sex, and more than 50% are located in the region of the jugular fossa. They are innervated by the glossopharyngeal nerve, whereas those along Arnold's nerve are thought to be innervated by the vagus nerve. Intravagal paraganglions, as scattered cell groups, occupy the epineurium of the vagus nerve. The paraganglions are well vascularized and are composed of clusters (Zellballen) of chief cells supported by sustentacular cells and small blood vessels.[9]

The ultrastructural appearance of paragangliomas mimics that of their paraganglions of origin.[6] Their chief cells contain cytoplasmic granules that store catecholamines.[7] Two types of chief cells, light and dark, are identified ultrastructurally.

Biochemistry

The chief cells of the paraganglions are 1 of 40 distinct cell types of the DNES, the cells of which have the capacity to produce catecholamines and neuropeptides that may serve as neurotransmitters, neurohormones, hormones, and parahormones.[9,10]

The metabolism of tyrosine is a key to the biochemistry of catecholamines.[6] Because paraganglions lack the enzyme phenylethanolamine-*N*-methyltransferase, usually norepinephrine accumulates[11]; however, a dopamine-secreting GT has been documented.[12] A GT secreting serotonin that provoked the carcinoid syndrome has been reported.[13] Neurohormones have been immunohistochemically documented in paraganglions and paragangliomas, including neuron-specific enolase (NSE), substance P, cholecystokinin, bombesin, chromogranin, vasoactive intestinal polypeptide, somatostatin, calcitonin, S-100 protein, melanocyte-stimulating hormone, and gastrin.[6]

Clinical Correlates

The biochemical capacity of the GT is indeed rich. Its potential to produce neuroendocrine secretory products permits anticipation of a variable clinical symptomatology, and those tumors that secrete sufficient quantities are known as "functional" tumors or "secretors."

Every patient with a GT (except those with small GTy tumors) undergoes measurement of serum catecholamine levels and urinary metabolites. Functioning paragangliomas occur in 1 to 3% of cases.[12] Norepinephrine levels elevated three to five times normal are generally required to produce the symptoms and signs of catecholamine secretion, such as headaches, excessive perspiration, palpitations, pallor, and nausea.[12] Rarely, the carcinoid syndrome may be encountered. The detection of

TABLE 41–1 Glasscock-Jackson glomus tumor classification

TYPE	PHYSICAL FINDINGS
Glomus tympanicum	
Type I	Small mass limited to the promontory
Type II	Tumor completely filling middle ear space
Type III	Tumor filling middle ear and extending into mastoid process
Type IV	Tumor filling middle ear, extending into mastoid or through tympanic membrane to fill external auditory canal; may extend anterior to internal carotid artery
Glomus jugulare	
Type I	Small tumor involving jugular bulb, middle ear, and mastoid process
Type II	Tumor extending under internal auditory canal; may have intracranial extension
Type III	Tumor extending into petrous apex; may have intracranial extension
Type IV	Tumor extending beyond petrous apex into clivus or infratemporal fossa; may have intracranial extension

elevated epinephrine levels mandates computed tomography (CT) of the adrenal glands or selective renal vein sampling to rule out pheochromocytoma.

Perioperative management is essential to safeguard against the mortal consequences of catecholamine overload on anesthesia induction or intraoperatively on tumor manipulation. Modern protocols for pharmacologic blockade employed for a pheochromocytoma are used. Alpha- and beta-blockade beginning 2 weeks preoperatively has been abandoned.

Paraneoplastic syndromes associated with other neurohormones (anemia, gastrointestinal symptoms, etc.) must be sought and identified.

The presence of immunoreactive peptides can be used to diagnostic advantage. Scanning incorporating the somatostatin analogue ^{123}I-labeled Tyr3-octreotide (octreotide scanning) has been useful.[14] Histochemical markers may provide insight into the biologic aggressiveness of a tumor. Aggressive tumors have been proposed to have scarce sustentacular cell populations and produce fewer neuropeptides when compared to more benign lesions. Tendency toward malignant character has been implied by immunohistochemical analysis of relative ratios of chief cells to sustentacular cells and marker reactivity in the latter.[6]

The chief cells of GTs, as members of the DNES, are grouped with other cells of neural crest derivation and their associated neoplasms. Tumors known to occur in association with GTs include pheochromocytoma, thyroid neoplasms, and parathyroid adenoma. Glomus tumors have been noted in association with the multiple endocrine neoplasia (MEN) syndromes.[6]

Glomus tumors are characteristically slow-growing and rarely metastasize. They spread from their sites of origin along tracts of least resistance, the most important of which are the air cell tracts of the TB. Vascular lumina, neurovascular foramina, the ET, and direct extension allow spread beyond the TB. Glomus tumors invade bone. Cochleovestibular destruction is caused by ischemic necrosis.[15,16] Spread along several fronts occurs simultaneously and is multidirectional. Intracranial extension into the posterior cranial fossa occurs directly through dura or along cranial nerve routes. The IAC is a frequent highway.

Cranial nerve paralysis occurs in 35% of jugulotympanic lesions and 57% of intravagal paragangliomas.[6] Cranial nerves VII through XII and the sympathetic trunk are most commonly involved.

Glomus tumors arise more often in Caucasians. Females are four to six times more commonly affected than males.[6] Tumors occur in infants and the elderly, but usually occur in the fifth and sixth decades. A heredofamilial tendency has been outlined with an autosomal dominant mode of transmission. In familial tumors, the incidence of associated lesions is 25 to 50%.

A remarkable characteristic of GTs is their tendency toward multiplicity. In 10% of nonfamilial cases, another GT can be expected.[17] The additional tumor(s) may be ipsilateral or contralateral and involve any of the branchiomeric paraganglions.[18] The most common combination is a carotid body tumor with an ipsilateral GTy or GJ tumor.

Jugulotympanic paragangliomas rarely exhibit malignant degeneration, defined by finding paraganglioma tissue in locations other than those in which paraganglioma otherwise occur. Histologic evidence of malignancy is indeed rare. Lattes and Waltner[19] first reported a metastatic GT (to the liver) in 1948. The fraction of GTs that are malignant ranges from 1 to 12%, with the commonly cited figure at 4%.[20] The most common locations for metastatic deposits are the lymph nodes, skeleton, lung, liver, and occasionally spleen.[21] Glomus vagale (GV) tumors have a higher malignancy rate, estimated at 19%.[22] Symptomatology tends to be more severe and rapidly progressive in malignant GTs; they present at a more advanced state with a higher incidence of cranial nerve deficits. Treatment morbidity and mortality are higher than that for nonmalignant GTs. Nonetheless, prolonged survival is possible in the face of metastatic disease.[23]

The biology of the GT is indeed rich.[6] Its clinical evaluation involves not only delineation of tumor type and extent but also a comprehensive assessment of its unique biologic capacity.

Diagnosis

Clinical

Early diagnosis is key to conservation surgery, which ensures a high-grade postsurgical functional outcome.[24] The diagnostic process must be regarded as a treatment planning tool.

The clinical features of GT serve to alert the physician to a disorder of the ear, TB, and jugular fossa (Table 41–2). The patient with a GT usually complains of pulsatile tinnitus and/or hearing loss. Tumor growth into the mesotympanum manifests as a conductive hearing loss, whereas the extent of labyrinthine invasion determines the degree of the sensorineural component. Tympanic membrane erosion and bleeding are late symptoms. Cranial neuropathy suggests a more extensive process. Neurological symptoms may, however, go unnoticed for a long time. Growth is slow, and neural degeneration occurs simultaneously with compensation. As cranial nerves are lost in aggregate, dysphagia, loss of airway protection, and shoulder, tongue, and voice weakness occur. "Idiopathic" cranial neuropathy, as it often reflects jugular or hypoglossal foramen disease, is an unacceptable diagnosis and mandates an aggressive search, with imaging studies, for a lateral skull base lesion. Facial paralysis is usually a late sign and an ominous omen for FN outcome. The aforementioned signs and symptoms of a "functioning" GT must be sought and differentiated from pheochromocytoma.

A mesotympanic vascular mass is characteristic but rarely may be absent. Superior mesotympanic masses can occur in GT but are rare and diagnostically confusing. Margins visible 360 degrees about the circumference of a mesotympanic mass permit the diagnosis of a tympanicum lesion (and its differential diagnoses). Without this physical finding, differentiation of a GTy tumor from a GJ tumor is insecure and impossible without imaging. When the margins of the mass are not clear, a GJ lesion should be expected until proven otherwise.

Myringotomy or tympanotomy for biopsy is mentioned in condemnation only. Such biopsy results in brisk bleeding that must be packed, risking damage to structures of the ear. Biopsy of an aberrant ICA cannot only be dramatic but also potentially catastrophic. Biopsy is rarely necessary in the face of good imaging. When indicated and unavoidable, a postauricular transmastoid approach, with all vital anatomy identified, is recommended.

TABLE 41–2 Presenting signs and symptoms among patients with glomus tumors

	TUMOR TYPE	
PRESENTING SYMPTOM	GLOMUS JUGULARE (n = 106)	GLOMUS VAGALE (n = 27)
Pulsatile tinnitus	84	8
Hearing loss	62	4
Otalgia	13	3
Aural fullness	32	3
Hoarseness	12	4
Dysphagia	8	5
Pharyngeal fullness	0	9
Vertigo	15	1
Facial weakness	15	1
Headache	5	0
Dysarthria	0	0
Aural bleeding	2	0

The GV presents as an enlarging cervical or parapharyngeal mass characterized by a vague fullness high in the neck. Although inferior vagal paralysis is invariable and presents as aspiration or hoarseness, Horner's syndrome, other cranial neuropathies, and nasal and oropharyngeal signs can also emerge. Middle-ear symptoms are rare.

Intracranial jugular foramen schwannomas may mimic some of the presenting manifestations of GTs or acoustic neuromas. Tumors that are limited to the jugular foramen may cause gradual onset of lower cranial nerve deficits without pulsatile tinnitus or clinical symptoms. Intradural or ICE of these tumors may mimic acoustic neuromas with superior displacement of cranial nerve VIII causing sensorineural hearing loss and tinnitus.[25]

The type and extent of tumor cannot be determined from physical examination alone.

Laboratory

Treatment planning requires achievement of the following objectives[26]:

- Determination of the tumor size, type, and extent
- Evaluation of histochemical or multicentric associated lesions
- Identification and assessment of ICE
- Assessment of major vasculature involvement
- Assessment of intracranial collateral circulation

Most of these objectives are satisfied by defining a soft tissue mass and/or its associated bony destruction. A GTy tumor must be differentiated from a GJ tumor. Disease extent is then defined. The mainstay of this diagnostic phase is radiologic imaging.

The identification of air and/or bone between the tumor mass and jugular bulb characterizes the mesotympanic mass as a GTy tumor and is best achieved by CT of TB with bone windows in both the axial and coronal planes. Computed tomography also defines the tumor extent relative to the bony anatomy of the TB (Figures 41–1 to 41–3).

It is important to examine the caroticojugular plate (or spine) that separates the jugular bulb from the ICA. This bony plate will be eroded very early in the progression of a GJ tumor but will be intact with GTy tumors. A mottled appearance to this plate is very characteristic for GJ tumors. Tumor extent, ICE, and the relationship of the tumor to neural and vascular structures are best evaluated by magnetic resonance imaging (MRI). Magnetic resonance imaging can also differentiate GTs that are characterized by multiple vascular flow voids (salt and pepper pattern) from schwannomas (homogeneous

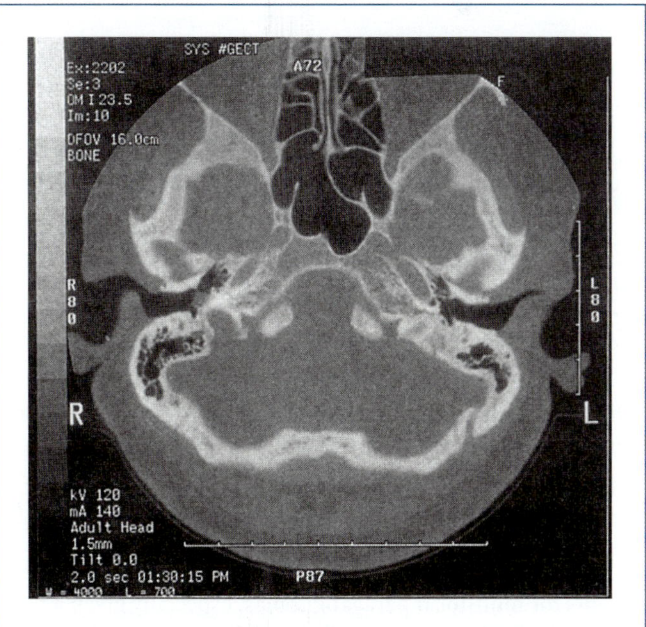

FIGURE 41–1 • Axial computed tomographic scan shows right glomus tympanicum tumor and an uninvolved jugular bulb.

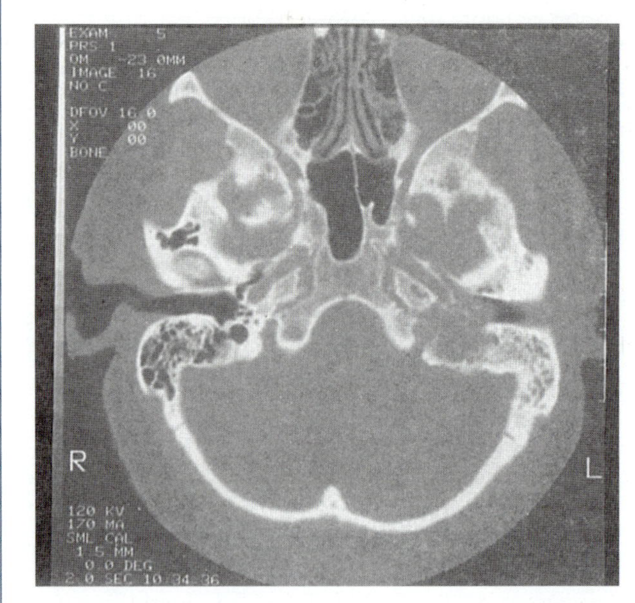

FIGURE 41–2 • Computed tomographic scan shows tumor extent within the temporal bone.

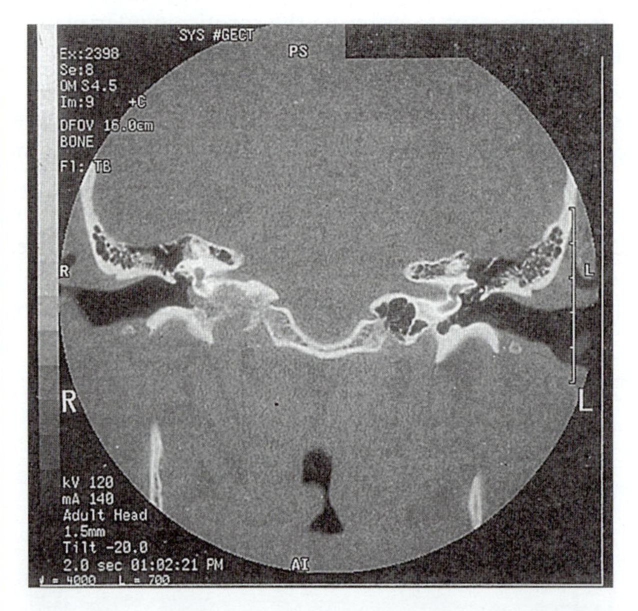

FIGURE 41–3 • Axial computed tomographic scan shows right glomus jugulare tumor and extent relative to the petrous internal carotid artery.

enhancement and possible cystic variations) of the jugular foramen[27] (Figure 41–4).

Magnetic resonance imaging of the head and neck of a known GJ tumor capably assesses for multicentricity (Figure 41–5 and Figure 41–6).

Radionuclide scintigraphy imaging is also used to screen patients for multifocal paragangliomas, especially given a family history of this occurrence. Paragangliomas have a high density of somatostatin type 2 receptors on the cell surface and somatostatin analogs, when coupled to radioisotopes, produce a scintigraphic image of endocrine tumors that express somatostatin type 2 receptors.

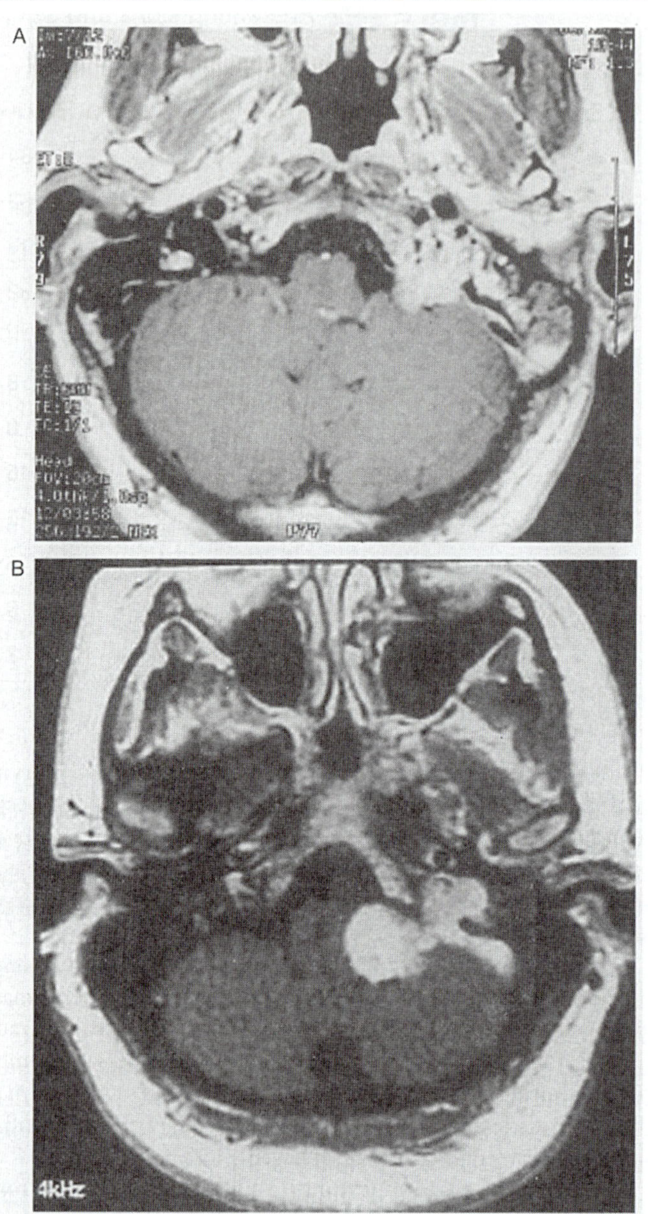

FIGURE 41–4 • *A*, Left glomus jugulare tumor with "salt and pepper" appearance on MRI. *B*, Left jugular foramen neuroma with homogeneous MRI enhancement. *From Eldevik OP, Gabrielsen TO, Jacobsen EA. Imaging findings in schwannomas of the jugular foramen. AJNR Am J Neuroradio 2000;21:1139–44.*

Some of the available imaging agents include ^{99m}Tc-methoxy-isobutyl-isonitrile (MIBI), indium III-octreotide, and iodine-131/132 meta iodobenzylguanidine. Octreotide has been shown to be both sensitive and specific for the diagnosis and localization of paragangliomas down to a resolution of 1 cm. It has also shown value in detecting recurrent lesions as the postoperative changes that interfere with other imaging modalities do not interfere with receptor expression and binding. Such scanning may also identify other endocrine tumors in the MEN syndrome and metastatic disease.[27–29]

FIGURE 41–5 • Magnetic resonance image shows typical appearance of a glomus jugulare tumor with flow voids of vessels within the tumor.

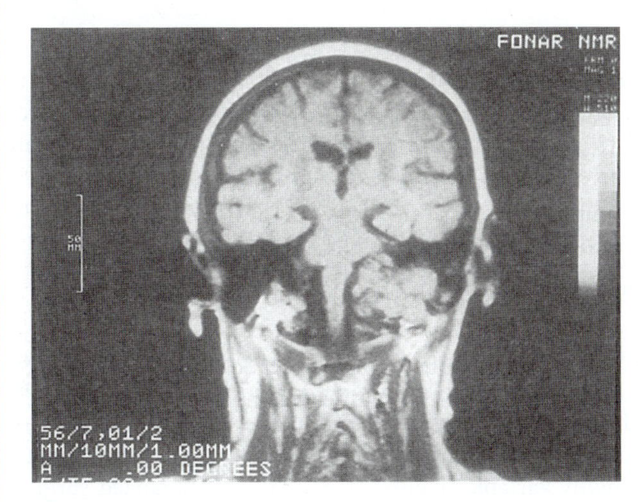

FIGURE 41–6 • Magnetic resonance image shows intracranial extension.

Computed tomography angiography (CTA) may be helpful in defining the vascular supply of the tumor and for evaluating ICA involvement, and CT venography can determine whether the jugular vein is occluded or patent. These tests can help in the decision-making process whether to follow a tumor for growth, advise STS, or plan surgical excision.

Bilateral carotid angiography is performed to evaluate ICA tumor involvement and is done preoperatively, at the time of tumor embolization. Angiography is particularly useful in determining tumor blood supply. This information is important in managing ICE, which can derive vascular supply from pial sources, the vertebral artery, the ICA, and anterior inferior cerebellar artery (AICA) and posterior inferior cerebellar artery (PICA), in addition to usual external carotid artery (ECA) sources. The utility of embolization in limiting operative blood loss is documented.[26,30–32] The risks today are predictably low (Figure 41–7A and B).

As ICA sacrifice is not done without revascularization, ICA sacrifice prediction testing is generally not done contemporarily.

The diagnostic laboratory evaluation of GT patient is completed by catecholamine screening.

Treatment Planning

Treatment is palliative or definitive (curative). For the purpose of this chapter, RT is considered a palliative therapy. Definitive treatment is surgical.

No lesion is technically unresectable. Each treatment plan is based on data generated by the diagnostic evaluation yet must consider patient factors such as age, tumor type and natural history, and general medical health. The issue is whether in the natural course of the patient's remaining life, the tumor is likely to cause significant morbidity or mortality.

Palliation is recommended for the elderly, medically infirm, or those select, multicentric lesions in which definitive treatment is otherwise contraindicated. "Elderly" is best defined physiologically, yet approximates 65 to 70 years. A small GT in a 75-year old is unlikely to cause concern in his/her remaining years as GTs are slow-growing. In contrast, slow-growth rate is not relevant to the typical 30-year-old woman in whom the GT is usually encountered. Surgery is offered to the latter and not typically recommended to the former. For the asymptomatic patient in whom palliation is elected, the GT is carefully observed with serial imaging. Tumors demonstrating growth or creating symptoms are irradiated.

In synchronous lesions, the most life-threatening lesion is operated on first. Neurological outcome determines subsequent recommendations. Bilateral GJ tumors are particularly challenging. If one is operated on and the patient emerges neurologically intact, contralateral surgery is planned in 6 months. Extensive cranial nerve loss mitigates against such a plan because of the extraordinary risk of laryngeal denervation and pharyngeal deafferentation. Such an outcome represents a serious assault on quality of life attended by permanent tracheostomy, tracheal diversion, and/or artificial alimentary support. In such a case, the residual lesion is followed and palliated as indicated. Often no right answer exists.

Radiation Therapy

Resection of GJ tumors for cure has always represented a primary objective.[26] Owing to the technical capacity of the day, issues of resection or resectability have been minimized. Virtually any lesion is "resectable." The perceived risk of functional incapacity that attends lateral skull base surgery is the most common reason for which surgery is criticized. Today the success of conservation surgery and the operative rehabilitation of existing or iatrogenic phonopharyngeal deficits have gone far to mitigate such criticism.

As an alternative, RT and STS are offered as a minimal, low-morbidity, low-cost conservation strategy. Recently, RT and particularly STS have received much attention.[33–35] They are reviewed in detail in Chapter 39. Under the influence of

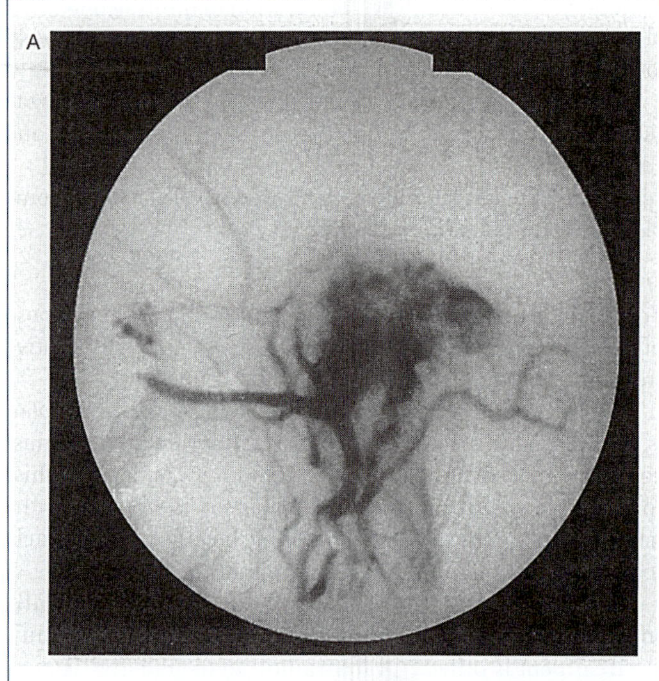

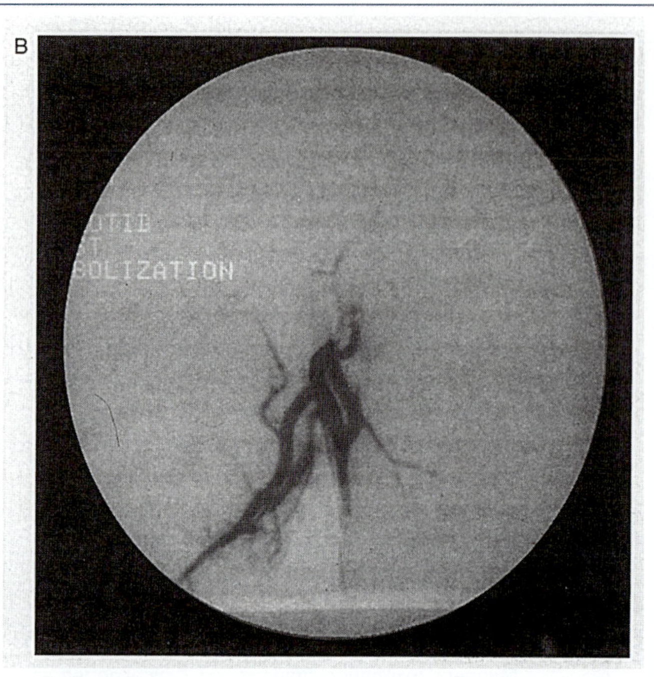

FIGURE 41–7 • *A*, Angiogram blush before embolization. *B*, Successful embolization of this same tumor shown.

managed care, it is expected that RT will continue to hold its prominent place in GT care.

As a result, a sharp controversy between surgeons and radiation therapists has emerged as to which modality is the best primary therapy for GT. The data to resolve this controversy do not exist. The RT position is summed by Cummings and colleagues,[36] who have noted "...the relief of symptoms and the failure of the tumor to grow during the remainder of the patient's lifetime is a practical measure of successful treatment." However, the assumption that irradiated tumor consists only of benign masses of inert cells is probably inaccurate.[37–39] Radiation therapy forces the patient to coexist with a biologically altered tumor. Because of the relative rarity of these tumors (which confounds statistical analysis), the protracted (15 to 20 years) natural history, and advancements in RT made over several decades, current data cannot support the contention of disease "control." The conceptual distinction between disease "control" and "cure" is more than semantic. In large tumors, no new cranial nerve deficits are generally created by GT tumor surgery, but in GJ tumor surgery, cranial nerve loss is a fact of life. Even though compensation and operative rehabilitation are effective, functional capacity is diminished. To the end of cure, the real risks of surgery are well defined, concurrent, and qualitatively documented.[40,41] Jackson and colleagues[40] reviewed the RT literature and compulsively sought the risks of RT with respect to hearing loss, central nervous system damage, osteoradionecrosis, and radiation-induced malignancy. They[40] concluded that the real risks of RT were ongoing, long term, and, as yet, undetermined.

The RT versus surgery debate continues to rage. In point of fact, RT as a minimally invasive protocol must continue to hold a prominent place in GT management. Glomus tumors are complicated treatment challenges. As data continue to be generated to properly quantify the risk/benefit ratio for each treatment modality, the patient's decision to tolerate coexistence with tumor or to seek freedom from it must be fully informed. Both options with available data need to be provided.

Surgical Treatment

Basic Principles: Routes of Extension

Glomus tumors originate from paraganglions that populate the ME and hypotympanum in the proximity of the jugular bulb. We have already discussed that from this regionally focused origin, routes of extension are along the lines of least resistance and are highly variable (Figure 41–8). An individualized surgical approach to each tumor and its ramifications within and beyond the TB must be represented by a coherent composition of surgical units as options (Figure 41–9). By definition, the strategy must be multidisciplinary and must accomplish the following:

- Exposure of all tumor margins
- Identification/control of vital regional anatomy
- Access to all margins of ICE

Following basic surgical principles,[26,41] the multidisciplinary approach maximizes the likelihood of complete tumor resection with the conservation of as much normal function as possible.

The Facial Nerve in Lateral Skull Base Surgery

In lateral skull base surgery, the FN is an impediment to the fundamental principle of exposure. For the neuro-otologist, the FN is a structure to be dealt with rather than used. This general topic has been reviewed in detail in the surgical literature.[26,42,43]

It is the vascular supply of the FN that allows its successful relocation and manipulation and comprises extrinsic and

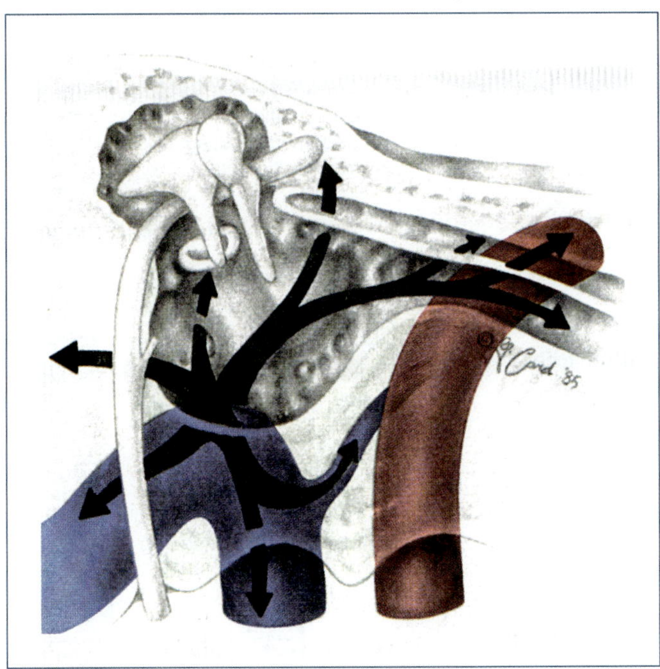

FIGURE 41–8 • Glomus tumor extension route.

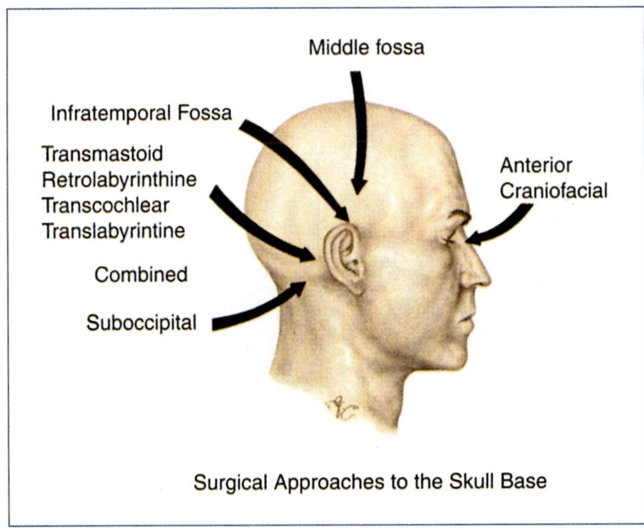

FIGURE 41–9 • The surgical team must combine a variety of approach options.

intrinsic components. Facial nerve neural integrity monitoring (FNNIM) educates FN mobilization so as to promote the maintenance of vascular and neural integrity.

Facial nerve options in GT surgery are simple exposure, short or long mobilization, segmental resection, and selective division. The fundamental factors that determine which FN option is selected are tumor size and how much distal ICA control the tumor extent requires. Much attention has been given to protocols that involve simple FN exposure only, working between the lateral process of C1 and FN. "Short" mobilization of the FN from the external genu laterally causes minimal morbidity and nearly normal postoperative FN function is the rule. In the event of some weakness, long-term House-Brackmann (HB) recovery is excellent (Grades 1 to 2). For larger tumors, "long mobilization," is required from GG distally. The vascular supply to the FN may be best preserved by leaving a wide cuff of skull base fascia around the FN from within the stylomastoid foramen and maintaining continuity with the parotid fascia anteriorly. The stylomastoid foramen segment can subsequently be pressed anteriorly yielding excellent exposure while reducing the risk of compromising the inferior vascular supply to the vertical segment of the FN. Long-term HB outcomes with this approach are also good. Selective division of the FN or its branches with reanastomosis is rarely necessary today. Segmental resection is required when the FN is inextricable from the tumor, but this is rarely the case despite apparent involvement at the time of surgery. When FN function is normal prior to surgery, dissection of the FN from GT should always be attempted. The presence of FN paralysis preoperatively bodes poorly for FN salvation without resection and end-to-end anastomosis or interpositional grafting for reanimation. An algorithm for management of the facial nerve in lateral skull base surgery is shown in Figure 41–10.

Internal Carotid Artery

The ICA is fundamental to lateral skull base surgery as in every case the GT relates or attaches to it. The rate-limiting step in all lateral skull base surgery is the dissection of tumor from the ICA. The basic principles of vascular surgery—proximal and distal control—must be applied. "Control" means circumferential access to normal vessel. Access to the tympanic, petrous, and intracranial segments of the ICA must complement the generally easy access to the proximal vessel in the neck.

Guidelines for ICA sacrifice remain insecure, and prediction of outcome therefrom is less secure. When tumor inextricably involves the ICA, ICA continuity is restored by interpositional vein graft. Tumor behavior relative to the ICA cannot be preoperatively determined. If possible, when the need to sacrifice the ICA is determined preoperatively, and construction is not possible, extracranial bypass is performed.[44]

Internal carotid artery spasm is a dreadful intraoperative occurrence and occurs in response to longitudinal stretching of the vessel. When spasm occurs, manipulation should cease immediately, pharmacological measures should be taken (topical or ICA wall injection with papaverine), and the vessel should be observed.[45] In extreme cases, manual dilatation or segmental resection is required.

Internal carotid artery sacrifice by detachable, intravascular balloon, intra- or preoperatively, is still recommended by Fisch.[46] This extreme solution should be entertained only for extreme problems.

Surgical Technique

Slomus Tympanicum Tumors

For a Class I tympanicum tumor (ie, a mesotympanic mass, the margins of which are visible 360 degrees, and with confirmatory imaging studies), complete resection can be accomplished by means of a transcanal tympanotomy. The mass is avulsed from the promontory, and bleeding is controlled by microbipolar coagulation or light packing.

For a Class II–IV GTy tumor, in which tumor margins cannot be visualized on otoscopy and in which radiologic differentiation from a GJ tumor has been accomplished, a transmastoid

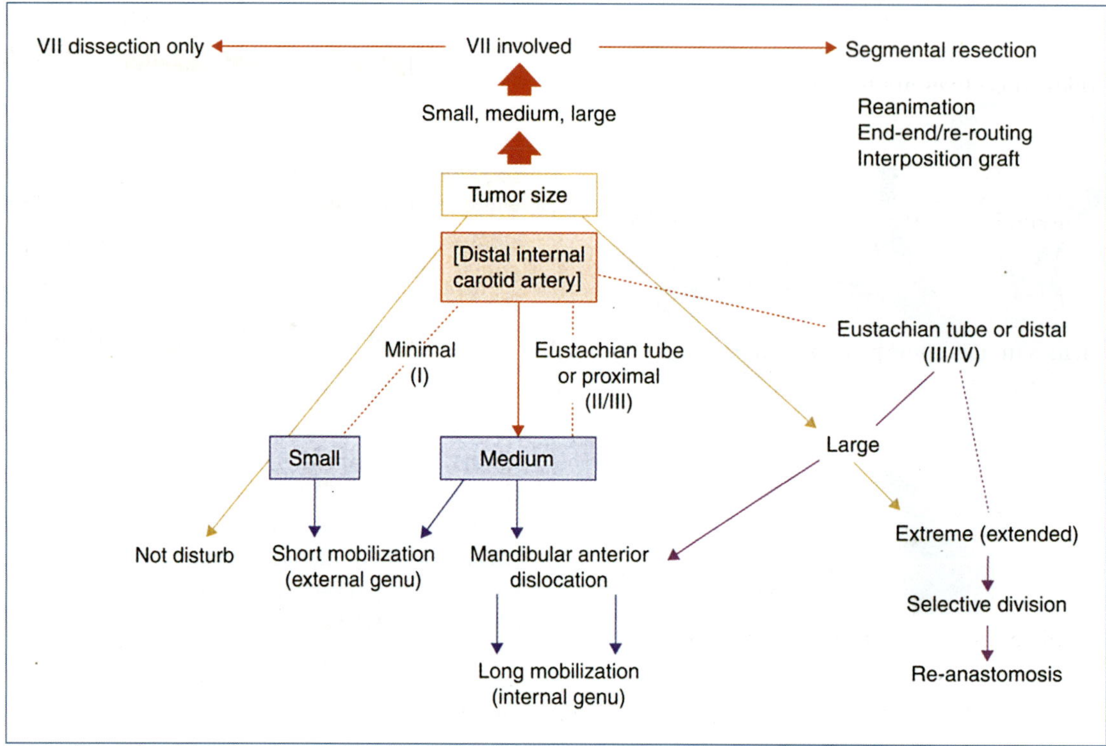

FIGURE 41–10 • Algorithm for management of the facial nerve.

approach is elected. If imaging is found to have been unreliable and it is determined that the tumor is a GJ tumor, the procedure is aborted and definitive lateral skull base surgery is planned for another day.

The transmastoid resection is performed on an outpatient basis and comprises a complete mastoidectomy with extended facial recess exposure.[40,47] Hypotympanic exposure permits visual assessment of the GTy relative to the jugular bulb, ICA, and the structures of the TB (Figure 41–11). Once the GTy tumor is removed, necessary tympanoplastic reconstruction can be done. The inferior EAC and inferior tympanic ring are often drilled substantially to yield adequate exposure of the hypotympanum. This bone can be reconstructed bone dust (pate) collected from the cortical bone of the mastoid at the beginning of the mastoidectomy.

New technology employs the laser.[42] The laser can be defocused to bloodlessly shrink the tumor and identify the feeding vessels. Small vessels can be shrunken and cauterized with the defocused laser. Larger vessels require microbipolar coagulation, light packing, or bone wax packing of the promontory or hypotympanic sources.

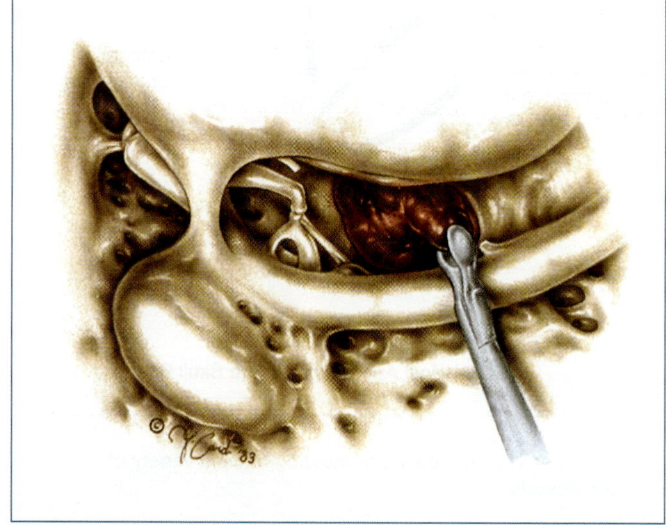

FIGURE 41–11 • Facial recess and extensions provide wide exposure into the hypotympanum for tumor removal.

Glomus Jugulare Tumor

The GJ tumor is removed by means of lateral skull base surgery and represents a multidisciplinary team effort.

Anesthetic goals in lateral skull base surgery include the following[26]:

- Maintenance of hemodynamic stability
- Prevention of increased intracranial pressure
- Maintenance of cerebral perfusion and oxygenation
- Maintenance of a still surgical field
- Facilitation of electrophysiologic monitoring
- Facilitation of surgical exposure and tumor removal
- Replacement of lost blood and prevention of transfusion-associated coagulopathies
- Provision of rapid emergence from anesthesia for the purpose of prompt establishment of a neurological baseline
- Postoperative airway management

Invasive monitoring provides data regarding hemodynamic status, which is especially important during tumor manipulation and the fluctuant release of catecholamines. Blood replacement must keep pace with loss, and autologous blood is used whenever possible. Preoperative identification and treatment of "secretors" permit controlled induction and administration of anesthesia.

The surgical objectives are total tumor removal, with the preservation of structure and function to the greatest extent possible, that is, conservation surgery.

Glomus Jugulare Tumor Class I and II (Small to Medium)

The tumors are confined to the infralabyrinthine chamber and involve the ICA only in its tympanic segment, and are amenable to a hearing conservation approach that conserves the EAC (provided that hearing is salvageable).[40]

The patient is in the supine position. An incision is outlined that permits access to the TB and neck and creates an anteriorly based flap (Figure 41–12). The vital neurovascular anatomy of the neck is isolated and controlled. Facial nerve extratemporal dissection is held to a minimum to protect vascular supply and neural integrity. The ICA is controlled and the internal jugular vein is ligated. Complete mastoidectomy, removal of the mastoid tip, inferior tympanic bone removal, and skeletonization of the inferior-anterior EAC allow access to the mesotympanum and complete dissection of the tympanic ICA to the ET for control (Figure 41–13). The FN undergoes "short" mobilization (Figure 41–14). Proximal control of the lateral venous sinus (LVS) is achieved by intraluminal or extraluminal packing, or with both. During the mastoidectomy, a shelf of bone is left overlying the proximal sinus with the intention that extraluminal packing will be placed between this shelf and the lateral wall of the proximal sinus. Excessive packing in a proximal direction deep into the transverse sinus risks the development of a retrograde propogating thrombus that could risk venous congestion with alteration in consciousness, aphasia, or other neurological deficits that are usually temporary if infarction is avoided. Occlusion of the vein of Labbé can be fatal.

With tumor dissected from the ICA, it is mobilized from the infralabyrinthine chamber. Within the jugular bulb, brisk bleeding from the multiple openings leading to the inferior petrosal sinus(es) is packed gently and with the minimal amount of material necessary to control the bleeding. Excessive pressure from packing is injurious to the lower cranial nerves passing through the pars nervosa just deep to the petrosal openings. Delicate dissection of GJ tumor from the contents of the pars nervosa of the jugular foramen and the hypoglossal canal is rewarded by cranial nerve preservation in the smaller lesions.

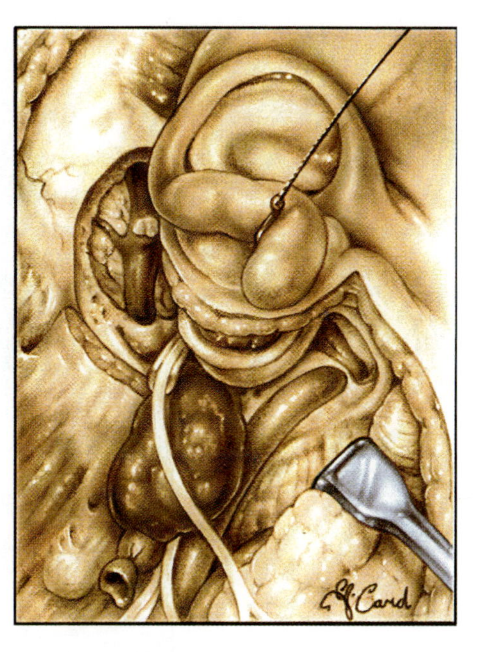

FIGURE 41–13 • The infratympanic extended facial recess approach provides distal control of the internal carotid artery and allows hearing conservation.

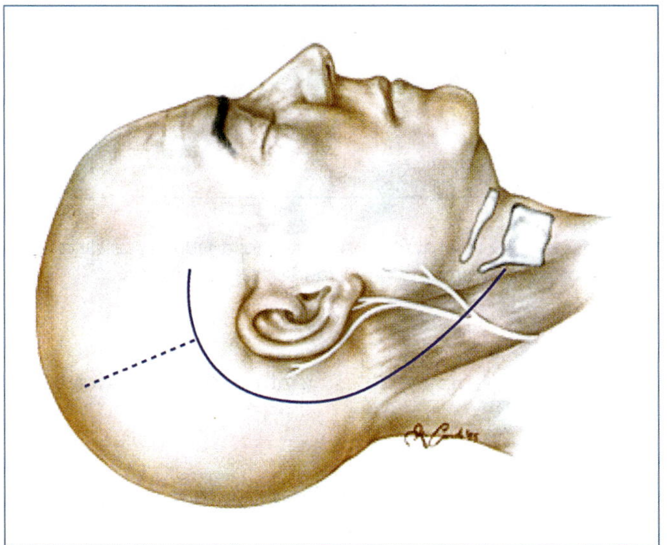

FIGURE 41–12 • Incision minimizes superior flap necrosis and allows cephalic access for temporoparietal fascia.

Glomus Jugulare Tumor Class III and IV (Medium to Large)

When the GT extends out of the TB into the IFTF or when control of the petrous portion of the ICA is required, a modified IFTF approach, or its extension, is necessary. These approaches offer not only access to the deep recesses of the TB and IFTF but also the clivus, the nasopharynx, cavernous sinus, and the posterior, middle, and anterior cranial fossae for removal of ICE. A complete conductive hearing loss is conceded.

The same incision is executed as for GJ tumor Class I/II excision, but the EAC is transected and oversewn (Figure 41–15). The EAC, TM, and the contents of the ME lateral to the stapes are resected. Access to the petrous ICA and IFTF requires anterior and inferior dislocation of the mandible by dividing its anteromedial ligamentous attachments. The FN undergoes "long mobilization" (Figure 41–16). More recent technique modifications leave the contents of the stylomastoid foramen and digastric attached to VII during translocation[48,49] (illustrations show the FN alone for illustrative clarity).

Retraction needs, to maintain exposure, are more formidable. The extirpation of tumor, with exposure achieved, proceeds as before.

When anterosuperior tumor extension or ICA dissection distally is extreme, this exposure is extended. By resecting the zygoma and TMJ unit and inferiorly reflecting the

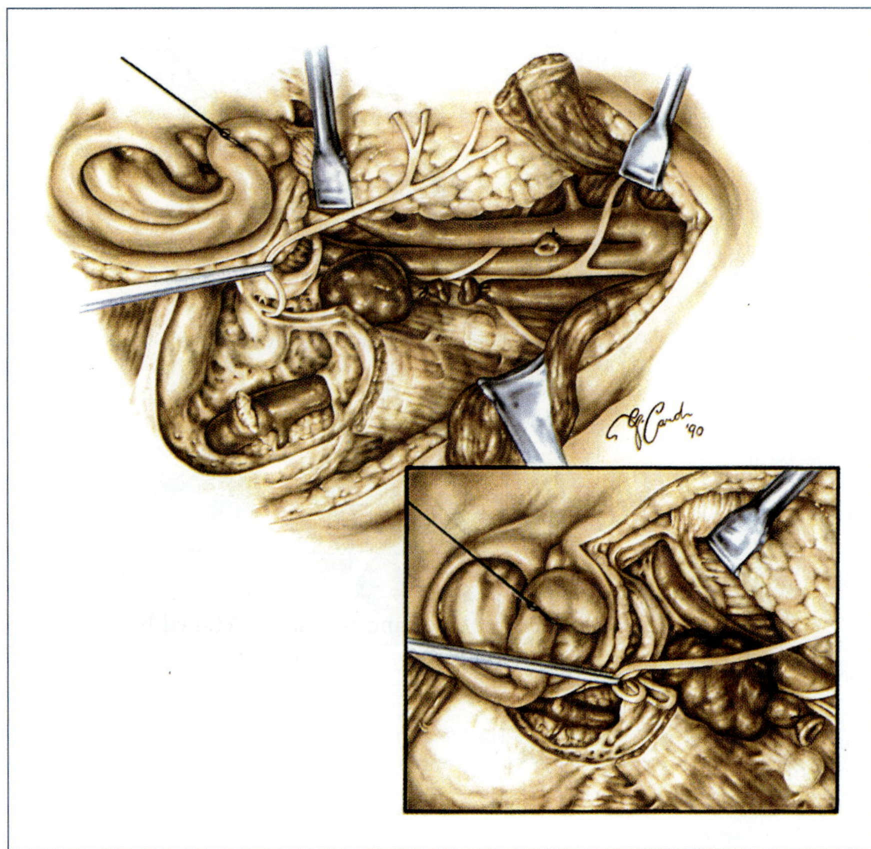

FIGURE 41–14 • Tympanic bone removal, skeletonization of the external auditory canal, and facial nerve mobilization are basic.

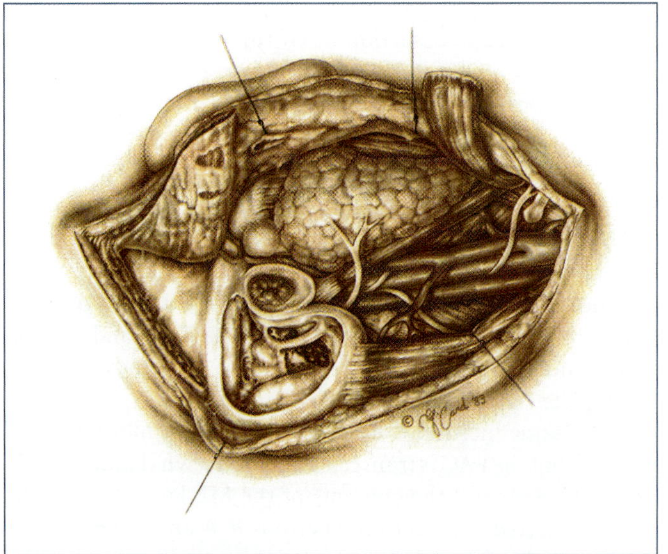

FIGURE 41–15 • The external auditory canal is transected and oversewn in the infratemporal fossa approach.

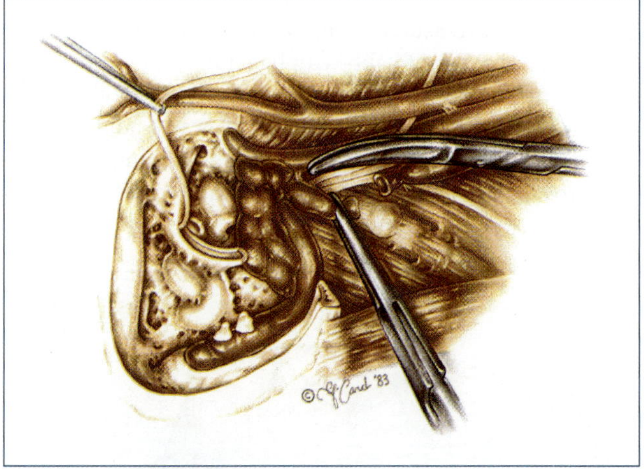

FIGURE 41–16 • Facial nerve mobilization and mandibular dislocation provide proximal petrous internal carotid artery exposure.

temporalis muscle with maximum anterior-inferior mandibular dislocation, the structures of the IFTF can be accessed (Figure 41–17). The ET is resected and the contents of the foramen spinosum managed on the way toward ICA dissection through the pterygoid region to its precavernous margin (Figure 41–18). Access to the middle cranial fossa, nasopharynx, foramen rotundum, clivus, posterior cranial fossa, and cavernous sinus is possible. Tumor resection proceeds as before.

Intracranial Extension

Intracranial extension is defined as the transdural spread of tumor through dura into the subarachnoid space. Intracranial extension was once regarded as a criterion for unresectability. The tumor and its ICE were often regarded as two separate lesions and managed as such. The modern trend is to correctly

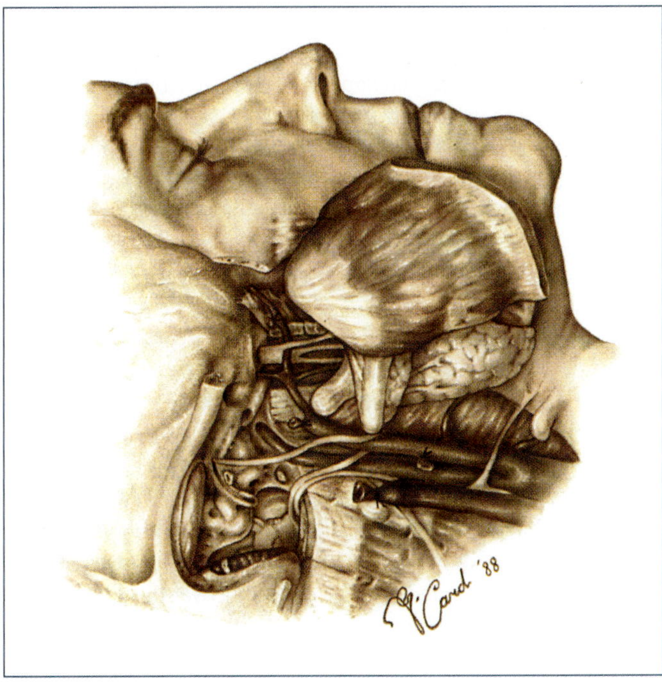

FIGURE 41–17 • The internal carotid artery exposure is developed. Middle cranial fossa exposure is excellent.

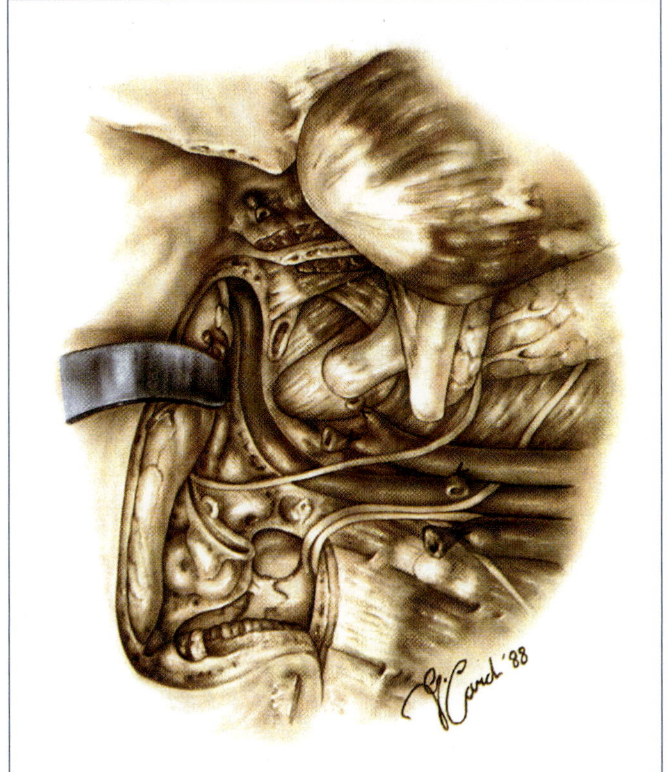

FIGURE 41–18 • The internal carotid artery exposure is completed. The maxillary division of cranial nerve V in the foramen rotundum is depicted.

consider them a single unit with management in an unstaged procedure.

The single-stage resection of ICE poses problems unique to lateral skull base surgery. Single-stage resection is complicated by problems of dural defect reconstruction and cerebrospinal fluid (CSF) management far more complex than those posed, for example, by the resection of an acoustic neuroma. In neurotologic lateral skull base surgery, the following obstacles are unique[24]:

- Wider bony and soft tissue defects
- Local tissue usually rendered unavailable for reconstruction
- CSF pressures enhanced by venous occlusion
- Regional devitalization by RT, ICA exposure, and regional ischemia as a result of EAC ligation

Reconstruction schemes have as fundamentals the need for wide capacity ranging from simple to complex.

Intracranial extension usually occurs through the posterior fossa dura or along cranial nerve roots to the posterior cranial fossa (Figure 41–19) and is reliably detailed by MRI (see Figure 41–6). The management of a GJ tumor with ICE follows this sequence:

- Tumor dissection from the ICA/IFTF
- Tumor debulking from the TB down to the dura
- Removal of the ICE
- Defect reconstruction

Tumor removal from the posterior cranial fossa is usually not difficult through the exposure available once the LVS has been resected. Translabyrinthine and transcochlear adjunctive dissection expands the posterior cranial fossa exposure.

Resection of ICE limited to the area of the pars nervosa usually results in a small dural defect.

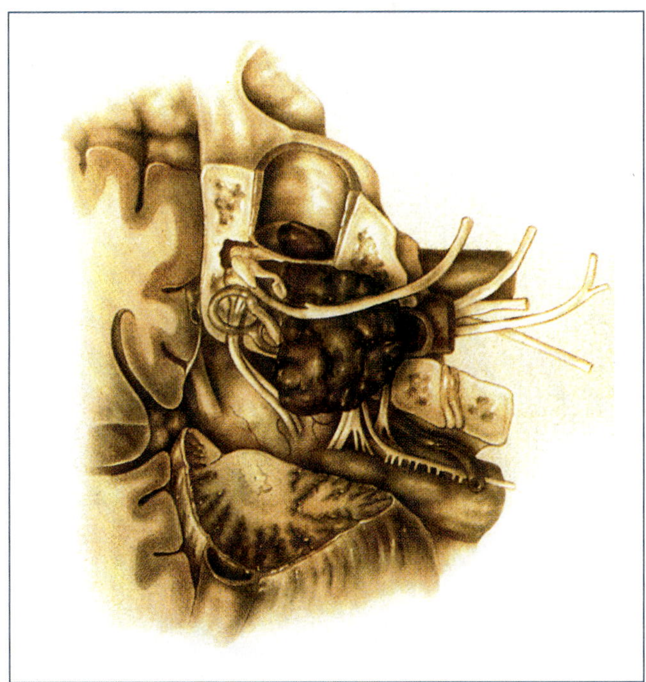

FIGURE 41–19 • Transdural extension of tumor occurs into the posterior cranial fossa.

Defect Reconstruction

The size of the defect determines the complexity of the repair, which is modified by associated complicating factors such as the effects of RT.

The following generalities apply[26]:

- Dural defect reconstruction by vascularized tissue
- Tissue bulk to reinforce the reconstruction and resist the CSF pressure head, also often vascularized
- CSF decompression by lumbar drain for 5 to 7 days
- Adherence to the basic principles of preservation and mobilization of local tissue to facilitate wound closure
- A prerequisite to successful resection of extensive tumors was the development of strategies to reconstruct the defects created and to prevent CSF leakage. In the face of significant tissue loss, the dura must be closed and ICA exposure addressed.

The successful reconstruction of these defects can be facilitated by the careful preservation and mobilization of tissues (Figure 41–20A to C). The skin incision is outlined for access to the superficial temporalis fascia, the TB, and the neck. The neck skin flap is elevated deep to the platysma; elevation over the mastoid is superficial and subcutaneous to create a strong sternocleidomastoid (SCM) fascial flap, which is created by cutting along the temporal line up to or beyond the EAC if it is to be sacrificed. The SCM fascial flap is then mobilized posteriorly and inferiorly. This flap greatly facilitates closure through the reattachment of this tissue to the deep temporal fascia superiorly and parotid fascia anteriorly when the EAC has been transected. When the EAC is preserved, this flap is closed to the bony-cartilaginous junction of the EAC.

To preserve regional blood supply, the EAC is not divided.

Small dural defects are closed with vascularized superficial temporal fascia and a free abdominal fat graft.[26,40,42] This flap, described by Abul-Hassan and colleagues,[50] is vascularized by the EAC and requires careful dissection in the zygomatic region to maintain viable blood supply. Often referred to as a temporoparietal fascia flap, it is extensive. The superficial temporal fascia is left attached to the skin flap until it is determined it is needed. It is then detached and rotated into the defect to cover the dural defect (Figure 41–21). Even when the EAC is left intact and the ME opens

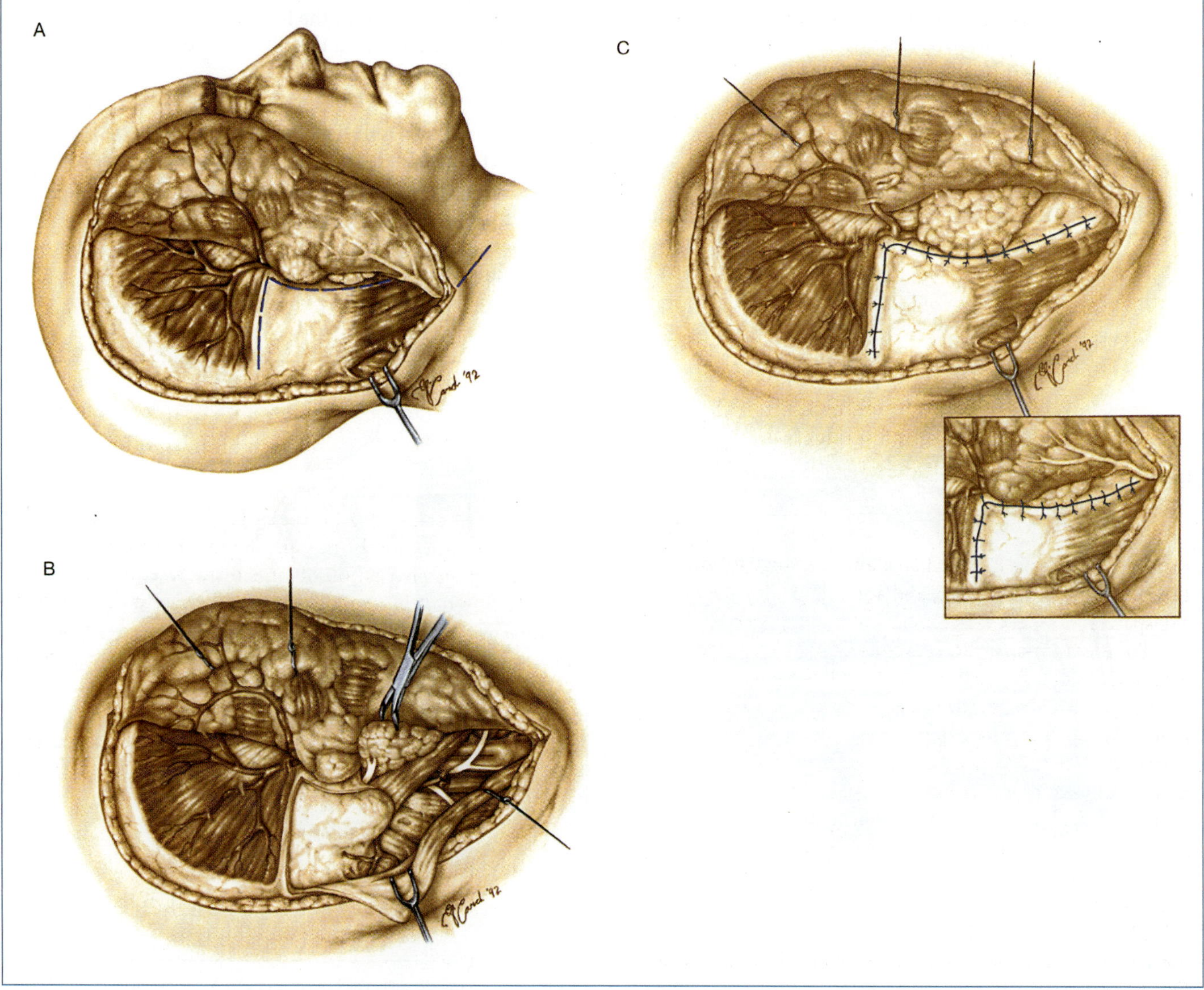

FIGURE 41–20 • Watertight closure after tumor resection.

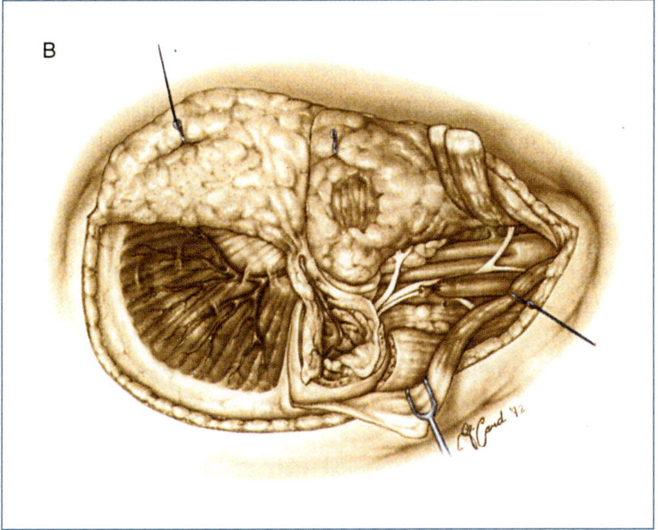

FIGURE 41–21 • Based on superficial temporal artery, the superficial temporoparietal fascia is used for repair after tumor ablation.

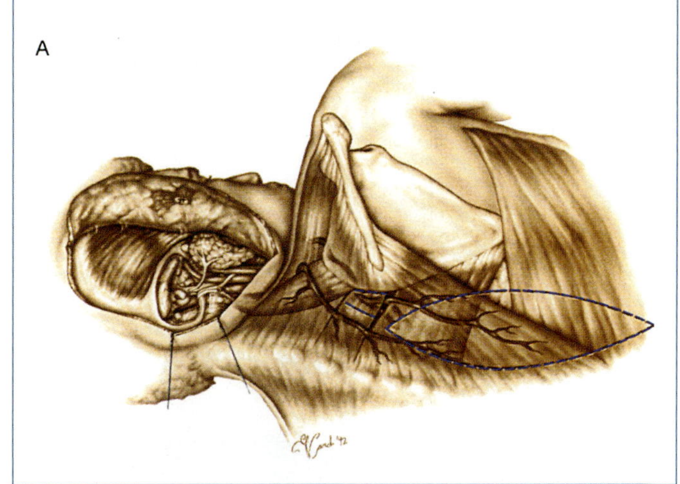

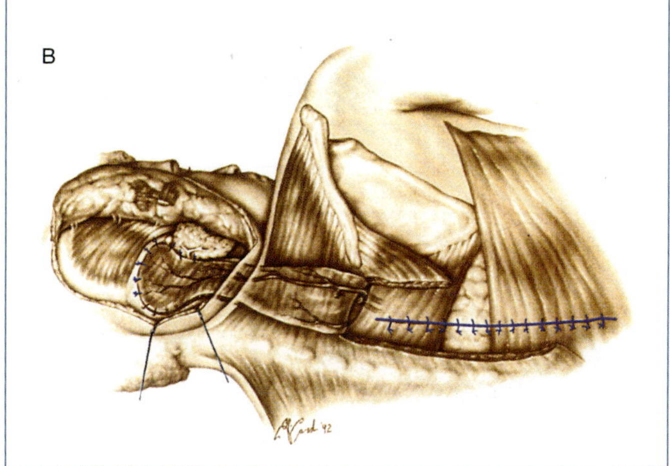

FIGURE 41–22 • The lower trapezius flap.

to CSF egress via the ET, this flap is ample enough to wrap around the intact EAC, facial recess, and antrum to allow for an aerated ME space. A lumbar drain remains indwelling for 5 to 7 days.

For medium-sized defects consequent to resection of more extensive lesions (more likely with malignancies of the TB, ear, parotid, or meningioma, rather than the GT), more bulk is required,[51] such as that provided by a myocutaneous flap. In a young woman, the typical GT patient, a pectoralis donor site is unappealing; rather, the lower trapezius myocutaneous flap is preferred (Figure 41–22). Small defects in previously operated on or irradiated tissue may require this type of reconstruction. The flap is hearty and provides excellent coverage while maintaining trapezius function.

More massive defects require alternative flaps. The latissimus dorsi myocutaneous flap can be employed, but free-flap reconstruction is preferred. Of the multiple flaps available, the rectus abdominis muscle and its overlying tissue are preferred for the largest defects (Figure 41–23). Significant atrophy (40%) can be expected and is a drawback. The flap should be intentionally oversized to overcompensate for the atrophy. Overcompensation that persists can easily be corrected, more easily than additional bulk can be added. This flap has the added advantage of operative efficiency as harvesting can begun by another team working in the abdomen as the final stages of lateral skull base surgery are completed.

The serratus muscle may also be utilized for microvascular free-flap reconstruction of large or radiated defects. Three or more slips of this muscle can be inserted into the nasolabial region when FN and muscular resection is necessary to accomplish total tumor removal. Proximal FN anastomosis to the motor nerve to the serratus muscle will provide natural, voluntary mid-facial movement. The gracilus muscle and radial forearm flaps can be used for combined defect reconstruction and facial reanimation.

It is emphasized that extreme solutions are applied only to extreme problems. The totipotential surgical capacity to customize resection and reconstruction ensures maximum possible functional outcome in these patients with dreadful lesions.

Rehabilitation of Cranial Nerve Loss

For small lesions, cranial nerve preservation can be achieved in over 90% of cases.[26,40–42] For preexisting cranial nerve deficits or for those created at surgery, a strategy must exist to

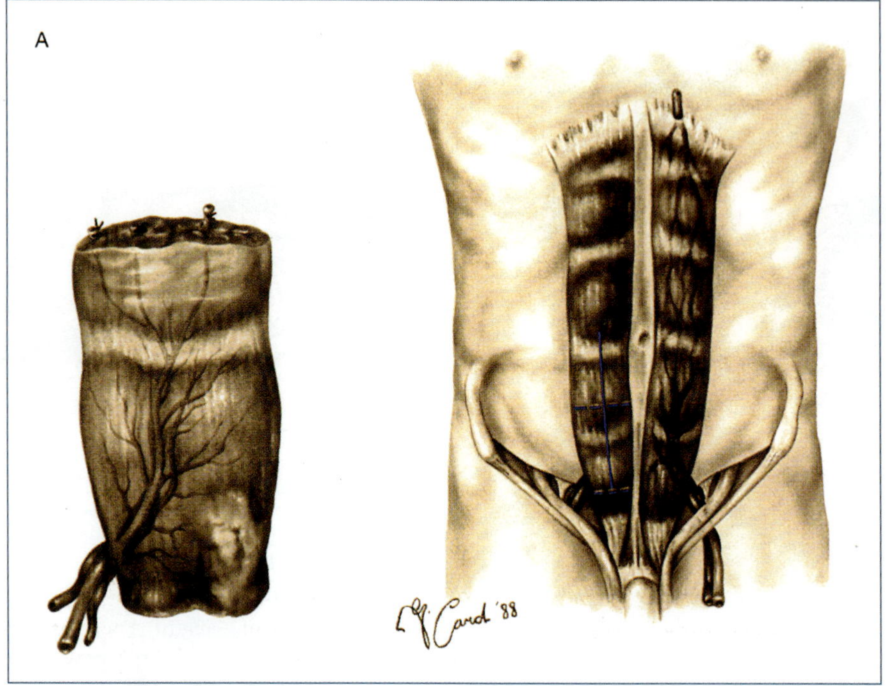

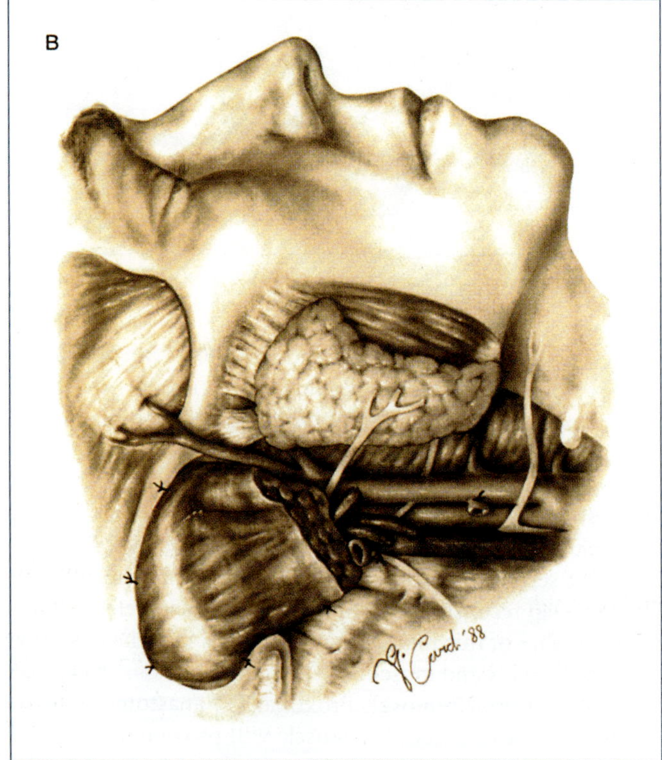

FIGURE 41–23 • The rectus abdominis free flap.

ensure postsurgical outcomes that are of high quality. The lower cranial nerves function as a unit orchestrating phonopharyngeal function (Figure 41–24). Single-nerve loss rarely causes a problem in airway protection, swallowing, or speech as most patients are able to compensate. Lateral skull base surgery exposes the patient to potential loss of cranial nerves IV through XII, as well as the sympathetic trunk. Acute loss of cranial nerves in aggregate is poorly tolerated but generally can be surgically rehabilitated. In the elderly, rehabilitation of swallowing may be impossible when combined cranial nerve loss occurs.

A detailed description of rehabilitation strategies for each cranial nerve is outlined by Netterville and Civantos.[51] Globally, however, primary Silastic® medialization of the vocal cord has obviated the need for tracheostomy, shortened the length of hospital stay, and reduced the time at which oral intake is resumed. It has revolutionized lateral skull base surgery.[52,53]

Surgical Treatment of Glomus Tumors: Long-Term Results

Glomus Tympanicum Tumors

Jackson and colleagues[54] recently published a review on the long-term control of GTy tumors that were treated surgically. The average length of follow-up was 55 months, and the average patient age was 53 years. Ninety-one percent of the patients were women. Thirty-four percent of the tumors were Stage I, 52% were Stage II, 3% were Stage III, and 11% were Stage IV. The extended facial recess approach was used in 73% of cases; 16% were removed via the transcanal approach. Eleven percent required a canal-wall-down procedure. Total tumor removal was accomplished in 95% of patients.

Postoperative complications were infrequent and included one wound infection, four TM perforations, one EAC stenosis, one cholesteatoma, one immediate postoperative FN paralysis, and one cerebrovascular accident.

Postoperative audiograms, available for 57 patients, are summarized in Figure 41–10. Four patients had high-frequency threshold drops exceeding 15 dB.

There were two recurrences. Long-term tumor control was accomplished in 92.5% of patients.

In this series,[54] GTy tumor was associated with other paragangliomas only once, in a patient with a history of familial

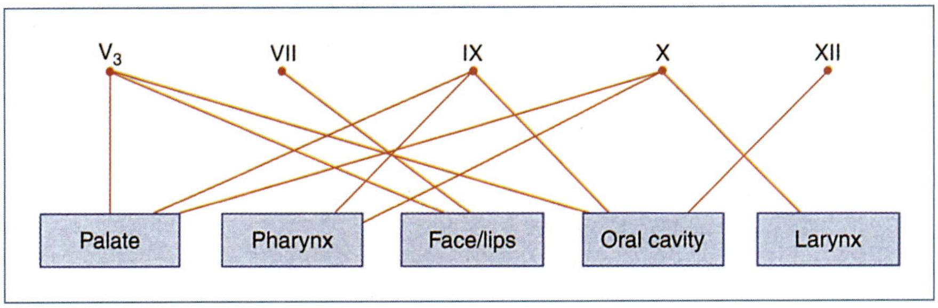

V3 VII IX X XII
Palate Pharynx Face/lips Oral cavity Larynx

FIGURE 41–24 • Interaction of lower cranial nerves in phonopharyngeal function.

paragangliomas. No patient exhibited symptoms of catecholamine, hormone, or parahormone secretion. Accordingly, we have modified our diagnostic protocol for GTy by eliminating routine biochemical analysis and urine sampling for catecholamines; biochemical survey is reserved for patients with GTy tumors with known multiple lesions and/or a family history of paragangliomas.

High-resolution CT of the TB, with and without contrast, is the definitive imaging study for GTy tumors. We employ MRI only when the diagnosis and/or the extent of the disease are in question. Extensive imaging evaluation is performed only in patients with GTy tumors with a known familial tendency and/or multiple lesions.

As one patient in this series developed a recurrence 14 years after surgery, long-term follow-up appears necessary. We follow our patients with GTy tumors yearly for 5 years and once every 5 years thereafter.

Skull Base Glomus Tumors

The long-term control of GTs managed by lateral skull base surgery has been recently reviewed.[55] This review contains current data regarding the incidence of major complications, surgical cranial nerve deficits, long-term surgical control rates, and recurrence risk of patients undergoing skull base resection for large paragangliomas using modern microsurgical techniques. Surgical control was defined as complete tumor removal with no evidence of recurrence over the follow-up period; coexistence with tumor was not considered control.

The review examined a total of 279 skull base procedures performed on 176 patients; 152 patients had GJ, 27 had GV, and 3 had carotid body tumors that extended to the base of the skull. The average patient age was 41 years, and there was a 2.59 to 1 female-to-male ratio. The average length of follow-up was 54 months (range 1 month to 23.25 years).

Using the Glasscock-Jackson classification system, there were 27 (21.4%) Class I, 26 (20.6%) Class II, 44 (34.9%) Class III, and 29 (23%) Class IV tumors. Seventeen patients (9.7%) exhibited symptoms of catecholamine secretion, whereas 9% had multicentric tumors. The incidence of malignant GT in this series was 3.3%. (Regional or distant tumor developing in known glomus locations was regarded as a manifestation of multiple lesions, whereas tumor appearing in regional or distant nonglomus locations was viewed as a metastasis.)

Ten patients had previously undergone RT, whereas 77 patients had previously undergone surgery.

Surgical control was obtained in 164 of 182 patients (85%) (Table 41–3). Eighteen patients (9.9%) experienced subtotal resection, four of which were palliative procedures in elderly individuals. In accordance with preoperative patient preference, 14 procedures were planned as subtotal resections to maximize the preservation of cranial nerves or the ICA.

Nine cases (4.9%) developed recurrent tumor, defined as the reappearance of tumor in the resection field. Time to recurrence averaged 8.17 years; for this reason, postoperative surveillance is emphasized as appropriate throughout the postoperative life of the patient. Five of these patients ultimately underwent successful resection of the recurrent tumor, one was irradiated, two are under surveillance, and one was lost to follow-up.

The nerve most commonly affected was cranial nerve X. Preoperative cranial nerve dysfunction was associated with a significantly higher incidence of ICE. For the whole series, ICE was acknowledged in 36%. When a preoperative deficit in cranial nerves IX, X, XI, or XII existed, there was an ICE incidence of 68%, 63%, 63%, and 56%, respectively. Intracranial extension resection was required, and accomplished in a single stage, in 36% of cases.

The most common site of lower cranial nerve involvement was the pars nervosa of the jugular bulb, and this involvement was typically multiple. Involvement at the pars nervosa resulted in resection of cranial nerves IX through XII in 34.6% of cases. Total tumor removal was possible without any cranial nerve resection in 31% of cases. In all cases of GV tumor resection, cranial nerve X was involved with tumor and was resected.

When ICE was present, 67% of cases had extensive pars nervosa tumor involvement resulting in resection of cranial nerves IX through XII. When there was a preoperative deficit of the lower cranial nerves, pars nervosa tumor invasion and resection occurred in 61%. When preoperative exhibition of lower cranial nerve deficits and ICE were present, the pars nervosa was involved with tumor and resected in 87% of cases. When neither preoperative lower cranial nerve deficits nor ICE was present, only 11% had tumor involvement of the pars nervosa requiring resection. Pars nervosa tumor involvement and complete resection of cranial nerves IX through XII occurred in 100% of Class IV, 54% of Class III, 15% of Class II, and 0% of Class I tumors. Cranial nerve IX was taken alone in 19% of cases, not because of tumor involvement but to achieve distal control of the ICA.

Preoperative FN paralysis bodes poorly for its preservation as the FN could not be salvaged in any such case.

Complications included mortality (5 cases, or 2.7%), CSF leakage (3 cases), tracheitis (1 case), wound infection (6 cases), meningitis (4 cases), ICA erosion and hemorrhage (1 case), CVA (4 cases), hematoma (3 cases), ileus (6 cases), aspiration

TABLE 41–3 Surgical control

		NUMBER OF PROCEDURES	PERCENTAGE OF TOTAL
Subtotal resection		18	9.9
Palliation in elderly	4		
Carotid preservation	11		
Pars nervosa preservation	3		
Tumor recurrence		9	4.9
Complete resection		164	85.0
Total		182	

(19 cases), pneumothorax (2 cases), pneumonia (5 cases), and TM perforation (4 cases).

Because of their propensity for late recurrence and multicentricity, postoperative MRI surveillance should be conducted 1 year, 3 years, 5 years, and then every 5 years postoperatively for the life of the patient.

Selected Neoplasms

Neuromas if the Jugular Foramen

Lower cranial nerve schwannomas of the jugular foramen are significantly less common than GJ tumors. Contralateral cranial nerve compensation accounts for the paucity of symptoms in patients with relatively large neuromas in the jugular foramen. Transcranial lesions can be resected by combining a retrosigmoid approach with the standard infratemporal access while extracranial growth requires transcervical or transparotid dissection. The majority of these tumors can be surgically resected in one procedure, although some surgeons prefer staging the intracranial and extracranial component procedures separately. Total tumor resection is an achievable goal in the vast majority of patients and anatomic preservation of unaffected cranial nerves is sometimes possible.

Radiographic surveillance with annual MRI is a wise option for elderly patients due to the inherent difficulties with swallowing and airway protection. While vocal cord injection or medialization can restore voice quality, post operative aspiration pneumonia, in this age group, can prove life-threatening. Intracranial, intradural tumor debulking of large tumors is also a viable option for elderly patients if it is planned that lower cranial nerve injury can be avoided. If irradiated, these large tumors may become cystic and demonstrate rapid medial growth with brainstem compression. Partial tumor resection with planned focused radiation may be considered in selected cases.[56,57]

The same IFTF approach as described for GTs can be utilized in the surgical resection of lower cranial nerve schwannomas confined to the jugular foramen. Extracranial extension of these tumors may require additional transparotid or transcervical exposure. Intracranial tumor growth can be managed with a petrosal, retrosigmoid, transcondylar, or combined lateral skull base approach.[58,59]

The transpetrosal approach may be useful in patients with intracranial lower cranial nerve schwannomas or meningiomas involving the medial aspect of the jugular foramen. This hearing-sparing approach involves a standard mastoidectomy with a retrosigmoid bone flap to allow posterior retraction of the lateral and sigmoid sinus following ligation of the superior petrosal sinus and incision of the tentorium. Meticulous transtemporal identification of the bony labyrinth, facial nerve (vertical segment), and the jugular bulb allows for maximal posterior fossa exposure following a vertical, pre-sigmoid dural opening. This retrolabyrinthine access may be limited by an anteriorly positioned sigmoid sinus and/or a high jugular bulb. Transdural adipose packing provides a better dural seal than primary closure of the pre-sigmoid dura.

The retrosigmoid or suboccipital approach can be utilized in patients with an anteriorly positioned sigmoid sinus or a very contracted mastoid cavity. A trans-sigmoid approach may be employed for any jugular foramen tumor that has occluded the blood flow through the jugular bulb. In such cases, however, extracranial veins, emissary veins, or an accessory occipital sinus may all play a significant role in the posterior fossa venous return on the ipsilateral (tumor) side.

The transcondylar approach (far-lateral) can be utilized in patients with intracranial or transcranial jugular foramen tumors with additional involvement of the clivus, hypoglossal canal, foramen magnum, or C_1-C_2 structures. This posterolateral to anteromedial route involves drill curettage of the mastoid bone and the retrosigmoid occipital bone prior to removal of the occipital condyle and involved clivus. Additional inferior exposure is gained by careful dissection and posteroinferior mobilization of the vertebral artery. The transcondylar (far-lateral) approach allows wide exposure for large extradural tumors and can also provide intradural access in patients with transcranial or dumbbell-shaped tumors.

Accurate tumor mapping from imaging results and surgical team planning ensures the selection of an operative approach or a combination of approaches that maximize exposure, enhance the tumor resectability, and minimize perioperative patient morbidity.

Defect Reconstruction

The principles of reconstruction are the same as for GTs and other skull base cases. In cases of extracranial, extradural jugular foramen tumors, surrounding rotation flaps of the temporalis muscle, extended temporoparietal fascia, the SCM muscle, and the parotid gland can all be reapproximated in a primary fashion. A free adipose tissue graft can be used as a deep filler to reduce the long-term caved-in appearance taking care to over pack the defect accounting for 50% tissue atrophy over 6 to 12 months. The same closure is utilized when the dura has been primarily repaired. If a presigmoid dural defect is present, the adipose strips are transdurally positioned prior to flap reapproximation.

In patients requiring removal of the ossicular chain, TM, and EAC, the ET is packed with pieces of temporalis muscle and the middle-ear ET orifice is occluded with bone wax mixed with previously collected bone pate, minimizing the possibility of postoperative CSF rhinorrhea.

Microvascular free tissue transfer reconstruction may be necessary in cases of large dural defects, radiated wounds, or revision surgery with vascular compromise of the surrounding soft tissues.

The rectus abdominus muscle is ideal for most lateral skull base defects as the patient is usually in the supine position allowing the reconstructive team to work on the donor flap elevation while the tumor ablative team works above. The donor vessels, which may include the deep inferior epigastric or the subscapular artery, easily reach a number of external carotid arterial branches in the superior cervical neck. The muscle alone serves as an excellent defect "filler" and a myocutaneous flap can be utilized in cases requiring skin resection or compromised blood supply due to prior radiation (Figure 41–25).

The serratus muscle is an excellent reconstructive option if the patient is in a lateral or semilateral position as in the far-lateral or transcondylar approach. The thoracodorsal arterial pedicle is rather long, and can easily reach the recipient arterial branches of the ECA. Patient positioning, however, makes simultaneous tumor resection and flap preparation.[60,61]

Endolymphatic Sac Tumors

In 1984, Hasserd and colleagues[62] reported the first endolymphatic sac tumor, which was discovered during endolymphatic sac surgery for presumed Meniere's disease; they described a highly vascular, lobular mass centered along the posterior portion of the TB. Both anatomic location and histopathology were highly suggestive of endolymphatic sac origin. Heffner,[63] based on microscopic (both light and electron) and immunochemical analysis of 20 similarly papillary-adenomatous tumors of the TB, proposed that the endolymphatic sac was indeed the site of tumor origin and that the tumor be designated as an "adenocarcinoma of the endolymphatic sac."

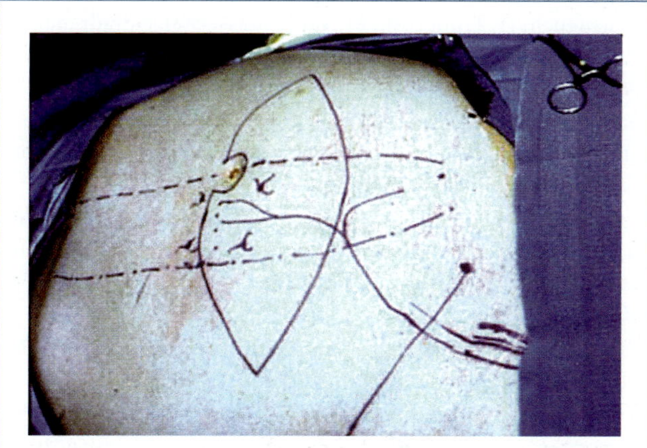

FIGURE 41–25 • Donor site for a rectus abdominus microvascular myocutaneous free flap.

It is now generally thought that the endolymphatic sac, rather than the mucosa of the tympanomastoid compartment, is the source of low-grade, aggressive papillary tumors of the TB. These highly destructive tumors are centered between the sigmoid sinus and the IAC in the region of the vestibular aqueduct and frequently extend intracranially.[63] Macroscopically, the tumors are red, vascular, and polypoid. Microscopically, the tumors demonstrate a papillary-cystic architecture, with villus formation, a cuboidal or columnar lining epithelium, an underlying spindle or myoepithelial cell layer, and glandular lumens simulating a thyroid neoplasm.[63,64]

Endolymphatic sac tumors must be differentiated from ME adenomas and adenocarcinomas (see Chapter 37), as well as carcinoid and choroid plexus tumors. Immunohistochemical analysis can help in the differential diagnosis. For example, Levin and colleagues[65] showed that, similar to normal endolymphatic sac tissue, endolymphatic sac tumors expressed cytokeratin, S-100 protein, NSE, and vimentin but not glial fibrillary acidic protein (GFAP). Mergerian and colleagues[66] found differential expression between choroid plexus papillomas and endolymphatic sac tumors for transthyretin, a known marker for choroid plexus epithelial tissue.

Endolymphatic sac tumors grow slowly and often are not diagnosed until extensive local destruction and ICE have occurred; however, no tumor has been reported to have metastasized. Typical clinical manifestations include (sudden or progressive) sensorineural hearing loss and facial paralysis, with the diagnosis of the hearing loss preceding the diagnosis of endolymphatic sac tumor by an average of 10.6 years.[67] Endolymphatic sac tumors may mimic Meniere's disease, provoking hearing loss, tinnitus, and episodic vertigo.[67]

Gaffey and colleagues[68] documented a highly significant association of endolymphatic sac tumors with von Hippel-Lindau (VHL) disease (VHL is an autosomal dominant, hereditary phakomatosis consisting of retinal and cerebellar angiomatosis). Accordingly, the monitoring of VHL patient should encompass a careful scrutiny of the endolymphatic sac region; early detection of an endolymphatic sac tumor may allow for tumor resection with hearing preservation.[69] Similarly, diagnosis of an endolymphatic sac tumor (if in conjunction with another major manifestation of VHL or VHL in at least one consanguineous relative) should prompt consideration of the diagnosis of VHL.[68]

On CT scanning, endolymphatic sac tumors appear as destructive lesions that are centered in the retrolabyrinthine portion of the TB and that contain areas of calcification.[70] Magnetic resonance imaging findings include areas of high signal intensity on T_1- and T_2-weighted images, as well as enhancement with gadolinium; tumors larger than 2 cm demonstrate flow voids.[69,70]

Complete surgical excision is the recommended management. Preoperative embolization of the tumor may expedite surgical excision.[71] Long-term follow-up is mandated as these tumors may recur as late as 10 years after resection.[67]

Choristoma

Choristomas consist of histologically normal rests of congenitally heterotopic tissue.[72] The most frequently reported choristoma of the ME[73] is made up of salivary gland tissue (~26 cases), but a neural choristoma has also been reported.[72]

Choristomas typically present with a unilateral, conductive hearing loss and a tympanic mass; branchial cleft and FN abnormalities are also often present.[73] Differentiating them from other ME tumors is difficult.

Surgical findings include ossicular abnormalities and FN involvement, with the latter finding complicating excision of the choristoma.[73] Attempts at tympanoplasty and ossicular reconstruction have uniformly failed. Because the choristoma is not a true neoplasm and has no aggressive potential, conservative management (surveillance) is usually recommended.

Fibrous Dysplasia

Fibrous dysplasia consists of fibrous tissue, bony spicules that are undergoing resorption and formation, and islands of cartilage replacing bone marrow; it generally leaves the cortex intact.[74] There are monostotic and polyostotic forms, the latter exemplified by McCune-Albright syndrome (polyostotic fibrous dysplasia with precocious sexual development).

Radiographically, fibrous dysplasia has a "groundglass" appearance. If it involves the TB, there may be progressive EAC occlusion,[75] as well as extension into the substance of the TB. Surgical excision may be indicated if there is progressive EAC obstruction, conductive hearing loss, recurrent infection, or EAC cholesteatoma.

Papilloma

Squamous papilloma is a benign neoplasm commonly occurring in the EAC. The lesion is typical of other papillomatous lesions and is usually exophytic and black or brown in color. It is believed to have a viral etiology. Excisional biopsy is often curative.

Schneiderian (inverting) papillomas, commonly encountered in the sinonasal tract, rarely involve the ME and mastoid.[76] Therapy for these papillomas of the ME is surgical. Conservative surgery uniformly fails as these lesions have a very high propensity for recurrence. Attention should be directed to the ET as a primary highway from which extension from the sinonasal tract into the ME can occur. The danger of the inverting papilloma lies in its propensity for malignant degeneration and represents the primary impetus for early and aggressive surgical management.

Aberrant Internal Carotid Artery

Although not neoplasms, arterial anomalies of the TB figure conspicuously in the differential diagnosis of an ME mass. The incidence of one such anomaly, the aberrant (intratympanic) ICA has been reported[77] to be approximately 1%. Its clinical presentation has few distinguishing features, and on otoscopy it appears as a red, pulsatile, anterior mesotympanic mass. More than 50% of reported cases of aberrant ICA were diagnosed at the time of tympanostomy or biopsy, during which severe arterial bleeding resulted. High-resolution CT (axial and coronal) is the diagnostic imaging procedure of choice; magnetic resonance angiography can also demonstrate the aberrant ICA.

CONCLUSION

Paragangliomas are the most common lesions involving the ME and TB. The differential diagnosis of benign lesions of the TB, however, is broad. Myringotomy and biopsy, traditional solutions to this problem, should rarely be necessary given the wonderful imaging capacity afforded by high-resolution CT and MRI. The broad-based embryology of the TB contributes a potentially rich diversity in the variety of pathology exhibited within. We have the tools available to us to determine the type and the extent of TB disease preoperatively. Only as the result of such detailed presurgical inquiry can treatment be individualized and postsurgical outcomes maximized.

References

1. Anson BJ, Donaldson JA. Surgical anatomy of the temporal bone. Philadelphia: WB Saunders; 1981.
2. Graham MD. The jugular bulb: its anatomic and clinical considerations in contemporary otology. Laryngoscope 1977;87:105–25.
3. Oldring D, Fisch U. Glomus tumors of the temporal bone: surgical therapy. Am J Otol 1979;1:7–18.
4. Fisch U. Carotid lesions at the skull base. In: Neurological surgery of the ear and skull base. Brackmann DE, editor. New York: Raven Press; 1982. p. 269–81.
5. Jackson CG, Glasscock ME, Harris PF. Glomus tumors: Diagnosis, classification and management of large lesions. Arch Otolaryngol 1982;108:401–10.
6. Gulya AJ. The glomus tumor and its biology. Laryngoscope 1993;103(Suppl 60):7–15.
7. Glenner GG, Grimley PM. Tumors of the extra-adrenal paraganglion system (including chemoreceptors). In: Atlas of tumor pathology. 2nd series. Fascicle 9. Washington (DC): Armed Forces Institute of Pathology; 1974. p. 1–90.
8. Guild SR. The glomus jugulare, a nonchromaffin paraganglion, in man. Ann Otol Rhinol Laryngol 1953;62:1045–71.
9. Pearse AGE. The cytochemistry and ultrastructure of polypeptide hormone-producing cells of the APUD series and the embryologic, physiologic and pathologic implications of the concept. J Histochem Cytochem 1969;17:303–13.
10. Pearse AGE. The diffuse neuroendocrine system: Historical review. Front Horm Res 1984;12:1–7.
11. Matsuguchi H, Tsuneyoshi M, Takeshita A, et al. Noradrenaline-secreting glomus jugulare tumor with cyclic change of blood pressure. Arch Intern Med 1975;135:1110–3.
12. Schwaber MK, Glasscock ME, Jackson CG, et al. Diagnosis and management of catecholamine secreting glomus tumors. Laryngoscope 1984;94:1008–15.
13. Farrior JB III, Hyams VJ, Benke RH, et al. Carcinoid apudoma arising in a glomus jugulare tumor: Review of endocrine activity in glomus jugulare tumors. Laryngoscope 1980;90:111–9.
14. Myssiorek MD, Palestro CJ. ^{111}Indium pentreotide scan detection of familial paragangliomas. Laryngoscope 1998;108:228–31.
15. Myers EN, Newman J, Kaseff L, et al. Glomus jugulare tumor—a radiographic-histologic correlation. Laryngoscope 1971;81:1838–51.
16. Kinney SE. Glomus jugulare tumor surgery with intracranial extension. Otolaryngol Head Neck Surg 1980;88:531–5.

17. Spector GJ, Ciralski R, Maisel RH, et al. Multiple glomus tumors in the head and neck. Laryngoscope 1975;85:1066–75.

18. Ervin DM, Osguthorpe JD. Multicentric paragangliomas. Ann Otol Rhinol Laryngol 1984;93:96–7.

19. Lattes R, Waltner JG. Nonchromaffin paraganglioma of middle ear (carotid-body-like tumor, glomus-jugulare tumor). Cancer 1949;2:447–68.

20. Borsanyi SJ. Glomus jugulare tumors. Laryngoscope 1962;72:1336–45.

21. Davis JM, Davis KR, Hesselink JR, et al. Malignant glomus jugulare tumor: a case with two unusual radiographic features. J Comput Assist Tomogr 1980;4:415–7.

22. Druck NS, Spector GJ, Ciralsky RH, et al. Malignant glomus vagale: report of a case and review of the literature. Arch Otolaryngol 1976;102:634–6.

23. Irons GB, Weiland LH, Brown WL. Paragangliomas of the neck: clinical and pathologic analysis of 116 cases. Surg Clin North Am 1977;57:575–83.

24. Jackson CG, Cueva RA, Thedinger BA, Glasscock ME. Conservation surgery for glomus jugulare tumors: The value of early diagnosis. Laryngoscope 1990;100:1031–6.

25. Leonetti JP, Anderson DE, Marzo SJ, Origitano TC, Shirazi M. Intracranial schwannomas of the lower cranial nerves. Otology and Neurotology 2006;27:1142–5.

26. Jackson CG, Marzo S, Ishiyama A, Lambert PR. Glomus and other benign tumors of the temporal bone. In: The ear: Comprehensive otology. Canalis RF, Lambert PR, editors. New York: Lippincott Williams & Wilkins; 2001. p. 813–34.

27. Nilssen E, Wormald PJ. The role of NIB6 scintigraphy in the management of a case of metastatic glomus jugulare tumour. J Laryngol Otol 1996;110:373–5.

28. Kav R, Arnold W. Somatostatin receptor scintigraphy and therapy of neuroendocrine (APUD) tumors of the head and neck. Acta Otolaryngo 1996;116:345–9.

29. Bustillo A, Telischi FF. Octreotide scintigraphy in the detection of recurrent paragangliomas. Otolaryngol Head Neck Surg 2004;130:479–82.

30. Lasjaunais P, Berenstein A. Endovascular treatment of craniofacial lesions. In: Surgical neuroangiography. Vol. 2. Berlin: Springer-Verlag; 1987.

31. Schick PM, Hieshima GB, White RA, et al. Arterial catheter embolization followed by surgery for large chemodectoma. Surgery 1980;87:459–64.

32. Valavanis A. Preoperative embolization of the head and neck: indications, patient selection, goals, and precautions. AJNR Am J Neuroradiol 1986;7:943–52.

33. Cole JM, Beiler D. Long-term results of treatment for glomus jugulare and glomus vagale tumors with radiotherapy. Laryngoscope 1994;104:1461–5.

34. de Jong AL, Coker NJ, Jenkins HA, et al. Radiation therapy in the management of paragangliomas of the temporal bone. Am J Otol 1995;16:283–9.

35. Carrasco V, Rosenman J. Radiation therapy of glomus jugulare tumors. Laryngoscope 1993;103(Suppl 60):23–7.

36. Cummings BJ, Beale FA, Garrett PG, et al. The treatment of glomus tumors in the temporal bone by megavoltage radiation. Cancer 1984;52:2635–40.

37. Brackmann DE, House WF, Terry R, et al. Glomus jugulare tumors: effect of irradiation. Trans Am Acad Ophthalmol Otolaryngol 1972;76:1423–31.

38. Spector GJ, Compagno J, Perez CA, et al. Glomus jugulare tumors: effects of radiotherapy. Cancer 1975;35:1316–21.

39. Spector GJ, Maisel RH, Ogura JH. Glomus jugulare tumors. II. A clinicopathologic analysis of the effects of radiotherapy. Ann Otol Rhinol Laryngol 1974;83:26–32.

40. Jackson CG, Haynes DS, Walker PA, et al. Hearing conservation surgery for glomus jugulare tumors. Am J Otol 1996;17: 425–37.

41. Jackson CG. Glomus tympanicum and glomus jugulare tumors. Otolaryngol Clin North Am 2001;34(5):941–70, vii.

42. Jackson CG. Surgical principles of neurotologic skull base surgery. Laryngoscope 1993;103(Suppl 60):29–44.

43. van Doersten PG, Jackson CG, Manolidis S, et al. Facial nerve outcome in lateral skull base surgery for benign lesions. Laryngoscope 1998;108:1480–4.

44. Awad IA, Spetzler RF. Extracranial-intracranial bypass surgery: A critical analysis in light of the International Cooperative Study. Neurosurgery 1986;19:655–64.

45. Smith PG, Killeen TE. Carotid artery vasospasm complicating extensive skull base surgery: Cause, prevention, and management. Otolaryngol Head Neck Surg 1987;97:1–7.

46. Zane RS, Aeschbacher P, Moll C, et al. Carotid occlusion without reconstruction: A safe surgical option in selected patients. Am J Otol 1995;16:353–9.

47. Jackson CG. Infratympanic extended facial recess approach for anteriorly extensive middle ear disease: A conservation technique. Laryngoscope 1993;103:451–4.

48. Brackmann DE. The facial nerve in the infratemporal approach. Otolaryngol Head Neck Surg 1987;97:15–7.

49. Leonetti JP, Brackmann DE, Prass RL. Improved preservation of facial nerve function in the infratemporal approach to the skull base. Otolaryngol Head Neck Surg 1989;101:74–8.

50. Abul-Hassan HS, von Drasek Ascher G, Acland RD. Surgical anatomy and supply of the fascial layers of the temporal region. Plast Reconstr Surg 1986;77:17–28.

51. Netterville JL, Civantos F. Defect reconstruction following neurotologic skull base surgery. Laryngoscope 1993;103(Suppl 60):55–63.

52. Netterville JL, Civantos F. Rehabilitation of cranial nerve deficits after neurotologic skull base surgery. Laryngoscope 1993;103(Suppl 60):45–54.

53. Netterville JL, Jackson CG, Civantos F. Thyroplasty in the functional rehabilitation of neurotologic skull base surgery. Am J Otol 1993;14:460–4.

54. Forest JA III, Jackson CG, McGrew BM. Long-term control of surgically treated glomus tympanicum tumors. Otol Neurotol 2001;22:232–6.

55. Jackson CG, McGrew BM, Forest JA, et al. Lateral skull base surgery for glomus tumors: Long-term control. Otol Neurotol 2001;22:377–82.

56. Crumley RL, Wilson C. Schwannomas of the jugular foramen. Laryngoscope 1984;94:772–8.

57. Samii M, Bini W. Surgical strategy for jugular foramen tumors. In: Surgery of cranial base tumors. Sekhar LN, Janecka IP, editors. New York: Raven Press; 1993. p. 379–87.

58. Maniglia A, Chandler J, Goodwin W. Schwannomas of the parapharyngeal space and jugular foramen. Laryngoscope 1979;89:1405–14.

59. Samii M, Babu RP, Tatagiba M. Surgical Treatment of jugular foramen schwannomas. J. Neurosurg 1995;82:924–32.

60. Izquierdo R, Leonetti JP, Origitano TC, Al-Mefty O, Anderson DE, Reichman OH. Refinements using free-tissue transfer for complex cranial base reconstruction. Plast Reconstr Surg 1993;92:567–74.
61. Leonetti JP, Zender CA, Vandevender D, Marzo SJ. Long-term results of microvascular free-tissue transfer reanimation of the paralyzed face. Ear Nose Throat J 2008;87:226–30.
62. Hassard AD, Boudreau SF, Cron CC. Adenoma of the endolymphatic sac. J Otolaryngol 1984;13:213–6.
63. Heffner DK. Low-grade adenocarcinoma of probable endolymphatic sac origin. A clinicopathologic study of 20 cases. Cancer 1989;64:2292–302.
64. Batsakis JG, El-Naggar AK. Papillary neoplasms (Heffner's tumors) of the endolymphatic sac. Ann Otol Rhinol Laryngol 1993;102:648–51.
65. Levin RJ, Feghali JG, Morganstern N, et al. Aggressive papillary tumors of the temporal bone: An immunohistochemical analysis in tissue culture. Laryngoscope 1996;106:144–7.
66. Megerian CA, Pilch BZ, Bhan AK, et al. Differential expression of transthyretin in papillary tumors of the endolymphatic sac and choroid plexus. Laryngoscope 1997;107:216–21.
67. Megerian CA, McKenna MJ, Nuss RC, et al. Endolymphatic sac tumors: histopathologic confirmation, clinical characterization, and implication in von Hippel-Lindau disease. Laryngoscope 1995;105:801–8.
68. Gaffey MJ, Mills SE, Boyd JC. Aggressive papillary tumor of middle ear/temporal bone and adnexal papillary cystadenoma. Manifestations of von Hippel-Lindau disease. Am J Surg Pathol 1994;18:1254–60.
69. Manski TJ, Heffner DK, Glenn GM, et al. Endolymphatic sac tumors: a source of morbid hearing loss in von Hippel-Lindau disease. JAMA 1997;277:1461–6.
70. Mukherji SK, Albernaz VS, Lo WW, et al. Papillary endolymphatic sac tumors: CT, MR imaging, and angiographic findings in 20 patients. Radiology 1997;202:801–8.
71. Mukherji SK, Castillo M. Adenocarcinoma of the endolymphatic sac: Imaging features and preoperative embolization. Neuroradiology 1996;38:179–80.
72. Gulya AJ, Glasscock ME III, Pensak ML. Neural choristoma of the middle ear. Otolaryngol Head Neck Surg 1987;97:52–6.
73. Buckmiller LM, Brodie HA, Doyle KJ, et al. Choristoma of the middle ear: A component of a new syndrome? Otol Neurotol 2001;22:363–8.
74. Schuknecht HF. Pathology of the ear. 2nd ed, Philadelphia: Lea & Febiger; 1993.
75. Nager GT, Kennedy D, Kopstein E. Fibrous dysplasia: a review of the disease and its manifestations in the temporal bone. Ann Otol Rhinol Laryngol 1982;91:1–52.
76. Wenig BM. Schneiderian-type mucosal papillomas of the middle ear and mastoid. Ann Otol Rhinol Laryngol 1996;105:226–33.
77. McElveen JT Jr, Lo WW, el Gabri TH, et al. Aberrant internal carotid artery: Classic findings on computed tomography. Otolaryngol Head Neck Surg 1986;94:616–21.

Surgery for Malignant Lesions 42

Keith A. Casper, MD / Myles Pensak, MD FACS

INTRODUCTION

Malignancy of the temporal bone is a rare entity. Despite the surgical and radiographic advancements over the last several decades, the prognosis remains guarded for extensive lesions. Delayed diagnosis is common with this malignancy and has been correlated with a poorer outcome.[1,2] The anatomic constraints of the temporal bone and lateral skull base complicate the management strategy of temporal bone malignancy. Significant morbidity and mortality is common from both the tumor itself and the treatment regimen. This chapter provides an overview for the physician treating patients with temporal bone malignancies; however, this chapter is unable to provide answers to many subjective concerns that come into play when deciding the most appropriate treatment option, if any, for each patient.

HISTORY

The surgical evolution of treatment for malignant lesions of the temporal bone coincides with the refinement of the field of skull base surgery over the last half-century. Temporal bone carcinoma was first reported histologically by Politzer in 1883 in the classic *Textbook of Disease of the Ear*.[3] The first attempted extirpation of a temporal bone malignancy was described by Heyer in 1899.[4] The surgical technique involved a piecemeal resection without the benefit of magnification. For the greater part of the early 20th century, the standard treatment was radical mastoidectomy followed by radiation therapy. It was not until the middle of the 20th century that the concept of en bloc removal of all or a portion of the temporal bone was formalized. Ward, Loch, and Lawrence as well as Campbell, Volk, and Burkland independently described the possibility of temporal bone resection in 1951, but it was Parsons and Lewis who reported the first successful single-stage temporal bone resection with preservation of the petrous apex in 1954.[5–7] In 1969, Hilding and Selker described the technique of resection of the petrous apex with preservation of the internal carotid artery via a preauricular, transcondylar approach.[8] Temporal bone resection with sacrifice of the internal carotid artery was described by Graham in 1984 and elaborated upon by Sataloff in 1987.[9,10] Over the ensuing years, there have been many independent adaptations to the concept of temporal bone resection.[9–17] Despite the many advances, however, extensive temporal bone malignancies still carry an ominous prognosis.

ANATOMY

The temporal bone is one of the most complex anatomic regions of the human body. It is a composite structure that resides at the junction of the cranial cavity, skull base, and neck. The temporal bone contains the sensory organs of hearing and balance, cranial nerves VII and VIII, the internal carotid artery, and the jugular bulb, which ultimately drains into the jugular vein. The complex anatomic configuration and numerous vital structures contained within or near the temporal bone demands considerable training and expertise when performing oncologic resections of temporal bone malignancies. In addition, these structures are at risk of injury by primary tumors of the temporal bone, locoregional spread of tumors from the surrounding area, and distant metastases. For a more detailed anatomic description of the temporal bone and skull base, see Chapter 1; pertinent anatomic features will be reviewed here. The temporal bone is composed of four relatively distinct regions: tympanic portion, squamous portion, petrous portion, and mastoid portion. Tumor extension (Figure 42–1) in each of these areas requires different surgical considerations and ultimately may determine different prognoses.

The external auditory canal (EAC) extends from the auricle to the tympanic membrane. The outer third of the canal is cartilaginous, whereas the medial two-thirds is formed by the tympanic bone. The lateral portion of the EAC contains subcutaneous tissue with associated cutaneous accessory organs, including sebaceous and ceruminous glands as well as hair follicles. The skin of the medial two-thirds is extremely thin with no subcutaneous tissue. The parotid gland and the infratemporal fossa are anterior to EAC, whereas the temporomandibular joint, which lies in the glenoid fossa, is in more inferior position. The foramen of Huschke is the result of incomplete

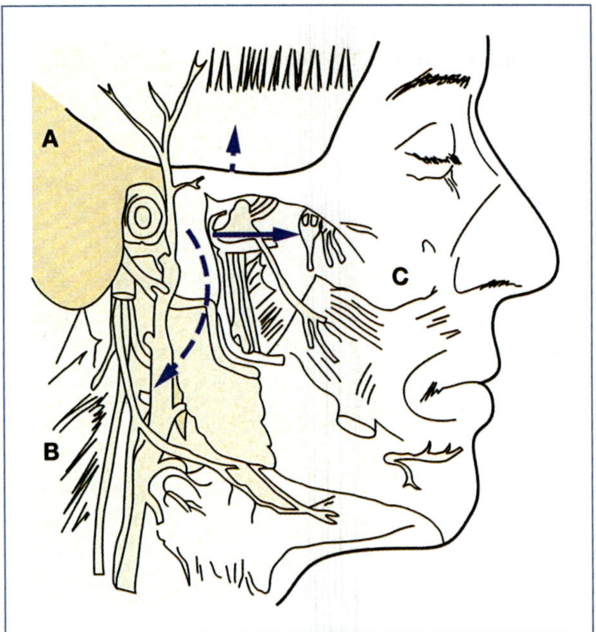

FIGURE 42–1 • Tumors in the external auditory canal can spread easily through anatomic fissures in the anterior wall of the external auditory canal. Once beyond the confines of the canal, tumors can extend into the infratemporal fossa (*A*), the glenoid fossa or pterygomaxillary fissure (*B*), and the parotid gland (*C*). These anterior pathways are often sites of persistent or recurrent disease.

closure of the tympanic bone anteriorly. The fissures of Santorini are small defects in the anterior cartilaginous canal. These defects of the anterior canal wall are potential routes for tumor extension into these regions. Medial to the EAC is the tympanic membrane that provides little resistance to invasion into the tympanic cavity and middle-ear space. The bony posterior canal wall and roof of the EAC provide a more consistent barrier to tumor spread, but a breach of either of these barriers will lead to mastoid cavity and potentially fallopian canal involvement posteriorly and middle cranial fossa involvement superiorly.

The middle ear space is composed of several spaces and contains the ossicles as well as the chorda tympani nerve. The middle ear space includes protympanum, hypotympanum, epitympanum, and mesotympanum. The lateral border of the middle ear space is the tympanic membrane. The jugular bulb and internal carotid artery comprise the floor. Anteriorly, the major structures include the horizontal portion of internal carotid artery and the eustachian tube. Superiorly is the middle fossa; posteriorly is the aditus ad antrum, which leads to the mastoid cavity. The medial wall is a complex region composed of several structures, including the otic capsule and the horizontal segment of the fallopian canal. The dense bone of the otic capsule theoretically protects it from direct tumor invasion; however, tumor may still extend to the inner ear via neurovascular channels, congenital fissures, or even the round window.

The mastoid cavity is variably pneumatized. Tumor involving the mastoid cavity can spread via preexisting air cell tracts. Tumor commonly extends from the central mastoid air cell tract into other pneumatized pathways, eg, the perilabyrinthine, retrofacial, perisinus, and subarcuate air cell tracts. The roof of the mastoid cavity is the tegmen. This barrier can be very thin and often provides minimal resistance to intracranial extension of tumor. The facial nerve courses in its fallopian canal, dehiscences in which are not uncommon and can facilitate tumor invasion of the facial nerve.

The petrous bone is the anterior component of the temporal bone. It contains the internal carotid artery. Numerous cranial nerves, including cranial nerves V and VI, lie in close approximation to the anteromedial aspect of the petrous apex. The petrous apex varies in its degree of pneumatization, ranging from highly pneumatized to nonpneumatized to sclerotic. Nonpneumatized petrous apices contain marrow, an important anatomic consideration because they may serve as a site for hematogenous spread of distant metastatic disease.

The lymphatic drainage of the EAC includes the parotid and preauricular nodes anteriorly, the deep upper jugular nodes inferiorly, and the postauricular nodes posteriorly. The lymphatics of the middle ear and mastoid cavity drain into the deep upper jugular nodes and the retropharyngeal nodes. The inner ear has no known lymphatic drainage.

PHYSIOLOGY

Malignancy of the temporal bone is a rare entity. The reported incidence is approximately 1 to 6 cases per 1,000,000.[18–20] The vast majority of otologic malignancies arise from the auricle; therefore, it is not unexpected that approximately 20 to 60% of all temporal bone cancers are attributed to advanced auricular neoplasms.[15,21] The EAC is the site of origin for more than 25% of temporal bone malignancies, and the middle ear and mastoid account for approximately 12%.[15] The average age of presentation depends upon the histologic type of tumor. Squamous cell carcinoma (SCCA) of the temporal bone typically presents between the fifth and seventh decade of life; rhabdomyosarcoma (RMS), however, is almost exclusively a pediatric malignancy.[10,14,16,19]

Squamous cell carcinoma accounts for 60 to 85% of all temporal bone malignancies.[17,22] The second most common malignancy is basal cell carcinoma (BCC) followed by a variety of other less common tumors. Table 42–1 is a compilation from several large series over the last few decades, documenting the frequency of particular histologic subtypes of temporal bone malignancies. The discrepancy in reporting most likely represents a selection bias based on the particular referral pattern of the reporting institution.

The risk factors for temporal bone malignancy are not well understood. The relative infrequency of these lesions precludes the ability to undertake appropriate prospective evaluation. Chronic otitis media, however, is frequently cited as a risk factor for temporal bone malignancy, particularly SCCA.[17,23] Despite the common association, no definitive correlation has ever been identified.[24] Many patients with carcinoma of the EAC or middle ear initially present with foul, purulent otorrhea. Differentiating between a chronically draining ear with associated inflammation as opposed to a malignancy can be

TABLE 42–1 Malignancies of the temporal bone

TYPE	NUMBER (%)
Epidermal	538 (82)
Squamous cell carcinoma	452 (69.2)
Basal cell carcinoma	74 (11)
Melanoma	12 (1.8)
Glandular	69 (10.6)
Adenocarcinoma*	28 (4.3)
Adenoid cystic carcinoma	25 (3.8)
Other†	16 (2.5)
Sarcomas 23	(3.5)
Rhabdomyosarcoma	9 (1.4)
Other‡	14 (2.1)
Other malignancies§	23 (3.5)
Total	653

Data compiled from Conley and Schuller,[5] Crabtree and colleagues,[6] Gacek and Goodman,[7] Lewis,[8] Kinney and Wood,[11] Pensak and colleagues,[12] Manolidis and colleagues,[17] Moody and colleagues,[19] Goodwin and Jesse,[21] Lesser,[22] and Pfreundner and colleagues.[23]
*Includes papillary cystadenocarcinoma.
†Includes mucoepidermoid and unspecified salivary malignancies.
‡Includes osteosarcoma, angiosarcoma, chondrosarcoma, and unspecified "sarcomas."
§Includes lymphoma, undifferentiated carcinoma, chordoma, malignant glioma, and metastatic renal cell carcinoma.

TABLE 42–2 Signs and symptoms of temporal bone malignancies

SIGN/SYMPTOM	FREQUENCY AT PRESENTATION (%)
Aural discharge	80
Otalgia	80
Hearing loss	71
Facial palsy	32
Canal mass/lesion	26
Tinnitus	26
Periauricular swelling	22
Pruritus	20–39*
Headache	17–46†
Vertigo	15
Aural bleeding	3–28‡

The data of 710 patients summarized from multiple series of temporal bone malignancies are presented above (Pensak and colleagues,[12] Manolidis and colleagues,[17] Moody and colleagues,[19] Kuhel and colleagues,[29] Liu and colleagues,[30] Leonetti and colleagues,[31] Kenyon and colleagues,[32] Zhang and colleagues[33]).
Because some symptoms (pruritus, headache, and bleeding) were reported only in a few studies, the range of frequencies of those symptoms in the studies is provided rather than an overall frequency calculated using the entire group of patients.
*Data from Pensak and colleagues[12] and Liu and colleagues.[30]
†Data from Pensak and colleagues[12] and Leonetti and colleagues.[31]
‡Data from Pensak and colleagues,[12] Manolidis and colleagues,[17] and Liu and colleagues.[30]

difficult, especially considering the infrequency of malignancy. In 1968, Whitehead was the first author to suggest a causal association between the two entities.[25] It has been theorized that carcinoma of the temporal bone may arise in a manner similar to Marjolin's ulcers, in which the mitotic activity of the epithelium is altered due to damage caused by chronic otorrhea or bacterial toxins. Additionally, cholesteatoma has been implicated in the development of malignant disease, but a definitive association has not been established.[2,26]

Ultraviolet radiation is not a significant etiologic factor in temporal bone malignancy in contrast to carcinoma of the auricle. There is a potential association between temporal bone malignancy and other forms of radiation, however. Radium exposure, particularly in dial workers in the 1940s and 1950s, is a well-known carcinogen, and a number of reported temporal bone malignancies have been linked to such exposure.[27] In addition, external beam radiation can induce future malignant transformation anywhere within the treatment field.[17,28] Human papillomavirus (HPV) is associated with the development of carcinoma in numerous areas of the body and has been detected in temporal bone carcinoma. A high prevalence of HPV has been demonstrated in carcinoma of the middle ear associated with chronic otitis media.[29]

DIFFERENTIAL DIAGNOSIS

The diagnosis of SCCA of the temporal bone is often delayed due to the nonspecific nature of the common presenting symptoms. Table 42–3 lists the most frequent signs and symptoms from several large series.[16,21,30–35] The initial manifestations of temporal bone carcinoma closely resemble those of chronic otitis externa or chronic suppurative otitis media, including purulent foul-smelling otorrhea, severe otalgia, bleeding, and pruritus. Patients with a chronic aural suppurative process unresponsive to antibiotic therapy should be evaluated carefully for malignancy. A high index of suspicion is often necessary given the low incidence of temporal bone malignancy. However, early detection can have a significant impact on outcome.

Other presenting symptoms of malignancy include hearing loss, headaches, tinnitus, vertigo, and aural fullness. Secondary bacterial infection often complicates the diagnosis. Cranial nerve involvement usually occurs late and is an ominous sign of more significant tumor extension. The facial nerve can be involved by invasion of tumor in the mastoid or tympanic segment, or by extratemporal extension into the parotid gland.

Involvement of other cranial nerves can cause a diffuse spectrum of symptoms, including facial paresthesia, hoarseness, visual disturbance, and dysphagia. Extension into the glenoid fossa can result in trismus, and dural involvement can produce severe pain and headache.

Nonmalignant Entities

A number of more common, benign entities often present in a fashion similar to temporal bone malignancies. These entities include chronic suppurative otitis media with or without cholesteatoma, EAC cholesteatoma, EAC exostosis or osteoma, and pseudoepitheliomatous hyperplasia (PH). Pseudoepitheliomatous hyperplasia is considered to be a result of chronic irritation to the epithelium, which is often associated with chronic infections. Pseudoepitheliomatous hyperplasia needs to be considered in all suspicious lesions of the EAC. There have been documented cases of PH initially diagnosed as SCCA; conversely, there have also been patients initially diagnosed as PH after appropriate surgical resection who present with SCCA years later.[36]

Squamous Cell Carcinoma

Squamous cell carcinoma is the most common histopathologic subtype of temporal bone malignancy. Squamous cell carcinoma is responsible for 60 to 85% of all malignant lesions.[17,22] The sites of origin include the EAC, the middle ear space or mastoid, and extensive auricular neoplasms. The most common presenting symptoms have been described earlier. Regional and distant metastases from the temporal bone are infrequent. The reported rates of regional metastases at time of presentation range from 9 to 18%.[6,19,37–39] When nodal disease is present, the upper jugulodigastric and parotid nodes are most commonly involved.

Basal Cell Carcinoma

Basal cell carcinoma accounts for approximately 11% of tumors of the temporal bone (see Table 42–1). Temporal bone involvement most commonly occurs as a result of tumor extension from the auricle to involve the EAC. This mode of extension is particularly common in lesions originating in the preauricular skin and the conchal bowl region. Basal cell carcinomas rarely metastasize but can be very locally aggressive. Basal cell carcinoma typically has a better prognosis than SCCA, and even extensive tumors are usually amenable to surgical excision.[16]

Melanoma

Melanoma originating in the EAC and temporal bone is rare. Unlike the auricle, which is exposed to a large amount of ultraviolet radiation, the EAC is shielded. When melanoma does involve the canal or temporal bone, it is typically advanced and caries an exceedingly poor prognosis. Treatment is surgical excision (when feasible) followed by radiation therapy.

Glandular Malignancies

Malignancies arising from the glandular structures of the EAC are rare entities, representing approximately 10 to 20% of all temporal bone malignancies (see Table 42–1). There has been considerable variability in the pathologic categorization of these malignant lesions. The literature is replete with various pathologic descriptions such as ceruminoma, apocrine carcinoma, papillary cystadenocarcinoma, and ceruminous adenocarcinoma. More recent publications have attempted to simplify these chaotic classifications. The literature currently identifies two primary malignant glandular tumors: adenoid cystic carcinoma and ceruminous adenocarcinoma.[40,41] There are other less common glandular malignancies of the temporal bone such as mucoepidermoid carcinoma; however, these are extremely rare lesions.

Adenoid cystic carcinoma is the most common glandular malignancy of the EAC.[41] This lesion is typically characterized by slow but relentless growth with a predilection for perineural spread. Histologically, the tumor consists of cords and islands of neoplastic epithelial cells. There are four distinct histologic patterns classically described: cribiform, tubuloglandular, solid, and hyaline. The solid pattern carries the worst prognosis. Treatment of adenoid cystic carcinoma is surgical resection with wide margins. The propensity of these tumors for neurotropic extension causes difficulty in defining truly negative surgical margins. "Skip" areas of involvement and noninvolvement have been identified along the length of nerves both proximal and distal to the site of the primary lesion.[42] Therefore, postoperative radiation therapy is typically recommended. Adenoid cystic can also extend along the haversian systems of bone without obvious cortical disruption.[42] Short-term eradication of tumor is often achieved; however, local recurrence is quite common and often occurs 8 to 10 years after the initial surgery. In addition to local recurrence, tumor may present proximally along the skull base or intracranially due to neural propagation. This pattern of late local recurrence complicates the interpretation of studies documenting 5-year survival rates for adenoid cystic carcinoma. Distant metastases, most commonly to the lung, occur as well.[41] Patients may live for many years with active recurrent or metastatic disease, and recurrences do not necessarily lead to a rapid demise.

Ceruminous adenocarcinoma is a less common glandular malignancy of the temporal bone. The Armed Forces Institute of Pathology has divided this malignancy into a low-grade form (papillary cystadenocarcinoma) and a high-grade undifferentiated type.[43] The low-grade subtype is often slow growing, rarely metastasizes, and often can be distinguished from a benign adenoma only by pathologic evidence of invasion of surrounding tissue or bone. The tumor typically consists of double-layered cuboidal or columnar epithelial cells arranged in a glandular pattern. A variable amount of atypia and pleomorphism is usually present. The high-grade variant, adenocarcinoma, is characterized by undifferentiated cells that often resemble metastatic disease from other sources. Wide surgical excision with postoperative radiation is the treatment of choice. These tumors have a propensity to extend in a subcutaneous plane, which often creates difficulty with margin analysis. Tumor extension beyond the EAC carries a poor prognosis.[41]

Sarcoma

Sarcomas are the most common temporal bone malignancy in the pediatric population. Nonetheless, sarcomas of the temporal bone are exceedingly rare, representing less than 5% of all temporal bone malignancies (see Table 42–1). Rhabdomyosarcoma is the most common variant; it is accounting for approximately 30% of all sarcomas of the temporal bone.[15] Other types include fibrosarcoma, osteogenic sarcoma, Ewing's sarcoma, Kaposi's sarcoma, chondrosarcoma, and undifferentiated sarcomas.

Rhabdomyosarcoma is the most common soft tissue sarcoma in children. The head and neck region is the most common primary site.[44] The rate of head and neck involvement varies depending on the study, but the most recent intergroup study (IRS-IV) reported a 16% rate in the head and neck region (including the eye) and a 25% rate for parameningeal sites.[45] Fewer than 10% of the lesions of the head and neck actually involve the temporal bone, however.[46] More than 70% of patients present prior to age of 10, and the median age is 5 years.[45] The majority of otologic lesions arise from the middle ear.[47] The primary presenting symptoms are similar to those of chronic otitis media and include purulent or bloody otorrhea, otalgia, canal polyps and granulation tissue, as well as hearing loss. However, RMS originating in the petrous bone may cause headaches and cranial nerve palsy without associated aural symptoms.

The natural history of RMS in the temporal bone comprises aggressive local destruction with a propensity for distant metastases. Up to 14% of patients with RMS in parameningeal sites present with distant metastases.[48] In the middle ear, the tumor quickly invades the fallopian canal, resulting in facial paresis or paralysis, and can then spread proximally to the internal auditory canal, other cranial nerves, and the meninges. It can also spread by destruction of the tegmen or along the eustachian tube.

Rhabdomyosarcomas arise from striated skeletal muscle cells. The primary subtypes of RMS are embryonal, alveolar, and undifferentiated. The previously described botryoid and spindle cell variants are now categorized as subtypes of embryonal.[45] In the IRS-IV data, 70% of tumors were embryonal/botryoid/spindle cell variants, 20% alveolar, 4% undifferentiated, and 6% other.[45] The embryonal variant accounts for the vast majority of the head and neck lesions. The type of RMS significantly affects prognosis. Embryonal subtypes overall have a more favorable outcome than the alveolar or undifferentiated subtype.[45] The classification system for RMS is more complex than most malignancies. There is a TNM staging system along with the IRS grouping system. The grouping system is composed of four groups and is based on tumor resectability. Group I has completely resected localized disease. Group II has grossly resected disease with microscopically positive margins or regional disease; the regional disease is then further divided into Group IIa through Group IIc. Group III has partially resected disease, and Group IV has metastatic disease.

Historically, the treatment of temporal bone RMS consisted of aggressive surgical extirpation, which resulted in excessive morbidity and low cure rates. Prior to the1970s, the cure rate for RMS of the head and neck was barely 20%.[48] Since the 1970s, the cure rate for localized RMS has nearly tripled from 25% to approximately 70% with multimodal therapy including surgery and multiagent chemotherapy with or without radiation therapy.[49] Some patients with favorable characteristics and nonmetastatic disease are expected to have a greater than 80% overall long-term survival.[49] Four Intergroup Rhabdomyosarcoma Studies (IRS) have been performed over the last several decades. The most recent trial, IRS-IV, enrolled patients from 1991 to 1997, and long-term data from this trial is now becoming available.[45,49] Currently, the standard treatment protocol is surgical biopsy for pathologic diagnosis followed by chemotherapy, and possibly radiation therapy, for cure. Using this approach, the 3-year survival rates for head and neck RMS have risen to greater than 75%.[45] The overall treatment outcome for patients enrolled in IRS-IV was similar to IRS-III; however, patients with local or regional tumors with alveolar histology fared significantly better in the more recent trial.[45]

Sarcomas other than RMS are rare in the temporal bone. Prior radiation therapy may place a patient at risk for the development of these other sarcomas. Ewing's sarcoma responds best to radiation and chemotherapy, similar to RMS. Other sarcomas, including osteogenic sarcoma, fibrosarcoma, Kaposi's sarcoma, chondrosarcoma, and liposarcoma, should be treated with wide en bloc excision possibly followed by radiation. Their rarity makes survival and prognostic data unreliable.[50]

Metastatic Disease

Metastases to the temporal bone are rare. Metastatic disease most commonly occurs via hematogenous spread to marrow-containing areas of the temporal bone. The most common cancers metastasizing to the temporal bone are the breast (25%), lung (11%), kidney (9%), stomach (6%), bronchus (6%), and prostate (6%).[51] The most common presenting symptoms include hearing loss, facial paralysis, and vertigo. The prognosis for patients with temporal bone metastasis varies depending on the histopathology but is typically poor. When treatment is pursued, it generally consists of palliative radiotherapy.

Other Malignancies

In addition to the malignant lesions described earlier, other malignancies that may involve the temporal bone include those directly spreading from adjacent areas. Tumors originating in the parotid, nasopharynx, auricle, and central nervous system can all invade the temporal bone. Treatment is dependent on the individual tumor but often entails aggressive surgical extirpation if the tumor is deemed resectable. Other rare tumors include extramedullary plasmacytoma, lymphoma, and hemangiopericytoma, all of which involve other areas of the head and neck much more frequently than the temporal bone.

Finally, mention should be made of Langerhans' cell histiocytosis (LCH), formerly called histiocytosis X. Although not truly a malignancy, LCH can present as a disseminated process with locally aggressive disease. Langerhans' cell histiocytosis typically affects children but can be seen in all age ranges. It consists of an abnormal proliferation and accumulation of Langerhans' cells, which are antigen-presenting cells located in the epidermis. Lesions grossly appear soft and granular with areas of necrosis and hemorrhage. Microscopically, there are clusters of Langerhans' cells, eosinophils, multinucleated giant cells, and other inflammatory cells. By electron microscopy, Birbeck granules, which are specific for LCH, can be identified in the Langerhans' cells.

Classically, LCH has been divided into three progressively more aggressive groups: eosinophilic granuloma, Hand-Schüller-Christian disease, and Letterer-Siwe disease. Currently, descriptive terms are used to characterize these three groups (localized, multifocal, and disseminated disease). Approximately 25% of people with LCH develop aural symptoms.[52] Patients may present with granulation tissue in the middle ear or EAC, otorrhea, and hearing loss owing to destruction of the ossicles. Associated symptoms include painful swelling of the calvarium, cervical adenopathy, and a rash resembling chronic dermatitis. Other bony sites may be involved, and disseminated disease can be seen in other organs, especially in infants. Skull films may show characteristic hypolucent areas that can aid in the diagnosis. Biopsy of the lesions is critical, and any child, especially if younger than 3 years, with granulomatous or polypoid disease in the middle ear should undergo biopsy of the abnormal tissue to rule out LCH.

Biopsy and conservative curettage are often all that is needed to treat limited disease, and such tumors generally have an excellent prognosis. There is no reason to perform an extensive mastoidectomy or resection of the lesion.[53] For patients with multifocal or disseminated disease, adjuvant chemotherapy and radiation therapy play a vital role. Survival for patients with multifocal disease is 65 to 100%, but infants with disseminated disease have a very poor prognosis.[53]

DIAGNOSTIC TECHNIQUES

A detailed history and physical examination are the most important initial steps in the appropriate diagnosis of a temporal bone malignancy. The most common presenting signs and symptoms have been detailed earlier and are listed in Table 42–2. A full neurotologic examination should be performed on any patient suspected of having a temporal bone malignancy. Microscopic debridement and examination of the EAC is mandatory. Any suspicious canal wall masses, ulcerations, or polyps should be biopsied and sent for pathologic examination. Testing for cranial nerve dysfunction, balance disturbance, trismus, and periauricular swelling can help predict clinically areas of tumor extension. Lymphadenopathy is uncommon with temporal bone malignancy, but a thorough palpation of the neck should be performed.

The use of imaging modalities is critical for the appropriate assessment of tumor extent. High-resolution computed tomographic (CT) scans reveal the bony anatomy of the temporal bone and demonstrate the extent of any bony erosion. Computed tomographic imaging of the neck may also reveal lymphadenopathy that was clinically undetected. Magnetic resonance imaging (MRI) complements CT scanning by providing a more detailed evaluation of the surrounding or involved soft tissue structures as well as the tumor itself. Magnetic resonance imaging is extremely helpful in evaluating for dural involvement or frank invasion of brain parenchyma. Arteriography is not routinely used in the evaluation of temporal bone malignancy. However, if there is a possibility of carotid artery involvement or a potential for carotid artery sacrifice, preoperative evaluation is warranted. This evaluation may include traditional arteriography as well as MR or CT angiography. Balloon occlusion studies with or without SPECT imaging are also used for planned surgical resection of the internal carotid artery.

Staging

There is no universally accepted staging system for temporal bone malignancies, and reported series have neither used an accepted staging system nor do they provide enough detail in their materials and methods section to determine appropriate tumor stage. This lack of uniformity makes comparison of data among studies difficult. The American Joint Committee on Cancer (AJCC) designates the same staging system for cutaneous neoplasms as for neoplasms of the temporal bone. The unique anatomy of the temporal bone makes this staging system inadequate and fails to provide valid prognostic information for tumors involving the temporal bone.

Numerous authors have proposed their own staging systems over the years. In 1980, Goodwin and Jesse described a staging system divided into three groups.[26] This system was based on the extent of temporal bone involvement. Group I included disease confined to the cartilaginous ear canal; group II was defined by involvement of the bony canal or mastoid cortex. Group III demonstrated invasion of the more medial structures of the temporal bone.[26] In 1985, Stell and McCormick proposed a similar system based on the degree of invasion[54]; this system was later modified by Clark et al. in 1991.[55] In this classification schema, T1 tumors were limited to the site of origin with no evidence of bony destruction. T2 tumors demonstrated further invasion (facial palsy, bony destruction) but did not extend beyond the temporal bone. T3 lesions extended beyond the

TABLE 42–3 Pittsburgh staging system for external auditory canal tumors

T1	Tumor limited to the external auditory canal without bony erosion or evidence of soft tissue extension
T2	Tumor with limited external auditory canal bony erosion (not full thickness) or radiographic finding consistent with limited (< 0.5 cm) soft tissue involvement
T3	Tumor eroding the osseous external auditory canal (full thickness) with limited (< 0.5 cm) soft tissue involvement or tumor involving the middle ear and/or mastoid or patients presenting with facial paralysis.
T4	Tumor eroding the cochlea, petrous apex, medial wall of the middle ear, carotid canal, jugular foramen, or dura or with extensive (> 0.5 cm) soft tissue involvement.
N status	Involvement of lymph nodes is a poor prognostic finding and automatically places the patient in an advanced stage (ie, stage III [T1N1] or stage IV [T2, T3, or T4, and N1])
M status	Distant metastasis indicates a poor prognosis and immediately places a patient in the stage IV category

TABLE 42–4 University of Cincinnati grading system for temporal bone tumors

Grade I	Tumor in a single site, 1 cm or less in size
Grade II	Tumor in a single site, greater than 1 cm in size
Grade III	Transannular tumor extension
Grade IV	Mastoid or petrous air cell invasion
Grade V	Periauricular or contiguous extension (extratemporal)
Grade VI	Neck adenopathy, distant anatomic site, or infratemporal fossa extension

confines of the temporal bone, including the parotid, temporomandibular joint, or underlying skin, and T4 tumors were defined as lesions involving the dura, base of the skull, or brain parenchyma.

Pensak and Arriaga have independently published more detailed staging systems. The Pittsburgh classification system (Arriaga et al.) is probably the most frequently used system. This system (see Table 42–3) is based on radiographic findings and has been correlated with both histopathologic examination of the involved temporal bones and clinical outcomes.[39,56]

The University of Cincinnati classification system (Pensak et al.) (see Table 42–4) incorporates radiographic and clinical findings for the staging of malignant lesions of the temporal bone.[16] This system has been successfully used as a guide for determining the extent of temporal bone resection required. Ultimately, each of these systems emphasizes the detrimental effect of bony invasion, middle ear involvement, and extratemporal spread on prognosis. Although a universally accepted system has not been determined, future reports should at the very least include detailed tumor descriptions so that data can be compared across reports and effective therapies identified for these rare malignancies.

MEDICAL TREATMENT (NONSURGICAL TREATMENT)

Radiation Therapy

Radiation therapy has had limited success in the curative treatment of temporal bone malignancy. The infrequency of these lesions has limited the ability to evaluate treatment regimens prospectively. However, Zhang et al. reported a 28.7% 5-year cure rate with radiation alone compared with 59.6% for patients receiving surgery followed by adjuvant radiation.[35] There are several factors that negatively affect the ability of radiation to exert a tumoricidal effect, including the inherently poor vascularity of the temporal bone, the existence of an infected tumor bed, and low oxygen tension levels. The proximity of the brainstem also affects treatment planning.

Radiation therapy is most often used in an adjuvant fashion after surgical resection or for cure in medically infirm patients. Radiation can also be used in a palliative capacity; however, as a palliative measure, radiation therapy may have limited efficacy.[57] In an adjuvant fashion, radiotherapy has been reported by several authors to improve survival and reduce the incidence of local recurrence.[15,19] Lewis et al., in a series of 132 patients, found that postoperative radiation increased the 5-year survival rate from 28.5 to 35.5%.[14] Prasad et al., in a review of several published series of temporal bone malignancies, concluded that radiation therapy offered no survival benefit for tumors confined to the EAC, but more extensive tumors involving the middle ear and mastoid demonstrated an improved survival over mastoidectomy alone with the addition of adjuvant radiation.[58] The review, however, could not make any conclusions regarding adjuvant radiotherapy with more extensive resections.[58]

The radiation protocol used for the treatment of temporal bone malignancy must be individualized for specific patient and tumor characteristics. In general, the cumulative dose is typically 70 Gy if radiation alone is used for cure. The maximal dose to the brain parenchyma is approximately 60 Gy. In an adjuvant (postoperative) setting, the surgical resection site typically receives approximately 60 Gy, 63 to 66 Gy if the surgical margins were positive. Currently, intensity-modulated radiation therapy (IMRT) is being used with greater frequency. This modality allows an appropriate dose to be delivered to regions specified while minimizing the dose to the more radiosensitive surrounding tissues such as the brain, contralateral parotid gland, and the orbits.

The side effects of radiation therapy are well recognized. These include desquamation, serous otitis media, hearing loss, eustachian tube dysfunction, and vestibular dysfunction, as well as more serious complications such as osteoradionecrosis, cartilage radionecrosis, facial nerve paralysis, and brain necrosis.[59] In addition, radiation of the temporal bone has been associated with the development of aggressive temporal bone sarcomas many years later, although this phenomenon is exceedingly rare. No studies have definitively determined the rate of malignant degeneration following radiation of the temporal bone; however, a review of radiation-induced sarcoma following radiotherapy for breast carcinoma determined a cumulative incidence of 0.2% at 10 years.[60]

SURGICAL THEORY AND PRACTICE

Indications for surgery

Malignancy of the temporal bone is a surgical disease. The extent of the malignancy dictates the surgical procedure appropriate for the individual patient. The indications for each type of resection are reviewed in the surgical technique section. The poor efficacy of primary radiotherapy limits the viable nonsurgical options. Therefore, the only absolute contraindications to surgical intervention are significant medical comorbidities, the presence of far advanced local disease, or metastatic spread.

Contraindications

Although there are a variety of options for surgical resection of temporal bone neoplasms as well as many opinions regarding resectability, often the most important decision is whether to operate at all. Despite the technical ability to resect advanced temporal bone and skull base neoplasms, it is our opinion that patients with malignant invasion of the cavernous sinus, internal carotid artery, infratemporal fossa, or paraspinous musculature are not candidates for a curative surgical resection. Tumor extension into the infratemporal fossa bodes poorly but does not preclude definitive resection. Similarly, although neck dissection can be performed for regional metastases, patients with distant metastases are not surgical candidates. Palliative radiation and limited surgical procedures may be used to reduce disease morbidity, but extensive surgery, with its substantial iatrogenic morbidity, is not in the best interest of the patient if there is very little hope of cure.

Preoperative Management

The preoperative phase of care is limited. Recognition and diagnosis of malignancy is often the most difficult aspect of initial care given the tendency of these lesions to masquerade as more benign conditions. Once the diagnosis of malignancy is made and appropriate imaging acquired, the next step in preoperative management is surgical planning.

Preoperative Planning

Meticulous preoperative planning is crucial for the effective treatment of temporal bone malignancies, and relies substantially on the extent of disease delineated by imaging studies. Once the extent of surgery required has been determined, necessary consultations should be obtained. Depending on the lesion, neurosurgical or reconstructive expertise may be required. It is important to identify expertise required preoperatively to minimize intraoperative complications.

Surgical Controversies

The extent of surgery appropriate is a controversial topic. Some surgeons advocate total en bloc removal of the temporal bone, whereas others recommend piecemeal removal of gross tumor, allowing preservation of vital neurovascular structures, followed by radiation therapy.[1,2,9–13,26,30–32,35] Historically, surgeons have used radical mastoidectomy to treat temporal bone carcinomas. As discussed previously, Parsons and Lewis initially demonstrated the successful use of more extensive resection for temporal bone malignancy.[7] Subsequent authors expanded on their thesis, but patient survival rates remained poor.[11]

In an effort to improve local control, more extensive resections were performed to obtain clear margins around the tumors. The en bloc resection, advocated by Parsons and Lewis, was limited by the petrous carotid artery; therefore, the anterior portion of the petrous bone was left intact. In 1984, Graham et al. reported the first successful total temporal bone resection with sacrifice of the internal carotid artery.[9] The proponents of total temporal bone resection argue that the morbidity inherent with an advanced temporal bone tumor, along with the poor outcomes previously achieved with more limited surgical resection, make this procedure worthwhile. Sataloff et al. and Moffat et al. have reported their own results with this procedure.[10,61] Moffat and colleagues reported a 47% 5-year survival rate for advanced, recurrent temporal bone malignancies requiring salvage radical temporal bone resection.[61] They believe that this survival rate, especially considering the tumors managed, suggests that more radical surgery and subsequent radiotherapy may offer better long-term survival rates than treatment with more conservative surgical resection; however, no patient with poorly differentiated disease survived greater than 1 year after surgery.[61]

In early-stage tumors, an en bloc resection can often be performed with limited morbidity, especially with tumors limited to the EAC. More extensive en bloc resections for advanced neoplasms have increasing morbidity; therefore, many surgeons have advocated a piecemeal approach to such tumors. Kinney et al. detailed the difficulty in correctly identifying the true extent of temporal bone tumors.[15] They reported that in the course of numerous attempted en bloc resections, preoperatively unrecognized tumor margins were transected, leading them to employ an en bloc resection of the EAC followed by piecemeal removal of tumor extending beyond this surgical margin. They contend: "the step by step procedures create less operative morbidity and mortality. The operation is sequential and allows for decision making and innovation. Often more bone is removed than in a classical temporal bone resection."[15]

Local recurrence is the most common manifestation of surgical failure.[58] Manolidis et al. demonstrated a high incidence of positive margins following resection of advanced disease; they demonstrated a 50% chance of positive margins with T3 tumors and 86% in T4 lesions.[20] Positive margins reduce survival by nearly 50%.[20,38,39] Proponents of en bloc excision argue that it allows for clearer surgical margins, thus improving survival. No randomized study exists comparing piecemeal with en bloc excision, and, given the rarity of the disease, such a study is likely infeasible. In a meta-analysis by Prasad et al., there was no statistically significant difference in survival when comparing mastoidectomy (50% 5-year survival), lateral temporal bone resection (48.6% 5-year survival), or subtotal temporal bone resection (50% 5-year survival) for lesions confined to the external canal. For lesions involving the middle ear and mastoid, there was a trend toward better cure rates with subtotal temporal bone resection (41.7% 5-year survival) versus lateral temporal bone resection (28.6%5-year survival) or radical mastoidectomy (17.1% 5-year survival); however, there was no statistically significance difference among the approaches.[58] Other authors have reported good results utilizing a piecemeal approach for extensive tumors.[15,16,30] Pensak et al. reported a disease-specific survival of 81.5% utilizing a lateral temporal bone resection combined with anterior and posterior petrosectomy for advanced lesions.[16] Hence, they advocate a modified lateral temporal bone resection for disease extending beyond the EAC.[16,17]

The controversy over these differing surgical approaches to temporal bone tumors remains unresolved. Given the rarity of the disease and the variety of techniques employed, a conclusive study is unlikely. However, a thorough understanding of all the potential operations available is a prerequisite for determining the most appropriate approach for each individual lesion. The classic operations include sleeve resection, lateral temporal bone resection, subtotal temporal bone resection, and total temporal bone resection. The following sections include a detailed description of these operations along with our own personal views of when each should be employed.

OPERATIVE TECHNIQUES

Sleeve Resection

The sleeve resection should be used only for those rare tumors truly confined to the skin and soft tissue of the cartilaginous portion of the EAC. An incision is first made medially to ensure that the bony cartilaginous junction is not involved. The lateral cut is made so that the resection encompasses the entire lesion. The involved skin and underlying cartilage are removed, resulting in a wide meatoplasty. The area can be reconstructed with a split-thickness skin graft.

Lateral Temporal Bone Resection

A lateral temporal bone resection can be performed for tumors that involve the cartilaginous and bony canal but have not violated the annulus, thus not encroaching on the tympanic cavity. The entire external canal is removed en bloc along with the tympanic membrane, malleus, and incus (Figure 42–2). First, the outer canal opening is outlined and an extended postauricular incision is made. The ear is reflected anteriorly and the resulting flap is extended to expose the parotid gland. The facial nerve is dissected from the stylomastoid foramen to the pes anserinus.

A cortical mastoidectomy with an extended facial recess approach is performed. The facial nerve should be skeletonized from its second genu to the stylomastoid foramen. The incudostapedial joint is disarticulated and the facial nerve is further exposed anteriorly along its horizontal segment. To remove the specimen en bloc, two surgical planes must be developed. The superior attachment of the osseous canal must be freed by opening the epitympanum and zygomatic root. The second plane is created in an anterior, inferior, and medial direction, transecting the tympanic bone medial to the tympanic annulus but lateral to the jugular bulb and facial nerve. This plane is continued anteriorly until the glenoid fossa is skeletonized. The specimen is now held by the anterior tympanic bone, which can be fractured free with an osteotome. An expanded radical mastoid cavity is produced. The specimen is left attached to the parotid gland and a superficial parotidectomy is performed. The eustachian tube can be plugged with muscle and the defect closed with split-thickness skin grafts.

Modified Lateral Temporal Bone Resection

If the tumor extends into the tympanic cavity or involves the mastoid air cells, further resection of involved areas is performed. The facial nerve, if involved, should be sacrificed and biopsies taken to assess for potential tumor extension medially along the nerve. A posterior petrosectomy can be done to ensure removal of adequate bony margins. The cochlea and labyrinth are not sacrificed unless they are directly involved with tumor. Such piecemeal removal of bone allows a more complete excision of tumors with transannular or mastoid/petrous air cell invasion without the associated morbidity of a subtotal or total temporal bone resection.

The canal and postauricular incisions are made in a manner similar to those of the classic lateral temporal bone resection. A cortical mastoidectomy with extended facial recess approach is performed. The posterior petrosectomy consists of bone removal posteriorly to the transverse/sigmoid sinus junction and the posterior fossa dura. Medially, the superior petrosal sinus is identified and exposed. The tegmen is removed below the temporal lobe. The perilabyrinthine and retrofacial air cells are opened inferiorly to the jugular bulb. The anterior dissection continues to the glenoid fossa as in the classic lateral temporal bone resection. The resulting specimen is removed in a piecemeal fashion as already described. Temporalis and/or sternocleidomastoid muscle flaps are used to obliterate the more extensive defect created by this approach.

Subtotal Temporal Bone Resection

Traditionally, subtotal temporal bone resection (Figure 42–3) is designed to remove the entire temporal bone lateral to the petrous carotid artery in an en bloc fashion. If necessary, portions of dura, sigmoid sinus, parotid gland, and mandible can be resected with the specimen. It is typically used for tumors that extensively encroach on the tympanic cavity or the mastoid air cells.

Canal and postauricular incisions are made as described earlier. The inferior portion of the incision is extended into the neck to allow adequate exposure for neck exploration. The great vessels and nerves of the neck are dissected and identified. The zygoma is transected, as is the ascending ramus of the mandible. The divided ramus and head of the mandible are removed and a subtotal or total parotidectomy is performed. The facial nerve is transected; the distal stumps may be tagged for subsequent nerve grafting. The sternocleidomastoid muscle and the posterior belly of the digastric muscle are separated from the mastoid tip. The styloid process is transected. The external carotid artery is identified and divided. A temporal craniotomy is performed to verify the absence of intracranial extension of tumor. The temporal lobe is retracted medially to expose the petrous bone. An expanded mastoidectomy is performed, and the sigmoid sinus is skeletonized to the jugular bulb. Continuing anteriorly and superiorly, the internal carotid artery is exposed anterior to the jugular bulb and separated from the temporal bone. The internal auditory canal is opened using a middle cranial fossa approach and the VII and VIII cranial nerves are divided. The eustachian tube is divided anteriorly and the horizontal segment of the internal carotid artery is exposed. The only remaining attachment of the temporal bone is its anterior segment along the vertical face of the internal carotid artery. These osseous attachments can be fractured free with gentle rocking and careful use of osteotomes.

The large defect created can be filled either with regional muscle flaps or a microvascular free tissue transfer. There are numerous options for reconstruction, including but not limited to a radial forearm fasciocutaneous flap, a rectus myofasciocutaneous flap, and a lateral thigh flap. These flaps provide vascularized coverage of a large bony defect as well as appropriate coverage and protection to underlying dura or vessels.

In lieu of an en bloc resection, we have used the modified lateral temporal bone resection with a posterior petrosectomy. Removal of the facial nerve, cochlea, and labyrinth is performed only when they are identified to be involved with tumor in the

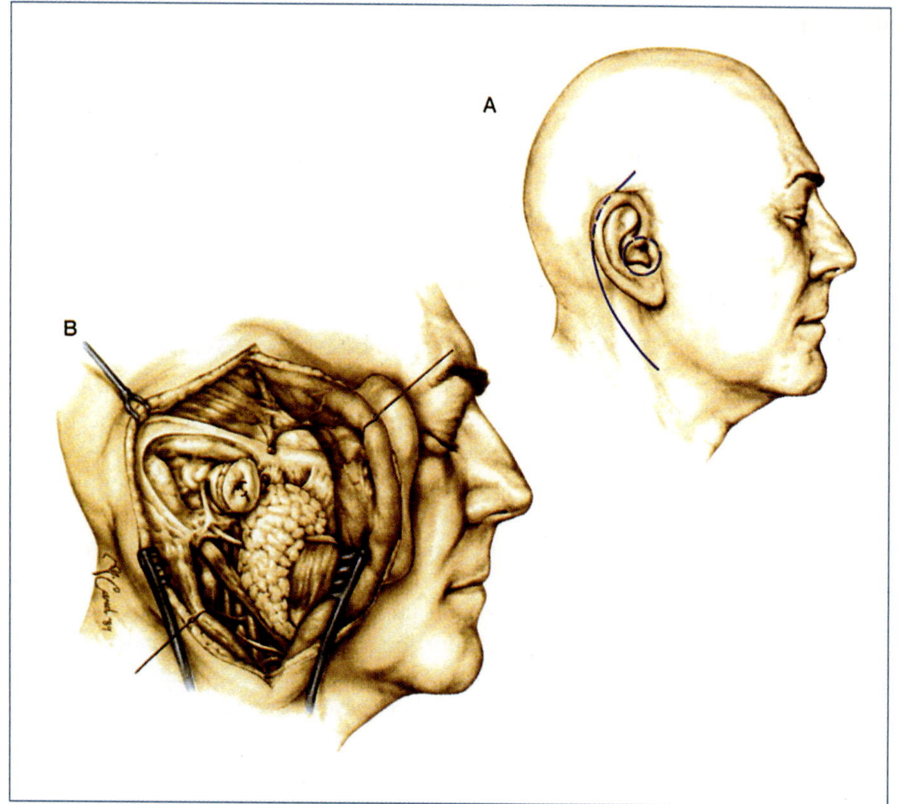

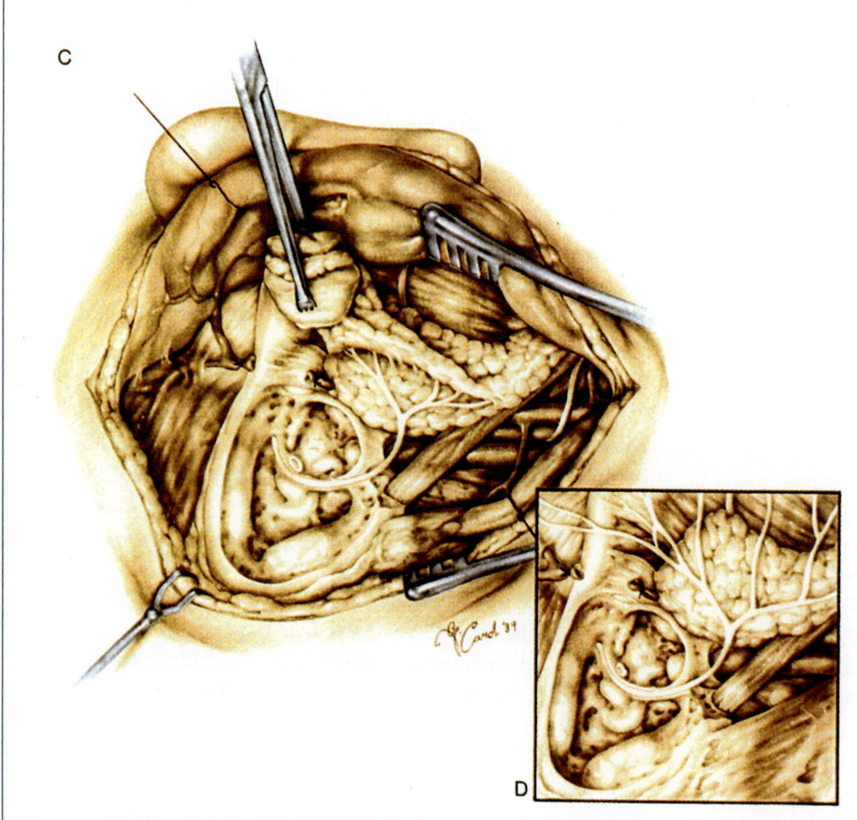

FIGURE 42–2 • Lateral temporal bone resection. *A*, Canal and extended postauricular incisions are carried out. Anterior and posterior flaps are developed, showing the exposed parotid gland and facial nerve at the stylomastoid foramen. *B*, A mastoidectomy with extended facial recess approach is performed. *C*, The external auditory canal and the tympanic membrane have been mobilized from the temporal bone. The specimen remains attached to the lateral lobe of the parotid gland. A lateral parotid lobectomy is completed. *D*, Appearance of a defect following removal of the specimen.

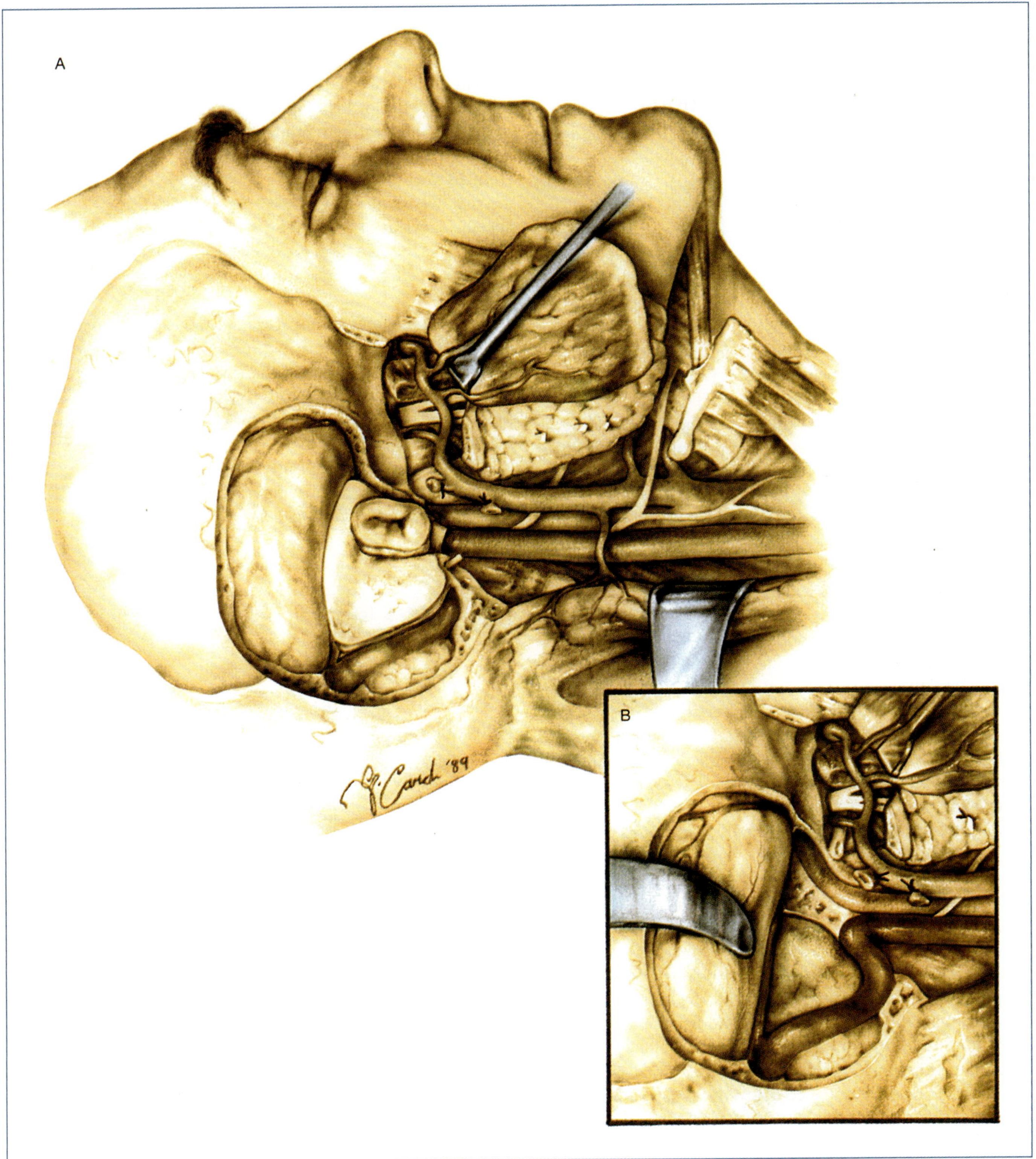

FIGURE 42–3 • Subtotal temporal bone resection. The major neurovascular structures of the neck have been identified. The ascending ramus of the mandible is removed, and a subtotal parotidectomy has been performed. The common carotid artery is isolated, and the branches of the external carotid artery are sacrificed. The posterior and middle fossa dura are exposed (*A*). Appearance following removal of the specimen. The internal carotid artery has been exposed throughout its intratemporal course. The eustachian tube is obliterated and the cavity can be lined with split-thickness skin grafts (*B*).

course of the procedure. In this manner, it is hoped that vital structures can be preserved, if at all possible, and morbidity can be minimized.

Total Temporal Bone Resection

As initially described by Graham et al., total temporal bone resection removes the entirety of the temporal bone and sacrifices the internal carotid artery.[9] This approach requires careful preoperative evaluation as previously described to determine if the patient can tolerate unilateral sacrifice of the internal carotid artery.

Auricular and cervical skin flaps are elevated and the great vessels and nerves in the neck identified. The parotid gland, facial nerve, and ascending ramus of the mandible are resected. The internal and external carotid arteries are divided, as well as cranial nerves IX (glossopharyngeal), X (vagus), and XI (spinal accessory) and the internal jugular vein. The pterygoid muscles are divided. The mandibular division of the trigeminal nerve (V3) is identified and preserved. A craniotomy is performed, and the middle and posterior fossa dura are exposed. The transverse sinus is ligated posterior to its junction with the sigmoid sinus. The superior petrosal sinus is divided anteriorly before it enters the cavernous sinus. Sataloff advocates ligation and division of the distal portion of the internal carotid artery intracranially between the cavernous sinus and the origin of the ophthalmic artery.[10]

A chisel is placed just inside the foramen ovale, directed toward the ligated portion of the superior petrosal sinus. It passes lateral to the cavernous sinus through the carotid canal, the skull base, and lateral skull wall, freeing the anterior portion of the middle fossa floor. A posterior cut is made, lateral to medial, directed anteriorly and stopping posteromedial to the mastoid tip and posterior to the jugular foramen. A connecting cut is made from the posterior-lateral cut, going medial to the jugular foramen and lateral to the foramen magnum. The inferior petrosal sinus is divided and the final connections severed allowing the specimen to be removed en bloc.

At the University of Cincinnati, we avoid use of total, en bloc temporal bone resection. If the entire petrous bone must be removed, we perform an anterior petrosectomy along with the posterior petrosectomy procedure described earlier. A temporal craniotomy is performed and the temporal lobe is retracted medially to expose V3, the middle meningeal artery at the foramen spinosum, the greater petrosal nerve, and the geniculate ganglion. The internal auditory canal is opened, and Kawase's triangle is drilled out to the posterior fossa dura subsequent to exposing the horizontal segment of the internal carotid artery. The remainder of the apex can then be removed in addition to the cochlea, with preservation of the cochlea, by following the internal carotid artery to its vertical segment. The reconstructive options are similar to the subtotal temporal bone resection.

PROGNOSIS

The prognosis for patients with temporal bone malignancy has improved over the last several decades. These modest gains are most likely to be attributable to improvements in temporal bone imaging, surgical technique, and radiotherapy.[1] Table 42–5 summarizes the overall results of several published series.[1,11,13,14,16,17,19,20,26,30,38] These series are all limited by small patient populations; therefore, given the heterogeneity of patients and tumor histology as well as the differing spectrum of disease and treatment modalities, it is difficult to determine a definitive treatment paradigm. Overall survival rates range from 28 to 66%.[1,11,13,14,16,17,19,20,26,30,38,39] A more recent study cited a 5-year overall survival of 77%[62]; however, its reported disease-specific survival of 79% and disease-free survival of 52% are comparable the date from previous studies.[1,11,13,14,16,17,19,20,26,30,38,39,62] Disease-specific survival rates typically range from 58 to 81.5%.[16,19,20]

These outcomes do not accurately reflect the poor prognosis for patients with extensive disease. The patient with disease limited to the EAC has a good chance of cure, with reported survival rates ranging from 80 to 100%, but disease is infrequently found to be limited. Disease extension into the middle ear and mastoid cavity reduces the 5-year survival rates to approximately 40 to 60%, and in the setting of gross tumor extension beyond the confines of the temporal bone, the 5-year survival is abysmal, ranging from 18 to 25%.[1,11,12,19,21,23,36]

TABLE 42–5 Temporal bone malignancies—survival

SOURCE	NO. OF PATIENTS	SURVIVAL (%)	MINIMUM FOLLOW-UP
Conley and Schuller[5]	61	61	2 yr
Gacek and Goodman[7]	31	61	2 yr
Lewis[8]	132	28	5 yr
Kinney and Wood[11]	30	69	6 mo (2.5 yr avg)
Pensak and colleagues[12]	39	51	5 yr
Austin and colleagues[16]	22	41	4 yr
Manolidis and colleagues[17]	81	58	3 yr
Moody and colleagues[19]	32	50	2 yr
Goodwin and Jesse[21]	136	46	5 yr
Pfreunder and colleagues[23]	27	61	2 yr
Arriaga and colleagues[36]	39	45	2 yr
Spector[38]	51	66	1.5 yr

Survival data reflect results regardless of staging, treatment modality, or pathology. Percentages are for overall survival, not disease-free or disease-specific survival.

CONCLUSIONS

Temporal bone malignancies are rare but potentially devastating tumors. Surgeons must be intimately familiar with the complex anatomy of the temporal bone and lateral skull base before attempting to surgical intervention. Although a great progress has been made in skull base surgery, heroic efforts at extirpation of an advanced temporal bone carcinoma often result in significant morbidity for the patient with little chance for a long-term survival. More conservative surgical approaches, combined with adjuvant therapies, may theoretically allow preservation of vital structures and important cranial nerve function while maintaining survival rates similar to those obtained with more radical resections. Physicians must consider social and emotional issues as well as surgical and oncologic concerns to define the most appropriate therapeutic regimen for the individual patient.

References

1. Spector JG. Management of temporal bone carcinomas: A therapeutic analysis of two grops of patients and long term follow-up. Otolarygol Head Neck Surg 1991;104:58–66.
2. Arena S. Tumor surgery of the temporal bone. Laryngoscope 1974;84:615–70.
3. Politzer A. Textbook of diseases of the ear. London: Balliere Tindall & Cox; 1883. p. 729–34.
4. Heyer H. Ueber einen Fall von Ohrencarcinoma, hehardelt mit Resection des Fesenbeines. Dtsch Z Chir 1899;50:552–3.
5. Ward GE, Loch WE, Burkland CW. Total resection of the temporal bone for malignancy of the middle ear. Ann Surg 1951;134:397–403.
6. Campbell EH, Volk RM, Burkland CW. Total resection of the temporal bone for malignancy of the middle ear. Ann Surg 1951;134:397–401.
7. Parsons H, Lewis JS. Subtotal temporal bone resection for cancer of the ear. Cancer 1954;7:995–1001.
8. Hilding D, Selker R. Total resection of the temporal bone for carcinoma. Arch Otolaryngol 1969;89:636–45.
9. Graham MD, Sataloff RT, Kemink JL, et al. Total en bloc resection of the temporal bone and carotid artery for malignant tumors of the ear and temporal bone. Laryngoscope 1984;94:528–33.
10. Sataloff RT, Myers DL, Lowry LD, et al. Total temporal bone resection for squamous cell carcinoma. Otolaryngol Head Neck Surg 1987;96:4–14.
11. Conley JJ, Schuller DE. Malignancies of the ear. Laryngoscope 1976;86:1147–63.
12. Crabtree JA, Britton BH, Pierce MK. Carcinoma of the external auditory canal. Laryngoscope 1976;86:405–15.
13. Gacek RR, Goodman M. Management of malignancy of the temporal bone. Laryngoscope 1977;87:622–34.
14. Lewis JS. Surgical management of tumors of the middle ear and mastoid. J Laryngol Otol 1983;97:299–311.
15. Kinney SE, Wood BG. Malignancies of the external ear canal and temporal bone: Surgical techniques and results. Laryngoscope 1987;97:158–64.
16. Pensak ML, Gleich LL, Gluckman JL, et al. Temporal bone carcinoma: contemporary perspectives in the skull base surgical era. Laryngoscope 1996;106:1234–7.
17. Kinney SE. Clinical evaluation and treatment of ear tumors. In: Comprehensive management of head and neck tumors. Vol 1. Thawley SE, Panje WR, Batsakis JG, et al., editors. Philadelphia, PA: WB Saunders; 1999. p. 380–94.
18. Arena S, Keen M. Carcinoma of the middle ear and temporal bone. Am J Otol 1988;9:351–6.
19. Austin JR, Stewart KL, Fawzi N. Squamous cell carcinoma of the external auditory canal: Therapeutic prognosis based on a proposed staging system. Arch Otolaryngol Head Neck Surg 1994;120:1228–32.
20. Manolidis S, Pappas D Jr, Von Doersten P, et al. Temporal bone and lateral skull base malignancy: Experience and results with 81 patients. Am J Otol 1998;Suppl 19:1–15.
21. Koriwchak M. Temporal bone cancer. Amer J Otolaryngology 1993;14:623.
22. Morton RP, Stell PM, Derrick PP. Epidemiology of cancer of the middle ear cleft. Cancer 1984;53:1612–7.
23. Chung SJ, Pensak ML. Chapter 60: Tumors of the temporal bone. In: Jackler RK, Brackman DE, editors. Neurotology. Philadelphia, PA: Elsevier Mosby; 2005. p. 1028–36.
24. Barrs DM. Temporal bone carcinoma. Otolaryngol Clin North Am. 2001;34(6):1197–218.
25. Whitehead AL. A case of primary epithelioma of the tympanum following chronic suppurative otitis media. Proc R Soc Med 1968;1:34–6.
26. Goodwin WJ, Jesse RH. Malignant neoplasms of the external auditory canal and temporal bone. Arch Otolaryngol 1980;106:675–9.
27. Beal D, Lindsay J, Ward PH. Radiation induced carcinoma of the mastoid. Arch Otolaryngol 1965;81:9–16.
28. Lustig LR, Jackler RK, Lanser MJ. Radiation-induced tumors of the temporal bone. Am J Otol 1997;18:230–5.
29. Jin YT, Tsai ST, Li C, et al. Prevalence of human papilloma virus in middle ear carcinoma associated with chronic otitis media. Am J Pathol 1997;150:1327–33.
30. Moody SA, Hirsch BE, Myers EN. Squamous cell carcinoma of the external auditory canal: an evaluation of a staging system. Am J Otol 2000;21:582–8.
31. Kuhel WI, Hume CR, Slesnick SH. Cancer of the external auditory canal and temporal bone. Otolaryngol Clin North Am 1996;29:827–53.
32. Liu F, Keane TJ, Davidson J. Primary carcinoma involving the petrous temporal bone. Head Neck 1993;15:39–43.
33. Leonetti JP, Smith PG, Kletzker GR, et al. Invasion patterns of advanced temporal bone malignancies. Am J Otol 1996;17:438–42.
34. Kenyon GS, Marks PV, Scholtz CL, et al. Squamous cell carcinoma of the middle ear: A 25 year retrospective study. Ann Otol Rhinol Laryngol 1985;94:273–7.
35. Zhang B, Tu G, Xu G, et al. Squamous cell carcinoma of temporal bone: reported on 33 patients. Head Neck 1999;21:461–6.
36. Gacek MR, Gacek RR, Gantz B, et al. Pseudoepitheliomatous hyperplasia versus squamous cell carcinoma of the EAC. Laryngoscope 1998;108:620–3.
37. Lesser RW, Spector GJ, Devineni VR. Malignant tumors of the middle ear and external auditory canal: A 20 year review. Otolaryngol Head Neck Surg 1987;96:43–7.
38. Pfreundner L, Schwager K, Willner J, et al. Carcinoma of the external auditory canal and middle ear. Int J Radiat Oncol Biol Phys 1999;44:777–88.

39. Arriaga M, Curtin H, Takahashi H, et al. Staging proposal for external auditory meatus carcinoma based on preoperative clinical examination and computed tomography findings. Ann Otol Rhinol Laryngol 1990;99:714–21.

40. Hicks GW. Tumors arising from the glandular structures of the external auditory canal. Laryngoscope 1983;93:326–40.

41. Chang CYJ, Cheung SW. Auditory canal: Glandular tumors. In: Tumors of the ear and temporal bone. Jackler RK, Driscoll CLW, editors. Philadelphia, PA: Lippincott, Williams & Wilkins; 2000. p. 84–102.

42. Foote RL, Olsen KD, Bonner JA, Lewis JE. Salivary Gland Cancer. In: Clinical radiation oncology. Gunderson LL, Tepper JE, editors. Philadelphia, PA: Elsevier; 2007. p. 781–99.

43. Hyams VJ, Batsakis JG. Pathology of tumors of the ear. In: Comprehensive management of head and neck tumors. Vol 1. Thawley SE, Panje WR, Batsakis JG, Lindberg RD, editors. Philadelphia, PA: WB Saunders; 1999. p. 380–94.

44. Wells SC. Embryonal rhabdomyosarcoma of the ear: A review of literature and case history. J Laryngol Otol 1984;98:1261–6.

45. Crist WM, Anderson JR, Meza JL, et al. Intergroup Rhabdomyosarcoma Study-IV: Results for patients with nonmetastatic disease. J Clin Oncol 2001;19:3091–102.

46. Sutow WW, Lindberg RD, Ruymann F, Soule EH. Three years relapse-free survival rates in childhood rhabdomyosarcoma of the head and neck, Cancer 1982;49:2217–21.

47. Wiatrak BJ, Pensak ML. Rhabdomyosarcoma of the ear and temporal bone. Laryngoscope 1989;99:1188–92.

48. Sutow WW, Sullivan MP, Reid HL. Three year relapse-free survival rates in childhood rhabdomyosarcoma of the head and neck: Report from the Intergroup Rhabdomyosarcoma Study. Cancer 1982;49:2217–21.

49. Meza JL, Anderson J, Pappo AS, Meyer WH. Children's Oncology Group. Analysis of prognostic factors in patients with nonmetastatic rhabdomyosarcoma treated on Children's Oncology Group. Analysis of prognostic factors in patients with nonmetastatic intergroup rhabdomyosarcoma studies III and IV: The Children's Oncology Group. J Clin Oncol 2006;24(24):3844–51.

50. Chandrasekhar SS. Temporal bone tumors in children: Sarcomas. In: Tumors of the ear and temporal bone. Jackler RK, Driscoll CLW, editors. Philadelphia, PA: Lippincott, Williams & Wilkins; 2000. p. 440–51.

51. Streitmann MJ, Sismanis A. Metastatic carcinoma of the temporal bone. Am J Otol 1996;17:780–3.

52. McCaffrey TV, McDonald TJ. Histiocytosis X of the ear and temporal bone: Review of 22 cases. Laryngoscope 1979;89: 1735–42.

53. Angeli SI, Alcalde J, Hoffman HT, et al. Langerhans' cell histiocytosis of the head and neck in children. Ann Otol Rhinol Laryngol 1995;104:173–80.

54. Stell PM, McCormick MS. Carcinoma of the external auditory meatus and middle ear: Prognostic factors and a suggested staging system. J Laryngol Otol 1985;99:847–50.

55. Clark LJ, Narula AQ, Morgan DA, et al. Squamous cell carcinoma of the temporal bone: A revised staging. J Laryngol Otol 1991;105:346–8.

56. Arriaga M, Curtin HD, Takahashi H, et al. The role of preoperative CT scans in staging external auditory meatus carcinoma: Radiologic-pathologic correlation study. Otolaryngol Head Neck Surg 1991;105:6–11.

57. Harwood AR, Keane TJ. Malignant tumors of the temporal bone and external ear: medical and radiation therapy. In: Otologic medicine and surgery. Vol 2. Alberti PW, Reuben RJ, editors. London: Churchill Livingstone; 1988. p. 1389–408.

58. Prasad S, Janecka IP. Efficacy of surgical treatments for squamous cell carcinoma of the temporal bone: A literature review. Otolaryngol Head Neck Surg 1994;110:270–80.

59. Smouha EE, Karmody CS. Non-osteitic complications of therapeutic radiation to the temporal bone. Am J Otol 1995;16: 83–7.

60. Taghian A, deVathaire F, Terrier P, et al. Long-term risk of sarcoma following radiation treatmaent for breast cancer. Int J Radiat Oncol Bio Phys 1991;21(2):361–7.

61. Moffat DA, Grey P, Ballagh RH, et al. Extended temporal bone resection for squamous cell carcinoma. Otolaryngol Head Neck Surg 1997;116:617–23.

62. Moore MG, Deschler DG, McKenna MJ, Varvares MA, Lin DT. Management outcomes following lateral temporal bone resection for ear and temporal bone malignancies. Otolarngol Head Neck Surg 2007;137:893–8.

Prevention and Management of Cerebrospinal Fluid Leaks

43

Roberto A. Cueva, MD, FACS / Christopher J. Danner, MD

INTRODUCTION

Cerebrospinal fluid (CSF) leak rates related to neurotologic surgery vary widely with a reported incidence from less than 2% to more than 20%.[1–8] Some authors have focused on different single "silver bullet" preventative measures ranging from prophylactic external CSF drainage, tissue glues, and bone cement in attempts to reduce the incidence of this relatively common complication. A retrospective meta-analysis of different preventative measures showed no significant change in leak rate with the isolated application of the above aforementioned techniques and the average leak rate in over 5,000 cases was 10%.[9] In 2004, Sanna et al. reported a CSF leak rate of 2.8% in 707 vestibular schwannoma patients, finding no correlation between CSF leak rate and tumor size. Furthermore, they attributed the low incidence of CSF leak to the meticulous application of multiple measures.[10,11] Supporting the contention that attention to multiple details of approach design, development of optimal tissue planes, and meticulous attention to details of wound closure can substantially lower CSF leak rate, Cueva and Mastrodimos reported a overall CSF leak rate of 1.2% in 343 patients undergoing cerebellopontine angle (CPA) surgery.[12]

Grotenhuis reported that postoperative CSF leaks increase medical costs by as much as 21.7% in a cohort of 412 elective craniotomy patients. This series had the highest incidence of CSF leak following infratentorial procedures (12.8%) and extensive skull base procedures (34.6%).[13] Patients with postoperative CSF leak are reported to require surgical repair in 50 to 75% of cases.[2,3] Meningitis continues to have high associated rates of morbidity and mortality. The risk of meningitis associated with postoperative CSF leak has been reported to be as high as 5%.[2] As Benjamin Franklin so aptly put it, when it comes to postoperative CSF leaks, "an ounce of prevention is worth a pound of cure."

We begin this chapter focusing on prevention of postoperative CSF leaks since doing so reduces patient morbidity, minimizes risk of meningitis, prevents revision surgery, shortens hospitalization, and speeds return to family and work. The next section will focus on diagnosis of CSF leak (postoperative and spontaneous). The last section addresses treatment of CSF leaks.

APPROACH DESIGN AND WOUND CLOSURE

Prevention of postoperative CSF leaks begins with approach design, anticipation of routes for CSF egress, application of measures to block the latter, and meticulous wound closure. This section will cover nuances specific to various common surgical approaches used for neurotologic skull base surgery.[12] The focus is on aspects of approach design and wound closure aimed at reducing CSF leak.

Translabyrinthine

The skin incision is placed approximately one-finger breadth above the ear and two-finger breadths behind the ear. As the incision approaches the mastoid tip, it is kept on the posterior surface to avoid the thin skin on the lateral aspect of the mastoid process. This provides a more robust layer for closure in this part of the skin incision. In the portion of the incision above the auricle, the dissection is taken through the periauricular muscles to the areolar temporalis fascia. As the cutaneous flap is developed, the plane of the flap is taken more superficial leaving the periauricular muscles attached to the underlying periosteum in the posterosuperior corner of the incision. This provides a thicker closure layer in this naturally thin part of the periosteum. Next, the muscular incision is offset from the cutaneous incision by approximately 1 cm. This offset creates an overlap of the skin and periosteal flaps, promoting tissue adhesion and avoiding an alignment of the muscle and skin incisions. The position of the muscle incision is usually beyond the margins of the bony resection, creating an overlap of the muscle flap onto the calvarium for another layer of tissue adhesion.

During the translabyrinthine exposure, a facial recess dissection is performed and the incus is removed. The long process of the incus is amputated and the body of the incus used to obstruct the middle-ear opening of the Eustachian tube. To more easily perform this maneuver, the tensor tympani tendon is cut and the tubal orifice visualized via the facial recess and attic exposure. The Eustachian tube may be first filled with periosteum from the deep cervical musculature. Then the short process of the incus is advanced firmly down the Eustachian tube to occlude the bony orifice with the incus body. Deep cervical muscle is harvested from the lower aspect of the soft-tissue exposure and is cut into small pieces. These are then used to fill the middle ear after the incus body has been placed in the Eustachian tube during the closure. If there are any significant air cells along the zygomatic root or around the internal auditory canal exposure, these should be waxed.

The dura that was opened in a "Y"-shaped incision with the bottom of the "Y" aimed at the sinodural angle is approximated as much as possible. Abdominal fat is cut into strips roughly the width of an index finger. The narrower end is positioned just through the dural defect with the wider end placed in the mastoid bony defect. Usually two to three such fat strips are required. The musculoperiosteal flap incision is closed in an interrupted fashion with 2–0 woven polyglactic acid sutures spaced approximately 1 cm (or less) apart. The deep cutaneous layer is closed with inverted interrupted sutures of the same material, which engage the deep dermis within the course of the stitch. Staple closure of the skin completes the closure. A compression dressing is applied and kept in place until the patient no longer has emesis or is discharged.

Presigmoid/Retrolabyrinthine

Incision planning is identical to the translabyrinthine approach but treatment of the middle ear and ossicles is radically different. Furthermore, during elevation of the cutaneous flap, an areolar temporalis fascia graft (measuring 5 to 6 cm in diameter) is harvested, pressed, and set aside to dry. The presigmoid/retrolabyrinthine approach is used to gain access to the posterior fossa while preserving hearing. Therefore, any manipulation of the middle-ear space is minimized and care is taken not to widely open the additus or facial recess. The dura is commonly opened with an incision paralleling the superior petrosal sinus and sigmoid sinus. Alternately, the dura may be opened with an incision that parallels the sigmoid sinus, extends onto the middle fossa dura, and entails division of the superior petrosal sinus. Either dural opening results in an anteriorly based dural flap, which is retracted over the labyrinth. If this flap is preserved during the surgery, it is used as part of the closure.

To start the closure, collagen sponge (Gelfoam, Pfizer Inc.) is placed into the epitympanum to prevent fixation of the ossicular chain. Then to isolate the middle ear from the intradural space, the broad sheet of fascia is carefully draped over the additus and open air cells along the course of the facial nerve and overlapping the bony labyrinth. The large continuous piece of fascia may often be folded to have a double layer covering the exposed air cells leading to the middle ear. Another technique for closing the air cells, using a calcium phosphate cement, Norian (Synthes Inc.) or Hydroset (Stryker Inc.) is effective in sealing the air cells while leaving the middle ear-space untouched. The junior author finds that Hydroset is less brittle and sets better in a wet environment.

Once the pathway to the middle ear and Eustachian tube has been dealt with if the dura posterior to the bony labyrinth has not been resected, it is reapproximated as much as possible and the temporal bone defect is then filled with abdominal fat. If a dural defect is present, it is packed as one would for a translabyrinthine approach. The muscle and skin layers are closed in the fashion described for translabyrinthine surgery.

Middle Fossa

The conventional middle fossa or extended middle fossa approaches are used to gain access to the internal auditory canal, superior and anterior CPA with hearing preservation in mind. Since hearing preservation is a major goal, care is taken to avoid opening the middle ear. Even when the middle ear is not directly opened, temporal bone air cells are commonly disrupted and may be a potential route for CSF escape. After the surgical objective has been completed, care is taken to seal the air cell system. If the air cells are only minimally opened, then one may seal them with a thin layer of bone wax. As the air cells become more disrupted, additional techniques are required to ensure that a proper CSF seal is achieved. A layer of areolar fascia harvested from the temporalis muscle, or commercially available dural substitute, is used to cover superior aspect of the exposed petrous bone and abdominal fat then placed on top of the fascia to firmly set it into place. This combined use of fascia and fat is very successful in preventing CSF leak when the air cell system has been extensively opened. Bacitracin soaked collagen sponge used in place of fat has also been successful.[12]

Retrosigmoid

Because of the thickness of the muscular tissues traversed during the retrosigmoid approach, offsetting the skin and muscular incisions is not necessary. The mastoid air cells opened while performing the retrosigmoid craniectomy(otomy) must be waxed to eliminate this route for CSF leak. Care is taken to make sure that the wax does not overhang the edges of bony dissection as manipulation of the surrounding soft tissue may dislodge the wax seal. Likewise, waxing the area of bony drilled during exposure of the internal auditory canal is routinely done even if no air cells are identified. To accomplish this, small pieces of bone wax are delivered into the area and then compressed onto the bone surrounding the internal auditory canal with a small cottonoid. The surgeon must avoid excess bone wax being inadvertently pushed into the distal internal auditory canal. Careful waxing the air cells is usually sufficient for preventing CSF otorhinorrhea. To facilitate closure of the opened dura at the end of surgery, it is beneficial to place saline soaked Gelfoam under the retraced dural leaflets to preventing desiccation during the procedure. If the dura is kept moist during the case, there is usually no difficulty closing the dural incisions. To further seal the dural suture lines, blood soaked microfibrillar collagen hemostat (Avitene, Davol Inc.) may be applied. Craniectomy may be performed with nothing to replace the skull defect other than Avitene. Other authors replace the bone flaps or fill the defect with a bone cement.[1]

Far Lateral/Transcondylar Approach

To approach the inferior aspect of the posterior fossa, foramen magnum, and upper spinal canal, the far lateral/transcondylar approach is often used. Proper planning and preservation of tissue planes helps minimize postoperative CSF leak. Overlapping tissue flaps with an anteriorly based skin flap and a posteriorly based periosteal flap keeps the incisions well separated to help prevent leak. Areolar temporalis fascia is harvested as discussed in earlier approach descriptions. Opened mastoid air cells are occluded with wax and the dura is reapproximated. The dura around the foramen magnum is difficult to close completely. A small cuff of tissue is purposely left on the transverse process of C1 and the mastoid process. This allows proper reapproximation of different tissue layers at the conclusion of the case. The areolar fascia graft is first placed over the dura. Then abdominal fat is packed into the areas of bone removal. These grafts are then held snugly in place by the overlying muscle tissue that is reattached to the transverse process of C1 and mastoid. The rest of the deep tissues are meticulously closed with interrupted suture placed about 1 cm apart. The skin is closed in a similar fashion with subcutaneous sutures. A pressure dressing is applied and left in place for approximately 5 days postoperatively.

DIAGNOSIS OF CSF LEAK

Postoperative, spontaneous, and post-traumatic CSF leaks may be diagnosed by careful history and physical exam. A defect in the dura around the temporal bone will transmit spinal fluid in to the mastoid air cells. The CSF may leak through a defect in the external ear canal, tympanic membrane, or percolate down the Eustachian tube into the nasopharynx. Patients may complain of unilateral nasal drainage that is worse after waking up or when bending over. Coughing or other exercises that increase intracranial pressure may also increase the flow of spinal fluid. Some cases of spontaneous CSF leak may eluded a rapid diagnosis, while others such as clear fluid seeping through the surgical incision pose little diagnostic dilemma.

Spinal fluid leaks not only occur as a consequence of surgery or trauma but may also occur spontaneously. Congenitally thin and dehiscent tegmen may be a source of spontaneous middle-ear effusion. Dehiscent tegmen may be a result of increase intracranial pressure or arachnoid granulations. Cerebrospinal fluid may also propagate along the fallopian canal and leak adjacent to the facial nerve.[14–17] Therefore, one needs to remain suspicious of a persistent middle-ear effusion and chronic clear tube otorrhea.[16] The cause of which may not be chronic otitis media but may be a persistent CSF leak.

Diagnosis of CSF leak may be done solely on clinic suspicion, radiologic imaging, and/or laboratory studies. At times a CSF leak is obvious and treatment may commence based solely on clinical findings. Other times leaks may be more insidious requiring multiple diagnostic tests before a firm diagnosis may be made. T2-weighted MRI cisternography is useful to localize the leak source. Computed tomography with intrathecal administration of contrast may also be used to locate the source of the leak.[18,19] If enough fluid can be collected, it can be sent for β_2-transferrin. However, β_2-transferrin is not the ideal confirmatory laboratory study for spinal fluid leak. Most medical centers do not perform the test on site since it requires gel electrophoresis. The specimen is commonly sent to a reference laboratory with results unavailable for several days. Other laboratory studies include CSF glucose and protein levels. Glucose and protein concentrations can be measured from the fluid suspected to be CSF. Glucose content needs to exceed 0.4 g/L and protein needs to be less than 1 g/L to a max of 2 g/L. However, unless the measured fluid contains almost pure CSF, rarely does the collected sample reach the specified diagnostic limits. A CSF leak of sufficient volume to collect almost pure CSF would be obvious and laboratory testing unnecessary. Therefore, glucose and protein concentrations are inherently inaccurate to definitively determine the presence of CSF.

Probably the most definitive laboratory test to evaluate the presence of spinal fluid is prostaglandin-D synthase. Prostaglandin-D synthase, β-trace protein, is produced in the epithelial cells of the choroid plexus and leptomeninges.[20] β-trace protein is one of the most abundant proteins in the CSF. The ratio between CSF and serum concentrations is about 35, the highest among all CSF-specific proteins. An automated assay has been developed which produces reliable results within 20 min.[21,22] Risch evaluated 107 patients with CSF leak and found a sensitivity of 98% and specificity of 100% when measuring β-trace protein. The fluid in question should have a β-trace protein level greater than 0.68 mg/L and the fluid to serum ratio should be 4.9 or greater. β_2-transferrin sensitivity was 84% comparatively in the same patients with known CSF leaks.[20]

Once the diagnosis of spinal fluid leak is made, one needs to determine the most efficient way of treating the leak.

POSTSURGICAL CEREBROSPINAL FLUID LEAK

Postoperative CSF leaks tend to occur in a bimodal chronological distribution. The first peak is within the first few days following surgery. This is less common than the second modal peak at 2 to 3 weeks postoperatively. Regardless of the timing of onset of the leak, it is treated in similar fashion. Any suspicion of meningitis (severe headache, photophobia, stiff neck, fever, etc) must be investigated. Infection not only reduces morbidity/mortality by early intervention but also increases intracranial pressure and can perpetuate a leak.

Transcutaneous/Incisional Leak

Incisional spinal fluid leaks may be treated by achieving a water-tight skin closure. This may be accomplished by over-sewing the wound. Another effective way of achieving a water-tight closure is applying a liberal amount of n-butyl-cyanoacrylate (Dermabond, Ethicon Inc.) to the wound. Either of these two procedures is usually effective in achieving a water-tight closure. A pressure dressing may also be applied to help counteract any increase in intracranial pressure that may be a consequence of body habitus or disruption in CSF absorption. If there are signs of infection or wound breakdown, the patient should return to the operating room for a formal would revision. In rare circumstances, lumbar drainage may also be required.

CSF Rhinorrhea

Postsurgical CSF rhinorrhea is a consequence of spinal fluid percolating through the mastoid air cells and reaching the nasopharynx via the Eustachian tube. Conservative management with bed rest may be attempted, but this is seldom effective. If the problem occurs in the first few days after surgery, then a lumbar drain is usually recommended for 5 days. Lumbar drainage is usually set to match the rate of CSF production. Cerebrospinal fluid production follows a circadian rhythm with an average production rate of 20 mL/h. A simple way to achieve this is to pin the lumbar drainage bag at the level of the patient's shoulder. To ambulate, the tubing is clamped. The patient will commonly have a headache while the lumbar drain is in place. Over drainage of CSF is to be avoided to reduce the possible complication of subdural hematoma. A pressure dressing is usually applied to the wound during this time. If spinal fluid leak persists after 5 days of a lumbar drain, then reoperation for internal sealing of CSF is usually required.

While revising a wound for a recalcitrant CSF leak, one's choice of surgical approach is dictated on the hearing status. If hearing is present, then reoperation proceeds through the existing soft-tissue approach and focuses on sealing the routes for CSF leak, paying particular attention to isolate all air cells from the intracranial cavity. If a fat graft had been used in the previous surgery, a new fat graft is harvested for repair of the CSF leak. Should a leak require reoperation for repair, then postoperative lumbar drain is commonly left in place for a few more days.

If hearing has been lost or sacrificed related to the prior surgery reentry into the intracranial compartment can be avoided. Friedman et al. advocate obliterating the Eustachian tube via a transcanal procedure. A circumferential incision is made in the ear canal skin. The deep-ear canal skin and tympanic membrane are resected. The Eustachian tube is packed tightly with fascia and/or muscle, which also fills the middle-ear and deep-ear canal. The ear canal skin is then everted and sewn shut.[23]

POSTTRAUMATIC CSF OTORRHEA/RHINORRHEA

In cases of blunt or penetrating head trauma that result in spinal fluid otorrhea, the patient is first stabilized. Treatment of a spinal fluid leak may be done in a parallel fashion while treating other neurologic injuries. In this setting, bed rest will often result in cessation of CSF leak as compared to the postoperative situation. A majority of temporal bone fractures with associated spinal fluid leaks will spontaneously stop leaking within 5 to 7 days. If the spinal fluid leak continues after 7 days of conservative management, then a lumbar drain should be considered. If the leak persists after 5 to 7 days of lumbar drainage, then surgical repair may be considered once the patient has stabilized from other injuries.

SPONTANEOUS CSF LEAK

Spontaneous CSF leaks occur from a congenitally thin or dehiscent tegmen or from arachnoid granulations. Typically leaks occur on and off until the anatomic disruption is surgically repaired. The repair may be performed either through the middle fossa or transmastoid approach. Repair of such tegmen defects uses a combination of soft tissue (fascia or perichondrium) and more rigid tissue such as cartilage or bone. The transmastoid approach can effectively reach tegmen defects posterior to the epitympanum. The middle fossa approach should be used to repair large (>1.5-cm diameter) tegmen defects or those anterior to the epitympanum.

CONCLUSION

The best way to manage CSF leaks is to prevent their occurrence. Keeping postoperative CSF leaks to a minimum can have a significant impact on reducing hospitalization costs related to treating skull base lesions. This is accomplished by using approach designs that respect tissue planes and offset cutaneous and muscular incisions. Attention to the potential routes for CSF escape into the temporal bone–air cell system must be occluded either with bone wax or soft tissue. In those approaches that sacrifice hearing, packing the Eustachian tube and middle ear with fibrous tissue further reduces the risk of a leak. Paying attention to these multiple factors is more effective than relying on a single "silver bullet" solution. Should, in spite of these preventative measures, a leak occur, then treatment begins with more conservative measures. Should conservative measures fail, then reoperation is required. Prevention and expeditious treatment of spinal fluid leaks helps prevent meningitis, reduces morbidity/mortality, decreases hospital stays, and speeds return of patients to their family and work place.

References

1. Arriaga MA, Chen DA, Burke EL. Hydroxyapatite cement cranioplasty in translabyrinthine acoustic neuroma surgery-update. Otol Neurotol 2007;28:538–40.
2. Bryce GE, Nedzelski JM, Rowed DW, Rappaport JM. Cerebrospinal fluid leaks and meningitis in acoustic neuroma surgery. Otolaryngol Head Neck Surg 1991;104:81–7.
3. Celikkanat SM, Saleh E, Khashaba A, et al. Cerebrospinal fluid leak after translabyrinthine acoustic neuroma surgery. Otolaryngol Head Neck Surg 1995;112:654–8.
4. Fishman AJ, Hoffman RA, Roland JT, Jr, Lebowitz RA, Cohen NL. Cerebrospinal fluid drainage in the management of CSF leak following acoustic neuroma surgery. The Laryngoscope 1996;106:1002–4.
5. Hardy DG, Macfarlane R, Baguley D, Moffat DA. Surgery for acoustic neurinoma. An analysis of 100 translabyrinthine operations. Journal Neurosurg 1989;71:799–804.
6. Kemink JL, LaRouere MJ, Kileny PR, Telian SA, Hoff JT. Hearing preservation following suboccipital removal of acoustic neuromas. The Laryngoscope 1990;100:597–602.
7. Leonetti J, Anderson D, Marzo S, Moynihan G. Cerebrospinal fluid fistula after transtemporal skull base surgery. Otolaryngol Head Neck Surg 2001;124:511–4.
8. Rodgers GK, Luxford WM. Factors affecting the development of cerebrospinal fluid leak and meningitis after translabyrinthine acoustic tumor surgery. The Laryngoscope 1993;103:959–62.
9. Selesnick SH, Liu JC, Jen A, Newman J. The incidence of cerebrospinal fluid leak after vestibular schwannoma surgery. Otol Neurotol 2004;25:387–93.

10. Sanna M, Rohit, Skinner LJ, Jain Y. Technique to prevent post-operative CSF leak in the translabyrinthine excision of vestibular schwannoma. J Laryngol Otol 2003;117:965–8.
11. Sanna M, Taibah A, Russo A, Falcioni M, Agarwal M. Perioperative complications in acoustic neuroma (vestibular schwannoma) surgery. Otol Neurotol 2004;25:379–386.
12. Cueva RA, Mastrodimos B. Approach design and closure techniques to minimize cerebrospinal fluid leak after cerebellopontine angle tumor surgery. Otol Neurotol 2005;26:1176–81.
13. Grotenhuis JA. Costs of postoperative cerebrospinal fluid leakage: 1-year, retrospective analysis of 412 consecutive nontrauma cases. Surg Neurol 2005;64:490–3; discussion 493–4.
14. Gubbels SP, Selden NR, Delashaw JB, Jr., McMenomey SO. Spontaneous middle fossa encephalocele and cerebrospinal fluid leakage: Diagnosis and management. Otol Neurotol 2007;28:1131–9.
15. Raghavan U, Majumdar S, Jones NS. Spontaneous CSF rhinorrhoea from separate defects of the anterior and middle cranial fossa. J Laryngol Otol 2002;116:546–7.
16. Gacek RR, Gacek MR, Tart R. Adult spontaneous cerebrospinal fluid otorrhea: Diagnosis and management. Amer J Otol 1999;20:770–6.
17. Schievink WI, Jacques L. Recurrent spontaneous spinal cerebrospinal fluid leak associated with "nude nerve root" syndrome: Case report. Neurosurgery 2003;53:1216–8; discussion 1218–9.
18. Liong WC, Constantinescu CS, Jaspan T. Intrathecal gadolinium-enhanced magnetic resonance myelography in the detection of CSF leak. Neurology 2006;67:1522.
19. Stone JA, Castillo M, Neelon B, Mukherji SK. Evaluation of CSF leaks: High-resolution CT compared with contrast-enhanced CT and radionuclide cisternography. AJNR Am J Neuroradiol 1999;20:706–12.
20. Risch L, Lisec I, Jutzi M, Podvinec M, Landolt H, Huber A. Rapid, accurate and non-invasive detection of cerebrospinal fluid leakage using combined determination of B-trace protein in secretion and serum. Clin Chim Acta 2005;351:169–6.
21. Bachmann G, Petereit H, Djenabi U, Michel O. Predictive values of beta-trace protein (prostaglandin D synthase) by use of laser-nephelometry assay for the identification of cerebrospinal fluid. Neurosurgery 2002;50:571–6; discussion 576–7.
22. Bachmann G. Beta-trace protein: An unknown marker for cerebrospinal fluid leaks. Laryngoscope 2005;115:756; author reply 756–7.
23. Friedman RA, Cullen RD, Ulis J, Brackmann DE. Management of cerebrospinal fluid leaks after acoustic tumor removal. Neurosurgery 2007;61:35–9; discussion 39–40.

APPENDIX Surgical Anatomy of the Temporal Bone and Dissection Guide

Dennis I. Bojrab, MD / Ben J. Balough, MD / Benjamin T. Crane, MD, PhD

INTRODUCTION: EXPANDING ON THE MATERIAL OF G. E. SHAMBAUGH JR., MD

It is easier to see today in the 21st century as we are on the shoulders of giants, with a much easier view of the terrain. The history of ear surgery is rich in dedication and resourcefulness. We owe much of our success to the many who have come before us, dedicated to ingenuity in research and development and teaching new generations of ear surgeons, allowing preceptorships and fellowships. All of the following otologists and many not mentioned encouraged and nurtured a collegial atmosphere of learning for all of us, many times through the relaxed atmosphere of a temporal bone laboratory. I would personally like to thank Dr. Michael E. Glasscock for my fellowship training and his encouragement to me in my endeavors. Dr. Howard House has too many achievements to cover in this format, but I would like to thank him for helping my career direction and for our many meetings during which he joyfully described to me the rich history of otologic surgery.

This Appendix is intended as an anatomic reference to the temporal bone and its structures, with a section on surgical dissection of the temporal bone. This resource is intended for the use of the otolaryngologist who wants a source that couples a basic guide to temporal bone anatomy, basic equipment knowledge of setting up a dissection bench (with microscope, drill, and suction irrigation), and a surgical dissection approach to the most common otologic procedures within the temporal bone.

The great pioneer otologist Bezold, in his *Textbook of Otology*, warned that "the danger to the patient of an incompetent operator, who does not know the many anatomical details crowded together in the narrow space of the temporal bone and their extreme variability, is much greater here than in any other region of the body." Only by cadaver dissections can the aspiring ear surgeon learn to safely traverse the perilous anatomy of the temporal bone so as to avoid injury to the many vital structures concealed in an area no larger than an olive.

Mastoid surgery was one of the most frequent surgeries in the 1930s for children with upper respiratory infections frequently developed acute otitis media followed by acute mastoiditis. Without antibiotics, mastoid surgery was required to combat disastrous complications such as meningitis, brain abscess, sinus thrombosis, and even death. The observation of Fleming, in 1928, of lysis of *Staphylococcus* colonies by *Penicillium* mold and the discovery by Domagk, in 1932, of the antistreptococcal effect of sulfanilamide progressively and dramatically reduced the mortality rate and indications for surgical intervention in acute ear infections. As the variety of antibiotics grew, ear surgery could evolve into a constructive rather than a destructive specialty.

In 1899, Körner suggested that in certain cases of chronic otitis, the tympanic membrane could be left in place during the radical operation, thus preserving useful hearing. In 1910, Bondy described the indication for and technique of a modification of the radical operation for cases of chronic otorrhea in which the pars flaccida perforation was accompanied by an intact pars tensa. Kessel, in 1879, performed stapes mobilization in an attempt to improve a conductive hearing loss. At the 1900 International Congress of Otology, leaders in the specialty united in condemning surgery for deafness as "not only useless, but dangerous to life." So complete was this rejection toward operations for improving hearing that earlier procedures such as stapes mobilization and stapedectomy for otosclerosis as well as operations for repair of tympanic membrane perforations and congenital aural atresia were discontinued. By 1919, Sir Charles Ballance's book *Surgery of the Temporal Bone* failed to mention any sort of operation to improve hearing. In 1930, with *Diseases of the Ear*, Kerrison devoted less than a page to "Surgical Measures for the Relief of Deafness," concluding that "these operations mentioned for their place in otologic history are quite obsolete today."

With considerable courage in the face of this concerted opposition, Bárány, in 1911, Jenkins, in 1912, and Holmgren, in 1914, began to operate to try to improve hearing in otosclerosis. Nylén, in 1921, a young assistant in Holmgren's clinic, first employed a monocular operating microscope to assist in a radical mastoidectomy. Holmgren immediately recognized the advantage of magnification and began to use a binocular operating microscope for his operations on otosclerosis. Holmgren demonstrated that by careful aseptic technique, a semicircular canal could be opened safely and a temporary hearing improvement achieved.

In 1924, Sourdille observed Holmgren's operations and returned to France to devise his two- or three-stage operations called the tympanolabyrinthopexy. With this operation, Sourdille created a fistula in the horizontal semicircular canal and covered it with a skin flap from the meatus. For the first time, permanent hearing improvements in otosclerosis were achieved. In 1937, Sourdille's lecture to the New York Academy of Medicine prompted Lempert to apply the technique, using the endaural approach (rather than the postauricular) and a dental drill, for his one-stage approach to fenestrate the semicircular canal in otosclerosis. In 1938, G. Shambaugh Jr. became his first pupil and performed more than 5,000 fenestration operations (Lempert and Sourdille relied on the loupe for magnification). In 1940, Shambaugh Jr innovated the use of the operating microscope, continuous irrigation, enchondralization, and a diamond drill for construction of the fenestra; lasting hearing improvements were achieved in 80% of fenestrations. With Rosen's reintroduction of stapes mobilization surgery in 1953, the approach to otosclerosis surgery became the oval window area rather than the ampullated end of the horizontal canal. In 1956, Dr. John Shea introduced the stapedectomy procedure that is now used worldwide.

With this success, operations for congenital meatal atresia and then tympanoplasty to rebuild a soundconducting system in the damaged ear began to rekindle. In 1950, Moritz used pedicled flaps to construct a closed middle ear cavity in cases of chronic otitis media, thus providing a sound shielding or protection for the round window preparatory to a later fenestration of the horizontal semicircular canal. In 1955, Dr. Fritz Zöllner and Dr. Horst Wullstein introduced their concept of myringoplasty and tympanoplasty, which was to allow restoration of hearing through reconstruction of ears with chronic disease or trauma. They reported the use of an oval strut of vinyl acrylic that acted as an acoustic transmitter between the mobile footplate and the tympanic membrane graft, but poor results with this material caused them to quickly abandon its use. They continued to enjoy great popularity in the United States for tympanoplasty and for connecting the incus to the oval window in stapedectomy. The use of ossicular repositioning by them and described by Hall and Rytzner became quite popular and are even to this day.

In 1958, Dr. William House applied the method of Clerc and Batisse of approaching the internal meatus and the geniculate ganglion from the middle cranial fossa. This led 3 years later to House's first operation to remove an acoustic neuroma by this approach. Soon House reported an impressive series of 47 acoustic neuroma operations without a fatality and with preservation of facial nerve function in the majority. Previous neurosurgical removals of similar tumors had carried a mortality rate of around 20% and permanent facial nerve paralysis in nearly all. House revived Portmann's operations for Meniere's disease and with Sheehy modified Jansen's operation for cholesteatoma without creating a radical cavity. House used the postaural approach to the temporal bone, whereas Lempert had taught that the endaural operation was best for nearly all ear surgery.

Temporal bone dissection has continued to play an important role in training the otolaryngologist to comprehend this complex anatomy. A foundation of normal anatomic dissection has become increasingly important in helping the surgeon coordinate the structural knowledge gained through dissection coupled with that of computed tomographic imaging to recognize and treat pathology. Anatomic knowledge provides the foundation for skillful and safe dissection of the temporal bone. The primary structure of interest in any dissection of the temporal bone is the facial nerve. Thus, locating and protecting this structure are essential aims in otologic surgery. The second key to achieving surgical proficiency is equipment knowledge. Understanding the mechanics and principles of the otologic drill and practice with that tool serves to facilitate dissection skills. Lastly, a road map that guides the surgeon through the dissections and provides a progressive course of more complex dissections built on familiar anatomy and procedures is the third step in mastering the temporal bone. Thus, this chapter will follow these guidelines and hopefully serve as a valuable bridge between the masters who came before and those who are just beginning their journey.

ANATOMY OF THE TEMPORAL BONE

External Anatomy

Lateral Surface

The lateral aspect of the temporal bone is the one most commonly encountered by the surgeon for operative procedures or during laboratory drilling. As such, special attention should be paid to the landmarks found here as they will be the ones identified during surgery after reflecting of the soft tissue. The tip of the mastoid process is easily palpated and is a landmark for the positioning of postauricular incisions. The zygomatic process is also readily identifiable. A prominent ridge known as the temporal line (linea temporalis) runs posteriorly and slightly superiorly from the root of the zygoma and defines the inferior border of the temporalis muscle. The temporal line also approximates the position of the floor of the middle cranial fossa. The squamous portion of the temporal bone (the squama) extends above the temporal line, whereas inferiorly and anteriorly is the tympanic ring and posteriorly the mastoid. Posterior and medial to the mastoid tip is a cleft for the posterior belly of the digastric muscle (digastric groove or mastoid incisure). The tympanomastoid fissure is anterior to the tip of the mastoid and can be traced medially to the stylomastoid foramen, which is the exit point of the facial nerve. Thus, caution must be exercised when dissecting anterior to the mastoid tip during mastoid surgery, particularly in young children in whom the tip is not well developed. Anteriorly, the tympanic ring separates the external auditory canal from the glenoid fossa, which lies beneath the root of the zygoma. The tympanosquamous suture line is located in the anterosuperior part of the ring, and the tympanomastoid suture is located posterosuperiorly. The spine of Henle is a prominence of variable size that is found at the posterosuperior rim of the external auditory canal. Macewen's triangle (the fossa mastoidea), which laterally overlies the mastoid antrum, is delimited by the temporal line superiorly, a tangent to the posterior external auditory canal posteriorly, and the posterosuperior rim of the canal. Macewen's triangle is characterized by the presence of multiple small perforating vessels and hence is also known as the cribrose (cribriform) area (Figure A–1).

Superior Surface

The superior surface (tegmen) of the temporal bone is the floor of the middle cranial fossa, separating the tympanomastoid compartment from the temporal lobe. The tegmen can be divided into an anterior tegmen tympani (covering the tympanic cavity) and a posterior tegmen mastoideum (covering the mastoid air cells). The petrotympanic suture line forms the medial boundary of the tegmen. Further medially, the dense petrous bone (petrosa) runs an oblique course from lateral to medial. The petrous portion of the temporal bone is marked by depressions and eminences corresponding to the convolutions of the brain and the internal structures of the temporal bone. The arcuate eminence, present in about 85% of temporal bones, approximates the position of the superior semicircular canal (SSCC) and is a key landmark in middle cranial fossa surgery. The greater petrosal nerve (GPN) separates from the geniculate ganglion and emerges through the facial hiatus to run in a groove that is slightly medial to the petrotympanic suture and that parallels the petrous ridge. Lateral to and paralleling the greater petrosal nerve is the lesser petrosal nerve, which runs in the petrosquamous suture (superior tympanic canaliculus). The tensor tympani muscle is inferior to the lesser petrosal nerve.

The foramen lacerum, located at the junction of the base of the greater wing of the sphenoid, the petrous apex, and the basiocciput, is a false foramen that is filled with fibrous connective tissue and that forms the roof of the carotid canal. The carotid canal also parallels the petrous ridge. The gasserian (semilunar) ganglion lies in a depression at the lateral aspect of the petrous apex. Anteriorly, proceeding medially to laterally, are the foramen ovale (for the mandibular division of the trigeminal nerve) and the foramen spinosum (for the middle meningeal vessels and a recurrent branch of the mandibular nerve); these structures serve as surgical landmarks for the anterior limit of the temporal bone (Figure A–2).

Posterior Surface

The posterior surface of the temporal bone forms the anterior border of the posterior cranial fossa. The sigmoid sulcus is an indentation at the lateral aspect of the posterior surface and accommodates the sigmoid sinus. Anterior to the sigmoid sulcus is the foveate fossa for the intradural portion of the endolymphatic sac. A ledge at the superior extent of the fossa, the operculum, covers the intraosseous portion of the endolymphatic sac. The vestibular aqueduct runs anteriorly, superiorly, and medially from the operculum to end at the medial wall of the vestibule. The superior petrosal sulcus, located at the interface of the posterior and middle cranial fossa plates of the temporal bone, carries the superior petrosal sinus from the sigmoid sinus to the cavernous sinus anteriorly.

The internal auditory canal penetrates the posterior surface of the petrous ridge, runs anteromedially to posterolaterally, and contains the cochlear, vestibular, and facial nerves, along with their blood supply. The canal extends approximately 1 cm from the porus medially to the fundus laterally. At the fundus, the canal is divided into an upper and a lower portion by the transverse crest (crista falciformis). The inferior compartment contains the cochlear nerve anteriorly and the inferior vestibular nerve inferiorly. A branch of the inferior vestibular nerve, the posterior ampullary nerve, which innervates the ampulla of the posterior semicircular canal, exits the internal auditory canal through the singular canal. A vertical crest of bone, Bill's

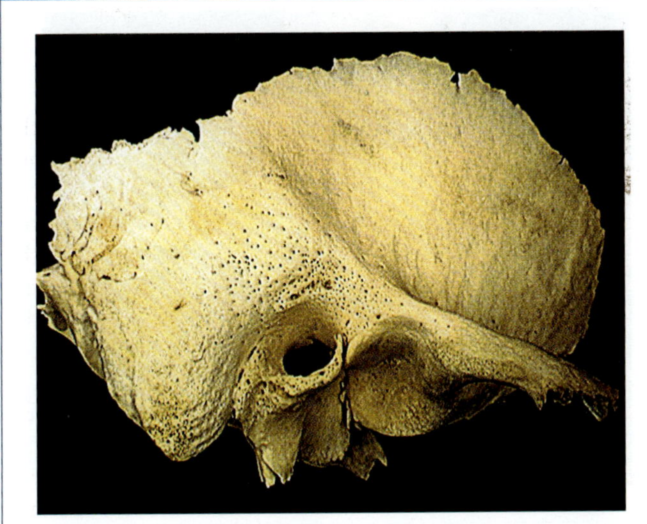

FIGURE A–1 • Lateral surface anatomy: note the zygomatic process, tympanic annulus, temporal line, and mastoid tip.

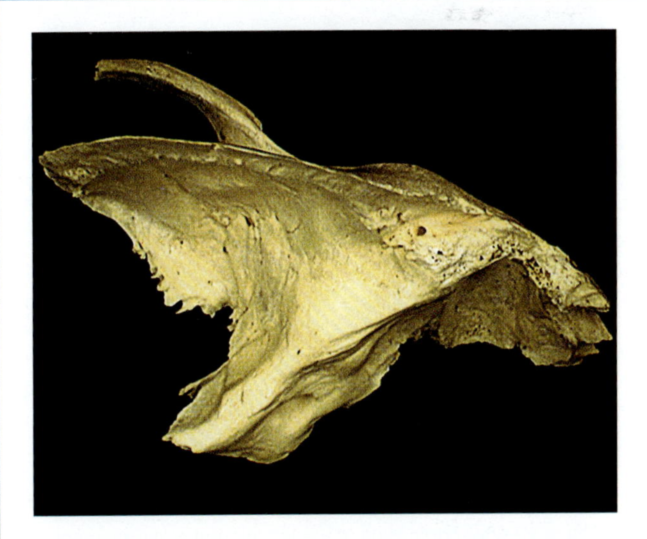

FIGURE A–2 • Superior surface anatomy: important landmarks for the middle fossa surgeon are the temporosquamous suture line, facial hiatus (greater superficial petrosal nerve), tympanic canaliculus (lesser petrosal nerve), arcuate eminence (relative position of superior semicircular canal), and foramen lacerum (carotid artery).

bar, separates the superior portion of the canal into an anterior compartment, occupied by the facial nerve, and a posterior compartment containing the superior vestibular nerve (Figures A–3 and A–4).

Inferior Surface

The inferior surface of the temporal bone separates the upper neck from the skull base. Accordingly, many vital neurovascular structures traverse this surface. Anteriorly and medially, the external carotid foramen is the point at which the internal carotid artery enters the temporal bone. Posteriorly, a ridge of bone, the jugulocarotid crest, separates the carotid canal from the jugular foramen. Classically, the jugular foramen has been thought of as being divided into a posterolateral pars venosa, which is occupied by the jugular vein, and an anteromedial pars nervosa, which is traversed by the glossopharyngeal, vagus, and spinal accessory nerves. The hypoglossal nerve exits the occipital bone by the hypoglossal canal, medial to the pars nervosa of the jugular foramen. Lateral to the jugular foramen is the styloid process. Immediately posterior to the styloid process is the stylomastoid foramen, by which the facial nerve exits the temporal bone. Medial to the mastoid tip is the digastric groove for the posterior belly of the digastric muscle. The triangular opening of the cochlear aqueduct is located medial to the jugular foramen. The inferior tympanic canaliculus runs in the jugulocarotid crest and carries the inferior tympanic artery (a branch of the ascending pharyngeal artery) and the tympanic branch of the glossopharyngeal nerve (Jacobson's nerve) into the tympanic cavity (Figure A–5).

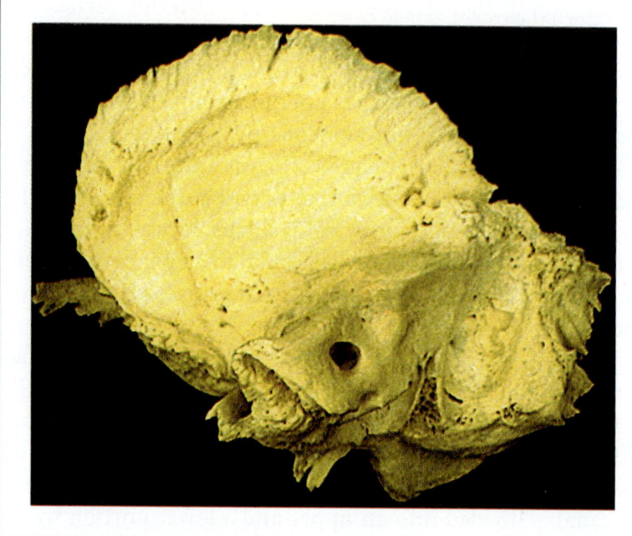

FIGURE A–3 • Posterior surface anatomy: the sigmoid sulcus forms a prominent depression on this surface. Anterior to the midportion of the sigmoid sinus is a lip of bone (operculum). Beneath the operculum is the opening for the vestibular aqueduct. Further anteriorly lies the internal auditory canal (IAC).

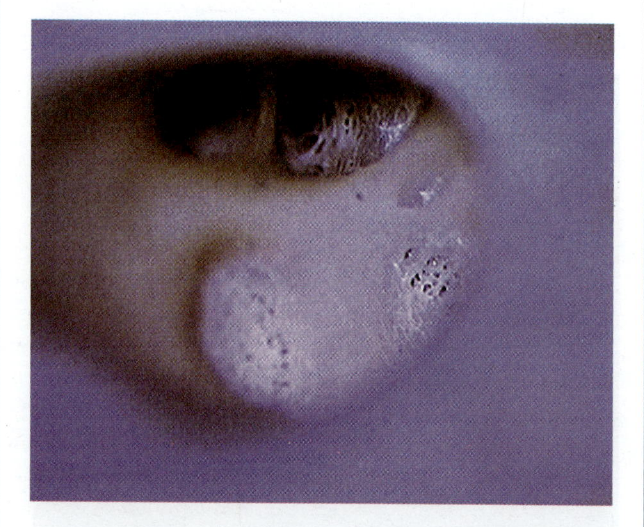

FIGURE A–4 • Endoscopic view of the left internal auditory canal (IAC). The transverse crest (crista falciformis) divides the lateral fundus of the IAC into superior and inferior compartments. The superior compartment is further divided by the vertical crest (Bill's bar), which separates the facial nerve anteriorly from the superior vestibular nerve posteriorly. The inferior compartment contains the cochlear nerve anteriorly and the inferior vestibular nerve posteriorly.

Anterior Surface

The petrous apex is the wedge of bone that separates the greater wing of the sphenoid from the occipital bone. The most prominent feature of this surface is the internal carotid foramen, through which the carotid artery exits the temporal bone. The impression for the trigeminal ganglion is located on the lateral surface of the petrous apex. The semicanal for the tensor tympani is lateral to the carotid canal; the bony portion of the eustachian tube runs inferior and parallel to the tensor tympani muscle. The thin medial wall of the eustachian tube forms the lateral wall of the carotid canal and is frequently dehiscent. Thus, the carotid canal is vulnerable to injury in the course of surgical manipulations in the anterior tympanic cavity and in the medial wall of the eustachian tube (Figure A–6).

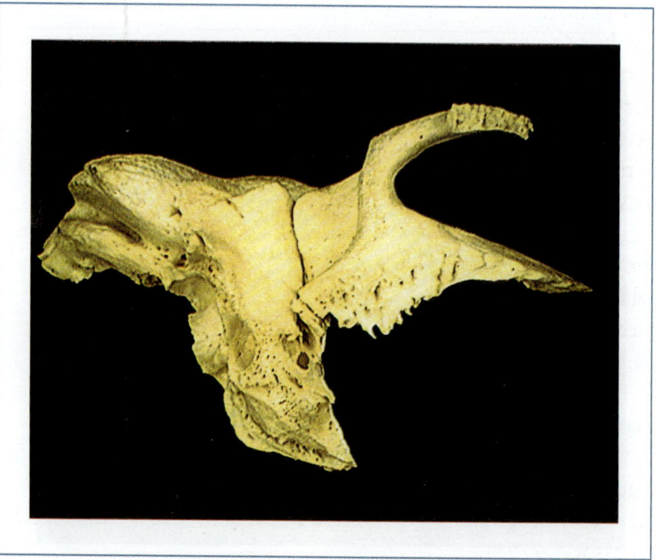

FIGURE A–5 • Inferior surface anatomy: crucial relationships here for the skull base surgeon include the jugular fossa, stylomastoid foramen, and carotid canal.

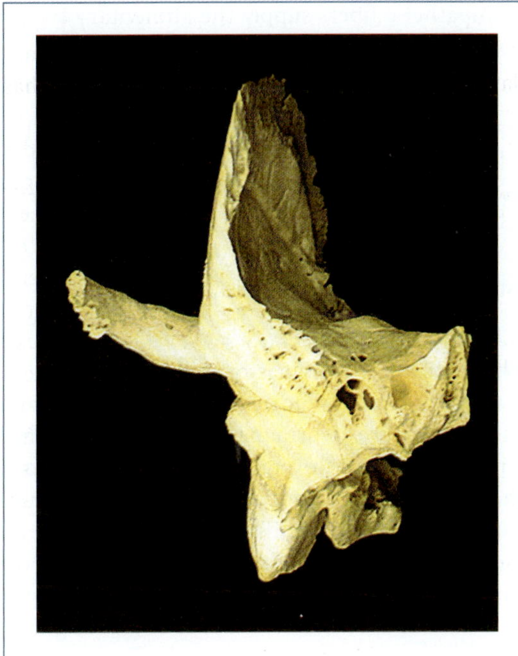

FIGURE A–6 • Anterior surface anatomy: note the relationships of the facial hiatus, carotid artery, semicanal of the tensor tympani, and eustachian tube.

Vascular Anatomy

Several large dural venous sinuses are intimately associated with the temporal bone and comprise the principal venous drainage of the brain and cranial vault. The superior sagittal sinus and straight sinus merge at the internal occipital protuberance. The right and left transverse sinuses extend beyond this junction. The right transverse sinus is primarily the continuation of the superior sagittal sinus and thus is generally larger in diameter than the left transverse sinus, which is primarily the continuation of the straight sinus. The transverse sinuses lie just inferior to the tentorium and parallel its course. Anteriorly, the superior petrosal sinus joins the transverse sinus, and this junction marks the beginning of the sigmoid sinus. The sigmoid sinus is the posterior boundary of the mastoid cavity. However, in particularly well-pneumatized bones, accessory air cells may extend posteriorly beyond the sigmoid sinus. The sigmoid sinus is most superficial (lateral) at its superior origin. The middle fossa dura approximates the superior portion of the sigmoid sinus at the sinodural angle of Citelli. From the sinodural angle, the sigmoid sinus runs inferiorly and medially, with a variable relationship to the bony labyrinth. At its inferior extent, the sigmoid sinus rises to the jugular bulb. The jugular bulb exhibits considerable variability in its height, location, and relationship to the labyrinth, internal auditory canal (IAC), and tympanic cavity. The inferior petrosal sinus arises from the medial aspect of the jugular bulb and runs anteromedially to the cavernous sinus. The jugular vein exits the skull through the jugular foramen, accompanied by the vagus, glossopharyngeal, and spinal accessory nerves.

Emissary veins are drainage routes of the dural venous sinuses through the skull that communicate with the superficial veins of the scalp. A fairly constant emissary vein, the mastoid emissary vein, can be found at the junction of the temporal and occipital bones and usually communicates with the occipital or postauricular vein.

The internal carotid artery also travels through the temporal bone. Its entrance, the external carotid foramen, is medial to the styloid process and anterior to the jugular foramen. The internal carotid artery travels superiorly until it encounters the dense bone of the cochlea, at which point it makes a 90-degree bend to run anteriorly and medially. The carotid canal forms the medial wall of the eustachian tube; the internal carotid artery may be dehiscent and vulnerable to injury here. Rarely, the internal carotid artery may encroach on the tympanic cavity proper.

Cranial Nerves

The majority of the cranial nerves are in close anatomic relationship to the temporal bone. Knowledge of their location is not only important in surgical dissection but also serves the astute clinician as a diagnostic aid when cranial nerve deficits are encountered.

Fifth Cranial (Trigeminal) Nerve

The trigeminal (gasserian, semilunar) ganglion lies on the lateral aspect of the anterior petrous apex and indents its surface. This nerve supplies sensory and motor innervation to the face. The sensory root (portia major) pierces the lateral surface of the pons at the superior aspect of the cerebellopontine angle. The first two divisions of the trigeminal nerve, the ophthalmic and the maxillary, are sensory only. The motor branch (portia minor) lies medial to the sensory branch and joins the third division, the mandibular, to supply the muscles of mastication; a small branch supplies the tensor tympani muscle within the middle ear.

Sixth Cranial (Abducens) Nerve

The abducens nerve innervates the ipsilateral lateral rectus muscle. It exits the brainstem from a groove between the superior medulla and inferior pons and then travels through Dorello's canal, which is formed by the petroclinoid (Gruber's) ligament and petrous apex. Inflammatory or neoplastic lesions in the petrous apex can present with lateral rectus palsy.

Seventh Cranial (Facial) Nerve

Preganglionic parasympathetic fibers destined for the pterygopalatine and submandibular ganglions and special sensory (taste) fibers comprise the nervus intermedius. This nerve joins the larger, motor root to form the facial nerve. In the cerebellopontine angle, the nervus intermedius lies between the facial and cochlear nerves. The facial nerve enters the temporal bone through the IAC, which it exits at the meatal foramen to travel anteriorly to the geniculate ganglion. This segment of the facial nerve, the labyrinthine segment, is the narrowest portion (0.61–0.68 mm) of the facial canal. At the geniculate ganglion, the GPN travels anteriorly, carrying parasympathetic fibers to the pterygopalatine ganglion. The main trunk of the facial nerve turns posteriorly, inferiorly, and laterally to continue in its tympanic (horizontal) segment. The nerve continues in this course until it turns inferiorly at the lateral semicircular canal (LSCC; the second genu), marking the terminus of the tympanic segment and the beginning of the mastoid segment. The facial nerve continues to travel inferiorly, posteriorly, and laterally until it exits the temporal bone at the stylomastoid foramen. For the majority of its course, the mastoid segment lies medial to the plane of the tympanic annulus; however, the nerve can cross the annular plane at any point as it travels inferiorly. Although the chorda tympani nerve usually separates from the mastoid segment of the facial nerve a few millimeters superior to the stylomastoid foramen, the exact location of this separation is quite variable. The chorda tympani nerve traverses the tympanic cavity to carry parasympathetic fibers to the submandibular ganglion and taste fibers to the anterior tongue. The motor component of the facial nerve supplies the stapedius, posterior digastric, and stylohyoid muscles, as well as the muscles of facial expression.

Eighth Cranial (Cochleovestibular) Nerve

The axons of the cochlear division of the eighth nerve arise from the bipolar cells of the spiral ganglion in the cochlea. From this ganglion, the fibers pass through the modiolus and the foramina of the tractus spiralis foraminosus and into the anterior-inferior portion of the fundus of the IAC, at which point they fuse to form the cochlear nerve. The vestibular portion of the eighth nerve divides into a superior and an inferior division in the IAC. The cell bodies for these nerves are in Scarpa's ganglion, also located in the canal. The superior vestibular nerve innervates the utricle, the SSCC and LSCC, and the superior saccule. The inferior vestibular nerve innervates the posterior semicircular canal and the inferior saccule.

Ninth Cranial (Glossopharyngeal) Nerve

The glossopharyngeal nerve exits the upper lateral medulla and passes through the jugular foramen, accompanied by the vagus and spinal accessory nerves. It carries preganglionic parasympathetic fibers to the otic ganglion and taste fibers from the posterior third of the tongue, general sensory afferents from the pharyngeal mucosa, and motor fibers to the stylopharyngeus muscle. After exiting the skull, the glossopharyngeal nerve descends between the internal jugular vein and the internal carotid artery and behind the styloid muscles before dividing into its several branches. One branch, the tympanic (Jacobson's nerve), is of particular interest to the otologist; this branch re-enters the temporal bone through the inferior tympanic canaliculus and emerges onto the promontory to merge with sympathetic fibers at the tympanic plexus, forming the lesser petrosal nerve. At the cochleariform process, the lesser petrosal nerve travels medial to the semicanal of the tensor tympani muscle to emerge on the floor of the middle cranial fossa.

Tenth Cranial (Vagus) Nerve

The vagus nerve is the longest of the cranial nerves. It arises as 8 to 10 rootlets from the medulla oblongata; these roots unite into the vagus nerve, which passes beneath the flocculus to the jugular foramen and exits the skull within a dural sheath shared with the spinal accessory nerve. Beyond its jugular and nodose ganglia, the vagus nerve travels through the neck and into the chest within the carotid sheath, between the internal jugular vein and common carotid artery. The vagus nerve carries sensory fibers from the hypopharynx and the larynx; its motor fibers supply the pharyngeal plexus and larynx. Additional sensory, motor, and parasympathetic fibers supply the alimentary tract to the splenic flexure of the colon.

Eleventh Cranial (Spinal Accessory) Nerve

Cranial and spinal rootlets combine to form the eleventh nerve. The spinal component extends to the level of C5 or C6. These rootlets ascend through the foramen magnum into the cranial cavity, cross the occipital bone, and exit through the jugular foramen. The spinal accessory nerve innervates the sternocleidomastoid and trapezius muscles.

Twelfth Cranial (Hypoglossal) Nerve

The twelfth nerve arises from the medulla and exits the brainstem as a series of rootlets located between the pyramid and olive. These rootlets fuse to form the hypoglossal nerve that exits the posterior cranial fossa through the hypoglossal canal of the occipital bone. The nerve then travels between the internal jugular vein and the internal carotid artery. Superior to the carotid bifurcation, the hypoglossal nerve passes lateral to both the internal and external carotid arteries and subsequently curves upward to innervate the intrinsic muscles of the tongue.

Tympanic Cavity

The tympanic cavity is divided into three portions: the attic (epitympanum), which lies above the tympanic annulus; the tympanic cavity proper (mesotympanum); and the hypotympanum, which is below the level of the tympanic annulus.

Superiorly, the middle ear cavity is separated from the brain by the tegmen tympani. Inferiorly, a thin bony covering separates the tympanic cavity from the jugular bulb. The tympanic membrane laterally delimits the tympanic cavity, and the inner ear is its medial boundary.

In adults, the tympanic membrane lies at a 45-degree angle to the long axis of the petrous pyramid. The ring of bone within which the tympanic annulus sits, the tympanic sulcus, is deficient superiorly at the notch of Rivinus. Two bands (the anterior and posterior malleal folds) extend from the notch and attach to the lateral process of the malleus. This notch and the malleal folds divide the tympanic membrane into two portions: superiorly, the pars flaccida (Shrapnell's membrane), and inferiorly, the main portion of the tympanic membrane, the pars tensa. The pars tensa averages 10 mm in diameter. The most medial portion of the eardrum, the umbo, lies at the tip of the handle (manubrium) of the malleus (Figure A–7).

Mesotympanum

The basal turn of the cochlea, in the form of its promontory, forms the majority of the medial wall of the mesotympanum. The tympanic plexus lies on the promontory. Superior to the promontory is the oval window (fenestra vestibuli), occupied by the footplate of the stapes. The round window (fenestra cochleae), sealed by the round window membrane (secondary tympanic membrane), is just inferior and leads to the scala tympani.

The tensor tympani tendon exits its semicanal at the cochleariform (spoon-shaped) process and inserts onto the malleus. Superior to the cochleariform process, the facial nerve makes a sharp bend (first genu) posteriorly and superiorly toward the IAC. The area superior to the cochleariform process

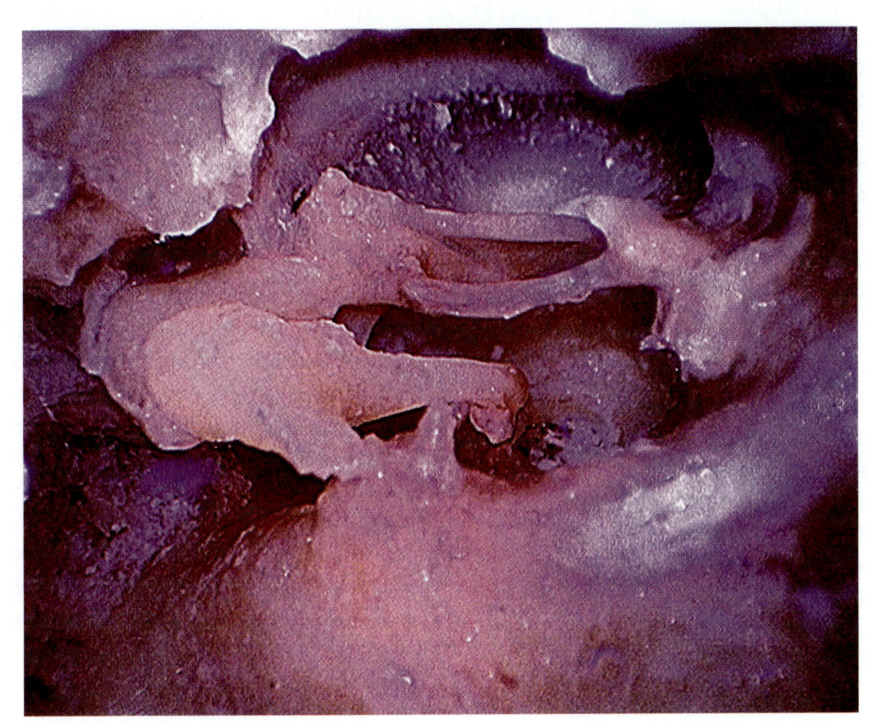

FIGURE A–7 • Surgeon's view of the ossicles and middle ear with the external auditory canal removed. Note the positions of the umbo, chorda tympani, and the relationship between the lateral semicircular canal, incus, and horizontal facial canal.

approximates the position of the geniculate ganglion on the superior aspect of the temporal bone. From the cochleariform process, the facial nerve courses posteriorly and slightly inferiorly in the tympanic (horizontal) segment of its fallopian canal. The horizontal segment ends at the second genu of the facial nerve, which curves posterior and superior to the oval window and anteroinferior to the LSCC. The horizontal segment of the facial nerve and the cochleariform process medially define the superior extent of the mesotympanum.

The chorda tympani nerve enters the tympanic cavity through its posterior iter, which usually is located lateral to the pyramidal eminence and medial to the annulus, at the level of the round window and cochlear aqueduct; the facial recess lies between the facial and chorda tympani nerves. The chorda tympani nerve passes lateral to the long process of the incus and medial to the neck of the malleus before it exits the tympanic cavity through its anterior iter (the canal of Huguier) and the petrotympanic fissure.

Traveling along the posterior wall of the tympanic cavity,the first structure encountered below the posterior end of the tympanic facial nerve is the pyramidal eminence, traversed by the tendon of the stapedius muscle. The sinus tympani lies in the posterior mesotympanum, medial to the pyramidal eminence. The medial wall of the posterior mesotympanum is divided by two ridges, the ponticulus and the subiculum. The ponticulus runs from the oval window to the sinus tympani and defines its superior extent. The subiculum defines the inferior extent of the sinus tympani as it runs from the round window to the sinus.

Jacobson's nerve (the tympanic branch of the glossopharyngeal nerve) is a landmark on the promontory of the cochlea and "points" to the cochleariform process. As the facial nerve runs immediately superior to the cochleariform process, Jacobson's nerve can be used to locate the facial nerve.

The semicanal of the tensor tympani muscle is located in the anterior wall of the middle ear cleft and runs almost parallel to the eustachian tube. The tensor tympani muscle originates from the cartilaginous portion of the eustachian tube, passes along the cochleariform process, and inserts via its tendon, on the manubrium of the malleus. The eustachian tube connects the tympanic cavity with the nasopharynx, allowing passage of air between the two. In the adult, the upper one-third of the eustachian tube is bony, whereas the lower two-thirds is cartilaginous. In addition, the eustachian tube follows an inferiorly angled course to the nasopharynx. In infants and children, a greater proportion of the tube is cartilaginous; the tube is much smaller in diameter and follows a more horizontal course. These anatomic differences are thought to underlie the increased incidence of eustachian tube dysfunction in infants and children.

Epitympanum

The epitympanum (attic) leads to the aditus ad antrum and the mastoid antrum, the first area to be aerated in the process of pneumatization. The antrum leads to the remainder of the mastoid air cell system. The head of the malleus and the body of the incus are in the epitympanum. The fossa incudis in the posterior epitympanum houses the short process of the incus and serves as an important surgical landmark for the facial nerve. The cog, a bony projection from the tegmen superior to the cochleariform process, serves as an approximate landmark for the facial nerve. The cog also separates the anterior epitympanic space (the supratubal recess) from the remainder of the epitympanum.

Hypotympanum

The most variable region of the tympanic cavity is the hypotympanum. The depth of the tympanic cavity is largely determined by the height of the jugular bulb as the anterior jugular bulb forms the inferior and posterior borders of the hypotympanum. A more inferiorly placed jugular bulb creates a deeper hypotympanic space. Often the bone overlying the jugular bulb is thin or absent and the bulb can be visualized otoscopically as a purple, retrotympanic mass. Anteriorly, the carotid canal runs in the floor of the hypotympanum. The promontory delimits the hypotympanum superiorly. The infralabyrinthine cell tract runs inferior to the cochlea, between the jugular bulb and carotid artery, and can be used as a route to the petrous apex.

Auditory Ossicles

The ossicular chain consists of three bones connected by delicate articulations and ligaments. Passing from lateral to medial, the first ossicle encountered is the malleus, which has a head, neck, and three processes (anterior, lateral, and the manubrium). The head articulates with the body of the incus in the epitympanum. The tympanic membrane attaches to the malleal periosteum at the short process and at the umbo (the tip of the malleus). The incus consists of a body and two processes, short and long. On the anterior surface of the body of the incus, there is a facet that articulates with the head of the malleus by a synovial joint. The short process of the incus is tethered in the fossa incudis by the posterior incudal ligament. The long process, by means of its lenticular process, articulates with the stapes. The stapes comprises a footplate, anterior and posterior crura, a neck, and a head (capitulum). The stapedius tendon attaches to the neck. The footplate is secured in the oval window by the annular ligament (Figure A–8).

DISSECTION GUIDE

Temporal Bone Station Setup

The temporal bone dissection laboratory should provide a comfortable working space that is easy to set up and clean, which facilitates frequent use of the laboratory for dissection. Ideally, the equipment within the laboratory should closely resemble what is used in the operating room to simulate the operative experience realistically. The space itself should be well ventilated and lit and provide sinks for cleaning the equipment. Any flat working space can serve as a dissection station. Custom-built tables provide amenities such as integrated suction and water lines, electrical outlets, and drawers and cabinets for storage. A comfortable, adjustable chair enhances the ergonomics of the dissection station, which, as in the operating room, facilitates prolonged work without undue fatigue. Personal protective equipment such as gowns, masks, and gloves should be readily available. A temporal bone holder is essential to secure the bone during dissection. A holder that allows for movement in several planes, such as the House-Urban temporal bone holder, more closely simulates the surgical environment than a stationary holder and is thus preferred. Considerable additional instrumentation is essential and should be kept within the laboratory separate from that used in the operating room. Periosteal elevators, dissecting scissors, and scalpel handles and blades are useful in removing soft tissue prior to dissection. Middle ear instruments, such as canal elevators, picks, alligators, cup

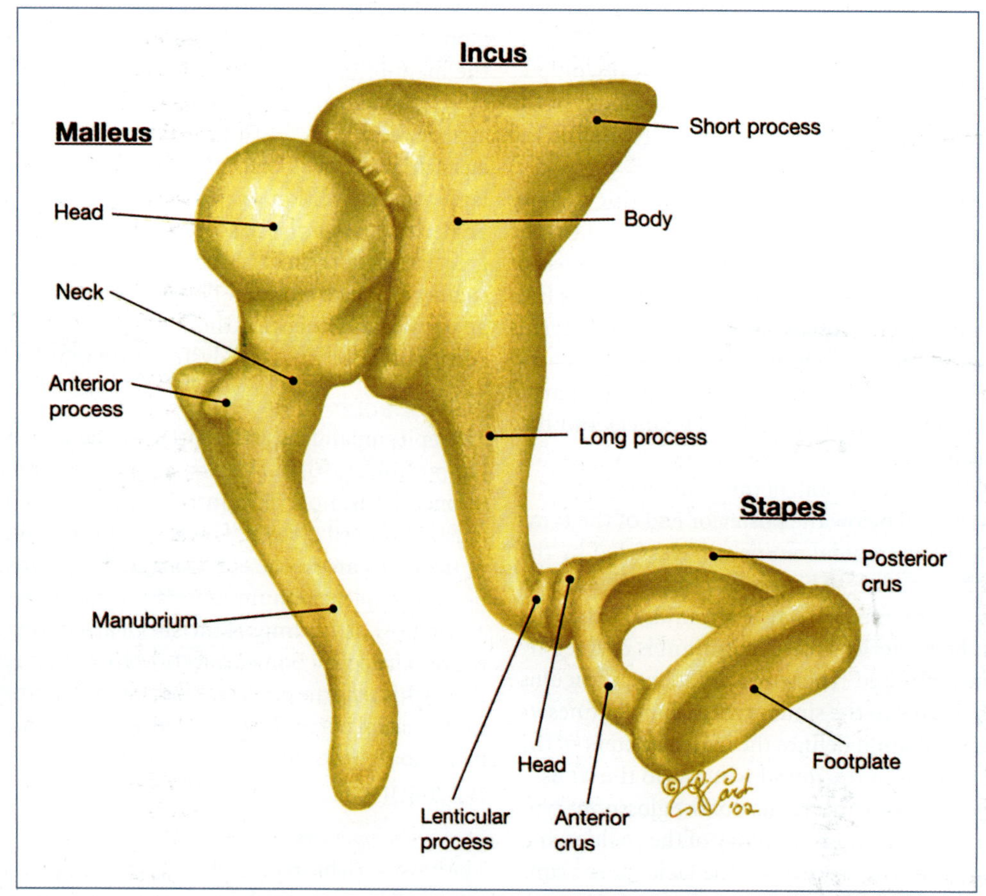

FIGURE A–8 • Artist's depiction of the auditory ossicles under high magnification.

forceps, and microscissors, are also required. Various sizes of plain and irrigating suction tips are essential to the dissection (Figures A–9 and A–10).

Operating Microscope

Carl Zeiss Inc (Oberkochen, Germany), working with Dr. Horst Wullstein, introduced the first operating microscope for otologic surgery in the late 1950s. Shortly afterward, Drs. Shambaugh and Kinney brought the first operating microscopes to the United States and, along with many other otologic surgeons, helped to popularize their use. Since the 1960s, operating microscopes have become an indispensable part of ear surgery. The microscope provides controlled magnification, stereoscopic vision, and coaxial illumination and protects the eyes during dissection. Modern amenities, such as video cameras and observer heads, expand the utility of the microscope for teaching and mainly were a result of the engineering genius of Jack Urban working with Drs. Howard and William House. Large, floor-mounted microscopes, such as those used in the operating room, are impractical for the laboratory. Many manufacturers provide microscopes that can be mounted to the workbench. The microscope selected should provide bright illumination, a variety of magnification settings, and adjustable binocular eyepieces. The eyepieces should offer adjustments for interpupillary distance and diopter setting. Optional items include exchangeable objective lenses with differing focal lengths or a variable focal length system and beam splitters to allow for the placement of teaching heads or cameras (Figure A–11).

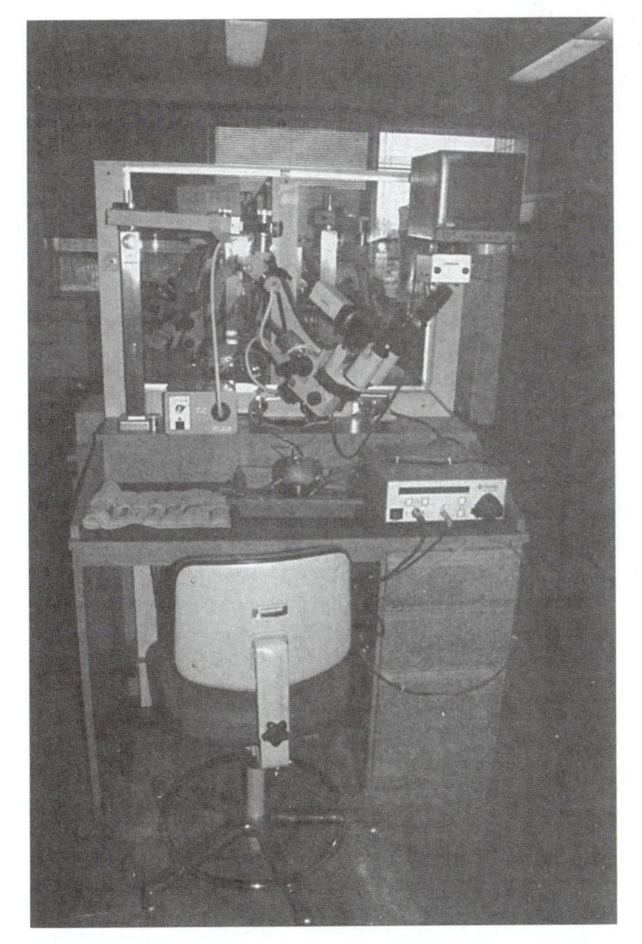

FIGURE A–9 • Temporal bone dissection station at the Michigan Ear Institute depicting a microscope with an observer arm and a video monitor, an electric otologic drill system, a temporal bone holder, and a selection of instruments.

The eyepieces contribute to the total magnification and compensate for operator visual acuity differences. It is very important that the eyepieces be correctly set and then locked, ensuring that the microscope is par focal. The major cause of eye fatigue, loss of convergence, and excessive refocusing is improper eyepiece settings. The eyepiece has a large diopter adjustment range, but the operator requiring correction for astigmatism should wear eyeglasses when using the microscope.

Par focal vision is achieved using the following procedures*:

1. Position the microscope over a steady flat surface.
2. Make a small crosshatch (#) mark on white paper to be used as a focusing target.
3. Confirm that eyepieces are fully inserted into binocular eyepiece tubes and set both eyepiece diopter settings to 0.
4. Focus the microscope on the crosshatch target with the magnification changer at maximum. The fine focus knobs are to be used for this setting. When this setting is achieved, lightly tighten all tension knobs, making sure that the microscope is stable and has not moved or changed focus.
5. Being careful not to change focus, revolve the magnification changer to the lowest magnification.
6. While closing one eye, adjust the other eyepiece for the best image possible. When this has been accomplished for both eyes, tighten the diopter locks and make a note of the right and left eye settings for future use.
7. Adjust the eyepiece interpupillary distance for convergence.
8. To ensure that the microscope is par focal, revolve the magnification changer through each setting while viewing the target through the eyepieces.

Drill System and Burs

The drill is an important instrument for temporal bone dissection. Two equally important factors, the drill system and the drill bits, determine the ease and safety of bone removal. Modern, high-speed otologic drill systems allow for rapid, safe bone removal with relative ease. Both gas-driven and electric systems are used in the operating room, and each has its advantages and advocates. Ideally, a drill should be easy to handle, lightweight, and provide high speed and power, with little torque of the handpiece on initiation or cessation of drilling. Some surgeons prefer a drill bur to have a forward and a reverse mode.

Gas-driven drills traditionally have provided more power and speed, which helps in more rapid bone removal. The primary disadvantages of gas-driven systems are the need for dedicated high-pressure lines in the operating room (or compressed gas cylinders), the bulkiness of the delivery cord, and the noise level of the device. Electric drill systems allow for rapid setup, a thinner delivery cord, lower noise level, and ready

* Courtesy of Lerry K. Kleinberg from Urban Engineering

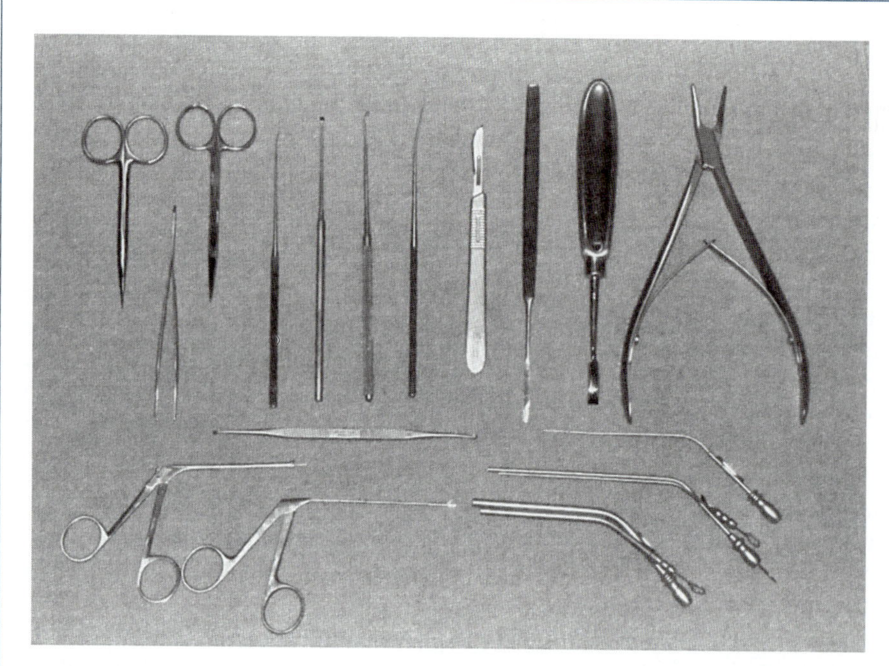

FIGURE A–10 • In addition to the drill system, a variety of instruments are useful in the laboratory including plain and suction irrigators, forceps, scalpel handle, periosteal elevators, a selection of otologic picks, curette, and alligator scissors and forceps.

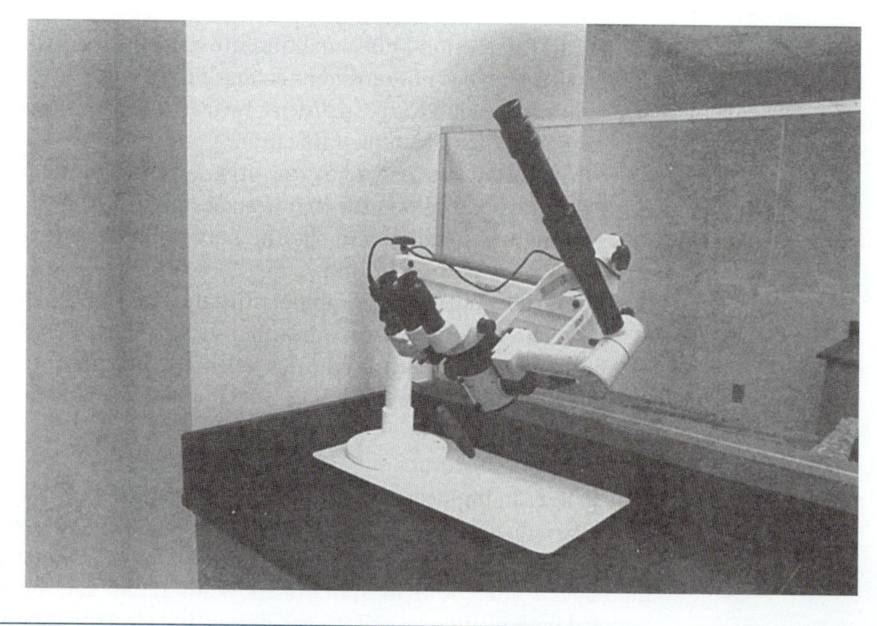

FIGURE A–11 • Leica™ temporal bone dissection microscope with a monocular observer arm and a video camera.

power availability. The limiting factors of electric drills have been their lack of speed and torque, resulting in less efficient bone removal. Also, the handpieces tended to become hot during heavy use, further impeding dissection by requiring pauses, while the drill cooled. Recent advances in electric motor design have overcome these limitations. Electrically powered otologic drill systems are now available that provide speed and torque closely equaling that of gaspowered drills. Further innovations such as water-cooled drills enable prolonged use without overheating (Figure A–12).

The otologic drill is a versatile tool that enables millimeter-precise dissection of bone while leaving intact delicate underlying structures. Factors that can be modulated during drilling include bur size and type, speed, direction, and pressure. The specifics of using these variables are discussed below, but general guidelines are discussed here. A thorough familiarity with these variables must be gained through practice in the temporal bone laboratory.

A large bur contacts a greater surface area than a smaller bur. Thus, larger burs are generally more efficient in bone removal. Furthermore, the large surface area distributes the pressure of the bur tip, thus reducing the likelihood of the bur penetrating and damaging underlying structures. Hence, not only are larger burs more efficient, they are also "safer" and, accordingly, should be used whenever practical. The danger of larger burs relates to their limitation of visibility and the possibility

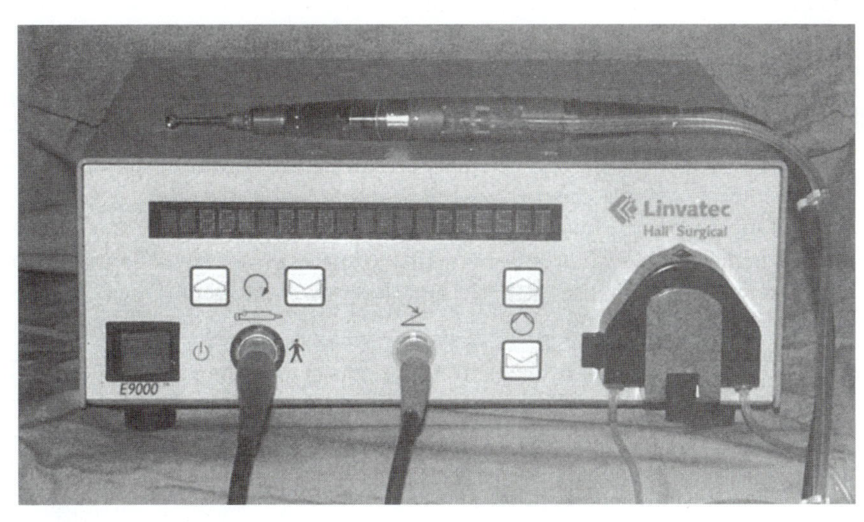

FIGURE A–12 • Hall™ Linvatec otologic drill system and power supply. This electric drill provides a maximum speed of 80,000 rpm and has a unique water-cooling system.

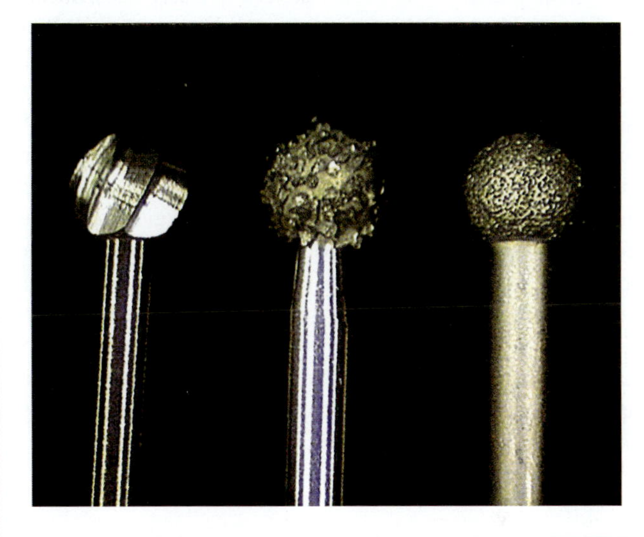

FIGURE A–13 • Otologic burs are available in a variety of styles and sizes. The bur on the left is a cutting bur. The bur in the middle is a cutting diamond bur (note the course texture). The bur on the right is a diamond bur.

of unintentionally contacting surfaces with the bur. As experience is gained, larger burs can be used more frequently. Cutting, diamond stone, and "rough cut" diamond burs are currently available. Cutting burs provide the most rapid removal of bone but are more likely to injure soft tissue and fracture thin bone. Flute design is important; there is an optimal interflute space that allows a safe cut without clogging with bone dust. Diamond burs have a variety of uses. Their primary function is in the removal of bone approximating delicate structures, such as the sigmoid sinus, dura, or facial nerve. They can also be used to smooth and polish bony surfaces after dissection with a cutting bur. An additional use is to stop bleeding from bone surfaces, which can best be achieved with a gentle, pushing stroke and minimal or no irrigation. With practice, this can effectively stop bleeding from small temporal bone vessels. Diamond burs require relatively more irrigation than cutting burs. The irrigation cools the bone and bur, preventing burning of tissue; without sufficient irrigation, the diamond bur quickly becomes clogged with bone dust, dramatically reducing its usefulness. A third type of bit, the rough cut diamond, contains coarse particles of diamond stone. This bit can be used as an intermediate between the easy bone removal of a cutting bur and the relative safety of a diamond bur.

Drill speed is also an important variable. High speed equates to more efficient bone removal with less pressure, resulting in less operator fatigue. Higher speed also increases the likelihood that the drill will "run" and result in unintentional dissection and potential injury. Slower speeds result in improved control but less efficient dissection and greater drill pressure, potentially increasing operator fatigue. As a general rule, slower speeds are best used for the final removal of bone over delicate structures and in confined spaces (Figure A–13).

DISSECTION MANUAL

Intact Canal Wall Mastoidectomy

The simple mastoidectomy is the basic approach to the temporal bone. As in soft tissue surgery, an intact canal wall mastoidectomy should provide adequate exposure to the deeper structures of interest, which are the antrum, the LSCC, and the incus. However, unlike soft tissue surgery, the structures of interest are located within dense bone that varies in thickness, shape, and pneumatization. Furthermore, other vital structures that occupy variable positions in the bone (eg, the sigmoid sinus and tegmen) can affect dissection and exposure. Therefore, the initial objective is to perform rapid, safe removal of bone to permit visualization of the antrum, LSCC, and incus.

Opening the Mastoid Antrum

After reflection of the soft tissues, the following landmarks are identified on the lateral surface of the bone: the root of the zygoma, the mastoid tip, and the external auditory canal (EAC). Using the largest cutting bur practical, a firm stroke is drawn posteriorly from the root of the zygoma paralleling the temporal line. By drawing the bur toward the surgeon, firm pressure can be applied in a controlled fashion. This cut roughly parallels the middle fossa dura and defines the superior limit of the dissection. The next stroke is perpendicular to the first and tangential to the EAC. This cut defines the anterior limit of dissection. As the area of dissection is roughly triangular in shape, only the posterior boundary remains to be defined. The extent of the posterior boundary varies depending on the position of the sigmoid sinus (Figures A–14 and A–15).

As the dissection progresses, the surgeon identifies the tegmen mastoideum, the sinodural angle, and the area of the sigmoid sinus. Often adequate exposure can be obtained without skeletonizing the sigmoid sinus. The mastoid cortex is removed in a systematic, saucerizing (ie, eliminating bony overhangs) fashion. The surgeon may encounter a bony plate (Körner's petrosquamous septum) of variable prominence. The antrum is the next landmark of importance and displays considerable interindividual variability in size.

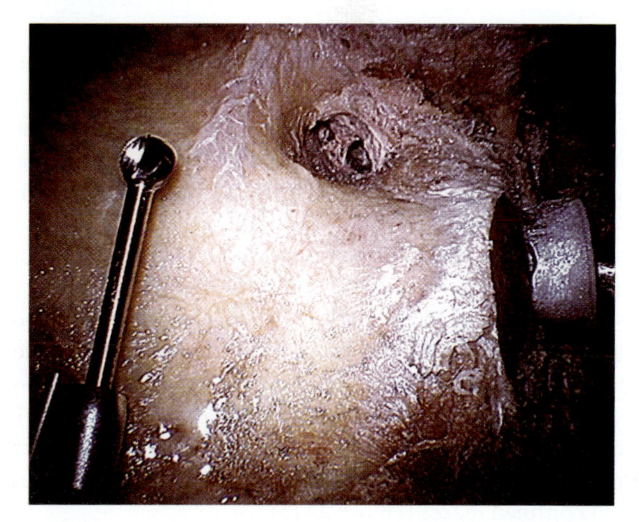

FIGURE A–14 • Dried temporal bone specimen placed in the surgical position within the temporal bone holder.

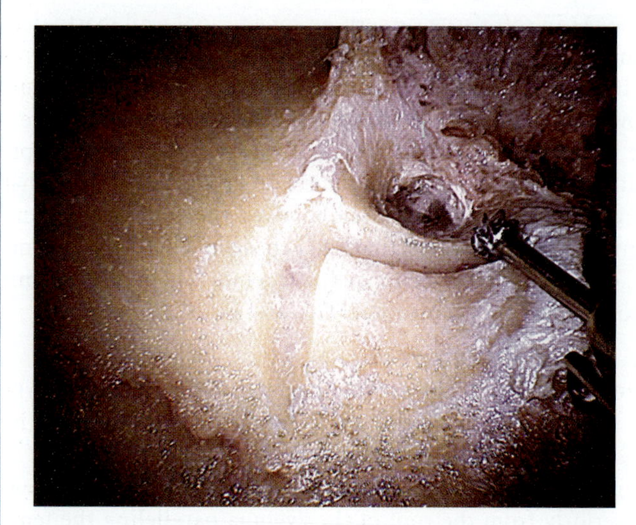

FIGURE A–15 • Initial two cuts along the temporal line and tangential to the external auditory canal.

The antrum is our personal most valuable "safe" landmark as it opens to the important landmarks for otologic surgery: medially, the compact bone of the LSSC that allows exposure of the fossa incudis; the epitympanum anteriorly and superiorly; and the external genu of the facial nerve. The dense bone of the LSSC extends posteroinferiorly to the posterior semicircular canal.

To open the antrum, we use a small bur and, staying superior, dissect from medial to lateral to saucerize the antrum and visualize the LSCC and the body of the incus (Figure A–16).

Fossa Incudis, Facial Recess, and Facial Nerve

The next exposure to be mastered through dissection of the temporal bone is the facial recess approach. The boundaries of this triangularly shaped region are the facial nerve medially, the chorda tympani nerve laterally, and the fossa incudis superiorly. Opening the facial recess allows for positive and safe identification of the facial nerve as well as access to the tympanic cavity.

Dissection begins just inferior to the short process of the incus, in the plane of the incus, generally using a 3-mm diamond bur, and is carried inferiorly, paralleling the vertical segment of the facial nerve. Drilling is *never* perpendicular to the facial nerve (or, for that matter, any structure one wishes to preserve). With the high-intensity illumination and magnification afforded by the modern operating microscope, the surgeon can detect vital structures, such as the facial nerve, while a protective bony covering remains. Preferred surgical technique reveals anatomic structures and does not penetrate them. Since the tympanic segment of the facial nerve is medial to the incus, safe dissection is in the plane of the incus. Even in very sclerotic bones, a "herald" air cell is generally encountered just lateral to the second genu of the facial nerve. Once the facial and chorda tympani nerves are identified, smaller burs can be used to open the recess fully (Figures A–17 and A–18).

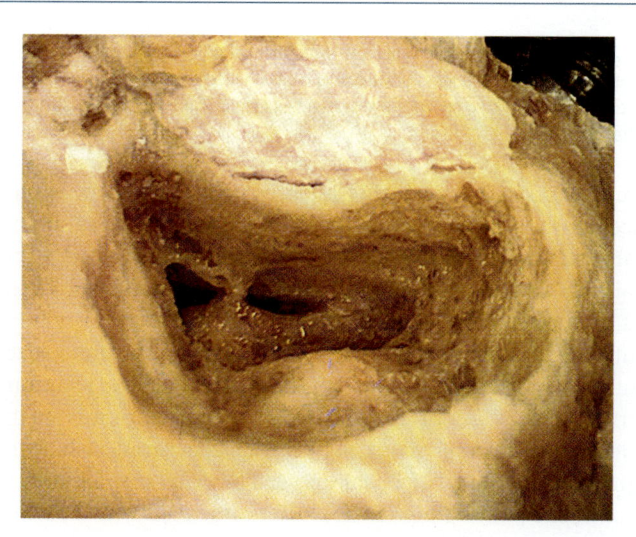

FIGURE A–16 • Basic mastoidectomy completed. Initial cuts define the superior and anterior borders of the dissection. The posterior dissection is continued until the sigmoid sinus is identified. Further bone removal continues medially until the lateral semicircular canal and incus are identified.

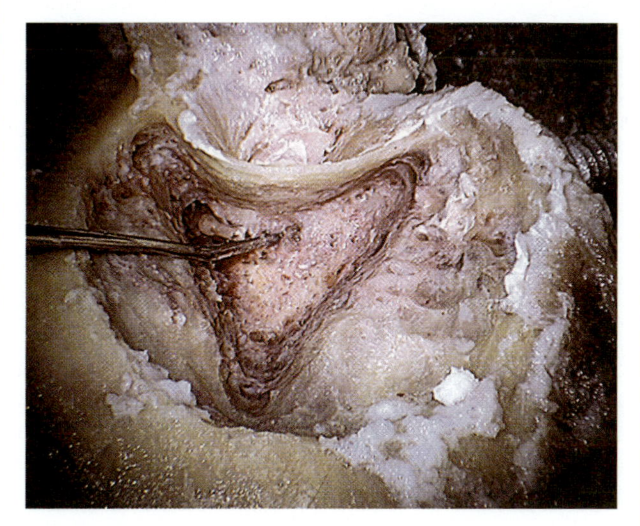

FIGURE A–17 • Dissection inferior to the lateral semicircular canal and lateral to the incus develops the facial recess. Here the probe identifies the "herald" air cell that can be found even in very sclerotic bones.

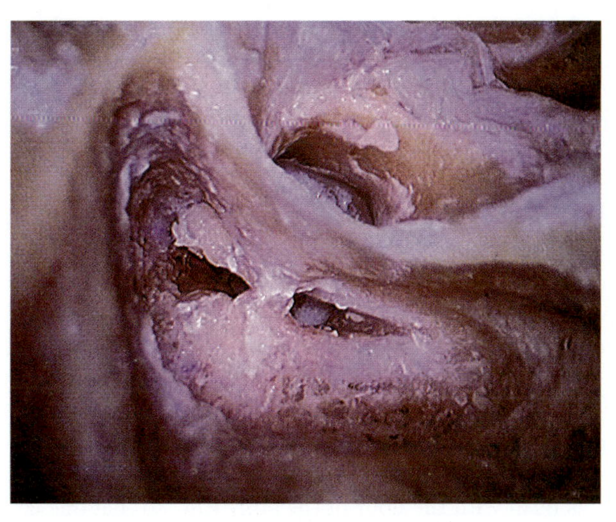

FIGURE A–18 • Facial recesses fully developed between the facial and chorda tympani nerves.

At the completion of the facial recess approach, the pyramidal process, stapedial tendon, stapes superstructure, long process of the incus, and oval and round windows can be visualized. This exposure provides access for dissection of cholesteatoma from the stapes and oval window, although the sinus tympani remains hidden. This approach also allows for accurate disarticulation of the incudostapedial joint and is used to provide access to the round window for cochlear implantation.

Caution: Care must be exercised when drilling close to the incus in the presence of an intact ossicular chain. Even slightly touching the incus with the bur can precipitate a substantial sensorineural hearing loss. The use of a small curette or pick to remove the last bit of bone can be quite useful in avoiding this complication.

Extended Facial Recess

Increased access to the hypotympanum can be obtained by extending the facial recess to the level of the tympanic annulus, which requires sacrifice of the chorda tympani nerve. The landmarks used in the dissection are the facial nerve, the chorda tympani nerve, the annulus, and the tympanic membrane. Inferiorly, the plane of the tympanic annulus tilts medially and the facial nerve courses laterally. Dissection begins at the point at which the chorda tympani nerve separates from the facial nerve. The chorda is transected at this site and the fallopian canal is followed inferiorly, carefully drilling with a small diamond bur. Occasionally, the facial nerve may pass lateral to the annulus before the inferior limit of the annulus is reached; by following the fallopian canal from a superior to inferior direction, facial nerve injury can be avoided. To avoid injury to the facial nerve, it is also important to use copious irrigation to cool the bur.

The extended facial recess approach can prove useful in accessing the hypotympanum and jugular bulb region (eg, for resection of a glomus tympanicum tumor) (Figure A–19).

Removal of the Incus and the Head of the Malleus

Dissection anteriorly and laterally from the mastoid antrum toward the root of the zygoma opens the attic. The limit of this space is the external canal wall inferiorly, and the tegmen tympani superiorly. Once completed, this dissection provides access to the body and short process of the incus, ossicular ligaments, and head of the malleus.

Removing the incus and head of the malleus affords access to the anterior epitympanic space and visualization of the entire tympanic segment of the facial nerve. This exposure also can provide access for decompression of the facial nerve lateral to the geniculate ganglion (Figure A–20).

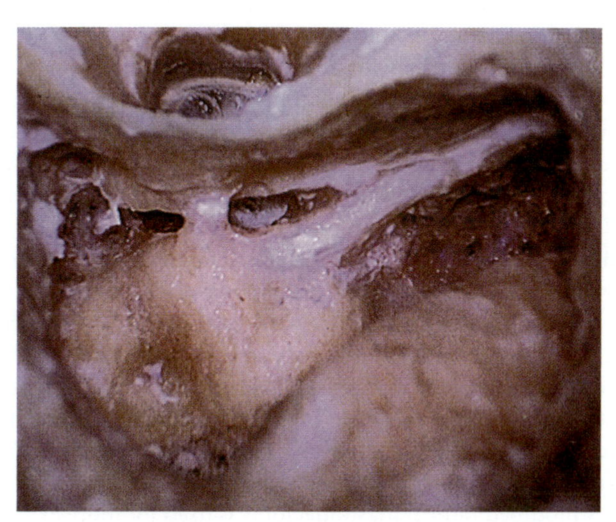

FIGURE A–19 • Further expansion of the dissection into the facial recess. Note the delineation of the horizontal and vertical facial nerve and the improved access to the middle ear.

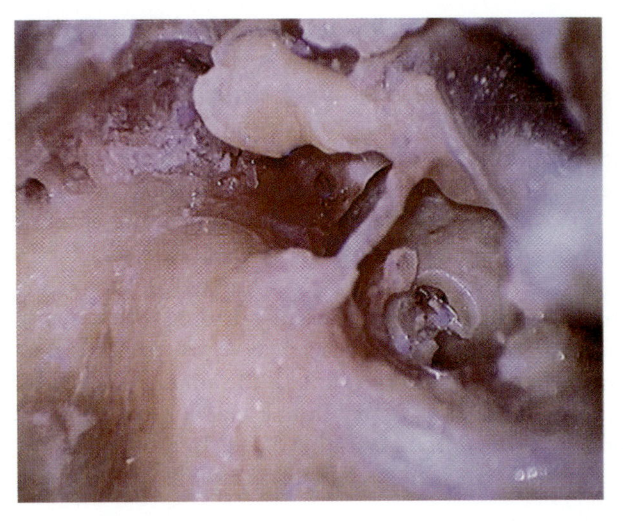

FIGURE A–20 • High-power view of the epitympanum with the incus removed. Further removal of the malleus head will provide access to the anterior epitympanum, petrous apex, and complete horizontal facial nerve segment including the geniculate ganglion.

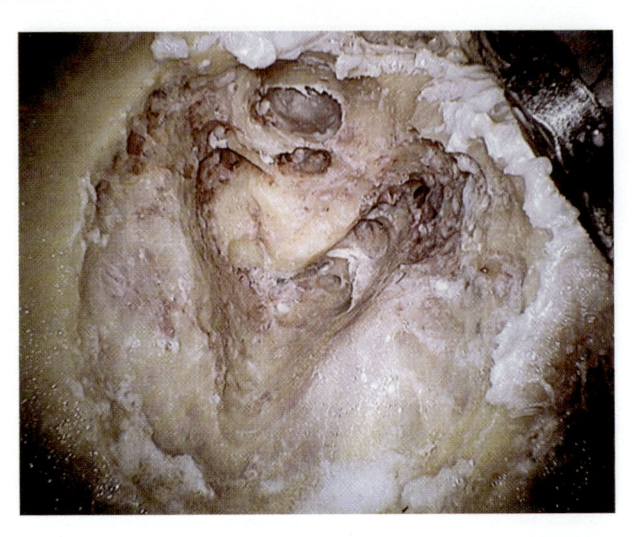

FIGURE A–21 • Bondy modified mastoid cavity demonstrating removal of the external canal wall with preservation of the tympanic membrane and ossicular chain.

Modified Radical (Canal-Wall-Down) Mastoidectomy

The modified radical mastoidectomy is used primarily to manage cholesteatoma, and the extent of the approach varies with the extent of disease encountered. Therefore, we describe a few specific approaches to be practiced in the temporal bone laboratory, recognizing that modification must be made for the individual patient. Furthermore, this approach can identify the extent of disease and simplify the surgical decision to continue with a more extensive procedure. Judicious dissection to provide adequate access to disease resection or exteriorization leaves a smaller cavity that better serves both the patient and surgeon. The dissection begins with the intact canal wall mastoidectomy already described. Identification of the antrum and LSSC gives a point of reference for the depth of the dissection.

Depending on the extent of disease, and if the ossicular chain is intact, a *Bondy mastoidectomy* (limited cavity) can be performed. In this procedure, a limited intact canal wall procedure is performed, staying superior in the dissection, identifying the antrum, and removing the superior and posterior canal wall until only a thin rim of bone remains over the ossicles. A medium-sized bur, drawn medially to laterally, facilitates bone removal. The final rim of bone is removed with a small curette to avoid traumatizing the intact ossicular chain. With experience, and in carefully selected patients, this procedure can be performed entirely from the canal side ("inside out"), thereby creating the smallest possible cavity. It is necessary to perform a meatoplasty to facilitate postoperative cleaning of the cavity (Figure A–21).

A modified radical mastoidectomy is used for more extensive disease and is designed to exteriorize all areas of the temporal bone. On occasion, the status of the tympanic cavity may allow for hearing preservation or reconstruction, that is, tympanoplasty. An important landmark is the anterior buttress (the point at which the posterior bony canal wall meets the tegmen), which is totally removed to achieve a smooth continuum between the mastoid tegmen and the tegmen tympani. The posterior buttress, which marks the meeting of the posterior canal wall and the floor of the EAC lateral to the facial nerve, is also removed.

In the dissection laboratory, an intact canal wall mastoidectomy is performed. Removal of the incus reduces the potential for trauma to the ossicular chain, facilitating both the safety of the procedure and the speed with which it can be performed. The chorda tympani nerve is sacrificed, and the posterior canal wall is lowered to the fallopian canal (the "facial ridge"), improving exposure of the sinus tympani and the hypotympanum. At the completion of the procedure, the anterior epitympanic cavity is flush with the mesotympanum, and the floor of the mastoid cavity is flush with the floor of the bony EAC so that one large cavity is created. On occasion, the mastoid tip extends below the level of the bony canal, creating the potential for a "sink trap." To avoid the sink trap effect, the lateral (to the digastric ridge) mastoid tip cells should be removed, resulting in a shallower mastoid cavity (Figure A–22).

A poorly performed modified radical mastoidectomy is characterized by incomplete removal of the posterior canal wall, superior canal wall, high facial ridge, and an inadequate meatoplasty.

Approach to the Endolymphatic Sac, Labyrinthectomy, and Translabyrinthine Exposure of the Internal Auditory Canal

This dissection begins with an extensively saucerized, intact canal wall mastoidectomy. Opening the facial recess to identify the facial nerve facilitates dissection. The fallopian canal is traced from the LSCC to the digastric ridge. The sigmoid sinus is followed to the jugular bulb, medial to the fallopian

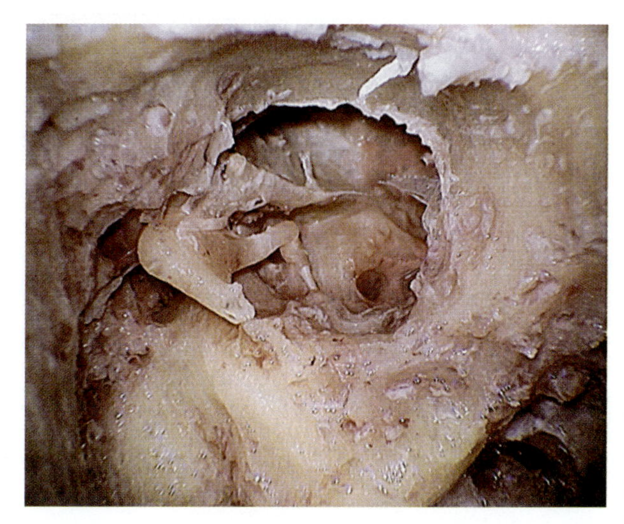

FIGURE A–22 • Modified radical mastoid cavity. Compared to Figure A-21, the tympanic membrane has been removed and the canal wall lowered to the vertical facial nerve. Further saucerization of the cavity has also been performed, particularly anterosuperiorly and posteroinferiorly. The ossicular chain has been left intact for reference.

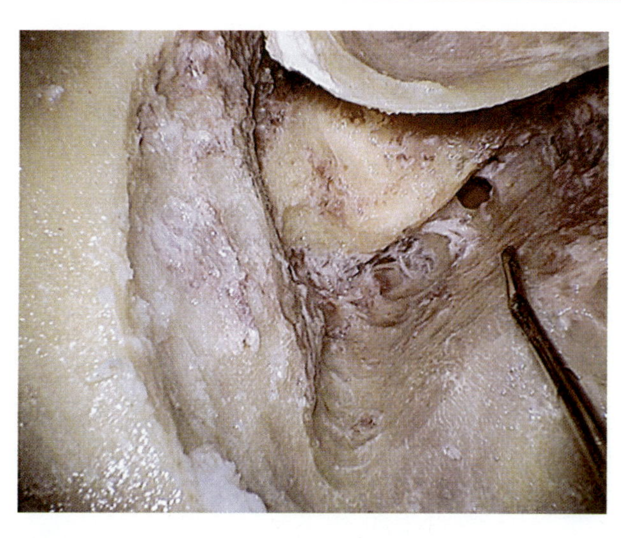

FIGURE A–23 • The basic mastoidectomy is extended by removing the bone behind and over the sigmoid sinus in preparation for accessing the posterior fossa dura, endolymphatic sac, and labyrinth. The sigmoid sinus can now be compressed, allowing better access to these structures.

canal. Air cells are removed and the semicircular canals are identified.

Access to the posterior fossa dura, endolymphatic sac, and labyrinth can be improved by decompressing the sigmoid sinus. Either complete or partial (leaving a bony island) removal of bone over the sinus works equally well. Having decompressed the sinus, the angle of approach to the semicircular canals is less acute, and broader strokes can be employed (Figure A–23).

Donaldson's line is an imaginary line drawn through the long axis of the LSCC, bisecting the posterior semicircular canal (PSCC). The endolymphatic sac is located inferior to this line and appears as a thickening of the posterior fossa dura. By opening the retrofacial air cells (medial to the facial nerve, inferior to the PSCC, and superior to the jugular bulb), the posterior fossa dura and the endolymphatic sac are exposed. Decompression (or drainage) of the endolymphatic sac is the only nondestructive surgical therapy for Meniere's disease (Figure A–24).

In addition to accessing the endolymphatic sac and jugular bulb, this posterior approach to the labyrinth can also be used for PSCC occlusion, used to treat BPPV. Soft, judicious strokes with a small diamond bur, paralleling the canal, provide wide exposure of the canal.

A transmastoid labyrinthectomy is performed systematically and begins with an intact canal wall mastoidectomy and a limited facial recess dissection to establish the position of the facial nerve. If necessary, the sigmoid sinus is decompressed to provide better exposure. The semicircular canals are defined by removal of surrounding cancellous bone. Using a medium-sized bur and opening the LSSC, drilling from anterior to posterior, to expose the membranous canal begins the labyrinthectomy. An instructive exercise in the temporal bone laboratory consists of carefully removing the bone of the labyrinth, noting the color transition from yellow-white to bluish-gray as the bone is

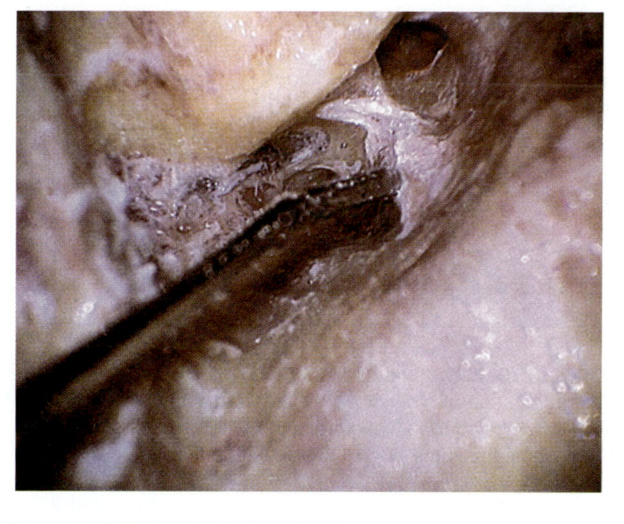

FIGURE A–24 • Higher-power view of Figure A–23. The bone over the posterior fossa dura has now been removed. The probe is passed between the layers of dura into the superior limit of the endolymphatic sac. Anterior to the probe lies the endolymphatic duct as it travels to the crus communis.

thinned. Familiarity with the varying appearance of the bone as it is thinned is useful in the operating room when trying to assess fistulization of the labyrinth in chronic otitis media. The open LSCC is followed to the PSCC, which is opened. The posterior canal is traced forward until the junction of the nonampullated ends of the posterior and superior canals is identified at the common crus (crus communis). The endolymphatic duct can be identified running from the endolymphatic sac to the common crus. A "cup" is formed, and drilling within this "cup" in a circular fashion is recommended to avoid bur slippage

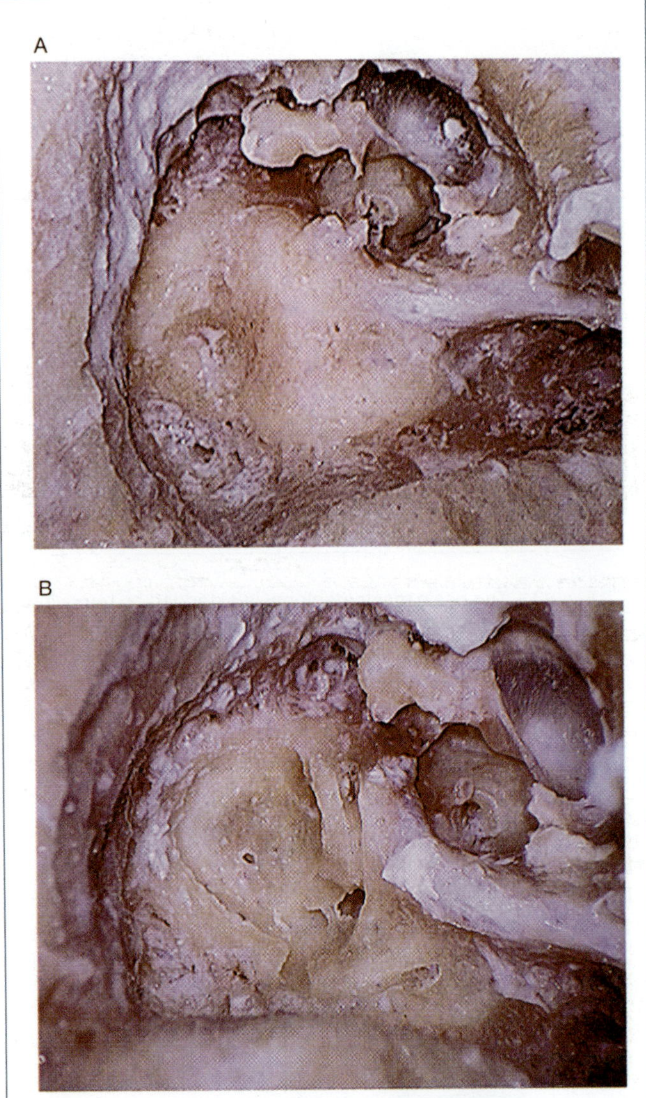

FIGURE A–25 • Labyrinthectomy part one. *A*, The bone of the lateral, posterior, and superior canals is skeletonized. Note the position of the facial nerve in relation to the lateral and posterior canals. *B*, Canals opened within the same bone to demonstrate their orientation.

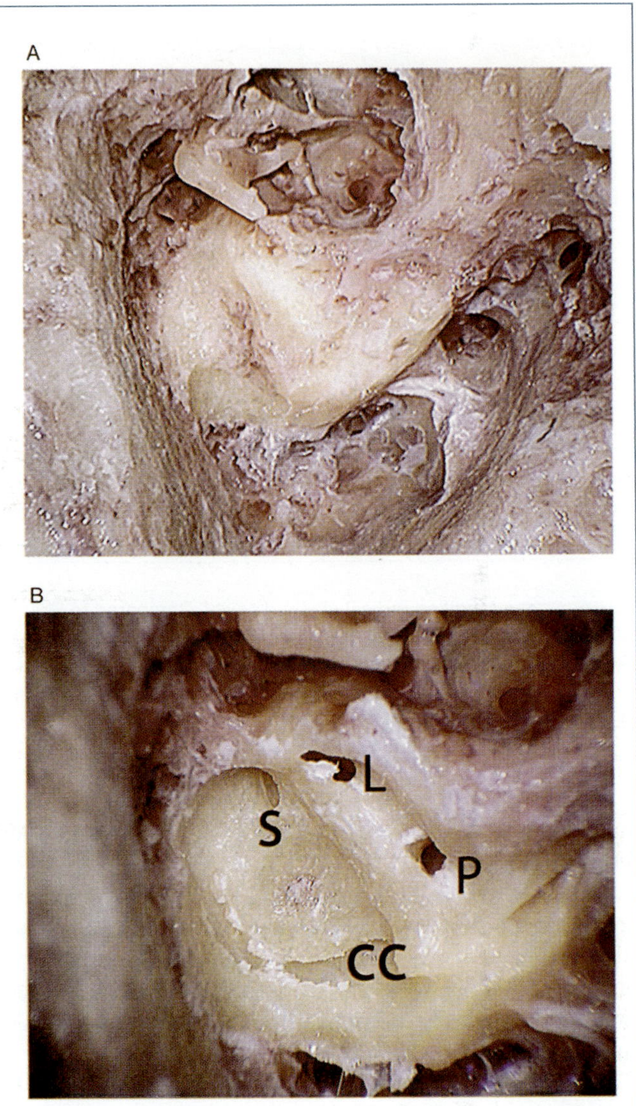

FIGURE A–26 • Labyrinthectomy part two. *A*, Positions of bony canals. *B*, Canals have been traced and opened. CC, crus communis joining superior and posterior canals; FN, facial nerve; S, L, P, relative positions of ampullae of superior, lateral, and posterior canals.

and consequent injury to the horizontal segment of the facial nerve. The superior canal is opened and followed anteriorly to its ampulla; the subarcuate artery is encountered as it courses within the arc of the superior canal. Lastly, the inferior portion of the PSCC is opened, taking care to avoid injuring the vertical segment of the facial nerve (Figures A–25 and A–26).

Each of the ampullae of the semicircular canals closely approximates a portion of the facial nerve. The labyrinthine portion of the facial nerve lies anterior to the ampulla of the superior canal. The ampulla of the lateral canal is just superior to the tympanic segment of the facial nerve. The posterior canal ampulla is just medial to the mastoid segment of the facial nerve.

Once all three canals are opened, drilling anteriorly from the ampulla of the posterior canal opens the vestibule. Within the vestibule, the elliptical recess (for the utricle) and the spherical recess (for the saccule) can be seen. The cribriform opening for the superior vestibular nerve (the macula cribrosa superior) is known as Mike's dot and serves as the landmark for the fundus of the IAC (Figures A–27 and A–28). Once the labyrinthectomy has been completed, exposure of the IAC can begin and is done using a medium-sized bur. The superior boundary of the IAC lies inferior to the subarcuate artery. Thus, bone superior to this plane can be removed safely. The inferior border of the canal lies superior to the jugular bulb. With further medial and inferior dissection, the cochlear aqueduct is encountered. The cochlear aqueduct not only marks the inferior boundary of the IAC, it marks the medial extent of the canal as well. The bony plate of the posterior fossa is thinned until the porus of the IAC is defined. With the fundus and the porus thus defined, the bone of the IAC can then be thinned throughout its length. Finally, when eggshell thin, the remaining bone can be removed with a small hook, revealing the dural sheath and nerves within (Figure A–29).

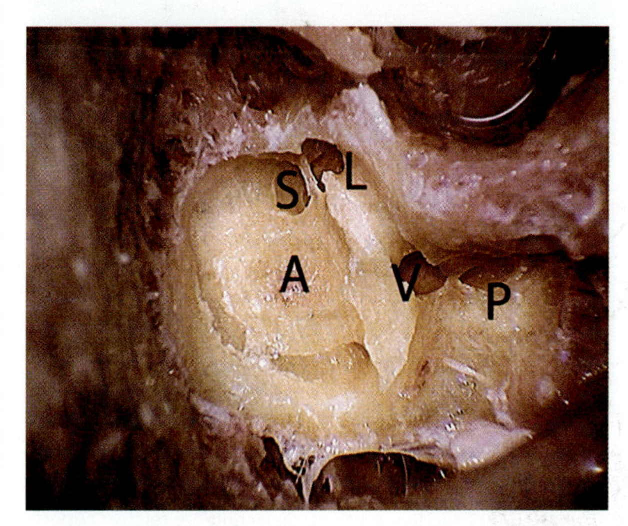

FIGURE A–27 • Labyrinthectomy part three: the semicircular canals have been removed and the vestibule opened. This completes the labyrinthectomy. A, subarcuate artery; S,L, and P, ampullae of superior, lateral, and posterior canals; V, vestibule.

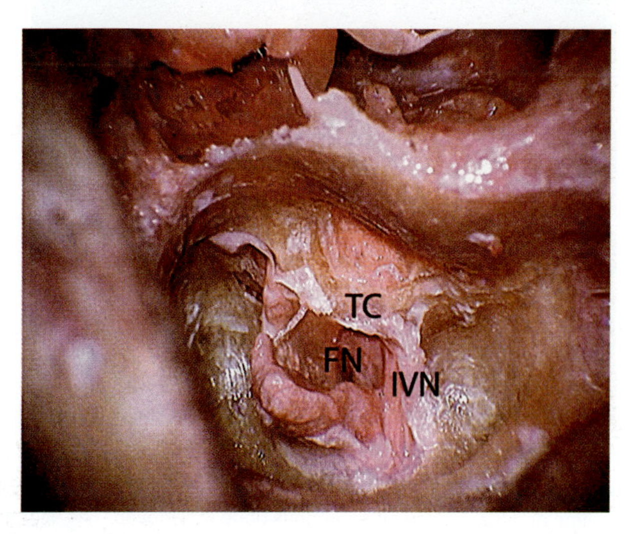

FIGURE A–29 • The bone overlying the internal auditory canal (IAC) has been removed, exposing the neural structures contained within. The superior vestibular nerve has been removed to reveal the facial nerve (FN) beneath. The inferior vestibular nerve is also visible (IVN). TC, transverse crest.

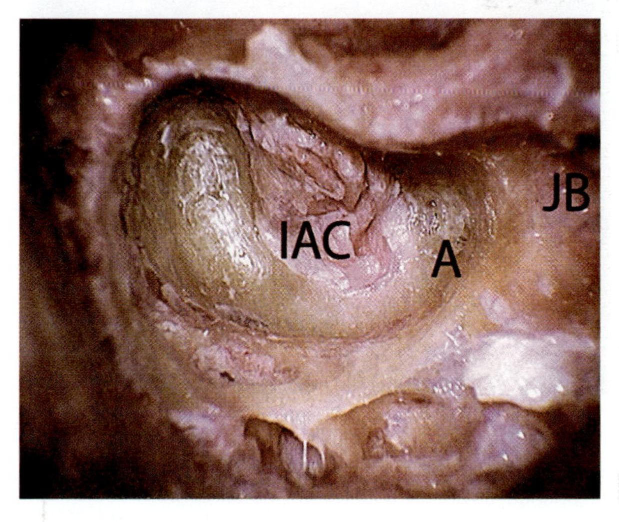

FIGURE A–28 • The superior and inferior limits of the internal auditory canal (IAC) have been defined. Inferiorly note the positions of the jugular bulb (JB) and cochlear aqueduct (A). Compare this view with Figure A-27B, and note the position of the vestibule with respect to the lateral IAC.

From the translabyrinthine approach, the first nerves encountered within the IAC are the superior and inferior vestibular nerves, separated by a variable projection of bone, the transverse crest. Medial to the superior vestibular nerve, another small bony projection, the vertical crest (Bill's bar), can be palpated with a small hook; Bill's bar separates the superior vestibular nerve from the facial nerve. The facial nerve may, in fact, be difficult to visualize until the superior vestibular nerve has been avulsed and reflected posteriorly. The facial nerve is then visible, and the bone surrounding its labyrinthine segment can be removed until the geniculate ganglion is reached. The cochlear nerve is in the anterior/inferior compartment of the IAC and can be seen inferior to the facial nerve. Reflecting the inferior vestibular nerve posteriorly improves visualization of the cochlear nerve (Figure A–29).

Middle Fossa Approach to the Internal Auditory Canal

The temporal bone positioning used for a middle fossa dissection differs from the typical placement and warrants special mention. For middle fossa procedures, the surgeon sits at the head of the patient looking toward the feet. In this position, the mastoid tip is pointing away from the surgeon. A 5-cm-square squamous craniectomy, centered on the zygomatic process and extending down to the linea temporalis (approximating the floor of the middle cranial fossa), is created. Dura is elevated in a posterior to anterior direction to avoid injuring an exposed geniculate ganglion and GPN (Figure A–30).

Middle fossa anatomic dissection, more so than transmastoid dissection, relies on the geometric relationships of critical anatomic structures. Proceeding medially, the first structure encountered is the tympanosquamous suture line, medial to which is the facial hiatus for the GPN. The course of the GPN parallels the petrous ridge. The SSCC lies approximately 10 mm posterior and 5 mm medial to the GPN. At this point, the bone is thinned carefully until the superior SCC is blue-lined. The SSSC forms a right angle to the petrous ridge, and the IAC runs at approximately a 60-degree angle from the SSSC. The GPN is traced posteriorly until the geniculate ganglion is encountered. Typically, only 4 mm separate the geniculate

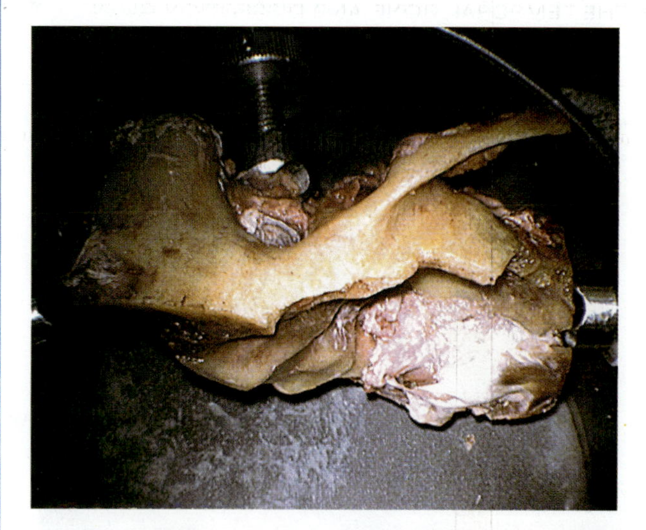

FIGURE A–30 • Middle cranial fossa 1: the bone is placed in the surgical position and the window of squamous bone is removed. The shape of the bone flap has been altered to accommodate the specimen.

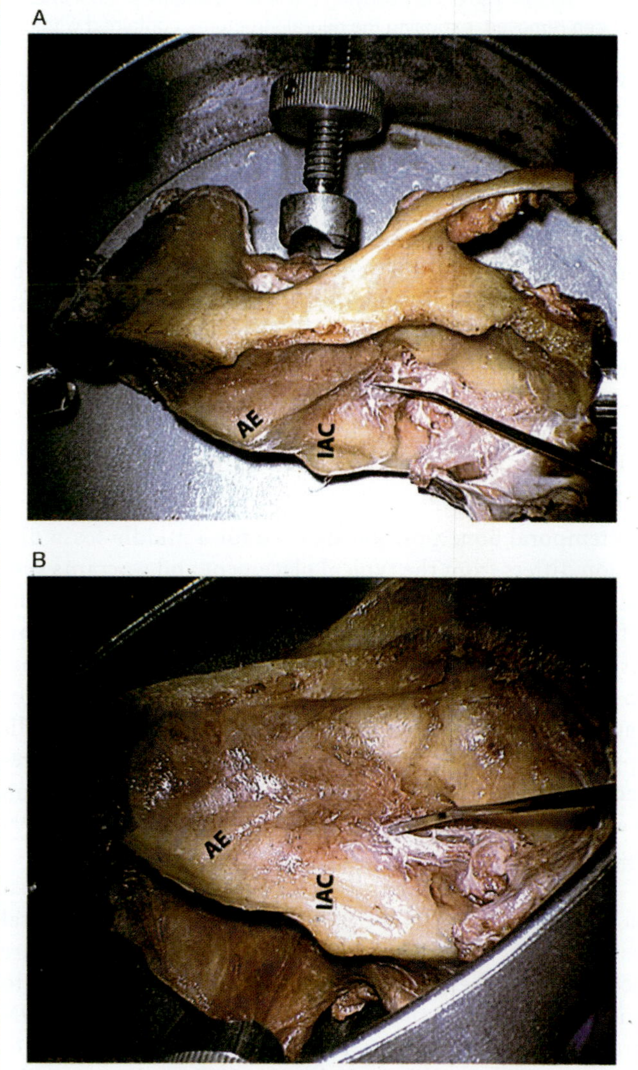

FIGURE A–31 • Middle cranial fossa 2: the probe marks the facial hiatus for the greater superficial petrosal nerve. The relevant landmark of the arcuate eminence is labeled (AE) and superior canal (SC) are labeled, and the relative position of the internal auditory canal (IAC) is noted. *A*, Surgical view and *B*, superior view.

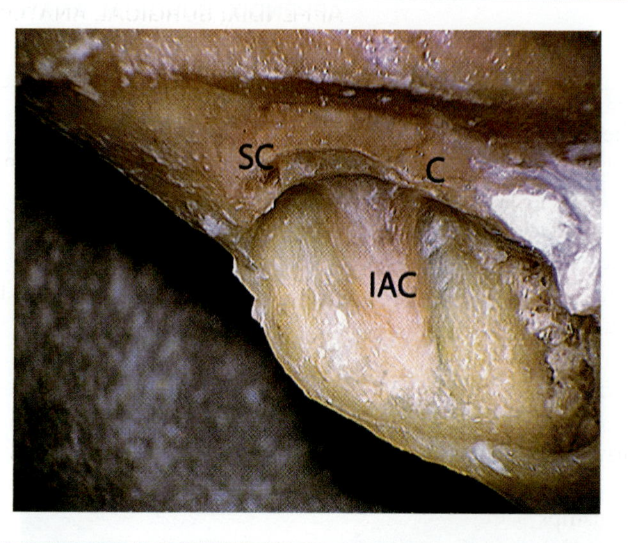

FIGURE A–32 • Middle cranial fossa 3: the internal auditory canal (IAC) is developed. Note the depth medially and the relative superficial placement laterally. C, otic capsule containing cochlea; IAC, internal auditory canal; SC, superior canal.

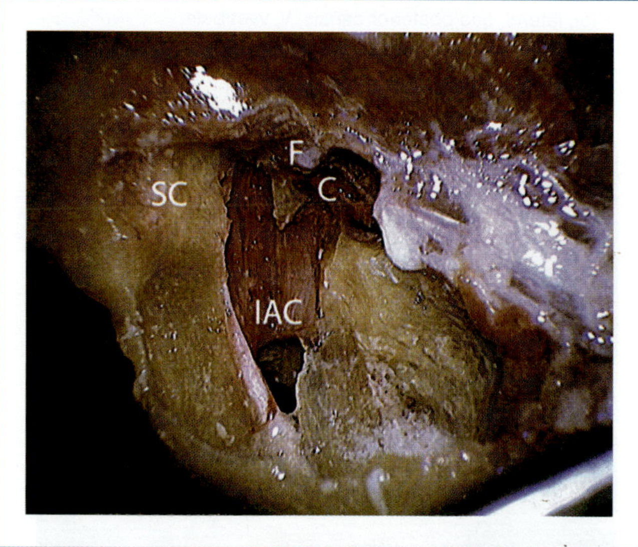

FIGURE A–33 • Middle cranial fossa 4: the internal auditory canal (IAC) is opened, as are the cochlea (C) and the ampulla of the superior canal (SC), for reference. Note the proximity of the meatal facial nerve (F) to the basal turn of the cochlea and the wedge of bone, Bill's bar, separating the superior vestibular nerve from the facial nerve.

ganglion from the ampulla of the SSSC. Between these two structures lies the fundus of the IAC. Laterally, the IAC is relatively superficial but becomes deeper within the petrous ridge as it is traced medially. Once the approximate location and direction of the IAC are determined by the geniculate ganglion, SSSC, and petrous ridge, the bone of the ridge is removed (Figure A–31).

The safest area for dissection is medially as the critical structures are nearest to one another at the fundus. The basal turn of the cochlea lies just anterior and medial to the labyrinthine segment of the facial nerve. Medially, 180 degrees or more of the IAC can be exposed. When the bone overlying the

IAC is sufficiently thinned, a small hook can be used to remove the final layer of bone and open the dural sheath. The vertical crest (Bill's bar) can be identified at the fundus as it separates the facial and superior vestibular nerves. The facial nerve can be traced from the meatal foramen, through the geniculate ganglion, and to the tympanic segment. The fibers to the SSCC, LSCC, and the utricle can be seen passing through the macula cribrosa superior. The nervus intermedius (Wrisberg's nerve) can be seen traveling just inferior and posterior to the facial nerve. Inferior to these nerves is the transverse crest. The cochlear nerve and inferior vestibular nerve travel anteriorly and posteriorly, respectively, through this compartment. Finally, to complete the understanding of the anatomic relationships of this area, the SSCC and cochlea can be opened. Note that the cochlea is relatively closer to the IAC than is the SSCC. Thus, it is safer to begin delineating the IAC on its posterior surface (Figures A–32 and A–33).

Selected Reading

Black B. Posterior geniculate artery: A surgeon's guide to the facial nerve. Am J Otol 1992;13:78–9.

Donaldson JA, Duckert LG, Lambert PM, et al. Surgical anatomy of the temporal bone. 4th edition. New York: Raven Press; 1992.

Gacek RR. Surgical landmark for the facial nerve in the epitympanum. Ann Otol Rhinol Laryngol 1980;89(3 Pt 1):249–50.

Gulya AJ, Schuknecht HF. Anatomy of the temporal bone with surgical implications. 2nd edition. New York: Parthenon; 1995.

Kartush JM, Kemink JL, Graham MD. The arcuate eminence. Topographic orientation in middle cranial fossa surgery. Ann Otol Rhinol Laryngol 1985;94(1 Pt 1):25–8.

Litton WB, Krause CJ, Anson BA, et al. The relationship of the facial canal to the annular sulcus. Laryngoscope 1969;79:1584–604.

Proctor B. Surgical anatomy of the ear and temporal bone. New York: Thieme Medical Publishers; 1989.

Index

Page numbers in italics indicate figures and those followed by "t" indicate